MURTAGH'S

GENERAL PRACTICE

To all our medical colleagues, past and present, who have provided the vast reservoir of knowledge from which the content of this book was made possible

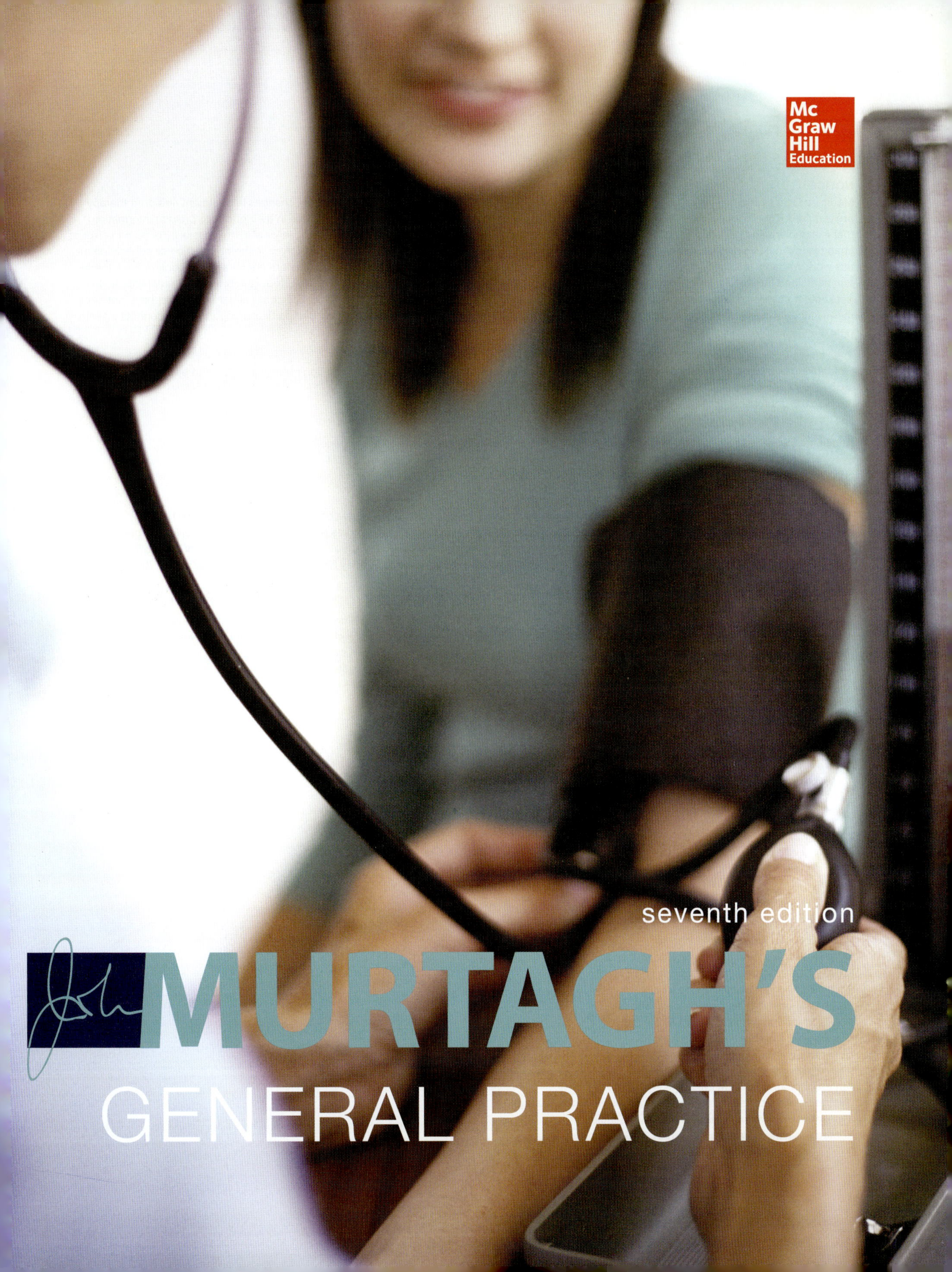
McGraw Hill Education
seventh edition
MURTAGH'S
GENERAL PRACTICE

NOTICE

Medicine is an ever-changing science. As new research and clinical experience broaden our knowledge, changes in treatment and drug therapy are required. The editors and the publisher of this work have checked with sources believed to be reliable in their efforts to provide information that is complete and generally in accord with the standards accepted at the time of publication. However, in view of the possibility of human error or changes in medical sciences, neither the editors, nor the publisher, nor any other party who has been involved in the preparation or publication of this work warrants that the information contained herein is in every respect accurate or complete. Readers are encouraged to confirm the information contained herein with other sources. For example, and in particular, readers are advised to check the product information sheet included in the package of each drug they plan to administer to be certain that the information contained in this book is accurate and that changes have not been made in the recommended dose or in the contraindications for administration. This recommendation is of particular importance in connection with new or infrequently used drugs.

This seventh edition published 2018
First edition published 1994, second edition published 1998, third edition published 2003, fourth edition published 2007, fifth edition published 2011, sixth edition published 2015

National Library of Australia Cataloguing-in-Publication Data:

A catalogue record for this book is available from the National Library of Australia

Authors:	John Murtagh, Jill Rosenblatt, Justin Coleman, Clare Murtagh
Title:	John Murtagh's General Practice
Edition:	7th edition
ISBN:	9781760422295

Published in Australia by
McGraw-Hill Education (Australia) Pty Ltd
Level 33, 680 George Street, Sydney NSW 2000
Publisher: Michael Weitz
Production editor: Genevieve MacDermott
Copyeditors: Laura Carmody and Ali Moore
Proofreader: Anne Savage
Cover design: Christa Moffitt, christabella designs
Internal design: David Rosemeyer
Author photograph: Gerrit Fokkema Photography
Illustrators: Alan Laver/Shelly Communications and John Murtagh
Typeset in STIX MathJax Main 10/11.5 by SPI, India
Printed in China on 70 gsm matt art by 1010 Printing Int. Ltd

The authors

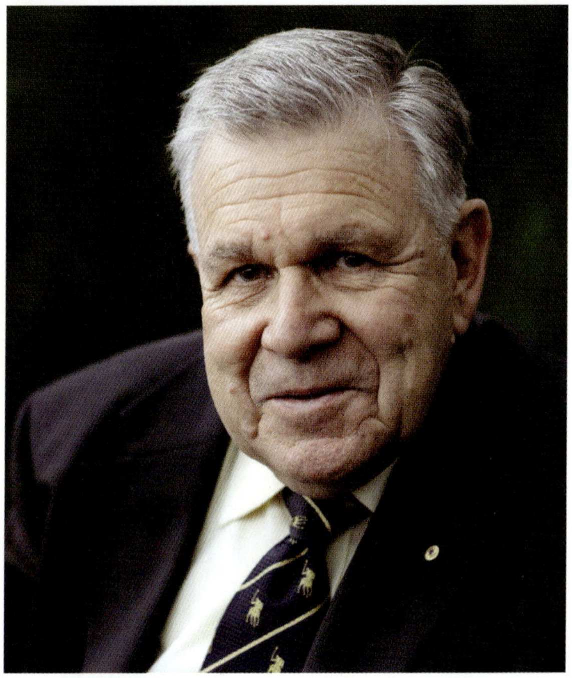

Professor John Murtagh AM

MBBS, MD, BSc, BEd, FRACGP, DipObstRCOG

Emeritus Professor in General Practice, School of Primary Health, Monash University, Melbourne

Professorial Fellow, Department of General Practice, University of Melbourne

Adjunct Clinical Professor, Graduate School of Medicine, University of Notre Dame, Fremantle, Western Australia

John Murtagh was a science master teaching chemistry, biology and physics in Victorian secondary schools when he was admitted to the first intake of the newly established Medical School at Monash University, graduating in 1966. Following a comprehensive postgraduate training program, which included surgical registrarship, he practised in partnership with his wife, Dr Jill Rosenblatt, for 10 years in the rural community of Neerim South, Victoria.

He was appointed Senior Lecturer (part-time) in the Department of Community Medicine at Monash University and eventually returned to Melbourne as a full-time Senior Lecturer. He was appointed to a professorial chair in Community Medicine at Box Hill Hospital in 1988 and subsequently as chairman of the extended department and Professor of General Practice in 1993 until retirement from this position in 2010. He now holds teaching positions as Emeritus Professor in General Practice at Monash University, Adjunct Clinical Professor, University of Notre Dame and Professorial Fellow, University of Melbourne. He achieved the Doctor of Medicine degree in 1988 for his thesis 'The management of back pain in general practice'.

He was appointed Associate Medical Editor of *Australian Family Physician* in 1980 and Medical Editor in 1986, a position he held until 1995. In 1995 he was awarded the Member of the Order of Australia for services to medicine, particularly in the areas of medical education, research and publishing.

One of his numerous publications, *Practice Tips,* was named as the British Medical Association's Best Primary Care Book Award in 2005. In the same year he was named as one of the most influential people in general practice by the publication *Australian Doctor.* John Murtagh was awarded the inaugural David de Kretser medal from Monash University for his exceptional contribution to the Faculty of Medicine, Nursing and Health Sciences over a significant period of time. Members of the Royal Australian College of General Practitioners may know that the honour of the namesake of the College library was bestowed upon him.

In 2018 he will host the 40th Annual John Murtagh Update Course for General Practitioners at Monash University.

Today John Murtagh continues to enjoy active participation with the diverse spectrum of general practitioners—whether they are students or experienced practitioners, rural- or urban-based, local or international medical graduates, clinicians or researchers. His vast experience with all of these groups has provided him with tremendous insights into their needs, which is reflected in the culminated experience and wisdom of *John Murtagh's General Practice.*

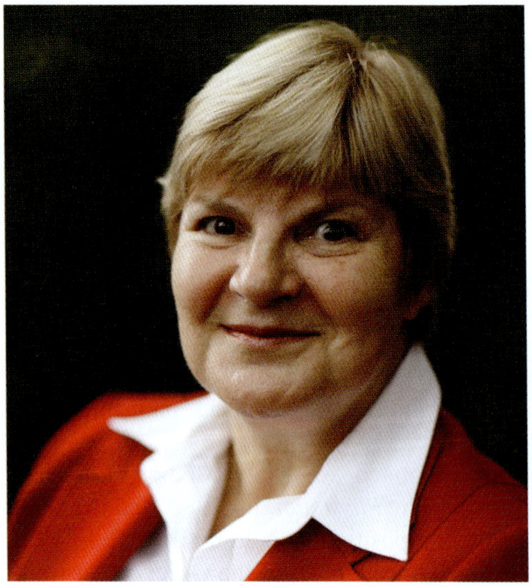

Dr Jill Rosenblatt

MBBS, FRACGP, DipObstRCOG, GradDipAppSci

Adjunct Senior Lecturer, School of Primary Health Care, Monash University, Melbourne

Jill Rosenblatt graduated in medicine from the University of Melbourne in 1968. Following terms as a resident medical officer she entered rural practice in Neerim South, Victoria, in partnership with her husband John Murtagh. She was responsible for inpatient hospital care in the Neerim District Bush Nursing Hospital and in the West Gippsland Base Hospital. Her special interests were obstetrics, paediatrics and anaesthetics. Jill has also had a special interest in Indigenous culture and health since she lived at Koonibba Mission in South Australia, where her father was Superintendent.

After leaving rural life she came to Melbourne and joined the Ashwood Medical Group, where she practised comprehensive general medicine, and care of the elderly in particular. She was appointed Adjunct Senior Lecturer in the Department of General Practice at Monash University in 1980 and a teacher in the GP registrar program.

She gained a Diploma of Sports Medicine (RACGP) in 1985 and a Graduate Diploma of Applied Science in Nutritional and Environmental Medicine from Swinburne University of Technology in 2001.

Jill Rosenblatt brings a wealth of diverse experience to the compilation of this textbook. This is based on 50 years of experience in rural and metropolitan general practice. In addition she has served as clinical assistant to the Shepherd Foundation, the Menopause Clinics at Prince Henry's Hospital and Box Hill Hospital and the Department of Anaesthetics at Prince Henry's Hospital. Jill has served as an examiner for the RACGP for 39 years and for the Australian Medical Council for 16 years. She was awarded a life membership of the Royal Australian College of General Practitioners in 2010 and a Distinguished Service award of the College in 2014.

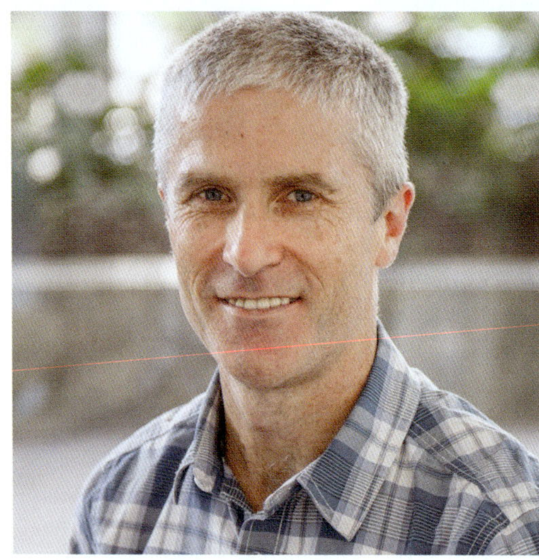

Dr Justin Coleman

MBBS, FRACGP, MPH

General Practitioner, Inala Indigenous Health Service, Brisbane

Senior Lecturer, Griffith University

Senior Lecturer, University of Queensland

Editor, Diabetes Management Journal

Chair of Choosing Wisely working group, RACGP

Justin Coleman graduated from Melbourne University medicine in 1992 and spent the next two decades as a rural GP in Victoria and the remote Northern Territory before settling in Brisbane, where he works in Aboriginal and Torres Strait Islander health.

Soon after graduating, Justin began writing for the GP newspaper *Medical Observer* and hasn't stopped since. One of his weekly columns, 'Handy Hints for GPs', ran for 13 years. He even wrote 40 humorous columns until the editors lost their sense of humour.

Justin is a prolific writer for medical and non-medical readerships; he has published well over 1,000 medical articles in around 50 different newspapers, magazines, books and journals. For five years he served as President of the Australasian Medical Writers Association and he regularly runs writing workshops for medical writers and academics.

Since completing a Master of Public Health (UQ 2011, first class hons), Justin has dedicated much of his career to educating other GPs about how to improve various aspects of medical practice. His interests include evidence-based medicine, the rational use of medical tests and treatments, and dealing with uncertainty during a GP consultation. He represents the RACGP on matters pertaining to conflicts of interest and fiercely guards his own independence, never having accepted payment from a pharmaceutical or medical device company.

For the past quarter of a century, Justin has supervised hundreds of medical students and GP registrars. He has taught in the medical schools of three universities and for a dozen medical education organisations.

Justin edited his first medical book 20 years ago and has remained a medical editor ever since. He completed a Writing and Editing program in 2010 (UQ, first class hons). He currently edits *Diabetes Management Journal*, writes and does peer reviews for the MJA, AJGP (formerly AFP) and BMJ, and is a member of the Australasian Health and Medical journal Editors' Network (AHMEN).

Justin was honoured to be invited by Professor John Murtagh to help edit Australia's seminal textbook on general practice. This represents the grand intersection of every one of his aforementioned interests.

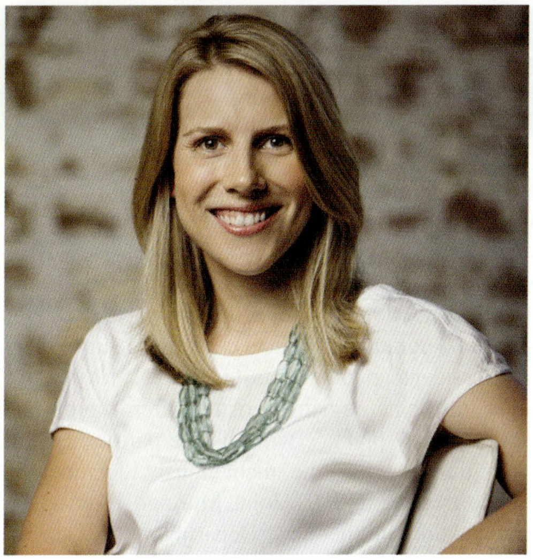

Dr Clare Murtagh

MBBS, FRACGP

General Practitioner, Your Doctors, Leichhardt

Clare Murtagh completed her medical studies at Monash University in 2007 and spent her early career working in hospitals in Geelong and rural Victoria. Following experience as a medical officer for trekkers in Nepal, she moved to Sydney where she completed her General Practice training in 2013.

A passionate generalist, Clare has special interest in dermatology, travel medicine, women's health and paediatrics. She holds a Diploma of Dermatology and Certificates in Sexual and Reproductive Health, and Medical Education. In her practice at Your Doctors in Sydney's inner west, she cares for a wide variety of patients and is an antenatal shared care provider.

In recent years, Clare has gained increasing experience in medical education as a supervisor of training GPs and as an examiner for the RACGP. She has worked as a medical educator at GP Synergy and is a lecturer on dermatology.

Clare has been an enthusiastic contributor to the 'Women's health', 'Sexual health' and 'Problems of the skin' sections of the sixth and seventh edition of *Murtagh's General Practice.* As the daughter of co-authors John Murtagh and Jill Rosenblatt, she has benefited from their mentorship and appreciates the genesis and philosophy of the editorial direction of the textbook.

Foreword

In 1960 a young schoolmaster, then teaching biology and chemistry in a secondary school in rural Victoria, decided to become a country doctor. He was part of the first intake of students into the Medical School of the newly established Monash University, and at the end of his six-year undergraduate medical course and subsequent intern and resident appointments his resolve to practise community medicine remained firm. After more than a decade in country practice with his life partner, Dr Jill Rosenblatt, during which he meticulously documented the cases he treated, in 1977 John Murtagh took up an academic position in the new Department of General Practice at Monash University. He subsequently moved through the ranks of Senior Lecturer, Associate Professor and Professor, now enjoying the title of Emeritus Professor.

Through his writing, pedagogy and research, John Murtagh became a national and international authority on the content and teaching of primary care medicine. It was during his tenure as Medical Editor of *Australian Family Physician* from 1986 to 1995 that the journal became the most widely read medical journal in Australia.

This textbook provides a distillate of the vast experience gained by a once rural doctor, whose career has embraced teaching; whose abiding interest is in ensuring that disease, whether minor or life-threatening, is recognised quickly; and whose concern is that strategies to match each contingency are well understood.

The first edition of this book, published in 1994, achieved remarkable success on both the national and international scene. The second and third editions built on this initial success and the book has become known as the 'bible of general practice' in Australia. In addition to being widely used by practising doctors, it has become a popular and standard textbook in several medical schools and also in the teaching institutions for alternative health practitioners, such as chiropractic, naturopathy and osteopathy. In particular, medical undergraduates and graduates struggling to learn English have found the book relatively comprehensible. The fourth and fifth editions were updated and expanded, retaining the successful, user-friendly format, including clinical photography and illustrations in colour. Dr Jill Rosenblatt joined John in authoring and editing the fifth, sixth and seventh editions. Now, almost 25 years since the launch of the first edition, the seventh edition introduces two new author/editors in Dr Justin Coleman and Dr Clare Murtagh.

Having known John and worked with him for more than three decades, I feel privileged to write this foreword to the seventh edition, adding to earlier forewords by the late Professor Schofield. During this 25-year period I have watched each edition blossom, only to be superseded by a bigger and better replacement. John Murtagh has become a legend nationally and internationally, and in a 2012 *Medical Observer* survey he was voted the most revered Australian doctor, ahead of Fred Hollows and Victor Chang. Most recently, in 2018 John was awarded the Australian Medical Association's highest honour, the AMA Gold Medal for his 'contribution to medicine and general practice as a doctor and educator'.

This edition retains the time-honoured framework that has made it the seminal text for GPs, GP registrars and students of general practice worldwide. It is to general practice what 'Harrisons' is to internal medicine.

Although this edition retains the same format, it has a number of significant changes and additions, including a strong emphasis on the diagnostic approach to the disturbed patient, as well as patients presenting with neurological symptoms and signs. Reflecting John's lifelong commitment to medical education, he has included more visual material, more practical tips for day-to-day clinical practice and importantly, more on therapeutics supported by references to *Therapeutic Guidelines*.

The expanded volume has necessitated a significant increase in references to original sources to substantiate the evidence base within this text. As expected in contemporary texts, there is also an abundance of online resources.

John Murtagh's works, including this text, have been translated into Italian by McGraw-Hill Libri Italia s.r.l., Portuguese by McGraw-Hill Nova Iorque and Spanish by McGraw-Hill Interamericana Mexico and also into Chinese, Greek, Polish and Russian. In 2009 *John Murtagh's General Practice* was chosen by the Chinese Ministry of Health as the textbook to aid the development of general practice in China. Now, 25 years since its beginning, the text is available in 13 languages, most recently adding Farsi and Turkish translations. A truly remarkable achievement.

GC SCHOFIELD
OBE, MD, ChB(NZ), DPhil(Oxon), FRACP, FRACMA, FAMA
Emeritus Professor of Anatomy
Dean of Medicine
Monash University, 1977–88

Leon Piterman AM (Foreword to the sixth and seventh editions)
MBBS, MD, MMed, MEdSt, FRCP(Edin), FRACGP
Professor of General Practice,
Monash University

Contents

Acknowledgments

Professor Murtagh would like to thank the Publication Division of the Royal Australian College of General Practitioners for supporting his past role as Medical Editor of *Australian Family Physician,* which provided an excellent opportunity to gather material for this book. Acknowledgment is also due to those medical organisations that have given permission to use selected information from their publications. They include the Preventive and Community Medicine committee of the RACGP (Guidelines for Preventive Activities in General Practice), Therapeutic Guidelines Limited (*Therapeutic Guidelines* series), the Hypertension Guideline Committee: Research Unit RACGP (South Australian Faculty) and the *Medical Observer,* publishers of *A Manual for Primary Health Care,* for permitting reproduction of Appendices I–IV.

Special thanks to the late Chris Sorrell for his art illustration, and to Nicki Cooper, Jenny Green and Caroline Menara for their skill and patience in typing the manuscript.

Many of the quotations at the beginning of chapters appear in either Robert Wilkins (ed), *The Doctor's Quotation Book,* Robert Hale Ltd, London, 1991, or Maurice B. Strauss (ed), *Familiar Medical Quotations,* Little, Brown & Co., New York, 1958.

Thanks also to Dr Bruce Mugford, Dr Lucie Stanford, Dr Mohammad Shafeeq Lone, Dr Brian Bedkobar, Dr Ebrahim Pishan, Dr Joseph Turner and Lesley Rowe for reviewing the manuscript, and to the publishing and production team at McGraw-Hill Education (Australia) for their patience and assistance in so many ways.

Finally, thanks to Dr Ndidi Victor Ikealumba for his expert review of *General Practice* sixth edition and his subsequent contribution.

Photo credits

Photographs appearing on the pages below are from *The Colour Atlas of Family Medicine* 2nd edn by RP Usatine, MA Smith, EJ Mayeaux Jr and H Chumley, McGraw-Hill Education US 2013, with the kind permission of the following people:

Dr Richard P Usatine: Fig 16.3, p 144; Fig 35.5, p 364; Fig 72.2, p 830; Fig 72.7, p 835; Figs 91.7 and 91.8, p 1011; Fig 91.9, p 1012; Fig 101.3, p 1112; Fig 106.5, p 1160; Fig 107.1, p 1164; Fig 119.5, p 1279; Fig 123.12, p 1324; Fig 126.20, p 1369; Fig 128.5 and 128.6, p 1391.

Dr William Clark: Fig 50.3, p 565; Fig 50.6, p 566; Fig 50.7, p 567; Fig 59.1, p 665.

Frontline Medical Communications: Fig 95.4, p 1059; Fig 125.6, p 1356.

Paul D. Comeau: Fig 51.6, p 582.

DEA: Fig 21.6, p 210.

Dr Nicolette Deveneau: Fig 100.2, p 1109.

Dr James L Fishback: Fig 138.3, p 1508.

Javier La Fontaine DPM: Fig 125.5, p 1355.

Reproduced from Gleason, in Tannenbaum: Fig 116.4, p 1245.

Dr Michelle Rowe: Fig 21.5, p 210.

Dr C. Blake Simpson: Fig 57.1, p 643.

Dr Marc Solioz: Fig 16.1, p 142.

Dr Eric Kraus: Fig 122.5, p 1305.

Preface

The discipline of general practice has become complex, expansive and challenging, but nevertheless remains manageable, fascinating and rewarding. *John Murtagh's General Practice* attempts to address the issue of the base of knowledge and skills required in modern general practice. Some of the basics of primary healthcare remain the same. In fact, there is an everlasting identity about many of the medical problems that affect human beings, be it a splinter under a nail, a stye of the eyelid, a terminal illness or simply stress-related anxiety. Many of the treatments and approaches to caring management are universal and timeless.

This text covers a mix of traditional and modern practice with an emphasis on the importance of clinical reasoning, early diagnosis, strategies for solving common presenting problems, continuing care, holistic management and 'tricks of the trade'. One feature of our discipline is the patient who presents with undifferentiated problems featuring an overlap of organic and psychosocial components. There is the constant challenge to make an early diagnosis and identify the ever-lurking, life-threatening illness. Hence the 'must not be missed' catch cry throughout the text. To reinforce this awareness, 'red flag pointers' to serious disease are included where appropriate. The general practice diagnostic model, which pervades all the chapters on problem solving, is based on the authors' experience, but readers can draw on their own experience to make the model work effectively for themselves.

This seventh edition expands on the challenging initiative of diagnostic triads (or tetrads), which act as a brief *aide-memoire* to assist in identifying a disorder from three (or four) key symptoms or signs. A particular challenge in the preparation of the text was to identify as much appropriate and credible evidence-based information as possible. This material, which still has its limitations, has been combined with considerable collective wisdom from experts, especially from the *Therapeutic Guidelines* series. To provide updated accuracy and credibility, the authors have had the relevant chapters peer reviewed by independent experts in the respective disciplines. These consultants are acknowledged in the reviewers section. The revised editions also have the advantage of co-authorship from experienced general practitioner Dr Jill Rosenblatt. With a view to the future and bringing a modern dimension, two authors have been added to the editorial team. They are Dr Clare Murtagh, a general practitioner with experience in medical education and Dr Justin Coleman, past president of the Australasian Medical Writers Association and editor of Diabetes Management Journal, among several appointments. His medical writing is legendary.

A comprehensive book such as this one, which presents a basic overview of primary medicine, cannot possibly cover all the medical problems likely to be encountered. An attempt has been made, however, to focus on problems that are common, significant, preventable and treatable. Expanded material on genetic disorders, infectious diseases and tropical medicine provides a glimpse of relatively uncommon presenting problems in first-world practice.

John Murtagh's General Practice is written with the recent graduate, the international medical graduate and the medical student in mind. However, all primary-care practitioners will gain useful information from the book's content.

Making the most of your book

Diagnostic strategy models

Diagnostic strategy models for common presenting problems form the backbone of this book. *General Practice* is renowned for this unique and powerful learning feature, which was introduced in the first edition.

Bruising and bleeding 431

The clinical approach

Differentiation of coagulation factor deficiencies and platelet disorders as the cause of a bleeding problem can usually be determined by a careful evaluation of the history and physical examination.

History

Factors that suggest the presence of a systemic bleeding defect include:

- spontaneous haemorrhage
- severe or recurrent haemorrhagic episodes, e.g. epistaxis
- bleeding from multiple sites
- bleeding out of proportion to the degree of trauma
- cutaneous bleeding
- gastrointestinal bleeding
- postpartum haemorrhage
- bleeding from tooth extraction/oral cavity
- menorrhagia
- muscle haematomas or haemarthrosis

If a bleeding diathesis is suspected it is essential to determine whether local pathology is contributing to the blood loss (e.g. postoperative bleeding, postpartum bleeding, gastrointestinal haemorrhage).

Diagnostic tips

- Platelet abnormalities present as early bleeding following trauma.
- Coagulation factor deficiencies present with delayed bleeding after initial haemostasis is achieved by normal platelets.
- A normal response to previous coagulation stresses (e.g. dental extraction, circumcision or pregnancy) indicates an acquired problem.
- If acquired, look for evidence of MILD: Malignancy, Infection, Liver disease, Drugs.
- A diagnostic strategy is outlined in TABLE 39.2.

Family history

A positive family history can be a positive pointer to the diagnosis:

- sex-linked recessive pattern: haemophilia A or B
- autosomal dominant pattern: vWD, dysfibrinogenaemias
- autosomal recessive pattern: deficiency of coagulation factors V, VII and X

Enquire whether the patient has noticed blood in the urine or stools and whether menorrhagia is present in women. A checklist for a bleeding history is

Table 39.2 Purpura: diagnostic strategy model
Probability diagnosis
Simple purpura (easy bruising syndrome)
Senile purpura
Corticosteroid-induced purpura
Immune thrombocytopenic purpura
Henoch–Schönlein purpura
Liver disease, especially alcoholic cirrhosis
Increased intravascular pressure, e.g. coughing, vomiting
Serious disorders not to be missed
Malignant disease:
• leukaemia
• myeloma
Aplastic anaemia
Myelofibrosis
Severe infections:
• septicaemia
• meningococcal infection
• measles
• typhoid
• dengue/chikungunya
Disseminated intravascular coagulation
Thrombotic thrombocytopenic purpura
Fat embolism
Pitfalls (often missed)
Haemophilia A, B vWD
Post-transfusion purpura
Trauma (e.g. domestic violence, child abuse)
Rarities:
• hereditary telangiectasia (Osler–Weber–Rendu syndrome)
• Ehlers–Danlos syndrome
• scurvy
• Fanconi syndrome
Seven masquerades checklist
Drugs: examples (see 'Medication Record')
• sodium valproate
• various antibiotics
• quinine/quinidine
• thiazide diuretics
• NSAIDs/salicylates
• cytotoxics
• oral anticoagulants/heparin
Anaemia:
• aplastic anaemia
Psychogenic factors
Factitial purpura

39

Key facts and checkpoints

Key facts and checkpoints provide accurate statistics and local and global contexts.

Key facts and checkpoints

- Cough is the commonest manifestation of lower respiratory tract infection.
- Cough is the cardinal feature of chronic bronchitis.
- Cough is a feature of asthma with sputum production, especially at night.
- Cough can have a psychogenic basis.
- Cough may persist for many weeks following an acute upper respiratory tract infection (URTI) as a result of persisting bronchial inflammation and increased airway responsiveness.[1]
- Postnasal drip is the commonest cause of a persistent or chronic cough, especially causing nocturnal cough due to secretions (mainly from chronic sinusitis) tracking down the larynx and trachea during sleep.
- The commonest causes of haemoptysis are URTI (24%), acute or chronic bronchitis (17%), bronchiectasis (13%), TB (10%). Unknown causes totalled 22% and cancer 4% (figures from a UK study).[2]

Vertebral dysfunction with non-radicular pain (non-specific back pain)

This outstanding common cause of low back pain is considered to be due mainly to dysfunction of the pain-sensitive facet joint. The precise pathophysiology is difficult to pinpoint.

The staff of Asclepius

The staff of Asclepius icon highlights diseases for when you are specifically searching for information on a particular disease.

Red and yellow flags

Red and yellow flags alert you to potential dangers. Red is the most urgent, but yellow also requires careful consideration.

Yellow flag pointers

This term has been introduced to identify psychosocial and occupational factors that may increase the risk of chronicity in people presenting with acute back pain. Consider psychological issues if:

- abnormal illness behaviour
- 'fear avoidance': concern re pain on activity
- compensation issues
- unsatisfactory restoration of activities
- failure to return to work
- unsatisfactory response to treatment
- treatment refused
- atypical presenting physical signs

Red flag pointers for low back pain

There are several so-called 'red flag' or precautionary pointers to a serious underlying cause of back pain (see TABLE 38.3). Such symptoms and signs should alert the practitioner to a serious health problem and thus guide selection of investigations, particularly appropriate imaging of the lumbar spine.

Clinical framework

Clinical framework based on major steps of clinical features, investigations, diagnosis, management and treatment reflects the key activities in the daily tasks of general practitioners.

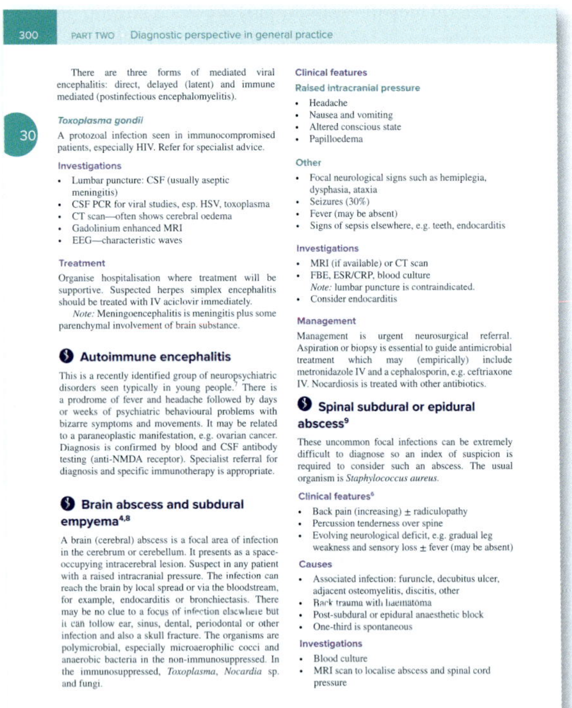
300 PART TWO Diagnostic perspective in general practice

There are three forms of mediated viral encephalitis: direct, delayed (latent) and immune mediated (postinfectious encephalomyelitis).

30

Toxoplasma gondii

A protozoal infection seen in immunocompromised patients, especially HIV. Refer for specialist advice.

Investigations

- Lumbar puncture: CSF (usually aseptic meningitis)
- CSF PCR for viral studies, esp. HSV, toxoplasma
- CT scan—often shows cerebral oedema
- Gadolinium enhanced MRI
- EEG—characteristic waves

Treatment

Organise hospitalisation where treatment will be supportive. Suspected herpes simplex encephalitis should be treated with IV aciclovir immediately.

Note: Meningoencephalitis is meningitis plus some parenchymal involvement of brain substance.

Autoimmune encephalitis

This is a recently identified group of neuropsychiatric disorders seen typically in young people.[7] There is a prodrome of fever and headache followed by days or weeks of psychiatric behavioural problems with bizarre symptoms and movements. It may be related to a paraneoplastic manifestation, e.g. ovarian cancer. Diagnosis is confirmed by blood and CSF antibody testing (anti-NMDA receptor). Specialist referral for diagnosis and specific immunotherapy is appropriate.

Brain abscess and subdural empyema[4,8]

A brain (cerebral) abscess is a focal area of infection in the cerebrum or cerebellum. It presents as a space-occupying intracerebral lesion. Suspect in any patient with a raised intracranial pressure. The infection can reach the brain by local spread or via the bloodstream, for example, endocarditis or bronchiectasis. There may be no clue to a focus of infection elsewhere but it can follow ear, sinus, dental, periodontal or other infection and also a skull fracture. The organisms are polymicrobial, especially microaerophilic cocci and anaerobic bacteria in the non-immunosuppressed. In the immunosuppressed, *Toxoplasma*, *Nocardia* sp. and fungi.

Clinical features

Raised intracranial pressure

- Headache
- Nausea and vomiting
- Altered conscious state
- Papilloedema

Other

- Focal neurological signs such as hemiplegia, dysphasia, ataxia
- Seizures (30%)
- Fever (may be absent)
- Signs of sepsis elsewhere, e.g. teeth, endocarditis

Investigations

- MRI (if available) or CT scan
- FBE, ESR/CRP, blood culture
  Note: lumbar puncture is contraindicated.
- Consider endocarditis

Management

Management is urgent neurosurgical referral. Aspiration or biopsy is essential to guide antimicrobial treatment which may (empirically) include metronidazole IV and a cephalosporin, e.g. ceftriaxone IV. Nocardiosis is treated with other antibiotics.

Spinal subdural or epidural abscess[9]

These uncommon focal infections can be extremely difficult to diagnose so an index of suspicion is required to consider such an abscess. The usual organism is *Staphylococcus aureus*.

Clinical features[6]

- Back pain (increasing) ± radiculopathy
- Percussion tenderness over spine
- Evolving neurological deficit, e.g. gradual leg weakness and sensory loss ± fever (may be absent)

Causes

- Associated infection: furuncle, decubitus ulcer, adjacent osteomyelitis, discitis, other
- Back trauma with haematoma
- Post-subdural or epidural anaesthetic block
- One-third is spontaneous

Investigations

- Blood culture
- MRI scan to localise abscess and spinal cord pressure

Seven masquerades checklist

This unique feature of the book reminds you of potential and hidden dangers underlying patient presentations.

Seven masquerades checklist

Depression, diabetes, drugs, spinal dysfunction and UTI can all cause abdominal pain although the pain may be more subacute or chronic. Abdominal pain and even tenderness can accompany diabetic ketoacidosis. Drugs that can cause abdominal pain are listed in TABLE 34.4.

Spinal dysfunction of the lower thoracic spine and thoracolumbar junction can cause referred pain to the abdomen. The pain is invariably unilateral, radicular in distribution, and related to activity. It can be confused with intra-abdominal problems such as biliary disease (right-sided), appendicitis and Crohn disease (right side), diverticular disorder (left-sided) and pyelonephritis.

Diagnostic triads

Key features that may discriminate between one disease and another are clearly presented.

DxT light-brown skin patches + skin tumours + axillary freckles ➜ NF1

Evidence-based research

Evidence-based research is recognised with a full chapter on research in general practice and evidence base, including more on qualitative models. In addition, substantial references are provided for every chapter.

Research and evidence-based medicine 13

Not the possession of truth, but the effort of struggling to attain it brings joy to the researcher.

GOFFHOLD LASSING (1729–81)

Effective research is the trademark of the medical profession. When confronted with the great responsibility of understanding and treating human beings we need as much scientific evidence as possible to render our decision making valid, credible and justifiable.

Research can be defined as 'a systematic method in which the truth of evidence is based on observing and testing the soundness of conclusions according to consistent rules'[1] or, to put it more simply, 'research is organised curiosity',[2] the end point being new and improved knowledge.

In the medical context the term 'research' tends to conjecture bench-type laboratory research. However, the discipline of general practice provides a fertile research area in which to evaluate the morbidity patterns and the nature of common problems in addition to the processes specific to primary health care.

There has been an excellent tradition of research conducted by GPs. Tim Murrell in his paper 'Nineteenth century masters of general practice'[3] describes the contributions of Edward Jenner, Caleb Parry, John Snow, Robert Koch and James MacKenzie, and notes that 'among the characteristics they shared was their capacity to observe and record natural phenomena, breaking new frontiers of discovery in medicine using an ecological paradigm'.

This tradition was carried into the 20th century by Australian GPs such as Clifford Jungfer, Alan Chancellor, Charles Bridges-Webb, Kevin Cullen and Trevor Beard,[4] and now the research activities of the new generation of GPs, academic-based or practice-based, have been taken to a higher level with the development of evidence-based medicine (EBM).

Based on the work of the Cochrane Collaboration and the initiatives of Chris Silagy, Paul Glasziou and Chris Del Mar in particular, research has moved from the relatively 'pure' hospital environment to 'real world' scenarios which better reflect the circumstances of patients living in the community. Plenty of interventions which seem to work well in sponsored clinical trials are less impressive when measured in general practice. Some other interventions such as lifestyle management turn out to be surprisingly effective once they are accurately measured.

The focus of EBM has been to improve health care and health economics. Its development has gone hand in hand with improved information technology. EBM is inextricably linked to research.

The aim of this chapter is to present a brief overview of research and EBM and, in particular, to encourage GPs, either singly or collectively, to undertake research—simple or sophisticated—and also to publish their work. The benefits of such are well outlined in John Howie's classic text *Research in General Practice*.[5]

Why do research?

The basic objective of research is to acquire new knowledge and justification for decision making in medical practice. Research provides a basis for the acquisition of many skills, particularly those of critical thinking and scientific methodology. The discipline of general practice is special to us with its core content of continuing, comprehensive, community-based primary care, family care, domiciliary care, whole-person care and preventive care. To achieve credibility and parity with our specialist colleagues we need to research this area with appropriate methodology and to define the discipline clearly. There is no area of medicine that involves such a diverse range and quantity of decisions each day as general practice, and therefore patient management needs as much evidence-based rigour as possible.

Our own patch, be it an isolated rural practice or an industrial suburban practice, has its own micro-epidemiological fascination. Thus, it provides a unique opportunity to find answers to questions and make observations about that particular community.

Increasingly, GPs are expected to be able to sift through mountains of information in order to reliably offer advice about how the evidence applies to the individual sitting in front of them. Much of the information available to patients and doctors is either dubious opinion, or skewed towards the interests of an entity providing the intervention, rather than to the patient. An understanding

Extensive coverage of paediatric and geriatric care, pregnancy and complementary therapies

Extensive coverage of paediatric and geriatric care, pregnancy and complementary therapies is integrated throughout, as well as devoted chapter content providing more comprehensive information in these areas.

102 PART ONE The basis of general practice

Analgesics in the elderly

Older patients have the highest incidence of painful disorders and also surgical procedures. As a general rule, most elderly patients are more sensitive to opioid analgesics and to aspirin and other NSAIDs but there may be considerable individual differences in tolerance. Patients over 65 years should receive lower initial doses of opioid analgesics with subsequent doses being titrated according to the patient's needs.[1]

Some general rules and tips[1,9]

- Start with 25–50% of the usual dose.
- Give analgesics at fixed times by the clock rather than 'prn' for ongoing pain.
- Regularly monitor your patient's analgesic requirements and modify according to needs and adverse effects.
- Start with a dose towards the lower end of the dose range and then titrate upwards depending on response.
- Avoid using compound analgesics and prescribe simple and opioid analgesics separately.
- Reserve the use of anti-emetics for the development of nausea and vomiting with opioids. Extrapyramidal reactions (dystonia and oculogyric crises) can be a problem with anti-emetics.
- Advise patients about the benefits of high-fibre foods if on analgesics. Prescribe a bulking agent (peristalsis stimulant) or lactulose if necessary.

Prescribing NSAIDs

12

NSAIDs have analgesic, antipyretic and anti-inflammatory activity. They inhibit synthesis of prostaglandins by inhibiting cyclo-oxygenase (COX) present in COX-1 and COX-2. They are very effective against nociceptive pain.

The prescribing of aspirin and other NSAIDs is an area of increasing concern to all GPs, especially in the elderly with their increasing propensity to the pain of arthritic conditions and demands for relief. About 15% of the patients on a GP's list in the UK will present with a locomotor problem.[10] A common response to the symptoms of rheumatic complaints is to prescribe NSAIDs; in the US 55% of all visits by patients with arthritis will lead to a prescription for a NSAID.[11]

Unfortunately, the use of NSAIDs involves a high incidence of side effects, ranging from the trivial to the lethal, with many deaths from bleeding ulcers, especially in the elderly. The NSAIDs 'epidemic' prevails because the agents continue to be perceived as the best available for the relief of arthritic symptoms. Of particular concern, however, is the widespread use of NSAIDs for common problems such as back pain when the main cause is dysfunctional or mechanical without evidence of inflammation. Surprisingly, many of these patients appear to achieve a good response to NSAIDs.

The choice of NSAIDs can be controversial. Some are claimed to have more adverse effects than others but there is little evidence of substantial differences.[2,11] There is no doubt that particular NSAIDs are of great value in specific rheumatic conditions. Both indomethacin and phenylbutazone are more effective for the spondyloarthropathies and gout.[11] It is worthwhile being mindful of their half-lives. NSAIDs with short half-lives include aspirin, diclofenac, tiaprofenic acid, ketoprofen, ibuprofen and indomethacin. NSAIDs with long half-lives include diflunisal, naproxen, sulindac, piroxicam and tenoxicam, and these are useful in the treatment of chronic pain such as bony metastases in cancer.

TABLE 12.3 shows the classification of NSAIDs.

Table 12.3 Classification of NSAIDs[1]

Action	Example
Non-selective inhibitors of COX-1 and COX-2, mainly in CNS	Paracetamol
Non-selective inhibitors of COX-1 and COX-2, acting in both CNS and periphery	Aspirin Ketorolac Other NSAIDs
Selective NSAIDs	
Specific inhibitors of COX-2	Celecoxib Etoricoxib Meloxicam Paracoxib
Preferential inhibitors of COX-2 over COX-1	Meloxicam

Note: COX = cyclo-oxygenase

Studies have identified certain patients who appear to have significant risk factors for the likely development of NSAID lesions (gastropathy). NSAID ulceration and its complications (see TABLE 12.4) are more prevalent in the elderly, particularly in females.

It is likely that NSAIDs have been prescribed too readily in Australia, particularly in general practice.[11] In a review,[12] a reduction of NSAID prescribing was recommended, particularly for conditions where inflammation is not a major feature (e.g. osteoarthritis and 'mechanical' back pain). Consumption has

Practice tips

Practice tips consist of key points that are of use in the clinical setting.

Practice tips

- Back pain that is related to posture, aggravated by movement and sitting, and relieved by lying down is due to vertebral dysfunction, especially a disc disruption.
- The pain from most disc lesions is generally relieved by rest.
- Plain X-rays are of limited use, especially in younger patients, and may appear normal in disc

Clinical photos

Clinical photos provide authentic, visual examples of many conditions and serve as either a valuable introduction or confirmation of diagnosis.

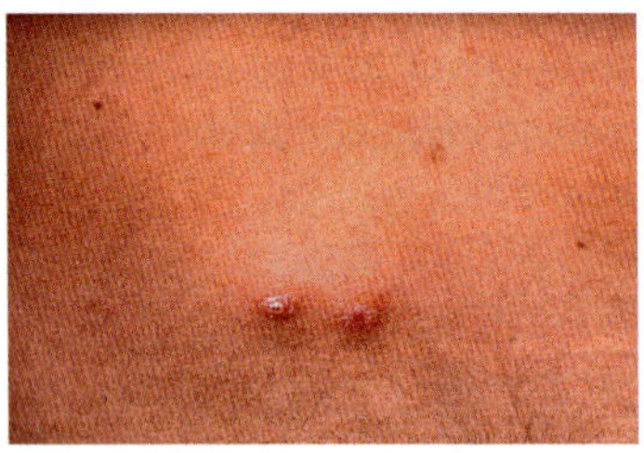

FIGURE 15.4 Cutaneous leishmaniasis in a serviceman after returning from the Middle East

Significantly enhanced index

The index has more sub-categories with bold page numbers indicating the main treatment of a topic, enabling you to quickly pinpoint the most relevant information. Page numbers in italics refer to figures and tables. Entries with '*see also*' have cross-references to related, but more specific information on the topic.

Index

Page numbers in **bold** indicate sections or extensive treatment of a topic.
Page numbers in *italics* indicate figures or tables.
Entries starting with numbers precede the alphabetical sequence, excepting numbers preceding the names of chemicals, which are ignored in filing. For example: 5-fluorouracil files as fluorouracil.

Full colour illustrations

Full colour illustrations are provided, with more than 600 diagrams in the clean, simple style that has proved so popular.

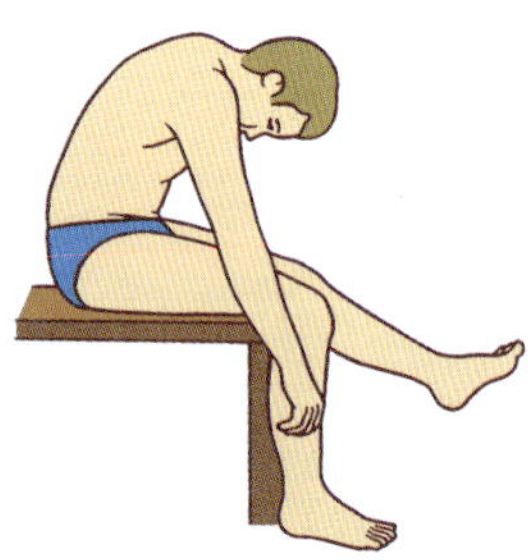

FIGURE 38.5 The slump test: one of the stages

Patient education resources

Indicates where you can find relevant information from *Murtagh's Patient Education*, seventh edition, to photocopy and hand out to patients.

Patient education resources

Hand-out sheets from *Murtagh's Patient Education* 7th edition:

- Backache
- Exercises for your lower back
- Sciatica
- Spondylosis

Reviewers

The sixth and seventh editions underwent a rigorous peer review process to ensure that *General Practice* remains the gold standard reference for general practitioners around the world.

To that end, the author and the publishers extend their sincere gratitude to the following people who generously gave their time, knowledge and expertise.

Content consultants

The authors are indebted to the many consultants who reviewed parts of the manuscript relevant to their areas of expertise and provided help and advice.

Dr Deborah Bateson	family planning
Dr Roy Beran	epilepsy; neurological dilemmas
Dr Peter Berger	a diagnostic and management approach to skin problems
Dr James Best	depression, anxiety, male health, child and adolescent health, communication skills
Professor Geoff Bishop	basic antenatal care
Dr John Boxall	palpitations
Dr Penny Burns	disaster medicine
Dr Jill Cargnello	hair disorders
Dr Paul Coughlin and Professor Hatem Salem	bruising and bleeding; thrombosis and thromboembolism
Mr Rod Dalziel	shoulder pain
Dr David Dunn and Dr Hung The Nguyen	the health of Indigenous peoples
Dr Robert Dunne	common skin wounds and foreign bodies
Professor Jon Emery	genetic disorders, malignant disease
Genetic Health Services, Victoria	genetic disorders
Dr Lindsay Grayson and Associate Professor Joseph Torresi	travel medicine, the returned traveller and tropical medicine
Dr Michael Gribble	anaemia
Mr John Griffiths	pain in the hip and buttock
Professor Michael Grigg	pain in the leg
Dr Gary Grossbard	the painful knee
Dr Peter Hardy-Smith	the red and tender eye; visual failure
Professor David Healy (deceased)	abnormal uterine bleeding
Assoc Professor Peter Holmes	cough; dyspnoea; asthma; COPD

Dr Ndidi Victor Ikealumba and Dr Cheng I-Hao	refugee health, tropical medicine (Dr Ikealumba)
Professor Michael Kidd, Dr Ron McCoy and Dr Alex Welborn	human immunodeficiency virus infection
Professor Gab Kovacs	abnormal uterine bleeding; the subfertile couple
Professor Even Laerum	research in general practice
Dr Barry Lauritz (deceased)	common skin problems; pigmented skin lesions
Mr Peter Lawson (deceased) and Dr Sanjiva Wijesinha	disorders of the penis; prostatic disorders
Dr Peter Lowthian	arthritis
Mr Frank Lyons	common fractures and dislocations
Dr John Mackellar	child abuse and domestic violence
Professor Barry McGrath	hypertension
Dr Joe McKendrick	malignant disease
Dr Luke Murtagh	pain and its management
Professor Robyn O'Hehir	allergic disorders, including hayfever
Dr Michael Oldmeadow	tiredness
Dr Frank Panetta	chest pain
Professor Roger Pepperell	basic antenatal care
Dr Geoff Quail	pain in the face, sore mouth and tongue
Mr Ronald Quirk	pain in the foot and ankle
Dr Ian Rogers	emergency care
Professor Avni Sali	abdominal pain, lumps in the breast, jaundice, constipation, dyspepsia, nutrition
Dr Hugo Standish	urinary tract infection, chronic kidney failure
Dr Richard Stark	neurological diagnostic triads
Professor Geoff Sussman	skin ulcers
Dr Paul Tallman	stroke and transient ischaemic attacks
Dr Alison Walsh	breastfeeding, post-natal breast disorders
Professor Greg Whelan	alcohol problems, drug problems
Dr Sanjiva Wijesinha	men's health, scrotal pain, inguinoscrotal lumps
Dr Alan Yung	fever and chills, sore throat
Dr Ronnie Yuen	diabetes mellitus, thyroid and other endocrine disorders

A substantial number of people were involved in reviewing this book through surveys; their invaluable contribution is acknowledged below. We also take the opportunity to thank the other participants who preferred not to be named in this collective.

Survey respondents

Ashraf Aboud
Mehdi Alzaini

Anne Balcomb
Jill Benson
Ibrahim K Botros
Chris Briggs
Kathy Brotchie
Shane Brun
Daniel Byrne

Paul Carroll
Louisa Case
Ercelle Celis
Peter Charlton
Tricia Charmer
Rudolph W M Chow
Patrick Clancy
Jennifer Cook-Foxwell
Barrie Coulson
Therese Cox
Roxane Craig
Gordana Cuk
Melita Cullen
Alice Cunningham

Fred De Looze
Rudi De Mulder
Gabrielle Dellit
Michael Desouza
Yock Seck Ding
Matthew Dwyer

Judith Ellis
Jon Emery
Say Poh Eng
Iain Esslemont
Marian Evans

Wes Fabb
N Fajardo
Cyril Fernandez
Danika Fietz
Clare Finnigan
Anthony Fok
Oliver Frank

Brett Garrett
Tarek Gergis
Ben Gerhardy
Elena Ghergori
Naomi Ginges
Jim Griffin
Ranjan Gupta

Hadia Haikal-Mukhtar
Pedita Hall
Nazih Hamzeh
Erfanul Haque
Abby Harwood
Mark Henschke
Edward C Herman
D Ho
David Holford
Sue Hookey
Elspeth Horn
Seyed Ebrahim Hosseini
Faline Howes
Brett Hunt
Rosalyn Hunt
Farhana Hussein
Robyn Hüttenmeister

Anwar Ikladios
John Inkwater

Daljit Janjua
Diosdado Javellana
Aravinda Jawali
Les Jenshel
Fiona Joske
Meredith Joslin
Gloria Jove

Mohammed Al Kamil
Inas Abdul Karim
Sophia Kennelly
George Kostalas
Jim Kourdoulos

Ivan S Lee
Mohammad Shafeeq
Lone
Christine Lonergan
Dac Luu

Justin Madden
Hemant Mahagaonkar
Meredith Makeham
Shahid Malick
Muhammad Mannan
Luke Manestar
Linda Mann
Cameron Martin
Kohei Matsuda
Ronald Mccoy
Mark McGrath
Robert Meehan
Scott Milan
Kirsten Miles
Vahid Mohabbati
Megha Mulchandani
Patrick Mulhern
Brad Murphy
Charles Mutandwa

Keshwan Nadan
Ching-Luen Ng
Mark Nelson
Harry Nespolon

Brent O'Carrigan
Christopher Oh

John Padgett
George Pappas
Peter Parkes
W J Patterson
Anoula Pavli
Matthew Penn
Satish Prasad

Tereza Rada
Jason Rajakulendran
Muhammad Raza
Kate Roe
Daniel Rouhead
Fiona Runacres

Safwat Saba
Amin Sauddin
Kelly Seach
Leslie Segal
Isaac Seidl
Rubini Selvaratnam
Theja Seneviratne
Karina Severin
Pravesh Shah
Mitra Babazadeh Shahri
Jamie Sharples
G Sivasambu
Russell Shute
Sue Smith
Jane Smith
Lucie Stanford
Sean Stevens
S Sutharsamohan

Hui Tai Tan
Marlene Tham
Heinz Tilenius
Judy Toman
Khai Tran
Joseph V Turner

Susan Wearne
Anthony Wickins
Kristen Willson
Melanie Winter
Jeanita Wong
Belinda Woo
Belinda Wozencroft

Laboratory reference values

These reference values and ranges are given in the system of international units (SI) and may vary from laboratory to laboratory.

An asterisk (*) indicates that paediatric reference ranges differ from the adult range given.

Electrolytes/renal	
Sodium	135–145 mmol/L
Potassium*	3.5–5.0 mmol/L
Chloride	95–110 mmol/L
Bicarbonate	23–32 mmol/L
Urea	3–8.0 mmol/L
Creatinine	♀ 50–110; ♂ 60–120 μmol/L
eGFR	>60 mL/min/1.72 m^2
Calcium*	2.10–2.60 mmol/L (total)
Phosphate	0.90–1.35 mmol/L
Magnesium*	0.65–1.00 mmol/L
Uric acid*	♀ 0.12–0.40; ♂ 0.15–0.45 mmol/L

Liver function/pancreas	
Bilirubin*	<20 μmol/L (total) <3 μmol/L (direct)
AST*	<40 U/L
GGT*	♀ <30; ♂ <50 U/L
Alkaline phosphatase (ALP)*	25–100 U/L
Total protein	60–80 g/L
Albumin	38–50 g/L
Amylase	30–110 U/L
Lipase	<100 U/L

Glucose	
Glucose fasting	3–5.4 mmol/L
Glucose random	3–7.7 mmol/L
HbA1c	4.7–6.1%

Haematology	
Hb*	♀ 115–165; ♂ 130–180 g/L
PCV*	♀ 37–47; ♂ 40–54%
MCV*	80–100 fL
Reticulocytes	0.5–2.0%
White cells	4.0–11.0 × 10^9/L
Platelets	150–400 × 10^9/L
ESR	<20 mm; <35mm if >70 years
Band neutrophils*	(0.05 × 10^9/L)
Mature neutrophils*	(2.0–7.5 × 10^9/L)
Lymphocytes*	(1.0–4.0 × 10^9/L)
Monocytes*	(0.2–0.8 × 10^9/L)
Eosinophils*	(0.0–0.4 × 10^9/L)
Folate	serum 7–45 nmol/L, red cell 360–1400 nmol/L
s Vitamin B12	(150–700 pmol/L)

Coagulation	
Bleeding time	2.0–8.5 min
Fibrinogen	2.0–4.0 g/L
Prothrombin time	sec.
Prothrombin ratio INR	1.0–1.2
APTT	25–35 sec
D-dimer	<500 mg/mL

Others	
s Creatine phospho kinase	<90 U/L
s Lead	<2 μmol/L
s C–reactive protein	<10 mg/L
Vitamin D	>75 mmol/L

Cardiac/lipids	
Troponin I or T	<0.1 ug/L
CK total	♀ <200; ♂ <220 U/L
CK-MB	<25 U/L
Cholesterol*	<5.5 mmol/L
Triglycerides*	<1.7 mmol/L
HDL cholesterol	♀ 1–2.2; ♂ 0.9–2.0 mmol/L
LDL cholesterol	2–3.4 mmol/L

Thyroid tests	
Free T_4	10.0–25.0 pmol/L
Ultra–sensitive TSH*	0.4–5.0 mU/L
Free T_3	3.3–8.2 pmol/L

Other endocrine tests	
s Cortisol	8 am 130–700 nmol/L
	4 pm 80–350 nmol/L
FSH	1–9 IU/L (adult ♀) 10–30 IU/L (ovulation) 4–200 IU/L (postmenopausal)
Oestradiol menopausal	<200 pmol/L
Testosterone	♀ <3.5; ♂ 10–35 nmol/L

Tumour markers	
PSA	0–1.0 mcg/L
CEA	<7.5 mcg/L
AFT	<10 mcg/mL
CA–125	<35 U/mL

Iron studies	
Ferritin	♀ 15–200; ♂ 30–300 mcg/L
Iron	10–30 μmol/L
Iron–binding capacity	45–80 μmol/L
Transferrin	2–3.5 g/L
Transferrin saturation	♀ 15–45%; ♂ 15–55%

Blood gases/arterial	
pH*	7.38–7.43
P_aO_2*	85–105 mmHg
P_aCO_2*	36–44 mmHg
Bicarbonate*	20–28 mmol/L
Base excess*	–3 to +3 mmol/L

Normal values: worth knowing by heart

The following is a checklist that can be used as a template to memorise normal quantitative values for basic medical conditions and management.

Vital signs (average)	< 6 months	6 months – 3 years	3 – 12 years	Adult
Pulse	120–140	110	80 – 100	60 – 100
Respiratory rate	45	30	20	14
BP (mmHg)	90/60	90/60	100/70	≤ 130/85

Children's weight	1–10 years
Rule of thumb:	Wt = (age + 4) × 2 kg

Fever—temperature (morning)[(a)]

(a) There is considerable diurnal variation in temperature so that it is higher in the evening (0.5–1°C). I would recommend the definition given by Yung et al. in *Infectious Diseases: a Clinical Approach*: 'Fever can be defined as an early morning oral temperature > 37.2°C or a temperature > 37.8°C at other times of the day'.

Oral	> 37.2°C
Rectal	> 37.7°C

Diabetes mellitus—Diagnostic criteria: blood sugar	
Random 1 reading if symptomatic 2 readings if asymptomatic	> 11.1 mmol/L
Fasting	> 7.0 mmol/L
or	the 2 values from an oral GTT

Hypokalaemia	
Serum potassium	< 3.5 mmol/L

Jaundice	
Serum bilirubin	> 19 μmol/L

Hyperkalaemia	
Serum potassium	> 5.0 mmol/L

Hypertension	
BP	> 140/90 mmHg

Alcohol excessive drinking	
Males	> 4 standard drinks/day
Females	> 2 standard drinks/day

Alcohol health guidelines	
Males and females	≤ 2 standard drinks/day < 4 standard drinks/occasion

Anaemia—haemoglobin	
Males	< 130 g/L
Females	< 115 g/L

Body mass index	Wt (kg)/Ht (m2)
Normal	20–25
Overweight	> 25
Obesity	> 30

Abbreviations

AAA	abdominal aortic aneurysm
AAFP	American Academy of Family Physicians
ABA	Australian Breastfeeding Association
ABC	airway, breathing, circulation
ABCD	airway, breathing, circulation, dextrose
ABFP	American Board of Family Practice
ABI	ankle brachial index
ABO	A, B and O blood groups
AC	air conduction
AC	acromioclavicular
ACAH	autoimmune chronic active hepatitis
ACE	angiotensin-converting enzyme
ACL	anterior cruciate ligament
ACR	albumin creatine ratio
ACTH	adrenocorticotrophic hormone
AD	aortic dissection
AD	autosomal dominant
ADHD	attention deficit hyperactivity disorder
ADT	adult diphtheria vaccine
AF	atrial fibrillation
AFI	amniotic fluid index
AFP	alpha-fetoprotein
AI	aortic incompetence
AICD	automatic implantable cardiac defibrillator
AIDS	acquired immunodeficiency syndrome
AIIRA	angiotension II(2) reuptake antagonist
AKF	acute kidney failure
ALE	average life expectancy
ALL	acute lymphocytic leukaemia
ALP	alkaline phosphatase
ALT	alanine aminotransferase
ALTE	apparent life-threatening episode
AMI	acute myocardial infarction
AML	acute myeloid leukaemia
ANA	antinuclear antibody
ANCI	antineutrophil cytoplasmic antibody
ANF	antinuclear factor
a/n/v	anorexia/nausea/vomiting
AP	anterior–posterior
APF	Australian pharmaceutical formulary
APH	ante-partum haemorrhage
APRI	ast to platelet ratio index
APTT	activated partial thromboplastin time
AR	autosomal recessive
ARB	Angiotension II receptor blocker
ARC	AIDS-related complex
ARDS	adult respiratory distress syndrome
ARR	absolute risk reduction
ART	anti retroviral therapy
ASD	atrial septal defect
ASIS	anterior superior iliac spine
ASOT	antistreptolysin 0 titre
AST	aspartate aminotransferase
ATFL	anterior talofibular ligament
AV	atrioventricular
AVM	arteriovenous malformation
AZT	azidothymidine
BC	bone conduction
BCC	basal cell carcinoma
BCG	bacille Calmette–Guérin
bDMARDs	biological disease modifying antirheumatic drugs
BMD	bone mass density
BMI	body mass index
BNP	B-type natriuretic peptide
BOO	bladder outlet obstruction
BP	blood pressure
BPH	benign prostatic hyperplasia
BPPV	benign paroxysmal positional vertigo
BSE	breast self-examination
Ca	carcinoma
CABG	coronary artery bypass grafting
CAD	coronary artery disease
CAP	community acquired pneumonia
CBE	clinical breast examination
CBT	cognitive behaviour therapy
CCB	calcium channel blocker
CCF	congestive cardiac failure

CCP cyclic citrinullated peptide
CCT controlled clinical trial
CCU coronary care unit
CD_4 T helper cell
CD_8 T suppressor cell
CDT combined diphtheria/tetanus vaccine
CEA carcinoembryonic antigen
CFL calcaneofibular ligament
CFS chronic fatigue syndrome
cfu colony forming unit
CHC combined hormonal contraception
CHD coronary heart disease
CHF chronic heart failure
CI confidence interval
CIN cervical intraepithelial neoplasia
CJD Creutzfeldt–Jakob disease
CK creatinine kinase
CK–MB creatinine kinase–myocardial bound fraction
CKD chronic kidney disease
CKF chronic kidney failure
CMC carpometacarpal
CML chronic myeloid leukaemia
CMV cytomegalovirus
CNS central nervous system
co compound
COAD chronic obstructive airways disease
COC combined oral contraceptive
COCP combined oral contraceptive pill
COMT catechol-O-methyl transferase
COPD chronic obstructive pulmonary disease
COX cyclooxygenase
CPA cardiopulmonary arrest
CPAP continuous positive airways pressure
CPK creatine phosphokinase
CPPD calcium pyrophosphate dihydrate
CPR cardiopulmonary resuscitation
CPS complex partial seizures
CR controlled release
CRD computerised reference database system
CREST calcinosis cutis; Raynaud's phenomenon; oesophageal involvement; sclerodactyly; telangiectasia
CRF chronic renal failure
CRFM chloroquine-resistant falciparum malaria
CRH corticotrophin-releasing hormone
CR(K)F chronic renal (kidney) failure
CRP C-reactive protein
CSF cerebrospinal fluid
CSFM chloroquine-sensitive falciparum malaria
CSIs COX-2 specific inhibitors
CSU catheter specimen of urine
CT computerised tomography
CTD connective tissue disorder
CTG cardiotocograph
CTS carpal tunnel syndrome
CVA cerebrovascular accident
CVS cardiovascular system
CXR chest X-ray

DAA direct acting antivirals
DBP diastolic blood pressure
DC direct current
DDAVP desmopressin acetate
DDH developmental dysplasia of the hip
DDP dipeptidyl peptidase
DEXA dual energy X-ray absorptiometry
DHA docosahexaenoic acid
DHEA dihydroepiandrosterone
DI diabetes insipidus
DIC disseminated intravascular coagulation
DIDA di-imino diacetic acid
DIMS disorders of initiating and maintaining sleep
DIP distal interphalangeal
dL decilitre
DMARDs disease modifying antirheumatic drugs
DNA deoxyribose-nucleic acid
DOM direction of movement
DRE digital rectal examination
DRABC defibrillation, resuscitation, airway, breathing, circulation
drug dosage bd—twice daily; tid, tds—three times daily; qid—four times daily
ds double strand
DS double strength
DSM diagnostic and statistical manual (of mental disorders)
DU duodenal ulcer
DUB dysfunctional uterine bleeding
DVT deep venous thrombosis
DxT diagnostic triad

EAR	expired air resuscitation
EBM	Epstein–Barr mononucleosis (glandular fever)
EBNA	Epstein–Barr nuclear antigen
EBV	Epstein–Barr virus
ECC	external chest compression
ECG	electrocardiogram
ECT	electroconvulsive therapy
ED	emergency department
EDD	expected due date
EEG	electroencephalogram
ELISA	enzyme linked immunosorbent assay
EMG	electromyogram
ENA	extractable nuclear antigen
EO	ethinyloestradiol
EPA	eicosapentaenoic acid
EPL	extensor pollicis longus
EPS	expressed prostatic secretions
ER	external rotation
ESRF	end-stage renal failure
ESR(K)F	end stage renal (kidney) failure
ERCP	endoscopic retrograde cholangiopancreatography
esp.	especially
ESR	erythrocyte sedimentation rate
ET	embryo transfer
ETT	endotracheal tube

FAD	familial Alzheimer disease
FAI	femeroacetabular impingement
FAP	familial adenomatous polyposis
FB	foreign body
FBE	full blood count
FDIU	fetal death in utero
FDL	flexor digitorum longus
FEV_1	forced expiratory volume in 1 second
FHL	flexor hallucis longus
fL	femto-litre (10^{-15})
FRAX	fracture risk assessment tool
FRC	functional residual capacity
FSH	follicle stimulating hormone
FTA–ABS	fluorescent treponemal antibody absorption test
FTT	failure to thrive
FUO	fever of undetermined origin
FVC	forced vital capacity
FXS	fragile X syndrome

g	gram
GA	general anaesthetic
GABHS	group A beta-haemolytic streptococcus
GBS	Guillain–Barré syndrome
GCA	giant cell arteritis
GESA	Gastroenterological Society of Australia
GFR	glomerular filtration rate
GGT	gamma-glutamyl transferase
GHJ	glenohumeral joint
GI	glycaemic index
GIFT	gamete intrafallopian transfer
GIT	gastrointestinal tract
GLP	glucagon-like peptide
GnRH	gonadotrophin-releasing hormone
GO	gastro-oesophageal
GORD	gastro-oesophageal reflux
GP	general practitioner
G-6-PD	glucose-6-phosphate
GSI	genuine stress incontinence
GU	gastric ulcer
GV	growth velocity

HAV	hepatitis A virus
anti-HAV	hepatitis A antibody
Hb	haemoglobin
HbA	haemoglobin A
anti-HBc	hepatitis B core antibody
HBeAg	hepatitis Be antigen
anti-HBs	hepatits B surface antibody
HBsAg	hepatitis B surface antigen
HBV	hepatitis B virus
HCG	human chorionic gonadotropin
HCV	hepatitis C virus
anti-HCV	hepatitis C virus antibody
HDL	high-density lipoprotein
HDV	hepatitis D (Delta) virus
HEV	hepatitis E virus
HFA	hydrofluoro alkane
HFM	hand, foot and mouth
HFV	hepatitis F virus
HGV	hepatitis G virus
HHC	hereditary haemochromatosis
HIDA	hydroxy iminodiacetic acid
HIV	human immunodeficiency virus

$HLA\text{-}B_{27}$	human leucocyte antigen
HMGCoA	hydroxymethylglutaryl CoA
HNPCC	hereditary nonpolyposis colorectal cancer
HPV	human papilloma virus
HRT	hormone replacement therapy
HSIL	high grade squamous intraepithelial lesion
HSP	Henoch–Schönlein purpura
HSV	herpes simplex viral infection
H	hypertension
IBS	irritable bowel syndrome
ICE	ice, compression, elevation
ICHPPC	International Classification of Health Problems in Primary Care
ICS	inhaled corticosteroid
ICS	intercondylar separation
ICSI	intracytoplasmic sperm injection
ICT	immunochromatographic test
IDDM	insulin dependent diabetes mellitus
IDU	injecting drug user
IgE	immunoglobulin E
IgG	immunoglobulin G
IgM	immunoglobulin M
IGRA	interferon gamma release assay
IHD	ischaemic heart disease
IHS	International Headache Society
IM, IMI	intramuscular injection
IMS	intermalleolar separation
inc.	including
INCS	intranasal corticosteroids
INR	international normalised ratio
IOC	International Olympic Committee
IOFB	intraocular foreign body
IP	interphalangeal
IPPV	intermittent positive pressure variation
IR	internal rotation *or* immediate release
ITP	idiopathic (or immune) thrombocytopenia purpura
IUCD	intrauterine contraceptive device
IUGR	intrauterine growth retardation
IV	intravenous
IVF	in-vitro fertilisation
IVI	intravenous injection
IVP	intravenous pyelogram
IVU	intravenous urogram
JCA	juvenile chronic arthritis
JVP	jugular venous pulse
KA	keratoacanthoma
KFT	kidney function test
kg	kilogram
KOH	potassium hydroxide
KUB-scan	kidney ureter bladder scan
LA	local anaesthetic
LABA	long acting beta agonist
LBBB	left branch bundle block
LBO	large bowel obstruction
LBP	low back pain
LCR	ligase chain reaction
LDH/LH	lactic dehydrogenase
LDL	low-density lipoprotein
LFTs	liver function tests
LH	luteinising hormone
LHRH	luteinising hormone releasing hormone
LIF	left iliac fossa
LLS	lumbar spinal canal stenosis
LMN	lower motor neurone
LNG	levonorgestrel
LPC	liquor picis carbonis
LRTI	lower respiratory tract infection
LSD	lysergic acid
LSIL	low grade squamous intraepithelial lesion
LUQ	left upper quadrant
LUT	lower urinary tract
LUTS	lower urinary tract symptoms
LV	left ventricular
LVH	left ventricular hypertrophy
MAIS	*Mycobacterium avium intracellulare* or *M. sacrofulaceum*
mane	in morning
MAOI	monoamine oxidase inhibitor
MAST	medical anti-shock trousers
MB	myocardial base
mcg	micrograms (also μg)
MCL	medial collateral ligament
MCP	metacarpal phalangeal
MCU	microscopy and culture of urine
MCV	mean corpuscular volume

MDI	metered dose inhaler
MDMA	methylenedioxymethamphetamine
MDR	multi-drug resistant TB
MG	myaesthenia gravis
MHT	menopause hormone therapy
MI	myocardial infarction
MIC	mitral incompetence
MID	minor intervertebral derangement
MMSE	mini mental state examination
MND	motor neurone disease
MRCP	magnetic resonance cholangiography
MRI	magnetic resonance imaging
MRSA	methicillin-resistant *staphylococcus aureus*
MS	multiple sclerosis
MSM	men who have sex with men
MSST	maternal serum screening test
MSU	midstream urine
MTP	metatarsophalangeal
MVA	motor vehicle accident

N	normal
N saline	normal saline
NAAT	nucleic acid amplification technology
NAD	no abnormality detected
NET	norethisterone
NF	neurofibromatosis
NGU	non-gonococcal urethritis
NHL	non-Hodgkin's lymphoma
NH&MRC	National Health and Medical Research Council
NIDDM	non-insulin dependent diabetes mellitus
NNT	numbers needed to treat
NOAC	new oral anticoagulants
nocte	at night
NR	normal range
NRT	nicotine replacement therapy
NSAIDs	non-steroidal anti-inflammatory drugs
NSCLC	non-small cell lung cancer
NSU	non-specific urethritis
NTT	nuchal translucency test
NVDPA	National Vascular Disease Prevention Alliance

(o)	taken orally
OA	osteoarthritis
OCP	oral contraceptive pill
OGTT	oral glucose tolerance test
OSA	obstructive sleep apnoea
OSD	Osgood–Schlatter disorder
OT	occupational therapist
OTC	over the counter

PA	posterior–anterior
PAN	polyarteritis nodosa
Pap	Papanicolaou
PBG	porphobilinogen
PBS	Pharmaceutical Benefits Scheme
pc	after meals
PCA	percutaneous continuous analgesia
PCB	post coital bleeding
PCI	percutaneous coronary intervention
PCL	posterior cruciate ligament
PCOS	polycystic ovarian syndrome
PCP	pneumocystitis pneumonia
PCR	polymerase chain reaction
PCV	packed cell volume
PD	Parkinson's disease
PDA	patent ductus arteriosus
PDD	pervasive development disorders
PEF	peak expiratory flow
PEFR	peak expiratory flow rate
PET	pre-eclamptic toxaemia
PET	positron emission tomography
PFO	patent foramen ovale
PFT	pulmonary function test
PGL	persistent generalised lymphadenopathy
PH	past history
PHR	personal health record
PID	pelvic inflammatory disease
PIP	proximal interphalangeal
PKU	phenylketonuria
PLISSIT	permission: limited information: specific suggestion: intensive therapy
PLMs	periodic limb movements
PMDD	premenstrual dysphoric disorder
PMS	premenstrual syndrome
PMT	premenstrual tension
PaO_2	partial pressure oxygen (arterial blood)
POP	plaster of Paris
POP	progestogen-only pill
PPI	proton-pump inhibitor

PPROM	preterm premature rupture of membranes
PR	per rectum
prn	as and when needed
PRNG	penicillin-resistant gonococci
PROM	premature rupture of membranes
PSA	prostate specific antigen
PSGN	post streptococcal glomerulonephritis
PSIS	posterior superior iliac spine
PSVT	paroxysmal supraventricular tachycardia
PT	prothrombin time
PTC	percutaneous transhepatic cholangiography
PTFL	posterior talofibular ligament
PU	peptic ulcer
PUO	pyrexia of undetermined origin
PUVA	psoralen + UVA
pv	per vagina
PVC	polyvinyl chloride
PVD	peripheral vascular disease

qds, qid	four times daily

RA	rheumatoid arthritis
RACGP	Royal Australian College of General Practitioners
RAP	recurrent abdominal pain
RBBB	right branch bundle block
RBC	red blood cell
RCT	randomised controlled trial
RF	rheumatic fever
Rh	rhesus
RIB	rest in bed
RICE	rest, ice, compression, elevation
RIF	right iliac fossa
RPR	rapid plasma reagin
RR	relative risk
RRR	relative risk reduction
RSD	reflex sympathetic dystrophy
RSI	repetition strain injury
RSV	respiratory syncytial virus
RT	reverse transcriptase
rtPA	recombinant tissue plasminogen activator
RUQ	right upper quadrant

s	serum
SABA	short-acting beta agonist
SAH	subarachnoid haemorrhage
SARS	severe acute respiratory distress syndrome
SBE	subacute bacterial endocarditis
SBO	small bowel obstruction
SBP	systolic blood pressure
SC/SCI	subcutaneous/subcutaneous injection
SCC	squamous cell carcinoma
SCFE	slipped capital femoral epiphysis
SCG	sodium cromoglycate
SCLC	small cell lung cancer
SERM	selective estrogen receptor modulator
SIADH	syndrome of secretion of inappropriate antidiuretic hormone
SIDS	sudden infant death syndrome
SIJ	sacroiliac joint
SL	sublingual
SLD	specific learning disability
SLE	systemic lupus erythematosus
SLR	straight leg raising
SND	sensorineural deafness
SNHL	sensorineural hearing loss
SNPs	single nucleotide polymorphisms
SNRI	serotonin noradrenaline reuptake inhibitor
SOB	shortness of breath
SLS	salt-losing state
sp	species
SPA	suprapubic aspirate of urine
SPECT	single photon emission computerised tomography
SPF	sun penetration factor
SR	sustained release
SSRI	selective serotonin reuptake inhibitor
SSS	sick sinus syndrome
statim	at once
STI	sexually transmitted infection
STD	sodium tetradecyl sulfate
SUFE	slipped upper femoral epiphysis
SVC	superior vena cava
SVT	supraventricular tachycardia

T_3	tri-iodothyronine
T_4	thyroxine
TA	temporal arteritis
TB	tuberculosis
TCA	tricyclic antidepressant
tds, tid	three times daily
TENS	transcutaneous electrical nerve stimulation
TFTs	thyroid function tests
TG	triglyceride
TIA	transient ischaemic attack
TIBC	total iron binding capacity
TM	tympanic membrane
TMJ	temporomandibular joint
TNF	tissue necrosis factor
TOE	transoesophageal echocardiography
TOF	tracheo-oesophageal fistula
TORCH	toxoplasmosis, rubella, cytomegalovirus, herpes virus
TPHA	Treponema pallidum haemaglutination test
TSE	testicular self-examination
TSH	thyroid-stimulating hormone
TT	thrombin time
TUE	therapeutic use exemption
TUIP	transurethral incision of prostate
TURP	transurethral resection of prostate
TV	tidal volume

U	units
UC	ulcerative colitis
U & E	urea and electrolytes
UGIB	upper gastrointestinal bleeding
μg	microgram
UMN	upper motor neurone
URT	upper respiratory tract
URTI	upper respiratory tract infection
US	ultrasound
UTI	urinary tract infection
U	ultraviolet

VAS	visual analogue scale
VBI	vertebrobasilar insufficiency
VC	vital capacity
VDRL	Venereal Disease Reference Laboratory
VF	ventricular fibrillation
VMA	vanillylmandelic acid
VPG	venous plasma glucose
VRE	vancomycin-resistant enterococci
VSD	ventricular septal defect
VT	ventricular tachycardia
VUR	vesicoureteric reflux
VVS	vulvar vestibular syndrome
vWD	von Willebrand's disease

WBC	white blood cells
WBR	white → blue → red
WCC	white cell count
WHO	World Health Organization
WPW	Wolff–Parkinson–White

XL	sex linked

Part 1

The basis of general practice

1 The nature, scope and content of general practice

Medical practice is not knitting and weaving and the labour of the hands, but it must be inspired with soul and be filled with understanding and equipped with the gift of keen observation; these together with accurate scientific knowledge are the indispensable requisites for proficient medical practice.

MOSES BEN MAIMON (1135–1204)

General practice is a traditional method of bringing primary health care to the community. It is a medical discipline in its own right, linking the vast amount of accumulated medical knowledge with the art of communication.

Definitions

General practice can be defined as that medical discipline which provides 'community-based, continuing, comprehensive, preventive primary care', sometimes referred to as the CCCP model. It is regarded as synonymous with primary care and family practice.

The Royal Australian College of General Practitioners (RACGP) uses the following definitions of general practice and primary care:

> General practice is that component of the health care system which provides initial, continuing, comprehensive and coordinated medical care for all individuals, families and communities and which integrates current biomedical, psychological and social understandings of health.
>
> A general practitioner is a medical practitioner with recognised generalist training, experience and skills, who provides and co-ordinates comprehensive medical care for individuals, families and communities.
>
> General/family practice is the point of first contact for the majority of people seeking health care. In the provision of primary care, much ill-defined illness is seen; the general/family practitioner often deals with problem complexes rather than with established diseases.

The RACGP has defined five domains of general practice:

- communication skills and the doctor–patient relationship
- applied professional knowledge and skills
- population health and the context of general practice
- professional and ethical role
- organisational and legal dimensions

Furthermore the RACGP has identified eight core characteristics of general practice:

1. whole person care
2. person centredness
3. continuity of care
4. comprehensiveness
5. diagnostic and therapeutic skills
6. a command of complexity and uncertainty
7. coordinated clinical teamwork
8. leadership, advocacy and equity

The American Academy of Family Physicians (AAFP) has expanded on the function of delivery of primary health care.[1,2]

> Primary care is a form of delivery of medical care that encompasses the following functions:
>
> 1. It is 'first-contact' care, serving as a point-of-entry for patients into the health care system.
> 2. It includes continuity by virtue of caring for patients over a period of time, both in sickness and in health.
> 3. It is comprehensive care, drawing from all the traditional major disciplines for its functional content.
> 4. It serves a coordinative function for all the health care needs of the patient.
> 5. It assumes continuing responsibility for individual patient follow-up and community health problems.
> 6. It is a highly personalised type of care.

General practice is fundamentally relational, based on the doctor having a deep understanding of the whole person, and the ability to manage complex conditions and circumstances. The general practitioner functions as a physician, counsellor, advocate and agent of change for individuals, families and their communities.[3]

General practice is not the summation of specialties practised at a superficial level and we must avoid the temptation to become 'specialoids'. In the current climate, where medicine is often fragmented, there is a greater than ever need for the generalist. The patient requires a trusted focal point in the often bewildering health service jungle. Who is to do this better than the caring family doctor taking full responsibility for the welfare of the patient and intervening on his or her behalf? Specialists also need highly competent generalists to whom they can entrust ongoing care.

Unique features of general practice

Anderson, Bridges-Webb and Chancellor[4] emphasise that 'the unique and important work of the general practitioner is to provide availability and continuity of care, competence in the realm of diagnosis, care of acute and chronic illness, prompt treatment of emergencies and a preventive approach to health care'.

The features that make general practice different from hospital- or specialist-based medical practices include:

- first contact
- compassion
- diagnostic methodology
- early diagnosis of life-threatening and serious disease
- continuity and availability of care
- personalised care
- care of acute and chronic illness
- domiciliary care
- emergency care (prompt treatment at home or in the community)
- family care
- palliative care (at home)
- preventive care
- scope for health promotion and patient education
- holistic approach to management
- health care coordination

The GP has to be prepared for any problem that comes in the door (FIG. 1.1).

Apart from these processes the GP has to manage very common problems including a whole variety of problems not normally taught in medical school or in postgraduate programs. Many of these problems are unusual yet common and can be regarded as the 'nitty gritty' or 'bread and butter' problems of primary health care.

In considering the level of care of symptoms, 25% of patients abandon self-care for a visit to the GP. Ninety per cent of these visits are managed entirely within primary care. Levels of care are represented in FIGURE 1.1.[5]

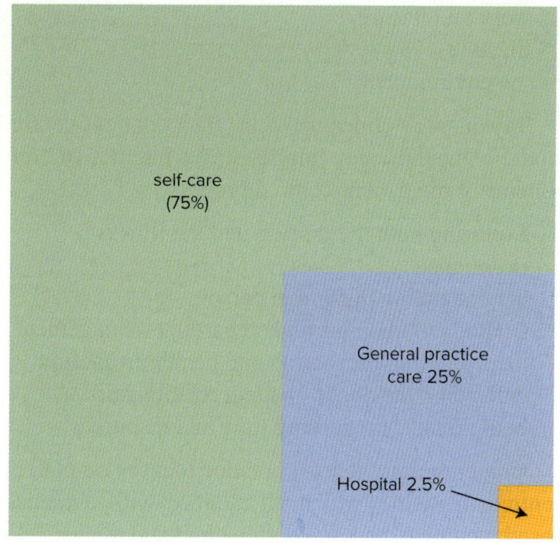

FIGURE 1.1 Degrees of care of symptoms

Holistic approach to management

The management of the whole person, or the holistic approach, is an important approach to patient care in general practice. Whole-person diagnosis is based on two components:

1 the disease-centred diagnosis
2 the patient-centred diagnosis

The disease-centred consultation is the traditional medical model based on the history, examination and special investigations, with the emphasis on making a diagnosis and treating the disease. The disease-centred diagnosis, which is typical of hospital-based medicine, is defined in terms of pathology and does not focus significantly on the feelings of the person suffering from the disease.

> Whole-person care—mind and body—is the hallmark of the good GP.

The patient-centred consultation not only takes into account the diagnosed disease and its management but also adds another dimension—that of the psychosocial hallmarks of the patient, including details about:

- the patient as a person
- emotional reactions to the illness
- the family
- the effect on relationships

- work and leisure
- lifestyle
- the environment

Taylor and colleagues, in their patient-centred model of health care, emphasise six interactive components of the patient-centred process:[6]

1. exploring both the disease and the illness experience
2. understanding the whole person
3. finding common grounds regarding management
4. incorporating prevention and health promotion
5. enhancing the doctor–patient relationship
6. being realistic regarding time and resources

Contemporary general practice focuses on patient-centred medicine, which, in alliance with evidence-based medicine, benefits both patient and doctor.

Continuing care

The essence of general practice is continuity of care. The doctor–patient relationship is unique in general practice in the sense that it covers a span of time that is not restricted to a specific major illness. The continuing relationship involving many separate episodes of illness provides an opportunity for the doctor to develop considerable knowledge and understanding of the patient, the family and its stresses, and the patient's work and recreational environment.

In 2008 the World Health Organization (WHO) reaffirmed the global importance of primary health care with its landmark report *Primary Health Care Now More Than Ever.* WHO[7] highlighted the evidence that continuity of care through general practice contributed to the following better outcomes:

- lower all-cause morbidity
- better access to care
- fewer rehospitalisations
- fewer consultations with specialists
- less use of emergency services
- better detection of adverse effects of medication interventions

Home visits

'You don't know your patient until you have seen them in their home.' Home visits are a goldmine of information about intra-family dynamics. They should cement the doctor–patient relationship if used appropriately. We are the only doctors who practise domiciliary care.

Common presenting problems

Common presenting symptoms in Australian general practices (BEACH study, 2013) are presented in TABLE 1.1[8] (note that the top 15 problems represent only one-third of all encounters).

Table 1.1 Most frequent presenting problems in Australian general practice

		Per cent of problems
1	Hypertension	5.7
2	Immunisation	4.2
3	URTI	3.3
4	Depression	2.9
5	Diabetes	2.3
6	Lipid disorders	2.1
7	General check-up	1.9
8	Osteoarthritis	1.7
9	Back pain	1.7
10	Prescription	1.6
11	Oesophageal (inc. GORD)	1.6
12	Female genital check-up	1.5
13	Acute bronchitis/bronchiolitis	1.5
14	Asthma	1.3
15	Anxiety	1.2
Cumulative top 15		34.6

Source: Cooke et al.[8]

To cover 75% of presenting problems, GPs must be able to diagnose and manage more than 100 different problems, and to cover 85% requires a good working knowledge of 167 problems.[8] The breadth of knowledge required to become a proficient GP is tremendous.

The content of this book reflects what is fundamental to the nature and content of general practice—that which is common but is significant, relevant, preventable and treatable.

Most frequent presenting symptoms in the author's practice

The most common presenting symptoms in the author's rural practice in the 1970s[9] were identified, with the emphasis being on pain syndromes:

- cough
- disturbance of bowel function
- pain in abdomen
- pain in back
- pain in chest
- pain in head

- pain in neck
- pain in ear
- pain in throat
- pain in joints/limbs
- rashes
- sleep problems
- tiredness/fatigue
- vaginal discomfort

Symptoms and conditions related to litigation

Medical defence organisations have highlighted the following areas as being those most vulnerable for management mishaps:

- acute abdominal pain
- acute chest pain
- breast lumps
- children's problems, especially the sick febrile child <2 years, groin pain and lumps
- dyspnoea ± cough (? heart failure, cancer, TB)
- headache

The most common reasons for claims against GPs are:

- diagnostic error 38%
- procedural complications 18%
- treatment issues 16%
- general duty of care 14%
- medication-related issues 9%
- legal issues 2%
- consent issues 1%
- medicolegal reports 1%
- anaesthesia 1%

Source: Bird S, MDA National

Chronic disease management

A study of international target conditions[10,11] in chronic disease management has highlighted the importance of the following (as common themes):

- ischaemic heart disease
- chronic heart failure
- cerebrovascular disease
- hypertension
- diabetes mellitus type 2
- chronic obstructive pulmonary disease
- asthma
- obesity
- epilepsy
- hypothyroidism
- chronic mental illness, especially depression
- medication monitoring
- arthritis

References

1 American Academy of Family Physicians. Official definition of Family Practice and Family Physician (AAFP Publication No. 303). Kansas City, Mo, AAFP, 1986.

2 Rakel RE. *Essentials of Family Practice.* Philadelphia: WB Saunders Company, 1993: 2–3.

3 RACGP. What is General Practice? Available from: <www.racgp.org.au/becomingagp/what-is-a-gp/what-is-general-practice>, accessed January 2018.

4 Anderson NA, Bridges-Webb C, Chancellor AHB. *General Practice in Australia.* Sydney: Sydney University Press, 1986: 3–4.

5 Fraser RC (ed). *Clinical Method: A General Practice Approach* (3rd edn). Oxford: Butterworth-Heinemann, 1999.

6 Taylor RJ, McAvoy BR, O'Dowd T. *General Practice Medicine.* Edinburgh: Churchill Livingstone, 2003: 6–7.

7 World Health Organization Geneva. *The World Health Report 2008; Primary Health Care: Now More Than Ever.* 2008.

8 Britt H, Sayer GP et al. *Bettering the Evaluation and Care of Health: General Practice in Australia* 1998–9. Sydney: University of Sydney & the Australian Institute of Health & Welfare, 1998–99.

9 Murtagh JE. *The Anatomy of a Rural Practice.* Melbourne: Monash University, Department of Community Practice Publication, 1980: 8–13.

10 Piterman L. *Chronic Disease Management OSP Report.* Melbourne: Monash University, 2004.

11 Rakel RE, Rakel DP. *Textbook of Family Medicine* (9th edn). Philadelphia: Elsevier Saunders, 2016: 16.

Resources

The World Organization of National Colleges, Academies and Academic Associations of General Practitioners/Family Physicians (WONCA). <www.globalfamilydoctor.com>, accessed January 2018.

2 The family

The family is the best department of Health, Education and Welfare ever devised.

PETER WESTMORE 2015

Working with families is the basis of family practice. Families living in relative harmony provide the basis for the good mental health of their members and also for social stability.

However, the traditional concept of the nuclear family, where the wife stays at home to care for the children, occurs in only about 15% of Australian families. Approximately 46% of Australian marriages end in separation. Families take many shapes and forms, among them single-parent households, de facto partnerships, same-sex couples and families formed by a partnership between two separated parents and their children. Psychosocial problems may occur in almost any family arrangement and family doctors need to know how to address such problems.

Family therapy is ideally undertaken by GPs, who are in a unique position as providers of continuing care and family care. It is important for them to work together with families in the counselling process and to avoid the common pitfalls of working in isolation and assuming personal responsibility for changing the family. We should understand that definitions of family vary greatly across cultures.

Bader[1] summarises working with families succinctly:

> From the perspective of family therapy, working with families means avoiding the trap of being too directive, too responsible for the family's welfare, with the result that the family becomes overly dependent on the general practitioner for its health and development. From the perspective of family education, working with families means developing the skills of anticipating guidance, helping families to prepare, not only for the normal changes occurring as the family develops, but also for the impact of illness on the family system.

Characteristics of healthy families

Successful families have certain characteristics, an understanding of which can give the family doctor a basis for assessing the health of the family and a goal to help set targets for change in disrupted families. Such characteristics are:

- *Healthy communication.* In this situation family members have freedom of expression for their feelings and emotions.
- *Personal autonomy.* This includes appropriate use of power sharing between spouses/partners.
- *Flexibility.* This leads to appropriate 'give and take' with adaptation to individual needs and changing circumstances.
- *Appreciation.* This involves encouragement and praise so that members develop a healthy sense of self-esteem.
- *Support networks.* Adequate support from within and without the family engenders security, resistance to stress and a healthy environment in general (see FIG. 2.1). The family doctor is part of this network.

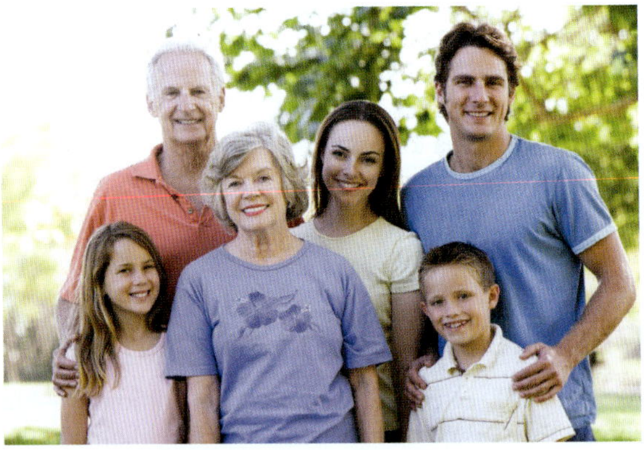

FIGURE 2.1 Three generations of a supportive family network

- *Family time and involvement.* Studies have shown that the most satisfying hallmark of a happy family is 'doing things together'.
- *Spouse/partner bonding.* The importance of a sound marital relationship becomes obvious when family therapy is undertaken.
- *Growth.* There needs to be appropriate opportunities for growth of individual family members in an encouraging atmosphere.

- *Spiritual and religious values.* An attachment to spiritual beliefs and values is known to be associated with positive family health.

Families in crisis

Doctors are closely involved with families who experience unexpected crises, which include illnesses, accidents, divorce, separation, unemployment, death of a family member and financial disasters.

The effect of illness

Serious illness often precipitates crises in individual members of the family, crises that have not previously surfaced in the apparently balanced family system. It is recognised, for example, that bereavement over the unexpected loss of a child may lead to marital breakdown, separation or divorce.

In the long term, other family members may be affected more than the patient. This may apply particularly to children and manifest as school underachievement and behaviour disturbances.

During the crisis the obvious priority of the doctor is to the patient but the less obvious needs of the family should not be ignored.

Guidelines for the doctor

- Include the family as much as possible, starting early in the acute phase of the illness. It may necessitate family conferences.
- Include the family on a continuing basis, especially if a long-term illness is anticipated. It is helpful to be alert for changes in attitudes, such as anger and resentment towards the sick member.
- Include the family in hospital discharge planning.
- If a serious change in family dynamics is observed, the use of experts may be needed.
- Offer a family conference at critical times.

Significant presentations of family dysfunction

The following presentations may be indicators that all is not well in the family, and so the doctor needs to 'think family':

- marital or sexual difficulties
- multiple presentations of a family member—'the thick file syndrome'
- multiple presentations by multiple family members
- abnormal behaviour in a child
- the 'difficult patient'
- inappropriate behaviour in the antenatal and/or postpartum period
- drug or alcohol abuse in a family member
- evidence of physical or sexual abuse in one of the partners (male or female) or a child
- psychiatric disorders, especially depression and psychosis
- susceptibility to illness
- increased stress/anxiety
- complaints of chronic fatigue or insomnia

It is important that the family doctor remains alert to the diversity of presentations and takes the responsibility for identifying an underlying family-based problem.

The patient and family dynamics

Family doctors see many patients who present with physical symptoms that have primarily an emotional or psychosocial basis with either little or no organic pathology. As many as 50–75% of patients utilising primary care clinics have a psychosocial precipitant as opposed to biomedical problems as the main cause of their visit.[2]

In order to understand the clinical manifestations of the sick role of patients, family doctors should first understand the individual's response to stress stimuli, which may come from external (family, work or sexual behaviour) or internal (personality trait or psychosocial) sources (see FIG. 2.2 and TABLE 2.1).

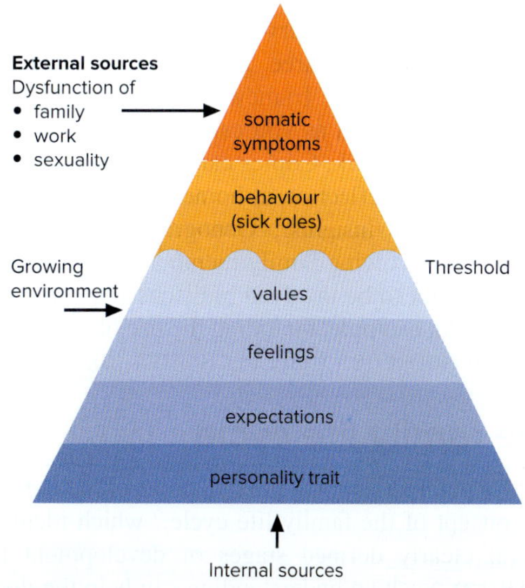

FIGURE 2.2 Family dynamics and psychosomatic illness iceberg

2

Table 2.1 Areas of possible biopsychosocial dysfunction

Work	Family	Sex
Type of work Workload Work environment Goals Work satisfaction	Present family (change of structure and function) Extended family (parents and relatives) Growing environment (family tree)	Sexual dysfunction Disharmony Deprivation Guilt

How to evaluate the family dynamics

- Carefully observe family members interacting.
- Invite the whole family to a counselling session (if possible).
- Visit the home: an impromptu home visit (with some pretext such as a concern about a blood test result) on the way home from work may be very revealing. This will be appropriate in some but not all family practice settings.
- Prepare a genogram (see FIG. 18.1, CHAPTER 18): family dynamics and behaviour can be understood by drawing a family map or genogram (a diagrammatic representation of family structure and relationships).[3,4]

The genogram

The genogram is a very valuable pedigree chart that usually covers three generations of a family tree.[3] Such a visual framework helps the general practice consultation as you can continue to build on that basic framework. Copies can be given to patients and families to reflect on at home and return to their GP for further insights.[5] Genograms are a useful strategy for involving family members who may have been reluctant to be involved in discussions on family matters.[4] An example, including the use of symbols, is shown in FIGURE 18.1 (refer to CHAPTER 18).

The family life cycle

Helpful in understanding the dynamics of the family is the concept of the family life cycle,[6] which identifies several clearly defined stages of development (see TABLE 2.2). Such an understanding can help the doctor form appropriate hypotheses about the problems patients are experiencing at a particular stage. Each stage brings its own tasks, happiness, crises and difficulties. This cycle is also well represented in FIGURE 2.3, which indicates the approximate length of time on each of the stages.

Table 2.2 The family life cycle[1]

Stage		Tasks to be achieved
1	Leaving home	Establishing personal independence. Beginning the emotional separation from parents.
2	Getting married	Establishing an intimate relationship with spouse. Developing further the emotional separation from parents.
3	Learning to live together	Dividing the various marital roles in an equitable way. Establishing a new, more independent relationship with family.
4	Parenting the first child	Opening the family to include a new member. Dividing the parenting roles.
5	Living with the adolescent	Increasing the flexibility of the family boundaries to allow the adolescent(s) to move in and out of the family system.
6	Launching children: the empty-nest phase	Accepting the multitude of exits from and entries into the family system. Adjusting to the ending of parenting roles.
7	Retirement	Adjusting to the ending of the wage-earning roles. Developing new relationships with children, grandchildren and each other.
8	Old age	Dealing with lessening abilities and greater dependence on others. Dealing with losses of friends, family members and, eventually, each other.

Family assessment

The assessment of families with problems can be formalised through a questionnaire that allows the collection of information in a systematic way in order to give an understanding of the functioning of the family in question.

The questionnaire[1]

1. Family of origin
    - Could each of you tell us something about the families you grew up in?
    - Where do you come in the family?
    - Were you particularly close to anyone else in the family?

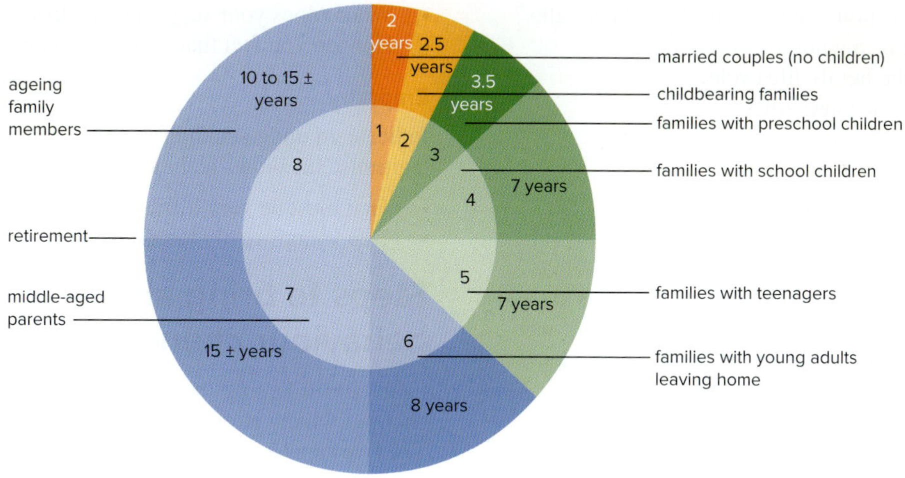

FIGURE 2.3 The family life cycle (approximate time in each stage)
Source: After McWhinney[7] and Duvall[8]

- Were there any severe conflicts between family members?
- Did anyone abuse you in any way?
- Do you have much contact with any of your family now?
- Have you tried to model (or avoid) any features for your own family?

2. History of the couple's relationship
   - How did you two meet?
   - What attracted you to each other?
   - Why did you choose this person rather than someone else?
   - How did your families react to your choice?
   - How did the birth of your children affect your relationship?
   - When was your relationship at its best? Why?
3. Experience in counselling and enrichment
   - Have any of you been to a marriage support program?
   - Have any of you been to any form of counselling?
   - Did you go alone or with another family member?
   - What did you like or dislike about the experience?
   - In what way was it helpful or unhelpful?
4. Expectations and goals
   - Whose idea was it to come here?
   - What was the reaction of other family members?
   - Why did you come now?
   - Was there any particular event that triggered the decision?
   - What does each of you hope to gain by coming for an assessment?
5. Family function[1]
   - What is it like for each of you to live in this family? (If children are present, they should be asked first.)
   - Do you have any difficulty in talking to other members of the family? (Again, children first.)
   - Do you have any difficulty in expressing appreciation to each other? (Mention here that studies on healthy families show that both communication and appreciation rank in the top qualities.)
   - How do you show appreciation in this family?
   - How do you show affection in this family? (Again, children first.)
   - How satisfied are you with the present arrangement? Are there any changes you would like to see?
   - What ways have you used to resolve disagreements or change the way the family functions?

Assessment based on the questionnaire

- Family members present in interview (names and ages)
- Missing members (names and ages)
- Presenting problems or reasons for family interview identified by whom? Any attempted solutions?
- Roles—structure, organisation (who is dominant and so on)
- Affect—predominant emotional tone and expressed emotions

- Communication—Who dominates? Who talks? Who listens to whom?
- Stage in the family life cycle
- Illness and sickness roles
- Coping mechanisms

Family-based medical counselling

There are several brief counselling models to assist the family doctor in probing and counselling, using a simple infrastructure such as the BATHE model.

The BATHE technique[9]

This really represents a diagnostic technique to identify sources of disharmony, which can act as a springboard for counselling.

The acronym BATHE stands for *background, affect, trouble, handling* and *empathy,* and can be summarised as follows.

Background

Enquire about possible areas of psychosocial problems to help elicit the context of the patient's visit.

- What is happening in your life?
- Is there anything different since before you got sick?
- How are things at home?

Affect

Affect is the 'feeling state' and includes anxiety, so it is wise to probe potentially sensitive areas.

- How do you feel about what is going on in your life?
- How do you feel about your home life?
- How do you feel about work/school?
- How do you feel about your (spouse/partner or daughter or . . .)?
- What is your mood like? Do you feel sad or happy?

Trouble

Enquire about how the patient's problems are troubling the patient.

- What about the situation troubles you most?
- What troubles or worries you most in your life?
- What worries you most at home?
- How stressed and upset are you about this problem?
- How do you think this problem affects you?

Handling

- How are you handling this problem?
- Do you think that you have mishandled anything?
- Do you get support at home to help handle the problem?
- Where does your support come from?
- How do you feel that you are coping?

Empathy

Indicate an understanding of the patient's distress and legitimise his or her feelings.

- That must be very difficult for you.
- That sounds really tough on you.

Steps to bring about behaviour change

Fabb and Fleming have introduced the model of change, which is fundamental to initiating therapy. The five steps are:

1. *Dissatisfaction.* There must be dissatisfaction with the present pattern of behaviour.
2. *Alternative.* There must be an acceptable alternative behaviour pattern available.
3. *Emotional commitment.* There must be an emotional commitment to the new pattern of behaviour over the old.
4. *Practice with feedback.* There must be practice of the new behaviour, with feedback, to establish the new pattern as an available behaviour.
5. *Habituation with support.* There must be installation of the new behaviour in the normal work/living situation with support.

All of these must be present for change to occur. Steps 4 and 5 are often neglected, with the result that change does not occur or is less successful.

Marital disharmony

Family doctors often have to provide marital counselling for one or both partners. The problems may be resolved quite simply or be so complex that marital breakdown is inevitable despite optimal opportunities for counselling.

Opportunities for prevention, including anticipatory guidance about marital problems, do exist and the wise practitioner will offer appropriate advice and counselling. Examples include an accident to a child attributable to neglect by a parent, or similar situation in which that parent may be the focus of blame, leading to resentment and tension. The practitioner could intervene from the outset to alleviate possible feelings of guilt and anger in that marriage.

Some common causes of marital disharmony are:

- selfishness
- unrealistic expectations
- financial problems/meanness

- not listening to each other
- sickness (e.g. depression)
- drug or alcohol excess
- jealousy, especially in men
- fault finding
- 'playing games' with each other
- driving ambition
- immaturity
- poor communication

Basic counselling of couples

The following text on basic counselling of couples,[10] which should be regarded as a patient education sheet, includes useful advice for couples:

> The two big secrets of marital success are caring and responsibility.

Some important facts

- Research has shown that we tend to choose partners who are similar to our parents and that we may take our childish and selfish attitudes into our marriage.
- The trouble spots listed above reflect this childishness; we often expect our partners to change and meet our needs.
- If we take proper care and responsibility, we can keep these problems to a minimum.
- Physical passion is not enough to hold a marriage together—'when it burns out, only ashes will be left'.
- While a good sexual relationship is great, most experts agree that what goes on *out* of bed counts for more.
- When we do something wrong, it is most important that we feel forgiven by our partner.

Positive guidelines for success (summary)[10]

1. Know yourself.
2. Share interests and goals.
3. Continue courtship after marriage.
4. Make love, not war.
5. Cherish your mate.
6. Prepare yourself for parenthood.
7. Seek proper help when necessary.
8. Do unto your mate as you would have your mate do unto you.

The BE Attitudes (virtues to help achieve success)	
BE honest	**BE** loyal
BE loving	**BE** desiring
BE patient	**BE** fun to live with
BE forgiving	**BE** one
BE generous	**BE** caring

Making lists—a practical task

Make lists for each other to compare and discuss.

- List qualities (desirable and undesirable) of your parents.
- List qualities of each other.
- List examples of behaviour each would like the other to change.
- List things you would like the other to do for you.

Put aside special quiet times each week to share these things.

Pitfalls[1]

The GP who is too closely attached to one or more members of the family can easily become trapped in the role of the 'rescuer' or 'saviour' of those members. The best defence against this trap is to respect the family's autonomy and work with the family to achieve the goals the family sets for itself, thus avoiding three major pitfalls for the GP in treating families:

1. assuming personal responsibility for changing the family
2. working alone, neglecting the assistance of the family
3. becoming a 'rescuer' or 'saviour'

Other pitfalls

- Conducting therapy in the absence of a significant family member
- Breaching confidentiality of individuals within the family
- Failing to recognise the 'ganging-up effect'
- Taking sides
- Failing to use available resources
- Overrelating to your own experiences

Possible solutions to avoid pitfalls[1]

- Let the patients do the work.
- Share the burden with a colleague or other resources.
- Ensure that the goals for therapy are realistic.
- Point out that all family members have to work together and that therapy works best when there is openness on all sides.

2

- Identify any tendency to look for scapegoats within the family.
- Look out for vulnerable family members—the 'hidden patient'.
- Avoid trying to achieve quick solutions.
- Obtain clear-cut agreements on confidential matters and record this in the history.
- Keep an open mind and avoid forcing your own values on to the family.

References

1 Bader E. Working with families. Aust Fam Physician, 1990; 19: 522–8.
2 Fabb W. *Handbook for Medical Students*. Hong Kong: Chinese University of Hong Kong, 1995: 31.
3 McGoldrick M, Gerson R. *Genograms in Family Assessment*. New York: WW Norton, 1985: chs 1–4.
4 Jackson L, Tisher M. Family therapy skills for general practitioners. Aust Fam Physician, 1996; 25: 1265–9.
5 Larner G, Lajorie M. Family therapy in general practice: how to treat. Australian Doctor, 2006; 10 December: 23–30.
6 Van Doorn H. *Common Problems Checklist for General Practice*. Melbourne: Royal Australian College of General Practitioners, 1989: 19.
7 McWhinney IR, Freeman T. *A Textbook of Family Medicine* (2nd edn). Oxford: Oxford University Press, 2009: 230–44.
8 Duvall EM. *Family Development* (5th edn). Philadelphia: Lippincott, 1977.
9 Stuart MR, Leiberman JA III. *The 15-Minute Hour: Applied Psychotherapy for the Primary Care Physician*. New York: Praeger, 1986.
10 Murtagh JE. *Patient Education* (7th edn). Sydney: McGraw-Hill, 2017: 2.

Resource

Australian Government, Institute of Family Studies. Family Matters No. 87, 2011. *Think Family: A new approach to Families at Risk*, <https://aifs.gov.au/sites/default/files/fm87e.pdf>, accessed January 2018.

Consulting skills 3

The essential unit of medical practice is the occasion when in the intimacy of the consulting room the person who is ill or believes himself (or herself) to be ill, seeks the advice of a doctor whom he (she) trusts. This is the consultation and all else in the practice of medicine derives from it.

Sir James Spence 1960

The *objectives of the consultation* are to:

- determine the exact reason for the presentation
- achieve a good therapeutic outcome for the patient
- develop a strong doctor–patient relationship

The skills of general practice

A successful outcome to the medical consultation depends on a whole array of skills required by the GP. Although interrelated, these skills, which can be collectively termed 'consulting skills', include interviewing skills, clinical skills, diagnostic skills, management skills, communication skills, educative skills, therapeutic skills, manual skills and counselling skills.

Communication skills, which are fundamental to consulting skills, are the key to the effectiveness of the doctor as a professional, and expertise with these skills is fundamental to the doctor–patient relationship. Communication skills are essential in obtaining a good history and constitute one of the cornerstones of therapy (see CHAPTER 4).

A skilled interviewer will succeed in transmitting his or her findings to the patient so that they are clearly understood, are not unduly disturbing, and inspire trust and confidence in the physician.

Models of the consultation

Several models that formalise the general practice consultation can be very useful for developing an understanding of the process of the consultation. Two classic models are those by Pendleton and colleagues,[1] and by Stott and Davis.[2] Pendleton and colleagues, in their landmark book *The Consultation: An Approach to Learning and Teaching,*[1] defined seven key tasks to the consultation, which serve as helpful guidelines:

1. To define the reason for the patient's attendance, including:
   - the nature and history of problems
   - their aetiology
   - the patient's ideas, concerns and expectations
   - the effect of the problems
2. To consider other issues:
   - continuing problems
   - risk factors
3. To choose, with the patient, an appropriate action for each problem
4. To achieve a shared understanding of the problems with the patient
5. To involve the patient in the management and encourage him or her to accept appropriate responsibility
6. To use time and resources efficiently and appropriately:
   - in the consultation
   - in the long term
7. To establish or maintain a relationship with the patient that helps to achieve the other tasks

The exceptional potential in each primary care consultation described by Stott and Davis,[2] which is presented in TABLE 3.1, also acts as an excellent aide-memoire to achieve maximal benefit from the consultation.

Table 3.1 The potential in each primary care consultation

A	B
Management of presenting problems	Modification of health-seeking behaviour
C	**D**
Management of continuing problems	Opportunistic health promotion

Source: Stott & Davis[2]

3

Phases of the consultation

The consultation can be considered in three phases, as follows:

1. Establishment of rapport (see FIG. 3.1)
2. Diagnostic phase
   - the interview and history
   - the physical and mental examination
   - investigations
3. Management phase
   - explanation and education
   - prescribing medication
   - procedural–therapeutic or extended diagnostic
   - referral
   - follow-up

> **Practice tip**
>
> Remembering the patient's preferred name and their basic past history creates powerful rapport.

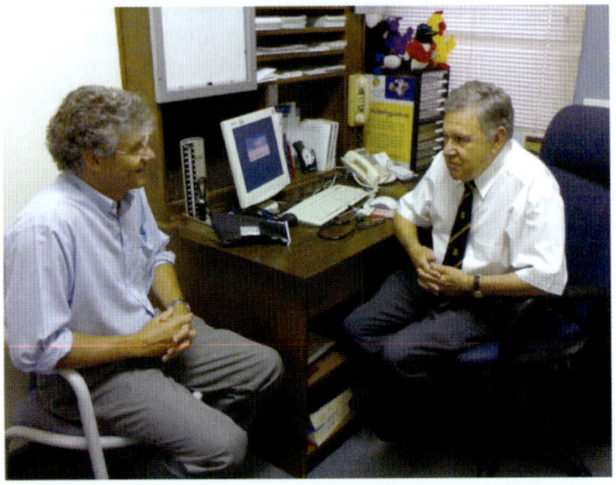

FIGURE 3.1 The consultation: establishment of good rapport is the foundation to successful consulting skills

The history

The doctor has four basic tasks to perform during the history-taking phase of the consultation. These are to determine:

1. the patient's stated reason for attending
2. why the patient is attending today, or at this particular time in the course of this illness
3. a list of problems or supplementary symptoms
4. any other initially unspoken or hidden reason for attending (e.g. the fear of cancer)

The old medical cliché that 'a good history is the basis of the clinical examination' is as relevant as always. The art of history taking, which is based on good communication, is the most fundamental skill in general practice and requires a disciplined approach.

A very good approach is that used by Professor Rita Charon of Columbia University: 'I'm going to be your doctor, so I need to know a great deal about your body, health and life. Please tell me what you think I should know about yourself and your situation.'

Guidelines include:[3]

- Commence by eliciting the presenting complaint.
- Permit an uninterrupted history.
- Use appropriate language—keep the questions simple.
- Use specific questions to clarify the presenting complaint.
- Write notes or use the keyboard to record information but maintain as much eye contact as possible.
- Enquire about general symptoms, such as fatigue, weight changes, fever, headache, sleep and coping ability (see TABLE 3.2). These are important since they uncover 'red flags' for serious, life-threatening disorders.

Table 3.2 Important general questions
Fatigue, tiredness or malaise
Fever, sweating, shakes
Weight change, especially loss
Pain or discomfort anywhere
Any unusual lumps or bumps
Any unusual bleeding
Skin problems—rash or itching

- Undertake a relevant systems review.
- A historical checklist includes past medical history, complete medication history, drug habits and sensitivities, family history, psychosocial history and preventive care history.
- Give feedback to the patient about your understanding of the problems and agenda, and correct any misconceptions.

Good questions

In order to determine any underlying agenda or significant psychosocial problems, it is very helpful to use analytical questions. Such opening questions and inviting statements could include:

- Why have you come to see me today?
- Do you have any particular concern about your health?

- That really interests me—tell me more—it seems important.
- What were you hoping I could do for you today?
- Where would you put your real feelings between 0 and 100%?
- What is it that's really upsetting or bothering you?
- What do you really think deep down is the cause of your problem?
- Are you basically satisfied with your life?
- Is there anything that I haven't asked you and that you should tell me about?
- Tell me about things at home.
- Tell me about things at work.
- Do you experience any bullying?
- Are you afraid that something bad is going to happen to you?
- Is your relationship with any particular loved one/person causing you stress? (This may lead to information about sensitive issues such as domestic violence or sexual problems.)
- Is there anything in your life that you would like to change?
- I'm concerned about what you are not telling me.

Basic interviewing techniques

A number of basic interviewing techniques[4] encourage communication. It is important to use the least controlling interview techniques before embarking on direct questioning.

Questions

When the patient is asked a question, the doctor tends to take control of the interview, and so directs it along the lines of his or her own thinking or hypothesis generation. The problem is that if questions are used too early in the interview, the amount of desirable information is restricted and may disrupt the true priorities of the patient's concerns.

Open-ended questions and direct questions are very useful at appropriate times, while other questions are very restrictive. Examples, using pain as the 'problem', are:

- Open-ended question: 'Tell me about the pain.'
- Direct question: 'Where is the pain?'
- Closed question: 'Is the pain severe?'
- Leading question: 'The pain is severe?'
- Reflective question: 'You want to know the cause of the pain?'

The open-ended question

The open-ended question is essential in initiating the interview. A question such as 'What kind of troubles have you been having?' says to the patient 'I'm interested in anything you may feel is important enough for you to tell me'.

The open-ended question gives the patient an opportunity to take temporary control of the consultation and to outline problems and concerns.

Ongoing interview strategies of listening and silence, facilitation and summarisation are outlined in CHAPTER 4, (section on Communication in the consultation).

Information from other sources

Sometimes it is important to obtain information from other sources, especially friends or relatives. Off-hand comments from others may be loaded with 'cues' and one should be listening intently.

Problem definition

Part of the diagnostic process is defining the patient's problem or problems. The more complex the presentation, the more necessary it is to have an orderly approach. It is clearly important to list the problems in a priority order. These problems may have been 'offered' by the patient, 'observed' by the doctor, 'derived' during the interview or 'known' from the past history. Problems can be conveniently considered as organic or physiological, and intrapersonal or social.[5]

Touching the patient

Sometimes a natural response is to touch the distressed patient as a reassuring gesture. It is best to adopt a caring-and-support gesture, such as offering tissues to the weeping patient, but it may be quite acceptable for most patients to give a reassuring, momentary touch somewhere between the shoulder and wrist on the arm nearest to you. Touching should be a natural gesture that is comfortable for both the doctor and patient. Touch elsewhere should generally be avoided.

The physical and mental examination

If a diagnostic hypothesis based on the history is being tested, the examination may be confined to one system or to one anatomical region. However, other regions, systems or a general examination may be undertaken for medicolegal or preventive reasons. Patients tend to feel vulnerable during the physical examination, so their sensitivity and modesty have to be respected. Generally, the examination is conducted in relative silence, with the doctor instructing the patient what to do.

Patients need to be warned of possible discomfort or pain that may accompany certain examinations, of the reason for the examination, and of its immediate results, particularly if normal. Continued silence on

3

the doctor's part is often interpreted by patients as being indicative of something serious or unusual being found. For the same reason the doctor's non-verbal behaviour is important.

Medicolegal guidelines for examinations[6,7]

The following guidelines have been recommended by the NSW Medical Board for consultations and physical examinations:

- Carefully explain the nature and purpose of the physical examination before you start. Take particular care with explanations before rectal, vaginal, breast and genital examination.
- Indicate when an examination may be uncomfortable and ask the patient to advise if you are causing pain.
- If a patient is required to disrobe, explain to what extent undressing is required and why.
- A patient's modesty should be preserved when undressing and dressing before and after a physical examination. Privacy screens, sheets and gowns should be provided as a matter of course. Clinic staff should not interrupt physical examinations.
- If the patient requests the presence of a chaperone or a friend, this should be respected.
- Do not lock the door of the consultation room. The setting should allow the patient confidence to terminate the consultation at any time if he or she is uncomfortable.
- Ask yourself 'Is what I am doing part of accepted medical practice?'.[8]

Investigations

It is often necessary to arrange for special tests to assist in the diagnostic process or to monitor the progress of certain illnesses or response to treatment. The informed consent of patients must be obtained. A collaborative decision for or against certain tests may be negotiated.

GPs have a responsibility (clinical and economic) to be very discerning and selective in the investigations that they choose. The questions that should be asked in decision making include:

- Is this investigation necessary?
- Will it change my management?

Richard Asher (1954) listed the questions a clinician should ask before requesting an investigation:[9]

- Why am I ordering this test?
- What am I going to look for in the result?
- If I find it, will it affect my diagnosis?
- How will this affect my management of the case?
- Will this ultimately benefit the patient?

In general, investigations should be performed only when the following criteria are satisfied:[9]

- The consequence of the result of the investigation could not be obtained by a cheaper, less intrusive method (e.g. taking a better history or using time).
- The risks of the investigation should relate to the value of the information likely to be gained.
- The result will directly assist in the diagnosis or have an effect on subsequent management.

The three strikes and you're out rule

A very useful rule is to bail out of the diagnosis and refer to a colleague if you have failed to make a diagnosis after three consultations.

Management phase of the consultation

The management phase of the consultation may immediately follow the information-gathering interview, or it may take place on review, after diagnostic tests or referral. It should be remembered that there are at least two people concerned in management: the doctor *and* the patient. Poor patient compliance with any proposed therapy can be a result of a poorly conducted management phase. It is necessary not only for the doctor to make statements concerning therapy and the reasons for the chosen therapy, but also for the information to be conveyed in a language appropriate to each patient's understanding. Negotiate a management plan.

Management includes immediate care, prevention and long-term care. Doctors generally tend to be authoritarian in their management proposals. Whole-person management, however, implies that the patient's views are listened to, explanations are offered where necessary by the doctor, and an educative approach is adopted to encourage the patient to actively participate in management and preventive behaviour, where possible.

The objectives of the management phase of the consultation are summarised in TABLE 3.3.

The sequence of the management interview[4]

The following, which represents an excellent teaching strategy, is a suggested *10-point plan* or sequence for conducting a management interview. These guidelines

Table 3.3 Objectives of the management phase of the consultation[4]

To make use of the doctor–patient relationship in therapy
To involve the patient as far as possible in the management of his or her own problem
To educate the patient about the illness
To promote rational prescribing
To achieve compliance in therapy
To emphasise preventive opportunities
To provide appropriate reassurance
To encourage continuity of ongoing care

will not always need to be applied in their entirety, and may need to be staged over a number of consultations. The use of this sequence should ensure identification of all the patient's problems by the doctor (including fears, feelings and expectations), adequate patient understanding of his or her problems, an acceptable and appropriate treatment plan being defined for each problem, preventive opportunities being addressed, and the patient being satisfied with the consultation and being clear about follow-up arrangements.

The sequence is as follows.

1 Tell the patient the diagnosis

2 Establish the patient's knowledge of the diagnosis

3 Establish the patient's attitude to the diagnosis and management

4 Educate the patient about diagnosis

- Correct any incorrect health beliefs recognised in point 2.
- Supplement the patient's existing knowledge to a level appropriate to the needs of the patient and the doctor.

5 Develop a management plan for the presenting problem

Develop precise instructions using three headings:

- *Immediate:* always included, even if no action is proposed
- *Long term:* for chronic, long-term or recurrent illnesses
- *Preventive:* sometimes specific measures apply—often patient education is the method required

The patient should be encouraged at this stage to participate in decision making regarding management and to make a commitment to the plans.

6 Explore other preventive opportunities

7 Reinforce the information

- Use the patient's own results (e.g. X-rays and ECGs).
- Encourage the patient to participate in the decision making and in accepting some degree of responsibility for his or her own management.

8 Provide take-away information

Examples of this important strategy include patient instruction leaflets and resource contacts.

9 Evaluate the consultation

10 Arrange follow-up

Closing the session

Good closure is an important strategy; ask 'Has this visit helped you and your problems—is there anything more I can do?'

A patient management strategy

Brian McAvoy, writing in Fraser's excellent book *Clinical Method: A General Practice Approach,* presents a helpful aide-mémoire in the approach to patient management:[9]

1. reassurance and/or explanation
2. advice
3. prescription
4. referral
5. investigation
6. observation (follow-up)
7. prevention

Prescriptions

It is worth emphasising that prescribing medicine is a relatively complex skill that requires considerable knowledge of the disease, patient's expectations, the drugs prescribed, their interactions and their adverse reactions. Part of this skill is making a decision not to prescribe medication when it is not absolutely necessary and then explaining the reasons and including non-pharmacological measures. This decision may be made in the context of a patient expecting a biochemical solution for his or her problem. As McAvoy points out, 'If in doubt whether or not to give a drug—don't'.[9]

Rational prescribing applies particularly to opioids, antibiotics and tranquillisers.

General guidelines for antibiotic prescribing

Rules of thumb

Choose the agent with the:

- narrowest spectrum that will cover the likely pathogens (based on culture/sensitivity)
- lowest cost if efficacy and safety are otherwise equal

3

- fewest serious side-effects
- duration as short as possible

Avoid wherever possible:

- prescribing antibacterial antibiotics for viral respiratory infections
- combinations if a single drug is likely to be effective
- topical antibiotics, as resistance is much more likely to develop (exceptions include eye infections and vaginitis)
- antibiotic combinations, except in proven clinical circumstances or when coverage is difficult with a single drug
- prophylactic antibiotics, unless they are of proven benefit (in general only in some elective surgery or dental procedures)

The common respiratory infections such as acute otitis media, pharyngitis, tonsillitis, acute bronchitis, bronchiolitis and influenza have commonly a viral cause and it is appropriate to treat symptomatically with a 'wait and see' surveillance.[10]

Referral

The decision to refer a patient is also another important skill. It is often difficult to find the right balance. Some practitioners refer excessively—others cling to their patients inappropriately. It is a mistake not to refer a patient with a serious chronic or life-threatening disease. Apart from consultants and hospitals, referral should be considered to GP colleagues or partners with special interests or expertise, support groups and other members of the primary health care team, such as physiotherapists, dietitians, chiropodists and social workers. At all times the GP should act as the focal reference point and maintain control of patient management.

The 'gatekeeper' role of the GP

A patient's GP is the obvious and ideal linchpin in the health care system to take responsibility for the patient's health concerns and management. The patient may become confused with the system, especially if his or her problems are many and complex. The patient's GP has a vital role in acting as a 'gatekeeper' between primary and secondary care, and between paramedical services. The GP should always act in the patient's best interests and intervene, if necessary, to ensure that the patient is getting the best possible care.

The healing art of the doctor

The counselling process in general practice is based on the therapeutic effect of the doctor. This well-recorded feature is reinforced if the doctor has a certain professional charisma, and is caring and competent. We cannot underestimate the dependency of our patients on this healing factor, especially where significant psychic factors are involved.

Key points on patient management[11]

- It is difficult, perhaps impossible, to reassure patients in the absence of an appropriate physical examination and certain investigations.
- Reassurance must always be appropriate and therefore based on a substantial foundation: inappropriate reassurance damages the credibility of both the doctor and his or her profession.
- The two key characteristics of the doctor in establishing the basis of a successful outcome for the doctor–patient relationship are caring and responsibility.
- Vital factors included in this relationship are good communication, genuine interest and trust.
- Listen to what the patient is saying and not saying.

References

1. Pendleton D et al. *The Consultation: An Approach to Learning and Teaching*. Oxford: Oxford University Press, 1984.
2. Stott N, Davis R. The exceptional potential in each primary care consultation. J R Coll Gen Pract, 1979; 29: 201–5.
3. Nyman KC. *Successful Consulting*. Melbourne: Royal Australian College of General Practitioners, 1996: 11–32.
4. Rose AT. Basic interview techniques. In Kidd M, Rose A. *An Introduction to Consulting Skills*. Community Medicine Student Handbook. Melbourne: Monash University, 1991: 32–40.
5. Gask L, Usherwood T. The Consultation. BMJ 2002; 324: 567.
6. Johnson P. Bedside manners: advice for doctors in training. UMP Journal, 1998; 2: 2.
7. *Guidelines for Medico-Legal Consultation and Examinations.* Sydney: NSW Medical Board, 1997.
8. Bird S. Managing professional boundaries. Aust Fam Physician, 2013, 42: 9: 666–8.
9. Fraser RC. *Clinical Method: A General Practice Approach* (3rd edn). Oxford: Butterworth-Heinemann, 1999: 6–72.
10. Scott AM, Del Mar C. Controlling antibiotic prescribing for lower respiratory tract infections. BMJ 2017; 357: j2398.
11. Tam M. Hints and tips in the medical consultation: The Medicine Box: Advice March 2007: 1–3.

Communication skills 4

Most people have a furious itch to talk about themselves and are restrained only by the disinclination of others to listen. Reserve is an artificial quality that is developed in most of us as a result of innumerable rebuffs. The doctor is discreet. It is his business to listen and no details are too intimate for his ears.

W SOMERSET MAUGHAM (1874–1965), *SUMMING UP*

Hippocrates wrote:

> In the art of medicine there are three factors—the disease, the patient and the doctor . . . It is not easy for the ordinary people to understand why they are ill or why they get better or worse, but if it is explained by someone else, it can seem quite a simple matter—if the doctor fails to make himself understood he may miss the truth of the illness.[1]

Francis Macnab, Doctor of Divinity and patient, wrote: 'The style of the doctor, the communication of the doctor and the person of the doctor at the level of primary contact and primary care can be crucial in a person's life.'[2]

Much of the art of general practice lies in the ability to communicate.

Research continues to focus the 'blame' for communication breakdown on the doctor, ignoring the role of the patient.[3]

Communication

Communication can be defined as 'the successful passing of a message from one person to another'.

There are five basic **elements** in the communication process:

- the communicator
- the message
- the method of communicating
- the recipient
- the response

Important **principles** facilitating the communication process are:

- the rapport between the people involved
- the time factor, facilitated by devoting more time
- the message, which needs to be clear, correct, concise, unambiguous and in context
- the attitudes of both the communicator and the recipient

These elements and principles can be seen emerging in various phases through the consultation, as illustrated in FIGURE 4.1.

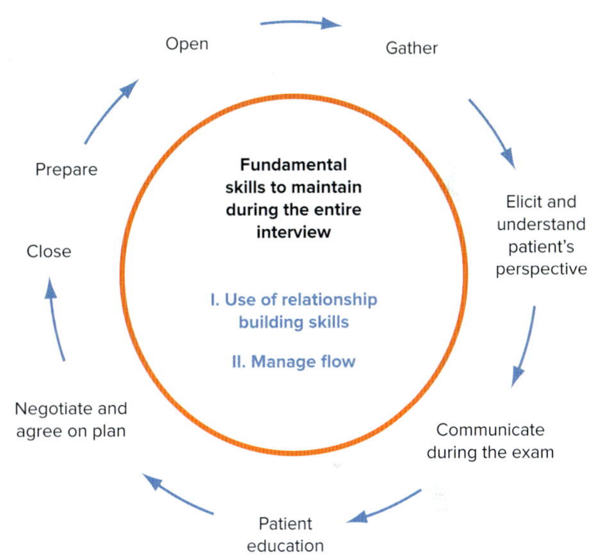

FIGURE 4.1 The sequence of communication in the consultation

Source: Courtesy of the New York University Macy Initiative on Health Communication

Communication in the consultation[3,4]

Communication in the consultation can be considered in the following sequence:

The doctor requires appropriate communication skills for complete diagnosis (physical, emotional and social) and competent management. It important to be aware of the patient's cultural background and educational level and allow for these factors. The majority of interaction between doctor and patient occurs in the traditional consultation. This involves both verbal and non-verbal communication.

4

Prepare

The 'prepare' phase includes preparation done both well before the consultation and then just prior to the consultation. Well before consulting, the doctor should think about and prepare the physical environment. Comfort and privacy should be maximised, and distractions and interruptions minimised. The patient should be physically positioned to feel empowered (e.g. avoid talking across a desk or talking down to a patient on a bed).

As well as reviewing the environment, doctors should review themselves. They should do some self-reflection to consider what personal qualities, assumptions and values they have that may influence a consultation.

Just prior to the consultation, a review of the patient's health record will improve the doctor's awareness of important facts about the patient. Opening the file is actually when the consultation starts. Here, crucial clues can be found, such as:

- what happened at the last consultation
- what are the important medical issues for this patient
- any recent test results or correspondence that have arrived
- even the names of partners, parents or children who may come into the room with the patient
- brief notes on personal characteristics, likes/dislikes (e.g. has needle phobia)

When a record is examined well, the reasons for the consultation can often be anticipated prior to the formal start of the consultation, giving the doctor a wonderful opportunity to improve communication.

Increasingly in general practice we see patients as part of a team. The patient may previously have been seen by a practice nurse or a more junior doctor or medical student. This 'teamlet model of primary care'.[5,6] has been shown to help elucidate patients' concerns, as have 'patient agenda forms', which patients fill out prior to the consultation, prompting them to list what is on their agenda for the consultation.[6,7]

At first contact, we usually call a patient from the waiting room into the consulting room. Having your eyes and ears ready and focused here can give you invaluable information. What is the person wearing? What is the significance of any badges, necklaces, rings or tatoos? What does his or her body language suggest? Who is accompanying the patient and how are they interacting with each other? Clues about their interests (e.g. a child's T-shirt reflecting a favourite TV character), their cultural and social backgrounds (e.g. dress and appearance) and even their medical issues at hand (e.g. a limp, a bandage or carrying an X-ray folder or hospital letter) abound in this 'pre-opener space'. Picking up on these clues early helps the doctor anticipate and reflect on issues before they emerge in the consultation, avoids communication breakdown, makes the patient feel that the doctor is interested in him or her and can make the doctor appear switched on and observant.

Open

When we get to the 'opener' (e.g. 'What can I do for you today?' or 'Why have you come to see me today?') and beyond, we should:[8]

- greet and address the patient by his or her preferred name (and anyone else entering the room)
- try to make the patient feel comfortable
- try to appear 'unhurried' and relaxed
- focus firmly on the patient
- use open-ended questions where possible
- make appropriate reassuring gestures

Gather

It is in the early stages of the consultation that silence (on the doctor's part) can be golden. In what is termed *active listening,* we listen to more than the words—we are also alert to the messages buried in the words. We listen to the tone and rhythm and we look for the context of what we are hearing. We listen with understanding, in a relaxed, attentive silence. Note-taking, whether written or typed, should not become a barrier to appearing to listen; as it is done, it can be verbalised by the doctor, so the patient knows he or she is being heard. The computer should not be allowed to be the intrusive third person in the room.

Allowing the patient to talk (without interruption), and even leaving a slightly prolonged pause, often provides enough space for the patient's concerns to emerge. This is especially the case with psychosocial issues.[9]

This ability to elicit patient concerns is unfortunately not one that doctors have always done well. Stewart[10] summarises the evidence in this area:

> 50% of psychosocial and psychiatric problems are missed, physicians interrupt patients an average of 18 seconds into the patient's description of the presenting problem . . . 54% of patient problems and 45% of patient concerns are neither elicited by the physician nor disclosed by the patient . . . patients and physicians do not agree on the main presenting problem in 50% of visits and . . . patients are dissatisfied with the information provided to them by physicians.

This evidence is of course in relation to doctors as a whole and not just general practitioners, but it does illustrate how important and at times difficult effective communication in medical consultations can be.

Three techniques that have been demonstrated[8,11] to improve how we elicit patient concerns are:

- facilitation
- the open-to-closed cone
- summarisation

Facilitation refers to comments or behaviours by the doctor that encourage the patient to keep talking. This could include a head-nod, a 'hmm' at the right time, or 'Tell me more about that'. The open-to-closed cone is a gradual narrowing of focus from an indirect non-directive exploration to a more direct exploration. It is often difficult to resist the urge to 'dive in' and explore the initial concern raised and narrow the cone too quickly.[6,12]

After each problem or concern is elicited, the doctor should continue to explore to ensure there are not any more. What are the patient's concerns (e.g. headache, depressed mood) and needs (e.g. a prescription, a referral or a form to be filled out)?[9] The doctor does not take too much control of the conversation, does not direct the topic away from the patient's concerns and hence helps to demonstrate empathy as well as a real interest in the patient. Using a patient-centred approach leads to improved patient trust and satisfaction, more appropriate prescribing and more efficient practice.[6]

Summarisation is when the doctor provides the patient with an explicit verbal summary of the information gathered thus far in the consultation.[11] This helps to orientate the patient, acknowledging to him or her that the doctor has taken on board what they have said, and reflecting back to the patient the doctor's understanding of it.

If we initially 'limit ourselves to triage questions' and wait until 'all the cards are on the table',[9] it reduces the chance of patient concerns being missed. The value of a question like 'Is there anything else today?', and repeatedly making such an enquiry until we receive a 'no' in response, will help ensure we have obtained a complete understanding of the patient's agenda.[9]

Non-verbal communication

Non-verbal communication or body language is a vital feature of the communication process. Human communication takes place through the use of gestures, postures, position and distances (non-verbal communication or *body language*) more than by any other method. Non-verbal cues comprise the majority of the impact of any communicated message (see TABLE 4.1).[13]

Table 4.1 Impact of the message

Cue	%
Words alone	7
Tone of voice	38
Non-verbal communication	55

4

Recognition of non-verbal cues in our communication is important, especially in a doctor–patient relationship. Charles Darwin in his 'Expression of the Emotions in Man and Animals' (1872) concluded that there is a unique pattern of non-verbal actions for each emotion, such as snarling as a sign of aggression. The ability to identify non-verbal cues improves communication, rapport and understanding of the patient's fears and concerns. Recognising body language can allow doctors to modify their behaviour, thus promoting optimum communication.

Interpreting body language

The interpretation of body language, which differs between cultures, is a special study in its own right, but there are certain cues and gestures that can be readily understood. Examples illustrated include: the depressed patient (see FIG. 4.2); barrier-type signals, often used as a defensive mechanism to provide comfort or indicate a negative attitude (see FIG. 4.3); and a readiness gesture, indicating a desire to terminate the communication (see FIG. 4.4).

Having noted the non-verbal communication, the doctor must then deal with it. This may require confrontation—that is, diplomatically bringing these cues to the patient's attention and exploring the associated feeling further.

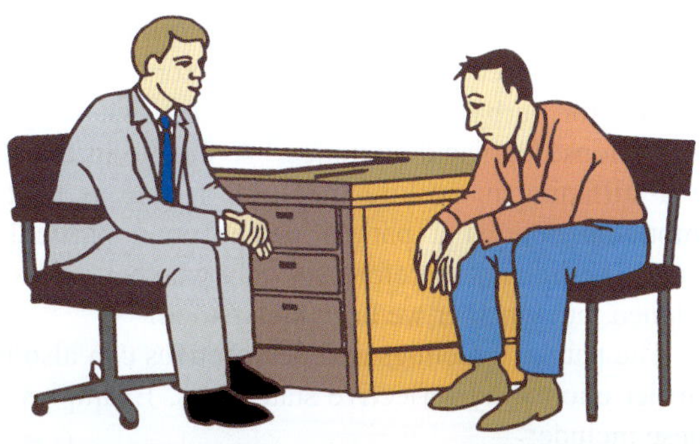

FIGURE 4.2 Posture of a depressed person: head down, slumped, inanimate; position of desk and people correct

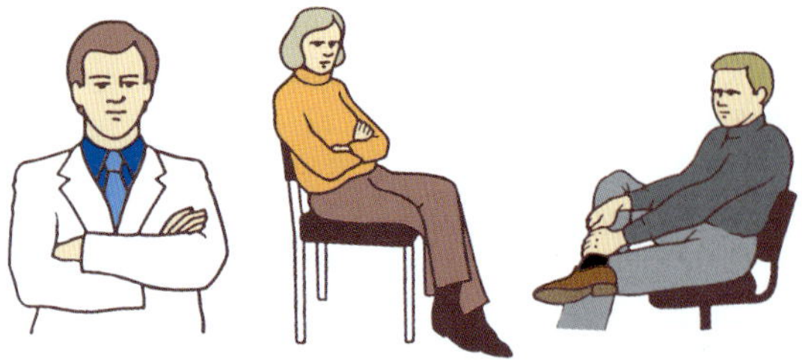

FIGURE 4.3 Body language barrier signals: (A) arms folded, (B) legs crossed, (C) 'ankle lock' pose

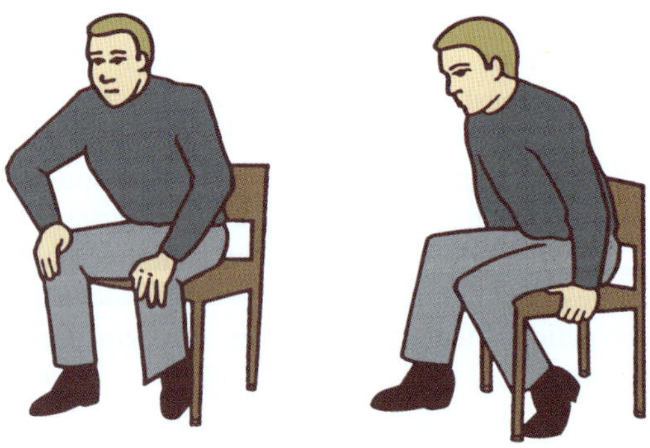

FIGURE 4.4 Body language: 'readiness to go' gestures

The patient's perspective

The treatment of disease must be completely impersonal; the treatment of a patient must be completely personal.

DR FRANCIS WELD PEABODY, HARVARD, 1926

To be truly patient-centred, it is not enough merely to find out the patient's concerns and needs—we also need to explore his or her ideas, beliefs and expectations.[8] What is the patient's *perspective* on his or her concerns and needs? What does the patient expect of you and from the consultation? What are the priorities?

To best meet this challenge, doctors should be vigilant for verbal and non-verbal cues that suggest frustrations, fears and anxieties.[3] A shuffle in a chair or a stiffening in posture may give a clue as to the emotional context a patient places on a particular issue. The issue is therefore not only whether we have listened, but whether we have understood.[9]

The patient's feelings and perspectives can also be further elicited by reflective statements. Examples of these include:

- you seem very sad today
- you seem upset about your husband
- it seems you're having trouble coping
- you seem to be telling me that . . .
- your main concern seems to me to be . . .

Discovering the patient's beliefs about illness will allow us to make statements to them that are congruent with those beliefs. This is especially important in mental health, where illness beliefs are often emotionally laden and unpredictable.

Understanding the patient's perspective also needs to be considered in a cultural context. Culture can have many dimensions, including ethnicity, age, gender, sexuality, community and religious beliefs. Being *culturally competent* by showing an interest in, respect for and sensitivity to that culture will help us achieve a shared understanding of where the patient is coming from and how he or she is seeing things.[8]

Communicating during the physical examination or procedure

In the same way that we obtain consent for surgical procedures, we should also fully inform the patient of what we plan to do and obtain consent in any physical interaction with the patient. Physical examination can be very confrontational for some patients and this can be underestimated by the doctor. There may be factors of which the doctor is unaware that may make examination particularly difficult for the patient, such as unpleasant previous experiences, cultural, gender or sexual issues surrounding touch, or phobias about medical procedures or needles.

As well as preparing the patient, explaining during the examination or procedure what is happening and what we are observing and finding will help the patient feel valued and respected. We should also continue to keep an ear out for any further patient concerns being raised.[3]

If we are fully eliciting the patient's concerns and needs and are consulting using a patient-centred approach, a point is reached in the consultation where the information flow will need to go in the opposite direction—from doctor back to patient (in fact, in most consultations this flow often moves repeatedly back and forth). How we deliver this information is critical to patient communication.

When we are communicating information to a patient, it will be best understood and accepted when the information is congruent with the patient's beliefs. If these beliefs are helpful, we should recognise them and reinforce them. For instance, 'I agree with you; I think stress might be contributing to your pain here.'

Four techniques that will help maximise patient understanding are:

- signposting
- 'chunk and check'
- avoiding jargon
- using visual and physical techniques to communicate[8]

Signposting is a technique whereby the doctor explicitly states what he or she has done and/or is about to do (e.g. 'Andrew, I have finished examining you, now I would like to explain what I think the issues are' or 'Mrs Jones, I have two matters I would like to discuss: first . . .'). Signposting helps orientate the patient, which further helps him or her to relax and focus better on what you are saying.

Chunk and check is where the doctor provides a chunk of information to the patient and then immediately checks the patient's understanding of what has been said. Chunk and check works best when the chunks are small, as this information is often new to the patient and best digested in small grabs. It is frequently surprising to find how far away the patient's understanding is from what we intended to communicate, so this technique informs the doctor of any misunderstanding and hence provides an early opportunity to correct this.

Jargon is a barrier to communication in many professions (think accountants or IT technicians) and medicine is rife with jargon. However, jargon is not a dirty word. The way we are educated and the way doctors and other health professionals continue to communicate with each other is expedited by using jargon—it makes our communication more efficient by having a technical language to use.

On the other hand, when dealing with patients, using jargon not only impairs the patient's understanding, but can also be alienating and intimidating. What actually constitutes jargon is also often underestimated. While a doctor will usually realise that 'acute myocardial infarction' or 'cholecystectomy' are jargon, more subtle forms of jargon could include words such as 'complication', 'rare' or 'tumour'. A patient's understanding of such words may be very different from the doctor's, so checking this understanding will help protect against this. What is jargon will also vary from patient to patient. Factors such as age, education, language skills and cultural background can affect which forms of language and words are beyond the patient's understanding. The patient needs to have the cognitive and communicative capacity to understand the message.[14]

Visual and physical methods of conveying information given (or plans made) can include diagrams, models, patient hand-outs or information sheets.[8] Having ready access to electronic visual materials or websites on a desktop computer can also help. Videos on websites such as YouTube can be used to illustrate how the body functions, how a disease manifests, or a particular medical procedure, and directing patients to reputable and reliable information sources on the web or elsewhere (before they find unreliable information themselves) will help avoid misinformation and extend the communication beyond the consultation.

4

Negotiate and agree on a plan

Looking beyond patient-centred communication, we can then think about planning: what do we intend to do, how we are going to decide this, who is going to do it? The preferred technique for this is *shared or collaborative decision making.*[14,15] The aim should be to have such collaboration at all stages of the consultation. But because patients can often feel intimidated, it is a challenge for the doctor to make the patient feel comfortable enough to do so.[16]

To enable this collaboration, the doctor and patient should treat each other's concerns with respect; this will lead to a shared responsibility for agenda setting.[9] Such collaboration, when done well, can lead to a coming-together of thinking that has been called a *shared mind.*[14] Strategies that will help achieve this include finding common ground, reaching consensus on a treatment plan and establishing a mutually acceptable follow-up plan.[13] 'This is what I would suggest, what do you think?' As a way of thinking, a shared mind involves a doctor being mindful of the patient's values, thoughts and feelings (as well as those of his or her own), and seeing where the two connect.[17]

This mindfulness of each other's position can help the negotiation of what happens in the consultation and also avoid communication breakdowns. For instance, what shall we deal with today, and what should be delayed or rolled over to another consultation?[9] It can also help repair a communication breakdown. For example, if a patient is heading off at a tangent, if we are mindful of where he or she is coming from and what is important to that person, it will enable us to gently bring him or her back to the topic we feel is more pressing.

One technique that uses this principle is called an *empathic bridge.*[9] This is where we anchor the conversation in the patient's experience by reflecting or paraphrasing. From this anchor, we then manoeuvre the conversation back to where it needs to be (e.g. 'It sounds like your pumpkin soup recipe is something special. It is a pity you managed to cut your finger while making it today. Now let's have a look at that cut').

Another aspect of the doctor–patient relationship that enhances collaborative decision making, particularly in general practice, is *shared experiences.*[18] GP–patient relationships evolve over time, and a shared experience such as helping a patient through a difficult pregnancy, a major illness or even doing a home visit can enrich the relationship, deepen the connection and trust between doctor and patient, and lead to greater collaborative decision making.

Close

How should we close a consultation? If we follow the principles of patient-centred communication and remember that we should keep our focus on the patient's concerns and needs, it soon becomes apparent.

First, is the patient aware of the imminent closure? Anxious and distressed patients may have no idea how long they have been ruminating about their concerns through the consultation, and be unaware that the waiting room full of people is actually starting to concern you. In such situations, letting them know in advance that closure is being planned (and why) will allow them to not feel pushed out of the room.

Secondly, making sure that there are no further disclosures of concerns or needs to come (yet again) will reduce the risk of what has been termed the 'doorknob presentation'—the raising of a patient concern that happens as the doctor puts his or her hand on the doorknob to leave the room (this has also been called the 'Oh, by the way doctor' syndrome in the USA, the 'à propos, docteur' in France, and 'tussen haakjes' in Denmark, which translates to 'between two brackets' or, as we may say, 'parenthetically').[9]

Thirdly, summarising the critical points of the consultation and planned actions and expectations will provide a final opportunity to identify gaps between what the doctor and patient are respectively thinking. We should also prepare a safety net by considering any possible unexpected outcomes to what is being planned (e.g. what a parent should watch out for and what to do if things worsen with the febrile infant patient).

Finally, we should thank and say farewell to the patient with an appropriate parting statement. Does this include a handshake? This may be determined by your style, the patient's style and cultural issues.

Use of relationship-building skills

During the consultation and throughout a doctor–patient relationship over many consultations (and potentially, in general practice, over decades), effective communication is underpinned by using skills that develop the interpersonal relationship between doctor and patient.[3,8]

These skills include the doctor paying attention to non-verbal behaviour on display, as mentioned above, such as appropriate eye contact, posture, position and movement. Verbal cues such as the speed of speech, volume and tone can also be used. If using a computer or taking written notes, the doctor should do so in a fashion that does not interfere with dialogue or rapport. Also, given that patients are often highly emotionally invested in what we say, consulting in a manner that reflects confidence (without stepping over into arrogance) will help build trust.

Rapport, which originates from an old French word that literally means 'to carry back', can be engendered by fostering connections back and forth with the patient. Displaying empathy for the patient's situation or feelings, acknowledging his or her view or efforts, and dealing sensitively with embarrassing or disturbing topics such as pain or grief, will engender rapport. We can show we are willing to provide emotional support by overtly expressing our concern or understanding, or a willingness to help or offer partnership.[8,16] An offer such as 'I am really keen to help you with this situation' can go a long way.

Connections that build rapport can also happen away from medical issues, and are often more powerful. This is where the 'clues' that we were looking for at the beginning of the consultation can come into play. If a short interplay can happen between doctor and patient about something the patient is passionate about or interested in, which has nothing to do with the medical issues at hand, the patient will feel that he or she is respected as a person, not just as a medical presentation to be solved. Examples of such clues that could be picked up and explored by the doctor could be a favourite toy being held by a child, a book that a patient carries into the room, or the doctor noticing that the occupation of the patient is something he or she is interested in asking about. It comes down to patients feeling that the doctor is actually interested in them. When such connections are made, any tension in the consultation room can be seen to evaporate.

Other rapport-building techniques

A person can develop a rapport with another by mimicking his or her body language, speech, posture, pace and other characteristics. Such techniques can be used to help the doctor communicate better with a patient and also to improve the patient's attitude by changing the patient's body language position.

Mirroring

Mirroring is a useful technique whereby the limb positions and body angles of the person you are talking to can be copied. A mirror image is formed of their position so that when they look at you they see themselves as in a mirror. It is not necessary to copy uncomfortable gestures or unusual limb positions, such as hands behind the head. A partial mirror is often sufficient.

Pacing

People exhibit a certain rhythm or pace that can be revealed through their breathing, talking, and movements of the head, hands or feet. If you can copy the pace of another person, it will establish a sense of oneness or rapport with them. Once this pace is established, you can change their pace by changing yours. This is called *leading*.

Vocal copying

Vocal copying is another way to develop rapport with people. It involves copying intonation, pitch, volume, pace, rhythm, breathing and length of the sentence before pausing.

Manage flow

At the end of the day, the doctor has a professional responsibility to appropriately meet the needs of the patient but also to keep control of a consultation so that it does not affect other consultations which follow. In most consultations, this is not difficult, but with a small proportion of patients, particularly those who have mental health and/or psychosocial issues to deal with, maintaining control and managing time can be challenging.[19]

A balance must be struck between maintaining control and not undermining the doctor–patient relationship.

The doctor having a 'wide-angle lens' on the consultation, so that he or she is mindful of where they are up to in the consultation and how much time has been taken up already, as well as the actual medical issues being discussed, will help anticipate a problem. Doing so subtly (e.g. not looking at a watch!) will help. It can be useful to have a wall clock situated behind the patient's chair or to be aware of where the consultation timer is on the computer screen. Being time aware can be particularly difficult for inexperienced doctors, who will be more focused on not making a mistake with the medical issues at hand. Naturally, even if the time is way over, it may be entirely appropriate to carry on if it is an important issue, such as with a suicidal or distressed patient.

If a consultation's flow is becoming problematic, the doctor should employ *appropriate use of power.*[18] This can be done with techniques such as setting rules in advance for patients where this is a problem (e.g. time limits for the consultation or limits on the number of concerns to be addressed). We can also use, if required, *blocking behaviours,* which can be verbal or non-verbal. These are behaviours that consciously block the flow of a consultation that is not being appropriately controlled. Examples include the doctor using body language that suggests he or she has something to say, or purposefully focusing on the (sometimes very short) space between a hyper-verbal patient's sentences to enable him or her to 'jump in' and take control of the consultation.

Practice tip

- Using a patient-centred approach leads to improved patient trust and satisfaction, more appropriate prescribing and more efficient practice.
- Undertaking the strategies of facilitation, the open-to-closed cone and summarisation will help us effectively elicit patient concerns.
- Associated with listening, observe non-verbal language, which may in many instances be the most significant part of the communication process.
- Techniques that will help maximise patient understanding are signposting, 'chunk and check', avoiding jargon and using visual and physical techniques to communicate.
- Collaborative decision making helps the negotiation of what happens in the consultation and also avoids communication breakdowns.

Key features of good communication[20]

- A patient-centred approach
- Eliciting all of the patient's concerns
- Exploring the patient's ideas, beliefs and expectations
- Showing empathy and respect
- Summarising
- Avoiding jargon
- Collaborative decision making
- Good closure

4

References

1 Elliott-Binns E. *Medicine: The Forgotten Art.* Tunbridge Wells, Kent: Pitman Books, 1978: 35.
2 Macnab F. Changing levels of susceptibility in sickness and in health. Aust Fam Physician, 1986; 15: 1370.
3 NYU Macy Initiative on Health Communication. *Overview of the Structure and Sequence of Effective Doctor Patient Communication* New York University, 2001. <http://nyumacy.med.nyu.edu/curriculum/model/m07.html>, accessed September 2013.
4 Makoul G. Essential elements of communication in medical encounters: the Kalamazoo consensus statement. Acad Med, 2001; 76: 390–3.
5 Bodenbeimer H, Laing B. The teamlet model of primary care. Ann Fam Med, 2007; 5: 457–61.
6 Epstein R, Carroll J. Have you really addressed your patient's concerns? Family Practice Management, 2008: 36–40.
7 Middleton R, McKinley R, Gillies C. Effect of patient completed agenda forms and doctor's education about the agenda on the outcome of consultations: randomised control trial. BMJ Online, 2006.
8 Calgary-Cambridge Guide to the Medical Interview—Communication Process. Available from: <www.gp-training.net/training/communication_skills/calgary/calgary.pdf>, accessed October 2013.
9 Baker L, O'Connell D, Platt F. 'What else?' Setting the agenda for the clinical interview. Ann Intern Med, 2005; 143: 766–70.
10 Stewart, M. Effective physician-patient communication and health outcomes: a review. CMAJ, 1995; 152(9): 1423–33.
11 Takemura Y, Atsumi R, Tsuda T. Identifying medical interview behaviors that best elicit information from patients in clinical practice. Tohoku J Exp Med, 2007; 213(2): 121–7.
12 Mausch L, Hillenberg L, Robins L. The established focus protocol: training for collaborative agenda setting and time management in the medical interview. Families, Systems and Health, 2001; 19(2): 147–57.
13 Mehrabian A. *Silent Messages* Belmont, CA: Wadsworth, 1971.
14 Politi M, Street R. The importance of communication in collaborative decision making: facilitating shared mind and the management of uncertainty. J Eval Clin Pract, 2011; 17: 579–84.
15 Wensing M, Elwyn G, Grol R. Deconstructing patient centred communication and uncovering shared decision making: an observational study. BMC, 2002; 2: 2.
16 Charles C, Whelan T, Gafni A. What do we mean by partnerships making decisions about treatment? BMJ, 1999; 319 (7212): 780–2.
17 Epstein R, Peters E. Beyond information: exploring patient preferences. JAMA, 2009; 302: 195–7.
18 Stewart M, Gilbert B. Reflections on the doctor-patient relationship: from evidence and experience. BJGP, 2005; 55(519): 793–801.
19 Elder N, Ricer R, Tobias B. How respected family physicians manage difficult patient encounters. J Am Board Fam Med, 2006; 19: 533–41.
20 Lloyd M, Bor R. *Communication skills in medicine.* Elsevier, 2017: 240–2.

Counselling skills 5

The doctor should have a kind disposition, great patience, self-possession, meticulous freedom from prejudice, an understanding of human nature resulting from an abundant knowledge of the world, adroitness in conversation and a special love of his calling.

G GRIESINGER 1840

The *Macquarie Dictionary* says that counselling is 'giving advice': that it is 'opinion or instruction given in directing the judgment or conduct of another'. In the clinical context counselling can be defined as 'the therapeutic process of helping a patient to explore the nature of his or her problem in such a way that he or she determines his or her decisions about what to do, without direct advice or reassurance from the counsellor'.

The counselling process in general practice is based on the therapeutic effect of the doctor. There is an enormous and ever-increasing need for people in the community to have many of their emotional and social problems addressed by the health profession. Modern medicine has acquired a much more scientific face over recent years at the expense of its once respected humanistic one. Medicine is primarily a humanitarian pursuit, not an economic or scientific one, and uses science as a tool. Many feel that medicine is losing sight of this, at the considerable expense of its standing in the community.[1]

The public perceives that GPs can and do counsel people because more people go to their GP for counselling than to any other group of health workers, including psychologists, psychiatrists, social workers, marriage guidance counsellors and clergy.[1] People do not generally tell the doctor or even realise that counselling is exactly what led them to come to the doctor in the first place. The GP is, therefore, ideally placed in the community to make the most significant contribution to fill the community's needs in this area.

The GP as an effective counsellor

GPs can be effective counsellors for the following reasons:[2]

- They have the opportunity to observe and understand patients and their environment.
- They are ideally placed to treat the whole patient.
- Their generalist skills and holistic approach permit GPs to have a broad grasp of a patient's problems and a multifaceted approach to treatment.
- They can provide treatment in comfortable and familiar surroundings, including the doctor's rooms and the patient's home.
- They are skilled at working as a member of a professional team and directing patients to more expert members of the team as necessary.
- They can readily organise 'contracts' with the patient.
- They often have an intimate knowledge of the family and the family dynamics.
- They fit comfortably into continuing patient care with appropriate follow-up treatment programs.

To be an effective counsellor the GP must prepare for this role, first by making a commitment to its importance, then by acquiring the knowledge and skills for basic counselling by reading, attending workshops and discussing cases with colleagues who are skilled in counselling.[2] Appropriate workshops are those based on the seminal model of therapy by Balint,[3] which aim to teach the patient new coping skills and so alleviate symptoms and improve the patient's functioning in social and occupational roles. Well-developed interviewing skills are essential, as is self-discipline to appreciate one's strengths and limitations.

Features of counselling

Doctors can respond to patients' problems and distress by a spectrum of behaviours from doctor-centred, directive behavior (directed psychotherapy) or advice at one end, to patient-centred, non-directive behaviour at the other, where the patient does most of the talking (expressive psychotherapy).[2] In handling psychosocial problems, advice-giving is at one end of the spectrum and psychotherapy at the other.

Counselling, as an activity in general practice, can be represented by a moving point between these two extremes.[1]

Patient-centred ⟷ Doctor-centred
Psychotherapy ↑ Advice
Counselling

Counselling can be seen as having the following features:[1]

- It is a clear-cut treatment option, like a course of antibiotics.
- It is a cooperative problem-solving process.
- It is an educational venture where patients learn new information and new activities.
- It is a developmental process for patients.
- It is a change process—often moving a patient from a 'stuck state'.
- It is a goal-directed activity.
- It is a process of energising patients and lifting their morale.
- It is a sensitive response to problems within a caring relationship.

A problem-solving approach

Defining the problem (what the matter really is) is the most important step in the process of patient care. The following outline is one approach to counselling that is applicable to a general practice context.[1]

1. Listen to the problem of first presentation: this involves listening not only to issues, events and experiences, but also to the patient's feelings and distress. The emphasis here is more on the communication skills of facilitation, silence, clarification, reflection, paraphrasing, confrontation and summary, than on questioning. In many cases this phase of the counselling constitutes the major part of the therapy; for example, in grief or bereavement counselling, the doctor supports the patient through a natural but distressing process.
2. Define the problem, if possible in behavioural terms:
   Beneath the feeling is the experience, beneath the experience is the event, the event is related to a problem.[4]
3. Establish a contract for counselling, with an agreed number of visits initially (e.g. weekly half-hour or hour appointments for 4 to 6 weeks).
4. Define short-term and long-term goals for action.
5. Decide on one option—'experimental action'.
6. Build an action program with the patient—negotiate 'homework' for the patient between visits.
7. Evaluate progress.
8. Continue action or select another option.
9. Evaluate progress.
10. Terminate or refer.

Counselling models

The PLISSIT model

The PLISSIT model, developed by Annon (1974)[5] as an aid in therapy for sexual problems, is a very useful model for problems presented as feelings where there is limited scope for intervention by the therapist.

The mnemonic PLISSIT stands for the following:

- P is for permission giving
- LI is for limited information
- SS is for specific suggestion
- IT is for intensive therapy

Annon emphasises that every primary care practitioner should be competent to offer 'permission giving' and 'limited information'.

The Colagiuri and Craig model

The medical counselling model was developed by Colagiuri and Craig (see FIG. 5.1)[6] as a useful tool for teaching contraceptive, abortion and sterilisation counselling. It can be applied in most situations as it empowers the patients to make their own decisions through facilitation as opposed to the directive and advisory learning model.

The value of patient-centred counselling

There is evidence that the use of non-directive counselling techniques leads to more accurate diagnosis and therefore to more appropriate management and an improved outcome.[7]

Jerome Frank wrote in 1967: 'The field of counselling and psychotherapy has for years presented the puzzling spectacle of unabating enthusiasm for forms of treatment where effectiveness could not be objectively demonstrated'.[8] Traux and Carkhuff[9] measured important aspects of the psychotherapeutic relationship and demonstrated what had long been recognised: the outcome was enhanced if practitioners had such qualities as accurate and sensitive awareness of the patient's feelings, deep concern for the patient's welfare (without attempting to dominate) and openness about their own reactions.

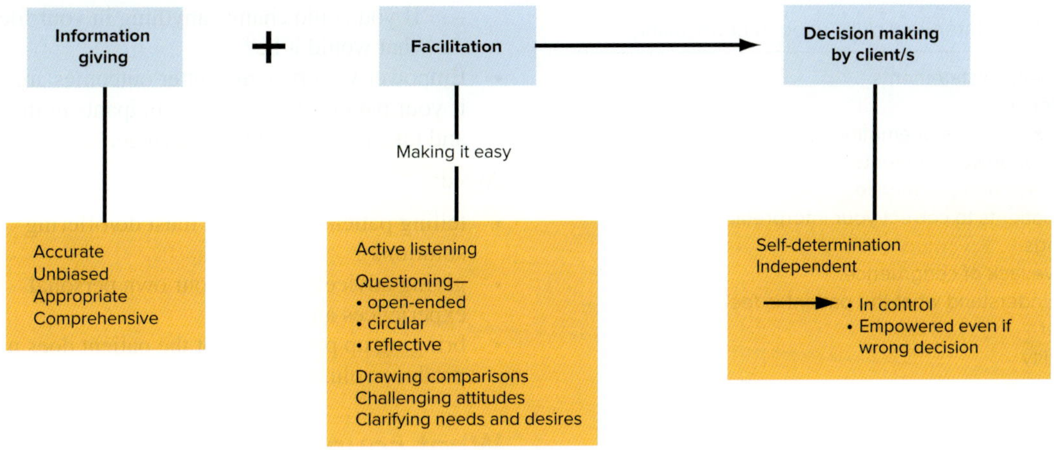

FIGURE 5.1 Medical counselling model
Source: After Colagiuri and Craig[6]

The essential feature of the patient-centred approach is that the counsellor is more like a facilitator; that is, by the asking of well-directed questions it is hoped that patients can realise their own solutions for their problems.[1] This encourages patients to attain understanding and personal growth themselves rather than just put their personal affairs in the hands of someone else. This does not mean to say that the facilitator is passive in the process of assessing the relative merit of various solutions produced by the patient. The doctor-centred approach is most applicable for patients who are so confused or distraught that their ability to reflect usefully is temporarily or permanently inaccessible. Here, taking a more active and authoritarian role may be just what is required. It is therefore important to be flexible and move between the two ends of the spectrum as needed.

Basics of counselling and psychotherapy

- Listening and empathy are the beginning of counselling.
- Good communication is the basis of counselling.
- The therapist must really care about the patient.
- Always be aware of the family context.
- It is important for therapists to handle and monitor their own feelings and emotions.
- Maintain eye contact.
- The therapist must tolerate and be comfortable with what the patient says.
- Confidentiality is essential.
- Counselling is easier if there is a good rapport with the patient, especially if a long-standing relationship exists.
- Counselling is difficult if a social relationship is present.
- Don't say to the patient 'I'm counselling you' or 'I'm giving you psychotherapy'—make it a natural communication process.
- The therapist must be versatile and adapt a counselling style to the clinical occasion.
- Characteristics of the effective counsellor have been demonstrated to be genuineness, non-possessive warmth for the patient, and accurate and empathetic understanding.

A fundamental feature of counselling is reflective listening to direct patients to think about and then resolve their problems.

Some useful interviewing skills used in counselling are summarised in TABLE 5.1.

Counselling strategies[4,7]

- The therapy should be patient-centred.
- Use gentle, clever, probing questions.
- Facilitate the discussion to draw out relevant areas.
- It is important to be non-judgmental.
- Counsel through intuition and base it on common sense.
- Do not tell the patient what to do.

Table 5.1 Interview skills used in counselling

Use reflective statements.
Use silence.
Allow expressions of emotion.
Offer supportive comments.
Paraphrase and summarise.
Allow patients to correct your interpretations of their feelings.
Observe lack of congruence.
Try to understand what the patient is feeling: • anger • hostility • fear • manipulation • seduction • insecurity
Make intelligent guesses to prompt patient to continue.
Don't reassure too soon.

- Do not try to rush patients into achieving a happy ending.
- Provide guidance to allow the patient to gain insight.
- Wherever possible, make therapy non-authoritarian and non-directional.
- Use appropriate 'gentle' confrontation to allow self-examination.
- Help patients to explore their own situation and express emotions, such as anxiety, guilt, fear, anger, hope, sadness, self-hate, hostility to others and hurt feelings.
- Explore possible feelings of insecurity and allow free expression of such feelings.
- Explore patients' belief systems and consider and respect their spiritual aspirations and conflicts.
- Ask key searching questions, such as:
  - 'What would be different in your life if you were well?'
  - 'Who are you mad at?'
  - 'If I understand you correctly you are telling me that . . .'
  - 'You seem to be telling me that . . .'
  - 'Correct me if I'm on the wrong track, but you are saying that . . .'
  - 'What do you think deep down is the cause of your problem?'
  - 'What does your illness do to you?'
  - 'Do you really worry about any things in particular?'
  - 'How do you think your problem should be treated?'
  - 'If you could change anything in your life, what would it be?'
- Empower your patient. Better outcomes are likely if your patients are active participants in their care and take responsibility for change.

Avoid:

- telling patients what they must do/offering solutions
- giving advice based on your own personal experiences and beliefs
- bringing up problems that the patient does not produce voluntarily

What counselling is not

- Giving information
- Giving advice
- Being judgmental
- Imposing one's own values, behaviour and practices
- The same as interviewing
- Handing out patient education material

Cautions[1]

- Individual doctors cannot be useful to all patients, so be selective.
- We cannot solve patients' problems for them.
- Patients' problems belong to them and not to their counsellors.
- Patients often have to change by only an inch in order to move a mile.
- If a counselling relationship is no longer productive, then terminate and refer.
- Most patients in primary care need information, support and a lift in morale, not long-term psychotherapy.

Patients unlikely to benefit

The following groups of patients are not likely to benefit from counselling therapy[1] (i.e. relative contraindications):

- psychotic patients
- patients who have had an unrewarding experience with psychiatrists and other psychotherapists
- people who are antagonistic to the notion of a psychosocial diagnosis, subsequently found to be organic
- patients with little awareness or language to express emotional difficulty
- patients who do not believe doctors can treat psychosocial problems

- patients with a vested interest in remaining unwell who are therefore resistant to change (e.g. patients with work-related disabilities awaiting legal settlement)
- patients with chronic psychosomatic tendencies who are willing to do almost anything to maintain the relationship
- those in an intractable life situation who are unable or unwilling to change

Types of psychotherapy[2,10]

- Interpersonal psychotherapy/counselling, ideal for primary care and the treatment of depression, is therapy for interpersonal problems.
- Mindfulness based on intervention therapy.
- Behaviour therapy (BT) is where the patient is directed to do something.
- Cognitive therapy (CT) is based on the identification of automatic thoughts that are invariably negative. Cognitions are thoughts, beliefs and perceptions.
- Cognitive behaviour therapy (CBT), which combines BT and CT.

The psychotherapy continuum is illustrated in FIGURE 5.2.[2]

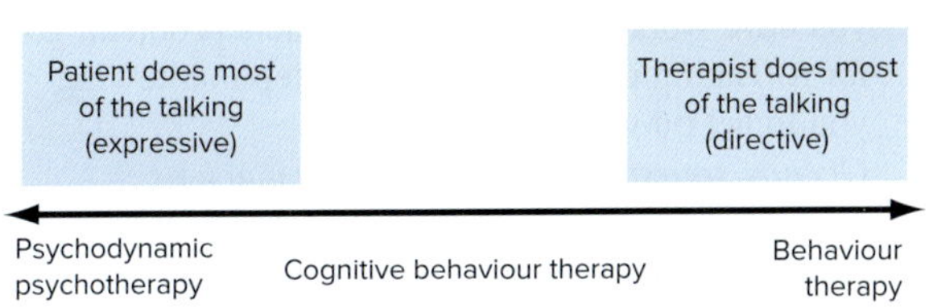
Patient does most of the talking (expressive)
Therapist does most of the talking (directive)
Psychodynamic psychotherapy
Cognitive behaviour therapy
Behaviour therapy

FIGURE 5.2 Psychotherapy continuum

Source: Selzer R, Ellen S. *Psych-lite: Psychiatry That's Easy to Read.* Sydney: McGraw Hill, 2010: 70–3.

Cognitive behaviour therapy

CBT is a form of non-pharmacologic treatment emphasising self-help and aiming to change perceptions and behaviour that may perpetuate symptoms and disability. It is basically a system of graded exposure (systematic desensitisation). It can be applied in any area of medical practice as a form of psychotherapy and is suitable in general practice for the treatment of depression, insomnia, eating disorders, delusions and hallucinations in psychotic disorders and anxiety in all forms, especially social anxiety disorder and phobias—in all of which CBT has proved to be better than a placebo.[11]

It is a relatively brief, active, directive and practical form of therapy. However, not all therapists or patients are suited to CBT.

The basic processes of CBT are to:

- define specific and concrete goals for functional activities and moods, e.g. pain control
- educate the patient
- teach basic skills for symptom control, relaxation and breathing control (especially for hyperventilation)
- identify, challenge and change maladaptive thoughts, feelings, perceptions and behaviour

Some basic principles and objectives of CBT are to:

- aim to bring about a desired change in patients' lives, i.e. aim to achieve desired goals
- assess, monitor and attempt to modify thoughts and behaviour
- reinforce positive behaviour and discourage negative behaviour
- educate about any misconceptions about a patient's illness
- encourage the patient to be an active participant (not a passive recipient)
- get patients to establish a problem list and hierarchy of problems
- aim for more realistic thinking and more adaptive responses

Mindfulness

Mindfulness, which is based on meditation, is the process about raising awareness and a special way of paying attention to help the person cope with the daily events in their life.

The basic processes of mindfulness are to:

- train people to focus on the positive aspects of their lives and shut out distraction and negativity, i.e. attention training
- learn to concentrate in a restful way and cope with stress
- emphasise attentiveness to the present moment
- voluntarily reign in a wandering attention time and again

Specific areas of counselling

Opportunities for basic counselling by the GP are ubiquitous in medical practice. Complex problems require referral but, even then, the GP still has an important role in continuing management.

Areas demanding counselling include:

- any crisis situation—breaking bad news
- bereavement or grief
- terminal illness/palliative care (CHAPTER 11)
- marital problems (CHAPTER 2)

- family problems (CHAPTER 2)
- sexual dysfunction (CHAPTER 116)
- chronic pain
- anxiety and stress (CHAPTER 81)
- depression (CHAPTER 19)
- intellectual handicap in a child
- infertility (CHAPTER 115)
- any disease or illness, especially severe illness
- sexual abuse/child abuse (CHAPTER 95)
- intimate partner violence (CHAPTER 118)
- insomnia and other sleep disturbances (CHAPTER 74)

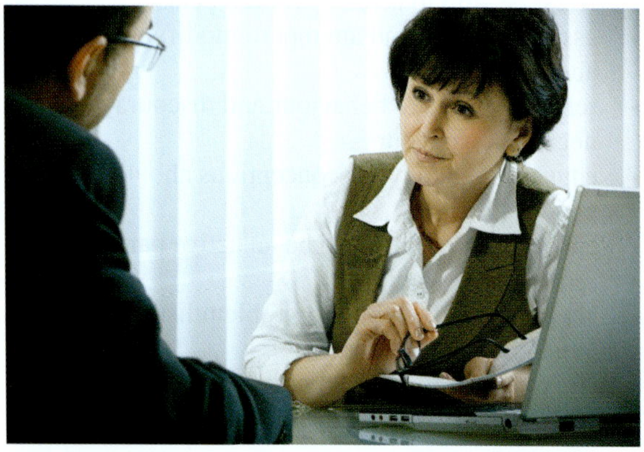

FIGURE 5.3 Counselling skills: these skills include good eye contact, listening, empathy and appropriate communication skills

Crisis management

Crisis situations are not uncommon in general practice and people in crisis are usually highly aroused and demanding. Examples include tragic deaths, such as children drowning or sudden infant death syndrome (SIDS), unexpected marital break-up and breaking bad news.

Aims of crisis intervention

- Resolve the crisis and restore psychological equilibrium as quickly and constructively as possible.
- Encourage the person in crisis to regain control and take appropriate action.

Principles of management

- Intervene early—actively and directly.
- Establish an empathetic alliance.
- Be accessible.
- Attend to family and social supports.
- Be prepared for the difficult phase of 24–48 hours.
- Do not carry the burden of crisis.
- Aim for brief, time-limited intervention (no more than six interviews over 6 weeks).
- When necessary, be prepared to provide short-term use of psychotropic drugs (e.g. a hypnotic), for two or three nights of good sleep.

Ten rules to help those in distress

The following rules are given to those in crisis (personal explanation followed by a take-home hand-out):

1 *Give expression to your emotions.* You need to accept your reactions as normal and not be afraid to cry or call out. Try not to bottle up feelings.
2 *Talk things over with your friends.* Try not to overburden them but seek their advice and listen to them. Do not avoid talking about what has happened.
3 *Focus on things as they are now—at this moment.* Aim not to brood on the past and your misfortune. Concentrate on the future in a positive way.
4 *Consider your problems one at a time.* Try not to allow your mind to race wildly over a wide range of problems. You can cope with one problem at a time.
5 *Act firmly and promptly to solve a problem.* Once you have worked out a way to tackle a problem, go for it. Taking positive action is a step in allowing you to get on with life.
6 *Occupy yourself and your mind as much as possible.* Any social activity—sports, theatre, cards, discussion groups, club activity—is better than sitting around alone. Many people find benefit from a holiday visit to an understanding friend or relative. Religious people usually find their faith and prayer life a great source of strength at this time.
7 *Try not to nurse grudges or blame other people.* This is not easy but you need to avoid getting hostile. In particular, endeavour not to get angry with yourself and your family, especially your spouse.
8 *Set aside some time every day for physical relaxation.* Make a point of doing something physical, such as going for a walk, swimming or enjoying an easy exercise routine.
9 *Stick to your daily routine as much as possible.* At times of crisis a familiar pattern of regular meals and chores can bring a sense of order and security. Avoid taking your problems to bed and thus ensuring sleepless nights. Try to 'switch off' after 8 pm. Taking sleeping tablets for those few bad nights will help.

10 *Consult your family doctor when you need help.* Your doctor will clearly understand your problem because stress and crisis problems are probably the commonest he or she handles. Consult your doctor sooner rather than later.

- Remember that there are many community resources to help you cope (e.g. your religious leader, social workers, community nurses, crisis centres and organisers within churches and other religious centres).
- Take care: do drive carefully and avoid accidents, which are more common at this time.

Bereavement

Bereavement or grief may be defined as deep or intense sorrow or distress following loss.[12] Raphael uses the term to connote 'the emotional response to loss: the complex amalgam of painful affects including sadness, anger, helplessness, guilt, despair'.[13]

The GP will see grief in all its forms over a wide variety of losses. Although the nature of loss and patient reaction to it varies enormously, the principles of management are similar.

Stages of normal bereavement

1 *Shock or disbelief.* Feelings include numbness and emptiness, searching, anxiety, fear and suicidal ideation, 'I don't believe it'. Concentration is difficult and spontaneous emotions, such as crying, screaming or laughing, tend to occur. There may be a sense of the deceased's presence, and hallucinations (visual and auditory) may occur.

2 *Grief and despair.* Feelings include anger, 'Why me?', guilt and self-blame, and yearning. Social withdrawal and memory impairment may occur. The feeling of intense grief usually lasts about 6 weeks and the overall stage of grief and despair for about 6 months, but it can resurface occasionally for a few years. The last few months involve feelings of sadness and helplessness.

3 *Adaptation and acceptance.* Features of the third stage include significant feelings of apathy and depression. This phase takes a year or more. Physical illness is common and includes problems such as insomnia, asthma, bowel dysfunction, headache and appetite disturbances.

Pathological bereavement

Pathological bereavement can occur and may manifest as intense emotion, particularly anger, and multiple visits with somatic complaints; the patient often gets around to long dissertations about the deceased and the circumstances surrounding death. Extreme anger is likely when the sense of rejection is great, as with divorce or sudden death. Guilt can also be intense.[12]

Raphael's classification of the patterns of pathological grief and its various resolutions are presented in TABLE 5.2.[13]

Table 5.2 Patterns and resolution of pathological grief

Morbid or pathological patterns

Absence, inhibition or delay of bereavement
Distorted bereavement
Chronic grief (intense anguish continues unabated)

Outcomes

- Normal resolution, satisfactory adjustment; reintegration in life, satisfying attachments
- General symptomatology (leading to increased care-eliciting behaviour)
- Depression, suicidal behaviour
- Other psychiatric disorders (anxiety state; phobia; mania; alcoholism; criminal activity, such as shoplifting)
- Altered relationship patterns
- Vulnerability to loss
- Anniversary phenomenon
- Death (more likely in the first 12 months)

The GP as counsellor[1]

Important rules to bear in mind:

- The bereaved may be feeling very guilty.
- They may be angry towards their doctor or the medical profession in general.
- They need a clear explanation as to the exact cause and manner of death. Autopsy reports should be obtained and discussed.
- The bereaved tend to view an apparent lack of concern and support as disinterest or guilt.[12]
- Early intervention averts pathological grief.

The GP probably had a close relationship with the deceased and the family. The GP will have a special awareness of those at risk and the nature of the relationships within the family. The family is likely to maintain the relationship with the GP, expressing the physical and psychological effects of grief and consulting about intercurrent problems.[12]

Working through the stages of grief with patients will allow GPs to reach some acceptance of their own emotions, as well as ensure that patients feel supported and cared for, rather than distanced by embarrassment.

Help from religious sources is highly valued as it can meet both spiritual and personal needs. Other resources include funeral directors, hospice (and other) counsellors, and support groups, such as those for SIDS.[12]

At least 30 minutes should be allowed for consultations.

Long-term counselling

Normal bereavement can persist for years. Ongoing counselling is indicated if it continues unabated or psychiatric referral sought if grief is extreme. Regular enquiries during routine consultations or meetings are important if the patient appears to be coping.

Breaking bad news

Good communication skills are fundamental to giving bad news appropriately. When bad news is broken insensitively or inadequately the impact can be distressing for both giver and recipient, leaving lasting scars for the latter. For the doctor it may represent professional failure, fear of people's reaction and feelings of guilt. Doctors should have a plan for this difficult process and learn how to cope with the recipient's reaction. Most of the circumstances described apply to unexpected death or anticipated death.[14]

Sharing bad news with a patient

This difficult task is based on sound communication skills and good dialogue. The meeting should be face to face, not over the phone or internet.

Basic guidelines

- Plan the consultation, review clinical data, set aside ample time.
- Meet in an appropriate room with privacy and no interruption.
- Ask the patient if they would like company (e.g. a relative or friend).
- Make good eye contact and be alert for non-verbal responses.
- Use simple, understandable language; avoid medical jargon, speak clearly and sensitively
- Be honest and diplomatically to the point (don't cover up the issue).
- Allow time, silence, tears or anger.
- Avoid inappropriate methods (refer to 'avoid' in TABLE 5.4) and don't give precise predictions about life expectancy.
- Write down significant points and use sketches or diagrams as appropriate.

Management

Follow the 10 basic steps of the management interview (see CHAPTER 3) with the emphasis on the patient's understanding of the message and his/her feelings about it (see TABLE 5.3). Offer ongoing support and arrangements for continuing involvement including allied health professionals.

Table 5.3 Seven-step protocol for breaking bad news

1. Assess the patient's interest in, and capacity for detailed information.
2. Establish the patient's beliefs about the illness, and what he or she wants to know.
3. Provide accurate information in small doses, checking regularly what has been understood.
4. Monitor how the patient feels about the problem and what has been said.
5. Repeat the messages as the illness progresses, especially after each new step of management and/or deterioration.
6. Involve family members as much as the patient wants.
7. Plan for continued involvement. An assurance of continuing contact between doctor and patient is important.

Source: After Buchanan[15]

Coping with patient responses

- The responses cover a wide range—stunned silence, disbelief, acute distress, anger, extreme guilt.
- Be prepared for any of these responses.
- Appropriate training using simulated patients, video replays and skilled feedback improves communication skills.
- Give permission and encouragement for reactions, such as crying and screaming.
- Have a box of tissues available.
- A comforting hand on the shoulder or arm or holding a hand is an acceptable comfort zone.
- Offer a cup of tea or a cool drink if available.
- Ask the patients or relatives how they feel, what they would like to do and if they want you to contact anyone.
- Arrange follow-up.
- Give appropriate patient education material.
- Provide information about support services.

Children

Remember that there are two 'patients'—child and family. The same 'bad news' principles apply. Talk in age-appropriate terms to the child with the aim of establishing their understanding of their illness and feelings.

Unexpected death

Some basic initial rules:[16]

- If relatives have to be contacted it is preferable for the doctor (if at all possible) or a sympathetic police officer to make the contact personally, rather than a relatively matter-of-fact telephone call from the hospital or elsewhere.
- If a telephone message is necessary, it should be given by an experienced person.
- The relatives or close friends should not drive to the clinic alone.

The setting for the interview:

- Use a suitable quiet private room if possible.
- See the recipients of the news alone in the room.
- Advise that the meeting should be undisturbed.

Guidelines for the doctor

- Be well prepared: check the facts and plan your approach.
- Always ask those involved if they have heard any news or know the reasons for the consultation.
- Always assess their understanding.
- Give information in an unhurried, honest, balanced, empathetic manner.[17]
- Look directly at the person you are talking to, be honest and direct, and keep information simple (avoid technical language).
- The sad news must be accompanied by positive support, understanding and encouragement.
- Give recipients time to react (offer time and moments of silence to allow the facts to sink in) and opportunities to ask questions.
- Avoid false reassurance.
- Remember that relatives appreciate the truth and genuine empathy.
- In the event of death, relatives should be given a clear explanation of the cause of death.

A list of guidelines for the interview is summarised in TABLE 5.4.[16]

Table 5.4 Breaking bad news for unexpected death: recommended actions during the interview

Allow
Time
Opportunities to react
Silence
Touching
Free expression of emotions
Questions
Viewing of a dead or injured body
Avoid
Rushing
Bluntness
Withholding the truth
Platitudes
Protecting own inadequacies
Euphemisms
The notion 'nothing more can be done'
Using medical jargon
Meeting anger with anger
Leaving the patient or loved one without a follow-on contact

Source: After McLauchlan[16]

The depressed patient

Studies have emphasised the importance and therapeutic efficacy of counselling in the management of the depressed patient.[17] The most practical approach by the GP to the depressed patient is empathy, support and a logical explanation of their malaise. The author gives the following explanation to the patient.

> Depression is a very real illness that affects the entire mind and body. It seriously dampens the five basic activities of humans, namely their energy for activity, sex drive, sleep, appetite and ability to cope with life. They cannot seem to lift themselves out of their misery or fight it themselves. Superficial advice to 'snap out of it' is unhelpful because the person has no control over it.
>
> The cause is somewhat mysterious but it has been found that an important chemical is present in smaller amounts than usual in the nervous system. It is rather like a person low in iron becoming anaemic.
>
> Depression can follow a severe loss such as the death of a loved one, a marital separation or financial loss. On the other hand it can develop for no apparent reason although it may follow an illness such as glandular fever or influenza, an operation or childbirth.

Emphasising the 'missing chemical' theory really helps patients and family come to terms with an illness that tends to have socially embarrassing connotations. It also helps compliance with therapy when antidepressant medication is prescribed.

Ongoing contact, support and availability are an important component of counselling with appropriate referral to someone with more expertise, should that be required. CBT is a most effective and important approach to the management of depressive illness.

Chronic pain

5

Patients suffering from long-term pain are a special problem, especially those with back pain who seem to be on a merry-go-round of failed multiple treatments and complex psychosocial problems. These patients are frequently treated in pain clinics. As family doctors we often observe an apparently normal, pleasant person transformed into a person who seems neurotic, pain-driven and doctor-dependent. The problem is very frustrating to the practitioner, often provoking feelings of suspicion, uncertainty and discomfort.

De Vaul and colleagues[18] list five subgroups of patients where perplexing pain presents as the major symptom:

1. pain as a symptom of depression
2. pain as a delusional symptom of psychosis
3. pain as a conversion symptom of hysterical neurosis
4. pain as a symptom of an unresolved bereavement reaction
5. pain as a symptom of a 'need to suffer'

Patients who somatise their symptoms present one of the most difficult challenges to our skills and usually require a multidisciplinary team approach.

Management involves:

- thorough medical assessment
- psychological assessment
- detailed explanations to the patient and family about treatment
- rational explanations about the cause of the pain
- management of associated problems (e.g. depression, sexual dysfunction)
- behavioural modification to encourage increased activity and a gradual return to normality

Problem gambling

Problem or pathological gambling is persistent and recurrent maladaptive gambling behaviour despite its detrimental effect (disruption of personal, family or work life). It is undoubtedly a dependence disorder similar to alcohol and other drugs with a similar approach to management. Refer to DSM-5 criteria for pathological gambling. Prevalence: 0.5–1.5% adult population.

Dangers

- Suicide risk (high)
- Major depression (up to 75%)
- Stress-related problems
- Domestic violence

Key warning

- Gambling >$200 week
- Chasing losses

Other telltale signs

- Spending many hours gambling
- Placing larger, more frequent bets
- Lying about behaviour
- Being secretive
- Promising cutting back, but not doing it
- Impulsive activity
- Mood swings
- Gambling at the expense of other pleasant social activities
- Growing debts
- Excessive drinking

First-line management

- Ask (as part of social history).
- Consider South Oaks Gambling screen to support provisional diagnosis.[19]
- Confront firmly if suspected.
- Consider using the Prochaska and Di Clemente model of change (CHAPTER 21).
- Provide education material.
- Look into the family (domestic violence?) and provide support.
- Advise the family not to provide 'rescue money'.
- There is no recommended pharmacological treatment.

Counselling approach

Problem gambling is a treatable condition and GPs can provide a central role in management. As for smoking and alcohol dependence, a brief intervention and education consultation session about the impact of excessive behaviour can be most effective. CBT is a very effective treatment for gambling. It combines systematic discussion and carefully structured behavioural assignments to help patients modify problematic thinking patterns and behaviours. 'CBT directed towards correcting erroneous perceptions, irrational beliefs and misunderstanding of concepts of randomness and independence of chance events is a fundamental element of any therapeutic approach.'[20]

It is appropriate to use specialist gambling counsellors when one's intervention is not proving effective or where there is evidence of disturbing gambling problems. (Refer www.gamblersanonymous.org.)

If one feels out of one's depth, then immediate referral to an expert is important. CBT is a most appropriate therapy for most conditions.

Summary: counselling skills strategies

- Provide guidance and facilitation to allow the patient to gain insight.
- Use appropriate 'gentle' confrontation to allow self-examination.
- Help patients to explore their own situation and express emotions such as anxiety, guilt, fear, anger, hostility and hurt feelings.
- Explore possible feelings of insecurity and allow free expression of such feelings.
- Ask key searching questions, such as:
  - What do you think deep down is the cause of your problem?
  - How do you think your problem should be treated?
- Provide 'okay' specific suggestions, such as:
  - I wonder if your basic problem is that you are a perfectionist?
  - Many people in your situation feel guilty about something that may even be trivial and need to feel forgiven.

Effective counselling comes from commitment, experience and a genuine caring compassionate feeling for patients and their ethos.

Key rules to counselling

- The patient must leave feeling better.
- Provide *insight* into their illness and/or behaviour.
- Address any feelings of *guilt* (people must feel okay or forgiven about any perceived transgression).

Patient education resources

Hand-out sheets from *Murtagh's Patient Education* 7th edition:

- Depression
- Coping with a crisis
- Bereavement
- Gambling: problem gambling

References

1 Hassed C. Counselling. In: *Final Year Handbook.* Melbourne: Monash University, Department of Community Medicine, 1992: 97–104.
2 Selzer R, Ellen S. *Psych-lite: Psychiatry That's Easy to Read.* Sydney: McGraw Hill, 2010: 70–3.
3 Balint M. *The Doctor, His Patient, and the Illness* (2nd edn). London: Pitman, 1964.
4 Harris RD, Ramsay AT. *Health Care Counselling.* Sydney: Williams & Wilkins, 1988: 68–95.
5 Annon JS. *The Behavioural Treatment of Sexual Problems.* Vols 1 and 2. Honolulu: Enabling Systems Inc, 1974.
6 Craig S. A medical model for infertility counselling. Aust Fam Physician, 1990; 19: 491–500.
7 Cook H. Counselling in general practice: principles and strategies. Aust Fam Physician, 1986; 15: 979–81.
8 Frank JF. Foreword. In: Traux CB, Carkhuff RR. *Toward Effective Counselling and Psychotherapy: Training in Practice.* New York: Aldine, 1967: ix.
9 Traux CB, Carkhuff RR. *Toward Effective Counselling and Psychotherapy.* New York: Aldine, 1967.
10 Expert group for Psychotropic guidelines. Psychotropic. In: eTG complete. Melbourne: Therapeutic Guidelines Ltd. Available from: <www.tg.org.au>, accessed January 2018.
11 Tiller JWG. Cognitive behaviour therapy in medical practice. Australian Prescriber, 2001; 24(2): 33–7.
12 Williams AS. Grief counselling. Aust Fam Physician, 1986; 15: 995–1002.
13 Raphael B. *The Anatomy of Bereavement: A Handbook for the Caring Professions.* London: Hutchinson, 1984: 33–62.
14 Gregg K, Vandekiett MD. Breaking Bad News. Am Fam Physician, 2001; Dec 15: 64(12): 1975–9.
15 Buchanan J. Giving bad news. Medicine Today. October 2001: 84–5.
16 McLauchlan CAJ. Handling distressed relatives and breaking bad news. In: Skinner D. *ABC of Major Trauma.* London: British Medical Association, 1991: 102–6.
17 Cunningham C, Morgan P, McGucken R. Down syndrome: is dissatisfaction with disclosure of diagnosis inevitable? Dev Med Child Neurol, 1984; 26: 33–9.
18 Williams CD. Overcoming depression and low mood: a five areas approach (3rd edn). London: Hodder Education, 2009.
19 De Vaul RA, Zisook S, Stuart HJ. Patients with psychogenic pain. J Fam Pract, 1977; 4(1): 53–5.
20 Lesieur HR, Blume S. The South Oaks Gambling Screen (SOGS): a new instrument for the identification of pathological gamblers. Am J Psychiatry, 1987; 144: 1184–8.
21 Blaszczynski A. How to treat: problem gambling. Australian Doctor, 2005; 12 August: 37–44.

6 Difficult, demanding and angry patients

There are patients in every practice who give the doctor and staff a feeling of 'heartsink' every time they consult.

THOMAS O'DOWD 1988[1]

Weston defines a 'difficult patient' as one with whom the physician has trouble forming an effective working relationship.[2] However, it is more appropriate to refer to difficult problems rather than difficult patients—it is the patients who have the problems while doctors have the difficulties.

The proportion of consultations that are taken up by *difficult patients* (also called *heartsink* or *hateful* patients) has been measured as being 15%.[2] While in the minority, by their nature they can often take up a disproportionate amount of the doctor's time, energy and emotional reserves. One difficult patient may disrupt an entire consulting session. The concept of the difficult patient was first popularised by the landmark paper by Groves in 1978,[3] and many difficult patient types have since been described. Four of the more common and better-known types[4] are as follows:

1. *The dependent clinger*
   Dependent clingers require constant reassurance, and have an unquenchable need for explanation, affection and attention. They may break social or professional barriers to meet this need, such as calling the doctor at home or continually making unplanned presentations at the surgery. The doctor can feel threatened by such patients, and if pushed away, dependent clingers can feel rejected, which may exacerbate their behaviour. They respond well to an empathic approach that needs to be delivered within clearly defined and enforced boundaries.
2. *The entitled demander*
   Entitled demanders attempt to control the doctor through intimidation and by inducing guilt or fear in the doctor. They project an air of superiority and entitlement, and may demand tests or consultation prioritisation, withhold payment and are often litigious. The doctor may understandably feel afraid and despairing in such situations, but this type of difficult patient is often driven by an underlying insecurity and is attempting to obtain control through bluster. The appropriate use of power is clearly required for such patients, but it is important (and often difficult) to stay in control and interact in a respectful and non-confrontational manner. This may include pointing out calmly but clearly when boundaries are being crossed.
3. *The manipulative help rejecter*
   Manipulative help rejecters are patients who are on a self-destructive path but refuse to take important medical advice. They crave the relationship with the doctor and solving or improving the medical situation may threaten that relationship. Substance abuse is a common manifestation of how manipulative help rejecters present and manipulate the relationship, as are non-compliance and chronic pain issues. The doctor can feel frustrated and even demoralised, and it is important to reflect on our own feelings and expectations with such patients.
4. *The self-destructive denier*
   Rather than wanting to cling to the doctor (like the manipulative help rejecter), self-destructive deniers appear to want to damage themselves, their motivation driven by self-loathing. They may induce feelings of indifference or hatred in the doctor because of their destructive behaviour and apparent refusal to change their ways. An empathic approach is the most useful here, but this may be emotionally draining for the doctor.

An inevitably poor consultation will follow if we allow feelings of hostility to affect our communication with the difficult patient, especially the demanding, angry or 'compo' patient.

However, it is important not to misdiagnose organic disease and also to consider the possibilities of various psychological disorders, which may be masked. Hahn and Kroenke identified six diagnoses:[3,5]

- generalised anxiety disorders
- multi-somatoform disorder

- dysthymia
- panic disorder
- major depression
- drug dependency/alcohol abuse

It is therefore appropriate to maintain traditional standards by continually updating the database, integrating psychosocial aspects, carefully evaluating new symptoms, conducting an appropriate physical examination and being discriminating with investigations.

Management of the violent and dangerous patient is presented in CHAPTER 45 on the disturbed patient.

Management strategies

Our professional responsibility is to rise above interpersonal conflict and facilitate productive communication by establishing a caring and responsible relationship with such patients. An appropriate strategy is to follow Professor Aldrich's precepts for the 'difficult' patients who do not have an organic disorder or a psychiatric illness:[6]

1. Give up trying to cure them—they are using their symptoms to maintain their relationship with you: accept them as they are.
2. Accept their symptoms as expressions of their neurosis. Make a primary positive diagnosis—only test if you have to.
3. Structure a program for them, for example, 'Mrs Jones, I have decided that we should meet for 15 minutes every second Wednesday at 10 am.'
4. During the consultation, demonstrate your genuine interest in the person's life, garden, work and so on; show less interest, even boredom, for the litany of complaints.

Other management guidelines include the following.

- Use reassurance with caution—it is insufficient by itself and should be soundly based.
- Be honest and maintain trust.
- Allow the patient a fair share of your time—this is your part of the contract. At the same time indicate that there are limits to your time (set rules).
- Be polite yet assertive.
- Avoid using labels of convenience and placebo therapy.
- Be honest about your understanding (or lack of understanding) of the problems.
- Remember that the consultation is often the therapy, without a prescription.
- Do not undermine other doctors. Avoid collusion.
- Have limited objectives—zealous attempts to cure may be inappropriate.
- Do not abandon the patient, however frustrating the relationship. Accept this as a legitimate role.
- Remain available if alternative therapies are sought by the patient.
- Take extra care with the 'familiar' patient and sometimes the patient who brings gifts. Maintain your professional role.
- If you are uncomfortable with counselling, consider early referral to a counsellor while maintaining contact in the future.
- You may have to accept that there are some people whom no one can help.

Complaints

Complaints from all groups of patients are common and disturbing. The main issues are usually a breakdown in communication or unmet expectations. This is likely to occur when something has gone wrong.

Tips to handle complaints include:[7]

- don't ignore them—deal with them as quickly as possible
- speak directly to the complaining patient, preferably face to face
- refer the complaint to the medical registration board or to your medical insurer for advice if there is a legal claim for negligence
- an appropriate strategy for other complaints is to acknowledge them in writing and follow up with a phone call
- recommend a meeting to discuss concerns
- check all facts surrounding the issue including detailed copies of reports and records of phone calls

An ABCDE of dealing with complaints is presented in TABLE 6.1.

Table 6.1 The ABCDE of dealing with complaints

A	**A**cknowledge the complaint.
B	Set **B**oundaries for the patient.
C	Show **C**ompassion and **C**aring.
D	**D**etermine the reason for the behaviour.
E	**E**scape or **E**xit, if there is an impasse.

A 'heartsink' survival kit

A pilot workshop of managing 'heartsink' patients described by Mathers and Gask[8] led to the formulation

6

of a 'heartsink survival' model for the management of patients with somatic symptoms of emotional distress.

The first part of the three-part model, which is called 'feeling understood', includes a full history of symptoms, exploration of psychosocial cues and health beliefs, and a brief, focused, physical examination. In the second stage, termed 'broadening the agenda', the basic aim is to involve discussion of both emotional and physical aspects during the consultation. It includes reframing the patient's symptoms and complaints to provide insight into the link between physical, psychological and life events.

In the third stage, 'making the link', simple patient education methods are used to explain the causation of somatic symptoms, such as the way in which stress, anxiety or depression can exaggerate symptoms. It also includes projection or identification techniques using other sufferers as examples.

The angry patient

Anger in patients and their relatives is a common reaction in the emotive area of sickness and healing. The anger, which may be concealed or overt, might be a combination of fear and insecurity. It is important to bear in mind that many apparently calm patients may be harbouring controlled anger. The practice of our healing art is highly emotive and can provoke feelings of frustration and anger in our patients, their friends and their relatives.

Anger is a normal and powerful emotion, common to every human being, yet with an enormous variety of expression. The many circumstances in medicine that provoke feelings of anger include:[9]

- disappointment at unmet expectations
- crisis situations, including grief
- any illness, especially an unexpected one
- the development of a fatal illness
- iatrogenic illness
- chronic illness, such as asthma
- financial transactions, such as high cost for services
- referral to colleagues, which is often perceived as failure
- poor service, such as long waits for an appointment
- problems with medical certificates
- poor response to treatment
- inappropriate doctor behaviour (e.g. brusqueness, sarcasm, moralistic comments, aloofness, superiority)

The patient's anger may manifest as a direct confrontation with the doctor or perhaps with the receptionist, with litigation or with public condemnation.

In an extreme example, a Melbourne doctor was shot and killed by an angry patient who had been denied a worker's compensation certificate for a claim considered unjustified.

When a patient expresses anger about the medical profession or our colleagues it may be directed at us personally and, conversely, if directed to us it may be displaced from someone else, such as a spouse, employer or other figure of authority.

What is anger?

Anger is a person's emotional response to provocation or to a threat to his or her equilibrium. If inappropriate, it is almost always the manifestation of a deeper fear and of hidden insecurity. Angry, abusive behaviour may be a veiled expression of frustration, fear, self-rejection or even guilt.

On the other hand, its expression may be a defence against the threat of feeling too close to the doctor, who could have an overfamiliar, patronising or overly friendly attitude towards the patient. Some patients cannot handle this threatening feeling.

Basically, anger may be a communication of fear and insecurity. The patient could be saying, 'I am afraid there is something seriously wrong with me. Are you doing everything to help me?'

Consulting strategies[10]

When one feels attacked unfairly, to react with anger is a natural human response. This response, however, must be avoided since it will damage the doctor–patient relationship and possibly aggravate the problem.

- The initial response should be to remain calm, keep still and establish eye contact.
- 'Step back' from the emotionally charged situation and try to analyse what is happening.
- Ask the patient to sit down and try to adopt a similar position (the mirroring strategy) without any aggressive pose.
- Address the patient (or relative) by the appropriate name, be it Mr or Mrs Jones or a first name.
- Appear calm, comfortable and controlled.
- Be interested and concerned about the patient and the problem.
- Use clear, firm, non-emotive language.
- Listen intently.
- Allow patients to ventilate their feelings and help to relieve their burdens.
- Allow patients to 'be themselves'.
- Give appropriate reassurance (do not go overboard to appease the patient).
- Avoid a judgmental approach

- Allow time (at least 20 minutes).
- For the threatening aggressive patient, sit closest to the door to allow escape should the patient turn violent.

Analysing the responses

- Search for any 'hidden agenda'.
- Recognise the relationship between anger and fear.

Recognising distress signals

It is important to recognise signs of deteriorating emotional distress:[11]

- body language (demonstrative agitated movements or closing in)
- speech (either becoming quiet or more rapid and louder)
- colour (either becoming flushed or pale)
- facial expression (as above, tense, tightening of muscles of eye and mouth, loss of eye contact)
- manner (impatient, threatening)

Skilful consulting strategies should then be employed. It is worthwhile having a contingency plan, such as memorising a telephone number to summon security help.

Questions to uncover the true source of anger

The following represent some typical questions or responses that could be used during the interview.

Rapport building

- 'I can appreciate how you feel.'
- 'It concerns me that you feel so strongly about this.'
- 'Tell me how I can make it easier for you.'

Confrontation

- 'You seem very angry.'
- 'It's unlike you to be like this.'
- 'I get the feeling that you are upset with . . .'
- 'What is it that's upsetting you?'
- 'What really makes you feel this way?'

Facilitation, clarification

- 'I find it puzzling that you are angry with me.'
- 'So you feel that . . .'
- 'You seem to be telling me . . .'
- 'If I understand you correctly . . .'
- 'Tell me more about this . . .'
- 'I would like you to enlarge on this point—it seems important.'

Searching

- 'Do you have any special concerns about your health?'
- 'Tell me about things at home.'
- 'How are things at work?'
- 'How are you sleeping?'
- 'Do you have any special dreams?'
- 'Do you relate to anyone who has a problem like yours?'
- 'If there's any one thing in your life that you would like to change, what would it be?'

Some important guidelines are summarised in TABLE 6.2.

Table 6.2 Guidelines for handling the angry patient

Do	Don't
Listen	Touch the patient
Be calm	Meet anger with anger
Be comfortable	Reject the patient
Show interest and concern	Be a 'wimp'
Be conciliatory	Evade the situation
Be genuine	Be overfamiliar
Allay any guilt	Talk too much
Be sincere	Be judgmental
Give time	Be patronising
Arrange follow-up	Be drawn into action
Act as a catalyst and guide	

The drug-dependent doctor shopper[12]

Nicholas Carr's five-step approach:

1. Elicit request for drug early:
   'In what way did you think I could help?'
   'What sort of thing did you have in mind?'
2. Respectful refusal and brief minimal explanation:
   'I don't prescribe Valium (or requested drug).'
   'Yes, I could but I choose not to.'
3. Avoid being drawn into the patient's agenda:
   'I understand this doesn't suit you, but I don't prescribe these drugs.'
4. Depersonalise:
   'It's nothing to do with you personally—this is the way I work.'
5. Offer alternative help:
   'I'm happy to talk about other ways of helping, but they don't involve a prescription.'

Management

When confronted with an angry patient, the practitioner should be prepared to remain calm, interested and concerned. It is important to listen intently and allow time for the patient to ventilate his or her feelings.

A skilful consultation should provide both doctor and patient with insight into the cause of the anger and result in a contract in which both parties agree to work in a therapeutic relationship. The objective should be to come to amicable terms which, of course, may not be possible, depending on the nature of the patient's grievance.

If the problem cannot be resolved in the time available a further appointment should be made to continue the interview.

Sometimes it may be appropriate to advise the patient to seek another opinion. If the angry patient does have problems with relationships and seeks help, it would be appropriate to arrange counselling so that the patient acquires a more realistic self-image, thus leading to improved self-esteem and effectiveness in dealing with people. In addition, it should lead to the ability to withstand frustration and cope with the many vicissitudes of life—a most rewarding outcome for a consultation that began with confrontation.

References

1 O'Dowd TC. Five years of 'heartsink' patients in general practice. BMJ, 1988; 297: 528–30.
2 McWhinney I. *A Textbook of Family Medicine.* New York: Oxford, 1989: 96–8.
3 Groves JE. Taking care of the hateful patient. N Engl J Med, 1978; 298: 883–7.
4 Strous R, Ulman A, Kotler M. The hateful patient revisited: relevance for 21st century medicine. Eur J Int Med, 2006; 17: 387–93.
5 Hahn SR, Kroenke K et al. The difficult patient. J Gen Intern Med, 1996; Jan 1, 11 (1): 1–8.
6 Elliott CE. 'How am I doing?' Med J Aust, 1979; 2: 644–5.
7 Avant handbook. Handling professional complaints against doctors. Sydney, Avant Advocacy 2015.
8 Mathers NJ, Gask L. Surviving the 'heartsink' experience. Fam Pract, 1995; 12: 176–83.
9 Murtagh JE. The angry patient. Aust Fam Physician, 1991; 20: 388–9.
10 Mongtomery B, Morris L. *Surviving: Coping with a Crisis.* Melbourne: Lothian, 1989: 179–86.
11 Lloyd M, Bor R. *Communication Skills for Medicine.* London: Churchill Livingstone, 1996: 135–7.
12 Carr N. I just want some Valium, doc. Monash University update course. November 2013.

Health promotion and patient education

7

Never believe what a patient tells you his doctor said.

SIR WILLIAM JENNER (1815–98)

Health promotion[1]

Health promotion is the motivation and encouragement of individuals and the community to see good health as a desirable state that should be maintained by the adoption of healthy practices. It is also the process of helping people to increase control over and improve their health (WHO definition 2009).

For those who feel healthy, the message may have little meaning, but it is reinforced by contact with others who become ill, particularly within the family.

The Lalonde report[1] highlighted the notion that all causes of death and disease had four contributing elements:

- inadequacies of the existing health care system
- environmental hazards
- behavioural factors and unhealthy lifestyles
- human biological factors

Health education

Health education is the provision of information about how to maintain or attain good health.

There are many methods, including the advertising of health practices, the provision of written information (e.g. about diet and exercise, immunisation, accident prevention and the symptoms of disease), and information about methods to avoid disease (e.g. sexually transmitted infection).

Illness education

A lot of so-called 'health' education is, in reality, information about the cause of particular illnesses. Clearly, the medical practitioner is in a pre-eminent position to provide his or her patients with specific information about the cause of an illness at the time, either individually or to the family. This educative strategy has a preventive objective that is often the modification of help-seeking behaviour.

Every consultation is an opportunity to provide information about the condition under care and this can be reinforced in written, diagrammatic or printed form. Patients' own X-rays can be similarly used to illustrate the nature of the problem.

Health promotion in general practice

GPs are ideally placed to undertake health promotion and prevention, mainly due to opportunity.

There are several reasons for this health promotion role:

- Population access: over 80% of the population visits a GP at least once a year.[2]
- On average, people visit a GP about five times each year.
- GPs have a knowledge of the patient's personal and family health history.
- The GP can act as leader or coordinator of preventive health services in his or her local area.
- The GP can participate in community education programs.
- GPs should undertake opportunistic health promotion—the ordinary consultation can be used not just to treat the presenting problem, but also to manage ongoing problems, coordinate care with other health professionals, check whether health services are being used appropriately and undertake preventive health activities.[2]

Opportunistic health promotion

The classic model by Stott and Davis (see TABLE 3.1 in CHAPTER 3) highlights the opportunities for health promotion in each consultation.[3] Since the consultation is patient-initiated, it is the doctor who needs to be the initiator of preventive health care. The potential in the consultation involves reactive and proactive behaviour by the doctor (see FIG. 7.1).[4]

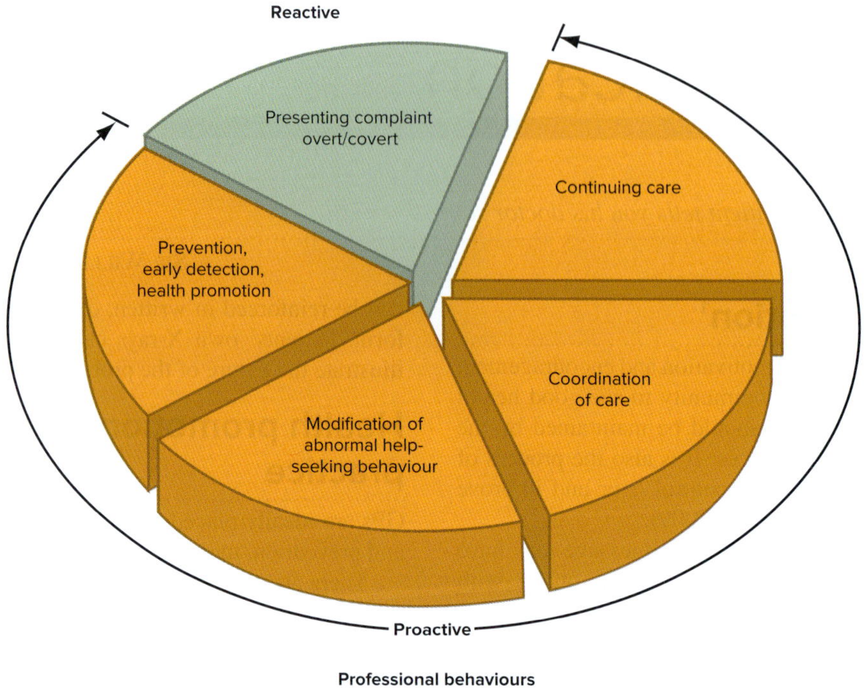

7

FIGURE 7.1 The potential in every general practice consultation
Source: Reproduced with permission from M Sales[4]

Reactive professional behaviour deals only with the presenting complaint. It may be performed with skill but if the practitioner is only trained to perform reactively then the opportunity for preventive and promotive health care will be lost.

Proactive behaviour is defined as professional behaviour that is necessary for the patient's well-being, but it is performed not merely as a response to the presenting problem and it is initiated by the doctor.[4] It includes health promotion, preventive care and screening and the early detection of disease, before it becomes symptomatic. Other aspects of proactive care are seen in FIGURE 7.1.

Proactive behaviour also includes:[4]

- continuing care of a previously treated problem (e.g. rechecking blood pressure, checking diabetic control, follow-up bereavement counselling)
- coordination of care by organising referral to appropriate agencies or specialists and maintaining adequate medical records
- the modification of abnormal or inappropriate help-seeking behaviour (e.g. the person who never attends is at risk from 'silent disease'; the too-frequent attender wastes resources and serious illness may be overlooked)

This mix of reactive and proactive behaviour is not appropriate in every consultation. It requires counselling skills and training in the delivery of quality general practice.

Methods

- Being informed and updated by maintaining continuing medical education, especially in preventive roles.
- Using health promotional material for patient education:
  - — handouts
  - — waiting room posters
  - — waiting room video systems
- Having an efficient medical record system.
- Operating a patient register and recall system.
- Encouraging regular health checks for at-risk groups.
- Providing regular advice on:
  - — nutrition
  - — exercise
  - — stress management
  - — weight control
- Providing personal health records to the parents of newborn babies.

Health goals and targets

Health goals and targets as determined by the Health Targets and Implementation Committee[5] were set in three areas—population groups, major causes of illness and death, and risk factors (see TABLE 7.1).

Table 7.1 Health promotion areas in which goals and targets have been set

Population groups
The socioeconomically disadvantaged, Indigenous Australians, refugees, migrants, women, men, older people, children and adolescents
Major causes of illness and death
Heart disease and stroke, cancers (including lung, breast, cervical and skin cancer), injury, communicable diseases, musculoskeletal disease, diabetes, disability, dental disease, mental illness, asthma
Risk factors
Drugs (including tobacco smoking, alcohol misuse, pharmaceutical misuse or abuse, illicit drugs and substance abuse), nutrition, physical inactivity, high blood pressure, high blood cholesterol, occupational health hazards, unprotected sexual activity, environmental health hazards

Source: Health Targets and Implementation Committee[5]

The seven priority health areas for Australians are:[5]

- asthma
- cancer control
- cardiovascular health
- obesity control
- diabetes mellitus
- injury prevention and control
- mental health

Promoting healthy lifestyle in general practice

GPs can provide a simple framework to encourage patients to adopt a healthy lifestyle whether they have a particular disorder or not. The acronyms act as a good aide-mémoire for practitioners for opportunistic health promotion.

The SNAP guide[6]

The SNAP guide was developed by the Royal Australian College of General Practitioners to address important risk factors with patients with a view to encouraging change if appropriate. The guide comes as a comprehensive booklet and includes the 'Estimation of absolute 5-year risk of cardiovascular events' tables.

The SNAP guide can be summarised by the following risk factors.

S = **S**moking
N = **N**utrition
A = **A**lcohol
P = **P**hysical activity

The guide emphasises that there are *health inequalities* in the community because the risk factors are far more prevalent in people from low-socioeconomic-status backgrounds and Indigenous Australians.

The guide focuses on the '5 As' as stages of change theory to promote change on lifestyle where appropriate (see TABLE 7.2).

Table 7.2 The '5 As'

1	**Ask**	Identify patients with risk factors
2	**Assess**	Level of risk factor and its relevance to the individual in terms of health Readiness to change/motivation
3	**Advise**	Provide written information Provide a lifestyle prescription
4	**Assist**	Pharmacotherapies Support for self-monitoring
5	**Arrange**	Referral to special services Social support groups Phone information/counselling services Follow-up with the GP

This information can be accessed at http://www.racgp.org.au/guidelines/snap.

The NEAT guide

The NEAT guide (see TABLE 7.3) is similar to the SNAP guide, but with a greater emphasis on counselling the patient about lifestyle and the importance of stress management.

Psychosocial health promotion

There is a tendency for health goals and targets to focus mainly on physical illness and not emphasise mental health. However, this area represents an enormous

Table 7.3 The NEAT guide

N = **N**utrition: optimal diet
E = **E**xercise/physical activity
A = **A**voidance or moderation of potential harmful substances (CATS):
- caffeine
- alcohol
- tobacco
- sugar, salt and social drugs

T = **T**ranquillity and promotion of recreation, relaxation techniques, meditation

opportunity for anticipatory guidance. It includes the important problems of stress and anxiety, chronic pain, depression, crisis and bereavement, sexual problems, adolescent problems, bullying, domestic abuse, child behavioural problems, psychotic disorders and several other psychosocial problems.

Time spent in counselling, giving advice and stressing ways of coping with potential problems such as suicide and deterioration in relationships is rewarding. GPs need to pay more attention to promoting health in this area, which at times can be quite complex.

Patient education/hand-outs

Evidence has shown that intervention by GPs can have a significant effect on patients' attitudes to a change to a healthier lifestyle. If we are to have an impact on improving the health of the community, we must encourage our patients to take responsibility for their own health and thus change to a healthier lifestyle. They must be supported, however, by a caring doctor who follows the same guidelines and maintains a continuing interest. Examples include modifying diet, cessation of smoking, reduction of alcohol intake and undertaking exercise.

In an American survey of 360 patients, 90% reported wanting a pamphlet at some or all of their office visits. Overall, 67% reported reading or looking through and saving pamphlets received, 30% read or looked through them and then threw them away, and only 2% threw them away without review. Only 11% of males and 26% of females reported ever asking a doctor for pamphlets. More patients desired pamphlets than received them.[7]

Patient education materials have been shown to have a beneficial effect. Giving patients a hand-out about tetanus increased the rate of immunisation against tetanus among adults threefold.[8] An education booklet on back pain for patients reduced the number of consultations made by patients over the following year and 84% said that they found it useful.[9] Providing systematic patient education on cough significantly changed the behaviour of patients to follow practice guidelines and did not result in patients delaying consultation when they had a cough lasting longer than 3 weeks or one with 'serious' symptoms.[10]

One form of patient education is giving hand-outs (either prepared or printed from a computer at the time of the consultation) to the patient as an adjunct to the verbal explanation which, it must be emphasised, is more important than the printed hand-out.

The patient education leaflets should be in non-technical language and focus on the key points of the illness or problem. The objectives are to improve the quality of care, reduce costs and encourage a greater input by patients in the management of their own illness. In modern society where informed consent and better education about health and disease is expected, this information is very helpful from a medicolegal viewpoint.

The author has produced a book called *Patient Education,* which has a one-page summary of each of 345 common medical conditions.[11] The concept is to photocopy the relevant problem or preventive advice and hand it to the patient or relative. Over the years the greatest demand (following a survey of requests for prints of the sheets) has been for the following (in order):

- exercises for your lower back (see FIG. 7.2)
- backache
- exercises for your neck
- your painful neck
- exercises for your knee
- breastfeeding and milk supply
- how to lower cholesterol
- breast self-examination
- testicular self-examination
- vaginal thrush
- menopause
- anxiety
- coping with stress
- depression
- bereavement

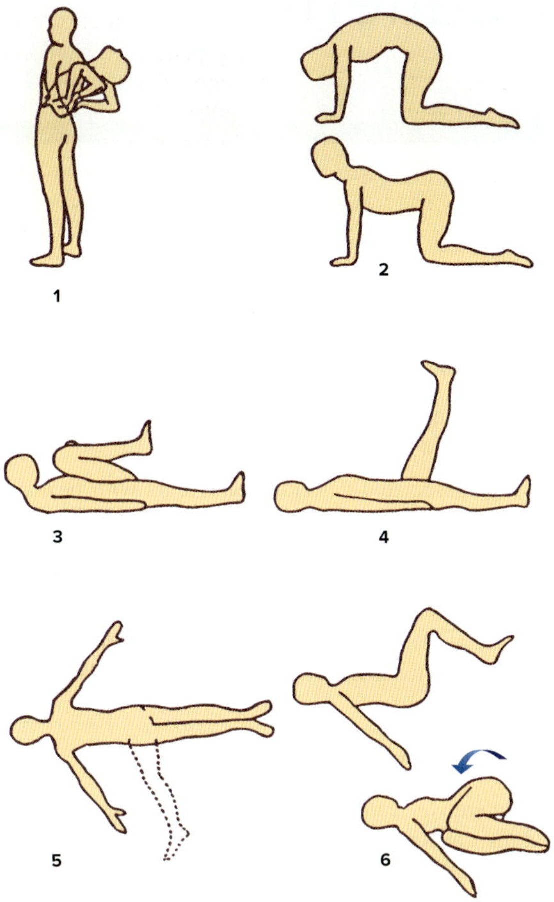

FIGURE 7.2 Patient education leaflet (diagrammatic part only): exercises for your lower back

Summary

Recommended target areas for health promotion in general practice include:

- nutrition
- weight control
- substance abuse and control
  - smoking
  - alcohol
  - other drugs
- exercise practices
- appropriate sleep, rest and recreation
- safe sexual practices
- promotion of self-esteem and personal growth
- stress management

Important health promotion recommendations are to encourage patients to:[12,13]

- cease smoking
- reduce alcohol intake to safe levels (for healthy men and women, no more than two standard drinks per day and no more than four standard drinks on any single occasion; young people under 15 years should avoid drinking and young people aged 15–17 years should delay drinking for as long as possible; when pregnant or breastfeeding, no alcohol is the safest option)
- limit caffeine intake to three drinks per day
- increase regular physical activity (at least 30 minutes per day for 3 days per week, sufficient to produce a sweat)
- reduce fasting plasma cholesterol to 4.0 mmol/L or less
- have a diastolic BP of less than 85 mmHg
- have a BMI of between 20 and 25 (see CHAPTER 9)
- reduce fat, refined sugar and salt intake in all food
- increase dietary fibre to 30 g/day
- build up a circle of friends who offer emotional support
- express their feelings rather than suppress them
- discuss their problems regularly with another person
- work continuously to improve their relationships with people
- not drive a car when angry, upset or after drinking
- follow cervical cancer screening guidelines
- practise safe sex
- have an HIV antibody check before entering a relationship

References

1 Lalonde, M. A *New Perspective for Health of Canadians. A Working Document.* Ottawa: Government of Canada, 1974.
2 National Health Strategy. *The Future of General Practice.* Issues paper No. 3. Canberra: AGPS, 1992: 54–169.
3 Stott N, Davis R. The exceptional potential in each primary care consultation. J R Coll Gen Pract, 1979; 29: 201–5.
4 Sales M. Health promotion and prevention. Aust Fam Physician, 1989; 18: 18–21.
5 Health Targets and Implementation (Health for All) Committee. *Health for All Australians.* Canberra: AGPS, 1988.
6 Harris M. *SNAP. A Population Guide to Behavioural Risk Factors in General Practice.* South Melbourne: RACGP, 2004.
7 Shank JC, Murphy M, Schulte-Mowry L. Patient preferences regarding educational pamphlets in the family practice center. Fam Med, 1991; 23(6): 429–32.
8 Cates CJ. A handout about tetanus immunisation: influence on immunisation rate in general practice. BMJ, 1990; 300(6727): 789–90.
9 Roland M, Dixon M. Randomised controlled trial of an educational booklet for patients presenting with back pain in general practice. J R Coll Gen Pract, 1989; 39(323): 244–6.
10 Rutten G, Van Eijk J, Beek M, Van der Velden H. Patient education about cough: effect on the consulting behaviour of general practice patients. Br J Gen Pract, 1991; 41(348): 289–92.
11 Murtagh J. *Patient Education* (7th edn). Sydney: McGraw-Hill, 2017.
12 Fisher E. The botch of Egypt: prevention better than cure. Aust Fam Physician, 1987; 16: 187.
13 Howland JS, Baker MG, Poe T. Does patient education cause side effects? A controlled trial. J Fam Pract, 1990; 31(1): 62–4.

8 The elderly patient

Last scene of all,
That ends this strange eventful history,
Is second childishness, and mere oblivion,
Sans teeth, sans eyes, sans taste, sans everything

WILLIAM SHAKESPEARE (1564–1616), *AS YOU LIKE IT*

The ageing (over 65 years) are the fastest growing section of the Australian population. The number of 'old-old' (over 85 years) is increasing at an even faster rate.[1] Life expectancy has risen to 84.4 years for women and 80.3 for men.[2]

The over-65s in 2014 made up 15% of the Australian population. It is expected that this group will make up at least 20% of the population in 2031. A similar trend is expected in the US with 18% in 2040.[2]

The over-65s use twice the number of health services per head of population. They account for 25% of all hospital costs and 75% of all nursing home costs. They represent 29.6% of all general practice consultations.[3] Many are affected by multisystem disease. All are affected to a greater or lesser extent by the normal physiological changes of organ ageing.

Ageing is characterised by the following:[1]

- decrease in metabolic mass
- reduction in the functional capacity of organs
- reduced capacity to adapt to stress
- increased vulnerability to disease
- increased probability of death

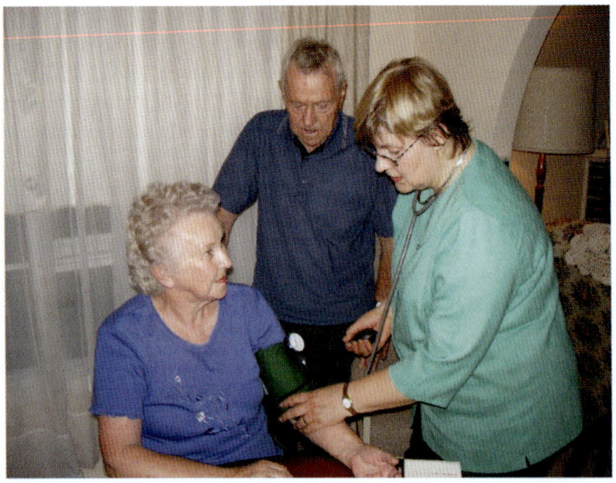

FIGURE 8.1 Establishing rapport and support through the home visit to the elderly patient is an important security gesture

Age-associated deterioration occurs with hearing, vision, glucose tolerance, systolic blood pressure, kidney function, pulmonary function, immune function, bone density, cognitive function, mastication and bladder function.

One of the main contributing factors is the problem of disuse. Encourage exercise, especially walking and water aerobics.

Ageing and disease

Degenerative cardiovascular disease emerges with ageing according to the following approximate guidelines:

Age	
40	Obesity
50	Diabetes
55	Ischaemic heart disease
65	Myocardial infarction
70	Cardiac arrhythmias
75	Heart failure
80	Cerebrovascular accidents

Deterioration in health and the 'masquerades'

Unexpected illness, including mental confusion (one of the major hallmarks of disease in the elderly), can be caused commonly by any of the so-called masquerades outlined in CHAPTER 17:

- depression
- drugs, including alcohol, anticholinergics
- diabetes mellitus
- anaemia
- thyroid disease
- urinary tract infection

- neurological dilemmas
  - Parkinson disease
  - cerebrovascular accident
- infections (e.g. bronchopneumonia)
- neoplasia
- giant cell arteritis/polymyalgia rheumatica

Common significant management disorders encountered in the elderly include:

- hypertension
- ischaemic heart disease and heart failure
- depression
- diabetes (type 2)
- dementia
- social and physical isolation
- osteoarthritis
- disorders of the prostate
- urinary incontinence
- locomotive (lower limb) disorders
  - neurological
  - peripheral neuropathy
  - ataxia
  - claudication due to vascular insufficiency
  - other peripheral vascular disease
  - claudication due to spinal canal stenosis
  - sciatica/nerve root paresis
  - osteoarthritis: hips, knees, feet
  - foot disorders (e.g. ingrown toenails)
  - leg ulceration
  - sarcopenia (loss of muscle mass)

Important problems affecting the elderly are presented in FIGURE 8.2.

The 'classic' triad[4]

Be mindful of the classic triad:

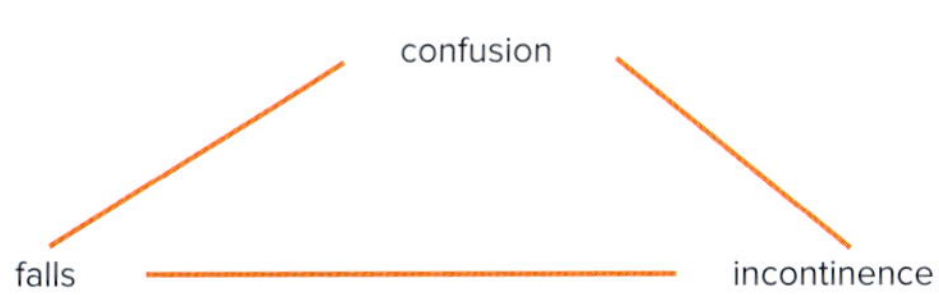

This can represent non-specific signs of acute illness, particularly infection. Aggressive antibiotic treatment is worth considering while awaiting the results of culture or clinical developments.

Changes in sensory thresholds and homeostasis

A clinically significant feature in some elderly patients is the raising of the pain threshold and changes in homeostatic mechanisms, such as temperature control. Consequently, these patients may have an abnormal response to diseases such as appendicitis, pyelonephritis, internal abscess, pneumonia and septicaemia. There may be no complaints of pain and no significant fever but simply general malaise and abnormal behaviour, such as delirium, agitation and restlessness.

Establishing rapport with the elderly patient

The elderly patient especially requires considerable support, understanding, caring and attention from a GP who can instil confidence and security in a patient who is likely to be lonely, insecure and fragile. This means taking time, showing a genuine interest and a modicum of humour, and always leaving detailed instructions.

One of the best ways to generate a good relationship is through home visits. The value of home visits can be considered under the precepts of the Royal Australian College of General Practitioners.[5]

1. Assessment, both initial and continuing: 'You don't know your patient until you've visited their home'.
2. Continuing care:
   - security to the patient
   - support for 'caring' family
   - effective monitoring/intervention role
   - effective liaison with patient/family
   - checking medication

Home visits can be considered in three categories:

1 an 'unexpected' visit (especially to a new patient)
2 a patient-initiated but routine request for a 'check-up and tablets'
3 the regular call—usually 2 to 4 weeks

These home visits are a 'security gesture' to the patient—evidence that they are supported in their desire to remain independent for as long as possible in their own home (FIG. 8.1). They strengthen the patient–doctor relationship as a position of trust, which is of special importance to frail, elderly people feeling increasingly insecure and threatened.

If the patient is being supported by a spouse or relative, the doctor can provide continuous reassurance and support to all concerned as well as their continual assessment, both physical and mental. Finally, the home visit may become part of the terminal care of a dying patient, something that is very important to the elderly patient. Home visits can enhance the quality of life, both physical and mental, of an ageing person.

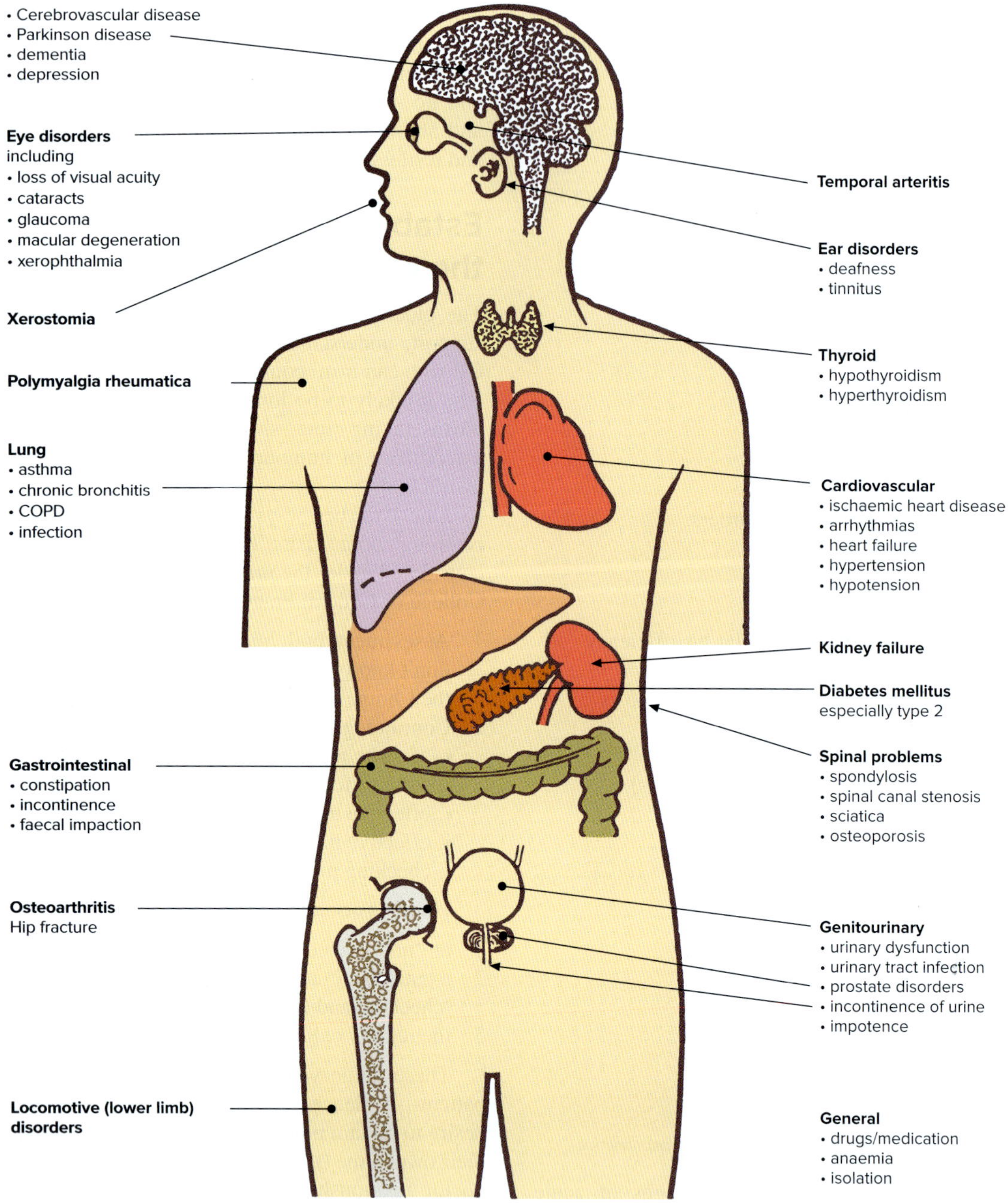

FIGURE 8.2 Significant problems affecting the elderly

8

Loneliness in the elderly

Forbes points out that at least one in three elderly people feel lonely.[6] It is more likely to affect the 'old-old', widows and widowers, and those affected by disability. They may tend to stay indoors, troubled by depression, agoraphobia, social phobia, sensory impairment or incontinence of urine or faeces.

Possible signs of loneliness include:

- verbal outpouring
- drab clothing
- dependence on television
- body language with a 'defeated' demeanour
- prolongation of visit including holding on to one's hand

Doctor behaviour that can irritate and confuse elderly patients

Ellard[7] has written a most interesting paper, based on a compendium of complaints by the elderly about their doctors, on behaviour that upsets the elderly:

- having a consulting room with slippery steps, poor lighting and inadequate handrails
- keeping them waiting
- having low soft chairs in the waiting room and surgery
- being overfamiliar, with addresses such as 'Pop' or first names for elderly females
- shouting at them on the assumption that they are deaf
- appearing rushed and keen to get the consultation over quickly
- forgetting their psychosocial problems and concentrating only on their physical problems (i.e. not treating the whole person)
- forgetting that they have several things wrong with them and using a different priority list from theirs
- failing to ask patients to give their understanding of what is wrong
- omitting to give printed patient education handouts about their problems and medications
- omitting to explain how the medication will work
- treating them as though they would have little comprehension of their health and treatment
- failing to respect their privacy, such as not knocking before entering the examination room
- failing to provide appropriate advice on various social services such as meals on wheels and other support groups
- failing to re-evaluate carefully their health and medication
- failing to take steps to reverse any deterioration in their health, including reluctance to refer

Assessment of the elderly patient

The initial consultation should include a thorough clinical examination on the traditional lines of history, physical examination and selective laboratory investigation. At regular intervals during continuing care this careful assessment may need to be repeated.

> **A golden rule**
>
> You don't know your patient until you've visited them at home.

History

The medical history may be difficult to obtain and the help of a family member is recommended. The use of questionnaires, which can be completed at leisure at home with the help of family members, is most helpful as complementary to the medical interview.

Important specific areas to focus on are:

- previous medical history and hospitalisation
- immunisation status
- medications, prescription and OTC drugs
- alcohol intake, smoking
- problem list of complaints
- dependence on others
- members of household
- household problems
- comforts: heating, cooling, bedding, etc.
- ambulation/mobility/use of frame or stick
- meals: diet
- hygiene: bathing
- toileting: continence
- teeth: condition, ?dentures
- vision
- hearing (always ask about this)
- systems review, especially:
  - genitourinary function
  - gastrointestinal
  - cardiorespiratory
- locomotion, including feet
- nervous system, ?falls, giddiness, loss of balance, faints
- emotional and mental health
- evidence of depression
- history of bereavement
- history of abuse by carers, family members
- financial/insurance status

A thorough family history and psychosocial history is of prime importance. At all times concentrate on a general assessment of the patients' ability to communicate by evaluating mental status, comprehension, hearing, vision, mood and speech.

Physical examination

The routine for the physical examination is similar to that of the younger adult but certain areas require more attention. The elderly patient expects to be examined adequately (especially having blood pressure measured) but requires appropriate dignity. It is recommended that the practice nurse supervises dressing and undressing and prepares the patient for examination.

Practice nurse

- Prepares for examination
- Helps with questionnaire
- Records weight and height
- Takes temperature, pulse and respiration
- Checks audiometry (if hearing problem)
- Checks ocular tension (if appropriate)
- Prepares cervical smear tray for female patient (if relevant)

Doctor

The following areas should be examined:

- general appearance, including skin, hair and face (evaluate nutritional status)
- mental state examination (see FIG. 8.3)
- eyes: visual acuity
- ears: simple hearing test; auroscopic examination
- oral cavity, including teeth and gums
- neck especially thyroid
- lungs: consider peak flow meter
- pulse and blood pressure (repeat)
- heart; breasts
- abdomen; hernial orifices
- spine
- lower limbs: joints; circulation; feet including nails
- gait
- men: rectal examination; scrotum and testes
- women: cervical smear if appropriate

8

'Rules of 7' for assessment of the non-coping elderly patient

If your elderly patient presents with non-specific symptoms, unexpected deterioration in health and/or an inability to cope with the activities of daily living, consider the checklist precented in TABLE 8.1 in your assessment. Apart from confusion, other non-specific symptoms include drowsiness, poor concentration, apathy, fatigue/weakness/tiredness/lethargy, anorexia, nausea, weight loss, dyspnoea, immobility, 'stuck in bed or chair', stumbles or falls. It is also important to consider infections including pneumonia and the masquerades (see CHAPTER 17). Dementia symptoms should be investigated as soon as possible.

Table 8.1 The 'rules of 7'

1	**Mental state**	?	Confusion/dementia Depression Bereavement, incl. pets Elderly abuse/bullying
2	**Eyes**	?	Visual acuity Cataracts/glaucoma
3	**Ears**	?	Deafness, e.g. wax Tinnitus
4	**Mouth**	?	Dentition Xerostomia Malnutrition
5	**Medication**	?	Polypharmacy Adverse reactions
6	**Bladder and bowels**	?	Incontinence Retention Urinary infection
7	**Locomotion**	?	Gait—antalgic; movement disorder, esp. Parkinson disease Arthritis—hips/knees Back/sciatica Feet—nails; neuropathy Circulation Leg ulcers

The mini-mental state examination

Evidence of memory difficulty remains the best single indicator of dementia and should always be evaluated by formal memory testing. However, memory problems may be due to factors other than dementia, and demonstrating failure in other areas of cognitive functioning (language, spatial ability, reasoning) is necessary to confirm the diagnosis of dementia.[8] A number of screening tests are available but the mini-mental state examination (MMSE), particularly the Folstein MMSE depicted in FIGURE 8.3, is commonly used and is the recommended test to use.

Another, somewhat simpler test is the 'Quick 10-step cognitive impairment test' (see TABLE 8.2).[9,10]

The clock-face drawing test

This relatively simple test provides a ready qualitative screening test to differentiate normal elderly from patients with cognitive impairment, particularly dementia.[11]

Mini mental state examination		
ASK the patient	INSTRUCTIONS for assessor	Score
Orientation		
What is the year, month, day and date? What is the season?	Ask specifically for omitted details, e.g. month, year. Score one point for each correct answer.	/5
Can you tell me where we are now?	Expect street no., road name, suburb, city, state. Ask in turn for each place (if necessary). Score one point for each correct answer.	/5
Registration		
'I am going to test your memory—I want you to repeat these three items after me, and hold them in your mind for when I ask you later.'	Name three unrelated objects (e.g. orange, camel, table) speaking clearly and slowly; repeat up to five times or until all three are learned, and ask to recall after each time. Only score after first attempt – 1 point for each correct answer.	/3
Attention and calculation		
'Beginning at 100, count backwards by 7' or, if patient is unable to perform this task, ask: 'Spell the word "WORLD" backwards'.	Stop after five answers—93, 86, 79, 72, 65; each correct answer scores one. Score equals number of letters before first mistake.	/5
Recall		
'What are the three words I asked you before?'	Score one point for each correct answer.	/3
Language		
'What is the name of this object?'	Show two objects. Point to a watch, and then a pen.	/2
'Please repeat this sentence "NO IFS, ANDS, OR BUTS".'		/1
Giving the patient a blank piece of paper, say: 'Take this paper in your right hand, fold it in half, and put it in your lap.'	Score one point for each step.	/3
Praxis (three tasks)		
On a blank piece of paper write 'CLOSE YOUR EYES' 1 Ask the patient 'Read and obey this task.'	Score only if patient closes eyes.	/1
2 'Write a sentence'	Sentence must be sensible and contain a verb and subject (noun).	/1
3 'Copy this design' 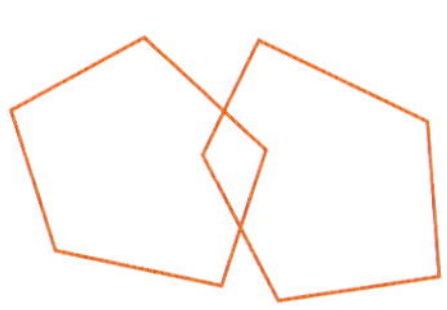	All 10 angles must be present with two intersecting (ignore tremor, scale and rotation).	/1
		/30
Scoring guide only: 19–23 (probable mild dementia); 10–18 (probable moderate impairment); <10 (severe impairment). A decline in score of greater than two points over 1 year may be significant. *Note:* These scores are used as a baseline to determine the criteria for prescribing anti-dementia drugs		Max score

FIGURE 8.3 A practical adaptation of the mini-mental state examination

Source: Adapted from MF Folstein, SE Folstein and PR McHugh. Mini-mental state. J Psych Res, 1975; 12: 189

Table 8.2 The quick 10-step cognitive impairment test

Scoring: questions 1 to 8: correct—0, incorrect—2; questions 9 and 10: correct—0, 1 error—2, >1 error—4

1	When were you born?
2	What year is it?
3	What month is it?
4	What is the date today?
Remember the following address: *25 Main Street, Newcastle*	
5	What is your telephone number? (or if no telephone) What is your street address?
6	What time is it (to nearest hour)?
7	Who is the Prime Minister of Australia?
8	What year did World War II end?
9	Count backwards from 20 to 1.
10	Repeat the memory test I gave you.

Evaluation: 0–8 not significant
9–12 probably significant
13–24 significant

Source: Adapted from Hodkinson[9] and Kingshill[10]

Method

- Give the patient a blank, A4-sized piece of paper.
- Ask the patient to draw the face of a round clock and put the numbers in their correct positions on the face of the clock to represent the hours (see FIG. 8.4).
- Ask the patient to draw in the hands of the clock, indicating 10 minutes after 11 (or some other suitable time) (see FIG. 8.4).
- Repeat the instructions if the patient does not understand them.

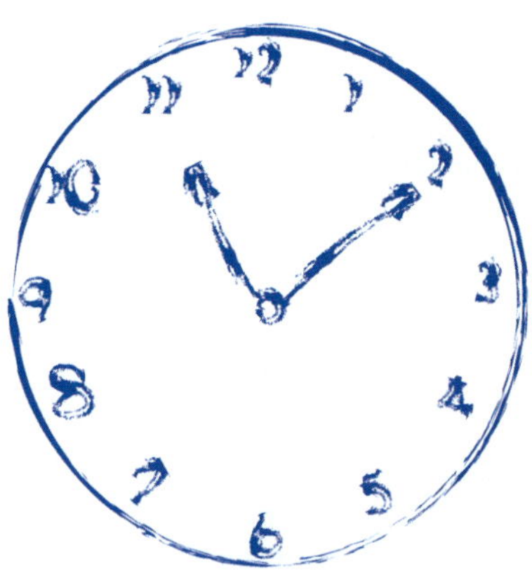

FIGURE 8.4 The clock-face drawing test

Scoring system

- A closed circle is drawn—3 points
- Numbers are in the correct position—2 points
- All correct numbers are included—2 points
- Clock hands are placed in the correct position—2 points

The maximum score is 9. A low score indicates the need for further evaluation and does not establish the criteria for dementia, being a pointer only.

Laboratory investigations

The laboratory tests should be selected according to the evaluation of the patient and to costs versus potential benefits.

Recommended investigations for suspected dementia include:[8,12]

- kidney function
- hepatic function
- thyroid function
- full blood screen
- blood glucose
- serum electrolytes (especially if on diuretics)
- serum calcium and phosphate
- urinalysis
- serum vitamin B12 and folate
- serum vitamin D
- syphilis serology (consider HIV)
- chest X-ray
- neuroimaging: computed tomography (CT), especially non-contrast CT, or magnetic resonance imaging (MRI) (preferably)
- positron emission tomography (PET) scan or single photo emission computed tomography (SPECT) scan—for further information

Behavioural changes in the elderly

As GPs, we are often called to assess abnormal behaviour in the elderly patient, with the question being asked, 'Is it dementia?' or 'Is it Alzheimer's, doctor?'.

There are many other causes of behavioural changes in people over the age of 65 years and dementia must be regarded as a diagnosis of exclusion. The clinical presentation of some of these conditions can be virtually identical to early dementia.

The clinical features of early dementia include:

- poor recent memory
- impaired acquisition of new information

- mild anomia (cannot remember names)
- personality change (e.g. withdrawn, irritable)
- minimal visuospatial impairment (e.g. tripping easily)
- inability to perform sequential tasks

The differential diagnosis for behavioural changes apart from dementia include several other common and important problems (which must be excluded) and can be considered under a mnemonic for dementia (see TABLE 8.3).[12]

Table 8.3 Mnemonic for DEMENTIA

D	=	**D**rugs and alcohol **D**epression
E	=	**E**ars **E**yes
M	=	**M**etabolic, e.g. hyponatraemia, diabetes mellitus, hypothyroidism
E	=	**E**motional problems (e.g. loneliness)
N	=	**N**utrition: diet (e.g. vitamin B group deficiency, teeth problems)
T	=	Tumours, Trauma } of central nervous system
I	=	**I**nfection
A	=	**A**rteriovascular disease → cerebral insufficiency

All these conditions should be considered with the onset of deterioration in health of the elderly person. Even apparently minor problems—such as the onset of deafness (e.g. wax in ears), visual deterioration (e.g. cataracts), diuretic therapy, poor mastication and diet, urinary tract intercurrent infection, boredom and anxiety—can precipitate abnormal behaviour.

Elder abuse

> Definition: 'Elder abuse is a single or repeated act or lack of appropriate action, occurring within any relationship where there is an expectation of trust, which causes harm or distress to an older person. It can include physical, sexual, financial, psychological and social abuse and/or neglect.' (Healthy Ageing Taskforce 2000)

It is important to keep in mind the possibility of abuse of the elderly, especially where there is a family history of abuse of members. The issue is as important as child and spouse abuse. Over one million elderly people are estimated to be the victims of physical or psychological abuse each year in the US.[4] We should keep in mind the occasional possibility of Munchausen syndrome by proxy. General practitioners should be alert to signs and symptoms of abuse and consider referral to an Aged Care Assessment/Service worker, e.g. ACAT team, Guardianship Tribunal or other responsible person or service. Ensure patient confidentiality and take care signing or witnessing forms for family members. Mandatory reporting law may vary from state to state.

Depression and dementia

The main differential diagnosis of dementia is depression, especially major depression, which is termed pseudodementia. The mode of onset is one way in which it may be possible to distinguish between depression and dementia. Dementia has a slow and surreptitious onset that is not clear-cut, while depression has a more definable and clear-cut onset that may be precipitated by a specific incident. Patients often have a past history of depression. Those with dementia have no insight; those with depression have insight, readily give up tasks, complain bitterly and become distressed by their inability to perform normal enjoyable tasks. It is vital to determine the cause of dementia.

In response to cognitive testing, the typical response of the depressed patient is 'don't know', while making an attempt with a near-miss typifies the patient with dementia (see TABLE 8.4).

Table 8.4 Comparison of dementia and pseudodementia (commonly severe depression)

	Dementia	Pseudodementia
Onset	Insidious	Clear-cut, often acute
Course over 24 hours	Worse in evening or at night	Worse in morning
Insight	Nil	Present
Orientation	Poor	Reasonable
Memory loss	Recent > remote	Recent = remote
Responses to mistakes	Agitated	Gives up easily
Response to cognitive testing (questions)	Near-miss! Difficulty understanding	'Don't know' Slow and reluctant but understands words (if cooperative)

It is vital to detect depression in the elderly as they are prone to suicide: 'Nothing to look back on with pride and nothing to look forward to.' The middle-aged and elderly may not complain of depression, which can be masked. They may present with somatic symptoms or delusions.

Note that depression occurs commonly in people with dementia, especially in the early stages.

Dementia (chronic organic brain syndrome)[13]

The incidence of dementia increases with age, affecting about 1 person in 10 over 65 years and 1 in 5 over 80 years. It doubles every 5 years from age 65 and is uncommon under 60 years. The important causes of dementia are:

- degenerative cerebral diseases, including
  - Alzheimer disease (about 60%)
  - dementia of frontotemporal type (up to 10%)
  - dementia with Lewy bodies (up to 10%)
- vascular (15%)
- alcohol excess (5%)
- Parkinson disease-associated dementia

Note: Mixed dementia should be considered.

Other causes of dementia:

- AIDS dementia
- corticobasal degeneration
- cerebral tumours
- Creutzfeldt–Jakob disease
- Pick disease
- neurosyphilis
- amyloidosis
- normal pressure hydrocephalus

In Alzheimer disease, there is insidious onset with initial forgetfulness progressing to severe memory loss (see FIG. 8.5). In frontal dementias the earliest manifestations are personality change and alteration of behaviour, including social dysfunction. Dementia with Lewy bodies is characterised by any two of visual hallucinations, spontaneous motor Parkinsonism and fluctuations in the mental state. Vascular dementia usually starts suddenly and is accompanied by focal neurological signs with evidence of cerebrovascular disease.

The characteristic feature of dementia is impairment of memory. Abstract thinking, judgment, verbal fluency and the ability to perform complex tasks also become impaired. Personality may change, impulse control may be lost and personal care deteriorate.

Risk factors for dementia include:

- family history
- increasing age
- late-onset depression
- hypothyroidism
- Down syndrome
- history of head injury
- HIV/AIDS
- generalised atherosclerosis
- Parkinson disease
- Aboriginal and Torres Strait Islander people

Differential diagnosis of dementia includes:

- normal cognitive impairment of ageing
- delirium
- major depression
- acquired brain injury
- drug abuse
- amnestic disorder
- various medical conditions (e.g. anaemia, thyroid/endocrine disorders)

The DSM-IV (TR) criteria for dementia are presented in TABLE 8.5 and clinical clues suggesting dementia in TABLE 8.6.

Table 8.5 DSM-IV (TR) criteria for dementia of Alzheimer type (modified)

Diagnosis of dementia requires evidence of:

A1	Clear evidence of decline in memory and learning
A2	At least one of the following cognitive disturbances: • Language = aphasia • Motor actions = apraxia • Recognition = agnosia • Executive functioning (e.g. organising)
B	Disturbance significantly interferes with social and work functions
C	Gradual onset and continuing cognitive decline
D	Not due to known organic causes (e.g. drugs, cerebrovascular disorders)
E	Not due to delirium
F	Not due to another axis 1 disorder (e.g. major depression)

(a) Classified with or without behavioural disturbance
(b) Also with early onset <65 years or late onset >65 years

Source: Diagnostic and Statistical Manual (4th edn, revised). Washington, DC: American Psychiatric Association, 2000.

Note: DCM-IV considered more explicit than DSM-5

Table 8.6 Clinical clues suggesting dementia

1 Patient presentations
New psychological problems in old age
Ill-defined and muddled complaints
Uncharacteristic behaviour
Relapse of physical disorders
Recurrent episodes of confusion
2 Problems noted by carers
'Not themselves'—change in personality (e.g. humourless)
Domestic accidents, especially with cooking and heating
Unsafe driving
False accusations
Emotional, irritable outbursts
Tendency to wander
Misplacing or losing items (e.g. keys, money, tablets, glasses)
Muddled on awakening at night
3 Mental state observations
Vague, rambling or disorganised conversation
Difficulty dating or sequencing past events
Repeating stock phrases or comments
Playing down obvious, perhaps serious, problems
Deflecting or evading memory testing

Source: After McLean[14]

The many guises of dementia can be considered in terms of four major symptom groups:[14]

1 Deficit presentations—due to loss of cognitive abilities, including:
- forgetfulness
- confusion and restlessness
- apathy (usually a late change)
- self-neglect with no insight
- poor powers of reasoning and understanding

2 Unsociable presentations—based on personality change, including:
- uninhibited behaviour
- risk taking and impulsive behaviour
- suspicious manner
- withdrawn behaviour

3 Dysphoric presentations—based on disturbed mood and personal distress, including:
- depression (hopeless and helpless)
- irritability with emotional outbursts
- lack of cooperation
- insecurity

4 Disruptive presentations—causing distress and disturbance to others, including:
- aggressive, sometimes violent, behaviour
- agitation with restlessness

The problem occasionally results in marked emotional and physical instability. It is sad and difficult for relatives to watch their loved ones develop aggressive and antisocial behaviour, such as poor table manners, poor personal cleanliness, rudeness and a lack of interest in others. Sometimes severe problems, such as violent behaviour, sexual promiscuity and incontinence, will eventuate.

There is always the likelihood of accidents with household items such as fire, gas, kitchen knives and hot water. Accidents at the toilet, in the bath and crossing roads may be a problem, especially if combined with failing sight and hearing. Such people should not drive motor vehicles.

8

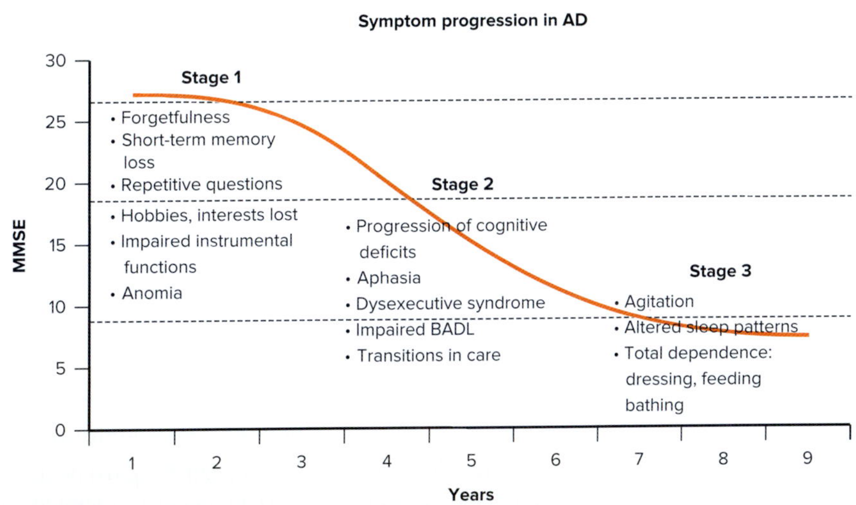

BADL = basic activities of daily living.
Source: Modified from Feldman et al. *Clinical Diagnosis and Management of Alzheimer's Disease* (1st edn), 1998

FIGURE 8.5 Symptom progression in Alzheimer disease

Without proper supervision they are likely to eat poorly, neglect their bodies and develop medical problems, such as skin ulcers and infections. They can also suffer from malnutrition and incontinence of urine or faeces. The median time to death after diagnosis is 3 years.

Management of suspected dementia

Exclude reversible or arrestable causes of dementia:

- full medical history (including drug and alcohol intake)
- mental state examination: select from several tools, e.g. Montreal Cognitive Assessment
- physical examination
- investigations (see Laboratory investigations, above, and CHAPTER 45)
- psychometric assessment

Management of dementia

Refer to a specialist to confirm the diagnosis and provide ongoing shared care. There is currently no cure for dementia—the best that can be offered to the patient is tender, loving care.

> Dementia is a terminal disease.

Education, support and advice should be given to both patient and family. Legal issues should be discussed such as enduring power of attorney, enduring guardianship and advanced care planning. Multidisciplinary evaluation and assistance are needed. Regular home visits by caring, sympathetic people are important. Such people include relatives, friends, GPs, district nurses, home help, members of a dementia self-help group, religious ministers and meals on wheels. People with dementia tend to manage much better in the familiar surroundings of their own home and this assists in preventing behaviour disturbance. Encourage the person to exercise, eat well and stay socially connected.

Special attention should be paid to organising memory aids, such as lists, routines and medication, and to hygiene, diet and warmth. Adequate nutrition, including vitamin supplements if necessary, has been shown to help. Provide ongoing support to carers.

Driving

Driving is a problem, especially as many are reluctant to give up their licence. Those with mild dementia are more likely to cause road accidents. In some states it is compulsory for doctors to report patients who are unfit to drive. If uncertainties arise or a patient is recalcitrant, refer to the local Road Traffic Authority. In Sweden it is recommended that those with moderate to severe dementia should not drive.

Comorbidity/associated problems[15]

The behavioural and neuropsychiatric problems are a major management issue. Depression can occur early in dementia and requires intervention. Demented patients are vulnerable to superimposed delirium, which is often due to:

- urinary tract infection
- other febrile illness
- prescribed medication
- drug withdrawal

Delirium should be suspected if a stable patient becomes acutely disturbed.

Dementia and Parkinson disease

A feature of Lewy body dementia, Parkinson disease is a very difficult yet common problem. One problem is that medication affects the mental processes. Lewy body dementia is extremely sensitive to the typical antipsychotics—typical agents should not be prescribed.[16] Quetiapine is the agent of choice. The choice of drugs is critical to care, so referral to an experienced team which can provide a good neuropsychiatric assessment is advisable. The best option appears to be the administration of:

- levodopa to maximum dose
- quetiapine at night

Medication[15]

Demented patients often do not require any psychotropic medication. Antidepressant drugs can be prescribed for depression. Citalopram is effective in treating agitation but tricyclic antidepressants (TCAs) tend to aggravate confusion.[16] Benzodiazepines are effective for short term use in agitated behaviours. The cholinesterase inhibitors donepezil, galantamine and rivastigmine appear to delay progression of dementia to a modest extent only. There appears to be no differences between the available agents. Beware of drugs that aggravate such as anticholinergics, opiates, TCAs, frusemide, prednisolone and salbutamol.[16]

Available drugs for Alzheimer disease

Cholinesterase inhibitors

- donepezil 5 mg (o) nocte for 4 weeks, increase to 10 mg nocte as tolerated
- galantamine prolonged release 8 mg (o) daily for 4 weeks, increase to 16 mg daily or 24 mg if tolerated

- rivastigmine 1.5 mg (o) bd for 2 weeks, increase gradually up to 6 mg bd as tolerated
  or
- rivastigmine 4.6 mg transdermal daily for 4 weeks, then 9.5 mg daily as tolerated

Aspartate (NMDA) antagonist

- memantine (Ebixa) 5 mg (o) mane for 1 week → 5 mg bd week two → 10 mg bd from week 4

Based on double-blind randomised trials of the two drugs donepezil and rivastigmine and using Cochrane data,[15,17] the following points emerge:

- only modest improvement overall
- greatest improvement with higher doses
- higher doses less well tolerated
- long-term efficacy unknown
- clinical effectiveness in severe disease has not been demonstrated[18]

The newer agent memantine appears to have similar outcomes and can be used in combination.

Using evidence-based medicine criteria on numbers needed to treat (see CHAPTER 13), the evidence shows that 13 patients must be treated with rivastigmine 6–12 mg/day for 6 months for one patient to display clinically meaningful improvement.[18,19]

To control psychotic symptoms or disturbed behaviour probably due to psychosis:[20]

olanzapine 2.5–10 mg (o) daily
or
risperidone 0.25–2 mg (o) bd, increasing to maximum of 2 mg daily

To control symptoms of anxiety and agitation use:

oxazepam 7.5 mg (o) one to three times daily

Benzodiazepines should be used only for short periods (maximum 2 weeks) as they tend to exacerbate cognitive impairment in dementia.

Complementary therapy[15]

As yet there is insufficient evidence for the efficacy of complementary medicines such as *Ginkgo biloba,*[21] vitamin E[22] and other antioxidants in treating (alleviating symptoms in) dementia, despite some epidemiological evidence, especially in the case of vitamin E. However, we should encourage our patients in preventive healthy lifestyle strategies, such as optimal nutrition rich in essential vitamins and exercise. Deficiencies of folate, vitamin B12 and vitamin D should be treated.

Dementia prevention strategies

This suggested program is based on the research work of Dr Michael Valenzuela.[23]

- Healthy blood pressure—'a healthy heart means a healthy brain'—the strongest evidence for dementia prevention.
- The three keys:

  A physical: walking 30–60 minutes 3–4 times a week, plus strength exercises, balance and stretching exercises—reportedly known to enhance brain cell growth, brain cell interconnections and angiogenesis

  B mentally stimulating activities

  C social activities in company that are both fun and rewarding.

- Alcohol control: avoid binge drinking and *always* promote a safe intake, i.e. 1–2 standard drinks with a meal for 3 days a week.
- Diet—Mediterranean in style, oily fish 2–3 times a week (consider Chia seed), 2 fruits and 5 vegetables daily.

Causes of mild neurocognitive impairment

- Early dementia
- Benign senescent forgetfulness
- Depression
- Anxiety
- Acquired brain injury
- Physical illness

Benign senescent forgetfulness[24]

This 'popular' term is also referred to as 'age-related memory loss' or 'mild cognitive impairment' of ageing. Features include:

- short-term forgetfulness
- inability to find the right word
- embarrassment about shortcomings
- feeling dithery
- inability to find items stored away
- forgetting to pay accounts

It is debatable whether these are truly benign cognitive impairment or early features of dementia.[25]

Late life depression and suicide

The risk of suicide increases with age in males. The risk factors for late life suicide are:[25]

- male
- single

- recent bereavement
- social isolation
- recent relocation
- poor pain control
- feeling helpless/hopeless
- anhedonia
- indicating a wish to die
- recent alcohol abuse

The principles of treatment include supportive care, regular visits, CAT team, interpersonal psychotherapy, cognitive behavioural therapy and family support/interventions.

Paraphrenia[26]

Paraphrenia, known as 'late onset' schizophrenia, is that condition where the symptoms and signs of paranoid psychosis appear for the first time in the elderly. In this apparent non-psychotic mental illness, the patient, who is usually an elderly female, presents with paranoid delusions, such as a feeling of being watched or persecuted and even hallucinations. These are usually associated with visual and hearing problems. Treatment is with an antipsychotic agent, e.g. risperidone or olanzapine.

Sarcopenia

Sarcopenia is degenerative loss of skeletal mass, strength and possibly function as a result of ageing, illness, sedentary lifestyle and poor diet. Features of significant frailty include poor hand grip strength, slow walking speed, exhaustion with activity and susceptibility to infection and falls. Treatment strategies include exercise, especially resistance training, protein supplements in diet, Vitamin D and reduction in polypharmacy.

Falls in the elderly

TABLE 8.7 presents the diagnostic strategy model. Falls in the elderly are a major problem as 30% of people over the age of 65 experience at least one fall per year, with 1 in 4 of these having significant injury. About 5% of falls result in fracture.[27] In 2002 in Australia, there were approximately 1200 deaths in people over 75 years of age following falls, which were responsible for 90% of hip fractures and 50% of vertebral fractures.

Table 8.7 Falls in the elderly: diagnostic strategy model

Probability diagnosis
Environmental hazards, e.g. slipping, tripping
Postural hypotension
Postural instability, e.g. knees, hips, Parkinson disease
Visual, e.g. glaucoma, macular degeneration
Alcohol use, acute or chronic
Medication, especially iatrogenic
Serious disorders not to be missed
Vascular
Cerebral insufficiency, incl. TIAs, stroke
Acute coronary syndromes
Cardiac arrhythmias, e.g. sick sinus syndrome
Subdural or extradural haematoma
Infection
Any systemic infection, esp. sepsis
Any febrile illness
Tumour/cancer
Cerebral tumour
Other
Kidney failure
Head injury
Cognitive impairment, e.g. dementia, delirium
Fluid and electrolyte disturbance
Pitfalls (often missed)
Parkinson disease, early
Peripheral neuropathy
Gait and foot disorders
Labyrinthine, e.g. BPPV, labyrinthitis
Rarities
Vitamin deficiency, esp. D
Cerebellar degeneration
Postprandial hypotension
Seven masquerades checklist
Depression
Diabetes: hypoglycaemia, neuropathy
Drugs; see history
Anaemia
Thyroid/endocrine: Addison disease, hypothyroidism
Spinal dysfunction, esp. myelopathy
Urinary tract infection: nocturia
Is the patient trying to tell me something?
Highly likely, consider conversion reaction

Assessment

The history should embrace the above causes and risk factors. In particular, a description of the fall by a witness, the perceived dysfunction at the time of the fall and whether there was loss of consciousness are particularly important.

The physical examination should include cardiac function, neurological status (including the mini-mental function test) and the musculoskeletal system (including assessment of gait). The 'get up and go' test (see TABLE 8.8) is useful.

Table 8.8 The 'get up and go' test: a brief test of postural competence

1	Get up from chair without use of arms.
2	Observe normal gait and 360° turn.
3	Carry out the Romberg test (slight push with eyes closed).
4	Observe tandem walking (heel toe, straight line).

As special investigations (especially for those proving difficult to evaluate), consider full blood examination and erythrocyte sedimentation rate (ESR), blood sugar, urea and electrolytes, vitamin D, thyroid function tests, cardiac investigations (e.g. ambulatory electrocardiogram [ECG] monitoring, ambulatory blood pressure monitoring), vestibular function testing, and CT scans or MRI scans.[28]

Management and prevention

Steps should be taken to correct any medical disorders and risk factors. It is appropriate to refer to a multidisciplinary team that includes occupational therapists and physiotherapists. Assessment of circumstances in the home is very helpful. This may lead to reducing environmental hazards and providing walking aids. Exercise training and medication reduction are also important strategies. (See www.racgp.org.au/redbook, section 5.2: Falls and physical activity.)

Prescribing and adverse drug reactions

Ageing is associated with increased rates of adverse drug reactions.[1] The rate of adverse drug reactions for a single medication rises from about 6% at age 20 years to about 20% at age 70 years.

For fewer than six medications taken concurrently, the rate of adverse drug reactions is about 6%. For more than six medications taken concurrently, the rate of adverse drug reactions jumps to 20%.[1] Approximately 15% of elderly patients admitted to hospital are suffering adverse drug reactions. Most adverse drug reactions are type A (dose related) rather than type B (idiosyncratic).[29]

Factors predisposing to adverse drug reactions in the elderly[1]

Most adverse drug reactions in the elderly are entirely predictable. Most are merely an extension of the pharmacological action of the drug (e.g. all antihypertensives will reduce blood pressure and have the capacity to cause hypotension and falls in a person with impaired baroreceptor function or poor homeostasis in their vascular tree). Very few adverse reactions are idiosyncratic or unexpected.

The five mechanisms of adverse drug reactions in the elderly are:

1 *Drug–drug interaction.* For example, beta blockers given concomitantly with digoxin increases the risk of heart block and bradycardia. Alcohol used in combination with antidepressants increases the risk of sedation.
2 *Drug–disease interaction.* For example, in the presence of kidney impairment, tetracyclines carry an increased risk of kidney deterioration.
3 *Age-related changes leading to increases in drug plasma concentration.* Decreased kidney excretion can extend the half-life of medication, leading to accumulation and toxicity.
4 *Age-related changes leading to increased drug sensitivity.* For example, there is some suggestion that the pharmacological response to warfarin, narcotics and benzodiazepines is increased in the elderly. Conversely, the pharmacological response to insulin, theophylline and beta-adrenergic blocking agents is thought to be decreased.
5 *Patient error.* Multiple medications can lead to patient error. The incidence and prevalence of dementia also increases with age. Other problems include failing eyesight and reduced manual dexterity.

8

Risk factors predisposing to medicine-related problems

Adverse drug effects in older people are influenced by multiple factors, with many exposed to more than one of these factors at a given time. Furthermore, their recovery from serious incidents such as a hip fracture is jeopardised, possibly ending in death.

Increasing the number of simultaneous medications increases the risk for all five mechanisms of adverse drug reactions.

In a study on adverse drug reaction in elderly patients the drugs most frequently causing admission to hospital were:[30]

- psychotropics and hypnotics
- diuretics
- antihypertensives (including beta blockers)
- anti-Parkinson drugs
- anti-convulsants
- analgesics and NSAIDs

The main drugs contributing to falls were:[31]

- antidepressants
- benzodiazepines
- antipsychotics
- antihypertensives
- anti-Parkinson
- diuretics
- hypnotics
- sedatives
- anti-convulsants

Drug regimens should be kept as simple as possible to aid compliance and avoid or minimise drug interactions.

The elderly may need much lower doses of anxiolytics and hypnotics than younger patients to produce the same effect, thus rendering them more susceptible to adverse effects and toxicity. The elderly are especially liable to accumulate the longer-acting benzodiazepines.

In particular, any drug or combination of drugs with anticholinergic properties (e.g. tricyclic antidepressants, anti-Parkinsonian agents, antihistamines, phenothiazines and some cold remedies) can precipitate a central anticholinergic syndrome.[14]

The elderly are very prone to adverse effects to most of the more potent drugs, especially those for cardiac dysfunction and hypertension. Both ACE inhibitors and calcium channel blockers have been shown to produce a greater fall in blood pressure in elderly compared with younger subjects, presumably related also to a reduced homeostatic response.[7]

8

Practice tip

Beware of the 'triple whammy': ACE inhibitor + diuretic + NSAID.

Starting medications[15]

The starting dose of a drug in the aged[14] should be at the lower end of recommended ranges. Dosage increments should be gradual and reviewed regularly.

That is, start low, go slow and monitor frequently. It is important to individualise doses for the elderly with the simplest dosage regimen.

Minimising medication problems

- Write simple instructions on all prescriptions.
- Individualise doses for the elderly.
- Give patients a list of their medications.
- Ask them to bring the list and their medications at each visit.
- Update this list as necessary.
- Keep medication regimen as simple as possible.
- Consider a Dosette box or Webster pack for polypharmacy.
- At home visits use the opportunity to inspect medications.
- Observe for drug interactions and toxicity.
- Keep detailed records of all medications prescribed.
- Carefully review medication after discharge from hospital.

Other tips for medication in the elderly

- Obtain relatives/carers' consent for medication, especially in the confused.

References

1 Harris E. *Prescribing for the Ageing Population.* Update Course Proceedings Handbook. Melbourne: Monash University Medical School, 1992.

2 Australian Institute of Health and Welfare. *Australia's Health 2014.* Canberra: Australian Government.

3 Valenti L, Britt H. Older patients. Aust Fam Physician, 2010; 39(10): 717.

4 Mold JW. Principles of geriatric care. American Health Consultants. Primary Care Rep, 1996; 2(1): 2–9.

5 Lang D. Home visits to the elderly. Aust Fam Physician, 1993; 22: 264.

6 Forbes A. Caring for older people: loneliness. BMJ, 1996; 313: 352–4.

7 Ellard J. How to irritate and confuse your elderly patients: 20 simple rules. Modern Medicine Australia, 1990; 7: 66–8.

8 Workman B. Early dementia: optimal management in general practice. Aust Fam Physician, 2010; 39(10): 722–6.

9 Hodkinson HM. Evaluation of a mental test score for assessment of mental impairment in the elderly. BMJ, 1972; 1: 233–8.

10 Kingshill 2000 <www.kingshill-research.org>.

11 Fredman M, Leach L, Kaplan E et al. *Clock Drawing: A Neuropsychological Analysis.* New York: Oxford University Press, 1994.

12 Bridges-Webb C. *Care of Patients with Dementia: General Practice Guidelines.* Sydney: NSW Health, 2003.

13 Ames D, Burns A, O'Brien J. *Dementia* (4th edn). London: Hodder Arnold, 2010.

14 McLean S. Is it dementia? Aust Fam Physician 1992; 21: 1762–76.

15 Expert group for Psychotropic guidelines. Psychotropic: dementia. In: eTG complete. Melbourne: Therapeutic Guidelines Ltd. Available from: <www.tg.org.au>, accessed August 2017.

16 Macfarlane S. Management of behavioural and psychological symptoms in dementia. Proceedings for Monash University

Update Course for GPs. Melbourne: November 2017 (notes available on request).
17 Birks JS et al. Donepezil for mild and moderate Alzheimer's disease (Cochrane Review). In: The Cochrane Library. Issue 1, 2001. Oxford: Update Software.
18 Birks JS et al. Rivastigmine for Alzheimer's disease (Cochrane Review). In: The Cochrane Library. Issue 1, 2001. Oxford: Update Software.
19 New Alzheimer's drugs show only modest benefit. NPS News, 2001; 16: 1–6.
20 Herman N, Lanctot K. Pharmacologic management of neuropsychological symptoms for Alzheimer's disease. Can J Psychiatry, 2007; 52(6): 630–45.
21 Le Bars PL et al. *Ginkgo biloba* and dementia. JAMA, 1997; 278: 1327–32.
22 Tabet N et al. Vitamin E for Alzheimer's disease (Cochrane Review). In: The Cochrane Library. Issue 1, 2001. Oxford: Update Software.
23 Valenzuela M. *Maintain Your Brain.* Sydney: Harper Collins, 2001.
24 Bamford KA, Caine ED. Does benign senescent forgetfulness exist? Clin Geriatr Med, 1988; Nov 4(4): 397–416.
25 Jeffreys D. Late-life depression. Medical Observer, 18 July 2003: 36–7.
26 Abrams WB, Beers M, Berkow W. *The Merck Manual of Geriatrics* (3rd edn). New Jersey: Merck Research Laboratories 2009: Chapter 36.
27 Hindmarsh JJ, Estes H. Falls in older persons: causes and intervention. Arch Intern Med, 1989; 149: 2217.
28 Quail GG. An approach to the assessment of falls in the elderly. Aust Fam Physician, 1994; 23: 873–83.
29 NPS News. Medicines and older people: an accident waiting to happen? NPS News, 2004; 34: 1–4.
30 Briant RH. Medication problems of old age. Patient Management, 1988; 5: 27–31.
31 Bell Js, Blacker N, Edwards et al. Osteoporosis: pharmacological prevention and management in older people. Aust Fam Physician, 2012; 41(3): 110–8.

Resources

Dementia Australia. <www.dementia.org.au>, accessed January 2018.
National Prescribing Service (NPS). Balancing the benefits and harms of antipsychotic therapy. Prescribing Practice Review, 2011; (PPR 55).

9 Prevention in general practice

When meditating over a disease, I never think of finding a remedy for it, but, instead, a means of preventing it.

Louis Pasteur 1884

Definitions[1]

Prevention may be defined as the means of promoting and maintaining health or averting illness.

It is concerned with removal or reduction of risks; early diagnosis; early treatment; limitation of complications, including those of iatrogenic origin; and maximum adaptation to disability.

The promotion of health concerns helping well people to learn healthy behaviours and to accept responsibility for their own well-being.

A preventive attitude implies that the doctor understands and can utilise the preventive potential in each primary care consultation by an 'opportunistic approach'. In addition to the traditional management of both presenting and continuing problems, the doctor takes the opportunity to modify the patient's health-seeking behaviour, to provide education about the illness, and to promote health by relating the patient's present condition to previous unhealthy behaviour.

A general reference for prevention is the RACGP red book—*Guidelines for preventive activities in general practice* (9th edition). www.racgp.org.au/your-practice/guidelines/redbook.

Primary prevention

Primary prevention includes action taken to avert the occurrence of disease. As a result there is no disease. Primary preventive strategies include:

1. education to bring about changes in lifestyle factors known to be associated with diseases (e.g. smoking cessation, healthy balanced diets, reduction in alcohol intake, exercise)
2. sterilisation of surgical instruments and other medical equipment
3. eradication, as with vector control of mosquitoes to prevent malaria
4. immunisation against infective diseases
5. sanitation, keeping our water supplies clean and disposing efficiently of sewage and industrial wastes
6. legislation to ensure that some of these primary preventive measures are carried out

Secondary prevention

Secondary prevention includes actions taken to stop or delay the progression of disease.

The term is usually applied to measures for the detection of disease at its earliest stage, i.e. in the presymptomatic phase, so that treatment can be started before irreversible pathology is present. The early recognition of hypertension through routine testing (screening) of patients allows treatment during the presymptomatic phase of the illness process. Screening for cervical cancer allows the treatment of cervical dysplasia, a premalignant condition. Other examples include mammography and endoscopy for polyps of the large bowel.

Tertiary prevention

Tertiary prevention includes the management of established disease so as to minimise disability.

The term is usually applied to the rehabilitation process necessary to restore the patient to the best level of adaptation possible when there has been damage of an irreversible nature. A patient who has suffered a stroke because of hypertension may be restored to a useful lifestyle with appropriate rehabilitation.

Relationship between types of prevention

It can be seen that there is a clearer demarcation between primary and secondary prevention than between secondary and tertiary prevention, although the latter term is particularly useful in dealing with the elderly and the handicapped. Conceptually, curative medicine falls within the definitions of secondary and tertiary prevention while public health measures are mainly concerned with primary prevention. Prevention is really wider than medical practice but because of the success of public health practices in the past, more attention is now being focused on prevention by doctors (see FIG. 9.1).[2]

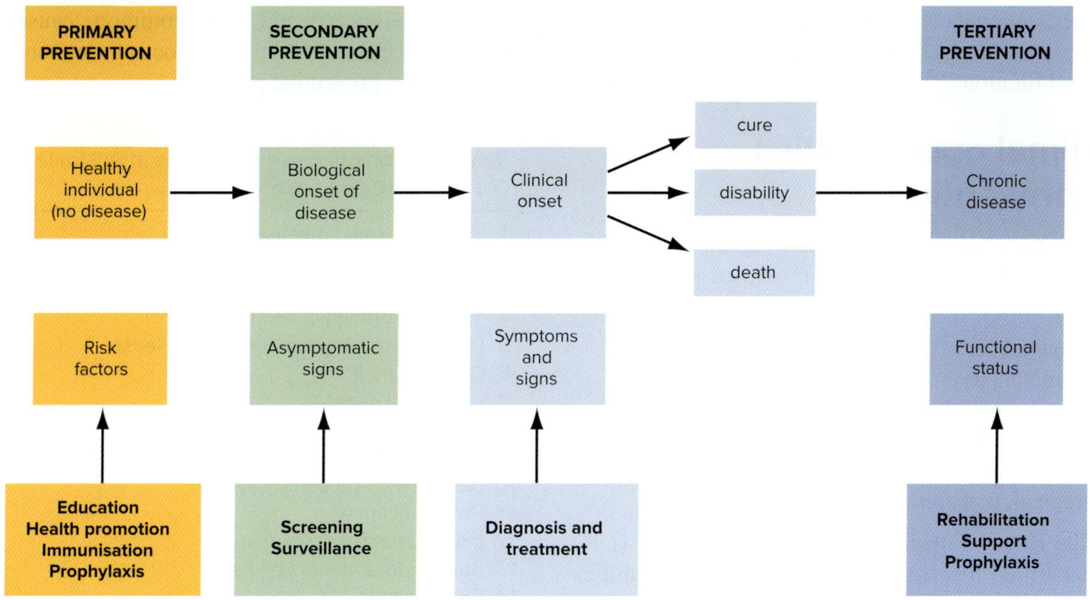

FIGURE 9.1 The phases of prevention in relation to the natural history of disease

As GPs our role in prevention is twofold.

1 First, we can recognise the preventable factors that are involved in an illness process and determine appropriate interventions.
2 Second, we can act to implement the preventive measure. In cases where the responsibility rests with the individual or the community, doctors can support prevention through education, applying political pressure or working with community agencies.

The practice of preventive medicine

What is preventable?

The first step in the implementation of prevention is to define which specific diseases can be prevented and to what extent, given certain restraints such as human resources, technology and the cost to the community. All diseases have a potential preventability but it may be unrealistic to try to achieve this.

Diseases that can be prevented can be grouped according to their aetiology. They fall into the following broad categories:

- genetic disorders
- conditions occurring during pregnancy and the puerperium
- developmental disorders
- accidents
- infections
- addictions
- behavioural disorders
- occupational disorders
- premature vascular disease
- neoplasms
- handicap in the disabled
- certain 'other' diseases (e.g. diverticular disease)

Mortality is the only reliable index by which the outcome of preventive activities can be judged. Conditions can be ranked in importance as causes of premature death according to the 'years of potential life lost before 78 years [of age]' as follows:[1]

- Accidents, poisoning, suicide and violence
- Neoplasms
- Circulatory diseases
- Perinatal conditions
- Congenital conditions
- Alzheimer disease

This gives quite a different perspective to prevention and explains why the efforts of public health authorities and practising doctors do not always coincide.

The interventions available to us in medical practice are as follows:

1 educational—health promotion, health education and illness education
2 screening
3 surveillance

4 interventional care—immunisation, behaviour modification and drug prophylaxis
5 rehabilitation

Optimal opportunities for prevention

Primary prevention par excellence can be practised in general practice under the opportunities provided by the following clinical circumstances:

- antenatal care
- postnatal care
- advising people travelling overseas
- visits by infants with their parents
- times of crisis or potential crisis
- pregnancy planning

The Royal College of General Practitioners (UK) has identified the seven most important opportunities for prevention as:

1 family planning
2 antenatal care
3 immunisation
4 fostering the bonds between mother and child
5 discouragement of smoking
6 detection and management of raised blood pressure
7 helping the bereaved

9

Mortality and morbidity considerations

An understanding of the mortality and morbidity patterns in the modern human being is essential to the planning of preventive programs. The great infectious diseases of the past, such as tuberculosis, syphilis, smallpox, influenza, diphtheria and streptococcal infections, have been largely contained but other diseases have become prominent as life expectancy increases. The great modern diseases are atherosclerosis (hardening of the arteries), malignant disease (cancer), HIV infection and iatrogenesis (doctor-induced illness). The two most common causes of death in Australia are cancer and cardiovascular disease, each accounting for approximately 29% of all deaths.[3]

By comparison, the ten leading causes of death in the world are (in order) ischaemic heart disease, stroke, lower respiratory tract infection, COPD, diarrhoeal disease, HIV/AIDS, cancer, diabetes mellitus, road injury and prematurity (WHO: Fact sheet 310; July 2013).

These diseases and the common causes of mortality (see TABLE 9.1) act as a focus for our energies in addressing preventive programs.

Table 9.1 Common causes of deaths in Australia in 2015 (in rank order)

1	Ischaemic heart disease
2	Dementia/Alzheimer
3	Cerebrovascular disease
4	Tracheal, bronchial and lung cancer
5	Chronic obstructive pulmonary disease
6	Diabetes mellitus
7	Colorectal cancer
8	Blood and lymph cancer
9	Heart failure
10	Diseases of the urinary system
11	Prostate cancer
12	Influenza and pneumonia
13	Suicide, intentional self-harm
14	Breast cancer

*Cancer is the no. 1 cause if grouped together

Source: Australian Bureau of Statistics, *Year Book Australia*, 2015

It is worth focusing on the changes in disease indices during the past generation in order to evaluate the effect of preventive and health promotion programs during this period (see TABLE 9.2).[3] The messages are to harness and promote with renewed vigour those strategies that are working, such as prevention of death from coronary artery disease and motor vehicle accidents, and to re-evaluate those important areas, such as Aboriginal mortality, HIV infection, cancer, suicide and asthma, which are bad news!

A global strategy for good health

The World Health Organization (WHO) defines good health as 'a state of dynamic harmony between the body, mind and spirit of a person and the social and cultural influences which make up his or her environment'.

A considerable amount of epidemiological information has emerged to support what GPs have known for a long time—that a commonsense, healthy lifestyle not only promotes good health but also reduces the risk of the main causes of mortality and morbidity in this country, including cardiovascular disease and cancer.

The common theme for virtually all disease is to follow the nutrition and lifestyle guidelines presented in CHAPTER 10.

Table 9.2 Major changes in public health in Australia, with trends in the two decades up to 2012

Improvements	Deterioration
Overall mortality	Alcohol-related diseases
Heart disease	Drug abuse
Stroke	Dementia
Smoking	Depression, mental health
Road safety	Health inequalities
Diseases controlled by immunisation	Obesity
Dental health	Diabetes
Cancer, overall especially	Arthritis/musculoskeletal problems
• cervix	Fall injuries
• stomach	Environmental pollution problems
• breast	
• testis	
• colorectal	
Pregnancy complications	
Congenital abnormalities	
HIV/AIDS	

Source: G Egger, R Spark, L Donovan, *Health Promotion Strategies and Method,* 2013

Behaviour modification

Lifestyle habits that have developed over many years can be very difficult to change even when the individual is well motivated to change. A variety of instructional, motivational and behavioural techniques can be used to initiate a lifestyle change program; GPs should be aware of these and use the resources of a multidisciplinary team to give support to motivated people who as a rule find behaviour modification difficult.

Vascular disease

Risk factors for vascular disease (atherosclerosis) are:

- hypertension
- smoking
- high cholesterol
- diabetes
- obesity
- sedentary lifestyle
- stress
- alcohol excess
- poor diet
- family history

The guidelines for good health given in CHAPTER 10, if followed, will help prevent the development of cardiovascular and cerebrovascular disease.

It is worth noting that the death rate from coronary heart disease is about 70% higher for smokers than for non-smokers and for very heavy smokers the risk is almost 200% higher. It has been shown that the incidence of heart disease falls in those who have ceased smoking.

GPs can estimate the absolute 5-year risks of cardiovascular events in their patients by referring to the New Zealand Guidelines Group Cardiovascular Risk Charts (www.nzgg.org.nz); see CHAPTER 85.

The parameters used are:

- gender and age
- smoking status
- diabetes status
- blood pressure
- total cholesterol/HDL ratio

Malignant disease

Primary prevention of cancer is an important objective and there is a need to focus on this vital factor as much as on secondary prevention.

Updated important facts about cancer in Australia* (current and immediate future)

- It continues to be more common in men than women overall; in 2017 more than half (54%) of all diagnosed cases were expected to be in men.
- Breast cancer (in women) is expected to be the most common type of cancer diagnosed, followed by colorectal cancer and prostate cancer.*
- The death rate from all cancers has fallen from 209 deaths per 100 000 people in 1982 to an estimated 161 per 100 000.
- Survival rates from all cancers have improved substantially, with five-year survival increasing from 48% in 1984–1988 to 68% in 2009–2013.
- Survival varied by cancer type, with the largest survival improvements seen in prostate cancer, non-Hodgkin lymphoma, kidney cancer and multiple myeloma.
- Pancreatic cancer and lung cancer showed only small improvements, while bladder cancer and cancer of the larynx actually had lower survival rates.
- Lung cancer is likely to be the leading cause of cancer death, followed by bowel cancer, prostate cancer, breast cancer in women and pancreatic cancer.

*Excluding basal and squamous cell carcinoma

Source: Cancer Council of Australia (www.cancer.org.au/about-cancer)

That environmental factors are involved in the aetiology of colorectal cancer and other cancers is indicated by wide variations in incidence between different countries.

Suspicion falls on diet and there is epidemiological evidence implicating diets high in animal fats and low in insoluble fibre, fruits and vegetables, and also high alcohol consumption. It is noted that there are higher incidence rates in people migrating from low-to high-risk countries, such as Japanese to Hawaii[5] and Greeks and Italians to Australia.[5]

Studies in the US indicate that at least 35% of all cancer deaths are related to diet. Obese individuals have an increased risk of colon, breast and uterine cancers. High-fat diets are a risk factor for prostate, breast and colon cancers. Salt-cured, smoked and nitrate-cured foods increase the risk of upper GIT cancers. Foods rich in vitamin A and folate (dark green and deep yellow vegetables and fruits) and vitamin C and cruciferous vegetables (cabbage, Brussels sprouts, broccoli and cauliflower) are all considered to have protective effects for various cancers.[6,7] Phytochemicals (plant chemicals) exist in these foods and in other vegetables and fruit that have a cancer-protective effect.[8]

Overall, diet, smoking, alcohol and occupational exposures (5%) appear to account for over 73% of all cancer mortality.[7]

Doll and Peto[9] considered that environmental factors were responsible for 80–90% of cancers and estimated that diet was a major factor in the cause of cancer in 40% of men and 60% of women.

The role of immunity in cancer

The development of a number of cancers appears to be related to a depression of the individual's immune system, particularly in relation to cellular immunity, in a similar way (albeit on a different scale) to the effect of HIV infection. Studies have shown that the immune system is adversely influenced by:[10]

- stress, especially bereavement
- depression
- ageing
- drugs
- pollutants
- cigarette smoke
- inappropriate diet
- alcohol
- radiation

On the other hand, a protective effect on the immune system may be provided by:

- food antioxidants (see TABLE 10.2 in CHAPTER 10)
- tranquillity
- meditation

In some instances malignancies appear to undergo unpredictable remissions with patients following an optimal diet, taking antioxidants, changing their lifestyle and practising meditation. However, an Australian study indicated that the enthusiasm for the value of antioxidants may be unjustified.[11]

Diet certainly appears to be a most important factor in the primary prevention of disease. If immune deficient diseases can respond in such a way, imagine what a powerful primary preventive force such a lifestyle represents for all disease.

Asthma and other respiratory diseases

The death rate and morbidity rate for asthma and other respiratory diseases is unacceptable and much of it can be prevented.[12] A report on the cost of asthma claimed that there is evidence that a significant proportion of diagnosed asthmatics are currently receiving treatment that does not provide the best possible control of the disease.[12]

Prevention means being better informed and treating such an 'irritable' disease as bronchial asthma aggressively. It means focusing on better assessment and monitoring (e.g. home use of the mini peak flow meter), better delivery of medication to the airways (e.g. use of spacers attached to inhalers and/or use of pumps and nebulisers) and appropriate management of the cause (inflammation of the bronchial tree) by the use of inhaled corticosteroids or sodium cromoglycate as the first-line treatment for significant asthma. An appropriate strategy is to follow the six-step asthma management plan (see TABLE 9.3) of the National Asthma Campaign.

Table 9.3 The six-step asthma management plan

1. Establish the severity of the asthma.
2. Achieve best lung function.
3. Maintain best lung function—identify and avoid trigger factors.
4. Maintain best lung function—follow an optimal medication program.
5. Develop an action plan.
6. Educate and review regularly.

Source: National Asthma Campaign: Australia, 2008

The protective effect for asthma and COPD of vitamin C, fish oils, a low-salt diet and other natural antioxidants is highlighted by Sridhar.[13]

Periodic health examination

Since 86% of the population visit a GP at some stage of the year,[3] and these people visit about five times each year (on average), GPs are in an ideal position to develop strategies for a periodic health examination. An emphasis should be placed on the history in addition to the physical examination and related basic investigations.

As for any smooth-running quality professional program, it is important to be organised with prepared practice staff, checklists and record systems. The Royal Australian College of General Practitioners (RACGP) has developed a College Record System, which has several leaflets covering all approaches to the patient 'check-up'.[14]

The following guidelines for the periodic health examination are adapted from those recommended by the Preventive and Community Medicine Committee of the RACGP.[14] This represents appropriate screening at the front line of primary health care.

Aims of screening

In practice, screening is not only to detect disease in asymptomatic people at its earliest stage, but also to find individuals at risk or those with established disease who are not receiving adequate care. There are three levels at which screening practice can be applied in general practice:

1. 'well' individuals with risk factors that predispose to disease (e.g. obesity, uncomplicated essential hypertension, hyperlipidaemia)
2. asymptomatic individuals with signs of early disease or illness (e.g. developmental dysplasia of the hip, ectopic testis, glaucoma, bacteriuria of pregnancy, carcinoma in situ of cervix)
3. symptomatic individuals whose irreversible abnormalities are unreported but the effects can be controlled or assisted (e.g. visual defects, deafness, mental handicap)

The history[14]

An appropriate history will allow the recognition of certain risk factors that may foreshadow future disease. Though established patients will have a previously acquired database, their history should be reviewed and updated. It is recommended that the following items be included in history taking in the appropriate age groups.

Family history. In particular, cardiovascular disease, some cancers (breast, bowel, melanoma with dysplastic naevi), diabetes, asthma, genetic disorders and bowel disease will alert the doctor to specific risk factors (and psychological factors) for these patients.

Suicide and accidents. Consider the risk factors predisposing to suicide and accidents, which are the major preventable causes of death in children and young adults.

Substance abuse. Tobacco and alcohol are the major causes of preventable death in adults, although other drugs contribute to a lesser extent. Counselling by GPs, about smoking in particular, has been shown to be effective.

Exercise and nutrition. These factors have a role to play in preventing cardiovascular disease and to a lesser extent in blood pressure control, cancer, diabetes and constipation. They have an even greater role to play in improving general well-being and preventing morbidity.

Occupational health hazards. Consider these in working adults, as occupational health hazards can significantly contribute to morbidity and mortality (e.g. exposure to toxic substances, unsafe work practices). Specific examples include:

- coal miners—pneumoconiosis
- gold, copper and tin miners—silicosis
- asbestos workers and builders—asbestosis, mesothelioma
- veterinarians, farmers, abattoir workers—zoonoses
- aniline dye workers—bladder cancer
- health care providers—hepatitis B

Physical functioning, home conditions and social supports. Consider these in elderly people, as physical function and social supports are of crucial importance in determining whether they can care for themselves—intervention can prevent accidents and death.

Sexuality/contraception. Sexually transmitted infections are all preventable, as are unwanted pregnancies. Opportunities should be sought to ask young people, in particular, about their sexuality, and to counsel them. The question 'Do you have any concerns about sex?' is very useful in this context.

Osteoporosis. Osteoporosis affects nearly a third of all postmenopausal women, most of whom suffer osteoporotic fractures. Fractures of the femoral neck have a particularly poor prognosis, with up to a third of these women dying within 6 months, and many more requiring continuing nursing home care. Bone loss accelerates at the time of the menopause, and can be reduced by hormone replacement therapy.

Women at risk of osteoporosis are short, slim, Caucasian; they drink coffee and alcohol, smoke, eat a high-protein and high-salt diet, and don't exercise.

Masquerades in general practice. It is worth considering the 'masquerades' (see CHAPTER 17, TABLES 17.4 and 17.5), which may present as undifferentiated illness, as a means of following the important medical principle of early detection of disease: engendering a certain awareness.

Primary masquerades to consider are:

- depression
- diabetes mellitus
- drug problems
- anaemia
- thyroid disorders, especially hypothyroidism
- urinary tract infection
- vertebral (spinal) dysfunction

Hypothyroidism has been estimated to exist in up to 15% of women aged 60 and above, and searching for clues may elicit subtle symptoms and signs previously attributed to ageing.

Relationships and psychosocial health. Consider the mental health of patients, particularly the elderly, by enquiring about how they are coping with life, how they are coping financially, about their peace of mind and how things are at home. Focus on the quality of their close relationships (e.g. husband–wife, father–son, mother–daughter, employer–employee). Enquire about losses in their life, especially family bereavements.

Screening for children[14]

Childhood health record books provide an excellent opportunity for communication between different health care givers; parents should be provided with the record books and encouraged to bring them to every visit. Various recommendations for screening are made under the following headings.

Height/weight/head circumference. Record length/height, weight and head circumference at regular intervals. Head circumference can be recorded until 2 years and should increase by 1 cm per month in the first 3 months, then 0.5 cm per month from 3–6 months. It provides further data about a child's growth. It is important to check the fontanelles. Calculate the BMI from 2 years. The adequacy of a child's growth cannot be assessed on one measurement and serial recordings on growth charts are recommended.

Hips. Screen for congenital dislocation at birth, 6–8 weeks, 6–9 months and 12–24 months (see CHAPTER 65).

The flexed hips are abducted, checking for movement and a 'clunk' of the femoral head forwards (the test is most likely to be positive at 3–6 weeks and usually negative after 8 weeks). Shortening or limited abduction is also abnormal. Ultrasound examination is more sensitive than the clinical examination especially up to 3–4 months. Observe gait when starting to walk.

Strabismus. Strabismus should be sought in all infants and toddlers by occlusion testing (not very sensitive), examining light reflexes and questioning parents, which must be taken very seriously. Amblyopia can be prevented by early recognition and treatment of strabismus by occlusion and surgery. Early referral is essential.

Visual acuity. At birth and 2 months, eyes should be inspected and examined with an ophthalmoscope with a 3+ lens at a distance of 20–30 cm to detect cataracts and red reflexes. At 9 months gross vision should be determined by assessing ability to see common objects. Visual acuity should be formally assessed at school entry using Sheridan Gardiner charts.

Hearing. Hearing should be tested by distraction at 9 months or earlier; also by pure tone audiometry at 1000 and 4000 hertz when a child is 4 years (preschool entry) and 12 years.

Note: Formal audiological evaluation should be carried out at any time if there is clinical suspicion or parental concern. No simple screening test is very reliable for sensorineural or conductive deafness.

Testes. Screen at birth, and 6–8 weeks, 6–9 months and 3 years for absence or maldescent. Those who have been treated for maldescent have a higher risk of neoplastic development in adolescence.

Oral health/dental assessment/fluoride. Advise daily fluoride drops or tablets, if water supply is not fluoridated. Children's teeth should be checked regularly, particularly if a school dental service is not available. Advice should be given on sugar consumption, especially night-time bottles, and tooth cleaning with fluoride toothpaste to prevent plaque.

Scoliosis. Screening of females by the forward flexion test, which is carried out around 12 years of age, is of questionable value because of poor sensitivity and specificity.

Congenital heart disease. The heart should be auscultated at birth, in the first few days, at 6–8 weeks and on school entry.

Femoral pulses. Testing for absence of femoral pulses or delay between brachial/femoral pulses at birth and 8 weeks will exclude coarctation of the aorta. Refer the child immediately if concerned.

Speech and language. A child's speech should be intelligible to strangers by 3 years. It is related to hearing.

General development

Apart from speech and language, check social and emotional development, toilet habits, behaviour and mood.

This includes 'parents' evaluation of developmental status' (PEDS) (see www.pedstest.com; www.rch.org.au/ccch).

For general checklists, see www.cdc.gov/actearly. Be alert to the 'red flags' of autism spectrum disorder (see CHAPTER 94).

Screening in the elderly

Refer to CHAPTER 8.

Screening for adults[14]

The following recommendations apply for adults.

Weight. Weight should be recorded at least every few years. Obesity is a major reversible health risk for adults, contributing to many diseases (e.g. heart disease, diabetes, arthritis). Body mass index (BMI) should ideally be between 20 and 25.

$$\text{BMI} = \text{weight (kg)} \div \text{height (m}^2\text{)}$$

Abdominal obesity is a major risk factor for adults. The waist:hip circumference ratio is regarded as a useful predictor of cardiac disease. Recommended waist:hip ratios are:

- males <0.9
- females <0.8

Blood pressure. Blood pressure should be recorded at least every 1–2 years on all people 16 years and over. There is no dispute that control of blood pressure results in reduced mortality from cerebrovascular accidents and, to a lesser extent, heart disease, kidney failure and retinopathy.

Cholesterol. All adults aged 45 and over should have a 5-yearly estimation of serum cholesterol. Total cholesterol is adequate for screening purposes. HDL levels give additional information. The National Heart Foundation recommends keeping cholesterol levels below 4.0 mmol/L. For most, dietary modification is sufficient to achieve these levels; some may require drug treatment.

Fasting blood glucose. Screen every 3 years for all patients >40 years of age.

Cervical cancer. From age 25 (to age 74), women who have ever been sexually active should commence cervical screening with a HPV test 2 years after their last Pap test. If negative, this can be performed every 5 years. If positive, cervical cytology will be checked with the sample and follow-up is determined according to the national guidelines. Women aged 70–74 should be offered a final 'exit test' and can cease screening if negative.

Breast cancer. Mammography should be performed at least every 2 years on women aged 50–74 years. It is not useful for screening prior to age 40 years due to difficulty in discriminating malignant lesions from dense tissue. Women aged 40–49 years may also choose to have a mammogram.[14] Mammography must not be used alone to exclude cancer if a lump is palpable. Such lesions require a complete appraisal since, even in the best hands, mammography still has a false-negative rate of at least 10%. Genetic testing should be considered in those at risk.

Colorectal cancer (CRC). A history should be taken, with specific enquiry as to family history of adenomas or colorectal cancer, past history of inflammatory bowel disease and rectal bleeding. Rectal examination should be performed as part of an examination. Faecal occult blood testing (FOBT) every 2 years is now recommended for screening for people over 50 years without symptoms and with average or slightly above average risk.

Should a positive history be elicited, then the following are recommended:

- past history of large bowel cancer or colonic adenomas—colonoscopy
- past or present history of ulcerative colitis—colonoscopy with biopsies
- familial polyposis, Gardner syndrome—sigmoidoscopy or colonoscopy

Prophylactic colectomy needs consideration in some individuals.

Apart from FOBT screening, the National Health and Medical Research Council (NHMRC) currently recommends 2-yearly colonoscopy for people from 25–30 years of age if there is a family history on the same side of the family of:

- three or more first or second degree relatives with CRC at any age
- two or more first or second degree relatives diagnosed as CRC <50 years of age
- a family member where genetic studies identify a high risk

Refer to the RACGP *Guidelines for Preventive Activities in General Practice*[14] for further information. Genetic testing should be considered in those at risk.

Prostate cancer. Screening is controversial. The RACGP guidelines do not recommend routine screening with DRE, PSA or transabdominal ultrasound. Patients should make their own decision after being fully informed of the potential benefits, risks and uncertainties of testing. Doctors should also use their clinical judgment for their individual male patients.

Skin cancer. All patients should be informed regularly about the need for protection of the skin and eyes from ultraviolet (UV) radiation, using hats, clothing, sunglasses and sunscreens, and avoiding exposure during peak UV periods (10 am to 3 pm).

Skin cancer, which is increasing in incidence, is common in Australia, particularly in more northern areas. Squamous cell carcinoma, and melanoma in particular, may be lethal. Detection and treatment of early lesions prevents mortality and morbidity. Prevention of skin cancer by reduction of sun exposure should be taught to all patients.

Oral hygiene/cancer. Patients should be counselled about cessation of smoking and alcohol consumption, and dental hygiene should be taught. The oral cavity should be inspected annually in patients over the age of 40 years.

Although oral cancer has a relatively low incidence, premalignant lesions may be detected by inspection of the oral cavity. Its incidence is highest in elderly people with a history of heavy smoking or drinking. Poor dental hygiene may result in poor nutrition, particularly among the elderly.

9

Cancer screening in summary[14]

- Screen for breast, cervical and colorectal cancer.
- Routine population-based screening is at this stage of evidence not recommended for lung, melanoma, ovarian, prostate and testicular cancers.

Immunisation

Children and adolescents should be immunised according to the current NHMRC recommended standard vaccination schedule (www.immunise.health.gov.au).

The NHMRC advises administering intramuscular and subcutaneous vaccines to the anterolateral thighs for children under 12 months, and to the deltoid region in older children and adults. Do not postpone immunisation for minor illnesses such as mild URTI.

All adults should receive an adult diphtheria and tetanus (ADT) booster every 10 years.

All women of child-bearing years should have their rubella antibody status reviewed. During pregnancy, it is recommended to have the seasonal influenza vaccination any time in the pregnancy and a pertussis booster in the final trimester.

Table 9.4 National Immunisation Program Schedule[15] (as from 2018)

Age	Immunisation
Birth	Hepatitis B
2 months	DTP, Hib, hepatitis B, polio, pneumococcus, rotavirus
4 months	DTP, Hib, hepatitis B, polio, pneumococcus, rotavirus
6 months	DTP, polio, Hib and hepatitis B
12 months	Measles/mumps/rubella (MMR), pneumococcus, meningococcal ACWY
18 months	DTP, varicella, measles, mumps, rubella (MMR), Hib
4 years	DTP, polio
School programs 10–15 years (contact state authorities)	HPV, DTP (adult), meningococcal ACWY, hepatitis B (if no first course)
From 65 years	Influenza (yearly), pneumococcal polysacharide (23vPPV)
70–79 years	Herpes zoster

Hib = Haemophilas influenza type b

HPV = human papilloma virus

DTP (triple antigen) = diphtheria, tetanus, pertussis

Note: Aboriginal and Torres Strait Islanders (ATSIP) and other at-risk groups have further recommended immunisations, including influenza, pneumococcus and hepatitis A.

Adverse effects of vaccination

Common adverse effects are irritability, malaise, fever and a local reaction to the injection. There is a very small risk of anaphylaxis. It is advisable to wait 15–30 minutes for observation after vaccination. Paracetamol is recommended for fever and local pain; however, routine use at the time of or immediately after vaccination is not recommended.[15]

Fever and illness. Children with minor illness (providing the temperature is <38.0ºC) may be vaccinated safely. Otherwise it should be delayed. A simple past febrile convulsion or pre-existing neurological disease is not a contraindication to pertussis vaccination. Absolute contraindications include encephalopathy within 7 days of a previous DTP or an immediate severe or anaphylactic reaction to DTP.

The case for vaccines

Influenza. The population needs to be immunised against this ever severe and constantly mutating endemic infection. Influenza immunisation is recommended on an annual basis for persons of all ages with chronic debilitating diseases, especially chronic cardiac, pulmonary, kidney and metabolic diseases, persons over 65 years of age, Indigenous Australian adults over 50 years of age and persons receiving immunosuppressant therapy. Health care personnel may wish to consider it for their own use.

Pneumococcal disease. This should be considered for the same risk groups as influenza vaccine. Those at higher risk of fatal pneumococcal infection (e.g. post-splenectomy or Hodgkin lymphoma), should receive a booster every 5 years. This is currently provided for all children.

Hepatitis A. Immunisation is recommended for:

- certain occupational groups at risk (e.g. health workers, child care workers, sewage workers)
- non-immune homosexual men
- those with chronic liver disease
- recipients of blood products
- travellers to hepatitis A-endemic areas

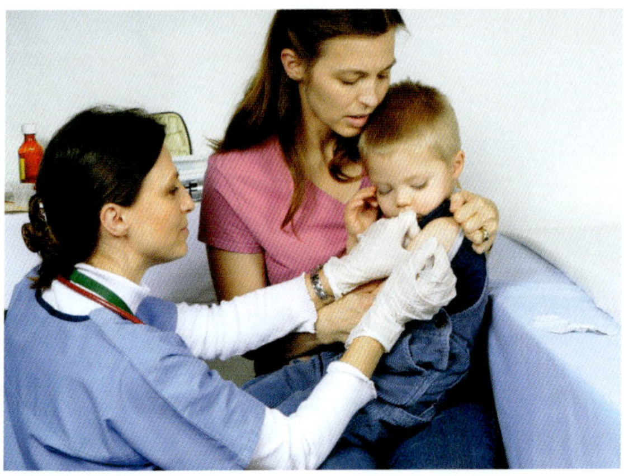

FIGURE 9.2 Immunisation of an older child: important continuing preventive care

Hepatitis B. Immunisation is recommended routinely for all children at birth, 2 months, 4 months and at either 6 or 12 months, and for individuals of all ages who, through work or lifestyle, may be exposed to hepatitis B and have been shown to be susceptible. Such groups would include health care personnel, personnel and residents of institutions, prisoners and prison staff, persons with frequent and/or close contact with high-risk groups, and persons at increased risk due to their sexual practices. Household contacts of any of the above groups should be considered for immunisation. Booster doses are not recommended for immunocompetent people but are recommended for immunosuppressed individuals. Universal vaccination represents a preventive step against hepatocellular cancer.

Haemophilus influenza type b. Hib immunisation is recommended for all children, especially those in child care. It is ideal to achieve immunity by the age of 18 months and preferably commencing at 2 months. Risk factors for Hib disease include day care attendance, presence of ill siblings under 6 years of age in the home and household crowding.

Q fever. People at reasonable risk from Q fever, particularly abattoir workers, should be given this vaccine, which is virtually 100% effective.

Measles-mumps-rubella. Both females and males should be immunised against measles, mumps and rubella at the age of 12 months and 4–5 years using the trivalent vaccine. All non-immune women who are postpartum or of child-bearing age should be immunised.

Varicella vaccine. This is available and one dose is given at 18 months. Those over 12 years have a course of two injections.

Meningococcal vaccine. Meningococcal disease is caused by *Neisseria meningitides,* which has 13 serogroups of which A, B and C account for over 90% of isolated cases, with serogroup B responsible for most cases. A vaccine against serogroup B is available but not yet as part of the recommended schedule as evaluation studies are being assessed. The main vaccine that is available is a quadrivalent polysaccharide vaccine against serogroups A, C, Y and W125 for use in individuals over 2 years as a single injection. Universal prevention by immunisation remains unsatisfactory. It is most useful when a community outbreak due to proven serogroup C occurs.

Rotavirus. A course of two (usually) or three oral live attenuated rotavirus vaccines is given to children to cover a common cause of childhood gastroenteritis. Inform parents of the risk of intussusception with the first dose.

Human papilloma virus. A course of two injections is provided by schools to all pupils aged 11–12 years.

Neonatal screening

Blood from a heel prick at 48–72 hours following birth checks 25 conditions including cystic fibrosis, phenyloketonuria and hypothyroidism.

Genetic screening

Genetic screening programs are presented in CHAPTER 18.

Key checkpoints

- Leading risk factors contributing to the burden of disease in Australia are tobacco, hypertension, excess weight/obesity, physical inactivity, hypercholesterolaemia, alcohol, and low fruit and vegetable consumption.
- Studies in the US conclude that healthy lifestyle consists of not smoking, BMI <30 kg/m2, five servings of fruit and vegetables a day, and about 150 minutes of exercise each week.

Resource

Australian Government. Australian Institute of Health and Welfare, 3 February 2017, Cat. No. OAN 100.

References

1 Silagy C. Prevention in general practice. In: McNeil J et al. (eds), *A Textbook of Preventive Medicine*, Melbourne: Edward Arnold, 1990: 269–77.

2 Piterman L, Sommer SJ. *Preventive Care.* Melbourne: Monash University, Department of Community Medicine, Final Year Handbook, 1993: 75–85.

3 Australian Bureau of Statistics. Commonwealth of Australia, Canberra, 2015 (<www.abs.gov.au/aus>, see Statistics).

4 Egger G, Spark R, Donovan L. *Health Promotion Strategies and Method.* Sydney, McGraw-Hill; 2013: 8.

5 Locke FB, King H. Cancer mortality risk among Japanese in the United States. National Cancer Institute, 1980; 65: 1149.

6 Potter JD, McMichael AJ. Diet and cancer of the colon and rectum: a case control study. National Cancer Institute, 1986; 76: 557–69.

7 Rakel RE, Rakel D. *Textbook of Family Medicine 9th edn.* Philadelphia. Elsevier. Saunders, 2016: 87–105.

8 Editorial. Position of the American Dietetic Association: photochemicals and functional foods. J Am Diet Assoc, 1993; 93: 493–6.

9 Doll R, Peto R. *The Causes of Cancer.* New York: Oxford University Press, 1981: 1197–219.

10 Sali A. Strategies for cancer prevention. Aust Fam Physician, 1987; 16: 1603–13.

11 Bury R. *Clinical Application of Antioxidant Nutrients. Melbourne:* Department of Human Services, 1996; 26.

12 Antic R. *Report on the Cost of Asthma in Australia.* Melbourne: National Asthma Campaign, 1992: 14–33.

13 Sridhar MK. Editorial. Nutrition and lung health. BMJ, 1995; 310: 75–6.

14 Royal Australian College of General Practitioners. *Guidelines for Preventive Activities in General Practice* (9th edn). Melbourne: RACGP, 2016.

15 Australian Government. National Health and Medical Research Council, Canberra. *The Australian Immunisation Handbook* (10th edn), 2015.

Nutrition in health and illness

10

On the 20th of May 1747 on board the Salisbury *at sea I took 12 patients in the scurvy with putrid gums, the spots and lassitude and weakness of their knees. They had a common diet—two were ordered a quart of cyder a day—two, elixir vitriol three times a day—two, 2 spoonfuls of vinegar three times a day—two were put on a course of sea water—two had 2 oranges and one lemon each day—two, nutmeg, garlic and other additives to barley water. The consequence was, that the most sudden and visible good effects were perceived from the use of the oranges and lemons with one being at the end of 6 days fit for duty.*

JAMES LIND 1747, *A (SUMMARISED) ACCOUNT OF SCURVY*

Good nutrition is fundamental to good health. It influences management in all branches of medicine. Modern people's health varies from the excesses of inappropriate nutrition, resulting in obesity and various degenerative disorders, to malnutrition and other deficiency states seen in those unfortunates deprived of nutrients.

The essential components of nutrition[1] can be classified as:

- macronutrients—proteins, fats and carbohydrates, which are interchangeable sources of energy and also water
- macrominerals—sodium, chloride, potassium, calcium, phosphate and magnesium
- micronutrients—water-soluble vitamins (e.g. C, B); fat-soluble vitamins (e.g. A, E, K); essential trace elements (e.g. copper, iodine, iron, zinc)

Nutritional factors may play a vital role in the causation of several of the major diseases, such as coronary artery disease, hypertension, diabetes and cancer.

Special diets are important in the management of many hereditary metabolic disorders, such as phenylketonuria and galactosaemia, and several other disorders such as coeliac disease.

Protein[2]

Proteins are composed of carbon, hydrogen, oxygen, nitrogen, phosphorus, sulphur and iron. They make up the greater part of plant and animal tissue and provide the amino acids essential for the growth and repair of tissue. Protein in the body in muscle, connective tissue and enzymes is constantly being broken down, while dietary protein is hydrolysed to amino acids that are both essential and non-essential. A complete protein is one that contains all the nine indispensable amino acids, namely, histidine, isoleucine, leucine, lysine, methionine, phenylalanine, threonine, tryptophan and valine.

Protein in animal products (fish, meat and milk) is of high quality and that in vegetable products is lower because of a limited supply of lysine (in cereals) and methionine and cysteine (in legumes).[3] Vegetarian diets are usually adequate in protein, especially if the combining vegetable groups complement each other in basic amino acid groups. Diets that exclude all animal products may be inadequate, especially in children. Infants and children require 2–2.2 g protein/kg/day.

- High protein content foods—lean beef and lamb, chicken, fish, eggs, milk, cheese, soy beans
- Medium protein content foods—bread, spaghetti, corn, potatoes (cooked), rice (cooked), cabbage, cauliflower

Protein

Energy malnutrition

This is a deficiency syndrome with a reduction in all macronutrients, energy (kilojoules) and many micronutrients due to an inadequate intake of protein and energy foodstuffs.

It is commonly found in infants and children in developing countries but can occur in persons of any age in any country.

Clinically, protein-energy malnutrition has three forms:

1. dry (thin, desiccated)—*marasmus*
2. wet (oedematous, swollen)—*kwashiorkor*
3. combined—*marasmic kwashiorkor*

Marasmus

Clinical features:

- grossly underweight
- gross muscle wasting
- abdominal distension
- no fat
- hungry
- 'old man's' face
- no oedema
- normal hair

Caused by a diet low in protein and calories.

Kwashiorkor

Clinical features:

- oedema (feet first then generalised)
- 'moon' face
- anorexia
- hair pale and thinned
- apathetic
- skin changes

Caused by a diet low in protein with some carbohydrate, leading to hypoalbuminaemia.

Carbohydrates

Dietary carbohydrates include simple sugars, complex carbohydrates (starches) and indigestible carbohydrate (dietary fibre). Carbohydrates are the main source of dietary energy. The two most important crops feeding the world are rice and wheat, which are rich in starch. Starch and sucrose account for the majority of carbohydrates consumed in all diets. Carbohydrates that are available in food are:

- sugars—sucrose, lactose, maltose, glucose, fructose
- polyols—sorbitol, xylitol, maltilol, lactilol
- starch—amylose, amylopectin
- dextrose

As long as adequate energy and protein are provided in the diet, there is no specific requirement for dietary carbohydrate. A small amount—100 g/day—is necessary to prevent ketosis.[3]

The glycaemic index (GI)

The GI, which applies to carbohydrate foods, is a numerical index based on a reference point of 100. It is a measure of the capacity to increase postprandial glucose levels compared to a glucose load. The standard food is glucose, which is given an arbitrary level of 100.

The higher the GI, then the higher the rise in blood glucose level and thus the greater the insulin response. Low-GI foods may improve glycaemic control.

Low-GI foods (<55) include dense wholegrain breads, porridge, most fresh fruits, yogurt and low-fat milk. High-GI foods (>70) include sweet breakfast cereals, potatoes, white bread, watermelon, ripe bananas, dates, white rice and biscuits.

Fat

Dietary fat, which is composed mainly of fatty acids and dietary cholesterol, is the most concentrated source of food energy.[2]

Fatty acids are classified according to the number of unsaturated double bonds:

- nil—saturated (e.g. butyric and stearic acids)
- one—monounsaturated (e.g. oleic acid)
- more than one—polyunsaturated (e.g. linoleic acid, eicosapentanoic acid [EPA], docosahexanoic acid [DHA])

Polyunsaturated fatty acids (two or more unsaturated bonds) can be subdivided into:

- n-6 (e.g. linoleic acid, 2 unsaturated bonds; arachidonic acid, 4 unsaturated bonds)
- n-3—omega-3 fatty acids (e.g. alpha-linolenic acid, 3 unsaturated bonds; EPA, 5 unsaturated bonds; DHA, 6 unsaturated bonds)

The n-3 and n-6 polyunsaturated fatty acids with chain lengths of 18 or more are called essential fatty acids because they are required for vital body functions and animals, including humans, are unable to synthesise them.[2]

The proportions of saturated, monounsaturated and polyunsaturated fatty acids in the diet are important determinants of health and disease.[2] The current strategy is to reduce total fat intake and reduce saturated fats and increase unsaturated fats, especially n-3 polyunsaturated fats.

Fish oil contains omega-3 fatty acids, which are considered more potent than the omega-3 fatty acids found in plants. The value of omega-3 fatty acids in preventing cardiovascular mortality has been well proven. They have no effect on cholesterol levels but have a well-documented potent hypotriglyceridaemic effect.[4]

Cholesterol, which is a major constituent of cell membranes, is synthesised by the body and is not an essential nutrient. The plasma cholesterol level, and hence the amount of cholesterol in the diet, has been related to the development of atherosclerosis.

However, other factors are related to the development and prevention of atherosclerosis. In the past decade, specific nutrients, especially plant sterols (phytosterols), soy protein and soluble fibre, have been shown to improve the plasma cholesterol profile, which has led to their appropriate inclusion in 'designer' foods targeting the health-conscious consumer market.[4]

Nutritional assessment

The first step in nutritional assessment is to identify the high-risk patient.[5] Those at high risk of nutritional insufficiency include those with a history of obesity, eating disorders, chronic illness, psychological disorders, the elderly, the institutionalised, trauma victims and those with long periods of hospitalisation, including major surgery. Of particular interest is the rate of growth and development in infants and children and the body composition in children and adults.

When taking the history it is appropriate to include a 24-hour recall of foods eaten and ideally get the patient to complete a symptom questionnaire that can then be linked to a computerised nutritional evaluation program, such as Nutricheck.[5] Evaluate sunlight exposure.

A nutritionally focused physical examination should be performed on each patient at risk, with the emphasis on body weight, waist size, muscle wasting, fat stores and signs of micronutrient deficiencies. Examples of the latter include zinc deficiency, which affects taste and smell and the skin. Deficiencies of vitamins B6 and B12 cause neurological disorders, such as peripheral neuropathy.[2] Alcoholism and malnutrition affect many systems, including the gastrointestinal system. The oral cavity, especially the gums, teeth and buccal mucosa, are affected by vitamin B complex and vitamin C deficiencies. Bones and joints are affected in scurvy, rickets, osteomalacia and osteoporosis. The important anthropometric measurements include height and weight, skin-fold thickness and waist:hip circumference ratio (refer to CHAPTER 78). Laboratory investigations depend on the clinical examination and should be selective.

The general principles of optimal nutrition

In order to help people make healthy choices, the health foundations of several countries have developed recommendations for eating a healthy diet.

The heart-healthy eating pyramid of the Australian Nutrition Foundation (2012)[2] has a simplified system, namely:

- Eat most—vegetables, dried peas, beans and lentils, cereals, bread, fruit and nuts
- Eat moderately—lean meat, eggs, fish, chicken (without skin), milk, yoghurt, cheese
- Eat in small amounts—oil, margarine, reduced-fat spreads, butter, sugar

The RACGP in its red book[6] outlines dietary recommendations based on national guidelines. For adults this is summarised as follows.

Enjoy a wide variety of foods each day:

- five serves of vegetables and two serves of fruit
- lean meat, fish, poultry, eggs, tofu, nuts and seeds and/or alternatives
- grains and cereals, mostly wholegrain or high-fibre varieties such as bread, rice, pasta, oats and couscous
- drink plenty of water

Take care to:

- limit saturated fat
- limit salt intake
- limit alcohol intake
- limit sugars and foods containing added sugars, including soft drinks and commercial juice
- limit red meat to 3–4 serves per week and limit or avoid processed meat
- care for food: prepare and store it safely
- encourage and support breastfeeding

What is a serving?[2]

The following guides represent one serve:

Milk and milk products group	1 cup (300 mL) milk 200 g yoghurt 40 g cheese (2 slices)
Meat group	60–100 g cooked lean meat, poultry or fish 2 small eggs 1 cup cooked or canned legumes
Vegetable group	1 cup raw leafy vegetables ½ cup other green or orange vegetables (cooked or raw) 1/2 medium potato or sweet potato
Fruit group	1 medium apple, banana, orange, pear 2 small apricots or plums ½ cup fruit juice (no added sugar) 1 cup chopped, cooked or canned fruit (no added sugar) ¼ medium melon

Note: a serve is a measured unit while a portion is what is actually eaten, e.g. 1, 2 or 3 serves.

The Lyon Heart Study[7]

This very impressive prospective, randomised, single-blinded, secondary prevention trial investigated the effects of a 'Mediterranean'-type diet containing a plant oil rich in omega-3 fatty acids on 605 subjects who had survived their first heart attack. The control group were given a low-cholesterol diet with a mix of unsaturated fats. The intervention group had a diet higher in oleic acid, omega-3 fatty acid, fibre and vitamin C (olive and canola oils were used in food preparation). In this group, the cardiovascular mortality was reduced by 73%. This was far greater than the control group and also for groups taking lipid-lowering agents, and the benefit was independent of any reduction in cholesterol or triglycerides. One explanation is that the antioxidants and phytochemicals in the plant-based diet stabilise the endothelium of arteries.

Some consequent lessons for people with a high-lipid profile are:[4,7]

- Eat more fish—at least 2–3 times a week.
- Switch to skim-based dairy products—low-fat milk and yoghurts.
- Eat plenty of fruit, vegetables, nuts and grain food.
- Use monounsaturated (olive) oils and perhaps margarine instead of butter. However, use these cooking oils lightly.
- Use alternative toast spreads, e.g. hummus, baked beans, lentils, salmon.
- Limit intake of dietary cholesterol (less than 300 mg/day). Eat less animal-based food, dairy products, eggs (limit two a week), saturated fats, bakery food, fast food.

Antioxidants

The antioxidant issue is still controversial and unclear. Empirical observation of healthy communities over the years indicates good health outcomes, especially with cardiovascular status, in people having an optimal diet containing high levels of vitamins and minerals (especially from fruit and vegetables).

Food antioxidants (see TABLE 10.1) appear to protect against free radicals, which can suppress immunity.

Prime sources of antioxidants in food[9]

- Vitamin C—citrus fruits, berries, papaya, green leafy vegetables
- Vitamin E—seed-like cereal grains, nuts and oils (plants), eggs

Table 10.1 Food antioxidants

Vitamin A, especially beta-carotene
Vitamin C
Vitamin E
Ubidecarenone (co-enzyme Q10)
Selenium, zinc, manganese and copper (nutrient cofactors)

Source: After Sali[8]

- Beta-carotene—orange-coloured and dark-green leafy vegetables
- Selenium—grains, meats, Brazil nuts, fish
- Copper—cocoa, wheat bran, yeast
- Ubiquinone—meats, fish, peanuts
- Phytochemicals—soy, tea, green tea, herbs, apples, onions, cocoa

Folate-containing foods

- Green leafy vegetables—broccoli, spinach
- Wheat grain
- Wholegrain cereals
- Starchy beans—kidney and butter
- Peas, corn, cauliflower
- Nuts
- Avocado
- Liver
- Folic acid fortified foods (e.g. breakfast cereals)

Vitamin deficiency disorders[10]

These are rare in our society but can occur sporadically and are not rare in children in some third world countries or in refugees from these countries. Deficiencies tend to be seen as a specific disorder or as a multivitamin effect.

- *Vitamin A (beta-carotene/retinol)* deficiency causes night blindness and eye disease, as well as dryness with keratinisation of the conjunctivae and cornea. It causes growth retardation in children. Toxicity from overdosage of vitamin A is a serious problem.
- *Vitamin B complex*
  - *Vitamin B1 (thiamine)* deficiency causes **beriberi** and also Wernicke–Korsakoff syndrome (typically in alcoholics).
  - *Vitamin B2 (riboflavin)* deficiency causes growth retardation, dry scaly skin and angular cheilitis.

- *Vitamin B3 (niacin, nicotinic acid)* deficiency causes **pellagra.**
- *Vitamin B6 (pyridoxine)* deficiency may cause oral soreness, anaemia and CNS dysfunction.
- *Vitamin B12 (cobalamin)* deficiency causes **pernicious anaemia** and memory dysfunction.

- *Vitamin C (ascorbic acid)* deficiency is responsible for **scurvy.** Clinical features: weakness, malaise, fatigue, bleeding swollen inflamed gums, atraumatic haemarthrosis, impaired wound healing, impaired bone growth. One sign is the hyperkeratotic hair follicle with surrounding hyperaemia. Diagnosis by decreased plasma ascorbic acid and X-rays of bones and joints.
- *Vitamin D (calciferols)* deficiency causes **rickets** in children and **osteomalacia** in adults. Clinical features (rickets): impaired growth, skeletal deformities (bow legs, pelvis, 'rachitic rosary'), inability to walk, bone pain (arms, legs, spine, pelvis), dental deformities, muscle weakness. In adults: muscle weakness, bone pain, bowing of long bones. Diagnosis: low plasma $25(OH)D_3$ and phosphate; elevated PTH and alkaline phosphatase; X-rays of joints and long bones of leg.
- *Vitamin E (tocopherol)* deficiency causes no specific disease but may result in vague, undifferentiated symptoms and anaemia.
- *Vitamin K (phylloquinone)* deficiency is rare and can lead to an increased bleeding tendency.
- *Folic acid* deficiency is responsible for pernicious anaemia and neural tube defects in the fetus.

Gout

Certain foods can aggravate gout. These include:

- tinned fish (e.g. sardines, anchovies)
- organ meats (e.g. liver, pancreas, brain, kidney)
- alcohol (the major one)
- fizzy, sugary soft drinks

Gout often occurs in males after they binge drink in their late 20s or 30s. Beer is particularly problematic. It is useful to recommend an increase in water consumption. Since gout and hyperuricaemia have a proven association with coronary artery disease, a healthy heart prevention diet is advisable.

Dietary control of diabetes

Diabetes is an endemic problem in many communities, particularly in Indigenous communities. It is thought that for every two people diagnosed with diabetes, there may be one who is not diagnosed. Prevention of diabetes is very important and diet can play a significant role in this.

As many as 30% of people who suffer from diabetes are now taking insulin and oral hypoglycaemic medications. However, if sufferers can maintain an ideal weight and control symptoms through diet, the need for medications is reduced. Exercise is also very important.

Dietary principles for preventing and control of diabetes include:

- Follow the healthy eating guidelines, especially in regard to fruit and vegetable intake.
- Keep to an ideal weight.
- Eat low-GI foods.
- Limit the consumption of fat and fatty products.
- Eat high-fibre, complex carbohydrates, such as starchy fibre foods, cereals and wholemeal bread.
- Avoid or limit simple carbohydrates (e.g. sugar, concentrated sweets).
- Spread the consumption of carbohydrates throughout the day.
- Make vegetables the main part of your diet.

In summary, the diet for both type 1 and type 2 diabetes is based on achieving ideal weight and following a diet of high-fibre carbohydrates with a low GI and low fat.

Obesity

Refer to CHAPTER 78 for information on management of obesity.

Anaemia and iron

Iron-deficiency anaemia is a common problem in our society, particularly in children from 6 months to 2 years who have been given a lot of cow's milk. In such cases it is important to educate people about iron-rich foods and the quantities they need (see CHAPTER 22).

Guidelines for safe consumption of alcohol (current NHMRC recommendations)[11]

Healthy males and females

- No more than two standard drinks per day
- No more than four standard drinks on any single occasion

Young people

- People aged under 15 years should avoid alcohol altogether.
- People aged 15–17 years should delay drinking for as long as possible.

Pregnancy and breastfeeding

- No alcohol is the safest option.

Refer to CHAPTERS 21 and 108 for alcohol guidelines.

Coeliac disease

Coeliac disease occurs as a result of sensitivity to gluten. It is quite common and often undiagnosed. In some cases, it can occur after a bout of gastroenteritis. It can be treated with a gluten-free diet.

- For breakfast, exclude wheat, barley, oats and rye.
- Any food containing gluten (e.g. flour and bread) should be avoided.
- Any food containing hidden ingredients (e.g. stock cubes) should be avoided.

Foods associated with migraine

Common ones include:

- wine, particularly red wine
- cheese
- oranges
- tomatoes
- caffeine in some people

Other culprit foods might include amine-rich foods, such as bananas and avocados. It is helpful to ask patients to keep a diary to see if they can find links between what they eat and their migraine attacks. Some varieties of migraine are not linked to diet.

Nutrition and chronic simple constipation

Important advice for treatment of constipation includes:

- Drink a lot of fluids, especially water and fruit juices.
- Eat foods with bulk and roughage (e.g. bran, fresh and dried fruits and wholemeal bread).

Foods that are high in roughage include (in order):

- bran
- carrots
- apples
- lettuce
- cabbage
- peas
- cauliflower
- bananas
- potatoes

Fruits are high in fibre and some are natural laxatives, such as:

- prunes
- figs
- rhubarb
- apricots
- pears

Studies show that most people do not eat enough fruit. According to a recent survey of Victorian schoolchildren, one-third did not have fruit during the day, one-third did have fruit and one-third only had it spasmodically.

Recurrent urinary calculi

The dietary advice for recurrent urinary calculi (CHAPTER 34) includes:

1. Drink at least 2 L of water every day, or more if there is increased fluid loss: this is the most important step.
2. Minimise consumption of foods that contain oxalate or uric acid. Foods that contain oxalate include:
   - chocolate
   - coffee
   - cola and similar 'soft' drinks
   - rhubarb
   - tea

   Foods that contain uric acid include:
   - beer
   - red wine
   - red meat
   - organ meats
3. Avoid milk in tea—calcium precipitates oxalate.
4. Avoid processed meats, organ meats (e.g. brain, kidney, liver and sweetbread), yeast spreads and other high-salt foods. Restrict salt intake.
5. Reduce animal protein consumption: restrict to one major meat meal a day (includes chicken and fish).
6. Add citrate-containing fruit juices to the diet, including grapefruit, apple and orange juice.
7. Eat a healthy diet of vegetables and fruit with a high fibre content.

Iodine deficiency

The body needs small amounts of iodine to maintain normal function of the thyroid gland—crucial for normal growth and development. In iodine-deficient areas (in soil and water) there is a high rate of stillbirths, congenital hypothyroidism and cretinism. In adults, deficiency causes goitre and hypothyroidism. The usual intake of iodine in healthy persons is 100–200 mcg day, mostly from iodised salt. An adequate intake is 150 mcg/day with higher requirements for pregnancy (220 mcg) and breastfeeding (290 mcg).[12] Measurement is by urinary iodine levels (WHO replete level standard ≥100 mcg/L and ≥150 mcg/L in pregnancy[12]).

Dietary guidelines for children and adolescents in Australia (NHMRC)[11]

(See www.nhmrc.gov.au)
Encourage and support breastfeeding.
Children and adolescents need sufficient nutritious foods to grow and develop normally.

- Growth should he checked regularly for young children.
- Physical activity is important for all children and adolescents.

Enjoy a wide variety of nutritious foods.
Children and adolescents should be encouraged to:

- eat plenty of vegetables, legumes and fruits
- eat plenty of cereals (including breads, rice, pasta and noodles), preferably wholegrain
- include lean meat, fish, poultry and/or alternatives
- include milks, yoghurts, cheese and/or alternatives

Reduced-fat milks are not suitable for young children under 2 years, because of their high energy needs, but reduced-fat varieties should be encouraged for older children and adolescents.

- Choose water as a drink

Alcohol is not recommended for children.
In addition, care should be taken to:

- limit saturated fat and moderate total fat intake
  - low-fat diets are not suitable for infants
- choose foods low in salt
- consume only moderate amounts of sugars and foods containing added sugars

Care for your child's food: prepare and store it safely.

Dietary guidelines for Australian adults (NHMRC)

(See www.nhmrc.gov.au)
Enjoy a wide variety of nutritious foods.

- Eat plenty of vegetables, legumes and fruits.
- Eat plenty of cereals (including breads, rice, pasta and noodles), preferably wholegrain.
- Include lean meat, fish, poultry and/or alternatives.
- Include milks, yoghurts, cheeses and/or alternatives. Reduced-fat varieties should be chosen, where possible.
- Drink plenty of water.

Also, take care to:

- limit saturated fat and moderate total fat intake
- choose foods low in salt
- limit your alcohol intake if you choose to drink
- consume only moderate amounts of sugars and foods containing added sugars.

Prevent weight gain:

- Be physically active and eat according to your energy needs.

Care for your food: prepare and store it safely.

Summary of general dietary guidelines for good health

- Keep to an ideal weight.
- Eat a high-fibre diet.
- Eat more fruits and vegetables, least-processed breads and cereals, preferably wholegrain.
- Eat fish at least twice a week (daily if possible).
- Choose a nutritious diet.
- Eat less saturated fat, refined sugar and salt.
- Use low-fat dairy products—milk and yoghurt.
- Avoid fast foods and deep-fried foods.
- Do not eat animal meat every day, and then only in small portions. Note that processed meats, such as sausages, have a very high fat content.
- Use monounsaturated (olive) oils and perhaps margarine instead of butter.
- Use olive oil for cooking rather than polyunsaturated oils.
- Always trim fat off meat.
- Limit alcohol intake to 2 standard drinks per day.
- Drink more water.
- Limit salt intake; pepper is okay.
- Limit caffeine intake (0–3 drinks a day maximum).

continued

continued

- Check plasma cholesterol level and, if it is elevated, aim to reduce it with diet.
- The appropriate diet is a low-carbohydrate, healthy-fat, mediterranean-based diet.

Patient education resources

Murtagh's Patient Education 7th edition:

- Diet guidelines for good health

Resource

American Society for Nutrition. <https://nutrition.org>

References

1 Porter RS, Kaplan JL. *The Merck Manual of Diagnoses and Therapy* (19th edn). New Jersey: Merck Research Laboratories, 2011: 2–7.
2 Wahlqvist ML. *Food and Nutrition.* Sydney: Allen & Unwin, 1997.
3 Crimmins B. *Nutrition.* Check Program 391. Melbourne: RACGP, 2004; 391: 1–30.
4 Howe P. Nutrition and cardiovascular risk. Medical Observer, 2001; 16 November: 36–7.
5 Sydney-Smith M. Nutritional assessment. Current Therapeutics, 2000; September: 13–22.
6 Royal Australian College of General Practitioners. *Clinical Guidelines for Preventive Activities in General Practice* (9th edn). Melbourne: RACGP, 2016: 73–4.
7 De Lorgeril M, Renaud S, Mamelle S et al. Mediterranean alpha-linoleic acid-rich diet in secondary prevention of coronary heart disease. Lancet, 1994; 343: 1001–29.
8 Sali A. Strategies for cancer prevention. Aust Fam Physician, 1987; 16: 1603–13.
9 Wahlqvist ML, Wattanapenpaiboon N. Antioxidant nutrients. Australian Prescriber, 1999; 22(6): 142–4.
10 Truswell AS. Nutrient supplements. How to treat. Australian Doctor, 2003; 21 March: I–VII.
11 National Health and Medical Research Council. *Australian Dietary Guidelines.* Canberra: Department of Health and Ageing, 2013.
12 Porter RS, Kaplan JL. *The Merck Manual of Diagnosis and Therapy* (19th edn). New Jersey: Merck Research Laboratories, 2011: 53.

Palliative care 11

Death should simply become a discreet but dignified exit of a peaceful person from a helpful society—without pain or suffering and ultimately without fear.

PHILIPPE ARIÈS 1977

To enable a person to live in dignity, peace and comfort throughout their illnesses means responding to physical, psychological, emotional, social and spiritual needs.[1]

E FAIRBANK, T BANKS, *PALLIATIVE CARE: THE NITTY GRITTY HANDBOOK*, 1993

Palliative care is comprehensive, continuing, multidisciplinary patient care that involves the patients and their carers, consultants, domiciliary nurses, social workers, clergy and other health professionals who are able to contribute to optimal team care.

The fundamental principles of palliative care are:[2]

- good communication
- management planning
- symptom control
- emotional, social and spiritual support
- medical counselling and education
- patient involvement in decision making
- support for carers

The diseases

Palliative care applies not only to incurable malignant disease but also to several other diseases, such as end-stage organ failure (heart failure, kidney failure, respiratory failure and hepatic failure) and degenerative neuromuscular diseases. Thirty per cent of the population will die from cancer.

The special role of the family doctor

The GP is the ideal person to manage palliative care for a variety of reasons—availability, knowledge of the patient and family, and the relevant psychosocial influences. A key feature is the ability to provide the patient with independence and dignity by managing palliative care at home. Someone has to take the responsibility for leadership of the team and the most appropriate professional is a trusted family doctor.

Most patients and their families require answers to the following six questions.[3]

- What is wrong?
- What can medical science offer?
- Will I suffer?
- Will you look after me?
- How long will I live?
- Can I be looked after at home?

Caring honesty is the best policy when discussing the answers to these questions with the patient and family. Never lie to a patient and always avoid thoughtless candour.

Support for patients and carers

Studies have indicated that the most common complaints of patients are boredom and fear of the unknown. This highlights the importance for the attending doctor of the following points.

- Give emotional support.
- Listen and be receptive to unexpressed 'messages'.
- Treat the sufferer normally, openly, enthusiastically and confidently.
- Show empathy and compassion.
- Employ good communication skills.
- Give honest answers without labouring the point or giving false hope.
- Provide opportunities for questions and clarification.
- Show an understanding of the patient's needs and culture.
- Adopt a whole-person approach: attend to physical, psychosocial and spiritual needs.
- Anticipate and be prepared for likely problems.

These next special points are worth emphasising.

- The patient needs a feeling of security.
- Provide reassurance that the patient will not suffer unnecessarily.
- Be prepared to take the initiative and call in others who could help (e.g. clergy, cancer support group, massage therapists).

- Patients must not be made to feel isolated or be victims of the so-called 'conspiracy of silence' in which families collude with doctors to withhold information from the patient.
- The worst feeling a dying patient can sense is one of rejection and discomfort on the part of the doctor.
- Always be prepared to refer to an oncologist or appropriate therapist for another opinion about further management. The family and patient appreciate the feeling that every possible avenue is being explored.

Note: Always establish what the patient knows and wants to know.

The Gold Standards Framework (UK)

This framework, which provides an optimal model for palliative care by the primary care team, focuses on seven key tasks:

1. optimal quality of care
2. advanced planning (including out of hours)
3. teamwork
4. symptom control
5. patient support
6. carer support
7. staff support

The strategy has been shown to increase the number of patients dying in their preferred place with improved quality of care.[4]

Symptom control

Common symptoms

- boredom (the commonest symptom)
- loneliness/isolation
- fear/anxiety
- pain
  - physical
  - emotional
  - spiritual
  - social
- anorexia
- nausea and vomiting
- constipation

The grief reaction

This follows five stages, as identified by Kübler-Ross:[5]

1. denial and isolation
2. anger
3. bargaining
4. depression
5. acceptance

This model provides a useful guideline in understanding the stages a patient and family will be experiencing.

The principles of symptom management are summarised in TABLE 11.1. The goals of treatment according to the different stages of cancer are presented in FIGURE 11.1.

11

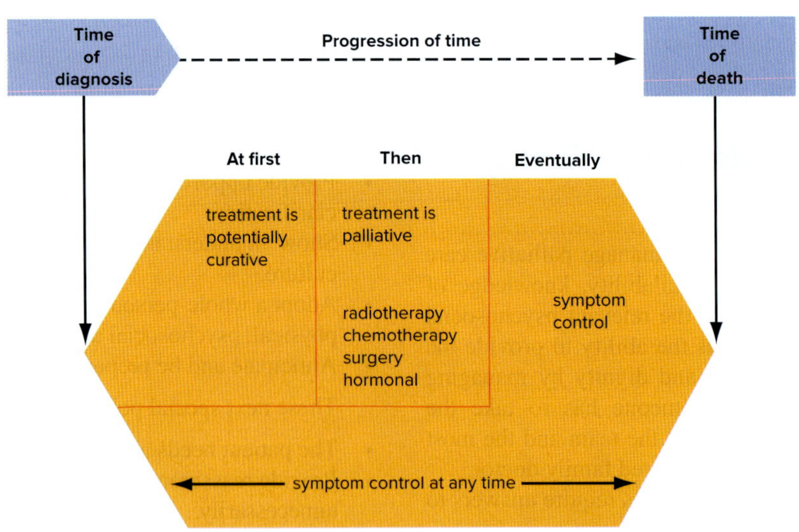

FIGURE 11.1 Stages of cancer management: the goals of treatment differ according to the different stages.
Source: After Buchanan et al.[6]

Table 11.1 Principles of symptom management[2]

Determine the cause.
Treat simply.
Provide appropriate explanation of symptoms and treatment.
Provide regular review.
Give medication regularly around the clock, not ad hoc.
Plan 'breakthrough' pain-relieving doses.
Provide physical treatment as necessary (e.g. paracentesis, pleural tap, nerve block).
Provide complementary conservative therapy (e.g. massage, physiotherapy, occupational therapy, dietary advice, relaxation therapy).
Provide close supervision.

Pain control in cancer

Pain is the commonest, most feared, but generally the most treatable symptom in advanced cancer. Achieving pain relief is one of the most important functions of palliative care and patients need reassurance that they can expect such relief. The principles of relief of cancer pain are:[1]

1 Treat the cancer.
2 Raise the pain threshold:
   - provide appropriate explanation
   - allow the patient to ventilate feelings and concepts
   - give good psychosocial support
   - use antidepressants or hypnotics.

Table 11.2 Treatment options for cancer pain[6,7] (based on aetiology)

Aetiology	1st line treatment	2nd line treatment	Other treatment modalities to consider
Nociceptive pain: stimulation of sensory nerves	Aspirin	Opioids Corticosteroids Antidepressants NSAIDs	Radiotherapy Neurosurgery
Neuropathic pain: direct nerve involvement (e.g. brachialgia, sciatica)	Opioids Antidepressants (e.g. amitriptyline) Antiepileptics (e.g. carbamazepine, gabapentin)		Spinal morphine Local anaesthetic Ketamine
Dysaesthesia: superficial burning pain	Antidepressants	Opioids	Local anaesthetic TENS
Pressure pain: tumour-associated oedema (e.g. raised intracranial pressure)	Corticosteroids (e.g. dexamethasone)	Opioids	Radiotherapy Neurosurgery
Bony metastases and other tissue destruction	NSAIDs Aspirin Paracetamol (if NSAIDs contraindicated) Orphrenadine	Opioids	Radiotherapy (the most effective) Bisphosphonates Hormones Orthopaedic surgery
Muscle spasm pain	Diazepam Clonazepam Baclofen	Opioids Dantrolene	
Viscus (hollow organ) obstruction (e.g. colic, tenesmus)	Antispasmodics (e.g. hyoscine)	Opioids Chlorpromazine Corticosteroids	Palliative surgery Radiotherapy
Metabolic effects: hypercalcaemia	Bisphosphonates (APD)		
Skin infiltration/ulceration	Aspirin Opioids	Corticosteroids	Treat infection Dressings Palliative surgery Radiotherapy

3 Add analgesics according to level of pain, for example, opioids (if necessary).
4 Use specific drugs for specific pain—not all pain responds to analgesics (refer TABLE 11.2).
5 Set realistic goals.
6 Organise supervision of pain control.

Note: The right drug, in the right dose, given at the right time relieves 80–90% of the pain.[1] Reports of the undertreatment of cancer pain persist.

Use of analgesics[7]

The World Health Organization (WHO) analgesic ladder is an appropriate guide for the management of cancer pain (see FIG. 11.2).

These should be given by the clock and administered according to the three-step method.

Step 1: Mild pain

Start with basic non-opioid analgesics:

aspirin 600–900 mg (o) 4 hourly (preferred)
or
paracetamol 1 g (o) 4 hourly or 1.32 g (o) 6–8 hourly ± NSAID (e.g. ibuprofen, celecoxib)

Step 2: Moderate pain

Use low dose or weak opioids (according to age and condition) or in combination with non-opioid analgesics (consider NSAIDs):

add morphine immediate release 5 to 10 mg (o) 4 hourly (2 to 5 mg in elderly)

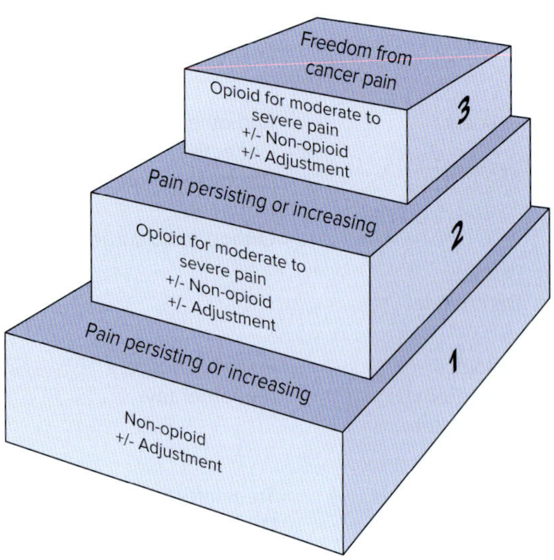

FIGURE 11.2 World Health Organization pain relief ladder

increase in increments of 30–50% up to 15–20 mg
or
tapentadol SR 50 mg (o) bd, can increase to max. 500 mg/day
or
oxycodone 2.5 mg (in elderly) up to 10 mg (o) 4 hourly or CR 10 mg (o) 12 hourly
or
oxycodone 30 mg, rectally, 8 hourly

Step 3: Severe pain

Maintain non-opioid analgesics. Larger doses of opioids should be used and morphine is the drug of choice:

morphine 10–15 mg (o) 4 hourly, increasing to 30 mg if necessary
or
morphine modified release tabs or caps (o) 12 hourly or once daily

- Give dosage according to individual needs (morphine CR/SR comes in 5, 10, 15, 20, 30, 50, 60, 90, 100, 120, 200 mg tablets or capsules).
- The proper dosage is that which is sufficient to alleviate pain.
- The usual starting dose is 20–30 mg bd.
- Give usual morphine 10 mg with first dose of morphine CR/SR and then as necessary for 'rescue dosing'.
- Gauge the probable dose of the long-acting morphine from the standard dosage.
- To convert to morphine CR/SR, calculate the daily oral dose of regular morphine and divide by 2 to get the 12 hourly dose.
- Do not crush or chew the tablets or capsules.
- Review doses after 1–2 days.

Guidelines

- Ensure that pain is likely to be opioid-sensitive.
- Use as few drugs as possible.
- Give morphine orally (e.g. Ordine) (if possible) either by mixture (preferred) or tablets (e.g. Sevredol, Anamorph).
- Starting doses are usually in the range of 5–20 mg (average 10 mg).
- If analgesia is inadequate, the next dose should be increased by 50% until pain control is achieved.
- Give it regularly, usually 4 hourly, before the return of the pain (see FIG. 11.3).
- Many patients find a mixture easier to swallow than tablets (e.g. 10 mg/10 mL solution).

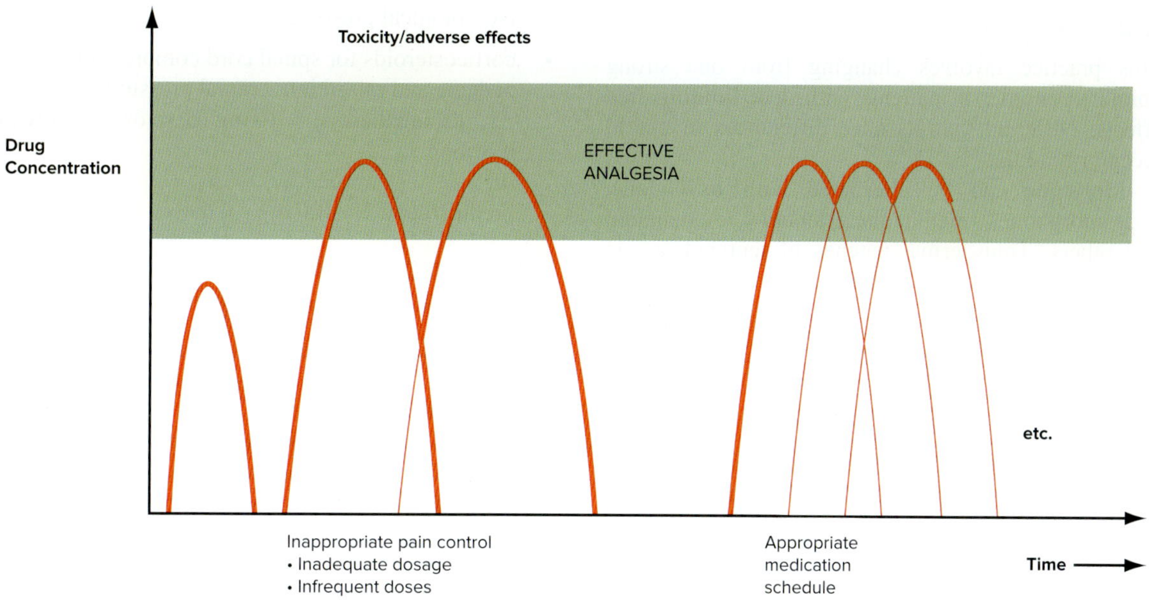

FIGURE 11.3 Appropriate schedule of analgesia to achieve optimal pain control[8]

- Constipation is a problem, so treat prophylactically with regular laxatives and carefully monitor bowel function.
- Consider oxycodone/naloxone (Targin) CR tablets for pain.
- Order a 'rescue dose' (usually 5–10 mg) for breakthrough pain or anticipated pain (e.g. going to toilet).
- Order antiemetics (e.g. haloperidol prn at first; usually can discontinue in 1–2 weeks as tolerance develops).
- Reassure the patient and family about the safety and efficacy of morphine (see TABLE 11.3). (Beware of opiophobia.)
- Using morphine as a mixture with other substances (e.g. Brompton's cocktail) has no particular advantage.
- Pethidine is not recommended (short half-life, toxic metabolites) and codeine and IM morphine (initially) should be avoided.
- Other opioids such as oxycodone, tapentadol and fentanyl are sometimes used instead of morphine and are an alternative to SC opioids but use with discretion (see CHAPTER 12).
- Fentanyl is a potent synthetic opioid which is available as a transdermal system. Effective and good for compliance. It is the least constipating opioid and can be used in kidney failure.
- Tapentadol is a new moderately strong opioid analgesic given orally, usually as a sustained release preparation. It is best avoided in severe kidney and liver impairment.
- Hydromorphone is a potent analgesic available as oral liquid, tablets and injection, and is now widely used in palliative care. It facilitates oral dosing when a high opioid dose is required and because of its short half-life (2–3 h) may reduce the incidence of side effects in the frail and elderly but like oxycodone may need to be given 4 hourly if used alone.
- Haloperidol is a first class adjuvant for morphine.

Table 11.3 Common myths about morphine[7]

Morphine is a last resort
This is not so, and there is no maximum dose.

The patient will become addicted
This is rare and probably irrelevant in the context of palliative care.

The patient will need ever-increasing amounts
The drug does not lose its effect but is usually increased according to disease progression.

Morphine will cause respiratory depression
This is rarely a problem and may even help those with dyspnoea. An overdose can be reversed with an injection of naloxone.

Morphine will shorten life
The reverse may in fact apply. It is not being used for euthanasia but to control pain.

11

Opioid rotation

This practice involves changing from one strong opioid to another in patients with dose-limiting side effects. Different opioids have differences in opioid receptor binding.

Morphine can be alternated with oxycodone, hydromorphone, methadone, fentanyl, tapentadol and others. Transdermal patches of fentanyl are an alternative to parenteral morphine.

Conversion rules (approximate potencies)[10,11]

- Divide oral dose morphine by 3 for equivalent SC dose,[10] e.g. 30 mg oral morphine = 10 mg SC/IM
- 10 mg morphine SC/IM = 150 mcg fentanyl SC/IM/IV *or* 2 mg hydromorphone SC/IM/IV *or* 10 mg oxycodone IV/SC or 20 mg (o) *or* 100 mg tramadol IM/IV or 150 mg (o)

Parenteral morphine

This is generally given subcutaneously (not IV or IM). Indications are:[6]

1 unable to swallow (e.g. severe oral mucositis; dysphagia; oesophageal obstruction)
2 bowel obstruction
3 severe nausea and vomiting
4 at high oral dose (i.e. above 100–200 mg dose) there appears to be no additional benefit from further dose increments

Adjuvant treatment

Refer to TABLE 11.2. In all three steps of pain control consider the use of adjuvant 'analgesics'; while not strictly speaking analgesics, they contribute to pain relief. Examples are corticosteroids, antidepressants, psychotropic agents and anticonvulsants.

11

Pain control

Bone pain:

- aspirin, paracetamol, NSAIDs are helpful co-analgesics, consider denusomab

Neuropathic pain (direct involvement of nerves):

- antidepressants (e.g. amitriptyline)
- anticonvulsants (e.g. carbamazepine, gabapentin)
- ketamine, an anaesthetic agent, is valuable for difficult pain but requires expertise in administration

Neurological pressure:

- corticosteroids for spinal cord compression, oedema and raised intracranial pressure
  e.g. dexamethasone 4–16 mg (o, sc or im) daily in morning
  or
  prednisolone 25–100 mg (o) daily

Continuous subcutaneous infusion of morphine

When the oral and/or rectal routes are not possible or are ineffective, a subcutaneous infusion with a syringe driver (pump) can be used.

It is also useful for symptom control when there is a need for a combination of drugs (e.g. for pain, nausea and agitation). It may avoid bolus peak effects (sedation, nausea or vomiting) or trough effects (breakthrough pain) with intermittent parenteral morphine injections.

Practical aspects

- Access to the subcutaneous space is via a 21 gauge butterfly needle, which is replaced regularly (1, 2, 3 or 4 days).
- Most regions are suitable. The more convenient are the abdomen, the anterior thigh, and the anterior upper arm (usually the anterior abdominal wall is used).
- The infusion can be managed at home.
- About one-half to two-thirds of the 24 hour oral morphine requirement is placed in the syringe.
- The syringe is placed into the pump driver, which is set for 24 hour delivery.
- Areas of oedema are not suitable.

Spinal morphine

Epidural or intrathecal morphine is sometimes indicated for pain below the head and neck, where oral or parenteral opioids have been ineffective. It is necessary to insert an epidural or intrathecal catheter (anaesthetist or neurosurgeon).[7]

Common symptom control

Common symptoms can be controlled as follows:[1]

Anorexia

metoclopramide 10 mg (o) tds
or
corticosteroids (e.g. dexamethasone 2–8 mg tds)
high-energy drink supplements

Constipation[6,7,9]

If opioids need to be maintained, the laxatives need to be peristaltic stimulants, not bulk-forming agents. Treat as for any patient in the GP setting. Aim for firm faeces with bowels open about every third day.

e.g. lactulose 20 mL bd
or
Movicol, one to two sachets, in 125 mL water, 1–3 times daily

Rectal suppositories, microenemas or enemas may be required (e.g. Microlax).

Shaw's (or PCU) cocktail is useful for severe constipation. With a small quantity of water melt one tablespoon of Senokot granules in a microwave oven. Add 20 mL Agarol and constitute to 100 ml with cold or warm milk or ice-cream.

Tip: Tilt the pelvis for defecation by sitting upright with books under feet for elevation.

Noisy breathing and secretions[7,11]

Conservative: repositioning to one side, reduced parenteral fluids and nasogastric suction.

For conscious patient:

- hyoscine butylbromide (Buscopan) 20 mg SC, 4 hourly or 60–80 mg daily by SC infusion
  or
- glycopyrrolate 0.2 mg SC as a single dose followed by 0.6–1.2 mg/24 hrs by continuous SC infusion

For unconscious patient, as above, also consider:

- hyoscine hydrobromide 0.4 mg SC, 4 hourly or 0.8–2.4 mg/24 hrs by continuous SC infusion
  or
- atropine 0.4–0.6 mg SC 4–6 hourly (be cautious of delirium)

These agents dry secretions and stop the 'death rattle'.

Dyspnoea

Identify the cause, such as a pleural effusion, and treat as appropriate. Pleural taps can be performed readily in the home (consider the PleurX® catheter). Adjust the patient's posture. Corticosteroids can be given for lung metastases. Oxygen may be necessary to help respiratory distress in the terminal stages and bedside oxygen can be readily obtained. Morphine can be used for intractable dyspnoea e.g. 2.5–5 mg (o) 4 hourly, together with haloperidol or a phenothiazine for nausea. Use a short-acting benzodiazepine (e.g. lorazepam 0.25–5 mg) sublingually if anxiety is a component.

Terminal distress/restlessness[7,11,12]

(Exclude reversal causes, e.g. drugs, fear, faecal impaction, urinary retention.)

1st choice:

clonazepam
0.5 mg SC bolus or 0.25–0.5 mg (o) 12 hourly (drops SL) (3 drops = 0.3 mg) or tabs[7]
1–4 mg over 24 hours in SC syringe driver
or
midazolam 2.5–5 mg SC 1–3 hourly prn or 2.5–10 mg sublingual or intranasal or 10 mg 4 hourly by SC infusion

If very severe:
add (with care because of fitting) haloperidol

Nausea and vomiting

If due to morphine:

haloperidol 1.5–5mg (o) daily or 0.5–1 mg (SC) 4 hourly prn (can be reduced after 10 days) or 1–2.5 mg over 24 hours via SC infusion
or
metoclopramide 10–20 mg (o) or SC 8 hourly prn

Alternatives: promethazine, cyclizine

If due to poor gastric emptying, use a prokinetic agent: metoclopramide, cisapride or domperidone.

Consider ondansetron or tropisetron for nausea and vomiting induced by cytotoxic chemotherapy and radiotherapy (see CHAPTER 60).

Wound dressings

To reduce pain, apply a mixture of 10 mg/mL topical morphine with 8 g/mL Intrasite hydrogel.

Cerebral metastases

Common symptoms are headache and nausea. Consider corticosteroid therapy (e.g. dexamethasone 4–16 mg daily). Analgesics and antiemetics such as haloperidol are effective.

Paraplegia

Paraplegia is especially prone to occur with carcinoma of the prostate, even when treated with LHRH analogues. The warning signs are the development of new back pain, paraesthesia in limbs or the recent development of urinary retention.[1] The objective is to prevent paraplegia developing. High-dose corticosteroids are given while arranging urgent hospital admission.

Hiccoughs[7,9]

Try a starting dose of:

clonazepam 0.25–1 mg (o) bd (consider oral liquid drops)

or

haloperidol 1–2.5 mg (o) bd

Swallowing granulated sugar with or without vinegar does not appear to be effective. Other drugs reported to be beneficial include baclofen, midazolam, chlorpromazine, nifedipine and metoclopramide.

Depression[11]

- mirtazapine 30 mg (o) daily, helpful for night-time sedation and appetite
- consider methylphenidate (psychostimulant) 5 mg (o) bd since evidence indicates an improvement in symptoms[13]

Weakness and weight loss

This problem may be assisted by a high-calorie and high-protein diet. Otherwise consider total parenteral nutrition. A list of high-energy drink supplements is provided in *Palliative Care: The Nitty Gritty Handbook.*[1]

Delirium

Determine the cause, including adverse opioid effect. Investigations include FBE, MCU, CXR, pulse oximetry. Consider treatment with olanzapine and haloperidol (refer to CHAPTER 45).

Hypercalcaemia

Consider hypercalcaemia in the presence of drowsiness, confusion, twitching and abdominal pain. It may be a paraneoplastic effect of myeloma and cancers (particularly lung and breast). It carries a poor prognosis—monitor serum calcium >3 mmol/L. Treat with rehydration, reduction of tissue mass and bisphosphonates.

The patient with AIDS

The same principles of management apply to the person suffering from the many manifestations of terminal AIDS, including pain. Many of these patients wish to die at home and there are excellent caring support groups to help. It is important to become acquainted with the service network. However, in Australia this service is thankfully becoming uncommon. Guidelines are included in CHAPTER 27. A very helpful guide to symptom control is presented in *Therapeutic Guidelines, Palliative Care: acquired immunodeficiency syndrome.*[7]

Palliative care in children

Principles of management

- Children should not be regarded as mini-adults.
- There is a different spectrum of illness apart from childhood cancer including congenital disorders such as cystic fibrosis, neurodegenerative disorders and cerebral palsy.
- The commonest malignancy is acute lymphatic leukaemia. Other important malignancies include: lymphomas, cerebral tumours, bone tumours and solid tumours.
- The focus of care is on the physical, mental and spiritual welfare of the child and the grieving family.
- Any pain must be accurately assessed.
- Morphine is the most commonly used opioid for pain although fentanyl and hydromorphone are now widely used.
- Nausea, vomiting and constipation require special attention.
- Avoid unpalatable medications and intramuscular injections.
- Adverse reactions to tranquillisers, corticosteroids, anti-emetics and aspirin are a special problem.
- Be prepared for home management, which is usually preferred by families.
- Pay attention to the impact on the vulnerable child, the parents and siblings. Consider support groups.

Dying and grieving

The stages of the grieving process as described by Kübler-Ross[5] may be experienced by both the patient and the family, albeit not exactly according to the five stages. The grieving process following the death of a loved one can vary enormously but many people are devastated.

The principles of care and counselling include:[1]

- Be available and be patient.
- Allow them to talk while you listen.
- Reassure them that their feelings are normal.
- Accept any show of anger passively.
- Avoid inappropriate reassurance.
- Encourage as much companionship as possible, if desired.

(See guidelines for crisis counselling given in CHAPTER 5.)

Communicating with the dying patient

Good communication is essential between the doctor and patient in order to inform, explain, encourage and show empathy. However, it can be very difficult, especially with the cancer patient.

Good communication is dependent on honesty and integrity in the relationship. Telling the truth can be painful and requires sensitivity, but it builds trust that enables optimal sharing of other difficult concerns and decisions, such as abandoning curative treatment, explaining the dying process and perhaps addressing thoughts on euthanasia.

Improved communication will lead not only to better 'spiritual' care but also to better symptom control.[1] Give patients every opportunity to talk about their illness and future expectations, and be available and patient in offering help and support.

Spiritual issues[1]

Spirituality is an important issue for all people, especially when faced with inevitable death. Many people are innately spiritual or religious and those with deep faith and a belief in 'paradise' appear to cope better with the dying process. Others begin to reflect seriously about spirituality and search for a meaning for life in this situation. Carers, including the attending doctor, should be sensitive to their needs and turmoil and reach out a helping hand, which may simply involve contacting a minister of religion.

Spiritual care builds on patients' existing resources to enable them to rise above the physical, emotional and social effects of their terminal illness.[1]

Advanced care planning (ACP)

ACP is a planning process where a patient, their family and carers, in consultation with a health care provider, makes decisions about his or her future health care, should he or she become incapable of making medical treatment decisions. Attention to ACP is not only important but rewarding to all parties.

The principles are:

- recognising the need to prepare for approaching death is an important medical skill
- the family needs to know that the patient is dying
- ACP is best when the patient is cognisant and involved in the decision making
- the health care is primarily patient-centred
- ensure the appointment of Medical Enduring Powers of Attorney and/or substitute decision maker for your patient
- ACP is best prior to or on admission to the caring facility or 6 months before anticipated death—then continuing review
- case conference, ideally with the GP, within this 6 months
- facilitate end-of-life pathway policy prior to death—certainly within the final week
- need for agreement for clear goals of end-of-life care, including resuscitation issues
- ACP only comes into effect when a patient is unable to make or communicate their own decisions

The question of euthanasia

This is a complex issue but will arise from time to time. It should be uncommonly encountered in the context of attentive whole-person continuing care. The non-use of life support systems, the use of 'round the clock' morphine, cessation of cytotoxic drugs, the use of ancillary drugs such as anti-depressants and anti-emetics, various nerve blocks and loving attention almost always help the patient cope without undue pain and suffering.[3]

Practice tips

- Morphine is the gold standard for pain.[14]
- Consider prescribing antidepressants routinely for patients in pain.
- Remember the 'sit down rule' whereby the home visit is treated as a social visit—sitting down with the patient and family, having a 'cuppa' and sharing medical and social talk.[3]
- Early referral of terminal patients with difficult-to-control problems, especially pain, to a hospice or multidisciplinary team can enhance the quality of care. However, the patient's family doctor must still be the focus of the team.

11

References

1 Fairbank E, Banks T. *Palliative Care: The Nitty Gritty Handbook.* Melbourne: RACGP Services Division, 1993: 1–18.
2 McGuckin R, Currow D, Redelman P. Palliative care: your role. Medical Observer, 1992; 27 November: 41–2.
3 Carson NE, Miller C. *Care of the Terminally Ill.* Melbourne: Monash University, Department of Community Medicine Handbook, 1993: 107–15.

4 National Institute for Health and Care Excellence (NICE) <www.nice.org.uk>.
5 Kübler-Ross E. *On Death and Dying*. London: Tavistock, 1970.
6 Buchanan J et al. *Management of Pain in Cancer.* Melbourne: Sigma Clinical Review, 1991; 18: 8–10.
7 Ravenscroft P (Chair) et al. *Therapeutic Guidelines: Palliative Care* (Version 3). Melbourne: Therapeutic Guidelines Ltd, 2010.
8 Portenoy RK, Ahmed E. Principles of opioid use in cancer pain. J Clin Oncol, 2014; 32(16): 1662–70.
9 Woodruff R. *Palliative Medicine* (3rd edn). Melbourne: Oxford University Press, 1999.
10 Waters A, Brooker C, Clayton JM. Cancer pain in palliative care. Australian Doctor, 2009; 12 June: 25–32.
11 Syrmis W, Good P et al. Opioid conversion ratios used in palliative care: is there an Australian consensus? Intern Med J, 2014; 44(5): 483–9.
12 Fischer J. Palliating symptoms other than pain. Aust Fam Physician, 2006; 35(10): 766–9.
13 Burke AL. Palliative care: an update on 'terminal restlessness'. Med J Aust, 1997; 166: 39–42.
14 Expert group for Palliative Care guidelines. In: eTG complete. Melbourne: Therapeutic Guidelines Ltd. Available from: <www.tg.org.au>, accessed January 2018.
15 Homsi J, Walsh D et al. Methylphenidate for depression in hospice practice. Am J Hosp Pall Care, 2000; 17: 393–8.
16 Mitchell GK. End-of-life care for patients with cancer. Aust Fam Physician, 2014; 43(8): 514–9.

Resource

National Institute for Health and Care Excellence (NICE). <www.nice.org.uk>, accessed January 2018.

Pain and its management 12

It is as much of the business of a physician to alleviate pain, and to smooth the avenues of death, when unavoidable, as to cure diseases.

JOHN GREGORY (1725–73), *LECTURES ON THE DUTIES AND QUALIFICATIONS OF A PHYSICIAN*

Pain is the capital symptom of humans—the great hallmark of disease—the signal par excellence to the patient and doctor that all is not well.

In modern medicine the successful management of chronic pain, in particular, still poses a great challenge. Its management or mismanagement is a yardstick of the excellence of that important bond—the doctor–patient relationship.

Pain is a multifactorial problem. The suffering patient must not only deal with the painful sensation itself but also cope with its possible serious significance.

- Does chest pain imply a pending heart attack?
- Does chronic ache or acute pain signify cancer?
- Does 'whiplash' imply neck pain to the grave?

Chronic pain is the most challenging problem. It must be emphasised that it always starts as an acute episode and that back pain accounts for the majority of cases of chronic pain encountered in general practice.

Golden rules

- Acute pain = acute anxiety
- Chronic pain = chronic depression

Definitions

Pain is defined as 'an unpleasant sensory and emotional experience associated with actual or potential tissue damage or described in terms of such damage'. The box below defines the variety of types of pain.

Glossary of terms[1]

Allodynia Pain due to a stimulus that does not normally provoke pain.
Mechanical—light touch feels painful.
Temperature—hot/cold stimulus (normally not painful) is painful.

Anaesthesia dolorosa Pain in an area or region that is anaesthetic.

Analgesia Absence of pain in response to stimulation that would normally be painful.

Breakthrough pain Pain which occurs between regular doses of analgesics and reflects increase in pain level above set baseline

Causalgia A syndrome of sustained burning pain, allodynia and hyperpathia after a traumatic nerve lesion, often combined with vasomotor and sudomotor dysfunction and later trophic changes (now known as complex regional pain syndrome II).

Central pain Pain associated with a lesion of the central nervous system.

Dysaesthesia An unpleasant abnormal sensation, whether spontaneous or evoked (e.g. formication—a feeling like ants crawling on the skin, burning, tingling).

Hyperaesthesia Increased sensitivity to stimulation, excluding the special senses.

Hyperalgesia An increased response to a stimulus that is normally painful (i.e. painful stimulus feels much more painful than expected, such as firm finger pressure).

Hyperpathia A painful syndrome, characterised by an increased reaction to a stimulus, especially a repetitive stimulus, as well as an increased threshold for sensory detection.

Hypoaesthesia Decreased sensitivity to stimulation, excluding the special senses.

Hypoalgesia Diminished pain in response to a normally painful stimulus.

Incident pain Pain that occurs on, or is exacerbated by, an activity (e.g. coughing, wound dressing, movement, weight-bearing).

Neuralgia Pain in the distribution of a nerve or nerves.

Neuritis Inflammation of a nerve or nerves.

Neuropathic pain Pain caused by a lesion or disease of the somatosensory nervous system (peripheral or central).

Neuropathy A disturbance of function or pathological change in a nerve.

continued

continued

Nociceptive pain Pain arising from stimulation of normal superficial or deep tissue pain receptors (nociceptors) from tissue injury or inflammation. From Latin 'nocere', to injure.

Paraesthesia Abnormal sensation, whether spontaneous or evoked.

Phantom pain The sensation of the presence of a missing body part.

Somatoform pain Pain that has the qualities of pain arising from a physical (somatic) cause but not attributable to any objectively demonstrable organic causation (i.e. the expression of psychological distress as physical symptoms).

Visceral pain A type of nociceptive pain that originates from activation of nociceptives of internal viscera (organs).

Origins of pain[1]

In general terms, the origin of conscious pain can be subdivided into three broad types—nociceptive, neuropathic or psychogenic.

1. *Nociceptive pain* is pain arising from stimulation of superficial or deep tissue pain receptors (nociceptors) in response to s noxious stimulus. It requires an intact nervous system. *Nociception* is stimulation of peripheral nociceptors (i.e. nerve endings sensitive to a noxious stimulus).
2. *Neuropathic pain* is pain caused or initiated by a primary lesion or dysfunction (i.e. damage) in the peripheral or central nervous system. It can be subdivided into central pain, when the primary lesion is in the central nervous system, or peripheral pain. Neuropathic pain is a form of neurogenic pain in which there is actual nerve cell or axonal damage due to inflammation, trauma or degenerative disease. It is typically a constant burning, episodic shooting or electric pain.
3. *Mixed nociceptive and neuropathic pain* e.g. some cancer related pain
4. *Psychogenic pain* is pain arising in the absence of any discernible injury and where the predominant aetiology is psychological or psychiatric. However, it is a real and distressing entity to the patient.

It should be emphasised that these types may overlap and patients may have more than one type of pain.

The features of the main types of pain are summarised in TABLE 12.1.

Table 12.1 Features of main types of pain[1]

Type of pain	Origin of pain	Symptoms and signs	Examples
Nociceptive			
1 Somatic	Skin mucosa Bones and joints Pleura and peritoneum	Localised stinging or burning Dull ache ± Pain on movement	Skin ulcers/abscess Aphthous ulcers Arthritis Minor fractures Pleurisy
2 Visceral	Solid or hollow organs	Deep, diffuse pain Poorly localised ± Colic ± Nausea and vomiting	Abdominal tumours Bowel obstruction Major surgery Ureteric/biliary colic
3 Muscle spasm	Skeletal muscle Smooth muscle	Pain worse on movement Severe colic Tenesmus	Acute low back pain (some) Ureteric/biliary colic Bowel obstruction Rectal dysfunction
Neuropathic			
1 Peripheral nerve	Nerve compression or peripheral nerve damage	Pain in nerve distribution ± Motor deficit ± Sensory deficit	Prolapse IV disc Limb amputation Peripheral neuropathies Post-herpetic neuralgia
2 Central pain	Cerebrovascular accident	Various pain syndromes (see text) ± Trophic changes	Stroke Spinal cord injury Multiple sclerosis

Components of pain[1]

A conceptual approach to the components of pain is illustrated in FIGURE 12.1.

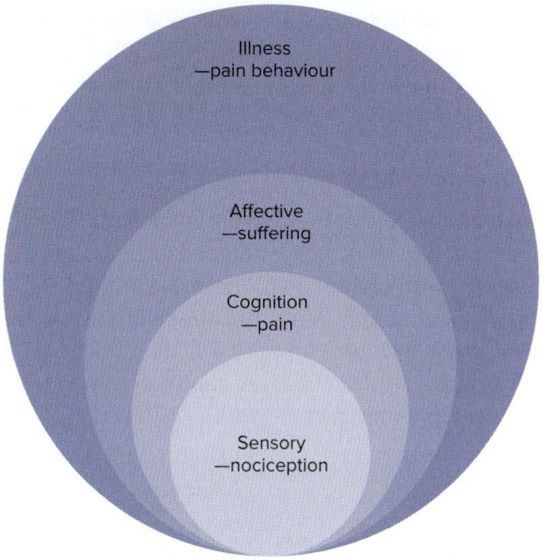

FIGURE 12.1 A conceptual approach to the components of pain: a biopsychosocial model

Developing an understanding of pain depends on the knowledge of relationships among nociception, pain, suffering and pain behaviour. The first three components cannot be measured or completely understood in individuals and only the pain behaviour can be observed and measured by parties other than the patient.

Categories of pain

Pain can be subcategorised as:

- acute pain
- cancer/palliative pain
- chronic non-cancer pain

Acute pain

Acute pain is pain of recent onset and short duration that usually has an obvious cause and a predictable duration. It is usually opioid sensitive. It is often due to nociception (e.g. postoperative pain).

Pain behaviour may be modified by socio-environmental factors (e.g. appropriate preparation for an operation results in lower postoperative analgesic requirements).

Early and appropriate interventions by GPs can have a major impact in improving the assessment and treatment of pain and helping to prevent the development of chronic pain, as in the chronic pain cycle. This applies particularly to acute musculoskeletal injury, such as acute neck and back pain and sporting injuries.

Problem areas in acute pain management include:

- acute back pain (CHAPTER 38)
- acute neck pain (CHAPTER 62)
- acute headache (CHAPTER 56)
- acute orofacial pain (CHAPTER 52)
- acute abdominal pain (CHAPTER 34)
- acute haemarthrosis (e.g. knee in haemophilia/sports injuries) (CHAPTER 67)
- acute chest pain (CHAPTER 40)
- sports injuries
- trauma
- burns
- neuropathic pain (e.g. herpes zoster)

Chronic pain

Chronic pain may be defined as pain present for a period greater than 3 months or pain present for 4 weeks more than the expected time of recovery.

Chronic pain is the classic 'heartsink' problem of practitioners as it is far more difficult to manage and is often unresponsive to agents effective in acute pain relief, such as opioids. It is, in itself, a type of disease state.

The management of chronic pain may require a multidisciplinary pain clinic strategy in which biological (pathological), psychological and social contributions to pain behaviour can be evaluated and managed.

Assessing and measuring pain

Pain is a subjective symptom and generates considerable emotion and frustration, and thus can be difficult to assess.

Four questions needed to assess any pain:

- What is the cause of the pain?
- What is the dominant mechanism—somatic, visceral or neuropathic?
- Is there a treatable cause and is the treatment of the cause optimal?
- Is there a significant incident factor?

12

The history

The classic historical approach is still the most important approach. Patients can use the PQRST approach to describe their pain,[1] namely, P—palliative and provocative factors, Q—quality, R—radiation, S—severity and T—timing. Most practitioners use the SOCRATES approach to pain, namely:

S **S**ite
O **O**nset and offset
C **C**haracter
R **R**adiation
A **A**ssociated symptoms
T **T**iming
E **E**xacerbating and relieving factors
S **S**everity

Use of body charts

To assist with diagnosis and ongoing management of pain, it is helpful to get patients to chart the site and radiation of their pain on body charts—either total body charts or regional charts (e.g. the head). This is particularly helpful for spinal pain with referral patterns and fibromyalgia.

Measurement of pain

Despite its subjective nature, it is good to record some type of repeatable measurement, especially for chronic pain requiring treatment outcomes. This involvement also helps the patient.

Unidimensional scales

Visual analogue scales (VAS), which are used as a research tool and well validated, can be useful in recording both acute and chronic pain levels. An example of a simple VAS linear scale on which the patient indicates the severity of their current pain is shown in FIGURE 12.2. A pictorial (faces) scale applicable to children is shown in FIGURE 12.3.

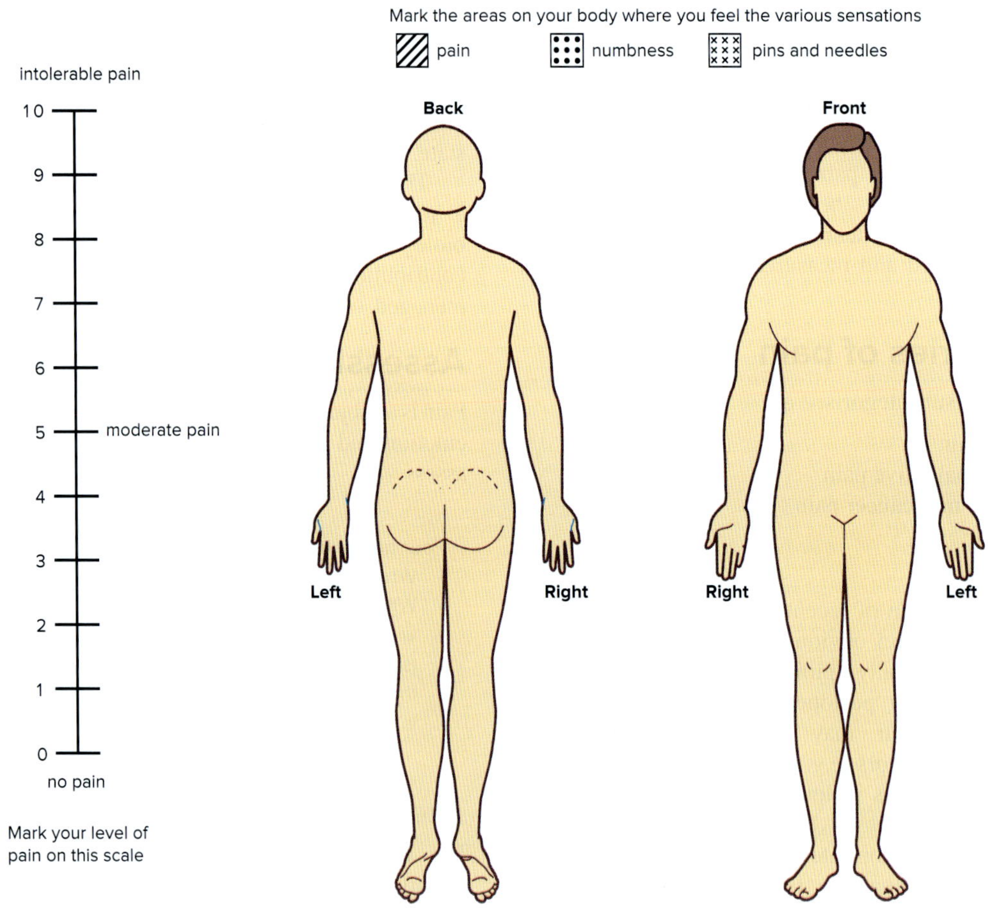

FIGURE 12.2 Assessing pain using a visual analogue scale and body chart: ideal for lumbosacral pain

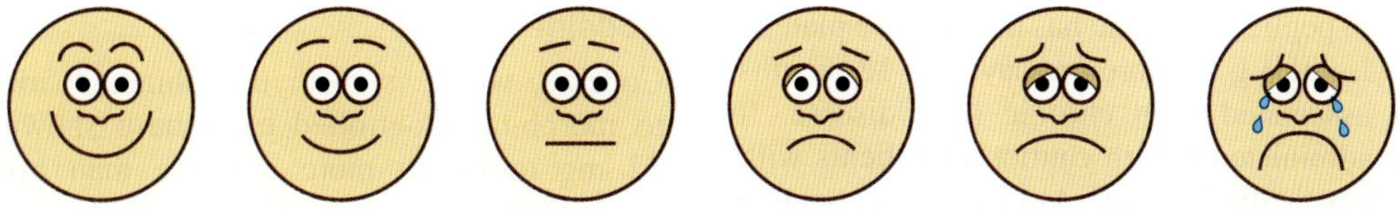
0
No hurt
1
Hurts little bit
2
Hurts little more
3
Hurts even more
4
Hurts whole lot
5
Hurts worst

FIGURE 12.3 Visual analogue scale: a faces pain rating scale ideal for children

Multidimensional scales

These scales, which are usually employed for chronic pain, take into account several aspects of pain perception in addition to assessing functional effects and levels of disability. Examples include the:

- McGill Pain Questionnaire
- Pain Disability Index
- Form 36 Health Survey (SF-36)
- Oswestry low-back pain questionnaire

The holistic approach to pain management

Doctors should assess not only the somatic basis of the pain but also the patient's psyche, mood, coping ability, attitude and family.

The pain threshold can be lowered by factors such as fatigue, anger, depression, loneliness, home or work environment. On the other hand, the factors that raise the pain threshold include a happy or contented disposition, drive to return to work, empathy, companionship, sleep, rest, pleasant diversions and good home support.[2]

Analgesic prescribing

The GP has an important responsibility not only to relieve patients' pain skilfully and completely (if possible) but to ensure that the appropriate drugs are prescribed without leading to dependence. This judicious drug use applies to opioids for non-palliative pain, in particular codeine, oxycodone and morphine.

The three categories of pain—nociceptive pain, neuropathic pain and psychogenic pain—each require different therapeutic agents.[2] For nociceptive pain the traditional analgesics are used: paracetamol, aspirin, other NSAIDs and opioids. Neuropathic pain is treated with antidepressants, antiepileptics and membrane stabilisers. Agents used to treat muscle pain are muscle relaxants and baclofen.

Medications used to treat pain include:

- 'simple' analgesics (aspirin, paracetamol)
- NSAIDS, cyclo-oxygenase-2 (COX-2) specific inhibitors
- opioids (weak and strong)
- antidepressants, TCAs (e.g. amitriptyline), SNRIs
- membrane stabilisers (anticonvulsants, antiarrhythmics)
- NMDA blockers (ketamine)
- $alpha_2$ agonists (clonidine)

Chronic pain, such as chronic low back pain, represents a challenge but the challenge is to manage acute pain skilfully and prevent chronicity. O'Reilly[3] has provided some useful guidelines for the role of the GP in the management of chronic pain:

- Emphasise that cure is unlikely.
- Encourage the patient to accept responsibility for pain management.
- Provide ongoing support and interest.
- Promote activity rather than rest.
- Educate patients about their condition: review X-rays and discuss drugs, especially the long-term disadvantages of opioids and sedatives.
- Encourage time-contingent versus pain-contingent use of medication.
- Withdraw unsuitable drugs (e.g. opioids and sedatives).
- Consider issue of undiagnosed depression or anxiety as amplifiers of pain perception and treat where necessary.
- Promote the use of relaxation, distraction and heat or ice packs rather than increased medication.
- Discuss strategy for management of flare-ups in advance.
- Refer for psychological support: mindfulness, acceptance–commitment therapy (ACT) and/or cognitive behaviour therapy recommended.

Analgesics in common use[1]

Paracetamol

Paracetamol has minimal anti-inflammatory activity but moderate analgesic (equipotent with aspirin) and antipyretic properties. It is metabolised by the liver and has an excretion half-life of approximately 4 hours. Adverse effects are uncommon but gastrointestinal discomfort such as dyspepsia and nausea can occur occasionally. It is well tolerated by patients with peptic ulcers and has no effect on platelet function. Use of 4 g or more per day over 12 months has been associated with chronic liver disease. It should be administered with caution in patients with kidney or hepatic dysfunction. Although less effective than NSAIDs for pain relief, its excellent safety in therapeutic doses makes it the first-line analgesic for mild to moderate pain.

Usual dosage:

1 g (o) 4 hourly (max. 4 g/day)

Formulations of paracetamol include:

- immediate release tablets and capsules
- oral solution and suspension
- chewable tablets
- soluble or effervescent tablets
- extended-action formulation—665 mg (may provide up to 8 hours pain relief)
- suppositories (125 mg, 250 mg, 500 mg forms)
- injectable formulation

NSAIDs

NSAIDs can be used instead of or in addition to paracetamol.

Aspirin

Aspirin has both analgesic and anti-inflammatory activity and is a very effective drug in adults for mild to moderate acute pain. It has an extremely short half-life and is metabolised to salicylic acid, which shares the above properties. The major problems with aspirin are gastrointestinal discomfort, ulceration and bleeding.

Usual dosage:

600 mg (o) 4 hourly (max. 4 g/day)

Opioid analgesics[4]

These agents are usually reserved for the treatment of severe pain and are more appropriate for palliative pain. Commonly used agents are the relatively weaker opioids—codeine, oxycodone, buprenorphine, tramadol—and the stronger ones—morphine, fentanyl, hydromorphone and methadone. Reviews show that opioids are no better than NSAIDs for back pain.[5]

12

Adverse effects, which are common, dose dependent and quite variable, include nausea and vomiting, constipation, respiratory depression and dysphoria, oral hygiene problems and hyperalgaesia. Ongoing assessment based on the 5As is recommended. These are: analgesic effect, activity, affect, abnormal behaviour, adverse effects.

Codeine

Codeine, which is methylmorphine, is metabolised to morphine. Controlled trials have shown codeine 32 mg to be no more effective than aspirin 600 mg.[3] Disturbing side effects include nausea and constipation. Its use is best avoided because of its variable metabolism secondary to cytochrome CYP 2D6 genotype polymorphism. This enzyme rapidly metabolises codeine to morphine causing sleepiness and confusion. Breastfed infants of mothers taking codeine require close monitoring.

Usual dosage:

30–60 mg (o) 4 hourly (max. 240 mg/day)

Oxycodone

Oxycodone is a synthetic opioid that is very effective orally. It is useful for moderate pain in bridging the gap between the simple analgesics and strong opioids.[2] The oral form has a duration of action of 4 hours.

Adverse side effects include nausea, constipation, confusion and itch. Dependency and abuse is a worldwide problem. It is available as an injection and is equianalgesic to morphine.

Usual dosage:

10 mg (o) 4 hourly (max. 60 mg/day),
controlled release, (various strengths) 12 hourly
30 mg rectally (8–12 hourly [Prolodone])
Examples: Endone, Oxycontin, OxyNorm, Targin

Dextropropoxyphene

This controversial drug is structurally related to methadone. Adverse effects include serious cardiac disorders, dysphoria, confusion, lightheadedness and constipation. It has been associated with relatively sudden death when taken in overdose, especially with alcohol.[1] Continuous use should be discouraged, particularly in elderly patients and those with cardiac disease.[1] Avoid prescribing it for new patients.

Morphine

Morphine is the most effective and 'gold standard' opioid for the relief of moderate to severe pain and cancer pain (see CHAPTER 11). It is worth noting that injections are not more effective than oral administration in achieving pain relief. It should be titrated according to patients' needs. Dose reduction may need to be made in patients with impaired liver or kidney function and in elderly or debilitated patients.

Note: Dose requirements vary considerably and patient response should be monitored frequently. There may be no upper limit to dosage in cancer patients.

Usual dosage:[2]

10 mg (o) 4 times daily
SC injection 5–10 mg
IV injection 5–10 mg
equipotent dose: 30 mg (o) = 10 mg parenteral

Tapentadol

Tapentadol (Palexia, Nucynta) is a new centrally acting opioid analgesic indicated for chronic moderate to severe pain not responding to non-narcotic analgesics, including palliative care and neuropathic pain. Similar benefits to oxycodone. Adverse effects are common and it should be avoided in severe kidney and liver disease. No known multi-equivalent dose to morphine 30 mg (o). Available as IR 50 mg, 75mg, 100mg ER: 50 mg, 100 mg, 150 mg, 200 mg, 250 mg.

Usual dosage:

initially ER 50 mg (o) every 12 hours, increasing as necessary (max. dose 500 mg/day).

Methadone[5]

Methadone is an effective oral analgesic with a long but variable half-life; it is given, preferably, once or at most twice a day. Relatively unsuitable for acute pain, it is valuable for chronic pain, although long-acting morphine preparations have displaced it. It should not be used in elderly patients or those with kidney dysfunction. Its place is in management of opioid dependency but it needs to be used with care because of the risk of respiratory depression and accumulation.

Pethidine

Pethidine is a synthetic opioid with a short duration of action. A problematic adverse effect is accumulation of its toxic metabolite (norpethidine), which can cause myoclonic and general seizures.[5] It has no place in the management of chronic pain, whether cancer or non-cancer, and possibly minimal use in acute pain.

Fentanyl[1]

Fentanyl is a very potent synthetic opioid which can be administered IV, IM, SC, intranasal (children), transdermal or by the epidural route. Its efficacy is similar to morphine but it has fewer side effects and is the drug of choice in renal failure. The conversion factor is: 10 mg (SC) morphine = 150–200 mcg (SC) fentanyl. Intranasal fetanyl has significant use in paediatric emergency care and also palliative care.

Usual dosage:

preoperation/postoperation pain, 50–100 mcg IM or slow IV
patches (various strengths, deliver over 72 hours), initial dose 12–25 mcg/hour
It takes about 8–12 hours before effecting analgesia.
A 25 mcg patch is equivalent to 30–35 mg IV or 100 mg oral morphine daily.

Hydromorphone

This is structurally similar to morphine but five times more potent. It is available for oral, parenteral and intraspinal use in moderate to severe pain. Like all opioids, the risk of drug dependence is high.

Usual dosage:

2–4 mg (o) every 4 hours
1–2 mg IM, SC or IV (slow) every 4–6 hours
4–8 mg daily of SR (sustained release) preparation

Tramadol

Tramadol is an atypical analgesic with both opioid and non-opioid features. Its use is suitable for mild to moderate mixed nociceptive and neuropathic pain. Its advantages include analgesia with minimal sedation or respiratory depression and low abuse/dependence potential. Side effects include the serotonin effect, dizziness, vertigo, nausea, vomiting, constipation, headache, somnolence, tremor, confusion and hypersensitivity reactions. Seizures have been reported.[6]

Usual dosage:

(as 50 mg caps or SR tabs—100, 150 or 200 mg)
50–100 mg (o) 2–4 times daily or 100–200 mg (SR) twice daily
injection 100 mg/2 mL: 50–100 mg 4–6 hourly IM or slow IV

Buprenorphine

This is a partial agonist opioid derived from the opium alkaloid thebaine. It is useful in pain management. Sublingual preparations (0.2 mg, 0.4 mg, 2 mg, 8 mg) are used for acute, chronic and cancer pain. It is also available as a transdermal patch (TD), e.g. Norspan and injection formulation. It is used in the treatment of opioid dependence.

The patches are available in 5, 10 and 20 mcg/24 hr patches (equivalent to 3, 6 and 12 mg morphine in a 24-hour period).

Combined analgesics

Combined analgesics are available for moderately severe pain. They now usually consist of a simple analgesic such as paracetamol combined with the NSAID ibuprofen. Combined analgesics have an additive effect because they act at different receptor sites. The use of combined preparations, especially with codeine, is generally not recommended but if both agents are needed it is advisable to prescribe them separately, thus enabling individual dose adjustments.[1] It is worth noting that codeine, either singularly or in combination, is not available over-the-counter (OTC) but only on prescription.

Ketamine

Ketamine (oral or IM use) can be used for induction and maintenance of anaesthesia and for pain relief. It should be used cautiously and by specialists. Neuropsychiatric adverse effects can be very disturbing for affected patients.

Methoxyflurane

This is a volatile anaesthetic agent that is administered as inhalational analgesia with the Penthrox Inhaler in emergency situations such as at the roadside. It can be used with oxygen or air. It provides pain relief after 8–10 breaths and it continues for several minutes. It should only be used if resuscitation facilities are available. Maximum adult dose is 6 ml/24 hours.

Prescribing guidelines for opioids[4,6]

- As a rule, restrict to SR morphine.
- SR oxycodone is more 'likeable' for patients and should be avoided for conditions such as back pain.
- TD buprenorphine is often a good starting agent.
- Restrict use of codeine and use with caution.
- Tramadol is useful but has a potential serotonin adverse effect and ceiling effect.
- Fentanyl is potent and its use questionable.
- Do not initiate with hydromorphone or fentanyl.
- Hydromorphone is very complex—best for palliative care.
- Methadone has complex kinetics so avoid initiating unless well informed.
- At least 80% of total daily opioid should be given as an SR formulation.
- Use immediate release (IR) as a guide to consolidate SR doses.
- Avoid IR-only regimens—use co-analgesics to limit dose and side effects.
- Do not use hydromorphone or transdermal fentanyl as first-line opioids in opioid-naive patients with chronic pain.
- Ensure that the pain syndrome is opioid sensitive.
- Good record keeping is mandatory.
- Beware of drug escalation.

Pain in children

The management of pain in children requires considerable sensitivity and wisdom. There are many clinical myths about this issue, especially that children have a high pain tolerance and analgesia is relatively dangerous. The inappropriate pain management of circumcision is a classic example.

Guiding principles[7]

- All children feel pain—as much as if not more than adults.
- Neonates do feel and remember pain—even the fetus feels pain.
- Children can localise and describe their pain.
- Pain in children can be masked and they often do not report pain.
- If a child complains of pain, they are serious and it is organic until proved otherwise.
- Consider other confusing factors (e.g. developmental delay).
- Consider children's fear of analgesic injections.
- Anxiety from anticipation of a procedure is a big issue—explanation, distraction and parental involvement help.
- Adverse effects of opioids, such as addiction, do not necessarily pose serious problems in children.[1]
- Analgesic medication should be dosed on a per-weight basis.
- Consider analgesic combinations with more severe pain (e.g. NSAID plus opioid).

Assessment of pain

This is very important in children of all ages and should involve a careful history and examination. Self-reporting of pain is reliable in children over 4 years of age. Close observation of non-verbal cues and behaviour is important (e.g. severe pain may be indicated by quiet withdrawal and whimpering; tachycardia).

Scaling strategies can be used—the modified faces pain scale (see FIG. 12.3) is useful in younger children, while older children and teenagers can use a visual analogue scale.

Analgesia in children[1,8]

The three most commonly used analgesics in children are paracetamol, NSAIDs and opioids. TABLE 12.2 lists the hierarchy of analgesics to be used in children.

Paracetamol (acetaminophen)

This is generally safe and effective even in asthmatics in therapeutic doses. It is rapidly absorbed orally within 30 minutes and well absorbed rectally.

Table 12.2 The analgesic hierarchy[7]

Paracetamol
NSAID (ibuprofen, naproxen)
Combination oral therapy: • paracetamol/codeine mixes • alternate and preferred: NSAID/paracetamol
Parenteral opioid: • bolus IM, IV; infusion; PCA
Combination parenteral therapy: • NSAID/opioid/ketamine • adjuvant clonidine

Usual dosage 1 month to 12 years of age:

15 mg/kg (o) every 4 hours prn (max. 4 doses/day)
20 mg/kg rectally, every 6 hours

Rules:

maximum daily dose:[8]
90 mg/kg to max. 4 g (for 2 days only)
60 mg/kg/day if aged <6 months
a dose of 10 mg/kg is no more effective than placebo
never exceed 1 g per dose

- Don't exceed recommended daily doses.
- Don't use continuously >48 hours without review.
- Don't double up, e.g. use cold and flu tablets with paracetamol. Be cautious of drug combinations.
- Don't use in a trivial fever.

Cautions:

- Jaundice
- Repeated doses over several days when febrile and/or dehydrated

Hepatotoxicity is rare and does not usually occur in doses below 150 mg/kg/day but acute paracetamol overdose (single doses of >100 mg/kg) is a potentially life-threatening event.

Aspirin

Aspirin is not in common use in children and should not be used <16 years since it has been associated with Reye syndrome.

For antiplatelet effects use low doses 2–5 mg/kg/day.

NSAIDs

NSAIDs have a proven safety and efficacy in children for mild to moderate pain and can be used in conjunction with paracetamol and opioids such as codeine and morphine. The advantage is their opioid-sparing effect. Contraindications include known hypersensitivity, severe asthma (especially if aspirin sensitive), bleeding diatheses, nasal polyposis and peptic ulcer disease.

Those commonly used for analgesia are:

- ibuprofen: 5–10 mg/kg (o) 6–8 hourly (max. 40 mg/kg/day)
- naproxen: 5–10 mg/kg (o) 12–24 hourly (max. 1 g/day)
- diclofenac: 1 mg/kg (o) 8 hourly (max. 150 mg/day)
- celecoxib 1.5–3 mg/kg (o) bd

The rectal dose is double the oral dose but only administered twice a day.

Opioid analgesics

Oral opioids[7]

These have relatively low bioavailability but can be used for moderate to severe pain when weaning from parenteral opioids, for ongoing severe pain (e.g. burns) and where the IV route is unavailable.

Codeine

Contraindicated <12 years. Usual dosage:

0.5–1 mg/kg (o), 4–6 hourly prn (max. 3 mg/kg/day)

There is no conclusive evidence that it is more effective if used combined with paracetamol or ibuprofen (see caution about variations in polymorphisms).

Morphine

Immediate release:

0.2–0.4 mg/kg (o) 4 hourly prn

Fentanyl

Fentanyl citrate can be administered orally (transmucosal) as 'lollipops', transcutaneously as 'patches', or intranasally via a mucosal atomiser device (for painful procedures).

Parenteral opioids[1,7]

These are the most powerful parenteral analgesics for children in severe pain and can be administered in intermittent boluses (IM, IV or SC) or by continuous infusion (IV or SC). Infants under 12 months are more sensitive and need careful monitoring (e.g. pulse oximetry). This management is invariably in the hospital. Administration of parenteral opioids should not be undertaken without the availability of oxygen, resuscitation equipment and naloxone to reverse overdose.

Analgesics in the elderly

Older patients have the highest incidence of painful disorders and also surgical procedures. As a general rule, most elderly patients are more sensitive to opioid analgesics and to aspirin and other NSAIDs but there may be considerable individual differences in tolerance. Patients over 65 years should receive lower initial doses of opioid analgesics with subsequent doses being titrated according to the patient's needs.[1]

Some general rules and tips[1,9]

- Start with 25–50% of the usual dose.
- Give analgesics at fixed times by the clock rather than 'prn' for ongoing pain.
- Regularly monitor your patient's analgesic requirements and modify according to needs and adverse effects.
- Start with a dose towards the lower end of the dose range and then titrate upwards depending on response.
- Avoid using compound analgesics and prescribe simple and opioid analgesics separately.
- Reserve the use of anti-emetics for the development of nausea and vomiting with opioids. Extrapyramidal reactions (dystonia and oculogyric crises) can be a problem with anti-emetics.
- Advise patients about the benefits of high-fibre foods if on analgesics. Prescribe a bulking agent (peristalsis stimulant) or lactulose if necessary.

Prescribing NSAIDs

NSAIDs have analgesic, antipyretic and anti-inflammatory activity. They inhibit synthesis of prostaglandins by inhibiting cyclo-oxygenase (COX) present in COX-1 and COX-2. They are very effective against nociceptive pain.

The prescribing of aspirin and other NSAIDs is an area of increasing concern to all GPs, especially in the elderly with their increasing propensity to the pain of arthritic conditions and demands for relief. About 15% of the patients on a GP's list in the UK will present with a locomotor problem.[10] A common response to the symptoms of rheumatic complaints is to prescribe NSAIDs; in the US 55% of all visits by patients with arthritis will lead to a prescription for a NSAID.[11]

12

Unfortunately, the use of NSAIDs involves a high incidence of side effects, ranging from the trivial to the lethal, with many deaths from bleeding ulcers, especially in the elderly. The NSAIDs 'epidemic' prevails because the agents continue to be perceived as the best available for the relief of arthritic symptoms. Of particular concern, however, is the widespread use of NSAIDs for common problems such as back pain when the main cause is dysfunctional or mechanical without evidence of inflammation. Surprisingly, many of these patients appear to achieve a good response to NSAIDs.

The choice of NSAIDs can be controversial. Some are claimed to have more adverse effects than others but there is little evidence of substantial differences.[2,11] There is no doubt that particular NSAIDs are of great value in specific rheumatic conditions. Both indomethacin and phenylbutazone are more effective for the spondyloarthropathies and gout.[11] It is worthwhile being mindful of their half-lives. NSAIDs with short half-lives include aspirin, diclofenac, tiaprofenic acid, ketoprofen, ibuprofen and indomethacin. NSAIDs with long half-lives include diflunisal, naproxen, sulindac, piroxicam and tenoxicam, and these are useful in the treatment of chronic pain such as bony metastases in cancer.

TABLE 12.3 shows the classification of NSAIDs.

Table 12.3 Classification of NSAIDs[1]

Action	Example
Non-selective inhibitors of COX-1 and COX-2, mainly in CNS	Paracetamol
Non-selective inhibitors of COX-1 and COX-2, acting in both CNS and periphery	Aspirin Ketorolac Other NSAIDs
Selective NSAIDs	
Specific inhibitors of COX-2	Celecoxib Etoricoxib Meloxicam Paracoxib
Preferential inhibitors of COX-2 over COX-1	Meloxicam

Note: COX = cyclo-oxygenase

Studies have identified certain patients who appear to have significant risk factors for the likely development of NSAID lesions (gastropathy). NSAID ulceration and its complications (see TABLE 12.4) are more prevalent in the elderly, particularly in females.

It is likely that NSAIDs have been prescribed too readily in Australia, particularly in general practice.[11] In a review,[12] a reduction of NSAID prescribing was recommended, particularly for conditions where inflammation is not a major feature (e.g. osteoarthritis and 'mechanical' back pain). Consumption has declined, probably in part because of media publicity. Haslock emphasises that those who both stop and start NSAIDs must recognise some clinical responsibilities.

Table 12.4 Persons at higher risk from NSAID-induced side effects[11]

Definite
Age >65 years
Prior ulcer disease or complication
High-dose, multiple NSAIDs
Concomitant corticosteroid therapy
Duration of therapy (>3 months)
Possible
Conditions necessitating NSAID treatment (e.g. RA)
Female sex
Ischaemic heart disease/hypertension
Kidney impairment
Smoking
Alcohol excess
Helicobacter pylori

Those who start the drug have obligations to:

- ensure there is an appropriate indication for it
- provide education about the drug to the patient—its purpose, side effects and dosage regimen
- monitor its continuing need, effectiveness and safety
- give the patient permission to telephone about any concerns
- be prepared to deal with side effects
- eradicate known *H. pylori* infection

Those who stop medication have an equal obligation to:

- ascertain whether there is still a need for its therapeutic action
- take the necessary steps, if the need exists, to provide an alternative

There is evidence that peptic ulcers that develop in patients taking NSAIDs heal faster if the NSAID is dropped.

An anti-inflammatory dose of fish oil should be considered as part of long-term treatment to minimise NSAID use.

A major advance has been the realisation that there are two forms of cyclo-oxygenase: cyclo-oxygenase 1 (COX-1) and cyclo-oxygenase 2 (COX-2). These both act as rate-limiting enzymes in prostaglandins and thromboxane synthesis. The respective roles of these two isoforms are depicted in FIGURE 12.4.

The coxibs are a group of NSAIDs synthesised to inhibit COX-2 specifically. They are on a par as an analgesic with the COX-1 inhibitors. Their gastrointestinal adverse reactions are less, but they have all the other adverse effects and drug interactions of COX inhibitors. The cardiovascular problems, including increased blood pressure, thrombosis (fatal myocardial infarction and stroke), and impairment of kidney function experienced with rofecoxib indicate the potential problems of these agents. If prescribed for patients at risk of thrombosis aspirin should be added.[13]

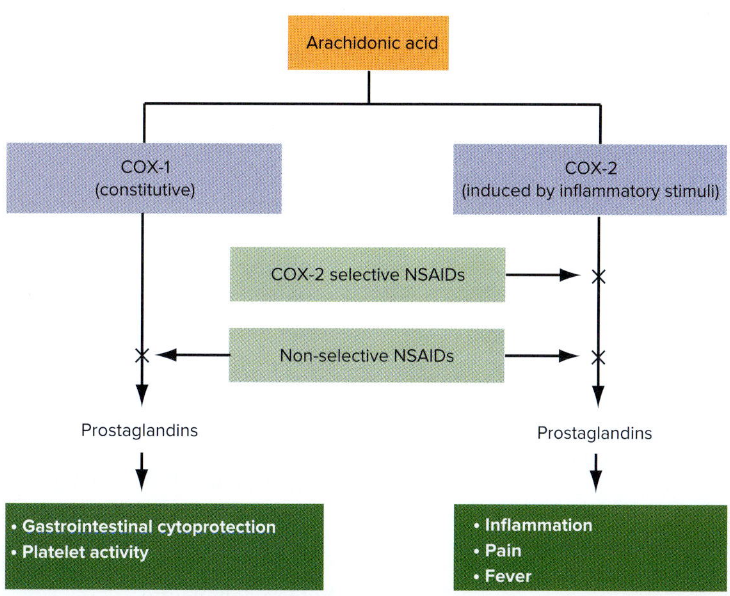

FIGURE 12.4 Synthesis of prostaglandins from arachidonic acid may be mediated by one of two forms of cyclo-oxygenase

12

Parecoxib is a COX-2 agent that is very effective for postoperative pain as an IM or IV injection. Newer agents include etoricoxib (Arcoxia).

All NSAIDs (i.e. selective and non-selective COX-2 inhibitors) produce their prime anti-inflammatory effect by blocking COX-2 function.

Topical NSAID gel formulations have doubtful effectiveness and although absorbed in small amounts can still cause gastrointestinal haemorrhage.[1]

NSAIDs and the elderly

NSAIDs with short half-lives (e.g. ibuprofen and diclofenac) may be safer in the elderly and all NSAIDs should be used in reduced dosage. Patients should be monitored for fluid retention and hypertensive control and kidney function.[1]

Prescribing recommendations

- Recommend intermittent use of NSAIDs based on appropriate patient education. Intermittent courses for 14 days can work well in chronic conditions, remembering that it takes about 10 days for NSAIDs to achieve maximal effectiveness. Ibuprofen is usually first choice.

Neuropathic pain[14]

Neuropathic pain can be defined as pain associated with injury, disease or surgical section of the peripheral or central nervous system. It is a common (affects about 1% of the population) although under-identified condition.[15]

Considerations regarding neuropathic pain include:

- essentially due to nerve damage
- frequently involves both peripheral (mainly) and central sensitisation
- has a multiplicity of clinical pain features
- many responsible mechanisms (e.g. neuroma, demyelination, loss of normal sensory input, enhanced sympathetic activity)

Clinical features[1,14]

12

- Burning, shooting, electric or stabbing pain
- Paroxysmal or spontaneous pain
- Pain in the absence of ongoing tissue damage
- Pain in an area of sensory loss (dolorosa)
- Allodynia (e.g. pain on light touch)
- Hyperpathia
- ± Hyperalgesia
- ± Dysaesthesia (e.g. 'ants crawling on skin')
- ± Delay in onset of pain after nerve injury
- Radiating electric shock-like pains in nerve distribution (e.g. Tinel's sign—tapping of neuroma or nerve)
- Often refractory to simple analgesics and NSAIDs
- Poor response to opioids
- ± Autonomic nervous system instability (e.g. pallor or cyanosis, excessive warmth or cold, sweating changes)

Examples of neuropathic pain states include:

- post-herpetic neuralgia
- trigeminal neuralgia ('tic douloureux')
- atypical facial pain
- phantom limb pain
- complex regional pain syndrome I (reflex sympathetic dystrophy)
- complex regional pain syndrome II (causalgia)
- other neuralgias
- diabetic/alcoholic peripheral neuropathy
- spinal cord injury pain
- late brachial/lumbar sacral plexus tumour infiltration
- post-stroke pain
- arachnoiditis

Treatment[14]

For initial pain relief, use aspirin or paracetamol or a NSAID. However, it is usual to depend on the use of analgesic adjuvants, either orally (mainly tricyclic antidepressants [TCAs] and anti-epileptics) or parenterally, such as lignocaine or ketamine. Adjuvants should be started in low doses and increased as necessary to the maximum tolerated level.

Antidepressants (first line)

TCAs:
amitriptyline 10–25 mg (o) nocte increasing every 7 days to 75–100 mg max.
Consider another TCA (e.g. nortriptyline 10 mg nocte or doxepin)[1]
SNRIs:
duloxetine (consider for peripheral diabetic neuropathy)
30 mg (o) daily (to max. 60 mg)
venlafaxine is another option
and/or

Anti-epileptic agents

carbamazepine 50–100 mg (o) bd initially increasing to 400 mg bd max.
or
gabapentin 100–300 mg (o) daily (nocte) initially, increasing as tolerated to three times daily (max. 2400 mg)

Note re gabapentin

- It is renally excreted, therefore caution in elderly and renally impaired.

- Try a test dose of 100 mg (o) at night in the elderly.
- Side effects include drowsiness, dizziness and generalised fatigue.

  or

  sodium valproate 200–600 mg (o) bd

  or

  pregabalin 75 mg (o) daily initially, up to 300 mg bd[15]

Ketamine infusions have been used for the central desensitisation of chronic neuropathic pain but evidence of benefit is limited.

Some guiding rules[1]

- TCAs may be better for constant burning pain.
- Anti-epileptics may be better for sharp shooting pain.
- Carbamazepine is the drug of choice for trigeminal neuralgia.
- Doses of TCAs are much smaller than those for treating depression.

Evidence base

- Level 1 evidence shows that about 70% of patients have a significant response to carbamezepine.[15,16]
- The newer anti-epileptic gabapentin has proven efficacy for diabetic neuropathy[17] and post-herpetic neuralgia.[17]

Painful diabetic neuropathy[18]

It is important to realise that painful diabetic neuropathy tends to occur in mild or even unrecognised cases of diabetes and sometimes may be a presenting symptom. Pain in the feet and legs is found in 11.6% of people with type 1 diabetes and in 31.2% of people with type 2 diabetes.

The classic complaint is burning in the feet with possible associated aching, cramping and tingling sensations. The symptoms are often worse during the night. Non-diabetic causes of painful neuropathy can include deficiency states associated with alcoholism and vitamin B12 deficiency, uraemia and ischaemic neuropathy associated with peripheral vascular disease. First-line treatment is TCAs and then duloxetine or gabapentin.

Somatoform pain disorder

In somatoform pain, which is sometimes referred to as psychogenic pain, the patient complains of severe and distressing pain that has the qualities of pain arising from a physical (somatic) cause, but which cannot be attributed to objectively demonstrable organic pathology.[1] Pain occurs in association with emotional conflict or psychosocial problems deep enough to point to their possible causation.

Differential diagnoses include occult organic pain, depression, substance abuse, malingering and rare disorders such as sickle cell anaemia and porphyria. Management is difficult and is based on caring support devoid of promoting the 'sick role'. Psychological treatments are directed towards helping the patient to cope and 'live with the pain'. The possibility of comorbid depression should be addressed and if it is possible an appropriate trial of antidepressants can be tried. Referral for CBT or similar psychotherapies or to a pain clinic are options.

Practice tips

- Stop opioids if not effective/not improving function and wean by 10% of daily dose per week (this may take months).
- Physiotherapy has an important role in the management of pain.

References

1. Expert group for Analgesic guidelines. Pain. In: eTG complete. Melbourne: Therapeutic Guidelines Ltd. Available from: <www.tg.org.au>, accessed January 2018.
2. Crammond T. Pain relief. In: *MIMS Disease Index* (2nd edn). Sydney: IMS Publishing, 1996: 380–5.
3. O'Reilly S. Treatment of chronic non-malignant pain in general practice. Aust Fam Physician, 1994; 23: 281.
4. Roxburgh A, Bruno R et al. Prescription of opioid analgesics and related harms in Australia. Med J Aust, 2011; 1985(5): 280–4.
5. Shaheed CA, Maher CA et al. Efficacy and dose dependent effects of opioid analgesia for low back pain: a systematic review and meta-analysis. JAMA Intern Med, May 23, 2016: 1251.
6. Mehta V, Langford PM. Acute pain management for opioid dependent patients. Anesthesia, 2006; 61(3): 269–76.
7. Thomson K, Tey D, Marks M. *Paediatric Handbook* (8th edn). Melbourne: Wiley-Blackwell, 2009: 54–70.
8. NSW Therapeutic Advisory Group Inc. Paracetamol use: a position statement. December 2008. Available from: <www.nswtag.org.au/wp-content/uploads/2017/07/paracetamol-use-dec-2008.pdf>, accessed February 2018.
9. Macintye PE, Scott DA et al. *Acute pain management: scientific evidence* (3rd edn). Melbourne: ANZ College, Faculty of Pain Medicine, 2010.
10. Baum C, Kennedy DL, Forbes MB. Utilisation of NSAIDs. Arthritis Rheum, 1985; 28: 686–92.
11. Ryan P. Pharmacology of musculoskeletal treatment agents. Monash Distance Education: Graduate Diploma in Family Medicine. Musculoskeletal Medicine Notes, 2001; 6(1): 10–13.
12. Brooks PM, Yeomans ND. NSAIDs gastropathy: is it preventable? Aust N Z J Med, 1992; 22: 685–91.

13 Day RO, Graham G. The vascular effects of COX–2 selective inhibitors. Australian Prescriber, 2004; 27: 142–5.

14 Expert group for Analgesic guidelines. Chronic pain; Neuropathic pain. In: eTG complete. Melbourne: Therapeutic Guidelines Ltd. Available from: <www.tg.org.au>, accessed January 2018.

15 Bashford GM. The use of anticonvulsants for neuropathic pain. Australian Prescriber, 1999; 22(6): 140–1.

16 Finnerup NB, Sindrup SH et al. The evidence for pharmacological treatment of neuropathic pain. Pain, 2010; 150(3): 573–581. Available from: <www.ncbi.nlm.nih.gov/pubmed/20705215>, accessed February 2018.

17 Backonja M, Beydoun A et al. Gabapentin for the symptomatic treatment of painful neuropathy in patients with diabetes mellitus. JAMA, 1998; 280: 1831–6.

18 Gouche R. Neuropathic pain. Part 1. Medical Observer, 2001; 22 June: 44–5.

Research and evidence-based medicine

13

Not the possession of truth, but the effort of struggling to attain it brings joy to the researcher.

GOFFHOLD LASSING (1729–81)

Effective research is the trademark of the medical profession. When confronted with the great responsibility of understanding and treating human beings we need as much scientific evidence as possible to render our decision making valid, credible and justifiable.

Research can be defined as 'a systematic method in which the truth of evidence is based on observing and testing the soundness of conclusions according to consistent rules'[1] or, to put it more simply, 'research is organised curiosity',[2] the end point being new and improved knowledge.

In the medical context the term 'research' tends to conjecture bench-type laboratory research. However, the discipline of general practice provides a fertile research area in which to evaluate the morbidity patterns and the nature of common problems in addition to the processes specific to primary health care.

There has been an excellent tradition of research conducted by GPs. Tim Murrell in his paper 'Nineteenth century masters of general practice'[3] describes the contributions of Edward Jenner, Caleb Parry, John Snow, Robert Koch and James MacKenzie, and notes that 'among the characteristics they shared was their capacity to observe and record natural phenomena, breaking new frontiers of discovery in medicine using an ecological paradigm'.

This tradition was carried into the 20th century by Australian GPs such as Clifford Jungfer, Alan Chancellor, Charles Bridges-Webb, Kevin Cullen and Trevor Beard,[4] and now the research activities of the new generation of GPs, academic-based or practice-based, have been taken to a higher level with the development of evidence-based medicine (EBM).

Based on the work of the Cochrane Collaboration and the initiatives of Chris Silagy, Paul Glasziou and Chris Del Mar in particular, research has moved from the relatively 'pure' hospital environment to 'real world' scenarios which better reflect the circumstances of patients living in the community. Plenty of interventions which seem to work well in sponsored clinical trials are less impressive when measured in general practice. Some other interventions such as lifestyle management turn out to be surprisingly effective once they are accurately measured.

The focus of EBM has been to improve health care and health economics. Its development has gone hand in hand with improved information technology. EBM is inextricably linked to research.

The aim of this chapter is to present a brief overview of research and EBM and, in particular, to encourage GPs, either singly or collectively, to undertake research—simple or sophisticated—and also to publish their work. The benefits of such are well outlined in John Howie's classic text *Research in General Practice.*[5]

Why do research?

The basic objective of research is to acquire new knowledge and justification for decision making in medical practice. Research provides a basis for the acquisition of many skills, particularly those of critical thinking and scientific methodology. The discipline of general practice is special to us with its core content of continuing, comprehensive, community-based primary care, family care, domiciliary care, whole-person care and preventive care. To achieve credibility and parity with our specialist colleagues we need to research this area with appropriate methodology and to define the discipline clearly. There is no area of medicine that involves such a diverse range and quantity of decisions each day as general practice, and therefore patient management needs as much evidence-based rigour as possible.

Our own patch, be it an isolated rural practice or an industrial suburban practice, has its own micro-epidemiological fascination. Thus, it provides a unique opportunity to find answers to questions and make observations about that particular community.

Increasingly, GPs are expected to be able to sift through mountains of information in order to reliably offer advice about how the evidence applies to the individual sitting in front of them. Much of the information available to patients and doctors is either dubious opinion, or skewed towards the interests of an entity providing the intervention, rather than to the patient. An understanding of how research is produced provides a basis for the ability to critically appraise medical evidence.

There are also personal reasons to undertake research. The process assists professional development, encourages clear and critical thinking, improves knowledge, and offers the satisfaction of developing new skills and opening horizons.

The author undertook many small studies on common, everyday problems during 10 years in country practice to determine the most effective treatments for which no or minimal evidence in the literature could be found. Many of these recommendations—for problems such as tennis elbow, cold sores, aphthous ulcers, ingrown toenails, hiccoughs, back pain, nightmares, temporomandibular dysfunction and warts—appear in this text. Although the numbers were relatively small, it was useful to compare treatments for about 10 or 20 cases to test hypotheses and allow trends to emerge. Subsequent results from a large controlled trial would, of course, take precedence over these recommendations if they differed. However, the exercise, albeit limited, added immense interest to one's practice, which at times can be tedious without such scholarly challenges.

An important reason to undertake research is to conform with quality assurance processes that are now being expected of practitioners. The significant processes evaluating our accountability for quality control include audits of our own records, studies of critical incidents and morbidity studies.

Who should do research?

Any GP searching for answers to questions and who has the opportunity should undertake research. Research is largely opportunistic; for some it may be an impulsive reaction to a fascinating observation, for others a carefully conceived plan.

The research question should be answerable, and that answer, whether positive or negative, should be useful to patients.

Research can be collaborative, and in fact a group practice is an excellent way to get started. Research can also be undertaken in solo practice where the ability for personalised supervision of outcomes in patients is unique but where double-blind controlled trials are almost impossible.

Many GPs who have started 'small' have progressed to great heights of research activity, especially if they enjoy analysing the raw data once it has been produced. In the process of posing questions and eventually finding the answers they frequently refer to the experience as 'good fun'.

The Royal Australian College of General Practitioners (RACGP) promotes and supports general practice research (visit www.racgp.org.au/support/research or email research@racgp.org.au).

Asking questions

We often ask questions during the course of managing patients and such questions can form the basis of a research project, however simple.

Typical questions might be:

- Is most night-time cough in children due to asthma?
- Is suicide or attempted suicide in adolescent males precipitated by sexual-orientation issues?
- Is recurrent migraine caused by cervical dysfunction?
- Should we use antibiotics to treat otitis media in children presenting in general practice?
- Does the distribution of leaflets by the receptionist in the waiting room lead to increased immunisation rates or cervical smears?
- Are my patients satisfied with the services they receive?
- Does the provision of patient information leaflets for the management of hypertension lead to better adherence?

Research on what?

General practice has its own unique characteristics including illness content, processes, epidemiology, health services, quality assurance and doctor–patient relationships. The special contact with patients provides opportunities to evaluate their perspectives on health service delivery, psychosocial issues and communication skills. The old saying 'dig where you are' is relevant to all of us. GPs invariably develop their own special interests and this is a logical area in which to conduct research. Conducting a morbidity and prescribing survey in a practice is a simple and fascinating study. If the results are added to a wider study, invaluable information about the nature of general practice is obtained.[5,6]

The World Organization of National Colleges and Assemblies of General Practice (WONCA) produced the first *International Classification of Primary Care* (ICPC) in 1987, since ratified by the WHO. This classification of presenting symptoms, diagnoses and treatments has greatly assisted the process of morbidity studies.[8]

Research in general practice obviously covers many clinical areas studied by other groups but we may ask different types of questions, study different populations and use different methodologies, especially qualitative methods.

It would be logical to conduct research on those common problems requiring continuing care by the GP. These include:

- alcohol problems
- anxiety and depression
- arthritis
- chronic back pain and neck pain
- cancer
- cardiovascular disorders
- diabetes mellitus
- epilepsy
- common acute infections
- migraine and other headache
- women's health

Special opportunities, such as the observation that certain diseases or conditions are linked with specific circumstances, present frequently in primary care. An example is the observation that a group of farmers who presented to their rural practitioner over a period of time with lymphosarcoma were all exposed to a specific herbicide to control blackberry growth on their farms. This led to further, statewide investigations of this association, which indicated a significant link between the agent and the disease.

Research in primary care populations often overturns long-held beliefs based on specialist research in high-risk populations, which was wrongly assumed to apply to general practice. Examples include screening for prostate cancer using the PSA test and the use of antibiotics in otitis media.

Understanding terminology

Validity and reliability

- An ideal method of collecting research material is one that is valid.
- A valid method is one that measures what it claims to measure.
- A reliable method is one that produces repeatable results.

Validity refers to the 'true' answer, which must be relevant, complete and accurate. Three significant questions that evaluate validity are:[1]

- Is the study useful or is the result inconclusive?
- Do you accept the results of this study as applied to the source population?
- Do the results apply to the population in which you would be interested?

Internal validity refers to the adequacy of the study methods in reference to the study population, while *external validity* refers to the generalisability of the results to the general population.

Reliability refers to the stability of question-and-answer response and is most successfully measured by testing and then retesting (repeatedly).

Sensitivity, specificity and predictive values

Sensitivity and specificity, which are integral to validity, are important considerations in decision making in medicine, particularly in choosing appropriate investigations for disease diagnoses. The method of calculation of sensitivity, specificity and predictive values is summarised in FIGURE 13.1.

The *sensitivity* of a test depends on the proportion of people with the characteristic (disease) in whom the test is positive (i.e. percentage positive with disease). For example, if the sensitivity for a sign is 90% then the sign will be detected in 90% of the people but not in 10%. The ultimate sensitive test is one that detects all true positive cases.

The *specificity* of a test depends on the proportion of people without the characteristic (disease) in whom the test is negative (i.e. percentage negative of healthy people). The ultimate specific test is one that detects all the truly negative (disease-free) cases. A *gold standard* test is one that is as close to 100% specificity and 100% sensitivity as possible.

Aide-mémoire tip

SPIN—Specific tests where a positive helps rule *IN* disease

SNOUT—Sensitive tests where a negative helps rule *OUT* disease

A clinical example of sensitivity and specificity is presented in TABLE 13.1.

Table 13.1 The predictability of signs and symptoms for carpal tunnel syndrome[9]

	Sensitivity (%)	Specificity (%)
Paraesthesia	97	4
Waking at night	91	14
Anaesthesia	57	61
Phalen's test	58	54
Tinel's test	42	63
Two point discrimination test	6	98

13

	Test positive	Test negative		
Condition present	A True positive	C False negative	A + C	Sensitivity $\frac{A}{A+C}$ %
Condition absent	B False positive	D True negative	B + D	Specificity $\frac{D}{B+D}$ %
	Positive predictive value $\frac{A}{A+B}$ %	Negative predictive value $\frac{D}{C+D}$ %		

Sensitivity:	How often a test shows pathology when it is present
Specificity:	How often a test is normal when no pathology present
Positive predictive value:	Indicates the likelihood of the patient having disease when the test is positive
Negative predictive value:	Indicates the likelihood of the patient not having disease when the test is negative

FIGURE 13.1 Definitions of sensitivity, specificity and predictive values

Predictive values express the proportion of positives that are 'true positives' and negatives that are 'true negatives'. They are markedly affected by the underlying risk of the disease in the population being studied. Because community patients usually have considerably lower rates of disease than hospitalised patients, positive predictive values (PPVs) are generally lower in general practice for any given test or symptom. This reduces the usefulness of ordering the test or relying on the symptom for a diagnosis.

For example, the presence of haematuria in a general practice patient gives a PPV of less than 5% for carcinoma being the cause, but the PPV is about 50% in the inpatient hospital setting.

Incidence and prevalence

The meanings of these two terms are easily confused:

- *Incidence* refers to the number of new cases of a disease (or factor of interest) occurring in a defined population within a specified period of time.
- *Prevalence* refers to the total number of individuals who have the disease (or factor of interest) at a particular time in a population. The number is divided by the number of people in the population at that time.
  - Examples: The prevalence of multiple sclerosis in temperate climates is 1 in 1000–2000 compared with 1 in 10 000 in the tropics. The incidence of multiple sclerosis in the Australian state of Victoria (population 5.8 million) is 8 per 100 000 per year.

Bias

This is any effect occurring during the research that tends to produce results that depart systematically from the true values. Varieties of bias include *measurement bias* (e.g. fault with a sphygmomanometer recording blood pressure), *confounding bias* (e.g. investigating the association between stress and hypertension without considering the influence of alcohol), *selection bias* (e.g. using hospital outpatients in a community-based study) and *publication bias* (around half of all research is not published, which skews the pool of evidence available for reading and analysis).

Confounding

This is a situation in which a measure of the effect of exposure on risk is distorted by the association of exposure with other (known or unknown) factors that influence the outcome.[1] A confounder is a factor that distorts the apparent magnitude of the effect of a study on risk.

Chance

One must question the probability that the results favouring the experimental intervention could have occurred by chance; therefore, we resort to statistical help in the form of a probability statement or significance level.

How is the research undertaken?

'Getting started' can be quite difficult for the beginner. However, assistance is available from several sources including individual GPs with research experience, university departments of general practice and the RACGP research committee. Seek out a suitable supervisor for the study. A chronological method follows.

1. *The idea.* Start with an idea or question, which needs to be interesting, relevant, significant and answerable.[10] It may be appropriate to develop a hypothesis at this stage.
2. *Float the idea.* Next, discuss the idea with colleagues or an appropriate accessible authority.
3. *Do a literature search.* Review the literature: for example, a Medline search or check with a central research 'bank'. Undertake a critical review.
4. *Prepare a plan.* This can be a short written plan outlining the methodology for the study.
5. *Evaluate the plan.* Then, contact a supervisor or appropriate authority to evaluate the study plan, which may be referred to a reference group or research committee.
6. *Methodology: develop a protocol.*
   - Prepare background; outline objectives and develop a hypothesis.
   - Select target population using clear criteria and appropriate numbers.
   - Design the research:
     - qualitative or quantitative?
     - questionnaire(s)
   - Assess internal validity.
   - Consider statistical implications early:
     - number of patients
     - method for data analysis
   - Recruit subjects and assistants.
   - Assess the timeframe.
   - Assess the ethical considerations → ethics approval committee.
7. *Consider a preliminary pilot study and project timetable.*
8. *Seek funding.* Solicit advice from appropriate funding bodies.
9. *Conduct the study.*
10. *Analyse the data/statistics.*
11. *Undertake interpretation and conclusions.*
12. *Prepare for publication.*

Research design

Hypothesis development

The reasoning process of the researcher is based on the null hypothesis—the default assumption that an experimental group does not differ from a control 'normal' group in outcome. The question to consider is: 'What is the probability that results from the experimental intervention would have occurred by chance?'. The answer is based on a probability statement: 'The probability that the positive results occurred by chance is less than 5% (p <0.05)'.[11]

Selecting a representative sample of appropriate size

Two basic components of subject selection are sample size and sample representativeness. The latter should be selected in a well-controlled manner.

A common question is: 'What is the ideal size of the sample?' There is no fixed answer but it must be adequate to produce statistically meaningful results, without being so large as to make the research impractical or unaffordable.

Recruitment of patients is a particular skill and often hard work, but it is easier if the researcher has a large pool of patients with whom he or she enjoys a good relationship. A useful rule is to aim to approach $3n$ patients if you wish to work with a sample size of n.

Some guidelines for choosing the sample size are:[11]

- the more the individuals in the population differ, the larger the required sample
- the more planned comparisons, the larger the size
- larger sample sizes allow detection of smaller differences

Types of research[1]

The two broad categories of research in general practice are qualitative research, which is based on observation and talking with people, and quantitative research, which is based on measurement and analysis of data collection.

Research can also be classified as primary research, which includes both qualitative and quantitative methods, and secondary research, which involves systematic reviews and meta-analysis.

Qualitative research[12]

This research is basically concerned with evaluating human behaviour from the subject's perspective. It is based on close observation and is expressed in a descriptive way. It addresses questions that begin 'Why?', 'How?', 'In what way does?', e.g. 'Why have so many people been dropping out of this fitness program?'.

Common qualitative approaches

- Phenomenology
- Ethnography
- Grounded theory
- Biography (life story, narrative enquiry)
- Case study

The methods used are:

- interviews (open-ended, semi-structured)
- focus groups
- participation observation
- document analysis

Qualitative research is an excellent method for generating hypotheses, and can lead to quantitative research.

Phenomenology

The central focus of this philosophy/method is the lived experience of the world of everyday life. It describes events, situations, experiences and concepts. It provides:

- detailed descriptions of an experience or event as it is lived
- deeper understandings and sensitivities
- improved thoughtful provision of care

Examples:

- effects of Viagra (and other agents) on marital/sexual relationships
- experience of carers in Alzheimer disease
- effects of workplace bullying on absenteeism

Ethnography (*ethnos* = a nation)

13

This examines cultures, peoples and societies including subgroups, e.g. adolescents. It is the basis of anthropology. The investigator usually identifies a number of key witnesses (informants) and interviews them to clarify observations.

Grounded theory

This is the development of new theory through the collection and analysis of data. It seeks to identify the core social processes within a given context in order to build theory that is grounded in the reality of those being studied.

Quantitative research

Quantitative research is research based on the collection of data in numerical quantities and asks a specific narrow question, such as 'What is the chance that . . .?' or 'What proportion of . . .?'. It is concerned with hypothesis testing, reliability and validity and is the cornerstone of epidemiology. It can be classified broadly as *observational,* which includes case control, cross-sectional and cohort studies, and *experimental,* which includes the classic controlled trial.[12]

- *Case control (or retrospective) study* is an observational study in which people with a disease (cases) are compared with those without it (control group). It is often used to determine a statistical association between an exposure and an outcome, particularly a rare outcome.
  - Examples: Patients with mesothelioma were investigated for exposure to asbestos or other agents; the mothers of children born with birth defects were investigated for an association with drug intake during pregnancy.
- *Cross-sectional or prevalence study* follows a correlation approach using existing databases. It is a survey of the frequency of disease, risk factors or other characteristics in a defined population at one particular time.
  - Example: The prevalence of diabetes mellitus (diagnosed and undiagnosed) was investigated in an Aboriginal community living in a particular area of metropolitan Sydney.
- *Cohort (or prospective) study* is also referred to as 'follow-up'. The study follows a group (cohort) of individuals with a specified characteristic or disease over a period of time. Comparisons may be made with a control group.
  - Example: 120 patients with chronic sciatica were followed over 10 years to determine the outcome of their pain and neurological deficit. These were compared with a matched group who had undergone laminectomy.
- *Randomised controlled trial* (RCT) is an experimental study that tests for hypothesised outcomes. Participants in the trial are randomly allocated to either receive the specific intervention or not receive it (the control group). The objective is to establish a causal relationship between the intervention and the hypothesised outcome. The ideal scientific trial is a **double-blind trial** where

neither staff nor the participating patient are aware whether the participant is in the intervention or control group. An RCT is the typical study when assessing the effect of a drug compared to a placebo.

Meta-analysis

Meta-analysis is the process that systematically assesses compatible randomised controlled trials by merging the data (usually from smaller and inconclusive trials) to draw a 'firmer' conclusion from larger numbers of subjects.

Evidence-based medicine

Evidence-based medicine (EBM) is a process of basing clinical practice on validated information. According to one of its modern architects, David Sackett, it is 'the explicit, judicious and conscientious use of current best available evidence in making decisions about the care of individual patients'.[13] According to Silagy and Haines, 'EBM is the integration of the best available scientific evidence with your clinical expertise and knowledge, your intuition, your wisdom'.[14]

The process of using EBM should be very comfortable for GPs because scientific methodology and evidence is second nature to us and has been the basis of our clinical decision making prior to and subsequent to graduation.

The proposed five steps of applying EBM are similar to basic research methodology:[14]

1 Construct a clinical question or define the problem.
2 Search for the evidence.
3 Appraise the quality and relevance of the evidence.
4 Apply it to the care of an individual patient.
5 Evaluate how effective it is.

The statistical methodologies used in EBM cover the traditional research methods but there is an emphasis on the methods of risk reduction, absolute and relative risk reduction, and number needed to treat (NNT). These definitions are included in the glossary of terms later in this chapter.

GPs have a responsibility to their patients to be well versed with the best evidence when making decisions about management (see TABLE 13.2), whether it be for a minor surgical procedure, selection of drugs, selection of an investigation, or referral to the most appropriate consultant. If the best evidence reveals that a certain practice we are using is of no value or is less efficacious than another method, then we should be prepared to change. On the other hand, if we find that a certain method works for us and there is no current evidence that it is inappropriate or the evidence is equivocal, then there is no compelling reason to change.

Table 13.2 Levels of evidencea

I	Evidence obtained from a systematic review of all relevant randomised trials.
II	Evidence obtained from at least one properly designed randomised controlled trial.
III	Evidence from well-controlled trials that are not randomised, or from well-designed cohort or case-control studies, or multiple time series (with and without the intervention).
IV	Opinions of respected authorities; opinion based on clinical experience; descriptive studies; or reports of expert committees.

Source: Modified from the NHMRC.

GPs need a healthy scepticism about what is best evidence and claims for treatment in addition to the skill of critical appraisal of research/evidence. We tend to be impressed by the perception that evidence is a numbers game. However, the great work of James Lind (see the introduction to CHAPTER 10) shows that facts do not necessarily involve large numbers.

For EBM to be accepted by GPs the information needs to be readily accessible, user friendly, significant, relevant and, perhaps, believable.

The strength of EBM is that it can provide the answers to very important everyday decisions, especially in screening and preventive medicine, where guidelines have fluctuated over the decades. The most recent RACGP guidelines for preventive activities in general practice (the red book)[15] highlight the value of current evidence (see www.racgp.org.au/your-practice/guidelines).

GPs are currently faced with important decisions about the effectiveness of complementary therapies, which are very tempting to embrace or trial when searching for ways to manage difficult problems, such as chronic fatigue syndrome, fibromyalgia, chronic asthma, chronic pain syndromes and other difficult-to-treat diseases. We are hopeful that EBM can provide the answers to best practice in addition to evaluating individual therapies.

Remember, however, that Bayes' theorem tells us that a positive trial result means less if the pre-existing chances of the treatment working were low to begin with. In other words, 'extraordinary claims require extraordinary evidence'.

Glossary of terms[18,19]

Apart from the terms and definitions used in preceding pages it is important to highlight the following terms used in EBM/research.

Absolute risk reduction (ARR) The absolute difference in event rates between two intervention or treatment groups. It gives an indication of the baseline risk and treatment effect. An *ARR* of 0 means no difference and thus the treatment has no effect.

Example: The *ARR* for prophylactic ciprofloxacin in the case cited is 10 – 2 = 8 per 100 (0.08) or 8%.

Accessing the evidence

- The Cochrane library is free to access in Australia. It includes:
  - Database of Systematic Reviews
  - Database of Abstracts of Reviews of Effectiveness
- www.thecochranelibrary.com

  or
- www.cochrane.org
- The TRIP database searches for all relevant research articles that answer your question (typed in plain English). See www.tripdatabase.com

Analysis of variance This allows comparisons between the means of two samples of similar populations with a normal distribution. The contribution to variance for each variable can be determined and tested for statistical significance.

Clinical significance Whether the benefit to people receiving an intervention compared to the control group is great enough to warrant the intervention. It is based on measure of effect.

Confidence interval A measure of the imprecision of the data results. The statistically derived range of values around a trial result in which the probability is that the true result will be within the range.

A 95% (standard) confidence interval for a sample indicates that there is a 95% chance that the interval includes the true population proportion whose circumstances comply with the evidence.

Control event rate (CER) The percentage of subjects in the control group that experienced the event of interest.

Experimental event rate (EER) The percentage of subjects in the intervention group that experienced the event of interest.

Kappa Cohen's *kappa* measures the agreement between the evaluations of two raters when both are rating the same object. A value of 1 indicates perfect agreement. A value of 0 indicates that agreement is no better than chance. It is an appropriate statistic for tables that have the same categories in the columns as in the rows (e.g. when measuring agreement between two raters).

Number needed to treat (NNT) The number of people who must be treated over a given period of time with the experimental therapy (specific intervention) to achieve one good outcome or prevent one adverse outcome. This incorporates the duration of treatment. It is a measure of the absolute relative risk. Obviously the lower the *NNT,* the better the treatment. It is calculated as 100/*ARR* (%); that is, the reciprocal of the *ARR.*

Note: The *NNT* will be different for different patient populations depending on their baseline risk for developing the outcome of interest.

Odds ratio The probability of the occurrence of an event compared to its non-occurrence.

Publications

- Clinical evidence: BMJ Publishing Group, refer to www.clinicalevidence.org
- Evidence-based medicine. BMJ Publishing Group

Probability (p) value A deceptively complex measure to understand. It is a statistical summary of the incompatibility between the observed data and what we would have expected to see if the treatment did not work in the slightest (i.e. if the 'null hypothesis' was true). The lower the p value, the less consistent it is that the experiment results can be explained by the null hypothesis. Confusingly, a p=0.05 does not at all equate to saying the treatment is therefore 95% likely to work. For the curious, a 2016 article offers a 14-page explanation.[20]

Relative risk (RR) The ratio of the risk of the outcome (e.g. disease or death) in the treatment/exposure group compared with the control/unexposed group. *RR* informs us how many times more likely an event is to occur in the treatment group compared with the control group.

Calculation: *RR* = *EER*/*CER*

RR = 1 means no difference, so treatment has no effect

RR > 1 means the treatment increases the risk of disease/death

RR < 1 means the treatment decreases the risk

Example: If the risk of death from people exposed to inhalation of anthrax spores is reduced from 10 in 100 cases to 2 in 100 cases with 60 days of prophylactic ciprofloxacin, the *RR* of death in this group is 0.20 or 20%.

Relative risk reduction (RRR) The proportional reduction of adverse events between the treatment/experimental and the control groups in a trial (i.e. *RRR* is the ratio of the absolute risk reduction to the risk of the outcome in the control group). An alternative way to calculate the *RRR* is to subtract the *RR* from 1 (i.e. *RRR* = 1 – *RR*).

In the example it is: 1 – 0.2 = 0.80 or 80% or:

$$RRR = \frac{APR}{10} = \frac{8}{10} = 0.80 \text{ or } 80\%$$

RRR is probably the most commonly reported measure of treatment effects, particularly when trying to emphasise the usefulness of a treatment, but the *ARR* gives a more realistic picture.

Risk (R) The probability that an event (death or disease) will occur.

Statistical significance The likelihood of a difference between two groups being real, based on the possibility that the difference may have occurred by chance alone. It is based on confidence intervals and p values.

Type I error A type I error occurs when a study concludes that there is a difference between two groups when there is no difference.

Type II error A type II error occurs when a study concludes that no difference exists between groups when there is a true difference.

To counterbalance the strengths (potential or real) of EBM there are concerns that it will be seized by bureaucrats to develop 'cook book' guidelines, Holy Writ or economic rationalisation. Others are concerned about the perceived lack of flexibility. A very interesting critical review, especially affecting psychiatry, was presented by John Ellard in his paper 'What exactly is evidence-based medicine?'.[16] He questioned the validity of the evidence underpinning EBM and the biases of both the proponents of 'science' and 'art' with the caution of Louis Pasteur: 'The greatest derangement of the mind is to believe in something because one wishes it to be so'.[17]

Critical appraisal of published research

The objective of critically appraising a paper is to determine whether the methods and results of the research have significant validity to produce useful information. The appraisal starts with a careful review of the abstract, which ideally should be presented in a structured format.

1 What were the objectives of the study?
2 Were the ethical aspects properly followed?
3 What was the study design?
4 Were there any potential problems associated with the design?
5 Were all the patients who entered the study properly accounted for at its conclusion?
6 What were the important results?
7 How would you interpret and explain these results?

Many studies, quite legitimately, are sponsored by a company that may benefit from a positive finding, and/or are authored by researchers who have received industry funding. This does not negate any finding, but does perhaps warrant a more thorough critical appraisal before applying that finding to your patients.

References

1 Schattner P. Introduction to research and research designs. In: Piterman L (ed). *Introduction to Research in Family Medicine MFM 2006,* 1996: 2–7.
2 Eimerl T. Organised curiosity. J R Coll Gen Pract, 1960; 3(1): 246–52.
3 Murrell TGC. Nineteenth century masters of general practice. Med J Aust, 1991; 155: 785–92.
4 Anderson NA, Bridges-Webb C, Chancellor A. *General Practice in Australia.* Sydney: Sydney University Press, 1986: 124–30.
5 Howie JGR. *Research in General Practice* (2nd edn). London: Chapman & Hall, 1992: 12–14.
6 Bridges-Webb C. The Australian general practice morbidity and prescribing survey, 1969–1976. Med J Aust (Suppl.) 1976; 2: 5–20.
7 Bridges-Webb C, Britt H, Miles DA et al. Morbidity and treatment in general practice in Australia 1990–1991. Med J Aust, 1992; 157: 51–7.
8 Lamberts H, Wood M. *ICPC: International Classification of Primary Care.* Oxford: Oxford University Press, 1987.
9 Buch-Jaeger N, Foucher G. Carpal tunnel syndrome: validity of clinical signs. J Hand Surg [Br], 1994; 19B: 72–4.
10 Silagy CA, Schattner P (eds). *An Introduction to General Practice Research.* Melbourne: Monash University, Department of Community Medicine, 1990.
11 Fowkes FGR, Fulton PM. Critical appraisal of published research: introductory guidelines. BMJ, 1991; 302: 1136–40.
12 McBride A, Hespe C. Research in general practice. Australian Doctor, 29 November 2013: 21–8.
13 Sackett DL et al. Evidence based medicine: what it is and what it isn't. BMJ, 1996; 312: 71–2.
14 Silagy C, Haines A. *Evidence Based Practice in Primary Care.* London: BMJ Books, 1998.
15 RACGP. *Guidelines for Preventive Activities in General Practice* (9th edn). Melbourne: RACGP, 2016.
16 Ellard J. What exactly is evidence-based medicine? Modern Medicine Australia, 1997; (September): 22–5.
17 Pasteur L. Speech to the French Academy of Medicine, July 18, 1876. In: Strauss MB (ed). *Familiar Medical Quotations.* Boston: Little Brown & Co., 1968: 502.
18 Rosser M, Shafir MS. *Evidence-based Family Medicine.* Hamilton: BC Decker Inc., 1998.
19 NPS News. Drug promotion: distinguishing the good oil from snake oil. NPS News, 2002; 25: 1–4.
20 Greenland, Sander et al. Statistical tests, P values, confidence intervals, and power: a guide to misinterpretations. European Journal of Epidemiology; 31(2016): 337–50.

Resources

Bowling A. *Research Methods in Health: Investigating Health and Health Services* (2nd edn). Milton Keynes: Open University Press, 2002.

Kristiansen I, Mooney G. *Evidence-based Medicine in its Place.* Oxfordshire: Routledge, 2004.

Sackett DL et al. *Evidence Based Medicine: How to Practice and Teach EBM.* London: Churchill Livingstone, 1997.

Glasziou P, Del Mar C, Salisbury J. *Evidence-based Medicine Workbook.* London: BMJ Books, 2003.

Silagy C, Haines A. *Evidence Based Practice in Primary Care.* London: BMJ Books, 1998.

Travel medicine

14

If you can't peel it, boil it or cook it—don't eat it.

ANON

Emporiatics—the science of travel medicine

With over 600 million international trips being taken annually, the health problems faced by travellers are considerable and variable depending on the countries visited and the lifestyle adopted by the traveller.[1] Travellers to North America, Europe and Australasia are usually at no greater risk of getting an infectious disease than they would be at home, but those visiting the less developed tropical and subtropical countries of Africa, Central and South America and South-East Asia are at significant risk of contracting infectious diseases. The immunocompromised are those at greatest risk.

Problems range in complexity from the most frequent and usually benign problems, such as traveller's diarrhoea, to more exotic and potentially fatal infections such as malaria, Japanese encephalitis and HIV. It must also be remembered that in some countries with volatile political changes there is the possibility of injury, incarceration or being left stranded. Travel means transport and thus the potential for accidents and crippled body and bank balance. Insurance for such contingencies is as important as preventive health measures.

Principles of pre-travel health care

- Advise the patient to plan early—at least 8 weeks beforehand.
- Register with Smartraveller (provided by the Australian Department of Foreign Affairs and Trade (DFAT)).
- Advise a dental check.
- Allow adequate time for consultation (e.g. 30–45 minutes).
- Individualise advice.
- Provide current information.
- Provide written as well as verbal advice.
- Provide a letter concerning existing medical illness and treatment.
- Encourage personal responsibility.

Key facts and checkpoints

- The main diseases facing the international traveller are traveller's diarrhoea (relatively mild) and malaria, especially the potentially lethal *Plasmodium falciparum* malaria.
- Register with Smartraveller (provided by the Australian Department of Foreign Affairs and Trade (DFAT)).
- Most cases of traveller's diarrhoea are caused by enterotoxigenic *Escherichia coli* and *Campylobacter* species.
- Enteroinvasive *E. coli* (a different serotype) produces a dysentery-like illness similar to *Shigella.*
- Traveller's diarrhoea is contracted mainly from contaminated water and ice used for beverages, washing food or utensils, or cleaning teeth.
- Poliomyelitis is endemic in at least 20 countries and thus immunisation for polio is still important.
- One bite from an infected mosquito during a single overnight stop in a malaria area can result in a possible lethal infection.
- Infections transmitted by mosquitoes include malaria, yellow fever, Rift Valley fever, Japanese B encephalitis, chikungunya, Zika and dengue fever. Avoiding their bites is excellent prevention.
- Every year approximately 1000 Australians catch malaria while travelling overseas.
- Malaria is a dusk-till-dawn risk only, but bites from daytime mosquitoes can cause dengue.
- *P. falciparum* malaria is steadily increasing, as is resistance to newer antimalarials.
- It is important for GPs to consult a travel medicine database to obtain specific information about 'at risk' countries.
- Avoid tattooing, ear-piercing, acupuncture or any skin puncturing while overseas.
- The commonest causes of death in travellers overseas are trauma (26%), particularly traffic accidents, and homicide (16.9%).
- Travellers visiting family and relatives (TVFR) in some countries are at risk of contracting preventable travel-related illnesses.

Gastrointestinal infections

The commonest problem facing travellers is traveller's diarrhoea but other important diseases caused by poor sanitation include hepatitis A, and worm infestations such as hookworm and schistosomiasis.

Contamination of food and water is a major problem, especially in third world countries.

Reputable soft drinks, such as Coca-Cola, should be recommended for drinking. Indian-style tea, in which the milk is boiled with tea, is usually safe, but tea with added milk is not. The food handlers can be infected and the water used to wash food may be contaminated.

Traveller's diarrhoea

Traveller's diarrhoea is a special problem in Mexico, Nepal, India, Pakistan, South-East Asia, Latin America, the Middle East and Central Africa and its many colourful labels include 'Bali Belly', 'Gippy Tummy', 'Rangoon Runs', 'Tokyo Trots' and 'Montezuma's Revenge'. It occurs about 6–12 hours after taking infected food or water.

The illness is usually mild and lasts only 2 or 3 days. It is unusual for it to last longer than 5 days. Symptoms include abdominal cramps, frequent diarrhoea with loose, watery bowel motions and possible vomiting. Very severe diarrhoea, especially if associated with the passing of blood or mucus, may be a feature of *Shigella* sp or *Campylobacter* sp infections and amoebiasis.

Most traveller's diarrhoea is caused by enterotoxigenic *E. coli (ETEC)*, *Campylobacter* sp, *Shigella* sp and *Salmonella* sp. Travellers are infected because they are exposed to slightly different types or strains of *E. coli* from the ones they are used to at home.[2]

The possible causes of diarrhoeal illness are listed in TABLE 14.1.

Table 14.1 Causes of diarrhoea in travellers

	Causative organism	Type of illness
Bacteria	*Escherichia coli*	Traveller's diarrhoea
	Shigella species	Dysentery
	Salmonella species	Typhoid fever, food poisoning
	Campylobacter jejuni	Traveller's diarrhoea, dysentery
	Vibrio cholerae	Cholera
	Vibrio parahaemolyticus	Traveller's diarrhoea
	Yersinia enterocolitica	Traveller's diarrhoea
	Aeromonas hydrophila	Traveller's diarrhoea
	Staphylococcus aureus (toxin)	Food poisoning
	Clostridium perfringens	Food poisoning
	Bacillus cereus	Food poisoning
Viruses	Rotavirus	Children's diarrhoea
	Norwalk virus	Traveller's diarrhoea
Protozoa parasites	Cryptosporidium	Amoebiasis
	Entamoeba histolytica	Giardiasis
	Giardia lamblia	Strongyloidiasis
	Strongyloides stercoralis	
	Schistosomiasis	
	Blastocystis hominis	
	Cyclosporiasis	
	Cryptosporidiosis	
	Isoporiasis	
	Blastocystitis hominis	
Chemicals	Capsicum (chilli)	

Treatment[3]

Refer to FIGURE 14.1.[2,3]

The key factor in treatment is rehydration.

Mild diarrhoea

- Maintain fluid intake—Gastrolyte.
- Antimotility agents (judicious use: if no blood in stools)—avoid in children.

loperamide (Imodium) 2 caps statim then 1 after each unformed stool (max. 8 caps/day)
or
diphenoxylate with atropine (Lomotil) 2 tablets statim then 1–2 (o) 8 hourly
Imodium is the preferred agent.

Moderate diarrhoea[3]

- Attend to hydration.
- Patient can self-administer antibiotic—e.g. single dose norfloxacin or azithromycin (especially in India, Nepal and Thailand).
- Loperamide in adults.

Severe diarrhoea (patient toxic and febrile)

- ?Admit to hospital.
- Attend to hydration—use an oral hydrate solution (e.g. Gastrolyte).
- Loperamide in adults.
- Antibiotic: norfloxacin (first choice), ciprofloxacin or azithromycin (usually 3 days).

Note: There is increasing resistance to doxycycline and cotrimoxazole, especially in South-East Asia.

Persistent diarrhoea

Any travellers with persistent diarrhoea after visiting less-developed countries, especially India and China, may have a protozoal infection such as amoebiasis

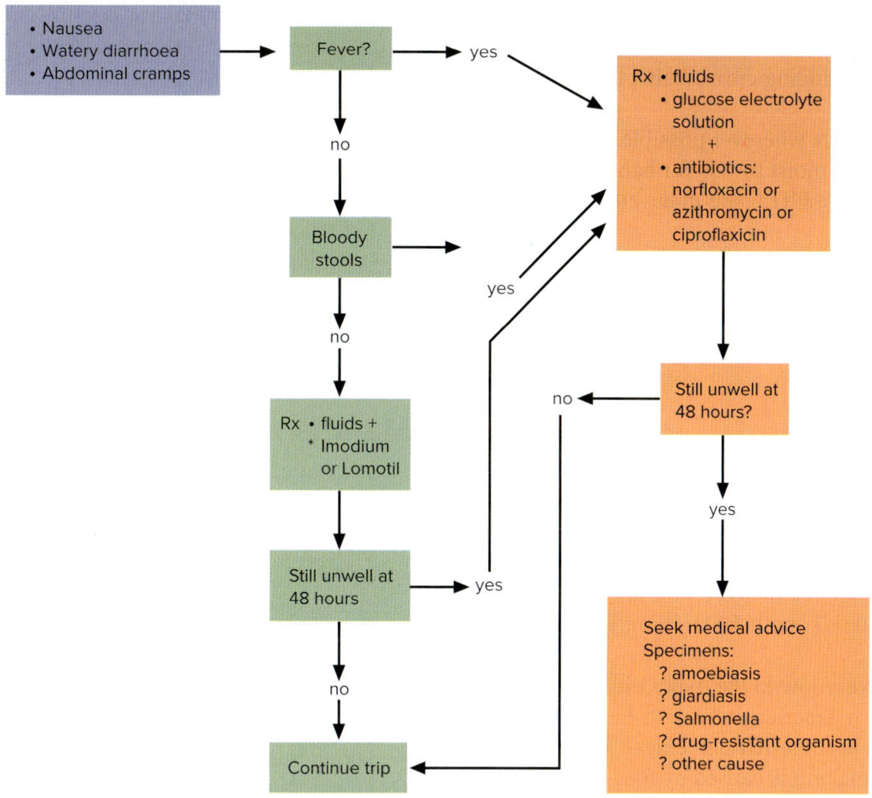

FIGURE 14.1 Algorithm for adult travellers with acute diarrhoea
Source: After Locke[2]

or giardiasis. If the patient has a fever and mucus or blood in the stools, suspect amoebiasis. Giardiasis is characterised by abdominal cramps, flatulence, and bubbly, foul-smelling diarrhoea persisting beyond 2 to 4 days. Take three specimens of faeces for analysis. In some cases serology may be helpful (e.g. amoebiasis).

Treatment

- Giardiasis: tinidazole or metronidazole
- Amoebiasis: metronidazole or tinidazole

Patients can self-administer these drugs and carry them if visiting areas at risk, but they can have a severe disulfram-like adverse reaction with alcohol.

Preventive advice

The following advice will help prevent diseases caused by contaminated food and water. These 'rules' need only be followed in areas of risk such as Africa, South America, India and other parts of Asia. Only drink purified water and only eat well-cooked food.

- Purify all water by boiling for 10 minutes. Adding purifying tablets is not so reliable, but if the water cannot be boiled some protection is provided by adding Puratabs (chlorine) or iodine (2% tincture of iodine), which is more effective than chlorine—use 4 drops of iodine to 1 litre of water and let it stand for 30 minutes.
- Avoid ice in your drinks unless known to be safe. Drink only boiled water (supplied in some hotels) or well-known bottled beverages (mineral water, 7-Up, Coca-Cola, beer).
- Brush your teeth using purified water.
- Avoid fresh salads or raw vegetables (including watercress). Salads or uncooked vegetables are often washed in contaminated water. Bananas and fruit with skins are safe once you have peeled and thrown away the skin but care should be taken with fruit that may possibly be injected with water.
- Be wary of dairy products such as milk, cream, ice-cream and cheese.

14

- Avoid eating raw shellfish and cold cooked meats.
- Avoid food, including citrus fruits, from street vendors.
- Drink hot liquids wherever possible.
- Use disposable moist towels for hand washing.
- Vaccines against ETEC are in development.

Golden rule for preventing diarrhoea

If you can't peel it, boil it or cook it—don't eat it.

Malaria

General aspects

- Travellers to all tropical countries are at some risk of this protozoal infection.
- Malaria is endemic in 102 countries;[4] 2.3 billion people are at risk, with 500 million affected every year.
- The risk is very low in the major cities of Central and Southern America and South-East Asia but can be high in some African cities.
- In humans malaria is caused by four species of plasmodium:
  - *Plasmodium vivax* and *P. ovale*—tertian malaria
  - *P. falciparum*—malignant tertian malaria
  - *P. malariae*—quartian malaria
  - *P. knowlesi*—presents like vivax and falciparum
- Malaria is either benign (vivax, ovale) or malignant (falciparum).
- Resistance to many drugs is increasing:
  - The lethal *P. falciparum* is developing resistance to chloroquine and the antifolate antimalarials (Fansidar and Maloprim).[4]
  - Resistance is now reported to mefloquine and artemether.
  - Resistance is common in South-East Asia, Papua New Guinea (PNG), northern South America and parts of Africa.
- Chloroquine is used infrequently as it is only effective in limited areas of the world but not PNG.
- The long-awaited vaccine will make all the complex drug management much simpler. However, it still appears to be many years away despite considerable research.
- Patients who have had splenectomies are at grave risk from *P. falciparum* malaria (PFM).
- People die from malaria because of delayed diagnosis, delayed therapy, inappropriate therapy and parasite–host factors.
- It is recommended that pregnant women and young children do not travel to malarious areas (if possible).
- Practitioners should follow updated recommended guidelines (e.g. WHO therapeutic guidelines (antibiotic)).

DxT fever + chills + headache → malaria

Malaria risk assessment

The risk of catching malaria is increased by:

- being in a malaria area, especially during and after the wet season
- a prolonged stay in a malaria area, especially rural areas, small towns and city fringes
- sleeping in unscreened rooms without mosquito nets over the bed
- wearing dark clothing with short-sleeved shirts and shorts
- taking inappropriate drug prophylaxis
- an incomplete course of prophylaxis

Malaria prevention

Travellers should be advised that malaria may be prevented by following two simple rules:

1. avoid mosquito bites
2. take antimalarial medicines regularly

In order to avoid mosquito bites, travellers are advised to:

- keep away from rural areas and avoid outdoor activities between dusk and darkness
- sleep in air-conditioned or properly screened rooms
- use insecticide sprays to kill any mosquitoes in the room or use mosquito coils at night
- smear an insect repellent on exposed parts of the body; an effective repellent is diethyl-m-toluamide (Muskol, Repellem, Rid)
- use mosquito nets (tuck under mattress; check for tears)
- impregnate nets with permethrin (Ambush) or deltamethrin
- wear sufficient light-coloured clothing, long sleeves and long trousers to protect whole body and arms and legs when in the open after sunset
- avoid using perfumes, cologne and after-shave lotion (also attract insects)

Important considerations in malaria prophylaxis

1 Minimise exposure to mosquitoes and avoid bites.
2 Know areas of risk:
   - tropical South America (southern Mexico to northern half South America)
   - tropical Africa (sub-Sahara to northern South Africa)
   - Nile region, including remote rural Egypt
   - Southern Asia, especially tropical areas
3 Know areas of widespread chloroquine resistance:
   - Asia, tropical South America (rare north of Panama Canal), sub-Sahara, East Africa
4 Consider several factors:
   - intensity of transmission
   - season and length of stay
   - itinerary

     urban—hotel
     urban—non-hotel
     rural—housing
     rural—backpacking
   - resistance patterns
   - host factors
     - age
     - pregnancy
     - associated illness
     - compliance
5 Know the antimalarial drugs (see TABLE 14.2).
6 Balance risk benefit of drug prophylaxis: drug side effects versus risk of PFM.
7 Visiting areas of PFM does not automatically require the use of potentially harmful drugs.[1]
8 Those at special risk are pregnant women, young children and the immunocompromised. Advise against travel.
9 No drugs give complete protection.

Drug prophylaxis

Refer to WHO guidelines (www.who.int/ith/en).

Guidelines

- Accommodation in large, air-conditioned hotels in most cities of South-East Asia (dusk–dawn) for <2 weeks: no prophylaxis required.
- For low-risk travel (urban: dusk–dawn) in areas of high resistance for <2 weeks: doxycycline is adequate; use a treatment course of Malarone if necessary (see TABLE 14.3).
- Chloroquine is no longer recommended because of the global spread of resistance.
- For short- and long-term travel to rural areas of high resistance (e.g. South-East Asia including Thailand, Kenya, Tanzania, Ecuador, Venezuela, Brazil): doxycycline daily alone or mefloquine (once a week). Atovaquone and proguanil (Malarone) is also very useful for short-term travel.

Table 14.2 Common drugs used for malarial prophylaxis[4,5,6]

	Adult dosage	Children's dose	Comments
Doxycycline*	100 mg each day, 1–2 days before, during, 4 weeks after	>8 years only 2 mg/kg/day up to 100 mg	Photosensitivity reactions
Mefloquine (Lariam)*	250 mg (1 tab) same day each week, 2–3 weeks before, during, 4 weeks after	Not recommended <45 kg; >45 kg as for adults	Avoid use in resistant areas, e.g. Greater Mekong Subregion Side effects: dizziness, 'fuzzy' head, blurred vision, neuropsychiatric Beware of beta blockers
Atovaquone+ proguanil (Malarone)*	250 mg/100 mg (1 tab) with food same day each week 2 days before, during, 7 days later	Junior tablets 62.5 mg/25 mg 11–20 kg: 1 tablet/day 21–30 kg: 2 tablets/day 31–40 kg: 3 tablets/day >40 kg: 1 adult tab/day	Avoid in pregnant women or women breastfeeding infants <11 kg Avoid in severe kidney impairment Side effects: GIT upset, headache, dizziness, myalgia—others

* chloroquine-resistant areas

Table 14.3 Drugs used for uncomplicated chloroquine-resistant malaria (presumptive breakthrough where professional medical care unavailable, i.e. emergency self-treatment)[5,6]

	Adult dose	Children's dose
Artemether/ lumefantrine (Riamet)	4 tablets at 0, 8, 24, 36, 48, 60 hours	Only if >12 years, >35 kg
Atovaquone/ proguanil (Malarone) (if not used for prophylaxis)	4 tablets daily for 3 days	11–20 kg: 1 tablet 21–30 kg: 2 tablets 31–40 kg: 3 tablets

Summary of malaria recommendations[5,6]

1 PFM area:
 mefloquine 250 mg/week
 or
 doxycycline 100 mg/day
 or
 atovaquone + proguanil
2 Multidrug-resistant area:
 Malarone for prophylaxis
 +
 standby treatment: Malarone or artemether + lumefantrine (Riamet)

Specific infectious diseases and immunisation

Protection from many types of infection is available through immunisation. All travellers should be immunised against tetanus, polio and diphtheria and measles. Protection against tetanus requires an initial course of three injections followed by a booster every 10 years.

Vaccinations are required for special circumstances. Yellow fever vaccination is a legal requirement for any travellers returning from a yellow fever endemic area. Cholera is not usually required.

Some travellers may be exposed to tuberculosis, hepatitis, plague, rabies, typhoid, typhus and meningococcal infection. Immunisation against these is available and recommended for those at risk. Smallpox has now been eradicated from the world and therefore smallpox vaccination is no longer required for any traveller.

Table 14.4 Summary of preventive measures and vaccinations[7]

All travellers, all destinations

Tetanus toxoid and diphtheria booster
if >10 years since last dose
if >5 years for third world travel
give DT <10 years of age and dT >10 years of age

Routine vaccination for all Australians (National Schedule)

Tetanus, diphtheria, pertussis
Hepatitis B
Haemophilus influenzae
Measles, mumps, rubella
Influenza**
Pneumococcal disease**
Poliomyelitis
Rotavirus
Varicella

Selected vaccinations based on risk

Cholera
Hepatitis A
Japanese encephalitis
Meningococcal disease*
Rabies
Tick-borne encephalitis
Tuberculosis (BCG if mantoux -ve)
Typhoid fever
Yellow fever*

DT = diphtheria/tetanus combined, diphtheria at a higher dose for children. dT = booster diphtheria/tetanus with a lower diphtheria tetanus for adolescents and adults.

Other: Preventive measures against gastrointestinal infections, mosquito bites, malaria (where applicable), sexually transmitted infections

* legal requirement in some countries
** recommended for older travellers

Japanese B encephalitis presents as a special problem to the traveller.

TABLE 14.4 outlines a summary of recommendations to consider.[7,8]

Compulsory immunisations

The two vaccinations that may be required before visiting 'at risk' areas are yellow fever and meningococcus.

Yellow fever

Yellow fever is a serious viral infection spread by *Aedes* mosquitoes and, like malaria, is a tropical disease.

Yellow fever vaccination, which is the only WHO-required vaccine, is essential for travel to or through equatorial Africa and northern parts of South America, and for re-entry to Australia from those countries.

> **DxT** fever + bradycardia + jaundice
> → yellow fever

One injection only is required and the immunisation is valid for 10 years. Children aged less than 9 months should not be given this vaccine. It should not be given within 3 weeks of cholera vaccine.

Note: It is important to check specific country requirements in the WHO book on vaccination requirements.[9]

According to the WHO a certificate against yellow fever is the only certificate that should be required for international travel. The requirements of some countries are in excess of international health regulations. However, vaccination against yellow fever is strongly recommended to all travellers who intend to visit places other than the major cities in the countries where the disease occurs in humans.

Meningococcal infection

Meningitis due to this organism is a contagious lethal disease. It is common in Nepal, Mongolia, Vietnam and parts of Africa and Asia, especially in the dry season. Travellers trekking through the Kathmandu valley of Nepal and those attending the Haj pilgrimage to Saudi Arabia are at special risk and should have the vaccine. However, some countries require immunisation for entry.

Voluntary immunisation

Precautions against the following diseases are recommended for those travellers who may be at special risk.[5]

Hepatitis A, B

Hepatitis A is a common problem in rural areas of developing countries. There is a declining level of antibodies to hepatitis A in developed countries and adults are at special risk so one or two doses of hepatitis A vaccine should be given. A blood test for hepatitis A antibodies can be carried out to determine a person's immunity.

Prevention

The rules of avoiding contaminated food and water apply (as for traveller's diarrhoea). Hepatitis A vaccine is given as a course of two injections.

Hepatitis B is endemic in South-East Asia, South America and other developing countries. Vaccination is recommended, especially for people working in such countries, particularly those in the health care area or those who may expect to have sexual or drug contact. If patients have a 'negative' HBV core IgG titre, then vaccination would be worthwhile (three doses: 0, 1 and 6 months). Hepatitis E has a high mortality rate in pregnant women.

The usual approach for non-immunised people is to give the combined hepatitis A and B vaccine (Twinrix) as a course of three injections.

Typhoid

Typhoid immunisation is not required for entry into any country but is recommended for travel to third world countries where the standards of sanitation are low. It should be considered for travellers to smaller cities, and village and rural areas in Africa, Asia, Central and South America and Southern Europe.

The parenteral (subcutaneous) vaccine can be used but the single dose typhi Vi vaccine or the oral vaccine, which have fewer side effects, are generally preferred. The oral vaccine, which is given as a series of three or four capsules, appears to afford protection for about 5 years but is contraindicated in the immunocompromised.

Cholera

Cholera vaccination is not officially recommended by the WHO because it has only limited effectiveness. It is advisable for health care workers or others at risk entering an endemic area. Cholera is given as an oral vaccine (Dukoral) over 1 week prior to exposure. It is not recommended in children under 5 years or pregnant women.

Japanese B encephalitis

This mosquito-borne flavivirus infection presents a real dilemma to the traveller and doctor because it is a very severe infection (mortality rate 20–40%) with high infectivity and high prevalence in endemic countries.

The disease is prevalent during the wet season in the region bounded in the west by Nepal and Siberian Russia and in the east by Japan and Singapore, especially in Nepal, Burma, Korea, Vietnam, Thailand, China, eastern Russia and the lowlands of India. Rice paddies and pig farms are areas of risk. The usual preventive measures against mosquito bites are important.

> **DxT** febrile illness + vomiting + stupor
> → Japanese B encephalitis

Rabies

Rabies vaccination is recommended for some international aid workers or travellers going to rabies-endemic areas for periods of more than 1 month or even for short periods of working with affected animals in those areas. The vaccination can be effective after the bite of a rabid animal, so routine vaccination is not recommended for the traveller. Affected animals include dogs, cats, monkeys, camels and feral (wild) animals. A traveller who sustains a bite or scratch or even is licked by an animal in countries at risk should wash the site immediately with soap or a detergent, and then seek medical help. The prebite vaccination does not remove the need for postexposure vaccination.

DxT painful bite + paraesthesia + hydrophobia (pain with drinking) → rabies

Plague

Plague is still prevalent in rodents in countries such as Vietnam, Brazil, Peru, Ecuador and Kenya. Although not compulsory, vaccination is recommended for those engaged in field operations in plague areas and rural health workers who may be exposed to infected patients. Two doses are given to adults (three to children <12 years) and a booster every 6 months.

Special problems

Prevention of sexually transmitted infections

Casual sexual contacts place the traveller at risk of contracting a serious, perhaps fatal, sexually transmitted infection (STI). The common STIs, especially prevalent in South-East Asia and Africa, are non-specific urethritis (NSU), gonorrhoea (especially penicillin-resistant strains), hepatitis B and syphilis. HIV infection is a rapidly increasing problem, with heterosexual transmission common in Africa and in South-East Asia. Unusual STIs such as lymphogranuloma venereum, chancroid and donovanosis are more common in tropical developing countries. A practical rule is to assume that all 'at risk' travellers are both ignorant and irresponsible and advise accordingly.

Rules for prevention

- Never permit blood, semen or vaginal fluids from a sexual partner to enter your body, unless you are absolutely certain they are not STI carriers.
- Abstain or take your partner (condoms and diaphragms do not give absolute protection).

Exposure to STIs

If a patient has had unprotected intercourse and is at definite risk of acquiring an STI, such as penicillin-resistant gonorrhoea or NSU, the following may be appropriate:[1]

- ceftriaxone 250 mg IM (as a single dose)
- doxycycline 100 mg (o) for 10 days or azithromycin 1 g (o) statim

Drugs

Possession of and trafficking in drugs is very hazardous and many people are held in foreign prisons for various drug offences. The penalty for carrying drugs can be death.

Countries that currently may enforce the death penalty are Burma, China, Indonesia, Malaysia, Singapore, Thailand and Turkey. Travellers should be warned about taking cannabis while in a foreign country, as it can cause profound personality changes in the user.

Drug addicts should under no circumstances travel. Young travellers should be wary about accepting lifts or hitchhiking in countries 'at risk'.

Pregnancy and travel

Most international airlines do not allow passengers to travel after the 36th week of pregnancy and may require a doctor's certificate after 28 weeks. Air travel is contraindicated in the last month of pregnancy and until the 7th day after delivery. The past obstetric history should be taken into account. The same health risks apply except that most antimalarial tablets and vaccinations are not recommended. Live vaccinations (measles, rubella, influenza) are generally contraindicated[9] but the WHO considers it safe to have polio vaccine. Administration of killed or inactivated vaccines, toxoids and polysaccharides is permitted during pregnancy. Yellow fever vaccine is considered safe after the 6th month. As a general rule pregnancy and travel to third world countries do not mix and pregnant women should be advised not to travel to these countries. Avoid travel if possible in Zika-affected areas.

Tetanus immunisation is important as protection is passed on to the child during early infancy. Immunoglobulin can be safely given as prevention against hepatitis.

The antimalarial drugs chloroquine, quinine and proguanil (with 5 mgm folic acid) may be given to pregnant women but all others mentioned in TABLE 14.2 are contraindicated.

Children and travel

Although children, including infants, are good travellers and adapt well, their resistance, especially to heat and infections, is lower. A child can suffer from acute dehydration very rapidly.[9] Air travel is not recommended for infants of less than 7 days or premature infants.

The change in atmospheric pressure on landing can cause distressing ear pain, so taking a bottle during descent is recommended.

In tropical areas it is important to keep children well hydrated and they should wear loose cotton clothing. A good guide to the health of children is the amount and colour of their urine. If it is scanty and concentrated they are not getting sufficient fluid.

Most vaccines (diphtheria, tetanus, poliomyelitis, BCG) can safely be given in the first few weeks of life. Measles is common overseas and it is worthwhile considering it even under 12 months. Yellow fever vaccine should not be given under 12 months, hence the importance of protection against mosquito bites. Malaria prophylaxis is important. Chloroquine, proguanil and quinine may be given safely to infants. However, as a rule young children should be discouraged from travel.

Air travel

Air travel is safe and comfortable, but jet lag and air sickness are problems that face many travellers.

Jet lag

This is the uncomfortable aftermath of a long flight in which the person feels exhausted and disoriented, and has poor concentration, insomnia and anxiety. The problem on arrival is poor concentration and judgment during the daytime.

Other symptoms that may occur include anorexia, weakness, headache, blurred vision and dizziness.

Jet lag is a feature of flying long distances east–west or west–east through several time zones, causing the person's routine daily rhythm of activity and sleep to get out of phase. The worst cases appear to be in those travelling eastbound from England to Australia. It can occur with travel in any direction, but the north–south flights are not so bothersome.

Factors influencing jet lag

Personal factors. These include age, state of health, tolerance to change, preparation for the long trip and, very importantly, the emotional and mental state.

General factors. Noise, vibration, air humidity and sitting still for long periods can influence jet lag.

Specific factors. Duration of the flight, time of departure, and changes in climate and culture at the destination affect the severity of jet lag. The problem is aggravated by:

- stress of the pretrip planning
- last-minute rushing and anxiety
- lack of sleep during the trip
- overeating and excessive alcohol during the flight
- smoking

How to minimise the problem (advice to patients)

Before the flight

- Allow plenty of time for planning.
- Plan a stopover if possible.
- If possible, arrange the itinerary so that you are flying into the night.
- Ensure a good sleep the night before flying.
- Ensure a relaxed trip to the airport.
- Take along earplugs if noise (75–100 decibels) is bothersome.

During the flight

- *Fluids.* Avoid alcohol and coffee. Drink plenty of non-alcoholic drinks such as orange juice and mineral water.
- *Food.* Eat only when hungry and even skip a meal or two. Eat the lighter, more digestible parts of your meals and avoid fatty foods and rich carbohydrate foods.
- *Dress.* Wear loose clothes (e.g. long skirts, comfortable jeans, light jumpers) and avoid restrictive clothing. Wear comfortable (not tight) shoes and take them off during the flight.
- *Sleep.* Try to sleep on longer sections of the flight (give the movies a miss). Close the blinds, wear special eye masks and ask for a pillow. Sedatives such as temazepam (Euhypnos or Normison) or antihistamines can help sleep.
- *Activity.* Try to take regular walks around the aircraft and exercise at airport stops. Keep feet up when resting, and exercise by flexing the major muscles of the legs. Avoid resting the calves of

legs against the seat for long periods. Rest without napping during daylight sectors.

- *Special body care.* Continually wet the face and eyes.

A wetting agent such as hypromellose 0.5% eye drops can help those with a tendency to sore eyes.

At the destination

Take a nap for 1–2 hours if possible.

Wander around until you are tired and go to bed at the usual time. It is good to have a full day's convalescence and avoid big decision making soon after arrival. Allow about 3 days for adjustment after the London to Australia flight.

Role of melatonin[10]

The importance of melatonin, a hormone secreted by the pineal gland, is somewhat controversial. However, a major review of trials by the Cochrane Library pointed to its efficacy for alleviating jet lag. Oral medication in a 2–5 mg dose close to the desired or usual bedtime decreased jet lag. One possible explanation is that it has a low-grade hypnotic effect.

Who is fit to fly?

Patients with these problems should avoid flying[9,11] or be assessed for fitness:

- upper airways congested by infection, including influenza, e.g. within 6 weeks of severe acute respiratory illness
- acute gastroenteritis
- severe respiratory disease (COPD, chronic bronchitis, pneumothorax)
- recent thoracic surgery
- cystic fibrosis
- pulmonary tuberculosis (people should not fly until rendered non-infective)
- past history of respiratory problems while flying (dyspnoea, chest pain, confusion)
- unstable heart failure
- severe anaemia (below 7.5 g/dL)
- pregnancy beyond 200 days (28 weeks) (up to 36 weeks if necessary)
- previous violent or unpredictable behaviour
- within 7 days of a myocardial infarction
- within 3 days of a cerebrovascular accident
- within 5–10 days of major surgery
- brain tumour or recent skull fracture
- recent eye surgery
- severe or poorly controlled hypertension
- poorly controlled epilepsy

Special precautions are required by travellers with the following problems:

- *Colostomy.* Patients should wear a large colostomy bag and take extra bags.
- *Varicose veins.* Such patients should wear supportive stockings and exercise frequently.
- *Plaster casts.* Those with broken limbs in plaster should be careful of swelling.
- *Pacemakers.* Those with pacemakers may have a problem with X-rays at some overseas airports. Mention it to security officials before passing through security equipment.
- *Epilepsy.* Medication should be increased on the day of travel.
- *Diabetics.* Diabetics should discuss their therapy and control with their doctor. They should carry sweets.

Prevention of DVT

There is a risk of DVT in any person flying on long international flights. Risk factors include: increasing age, clotting tendency, i.e. thrombophilia, past history of DVT, family history of DVT, smoking, obesity, varicose veins, dehydration, significant illness, recent major surgery and oestrogen therapy (see CHAPTER 131).

Prevention is by:

- keeping hydrated—drink ample fluids but avoid alcohol and caffeine drinks
- in-flight exercises, such as foot pumps, ankle circles, knee lifts
- compression stockings (class 18–20)
- medication for those at risk, e.g. thrombophilia, Clexane 80 mg SC 12 to 24 hourly (if no contraindication and normal renal function) use one dose for travel to South-East Asia and two doses for travel to Europe

Travel sickness

Almost everyone is sick when sailing on rough seas. However, some people, especially children, suffer sickness from the effect of motion on a boat, in a car or in a plane. The larger the boat, plane or car, the less the likelihood of sickness; travel by train rarely causes sickness. Nearly all children grow out of the tendency to have travel sickness, but many adults remain 'bad' sailors.

The problem is caused by sensitivity of the semicircular canals of the inner ear. They are affected by the movement and vibration of travel. Some people have sensitive inner ear canals and are prone to sickness, especially on certain types of journeys (e.g. winding roads through hills) and in certain vehicles.

The main symptoms of travel sickness are nausea, vomiting, dizziness, weakness and lethargy. Early signs are pallor and drowsiness, and sudden silence from an active, talkative child.

Medication for travel sickness

Many medicines are available for travel sickness. They include hyoscine, various antihistamines and other phenothiazine derivatives, all of which can cause drowsiness; although a problem for drivers, this sedative effect may be helpful for children or for those travelling long distances by plane.

Phenothiazine derivatives that provide appropriate anti-labyrinthine activity include prochlorperazine (Stemetil), promethazine hydrochloride (Phenergan) and promethazine theoclate (Avomine).

Combination antihistamine and hyoscine preparations for travel sickness include Travacalm and Benacine.

Hyoscine comes in tablet form, either alone or in combination and in the popular adhesive patches.

Recommended medications

Car travel: adult passengers and children

- dimenhydrinate (Dramamine)
  or
  promethazine theoclate (Avomine)
  or
  hyoscine (Kwells)

These preventive oral preparations should ideally be taken 30–60 minutes before the trip and can be repeated 4–6 hourly during the trip (maximum 4 tablets in 24 hours).

- hyoscine dermal discs (Scop)

If available, one of these adhesive patches should be applied to dry, unbroken, hairless skin behind the ear, 5–6 hours before travel and left on for 3 days. Wash the hands thoroughly after applying and removing the disc—be careful of accidental finger-to-eye contact.

Sea travel

Sea travel generally poses no special problems apart from motion sickness and the possibility of injuries in the aged. The larger the ship, the less likely the problem. Those prone to sea sickness are advised to take anti-emetics 60 minutes before sailing and for the first 2 days at sea until they obtain their 'sea legs'. However, the use of hyoscine transdermal delivery systems is recommended for convenience.

Experienced seamen's 'tricks':

- always keep looking to the horizon
- plug one ear with cotton wool or Blu-Tack
- drink ginger drinks, e.g. 'dry ginger', ginger beer
- chew gum

Severe sea sickness

The standard treatment is promethazine (Phenergan) 25 mg IM injection. If injections are not possible, prochlorperazine (Stemetil) suppositories can be used.

The aged

Generally the elderly travel well but should take safeguards to avoid falls. The chief surgeon on P&O's flagship recommends that elderly people should bring the following:

- a letter from their doctor stating diagnosis and medication
- a spare set of spectacles
- a spare set of dentures
- a walking stick (if appropriate)

Altitude sickness[12]

High altitudes pose special problems for people who live at low altitude, especially if they have heart and lung disease. The severity depends on altitude, the speed of ascent, the temperature and level of activity. The high altitudes of Africa (Kilimanjaro, Kenya), India, Nepal (Himalayas), the Rockies of Canada and the US, and the Andes of South America provide such problems. It is usually safe to trek under 2500 m altitude but rapid ascent beyond this commonly precipitates altitude sickness. Serious altitude sickness occurs at 3500–5800 m.

Forms

1. Acute mountain sickness (mild to severe)
2. High-altitude pulmonary oedema
3. High-altitude cerebral oedema

Clinical features

- Usually within 8–24 hours of exposure
- Frontal headache (worse in morning and when supine)
- Malaise, fatigue, anorexia, nausea, insomnia

More severe: fluid retention (peripheral or facial oedema), dyspnoea, vomiting, dry cough, dizziness

Serious: marked dyspnoea, neurological symptoms and signs

Prevention

- Careful acclimatisation with gradual ascent[11]
- Spend 2–3 days at intermediate altitudes
- Ascent rate less than 300 m per day above 3000 m (that is, try not to sleep at an altitude 300 m higher than that of the previous day)
- Ample fluid intake (more water than usual)
- Avoid alcohol
- Acetazolamide (Diamox) 250 mg 8 hourly the day before ascent; continue 3–6 days (deaths from mountain sickness have still occurred while on this drug)

Treatment

- Immediate (urgent and rapid) descent to below 2000 m
- Oxygen
- Dexamethasone (e.g. 4 mg, 6 hourly)

Travellers' medical kit

If a person intends to travel for a long time the following represents a comprehensive medical kit. It should not be regarded as an alternative to seeking appropriate medical help if it is available. Typical examples of general items are included in brackets.

Materials

- Alcohol swabs
- Bandaids and Elastoplast dressing strip
- Bandages (2 cotton gauze, 2 crepe × 10 cm)
- Pocket torch
- Steristrips or 'butterfly strips' (to patch small cuts)
- Sterile gauze and cotton wool
- Sterile gloves
- Thermometer
- Scissors and tweezers
- Safety pins
- Water purification tablets or iodine solution

Topical items

- Antifungal cream
- Chlorhexidine/cetrimide antiseptic cream (Savlon)
- Condoms
- Corticosteroid cream (e.g. hydrocortisone)
- Insect repellent containing diethyl-m-toluamide (DEET, Muskol, Repellem or Rid)
- Insecticide spray
- Mosquito net repellent solution: permethrin (Ambush—ICI)
- Nasal spray or drops
- Stingose spray (for bites and stings)
- Strepsils
- UV antisunburn cream (factor 30+)

Medication checklist

The medications below marked with * usually require a prescription.

- Antibiotics*
  - amoxycillin + clavulanate forte
  - norfloxacin 400 mg (6 tablets for 3 days)
  - azithromycin (for children)
- Antacid tablets—for heartburn or indigestion
- Antimalarials*—where appropriate (including malaria emergency self-treatment)
- Diamox tablets* for acute mountain sickness
- Fasigyn* 2 g or Flagyl* 2.4 g—for amoebiasis or giardiasis
- Laxative (Senokot)
- Imodium* or Lomotil*—for diarrhoea
- Motion sickness tablets (Avomine, Kwells or Phenergan)
- Paracetamol tablets—for fever or pain
- Sleeping tablets* (temazepam, promethazine)
- Rehydration mixture (Gastrolyte)
- Throat lozenges
- EpiPen—if history of anaphylaxis

General tips for the traveller

Checklist for at-risk countries

- If you can't peel it, boil it or cook it, don't eat it.
- Boil or purify water, avoid dairy products, ice-cream, shellfish, food left in open, salads, raw fruit and vegetables, ice and recooked or reheated food.
- Never walk around barefoot at night in snake areas (and use a torch).
- Always shake your shoes before putting them on.
- Never wear nylon items in hot tropical areas.
- Never bathe, wade or drink in rivers, lakes or harbours unless you know they are bilharzia free.
- Keep yourself well covered after dark and use a mosquito net.
- Use insect repellent on skin frequently.
- Use an insecticide spray in your bedroom.
- Seek medical help if bitten by an excited dog, after washing bite.

Other tips

- Organise a dental check before departure.
- Arrange stopovers on a long flight (if possible).
- Take along a spare pair of spectacles and adequate medication.

- Arrange health and travel insurance.
- Check out your nearest embassy/consulate when visiting remote areas or politically unstable countries.
- Take a letter from your doctor with your medical record.
- Consider a traveller's medical kit.
- Never carry a parcel or luggage through Customs to oblige a stranger or recent acquaintance.
- Abstain from sex with a stranger.
- Have a credit card that allows a quick cash advance or an airline ticket purchase (for many countries a policy of 'if you get sick, then get out' is necessary).
- Most death and injury among travellers is caused by motor accidents. Avoid overcrowded long-distance buses in African and South Asian countries (and elsewhere)—trains are safer.

Patient education resources

Hand-out sheets from *Murtagh's Patient Education* 7th edition:

- Travel: air travel
- Travel: guide for travellers
- Travel sickness

References

1 Bayram C, Pan Y, Miller G. Management of travel related problems in general practice. Aust Fam Physician, 2007; 36(5): 298–9.
2 Locke DM. Traveller's diarrhoea. Aust Fam Physician, 1990; 19: 194–203.
3 Expert group for Gastrointestinal guidelines. Travellers diarrhoea. In: eTG complete. Melbourne: Therapeutic Guidelines Ltd. Available from: <www.tg.org.au>, accessed December 2017.
4 Yung A, Ruff T, Torresi J, Leder K, O'Brien D. *Manual of Travel Medicine* (2nd edn). Melbourne: IP Communications, 2004: 139–80.
5 Expert group for Antibiotic: Malaria guidelines. In: eTG complete. Melbourne: Therapeutic Guidelines Ltd. Available from: <www.tg.org.au>, accessed December 2017.
6 Buckley N (Chairman). *Australian Medicines Handbook.* Adelaide, 2016: 227.
7 Cohen J. Travel health for GPs. Medical Observer, 14 March 2014: 21–6.
8 Lau S, Gherardin T. Travel vaccination. Aust Fam Physician, 2007; 36(5): 304–11.
9 World Health Organization. International Health for Travellers, 2001. In: The Cochrane Library, Issue 1, 2001. Oxford: Update software.
10 Herxheimer A. Melatonin and jet lag. In: The Cochrane Library, Issue 1, 2001, CD 001520. Oxford: Update software.
11 Fenner P, Fitness to travel. Aust Fam Physician, 2007; 36(5): 312–15.
12 Short B. *Altitude Medicine.* In RACGP Check Program: Travel Medicine Unit 387, 2004.

Resources

World Health Organization, International travel and health: <www.who.int/ith/en>

Travel Doctor-TMVC: <www.traveldoctor.com.au>

Smartraveller (country-specific information provided by the Australian Government): <http://smartraveller.gov.au>

Centers for Disease Control and Prevention: <www.cdc.gov/travel>

15 Tropical medicine and the returned traveller

Our lot is a perilous age . . . but where shall we fly to escape from pestilences that come and pestilences that do not come, from ships that bring us yellow fever, from cattle diseases that can only be exterminated by exterminating the cattle, from infectious patients whose pulses must be felt with a pair of tongs and their chests explored with tarred stethoscopes.

JACOB BIGELOW 1860

Doctors in western countries—including Australia, with its own tropical diseases in the far north—are more likely to encounter tropical diseases in the traveller returning from countries where these disorders are endemic. Many of these diseases are likely to be encountered in newly arrived refugees (see CHAPTER 135). The diseases include bacterial infections such as tuberculosis (a huge problem), plague, melioidosis, leprosy, typhoid/cholera, zoonoses. Other infections to be considered are parasitic, *Rickettsia* and myriad viral infections including haemorrhagic fevers, various types of encephalitis, yellow fever, polio, trachoma, hepatitis, lyssavirus such as rabies and bat bite infections, dengue and influenzas.

It is worth reviewing the various protozoal and helminthic parasitic infections that need to be considered in the sick returned traveller.[1] The helminths (worms) include cestodes (tapeworms), trematodes (flukes) and nematodes (roundworms).

- *Protozoal infections:* African trypanosomiasis (sleeping sickness), American trypanosomiasis (Chagas disease), amoebiasis, babesiosis, coccidiosis and microsporodiosis, cryptosporidiosis, giardiasis, leishmaniasis—cutaneous and visceral (kala-azar), malaria, toxoplasmosis, trichomonas
- *Cestodes (tapeworms):* Cysticercosis (*Taenia solium, T. saginata*), echinococcus (hydatid disease)
- *Trematodes (flukes):* Schistomiasis (bilharziasis), clonorchiasis, paragonimiasis
- *Nematodes (roundworms):* Ascariasis, enterobiasis (pinworm), *Dracunculus medinensis* (Guinea worm), filariasis, hookworm, larva migrans (cutaneous and visceral), strongyloidiasis, trichinosis (*Trichinella spiralis*), trichuriasis (whipworm)

Problems in the returned tropical traveller

- Most will present within 2 weeks except HIV seroconversion infection.
- Common infections encountered are dengue fever, giardiasis, hepatitis A and B, gonorrhoea or *Chlamydia trachomatis,* malaria and helminthic infestations.
- An important non-infection problem requiring vigilance is deep venous thrombosis (DVT) and thromboembolism.
- The asymptomatic traveller may present for advice about exposure (without illness) or about an illness acquired such as rabies, malaria, schistosomiasis and STIs.

Red flags in the returned traveller

- mental confusion/other CNS signs
- respiratory distress
- appears 'septic'
- hypotension
- haemorrhagic features
- pallor/anaemia

Gastrointestinal symptoms

Mild diarrhoea

- Stool microscopy and culture
- Look for and treat associated helminthic infestation (e.g. roundworms, hookworms)

Moderate or prolonged (>3 weeks) diarrhoea

Usually due to *Giardia lamblia, Entamoeba histolytica, Campylobacter jejuni (especially South-East Asia), Salmonella, Yersinia entero-colitica* or *Cryptosporidium.*[2]

- Stool examination (three fresh specimens):
  - microscopy
  - wet preparation
  - culture
- Faecal Multiplex PCR (if available)
- Treat pathogen (see guidelines under diarrhoea in CHAPTERS 14 and 44)

Non-pathogens such as *Escherichia coli* and *Endolimax nana* are often reported but do not treat specifically.

Note: Consider exotic causes such as schistosomiasis, strongyloidiasis and ciguatera in unusual chronic post-travel 'gastroenteritis'.

Persistent abdominal discomfort

This common syndrome includes bloating, intestinal hurry and borborygmi, and often follows an episode of diarrhoea. Usually no pathogens are found on stool examination. However, giardiasis can be difficult to detect and an empirical course of tinidazole (2 g statim) is worthwhile. Any persistent problem then is a type of postinfective bowel dysfunction or irritable bowel. Reassurance is important.

Rash/other skin lesions

- Maculopapular: consider dengue, HIV, typhus, syphilis, arbovirus infections, leptospirosis, Q fever
- Petechiae: viral haemorrhagic fevers, leptospirosis, dengue
- Rose spots: typhoid
- Eschar: typhus (tick and scrub), anthrax
- Chancre: African trypanosomiasis, syphilis

Fever

- Causes range from mild viral infections to potentially fatal cerebral malaria (see TABLE 15.1) and meningococcal septicaemia.
- An Australian study of fever in returned travellers[3] revealed the most common diagnosis was malaria (27%) followed by respiratory tract infection (24%), gastroenteritis (14%), dengue fever (8%) and bacterial pneumonia (6%). The commonness of malaria was supported by results from the GeoSentinel Surveillance Network.[4]
- The common serious causes are malaria, typhoid, hepatitis (especially A and B), dengue fever and amoebiasis.
- Most deaths from malaria have occurred after at least 3 or 4 days of symptoms that may be mild. Death can occur within 24 hours. Factors

Table 15.1 Fever and malaise in the returned traveller: diagnostic strategy model

Note: All fever in a returned traveller is malaria until proved otherwise!
Probability diagnosis
Viral respiratory illness (e.g. influenza)
Malaria
Hepatitis (may be subclinical)
Gastroenteritis/diarrhoeal illness
Dengue
Serious disorders not to be missed
Malaria
Tuberculosis
Typhoid
Encephalitis
Viral haemorrhagic diseases
Meningococcal meningitis
Melioidosis
Amoebiasis (liver abscess)
HIV seroconversion illness
Pitfalls (often missed)
Ascending cholangitis
Infective endocarditis
Cytomegalovirus
Epstein–Barr virus
Dengue fever
Lyme disease
Bronchopneumonia
Ross River fever
Rarities
Chikungunya
Legionnaire disease
Schistosomiasis
African trypanosomiasis
Typhus
Yellow fever
Zika virus
Rift Valley fever
Spotted fever
Lassa fever, Hantavirus, Marburg, Ebola and other haemorrhagic fevers
Note: Three causes of a dry cough (in absence of chest signs) are malaria, typhoid and amoebic liver abscess.
Seven masquerades checklist
Drugs (reaction to antimalarials)
Urinary infection
Investigations (if no obvious cause)
Full blood examination
Chest X-ray
Thick and thin blood films
Blood culture
Liver function tests
Urine—micro and culture

continued

continued

Stool—micro and culture
ESR, CRP
New malaria tests, e.g. rapid diagnostic test
Acute phase serology (hold pending convalescent serology)

responsible for death from malaria include delayed presentation, missed or delayed diagnosis (most cases), no chemoprophylaxis and old age.

- Refer immediately to a specialist unit if the patient is unwell.
- Be vigilant for meningitis and encephalitis.
- Be vigilant for amoebiasis—can present with a toxic megacolon, especially if antimotility drugs are given.
- If well but febrile, *first-line screening tests:*
  - full blood examination and ESR
  - thick and thin films
  - liver function tests
  - urine for micro and culture
- Refer immediately if malaria is proven or if fever persists after a further 24 hours.

Malaria

See FIGURE 15.1.

- Incubation period: *P. falciparum* 7–14 days; others 12–40 days
- Most present within 2 months of return
- Can present up to 2 or more years
- Can masquerade as several other illnesses

Clinical features

See CHAPTER 14.

- High fever, chills, rigor, sweating, headache
- Usually abrupt onset
- Can have atypical presentations (e.g. diarrhoea, abdominal pain, cough)

Other features

- Beware of modified infection.
- Must treat immediately. Delay may mean death.
- Typical relapsing patterns often absent.
- Thick smear allows detection of parasites (some laboratories are poorly skilled with thick films).
- Thin smear helps diagnose malaria type.
- If index of suspicion is high, repeat the smear ('No evidence of malaria' = 3 negative daily thick films). Newer tests (e.g. polymerase chain reaction [PCR] tests and immune chromatographic test [ICT] card tests for PFM) show promise. Cerebral malaria and blackwater fever are severe and dramatic. The Para check V test (a desktop test) is accurate and needs to be positive before prescribing artemether in some areas.

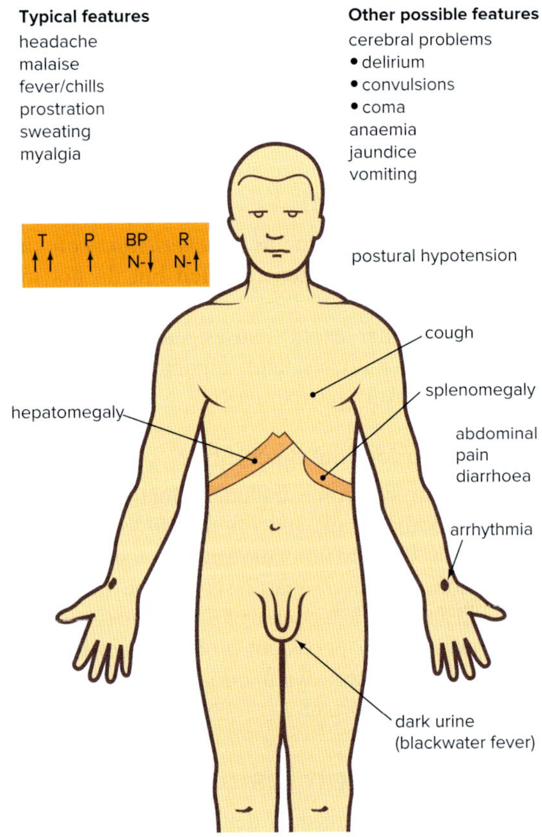

FIGURE 15.1 Clinical features of malaria

Treatment[5,6]

- Admit to hospital with infectious disease expertise. Rule out G6PD deficiency
- Supportive measures, including fluid replacement
- Avoid the same drugs used for prophylaxis
- *P. vivax, P. ovale, P. malariae*[5]
  artemether + lumefantrine 20 mg + 120 mg (Riamet)
  4 tablets with food at 0, 8, 24, 36, 48, 60 hours (i.e. 24 tablets) in 60 hours
  +
  primaquine dose by weight to achieve a total dose of 6 mg/kg

- *P. falciparum*[5] *uncomplicated*
  Riamet (as above)
  or
  atovaquone + progunail
  or
  quinine sulphate 600 mg (o) 8 hourly, 7 days + doxycycline 100 mg (o) 12 hourly, 7 days
  or
  clindamycin 300 mg (o) tds, 7 days (children, pregnancy)
  complicated (severe):
  artesunate 2.4 mg/kg IV statim, 12 hours, 24 hours, then once daily until oral therapy (Riamet) is possible
  or
  quinine dihydrochloride 20 mg/kg up to 1.4 g IV (over 4 hours) then after 4-hour gap 7 mg/kg IV 8 hourly until improved (ECG/cardiac monitoring)
  then
  quinine (o) 7 days
  Note: Check for hypoglycaemia. Beware if antimalarial use in previous 48 hours.

Typhoid fever

Incubation period 10–14 days

Clinical features

- Insidious onset
- Headache prominent
- Dry cough
- Fever gradually increases in 'stepladder' manner over 4 days or so
- Abdominal pain and constipation (early)
- Diarrhoea (pea soup) and rash—rose spots (late)
- ± splenomegaly

DxT 'stepladder' fever + abdominal pain + relative bradycardia ➜ typhoid (early)

Diagnosis

- On suspicion—blood and stool culture
- Serology not very helpful

Treatment

- Azithromycin 1 g (o) for 7 days
  or
- Ciprofloxacin 500 mg (o) bd for 7–10 days

Cholera

Incubation period a few hours–5 days

Clinical features

Variable

- Subclinical
- Mild, uncomplicated episode of diarrhoea
- Fulminant lethal form with severe water and electrolyte depletion, intense thirst, oliguria, weakness, sunken eyes and eventually collapse

DxT fever + vomiting + abrupt onset 'rice water' diarrhoea ➜ cholera

Diagnosis

Stool microscopy and culture (*Vibrio cholerae*)

Treatment

- In hospital with strict barrier nursing
- IV fluid and electrolytes
- Doxycycline

VIRAL HAEMORRHAGIC FEVERS

These include: yellow fever, Lassa fever, etc., plus dengue fever and chikungunya.

Yellow fever

Milder cases may present with flu-like symptoms and relative bradycardia (Faget's sign) and albuminuria. Severe cases experience these symptoms with abrupt fever then prostration, jaundice and abnormal bleeding from the gums and possibly haematemesis. Diagnosis is by ELISA testing.

DxT fever + bradycardia + jaundice + bleeding ➜ yellow fever

Lassa fever, Ebola virus, Marburg virus, Hanta virus

These rare but deadly tropical diseases usually commence with a flu-like illness, gastrointestinal symptoms with thrombocytopenia, anaemia and, if severe, findings consistent with disseminated intravascular coagulation leading to bleeding and possibly shock and frank haemorrhage. Hanta virus tends to cause respiratory symptoms, including cough, progressing to respiratory difficulty. Seek urgent expert help.

Ebola

- Incubation period: 2–16 days
- Transmission: direct body contact (body fluids, esp. blood, vomit from affected or dead person),

infected animals, contaminated objects (needles, medical equipment)
- Early symptoms: constitutional (fever, malaise, headache), upper respiratory (flu-like, cough, etc.), abdominal (pain, nausea, vomiting, diarrhoea)
- May progress to severe symptoms as above then multiorgan failure
- Diagnosis: PCR, histopathology
- Treatment is supportive, esp. IV fluids

Dengue fever[7]

Also known as 'breakbone' fever, it is widespread in the south-east Pacific and endemic in Queensland. A returned traveller with myalgia and fever <39°C is more likely to have dengue than malaria. It is commonly misdiagnosed.

Clinical features

- Mosquito-borne (*Aedes aegypti*) viral infection
- Incubation period 5–6 days
- Abrupt onset fever, malaise, headache, nausea, pain behind eyes, severe backache, prostration
- Sore throat
- Severe aching of muscles and joints
- Fever subsides for about 2 days, then returns
- Maculopapular rubelliform rash on limbs → trunk (hand pressure for 30 seconds causes blanching)
- Petechial rash common (even in absence of thrombocytopenia)
- Generalised erythema with 'islands of sparing'
- ± Diarrhoea
- The rare haemorrhagic form is very severe; may present with shock, which is usually fatal
- Later severe fatigue and depression (prone to suicide)

Note: A large-scale survey of dengue patients showed the symptoms as fever 100%, myalgia 79%, rash 74%, headache 68%, nausea 37%.

DxT fever + severe aching (especially headache) + rash ➜ dengue fever

Diagnosis

- Dengue-specific IgM serology—best on day 5
- PCR
- FBE: leukopenia; thrombocytopenia in haemorrhagic form

Treatment

- Symptomatic with rest, fluids and analgesics (paracetamol). Avoid antibiotics, aspirin, NSAIDs and corticosteroids

Prevention

- Avoid mosquito bites—no vaccine available

Zika virus

Also transmitted by *Aedes aegypti,* it is more common in Central and South America. Most infections are asymptomatic but common symptoms are fever, rash, arthralgia and conjunctivitis with a dengue-like syndrome. Can cause a Guillain–Barré-like syndrome or cerebral damage (microcephaly) in infants of infected mothers. Diagnosis is confirmed by serology and PCR. Treatment is symptomatic.

Chikungunya

This is an alpha-viral mosquito-borne infection with a similar clinical picture to dengue fever; it can cause haemorrhagic fever. It is encountered in tropical South-East Asia, Indian Ocean islands and parts of Africa.

Diagnosis

- Positive serology

Encephalitis

Encephalitis presents with fever, nausea and vomiting then progressing to stupor, coma and convulsions. Mosquito-borne cases include Japanese B encephalitis and West Nile fever.

Consider mosquito-borne encephalitis and meningococcal meningitis in a patient presenting with headache, fever and malaise before neurological symptoms such as delirium, convulsions and coma develop.

Melioidosis

This serious disease with a high mortality is caused by the Gram-negative bacillus *Burkholderia pseudomallei,* a soil saprophyte that infects humans mainly by penetrating through skin wounds, especially abrasions. It is mostly acquired while wading in rice paddies. It is mainly a disease of third world countries and occurs between 20° North and 20° South of the equator, mainly in South-East Asia and including northern Australia. It may manifest as a focal infection or as septicaemia with abscesses in the lung, kidney, skin, liver or spleen. It is called the 'Vietnamese time bomb' because it can present years after the initial infection, as seen in Vietnamese war veterans.

Clinical features

- Fever, headache, cough, pleuritic pain and generalised myalgia

> **DxT** fever + pneumonia + myalgia → melioidosis

Diagnosis

- Blood culture, swabs from focal lesions, haemagglutination test

Treatment (adults)[8]

- Ceftazidime 2 g IV, 6 hourly
  or
- Meropenem 1 g IV, 6 hourly
  or
- Imipenem 1 g IV, 6 hourly
- All for at least 14 days, followed by oral cotrimoxazole ± doxycycline bd + folic acid for 3 months

Prevention

- Traumatised people with open wounds (especially diabetics) in endemic areas (tropical South-East Asia) should be carefully nursed.

Plague

Plague (Black Death), which is caused by the Gram-negative bacterium *Yersinia pestis,* is endemic in parts of Asia, Africa and the Americas. It has been presumed to be transmitted by the flea: 'the flea bites the infected rat and then bites the human', but spread from person to person is now considered more likely.

Clinical features

There are basically two forms:

1 bubonic plague—painful suppurating inguinal or axillary lymphadenitis (buboes) (see FIG. 15.2)

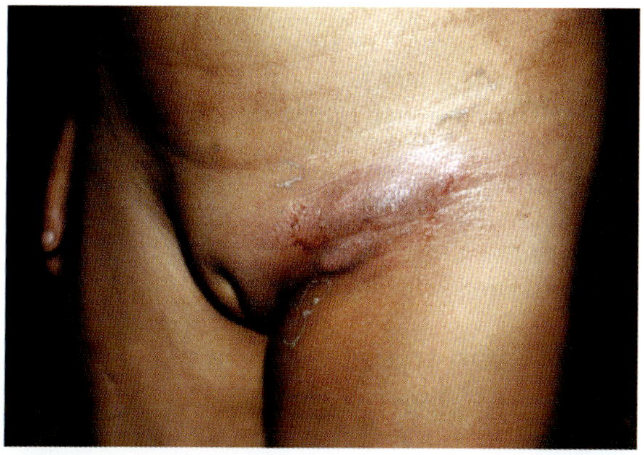

FIGURE 15.2 Young Vietnamese woman with a left inguinal bubo
Photo courtesy Dr RA Cooke

2 pneumonic plague—flu-like symptoms with haemoptysis, septicaemia and a fatal haemorrhagic illness (± buboes)

There is a rapid onset of high fever and prostration with black patches of skin due to subcutaneous haemorrhage.

Diagnosis

- Serology and smear/culture of buboes

Treatment

- Streptomycin and doxycycline

Rabies

Rabies is a rhabdovirus acquired by bites from an infected mammal, for example, a dog, cat, monkey, fox or bat.

Clinical features

Prodromal symptoms can include malaise, headache, abnormal behaviour including agitation and fever. It progresses to either paralytic 'dumb rabies' or encephalitic 'furious rabies', which involves excessive salivation and excruciating spasms of the pharyngeal muscles on drinking water (in particular). The patient is terrified of drinking water despite a great thirst (hydrophobia).

> **DxT** painful/itchy bite + agitation + hydrophobia → rabies

Diagnosis

- Viral testing

Treatment

- Post-bite prophylaxis (endemic area)

Wash the wound immediately then clean it. Administer rabies vaccine (if unimmunised) and rabies immune immunoglobulin ASAP (within 48 hours).

Ciguatera

This is a type of food poisoning caused by eating tropical fish, especially large coral trout and large cod, caught in tropical waters (e.g. the Caribbean and tropical Pacific). The problem is caused by a type of poison that concentrates in the fish after they feed on certain micro-organisms around reefs. Ciguatera poisoning presents within hours as a bout of 'gastroenteritis' (vomiting, diarrhoea and stomach pains) and then symptoms affecting the nervous system, such as muscle aching and weakness, paraesthesia and burning

15

sensations of the skin, particularly of the fingers and lips. There is no cure for the problem but it can be treated with IV fluids and possibly mannitol infusion or gammaglobulin. It is unwise to eat large predatory reef fish, especially their offal (mainly the liver).

Hansen's disease (leprosy)

Hansen's disease (Gerhard Hansen, 1869) is caused by the acid-fast bacillus *Mycobacterium leprae*. It is a disorder of tropical and warm temperate regions, especially South-East Asia. It is considered to be transmitted by nasal secretions with an incubation period of 2–6 years. It affects the skin and nerves, especially of the extremities.

Clinical features

(WHO 1999)
Diagnosis is one or more of:

- Skin lesions—usually anaesthetic; hypopigmented or reddish maculopapules or annular lesions (see FIG. 15.3)
- Thickened peripheral nerves with loss of sensation, e.g. ulnar (elbow), median (wrist), common peroneal (knee) and greater auricular (neck); also peripheral neuropathy or motor nerve impairment

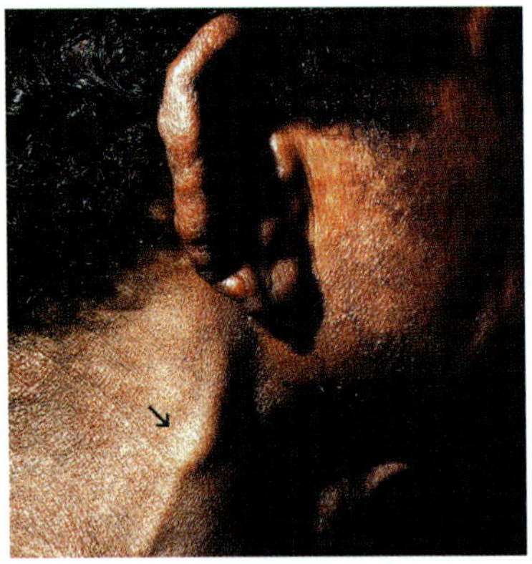

FIGURE 15.3 Advanced lepromatous leprosy. This patient has multiple nodules on his ear and the greater auricular nerve is markedly thickened.
Courtesy Dr RA Cooke

- Demonstration of acid-fast bacilli in a skin smear or on biopsy
- It can be localised (tuberculoid) or generalised (lepromatous)

Diagnosis

- Diagnosis is by biopsy, the lepromin test, cultivation of the organisms or by PCR tests.

Treatment

- Referral to specialists or a specialist centre is advisable for shared care.
- WHO treatment recommendations are multiple drug therapy, e.g. rifampicin, clofazimine and dapsone, but therapy is constantly being evaluated (see www.who.int/lep).

Scrub typhus

Scrub typhus is found in South-East Asia, northern Australia and the western Pacific. It is caused by *Rickettsia tsutsugamushi,* which is transmitted by mites.

Clinical features

- Abrupt onset febrile illness with headache and myalgia
- A black eschar at the site of the bite with regional and generalised lymphadenopathy
- Short-lived macular rash
- Can develop severe complications (e.g. pneumonitis, encephalitis)

Diagnosis

- Serological assays

Treatment

- Doxycycline 100 mg bd for 7–10 days

Queensland tick typhus

Queensland tick typhus, which is caused by *Rickettsia australis,* is directly related to a tick bite. The symptoms are almost identical to scrub typhus, although less severe, and the treatment is identical.

Tropical parasitic infections[1]

Travellers to tropical or subtropical areas are at risk of more unusual infections. Most of these infections are contracted through contaminated food and water, insect bites and walking barefoot on contaminated soil. The risk of such infections is highest in rural areas of countries other than Europe, North America and Australasia. Parasitic infections other than malaria include the following.

African trypanosomiasis (sleeping sickness)

Clinical features

Stage 1 (haemolymphatic)

- Incubation period about 3 weeks

- Fever, headache and a skin chancre or nodule
- Lymphadenopathy, hepatosplenomegaly

Stage 2 (meningoencephalitic)

- weeks or months later
- cerebral symptoms including hypersomnolence

Diagnosis

- Demonstrating trypomastigotes in peripheral blood smear or chancre aspirate

Treatment

- Suramin IV
- Infectious disease consultation essential

Prevention

- Avoid bites of the tsetse fly. If visiting areas of East, Central and West Africa, especially the safari game parks, travellers should use insect repellent and wear protective light-coloured clothing, including long sleeves and trousers.

Leishmaniasis

Visceral leishmaniasis (kala-azar)

The parasitic Leishmania which is transmitted by bites of sand flies and by blood transfusions and IV drug use, is endemic in 88 countries.

Clinical features

- The haemopoietic system is targeted and presenting features include fever; wasting; ulceration of the skin, mouth and nose; hepatosplenomegaly; and lymphadenopathy
- Among other signs is hyperpigmentation of the skin, hence the Hindu name kala-azar ('black fever')
- Most cases are subclinical

Diagnosis

- Serology and tissue biopsy

Cutaneous leishmaniasis

This may be encountered in travellers and servicemen and servicewomen returning from the Middle East, especially the Persian Gulf, and also travellers returning from Central and South America. The protozoa is transmitted by a sandfly and has an average incubation period of 9 weeks.

Clinical features

The key clinical finding is an erythematous papule (see FIG. 15.4).

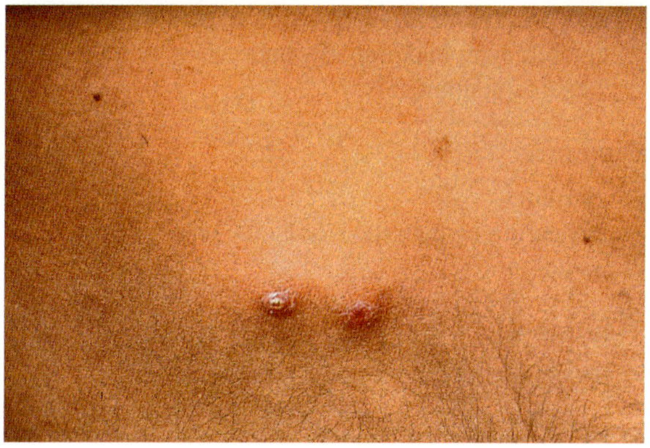

FIGURE 15.4 Cutaneous leishmaniasis in a serviceman after returning from the Middle East

Diagnosis

- Performing a punch biopsy and culturing tissue in a special medium

Treatment

- Treatment for extensive lesions is with high-dosage ketoconazole for 1 month.
- Smaller lesions should be treated topically with 15% paromomycin and 12% methyl benzethonium chloride ointment applied bd for 10 days.[9]
- A special vaccine is available in some Middle Eastern countries (e.g. Israel).

Schistosomiasis (bilharzia)

The infestation is caused by parasite organisms (schistosomes) which target the vasculature of the GIT or genitourinary tract. Its eggs are passed in human excreta, which contaminates watercourses (notably stagnant water) and irrigation channels in Egypt, other parts of Africa, South America, some parts of South-East Asia and China. Freshwater snails are the carriers (vectors).[10]

Clinical features

- The first clinical sign is a local skin reaction at the site of penetration of the parasite (it then invades liver, bowel, vulva and bladder). This site is known as 'swimmer's itch'.
- Within a week or so there is a generalised allergic response, usually with fever, malaise, myalgia, abdominal pain and urticaria.
- A gastroenteritis-like syndrome can occur (nausea, vomiting, diarrhoea) and respiratory symptoms, particularly cough.

- Clinical findings, such as in trypanosomiasis, include lymphadenopathy and hepatosplenomegaly.

Diagnosis

- Serology
- Detecting eggs in the stools, the urine or in a rectal biopsy

Treatment

- Praziquantel (may need retreatment)

Prevention

- Travellers should be warned against drinking from, or swimming and wading in, dams, watercourses or irrigation channels, especially in Egypt and other parts of Africa.

Amoebiasis

Amoebiasis (*Entamoeba histolytica*) can be diagnosed in a sick traveller returning from an endemic area with severe diarrhoea characterised by blood and mucus. Complications include fulminating colitis, amoebomas (a mass of fibrotic granulation tissue) in the bowel and liver abscess. Acute amoebic dysentery is treated with oral tinidazole or metronidazole.

Amoebic liver abscess

Clinical features

- High swinging fever
- Profound malaise and anorexia
- Tender hepatomegaly
- Effusion or consolidation of base of right chest

There is often no history of dysentery, and jaundice is unusual.

Diagnosis

- Serological tests for amoeba and by imaging (CT scan)

Treatment

- Metronidazole and by percutaneous CT-guided aspiration

Giardiasis

Giardia lamblia infection is usually acquired from contaminated drinking water.

Clinical features

- Often asymptomatic
- Symptoms include abdominal cramps, bloating, flatulence and bubbly, foul-smelling diarrhoea, which may be watery, explosive and profuse.

Diagnosis

- Three specimens of faeces for analysis (cysts and trophozoites): ELISA/PCR

Treatment

- Scrupulous hygiene: metronidazole or tinidazole

Cutaneous myiasis

Myiasis, which refers to the infestation of body tissues by the larvae (maggots) of flies, often presents as itchy 'boils'. Primary myiasis invariably occurs in travellers to tropical areas such as Africa (Tumbu fly) and Central and South America (bot fly), whereby the fly can introduce the larvae into the skin, or it can be due to secondary invasion of pre-existing wounds. All cutaneous bot fly lesions look like an unusual boil but with a small circular hole. Close inspection of lesions may reveal part or all of the larva. The simplest treatment is lateral pressure and tweezer extraction or place paraffin jelly (Vaseline) or thick ointment over the lesion to induce emergence by restricting oxygen, then apply a topical antibiotic.

Worms (helminths)

Worms that inhabit the human intestine can be classified into nematodes (roundworms), cestodes (tapeworms) and trematodes (flukes).

The roundworms, which include pinworm (*Enterobius vermicularis*), whipworm (*Trichuris trichiura*), human roundworm (*Ascaris lumbricoides*), human threadworm (*Strongyloides stercoralis*), hookworm (*Ankylostomiasis*), filariasis and larva migrans are the most prevalent worldwide and are usually asymptomatic in infected people.

Pinworm

Also known as 'threadworm', this is a ubiquitous parasite infesting mainly children of all social classes. They are tiny white worms about 1 cm long that multiply profusely and are spread readily between individuals by close contact (see FIG. 15.5). Virtually all children have been infected by the time they reach high school but at any one time approximately 50% of the 5–10 years age group will harbour pinworms.

Clinical features (usually asymptomatic)

- Pruritus ani (in about 30% of cases)
- Diarrhoea (occasionally)
- Abdominal pain, mimicking appendicitis

Diagnosis

- Inspect anus in child about 1 hour after going to sleep (see FIG. 15.5)
- Collect eggs with adhesive tape on perianal skin early morning—send to laboratory

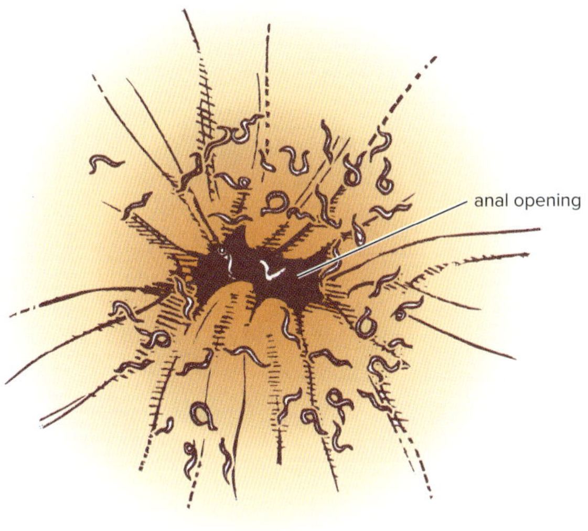

FIGURE 15.5 Pinworms: female worms appearing soon after sleep to lay eggs

Treatment

Management (troublesome cases)

- Scrupulous hygiene by family
- Hands should be washed thoroughly after toileting and before handling food
- Clip fingernails short (eggs lodge under nails)
- Patient should wear pyjamas (not nightgowns) and shower each morning
- Bed linen, nightwear and underwear changed and washed in very hot water daily for several days
- Vacuum room of affected person daily
- Have a veterinarian check any pets, especially dogs

Medication

- Any one of pyrantel, albendazole or mebendazole—as single dose orally
  pyrantel 10 mg/kg up to 750 mg
  or
  mebendazine 100 mg (child <10 kg: 50 mg)
  or
  albendazole 400 mg (child <10 kg: 200 mg)
- Repeat in 2–3 weeks—both patient and household contacts

Human roundworm

Adult worms are about 20–40 cm long and are usually acquired from contaminated food and water overseas. Many cases are asymptomatic but come to notice when they emerge from the anus, mouth or nostril (causing anxiety in the family!). Some will present with abdominal discomfort, failure to thrive, intestinal obstruction, cough, anaemia or biliary disease. They may be seen in radiological contrast examinations.

Diagnosis

- By finding eggs in the faeces. The worm is very sensitive to any of the three agents used for pinworm. May give positive faecal occult blood test.

Treatment

- A first-line option is pyrantel 20 mg/kg up to 750 mg orally, as a single dose—to be repeated after 7 days if a heavy infestation.

Whipworm

These used to be common in Indigenous communities, possibly causing failure to thrive, anaemia, abdominal pain and diarrhoea and rectal prolapse with heavy chronic infestation. The worms are about 1–2 cm long.

Diagnosis

- Faecal microscopy

Treatment

- Single large doses of mebendazole or albendazole

Hookworm

These are found in humid tropical regions but are now uncommon in northern Australia. About 1–1.5 cm long, the parasites are acquired by walking barefoot (or wearing thongs or sandals) on earth contaminated by faeces. The larvae penetrate the skin, travel through the lungs and settle in the small intestine.

Clinical features

The first sign is local irritation or 'creeping eruption' at the point of entry, known as 'ground itch', which is often unnoticed. This subsides within 2 days or so followed 1–2 weeks later by respiratory symptoms, which may be associated with bronchitis and bronchopneumonia. They can cause iron/protein deficiency anaemia in chronic infestation. Hookworm infection is the commonest cause of iron deficiency anaemia in the world.

Diagnosis

- As with other helminths, diagnosis is by finding eggs on microscopy of faeces

Treatment

- A single dose of mebendazole 100 mg bd for 3 days or 400 mg single dose pyrantel

Prevention

- Travellers should be warned to wear shoes and socks in endemic areas to prevent the entry of the larvae into the skin of the feet.

Human threadworm (*Strongyloides*)

These are tiny parasites (2 mm or so) and have a worldwide distribution. Infestation can cause symptoms such as recurrent abdominal pain and swelling and diarrhoea, skin and respiratory symptoms, with blood eosinophilia. Strongyloides can live and reproduce in the body for many years. The problem is aggravated by corticosteroid therapy and may present with a severe infection, such as septicaemia. High-risk people include migrants and refugees from tropical developing countries, returned soldiers, former prisoners of war from South-East Asia and workers or residents in northern Indigenous communities.

DxT abdominal pain (low grade) + recurrent diarrhoea + blood eosinophilia ➜ strongyloides

Diagnosis

- Detecting faecal larvae or duodenal biopsy
- ELISA: highly specific, sensitive

Treatment

- Ivermectin 200 mcg/kg (o) two doses 2 weeks apart (not in children < 5 years) or albendazole 200 mg bd for 3 days

  Adverse effects are common. Beware of these drugs in pregnancy and children.

Cutaneous larva migrans

Cutaneous larva migrans (creeping eruption) (see FIG 15.6) should be suspected in any pruritic, erythematous lesion with a serpiginous eruption on the skin, especially the hands, legs and feet of a person from a subtropical or tropical area. It is caused by the larvae of dog or cat hookworms penetrating and migrating throughout human skin, the larva always being just ahead of the lesion it causes. The diagnosis is based on the classic clinical appearance and by eosinophilia. Biopsy is usually not indicated. The problem is usually self-limiting.

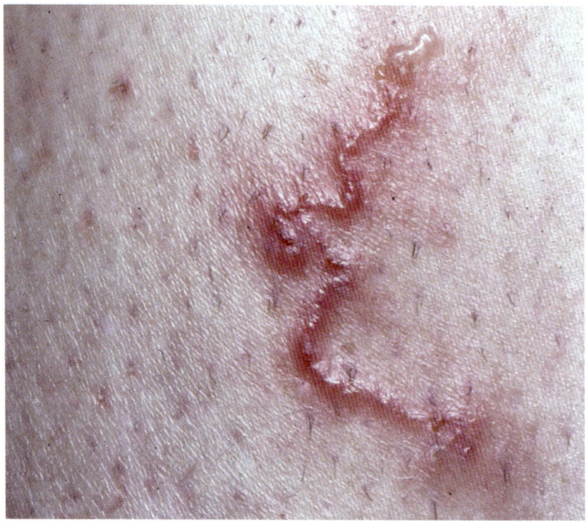

FIGURE 15.6 Cutaneous larva migrans on the leg: close-up of a serpiginous burrow

Diagnosis

- Clinical (characteristic appearance), eosinophilia (biopsy usually not indicated)

Treatment

- Ivermectin (single dose)
  or
  Albendazole
  Antihistamines for pruritus

  Note: This is usually a self-limiting problem.

Prevention

- As for hookworm. Moist sandy soil contaminated with dog or cat faeces is a common source.

Filariasis

This nematode infection has three main forms which are spread by mosquitoes, biting black flies and tabanid flies respectively.

1 Lymphatic filariasis causes acute adenolymphangitis and chronic lymphoedema with obstruction of lymph flow. The latter can manifest as a hydrocele, scrotal oedema or elephantiasis, especially of the extremities, genitals and breasts. Diagnosis is by blood film and serology.

2 Onchocerciasis (river blindness) starts as a nodule at the bite site followed by chronic skin disease and eye lesions such as uveitis and optic atrophy. It is the second leading cause of blindness worldwide. Diagnosis is by PCR testing, treatment by ivermectin.

3 Loiasis (tropical eye worm) due to the *Loa loa* worm causes conjunctivitis, localised angio-oedema and Calabar swellings. Diagnosis is by microscopic examination—microfilariae in blood.

Hydatid disease

Hydatid disease is acquired by ingesting eggs of the dog parasite *Echinococcus granulosus*, which is found in sheep farming areas here and in several countries in Asia. The parasites can migrate anywhere but usually form hydatid cysts in the liver and lungs.

Clinical features

There may be no symptoms although the patient may complain of abdominal discomfort or cystic lesions on the skin and other sites. Rupture of a cyst (usually hepatic) can cause severe anaphylaxis with possible death.

Diagnosis

- Serological tests and ultrasound

Treatment

- Usually surgical removal of a cyst and albendazole

Dracunculus medinensis (Guinea worm)

This is the longest nematode. It is transmitted by tiny crustaceans in water.

Clinical features

- Local symptoms include pain and intense itching at the skin ulcer or blister as the worm emerges into the skin

Treatment

- Slow extraction of pre-emerging worms as they exit the skin
- Metronidazole ± corticosteroids

References

1 Cooke RA. *Infectious Diseases.* Sydney: McGraw-Hill, 2008: 287–446.

2 Goldsmid JM, Leggat PA. The returned traveller with diarrhoea. Aust Fam Physician, 2007; 36(5): 322–7.

3 O'Brien D, Tobin S et al. Fever in returned travellers: review of hospital admissions for a 3-year period. Clinical Infectious Diseases, 2001; Sept 1, 33(5): 603–9.

4 Wilson ME, Weld LH et al. Fever in returned travellers: results from the GeoSentinel Surveillance Network. Clinical Infectious Diseases, 2007; 44: 1560–8.

5 Expert group for Antibiotic guidelines. Malaria. In: eTG complete. Melbourne: Therapeutic Guidelines Ltd. Available from: <www.tg.org.au>, accessed January 2018.

6 Buckley N (Chairman). *Australian Medicines Handbook.* Adelaide, 2016: 227.

7 Yung A, Ruff T, Torresi J, Leder K, O'Brien D. *Manual of Travel Medicine* (2nd edn). Melbourne: IP Communications, 2004: 203–5.

8 Expert group for Antibiotic guidelines. Systemic infection. In: eTG complete. Melbourne: Therapeutic Guidelines Ltd. Available from: <www.tg.org.au>, accessed January 2018.

9 Amichai B, Finkelstein E et al. Think cutaneous leishmaniasis. Aust Fam Physician, 1993; 22: 1213–17.

10 Colley DG et al. Human schistomiasis. Lancet, 2014; 383: 2253–64.

16 Inspection as a clinical skill

More mistakes, many more, are made by not looking than by not knowing.

SIR WILLIAM JENNER (1815–98)

GPs have an ideal opportunity to practise the art of careful observation and to notice all the signs and features characteristic of a patient from the time seen in the waiting room until the physical examination. We should be 'like Sherlock Holmes' in our analysis of the patient and accept the challenge of being astute diagnosticians and proud members of a noble profession.

It is important to stand back (so to speak) and look at the patient's general appearance and demeanour. We should be assessing their mood and affect as much as their physical appearance. The first assessment to make is 'Does the patient look sick?'.

First impressions

The first impression of the patient is always striking in some way and we should discipline ourselves to be as analytical as possible.

A rapid inspection from a trained observer may be all that is necessary to allow the observer to pinpoint specific disorders, such as anaemia, hyperthyroidism, jaundice, acromegaly and alcohol abuse. Such 'spot' diagnosis is not justifiable unless the original signs are supported by further examination, which must be comprehensive.

The following observations should therefore be made:

- facial characteristics
- abnormalities of the head and neck
- examination of the mouth
- character and distribution of hair
- examination of the skin (in general)
- height and weight
- posture and gait
- genitalia
- examination of extremities (hands, feet, nails, etc.)

Physiognomy

Physiognomy, from the Greek *physiognomonia,* meaning the judging of one's nature, is the art of judging character from the features of the face. It flourished during the Middle Ages. According to Addison,[1] 'everyone is in some degree a master of that art which is physiognomy; and naturally forms to themselves the character of a stranger from the features of the face'. In reality, all doctors use a physiognomical approach to diagnose many medical conditions, although we may not be as expert at the art as we should be.

The face is a person's most immediate means of communicating with others; it is a shield and banner, a mask and a mirror. It reveals mental faculties and emotional turmoil. It is the first perspective gained of patients as they walk into the consulting room.

The face as a mirror of disease

A fascinating aspect of the art of clinical medicine is the clinical interpretation of the patient's facies. Not only are specific skin lesions common on the face but the face may also mirror endocrine disorders and organ failure such as respiratory, cardiac, kidney and liver failure.

Jaundice may be masked by the natural colour of the cheeks but the yellow conjunctivae will be distinctive. A marked plethoric complexion may be seen in chronic alcoholics (alcohol may produce a pseudo-Cushing syndrome), in Cushing disease or in polycythaemia. Thickening of the subcutaneous tissues may be seen in chronic alcoholism, acromegaly and myxoedema, and the puffiness of the eyelids in the latter condition may simulate the true subcutaneous oedema of kidney disease.

An individual's personality and mood rarely fail to leave an impression on the facial characteristics.[2] This is partly due to the alteration in facial lines and wrinkles, which may become modified in anger, irritability, anxiety and stress. More profound changes occur with mental disease. Various CNS diseases, such as Parkinson disease and myopathies, can affect facial expression (e.g. the immobile face of the patient with Parkinson disease).

The appearance of the eyes can also be very significant and may reflect underlying systemic disease (see FIG. 16.1).

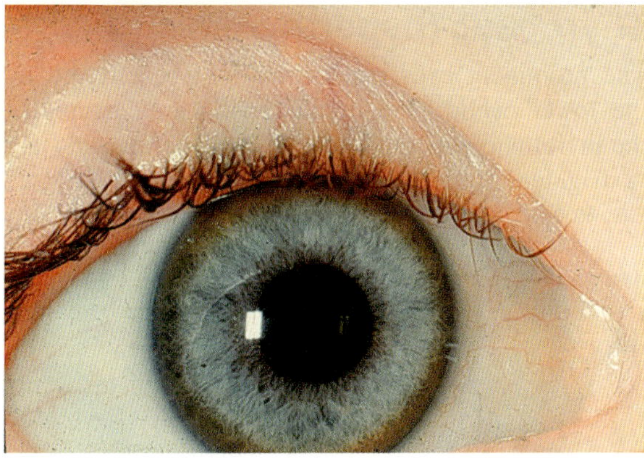

FIGURE 16.1 Kayser–Fleischer ring around the cornea in a patient with Wilson disease

Diagnostic facies[3]

Acromegalic

The enlarged characteristic face is due to a large supra-orbital ridge that causes frontal bossing, a broad nose and a prominent broad and square lower jaw. Other features include an enlarged tongue and soft tissue swelling of the nose, lips and ears (CHAPTER 23).

Adenoidal

Due to mouth breathing in children: a narrow nose/nares, a high-arched palate (the 'Gothic' palate), prominent incisor teeth, undershot jaw with a perpetually open mouth and 'stupid' expression.

Alcoholic (due to chronic use)

It is important to recognise the characteristic changes as early as possible—a plethoric face, thickened 'greasy' skin, telangiectasia, suffused conjunctivae and rosacea. Other features may include rhinophyma, parotid swelling and characteristic changes to the lips and corners of the mouth.

Bird-like (systemic sclerosis: CREST syndrome)

The bird-like features—beaking of the nose, limitation of mouth opening, puckering or furrowing of the lips and a fixed facial expression—are due to binding down of facial skin. Other features include telangiectasia on the face and hands.

Chipmunk (thalassaemia major)

There is bossing of the skull, hypertrophy of the maxillae (which tends to expose the upper teeth), prominent malar eminences and depression of the bridge of the nose. The major haemoglobinopathies cause hyperplasia of the skull and facial bones because of an increase in the bone marrow cavity.

Choleric

The patient with cholera has a pale face with cold clammy skin, sunken eyes, hollow cheeks and a forlorn, apathetic look (similar to the Hippocratic facies).

Cushingoid

The face has a typical 'moon shape', plethora, hirsutism (more obvious in women), acne (CHAPTER 23).

Facial nerve palsy

Features include unilateral drooping of the corner of the mouth and flattening of the nasolabial fold (CHAPTER 33).

- Upper motor neurone (UMN) type: the forehead movement is spared
- Lower motor neurone (LMN) type (e.g. Bell palsy, Ramsay–Hunt syndrome): lack of forehead muscle tone

Hippocratic

This describes the deathly, mask-like features of advanced peritonitis—sunken eyes; 'gaunt' face; 'collapsed' temples; dry, crusty lips; and clammy forehead.

Marfanoid (Marfan syndrome)

The typical tall stature, arachnodactyly and chest deformities, combined with the facial features of a subluxation of the lens of the eye and high-arched palate, help to pinpoint the diagnosis (CHAPTER 18).

Mitral (mitral valve disease, especially mitral stenosis)

This is typically shown in flushed or rosy cheeks with a bluish tinge due to dilatation of the malar capillaries. It is associated with pulmonary hypertension.

Mongoloid (Down syndrome)

The facial features include a flat profile, with crowded features, a round head, dysplastic lowset ears, protruding tongue, mongoloid slant of the eyes with epicanthic folds, mouth hanging open and peripheral silver iris spots (Brushfield's spots) (CHAPTER 18).

Myopathic (myopathy/myasthenia gravis)

Facial characteristics include an expressionless, 'tired'-looking face with bilateral ptosis.

Myotonic (dystrophia myotonia)

Typical features include frontal baldness, expressionless triangular facies, partial ptosis, cataracts and temporal muscle atrophy.

Myxoedemic (hypothyroidism)

The face usually has an apathetic look and is 'puffy' with possible periorbital oedema. There is broadening of the lower part of the face. The skin (not the sclera) may appear yellow (due to hypercarotenaemia) and is generally dry and coarse. Other features may include thin, coarse, listless hair and loss or thinning of the outer third of the eyebrows. The tongue is usually enlarged and the patient speaks with a 'thickened', croaking, slow speech (CHAPTER 23).

Obese

The distinguishing feature from the 'moon face' of Cushing disease is the general roundness and uniform fatness of the face.

Pagetic (Paget disease)

The main feature is skull enlargement, notably of the frontal and parietal areas (the head circumference is usually greater than 55 cm, which is abnormal)—the 'hat doesn't fit any more' hallmark. Other features include increased bony warmth and deafness (CHAPTER 69).

Parkinsonian

Characteristic is the mask-like facies with lack of facial expression and fixed unblinking stare. There is immobility of the facial muscles (CHAPTER 33).

Peutz–Jeghers

Pigmented macules (1–5 mm in diameter) occur on lips, buccal mucosa and fingers.

Risus sardonicus

A grin-like appearance of hypertonic facial muscles (typical of tetanus).

Smoker's

A face older than the years with premature gross wrinkling of the skin, stained teeth, deep raspy voice, 'loose' cough, smell of tobacco.

Thyrotoxic (hyperthyroidism)

The prominent eyes (sclera may not be covered by the lower eyelid) and conjunctivitis are features of the thyrotoxic patient (CHAPTER 23). The thyroid stare (a frightened expression) may also be present (see FIG. 16.2).

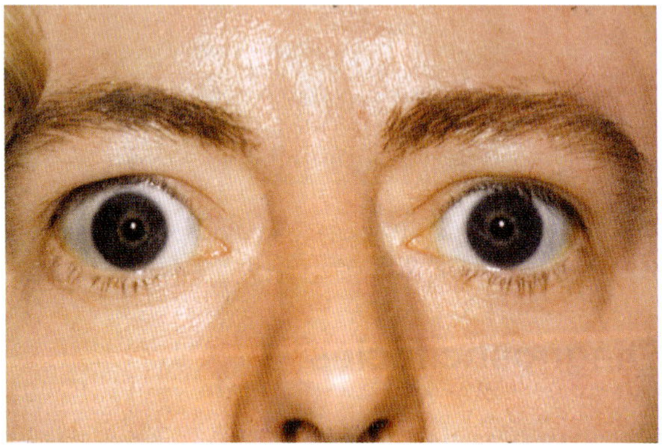

FIGURE 16.2 Thyrotoxicosis illustrating a typical thyroid stare

Turner syndrome

The facial characteristics include ptosis—'fishlike' mouth, small chin (micrognathia), low-set ears and deafness. Cardiac lesions include coarctation of the aorta and pulmonary stenosis. Webbing of the neck is the classic sign (CHAPTER 18).

Uraemic

A sallow 'muddy' complexion with uraemic fetor—an ammoniacal halitosis.

Other classic facies (similes)

Bulldog	Congenital syphilis
Chipmunk	Thalassaemia major
Elfin	William syndrome
Fish-like mouth	Turner syndrome
Hatchet	Dystropia myotonia
Death mask	Peritonitis; cholera
Long face	Fragile X syndrome
Mask	Parkinson: Wilson disease
Monkey	Hypopituitarism
Moon	Cushing syndrome
Old man in child	Marasmus
Raccoon	Basilar skull fracture
Toad	Hypothyroidism

Specific characteristics

Various facial signs may be present. The causes of these signs are listed below.

Butterfly 'rash'

- SLE
  Erythema, scaling with a discrete red advancing edge on the cheeks and bridge of the nose; the sharp border, lack of pustules and adherent scale make it differ from rosacea
- Rosacea
  Papules, pustules and telangiectasia on an erythematous background on cheeks, forehead and chin
- Erysipelas
  Painful, erythematous, indurated skin infection with a well-defined raised edge
- Seborrhoeic dermatitis
  Red and scaly rash involving eyebrows, eyelids, nasolabial folds
- Photosensitivity eruptions
  Erythematous on areas that are exposed to the sun

Chloasma/melasma

Increased browning pigmentation, usually confined to symmetrical areas of the cheeks (FIG. 16.3). Common in pregnancy and caused by drugs:

- combined oral contraceptive pill
- hydroxychloroquine (Plaquenil)
- diphenylhydrazine

Malar flush

- Mitral stenosis
- Pulmonary stenosis
- Rosacea
- SLE
- Mesenteric adenitis

Spider naevi

- Pregnancy
- Liver disease
- Vitamin B deficiency in normal people

Enlarged tongue

- Acromegaly
- Hypothyroidism
- Amyloidosis
- Down syndrome

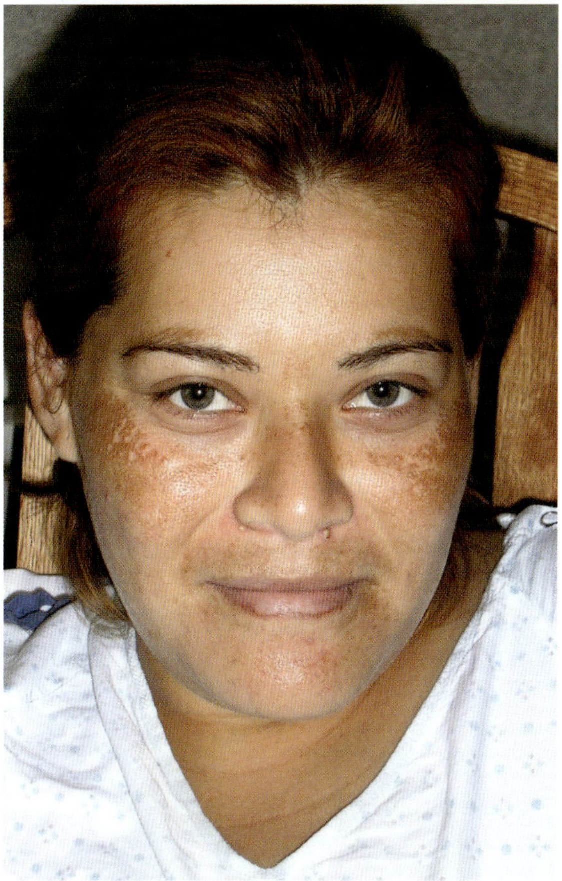

FIGURE 16.3 Melasma (chloasma) in the typical distribution soon after the birth of the second child. Sometimes called the mask of pregnancy.

Cataracts: risk factors

- Ageing
- Senility
- Corticosteroid therapy
- Diabetes
- Hypoparathyroidism
- Dystrophia myotonia
- Trauma (may be delayed)
- Ocular disease (e.g. glaucoma)
- Smoking

Telangiectasia

- Systemic sclerosis
- CREST syndrome
- Liver disease (e.g. alcoholism)

Cyanosis

Cyanosis is a bluish discolouration of the skin and mucous membranes due to deoxygenated haemoglobin concentrated in the superficial blood vessels. The arterial oxygen saturation is 80–85% before it is clinically apparent. It is classified as central or peripheral.

Central

Cyanosis is present in parts of the body with good circulation, such as the lips and tongue. The areas feel warm. The main causes are pulmonary disease, pulmonary oedema, cyanotic congenital heart disease (right to left shunt), respiratory depression, polycythaemia (see FIG. 16.4).

Peripheral

Cyanosis is in the extremities, such as the outer surface of the lips, finger tips, nose and ears. The areas feel cold. The main causes are peripheral vascular disease, cardiac failure, 'shock', exposure to cold, left ventricular failure and all causes of central cyanosis.

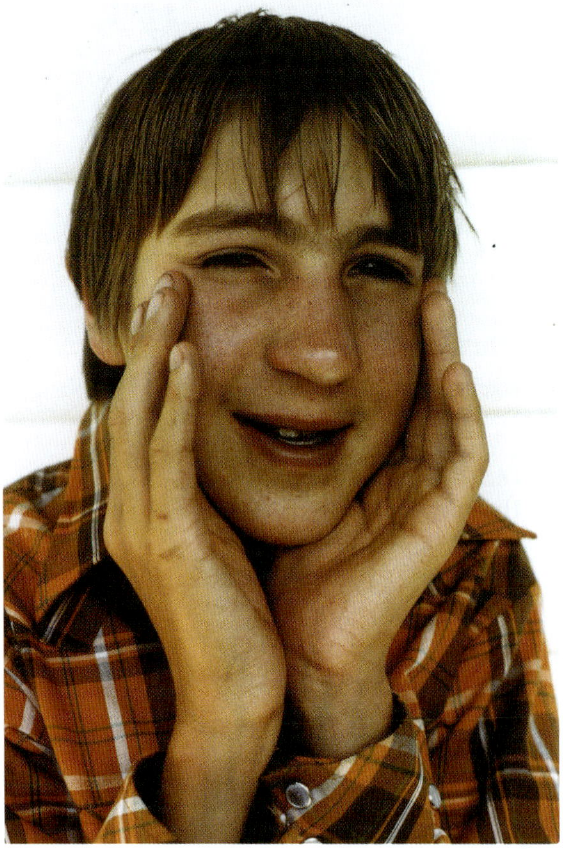

FIGURE 16.4 Adolescent patient with central cyanotic heart disease and associated clubbing of the fingers

Clubbing of fingers

Features

- Loss of usual angle between base of nail and nail fold
- Curvature in two planes
- Increased sponginess in base of nail
- Increased convexity of nail
- Mainly caused by respiratory disease

Causes

1 Lung disease:
   - carcinoma
   - bronchiectasis
   - cystic fibrosis
   - abscess/empyema
   - pulmonary fibrosis

2 Heart disease:
   - infective endocarditis
   - cyanotic congenital heart disease (see FIG. 16.4)

3 Liver disease:
   - cirrhosis

4 Gastrointestinal disease:
   - ulcerative colitis
   - Crohn disease
   - coeliac disease

5 Congenital

Increased general pigmentation

Increased pigmentation is not common but if obvious in areas exposed to the sun, look for 'hidden' areas, such as the inner aspect of the forearms. Causes include those listed below.

Increased melanocyte-stimulating hormone (MSH)

- Addison disease (see CHAPTER 23)
- Cushing syndrome
- Ectopic ACTH syndrome
- AIDS

Metabolic

- Hyperthyroidism
- Haemochromatosis (see FIG. 16.5)
- Cirrhosis of the liver
- Porphyria cutanea tarda
- Chronic kidney failure
- Malnutrition/malabsorption
- Pregnancy

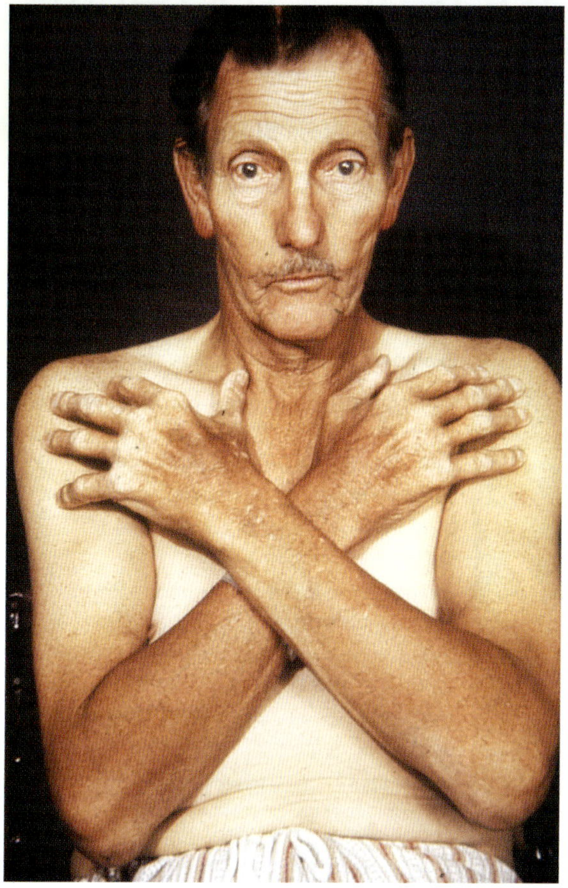

FIGURE 16.5 Patient showing pigmentation of primary haemochromatosis and associated arthritis of fingers

Drugs

- Amiodarone
- Antibiotics (busulphan, bleomycin, minocycline)
- Antimalarials (chloroquine/hydroxychloroquine)
- Arsenic, gold, silver
- Chemotherapy
- Dapsone
- Oral contraceptive pill (OCP)
- Phenothiazines
- Photochemotherapy (PUVA)
- Psoralens
- Thiazides

Tumours

- Lymphomas
- Acanthosis nigricans
- Metastatic melanoma

References

1 Addison T. *A Collection of the Published Writings of Thomas Addison MD.* New Sydenham Soc, 1818.

2 Bates B, Cleese J. *The Human Face*. London: BBC, 2001.

3 Talley NJ, O'Connor S. *Clinical Examination: A Systematic Guide to Physical Diagnosis.* (7th edn). Sydney: Elsevier, 2014: 30–3.

17 A safe diagnostic strategy

For most diagnoses all that is needed is an ounce of knowledge, an ounce of intelligence, and a pound of thoroughness.

ANON (1951), *LANCET*

The discipline of general practice is probably the most difficult, complex and challenging of all the healing arts. Our field of endeavour is at the very front line of medicine and as practitioners we shoulder the responsibility of the early diagnosis of very serious, perhaps life-threatening, illness in addition to the recognition of anxiety traits in our patients.

The teaching of our craft is also an exciting challenge and presupposes that we have a profound comprehension of our discipline.

Our area is characterised by a wide kaleidoscope of presenting problems, often foreign to the classic textbook presentation and sometimes embellished by a 'shopping list' of seemingly unconnected problems or vague symptoms—the so-called undifferentiated illness syndrome.[1] Common undifferentiated symptoms include tiredness or fatigue, sleeping problems, anxiety and stress, dizziness, headache, indigestion, anorexia and nausea, sexual dysfunction, weight loss, loss of interest, flatulence, abdominal discomfort and chest discomfort.[2] It is important, especially in a busy practice, to adopt a fail-safe strategy to analyse such presenting problems. Such an approach is even more important in a world of increasing medical litigation and specialisation.

To help bring order to the jungle of general practice problems, the principal author has developed a simple model to facilitate diagnosis and reduce the margin of error.

The concept of diagnostic triads

A most useful guide to learning or memorising diagnoses, especially of elusive and uncommon conditions, is to remember three key points to the condition. The cognitive process of learning these so-called 'triads' and even 'tetrads' provides a useful template for the diagnostic methodology required in general practice. Some simple examples are shown below.

Examples such as these are interspersed throughout the text, especially in this chapter, and are prefixed by the symbol DxT.

Examples of diagnostic triads

DxT angina + dyspnoea + blackouts ➜ aortic stenosis

DxT menstrual dysfunction + obesity + hirsutism ➜ polycystic ovarian syndrome

DxT malaise + night sweats + pruritus ➜ Hodgkin lymphoma

DxT abdominal pain + diarrhoea + fever ➜ Crohn disease

DxT vertigo + vomiting + tinnitus ➜ Ménière syndrome

DxT dizziness + hearing loss + tinnitus ➜ acoustic neuroma

DxT fatigue + muscle weakness + cramps ➜ hypokalaemia

The basic model

The use of the diagnostic model requires a disciplined approach to the problem with the medical practitioner quickly answering five self-posed questions. The questions are shown in TABLE 17.1.

This approach, which is based on considerable experience, requires the learning of a predetermined plan which, naturally, would vary in different parts of the world but would have a certain universal application in the so-called developed world.

Table 17.1 The diagnostic model for a presenting problem

1	What is the probability diagnosis?
2	What serious disorders must not be missed?
3	What conditions are often missed (the pitfalls)?
4	Could this patient have one of the 'masquerades' in medical practice?
5	Is this patient trying to tell me something else?

Each of the above five questions will be expanded.

17

An excellent acronym on this theme, 'PROMPT', was devised by a reader, Dr Kelly Teagle:

- **P** **P**robability
- **R** **R**ed flag
- **O** **O**ften missed
- **M** **M**asquerades
- **P** **P**atient wants to
- **T** **T**ell me something

Another contribution is by Flinders University medical student, Judah:

Things are not always cut and dried:

- **C** **C**onnective tissue disorders
- **U** **U**TIs, particularly in very old and very young
- **T** **T**hyroid disease

and

- **D** **D**epression
- **R** remember to **R**ule out serious and **R**are causes
- **I** **I**atrogenic causes
- **E** **E**motional needs
- **D** **D**iabetes

1 The probability diagnosis

The probability diagnosis is based on the doctor's perspective and experience with regard to prevalence, incidence and the natural history of disease. GPs acquire first-hand epidemiological knowledge about the patterns of illness apparent in individuals and in the community, which enables them to view illness from a perspective that is not available to doctors in any other disciplines. Thus, during the medical interview, the doctor not only is gathering information, allocating priorities and making hypotheses, but also is developing a probability diagnosis based on acquired epidemiological knowledge.

2 What serious disorders must not be missed?

While epidemiological knowledge is a great asset to the GP, it can be a disadvantage in that he or she is so familiar with what is common that the all-important rare cause of a presenting symptom may be overlooked. On the other hand, the doctor in the specialist clinic, where a different spectrum of disease is encountered, is more likely to focus on the rare at the expense of the common cause. However, it is vital, especially working in the modern framework of a litigation-conscious society, not to miss serious, life-threatening disorders.

To achieve early recognition of serious illness, the GP needs to develop a 'high index of suspicion'. This is generally regarded as largely intuitive, but this is probably not the case, and it would be more accurate to say that it comes with experience.

The serious disorders that should always be considered 'until proven otherwise' include malignant disease, acquired immunodeficiency syndrome (AIDS), coronary disease and life-threatening infections such as meningitis, meningococcal infection (see FIG. 17.1), *Haemophilus influenza* b infections, septicaemia and infective endocarditis (see TABLE 17.2).

Myocardial infarction or ischaemia is extremely important to consider because it is so potentially lethal and at times can be overlooked by the busy practitioner. It does not always manifest as the classic presentation of crushing central pain but can present as pain of varying severity and quality in a wide variety of sites.

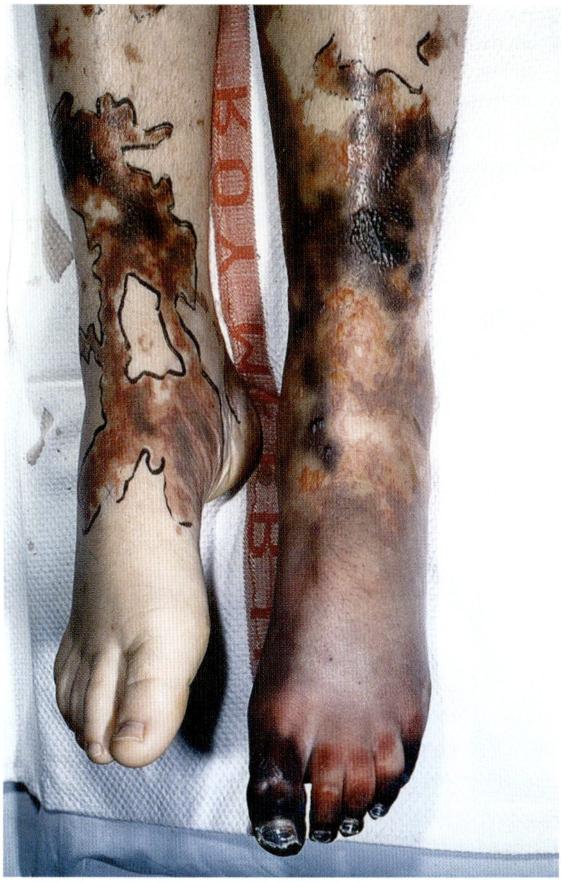

FIGURE 17.1 Meningococcal infection: complications of infarction (DIC) including gangrene from meningococcaemia

These sites include the jaw, neck, ear, arm, epigastrium and interscapular region. Coronary artery disease may manifest as life-threatening arrhythmias that may present as palpitations and/or dizziness. A high index of suspicion is necessary to diagnose arrhythmias.

Table 17.2 Serious 'not to be missed' conditions

Neoplasia, especially malignancy

HIV infection/AIDS

Asthma/anaphylaxis

Severe infections, especially:

- meningoencephalitis
- septicaemia
- meningococcal infection (see FIG. 17.1)
- epiglottitis
- infective endocarditis
- pneumonia/influenza/SARS
- clostridia infections, e.g. tetanus, botulism, gas gangrene

Coronary artery disease

- myocardial infarction
- unstable angina
- arrhythmias

Imminent or potential suicide

Intracerebral lesions (e.g. subarachnoid haemorrhage)

Ectopic pregnancy

Diagnostic triads for life-threatening conditions (examples)

DxT fever + rigors + hypotension ➔ septicaemia

DxT fever + vomiting + headache ➔ meningitis

DxT fatigue + dizziness ± syncope ➔ cardiac arrhythmia

DxT fever + drooling + stridor (child) ➔ epiglottitis

DxT headache + vomiting + altered consciousness ➔ subarachnoid haemorrhage (SAH)

DxT abdominal pain + amenorrhoea + abnormal vaginal bleeding ➔ ectopic pregnancy

DxT fatigue + dyspnoea on exertion + dizziness ➔ cardiomyopathy

Consider M^2I^2

A traditional way of classifying serious diseases is the pathology aide-mémoire:

- Malignancy
- Metabolic
- Infarction
- Infection

Danger: think VIC

V = **V**ascular
I = **I**nfection (severe)
C = **C**ancer

Red flags

Red flags (alarm bells) are symptoms or signs that alert us to the likelihood of significant harm. Such underlying disease *must not be missed* and demands careful investigation. Examples include weight loss, vomiting, altered cognition, fever >38°C, dizziness, and/or syncope at the toilet and pallor. Red flags will be outlined under presenting symptoms throughout the text.

3 What conditions are often missed?

This question refers to the common 'pitfalls' so often encountered in general practice. This area is definitely related to the experience factor and includes rather simple, non-life-threatening problems that can be so easily overlooked unless doctors are prepared to include them in their diagnostic framework.

Classic examples include smoking or dental caries as a cause of abdominal pain, allergies to a whole variety of unsuspected everyday contacts, foreign bodies, occupational or environmental hazards as a cause of headache, respiratory discomfort or malaise, and faecal impaction as a cause of diarrhoea. We have all experienced the 'red face syndrome' from a urinary tract infection, whether it is the cause of fever in a child, lumbar pain in a pregnant woman or malaise in an older person. The dermatomal pain pattern caused by herpes zoster prior to the eruption of the rash (or if only a few sparse vesicles erupt) is a real trap.

A typical pitfall is Addison disease, where some patients can wait up to 15 years before being diagnosed. The absence of subdued classic pigmentation (see FIG. 17.2) can mask the early diagnosis.

Haemochromatosis can be a surprise diagnosis, often discovered by serendipity following a screening blood test for unexplained fatigue. Coeliac disease is a classic master of disguise in both children and adults. It now ranks as one of the most common, widespread and undiagnosed illnesses affecting humans. In Australia, 1.5% of the population are affected but 80% remain undiagnosed.[4] Research by dermatologists[5] has highlighted that it can present in a number of ways that can affect the skin and hair. Apart from typical gastrointestinal symptoms, such as chronic diarrhoea,

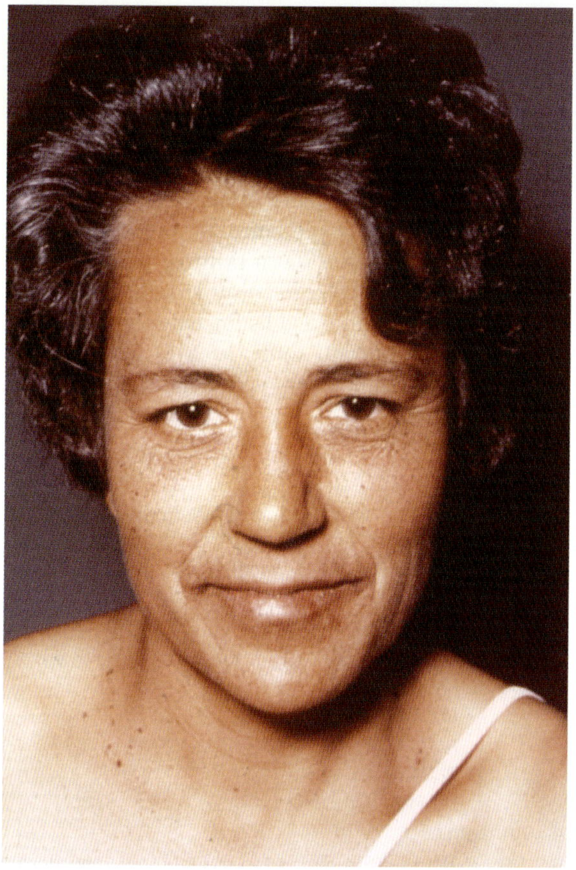

FIGURE 17.2 Woman with Addison disease showing facial pigmentation

steatorrhoea, weight loss, anorexia and abdominal distension, the following atypical symptoms have been described:

- nutritional presentations, including folate, zinc or iron (in particular) deficiency
- grouped blisters around the knees, elbows and buttocks (dermatitis herpetiformis)
- hair loss and mouth ulcers

Menopausal symptoms can also be overlooked as we focus on a particular symptom. Some important pitfalls are given in TABLE 17.3.

Diagnostic triads for some 'pitfalls'

DxT fatigue + weight loss + diarrhoea ➜ coeliac disease

DxT anorexia/nausea + faecal leaking + abdominal bloating ➜ faecal impaction

DxT abdominal cramps + flatulence + profuse diarrhoea ➜ giardiasis

DxT lethargy + tiredness + arthralgia ➜ haemochromatosis

DxT lethargy + abdominal pains + irritability (in child) ➜ lead poisoning

DxT aching bones + waddling gait + deafness ➜ Paget disease

DxT malaise + cough + fever (± erythema nodosum) ➜ sarcoidosis

DxT (male child) snorting, blinking + oral noises (e.g. grunts) ± loud expletives ➜ Tourette syndrome

Table 17.3 Classic pitfalls
Abscess (hidden)
Addison disease
Allergies
Candida infection
Chronic fatigue syndrome
Coeliac disease
Domestic abuse, including child abuse
Drugs (see TABLE 17.4)
Endometriosis
Faecal impaction
Foreign bodies
Giardiasis
Haemochromatosis
Herpes zoster
Lead poisoning
Malnutrition (unsuspected)
Menopause syndrome
Migraine (atypical variants)
Paget disease
Pregnancy (early)
Sarcoidosis
Seizure disorders
Tourette syndrome
Urinary infection

4 The masquerades ('chameleons')

It is important to utilise a type of fail-safe mechanism to avoid missing the diagnosis of these disorders. Some practitioners refer to consultations that make their 'head spin' in confusion and bewilderment, with patients presenting with a 'shopping list' of problems. It is in these patients that a checklist is useful. Consider the apparently neurotic patient who presents with headache, lethargy, tiredness, constipation, anorexia, indigestion, shortness of breath on exertion, pruritus, flatulence, sore tongue and backache. In such a patient we must consider a diagnosis that links all these symptoms, especially if the physical examination is inconclusive; this includes iron deficiency anaemia, depression, diabetes mellitus, hypothyroidism (see FIG. 17.3) and drug abuse.

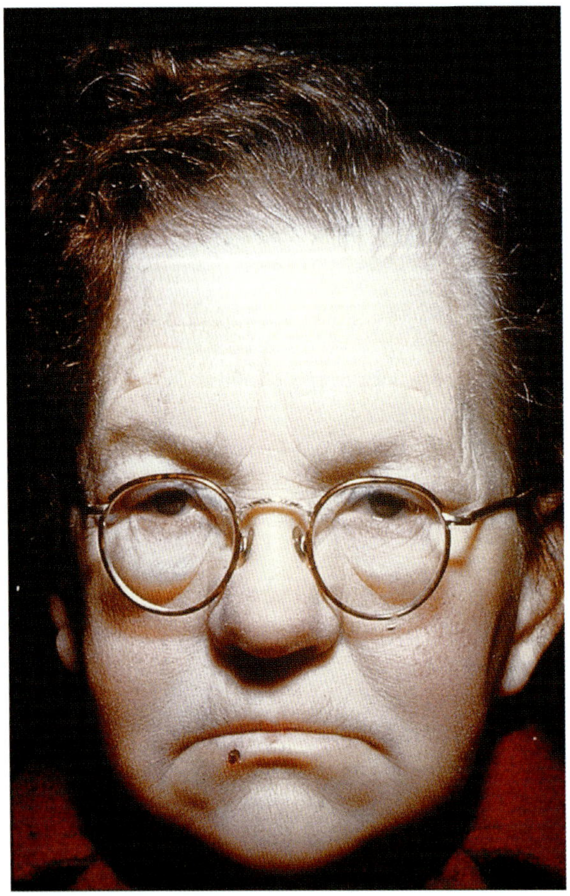

FIGURE 17.3 Hypothyroidism in a 60-year-old woman, a classic masquerade, with a slow subtle onset of facial changes

A century ago it was important to consider diseases such as syphilis and tuberculosis as the great common masquerades, but these infections have been replaced by iatrogenesis, malignant disease, alcoholism, endocrine disorders and the various manifestations of atherosclerosis, particularly coronary insufficiency and cerebrovascular insufficiency.

If the patient has pain anywhere it is possible that it could originate from the spine, so the possibility of spinal pain (radicular or referred) should be considered as the cause for various pain syndromes, such as headache, arm pain, leg pain, chest pain, pelvic pain and even abdominal pain. The author's experience is that spondylogenic pain is one of the most underdiagnosed problems in general practice.

A checklist that has been divided into two groups of seven disorders is presented in TABLES 17.4 and 17.5. The first list, 'the seven primary masquerades', represents the more common disorders encountered in general practice; the second list includes less common masquerades—although some, such as Epstein–Barr mononucleosis, can be very common masquerades in general practice.

Table 17.4 The seven primary masquerades

1 Depression
2 Diabetes mellitus
3 Drugs
- iatrogenic
- self-abuse
  - alcohol
  - narcotics
  - nicotine
  - others

4 Anaemia
5 Thyroid and other endocrine or metabolic disorders
- hyperthyroidism
- hypothyroidism
- Addison disease

6 Spinal dysfunction
7 Urinary tract infection (UTI)

Neoplasia, especially malignancy of the so-called 'silent areas', can be an elusive diagnostic problem. Typical examples are carcinoma of the nasopharynx and sinuses, ovary, caecum, kidney and lymphoietic tissue. Sarcoidosis is another disease that can be a real masquerade (see CHAPTER 49).

Systemic lupus erythematosus (SLE) has been described as 'the great pretender'.[6] The two most common symptoms are joint pain and fatigue but it is a multisystem disease that may present with involvement of any of these organ systems and may not initially be recognised as such.

As a practical diagnostic ploy, the author has both lists strategically placed on the surgery wall immediately behind the patient. The lists are rapidly perused for inspiration should the diagnosis for a particular patient prove elusive.

Table 17.5 The seven other masquerades

1 Chronic kidney failure
2 Malignant disease
- lymphomas
- lung
- caecum/colon
- kidney
- multiple myeloma
- ovary
- pancreas
- metastasis

3 HIV infection/AIDS
4 Baffling bacterial infections
- syphilis
- tuberculosis
- infective endocarditis
- the zoonoses
- *Chlamydia* infections
- atypical pneumonias (e.g. Legionnaire disease)
- others

5 Baffling viral (and protozoal) infections
- Epstein–Barr mononucleosis
- TORCH organisms (e.g. cytomegalovirus)
- hepatitis A, B, C, D, E
- mosquito-borne infections
  - malaria
  - Ross River fever
  - dengue fever
  - others

6 Neurological dilemmas
- Parkinson disease
- Guillain–Barré syndrome
- seizure disorders
- multiple sclerosis
- myasthenia gravis
- space-occupying lesion of skull
- migraine and its variants
- others

7 Connective tissue disorders and the vasculitides
- Connective tissue disorders
  - systemic lupus erythematosus (SLE)
  - systemic sclerosis
  - dermatomyositis
  - overlap syndrome
- Vasculitides
  - polyarteritis nodosa
  - giant cell arteritis/polymyalgia rheumatica
  - granulomatous disorders

5 Is the patient trying to tell me something?

The doctor has to consider, especially in the case of undifferentiated illness, whether the patient has a 'hidden agenda' for the presentation.[7] Of course, the patient may be depressed (overt or masked) or may have a true anxiety state. However, a presenting symptom such as tiredness may represent a 'ticket of entry' to the consulting room.[3] It may represent a plea for help in a stressed or anxious patient. We should be sensitive to patients' needs and feelings, and, as listening, caring, empathetic practitioners, provide the right opportunity for the patient to communicate freely.

Deep sexual anxieties and problems, poor self-esteem, and fear of malignancy or some other medical catastrophe are just some of the reasons patients present to doctors.

The patient with a self-induced bruising (see FIG. 17.4) was a health professional who was deeply attracted to an inpatient haematologist (Munchausen syndrome).

The author has another checklist (see TABLE 17.6) to help identify the psychosocial reasons for a patient's malaise.

Diagnostic triads for some 'masquerades'

DxT malaise + fever + cough (± erythema nodosa) ➜ TB *or* sarcoidosis

DxT fever + sore throat + cervical lymphadenopathy ➜ EB mononucleosis

DxT fatigue + a/n/v + sallow skin ➜ chronic kidney failure

DxT polyuria + polydipsia + skin/orifice infections ➜ diabetes mellitus

DxT FUO + cardiac murmur + embolic phenomena ➜ infective endocarditis

DxT fatigue + polyarthritis + fever or skin lesions ➜ SLE

DxT loin pain + haematuria + palpable loin mass ➜ kidney carcinoma

DxT malaise + weight loss + cough ➜ lung carcinoma

DxT fever + myalgia/headache + non-productive cough ➜ atypical pneumonia

DxT malaise + night sweats + painless lymphadenopathy ➜ non-Hodgkin lymphoma

DxT arthralgia + Raynaud phenomenon + GORD (± skin changes) ➜ systemic sclerosis

DxT fatigue + headache + jaw claudication ➜ temporal arteritis

DxT weakness + back pain + weight loss ➜ multiple myeloma

DxT lethargy + physical/mental slowing + constipation ➜ hypothyroidism

Note: Diagnostic triads for neurological dilemmas are included in CHAPTER 33.

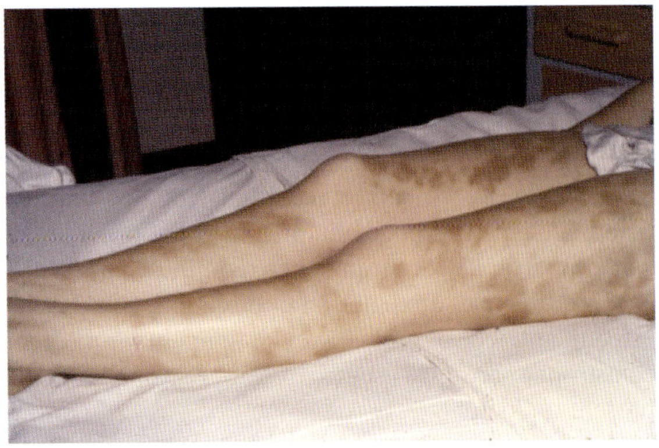

FIGURE 17.4 Artefactual purpura showing an unusually symmetrical distribution in sites that can be reached by the patient (a 'ticket of entry')—Munchausen syndrome

In the author's experience of counselling patients and families, the number of problems caused by interpersonal conflict is quite amazing and makes it worthwhile to specifically explore the quality of close relationships, such as those of husband–wife, mother–daughter and father–son.

Another common yet overlooked stressor is bullying,[8] whether it is in the workplace, school, university, home, internet or elsewhere. It is a significant public health issue. The current fashion for tough, dynamic, 'macho' management styles has created a culture in which bullying can thrive. As GPs we should be more aware of the possibility that workplace bullying may be contributing to the stresses with which many patients present. A simple, direct, routine question such as 'How are things at work?' can create an opportunity to raise the issue.

Table 17.6 Underlying fears or image problems that cause stress and anxiety

1	Interpersonal conflict in the family
2	Identification with sick or deceased friends
3	Fear of malignancy
4	STIs, especially AIDS
5	Impending 'coronary' or 'stroke'
6	Sexual problem
7	Drug-related problem
8	Crippling arthritis
9	Financial woes
10	Other abnormal stresses

Identification and transference of illness, symptoms and death, in particular, are important areas of anxiety to consider. Patients often identify their problems with relatives, friends or public personalities who have malignant disease. Other somatoform disorders and the factitious disorders, including the fascinating Munchausen syndrome, may be obvious or extremely complex and difficult to recognise. Consider also 'Munchausen by proxy' where carers intentionally produce or feign symptoms in the person (child or elderly patient) in their care. These subtle psychosocial issues are usually termed 'yellow flags'.

Yellow flags[3]

Yellow flags are signs or behaviours that flag or indicate a psychosocial barrier to recovery. They have been described originally within the framework of chronic pain and disability, especially chronic back pain, and require a shift in our focus of care. Conditions to consider are anxiety, depression, adjustment disorder and personality disorder. Typical yellow flags are presented in TABLE 17.7.

Table 17.7 Yellow flags: examples

Abnormal illness behaviour
Devious behaviour
Cancelling appointments
Treatment non-compliance/refusal
Somatisation
Absenteeism from work
Poor work performance
Personal neglect
Relationship breakdown
Law and order incidents

A survey by researchers at Melbourne's Centre for Behavioural Research[9] revealed that the three most feared diseases are cancer (81%), heart disease (32%) and HIV/AIDS (21%).

The bottom line is that patients are often desperately searching for security and we have an important role to play in helping them.

Some examples of application of the model

Hiccough

1	**Probability diagnosis** Food and alcohol excess Psychogenic/functional Postoperative • gastric distension • phrenic nerve irritation
2	**Serious disorders not to be missed** Neoplasia • CNS • neck • oesophagus • lung Subphrenic abscess Myocardial infarction/pericarditis CNS disorders (e.g. CVA infection) Chronic kidney failure
3	**Pitfalls** Alcohol excess Smoking Aerophagy Gastrointestinal disorders • oesophagitis • peptic ulcer • hiatus hernia • cholecystitis • hepatomegaly *Rarities* Sudden temperature change Neck cysts and vascular abnormalities
4	**Seven masquerades checklist** Drugs
5	**Is the patient trying to tell me something?** Emotional causes always to be considered.

Halitosis

(see CHAPTER 72)[10]

1	**Probability diagnosis** Dietary habits—odour-causing foods, e.g. garlic Poor oral hygiene Orodental disease, e.g. gingivitis, dental abscess Dry mouth (e.g. on waking) Smoking/alcohol
2	**Serious disorders not to be missed** Malignancy: lung, oropharynx, larynx, stomach, nose, leukaemia Pulmonary tuberculosis Quinsy Oral candidiasis Lung abscess Blood dyscrasias/leukaemia Uraemia Hepatic failure
3	**Pitfalls** Nasal and sinus infection Systemic infection Appendicitis Bronchiectasis Hiatus hernia Starvation *Rarities* Pharyngeal and oesophageal diverticula Sjögren syndrome Scurvy
4	**Seven masquerades checklist** Depression Diabetes: acidosis (acetone) Drugs
5	**Is the patient trying to tell me something?** Possible manifestation of psychogenic disorder Halitophobia

17

Practice tips

- Follow the 'baseball rule' for a delayed or puzzling diagnosis: 'Three strikes and you're out'.
- Infarction—think fast!
  - acute coronary events: 60–90 minutes
  - stroke: 3–4 hours
  - femoral artery: 4 hours
  - torsion of testis: 4–6 hours

Patient education resources

Hand-out sheets from *Murtagh's Patient Education* 7th edition:

- Bullying of children
- Bullying in the workplace

References

1 Murtagh J. Common problems: a safe diagnostic strategy. Aust Fam Physician, 1990; 19: 733–42.
2 Frith J, Knowlden S. Undifferentiated illness. Med J Aust, 1992; 156: 472–6.
3 Main CJ, Williams AC. ABC of psychological medicine. BMJ, 2002 (Sept 7); 325: 534–7.
4 Tye-Din J. Finding the hidden coeliac chameleon. MJA Insight. 27 March 2017; 11: 1–8.
5 Nixon R. Cutaneous manifestations of coeliac disease. Australas J Dermatol, 2001; 42: 136–8.
6 Hanrahan P. The great pretender: systemic lupus erythematosus. Aust Fam Physician, 2001; 30(7): 636–40.
7 Levenstein JH, McCracken EC, McWhinney IR et al. The patient-centred method. I. A model for the doctor–patient interaction in family medicine. Fam Pract, 1986; 3: 24–30.
8 McAvoy BR, Murtagh J. Workplace bullying: the silent epidemic. Editorial. BMJ, 2003; 326: 776–7.
9 Borland R et al. Illnesses that Australians fear most in 1986 and 1993. Australian Journal of Public Health, 1994; 18: 366–9.
10 Expert group for Oral and Dental guidelines. In: eTG complete. Melbourne: Therapeutic Guidelines Ltd. Available from: <www.tg.org.au>, accessed January 2018.

Genetic conditions 18

People love to oversimplify genetics, saying we have a 'gene for cancer' or a 'gene for diabetes'. But the fact is, genes determine only so much. Identical twins are identical genomes, yet one may develop juvenile diabetes and the other typically doesn't. Understanding the role of genes should help pinpoint environmental factors . . . The genome is a history book showing the entire 6 billion-member human species traces back 7000 generations to a tiny founding population of some 60 000 people. Our species has only a modest amount of genetic variation—the DNA of any two humans is 99.9% identical.

ERIC LANDER, HUMAN GENOME PROJECT, 2000[1]

The family doctor has an important role to play in the exciting and rapidly expanding world of medical genetics. The role includes routine diagnosis, early detection, and community and ethical guidance. Virtually all of the three billion nucleotides of the human genome have been sequenced and the knowledge of their organisation into the known 30 000–35 000 functional units or genes continues to become more sophisticated.[2]

The genome project has commenced mapping out 'single nucleotide polymorphisms' (SNPs) as signposts throughout the genome to assist in locating disease-associated genes and studying variations between individuals.[3] Any two unrelated individuals differ by one base per every thousand or so—these as SNPs—and it is believed that SNPs contribute to the risk of common disease rather than directly cause disease. If we carry the wrong set of SNPs, we can be predisposed to various diseases.

Genetic testing is now available for many common hereditary disorders, such as the *HFE* genes for haemochromatosis, presymptomatic DNA tests are available for the hereditary neurological disorders, such as Huntington disease, and predictive DNA testing is available for some forms of hereditary cancer, such as breast and colon cancer, and in the future for cardiovascular disease and diabetes.[4] Also in the future, pharmacogenetics, which predicts genetically determined responses to pharmaceuticals, will greatly assist rational prescribing, and gene therapy is a futuristic treatment modality.[5]

An important recent development in gene expression has been advances in DNA technology, with the detection of fetal DNA in maternal plasma, thus allowing an excellent screening test for Down syndrome.[6]

Epigenetics

Epigenetics, meaning 'on top of' traditional genetic inheritance, is a study of changes in genetic expression or cellular phenotype caused by mechanisms other than changes in the DNA sequence. These factors, which include environment, lifestyle, nutrition and psychosocial influences, can influence the outcomes of chronic illness such as cancer, diabetes, autoimmune disorders and ageing. The incurred changes are heritable. This is an expanding development.

A summary of the prevalence of genetic disease is presented in TABLE 18.1.

Table 18.1 Prevalence of genetic disease (after Kingston)[7]

Type of genetic disease	Estimated prevalence per 1000 population
Single gene	2–10
Autosomal dominant	2
Autosomal recessive	1–2
X-linked recessive	
Chromosomal abnormalities	6–7
Common disorders with appreciable genetic component	7–10
Congenital malformations	20
Total	38–51

18

Key facts and checkpoints

- All people carry a small number of recessive genes, which are carried asymptomatically.
- The background risk that any couple will bear a child with a birth defect is about 4%. This risk is doubled for a first-cousin (consanguineous) couple.[8]
- Although the majority of cancers are not inherited, some people carry inherited genetic mutations for certain cancers, notably breast and ovarian (linked), colorectal and others on a lesser scale, such as prostate cancer and melanoma.
- GPs should look out for a family history of cancer, including the number of people with cancer on both sides of the family, the type of cancer and the age and onset of primary cancers.
- A GP caring for 1000 patients would expect to have 15–17 patients with a hereditary cancer predisposition.
- As genetic testing becomes more accessible it is prudent to be aware of the psychological consequences to patients of predictive or presymptomatic testing. Specialised genetic counselling is advisable.
- Carrier screening is now widely used for thalassaemia, Tay–Sachs disorder and cystic fibrosis.
- Prenatal screening and testing for genetic disorders is also a reality, especially for Down syndrome, fetal abnormalities and the haemoglobinopathies. Once again, careful selection, screening and counselling is important.
- Genetic services and familial cancer clinics provide an excellent service for referral, especially for genetic counselling expertise and advice about appropriate services and genetic testing.
- Pharmacogenetics and gene therapy are the future hope for targeted treatments based on a person's genetic profile.

The spectrum of genetic disorders

The list of inherited disorders continues to grow as evidence supports intuition that certain conditions are hereditary. It is important for the family doctor to be aware of this potential. We are familiar with the more common classic disorders, such as cystic fibrosis, thalassaemia, Down syndrome and haemochromatosis, but it is incumbent on us to be conversant with the genetic basis of diseases such as cancer, particularly breast, ovarian and bowel cancer, in addition to the childhood chromosomal/microdeletion syndromes, various inborn errors of metabolism and the ever-emerging rare mutations, such as the mitochondrial disorders.

The genogram

The genogram is a valuable pedigree chart that usually covers at least three generations of a family tree. It is a simple and disciplined means of gathering data about an individual couple or family to determine inheritance patterns. The data have to be gathered with tact and care. A useful strategy is to encourage patients to develop their own family genogram using charts as templates (resource: Centre for Genetic Education, NSW Health, www.genetics.edu.au).

An example including the use of symbols is shown in FIGURE 18.1.

Specific important genetic disorders

Haemochromatosis

Hereditary haemochromatosis (HHC), which is a disorder of iron overload, is the most common serious single gene genetic disorder in our population.

It is a common condition in which the total body iron concentration is increased to 20–60 g (normal 4 g). The excess iron is deposited in and can damage several organs:

- liver—cirrhosis (10% develop cancer)
- pancreas—'bronze' diabetes
- skin—bronze or leaden grey colour
- heart—restrictive cardiomyopathy
- pituitary—hypogonadism, impotence
- joints—arthralgia (especially hands), chondrocalcinosis

It is usually hereditary (autosomal recessive = AR) or may be secondary to chronic haemolysis and multiple transfusions.

Note: Hereditary haemochromatosis is the genetic condition; haemosiderosis is the secondary condition.

Genetic profile[8]

Being an autosomal recessive disorder, the patient must inherit two altered (mutated) copies of the gene (see FIG. 18.2 for a thalassaemia example). It is a problem mainly affecting Caucasians, usually from middle age onwards. About 1 in 10 people are silent carriers of one mutated gene, while 1 in 200 are homozygous and are at risk of developing haemochromatosis. These people can have it to a variable extent (the penetrance

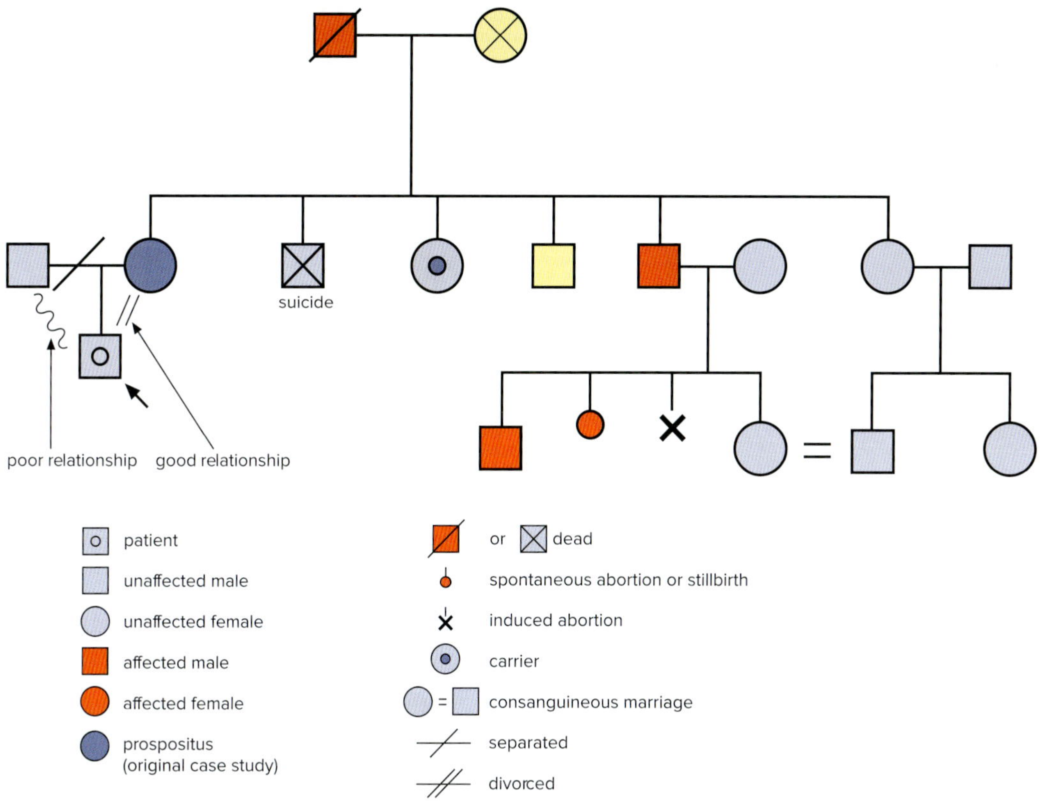

FIGURE 18.1 Genogram: illustration of a family tree for an inherited disorder

factor), and some are asymptomatic while others have a serious problem. It is rare for symptoms to manifest before the third decade.[9]

The two common identified specific mutations in the *HFE* gene are C282Y and H63D (another is S65C):

- homozygous C282Y—high risk for HHC
- homozygous H63D—unlikely to develop clinical HHC
- heterozygous C282Y and H63D—milder form of HHC

The key diagnostic sensitive markers are serum transferrin saturation and the serum ferritin level. The serum iron level is not a good indicator. An elevated ferritin level is not diagnostic of HHC but is the best serum marker of iron overload.

Clinical features

Most patients are asymptomatic but may have extreme lethargy, abdominal discomfort, signs of chronic liver disease, polyuria and polydipsia, arthralgia, erectile dysfunction, loss of libido and joint signs.

Signs: look for hepatomegaly, very tanned skin, cardiac arrhythmias, joint swelling, testicular atrophy.

Diagnosis

- Increased serum transferrin saturation >45%
- Increased serum ferritin level (see CHAPTER 22)
- CT, MRI or FerriScan—increased iron deposition in liver
- Liver biopsy (if liver function test enzymes are abnormal or ferritin >1000 mcg/L or hepatomegaly)—FerriScan now preferred
- Genetic studies: *HFE* gene—a C282Y and/or H63D mutation
- Screen first-degree relatives (serum ferritin levels and serum transferrin saturation in older relatives and genetic testing in younger ones). No need to screen before adulthood.

Note: Full blood count (FBE) and erythrocyte sedimentation rate are normal.

Management

- Refer for specialist care
- Weekly venesection 500 mL (250 mg iron) until serum iron stores are normal (may take at least 2 years), then every 3–4 months to keep serum ferritin level <100 mcg/L (usually 40–80 mcg/L),

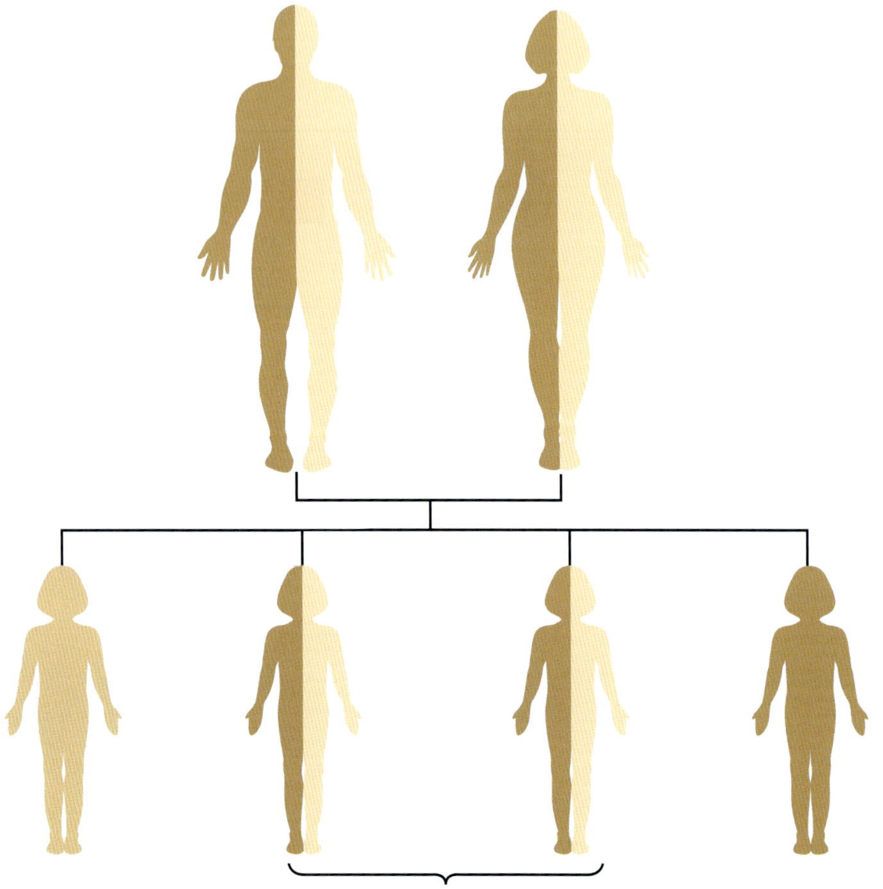

FIGURE 18.2 Typical genogram of inheritance of an autosomal recessive disorder: thalassaemia

serum transferrin saturation <50%, and iron levels normal

- Desferrioxamine can be used but not as effective as venesection
- Normal, healthy low-iron diet
- Avoid or limit alcohol
- Avoid iron tablets and vitamin C
- Life expectancy is normal if treated before cirrhosis or diabetes develops

Thalassaemia

The thalassaemias, the most common human single-gene disorders in the world, are a group of hereditary disorders characterised by a defect in the synthesis of one or more of the globin chains (α or β)—there are two of each (α2, β2). This causes defective haemoglobin synthesis leading to hypochromic microcytic anaemia. α-thalassaemia is usually seen in people of Asian origin while β-thalassaemia is seen in certain ethnic groups from the Mediterranean, the Middle East, South-East Asia and the Indian subcontinent. However, in our multicultural communities one cannot assume a person's origins. It is recommended that all women of child-bearing age be screened for thalassaemia. The thalassaemias are described as 'trait' when there are laboratory features without clinical expression.

Genetic profile[8]

α-thalassaemia is usually due to the deletion of one or more of the four genes for α-globin, the severity depending on the number of genes deleted: deletion of all four genes—α-thalassaemia (hydrops fetalis); of three genes—haemoglobin H disease, which results in lifelong anaemia of mild-to-moderate degree; of one or two genes—a symptomless carrier.

In β-thalassaemia, the β-chains are produced in decreased quantity rather than having large deletions. People who have two mutations (one in each β-globin gene) have β-thalassaemia major.

- β-thalassaemia minor—a single mutation (heterozygous)—the carrier or trait state
- β-thalassaemia major—two mutations (homozygous)—the person who has the disorder

Inheritance is illustrated in FIGURE 18.2. If both parents are carriers, there is a 1 in 4 chance that their child will have the disorder.

Clinical features

Carriers are clinically asymptomatic and do not need treatment apart from counselling. Patients with thalassaemia major present with symptoms of severe anaemia (haemolytic anaemia). Without treatment, children with thalassaemia major are lethargic and inactive, show a failure to thrive or to grow normally, and delayed puberty, hepatosplenomegaly and jaundice. Signs usually appear after 6 months and death from cardiac failure used to be common but with regular blood transfusions and iron-chelating treatment people can now live in good health.

DxT pallor + jaundice + hepatosplenomegaly → thalassaemia major

Diagnosis[9]

- FBE: in most carriers the mean corpuscular haemoglobin/mean corpuscular volume is low but can be normal. There is usually mild hypochromic microcytic anaemia but this is severe with the homozygous type.
- Haemoglobin electrophoresis: measures relative amounts of normal adult haemoglobin (HbA) and other variants (e.g. HbA_2, HbF). This will detect most carriers.
- Serum ferritin level: helps distinguish from iron deficiency, which has a similar blood film.
- DNA analysis: for mutation detection (mainly used to detect or confirm carriers).

Treatment for thalassaemia major

Treatment is based on a regular blood transfusion schedule for anaemia. Avoid iron supplements. Folate supplementation and a low-iron diet are advisable. Excess iron is removed by iron chelation (e.g. desferrioxamine). Allogenic bone marrow transplantation has been used with success.[10] Splenectomy may be appropriate.

Cystic fibrosis[9]

Cystic fibrosis is the result of a defect in an ion channel protein, the cystic fibrosis transmembrane receptor, which is found in the membranes of cells lining the exocrine ducts. The defect affects the normal transport of chloride ions, leading to a decreased sodium and water transfer, thus causing viscid secretions that affect the lungs, pancreas and gut.

18

Genetic profile[7,11]

- The most common AR paediatric illness
- About 1 in 2500 Caucasians affected
- About 1 in 20–25 are carriers
- A mutation (δ-F508) of chromosome 7 is the most common of some 500 possible mutations of the gene. This deletes a single phenylalanine residue from a 1480-aminoacid chain.

Clinical features

- General: malaise, failure to thrive, exercise intolerance
- Chronic respiratory problems: cough, recurrent pneumonia, bronchiectasis, sinus tenderness, nasal polyps
- Gastrointestinal: malabsorption, pale loose bulky stools, jaundice (pancreatic effect), meconium ileus (10% of newborn babies)
- Infertility in males (atrophy of vas deferens)
- Pancreatic insufficiency
- Early mortality but improving survival rates (mean age now 31 years)

DxT failure to thrive + chronic cough + loose bowel actions → cystic fibrosis

Diagnosis

- Screening for immunoreactive trypsin/trypsinogen in newborns detects 75%
- Sweat test for elevated chloride and sodium levels
- DNA testing for carriers identifies only the most common mutations (70–75%)

Treatment

- Early diagnosis and multidisciplinary team care are important
- Physiotherapy for drainage of airway secretions
- Hypertonic saline solution (by nebuliser) preceded by a bronchodilator

- Treatment of infections: therapeutic and prophylactic antibiotics
- Oral pancreatic enzyme replacement
- Dietary manipulation
- Lung and liver transplantation are considerations

There is currently no cure for cystic fibrosis; treatment is based on correcting the nutritional deficiencies and minimising chest infections.

Neurofibromatosis

- NF1—peripheral neurofibromatosis (von Recklinghausen disorder)
- NF2—central type, bilateral acoustic neuromas (schwannomas) (rare)

The gene for NF1 is carried on chromosome 17 and NF2 on chromosome 22. Diagnostic genetic testing is not routinely available. Diagnosis is by clinical examination.

DxT light-brown skin patches + skin tumours + axillary freckles ➜ NF1

Clinical features of NF1[8]

- Six or more café-au-lait spots (increasing with age)
- Freckling in the axillary or inguinal regions
- Flesh-coloured cutaneous tumours (appear at puberty)
- Hypertension
- Eye features (iris hamartomas)
- Learning difficulty
- Musculoskeletal problems (e.g. scoliosis, fibrous dysplasia, pseudoarthrosis)
- Optic nerve gliomas

General rule

- One-third asymptomatic, only have skin stigmata
- One-third minor problems, mainly cosmetic
- One-third significant problems (e.g. neurological tumours)

Management

- No special treatment available
- Surgical excisions of neurofibromas as appropriate
- Refer to a special clinic, including neurofibroma clinic
- Careful surveillance—report new symptoms
- Yearly examination for children and adults, including blood pressure, neurological, skeletal and ophthalmological examination

Duchenne muscular dystrophy (DMD)

DMD is a progressive proximal muscle weakness disorder with replacement of muscle by connective tissue. Becker muscular dystrophy is a less severe variant. Early diagnosis is important. First signs are delayed motor development, speech and language.

Genetic profile

DMD is an X-linked recessive condition. It is caused by a mutation in the gene coding for dystrophin, a protein found inside the muscle cell membrane.

Clinical features[8]

- Usually diagnosed from 2–5 years
- Weakness in hip and shoulder girdles
- Walking problems: delayed onset or starting in boys aged 3–7
- Waddling gait, falls, difficulty standing and climbing steps
- Pseudohypertrophy of muscles, especially calves
- Most in wheelchair by age 10–12
- ± Intellectual retardation/learning difficulties
- Most die of respiratory problems by age 25
- Gowers sign: patient uses 'trick' method by using hands to climb up his or her legs when rising to an erect position from the floor

DxT male child + gait disorder + bulky calves ➜ DMD

Diagnosis (initiate at first suspicion)

- Elevated serum creatinine kinase level
- Electromyography
- Direct dystrophin gene testing
- Muscle biopsy

Treatment

- Counselling, especially genetic counselling, education, screening (especially mother)
- No specific treatment available; support; corticosteroids delay progression

Spinal muscular atrophy (SMA)

Claimed to be the leading genetic cause of infant death, SMA includes several types, all manifesting as progressive muscle wasting and leading to early death in the more severe types.

Genetic profile

SMA is autosomal recessive and due to mutation in SMN1 gene on chromosome. Prevalence 1 in 6000-10000; carriers 1 in 40.

Clinical features

- muscle weakness, poor tone and floppiness
- feeding difficulties and feeble cry in babies
- weak swallowing, coughing and breathing
- normal intelligence and sensory modalities

Diagnosis is by DNA screening at birth and EEG studies. There is no cure at present and treatment is supportive. Intrathecal injections of nusinersen are available.

Dystrophia myotonica

Genetic profile: AD disorder.

Clinical features

- Typically presents 20–30 years as myotonia (tonic muscle spasm)
- Muscle weakness, esp. hands, legs, face, neck
- Slow relaxation of hand grip
- 'Hatchet face'—long haggard look with atrophy of facial muscles
- Frontal baldness in men
- Cataracts
- Mental impairment
- Cardiac disturbances, e.g. cardiomyopathy
- Endocrine abnormalities, e.g. diabetes

Investigation: electromyography.

Familial periodic paralysis

See CHAPTER 33.

Inherited adult onset neurological disorders[11,12]

These disorders have the following common features.

- They are serious and usually eventually fatal.
- Onset is in adulthood.
- They are currently incurable.
- They affect successive generations.
- Most are inherited from a parent in an autosomal dominant fashion.
- Specific genetic testing is usually available.

Examples of inherited adult onset neurological conditions are:

- Huntington disease
- Creutzfeldt–Jakob disease and other prion diseases
- familial Alzheimer disease
- familial epilepsy
- familial motor neurone disease
- Friedreich ataxia
- hereditary peripheral neuropathies (Charcot–Marie–Tooth disease)
- mitochondrial disorders
- hereditary spastic paraparesis
- muscular dystrophies
- myotonic dystrophy
- spinal muscular atrophy
- spinocerebellar ataxias

A minority of these conditions are due primarily to a dominantly inherited genetic alteration (mutation), e.g. Huntington disease, and are usually more accessible to genetic testing. Some gene alterations (polymorphism) may be associated with a higher risk of developing certain neurological conditions. Testing for polymorphisms is more complex. If concerned about a hereditary basis, GPs should refer their patients with these disorders to a neurologist or a neurogenetics clinic.

18

Huntington disease[9]

Genetic profile

- Inherited as an AD disorder.
- The responsible mutant gene has been located on the short arm of chromosome 4.
- One genetic mutation accounts for the vast majority of cases, which means that there is an accurate diagnostic test.
- Both sexes are equally affected.

DxT chorea + abnormal behaviour + dementia + family history → Huntington disease

Clinical features

- Insidious onset and progression of chorea
- Onset most often between 35 and 55 years
- Mental changes—change in behaviour (can be as early as childhood or in very late life), intellectual deterioration leading to dementia
- Family history present in the majority
- Motor symptoms: flicking movements of arms, lilting gait, facial grimacing, ataxia, dystonia
- Usually a fatal outcome 15–20 years from onset

Treatment

- There is no cure or specific treatment
- Supportive treatment with agents such as haloperidol

Genetic testing and counselling

This is available, sensitive and important because offspring have a 1 in 2 risk and the onset may be late—after childbearing years. It is appropriate to refer to expert centres for those seeking it. Of interest is that only 20% have undergone testing since it became available, indicating that those at risk generally prefer the uncertainty of not knowing the reality.

Familial Alzheimer disease (FAD)

Early onset familial Alzheimer disease (EoFAD), which accounts for less than 1% of all Alzheimer disease, is defined as the presence of two or more affected people with onset age <65 years in more than one generation of a family, with postmortem pathologically proven Alzheimer disease in at least one person. Mutations in any one of three different forms (alleles) of the susceptible *APOE* gene are known to cause FAD.[9,13]

Parkinson disease

Most cases are sporadic, and the majority of cases with a family history do not have a clear inheritance pattern and could be the result of several factors including a genetic predisposition or simply a chance aggregation. Consider referral to a neurogenetics clinic for families with unusual features, such as familial aggregation and/or early onset Parkinson disease.

Motor neurone disease (MND) (amyotrophic lateral sclerosis)

Five to 10% of motor neurone disease is inherited, with an autosomal dominant inheritance pattern. Inherited MND shows familial aggregation and an earlier age of onset than average (40s or younger); otherwise clinical features are essentially the same as the sporadic form (see CHAPTER 33). If more than one family member presents with MND consider referral to a neurogenetic clinic.

Mitochondrial disorders

Mitochondrial disease is usually caused by mutations of the genes or DNA. Since mitochondria are the 'power plants of the cells', disorders cannot convert food into energy so high energy tissues such as muscle and the brain are particularly at risk. The variety of disorders include neuromuscular diseases (referred to as mitochondrial myopathies), Leber's hereditary optic neuropathy, varieties of Parkinson disease, myoclonic epilepsy, chronic progressive external ophthalmoplegia, and the deadly MELAS syndrome (myopathy, encephalopathy, lactic acidosis and stroke-like episodes). Suspected cases should be referred for diagnosis which includes muscle testing. Treatment is supportive.

The epilepsies

The epilepsies comprise a group of disorders with differing genetic components and the inheritance or genetic contribution relates to each specific disorder. Further studies on this subject are in progress. If there are two or more individuals in a family with epilepsy, referral for advice about the nature and inheritance about their form of epilepsy may be appropriate.

Psychiatric conditions

Serious psychotic and mood disorders can run in families, especially schizophrenia and bipolar disorder, which have a clear genetic component that appears to be complex and poorly understood (see TABLE 18.2). To date no genes causing schizophrenia have been identified, but large regions on some chromosomes have been associated with schizophrenia. Individuals with a first-degree relative with bipolar disorder or purely depressive (unipolar) disorder have an increased risk of a mood disorder, but the genetics are not understood. Tourette syndrome is another psychological disorder that has a hereditary basis through an autosomal dominant gene with variable expression (penetrance).

TABLE 18.2 Genetic risks (approximate) in schizophrenia and bipolar disorder

Affected relative	Schizophrenia (% risk)	Bipolar (% risk)
Nil (general population)	1	2–3
Parent	13	15
Both parents	45	50
Sibling	9	13
Monozygotic twin	40	70
Dizygotic twin	10	20

Source: Harper P. *Practical Genetic Counselling.* Oxford: Butterworth Heinemann, 1988

HEREDITARY HAEMOGLOBINOPATHIES, HAEMOLYTIC DISORDERS, AND BLEEDING AND CLOTTING DISORDERS[9,14]

The commonest haemoglobinopathies are the thalassaemias (see earlier in this chapter), which are caused by a deficiency in the quality of globin chains, whereas other haemoglobinopathies are caused by structural variations in the globin chain. These conditions include HbS (sickle cell), HbC, HbD, HbE, HbO and HbLepore.

Other inherited conditions that can cause haemolytic anaemia are those with a red cell membrane defect and include hereditary spherocytosis, hereditary elliptocytosis and hereditary stomatocytosis.

Sickle cell disorders

The most important abnormality in the haemoglobin (Hb) chain is sickle cell haemoglobin (HbS), which results from a single base mutation of adenine to thymine leading to a substitution of valine for glutamine at position 6 on the β-globin chain. The defective Hb causes the red cells to become deformed in shape—'sickled'. The sickled cells tend to flow poorly and clog the microcirculation, resulting in hypoxia, which compounds the sickling. Such attacks, which result in tissue infarction, are called 'crises'. Sickling is precipitated by infection, hypoxia, dehydration, cold and acidosis, and may complicate operations. The autosomal recessive disorder occurs mainly in Africans (25% carry the gene), but it is also found in India, South-East Asia, the Middle East and southern Europe.

- Heterozygous state for HbS = sickle cell trait
- Homozygous state = sickle cell anaemia/disease

Sickle cell anaemia

This varies from being mild or asymptomatic to a severe haemolytic anaemia and recurrent painful crises. It may present in children with anaemia and mild jaundice. Children may develop digits of varying lengths from the hand-and-foot syndrome due to infarcts of small bones.

Features of infarctive sickle crises include:

- bone pain (usually limb bones)
- abdominal pain
- chest—pleuritic pain
- kidney—haematuria
- spleen—painful infarcts
- precipitated by cold, hypoxia, dehydration or infection

Hb electrophoresis is needed to confirm the diagnosis.

Long-term problems include chronic leg ulcers, susceptibility to infection, aseptic necrosis of bone (especially head of femur), blindness and chronic kidney disease. The prognosis is variable. Children in Africa often die within the first year of life. Infection is the commonest cause of death.

Sickle cell trait

People with this usually have no symptoms unless they are exposed to prolonged hypoxia, such as anaesthesia and flying in non-pressurised aircraft. The disorder is protective against malaria.

Hereditary spherocytosis

This is the commonest cause of inherited haemolytic anaemia in northern Europeans. It is an autosomal dominant disorder of variable severity, although in 25% of patients neither parent is affected, suggesting spontaneous mutation in some instances. Jaundice may present at birth or be delayed or occur not at all. Splenomegaly is a feature and splenectomy is considered to be the treatment of choice in severe cases. Maintenance of folic acid levels is important.

Bleeding disorders

In inherited bleeding deficiency disorders, there are deficiencies of vital factors (see CHAPTER 39). The common significant disorders are:

- haemophilia A (factor VIII deficiency)—X-linked recessive
- haemophilia B (factor IX deficiency)—X-linked recessive
- von Willebrand disease (deficiency of factor VIII:C + defective platelet factor)—autosomal dominant

Others to consider are:

- hereditary haemorrhagic telangiectasia (Osler–Weber–Rendu disease)
- inherited thrombocytopenia

Thrombophilia

This should be considered in patients with a past and/or family history of DVT or other thrombotic episodes (see CHAPTER 131). There are several causes, including important inherited factors, which are:

- factor V Leiden gene mutation (activated protein C resistance)
- prothrombin gene mutation
- protein C deficiency
- protein S deficiency
- antithrombin deficiency

It is important to be aware of these factors, especially in people with a past history of unexplained thrombotic episodes. Prescribing the oral contraceptive pill (OCP) is an issue but preliminary screening for thrombophilias is not recommended. In factor V Leiden, the most

18

common factor in this group, there is a 35-fold increased risk of thrombosis for those taking the OCP.

CHROMOSOMAL/MICRODELETION SYNDROMES (CHILDHOOD EXPRESSION)[9]

The following disorders, whose clinical features manifest in children, present with developmental and intellectual disability.

Down syndrome[15]

18

Down syndrome (trisomy 21) is based on typical facial features (flat facies, slanting eyes, prominent epicanthic folds, small ears), hypotonia, intellectual disability and a single palmar crease.

DxT typical facies + hypotonia + single palmar crease ➜ Down syndrome

Facts

- 95% have extra chromosome of maternal origin (trisomy 21)
- Remainder due to either unbalances, translocations or mosaicism
- Prenatal screening tests include early ultrasound (nuchal lucency) and maternal serum screening in first trimester (serum maternal and fetal DNA). Karyotyping of chorionic villus sampling on amniocytes for pregnancies at risk is available.
- Prevalence 1 in 650 live births

Associated disorders

- Seizures (usually later onset)
- Impaired hearing
- Leukaemia
- Hypothyroidism
- Congenital anomalies (e.g. heart, duodenal atresia, Hirschsprung, TOF)
- Alzheimer-like dementia (fourth–fifth decade)
- Atlantoaxial instability
- Coeliac disease
- Diabetes

Management

- Assess child's capabilities
- Refer to agencies for assessment (e.g. hearing, vision, developmental disability unit)
- Advise on sexuality, especially for females (i.e. menstrual management, contraception) as fertility must be presumed
- Genetic counselling for parents

Edward syndrome[9]

Trisomy 18

Clinical features

These include:

- incidence 1 in 2000 live births (approx.)
- microcephaly
- facial abnormalities, e.g. cleft lip/palate
- malformations of major organs
- malformations of hands and feet—clenched hand posture
- neural tube defect

Prognosis is poor—about one-third die in first month, <10% live beyond 12 months.

Prenatal diagnosis is available.

Patau syndrome[9]

Trisomy 13

Clinical features

These include:

- incidence 1 in 7000 (approx.)
- microcephaly
- brain and heart malformation
- cleft lip/palate
- polydactyly
- neural tube defect

Prognosis is poor—50% die within first month.

Fragile X syndrome (FXS)[15]

FXS presents as a classic physical phenotype with large prominent ears, long narrow face, macro-orchidism and intellectual disability. It is the most common inherited cause known of developmental disability and should always be considered. The cause is the result of an increase in the size of a trinucleotide repeat in the *FMR-1* gene on the X chromosome (the number of sequences determines carrier or full mutant status). Any individual with significant development delay should be tested for FXS.

DxT characteristic facies + intellectual disability + large testes ➜ FXS

Facts

- M:F ratio 2:1
- Prevalence of full mutation 1 in 4000
- Variable spectrum of characteristic features, making detection difficult in some cases

- 1 in 250 are pre-mutation carriers
- Family history of intellectual disability
- Affects all ethnic groups
- Females may appear normal but may be affected

Diagnosis

- Cytogenetic testing (karyotyping)
- DNA test (specific for full mutation as well as carriers)

Associated disorders[16]

- Intellectual disability (IQ <70)
- Autism or autistic-like behaviour
- Attention deficit in 10% (with or without hyperactivity)
- Seizures (20%)
- Connective tissue abnormalities
- Learning disability and speech delay
- Coordination difficulty
- Primary ovarian insufficiency
- Late onset tremor/ataxia syndrome

Management

- Careful genetic appraisal and counselling
- Assessment of child's capabilities
- Multidisciplinary assessment, including developmental disability unit
- Referral for integration of speech and language therapy, special education, behaviour management
- Pharmacological treatment of any epilepsy, or attention or mood behaviour disorders
- Medications may determine whether the child remains in the community or not

Prader–Willi syndrome

This uncommon disorder (1 in 10000–15000) has classic features, especially a bizarre appetite and eating habits, of which the GP should be aware. It is probable that there are many undiagnosed cases in the community. The most common cause is a deletion of the short arm of chromosome 15.

DxT neonatal hypotonia + failure to thrive + obesity (later) ➜ Prader–Willi syndrome

Clinical features

- Hypotonic infants with weak suction and failure to thrive, then voracious appetite causing morbid obesity
- Usually manifests at 3 years
- Intellectual disability
- Narrow forehead and turned-down mouth
- Small hands and feet
- Hypogonadism

Management

- Early diagnosis and referral
- Multidisciplinary approach
- Expert dietetic control

With proper care and support, longevity into the eighth decade is a reality.[14]

Williams syndrome

Williams syndrome (idiopathic hypercalcaemia or elfin face syndrome) is due to a microdeletion on chromosome 7, a deletion in the elastin gene.

Children have a distinctive elfin facial appearance, mild pre- and postnatal growth retardation, mild microcephaly and mild-to-moderate developmental delay. In the first 2 years of life, feeding problems, vomiting, irritability, hyperacusis, constipation and failure to thrive may lead to presentation, but children are rarely diagnosed at this stage.

DxT 'elfin' face + intellectual disability + aortic stenosis ➜ Williams syndrome

Marfan syndrome[9]

This is a systemic connective tissue disorder characterised by abnormalities of the skeletal, cardiovascular and ocular systems. It has variable expressions and is a potentially lethal disorder. If untreated, death in the 30s and 40s is common.

DxT tall stature + dislocated lens and myopia + aortic root dilatation ➜ Marfan syndrome

Genetic profile

- Mutations in the fibrillin gene on chromosome 15
- Autosomal dominant
- Prevalence about 5 per 100 000
- No specific laboratory test to date

Clinical features

- Disproportionally tall and thin
- Long digits—arachnodactyly
- Kyphoscoliosis
- Joint laxity (e.g. genu recurvatum)

- Myopia and ectopic ocular lens
- High arched palate
- Aortic dilatation and dissection
- Mitral valve prolapse

Management

- Needs surveillance of eyes, heart and thoracic aorta
- Echocardiography, possibly aortic root dilatation
- Long-term beta blockade therapy reduces rate of dilatation
- Consider prophylactic cardiovascular surgery
- Genetic counselling for the family

Tuberous sclerosis (epiloia)

This is an autosomal dominant disorder due to mutations in one of two genes located on chromosomes 9 and 16. A feature is tube-like growths that affect multiple systems including the brain.

> **DxT** facial rash + intellectual disability + seizures ➜ tuberous sclerosis

The above triad of features is classic but not applicable to all cases.

Noonan syndrome[15]

This is an AD disorder with mutation of chromosome 11. It has been described as a male Turner syndrome but affects both sexes.

> **DxT** facies + short stature + pulmonary stenosis ➜ Noonan syndrome

Clinical features[15]

- Characteristic facies—down-slanting palpebral fissures, widespread eyes, low-set ears ± ptosis
- Short stature
- Pulmonary valve stenosis
- Webbed neck
- Failure to thrive, usually mild
- Abnormalities of cardiac conduction and rhythm
- ± Intellectual disability

Treatment

- Refer to genetic service
- Evaluation of cardiac status
- Consider vision, hearing, clotting status, possible epilepsy

Angelman syndrome

Genetic profile

- Abnormal chromosome 15

Clinical features (a wide spectrum)

- Hand flapping
- 'Puppet'-like ataxia
- Frequent laughter/smiling
- Microcephaly by age 2 years
- Developmental delay
- Speech impairment
- Seizures
- Cannot live independently

Diagnosis based on clinical features and genetic studies.

Treatment with minocycline is promising.

Progeria

Sporadic mutation of LMA gene that codes for a protein leads to early cell death.

Accelerated ageing—manifests in early childhood causing premature death (median age 12 years) from vascular disease. No known treatment.

SEX CHROMOSOME ABNORMALITIES

Klinefelter syndrome[9]

This is due to an extra X chromosome, resulting in a male phenotype and occurring in 1 in 800 live births. Approximately 2 out of 3 are never recognised.

> **DxT** lanky men + small testes + infertility ➜ Klinefelter syndrome

Genetic profile

- XXY genotype
- The extra X chromosome is usually of maternal origin
- About 30 or more variants of the disorder

Clinical features

Marked variation but usually:

- tall men with long limbs
- small firm testes ≤2 cm (10 ml)
- infertility (azoospermia)

There may be:

- sparse facial hair
- reduced libido

- learning difficulties, especially reading
- intellectual ability may range from normal to disability
- gynaecomastia
- increased risk of breast cancer and diabetes

Diagnosis

Increased gonadotrophin, low to normal testosterone

Treatment

- Transdermal testosterone

Turner syndrome (gonadal dysgenesis)

This is due to only one X chromosome, occurring in 1 in 4000 live female newborns; 99% of conceptions are miscarried.[15]

DxT short stature + webbed neck + facies ➜ Turner syndrome

Genetic profile

- 45 chromosomes of XO karyotype (typical Turner's karyotype in 50% of cases)
- Many are mosaics (e.g. 45X/46XX chromosomes)
- Phenotypes vary

Clinical features of typical XO karyotype

- Short stature—average adult height 143 cm
- Primary amenorrhoea in XO patient; infertility
- Webbing of neck
- Typical facies: micrognathia, low hairline
- Lymphoedema of extremities
- Cardiac defects (e.g. coarctation of aorta)

Mental deficiency is rare.

Treatment

- Hormone-based (e.g. growth hormone, hormone replacement therapy)

Intersex states

These are uncommon chromosomal disorders of sexual development (DSD) in which the appearance of the external genitalia is either ambiguous or at variance with the individual's chromosomal sex. The inappropriate term 'hermaphrodite' should be avoided.

The conditions include:

- mixed gonadal dysgenesis
- ovotesticular disorder DSD
- 46, XX DSD (androgenised females)
- 46, XY DSD (underandrogenised males)

The latter may be caused by inadequate production of androgen or inadequate response to androgen, which includes the 'androgen insensitivity syndrome'. This syndrome, made prominent through athletes with a male genotype but female phenotype, results from a mutation of the gene encoding the androgen receptor.

Congenital adrenal hyperplasia

See CHAPTER 23.

18

FETAL ALCOHOL SYNDROME (FAS)[18]

FAS is the most severe form of the fetal alcohol spectrum disorders. These are caused by the tetrogenic effects of alcohol (not a chromosomal abnormality) and is estimated to involve 2 in 1000 live births. The phenotype varies with the dosage and gestational timing of the alcohol exposure.[16] Caution is needed not to overdiagnose.

DxT abnormal facies + growth retardation + microcephaly ➜ fetal alcohol syndrome

Clinical features of FAS

See FIGURE 18.3.

- Markedly underweight until puberty
- Learning difficulties
- Microcephaly

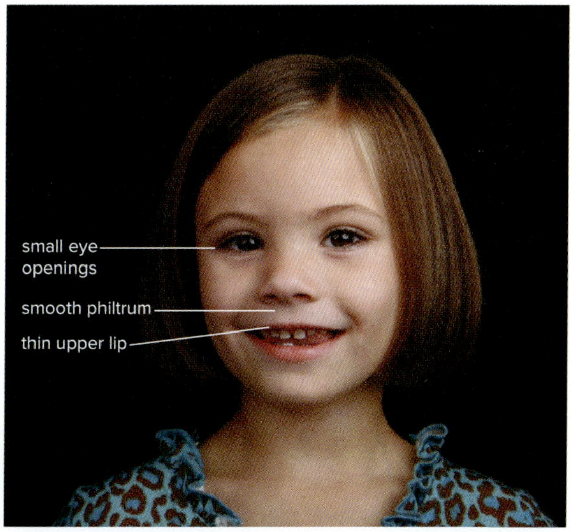

FIGURE 18.3 Fetal alcohol syndrome: facial features
Source: Shutterstock.com

- Characteristic facies (needs 2 of *)
  - shortened palpebral fissures*
  - long, smooth featureless philtrum*
  - thin upper lip*
  - upturned nose
- Hyperactivity
- Congenital heart disease often seen
- Skeletal abnormalities

Diagnosis based on alcohol history in pregnancy.

Management

- By preventive strategies with community education about the harmful effects of drinking, especially in early pregnancy

OTHER TYPES OF HEREDITARY DISORDERS

The many examples include familial hypercholesterolaemia (AD) and the AR disorders for which genetic testing is available, namely Gaucher disease, Tay-Sachs disease, glycogen storage disease, phenylketonuria, galactosaemia, homocystinuria, the porphyrias, glucose-6-phosphate dehydrogenase (G-6-PD) deficiency and the mitochondrial disorders.

Glucose-6-phosphate dehydrogenase deficiency

G-6-PD deficiency is a common disorder affecting over 400 million people worldwide. It is the most common red-cell enzyme defect that causes episodic haemolytic anaemia because of the decreased ability of red blood cells to cope with oxidative stresses. It is an X-linked recessive inherited disorder with a high prevalence among people of African, Mediterranean or Asian ancestry. In some countries such as Malaysia there is a national screening program. Consider the disorder in male black people (see CHAPTER 135).

The important clinical features are:

- asymptomatic in many
- neonatal jaundice—infants at risk should be observed after delivery (at least 5 days)
- episodic acute haemolytic anaemia—triggered by antioxidants and infections, and drugs, especially antimalarials, sulphonamides, nitrofurantoin, quinolones, traditional medicines, vitamins C and K, high dose aspirin, fava (broad) beans and naphthalene (e.g. moth balls)

There is no specific treatment. Known precipitants should be avoided. Avoid penicillin and probenecid.

Diagnosis is by G-6-PD assay and a blood film during an attack.

Hereditary haemorrhagic telangectasia

This is an autosomal dominant disorder of the development of vasculature. A strong family history aids diagnosis.

Key features:

- mucocutaneous telangiectasia (Osler–Weber–Rendu syndrome)
- recurrent epistaxis in children and adolescents
- visceral arteriovenous malformations, e.g. GIT, lips
- diagnosis is clinical, aided by imaging to detect AVMs

Gaucher disease

Gaucher disease, which is due to a deficiency of the lysosomal enzyme glucocerebrosidase, leads to anaemia and thrombocytopenia as a result primarily of hypersplenism. There is chronic bone pain and 'crises' of bone pain. Consider it in children with fatigue, bone pain, delayed growth, epistaxis, easy bruising and hepatosplenomegaly. Replacement enzyme therapy is available.

Galactosaemia[9]

Galactosaemia is an inborn error of metabolism in which the body is unable to metabolise galactose to glucose. There are three clinical syndromes caused by differing enzyme deficiencies, one of which is galactose-1-phosphate uridyl transferase, which causes the classic syndrome. It is an autosomal recessive disorder with an incidence of about 1 in 60 000 births. As lactose is the major source of galactose, the infant becomes anorexic and jaundiced within a few days or weeks of taking breast milk or lactose-containing formula. It can be rapidly fatal. Management is with a galactose (mainly lactose)-free formula such as soy with added calcium and vitamins.

Phenylketonuria (PKU)[9]

This autosomal recessive disorder of the catabolism of the amino acid, phenylalanine, is caused by a deficiency of phenylalanine hydroxylase activity, leading to an elevation of plasma phenylalanine, which if untreated can cause intellectual disability (often very severe) and other neurological symptoms, such as seizures. Neonatal screening for high blood phenylalanine levels (the Guthrie test) is performed routinely.

Treatment aims to limit phenylalanine intake so that essential amino acid needs are met but not exceeded. Diet therapy must commence as soon as possible. Females who have been treated for PKU need pre-pregnancy counselling and dietary management during pregnancy to prevent damage to the fetus by high phenylalanine levels.

The porphyrias

The three most common porphyrias are acute intermittent porphyria, porphyria cutanea tarda (the commonest) and erythropoietic protoporphyria, which are caused by deficiencies of the third, fifth and eighth enzymes, respectively, of the haem biosynthesis pathway. Their clinical features are quite different.

Acute intermittent porphyria

This autosomal dominant disorder is the most serious of the porphyrias although it remains clinically silent in the majority of patients who carry the trait. It is due to a deficiency of porphobilinogen (PBG) deaminase.

Clinical features

- Recurrent unexplained abdominal pain crises
- Usually young women (teens or 20s)
- Recurrent psychiatric illnesses, abnormal behaviour
- Acute peripheral or nervous system dysfunction (e.g. peripheral neuropathy, hypotonia)
- PBG in urine during attack
- Hyponatraemia
- Attacks precipitated by various drugs (e.g. anti-epileptics, alcohol, sulphonamides, barbiturates)

DxT severe abdominal pain + abnormal illness behaviour + 'red' urine ➜ acute intermittent porphyria

Diagnosis

- Urine PBGs (high) and serum sodium (very low) during 'attack'
- Erythrocyte PBG deaminase testing to screen relatives

Treatment

- Eliminate triggers and avoid 'unsafe' drugs
- High-carbohydrate diet, glucose oral or IV for attacks
- IV haemetin (haemarginate)

Glycogen storage disease (liver glycogenoses)

This is a group of inherited disorders caused by a deficiency of one or more enzymes involved in glycogen breakdown, leading to the deposition of abnormal amounts of glycogen in tissues, especially the liver. The best-known type is 1A (von Gierke disorder), an autosomal recessive disorder due to deficiency of glucose-6-phosphatase (G-6-P). It is seen in several ethnic groups. It typically causes growth retardation, hepatomegaly, renomegaly, hypoglycaemia (can be severe), lactic acidosis and hyperlipidaemia. Children have characteristic morphological features—short, doll-like facies with fat cheeks, thin extremities and large abdomen (hepatomegaly).

Diagnosis is by abnormal plasma lactate and lipid levels, liver biopsy and recently by gene analysis for the G-6-P gene.

Treatment is aimed to prevent hypoglycaemia and lactic acidosis via frequent carbohydrate feedings, such as uncooked cornstarch and overnight nasogastric glucose infusion. The prognosis is poor.

Tay–Sachs disease

About 1 in 25 Ashkenazi Jews is a carrier of Tay–Sachs disease (gangliosidosis), an AR disorder caused by a total deficiency of hexosaminidase A resulting in an accumulation of gangliosides in the brain.

The infantile form is fatal by age 3 or 4 with early progressive loss of motor skills, dementia, blindness, macrocephaly and cherry-red retinal spots. The juvenile onset form presents with dementia and ataxia, with death at age 10–15. The adult form has progression of neurological symptoms following clumsiness in childhood and motor weakness in adolescence. Carrier testing is available and prenatal diagnosis is available.

SINGLE GENE CARDIAC DISORDERS

Includes:

- cardiomyopathies
- arrhythmia syndromes, e.g. long QT syndrome
- sudden cardiac death families

Congenital long QT syndrome

This is an autosomal dominant condition with predisposition to ventricular arrhythmias, syncopal/fainting spells and sudden death, particularly during exercise. Confirm or exclude by ECG when suspected—interval 0.5–0.7 seconds. Management includes sports restrictions, beta blockers and pacemaker or AICD.

18

Hypertrophic cardiomyopathy

This is an AD disorder with several genetic mutations. It is the most common cause of sudden cardiac death among athletes.

Clinical features

- Fatigue
- Exertional dyspnoea and chest pain
- Palpitations
- Dizziness/syncope

Diagnosis by ECG (LV hypertrophy) and doppler echocardiography.

Insertion of AICD may prevent sudden death.

Familial hyperlipoproteinaemia[19]

There are several types of genetic disorder of lipid metabolism including the better-known familial hypercholesterolaemia and familial combined hyperlipidaemia. The former is identified by elevated cholesterol, corneal arcus juvenalis, tendon xanthomas in the patient or their first- and second-degree relatives and also by a DNA mutation. Homozygous patients present with atherosclerotis disease in childhood and early death from myocardial infarction. Heterozygotes may develop the disorder in their 30s or 40s.

This is common, being 1 in 500 Caucasians, 1 in 70 in Lebanese and Afrikaners. Eighty per cent are undiagnosed and missing out on preventive treatments. GPs have an important role in screening people with premature ischaemic heart disease to look for phenotype characteristics of the condition.

Familial cancer[20]

The majority of cancer is not inherited; rather it is acquired because of genetic mutations in several genes of a cell in a specific tissue during an individual's lifetime. Twenty to twenty-five individuals in a population of 1000 have a family history of bowel or breast cancer.[9]

However, some people carry inherited genetic mutations from conception that predispose them to developing certain cancers, particularly colorectal, breast and ovarian cancer, at a relatively young age. Up to 5% of some cancers are considered familial and the genetic basis of some of these is now understood. Most are AD with 50% of offspring being affected.

The three most significant familial cancer inherited susceptibility syndromes are:

- hereditary breast–ovarian cancer syndrome (*BRCA*$_1$ and *BRCA*$_2$ genes)
- hereditary non-polyposis colorectal cancer (HNPCC)
- familial adenomatous polyposis (FAP)

Features of breast–ovarian cancer syndrome[8,9]

- Mutations in either of the two genes—*BRCA*$_1$ and *BRCA*$_2$—result in a strong predisposition for both breast and ovarian cancer
- Mutations present in about 1 in 800 of the general population (male and female), who are carriers
- Dominant inheritance
- The risk of developing breast cancer is 10-fold and 40–80% of cases occur before the age of 70 years[17]
- The prognosis in these women is the same as for sporadic cases
- Early age of onset of breast cancer
- Male breast cancer (6% in males with *BRCA*$_2$ gene mutation)
- Coexistence of ovarian and breast cancer in the same family
- Carriers of mutations *may* be at an increased risk of prostate cancer, pancreatic cancer and colorectal cancer, although this is controversial for the latter two

Risk indicators for familial breast–ovarian cancer

- Two first-degree or second-degree relatives on one side of the family with cancer
- Individuals with age of onset of cancer <50 years
- Individuals with bilateral or multifocal breast cancer
- Individuals with ovarian cancer
- Breast cancer in a male relative
- Jewish ancestry

Colorectal cancer[20]

Both sexes have a risk of approximately 5% of developing bowel cancer in their lifetime. In some this risk is increased due to an inherited predisposition.

The two key disorders are HNPCC and FAP.

Lynch syndrome (hereditary non-polyposis colorectal cancer)

- Caused by a defect in one of the genes responsible for DNA mismatch repair
- Affects 1 in 1000 individuals
- Autosomal dominant
- Early age of onset
- Increased risk of certain extracolonic cancers, including endometrial, stomach, ovary and kidney tract cancers

- Screening should occur every 1–2 years from 25 years of age or 5 years earlier than affected family member developed it

Familial adenomatous polyposis

- Less common than HNPCC; affects about 1 in 10 000
- Caused by a mutation in the *APC* gene
- Usually hundreds or thousands of polyps
- Eventually almost 100% of cases develop colon cancer without prophylactic colectomy
- Median age of diagnosis 40 years
- Small increased risk of other cancers (e.g. thyroid, cerebral)
- Screening should occur annually from between 12–15 and 30–35 years of age, and then every 3 years

Individuals at risk

For Lynch syndrome (HNPCC):

- Three or more close relatives with bowel cancer
- Two or more close relatives with bowel cancer and:
  - more than one bowel cancer in same relative
  - onset of bowel cancer before 50 years
  - a relative with endometrial cancer or ovarian cancer

  (Refer: www.ncbi.nlm.nih.gov/pubmed/14970275.)

  For FAP:
- A relative with bowel cancer with polyposis
- Individuals with multiple polyposis

Other cancers where family history is significant

- Melanoma: an inherited mutation in certain genes (e.g. *BRAF* gene) is considered to be involved in up to 5% of melanomas.
- Prostate: family history is a risk factor; some genes are susceptible.
- Several other cancers can develop as a mutation, e.g. stomach, pancreas, kidney, thyroid, uterus (Cancer Council Australia, family cancer clinics helpline: 13 11 20).

The role of the GP in familial cancer[20]

The GP has an important role in identifying potential high-risk patients and families and in addressing their concerns.

- Take a family history and involve at least three generations.
- Map a family tree: include any diagnosed breast, ovarian or colorectal cancers in any relative and *any* type of cancer in first-degree or second-degree relatives on either side of the family.
- Record the age of onset and site of cancer in first-degree relatives.
- Confirm reports of cancer from medical records.
- Assess risk (high, low or intermediate) using guidelines from your country's national cancer guidelines, e.g. the NHMRC guidelines in Australia.
- Reassure low-risk patients but provide general preventive and screening guidelines.
- Refer all patients at potentially high risk to a familial cancer clinic.

  Services at these clinics involve:

- risk assessment
- genetic testing
- counselling, including pre- and post-testing
- surveillance advice

Management is based on early detection and potential prophylactic methods, for example:

- for breast cancer—regular imaging and clinical examination
- for ovarian cancer—transvaginal ultrasound and serum CA-125 detection
- for FAP and HNPCC—annual colonoscopy, faecal occult blood test

Patients at high risk will ask about prophylactic colectomy, mastectomy and oophorectomy, for which there are reasonable indications, but it is necessary to refer to a cancer geneticist for expert evaluation before such decisions are made.

Predictive genetic testing

The Human Genetics Society of Australia strongly advises against predictive or presymptomatic genetic testing of children for disease where there is no pre-emptive treatment in childhood. It should only be carried out in children if an effective treatment or preventive strategy is available. It raises issues of confidentiality, informed consent and harmful effects on self-esteem.[9]

Routine genetic testing is only advisable for high-risk individuals, such as those with a family history.

The ethical issues for adults are also considerable and for the individual the decision is difficult and requires considerable counselling via a clinical genetics service. This applies particularly to those at risk of Huntington disease and other adult-onset neurodegenerative conditions for which no preventive treatment exists.

Reproductive genetic screening[21]

The triple test is often used for sub-fertility screening. It tests for cystic fibrosis, fragile X syndrome and spinal muscular atrophy. A survey by the Murdoch Children's Research Institute identified one in 20 carriers in a study of prospective parents.

Newborn screening

With parental consent, blood from the infant's heel is usually screened for 25 conditions including cystic fibrosis, phenylketonuria (compare the Guthrie test), congenital hypothyroidism, galactosaemia and other rare disorders of metabolism. This test has the potential for global screening of disorders.

Prenatal screening and diagnosis of genetic disorders[22]

Approximately 2% of births are associated with congenital abnormalities, of which 1 in 7 are chromosomal, the most common of which is Down syndrome (trisomy 21). Antenatal screening tests that can now be performed for several conditions are mainly:

- screening tests for Down syndrome and other trisomies
- screening tests for thalassaemias/ haemoglobinopathies
- second-trimester ultrasound scans for fetal abnormalities, such as neural tube defects (NTD) and abdominal wall defects (AWD)

Screening for Down syndrome

This has a live birth incidence of 1.4 per 1000 in Australia.[19] The risk of conceiving a child with Down syndrome increases proportionally with age. For a woman aged 21, it is 1 in 1000, while for a woman aged 35, it is 1 in 275 and for a woman aged 45, it is 1 in 20.

The tests available to test for Down syndrome include the following:[5,23]

1. combined first-trimester screening tests (maternal serum screening/MSST; free fetal DNA at 10–12 weeks gestation; nuchal transparency ultrasound at 11–14 weeks)
2. second trimester MSST (4 analytes): alpha fetoprotein, oestriol, free beta hCG, inhibin A. A final risk is calculated by a computer program which combines other factors such as EDD age and age of gestation
3. non-invasive prenatal test (NIPT) from 10 weeks maternal serum. This anuploidy test usually covers three trisomies: 21 Down syndrome, 18 Edward syndrome, 13 Patau syndrome. It has the potential to screen multiple disorders
4. diagnostic tests (chorionic villus sampling, amniocentesis). The most reliable method is obtaining fetal tissue by these last means but there is a significant risk of miscarriage (1 in 100 for chorionic villus sampling and 1 in 200 for amniocentesis)

Consanguinity

Consanguinity is the situation where a couple shares one or more common ancestors. Consanguineous relationships occur in most societies and in some cultures are associated with particular advantages and religious traditions.[8]

The concern about the issue has been questioned by a study in the *Journal of Genetic Counselling,* which suggested 'aside from a thorough history, there is no need to offer genetic testing on the basis of consanguinity alone'. In a comment on this study which indicated that 'cousins run few risks in mating', the author pointed out that people like Charles Darwin, Queen Victoria and Albert Einstein married first cousins, and Darwin's children, in particular, were brilliant. In parts of Saudi Arabia 39% of all marriages are between first cousins.[24] On the other hand, there are substantiated records of problems with inherited disorders. Twenty-four US states ban the marriage of first cousins and the Catholic Church, with 2000 years of experience, has opposed cousin marriages for over 1000 years.

First cousins share a pair of grandparents and are statistically at an increased risk for autosomal recessive conditions. The baseline risk that any couple will have a baby with a birth defect is 3–4%.[8] In addition, empirical data show that for first cousin marriage there is an additional 4% risk of having a child with a birth defect—this includes malformations such as intellectual impairment and many rare autosomal recessive disorders. So the combined risk is 8% irrespective of a positive family history, which is an important consideration in counselling these people.[8]

For siblings the risk of increase in birth defects is 30% and 19% for second cousins.

Rare but helpful diagnostic tips

- Dark black urine on exposure = alkaptonuria

DxT arthritis + pigmentation of ear cartilage + grey–black urine with alkalisation ➔ alkaptonuria

- Red urine on exposure = porphyria
- Blue diapers = tryptophan malabsorption syndrome
- Maple syrup odour (urine and perspiration) = maple syrup urine disease (AR) (an amino acid metabolic disorder)

DxT odour + hypertonicity + seizures (infancy) → maple syrup urine disease

- Mousy body odour = phenylketonuria
- 'Fish-like' mouth with micrognathia = Turner syndrome
- 'Chipmunk' facies = thalassaemia major
- 'Doll-like' facies = glycogen storage disease (G-6-P deficiency)
- Elfin face = Williams syndrome
- Butterfly-like facial rash in children = tuberous sclerosis
- Weak suction + delayed sitting and crawling = Prader–Willi syndrome
- 'Happy puppet' features = Angelman syndrome
- Characteristic eyes: wide-spaced, down-slanting openings, ptosis = Noonan syndrome
- Long fingers and limbs = Marfan syndrome
- High-pitched meowing cry, low-set ears, mental retardation = 'cat-cry' syndrome (maladie du cri du chat)
- Blue sclera = osteogenesis imperfecta

References

1 Golden F, Lemonick M. The race is over. Time (Asia Pacific edn), 2000; 3 July: 56–61.

2 Tierney LM et al. *Current Medical Diagnosis and Treatment* (41st edn). New York: The McGraw-Hill Companies, 2002: 1645.

3 Warner BJ, McArthur GA. Cancer and the genetic revolution. Aust Fam Physician, 2001; 30: 933–5.

4 Newstead J, Metcalfe S. Getting the gene into genetic practice. Aust Fam Physician, 2001; 30: 927.

5 Singh A. Pharmacogenomics: the potential of genetically guided prescribing. Aust Fam Physician, 2007; 36(10): 821–4.

6 Hyett J. Non-invasive prenatal testing for Down syndrome. Aust Prescr, 2014; 37: 51–5.

7 Kingston H. Clinical genetic services. BMJ, 1989; 298: 306–7.

8 Craig J, Amor D, Macciocca I et al. Genetics. Check Program, 2001; issue 349.

9 Barlow-Stewart K, Emery J, Metcalfe S. *Genetics in Family Medicine: The Australian Handbook*. Canberra: Australian Government, NHMRC, 2007.

10 Lucarelli G. Bone marrow transplantation in adult thalassaemia patients. N Engl J Med, 1999; 93: 1164.

11 Ioannou L, McClaren BJ, Massie J et al. Population based carrier screening for cystic fibrosis: a systematic review of 23 years of research. Genet Med 2014; 16(3): 207–16.

12 Delatycki M, Tassicker R. Adult onset neurological disorders. Predictive genetic testing. Aust Fam Physician, 2001; 30(10): 948–52.

13 Levy-Lahad E, Bird T. Alzheimer's disease: genetic factors. In: Pulst SM (ed). *Neurogenetics*. New York: Oxford University Press, 2000.

14 Metcalfe S, Barlow-Stewart K et al. Genetics and blood haemoglobinopathies and clotting disorders. Aust Fam Physician, 2007; 36(10): 812–19.

15 Lennox N (Chairman). *Management Guidelines: People with Development and Intellectual Disabilities* (2nd edn). Melbourne: Therapeutic Guidelines Ltd, 2005.

16 Kidd SA, Lachiewicz A et al. Fragile X syndrome: a review of associated medical problems. Paediatrics, November 2014; 134(5): 995–1005.

17 Porter RS, Kaplan JL. *The Merck Manual* (19th edn). New Jersey: Merck Research Laboratories, 2011: 3003–4.

18 Bankier A. Syndrome Quiz. Fetal alcohol syndrome. Aust Fam Physician, 1990; 19: 1297.

19 Emery J, Barlow-Stewart K. Genetics and preventive health care. Aust Fam Physician, 2007; 36(10): 808–11

20 Amor D. Familial cancers. Aust Fam Physician, 2001; 30: 937–45.

21 Woolcock J, Grivell R. Noninvasive prenatal testing. Aust Fam Physician, July 2014; 43(7): 432–4.

22 Metcalfe S, Barlow-Stewart K. Population health screening. Aust Fam Physician, 2007; 36(10) 794–800.

23 The Royal Australian and New Zealand College of Obstetricians and Gynaecologists. Prenatal screening and diagnosis of chromosomal and genetic conditions in the fetus in pregnancy (C-Obs59) [under review]. East Melbourne: RANZCOG, 2011. Available from: <www.ranzcog.edu.au/Statements-Guidelines>, accessed February 2018.

24 Corliss R. Cousins: a new theory of relativity. Time, 2002; 15 April: 43.

Part 2

Diagnostic perspective in general practice

19 Depression

I am ignorant and impotent and yet, somehow or other, here I am, unhappy, no doubt, profoundly dissatisfied . . . In spite of everything I survive.

ALDOUS HUXLEY (1894–1963)

Depressive illness, which is probably the greatest masquerade in general practice, is one of the commonest illnesses in medicine and often confused with other illness. Untreated, depression can result in disability and death.[1] It is present in at least 17% of patients who present to GPs[2] and has a 12-month prevalence of 5% and a lifetime risk of 15%.[3] It is often unrecognised,[1] yet moderate to severe depression is as disabling as congestive heart failure[1] and with a morbidity comparable to coronary heart disease. Further, depression is the *leading* cause of disability for all conditions among both sexes, both in Australia and worldwide.[4,5] The lifetime risk of suicide in patients diagnosed with depression is 6% and treatment halves this risk.[1]

Despite being treatable, 60% of sufferers have not used any form of health service in the previous months.[4] Lack of awareness, stigma and shame on behalf of the patient contribute to this. Of those receiving treatment, three-quarters will be managed in general practice.[5,6] As Whitford[4] notes:

> It is clear that the main focus of activity aimed at reducing the burden of common mental health disorders in Australia is in primary care. Specialist mental health services play a supporting, but not central, role.

Depression is a chronic relapsing organic brain disease. Its mean onset is at 27 years of age. However, 40% of sufferers present by 20 years of age.[7] The average duration of episodes is 3–4 months and 40% of patients will relapse within a 12-month period.[7]

The cause of depression is multifactorial, having biological, psychological and social factors. Mood disorders in general have a strong familial tendency, and the risk of developing a depressive disorder can be thought of in terms of a 'stress-vulnerability model'. That is, an individual may have a genetically determined vulnerability and if enough stress is endured a mood disorder may result. Those who are more genetically vulnerable require less stress, but if enough stress is applied, any individual can develop a mood disorder.

There are six clusters of depressive symptoms:

- mood, e.g. sadness, anhedonia, irritability
- vegetative, e.g. sleep, appetite, sexual drive
- cognitive, e.g. attention, memory, self-worth
- impulse control, e.g. suicide, anger, homicide
- behavioural, e.g. motivation, interests, tiredness
- physical, e.g. headaches, constipation

A useful working rule is to consider depression as an illness that dampens the five basic innate activities of humans:

- energy for activity
- sex
- sleep
- appetite and thirst
- elimination of waste

Classifications

- The DSM-5 classification divides depressive disorders into major depressive disorder (MDD), disruptive mood dysregulation disorder, persistent depressive disorder (PDD) and premenstrual dysphoric disorder. Other 'specified' and 'unspecified' disorder categories allow for diagnosis of those patients who fall short of the various diagnostic criteria.
- MDD includes those disorders with one or more major depressive episodes. Excluding criteria include any previous mania or hypomania, and the episode not being attributable to a psychotic disorder, or a substance or medical condition.
  - MDD is subclassified with coded course and severity specifiers. These include mild, moderate and severe, with psychotic features, in partial remission and in full remission.
  - Non-coded specifiers can also be used, including 'with anxious distress', 'with mixed features', 'with melancholic features', 'with atypical features', 'with mood-congruent psychotic features', 'with catatonia', 'with peripartum onset' and 'with seasonal pattern'.

- Persistent depressive disorder (PDD) refers to long-standing (2 years or more) depression of mild severity.
- Adjustment disorder with depressed mood is a less severe form of depression without sufficient criteria for major depression. It is very common and occurs in response to identifiable stressors ('reactive depression', e.g. loss of employment). Its duration is usually no longer than 6 months.

The two key criteria for major depressive disorder (MDD) in the DSM-5 are a pervasive depressed mood and marked loss of interest or pleasure (otherwise referred to as anhedonia) persisting for at least 2 weeks. Other criteria (listed below) include sleep issues, fatigue, lack of energy, poor concentration and feelings of worthlessness.

In a general practice setting, having a checklist of these symptoms to work through with a patient can be a useful part of the assessment of the depressed patient. However, the DSM criteria can be too rigid for general practice, with many patients whom GPs recognise as having psychological issues not meeting DSM-5 criteria.[3] As Ian Hickie puts it, 'Primary care psychiatry is not specialist psychiatry in general practice.'[8]

Questions to assess level of depression

- What do you think is the matter with you?
- Do you think that your feelings are possibly caused by nerves, anxiety or depression?
- Can you think of any reason why you feel this way?
- Do you feel down in the dumps?
- Do you feel that you are coping well?
- Do you have any good times?
- Has anything changed in your life?
- How do you sleep? Do you wake early?
- What time of the day do you feel at your worst?
- Where would you put yourself between 0% and 100% (a visual analogue scale is useful here)?
- Have you felt hopeless?
- Do you brood about the past?
- What is your energy like?
- What is your appetite like?
- Are you as interested in sex as before?
- Do you feel guilty about anything?
- Do you feel that life is worthwhile?
- Has the thought of ending your life occurred to you?
- Do you cry when no one is around (especially useful for children)?

Two particularly good questions are:

- In the past month, have you been bothered by the fact that you feel down, depressed or hopeless?
- In the past month, have you often been bothered by the fact that you have little interest or pleasure in doing things?

DSM-5 diagnostic criteria for major depressive disorder

At least five of the following symptoms nearly every day for 2 weeks (criterion 1 or 2 essential):

1. depressed mood or irritability (subjective or objective) most of the day
2. loss of interest or pleasure
3. change in weight (5% change over 1 month) or appetite
4. change in sleep: insomnia or hypersomnia
5. psychomotor agitation or retardation
6. loss of energy or fatigue
7. worthlessness or guilt
8. impaired concentration or indecisiveness
9. suicidality: recurrent thoughts of death or suicide ideation or any suicide attempt

Source: Diagnostic and Statistical Manual (5th edition). Washington, DC: American Psychiatric Association, 2013

19

Depression scales

Depression scales are useful both to detect potential mood disorders (i.e. screening) and to monitor an individual patient over time. Scales commonly used include K10 (a distress score) and DASS 21 or 42 (for depression and anxiety symptoms).

Somatisation

Another issue with depression in the primary care setting is recognising somatising patients who present without obvious psychological symptoms. Non-specific symptoms such as insomnia, prolonged fatigue, headache, nausea and musculoskeletal pain are common presentations in people with depression.[9] Studies suggest GPs find it challenging to identify these patients, and that using self-reporting patient-screening tools can help with identification.[3]

Key facts and checkpoints

- Depression is common, serious and treatable.
- Depression is a chronic relapsing organic brain disease.

- The cause of depression is multifactorial, and can be thought of in terms of a 'stress-vulnerability model'.
- Somatising patients without obvious psychopathology are common and difficult to recognise and manage.

Depression in the elderly

The rate of antidepressant prescribing for Australians over 80 years of age is higher than for any other age group.[10] Despite this, depression in the elderly is underdiagnosed.[11] Depression can have bizarre features in the elderly and may be misdiagnosed as dementia or psychosis. Agitated depression is the most frequent type of depression in the aged. Features may include histrionic behaviour, delusions and disordered thinking.

Depression is often missed in the elderly because it is atypical and less expressive, and patients tend to be ashamed and reluctant to admit it.

A useful clue can be a change in sleep pattern. Medical illness is also an important precipitant of depression in the elderly.

Older patients may have more side effects from medications (especially nausea, dizziness, falls and hyponatraemia).[11] They also tend to have only a modest response to antidepressants, and, if medication is used, a low initial dose and slow increase is recommended.[1] Psychological therapies can be useful, but tend to be underused.[11]

Depression in children and adolescents

Sadness is common in children, but depression, although not as common, does occur and is characterised by feelings of helplessness, worthlessness and despair. Parents and doctors both tend to be unaware of depression in children.[12]

Major depression in children and adolescents may be diagnosed using the same criteria as for adults, namely loss of interest in usual activities and the presence of a sad or irritable mood, persisting for 2 weeks or more. In children, irritability may be more prominent than sadness.[13] The other constellation of depressive symptoms, including somatic complaints, may be present. Examples include difficulty in getting to sleep, not enjoying meals, poor concentration and low self-esteem. Poor motor skills and family instability are an association. Depression can present as antisocial behaviour or as a separation anxiety (e.g. school refusal). Although suicidal thoughts are common, suicide is rare before adolescence.

Depressed adolescents are a difficult challenge for the general practitioner. Effective engagement and establishing rapport in a 'youth-friendly' environment is critical.[14]

See CHAPTER 97 for the evaluation and treatment of depression in adolescents.

Perinatal depression

This term refers to depression occurring either in the antenatal period or in the 12 months after delivery. It affects 9% of women during pregnancy and 16% after the birth[15] and affects the well-being of the woman, the baby and significant others. Anxiety is likely to be as or more common.[15] Women at risk of perinatal depression include those with previous mental health problems, those who do not have support, those who have been through difficult times (e.g. family problems, abuse or loss), or who feel isolated either by distance or culture or both.

Because it is so prevalent, routine screening is recommended by the beyondblue guidelines. This involves implementing the use of the Edinburgh Postnatal Depression Scale (EPNDS), a validated screening tool, at least once, preferably twice, both antenatally and postnatally. Asking permission and explaining the process before implementing the screening is helpful. Women at higher risk will require more intense screening and monitoring.

If perinatal depression is identified, the GP should take into account the individual woman's context, her family and cultural setting, and use a family-centred approach. Because of the intense emotions involved in having a baby, establishing a strong therapeutic relationship, using an open collaborative approach and active listening techniques, will help to develop trust, confidence, mutual respect and empowerment. Psycho-education should be provided and appropriate follow-up and continuity of care, with (if appropriate) a co-ordinated team approach.

If a woman or a baby is at risk, urgent referral is recommended. Pharmacological therapies can be used in pregnancy, but the benefits need to be balanced against the risks to both mother and fetus. Psychosis in perinatal depression is fortunately rare but does occur, and requires urgent psychiatric assessment. Refer to CHAPTER 109.

Recurrent brief depression

There is a high prevalence in general practice of patients presenting with recurrent episodes of depression of short duration, about 3 to 7 days, as often as monthly. Premenstrual dysphoria may be a factor.

As a rule antidepressants are ineffective. Lithium is an alternative medication for long-term use. Management is based on psychotherapy, especially CBT.

Seasonal affective disorder

SAD or 'winter blues' is a recurrent depressive disorder seen in people living in cold climates where the winters are bleak and dark. Features of depression include sleeping difficulty, sadness, lethargy, irritability and anxiety while atypical symptoms include somnolence and increased appetite (carbohydrate craving). Treatment is based on psychotherapy, phototherapy and medication such as the SSRIs. Refer to www.sada.org.uk.

Management of depression

Important considerations from the outset are:

- Is the patient a suicide risk?
- Does the patient require inpatient assessment?
- Is referral to a specialist psychiatrist indicated?

Suicide assessment

The rules of seven:

- 1 in 7 people with recurrent depression die by suicide
- 70% of suicides have depression
- 70% of patients who suicide have seen a GP within the last 7 weeks
- Suicide is the 7th leading cause of death

If the symptoms are major and the patient appears in poor health or is a suicide risk, referral is appropriate.

The importance of putting these safety issues at the beginning of the management process is reflected in the SET A PACE[7] model of treatment, proposed by Mahli et al.

To clarify the risk of suicide and appropriate response, ask about:[14]

- suicidal thoughts
- plan
- lethality
- means
- past history
- suicide of family member or peer

Low risk (fleeting thoughts of self-harm or suicide but no current plan or means):

- Discuss availability of support and treatment options.
- Arrange follow-up consultation (timing of this will be based on clinical judgment).
- Identify relevant community resources and provide contact details.

Medium risk (suicidal thoughts and intent but no current plan or immediate means):

- Discuss availability of support and treatment options.
- Organise reassessment within 1 week.
- Have contingency plan in place for rapid reassessment if distress or symptoms escalate.
- Develop a safety plan (a prioritised written list of coping strategies and sources of support to use when experiencing suicidal thinking).

High risk (continual/specific suicidal thoughts, intent, plan and means):

- Ensure that the person is in an appropriately safe and secure environment.
- Organise reassessment within 24 hours and monitoring for this period.
- Follow-up outcome of assessment.

After safety is established (and this will need to be continually reassessed at each consultation), the two other aspects that need to be developed early in the process (and also continue on through the long-term management of the patient) are **educating** the patient about his or her condition and individual situation, and establishing a **therapeutic relationship**.

Assessment includes:

- **characterising** the symptom profile
- **calibrating** the severity and chronicity—rating scales can be employed here
- **corroborating** (if possible and appropriate) medical and psychiatric comorbidities and context. Significant psychiatric, physical and social comorbidities of depression are common. These include 49% suffering an anxiety disorder, 40% reporting child sexual abuse, 57% child physical abuse, 42% having been at some stage afraid of their partner and 72% reporting a chronic physical condition.[16] Putting the patient's condition into his or her individual psychosocial and medical context will improve the assessment
- **considering** coping styles, and the social, financial and occupational consequences of the patient's condition and situation

This assessment is often spread over multiple consultations.

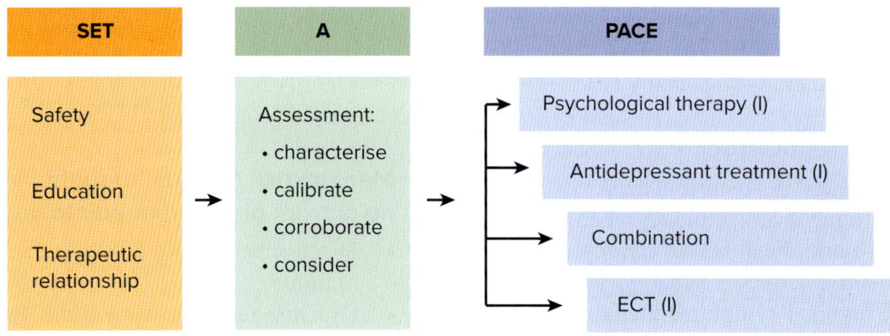

FIGURE 19.1 The SET A PACE model of treatment of depression
Source: Adapted from G Mahli et al.[7]

Treatment

The basic treatments are outlined by the acronym **PACE** (which purposefully places priority on the psychological treatments—see FIG. 19.1). These are:

- **Psychological,** including basic psychological treatments, such as advice on lifestyle changes, problem solving, guided self-help, structured supervised exercise and supportive counselling.[1,6] All patients with depression should be offered these types of support.[1,14] More sophisticated techniques, such as cognitive behaviour therapy (CBT) or interpersonal therapy (IPT) may be used for selected patients[7] and should be undertaken only by appropriately trained doctors or therapists.[6] Another option that some patients may prefer is computer-based cognitive behaviour therapy (CBT) programs.[11] CBT involves teaching patients new ways of positive thinking, which have to be relevant and achievable for the patient (see CHAPTER 5). Patients need to be able to recognise their own negative cognitions, including their anxieties and worries.
- **Antidepressants:** antidepressant medication is useful in moderate to severe depression (TABLE 19.1), or when depression has an anxiety disorder codiagnosis.[11] Antidepressant therapy should be avoided if bipolar disorder is suspected, and screening should be actively conducted for symptoms of past or previous mania.[11]
  - In terms of which drug to use, there is no single drug that is preferred. However, selective serotonin reuptake inhibitors (SSRIs) are considered to have the most favourable balance of benefit to harm in moderate to severe depression.[11] Sexual dysfunction and gastrointestinal side effects are common.[7]

TABLE 19.1 First-line pharmacological treatment options for depression[13]

Drug	Usual initial dose	Maximum dose
SSRIs		
citalopram	20 mg (10 mg >65 years)	40 mg (20 mg >65 years)
escitalopram	10 mg	20 mg
fluoxetine	20 mg	80 mg
fluvoxamine	50 mg (at night), then 100 mg after 5–7 days	300 mg
paroxetine	20 mg	60 mg
sertraline	50 mg, then 100 mg after 5–7 days	200 mg
SNRIs		
desvenlafaxine (controlled-release)	50 mg	200 mg
duloxetine	60 mg	120 mg
venlafaxine (controlled-release	75 mg	375 mg
Other		
mirtazepine	15–30 mg (at night)	60 mg

Other suitable first-line agents are reboxetine (common side effects include hypersomnia, fatigue and nausea) and mirtazepine (which can cause weight gain and drowsiness).[7] SSRIs have a relatively flat dose response curve, but dose increase within the recommended range is reasonable if there is a partial response at a lower dose and no troublesome side effects.

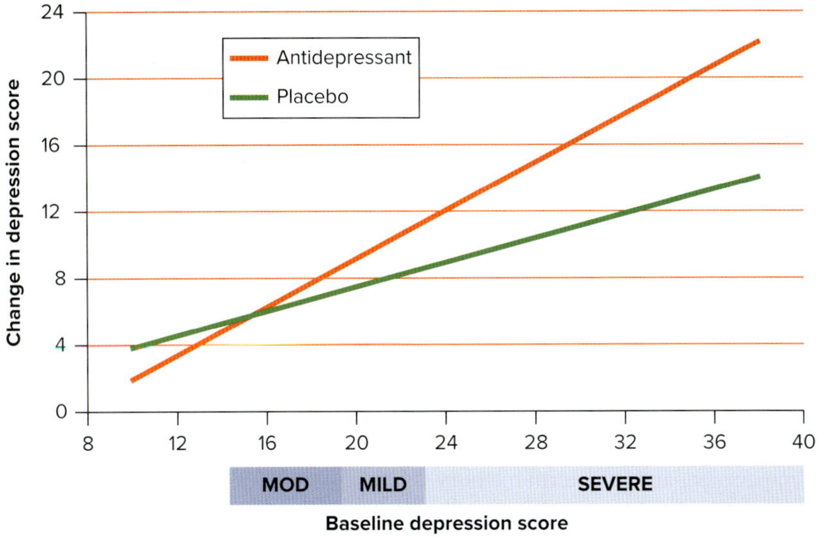

FIGURE 19.2 Antidepressant vs placebo drug effect on depression

Source: Adapted from Fournier et al. Antidepressant drug effect and depression severity: a patient-level meta-analysis. JAMA, 2010; 303: 47–53

- Combining different antidepressants or augmentation with lithium or antipsychotics should be done with psychiatrist supervision.[7]
- Seretonin and noradrenaline reuptake inhibitors (SNRIs) appear to be more effective in treating severe depression symptoms (and may be a suitable first-line option here) but otherwise adverse effects may limit them to second-line treatment.[7] Tricyclic antidepressants (TCAs) and monoamine oxidase inhibitors (MAOIs) are considered second-line because of their side effect profiles.[13]

The benefit of medication in moderate depression is equivalent to psychological therapies such as CBT/IPT and both of them are around 20% more likely to achieve remission than placebo.[1] In severe depression, medication is more effective than psychological therapies (see FIG. 19.2), though the latter in addition may help reduce relapse rates once remission is achieved by medication.[1,6]

The aim of treatment of depression is to achieve and maintain remission (see FIG. 19.3).[1] Remission is defined as having minimal or no symptoms of depression,[7] and a good way of asking patients about this is to ask 'Do you think you are back to your normal self?'.

When using antidepressants, if a response is not evident in the first 2 weeks or there is an inadequate response in 6 weeks, then it is unlikely that this medication will work for this patient, and a treatment

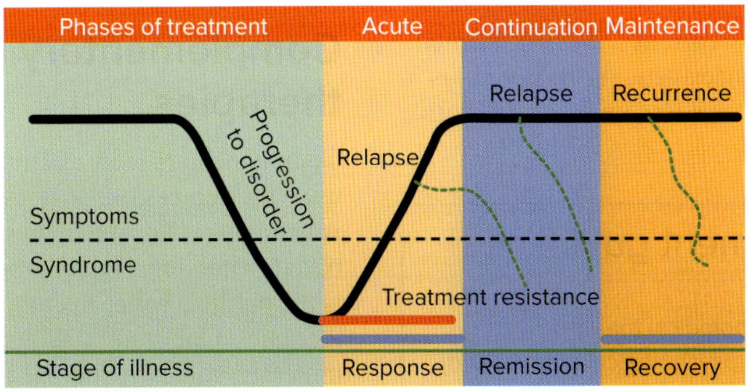

FIGURE 19.3 Terminology used in depression and treatment

(Response is defined as a significant reduction in symptoms and signs, and remission is the state of minimal or no symptoms/signs, but lacking full functional recovery.)

Source: Adapted from Kufper et al. Long term treatment of depression. J Clin Psychiatry, 1991; 52: 28–34

change is recommended.[7] A washout period will be required before a second medication is tried. Patients need close monitoring early on in the course of treatment, and weekly monitoring may be helpful.[11] If remission is not achieved in 3 months, then consider a second opinion and continue active treatment.[7]

- **A combination** of antidepressants and psychological therapy can be considered if there is an inadequate response to either therapy alone. Combining medication with psychological therapy is more effective than either therapy alone in moderate or severe depression.[7]
- **ECT (electroconvulsive therapy)** is a relatively safe and effective therapy for severe or resistant depression. There is some risk of transient short-term cognitive impairment and long-term memory impairment, and this therapy is reserved for severe depression when pharmacotherapy has failed;[7] it is administered under the supervision of a psychiatrist.

  Possible indications include:

  - psychotic depression (e.g. delusions, hallucinations)
  - melancholic depression unresponsive to antidepressants
  - severe postnatal depression and psychosis
  - substantial suicide risk
  - ineffective antidepressant medication and/or previous response to ECT
  - severe psychomotor depression: refusal to eat or drink, depressive stupor, severe personal neglect

Immediate referral for hospital admission is necessary in most of these circumstances. The course, which is highly variable and individually tailored, is about 8–12 sessions given at 1–3 sessions a week. The most common initial ECT method is unilateral therapy.[1]

Transcranial direct current electro-magnetic stimulation, where no anaesthetic is required, is a procedure being explored as a less invasive alternative to ECT.[17]

Useful management guidelines

- **Mild depression:** psychological therapy
- **Moderate depression:** psychological therapy and/or antidepressants
- **Severe depression:** antidepressants, and consider addition of psychological therapy to maintain remission. Consider psychiatric review, ECT.

When to refer

- Uncertainty about diagnosis
- Inpatient care obviously necessary
- Severe depression
- Inability to cope at home
- Psychotically depressed (with delusions or hallucinations)
- Substantial suicide risk
- Failure of response to routine antidepressant therapy
- Associated psychiatric or physical disorders
- Depression in the elderly can be a difficult problem—where diagnosis including dementia is doubtful
- Children with apparent major depression

Choice of treatment

The choice of treatment should be determined together by doctor and patient, and the best outcomes are likely when a good therapeutic alliance is formed[6] and patient preferences are taken into account.[11] To quote the RANZCP guidelines: 'Of greatest benefit is the therapeutic relationship, which enables agreement on treatment selection and continuation.'[1] A strong determining factor on patient preference may be the patient's own previous experience of treatments, or his or her perceptions of treatment results in other people they know or potential adverse effects of the proposed treatment.[11]

Whatever treatment is chosen by the doctor and patient working together, the choice is less important than persisting with treatment. As the beyondblue guidelines state, it is 'not so much what you do but that you keep doing it'.[6] This is why consistent follow-up and monitoring is so beneficial.

Complementary and alternative therapies

Complementary and alternative therapies are widely used for depression. It is estimated that only 50% of Australians who are depressed receive an evidence-based professional intervention.[18] A large driver for this is the public's belief in complementary and alternative therapies. One study[19] showed 57% regarded vitamins, minerals, tonics or herbal medicines as likely to be helpful for treating depression, compared with 29% who regarded antidepressants as likely to be helpful.

Despite this, none of these therapies is supported by evidence, though some warrant further evaluation.[20]

Because of their common usage (nearly half of Australians have used a complementary medicine in the previous 12 months),[20] actively enquiring about use of any complementary and alternative therapies in patients with depression is advised.

One of the more commonly used and extensively researched alternative therapies is St John's wort (*Hypericum perforatum*), which has had mixed results in the research on its effectiveness. One review of the literature suggests it is effective in mild to moderate depression,[21] though two others suggest it is not.[22,23]

Regardless of its effectiveness (or not), it has a lot of medication interactions. These include HIV medicines, warfarin, digoxin, anticonvulsants, oral contraceptives and triptans. Because of this, care needs to be taken with using St John's wort, including when switching between different preparations that may contain different amounts of active compound.

Serotonin syndrome

- While rare, serotonin syndrome is a serious adverse reaction to the use of SSRIs and other serotonergic medications, including St John's wort.
- Symptoms must coincide with the introduction or dose increase of a serotonergic agent. Drugs to be considered here include antidepressants, opioids (especially tramadol), stimulant drugs, illicit drugs, anti-emetics, lithium and selegiline.
- Other causes, such as infection, substance abuse or withdrawal, must be excluded.
- At least three of the symptoms or signs attributed to the syndrome must be present, e.g.:
  - mental status/behaviour changes (e.g. agitation, confusion, hypomania, seizures)
  - altered muscle tone (e.g. tremor, shivering, myoclonus, hyper-reflexia)
  - autonomic instability (e.g. hypertension or hypotension, tachycardia, fever, diarrhoea)

The offending agents should be withdrawn immediately and supportive therapy initiated; refer to an emergency department.

Continuing treatment

If antidepressant medication is used and remission achieved, it is recommended that it be continued for a minimum of 12 months for an initial episode, and for 2–3 years in subsequent episodes or in those at high risk of relapse.[1,11] Risk factors for relapse include:[7,11]

- residual depressive symptoms
- 2 or more prior episodes in the past 5 years
- 3 or more prior episodes
- history of severe or prolonged depression (especially with psychosis or attempted suicide)
- comorbid medical problems
- life stressors

When remission is achieved, and the treatment is in the maintenance phase, ongoing monitoring of treatment effectiveness, tolerability and adherence is recommended.[7] Encouragement to persist with the treatment will improve compliance.[1] When ceasing medication, withdrawal reactions are common, so a gradual withdrawal by halving the dose each week may help reduce these.[1]

References

1. Australian and New Zealand clinical practice guidelines for the treatment of depression. Australian and New Zealand Journal of Psychiatry, 2004; 38: 389–407.
2. Goldberg D. Epidemiology of mental disorders in primary care settings. Epidemiol Rev, 1995; 17: 182–90.
3. Wilhelm K, Finch A, Davenport T et al. Who can alert the general practitioner to people whose common mental health problems are unrecognised? Med J Aust, 2008; 188 (12): 114–18.
4. Whitford H-A. Depression in primary care: expanding the evidence base for diagnosis and treatment. Med J Aust, 2008; 188 (12): 101–2.
5. Slade T, Johnston A, Teesson M et al. *The Mental Health of Australians 2. Report on the 2007 National Survey of Mental Health and Wellbeing*. Canberra: Department of Health and Ageing, 2009.
6. Ellis P, Smith D. Treating depression: the *beyondblue* guidelines for treating depression in primary care. Med J Aust, 2002; 176: S77–S83.
7. Mahli G et al. Clinical practice recommendations for depression. Acta Psychiatr Scand, 2009; 119 (439): 8–26.
8. Hickie I. Primary care psychiatry is not specialist psychiatry in general practice. Med J Aust, 1999; 170: 171–3.
9. Goldman L, Nielson N, Champion H. Awareness, diagnosis and treatment of depression. J Gen Intern Med, 1999: 14; 569–80.
10. Hollingworth S, Burgess P, Whiteford H. Affective and anxiety disorders: prevalence, treatment and antidepressant medication use. Aust N Z J Psychiatry, 2010; 44: 513–19.
11. NPS News 78, April 2012. Depression—challenges in primary care. <www.nps.org.au/publications/health-professional/nps-news/2012/depression-challenges-in-primary-care> (accessed 31/12/2013).
12. Thomson K, Tey D, Marks M. *Paediatric Handbook* (RCH) (8th edn). Oxford: Wiley-Blackwell, 2004: 192–6.
13. Psychotropic therapeutic guidelines (revised July 2013). In: eTG complete (online). Melbourne: Therapeutic Guidelines Limited, 2013. <www.online.tg.org.au/ref/tablet/tgc/ptg71/ptg_topics.htm> (accessed 31/12/2013).
14. McDermott B, Baigent M, Chanen A et al. Clinical practice guidelines: depression in adolescents and young adults. Melbourne: beyondblue: the national depression initiative, 2011: 143.

15 Austin M-P, Highet N and the Guidelines Expert Advisory Committee. Clinical practice guidelines for depression and related disorders—anxiety, bipolar disorder and puerperal psychosis—in the perinatal period. A guideline for primary care health professionals. Melbourne: beyondblue: the national depression initiative, 2011.
16 Gunn J et al. Who is identified when screening for depression is undertaken in general practice? Baseline findings from the Diagnosis, Management and Outcomes of Depression in Primary Care (diamond) longitudinal study. Med J Aust, 2008; 188 (12): S199–25.
17 Fitzgerald P. Transcranial direct current stimulation. Med J Aust open 2012: Supplement 4:148–151
18 Andrews G et al. Why does the burden of disease persist? Relating the burden of anxiety and depression to effectiveness of treatment. Bulletin of the World Health Organization, 2000; 78: 446–54.
19 Jorm A et al. 'Mental health literacy': a survey of the public's ability to recognise mental disorders and their beliefs about the effectiveness of treatment. Med J Aust, 1997; 166: 182–6.
20 Jorm A et al. Effectiveness of complementary and self-help treatments for depression. Med J Aust, 2002; 176: S84–96.
21 Linde K. St John's wort—an overview. Forschende Komplementärmedizin: Research in Complementary Medicine, 2009; 16 (3): 146–55.
22 Linde K, Berner M, Kriston L. St John's wort for major depression. Cochrane Database Syst Rev. 2009; (4): CD000448. <www.thecochranelibrary.com> (accessed 11/1/2014).
23 National Institute of Mental Health. Depression. <www.nimh.nih.gov/health/publications/depression/index.shtml> (accessed 11/1/2014).

Diabetes mellitus

20

Those labouring with this Disease, piss a great deal more than they drink. Authors who affirm the drink to be little or nothing changed are very far from the truth, because the urine very much differed both from the drink taken in and also in being wonderfully sweet as if it were imbued with honey or sugar.

THOMAS WILLIS (1621–75), *THE PISSING EVIL*

Diabetes comes from a Greek word meaning 'to pass or flow through' (i.e. excessive urination) and *mellitus* means 'sweet'. It is a disease caused by a relative or absolute deficiency of insulin.

There are two main types of diabetes (see TABLE 20.1).

- Type 1 is also known as juvenile onset diabetes or insulin dependent diabetes mellitus (IDDM).
- Type 2 is also known as maturity onset diabetes or non-insulin dependent diabetes mellitus (NIDDM).

Type 1 has an autoimmune causation which is also responsible for a late-onset form known as late onset autoimmune diabetes in adults (LADA).

Table 20.1 Clinical differentiation between type 1 and type 2 diabetes

	Type 1	Type 2
Relative frequency (approx.)	10–15%	85–90%
Peak age incidence	10–30 years	>40 years
Age of onset	Usually young <20	Usually middle-aged >40
Onset	Rapid	Insidious/slow
Presentation	Polyuria, polydipsia weight loss	Milder symptoms, often asymptomatic
Weight at onset	Low (thin)	High (obese)
Ketoacidosis	Yes	Rare
Familial	Weak	Strong
Insulin status	Deficient	Resistant

Note: These are generalisations and the clinical features may vary (e.g. patients with type 2 diabetes may be thin and have a rapid onset, or present at an earlier age).

Diabetes: a real masquerade

The onset of type 2 diabetes can be subtle and by stealth. Studies have demonstrated that it takes, on average, 7–9 years before a patient is diagnosed.[1] At any one given time almost half of patients with type 2 diabetes are undiagnosed. In 2014–15, around 5% of Australians had diabetes.[2] A further 16% have impaired fasting glucose or impaired glucose tolerance.[3] Very importantly, about 35% of newly diagnosed diabetic patients are already harbouring complications of diabetes.[1] The challenge for GPs is to be on constant lookout for these patients, especially those at risk. Type 2 diabetes is becoming more prevalent in industrial countries—partly due to the ageing population and partly because our lifestyle encourages us to 'eat more and walk less'.[3] Furthermore, 60% of our population are overweight or obese.

Complications occur in type 2 diabetes as well as in type 1.

- Several causes of secondary diabetes are uncommon (pancreatic disease; approx. 2.5%) or very uncommon (see TABLE 20.2).

Key facts and checkpoints

- In Australians older than 25 years the prevalence of diabetes is 7.5%, with another 10.6% having impaired glucose tolerance.[2]
- About 30% of these people will develop clinical diabetes within 10 years.[3]
- Many people with type 2 diabetes are asymptomatic.
- Diabetes can exist for years before detection and complications may be evident.
- Type 2 diabetes is not a mild disease. About one-third of those surviving 15 years will require insulin injections to control symptoms or complications.[4]
- Blood glucose may be temporarily elevated during acute illness, after trauma or surgery.

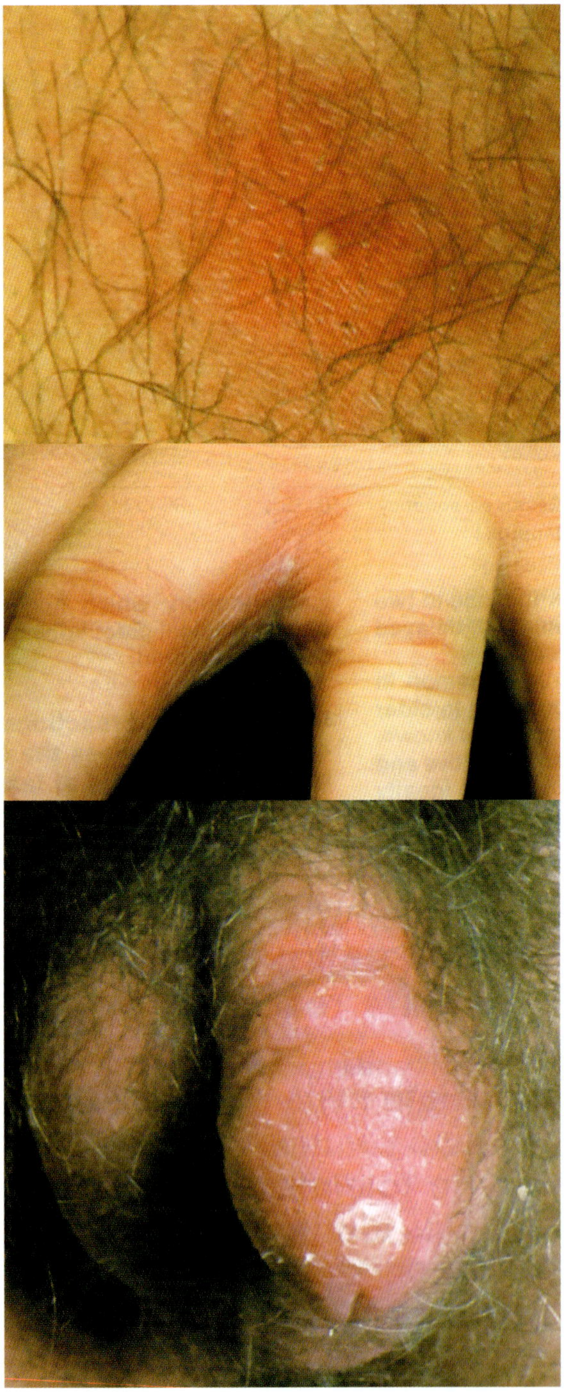

FIGURE 20.1 Skin signs of diabetes: **(a)** Recurrent staphylococcus folliculitis **(b)** *Candida albicans* erosio interdigitalis **(c)** *Candida albicans* balanitis

- Asymptomatic people at high risk of undiagnosed diabetes should be screened by blood glucose or HbA1c measurement.

Table 20.2 Causes of secondary diabetes

Pancreatic disorders (also called 'Type 3c diabetes')
Chronic pancreatitis
Endocrine disorders
Cushing syndrome
Acromegaly
Phaeochromocytoma
Polycystic ovarian syndrome
Haemochromatosis
Drug-induced diabetes (transient)
Thiazide diuretics
Oestrogen therapy (high dose—not with low-dose HRT)
Corticosteroids
Other transient causes
Gestational diabetes
Medical or surgical stress

Clinical features

The classic symptoms of uncontrolled diabetes are:

- polyuria
- polydipsia
- loss of weight (type 1)
- tiredness and fatigue
- propensity for infections, especially of the skin and genitals (vaginal thrush)

The young person with type 1 diabetes typically presents with a brief 2–10 week history of the classic triad of symptoms:

DxT thirst + polyuria + weight loss → type 1 diabetes

Other possible symptoms are:

- vulvovaginitis } due to *Candida albicans*
- pruritus vulvae } due to *Candida albicans*
- balanitis } due to *Candida albicans*
- nocturnal enuresis (type 1)
- blurred vision/visual changes

Symptoms of complications (may be presenting feature) include:

- staphylococcal skin infections
- polyneuropathy: tingling or numbness in feet, pain (can be severe if present)
- impotence
- arterial disease: myocardial ischaemia, peripheral vascular disease

History

The history of a suspected or known diabetic patient should cover the following features including assessment of cardiovascular risks and end-organ damage.

- Specific symptoms:
  - polyuria
  - polydipsia
  - loss of weight
  - polyphagia
  - tiredness/malaise/fatigue
  - nocturia
- Related general symptom review:
  - cardiovascular (e.g. chest pain, dyspnoea)
  - urinary function
  - sexual function
  - neurological (e.g. tingling in feet/hands)
  - vision (e.g. blurred)
  - infection tendency (e.g. skin, urine, genital)
  - genital itching
- General:
  - family history
  - medication
  - smoking and alcohol
  - obstetric history (where applicable)
  - physical activity
  - nutrition/eating habits

Examination

The physical examination should ideally follow the protocol for annual review.

Initial screening for suspected diabetes should include:

- general inspection, including skin
- BMI (weight/height)
- waist circumference
- visual acuity
- blood pressure—lying and standing
- test for peripheral neuropathy: tendon reflexes, sensation (e.g. cotton wool, 10 g monofilament, Neurotips)
- urinalysis: glucose, albumin, ketones, nitrites

Investigations

- Initial: fasting or random blood sugar, follow-up oral glucose tolerance test (OGTT) or glycated haemoglobin (HbA1c) if indicated
- Other tests according to clinical assessment (e.g. lipids, kidney function, urine albumin-creatinine ratio (ACR), ECG)

Risk factors

- Age >40 years
- Family history
- Overweight/obesity
- Sedentary lifestyle
- History of gestational diabetes
- Women with polycystic ovarian syndrome (PCOS)
- Hypertension/ischaemic heart disease
- Medication causing hyperglycaemia
- Ethnic/cultural groups: Aboriginal and Torres Strait Islanders, Pacific Islanders, people from Indian subcontinent, Chinese, Afro-Caribbeans

Screening (type 2)[5]

- People with impaired fasting glucose/impaired glucose tolerance ('prediabetes')
- Age >40 years
- Younger age (e.g. >30 years) with: family history (first-degree relative with type 2), obesity (BMI >30), high-prevalence ethnic groups
- Age >18 years in Aboriginal and Torres Strait Islander people
- Previous gestational diabetes
- People on long-term steroids
- People on antipsychotic medication
- Polycystic ovarian syndrome, especially if overweight
- Previous cardiovascular event

The optimal frequency is every 3 years from age 40 years using AUSDRISK (www.diabetesaustralia.com.au/are-you-at-risk-type-2) and annually in very high-risk groups, including Aboriginal and Torres Strait Islander people and those with 'prediabetes'.[6]

Diagnosis

Diabetes is diagnosed as follows:[3,5]

1 If symptomatic (at least two of polydipsia, polyuria, frequent skin infections or frequent genital thrush):
  - fasting venous blood glucose (VBG) ≥7.0 mmol/L

    or
  - random VBG (at least 2 hours after last eating) ≥11.1 mmol/L

    or
  - HbAlc >6.5% (>48 mmol/mol)

2 If asymptomatic:
  - at least two separate elevated values, either fasting, 2 or more hours post-prandial, or the two values from an oral glucose tolerance test (OGTT)

Note: If random or fasting VBG lies in an uncertain range (5.5–11.0 mmol/L) in either a symptomatic patient or a patient with risk factors (over 50 years, overweight, first-degree relative with T2D), perform an OGTT. The cut-off point for further testing is 5.5 mmol/L.[5,7]

The 2-hour blood sugar on an OGTT is still the gold standard for the diagnosis of uncertain diabetes, i.e. >11.1 mmol/L.

The OGTT should be reserved for true borderline cases and for gestational diabetes. A screening (oral glucose challenge) test at 26–30 (usually 28) weeks gestation is sometimes used during pregnancy.

Prediabetes

This is the condition where the VPG is elevated above the normal range (i.e. 6.1–6.9) but does not satisfy the type 2 diagnostic criteria. It includes two states:

- impaired fasting glucose (IFG)
- impaired glucose tolerance (IGT)

A diagnosis of prediabetes is not a call to start medication, but it increases the urgency of promoting lifestyle changes such as weight reduction and increased physical activity.

Urinalysis is unreliable in diagnosis since glycosuria occurs at different plasma glucose values in patients with different kidney thresholds.

For a summary of diagnosis of diabetic states refer to FIGURE 20.2.

Diabetes in children

A study by Sinah and colleagues detected impaired glucose tolerance in 25% of 55 obese children (4 to 10 years of age) and 21% of 112 obese adolescents

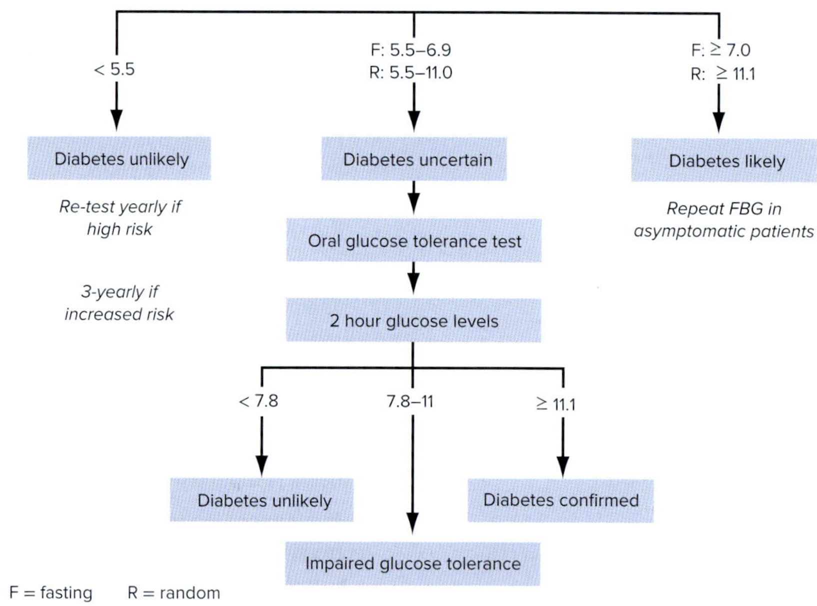

FIGURE 20.2 Blood glucose levels—venous plasma (mmol/L)

Source: Reproduced with permission from *Diabetes Management in General Practice. Guidelines for Type 2 Diabetes.* Melbourne: RACGP[5]

Table 20.3 Interpreting diagnostic tests for diabetes[8]

Test		Normal	Intermediate hyperglycaemia	Diabetes
Venous blood glucose concentration	fasting	up to 6 mmol/L	6.1–6.9 mmol/L	≥7 mmol/L
	random	up to 6 mmol/L		≥11.1 mmol/L
Oral glucose tolerance test	2-hour venous blood glucose concentration	up to 7.7 mmol/L	7.8–11 mmol/L	≥11.1 mmol/L
HbA1c				≥48 mmol/mol (6.5%)

(11 to 18 years of age).[9] Type 2 diabetes was identified in 4% of obese adolescents. However, over 30% of newly diagnosed diabetes in children and adolescents is upon presentation with diabetic ketoacidosis. Children with type 1 diabetes usually exhibit the classic features of polyuria, polydipsia, weight loss and lethargy. Be aware of unusual presentations such as urinary disorders including enuresis or daytime wetting accidents when a misdiagnosis of urinary infection or some other condition is sometimes forthcoming. The diagnosis can be made by an elevated random or fasting blood sugar. Oral glucose tolerance tests are inappropriate in the very young. Upon diagnosis it is appropriate to refer the child or adolescent to a multidisciplinary diabetes team.

Gestational diabetes

Gestational diabetes is the new onset of abnormal glucose tolerance during pregnancy. Pregnancy is diabetogenic for those with a genetic predisposition. All pregnant women should be screened at 24–28 weeks with an oral glucose tolerance test (OGTT). The definition of gestational diabetes mellitus (GDM) by the Australasian Diabetes in Pregnancy Society has widened considerably in the past decade and far more women are captured by the lower thresholds.[10] The 2014 consensus definition of gestational diabetes is a fasting plasma glucose of ≥5.1 mmol/L, or a post-75 g oral glucose load at 1 hour ≥10.0, or at 2 hours 8.5–11.0. Refer to CHAPTER 108.

Diabetes in the elderly

The incidence of diabetes rises with age. The elderly have increased mortality and morbidity from the disease and require careful monitoring, especially with adverse drug effects aggravated by polypharmacy and comorbidities. Special issues include diet, foot care and postural hypotension.

Complications of diabetes

Complications may occur in patients with both type 1 and type 2 diabetes, even with early diagnosis and treatment (see FIG. 20.3).

People with type 1 diabetes still have a significantly reduced life expectancy. The main causes of death are diabetic nephropathy and vascular disease (myocardial infarction and stroke).

Diabetes causes both macrovascular and microvascular complications but microvascular disease is specific to diabetes. Special attention should be paid to the association of type 2 diabetes with obesity, hypertension and dyslipidaemia—the 'deadly quartet'.[7,11]

Macrovascular complications include:

- ischaemic/coronary heart disease
- cerebrovascular disease
- peripheral vascular disease

An analysis of patients with type 2 diabetes in the HOPE study[12,13] showed a benefit of ramipril to reduce the risk of:

- death (24%)
- myocardial infarction (22%)
- stroke (33%)
- cardiovascular death (37%)
- overt nephropathy (24%)

Consider organs/problems affected by diabetes under the mnemonic 'KNIVES':

- **K**idney
- **N**erves
- **I**nfection
- **V**essels
- **E**yes
- **S**kin

20

Microvascular disease

The small vessels most affected from a clinical viewpoint are the retina, nerve sheath and kidney glomerulus. In younger patients it takes about 10 to 20 years after diagnosis for the problems of diabetic retinopathy, neuropathy and nephropathy to manifest.

Nephropathy

Prevention of diabetic nephropathy is an essential goal of treatment. Early detection of the yardstick, which is microalbuminuria, is important as the process can be reversed with optimal control, particularly of blood pressure. The dipstick method is unreliable and the preferred hospital method of 24-hour urine collection is considered impractical in general practice. Screening is done simply by a first morning urine sample to determine the albumin/creatinine ratio (see CHAPTER 31).

ACE inhibitors (or angiotensin II receptor blockers if a cough develops) should be used for evidence of hypertension.

Retinopathy and maculopathy

Retinopathy develops as a consequence of microvascular disease of the retina. Its prevalence is related to the duration of illness but up to 20% of people with type 2 diabetes have diabetic retinopathy at the time of diagnosis. The

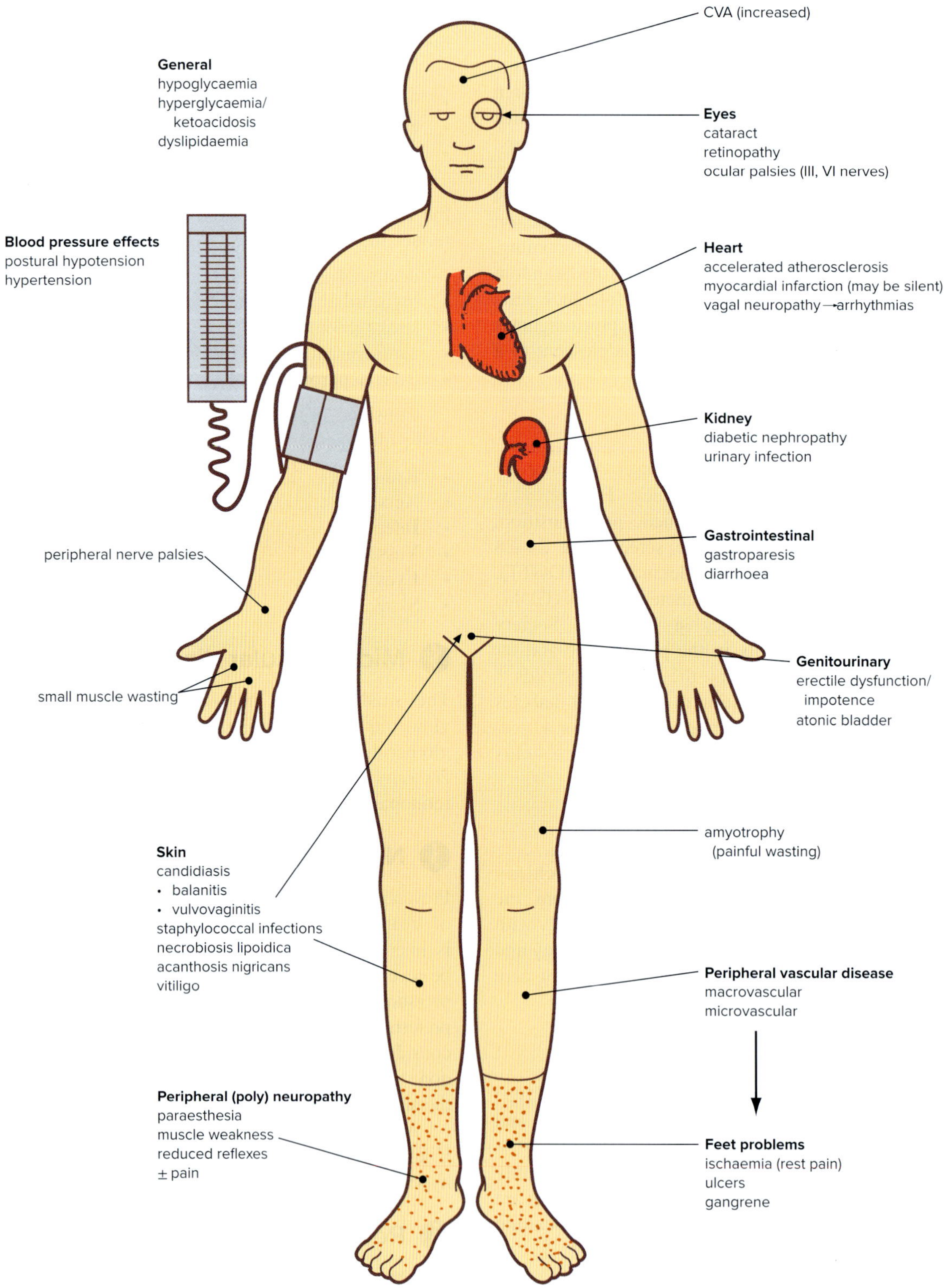

FIGURE 20.3 The complications of diabetes

European multicentre study[14,15] showed that diabetes is the single most common cause of blindness in European adults in the 16–64 years age groups. It is recommended that patients undergo fundoscopy each year by an expert. Assessment is by direct ophthalmoscopy (with dilated pupils), retinal photography or, if necessary, fluorescein angiography (depending on the state of the patient's fundi). Early diagnosis of serious retinopathy is vital since the early use of laser photocoagulation may delay and prevent visual loss.

Neuropathy

The following types of neuropathy may occur:

- radiculopathy (diabetic lumbosacral radiculoplexopathy)
- sensory polyneuropathy
- isolated mononeuropathy and multiple mononeuropathy
  - isolated peripheral nerve lesions (e.g. median nerve)
  - cranial nerve palsies (e.g. III, VI)
  - amyotrophy
- autonomic neuropathy, which may lead to:
  - erectile dysfunction
  - postural hypotension and syncope
  - impaired gastric emptying (gastroparesis)
  - diarrhoea
  - delayed or incomplete bladder emptying
  - loss of cardiac pain → 'silent' ischaemia
  - hypoglycaemic 'unawareness'
  - sudden arrest, especially under anaesthetic

Infections

People with poorly controlled diabetes are prone to infections, especially:

- skin: mucocutaneous candidiasis (e.g. balanitis, vulvovaginitis), staphylococcal infections (e.g. folliculitis)
- urinary tract: cystitis (women), pyelonephritis and perinephric abscess
- lungs: pneumonia (staphylococcal, streptococcal pneumonia), tuberculosis

Diabetic metabolic complications

- Hypoglycaemia
- Diabetic ketoacidosis
- Hyperosmolar hyperglycaemia
- Lactic acidosis

Other complications

- Cataracts
- Refractive errors of eye
- Sleep apnoea
- Depression
- Musculoskeletal: neuropathic joint damage (Charcot type arthropathy), tendon rupture
- Foot ulcers (related to neuropathy)

Prevention of diabetes

Several large studies have demonstrated it is possible to prevent or delay the onset of diabetes in those at risk.[14,15] This involves intensive lifestyle intervention in individuals who are overweight with impaired glucose tolerance or raised fasting blood glucose. One strategy is to follow the SNAP guidelines (Smoking, Nutrition, Alcohol, Physical activity). The essentials are healthy eating, weight loss and physical activity. This represents an important approach that GPs can recommend to their patients at risk. The enormous health gains which can be made in this prediabetic population by concentrating on SNAP outweigh any later health gains from diabetes medication.

Management of diabetes mellitus

The main objectives for the GP are to prevent the development of cardiovascular disease and other complications. Aim to achieve:[5]

1. reduction of 'lifestyle' risks—weight, smoking, low physical activity
2. strict glycaemic control as measured by HbA1c (target varies with circumstance, but usually ≤7%)
3. blood pressure control (≤130/80 mmHg, supine)
4. control of blood lipid levels

Note: Refer to the estimations of cardiovascular risk (see FIGs. 85.1 and 85.2 in CHAPTER 85).

Management principles

- Provide detailed and comprehensive patient education, support and reassurance.
- Achieve control of presenting symptoms.
- Achieve blood pressure control (≤130/80 mmHg supine).
- Develop a diabetes care plan.
- Emphasise the importance of the diet: good nutrition, adequate complex carbohydrates, protein, restricted fats and sugars.
- Promptly diagnose and treat urinary tract infection.
- Treat and prevent life-threatening complications of ketoacidosis or hyperosmolar coma.

- Treat and prevent hypoglycaemia in those taking insulin and oral hypoglycaemic agents.
- Organise self-testing of blood glucose for those on insulin.
- Detect and treat complications of diabetes—neuropathy, nephropathy, retinopathy, vascular disease.
- Ensure immunisation schedule, including influenza and pneumococcus, is updated.

Metabolic syndrome[8]

Beware of the deadly metabolic syndrome (syndrome X or insulin resistance syndrome).

- Upper truncal obesity (waist circumference) >102 cm ♂: >88 cm ♀ (European population) *plus* any 2 or more of the following
- ↑ triglycerides >1.7 mmol/L
- ↓ HDL cholesterol <1.0 ♂: <1.3 mmol/L ♀
- fasting glucose ≥5.5 mmol
- BP ≥130/85

This syndrome is associated with increased risk for the development of type 2 diabetes and atherosclerotic vascular disease. Aggressive treatment is required.

Monitoring techniques

- Blood glucose estimation (fasting and post-prandial)
- Urine glucose (of limited usefulness)
- Urine ketones (for type 1 diabetes)
- Glycated haemoglobin (HbA1c) (3-monthly)
- Microalbuminuria (usually urine ACR, regarded as an early and reversible indicator of nephropathy)
- Blood pressure
- Serum lipid levels
- Kidney function (serum urea/creatinine eGFR)
- ECG

Control guidelines are summarised in FIGURE 20.4 and TABLE 20.4.

The reference ranges vary in different laboratories.

Blood glucose monitoring at home

This is done using a glucose meter (glucometer). A wide variety of meters and smart phone apps are available: patients will require advice about what suits them.

How often and when?

- Type 1 diabetes:
  - four times a day (before meals and before bedtime) at first and for problems
  - twice a day (at least once)
  - may settle for 1–2 times a week (if good control)

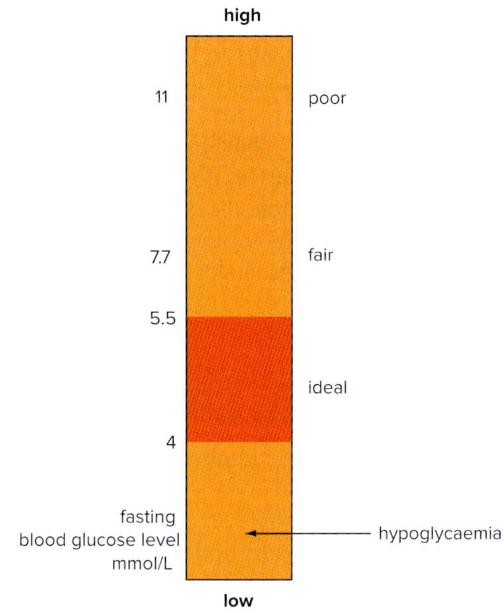

FIGURE 20.4 Control guidelines for diabetic management

Table 20.4 Suggested guidelines for glycaemic control (blood glucose mmol/L)[5,6,16]

	Ideal	Suboptimal or unacceptable
Before meals (fasting)	<5.5	>7.7
After meals (2 hours post-prandial)	<7	>11
HbA1c %*	<7	>11

*HbA1c is an index of the mean plasma glucose levels over the preceding 2–3 months (assume a reference range of 4.5–8%).

Goals of management[5,6]

All people with diabetes should be encouraged to maintain the following goals for optimum management of their diabetes:

• Blood glucose (fasting)	ideal 4–6 mmol/L NHMRC 6–8 mmol/L
• Blood glucose (postprandial)	8–10 mmol/L
• HbA1c	≤7% (53 mmol/mol)
• Total cholesterol	<4.0 mmol/L
• LDL cholesterol	<2.0 mmol/L
• HDL cholesterol	≥1.0 mmol/L
• non-HDL-C	<2.5 mmol/L
• triglycerides	<2.0 mmol/L
• Blood pressure	<130/80 mmHg without proteinuria ≤125/75 mmHg with proteinuria (1 g/day)

• BMI	18–25 where practicable
• Urinary albumin excretion	<20 mcg/min timed overnight collection <20 mg/L spot collection
• Albumin creatinine ratio	<2.5 mg/mmol—men <3.5 mg/mmol—women
• Cigarette consumption	zero
• Alcohol intake	≤2 standard drinks, 20 g/day (men and women)
• Exercise	at least 30 minutes walking (or equivalent) 5 or more days/week (total 150 minutes/week)

- Type 2 diabetes:
  - important for those on insulin, less important for oral medication (where monitoring HbA1c, gives similar outcomes in most circumstances)
  - more useful for pregnant women, frail elderly, heavy machinery operators or symptomatic hypoglycaemia

Note:

- Capillary blood glucose is approximately 7% higher than venous blood.
- Glucometer error is usually ± 5%.

Glycated haemoglobin

Glycated haemoglobin is abnormally high in diabetics with persistent hyperglycaemia and is reflective of their metabolic control. The major form of glycohaemoglobin is haemoglobin A1c, which normally comprises 4–6% of the total haemoglobin.[4] Glycohaemoglobins have a long half-life and their measure reflects the mean plasma glucose levels over the past 2–3 months and hence provides a good method of assessing overall diabetic control. It should be checked every 3–6 months.

Type 1 diabetes

The three main objectives of the treatment of type 1 diabetes are:

- maintain good health, free from the problems of hyperglycaemia and hypoglycaemia
- achieve proper growth and maturation for children and protect the fetus and mother in a mother with type 1 diabetes
- prevent, arrest or delay long-term macrovascular and microvascular complications

Insulin regimens for type 1 diabetes[5,8]

The most commonly used insulin injection preparations are the 'artificial' human insulins. Insulins are classified according to their time course of action:

- rapid-acting and short duration (ultra-short)—insulin lispro, insulin aspart
- short-acting—neutral (regular, soluble)
- intermediate-acting—isophane (NPH) or lente
- long-acting—ultralente, insulin detemir, insulin glargine
- pre-mixed short/intermediate—biphasic (neutral + isophane)

Also: continuous subcutaneous insulin infusion.

Starting insulin[8]

For less experienced GPs, shared care with an endocrinologist is recommended.

It is important to use the simplest regimen for the patient and to provide optimal education about its administration and monitoring. Full replacement of insulin is achieved by using 2, 3 or 4 injections per day. See TABLE 20.5 for available insulins.

1 *The pre-mixed 2 injection (biphasic) system*
Give twice daily, 30 minutes before breakfast and before evening meal (e.g. Mixtard 30/70, Humulin 30/70—the most common)
   - Typical starting dose: 0.3 IU/kg/day—for a 70 kg person use 10 units bd

2 *3 injections per day*
   - Short-acting insulin before breakfast and lunch
   - Intermediate- or long-acting insulin before evening meal

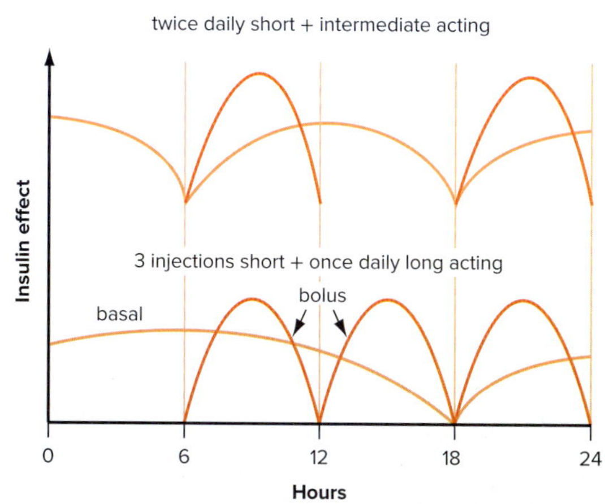

FIGURE 20.5 Illustration of time course of insulin injections regimens

3 *4 injections (basal-bolus) system*
- Short-acting insulin before breakfast, lunch and dinner (bolus)
- Intermediate-acting or long-acting insulin at bedtime (basal)

Insulin requirements often vary significantly even in the same individual under different lifestyle conditions. The rapid-acting analogues can be taken with meals.

Methods of giving insulin injections

When

Get the patient to develop a set routine, such as eating meals on time and giving the injection about 30 minutes before the meal.

Where

Into subcutaneous tissue—the best place is the abdomen. The leg is also acceptable. It is advisable to keep to one area such as the abdomen and avoid injections into the arms, near joints and the groin. The injection should be given at a different place each time, keeping a distance of 3 cm or more from the previous injection. This reduces the risk of the development of lipodystrophy. The means of delivery is the insulin syringe or the insulin delivery pen.

How

Pinch a large area of skin on the abdomen between the thumb and fingers and insert the needle straight in. After withdrawing the needle, press down firmly (do not rub or massage) over the injection site for 30 seconds. Alcohol swabs are unnecessary.

Guidelines for the patient[5]

- Take your insulin every day, even if you feel ill.
- Do not change your dose unless instructed by your doctor or you are competent to do so yourself.

Problems

Injection sites should be inspected regularly because lipohypertrophy or lipoatrophy can occur.

Sick days

Have a prearranged action plan.

Never omit the insulin dose even if the illness is accompanied by nausea, vomiting or marked anorexia. More top-up insulin is usually required (rapid/fast acting).

Maintain glucose. Keep regular blood glucose checks (a concern if >15 mmol/L).

Seek support and help.

Table 20.5 Available insulins[5,8]

Type	Brand name
Ultra-short-acting (peak 1 hour, duration 3.5–4.5 hours)	
Insulin lispro	Humalog*
Insulin aspart	NovoRapid**
Insulin glulisine	Apidra*
Short-acting (peak 2–5 hours, duration 6–8 hours)	
Neutral (regular)	Actrapid**
	Humulin R*
	Hypurin Neutral*
Intermediate-acting (duration 12–24 hours)	
Isophane (NPH)	Humulin NPH*
	Protaphane**
	Hypurin Isophane
Long-acting (analogues)	
Insulin glargine (duration 24–36 hours)	Lantus
Insulin detemir (duration up to 24 hours)	Levemir
Premixed (short- and intermediate or long-acting)	
Lispro 25%/Protamine 75%	Humalog Mix 25*
Lispro 50%/Protamine 50%	Humalog Mix 50*
Insulin aspart 30%/Protamine 70%	NovoMix 30**
Neutral 30%/Isophane 70%	Humulin 30/70*
	Mixtard 30/70**
Neutral 50%/Isophane 50%	Mixtard 50/50**

*Available in cartridges for use in pen injectors

**Available in cartridges for use in pen injectors or in disposable insulin pens

Sport

Encourage sporting activities. Careful planning (use expert help) and monitoring of blood sugar is required. Insulin doses may need to be adjusted before activities.

Additional carbohydrate may be needed.

Glycaemic targets for adults with type 1 diabetes

- HbA1c – 7% (53 mmol/mol)
- Blood glucose – fasting preprandial 4–7 mmoL/L
  – postprandial 5–10 mmoL/L

Type 2 diabetes[8,16]

First-line treatment (especially if obese):

- diet therapy
- exercise program

Most symptoms improve within 1–4 weeks on diet and exercise.[3] Prescribe and ask about exercise at every visit. Aim for an average of 20–30 minutes a day. Suggest variations such as social-type exercises. The secret to success is patient adherence through good education and supervision. The role of a diabetic education service, especially with a dietitian, can be invaluable. If unsatisfactory control persists after 3–6 months, consider adding an oral hypoglycaemic agent (see TABLE 20.6). The usual first-line agent is metformin, which reduces insulin resistance. If glycaemic targets are not achieved on monotherapy,

Table 20.6 Commonly prescribed oral hypoglycaemic agents[8] (with examples)

Drug	Duration of action (hours)	Daily dose range	Notes including main generic adverse effects
Metformin (a biguanide)	12 (also slow-release daily dosage)	0.5–3 g	Side effects: • GIT disturbances (e.g. diarrhoea, a/n/v) • avoid in cardiac, hepatic and kidney disease (eGFR <30) • lactic acidosis, a rare but serious complication
Sulfonylureas			
Gliclazide	18–24	40–320 mg	Hypoglycaemia most common side effect Others: weight gain (common), rash and GIT (rare) Shorter acting sulfonylurea is preferred in elderly
Glipizide	16–24	2.5–40 mg	Longer acting potent ones cause troublesome hypoglycaemia in elderly
Glibenclamide	18–24	2.5–20 mg	
Glimepiride	>24	1–4 mg	
α-glucosidase inhibitors			
Acarbose	3	150–600 mg	Flatulence, skin rashes, diarrhoea, liver effects
Thiazolidinediones (glitazones)			Dubious mortality benefit. Caution with heart failure.
Pioglitazone	24	15–45 mg	Oedema, weight gain, heart failure
Rosiglitazone	24	4–8 mg	Hepatic effects, fracture risks
DPP-4 inhibitors (gliptins)			Slight pancreatitis risk
sitagliptin	>24	25–100 mg	Rhinorrhoea, headache hypersensitivity, e.g. urticaria
linagliptin	>24	5 mg	
saxagliptin	24	5 mg	
vildagliptin	>24	50–100 mg	Dizziness, fatigue
$SGLT_2$ inhibitors			Modest short-term efficacy
canagliflozin	24	100–300 mg	A type of diuretic, beware kidney failure
dapagliflozin	24	5–10 mg	• genitourinary infections • dehydration, dizziness, hypoglycaemia

20

usual practice is to add in a secretagogue, such as a sulfonylurea, which increases insulin production. Newer agents include DPP-4 inhibitors (oral gliptins), SGLT2 inhibitors (the gliflozins) and incretin mimetics (by injection).

Consider metformin as the first-line agent for all patients with type 2 diabetes, irrespective of their weight, unless contraindicated. The usual starting dose is 500 mg once or twice daily. It has proven benefits over the sulphonylureas, especially in those that are overweight. Other benefits include no significant weight gain, no hypoglycaemia and an improved lipid profile. If monotherapy does not provide adequate glycaemic control, a combination of metformin with a sulfonylurea or other agent (see FIG. 20.6) is recommended.[17]

When the first oral hypoglycaemics fail (secondary failure) one of the new agents can be added (e.g. a gliptin, acarbose, one of the glitazones). The glitazones can be used as monotherapy but are used more often in combination with metformin, sulfonylureas or insulin

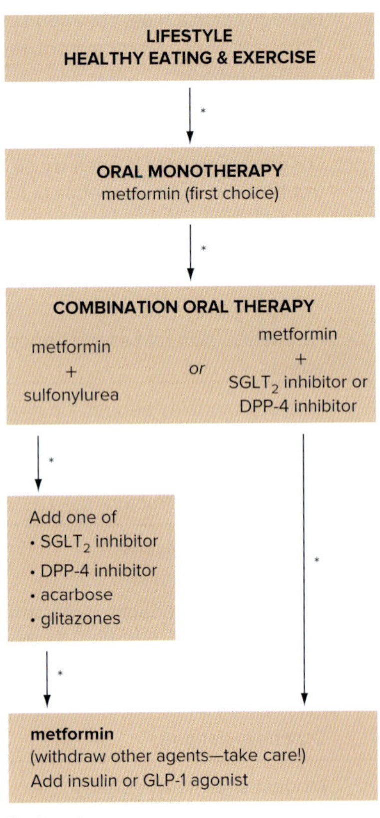

FIGURE 20.6 Step-up approach to management of type 2 diabetes[8]

but not rosiglitazone.[16] The newest treatment options in type 2 diabetes include:[17]

- dipeptidyl peptidase-IV (DDP-IV) inhibitors known as gliptins, such as sitagliptin
- sodium glucose cotransporter 2 (SGLT2) inhibitors taken orally, e.g. dapagliflozin, canagliflozin
- glucagon-like peptide-1 receptor (GLP-1) agonist (e.g. exanatide—twice daily dosing, liraglutide—daily dosing) given by SC injection. These improve satiety and are associated with weight loss. Nausea is fairly common, but tends to settle. Pancreatitis is a rare but important side effect.

The classic symptoms of hyperglycaemia may be present but more commonly patients experience general disability. Approximately 30% of type 2 patients eventually require insulin even after years of successful oral therapy. An algorithm for the management of type 2 diabetes is presented in FIGURE 20.6.

It is important not to delay the introduction of insulin. However, insulin will not substitute for healthy eating and activity.

Starting insulin in type 2 diabetes[14,18]

More than 30% of patients will eventually require insulin, often after 10–15 years of successful oral therapy.[8] Before commencing insulin one should be assured that the patient's lifestyle activities are being adequately addressed and that oral medication (at recommended maximum dose) is appropriate. There is no clear-cut rule about when to start insulin for patients with HbA1c >7%, but this can be as early as when drug therapy does not provide adequate control. Two golden rules are 'don't delay initiating basal insulin' and then 'start low and go slow'.[18]

When commencing patients on insulin, reassure them that the injections are not as uncomfortable as finger pricks and that they will feel much improved with more energy.

It is appropriate to refer to your diabetic team for shared care at this point—when starting insulin.

Suggested stepwise approach[14,16]

Step 1

- Continue oral agents: metformin + sulfonylurea ± glitazone or acarbose or DPP-4 inhibitor (limited to 3).
- Add 10 units isophane insulin at bedtime.

Step 2

- Titrate insulin therapy according to fasting blood glucose (6 mmol/L).
- Increase insulin in about 4–5 U increments every 3–4 days (or more gradually).
- Cease glitazone, acarbose, gliptin or $SGLT_2$ inhibitor (if used).

Step 3

If larger doses of insulin are required (NPH or mixed regimen), gradually withdraw sulfonylurea, continue metformin and review.

Note: The combination of a glitazone and insulin has been shown to improve control of diabetes sometimes to the extent of being able to reduce insulin dosage. In patients with type 2 diabetes needing relatively high doses of insulin, the addition of a glitazone is worth considering.

The importance of diet and nutrition

Nutrition management is based on controlling weight, having a healthy eating plan and supplementing it with exercise. It is recommended to eat a wide variety from all food groups:

- protein 10–20%, fat 20–40%, carbohydrate 35–60%
- reduce fat, especially saturated fats, sugar and alcohol

People with type 1 diabetes often require three meals and sometimes regular snacks each day. People with type 2 usually require less food intake and restriction of total food intake.

Principles of dietary management

- Keep to a regular nutritious diet.
- Achieve ideal body weight.
- Reduce calories (kilojoules), particularly:
  - added sugar
  - dietary fat
- Follow the glycaemic index values (see www.glycaemicindex.com).
- Increase proportions of vegetables, fresh fruit and cereal foods.
- Special diabetic foods are not necessary
- 'Whole foods' are preferred to supplements
- Qualitative diets are often more sustainable than quantitative diets (such as 'exchanges' or 'portions')

The importance of exercise[5,16]

Exercise is fundamental to good management. Exercise is any physical activity that keeps you fit. Good examples are brisk walking (e.g. 2 km per day), jogging, tennis, skiing and aerobics. Aim for at least 30 minutes three times a week, but daily exercise is ideal. Go slow when you start and increase your pace gradually.

Psychosocial considerations

The psychological and social factors involving the patient are very influential on outcome. Considerable support and counselling is necessary to help both patient and family cope with the 'distress' of the diagnosis and the discipline required for optimal control of their blood glucose. Reasons for poor dietary compliance and insulin administration must be determined and mobilisation of a supportive multidisciplinary network (where practical) is most helpful. The GP should be the pivot of the team. Encourage joining a self-support group where available.

Foot care

Foot problems are one of the commonest complications that need special attention; prevention is the appropriate approach. Pressure sores can develop on the soles of the feet from corns, calluses, ill-fitting footwear, and stones and nails. Minor injuries such as cuts can become a major problem through poor healing. Infection of wounds is a major problem. Check the patient's footwear.

Control of hypertension

Studies have highlighted the importance of blood pressure control to reduce macrovascular and microvascular complications in diabetes patients.[19] Their blood vessels (both macro and micro) are more susceptible to hypertensive, namely >130/85 mmHg, damage. Try non-pharmacological measures first.

Preferred pharmacological agents are ACE inhibitors or ARBs and calcium-channel blockers.[6,16]

Current recommendations are for tight control of blood pressure to below a threshold of 130/80 mmHg in patients with uncomplicated diabetes.[16]

However, this may be an inappropriately low target for those at risk of postural hypotension, particularly the elderly.

Getting to target blood pressure (<130/80 mmHg)*

Step 1: Diet, exercise, weight control
Step 2: ACEI or ARB
Step 3: ACEI/ARB and diuretic
Step 4: Beta blocker
ARB = angiotensin II receptor blocker

* <125/75 mmHg if proteinurea >1 g/day (ACR >70) present

Control of dyslipidaemia[5,16]

Mixed hyperlipidaemia is a common finding in patients with diabetes. Dyslipidaemia (especially hypercholesterolaemia) is an independent risk factor for the macrovascular complications of diabetes, and proper control is important. Non-pharmacological measures should be tried first. The preferred agents are HMG-CoA reductase inhibitors and resins for hypercholesterolaemia, and fibrates and resins for mixed hyperlipidaemia.

Targets should be:

- total cholesterol: <4 mmol/L
- triglycerides: <1.5 mmol/L
- HDL cholesterol: ≥1 mmol/L
- LDL cholesterol: <2.0 mmol/L

Management in summary[19]

The ABC of diabetic care is summarised in TABLE 20.7. A key to ongoing control of diabetes is to maintain the HbA1c at or below 7%, and recognising that it is cardiovascular disease that causes most of the complications and excess mortality in type 2 diabetes. In patient review, the National Health and Medical Research Council (NHMRC) guidelines emphasise lifestyle review as step one.[16] A useful lifestyle evaluation mnemonic is NEAT:

- **N**utrition—eat less, reach ideal weight, healthy low fat/complex carbohydrate diet
- **E**xercise—including 'walk more', interesting physical activities
- **A**voidance of toxins—alcohol, tobacco, salt, sugar, illicit drugs
- **T**ranquillity—rest, recreation and stress reduction

Antihypertensives and statins have an important role in management. A meta-analysis of the use of low-dose aspirin (acetyl salicylic acid 75–150 mg/day) showed secondary risk reduction in people with diabetes and a history of a cardiovascular event (AMI or CVA).[20]

Table 20.7 The ABC of diabetes care[3]

Risk factor	Target
Hb**A**1c	<7%
BP	<130/80*
Cholesterol	<4 mmol/L**
Smoking	Quit

* <125/75 if proteinuria exists
** corresponding to LDL cholesterol <2.0 mmol/L

A type 2 diabetes 'polypill' has been advocated for most people with diabetes.[21] The suggested pill mix is *metformin, an ACE inhibitor, a statin and aspirin.*

Metabolic complications of diabetes

Hypoglycaemia

Hypoglycaemia[5,8] occurs when blood glucose levels fall to less than 3.0 mmol/L. It is more common with treated type 1 diabetes but can occur in type 2 diabetes patients on oral hypoglycaemic drugs, notably sulfonylureas (metformin hardly ever causes hypoglycaemia). It is appropriate to ask often about symptoms of hypoglycaemia: 'recurrent hypoglycaemia begets hypoglycaemic unawareness'.

Clinical variations

1. Classic warning symptoms: sweating, tremor, palpitations, hunger, peri-oral paraesthesia. Usually treated with refined carbohydrate (e.g. glucose; sugar or honey in the mouth).
2. Rapid loss of consciousness, usually without warning
3. Coma: stuporose, comatose or 'strange' behaviour

For mild cases give something sweet by mouth, followed by a snack.

Treatment of hypoglycaemia requires one dose of carbohydrate.

Dose: (one of)

- 2 barley sugars
- 6 jelly beans
- glass of lemonade
- teaspoon of honey

Take one dose, and don't repeat unless still unwell 10 minutes later. Follow with a complex carbohydrate meal.

Treatment (severe cases or patient unconscious)

Treatment of choice

20–30 mL 50% glucose IV until fully conscious (instil rectally using the nozzle of the syringe if IV access difficult). Usually 10 mL in children.

or

(alternative) 1 mL glucagon IM or SC

Admit to hospital if concerned (rarely necessary). Ascertain cause of the hypoglycaemia and instruct the patient how to avoid a similar situation in the future.

Diabetic ketoacidosis[5]

This life-threatening emergency requires intensive management. It usually occurs during an illness (e.g. gastroenteritis) when insulin is omitted. It can also occur in Type 2 diabetes.

Clinical features

- Develops over a few days, but may occur in a few hours in 'brittle' diabetics
- Preceded by polyuria, polydipsia, drowsiness
- Vomiting and abdominal pain
- Hyperventilation—severe acidosis (acidotic breathing)
- Ketonuria

Management

- Arrange urgent hospital admission.
- Give 10 units rapid-acting insulin IM (not SC).
- Commence IV infusion of normal saline.

Tip: The comatose patient requires water, sodium (3L N saline), potassium (KCl) and insulin.

Hyperosmolar hyperglycaemia[5]

Patients with this problem may present with an altered conscious state varying from stupor to coma and with marked dehydration. The onset may be insidious over a period of weeks, with fatigue, polyuria and polydipsia. The key features are marked hyperglycaemia and dehydration without ketoacidosis. It occurs typically in uncontrolled type 2 diabetes, especially in elderly patients. Sometimes they have previously undiagnosed diabetes. There may be evidence of an underlying disorder such as pneumonia or a urinary infection. The essential findings are extreme hyperglycaemia and high plasma osmolarity. The condition has a high mortality—even higher than ketoacidosis.

Treatment

- IV fluids, e.g. normal to ½ normal saline, given slowly
- Insulin—relatively lower doses than acidosis

Lactic acidosis[5,8]

Patients with lactic acidosis present with marked hyperventilation 'air hunger' and confusion. It has a high mortality rate and must be considered in the very ill diabetic patient taking metformin, especially if kidney function is impaired. The risk of lactic acidosis is low if the therapeutic dose of metformin is not exceeded. The investigations reveal blood acidosis (low pH), low bicarbonate, high serum lactate, absent serum ketones and a large anion gap. Treatment is based on removal of the cause, rehydration and alkalinisation with IV sodium bicarbonate.

Other issues in diabetic patients

Erectile dysfunction[8]

The prevalence of erectile dysfunction in men with type 2 diabetes over 40 years may be as high as 50%. It may be caused by macrovascular disease, pelvic autonomic neuropathy or psychological causes. Those with organic-based ED may benefit from appropriate counselling and (if not taking nitrates) one of the phosphodiesterase inhibitors, starting with a low dose. The risk of cardiovascular disease needs to be evaluated.

Female sexual dysfunction

Autonomic dysfunction may result in reduced vaginal lubrication with arousal in women, but not the degree of sexual dysfunction that affects men. Appropriate education, reassurance and the use of lubricants should be helpful.

20

Postural hypotension[8]

Autonomic neuropathy-related postural hypotension may be compounded by medication, including antihypertensives and anti-angina agents. The usual strict blood pressure targets may need to be relaxed, particularly in the elderly. Persistent problems may be helped by graduated compression stockings to decrease venous pooling. If it continues to be a severe problem, the use of oral fludrocortisone may be helpful.

Gastroparesis

Symptoms of gastroparesis (due to autonomic neuropathy) with decreased gastric emptying include a sensation of fullness, dysphagia, reflux or recurrent nausea and vomiting, especially after meals. Treatment options include medication with domperidone, cisapride or erythromycin. Injections of botulinum toxin type A into the pylorus via gastroscopy may facilitate gastric emptying.

Diabetes and driving[5]

Diabetes may impair driving via hypoglycaemia (due to medication) or complications (particularly visual impairment). *Assessing Fitness to Drive 2016* outlines the specific legal obligations of medical practitioners for assessing drivers of private and commercial vehicles. Patients are obligated to provide details to the driver licensing authority and to their vehicle insurance company. In general terms, people controlled by diet alone have no restrictions for driving whereas those on insulin may obtain a conditional licence subject to annual or 2-yearly review. The main specific risk is hypoglycaemic episodes. Further details can be found at: www.austroads.com.au/drivers-vehicles/assessing-fitness-to-drive.

Contraception

Long-acting reversible contraceptives (e.g. Implanon, Mirena) or the combined oral contraceptive pill are appropriate options for birth control in women not interested in permanent sterilisation. Bear in mind the possibility of polycystic ovarian syndrome.

The future[5,17]

- Use of immunosuppressants and immunomodulators for type 1 diabetes
- Increased availability of glucagon-like and amylin-like peptides for type 2 diabetes
- Continuous implantable venous glucose monitoring
- Closed-loop sensor-and-insulin-delivery devices ('the artificial pancreas')
- Combination 'type 2 polypill'
- Inhaled insulin
- Transplantation:
  - combined kidney/pancreas
  - islet cells

Treatment errors and pitfalls[16]

- Avoid prescribing oral hypoglycaemic agents prematurely. Allow a reasonable trial of diet and exercise for type 2 patients, especially if they are overweight.
- Review the need for continued oral therapy after 3 months of treatment.
- Glucose tolerance tests should be avoided if the diagnosis can be made on the basis of symptoms and fasting, or random blood sugar or HbA1c (a glucose load carries a small risk of hyperosmolar coma).
- Keep an eye on the development of ketones in type 1 patients by checking urinary ketones and, if present, watch carefully because diabetic ketoacidosis is a life-threatening emergency.

When to refer[8]

- Type 1 diabetic patients for specialist evaluation and then 1- to 2-yearly review
- Type 2 diabetic patients: will depend on the GP's comfort level and experience. Particularly consider:
  - young patients
  - those requiring insulin
  - those with complications
- For ophthalmological screening: every 2 years to inspect retina (or use retinal photography)
- Diabetics with treatable complications, including:
  - retinopathy
  - nephropathy
  - neuropathy: test annually

Shared care

The management of the diabetic patient provides an ideal opportunity for shared care between a cooperative team comprising the patient, the GP and the specialist diabetic team. The objective is to encourage patients to attend their own doctor for primary care and be less reliant on hospital outpatient services or the diabetic clinics. A well-coordinated arrangement with good communication strategies provides optimal opportunities for the ongoing education of the patient, the GP and the specialist diabetic team.

Practice tips

- Many cases of type 2 diabetes remain undiagnosed, so vigilance is important.
- Follow-up programs should keep to a prepared format. Example formats are presented in TABLES 20.8 and 20.9.
- Hyperglycaemia is a common cause of tiredness. If elderly people with type 2 diabetes are very tired, think of hyperglycaemia and consider giving insulin to improve their symptoms.
- The management of the diabetic patient is a team effort involving family members, a nurse education centre, podiatrists, domiciliary nursing service, GP and consultant.
- If a person with diabetes (particularly type 1) is very drowsy and looks sick, consider first the diagnosis of ketoacidosis.
- Foot care is vital: always examine the feet when the patient comes in for review.
- Treat associated hypertension with ACE inhibitors or a calcium-channel blocker (also good in combination).
- Use a team approach and encourage joining special support groups (e.g. Diabetes Australia).
- 'Never let the sun go down on pus in a diabetic foot'—admit to hospital.[17]

- If a foot ulcer hasn't healed in 6 weeks, exclude osteomyelitis. Arrange for an MRI and investigate the vasculature.
- Prevention/detection of coronary heart disease should be an integral part of all consultations.

Table 20.8	Diabetes control: 3-monthly review

Discourage smoking and alcohol.
Review symptoms.
Review nutrition.
Check weight (BMI), BP, urine.
Review self-monitoring.
Review exercise and physical activity.
Review HbA1c (test at least every 6 months).
Review lipid levels (test every 12 months).

Table 20.9	Diabetes control: an annual review program[5]

1 History

Smoking and alcohol use
Symptoms of hypoglycaemia, hyperglycaemia
Check symptoms relating to eyes, circulation, feet*
Immunisation

2 Examinations

Weight, height, BMI
Blood pressure—standing and lying
Examine heart*
Carotid and peripheral pulses*
Eyes:
- visual acuity (Snellen chart)
- ? cataracts
- optic fundi (or ophthalmologist referral)*
- ? diabetic retinal photography

Tendon reflexes and sensation for peripheral neuropathy*
Skin (general)
Foot examination including footwear*
Check injection sites
Urine examination: albumin, ketones, glucose

3 Review biochemical levels

* These items comprise a program for detection of long-term complications. They should be conducted annually, commencing 5 years after diagnosis.

Patient education resources

Hand-out sheets from *Murtagh's Patient Education* 7th edition:
- Diabetes
- Diabetes: blood glucose monitoring at home
- Diabetes: foot care for diabetics
- Diabetes: healthy diet for diabetes
- Diabetes: insulin injections
- Diabetes: type 1
- Diabetes: type 2

References

1 UKPDS Group. Complications in newly diagnosed type 2 diabetic patients and their association with different clinical and biochemical risk factors. Diabetes Res, 1990; 13: 1–11.
2 Australian Bureau of Statistics. *National Health Survey: First Results, 2014–15*. December 2015. Available from: <www.abs.gov.au/ausstats/abs@.nsf/PrimaryMainFeatures/4364.0.55.001?OpenDocument>, accessed February 2018.
3 Phillips P. Diabetes. Check Program, Unit 401. Melbourne: RACGP, 2005: 4–20.
4 Welborn TA. Diabetic mellitus. In: *MIMS Disease Index* (2nd edn). Sydney: IMS Publishing, 1996: 149–52.
5 RACGP. *General Practice Management of Type 2 Diabetes: 2016–18*. East Melbourne, 2016 (book available from <www.diabetesaustralia.com.au> or <www.racgp.org.au>).
6 RACGP. *Guidelines for Preventive Activities in General Practice* (the red book) (9th edn). East Melbourne, 2016: 8.4. Available from: <www.racgp.org.au/guidelines/redbook>, accessed February 2018.
7 Welborn T et al. National Diabetic Study. Metabolism, 1997; 1: 1–3.
8 Moulds R (Chairman). *Therapeutic Guidelines: Endocrinology* (Version 5). Melbourne: Therapeutic Guidelines Ltd, 2013.
9 Sinah R et al. Diabetes in childhood obesity. N Engl J Med, 2002; 346: 802–10.
10 Nankervis A et al. ADIPS Consensus Guidelines for the Testing and Diagnosis of Hyperglycaemia in Pregnancy in Australia and New Zealand. Modified November 2014. Available from: <www.ranzcog.edu.au/RANZCOG_SITE/media/RANZCOG-MEDIA/Women%27s%20Health/ADIPS-GDM-Guidelines-2014.pdf?ext=.pdf>, accessed February 2018.
11 UK Prospective Diabetes Study Group. Tight blood pressure control and risk of macrovascular and microvascular complications in type 2 diabetes (UKPDS 38). BMJ, 1998; 317: 703–13.
12 Hypertension Expert Working Group. Evidence based guideline for the diagnosis and management of hypertension in type 2 diabetes. National evidence based guidelines for the management of type 2 diabetes mellitus. Draft for public consultation. Sydney: Australian Centre for Diabetes Strategies, Prince of Wales Hospital, January 2001.
13 Heart Outcomes Prevention Evaluation (HOPE) Study Investigators. Effects of ramipril on cardiovascular and microvascular outcomes in people with diabetes mellitus: results of the HOPE study and MICRO-HOPE substudy. Lancet, 2000; 355: 253–9.
14 Managing type 2 diabetes. NPS News, 2005; 39: I–VI.
15 Vaag A et al. Metabolic impact of a family history of type 2 diabetes. Results from a European multicentre study. Sisätautien Klinikka, 2001: 65.
16 National Health and Medical Research Council. *Evidence based Guidelines for the Management of Type 2 Diabetes Mellitus*. Canberra: NHMRC, 2005.

17 Newnham H. Diabetes in motion. Proceedings of the 27th Annual Update Course for General Practitioners. Monash University, 2005.

18 Goudswaard AN, Furlong NJ, Rutten GE et al. Insulin monotherapy versus combinations of insulin with oral hypoglycaemic agents in patients with type 2 diabetes mellitus. *Cochrane Database Syst Rev.* October 2004; 18(4): CD003418.

19 New Zealand Guidelines Group. Evidence-based best practice guidelines. Management of type 2 diabetes. Wellington: New Zealand Guidelines Group, 2003.

20 Colwell JA. Aspirin therapy in diabetes. Diabetes Care, 2001; 24: 62–3.

21 Phillips P, Braddon J. The type 2 tablet. Evidence-based medication for type 2 diabetes. Aust Fam Physician, 2003; 32: 431–6.

Drug and alcohol problems

21

A custome loathsome to the eye, hateful to the nose, harmeful to the braine, dangerous to the lungs and the blacke stinking fume thereof, neerest resembling the horrible Stigian smoke of the bottomless pit.

JAMES I (1566–1625), *ON SMOKING*

Ecstasy: a drug so strong it makes white people think that they can dance.

LENNY HENRY (1958–)

If you want to keep a dead man, put him in whisky; if you want to kill a live man put whisky in him.

THOMAS GUTHRIE (1803–73)

Drug-related problems are true masquerades in family practice. This includes prescribed drugs, over-the-counter drugs and social or illegal street drugs. It is important therefore that all prescribing doctors maintain a high index of suspicion that any clinical problem may be associated with their treatment of the patient.

Adverse drug reactions

An adverse drug effect is defined as 'any unwanted effect of treatment from the medical use of drugs that occurs at a usual therapeutic dose'. Almost every drug can cause an adverse reaction, which must be elicited in the history. Any substance that produces beneficial therapeutic effects may also produce unwanted, adverse or toxic effects. The severity of the reaction may range from a mild skin rash or nausea to sudden death from anaphylaxis. A study has shown that the incidence of adverse reactions increases from about 3% in patients 10–20 years of age to about 20% in patients 80–89 years of age.[1]

Reactions can be classified in several ways—side effects, overdosage, intolerance, hypersensitivity and idiosyncrasy. However, a useful classification of unwanted effects is divided into type A and type B.

Type A reactions are the most common and involve *augmented pharmacology;* that is, they are caused by unwanted, albeit predictable, effects of the drug. Examples include:

- constipation due to verapamil
- blurred vision and urinary outflow problems due to tricyclic antidepressants
- hyperuricaemia due to thiazide diuretics

Type A reactions are dose-dependent.

Type B reactions are idiosyncratic. The reactions are unpredictable from known properties of the drug. Examples include hepatotoxicity and blood dyscrasias.

Golden rules for prevention of adverse effects

Before prescribing any drug the prescriber should consider the following rules:

1. Is the drug really necessary?
2. What will happen if it is not used?
3. What good do I hope to achieve?
4. What harm may result from this treatment?

Common adverse effects

There is an extensive list of clinical problems caused by drugs as side effects or interactions that are highlighted throughout this book. Common side effects include:

- CNS—malaise, drowsiness, fatigue/tiredness, headache, dizziness
- CVS—palpitations, peripheral oedema, hypotension
- GIT—nausea, vomiting, dyspepsia, change in bowel habit (diarrhoea, constipation)
- skin—rash, pruritus, flushing
- psychiatric/emotional—insomnia, irritability, anxiety, depression, agitation

Drugs that commonly produce adverse effects

- Antidepressants (number 1 cause): tricyclics, MAOIs, SSRIs
- Antimicrobials: penicillin/cephalosporins, sulphonamides, tetracyclines, streptomycin, ketoconazole
- Anticonvulsants: carbamazepine, phenobarbitone, phenytoin, sodium valproate

- Anti-inflammatories and analgesics: aspirin/salicylates, opioids (e.g. codeine, morphine), NSAIDs, gold salts, DMARDs, bDMARDs
- Antihypertensive agents: several
- Cardiac agents: digoxin, quinidine, amiodarone, other antiarrhythmics
- Diuretics: thiazides, frusemide
- Tranquillisers: phenothiazines, benzodiazepines, barbiturates, chlordiazepoxide
- Other drugs: cytotoxics, hormones, allopurinol, warfarin

Tobacco use

'Smoking is good for you', according to an old Arab proverb. 'The dogs will not bite you because you smell so bad; thieves will not rob you at night because you cough in your sleep and you will not suffer the indignities of old age because you will die when you are relatively young.'

Tobacco smoking is the largest single, preventable cause of death and disease in Australia. It has been estimated to have caused approximately 15 000 deaths in 2004–05, over six times the number of deaths from road accidents.[2] Diseases attributed to smoking are summarised in FIGURE 21.1. Signs of major dependence are smoking within 30 minutes of waking and ≥20 cigarettes a day.

Advice to patients (quitting)

Several studies have highlighted the value of opportunistic intervention by the family doctor. It is important not only to encourage people to quit but also to organise a quitting program and follow-up. In Australia 80% of smokers (representing about 30% of the adult population) have indicated that they wish to stop smoking. Point out that it is not easy and requires strong will power. As Mark Twain said, 'Quitting is easy—I've done it a thousand times.'

- Educate patients about the risks to their health and the many advantages of giving up smoking, and emphasise the improvement in *health, longevity, money savings, looks* and *sexuality.*
- Point out the following advantages to quitting:
  - food tastes better
  - sense of smell improves
  - exercise tolerance is better
  - sexual pleasure is improved
  - bad breath improves
  - risk of lung cancer drops: after 10–15 years of quitting it is as low as someone who has never smoked
  - early COPD can be reversed
  - decreases URTIs and bronchitis
  - chance of premature skin wrinkling and stained teeth is less
  - removes effects of passive smoking on family and friends
  - removes problem of effects on pregnancy
- The extent of nicotine dependence can be assessed using a questionnaire (based on the Fagerstrom Test) and scoring system.[3] As a baseline ask about the number of cigarettes smoked per day, how soon after waking to smoking the first cigarette of the day and any difficulties with coping with antismoking venues (e.g. cinemas, plane travel).

Intervention: the 5A framework[3]

- *Ask* about and document tobacco use at every opportunity.
- *Assess* motivation and confidence to quit: 'Are you interested in quitting?'
- *Advise* all smokers to quit (in a diplomatic way).
- *Assist* the smoker to stop with counselling and pharmacotherapy.
- *Arrange* follow-up to maintain quit advice or non-smoking.

- Ask them to keep a smoker's diary.
- If they say no to quitting, give them motivational literature and ask them to reconsider.
- If they say yes, make a contract (example below).

A contract to quit

'I .... agree to stop smoking on ....
I understand that stopping smoking is the single best thing I can do for my health and that my doctor has strongly encouraged me to quit.'
.... (Patient's signature)
.... (Doctor's signature)

- These motivated patients will require educational and behavioural strategies to help them cope with quitting. Ongoing support by their GP is very important.
- Organise joining a support group.
- Contact your local Quitline (or similar service) for information about and support for quitting, especially if smoking ≥20 cigarettes a day.

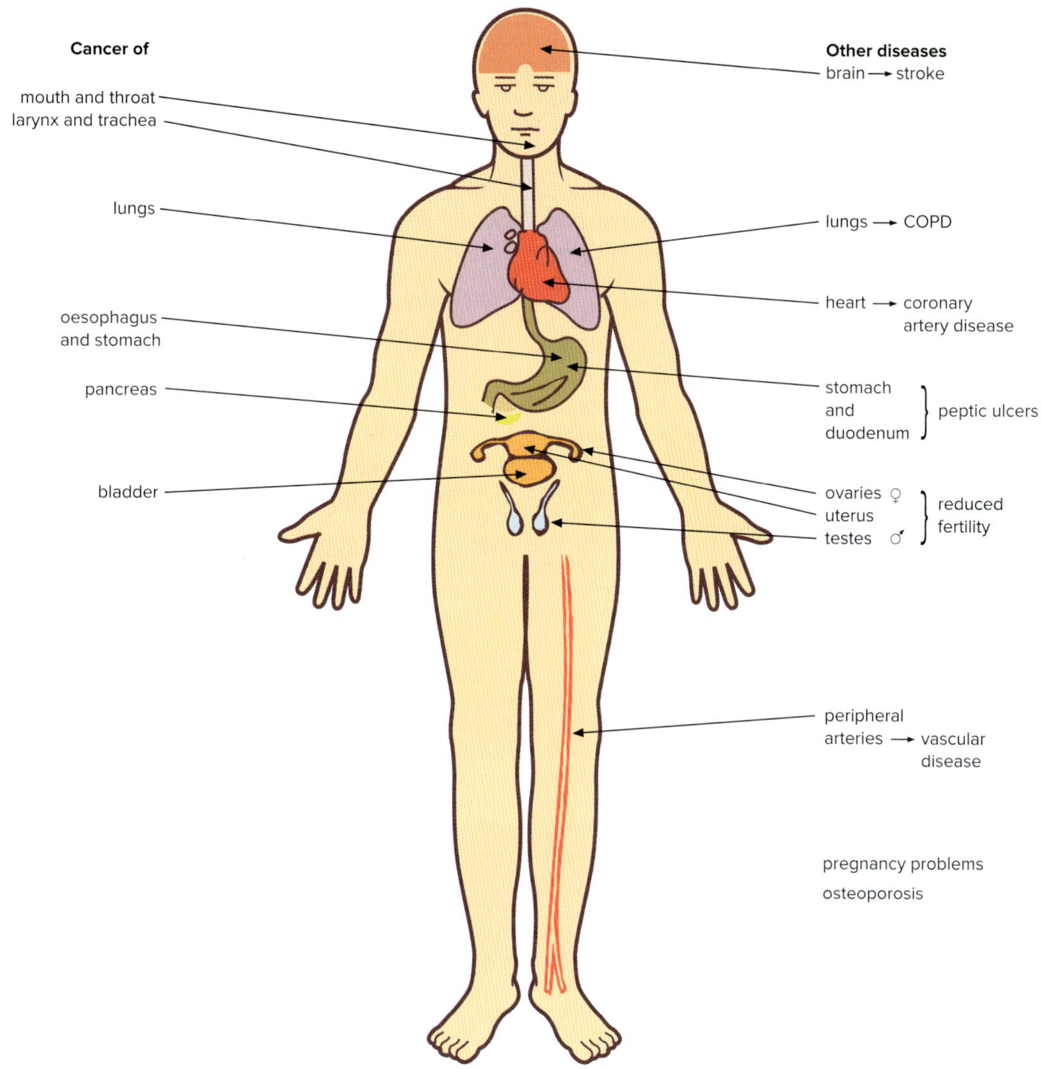

FIGURE 21.1 Possible serious adverse effects of nicotine smoking

- Arrange follow-up (very important), at least monthly, especially during first 3 months.
- Going 'cold turkey' (stopping completely) is preferable but before making the final break it can be made easier by changing to a lighter brand, inhaling less, stubbing out earlier and reducing the number. Changing to cigars or pipes is best avoided.

Withdrawal effects[3]

The initial symptoms are restlessness, cravings, hunger, irritability, poor concentration, headache and frustration (refer TABLE 21.1). After about 10 days most of these effects subside but it takes about three months for a smoker to feel relatively comfortable with not smoking any more. Nicotine replacement therapy certainly helps patients cope.

Table 21.1 Nicotine withdrawal symptoms (DSM-5)

1	Irritability, frustration or anger
2	Anxiety
3	Difficulty concentrating
4	Increased appetite
5	Restlessness
6	Depressed mood
7	Insomnia

Treatment

Pharmacological[3]

Nicotine replacement therapy (NRT), which should be used in conjunction with an educational support program, has been proved to be effective and is available as chewing gum, inhaler, oral spray, lozenges, sublingual tablets or transdermal patches (the preferred method). Ideally the nicotine should not be used longer than 3 months. Eight weeks of patch therapy is as effective as longer courses.

NRT should be directed at smokers with a moderate to high nicotine dependency who are motivated to quit. There is little evidence that drug treatment will benefit individuals with low levels of nicotine dependence who smoke fewer than 10 cigarettes a day.[4]

All forms of NRT are effective: a pooled analysis of all NRT trials showed an absolute increase in cessation at 1 year of 7% compared to placebo.[4]

NRT should start at the quit date, not while still smoking.

Nicotine gum[3]

This is available as 2 mg and 4 mg.

- Low dependence (less than 10 cigarettes per day, not needing to smoke within 30 minutes of waking): use non-pharmacological methods rather than replacement
- Moderate dependence (10–20 cigarettes per day, smoking within 30 minutes of waking): 2 mg every 1–2 hours, chew max. 8–12 pieces daily
- High dependence (>20 per day, waking at night to smoke or first thing after waking): 4 mg initially, 6–10 pieces chewed daily changing to 2 mg after 4–8 weeks (max. 12 pieces/24 hours)

Useful points:

- Chew each piece slowly for about 30 minutes.
- Ensure all the nicotine is utilised.
- Chew at least 6 pieces per day, replacing at regular intervals (not more than 1 piece per hour).
- Use for 3 months, weaning off before the end of this period.

Transdermal nicotine[3]

This is available as 16-hour or 24-hour nicotine patches in three different strengths. The patients should stop smoking immediately on use.

Recommendations:

- low to moderate dependence (10–20 cigarettes/ day): 15 mg/24 hour or 10 mg/16 hour patch, daily; aim to cease within 12 weeks
- high dependence (>20/day): 21 mg/24 hour or 15 mg/16 hour patch; change to 15 mg or 10 mg patch after 4–6 weeks; aim to cease within 12 weeks; use lower dose if patient is <45 kg or has CVS disease

Apply to non-hairy, clean, dry section of skin on upper outer arm or upper chest and leave in place for 24 hours. Rotate sites with a 7-day gap for reuse of a specific site.

Nicotine inhaler

Uses cartridges in a mouthpiece resembling smoking.

- 6–12/day for 12 weeks then taper

Nicotine oral spray

- 1 mg/spray: 1–2 sprays into mouth orally (max. 64 sprays/24 hours)

Nicotine lozenges and sublingual tablets

These are available in 2 mg and 4 mg strengths, the strength used according to the level of dependence, e.g. high dependence: suck 4 mg lozenges (max. 15/24 hours).

Combination therapy

Controlled trials have shown enhanced outcomes when nicotine patches are combined with gum or inhaler. Consider it for highly addicted smokers.

Other agents for smoking cessation[5]

Bupropion (Zyban)

This oral agent has a similar effectiveness to NRT.

Adverse effects include insomnia and dry mouth (both common), with serious effects, such as allergic reactions and increased seizure risk.[6] It is contraindicated in persons with a history of epilepsy.

Recommended dose: 150 mg (o) daily for 3 days then bd for 8 weeks.

Varenicline tartrate (Champix)[3,5]

- Commence with 0.5 mg (o) daily with food for 3 days titrating slowing to 1 mg bd by day 7 until the end of the 9-week course

It is an effective agent but there are several adverse side effects, especially nausea with a concern about neuropsychiatric effects.[6] Avoid in end-stage kidney disease and take care with diabetics.

Nortriptyline

- Start with 25 mg (o), increasing gradually to 75 mg (o) daily, starting 14 days before quit date then continue for 12 weeks

Note: Regular follow-up for all methods is essential for outcome.

Vaping

This involves inhaling and exhaling the vapour from 'electronic cigarettes' (no nicotine). Its use is controversial. There is a concern that it could be a 'gateway' to smoking in young people but there is currently no evidence for this impression. Banned by the Australian Government's Therapeutic Goods Administration (www.tga.gov.au) but legal in some countries.

Alcohol problems

Excessive drinking of alcohol is one of the most common and socially destructive problems in the world. One survey found that 5% of Australian men and 1% of women were alcohol-dependent. It also showed that 86% of men and 79% of women drink alcohol, with 8.3% of the population drinking alcohol every day.[6]

- Alcohol is estimated to have a harmful effect on about 1 in 10 people.
- At least 20–40% of acute general and psychiatric hospital admissions have an alcohol-related illness.
- About 20%-plus of fatal traffic accidents involve alcohol.
- The author's study[8] identified alcohol dependence in 9.7% of the population studied and a further group of problem drinkers that included the 'explosive' or binge drinker (see FIG. 21.2). Problem drinkers represent about 15–20% of the population.

Excessive and harmful drinking

National Health and Medical Research Council (NHMRC) revised guidelines addressing harmful drinking are presented in TABLE 21.2.[3,7]

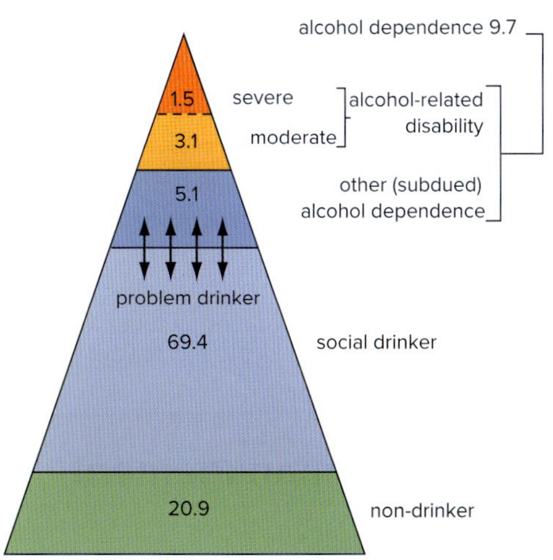

FIGURE 21.2 Prevalence of alcohol drinking patterns in the adult population (figures expressed as a percentage)

Table 21.2 Recommended guidelines to reduce health risks from drinking alcohol, NHMRC 2016[7]

Guideline 1 Reducing the risk of alcohol-related harm over a lifetime

For healthy men and women, drinking no more than 2 standard drinks on any day reduces the lifetime risk of harm from alcohol-related disease or injury.

Guideline 2 Reducing the risk of injury on a single occasion of drinking

For healthy men and women, no more than 4 standard drinks on a single occasion reduces the risk of harm arising from the occasion.

Guideline 3 For children and young people under 18 years of age not drinking alcohol is the safest option

a. Parents and carers should be advised that children <15 years are at the greatest risk of harm from drinking and that for this age group, not drinking alcohol is especially important.
b. For young people 15–17 years, the safest option is to delay the initiation of drinking for as long as possible.

Guideline 4 Maternal alcohol consumption can harm the developing fetus or breastfeeding baby

a. For women who are pregnant or planning a pregnancy not drinking is the safest option.
b. For women who are breastfeeding not drinking is the safest option.

High-risk and harmful drinking occurs at >6 standard drinks (SDs) a day (average) for men and >4 SDs for women.

The main causes of alcohol-related deaths are road trauma, cancer and alcoholic liver disease.[7]

Clinical pointers to alcohol abuse

Facial features of the patient can be a helpful pointer, albeit of the more advanced drinker. These include:

- plethoric facies
- puffy 'greasy' facies
- telangiectasia
- rosacea + rhinophyma
- suffused ('bloodshot') conjunctivae
- prominent lower lip with chelitis of corners of mouth
- smell of stale alcohol or very 'minty' sweet breath (masking effect)

Taking a drinking history

This requires tact and skill and it must be noted that many problem drinkers considerably understate the level of their intake.

21

Useful strategies[8]

- Ask questions as part of a matter-of-fact enquiry into health risk factors, such as smoking and diet.
- Place the onus of denial on the patient by asking questions such as 'When did you last drink alcohol?' rather than 'Do you ever drink alcohol?'
- Record your patient's intake quantitatively in terms of standard drinks or grams of alcohol.
- Confirm the history by enquiring about the time spent drinking per day and expenditure on alcohol.

Useful questionnaires

There are several questionnaires that can be most helpful, assuming the patient is fully cooperative. Two or more positive replies for the CAGE questionnaire[9] are suggestive of a problem drinker.

1. Have you ever felt you should CUT down on your drinking?
2. Have people ANNOYED you by criticising your drinking?
3. Have you ever felt bad or GUILTY about your drinking?
4. Have you ever had a drink first thing in the morning to steady your nerves or get rid of a hangover? (an EYE-OPENER)

Another very practical questionnaire is AUDIT (the Alcohol Use Disorders Identification Test) developed by the World Health Organization (www.who.int/substance_abuse/publications/audit/en) to facilitate the early detection of problem drinkers in primary care.

Laboratory investigations

The following blood tests may be helpful in the identification of excessive chronic alcohol intake:

- blood alcohol
- serum GGT: elevated in chronic drinkers (returns to normal with cessation of intake)
- MCV: >96 fL

Other changes:

- abnormal liver function tests (other than GGT)
- carbohydrate deficient transferrin (quite specific—dependent on an enzyme induced by alcohol)
- HDLs elevated
- LDLs lowered
- serum uric acid elevated

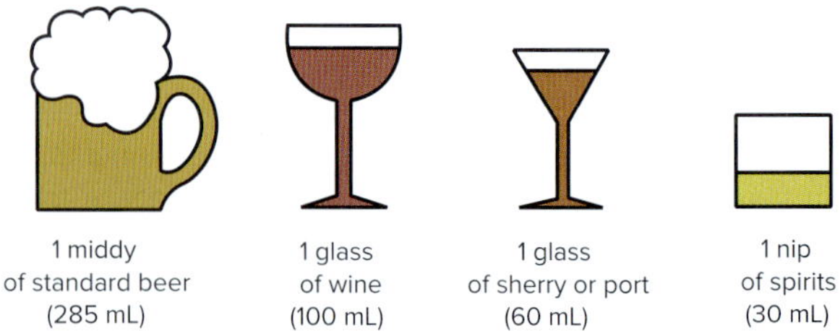
1 middy
of standard beer
(285 mL)
1 glass
of wine
(100 mL)
1 glass
of sherry or port
(60 mL)
1 nip
of spirits
(30 mL)

FIGURE 21.3 Standard drinks

Measuring alcohol intake

One standard drink contains 10 g of alcohol, which is the amount in one middy (or pot) of standard beer (285 mL), two middies of low-alcohol beer or five middies of super-light beer. These are equal in alcohol content to one small glass of table wine (122 mL), one glass of sherry or port (60 mL) or one nip of spirits (30 mL) (see FIG. 21.3).

- 1 stubbie or can of full-strength beer = 1.4 standard drinks
- 1 light beer = 0.9 standard drinks
- 1 × 750 mL bottle of beer = 2.6 standard drinks
- 1 × 750 mL bottle of wine = 7 standard drinks

Alcohol dependence

Alcohol dependence is a syndrome in which an individual demonstrates clinically significant impairment or distress as manifested by three or more of the following, occurring at any time in the same 12-month period:

1. tolerance
2. withdrawal
3. drinking in larger amounts or for a longer period than intended
4. unsuccessful attempts to cut down or control drinking
5. a great deal of time spent in activities necessary to obtain, use or recover from the effects of alcohol
6. important social, occupational or recreational activities reduced or given up because of drinking
7. continued drinking despite knowledge of having persistent or recurrent problems caused by or exacerbated by drinking

Approach to management

The challenge to the family doctor is early recognition of the problem. There are specific target areas which should be considered carefully by the GP. Several studies have shown that early intervention and brief counselling by the doctor are effective in leading to rehabilitation.[10] Some of the results are very revealing.

- Patients expect their family doctor to advise on safe drinking levels.
- They will listen and act on our advice.[11]
- Treatment is more effective if offered before dependence or chronic disease has developed.[11]

Of prime concern to the GP is the assessment of whether the patient is interested in changing his or her excessive drinking behaviour. The proposed model of change by Prochaska and Di Clemente helps identify the stage reached by the patient (see FIG. 21.4).[12]

Precontemplators are satisfied users who are either unconcerned about their drinking or have no desire to change. However, if there is any evidence of ambivalence or concern about drinking then the opportunity exists for motivational interviewing techniques.

Patients are not likely to offer concern about their drinking problem spontaneously but are often receptive to the initiative coming from their doctor.

The family doctor is ideally placed to identify and treat the problem of alcohol because the individual who abuses alcohol will tend to surface at some point in the provision of primary health care.

A brief practical management plan[13]

Giving patients feedback about their level of alcohol consumption, presenting objective evidence of harm and setting realistic goals for reducing alcohol intake induces many to change their drinking behaviour.

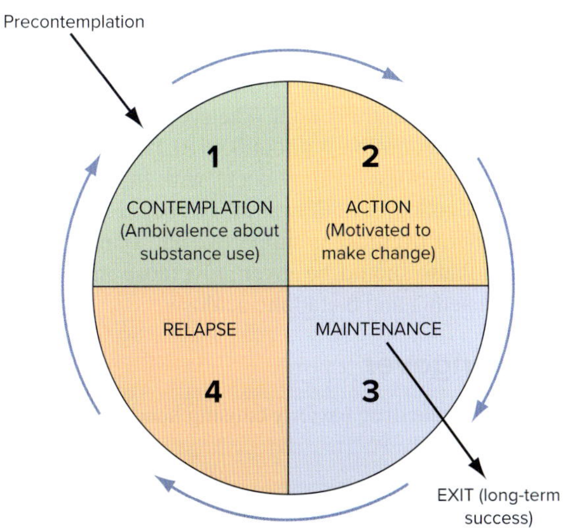

FIGURE 21.4 Prochaska's and Di Clemente's[12] proposed model of change to facilitate the identification of behavioural stages and the provision of counselling for treating dependence on alcohol, tobacco and other drugs

A six-step management plan, which has been employed in a general-practice early intervention program, is as follows:

1. Feed back the results of your assessment and specifically the degree of risk associated with their daily alcohol intake and bout drinking. Emphasise any damage that has already occurred.
2. Listen carefully to their reaction. They will need to ventilate their feelings and may respond defensively.
3. Outline the benefits of reducing drinking (e.g. save money, better health, weight loss).
4. Set goals for alcohol consumption that you both agree are feasible. In most cases this will involve reduction to below certain 'safe limits'.
   - For men: aim for fewer than 12 SDs per week.
   - For women: aim for fewer than 8 SDs per week. It is best for pregnant women not to drink.
   - For patients with illness who are physically dependent on alcohol, long-term abstinence is advisable.
5. Set strategies to keep below the upper safe limits, e.g.:
   - quench thirst with non-alcoholic drinks before having an alcoholic one
   - switch to low-alcohol beer
   - take care which parties you go to: avoid constant parties and other high-risk situations
   - explore new interests—fishing, cinema, social club, sporting activity
6. Evaluate progress by having patients monitor their drinking by using a diary; check that any abnormal blood test results are returning to normal. Make a definite appointment for follow-up and give appropriate literature such as *Alcohol: Harmful Use of Alcohol.* Obtain consent for a telephone follow-up. A useful minimum intervention plan is presented in TABLE 21.3.

Follow-up (long consultation 1 week later)

Review the patient's drinking diary. Explore any problems, summarise, listen and provide support and encouragement. If appointment is not kept, contact the patient.

Table 21.3 Minimum intervention technique plan (5–10 minutes)

1. Advise reduction to safe levels
2. Outline the benefits
3. Provide a self-help pamphlet
4. Organise a diary or other feedback system
5. Obtain consent for a telephone follow-up
6. Offer additional help (e.g. referral to an alcohol and drug unit or to a support group)

21

Specialist services

According to progress and the patient's wishes and consent, specialist treatment units, group therapy and attendance at meetings of Al-Anon or AA are potential sources of help to keep the alcohol-dependent person abstinent and coping.

'Anti-craving' drugs

The following show a modest effect on assisting abstinence:

- acamprosate 666 mg (o) tds
- naltrexone 50 mg (o) daily (under close supervision)
- consider a combination of the above 2 drugs

Note: Disulfiram can be helpful in highly motivated people but its use is recommended under specialist advice.

Withdrawal symptoms

Symptoms of a 'hangover' include headache, nausea, irritability, malaise and a mild tremor. Withdrawal from alcohol in a chronic problem drinker includes:

- agitation
- prominent tremor
- sweating
- insomnia
- seizures
- delirium tremens (DTs)

The aim of treatment for acute withdrawal symptoms is to prevent development of DTs. Maintain fluid, electrolytes and nutrition. Add vitamin B complex, including thiamine, because the patient is invariably thiamine deficient.

If medication is required (specialised advice):

- diazepam 20 mg (o) every 2 hours (up to 100 mg (o) daily) titrated against clinical response (taper off after 2 days) in the hospitalised or well-supervised patient
- thiamine 100 mg IM or IV daily for three days, then 300 mg (o) daily for several weeks
- vitamin B group supplement (o) or IM daily
- for psychotic features add haloperidol 1.5–5 mg (o) bd or 5 mg IM as single dose if necessary

Alcohol withdrawal delirium (delirium tremens)

DTs is a serious life-threatening withdrawal state. It has a high mortality rate if inadequately treated and hospitalisation is always necessary.

Clinical features

- May be precipitated by intercurrent infection or trauma
- 1–5 days after withdrawal (usually 3–4 days)
- Disorientation, agitation
- Clouding of consciousness
- Marked tremor
- Visual hallucinations (e.g. spiders, pink elephants)
- Sweating, tachycardia, pyrexia
- Signs of dehydration

Treatment[14]

- Hospitalisation with alcohol specialist advisory service
- Correct fluid and electrolyte imbalance with IV therapy
- Treat any systemic infection
- Thiamine (vitamin B1 300 mg IM or IV daily for 3–5 days, then thiamine 300 mg (o) daily
- Diazepam 20 mg (o) every 2 hours (up to max. 60 mg daily) until symptoms subside. This dose is usually required for 2–3 days, then should be gradually reduced till finished. If psychotic features (e.g. hallucinations and delusions) add haloperidol 0.5–2 mg (o) bd every 2 hours, titrated to clinical response (max. 10 mg/24 hours).

Note: Chlorpromazine is not recommended because of its potential to lower seizure threshold. Diazepam and haloperidol may worsen the symptoms of hepatic toxicity.

Alcohol overdose[14]

Overdose is potentially fatal. The average lethal blood alcohol concentration is about 0.45–0.5%. Death from a lower concentration may occur with other sedative drugs. Alcohol withdrawal may begin at 0.1%. Treatment of overdose is supportive and symptomatic. No stimulants should be given. Overdose may cause hypoglycaemia and metabolic acidosis.

Hangover

A type of acute drug toxicity causing headache, nausea and fatigue.

Prevention

- Drink alcohol on a full stomach.
- Select alcoholic drinks that suit you: avoid champagne.
- Avoid fast drinking—keep it slow.
- Restrict the quantity of alcohol.

- Dilute your drinks.
- Avoid or restrict smoking while drinking.
- Drink three large glasses of water before retiring.

Treatment

- Drink ample fluids especially water because of relative dehydration effect of alcohol.
- Take two paracetamol tablets for headache.
- Drink orange juice or tomato juice, with added sugar.
- A drink of honey in lemon juice helps.
- Tea is a suitable beverage.
- Have a substantial meal but avoid fatty food.

Illicit drugs

Several psychotropic substances are used for their effects on mood and other mental functions. Many of the severe problems are due to withdrawal of the drug. Symptomatic behaviour common to illicit drugs includes:

- rapid disappearance of clothing and personal belongings from home
- signs of unusual activity around hang-outs and other buildings
- loitering in hallways or in areas frequented by addicts
- spending unusual amounts of time in locked bathrooms
- inability to hold a job or stay in school
- rejection of old friends
- using the jargon of addicts

The drug list

Illicit drugs taken by injecting drug users in Victoria, Australia in 2005 were:

- heroin 89%
- cannabis 87%
- speed 75%
- ice 29%
- cocaine 15%
- base 13%

Source: Illicit drug reporting system

A summary of the effects of illicit or hard street drugs is presented in TABLE 21.4.

A list of street drugs and their slang names is presented in TABLE 21.5.

Opioid (narcotic) dependence

This section will focus on heroin dependence, although opioids such as codeine and controlled dose agents such as oxycodone and morphine are problematic.

Typical profile of a heroin-dependent person[15]

- Male or female: 16–30 years
- Family history: often severely disrupted, such as parental problems, early death, separation, divorce, alcohol or drug abuse, sexual abuse, mental illness, lack of affection
- Personal history: low threshold for toleration, unpleasant emotions, poor academic record, failure to fulfil aims, poor self-esteem
- First experiments with drugs are out of curiosity, and then regular use follows with loss of job, alienation from family, finally moving into a 'drug scene' type of lifestyle

Methods of intake

1. Oral ingestion
2. Inhalation (see FIG. 21.6)
    - intranasal
    - smoking
3. Parenteral
    - subcutaneous
    - intramuscular
    - intravenous (see FIG. 21.5)

Opioid withdrawal effects[14,15]

These develop within 12 hours of ceasing regular usage. Maximum withdrawal symptoms usually occur between 36 and 72 hours and tend to subside after 10 days.

- Anxiety and panic
- Irritability
- Chills and shivering
- Excessive sweating
- 'Gooseflesh' (cold turkey)
- Loss of appetite, nausea (possibly vomiting)
- Lacrimation/rhinorrhoea
- Tiredness/insomnia
- Muscle aches and cramps
- Abdominal colic
- Diarrhoea

A secondary abstinence syndrome is identified[15] at 2–3 months and includes irritability, depression and insomnia.

Complications of opioid dependence

Medical

- Overdose reaction: agitation, respiratory depression—may include fatal cardiopulmonary collapse. Since the early 2000s opioid deaths have fallen from peak levels of the 1990s, when there was a glut of heroin.

Table 21.4 Illicit substance abuse: a summary of hallmarks

Drug	Physical symptoms	Look for	Dangers
Amphetamines including methamphetamines (3 forms) • speed—powder • base—oily paste • ice—crystalline	Aggressive or agitated behaviour, giggling, silliness, euphoria, rapid speech, fever, confused thinking, anorexia, insomnia, extreme fatigue, dry mouth, shakiness, anxiety	Jars of pills of varying colours, chain smoking; white powder and crystals can also be snorted or injected	Hypertension, death from overdose, hallucinations, paranoia, may cause temporary psychosis, stroke, cardiac arrest
Ecstasy (methylene-dioxymethamphetamine)	Anxiety, panic, sweating, 'loving' feelings, jaw clenching, teeth grinding, bizarre overactive behaviour, hallucinations, increased heart rate, BP and body temperature, confidence, feelings of happiness and love	Small tablets of various colours, shapes, sizes and designs, also comes in powder and capsules	Convulsions, risk of death from heart attack, cerebral haemorrhage, hyperthermia, fluid imbalance with hyponatraemia, acute kidney failure, DIC, liver toxicity, hangover, depression
Fantasy (gamma-hydroxybutyrate)	Relaxation and drowsiness, dizziness, relaxed inhibition/euphoria, increased sexual arousal, impaired mobility and speech	Colourless, odourless liquid Also powder and capsules	Tremors and shaking, amnesia, coma, convulsions, death from high doses
Barbiturates	Drowsiness, stupor, dullness, slurred speech, drunk appearance, vomiting	Pills of various colours	Death from overdose or as a result of withdrawal, addictions, convulsions
Cannabis/marijuana	Initial euphoria, floating feeling, sleepiness, lethargy, wandering mind, enlarged pupils, lack of coordination, craving for sweets, changes of appetite, memory difficulty	Strong odour of burnt leaves, small seeds in pocket lining, cigarette paper, discoloured fingers	Inducement to take stronger narcotics, recent medical findings reveal that prolonged usage causes cognitive defects, precipitates or exacerbates schizophrenia
Glue sniffing	Aggression and violence, drunk appearance, slurred speech, dreamy or blank expression	Tubes of glue, glue smears, large paper or plastic bags or handkerchiefs	Lung/brain/liver damage, death through suffocation or choking
LSD (lysergic acid diethylamide)	Severe hallucinations, feelings of detachment, incoherent speech, cold hands and feet, vomiting, laughing and crying	Cube sugar with discolouration in centre, strong body odour, small tube of liquid	Suicidal tendencies, unpredictable behaviour, chronic exposure causes brain damage, LSD causes chromosomal breakdown
Narcotics (a) opioids (e.g. heroin)	Stupor/drowsiness, marks on body, watery eyes, loss of appetite, running nose, constricted pupils, loss of sex drive, agitation	Needle or hypodermic syringe, cotton, tourniquet—string, rope, belt, burnt bottle, caps or spoons, bloodstain on shirt sleeve, glass in envelopes	Death from overdose, mental deterioration, destruction of brain and liver, hepatitis, embolisms
(b) cocaine	Similar effects to amphetamines—muscle pains, irritability, paranoia, hyperactivity, jerky movements, euphoria, dilated pupils	Powder: in microwave ovens; inhaled, snorted or injected	Hallucinations, death from overdose—sudden death from arrhythmias, seizures, mental disorders, severe respiratory problems

Table 21.5 A street drug dictionary

Amphetamines or uppers	
Benzedrine	Roses, beanies, peaches
Dexedrine	Dexies, speed, hearts, pep pills, fast, go-ee, uppers, sulphate
Methamphetamines	Meth, crystals, white light, ice, whiz
Drinamyl	Purple hearts, goof balls
Amphetamine derivatives	
Ecstasy	E, eggs, eckies, XTC, 'the love drug', Mitsubishis, MDMA, vitamin E, X, Adam, death
Crank	Crystal M, crank
Hallucinogens	
LSD	Acid, blue cheer, strawberry fields, barrels, sunshine, pentagons, purple haze, peace pills, blue light, trips
Cannabis (Indian hemp)	
1 Hashish (the resin)	Hash, resin
2 Marijuana (from leaves)	Pot, tea, grass, hay, weed, locoweed, Mary Jane, rope, bong, jive, Acapulco gold
Cigarettes	Reefers, sticks, muggles, joints, spliffies, head, smoko, ganga
Smoking pot	Blow a stick, blast a joint, blow, get high, get stoned
Narcotics	
Morphine	Morph, Miss Emma
Heroin	H, Big H, Big Harry, GOM (God's own medicine), crap, junk, horse dynamite (high-grade heroin), lemonade (low-grade heroin). Injection of dissolved powder: mainlining, blast, smack. Inhalation of powder: sniffing
Cocaine	Coke, snow, lady of the streets, nose candy, ICE, snort, C, flake, rock, blow, vitamin C, crack, shabu, baby
H & C	Speed balls
Oxycontin	Hillbilly heroin
Miscellaneous	
Fantasy	GBH (grievous bodily harm), liquid G, liquid E, liquid ecstasy, liquid X, fantasy
Barbiturates	Devils, barbies, goof balls
Benzodiazepines	Rowies, moggies
Ketamine	'K', vitamin K, special K, K hole
Solvents	Chroming

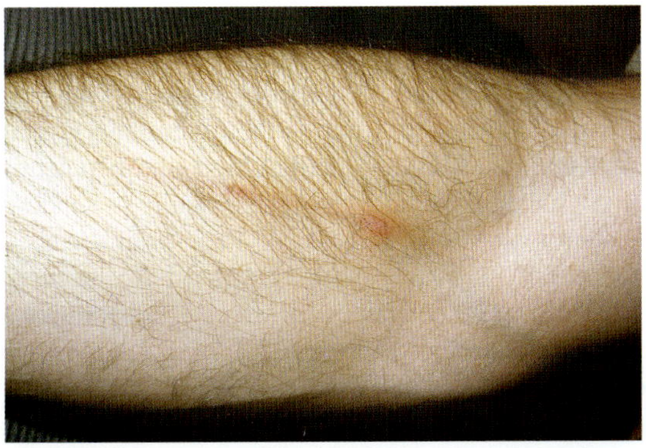

FIGURE 21.5 Intravenous heroin injection signs: linear tracks and scarring from repeated venepunctures along the course of a vein. Less common sites are the lower leg, dorsum of foot, neck and dorsal vein of penis.

Photo courtesy John Jagoda

- Injection site: scarring, pigmentation, thrombosis, abscesses, ulceration (especially with barbiturates)
- Distal septic complications: septicaemia, infective endocarditis, lung abscess, osteomyelitis, ophthalmitis
- Viral infections: hepatitis B, hepatitis C (refer to CHAPTER 58), HIV infection (refer to CHAPTER 27)
- Neurological complications: transverse myelitis, nerve trauma
- Physical disability: malnutrition

Social

- Alienation from family, loss of employment, loss of assets, criminal activity (theft, burglary, prostitution, drug trafficking)

Management

Management is complex because it includes the medical management not only of physical dependence and withdrawal but also of the individual complex social and emotional factors. The issues of impaired liver function, hepatitis B and C and HIV prevention also have to be addressed. Sociological tests for these illnesses should be considered.

Patients should be referred to a treatment clinic and then a shared-care approach can be used. The treatments include cold turkey (abrupt cessation) with pharmacological support, acupuncture, high doses of vitamin C, methadone substitution and drug-free community education programs.

Maintenance programs that include counselling techniques are widely used for heroin dependence. Acute toxicity requires injections of naloxone.

Opioid withdrawal[14]

Buprenorphine controlled withdrawal (short term) is used to prevent the emergence of a withdrawal syndrome in contradistinction from buprenorphine maintenance, where there is an extended treatment period.

21

Initial dose

- buprenorphine 4–8 mg (sublingual) as a single daily dose, increasing to 12 mg (max) on day 3, then reduce gradually over the next 3–5 days

Note: If autonomic signs, use clonidine 5–15 mg/kg/day (o) in 3 divided doses for 7–10 days then taper off. If anxiety and agitation, use diazepam 5–20 mg (o) qid (with care). Clonidine can be used as first-line treatment because of relative safety but buprenorphine is preferred to clonidine and methadone for the management of opioid withdrawal. Avoid benzodiazepines unless supervision is available.

Maintenance programs for long-term opioid dependence[14]

There are currently three alternative programs—methadone, buprenorphine and naltrexone—which are substitutes for heroin and other opioids.

Methadone

Seek specialist advice before starting treatment. The dose needs to be determined individually according to past use and initial response to methadone.

- Methadone 20 mg (o) daily initially. Stabilise dose over 3 weeks. Beware of doses >40 mg, especially in unwell patients. Maintenance 50–80 mg (o) daily.

Buprenorphine

- Buprenorphine 2–8 mg sublingual, once daily initially, increase to 8–24 mg daily or alternative days once stabilised. It is less dependent and prone to overdose than methadone but can precipitate withdrawal if used too soon.

Naltrexone

Care is required in giving naltrexone to a person physically dependent on opioids. A naloxone challenge test is used.[14] If no evidence of withdrawal give:

- Naltrexone 25 mg (o) initially increasing to 50 mg daily on day 2 if tolerated. Careful supervision with appropriate counselling is required.

The natural history of opioid dependence indicates that many patients do grow through their period of dependence and, irrespective of treatments provided, a high percentage become rehabilitated by their mid-30s.

Stimulant substance abuse

The stimulants include amphetamines and their analogues, ephedrine, designer drugs such as MDMA and 'fantasy', cocaine and certain appetite suppressants. The amphetamines include the common methamphetamine, dexamphetamine and the original amphetamines.

The drugs also include crack, which is a cocaine base where the hydrochloride has mostly been removed, usually in a microwave oven. Crack can be inhaled or smoked (see FIGS 21.6 and 21.7). Ice is the crude form of methamphetamine, a derivative of amphetamine (FIG. 21.7). Speed is dexamphetamine.

Party drugs

Ecstasy is another 'designer' drug which is an amphetamine derivative—methylenedioxy-methamphetamine (MDMA). It has high abuse potential, some hallucinogenic properties and a tendency to neurotoxicity, as proved on PET brain scans. It is popular in rave parties. Deaths have occurred, reportedly in association with relative dehydration or excessive hydration. Treatment for overdosage involves correction of fluid and electrolyte disturbances. An increasingly popular drug is fantasy (gamma-hydroxybutyrate), which has sedative and anaesthetic effects similar to alcohol. A popular party drug, it is implicated as a 'date rape' drug. There is no specific antidote.[13] Another party drug is ketamine, which is a

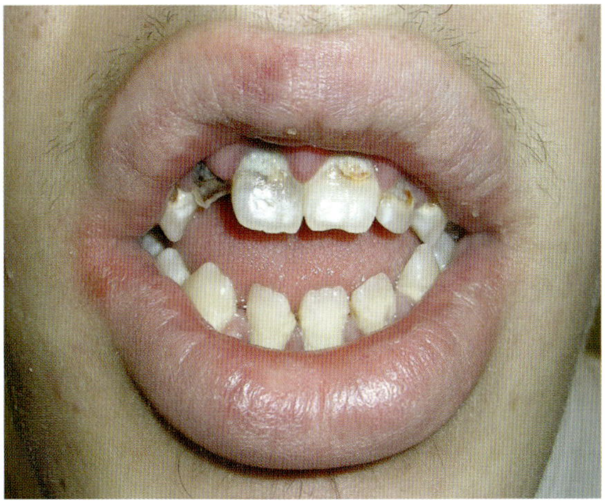

FIGURE 21.6 'Meth mouth' in a young man actively smoking methamphetamine

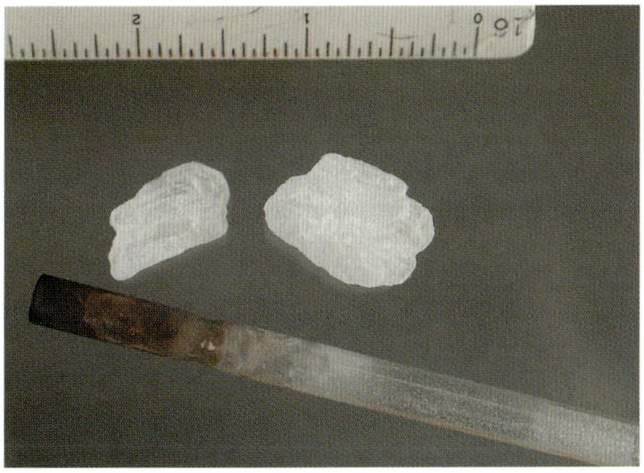

FIGURE 21.7 Methamphetamine ice with pipe

short-acting anaesthetic with hallucinogenic properties. It can produce nausea and vomiting if used with alcohol. Like fantasy, treatment of overdosage is symptomatic. Local anaesthetics can be dangerous in amphetamine users because of cardiotoxicity.

Stimulant-induced syndrome[14]

- Aggressive behaviour
- Paranoid behaviour
- Irritability
- Transient toxic psychosis
- Delirium
- Schizophrenic-like syndrome
- Increased sexual behaviour

Treatment

- Withdrawal of drugs
- Cognitive behaviour therapy
- No firm evidence on effectiveness of drugs

Stimulant-withdrawal syndrome[14]

This syndrome should be suspected in people whose occupation involves shift work, interstate transport driving or multiple jobs presenting with the following symptoms:

- drowsiness
- hypersomnia, then insomnia
- irritability
- hyperphagia
- aggressive behaviour
- depression/dysphoria
- urge to resume drugs

Treatment

- Psychological support and encouragement, e.g. CBT
- Desipramine (or similar tricyclic antidepressant) 75 mg (o) nocte (increasing as necessary)
- Bromocriptine 1.25 mg (o) bd has also been used for cocaine withdrawal

Hallucinogen abuse

Hallucinogens in use include lysergic acid diethylamide (LSD), phencyclidine (angel dust), the tropical plant products (Kava and Betel nuts) and many synthetics. Symptoms include psychotic behaviour, including severe hallucinations. Withdrawal from these drugs is not usually a problem but 'flashbacks' can occur. Treatment, especially where there is fear or anxiety, is diazepam 10–20 mg (o) statim.

Treatment (medication to counter symptoms)[14]

- haloperidol 2.5–10 mg (o) daily
  or
- diazepam 10–20 mg (o) repeated every 2 hours prn (to max 120 mg daily)

Cannabis (marijuana) use

Cannabis is a drug that comes from the plant *Cannabis sativa,* the Indian hemp plant. It is a stimulant and a hallucinogen. It contains the chemical tetrahydrocannabinol, which makes people get 'high'. It is commonly called marijuana, grass, pot, dope, hash or hashish. Other slang terms are Acapulco gold, ganga, herb, J, jay, hay, joint, reefer, weed, locoweed, smoke, tea, stick, Mary Jane, Panama red and spliffy (see TABLE 21.5). Marijuana comes from the leaves, while hashish is the concentrated form of the resinous substances from the head of the female plant and can be very strong (it comes as a resin or oil). The drug is usually smoked as a leaf (marijuana) or a powder (hashish), or hashish oil is added to a cigarette and then smoked. The effects of taking cannabis depend on how much is taken, how it is taken, how often, whether it is used with other drugs and on the particular person.[16] The effects vary from person to person. The effects of a small-to-moderate amount include:

- feeling of well-being and relaxation
- decreased inhibitions
- woozy, floating feeling
- lethargy and sleepiness
- talkativeness and laughing a lot
- red nose, gritty eyes and dry mouth
- unusual perception of sounds and colour
- nausea and dizziness
- loss of concentration
- looking 'spaced out' or drunk
- lack of coordination
- delusions and hallucinations (more likely with larger doses)
- a form called skunk or mad weed causes paranoia

21

The effects of smoking marijuana take up to 20 minutes to appear and usually last 2 to 3 hours and then drowsiness follows.[16] The effect on psychomotor function is similar to alcohol and this can impair driving skills. The main problem is habitual use with the development of dependence; dependence (addiction) is worse than originally believed.

Long-term use and addiction

The influence of pot has a severe effect on the personality and drive of the users. They lose their energy, initiative and enterprise. They become bored, inert, apathetic and careless. A serious effect of smoking pot is the inability to concentrate and loss of memory. Some serious problems include:

- deterioration of academic or job performance
- anxiety and paranoia
- respiratory disease (more potent than tobacco for lung disease): causes COPD, laryngitis and rhinitis
- often prelude to taking illicit drugs
- becoming psychotic (resembling schizophrenia): the drug appears to unmask an underlying psychosis[16]
- impaired ability to drive a car and operate machinery

Withdrawal

Sudden withdrawal produces insomnia, night sweats, nausea, depression, myalgia, irritability and maybe anger and aggression. However, the effects are often mild with recovery within a few days in many, but heavy users have a severe withdrawal.

Management

No specific pharmacological treatment is available. CBT is advisable.

The best treatment is prevention. People should either not use it or limit it to experimentation. If it is used, people should be prepared to sleep it off and not drive.

Anabolic steroid misuse

The apparent positive effects of anabolic steroids include gains in muscular strength (in conjunction with diet and exercise) and quicker healing of muscle injuries. However, the adverse effects, which are dependent on the dose and duration, are numerous.

Adverse effects in women are:

- masculinisation—male-pattern beard growth
- suppression of ovarian function
- changes in mood and libido
- hair loss

In adult men, adverse effects are:

- feminisation: enlarged breasts, high-pitched voice
- acne
- testicular atrophy and azoospermia
- libido changes
- hair loss

Severe effects with prolonged use include:

- liver function abnormalities, including hepatoma
- tumours of kidneys, prostate
- heart disease

In prepubescent children there can be premature epiphyseal closure with short stature.

Drugs in sport[17]

It is important for GPs to have a basic understanding of drugs that are banned and those that are permissible for elite sporting use. The guidelines formulated by the International Olympic Committee (IOC) Medical Commission and the World Anti-Doping Agency (WADA) are generally adopted by most major sporting organisations.[10] TABLES 21.6 and 21.7 provide useful guidelines. The IOC's list of prohibited

Table 21.6 Prohibited list: World Anti-Doping Guide (valid 1 January 2014)[17]

Classes	Examples
Prohibited substances at all times	
S1 Anabolic agents	Methandienone, nandrolone, stanozolol, testosterone, oxandrolone, DHEA, tetrahydrogestrinone, clenbuterol, zeronol, androstenediol, tibolone
S2 Peptide hormones, growth factors and related substances	Growth hormone, corticotrophin, chorionic gonadotrophin and LH (in males), erythropoietin (EPO), darbepoietin (dEPO), SERMS, insulin
	Note: masking agents such as probenecid, epitestosterone, diuretics and plasma expanders are banned.
S3 Beta-2 agonists	All beta-2 agonists, including both optical isomers (except inhaled salbutamol and salmeterol according to recommended guidelines)
S4 Hormone antagonists and modulators	Aromatase inhibitors, e.g. anastrozole, letrozole; SERMS, e.g. raloxifene, tamoxifen; other anti-oestrogenic substances, e.g. clomiphene; myostatin inhibitors; metabolic modulators—insulins
S5 Diuretics and other masking agents	Acetazolamide, frusemide, hydrochlorothiazide, triamterene, indapamide, spironolactone (and related substances)
Prohibited substances in competition	
S6 Stimulants	Amiphenazole, amphetamines, cocaine, ephedrine, ephedra, meldonium, mesocarb, terbutaline,* adrenaline, salmeterol,* salbutamol,* selegiline, pseudoephedrine, phenylpropanolamine, modafinil, phentermine
S7 Narcotics**	Diamorphine (heroin), methadone, morphine, pethidine, pentazocine, buprenorphine, hydromorphone, oxycodone, oxymorphone, fentanyl
S8 Cannabinoids	Natural (e.g. cannabis, hashish, marijuana) or synthetic THC and cannabimimetics (e.g. 'spice')
S9 Glucocorticosteroids	All glucocorticosteroids are prohibited when administered by oral, IV, IM or rectal routes
Substances prohibited in particular sports	
P1 Alcohol	Prohibited in competition only—aeronautic, archery, automobile, karate, motorcycling, power boating (doping threshold 0.10 g/L)
P2 Beta blockers	Prohibited in competition only, e.g. atenolol, carvedilol, metroprolol, propranol, timolol
	(Check list and sports, e.g. archery, shooting, golf, skiing)
Prohibited methods	
MI Enhancement of oxygen transfer	
M2 Chemical and physical manipulation	
M3 Gene doping	

* Permitted by inhaler but only with therapeutic use exemption (TUE).
** Caffeine, codeine, dextromethorphan, dextropropoxyphene, dihydrocodeine, tramadol, diphenoxylate and pholcodeine are permitted.
See www.wada-ama.org (World Anti-Doping Agency) or https://checksubstances.asada.gov.au for updated information.

Table 21.7 Guidelines for treatment of specific conditions: International Olympic Committee Medical Code 2008

Asthma	
Allowed	Salbutamol inhaler, salmeterol inhaler, terbutaline inhaler, formoterol inhaler
Banned	Sympathomimetic products (e.g. ephedrine, pseudoephedrine, isoprenaline, systemic beta-2 agonists), oral corticosteroids
Cough	
Allowed	All antibiotics, steam and menthol inhalations, cough mixtures containing antihistamines, pholcodine, dextromethorphan, dihydrocodeine
Banned	Sympathomimetic products (e.g. ephedrine, phenylpropanolamine)
Diarrhoea	
Allowed	Diphenoxylate, loperamide, products containing electrolytes (e.g. Gastrolyte)
Banned	Products containing opioids (e.g. morphine)
Hayfever	
Allowed	Antihistamines, nasal sprays containing a corticosteroid or antihistamine, sodium cromoglycate preparations
Banned	Products containing ephedrine, pseudoephedrine
Pain	
Allowed	Aspirin, codeine, dihydrocodeine, ibuprofen, paracetamol, tramadol, all NSAIDs, dextropropoxyphene
Banned	Products containing opioids (e.g. morphine) or caffeine
Vomiting	
Allowed	Domperidone, metoclopramide

drugs is regularly revised. Banned drug groups include stimulants, narcotics, cannabinoids (e.g. marijuana), anti-oestrogen agents (e.g. tamoxifen), glucocorticosteroids (e.g. prednisolone), anabolic agents, diuretics and various hormones. Banned methods include blood doping (the administration of blood, red blood cells and related blood products), enhancement of oxygen transfer (e.g. erythropoietin, efaproxiral), gene doping and pharmaceutical, chemical and physical manipulation (substances or methods that alter the integrity and validity of the urine testing).

Restricted drugs include alcohol, marijuana, local anaesthetics, corticosteroids and beta blockers. Practitioners can check the guidelines and provide written notification to the relevant authority. Be cautious of anorectics and weight-reducing agents.

Other drug groups permitted by WADA:

- antidepressants
- antihypertensives (excluding beta blockers)
- caffeine
- eye medications
- oral contraceptives
- skin creams and ointments
- sleeping tablets

Check websites including www.olympic.org.

Patient education resources

Hand-out sheets from *Murtagh's Patient Education* 7th edition:

- Alcohol: harmful use of alcohol
- Amphetamines
- Cocaine
- Ecstasy
- Heroin
- Smoking: quitting
- Cannabis (marijuana)

Further resources

- Global DRO, Athletes, check your medications! (country-specific), <www.globaldro.com>
- Department of Health, National drug campaign, <www.campaigns.health.gov.au/drughelp>
- <www.usada.org/substances/prohibited-list>

References

1 Kumar PJ, Clark ML. *Clinical Medicine* (1st edn). London: Elsevier Saunders, 2009: 927–8.
2 Professor Greg Whelan, personal communication.
3 Expert Group for Cardiovascular guidelines. Behavioural risk factor modification; Smoking and cardiovascular risk. In: eTG complete. Melbourne: Therapeutic Guidelines Ltd. Available from: <www.tg.org.au>, accessed September 2017.
4 Silagy C et al. Nicotine replacement therapy for smoking cessation (Cochrane review). In: The Cochrane Library, Issue 1, 2002. Oxford: Update software.

5 Mendelsohn C. Smoking cessation. Medical Observer, 28 February 2014: 21–6.

6 Australian Institute of Health and Welfare. *Alcohol and Other Drug Use in Australia.* Australian Government, Canberra: AIHW, 2004: 23–5.

7 National Health and Medical Research Council. *Australian Guidelines to Reduce Health Risks from Drinking Alcohol.* Canberra: NHMRC, 2009: 2–5. Available from: <www.nhmrc.gov.au/_files_nhmrc/publications/attachments/ds10-alcohol.pdf>, accessed February 2018.

8 Murtagh JE. Alcohol abuse in an Australian community. Aust Fam Physician, 1987; 16: 20–5.

9 Mayfield D, McLeod G, Hall P. The CAGE questionnaire. Am J Psychiatry, 1974; 131: 1121–3.

10 National Health and Medical Research Council. Guidelines on Preventive Interventions in Primary Health Care: Cardiovascular Disease and Cancer. No. 6. *Alcohol Overuse.* Canberra: NHMRC, 1996.

11 Wallace P, Cutler S, Haines A. Randomised controlled trial of general practitioner intervention in patients with excessive alcohol consumption. BMJ, 1988; 297: 663–8.

12 Prochaska JO, Di Clemente CC. Towards a comprehensive model of change. In: Miller WRJ, Heath N (eds). *Treating Addictive Behavior.* New York: Plenum, 1986: 3–27.

13 Saunders JB, Roche AM. One in six patients in your practice. NSW medical education project on alcohol and other drugs. A drug offensive pamphlet. Sydney, 1989: 1–6.

14 Expert Group for Psychotropic guidelines. Alcohol and other drug problems. In: eTG complete. Melbourne: Therapeutic Guidelines Ltd. Available from: <www.tg.org.au>, accessed August 2017.

15 Jagoda J. *Drug Dependence and Narcotic Abuse: Clinical Consequences.* Course Handbook. Melbourne: Monash University of Community Medicine, 1987: 66–71.

16 Semple DM, McIntosh AM, Lawrie SM. Cannabis as a risk factor for psychosis: systematic review. J Psychopharmacol, 2005; 19 (2): 187–94.

17 WADA. 2018 Prohibited List. Available from: <www.wada-ama.org/en/what-we-do/prohibited-list>, accessed February 2018.

22 Anaemia

There's never none of these demure boys come to any proof; for their drink doth so over cool their blood, and making many fish-meals, that they fall into a kind of male green-sickness.

William Shakespeare (1564–1616), *King Henry IV*

Anaemia is a label, not a specific diagnosis. Anaemia is defined as a reduction in red blood cell numbers or a haemoglobin (Hb) level below the normal reference level for the age and sex of that individual.

The WHO defines anaemia as haemoglobin <130 g/L for men, <120 g/L for women and <110 g/L in pregnant women and school-aged children.

Anaemia: a masquerade

Anaemia is regarded as a masquerade because the problem can develop surreptitiously and the patient may present with many seemingly undifferentiated symptoms before the anaemia is detected. Once identified, a cause must be found.

Key facts and checkpoints

- In Australia, most people with anaemia will have iron deficiency ranging from up to 5% for children to 20% for menstruating females.[1]
- The remainder will mainly have anaemia of chronic disorders.
- The incidence of haemoglobinopathy traits, especially thalassaemia, is increasing in multicultural Western societies.
- If a patient presents with precipitation or aggravation of myocardial ischaemia, heart failure or intermittent claudication, consider the possibility of anaemia.
- The serum ferritin level, which is low in cases of iron-deficiency anaemia, is probably the best test to monitor iron-deficiency anaemia as its level reflects the amount of stored iron.
- Normal reference values for peripheral blood are presented in TABLE 22.1.

DxT fatigue + palpitations + exertional dyspnoea ➜ anaemia

Table 22.1 Normal reference values for peripheral blood: adults

	Male	Female
Haemoglobin (g/L)	130–180	115–165
Red cells ($\times 10^{12}$/L)	4.5–6	4–5.5
PCV (haematocrit)	40–53	35–47
MCV (fL)	80–100	
Platelets ($\times 10^{9}$/L)	150–400	
White cell count ($\times 10^{9}$/L)	4–11	
Neutrophils	2.5–7.5	
Lymphocytes	1.5–4	
Monocytes	0.2–1	
Eosinophils	<0.5	
Reticulocytes (%)	0.5–2	
ESR (mm/hour)	<20 mm <35 mm if >70 years	

Source: Reproduced with permission from Dr M Gribble[2]

Clinical features

Patients with anaemia may be asymptomatic. When symptoms develop they are usually nonspecific. Symptoms can include:

- tiredness/fatigue
- muscle weakness
- headache and tinnitus
- lack of concentration
- faintness/dizziness
- dyspnoea on exertion
- palpitations
- angina on effort
- intermittent claudication
- pica—usually brittle and crunchy food, e.g. ice (iron-deficiency anaemia)

Signs

Non-specific signs include pallor, tachycardia, systolic flow murmur and angular cheilosis.

If severe, signs can include ankle oedema and cardiac failure.

Specific signs include jaundice—haemolytic anaemia, and koilonychias (spoon-shaped nails)—iron-deficiency anaemia.

History

The history may indicate the nature of the problem:

- iron deficiency: inadequate diet, pregnancy, GIT loss, menorrhagia, NSAID and anticoagulant ingestion
- folate deficiency: inadequate diet especially with pregnancy and alcoholism, small bowel disease
- vitamin B12 deficiency: previous gastric surgery, ileal disease or surgery, pernicious anaemia, selective diets (e.g. vegetarian, fad)
- haemolysis: abrupt onset anaemia with mild jaundice
- possibly lead toxicity, especially in children

Classification of anaemia

The various types of anaemia are classified in terms of the red cell size—the mean corpuscular volume (MCV):

- microcytic—MCV ≤ 80 fL
- macrocytic—MCV >100 fL
- normocytic—MCV 80–100 fL

Note: Upper limit of MCV varies from 95–100 fL depending on age and laboratory.

TABLE 22.2 outlines a classification of some of the more common causes of anaemia encountered in general practice. There can be an interchange of disorders between the above groups, for example, the anaemia of chronic disorders (chronic infection, inflammation and malignancy) can occasionally be microcytic as well as normocytic; the anaemia of hypothyroidism can be macrocytic in addition to the more likely normocytic; the anaemia of bone marrow disorder or infiltration can also be occasionally macrocytic.

MICROCYTIC ANAEMIA—MCV ≤ 80 FL

The main causes of microcytic anaemia are iron deficiency and haemoglobulinopathy, particularly thalassaemia. Consider lead poisoning.

Iron-deficiency anaemia[3]

Iron deficiency is the most common cause of anaemia worldwide. It is the biggest cause of microcytic anaemia, with the main differential diagnosis of microcytic anaemia being a haemoglobinopathy such as thalassaemia.

An understanding of the interpretation of iron studies is important in management.

Clinical features

- Microcytic anaemia
- Serum ferritin level low (NR: F 15–200 mcg/L: M 30–300 mcg/L)
- Serum iron level low
- Increased transferrin level
- MCV ↓, MCH ↓, MCHC ↓
- Reduced transferrin saturation
- Response to iron therapy

Non-haematological effects of chronic iron deficiency

- Angular cheilosis/stomatitis
- Glossitis
- Oesophageal webs
- Atrophic gastritis
- Brittle nails and koilonychias

Causes[1]

Blood loss

- Menorrhagia
- Gastrointestinal bleeding (e.g. carcinoma, haemorrhoids, peptic ulcer, hiatus hernia, GORD, NSAID therapy)
- Frequent blood donations
- Malignancy
- Hookworm (common in tropics)

Increased physiological requirements

- Prematurity, infant growth
- Adolescent growth
- Pregnancy

Malabsorption

- Coeliac disease
- Postgastrectomy

Dietary

- Inadequate intake
- Special diets (e.g. fad, vegetarianism)
- Pica—eating unnatural food, e.g. dirt, ashes

Table 22.2 Selected causes and investigations of anaemia

Causes/classification	Primary diagnostic features	Secondary investigations
Microcytic (MCV <80 fL)		
Iron deficiency	s.Fe ↓; s.ferr ↓; transferrin ↑	Therapeutic trial of iron; GIT evaluation for blood loss
Haemoglobinopathy (e.g. thalassaemia)	s.Fe N or ↑; s.ferr N or ↑	Haemoglobin investigation, e.g. electrophoresis
Sideroblastic anaemia (hereditary)	s.Fe N or ↑; s.ferr N or ↑	Bone marrow examination
Occasionally microcytic		
Anaemia of chronic disease (sometimes microcytic)	s.Fe ↓; s.ferr N or ↑; transferrin ↓	Specific for underlying disorder
Macrocytic (MCV >100 fL)		
(a) With megaloblastic changes		
Vitamin B12 deficiency	s.B12 ↓; rc.Fol N or ↑	IF antibody assay; Schilling test
Folate deficiency	s.B12 N; rc.Fol ↓	Usually none
Cytotoxic drugs	Appropriate setting; s.B12 N; rc.Fol N	None
(b) Without megaloblastic changes		
Liver disease/alcoholism	Appropriate setting; uniform macrocytosis; s.B12 N; rc.Fol N	Liver function tests
Myelodysplastic disorders (including sideroblastic anaemia)	Specific peripheral blood findings; s.B12 N; rc.Fol N	Bone marrow examination
Normocytic (MCV 80–100 fL)		
Acute blood loss/occult	Isolated anaemia; Retic ↑	Dictated by clinical findings
Anaemia of chronic disease[1]	Appropriate setting; Retic ↓	s.Fe ↓ and s.ferr N or ↑
Haemolysis	Specific red cell changes; Retic ↑	s.Bil and s.LDH ↑; s.hapt ↓ specific tests for cause
Chronic kidney disease	Isolated anaemia; Retic ↓	Kidney function
Endocrine disorders (e.g. hypothyroidism)	Appropriate setting; isolated anaemia; Retic ↓	Specific endocrine investigation

Abbreviations: MCV = mean corpuscular volume; s.Fe = serum iron; s.ferr = serum ferritin; s.B12 = serum vitamin B12; rc.Fol = red cell folate; IF = intrinsic factor; Retic = reticulocyte count; s.Bil = serum bilirubin; s.LDH = serum lactate dehydrogenase; s.hapt = serum haptoglobin; N = normal; ↓ = reduced; ↑ = elevated; GIT = gastrointestinal

Source: Adapted from 'Anaemia', *MIMS Disease Index,*[1] with permission of MIMS Australia, a division of MediMedia Australia Pty Limited[1]

22

Investigations

Investigations are based on the history and physical examination, including the rectal examination. If GIT bleeding is suspected the faecal occult blood test is not considered very valuable but appropriate investigations include gastroscopy and colonoscopy, small bowel biopsy and small bowel enema.

Haematological investigations: typical findings

- Microcytic, hypochromic red cells
- Anisocytosis (variation in size), poikilocytosis (shape)—pencil-shaped rods
- Low serum iron level
- Raised iron-binding capacity
- Serum ferritin level low (the most useful index)
- Soluble transferrin receptor factor—this factor is increased in iron deficiency, but not in chronic disease. It is very helpful therefore in differentiating iron deficiency from other forms. It is an indirect marker of what is happening in the bone marrow.[4]

The state of the iron stores is assessed by considering the serum iron, the serum ferritin and the serum transferrin levels in combination. Typically, in iron deficiency, the serum iron and ferritin levels are low and the transferrin high, but the serum iron level is also low in all infections—severe, mild and

Table 22.3 The interpretation of iron studies[2]

Condition	Serum Fe	TIBC	% Transferrin saturation	Ferritin
Iron deficiency	↓	N or ↑	↓	↓↓
β-thalassaemia	N or ↑	N	N or ↑	N or ↑
Anaemia of chronic disease	↓	N or ↓	↓	N or ↑
Sideroblastic anaemia	N or ↑	N	N or ↑	↑
Haemochromatosis	↑	↓	↑↑	↑↑

N = normal

even subclinical—as well as in inflammatory states, malignancy and other chronic conditions. Serum ferritin estimations are spuriously raised in liver disease of all types, chronic inflammatory conditions and malignancy; transferrin is normally raised in pregnancy. Since each of these estimations can be altered in conditions other than iron deficiency, all three quantities have to be considered together to establish the iron status (see TABLE 22.3).[2]

Treatment[4,5]

- Correct the identified cause.
- Diet—iron-rich foods, vitamin C-rich foods (see TABLE 22.4). Iron is present in meat and legumes as Fe^{+++} and therefore requires gastric acid for conversion to Fe^{++}.
- Iron preparations:
  - oral iron (ferrous sulphate 1–2 tablets daily between meals for 6 months), e.g. Ferro-Gradumet with orange juice or ascorbic acid until Hb is normal
  - parenteral iron preferably by IV infusion is probably best reserved for special circumstances such as a failed trial of oral iron for symptomatic iron deficiency anaemia (there is a risk of an allergic reaction and post-infusion skin staining around the cannula site). Infusion is best with ferric carboxymaltose in 0.9% (N) saline.[6] Avoid blood transfusions if possible.

Response

- Anaemia responds after about 2 weeks and is usually corrected after 2 months (if underlying cause addressed).[1]
- Oral iron is continued for 3 to 6 months to replenish stores.
- Monitor progress with regular serum ferritin levels.
- A serum ferritin level >50 mcg/L generally indicates adequate stores.

Table 22.4 Optimal adult diet for iron deficiency

Adults should limit milk intake to 500 mL a day while on iron tablets. Avoid excess caffeine, fad diets and excess processed bread. Eat ample iron-rich foods (especially protein).
Protein foods Meats—beef (especially), veal, pork, liver, poultry Fish and shellfish (e.g. oysters, sardines, tuna) Seeds (e.g. sesame, pumpkin) Eggs, especially egg yolk
Fruits Dried fruit (e.g. prunes, figs, raisins, currants, peaches) Juices (e.g. prune, blackberry) Most fresh fruit
Vegetables Greens (e.g. spinach, silver beet, lettuce) Dried peas and beans (e.g. kidney beans) Pumpkin, sweet potatoes
Grains Iron-fortified breads and dry cereals Oatmeal cereal For better iron absorption, add foods rich in vitamin C (e.g. citrus fruits, cantaloupe, Brussels sprouts, broccoli, cauliflower)

Failure of iron therapy

Consider:

- poor compliance
- continuing blood loss
- malabsorption (e.g. severe coeliac disease)
- incorrect diagnosis (e.g. thalassaemia minor, chronic disease)
- bone marrow infiltration

Thalassaemia

This inherited condition is seen mainly (although not exclusively) in people from the Mediterranean basin, the Middle East, north and central India and South-East

Asia, including south China. The heterozygous form is usually asymptomatic; patients show little if any anaemia and require no treatment. The condition is relatively common in people from these areas. The homozygous form is a very severe congenital anaemia needing lifelong transfusional support but is comparatively rare, even among the populations prone to thalassaemia (refer to CHAPTER 18).[2]

The key to the diagnosis of heterozygous thalassaemia minor is significant microcytosis quite out of proportion to the normal Hb or slight anaemia, and confirmed by finding a raised HbA_2 on Hb electrophoresis. DNA screening analysis is now available. The importance of recognising the condition lies in distinguishing it from iron-deficiency anaemia, for iron does not help people with thalassaemia and is theoretically contraindicated. Even more importantly, it lies in recognising the risk that, if both parents have thalassaemia minor, they run a one in four chance of having a baby with thalassaemia major in every pregnancy, with devastating consequences for both the affected child and the whole family.

Treatment of thalassaemia major is transfusion to a high normal Hb with packed cells plus desferrioxamine.

Haemoglobin E

22

This Hb variant is common throughout South-East Asia.[4] It has virtually no clinical effects in either the homozygous or heterozygous forms, but these people have microcytosis, which must be distinguished from iron deficiency; moreover, if the *HbE* gene is combined with the thalassaemia gene, the child may have a lifelong anaemia almost as severe as thalassaemia major. Both genes are well established in the South-East Asian populations in Australia as well as in their own countries.

MACROCYTIC ANAEMIA—MCV >100 FL

Alcohol and liver disease

Each individually, or in combination, leads to macrocytosis with or without anaemia. The importance of this finding lies in its often being the first indication of alcohol abuse, which can so frequently go unnoticed unless there is a firm index of suspicion. Chronic liver disease due to other causes may also be late in producing specific clinical symptoms.

Drug toxicity

Cytotoxic drugs, anticonvulsants in particular, and various others (see TABLE 22.5) may cause macrocytosis. This is of little clinical significance and does not need correction unless associated with anaemia or other cytopaenia.

Table 22.5 Drugs causing macrocytosis[2,5]

Alcohol	
Cytotoxics/ immunosuppressants	Azathioprine Methotrexate, 5-fluorouracil
Antibiotics	Cotrimoxazole, Pyrimethamine (incl. Fansidar and Maloprim) Zidovudine
Anticonvulsants	Phenytoin Primidone Phenobarbitone

Myelodysplastic syndromes

These conditions have been recognised under a variety of names, such as 'refractory anaemia' and 'preleukaemia', for a long time, but only relatively recently have they been grouped together. They are quite common in the elderly but may be seen in any age group (refer TABLE 22.2).

These conditions frequently present as a macrocytic anaemia with normal serum vitamin B12 and red cell folate, and are unresponsive to these or any other haematinics. They are usually associated with progressive intractable neutropaenia or thrombocytopenia or both, and progress slowly but relentlessly to be eventually fatal, terminating with infection, haemorrhage or, less often, acute leukaemia.

Vitamin B12 deficiency (pernicious anaemia)

Although well recognised, this is a much less common cause of macrocytosis than the foregoing conditions. It is usually caused by lack of intrinsic factor due to autoimmune atrophic changes and by gastrectomy. Anaemia does not develop for about 3 years after total gastrectomy. Vitamin B12 deficiency may also be seen together with other deficiencies in some cases of malabsorption and Crohn disease.

Vitamin B12 (cobalamin) is found in the normal diet but only in foods of animal origin and consequently very strict vegetarians may eventually develop deficiency. Causes of food vitamin B12 deficiency are:[4]

- atrophic gastritis
- *H. pylori* infection
- H_2 receptor blockers
- PPI drugs
- other drugs, e.g. OCP, metformin

- chronic alcoholism
- HIV
- strict vegan diet

The clinical features are anaemia (macrocytic), weight loss and neurological symptoms, especially a polyneuropathy. It can precipitate subacute combined degeneration of the cord. The serum vitamin B12 is below the normal level (normal range 150–700 pmol/L).

B12 >220 pmol/L = deficiency unlikely
<148 pmol/L = deficiency

Intrinsic factor antibody level is diagnostic.

Treatment (replacement therapy)[1]

- Vitamin B12 (1000 mcg, i.e. 1 mg) IM injection; body stores (3–5 mg) are replenished after 10–15 injections given every 2 to 3 days
- Maintenance with 1000 mcg injections every third month
- Can use crystalline oral B12
- Co-therapy with oral folate 5 mg/day (initially) is indicated.[9,10]
- Transfusion is best avoided. May need additional iron.

Folic acid deficiency

Diagnostic test: serum folate (normal range 7–45 nmol/L) and red cell folate—best test (normal >630 nmol/L).[7]

The main cause is poor intake associated with old age, poverty and malnutrition, usually associated with alcoholism. It may be seen in malabsorption and regular medication with anti-epileptic drugs such as phenytoin.[9] It is rarely, but very importantly, associated with pregnancy, when the demands of the developing fetus together with the needs of the mother outstrip the dietary intake—the so-called 'pernicious anaemia of pregnancy' which, if not recognised and treated immediately, can still be a fatal condition. Unlike vitamin B12, folic acid is not stored in the body to any significant degree and requirements have to be satisfied by the daily dietary intake, which invariably meets the requirement of 5–10 mcg/day. Folic acid is present in most fruit and vegetables, especially citrus fruits, nuts and green leafy vegetables (see CHAPTER 10).

Treatment (replacement therapy)

Oral folate 5 mg/day to replenish body stores (5–10 mg). This takes about 4 weeks but continue for 4 months. Vitamin B12 is usually given unless levels normal.

NORMOCYTIC ANAEMIA[2] (ANAEMIAS WITHOUT CHANGE IN THE MCV)

Acute haemorrhage

This is the most common cause of normocytic anaemia and is usually due to haematemesis and/or melaena.

Chronic disease

Chronic inflammation

Intercellular iron transport within the marrow is suppressed in inflammation so that, despite normal iron stores, the developing red cells are deprived of iron and erythropoiesis is depressed. If the inflammation is short-lived, the fall in Hb is not noticeable but, if it continues, an anaemia may develop that responds only when the inflammation subsides.

Malignancy

Anaemia may develop for the same reasons that apply to chronic inflammation.

Kidney failure

This is often associated with anaemia due to failure of erythropoietin secretion and is unresponsive to treatment, other than by alleviating the insufficiency or until erythropoietin is administered.

Haemolysis

Suspect haemolytic anaemia if there is a reticulocytosis, mild macrocytosis, reduced haptoglobin, increased bilirubin and urobilinogen. Haemolytic anaemias are relatively infrequent. The more common of the congenital ones are hereditary spherocytosis, sickle cell anaemia and deficiencies of the red cell enzymes, pyruvate kinase and G-6-PD, although most cases of G-6-PD deficiency haemolyse only when the patient takes oxidant drugs such as sulphonamides or eats broad beans—'favism'.

Acquired haemolytic anaemias include those of the newborn due to maternal haemolytic blood group antibodies passing back through the placenta to the fetus, and adult anaemias due to drug toxicity or to acquired auto-antibodies. About half of the latter are idiopathic and half associated with non-Hodgkin lymphomas, and the anaemia may be the presenting sign of lymphoma. Some of these antibodies are active only at cool temperatures—cold agglutinin disease; others act at body temperature and are the more potent cause of autoimmune haemolytic anaemia.

Keep in mind the rare acquired genetic disorder of paroxysmal nocturnal haemoglobinuria if dark morning urine is observed in the presence of anaemia. Flow cytometry is required for diagnosis.

Bone marrow replacement

This may be due to foreign tissue, such as carcinomatous metastases or fibrous tissue as in myelofibrosis; it may also be due to overgrowth by one or other normal elements of the bone marrow, as in chronic myeloid leukaemia, chronic lymphocytic leukaemia and lymphoma, as well as by acute leukaemic tissue. A leuco-erythroblastic picture, in which immature red and white cells appear in the peripheral blood, is often seen when the marrow is replaced by foreign tissue.

Anaemia in children

Haemoglobin reference range

Infant	Term (cord blood)	135–195 g/L
	3–6 months	95–135 g/L
Child	1 year	105–135 g/L
	3–6 years	105–140 g/L
	10–12 years	115–145 g/L

Important causes of anaemia in childhood include iron-deficiency anaemia (quite common), thalassaemia major, sickle-cell anaemia and drug-induced haemolysis. Consider one of the haemoglobinopathies in children of Mediterranean, South-East Asian, Arabic or African–American descent, especially with a family history, normal ferritin level or anaemia resistant to iron therapy. Investigate with Hb electrophoresis.

Drugs that can cause haemolysis (the film will have reticulocytosis, spherocytosis and fragmented red cells) include some antibiotics (e.g. sulfamethoxazole, antimalarials and some anti-inflammatories).

Think of anaemia in adolescents, especially females with a rapid growth spurt at the menarche and a relatively poor diet.

Iron deficiency in children[10]

- Iron deficiency is present in up to 10–30% of children in high-risk groups.
- It is often subclinical and anaemia develops in relatively few.
- It can lead to reduced cognitive and psychomotor performance (even without anaemia).
- High-risk groups include those infants <6 months who are premature and/or with low birthweight; toddlers 6–36 months with a diet high in cow's milk and low in iron-containing foods; those exclusively breastfed after 6 months; those with delayed introduction of solids; those with general poor food intake; and those with lack of vitamin C in their diet. Bottle-feeding encourages a high milk intake and reduces the appetite for solid food.
- Possible clinical features include irritability, lethargy, minor behavioural changes, poor growth, dyspnoea and pallor.

Prevention

- Give iron and multivitamin supplements to very premature and low birthweight (<1000 g) infants.
- Introduce iron-containing solids early—at 4 to 5 months, e.g. cereals, vegetables, egg and meat.
- Encourage breastfeeding and avoid cow's milk in the first 12 months.[9]
- Avoid excessive cow's milk up to 24 months.
- Use iron-fortified formulas and cereals.

Important sources of iron

Infant milk formulas, meat (especially red meat, and also fish and chicken), green vegetables and legumes, dried fruit, juices, fortified cereals, egg yolk.

Treatment

Treatment is mainly with ferrous gluconate (1 mL/kg of 300 mg/5 mL mixture). Continue for 3 months after Hb has normalised.

Practice tips

- Iron-deficiency anaemia is blood-loss anaemia until proved otherwise.
- It is possible to be tired from iron deficiency without anaemia.
- Blood-loss anaemia is usually due to menorrhagia or gastrointestinal loss until proved otherwise.
- Investigations for suspected anaemia should include FBE, ESR and iron studies. Others to consider are Hb electrophoresis, vitamin B12 and folate levels and kidney function tests.
- Hypothyroidism can cause a normocytic or a macrocytic anaemia.
- A therapeutic trial of iron (without investigations) is indefensible.
- Intramuscular injections of iron can tattoo so use with care: an IM iron dose is not 'stronger' than an oral iron dose.
- If microcytic anaemia is not responding to anaemia, consider sideroblastic anaemia.

Patient education resources

Hand-out sheets from *Murtagh's Patient Education* 7th edition:

- Iron deficiency anaemia

References

1 Van Der Weyden M. Anaemia. In: *MIMS Disease Index* (2nd edn). Sydney: IMS Publishing, 1996: 26–9.

2 Gribble M. Haematology. Check Program 188. Melbourne: RACGP, 1987: 3–12.

3 Hang W, Gibson J. Iron deficiency anaemia. Medical Observer, 4 April 2014: 21–6.

4 Coghlan D, Campbell P. Anaemia: how to treat. Australian Doctor, 8 November 2002: I–VIII.

5 Powers JM et al. Diagnostic and management of iron deficiency anaemia. Hematol Oncol Cln North Am, August 2014; 28(4): 729–45. [PMID: 26289639]

6 Avni T. The safety of intravenous iron preparations: systemic review and meta-analysis. Mayo Clin Proc, January 2015; 90(1): 12–23. [PMID: 25572192]

7 Farrell CT et al, Red cell or serum folate: what to do in clinical practice. Clin Chem Lab Med, March 2013; 51(3): 555–69. [PMID: 23449524]

8 Dickinson M et al. Haematology. Check Program 439. Melbourne: RACGP, 2008: 4–10.

9 Schrier S. UpToDate. Macrocytosis (16.1 edn). UpToDate, 2008.

10 Thomson K et al. *Paediatric Handbook* (8th edn). Melbourne: Wiley-Blackwell Science, 2009: 360–3.

23 Endocrine and metabolic disorders

It would indeed be rash for a mere pathologist to venture forth on the uncharted sea of the endocrines, strewn as it is with the wrecks of shattered hypotheses, where even the most wary mariner may easily lose his way as he seeks to steer his bark amid the glandular temptations whose siren voices have proved the downfall of many who have gone before.

William Boyd (1885–1969)

Endocrine, particularly thyroid, disorders can be a diagnostic trap in family practice and early diagnosis is a real challenge. A family practice of 2500 patients can expect one new case of thyroid disorder each year and 10 'cases' in the practice.[1] The diagnosis of an overactive or underactive thyroid can be difficult as the early clinical deviations from normality can be subtle.

The clinical diagnosis of classical Graves disease is usually obvious with the features of exophthalmos, hyperkinesis and a large goitre but if the eye and neck signs are absent it can be misdiagnosed as an anxiety state. Elderly patients may present with only cardiovascular signs, such as atrial fibrillation and tachycardia, or with unexplained weight loss.

The hypothyroid patient can be very difficult to diagnose in the early stages, especially if the patient is being seen frequently. Hypothyroidism often has a gradual onset with general symptoms such as constipation and lethargy.

If suspected, serum thyroid stimulating hormone (TSH) or thyrotropin should be requested.

Other common endocrine disorders include diabetes mellitus, hyperprolactinaemia, calcium metabolic disorder, PCOS, sexual dysfunction and subclinical hypogonadism. They may be difficult to diagnose in the early stages of development. The pituitary is the master gland and its regulating hormones are depicted in FIGURE 23.1.[2,3]

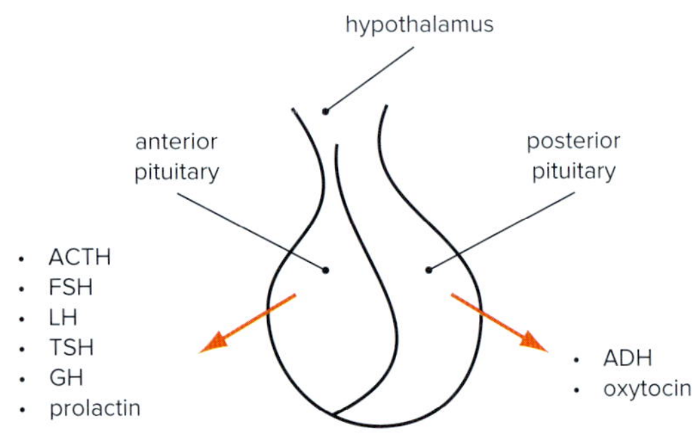

FIGURE 23.1 Pituitary hormones

Tests for thyroid disorders[2,3]

Thyroid function tests

Advances in technology have allowed the biochemical assessment of thyroid function to change dramatically in recent years with the introduction of the serum free thyroxine (T_4) and the monoclonal TSH assays. With the highly sensitive TSH assays it is now possible to distinguish suppressed TSH levels (as in hyperthyroidism) from low and normal levels of TSH. However, the new assays are not foolproof and require interpretation in the context of the clinical picture. The serum TSH level is the most sensitive index of thyroid function and is the preferred test for suspected thyroid dysfunction. If necessary repeat TSH in 3–6 months.

Serum tri-iodothyronine (T_3) measurement and serum free thyroxine (T_4) can be useful in suspected T_3 toxicosis where serum T_4 level may be normal, and for monitoring patients with treated thyroid dysfunction.

The relative values are summarised in TABLE 23.1.

Thyroid auto-antibodies

Raised auto-antibodies (antimicrosomal or antithyroid peroxidase) are suggestive of Hashimoto thyroiditis (autoimmune thyroiditis). Antithyroglobulin, anti-thyroid peroxidase and TSH receptor antibodies are elevated in Graves disease, the TSH receptor antibody being very specific for Graves disease.

Fine needle aspiration

This is the single most cost-effective investigation in the diagnosis of thyroid nodules. It is the best way to assess a nodule for malignancy. Care needs to be taken in the interpretation of the cytology results in conjunction with an experienced cytologist/pathologist.

Table 23.1 Summary of thyroid function tests[2]

	TSH	free T^4	free T^3	Antithyroid antibodies
Normal range	0.4–4.5 mU/L	10–22 pmol/L	3.3–8.0 pmol/L	
Hypothyroidism				
Primary	↑*	↓*	N or ↓ (not useful)	N or ↑
Secondary (pituitary dysfunction)	N or ↓	↓	N or ↓ (not useful)	N
Hyperthyroidism	↓*	↑*	↑*	N or ↑
Sick euthyroid	N or ↓	N or ↓	N or ↓	N

Notes: Results similar to hyperthyroidism can occur with acute psychiatric illness.

Normal ranges vary between laboratories.

* Main tests

Thyroid isotope scan

The scan may help in the differential diagnosis of thyroid nodules and in hyperthyroidism. A functioning nodule is said to be less likely to be malignant than a non-functioning nodule (cyst, colloid nodule, haemorrhage are non-functioning; carcinoma is usually non-functioning).

Thyroid ultrasound

A thyroid ultrasound is usually more sensitive in the detection of thyroid nodules. A multinodular goitre may be diagnosed on ultrasound while the clinical impression may be that of a solitary nodule (the other nodules not being palpable clinically). A multinodular goitre is said to be less likely to be malignant than a solitary thyroid nodule. An ultrasound allows for follow-up of thyroid nodule(s) to note if there are any changes in size over a period of time and to then discuss appropriate intervention with the patient. It can also differentiate a solid from a cystic mass.

CT scan

CT scan of the thyroid may be used particularly to determine if there is significant compression in the neck from a large multinodular goitre with retrosternal extension. Again follow-up CT scans may allow one to determine the progression or otherwise of such a goitre.

Hypothyroidism (myxoedema)

Hypothyroidism, which is relatively common, is more prevalent in elderly women (up to 5%).[4] The term *myxoedema* refers to the accumulation of mucopolysaccharide in subcutaneous tissues. The early changes are subtle and can be misdiagnosed, especially if only a single symptom is dominant.

Patients at risk include those with:

- previous Graves disease
- autoimmune disorders (e.g. rheumatoid arthritis, type 1 diabetes)
- Down syndrome
- Turner syndrome
- drug treatment: lithium, amiodarone, interferon
- previous thyroid or neck surgery
- previous radioactive iodine treatment of the thyroid

Clinical features

The main features are:

- constipation
- cold intolerance
- tiredness/lethargy/somnolence
- physical slowing
- mental slowing
- depression
- huskiness of voice
- puffiness of face and eyes
- pallor
- loss of hair
- weight gain

DxT tiredness + husky voice + cold intolerance → myxoedema

Physical examination

See FIGURE 23.2. The main signs are:

- sinus bradycardia
- delayed reflexes (normal muscular contraction, slow relaxation)

23

- coarse, dry and brittle hair
- thinning of outer third of eyebrows
- dry, cool skin
- skin pallor or yellowing
- obesity
- goitre

Other diverse presentations of thyroid disorders are given in TABLE 23.2.

Hashimoto thyroiditis (autoimmune thyroiditis)

Hashimoto thyroiditis, or lymphocytic thyroiditis, which is an autoimmune thyroiditis, is the commonest cause of bilateral non-thyrotoxic goitre in Australia. Features are:

- bilateral goitre
- classically described as firm and rubbery

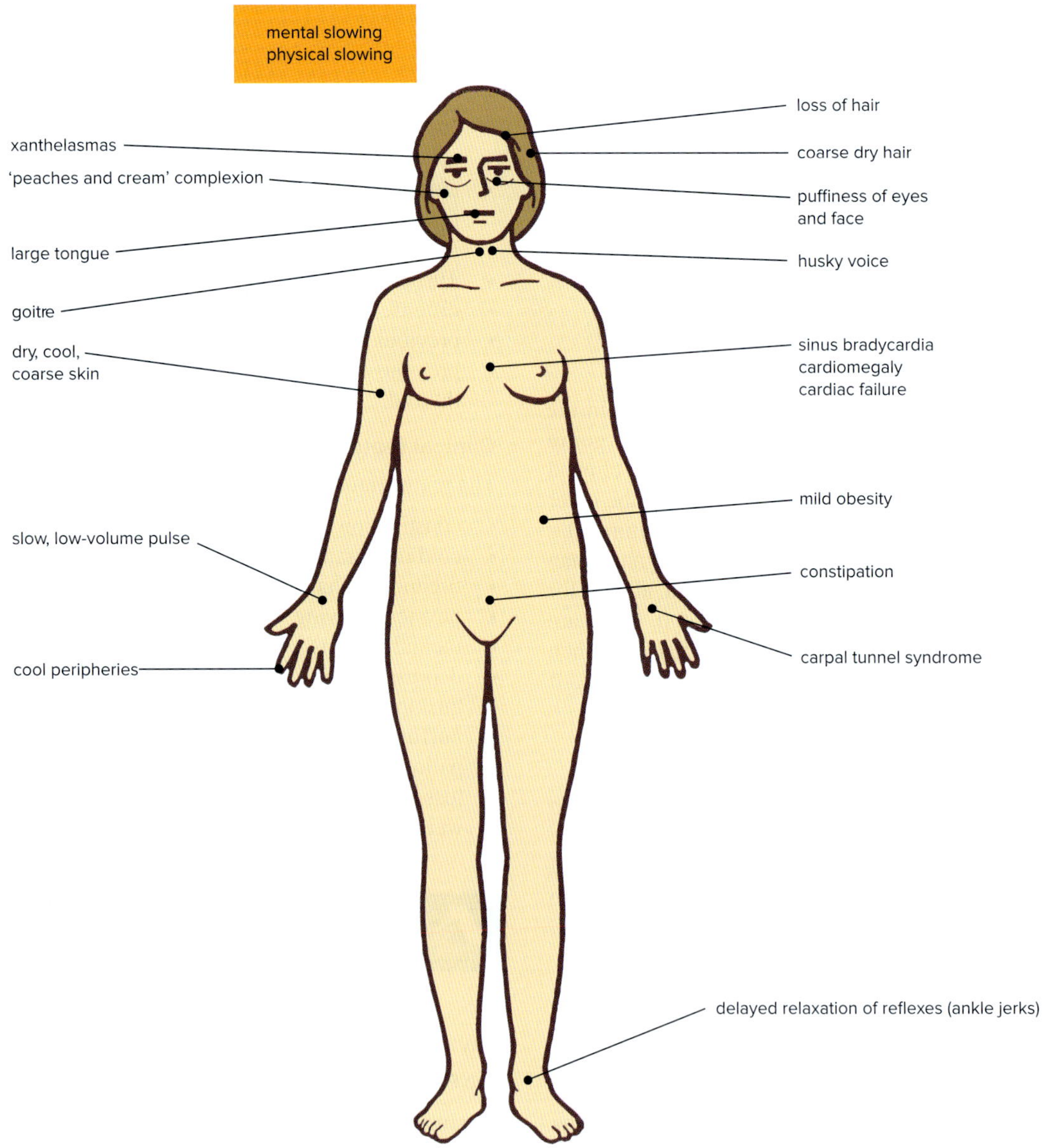

FIGURE 23.2 Clinical features of hypothyroidism

Table 23.2 Various diverse presentations of thyroid disorders[2,4]

	Hypothyroidism	Hyperthyroidism
General	Lethargy, tiredness Dry skin Husky voice	Weakness Sweaty skin, especially hands
Psychiatric	Depression Dementia Psychosis (myxoedema madness)	Anxiety/irritability Hyperkinesis Psychosis
Musculoskeletal	Myofibrositis Myalgia Joint effusions	Muscle weakness Proximal myopathy
Skin	Dry, cool skin Vitiligo	Warm, thin, soft, moist skin Vitiligo Pretibial myxoedema
Cardiovascular	Ischaemia Cardiomegaly Pericardial effusion Bradycardia Hyperlipidaemia	Tachycardia Atrial fibrillation Heart failure Systolic hypertension
Endocrine	Galactorrhoea Goitre Infertility	Goitre Gynaecomastia
Gynaecological	Menstrual irregularity Menorrhagia (mainly) Oligomenorrhoea	Oligomenorrhoea
Neurological	Neuropathy Nerve entrapment (e.g. carpal tunnel) Ataxia	Periodic paralysis Tremor
Haematological	Anaemia	–
Emergency	Myxoedema coma Postanaesthetic hypoventilation	Thyroid crisis
Other	Reduced libido Weight gain Cold intolerance Constipation	Reduced libido Eye signs Fever (uncommon) Onycholysis Premature grey hair Weight loss

- patients may be hypothyroid or euthyroid with a possible early period of thyrotoxicosis

Diagnosis is confirmed by a strongly positive antithyroid microsomal antibody titre and/or fine needle aspiration cytology.[3]

Hashimoto thyroiditis may present as postpartum hypothyroidism. The hypothyroidism may resolve in 6–12 months or may be permanent.[3]

Laboratory diagnosis of hypothyroidism

Thyroid function tests (see TABLE 23.1):

- T_4—subnormal
- TSH—elevated (>10 is clear gland failure)

If T_4 is low and TSH is low or normal, consider pituitary dysfunction (secondary hypothyroidism) or sick euthyroid syndrome. A raised TSH and T_4 in normal range denotes 'subclinical' hypothyroidism and treatment is appropriate albeit controversial.[2,5]

Interpretation of TFTs can be difficult but requires matching to the clinical 'picture' and consultant advice.

Other tests

- Serum cholesterol level elevated
- Anaemia: usually normocytic; may be macrocytic
- ECG: sinus bradycardia, low voltage, flat T waves

Management[7,8,9]

Confirm the diagnosis, provide appropriate patient education, and refer the patient where appropriate.

Exclude coexisting hypoadrenalism and ischaemic heart disease before T_4 replacement.

Note: Treatment as primary hypothyroidism when hypopituitarism is the cause may precipitate adrenal crisis.

Thyroid medication

- Thyroxine 50–100 mcg daily, increasing by 25–50 mcg up to 100–200 mcg if required

Note: Start with low doses (25–50 mcg daily) in elderly and those with ischaemic heart disease and 50–100 mcg in others. Avoid overdosage.

- Aim to achieve TSH levels of 0.5–2 mU/L.
- Monitor TSH levels monthly at first. As euthyroidism is achieved, monitoring may be less frequent (e.g. 2–3 months). When stable on optimum dose of T_4, monitor every 2–3 years. Treatment is usually lifelong.

Special treatment considerations

- *Ischaemic heart disease.* Rapid thyroxine replacement can precipitate myocardial infarction, especially in the elderly.
- *Pregnancy and postpartum.* Continue thyroxine during pregnancy; watch for hypothyroidism (an increased dose of T_4 is often required).
- *Elective surgery.* If euthyroid, can stop thyroxine for one week. If subthyroid, defer surgery until euthyroid.
- *Myxoedema coma.* Urgent hospitalisation under specialist care is required. Intensive treatment is required, which may involve parenteral T_4 or T_3 as liothyronine or thyroxine by slow IV injection.

23

Neonatal hypothyroidism

Misdiagnosing this serious condition leads to failure to thrive, retarded growth and poor school performance. If untreated it leads to permanent intellectual damage (cretinism). The clinical features of the newborn include coarse features, dry skin, supra-orbital oedema, jaundice, harsh cry, slow feeding and umbilical hernia. It is detected by routine neonatal heel prick blood testing. Thyroxine replacement should be started as soon as possible, at least before 2 weeks of age to avert intellectual retardation.

When to refer—hypothyroidism[4,8]

- Doubt about diagnosis, diagnostic tests or optimum replacement dosage
- Apparent secondary hypothyroidism, severe illness and associated ischaemic heart disease
- Concurrent autoimmune disease
- Hypothyroidism with goitre, postpartum thyroid dysfunction and in the neonate
- Myxoedema coma

Hyperthyroidism (thyrotoxicosis)

Hyperthyroidism is also relatively common and may affect up to 2% of women, who are affected four to five times more often than men (see FIG. 23.3). Graves disease is the most common cause followed closely by nodular thyroid disease.

Causes[3,10]

- Graves disease (typical symptoms with a diffuse goitre and eye signs)
- Autonomous functioning nodules/toxic adenoma
- Subacute thyroiditis (de Quervain thyroiditis)—viral origin (suspect if painful thyroid and malaise)

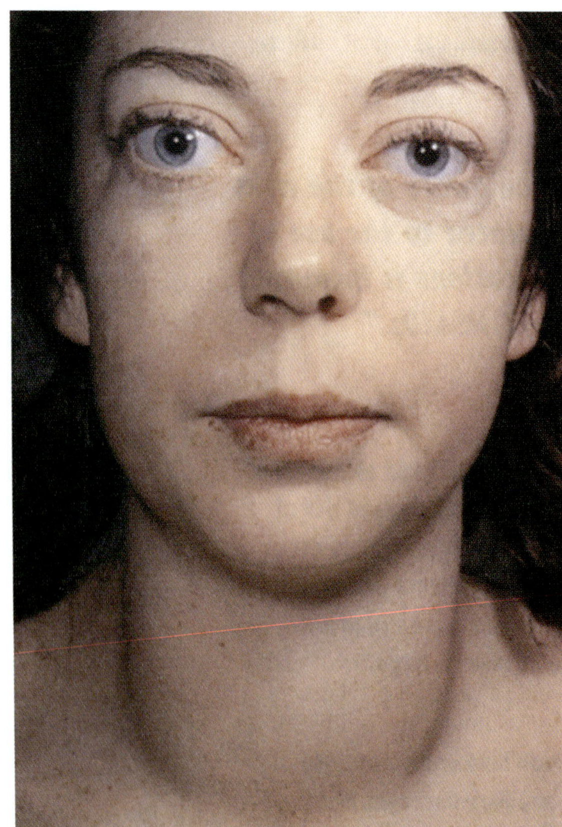

FIGURE 23.3 Thyrotoxicosis patient with exophthalmos and goitre
Photo courtesy Duncan Topliss

- Excessive intake of thyroid hormones—thyrotoxicosis factitia
- Exogenous iodine excess, e.g. food contamination
- Amiodarone (beware of this drug)

Key facts and checkpoints

- The classic symptoms may be lacking in elderly patients who may have only cardiovascular manifestations (e.g. unexplained heart failure or cardiac arrhythmias).
- Care has to be taken not to dismiss hyperthyroidism as severe anxiety.

Clinical features

- Heat intolerance
- Sweating of hands
- Muscle weakness
- Weight loss despite normal or increased appetite
- Emotional lability, especially anxiety, irritability
- Palpitations
- Frequent loose bowel motions

DxT anxiety + weight loss + weakness → thyrotoxicosis

Physical examination

See FIGURE 23.4. Signs are (usually):

- agitated, restless patient
- warm and sweaty hands
- fine tremor (place paper on hands)
- goitre
- proximal myopathy
- hyperactive reflexes
- bounding peripheral pulse
- ± atrial fibrillation

Eye signs

- Lid retraction (small area of sclera seen above iris)
- Lid lag
- Exophthalmos
- Ophthalmoplegia in severe cases

Investigations

- T_4 (and T_3) elevated
- TSH level suppressed
- Radioisotope scan
- Antithyroid peroxidase

The isotope scan enables a diagnosis of Graves disease to be made when the scan shows uniform increased uptake. Increased irregular uptake would suggest a toxic multinodular goitre, while there is poor or no uptake with de Quervain thyroiditis and thyrotoxicosis factitia.

Management

- Establish the precise cause before initiating treatment.
- Refer to an endocrinologist to guide treatment.
- Educate patients and emphasise the possibility of development of recurrent hyperthyroidism or hypothyroidism and the need for lifelong monitoring.
- Monitor for cardiovascular complications and osteoporosis.

Treatment[6,8,9]

- Radioactive iodine therapy (^{131}I)
- Thionamide antithyroid drugs (initial doses)
  - carbimazole 10–45 mg (o) daily starting with 10–20 mg in divided doses depending on disease activity

  or

  - propylthiouracil 200–600 mg (o) daily in divided doses or methimazole
- Adjunctive drugs
  - beta blockers (for symptoms in acute florid phase, e.g. propranolol 10–40 mg, 6 to 8 hourly); diltiazem or atenolol are alternatives
  - lithium carbonate (rarely used when there is intolerance to thionamides)
  - Lugol's iodine: mainly used prior to surgery
- Surgery
  - subtotal thyroidectomy

  or

  - total thyroidectomy

23

Treatment (Graves disease)

There is no ideal treatment, and selection of antithyroid drugs, radioiodine or surgery depends on many factors, including age, size of goitre, social and economic factors and complications of treatment.

Guidelines[6,9]

- Younger patients with small goitres and mild case—18-month course antithyroid drugs
- Older patients with small goitres—as above or radioiodine (preferably when euthyroid)
- Large goitres or moderate-to-severe cases—antithyroid drugs until euthyroid, then surgery or ^{131}I
- In Australia (as in the US) ^{131}I is being increasingly used

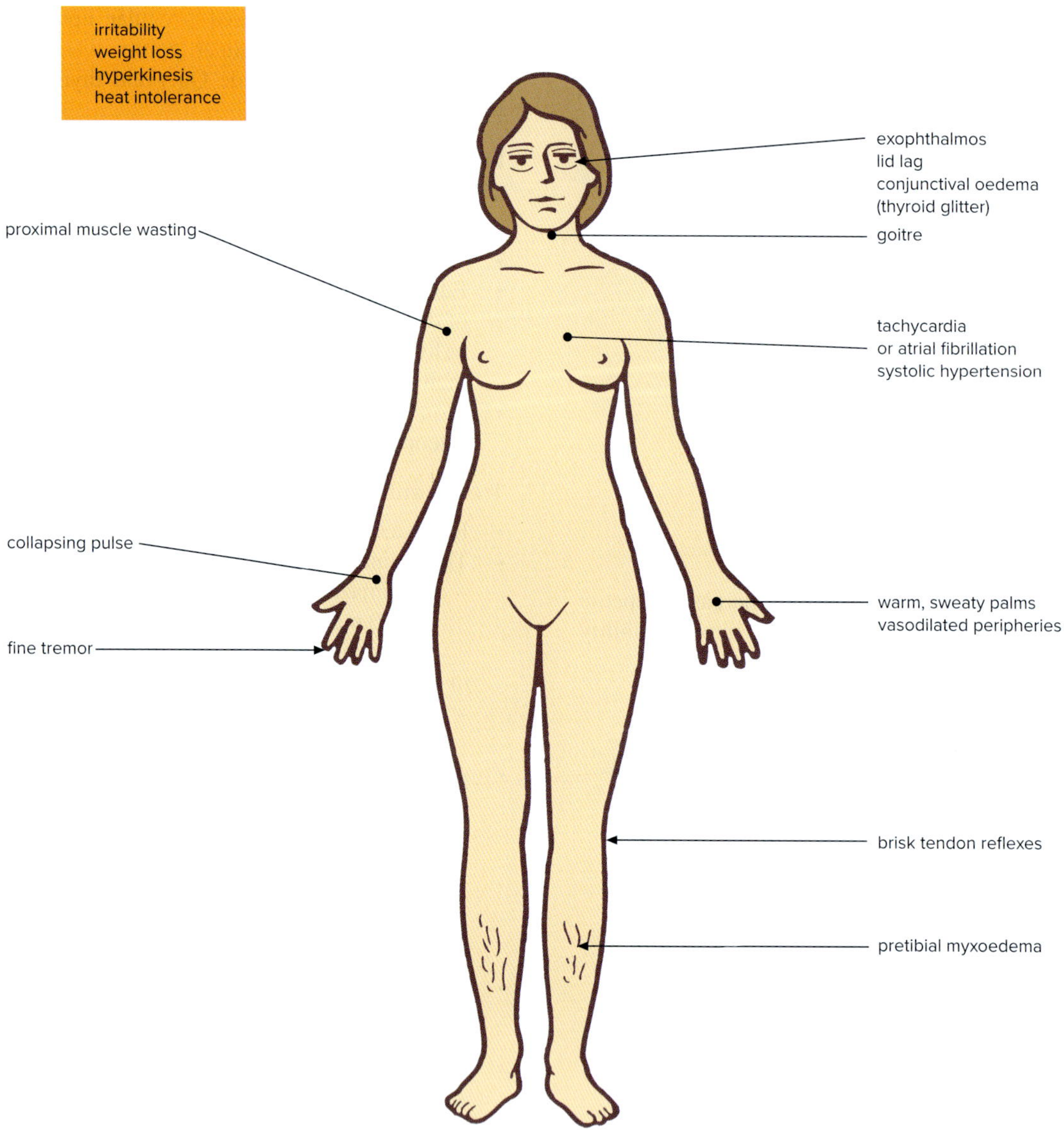

FIGURE 23.4 Clinical features of hyperthyroidism

Treatment (autonomous functioning nodules and toxic adenoma)

Control hyperthyroidism with antithyroid drugs, then surgery or ^{131}I. Long-term remissions on antithyroid drugs in a toxic nodular goitre are rare.

Treatment (subacute thyroiditis)[7]

Hyperthyroidism is usually transient and follows a surge of thyroxine after a viral-type illness. Symptoms include pain and/or tenderness over the goitre (especially on swallowing) and fever. In the acute phase treatment is based on rest, analgesics (aspirin 600 mg (o) 4–6 hourly) or ibuprofen 200–400 mg (o) and soft foods. Rarely, when pain is severe, corticosteroids may be used. Antithyroid drugs are not indicated but beta-blockers can be used to control symptoms.

Thyroid crisis (thyroid storm)[9]

Clinical features are marked anxiety, weight loss, weakness, proximal muscle weakness, hyperpyrexia, tachycardia (>150 per minute), heart failure and arrhythmias. It is usually precipitated by surgery or an infection in an undiagnosed patient.

It requires urgent intensive hospital management with antithyroid drugs; IV saline infusion, IV corticosteroids, anti-heart failure and antiarrhythmia therapy, especially beta-blockers.

When to refer—hyperthyroidism[10]

- Doubt about the diagnosis
- Severe hyperthyroidism, especially if there is coexisting thyrocardiac disease
- Pregnant patients with hyperthyroidism
- Progression of exophthalmos
- Ideally all cases

Thyroid nodules

A thyroid nodule is defined as a discrete lesion on palpation and/or ultrasonography that is distinct from the rest of the thyroid gland.

Causes

- Dominant nodule in a multinodular goitre (most likely)
- Colloid cyst
- True solitary nodule: adenoma, carcinoma (papillary or follicular)

Investigations

- Ultrasound imaging
- Fine-needle aspiration cytology
- Thyroid function tests

Thyroid carcinoma[9]

The main presentations are a painless nodule, a hard nodule in an enlarged gland or lymphadenopathy. Papillary carcinoma is the most common malignancy. Although rare compared with non-malignant lesions (such as colloid nodules, cysts, haemorrhage and benign adenomas), it is important not to miss carcinoma because of the very high cure rate with treatment. This often involves total thyroidectomy, ablative ^{131}I treatment, thyroxine replacement and follow-up with serum thyroglobulin measurements, ^{131}I/thallium scanning and neck ultrasound. Fine-needle aspiration is the investigation of choice.

PITUITARY DISORDERS

Pituitary tumours[10]

These are invariably benign adenomas. They can present with hormone deficiencies, features of hypersecretory syndromes (e.g. prolactin, GH, ACTH) or by local tumour mass symptoms (e.g. headache, visual field loss).

Hyperprolactinaemia[13]

The main causes (of many) are a pituitary adenoma (micro- or macro), pituitary stalk damage, drugs—such as antipsychotics, various antidepressants, metoclopramide, cimetidine, oestrogens, opiates, marijuana—and physiological causes such as pregnancy and breastfeeding.

Clinical features

- Symptoms common to males and females: reduced libido, subfertility, galactorrhoea (mainly females)
- Females: Amenorrhoea/oligomenorrhoea
- Males: erectile dysfunction, reduced facial hair

Diagnosis

- Serum prolactin and macroprolactin assays
- MRI: consider if headache, etc

Refer for management, which may include a dopamine agonist such as cabergoline or bromocriptine.

Acromegaly

Symptoms suggestive of acromegaly include:

- excessive growth of hands (increased glove size)
- excessive growth of tissues (e.g. nose, lips, face)
- excessive growth of feet (increased shoe size)
- increased size of jaw and tongue; kyphosis
- general: weakness, sweating, headaches
- sexual changes, including amenorrhoea and loss of libido
- disruptive snoring (sleep apnoea)
- deepening voice

DxT nasal problems + fitting problems (e.g. rings, shoes) + sweating ➜ acromegaly

Diagnosis[9,12]

- Plasma growth hormone excess
- Elevated insulin-like growth factor 1 (IGF-1) (somatomedin)—the key test
- X-ray skull and hands
- MRI scanning pituitary
- Consider associated impaired glucose tolerance/ diabetes

Obtain old photographs (if possible).
Treatment: pituitary microsurgery.

Diabetes insipidus and SIADH

Impaired secretion of vasopressin (antidiuretic hormone) from the posterior pituitary leads to polyuria, nocturia and compensatory polydipsia resulting in the passage of 3–20 L of dilute urine per day. There are several causes of diabetes insipidus (DI), the commonest being postoperative (hypothalamic-pituitary), which is usually transient only. Other causes of cranial DI include tumours, infections and infiltrations. In nephrogenic DI the kidney tubules are insensitive to vasopressin. Differential diagnosis includes compulsive (psychogenic) water drinking. The syndrome of secretion of inappropriate antidiuretic hormone (SIADH) is caused by cancer (e.g. lung, lymphomas, kidney, pancreas), pulmonary disorders, various intracranial lesions and drugs such as carbamazepine and many antipsychotic agents. Management of SIADH is essentially fluid restriction.

The treatment of DI is desmopressin, usually given twice daily intranasally.

> **DxT** weakness + polyuria + polydipsia ➜ diabetes insipidus

Hypopituitarism[9]

This rare disorder should be considered with:

- a history of postpartum haemorrhage
- symptoms of hypothyroidism
- symptoms of adrenal insufficiency
- symptoms suggestive of a pituitary tumour
- thin, wrinkled skin: 'monkey face'
- pale 'alabaster' skin/hairlessness

> **DxT** (female): amenorrhoea + loss of axillary and pubic hair + breast atrophy ➜ hypopituitarism
> **DxT** (male): ↓ libido + impotence + loss of body hair ➜ hypopituitarism

Investigate with serum pituitary hormones, imaging and triple stimulation test.

ADRENAL DISORDERS

The primary zones of the adrenal gland and their secretions

Cortex

- zona glomerulosa—mineral corticoids, especially aldosterone
- zona fasciculata—glucocorticoids
- zona reticularus—androgens, especially DHEA

Medulla

- catecholamines—epinepherine, norepinephrine

It is worth keeping in mind these uncommon disorders of the adrenal gland which can be difficult to diagnose in the early stages, namely:

- chronic adrenal insufficiency (Addison disease)—deficiency of cortisol and aldosterone
- Cushing syndrome—cortisol excess
- primary hyperaldosteronism (refer to CHAPTER 86)

Addison disease[9,14]

Autoimmune destruction of the adrenals is the most common cause.

Clinical features

- Lethargy/excessive fatigue/weakness
- Anorexia and nausea
- Diarrhoea/abdominal pain
- Weight loss
- Dizziness/funny turns, syncope: hypoglycaemia (rare); postural hypotension (common)
- Hyperpigmentation, especially mucous membranes of mouth and hard palate, skin creases of hands

If Addison disease remains undiagnosed, wasting leading to death may occur. Severe dehydration can be a feature. Delayed diagnosis is a huge problem. Hypertension and heart failure requires careful monitoring.

> **DxT** fatigue + a/n/v + abdominal pain (± skin discolouration) ➜ Addison disease

Diagnosis

- Elevated serum potassium, low serum sodium
- Low plasma cortisol level (fails to respond to synthetic adrenocorticotropic hormone [ACTH])
- The short synacthen stimulation test is the definitive test
- Consider adrenal auto-antibodies and imaging ? calcification of adrenals

Treatment: corticosteroid replacement—hydrocortisone/fludrocortisone acetate, other options.

Addisonian crisis[9,14]

An Addisonian crisis develops because of an inability to increase cortisol in response to stress, which may include intercurrent infection, surgery or trauma.

Clinical features

- Nausea and vomiting
- Acute abdominal pain
- Severe hypotension progressing to shock
- Weakness, drowsiness progressing to coma

Urgent management[14]

- Establish IV line with IV fluids
- Hydrocortisone sodium succinate 100 mg IV initially and 50–100 mg 4–6 hourly until stable
- Arrange urgent hospital admission

Cushing syndrome[9]

The five main causes are:

- iatrogenic—chronic corticosteroid administration
- pituitary ACTH excess (Cushing disease)
- bilateral adrenal hyperplasia
- adrenal tumour (adenoma, adenocarcinoma)
- ectopic ACTH or (rarely) corticotrophin-releasing hormone (CRH) from nonendocrine tumours (e.g. oat cell carcinoma of lung)

The clinical features (see FIG. 23.5) are caused by the effects of excess cortisol and/or adrenal androgens.

Clinical features

- Proximal muscle wasting and weakness
- Central obesity, buffalo hump on neck
- Cushing facies: plethora, moon face, acne
- Weakness
- Hirsutism
- Abdominal striae
- Thin skin, easy bruising
- Hypertension
- Hyperglycaemia (30%)
- Menstrual changes (e.g. amenorrhoea)
- Osteoporosis
- Psychiatric changes, especially depression
- Backache

DxT plethoric moon face + thin extremities + muscle weakness ➜ Cushing syndrome

Diagnosis (apart from iatrogenic cause)

- Cortisol excess (plasma or 24-hour urinary cortisol)
- Dexamethasone suppression test
- Inferior petrosal sinus sampling
- Serum ACTH
- Radiological localisation: MRI for ACTH-producing pituitary tumours; CT scanning for adrenal tumours

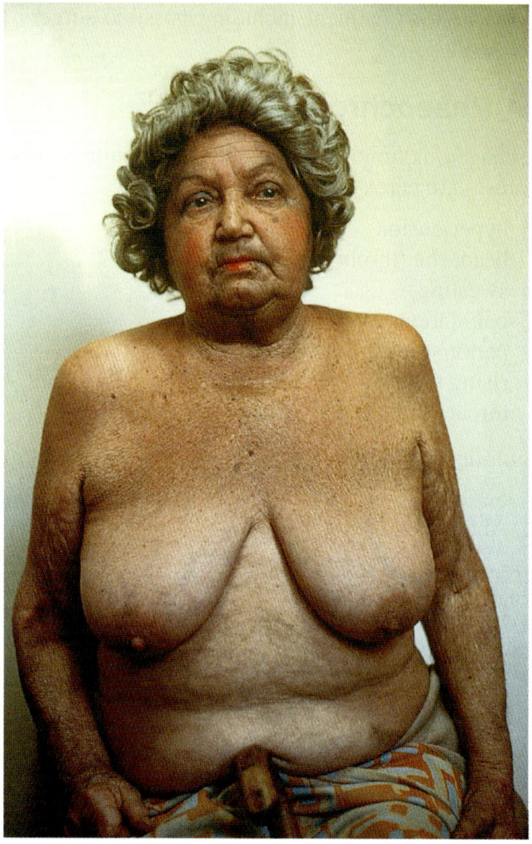

FIGURE 23.5 62-year-old woman with Cushing syndrome, showing centripetal obesity, hirsutism and virilisation (wearing a wig), 'moon' face, thin extremities and plethoric appearance

Photo courtesy David Dammery

23

Primary hyperaldosteronism[9]

Most commonly due to an adrenal adenoma.

Conn syndrome

Usually asymptomatic and hypertensive but any symptoms are features of hypokalaemia:

- weakness
- cramps
- paraesthesia
- polyuria and polydipsia

Investigations

- aldosterone (serum and urine) ↑
- plasma renin ↓
- Na ↑, K ↓, alkalosis
- imaging (MRI or CT scan) of adrenals

Refer for treatment including possible surgery to excise adenoma.

Phaeochromocytoma[9,12]

A dangerous tumour of the adrenal medulla. Clinical features are paroxysms or spells of:

- hypertension
- headache (throbbing)
- sweating
- palpitations
- pallor/skin blanching
- rising sensation of tightness in upper chest and throat (angina can occur)

Investigations

- Series of three 24-hour free catecholamines ↑ VMA
- Abdominal CT or MRI scan

Treatment

- Excise tumour, cover with alpha and beta blockers

Congenital adrenal hyperplasia (adrenogenital syndrome)[7,9]

An AR condition with 21-hydroxylase deficiency being the most common of several forms. There is inadequate synthesis of cortisol and aldosterone with increased androgenisation. Major problem is adrenal failure ± salt-losing state (SLS). In females, ambiguity of external genitalia and hirsutism before puberty usually occurs. Males may have normal urogenital development but SLS is a concern. Infants of either sex may present with failure to thrive or vomiting and dehydration (SLS). Lifelong glucocorticoid treatment is required. Wearing an alert bracelet or necklace is strongly recommended for these patients (www.medicalert.org.au).[7]

23

Adrenal tumours[10]

Most of those detected by abdominal imaging are benign and termed 'incidentalomas' but serious tumours include adrenal carcinoma, phaeochromocytoma, neuroblastoma, glucocorticoid or a mineral corticoid secreting tumour.

Rule: tumours >4 cm require thorough assessment as malignant tumours are large. Excision is usually advisable.

Incidentalomas

An important issue is malignancy, and if this is the case, whether it is primary, secondary or functional (hormone secreting).

Investigations to consider include electrolytes, aldosterone/rennin ratio, catecholamines, testosterone, DHEAs, dexamethasone suppression test, CT scan. Surgical excision should be considered under specialist guidance.

CALCIUM DISORDERS

Hypercalcaemia[12,15]

Suspect hypercalcaemia if there is weakness, tiredness, malaise, anorexia, nausea or vomiting, abdominal pain, loin pain, constipation, thirst, fever, polyuria, drowsiness, dizziness, personality changes, muscle aches and pains, visual disturbances. Measure urea and electrolytes (especially calcium), creatinine, albumin.

Primary hyperparathyroidism, familial hypercalciuric hypercalcaemia and neoplasia, especially lung and breast (with metastases to bone), account for over 90% of cases. Other causes include Paget disease, Williams syndrome, prolonged immobilisation, sarcoidosis and milk-alkali syndrome. Investigations include ESR, serum parathyroid hormone (N: 1.0–7 pmol/L), serum ACE levels, serum alkaline phosphatase, chest X-ray, Sestamibi scan and bone scan. Requires specialist referral.

DxT weakness + constipation + polyuria → hypercalcaemia
DxT cramps + confusion + tetany → hypocalcaemia

Primary hyperparathyroidism[12]

Hyperparathyroidism is caused by an excessive secretion of parathyroid hormone and is usually due to a parathyroid adenoma. The classic clinical features of hyperparathyroidism are due to the effects of hypercalcaemia. Rarely, a parathyroid crisis in a misdiagnosed patient may result in death from severe hypercalcaemia.

Classic mnemonic: bones, moans, stones, abdominal groans.

Diagnosis

- Exclusion of other causes of hypercalcaemia
- Serum parathyroid hormone (elevated)
- TC-99m Sestamibi scan to detect tumour

Hypocalcaemia[9,15]

Causes include parathyroid injury, autoimmune hyperparathyroidism, severe vitamin D deficiency and neonates of mothers with hypercalcaemia. This usually presents with tetany or more generalised neuromuscular hyperexcitability and neuropsychiatric manifestations. The sensory equivalents are paraesthesia in the hands, feet and around the mouth (distinguish from tetany seen in the respiratory alkalosis of hyperventilation). There may be seizures and cramps. The diagnosis is by measurement of serum total calcium concentration in relation to serum albumin (s. calcium <2.10 mmol/L).

Two important signs are:

- Trousseau sign: occlusion of the brachial artery with BP cuff precipitates carpopedal spasm (wrist flexion and fingers drawn together)
- Chvostek sign: tapping over parotid (facial nerve) causes twitching in facial muscles

Treatment involves careful adjustments in dosage of calcitriol and calcium to correct hypocalcaemia and avoid hypercalcaemia and hypercalciuria (the latter may lead to kidney impairment).

Hypoparathyroidism

Hypoparathyroidism is the most common cause of hypocalcaemia. Causes include postoperative thyroidectomy and parathyroidectomy, congenital deficiency (DiGeorge syndrome) and idiopathic (autoimmune) hypoparathyroidism. The main features are neuromuscular hyperexcitability, tetany and neuropsychiatric manifestations.

Other electrolyte disturbances

Hypernatraemia Na^+ >145 mmol/L

Causes

- water depletion (e.g. diabetes insipidus)
- water and sodium depletion (e.g. diarrhoea)
- corticosteroid excess (e.g. Cushing syndrome, Conn syndrome)
- iatrogenic: excess IV hypertonic Na solutions

Clinical features

- thirst, confusion, lethargy, weakness, irritability, oliguria
- orthostatic hypotension
- muscle twitching or cramps
- signs of dehydration
- severe: seizures, delirium, hyperthermia, coma

Hyponatraemia Na^+ <135 mmol/L

Causes

- water retention (e.g. CCF, hypoalbuminaemia)
- kidney failure to conserve salt (e.g. nephritis, diabetes mellitus, Addison disease)
- gastrointestinal loss of Na^+ (e.g. vomiting, diarrhoea)
- drugs (e.g. diuretic excess, ACE inhibitors)

Clinical features

- anorexia, nausea, lethargy, confusion, headache, mental changes (e.g. in personality)
- severe: convulsions, coma, death

Hyperkalaemia K^+ >5.5 mmol/L

The first sign of hyperkalaemia (e.g. >6) may be a cardiac arrest. A medical emergency if >6.5.

Causes

- oliguria, kidney failure
- acidosis (especially metabolic)
- mineralocorticoid deficiency: Addison disease, aldosterone antagonists
- excessive intake of K^+ (e.g. IV fluids with K)
- drugs (e.g. spironolactone, ACE inhibitors, NSAIDs, suxamethonium)
- Consider artefact, e.g. haemolysed sample

Clinical features

- malaise, muscle weakness, flaccid paralysis (rare)
- may be asymptomatic until cardiac toxicity
- may cause cardiac arrest—asystole or fibrillation
- ECG: peaked T waves, ↓ QT, ↑ PR interval → arrhythmias

Hypokalaemia K^+ <3.5 mmol/L

If <2.5 severe symptoms, seek urgent attention.

Causes

- kidney disease
- gastrointestinal loss: vomiting, diarrhoea
- alkalosis
- mineralocorticoid excess
- loss of extracellular fluid to intracellular (e.g. burns, other trauma, pyloric stenosis)
- drugs (e.g. diuretics: frusemide, thiazides), purgatives, liquorice abuse
- reduced intake of K^+

Clinical features

- lethargy, muscle weakness and cramps, mental lethargy and confusion

- severe flaccid paralysis, tetany, coma
- ECG: prominent U waves, depressed ST segment, T waves, arrhythmias

Patient education resources

Hand-out sheets from *Murtagh's Patient Education* 7th edition:

- Hyperthyroidism
- Hypothyroidism
- Goitre (thyroid swelling)

References

1 Fry J. *Common Diseases* (4th edn). Lancaster: MTP Press Limited, 1985: 358–61.
2 Stockigt J. Thyroid disorders: how to treat. Australian Doctor, 4 February 2005: 21–27.
3 Topliss DJ, Eastman CJ. Diagnosis and management of hyperthyroidism and hypothyroidism. Med J Aust, 2004; 180(4): 186–93.
4 Stockigt J, Topliss DJ. Hypothyroidism. In: *MIMS Disease Index* (2nd edn). Sydney: IMS Publishing, 1996: 267–9.
5 Need A. Thyroid function. IMVS Newsletter Issue 43, 2001 (available at <www.imvs.sa.gov.au>).
6 Walsh JP. Managing thyroid disease in general practice. Med J Aust, 2016; 205(4): 179–84.
7 Klaas J et al. Guidelines for the treatment of hypothyroidism: American Thyroid Association Task Force on Thyroid Hormone Replacement. Thyroid, December 2014; 24(12): 1670–5. [PMID: 25206247]
8 Stockigt J, Topliss DJ. Hypothyroidism: current drug therapy. Drugs, 1989; 37(3): 37–51, 186–93.
9 Expert Group for Endocrine guidelines. Thyroid disease. In: eTG complete. Melbourne: Therapeutic Guidelines Ltd. Available from: <www.tg.org.au>, accessed August 2017.
10 Bahn RS, Burch HB et al. Hyperthyroidism and other causes of thyrotoxicosis: management guidelines of the American thyroid association and American Association of Clinical Endocrinologists. Thyroid, 2011; 21(6): 593–646.
11 Boyages SC. Thyrotoxicosis. In: *MIMS Disease Index.* Sydney: IMS Publishing, 1996: 507–10.
12 Phillips P, Torpy D. Endocrinology 'pot pourri'. Check Program. Melbourne: RACGP, 2001: 347–8.
13 Donadio F, Barbiera A et al. Patients with macroprolactinaemia: clinical and radiological features. Eur J Clin Invest, 2007; 37(7): 552–7.
14 Debono M, Ross RJ. What is the best approach to tailoring hydrocortisone dose to meet patient needs in 2012? Clin Endcrinol (Oxf), 2013; 78(5): 659–64.
15 The Royal College of Pathologists of Australasia. Calcium: plasma or serum. Sydney, 2015.

Spinal dysfunction 24

The spine is an ordered series of bones running down your back. You sit on one end of it, sometimes too hard with ill effect, and your head sits on the other. Poor spine—what a load.

ANON, 19TH CENTURY

Spinal or vertebral dysfunction can be regarded as a masquerade mainly because the importance of the spine as a source of various pain syndromes has not been emphasised in medical training. Practitioners whose training and treatment are focused almost totally on the spine may swing to the other extreme and some may attribute almost every clinical syndrome to dysfunction of spinal segments. The true picture lies somewhere in between.

The diagnosis is straightforward when the patient is able to give a history of a precipitating event such as lifting, twisting the neck or having a motor vehicle accident, and can then localise the pain to the midline of the neck or back. The diagnostic problem arises when the pain is located distally to its source, whether it is radicular (due to pressure on a nerve root) or referred pain. The problem applies particularly to pain in anterior structures of the body.

If a patient has pain anywhere it is possible that it could be spondylogenic and practitioners should always keep this in mind.

The various syndromes caused by spinal dysfunction will be presented in more detail under neck pain, thoracic back pain and lumbar back pain.

Cervical spinal dysfunction[1]

The cervical spine is the origin of many confusing clinical problems and syndromes.

Clinical problems of cervical spinal origin

Pain originating from disorders of the cervical spine is usually, although not always, experienced in the neck. The patient may experience headache, or pain around the ear, face, arm, shoulder, upper anterior or posterior chest.[2]

Possible symptoms:

- neck pain
- neck stiffness
- headache
- 'migraine'-like headache
- facial pain
- arm pain (referred or radicular)
- myelopathy (sensory and motor changes in arms and legs)
- ipsilateral sensory changes of scalp
- ear pain (peri-auricular)
- scapular pain
- anterior chest pain
- torticollis
- dizziness/vertigo
- visual dysfunction

FIGURE 24.1 indicates typical directions of referred pain from the cervical spine. Pain in the arm (brachialgia) is common and tends to cover the shoulder and upper arm as indicated.

If the cervical spine is overlooked as a source of pain (such as in the head, shoulder, arm, upper chest—anterior and posterior—and around the ear or face) the cause of the symptoms will remain masked and mismanagement will follow.

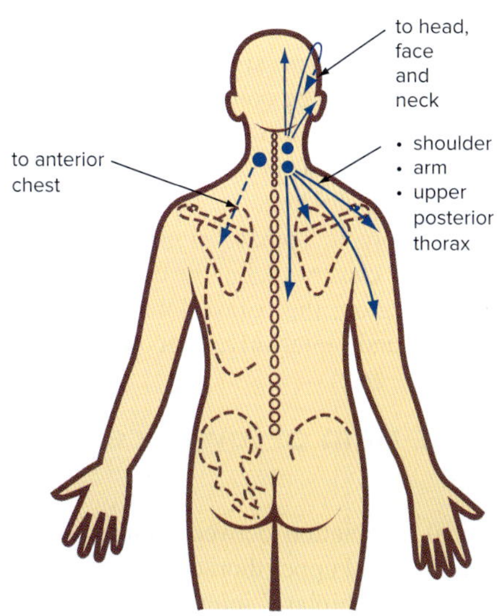

FIGURE 24.1 Possible directions of referred pain from the cervical spine

Dysfunction of the cervical spine can cause many unusual symptoms such as headache and vertigo, a fact that is often not recognised. Despite teaching to the contrary from some, the cervical spine is a common cause of headache, especially dysfunction of the facet joints at the C1–2 and C2–3 levels. The afferent pathways from these levels share a common pathway in the brain stem as the trigeminal nerve, hence the tendency for pain to be referred to the head and the face (see CHAPTER 52).

Manipulation of the cervical spine can be a dramatically effective technique, but it should be used with care and never used in the presence of organic disease and vertebrobasilar insufficiency. It should, therefore, be given only by skilled therapists. Two groups at special risk from quadriplegia are those with rheumatoid arthritis of the neck and Down syndrome, because of the instability of the odontoid process.

However, good results can be achieved by gentler techniques, such as mobilisation and muscle energy therapy (refer CHAPTER 62).

Thoracic spinal dysfunction

The most common and difficult masquerades related to spinal dysfunction occur with disorders of the thoracic spine (and also the low cervical spine), which can cause vague aches and pains in the chest, including the anterior chest. This applies particularly to unilateral pain.

Pain in the thoracic spine with referral to various parts of the chest wall and upper abdomen is common in all ages and can closely mimic the symptoms of visceral disease, such as angina pectoris and biliary colic (TABLE 24.1). If a non-cardiac cause of chest pain is excluded, then the possibility of referral from the thoracic spine should be considered in the differential diagnosis.[3] People of all ages can experience thoracic problems and it is surprisingly common in young people, including children.

Pain of thoracic spinal origin may be referred anywhere to the chest wall, but the commonest sites are the scapular region, the paravertebral region 2–5 cm from midline and, anteriorly, over the costochondral region (see FIG. 24.2).

Thoracic pain of lower cervical origin[4]

The clinical association between injury to the lower cervical region and upper thoracic pain is well known, especially with 'whiplash' injuries. It should be noted that the C4 dermatome is in close proximity to the T2 dermatome.

Table 24.1 Conditions mimicked by thoracic spinal dysfunction (usually unilateral pain)

Cardiovascular
Acute coronary syndromes
Angina
Pericarditis
Dissecting aneurysm
Chest/respiratory
Pleurisy
Pneumothorax
Carcinoma lung, esp. mesothelioma
Pulmonary infarction
Tuberculosis
Fractured rib, esp. cough fracture
Renal
Renal colic
Urinary infection/pyelonephritis
Gastrointestinal
Biliary colic
Appendicitis
Diverticulitis
Others
Herpes zoster
Epidemic pleurodynia (Bornholm disease)
Precordial catch (stitch in side)
Costochondritis
Hernia (symptomatic)
Muscular tears

The T2 dermatome appears to represent the cutaneous areas of the lower cervical segments, as the posterior primary rami of C5, C6, C7, C8 and T1 innervate musculature and have no significant cutaneous innervation.

The pain from the lower cervical spine can also refer pain to the anterior chest, and mimic coronary ischaemic pain. The associated autonomic nervous system disturbance can cause considerable confusion in making the diagnosis.

The medical profession tends to have a blind spot about various pain syndromes in the chest, especially the anterior chest and upper abdomen, caused by the common problem of dysfunction of the thoracic spine. Doctors who gain this insight are amazed at how often they diagnose the cause that previously did not enter their 'programmed' medical minds.

Physical therapy to the spine can be very effective when used appropriately. An example of this therapy is shown in FIGURE 37.8 in CHAPTER 37, and for the lumbar spine refer to FIGURES 38.15 and 38.16 in CHAPTER 38. Unfortunately, many of us associate it with quackery. It is devastating for patients to create

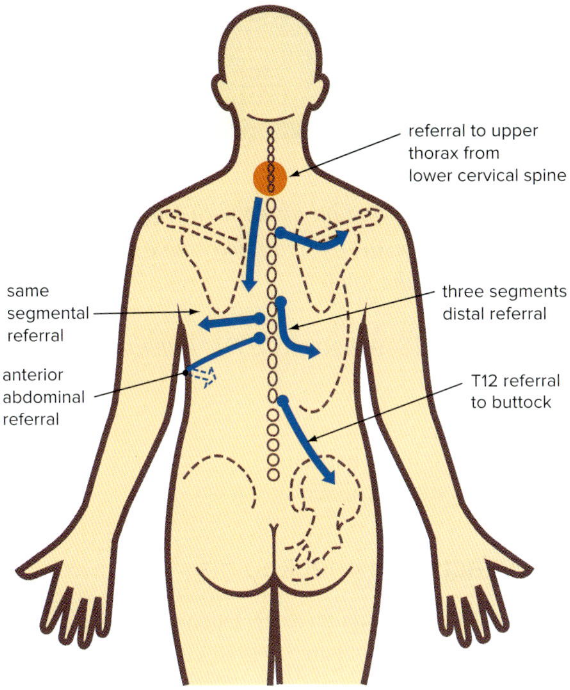

FIGURE 24.2 Examples of referral patterns for the thoracic spine

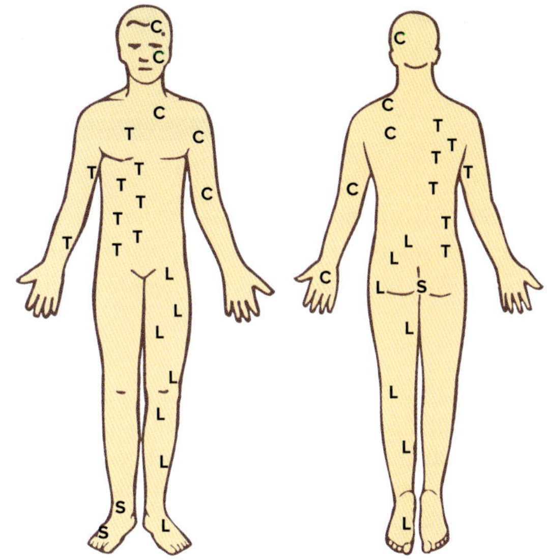

FIGURE 24.3 Examples of referred and radicular pain patterns from the spine (one side shown for each segment)

doubts in their minds about having a 'heart problem' or an 'anxiety neurosis' when the problem is spinal and it can be remedied simply (see CHAPTER 38).

Lumbar-sacral spinal dysfunction

The association between lumbar dysfunction and pain syndromes is generally easier to correlate. The pain is usually located in the low back and referred to the buttocks or the backs of the lower limbs. Pain manifestations of radiculopathy (sciatica) may follow dermatome patterns (see FIG. 66.1 in CHAPTER 66). Problems arise with referred pain to the pelvic area, groin and anterior aspects of the leg. Such patients may be diagnosed as suffering from inguinal or obturator hernial and nerve entrapment syndromes.

Typical examples of referral and radicular pain patterns from various segments of the spine are presented in FIGURE 24.3.

Management of lumbar spinal dysfunction[5]

This is best managed conservatively under medical supervision with collaboration between the general practitioner and skilled physiotherapist. The patient should continue their normal activities even if uncomfortable, avoid painful aggravating activities, and take basic analgesics such as paracetamol and ibuprofen. Evidence supports the value of prescribed exercises and physical interventions such as traction and spinal mobilisation or manipulation for persistent pain (refer CHAPTERS 37 and 38).

24

References

1 Murtagh J. *Cautionary Tales* (2nd edn). Sydney: McGraw-Hill, 2011: 193–5.
2 Sloane PD, Slatt LM, Baker RM. *Essentials of Family Medicine*. Baltimore: Williams & Wilkins, 1988: 236–40.
3 Murtagh J. *Cautionary Tales* (2nd edn). Sydney: McGraw-Hill, 2011: 49–51.
4 Kenna C, Murtagh J. *Back Pain and Spinal Manipulation* (2nd edn). Oxford: Butterworth Heinemann, 1997: 213–18.
5 Qaseem A, Wilf TG et al. Noninvasive treatments for acute, subacute and chronic low back pain: A clinical practice guideline from the American College of Physicians. Clinical Guidelines, 4 April 2017: 514–30.

25 Urinary tract infection

Experience has taught them, as mine has me, that one must listen to reason and agree with Hippocrates, Galen, Avicenna and many others, ancient and modern, that there is no surer way to determine the temperaments and constitutions of people of either sex than to look at the urine.

DAVACH DE LA RIVIÈRE (18TH CENTURY), *THE MIRROR OF URINES*

Urinary tract infection (UTI) is a common problem affecting all ages and accounts for approximately 1% of all attendances in general practice. It is very common in sexually active women but uncommon in men and children.

Organisms causing UTI in the community are usually sensitive to most of the commonly used antibiotics. Of great concern is the worldwide emergence of multidrug-resistant strains of *Escherichia coli* (*E. coli*). The important decision to make is whether to proceed with further investigation of the urinary tract. The morbidity of urinary infections in both children and adults is well known but it is vital to recognise the potential for progressive kidney damage, ending in chronic kidney failure. The main task in the prevention of chronic pyelonephritis is the early identification of patients with additional factors, such as reflux or obstruction, which could lead to progressive kidney damage.

UTI as a masquerade

UTI can be regarded as a masquerade when it presents with a constitutional problem or general symptoms, without symptoms suggestive of a urinary infection such as frequency, dysuria and loin pain. This applies particularly to infants and young children and the elderly but is not uncommon in adult women and in pregnancy. Acute UTI may occasionally present as acute abdominal pain. The causes of dysuria are outlined in the diagnostic strategy in CHAPTER 76.

In infants and children, presenting non-specific symptoms include:

- fever
- lethargy and irritability
- poor feeding
- failure to thrive
- vomiting
- abdominal pain
- diarrhoea

In the elderly:

- confusion
- behaviour disturbance
- fever of undetermined origin

Key facts and checkpoints

- As always, a thorough examination of the patient presenting with urinary symptoms and their history is important.
- Screening of asymptomatic women has shown that about 5% have bacterial UTI.[1]
- About 1% of neonates and 1–2% of schoolgirls have asymptomatic bacteriuria.[2]
- About one-third of women have been estimated to have symptoms suggestive of cystitis at some stage of their life.
- The vast majority of these women have anatomically normal kidney tracts, are at no significant risk from the UTI and respond quickly to simple therapy. The prevalence of underlying abnormalities is estimated at around 4%.[3]
- UTIs are largely caused by organisms from the bowel that colonise the perineum and reach the bladder via the urethra. In many young women infections are precipitated by sexual intercourse. Ascending infection accounts for 93% of UTIs.
- Haematogenous infection can occur sometimes, especially with the immunocompromised patient.
- All males and females less than 5 years old presenting with a UTI require investigation for an underlying abnormality of the urinary tract.
- In the presence of a normal urinary tract there is no evidence that UTI leads to progressive kidney damage.
- Always consider any family history of urinary tract abnormalities.
- Infants less than 6 months old with a UTI have a significant risk of bacteraemia.
- Consider the NSAID tiaprofenic acid as a cause of non-infective cystitis.

- Cloudy or malodorous urine does not usually require investigation or treatment unless the person has other signs of a UTI.[2,4]
- Care should be exercised in deciding the need for dipstick urinalysis and microscopy, culture and sensitivity (MCU) tests in elderly patients including residential aged care facilities to ensure appropriate diagnosis and avoidance of unnecessary antibiotic use.[2]

Risk factors

- Female sex
- Sexual intercourse
- Sexually transmitted infection
- Diabetes mellitus
- Diaphragm contraception or spermicidal exposure
- Pregnancy
- Immunosuppression
- Menopause
- Urinary tract obstruction/malformation/stricture
- Instrumentation
- Bladder polyps, carcinoma, diverticula, stones
- Diverticulitis with colo-vesical fistula (? pneumaturia)

Classification and clinical syndromes

Sterile pyuria

This is defined as the presence of pus cells but a sterile urine culture.[2] The common causes of sterile pyuria are:

- contamination of poorly collected urine specimens
- urinary infections being treated by antibiotics, i.e. inadequately treated infections
- analgesic nephropathy
- staghorn calculi
- other kidney disorders (e.g. polycystic kidney)
- bladder tumours
- tuberculosis
- chemical cystitis (e.g. cytotoxic therapy)
- appendicitis

Asymptomatic bacteriuria[4]

This is defined as the presence of a significant growth of bacteria in the urine (concentration $>10^8$ colony-forming units/L), which has not produced symptoms requiring consultation.[1]

Screening for and treatment of asymptomatic bacteriuria is not recommended except for:

- pregnant women because of the risk of pyelonephritis and pregnancy complications (see CHAPTER 108)
- patients before urological procedures (e.g. TURP)

Symptomatic bacteriuria

This is defined as the presence of frequency, dysuria and loin pain alone or in combination, together with a significant growth of organisms on urine culture.[2]

The clinical differentiation between cystitis or lower UTI and kidney or upper UTI cannot be made accurately on the basis of symptoms, except in those patients with well-defined loin pain and/or tenderness.

Acute cystitis (dysuria-frequency syndrome)[1]

- Inflammation of the bladder and/or urethra is associated with dysuria (pain or scalding with micturition) and/or urinary frequency.
- In severe cases, haematuria may be present, and the urine may have an offensive smell.
- Constitutional symptoms are minimal or absent.
- Other causes of dysuria and frequency include urethritis, prostatitis and vulvovaginitis, all of which can normally be distinguished clinically.

Acute pyelonephritis[1]

- Acute bacterial infection of the kidney produces loin pain and constitutional upset, with fever, rigors, nausea and sometimes vomiting.
- The symptoms of acute cystitis are often also present.
- The differential diagnosis includes causes of the acute abdomen, such as appendicitis, cholecystitis and acute tubal or ovarian diseases. The presence of pyuria and absence of rebound tenderness are helpful in distinction.

The clinical manifestations of UTI are summarised in FIGURE 25.1.

Uncomplicated urinary tract infection

This is cystitis occurring in the uninstrumented non-pregnant female without structural or neurological abnormalities. Acute infection is most commonly caused by *E. coli* and *Staphylococcus saprophyticus.*

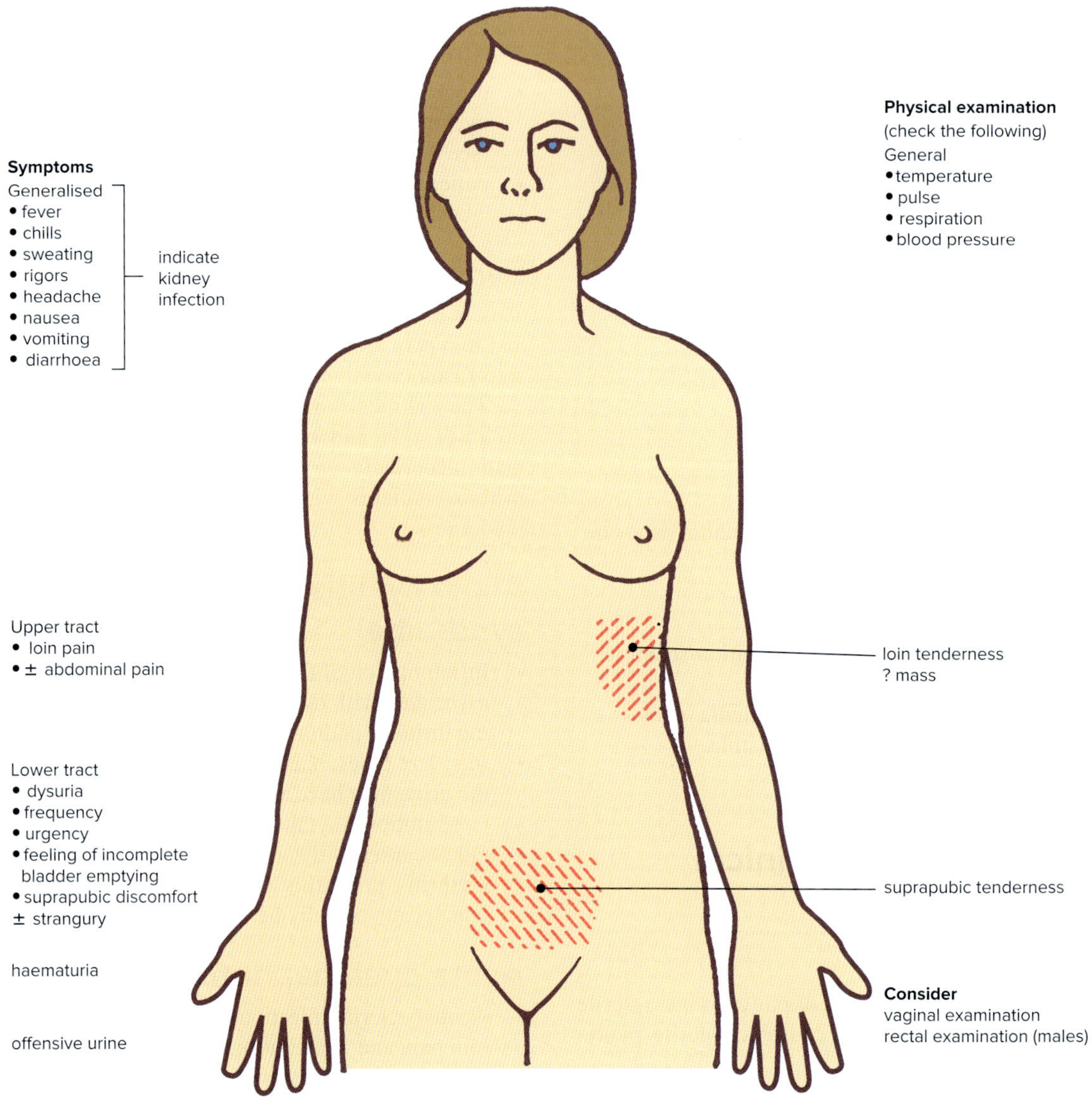

FIGURE 25.1 Clinical manifestations of urinary tract infection

Complicated urinary tract infection[4]

This is associated with anatomical or functional abnormalities (e.g. diabetes, urinary calculi) that increase the risk of serious complications or treatment failure.

Urethral syndrome

The urethral syndrome (sometimes termed abacterial cystitis) is that where the patient presents with dysuria and frequency and even abdominal pain but does not show a positive urine culture.[3]

- 30–40% of adult women with urinary symptoms have this syndrome.[3]
- Many actually have bacterial cystitis but a negative culture.
- The organisms may be anaerobic or fastidious in their culture requirements.
- The organisms may include *Ureaplasma, Mycoplasma genitalium, Chlamydia* and viruses.
- The urine may have antiseptic contamination or residual antibiotic.
- The infection may be undergoing spontaneous resolution at the time of the culture.

Interstitial cystitis[3]

This is an uncommon but important cause of the urethral syndrome.

- The classic symptoms are frequency day and night and a dull suprapubic ache relieved briefly by bladder emptying.
- The feature is small haemorrhages on distension of the bladder.
- Treatment is hydrodistension ± a course of tricyclics, for example amitriptyline.

Laboratory diagnosis

The laboratory diagnosis of UTI depends on careful collection, examination and culture of urine. This is recommended for the people listed in TABLE 25.1. It is not mandatory for non-pregnant women with suspected cystitis when empirical treatment may be appropriate.

Collection of urine[1]

It is best to collect the first urine passed in the morning, when it is highly concentrated and any bacteria have been incubated in the bladder overnight. Preferably the urine should be taken to the laboratory immediately, but it can be stored for up to 24 hours at 4°C to prevent bacterial multiplication.

- *Clean catch midstream specimen of urine (MSU).* This is best collected from a full bladder, to allow at least 100 mL of urine to be passed before collection of the MSU. It is important that the urine flow is continuous, and the container is moved in and out of the stream collecting at least 20 mL.
  - In women, a tampon should first be inserted and the vulva washed with clean water (to avoid contamination with vaginal and vulval organisms). Sit on the toilet and swing one knee to the side as far as possible. The labia are then held apart with the fingers of one hand to prevent contact with the urinary stream while the specimen is collected after passing a small amount of urine into the toilet.
  - In males, the foreskin (if present) is retracted and the glans washed with clean water.
  - In children, a midstream clean catch (MCC) is useful (although prone to contamination) especially in the hands of experienced collectors. The parent holds the child over a sterile bowl placed under cleansed genitalia.
  - In infants, the three-person French technique is useful. This is where the child is held in a 'frog leg' position or with arms and legs dangling. Another person holds a sterile urine container to catch the urine. A trained person stimulates the bladder by tapping over it at 100 light taps per minute for 30 seconds then massages the paravertebral area for up to 3 minutes or until voiding.
- *Catheter specimen of urine (CSU).* In women who have difficulty with collecting an uncontaminated MSU (as is commonly the case in the elderly, the infirm and the grossly obese), a short open-ended catheter can be inserted and a specimen collected after 200 mL has flushed the catheter.
- *Suprapubic aspirate of urine (SPA).* This is an extremely reliable way to detect bacteriuria in neonates and in patients where UTI is suspected but cannot be confirmed because of low colony counts or contamination in an MSU. Under local anaesthetic, a needle (lumbar puncture needle in adults) is inserted into the very full bladder about 1–2 cm above the pubic symphysis, and 20 mL is collected by a syringe. Any organisms in an SPA specimen indicate UTI (see FIG. 25.2).

Urine specimen collection in children

All children with a first UTI require investigation. It is diagnosed by significant growth on MSU, CSU, MCC or SPA.

- Bag specimen: cannot diagnose UTI
- MSU—usually by 3–4 years when cooperative
- MCC—practical and reliable
- SPA—reliable and the best option
- CSU—for failed SPA or those unable to void on request

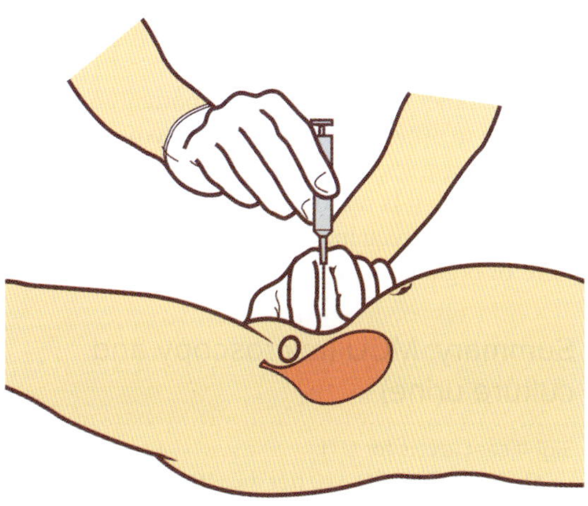

FIGURE 25.2 Suprapubic aspiration of urine in a child

25

Dipstick testing

Dipstick findings of urinary leucocytes or nitrite are suggestive of UTI and may be an indication for empirical treatment if asymptomatic. The reagents in dipstick testing are generally sensitive but have to be interpreted with care. Leucocyte esterase dipsticks are useful in detecting pyuria and give a good guide to infection with a specificity of 94–98% (2–6% false positive) and 74–96% sensitivity (4–26% false negatives).[5] Positive nitrite dipsticks give a useful guide to the presence of bacteria. Unexplained haematuria detected by dipstick analysis needs investigation.

Microscopic examination

The urine is examined under a microscope to detect pyuria (more than 10 pus cells—WBCs—per high-powered field) but should be examined in a counting chamber to calculate the number of WBCs/mL of urine. In the counting chamber pyuria is >8000 WBC/mL in phase-contrast microscopy. Pyuria is a very sensitive sign of UTI.

Vaginal squames and debris indicate contamination.

Culture of the urine

The nature and number of organisms present in the urine are the most useful indicators of UTI.[1]

- Most common are enteric organisms. *E. coli* (especially) and *Staphylococcus saprophyticus* are responsible for over 90% of UTIs, with other Gram-negative organisms (*Klebsiella* sp. and *Proteus* sp.), *enterococci* sp. and Gram-positive cocci (*Streptococcus faecalis* and other staphylococci) also responsible.
- Infections due to organisms other than *E. coli* (e.g. *Pseudomonas* sp.) are suggestive of an underlying kidney tract abnormality.
- If $>10^5$ colony forming units (cfu) per mL of bacteria are present in an MSU, it is highly likely that the patient has a UTI.
- On the other hand, it is most important to realise that up to 30% of women with acute bacterial cystitis have less than 10^5 cfu/mL in the MSU. For this reason, it is reasonable to treat women with dysuria and frequency even if they have $<10^5$ cfu/mL of organisms in an MSU.

25

Summary: MCU (microscopy and culture urine)

Significant levels for UTI:

- Microscopy: WBC >10 per mL (10×10^6/L)
- Culture: counts $>10^5$ cfu/mL (10^8/L)

Other investigations

- FBE, ESR/CRP, blood culture (if febrile and unwell), consider U&E, PSA (men)

Acute uncomplicated cystitis

Advice to women (especially if recurrent attacks):

- Keep yourself rested.
- Drink a lot of fluid: 2–3 cups of water at first and then 1 cup every 30 minutes.
- Try to empty your bladder completely each time.
- Gently wash or wipe your bottom from front to back with soft, moist tissues after opening your bowels (for prevention in recurrent attacks).
- Use analgesics such as paracetamol for pain.
- Make the urine alkaline by taking sodium citrotartrate (4 g orally 6 hourly)—not if taking nitrofurantoin.

UTI: basic management

- Urine dipstick
- Microculture (clean catch)
- First-line antibiotics—trimethoprim or cephalexin
- Alkaliniser for severe dysuria
- High fluid intake
- Check sensitivity—leave or change ABs
- Repeat MCU within 48 hours after AB course

Consider further investigation (see TABLE 25.1)

Treatment (non-pregnant women)[3,7]

Multiple dose therapy is preferred to single dose therapy.

Use for 5 days in women (trimethoprim—3 days).

Use for 10 days in women with known urinary tract abnormality:

- trimethoprim 300 mg (o) daily for 3 days (first choice)

  or
- cephalexin 500 mg (o) 12 hourly for 5 days

  or
- amoxycillin/+ clavulanate 500/125 mg (o) 12 hourly for 5 days

  or
- nitrofurantoin 100 mg (o) 12 hourly for 5 days

  or
- norfloxacin 400 mg (o) 12 hourly for 3 days (if resistance to above agents proven and if susceptible)

  Caution about tendonopathy, including rupture.

  Follow-up: MCU 1–2 weeks later.

Table 25.1 Investigation of symptomatic urinary tract infections

Investigations are indicated in:
All children
All males
All women with: • acute pyelonephritis • recurrent infections: >2 per year • confirmed sterile pyuria • other features of kidney disease, e.g. haematuria • pregnancy Others: • with failed antibiotic treatment • with recent international travel • aged care facility residents
Basic investigations include:
MCU—microscopy and culture (post-treatment)
Kidney function tests: plasma urea and creatinine, eGFR
Intravenous urogram (IVU) and/or ultrasound
Special considerations:
In children: micturating cystogram
In adult males: consider prostatic infection studies if IVU normal
In severe pyelonephritis: ultrasound or IVU (urgent) to exclude obstruction
In pregnant women: ultrasound to exclude obstruction

Note:

- Avoid using important quinolones—norfloxacin or ciprofloxacin—as first-line agents.
- Cotrimoxazole is not first line because it has no advantage over trimethoprim and has more side effects.
- Treatment failures are usually due to a resistant organism or an underlying abnormality of the urinary tract.

Pregnant women[4,9]

UTI in pregnant women requires careful surveillance. Asymptomatic bacteriuria should always be excluded during early pregnancy because it tends to be blown into a full infection. Seek expert advice.

Treatment of acute cystitis (empirical):

- cephalexin 500 mg (o) 12 hourly for 5 days
  or
- nitrofurantoin 100 mg (o) 12 hourly for 5 days
  or
- amoxycillin + clavulanate 500/125 mg (o) 12 hourly for 5 days

Repeat MCU at least 48 hours after completion. Asymptomatic bacteriuria should be treated with a week-long course. Refer to CHAPTER 108.

Adult males[4]

Consider the cause (see risk factors above).

Investigations: MCU, U&E, ultrasound.

Treatment (empirical, while awaiting investigation):

- trimethoprim 300 mg (o) daily for 7 days
  or
- cephalexin 500 mg (o) 12 hourly for 7 days
  or
- amoxycillin + clavulanate 500/125 mg (o) 12 hourly for 7 days
  or
- nitrofurantoin 100 mg (o) 12 hourly for 7 days

Note: all males with a UTI should be investigated to exclude an underlying abnormality, e.g. prostatitis, obstruction.

$ Acute pyelonephritis[4,6]

Urine microscopy and culture is mandatory. Mild cases can be treated with oral therapy alone using double the dosage of drugs recommended for uncomplicated cystitis, except for trimethoprim when the same dosage is recommended. Treatment should be continued for 14 days. Ciprofloxacin (500 mg (o) 12 hourly) or norfloxacin (400 mg (o) 12 hourly) is used for 7 days if resistance to these drugs is proven.

For severe infection with suspected septicaemia, admit to hospital and treat initially with parenteral antibiotics for 2 to 5 days after taking urine for microscopy and culture, and blood for culture. It is a particular problem if acquired in pregnancy.

- amoxycillin 2 g IV 6 hourly[4]
  plus
- gentamicin 4–6 mg/kg/day, single daily IV dose

Follow with oral therapy for a total of 14 days.

Drug levels of gentamicin require monitoring. Gentamicin can be replaced with IV cefotaxime or ceftriaxone.

All patients should be investigated for an underlying urinary tract abnormality.

$ Recurrent or chronic urinary tract infections[7,8]

Recurrent infections occur as a relapse of a previously treated infection or because of re-infection, often with differing organisms. Persistent (chronic) UTIs indicate that the organism is resistant to the antimicrobial agents employed or that there is an underlying abnormality such as a kidney stone or a chronically infected prostate in the male patient. MCSU is mandatory. Such infections may be treated with prolonged courses of an appropriate antibiotic or removal of the focus of infection.[6]

In men and children, an anatomical abnormality is usual, while recurrent cystitis in women often occurs despite a normal tract. In men, instruction on perineal hygiene, more frequent bladder emptying and post-intercourse voiding may assist in the prevention of re-infection.

Treatment[4]

The treatment is as for cystitis and pyelonephritis.

Prevention including antibiotic prophylaxis[4]

In some female patients with recurrent UTI a single dose of a suitable agent within 2 hours after intercourse is adequate but, in more severe cases, courses may be taken for 3–6 months or on occasions longer. Drinking more water is recommended. Adult doses given:

- trimethoprim 150 mg (o) nocte
  or
- cephalexin 250 mg (o) nocte

Cranberries

A recent Cochrane review on the use of cranberries (*Vaccinium macrocarpon*) for the prevention of UTI concluded that there was evidence to recommend cranberry juice or tablets for the prevention of recurrent symptomatic UTIs in women, but poor evidence for its use in the treatment of UTI, in the management of asymptomatic bacteriuria, or in the prevention of UTIs in children.[10,11]

An appropriate regimen is 150 mL cranberry juice or one tablet (1:30 parts concentrated juice) twice daily.

Urinary tract infection in children

By the age of 10 years, about 3% of boys[12] and 10% of girls will have had at least one episode of a urinary tract infection.

UTI in infants and very young children is often kidney in nature and may be associated with generalised symptoms such as fever, vomiting, diarrhoea and failure to thrive. Offensive urine may be noted. Causes of 'smelly' urine in children are urinary infection and/or dehydration especially with gastroenteritis. Symptoms of dysuria and frequency appear only after the age of 2 years when the child is able to indicate the source of the discomfort. In a girl or boy (rare presentation) with symptoms of dysuria and frequency an underlying abnormality is likely to be present with a reported incidence of vesicoureteric reflux (VUR) as high as 40% and scarred kidneys (reflux nephropathy) in 27%.[3]

Thus the early detection of children with VUR and control of recurrent kidney infection could prevent the development of scars, hypertension and chronic kidney failure. Radiological investigation of children with UTIs shows normal kidneys in approximately 66% and reflux in approximately 33%.

It is best to perform the ultrasound first and within the first 3 days for a febrile UTI. A urine specimen is essential before antibiotics are given.

Guidelines for investigation[12,13]

- <1 year—ultrasound; consider micturating cystourethrogram (MCUG) if US abnormal
  - if both negative, no further investigation
  - if abnormal, follow up referral/investigation
- >1 year—ultrasound

The dimercaptosuccinic acid scintigraph scan is occasionally indicated.

Treatment (mild infection in children)[4,12]

Empirical treatment in children one month or more while awaiting culture results. If less than one month, treatment with IV antibiotics is advisable.

Treatment should be taken orally for 7 days:

- trimethoprim 4 mg/kg (max. 150 mg) bd (suspension is 50 mg/5 mL)
  or
- cephalexin 12.5 mg/kg (max. 500 mg) bd
  or
- cotrimoxazole 4/20 mg/kg, (max. 160/800 mg) 6 hourly
  or
- amoxycillin/potassium clavulanate 22.5/3.2 mg/kg (max. 500/125 mg) orally bd

Norfloxacin and ciprofloxacin should be avoided routinely in children unless required on MCU.

Check MCU in 48 hours.

Severe infections in children[4]

For empirical treatment in those ≥12 months who appear septic or are vomiting, and infants <12 months, give gentamicin IV + amoxy/ampicillin IV. Subsequent treatment should be guided by culture results and clinical results with early change to oral therapy.

Duration of therapy: usually 10–14 days.

Vulvovaginitis in children

Although vulvovaginitis can affect women of any age, it is more prevalent in girls between 2 and 8 years. It can be confused with a UTI where there is dysuria, which is a common symptom in this type of dermatitis (see CHAPTER 107).

Urinary infections in the elderly

The typical settings in which UTIs occur in the elderly are in the frail, those who are immobilised, and those with faecal incontinence and inadequate bladder emptying. It is a particular problem in aged care facility residents. The presenting symptoms may be atypical, especially with upper UTI where fever of undetermined origin and behaviour disturbances may be a feature. In men, obstructive uropathy from prostatism should be excluded by ultrasound.

Uncomplicated infections should be treated the same way as for other age groups but no anti-microbial treatment is recommended for asymptomatic bacteriuria.

Genitourinary tuberculosis

The genitourinary tract is involved in 3–5% of cases of tuberculosis.[14] The genital and urinary tracts are often involved together as a result of miliary spread.

The commonest presenting complaints are dysuria and frequency, which can be severe. Other symptoms include strangury when the bladder is severely affected, loin pain and haematuria. Routine urine culture shows sterile pyuria.

Diagnosis is made on specific urine culture for myco-bacterium, ESR/CRP (high) or biopsy of bladder lesions or the typical X-ray appearance of distorted calyces and medullary calcification. Treatment is with antituberculosis drugs.

Candiduria[4]

The presence of *Candida albicans* in the urine is common. Antifungal therapy is not recommended if associated with indwelling catheters but is recommended if associated with upper UTIs and/or systemic candidiasis. Consider removal of catheter and stents.

Use fluconazole 200 mg (o) daily for 7 days.

Prostatitis

Consider bacterial prostatitis in men with few urinary symptoms (frequency, urgency and dysuria), flu-like illness, fever, low backache and perineal pain. The prostate is exquisitely tender on rectal examination. For mild to moderate infection, give the same oral antibiotics as for cystitis: amoxycillin + clavulanate 500/125 mg (o) bd for 4–6 weeks. If severe, use amoxy/ampicillin 2 g IV 6 hourly plus gentamicin (see CHAPTER 114).

Common treatment errors[1]

- Not treating women with dysuria and frequency merely because there are $<10^5$ cfu/mL in an MCU
- Overtreating women with acute cystitis and normal urinary tracts; single-dose therapy is effective in 70–80% of cases, and overtreatment often leads to vaginal candidiasis or antibiotic-induced diarrhoea
- Using single-dose therapy in patients with known anatomical abnormalities
- Failing to consider chronic prostatic infection in men with recurrent UTI and a normal IVU

When to refer

- It is wise to refer all patients with urinary tract abnormalities to a nephrologist or urologist for advice on specific management.
- Refer also if the simple methods outlined above do not control recurrent UTI.
- Refer males with urinary infections that are not clearly localised to the prostate.
- Refer patients with impaired kidney function.

Practice tips

- Most symptomatic UTIs are acute cystitis occurring in sexually active women with anatomically normal urinary tracts.
- A clinical diagnosis based on experience, plus a positive nitrite dipstick test and the finding of pyuria by office microscopy, will generally enable immediate curative treatment.
- A 3-day course of trimethoprim 300 mg daily is a suitable first choice for acute uncomplicated cystitis in women.
- Avoid overinvestigation of patients in whom there is a low likelihood of demonstrating structural abnormalities.
- The ultrasound examination may not detect calculi, small tumours, clubbed calyces and papillary necrosis.
- In males the prostate is the most common source of recurrent UTI.

continued

- UTI is commonly associated with microscopic haematuria (occasionally macroscopic haematuria).
- Persisting haematuria should be investigated, e.g. US, CT-IVP, TB.
- Due to the rising level of *E. coli* resistance, amoxycillin is no longer recommended unless susceptibility of the organism is proven.[3]

Patient education resources

Hand-out sheets from *Murtagh's Patient Education* 7th edition:

- Cystitis in women
- Urine infection in children

References

1 Becker GJ. Urinary tract infection. In: *MIMS Disease Index* (2nd edn). Sydney: IMS Publishing, 1996: 545–7.

2 NPS Medicine Wise 2017. <https://www.nps.org.au/medical-info/consumer-info/urinary-tract-infections-utis>, accessed February 2018.

3 Kincaid-Smith P, Larkins R, Whelan G. *Problems in Clinical Medicine.* Sydney: MacLennan & Petty, 1990: 280–3.

4 Expert group for Antibiotic guidelines. Urinary tract infections. In: eTG complete. Melbourne: Therapeutic Guidelines Ltd. Available from: <www.tg.org.au>, accessed January 2018.

5 Devillé WLJM et al. The urine dipstick test useful to rule out infections. A meta-analysis of the accuracy. BMC Urology, 2004; 4: 4.

6 Little P, Moon MV et al. Effectiveness of five different approaches in management of urinary tract infection: randomised controlled trial. BMJ, 2010; 340: c199.

7 Kerr PG, Blair S. How to investigate recurrent urinary tract infections. Medicine Today, 2008; 9(7): 53–61.

8 Epp A, Larochell A et al. Recurrent urinary infection. J Obst Gynaecol Can, 2010; 32(110): 1082–101.

9 Vazguez SC, Abatos E. Treatments for symptomatic urinary tract infections during pregnancy. Cochrane Database Systematic Review, 2011; (1): CD002256.

10 Jepson RG et al. Cranberries for preventing urinary tract infections. Cochrane Database Systematic Review, 2008; (1): CD001321.

11 Wyndam R. Cranberry juice and urinary tract infections. Medicine Today, 2006; 7(5): 72–3.

12 Turner P, Moran K. Urinary tract infections in children. Medical Observer, 29 February 2008: 27–30.

13 Thomson K et al. *Paediatric Handbook* (8th edn). Melbourne: Wiley-Blackwell, 2009: 488–93.

14 Bullock N, Sibley G, Whitaker R. *Essential Urology.* Edinburgh: Churchill Livingstone, 1989: 126–9.

Malignant disease 26

Cancers of the tongue and mouth begin with a small hard lump, and sometimes with a little sore; both of which are attended with pricking pains, and they spread in the same manner with cancerous sores in other parts. It is so great an evil, that the slightest suspicion of it occasions very great uneasiness.

WILLIAM HEBERDEN (1710–1801)

The terms *malignancy, cancer* and *neoplasia* are usually used interchangeably. The differences between a malignant tumour and a benign tumour are summarised in TABLE 26.1.

Table 26.1 Different characteristics of benign and malignant tumours

Benign	Malignant
Well-differentiated	Undifferentiated
Non-invasive	Invasive
Slow growth	Rapid growth
Not anaplastic	Anaplastic
Not metastatic	Metastatic

Malignant disease accounts for 1 in 8 deaths of people under 35 years in Australia and 3 in every 10 (29%) of deaths in those over 45 years.[1] Cancer is the only major cause of death in Australia that is increasing in both sexes. At current rates about 1 in 3 males and 1 in 4 females will develop a cancer, excluding non-melanoma skin cancers, by the age of 75.[1]

The six most common causes of death from cancer in Australia and the US are cancer of the lung, bowel, breast, prostate, lymphoma and pancreas.

Neoplasia, especially malignancy of the silent areas, can present as undifferentiated illness and be a real masquerade. The so-called 'silent' malignancies that pose a special problem include cancer of the ovary, pancreas, kidney, caecum and ascending colon, liver (hepatoma), melanoma and haematological tissue.

This chapter focuses on the general features of several of these malignancies in order to promote early diagnosis and urgent referral at the primary care level. Specific common cancers are discussed in other chapters.

Acute emergency problems that can develop with various malignancies include spinal cord compression, malignant effusions, disseminated intravascular coagulation and hypercalcaemia.

Cancer in children[2,3]

Although uncommon in children under 15 years, cancer is the second most common cause of death in this age group. The most common cancers (in order) are leukaemias, especially acute lymphocytic leukaemia (34%); brain tumours, especially astrocytoma (20%); lymphomas, especially non-Hodgkin (13%); neuroblastoma; Wilms tumour; soft tissue tumours, especially rhabdomyosarcoma; and bone tumours.

Survival has improved dramatically in recent decades, indicating the value of early diagnosis and referral for expert treatment.

Studies have highlighted the importance of GPs responding to concerns of parents even if they could find no abnormality after examination. Parents of children eventually diagnosed with cancer and who were in dispute with their GP were alerted by signs and symptoms which were often vague, non-specific and common, or unusual or 'scary'. They felt that their child 'wasn't right'.[2]

Red flags for childhood cancer

- lump or mass, especially neck or stomach
- unusual bleeding, bruising or rash
- white eye
- persistent nausea and vomiting
- constant illness
- constant tiredness and/or pallor
- headache, especially early morning
- continuing unexplained weight loss
- recurrent or persistent fever
- changes which occur suddenly and persist
- increased swelling or persistent pain in bone

Clinical manifestations

The clinical manifestations of malignancy are usually due to:

- pressure effects of the growth
- infiltration or metastases in various organs (e.g. liver, brain, lungs, bone, blood vessels)
- systemic symptoms, including paraneoplastic effects

Systemic symptoms

These can be divided into general non-specific effects and paraneoplastic syndromes, which are the remote effects caused by the tumour.

Undifferentiated general symptoms

- Tiredness/fatigue/weakness
- Anorexia and nausea
- Weight loss
- Fever
- Thirst (hypercalcaemia)
- Drowsiness (hyponatraemia)

Paraneoplastic effects

The paraneoplastic effects or syndromes are very important clinically because they may provide an early clue to the presence of a specific type of cancer, in addition to the possible lethal effect of the metabolic or toxic effect (e.g. hyponatraemia). These effects include:

- ectopic hormone production
- skin abnormalities
- metabolic effects: fever/sweats, weight loss/cachexia
- haematological disorders: anaemia, erythrocytosis/polycythemia, coagulation disorder, others
- neuropathies and CNS abnormalities
- collagen vascular disorders
- nephrotic syndrome

A summary of various paraneoplastic syndromes is presented in TABLE 26.2.

Clinical approach

A history of constitutional symptoms that are often quite undifferentiated (often bizarre) may provide the clue to the possibility of an underlying malignancy.

Table 26.2 Paraneoplastic syndromes and associated tumours: more common examples

Hormone excess syndrome	Tumour
Cushing	Lung, kidney, adrenal, thymoma, pancreas
ACTH	Lung, kidney, thymoma, thyroid
Gonadotrophins	Lung, hepatoma, choriocarcinoma
Other syndromes	
Hypercalcaemia	Lung, breast, kidney, multiple myeloma, prostate, pancreas, adrenal, hepatoma
Fever	Kidney, hepatoma, lymphoma, pancreas, thymoma
Neurologic	Lung, breast, thymoma, Hodgkin, prostate
Coagulopathy	Lung, breast, hepatoma, prostate, pancreas
Thrombophlebitis	Kidney, pancreas, prostate
Polycythaemia	Kidney, hepatoma
Dermatomyositis	Lung, breast, pancreas

An occupational history may be relevant to the clinical problem (see TABLE 26.3).

Table 26.3 Occupational causes of cancer

Agent	Occupation	Cancer
Arsenic	Chemical industry	Lung, skin, liver
Asbestos	Insulation worker	Mesothelioma
Benzene	Glue worker, varnisher	Leukaemia
Radiation	Mining	Various
Soot, coal tar	Chimney sweep	Skin
Ultraviolet light	Farmer, sailor, outdoor worker	Skin
Vinyl chloride	PVC manufacturing	Liver (angiosarcoma)

Familial cancer

Although the great majority of cancer is not inherited, some individuals carry inherited genetic mutations from conception that predispose them to developing certain cancers, particularly colorectal, breast and ovarian cancers. Refer to CHAPTER 18.

Tumour markers[4]

A tumour marker is an abnormal characteristic that is specific for a particular type of malignancy (e.g.

26

the Philadelphia chromosome for chronic myeloid leukaemia). Other examples include human chorionic gonadotrophin (HCG) (elevated in trophoblastic tumours and germ cell neoplasms of the testes and ovaries) and the oncofetal antigens—carcinoembryonic antigen (CEA) and alpha-fetoprotein (AFP).

CEA and AFP are not specific markers but are elevated in certain tumours and are very useful in monitoring tumour activity.

Tumour markers have a limited role in diagnosis of malignant disease because several have low sensitivity and specificity. The most valuable are those associated with testis cancer—AFP and beta-HCG. Markers may be an adjunct to diagnosis of certain malignancies, including the rather inaccurate CEA for bowel cancer and CA-125 for ovarian cancer. These markers are summarised in TABLE 26.4.

Table 26.4 Common tumour markers

Tumour marker	Condition
AFP	Testicular cancer (non-seminomatous)
	Hepatocellular carcinoma
	GIT cancers with and without liver metastases
CA-125	Ovarian cancer (non-mucinous), breast
CA-15-3	Breast
CA-19-9	Pancreas, colon, ovary
CEA	Colorectal cancer
	Pancreatic, breast, lung, small intestine, stomach, ovaries
PSA*	Prostate cancer
hCG	Choriocarcinoma
	Hydatidiform mole
	Trophoblastic diseases
b_2-microglobulin	Multiple myeloma, some lymphomas, CLL

* PSA = prostate-specific antigen

Lung cancer

Apart from non-melanoma skin cancer, lung cancer is the most common cancer in Australia in terms of both incidence and death, accounting for at least 20% of cancer deaths.[1] In the US it accounts for 28% of cancer deaths in men and 24% of deaths in women. Only 10–25% are asymptomatic at the time of diagnosis but lung cancer can cause an extraordinary variety of clinical symptoms and signs with a reputation for several paraneoplastic syndromes. Refer to CHAPTERS 42 and 49.

The paraneoplastic syndromes include hypercalcaemia, Cushing syndrome, carcinoid syndrome, dermatomyositis, visual loss progressing to blindness from retinal degeneration, cerebellar degeneration and encephalitis.

The presentation of cough and chest pain renders it less of an 'occult' malignancy than several other types.

DxT malaise + weight loss + cough → lung cancer

Kidney tumours

The most important tumours of the kidney are adenocarcinoma (80% of all kidney tumours)[3] and nephroblastoma (Wilms tumour).

Kidney cell cancer

Kidney cell cancer (adenocarcinoma, hypernephroma) has a great diversity of presenting symptoms, including:

- general symptoms of neoplasia, e.g. malaise, FUO
- haematuria (60%)
- loin pain (40%)
- loin mass (palpable kidney)
- signs of anaemia
- left supraclavicular lymphadenopathy (Virchow node)
- varicocele (left side)
- hypertension
- symptoms of metastases (to liver, lungs, brain, bones): respiratory symptoms, neurological symptoms and signs, bone pain, pathological fracture (vertebral collapse)
- urinalysis—67% positive for blood

Diagnosis is confirmed by imaging, e.g. CT MRI. Refer for radical nephrectomy.

The classic triad of symptoms, although in a small percentage of patients, is as follows.

DxT haematuria + loin pain + palpable kidney mass → kidney cell cancer

Wilms tumour (nephroblastoma)

Wilms tumour is responsible for 10% of all childhood malignancies. Clinical features include:[3]

- peak incidence 2–3 years
- general symptoms of neoplasia
- palpable mass 80%
- abdominal pain 30%
- haematuria 25%

Diagnosis is confirmed by urine cytology, ultrasound or CT/MRI scan.

Early diagnosis with nephrectomy and chemotherapy leads to a very favourable prognosis (90% 5-year survival).

DxT haematuria + abdominal mass + malaise ➜ Wilms tumour

Neuroblastoma[5]

Probably the most common cancer in infancy (usually <2–3 years). 90% present under 5 years. It is a tumour of the adrenal medulla (50%) and sympathetic nervous system, especially retroperitoneal neural tissue in abdomen (30%) but also in chest and neck.

First symptoms often vague:

- fatigue, anorexia, nausea, fever
- abdominal pain, abdominal swelling
- anaemia and weight loss

May present with metastases, e.g. bone pain.

Diagnosis: CT scan, skeletal survey; biopsy required.

Treatment is based on surgical resection then chemotherapy ± localised radiotherapy. Good response to therapy especially if <18 months.

Ovarian cancer[6]

Ovarian cancer has the highest mortality rate of all the gynaecological cancers because the majority of patients present in the late stage of the disease. It is responsible for 5% of deaths in females. It is usually asymptomatic prior to the development of metastases. Epithelial tumours are the most common of malignant ovarian tumours. They are uncommon under 40 years of age and the average age of diagnosis is 50 years.

The most common presentation is abdominal swelling (mass and/or ascites), abdominal bloating or discomfort. Non-specific symptoms, which may be present for a long time before diagnosis, include abnormal uterine bleeding, urinary frequency, weight loss, abdominal discomfort, reduced capacity for food, diarrhoea, anorexia, nausea and vomiting (refer to CHAPTER 103).

Diagnosis is supported by pelvic ultrasound and serum CA-125 tumour marker. A new test is the OvPlex™ serum test, which measures five serum markers.

DxT abdominal discomfort + anorexia + abdominal bloating/distension ➜ ovarian cancer

26

Carcinoma of caecum and ascending colon[4]

Malignancy in this area is more likely to present with symptoms of anaemia without the patient noting obvious blood in the faeces or alteration of bowel habit. Refer to CHAPTER 41.

DxT blood in stools + abdominal discomfort + change in bowel habit ➜ colon cancer

Pancreatic cancer

This is another cancer with vague symptoms, metastasising early and late presentation. It is mainly ductal adenocarcinoma, which, if in the head of the pancreas, presents with painless jaundice and if in the body and/or tail presents with epigastric pain radiating to the back, relieved by sitting forward (refer to CHAPTER 58).

DxT jaundice + anorexia + abdominal discomfort/pain ➜ pancreatic cancer

The leukaemias[7]

The leukaemias are caused by an acquired malignant transformation in the stem cell in the haemopoietic system. Acute leukaemia has a rapidly fatal course if untreated, while chronic leukaemia has a variable chronic course with an inevitable fatal outcome. See FIGURE 26.1. The main features of each type are as follows.

The usual age range for acute lymphatic leukaemia (ALL) is 2–10 years with a second peak at about 40 years. The median age of presentation of acute myeloid leukaemia (AML) is 55–60 years.

Acute leukaemia

Symptoms

- General constitutional (e.g. malaise)
- Symptoms of anaemia
- Susceptibility to infection (e.g. sore throat, mouth ulceration, chest infection)
- Easy bruising and bleeding (e.g. epistaxis, gingival bleeding)
- Bone pain (notably in children with ALL) and joint pain
- Symptoms due to infiltration of tissues with blast cells (e.g. gingival hypertrophy in AML)

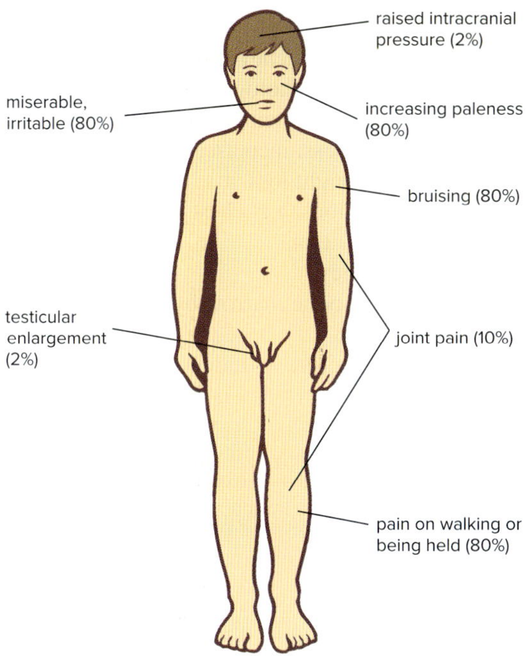

FIGURE 26.1 Clinical features of a child with leukaemia[6]

> **DxT** malaise + pallor + bone pain ➜ ALL
> **DxT** malaise + pallor + oral problems ➜ AML

Signs

- Pallor of anaemia
- Petechiae, bruising
- Gum hypertrophy/gingivitis/stomatitis
- Signs of infection
- Variable enlargement of liver, spleen and lymph nodes
- Bone tenderness, especially sternum

Diagnosis

- FBE and film: normochromic/normocytic anaemia; pancytopenia with circulatory blast cells; platelets: usually reduced
- Bone marrow examination
- PCR studies
- Cytogenetics

Treatment: chemotherapy, immunotherapy, stem cell therapy.

Note: As a rule, relapse of acute leukaemia means imminent death unless bone marrow transplantation is successful. The mean 5-year survival rate for childhood ALL is about 75–80%, for adult ALL 30%; for AML it varies with age with poorer survival, about 20%, over 55 years of age.

Chronic myeloid leukaemia (CML)

Clinical features

- A disorder of middle age, typically 40–60 years
- Insidious onset
- Constitutional symptoms: malaise, weight loss, fever, night sweats
- Symptoms of anaemia
- Splenomegaly (very large); abdominal discomfort
- Priapism
- Gout
- Markedly elevated white cell count (granulocytes)
- Marked left shift in myeloid series
- Presence of Philadelphia chromosome

> **DxT** fatigue + fever/night sweats + abdominal fullness (splenomegaly) ➜ CML

Chronic lymphocytic leukaemia (CLL)

Clinical features

- A disorder of late middle age and elderly
- Insidious onset
- Constitutional symptoms: malaise, weight loss, fever, night sweats
- Lymphadenopathy (large rubbery nodes)—neck, axilla, groin (80%)
- Moderately enlarged spleen and liver (about 50%)
- Mild anaemia
- Lymphocytosis $>15 \times 10^9$/L
- 'Mature' appearance of lymphocytes
- Consider cytogenetics

Note: Most cases, especially early indolent CLL, require no specific therapy but observation.

> **DxT** fatigue + weight loss + fever/night sweats + lymphadenopathy ➜ CLL

THE LYMPHOMAS[4]

Lymphomas, which are malignant tumours of lymphoid tissue, are classified as Hodgkin lymphoma and non-Hodgkin lymphoma on the basis of histological appearance of the involved lymph tissue.

Hodgkin lymphoma

Clinical features

- Painless (rubbery) lymphadenopathy, especially cervical nodes

- Constitutional symptoms (e.g. malaise, weakness, weight loss)
- Fever and drenching night sweats—undulant (Pel–Ebstein) fever
- Pruritus
- Alcohol-induced pain in any enlarged lymph nodes
- Possible enlarged spleen and liver

Diagnosis is by lymph node biopsy with histological confirmation. Other tests: FBE, CXR, CT/MRI (to stage), bone marrow biopsy, functional isotopic scanning. Staging is by using Ann Arbor nomenclature (IA to IVB). Treatment includes chemotherapy, immunotherapy and radiotherapy.

> **DxT** malaise + fever/night sweats + pruritus → Hodgkin lymphoma

Non-Hodgkin lymphomas

Non-Hodgkin lymphomas are a heterogeneous group of cancers of lymphocytes derived from the malignant clones of B or T cells.

Clinical features

- Painless lymphadenopathy—localised or widespread
- Constitutional symptoms possible, especially sweating
- Pruritus is uncommon
- Extra nodal sites of disease (e.g. CNS, bone, skin, GIT)
- Possible enlarged liver and spleen
- Possible nodular infiltration of skin (e.g. mycosis fungoides)

Diagnosis is by lymph node biopsy.
CXR and CT abdomen to stage.

> **DxT** malaise + fever/night sweats + lymphadenopathy → non-Hodgkin lymphoma

Multiple myeloma

Multiple myeloma is a clonal malignancy of the differentiated β lymphocyte—the plasma cell. It is regarded as a disease of the elderly, the mean age of presentation being 65 years.[8] It is asymptomatic in 20% of patients. The classic presenting triad in an older person is anaemia, back pain and elevated ESR which helps to differentiate it from monoclonal gammopathy of uncertain significance (MGUS).

Other investigations include serum protein electrophoresis and immunofixation, Sestamibi scan.

Clinical features

- Bone pain (e.g. backache)—in more than 80% of patients (possible pathological fracture)
- Bone tenderness, e.g. femur, ribs, spine
- Weakness, tiredness, increased thirst
- Anorexia and weight loss
- Recurrent infections, e.g. chest infection
- Symptoms of anaemia
- Bleeding tendency
- Replacement of bone marrow by malignant plasma cells
- Impaired renal failure → kidney failure
- Associated with amyloidosis and hypercalcaemia

> **DxT** weakness + unexplained back pain + susceptibility to infection → multiple myeloma

Diagnosis

Diagnostic criteria comprise the presence of:[6]

- paraprotein in serum (on electrophoresis)
- Bence–Jones protein in urine
- bony lytic lesions on skeletal survey

Treatment is with chemotherapy including thalidomide or lenalidomide: 5-year median survival. The younger patient may be given a stem cell transplant.[9]

MGUS

Monoclonal gammopathy of undetermined significance (MGUS) involves the production of paraprotein (M protein) by non-cancerous cells in the absence of other clinical manifestations of multiple myeloma. It is associated with various disorders. MGUS is usually asymptomatic but peripheral neuropathy can occur. No chemotherapy treatment is recommended.

Amyloidosis

This uncommon but difficult-to-diagnose disorder caused by the deposition of amyloid protein is classified as primary, familial or secondary (from chronic infection, e.g. TB, inflammation, RA, some cancers, others). It may be localised or generalised. Clinical features depend on the organ targeted such as the heart (CCF), kidney (nephrotic syndrome), GIT (malabsorption), brain (dementia) and peripheral nerves (e.g. CTS). Diagnosis is by tissue biopsy. Treatment, which varies with the type, is basically symptomatic and specialised. In primary amyloid it resembles the treatment for myeloma.

Carcinoid syndrome

Hormone secretion by carcinoid cells causes the characteristic carcinoid syndrome long before local growth or metastatic spread of the tumour is apparent (80% metastasise). Most carcinoid tumours are asymptomatic.

Clinical features

- Classic triad: skin flushing (especially face), diarrhoea (with abdominal cramps), valvular heart disease
- Other possible features: wheezing, telangiectasia, hypotension, cyanosis
- Sites of tumours: appendix/ileum, stomach, bronchi

Diagnosis

- 24-hour urine 5-hydroxyindoleacetic acid
- plasma chromogranin A/hepatic ultrasound

Polycythaemia vera

This is a malignant proliferation of RBCs and also WBCs and platelets.

Clinical features

- Older person
- Fatigue
- Headache, dizziness, tinnitus
- Pruritus after hot bath, shower
- Epistaxis
- Facial plethora
- Splenomegaly
- Thrombosis

Investigations

- FBE and haematocrit
- Bone marrow biopsy
- Genetic mutations—JAK2 mutation

Potentially curable malignant tumours

Several tumours are curable by chemotherapy even in the advanced stage. Such tumours are as follows.

Haematological tumours

- Some lymphomas
- Hodgkin lymphoma
- Acute lymphatic leukaemia
- Acute myeloid leukaemia

Solid tumours

- Choriocarcinoma
- Testicular teratoma
- Neuroblastoma
- Wilms tumour (nephroblastoma)
- Burkitt tumour
- Embryonal rhabdomyosarcoma

Tumours curable by adjuvant chemotherapy

- Breast cancer (especially up to stage 2)
- Osteogenic cancer
- Soft tissue cancer
- Colorectal cancer

Survival rates

Common cancers and their 5-year survival rates over a 15-year period (1982–2007) have been published by the Cancer Council Victoria (see TABLE 9.3, CHAPTER 9, and TABLE 26.5, below). These show improving trends for many cancers. The lowest survival rate was for mesothelioma at 4%. Updated statistics reveal that the overall 5-year survival has increased from 48% in 1984–1988 to 68% in 2009–2013.[11]

Table 26.5 Common cancers and their 5-year survival rates (a collation of surveys)[10]

Cancer	%
Testicular	98
Melanoma	91
Thyroid	92
Hodgkin lymphoma	86
Breast	89
Uterus	84
Prostate	89
Bladder	51
Non-Hodgkin lymphoma	69
Colon	63
Ovary	41
Stomach	25
Lung	12
Liver	10
Pancreas	5

Metastatic tumours

It is very helpful for the practitioner to have a working knowledge of possible primary sources of tumour when metastatic lesions are detected in various organs.

Common sites of metastatic presentation are the lymph nodes, liver, lung, mediastinum and bone. Other sites include the brain, bone marrow, peritoneum, retroperitoneum, skin and the spinal cord.

These important sites (listed below) are followed by likely primary sources with the most likely listed first.

- *Bone.* Breast, prostate, lung, Hodgkin lymphoma, kidney, thyroid, melanoma
- *Brain.* Breast, lung, colon, lymphoma, kidney, melanoma, prostate
- *Liver.* Colon, pancreas, liver, stomach, breast, lung, melanoma
- *Lung and mediastinum.* Breast, lung, colon, kidney, testes, cervix/uterus, Hodgkin lymphoma, melanoma
- *Lymph nodes:*
  - *High cervical.* Hodgkin lymphoma, lymphoma, squamous cell carcinoma, oropharynx, nasopharynx
  - *Low cervical.* Lung, stomach, lymphoma, Hodgkin lymphoma, oropharynx, larynx, skin, tongue
  - *Axillary.* Breast, lung, lymphoma
  - *Inguinal.* Lymphoma, ovary, uterus, vulva, prostate, skin
- *Retroperitoneum.* Lymphoma, Hodgkin lymphoma, ovary, uterus, testes, prostate
- *Skin.* Lung, colon, melanoma, Kaposi sarcoma

It is important to keep in mind those malignancies that are potentially curable and to refer as soon as possible.

Cancer with an unknown primary

Cancer without a clear primary source is present in about 5% of all cases. If the diagnosis cannot be made on the history, physical examination and baseline tests, then the key to excluding treatable primaries is adequate immunohistological staining on a tissue biopsy. It is worth referring for investigation as these could be treatable primaries. Adenocarcinoma is common in 40% resulting from lung, colorectal and pancreatic cancer. Poorly differentiated neoplasms include lymphoma, melanoma and sarcoma. The mean survival time in patients with an unknown primary is 6 months.[12]

Prevention

Preventive measures for malignant disease are addressed in more detail in CHAPTER 9. The significant decrease in deaths from cancer of the stomach in this country in recent years is probably reflected in our improved diet with more fresh fruit and vegetables. Important preventive measures include an appropriate healthy diet, no smoking, sun protection, HPV vaccination and perhaps safe sex measures. Of concern is the rapid increase in the incidence of prostate cancer, chronic myeloid leukaemia, myeloma and non-Hodgkin lymphoma and adenocarcinoma of the oesophagus.

Triads to consider

DxT anorexia + weight loss + jaundice (± epigastric pain) ➜ pancreatic cancer

DxT fatigue + dysphagia + weight loss ➜ oesophageal cancer

DxT anorexia + dyspepsia + weight loss ➜ stomach cancer

DxT headache + a/n/v + ataxia ➜ medulloblastoma (children)

DxT fever + malaise (extreme) + a/n/v (± anaemia) ➜ neuroblastoma

DxT mental dysfunction + vomiting + (waking) headache ➜ cerebral tumour (late)

DxT indrawn eye + small pupil + ptosis (± anhydrosis) ➜ Horner syndrome (? lung cancer)

Patient education resources

Hand-out sheets from *Murtagh's Patient Education* 7th edition:

- Bladder cancer
- Bowel cancer
- Breast cancer/lumps
- Cancer
- Leukaemia
- Lung cancer
- Lymphoma
- Melanoma
- Prostate (various)
- Testicle (various)
- Skin (various)

Other resources

Optimal cancer care pathways (prevention, early detection, screening recommendations): <jon.emery@unimelb.edu.au>

Royal Australian College of General Practitioners. Early detection of cancers. In: *Guidelines for Preventive Activities in General Practice* (9th edn). Melbourne: RACGP, 2016.

References

1. Australia's Health. Causes of Death. Canberra: Australian Institute of Health, 2007.
2. Halliday J. Malignant disease in children: the view of a general practitioner and parent. In: Baum J, Dominica F, Woodward R. *Listen My Child Has a Lot of Living to Do.* Oxford: Oxford University Press, 1990: 19–27.

3 Trahair T. Cancer in children: how to treat. Australian Doctor; 15 August 2008: 31–8.
4 Hamilton W, Peters TJ. *Cancer Diagnosis in Primary Care.* Oxford: Elsevier, 2007.
5 Robinson MJ, Roberton DM. *Practical Paediatrics* (5th edn). Edinburgh: Churchill Livingstone, 2003: 535.
6 Hamilton W, Peters TJ, et al. Risk of ovarian cancer in women with symptoms in primary care: population based case–control study. BMJ, 2009: 339.
7 Vowels MR. Common presentations and management of leukaemia in childhood. Aust Fam Physician, 1994; 23: 1519–21.
8 Davey P. *Medicine at a Glance* (3rd edn). Oxford: Blackwell Publishing, 2010: 36–7.
9 Moreau P et al. Frontline therapy of multiple myeloma. Blood, 14 May 2015; 125(20): 3076–84. [PMID 25838345]
10 Giles G. *Cancer Survival in Victoria.* Melbourne: Cancer Council Victoria, 2009.
11 Australian Institute of Health and Welfare 2017. Cancer in Australia 2017. Cancer series no.101. Cat. no. CAN 100. Canberra: AIHW, 2017: 72.
12 Davey P. *Medicine at a Glance* (3rd edn). Oxford: Blackwell Publishing, 2010: 380.

27 HIV/AIDS—could it be HIV?

The red ribbon is a symbol of solidarity with HIV positive people and those living with AIDS.

WHO 2015

HIV: a modern masquerade

HIV, the cause of the well-known AIDS, can rightly be included as one of the clinical masquerades of modern medicine. Public health measures in the Western world have limited the spread of the infection. By contrast, the incidence in Africa and Asia continues to rise at an alarming rate. The World Health Organization estimated that in 2010,[1] 34 million adults and children were living with HIV, including 23 million in sub-Saharan Africa and 25 000 in Australia, with 2.7 million newly infected and increasing, while 1.8 million people with HIV died. However, this figure reduced to 1.1 million in 2015.

In 2012, the average age of people newly diagnosed with HIV infection was 37 years and about 86% were male; most infections are in men who have sex with men (MSM). The conversion rate of HIV to AIDS has been 33% but it is improving with antiretroviral therapy (ART), which has dramatically changed people's lives. HIV is now a chronic disease management problem. The introduction of combination treatment with the protease inhibitors in November 1995 changed the previously understood natural history of the disease.

The benefit of early diagnosis has become even more impressive since the discovery that HIV is not a latent infection throughout most of its course. Soon after initial infection, an explosive replication of HIV occurs, which is brought under control by the immune system in 6 to 8 weeks as the host-versus-virus interaction reaches an active and dynamic equilibrium. This dynamic situation continues throughout a person's lifetime, with as many as 10 billion new viroids produced and up to 2 billion CD_4 T lymphocytes destroyed and replaced daily. Clinical immunodeficiency develops when the body's ability to replace CD_4 cells is finally exhausted, resulting in further uncontrolled viral replication. Viral load assays based on molecular techniques have revolutionised our understanding of the natural history of HIV disease. These advances make it imperative to make the diagnosis early in the course of the disease in order to start combination treatment to lessen the viral load.

The management of HIV infection is a specialised field but the GP is central in prevention, diagnosis, counselling, monitoring and shared management of HIV disease. The GP must be alert to the benefits of early diagnosis as summarised in TABLE 27.1.

Table 27.1 The benefits of early HIV diagnosis

To individual patients
Prolongation of the asymptomatic period
Delayed disease progression
Prevention of opportunistic infections
Optimal maintenance of health through patient education and counselling
Cures are only likely with early intervention
To the cohort of HIV-positive individuals
Monitoring of advances in treatment
Increased participation in research and clinical trials
Development of new services to meet changing patient needs
To the community
Documentation of changes in epidemiology
Reduced high-risk activities
Contact tracing
Control of HIV transmission
To the doctors
Time to influence the course of disease
Time to counsel the patient

Source: Penny R. Could it be HIV? 2. Benefits of early diagnosis of HIV infection. Med J Aust, 1993; 158: 35–6. © Copyright 1993, *The Medical Journal of Australia*—reproduced with permission

Key facts and checkpoints

- HIV is a retrovirus with two known strains that cause a similar spectrum of syndromes: HIV-1 and HIV-2 (mainly confined to West Africa). It infects T-helper cells bearing the CD_4 receptor.
- Always consider HIV in those at risk: enquire about history of STIs, injection of illicit drugs, past blood transfusions, sexual activities and partners.
- About 50% of patients develop an acute infective illness similar to glandular fever within weeks of acquiring the virus (the HIV seroconversion illness).[1] The main features are fever, lymphadenopathy, lethargy and possibly sore throat, and a generalised rash.
- If these patients have a negative infectious mononucleosis test, perform an HIV antibody test, which may have to be repeated in 4 weeks or so if negative.
- Patients invariably recover to enter a long period of good health for 5 years or more.[2]
- The so-called 'set point' is where the plasma viral load drops to a steady level for many years.
- *Pneumocystis jiroveci* (ex *carinii*) pneumonia (PJP) is the commonest presentation of AIDS.
- Approximately 15–40% of HIV-positive children are infected from HIV-infected mothers.[3]
- Infants born to these mothers may develop the disease within a few months, with 30% affected by the age of 18 months.
- The time for the onset of AIDS in HIV-affected adults varies from 2 months to 20 years or longer; the median time is around 10 years.
- In family practice the most common presentation of HIV-related illness is seen in the skin/oral mucosa, for example, candidiasis and herpes.[4]
- TB is a common, serious but treatable complication of HIV.
- HIV antibody testing is a two-stage process: the antigen–antibody test for screening followed by another method (e.g. Western blot) if positive.
- New rapid HIV tests or point of care HIV tests will overcome barriers, including delays to diagnosis.
- The seroconversion period from acquiring HIV infection to a positive antibody test varies between individuals: this period is known as the 'window period'.
- All HIV-infected patients require regular monitoring for immune function and viral load. The viral load test monitors viral activity.
- The level of immune depletion is best measured by the CD_4 positive T-lymphocyte (helper T-cell) count—the CD_4 cell count. The cut-off points for good health (asymptomatic) and severe disease appear to be 500 cells/μL and 200 cells/μL respectively.[2]
- Most patients with AIDS will need lifelong[1] daily medication with a combination of antiretroviral drugs.
- Current management focuses on treating HIV as a chronic disease.
- A leading concerning cause of death is cardiovascular disease.

Occurrence and transmission

HIV can be isolated from blood, tissues, semen, saliva, breast milk, cervical and vaginal secretions and tears of infected persons. HIV is transmitted in semen, blood and vaginal fluids, transplanted organs and breast milk through:

- unprotected sexual intercourse (anal or vaginal) and in rare cases oral sex with an infected person
- infected blood entering the body (through blood transfusion or by IV drug users sharing needles/ syringes)
- needle-stick injury
- artificial insemination, organ transplantation
- infected mothers (to babies during pregnancy, at birth or in breast milk)

Infection with HIV can occur via the vagina, rectum or open cuts and sores, including any on the lips or in the mouth. Social (non-sexual) contact and insect vectors have not been implicated in transmission.

Stages[5]

The clinical stages of HIV disease are summarised in TABLE 27.2.[6]

Acute (seroconversion) illness

At least 50% of patients have an acute illness associated with seroconversion. The illness usually occurs within 6 weeks of infection and is characterised by fever, night sweats, malaise, severe lethargy, anorexia, nausea, myalgia, arthralgia, headache, photophobia, sore throat, diarrhoea, lymphadenopathy, generalised maculoerythematous rash and thrombocytopenia. The main symptoms are headache, photophobia and malaise/fatigue. Neurological manifestations, including meningoencephalitis and peripheral neuritis, can occur. Acute HIV infection should be considered in the differential diagnosis of illnesses resembling glandular fever. This illness, which resembles infectious mononucleosis, is self-limiting and usually resolves within 1 to 3 weeks. However, chronic

Table 27.2 Clinical stages of HIV disease[6]

Clinical stage	Common clinical features	CD_4 count
Seroconversion illness (self-limited 1–3 weeks)	Fever, headache (may have aseptic meningitis), sore throat, maculopapular rash, lymphadenopathy, splenomegaly Atypical lymphocytes on FBE cells	Transient decrease, commonly followed by a return to near-normal levels
Asymptomatic	Headaches Persistent generalised lymphadenopathy	Usually >500 cells/μL Gradual decrease of 50–80 cells/μL
Symptomatic—early	Oral and vaginal candidiasis, oral hairy leukoplakia, seborrhoeic dermatitis, psoriasis, recurrent varicella zoster infection, cervical dysplasia, unexplained fever, sweats, weight loss, diarrhoea, tuberculosis	Usually 150–500 cells/μL
Symptomatic—late	PJP, Kaposi sarcoma, oesophageal candidiasis, cerebral toxoplasmosis, lymphoma, HIV-1 associated dementia complex, cryptococcal meningitis	Usually <150 cells/μL
Advanced	CMV retinitis, cerebral lymphoma, *Mycobacterium avium* complex (MAC) infection	Usually <50 cells/μL

Reproduced with permission[6]

lethargy, depression and irritability may persist after the acute illness. Non-specific viraemic sequelae such as mucosal ulceration, desquamation, exacerbation of seborrhoea and recurrences of herpes simplex may occur (see FIG. 27.1).

Acute illness may be accompanied by neutropenia, lymphopenia, thrombocytopenia, and mildly elevated ESR and serum transaminases. During recovery lymphocytosis may occur with appearance of atypical mononuclear cells and an inversion of the $CD_4^+:CD_8^+$ ratio due to elevation of CD_8^+ cells. It is seronegative for EBV.

Differential diagnoses are given in TABLE 27.3.

Table 27.3 Differential diagnoses of primary HIV infection

Epstein–Barr mononucleosis
Syphilis: secondary
TORCH organisms:
- toxoplasmosis
- rubella
- CMV (especially)
- herpes simplex

Disseminated gonococcal infection
Hepatitis A, B, C, D or E
Influenza
Other virus infections

DxT fever + severe malaise + lymphadenopathy ➜ acute HIV

Subsequent stage

After the acute illness, HIV disease passes into an asymptomatic stage of variable length, up to several years, but 30% have persistent generalised lympathenopathy.

Later constitutional symptoms develop along with minor opportunistic infections such as oral candidiasis, herpes simplex and herpes zoster. This early symptomatic stage is referred to as AIDS-related complex and is regarded as a prodromal to AIDS.

AIDS-defining conditions

The original US Centers for Disease Control (CDC) classification has been modified with time to provide a more simplified scheme for defining AIDS. The HIV/AIDS case surveillance system simply specifies a list of clinical conditions associated with the late stages of HIV infection as being 'AIDS-defining'.[7]

The AIDS-defining conditions are:

- candidiasis of bronchi, trachea or lungs
- candidiasis, oesophageal
- cervical cancer, invasive
- coccidioidomycosis, disseminated or extrapulmonary
- cryptococcosis, extrapulmonary
- cryptosporidiosis, chronic intestinal (>1 month's duration)
- cytomegalovirus (CMV) disease (other than liver, spleen or nodes)
- CMV retinitis (with loss of vision)
- encephalopathy, HIV-related

- herpes simplex virus (HSV): chronic ulcer(s) (>1 month's duration); or bronchitis, pneumonitis or oesophagitis
- histoplasmosis, disseminated or extrapulmonary
- isosporiasis, chronic intestinal (>1 month's duration)
- Kaposi sarcoma
- lymphoma, Burkitt (or equivalent term)
- lymphoma, immunoblastic (or equivalent term)
- lymphoma, primary, of brain
- *Mycobacterium avium* complex of *M. kansasii,* disseminated or extrapulmonary
- *Mycobacterium tuberculosis,* any site (pulmonary or extrapulmonary)
- *Mycobacterium,* other species or unidentified species, disseminated or extrapulmonary
- *Pneumocystis jiroveci* pneumonia (PJP)
- *Salmonella* septicaemia, recurrent
- toxoplasmosis of brain
- wasting syndrome due to HIV

The Australian AIDS surveillance case definition does not refer to the CD_4 cell count although in the US AIDS is also defined by a CD_4 cell count of <200/μL, regardless of clinical condition. At levels below this, people will become increasingly vulnerable to AIDS-defining conditions.

Clinical features

There is a multiplicity of clinical findings in HIV infection (see FIG. 27.1).

Fever

- Usually this is of unknown origin.

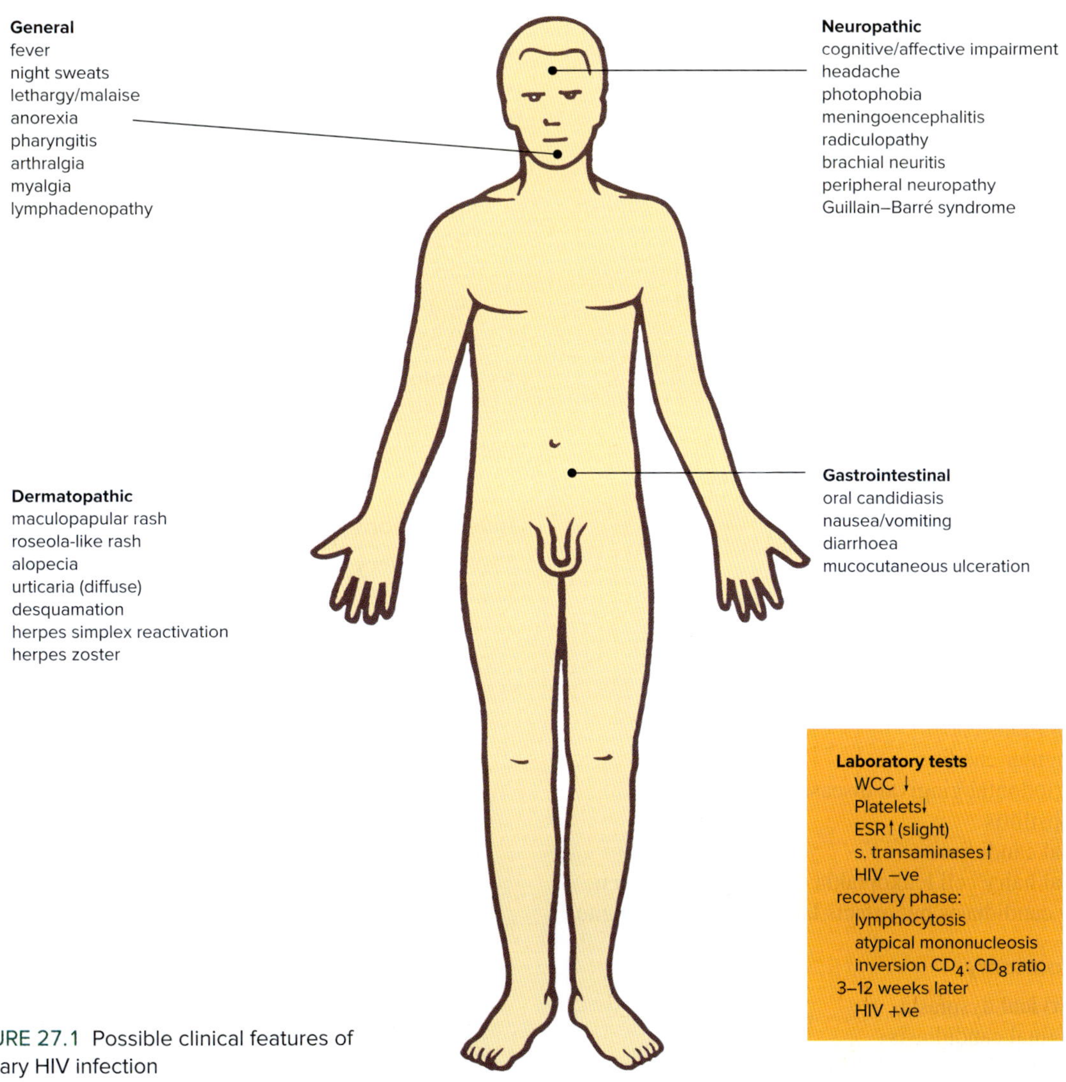

FIGURE 27.1 Possible clinical features of primary HIV infection

Weight loss

- Usually severe and muscle wasting

Respiratory

- Sinusitis
- Non-productive cough, increasing dyspnoea and fever: due to opportunistic pneumonias

More than 50% of patients present with PJP which may have an abrupt or insidious onset.[6] With the insidious type of onset, examination and chest X-ray are often normal early. Many other agents (e.g. CMV, cryptococcosis and TB) can be responsible. Exclusion of PJP is important as this condition carries a high mortality if untreated.[6]

> **Practice tip**
>
> Severe PJP can have little or no chest signs, and, unless treated, patients can rapidly deteriorate and die.

Gastrointestinal

- Chronic diarrhoea (many causes) with weight loss or dehydration

Neurological

- Headache
- Progressive dementia (HIV encephalopathy)
- Ataxia due to myelopathy
- Seizures
- Mononeuritis
- Guillain–Barré type mononeuropathy
- Toxoplasma encephalitis
- Cryptococcal meningitis
- Peripheral neuropathy
- Progressive visual loss (CMV retinitis)
- CNS lymphoma

Oral cavity

- Aphthous ulcers
- Angular cheilitis
- Periodontal/gingival disease
- Tonsillitis
- Oral candidiasis
- Oral hairy cell leukoplakia (frequently mistaken for candidiasis but affects lateral border of tongue)

Genitourinary

- Cervical dysplasia
- Vaginal candidiasis
- Various STIs (e.g. HSV, HPV)

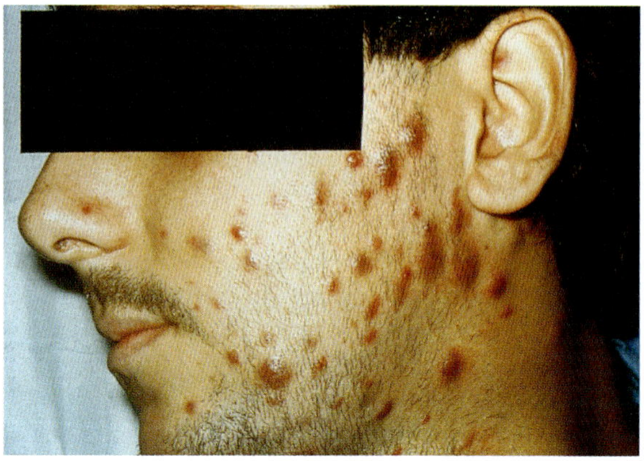

FIGURE 27.2 Kaposi sarcoma of the skin on the face of a man with AIDS

Photo courtesy Hugh Newton-John

Skin

- Impetigo
- Warts
- HSV
- Shingles, especially multidermatomal
- Seborrhoeic dermatitis
- Cutaneous mycoses
- Kaposi sarcoma (painless red-purple lesions on any part of the body including palms, soles, oral cavity and other parts of the GIT) (see FIG. 27.2).

Psychological

FIGURE 27.3 presents the chronology of HIV-induced disease correlated with time since infection and CD_4 cell levels.

Investigations and diagnosis[6]

The laboratory investigation of AIDS covers three broad areas:

1 Tests for HIV infection:
  - antigen–antibody test (ELISA screen) or HIV rapid test (at point of care). If positive—western blot technique (used for confirmation)
2 Tests of immune function:
  - CD_4 lymphocyte counts—the strongest predictor of possible clinical manifestations of HIV infection
  - low CD_4 cells (counts <500 cells/μL) = defective cell immunity[2,4]
  - counts <200 cells/μL = severe immunodeficiency
3 Plasma HIV RNA (viral load): a measure of the serum level of RNA of the HIV virus—correlates with response to treatment and progression to AIDS and death

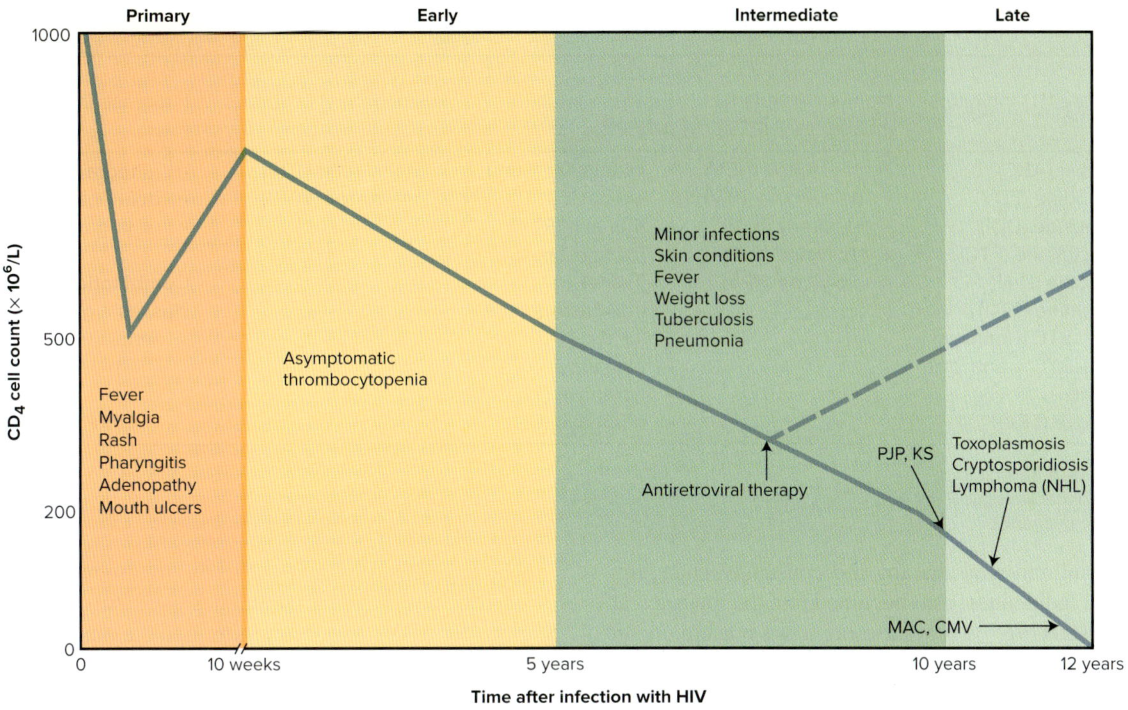

FIGURE 27.3 Chronology of HIV-induced disease correlated with time since infection

Abbreviations: CMV = cytomegalovirus; HIV = human immunodeficiency virus; KS = Kaposi sarcoma; MAC = *Mycobacterium avium* complex; NHL = non-Hodgkin lymphoma; PJP = *Pneumocystis jiroveci* pneumonia.

Source: HIV infection as a chronic disease. *MedicineToday,* 2014; 15 (2): 18. Courtesy of the Australasian Society for HIV Medicine (ASHM).

4 Genotype resistance (HLA B5701 if treatment with abacavir planned)
5 Tests for opportunistic infections and other problems, e.g. other STIs, EBV, CMV, hepatitis, Mantoux test
6 Routine general health tests, e.g. FBE, U&E, blood glucose, lipids, eGFR, LFTs

Management

Patients with HIV infection who invariably have to cope with profound psychological stress require considerable psychosocial support, counselling and regular assessment from a non-judgmental, caring practitioner. Best practice is referral to a specialist clinic for shared care.

The holistic approach

Most people with HIV infection will take 'natural therapies'. This should be viewed as being complementary to the management suggested by the GP, and the patient should be encouraged to tell his or her doctors of the alternative medicines being taken. Anecdotal reports suggest that 75% of people with HIV regularly use 'natural therapies',[8] and in the setting of the long-term nature of the condition it is important for doctors to be supportive and create a climate of acceptance around these practices.

Positive lifestyle factors include:

- a very healthy balanced diet: high fruit and vegetable intake, pure fruit juices, high fibre, low fat, high complex carbohydrates
- toxic avoidance: processed foods, caffeine, illicit drugs, alcohol, cigarettes
- relaxation and meditation (reduction and self-monitoring of stress levels)
- appropriate sleep and exercise
- consider supplementary antioxidants
- support groups and continuing counselling

Treatment (medication)[8,9,10]

Optimal antiretroviral therapy (ART), which has dramatically changed the outlook, now depends on the use of combinations of drugs. Monotherapy is no longer accepted practice. The recommendations for the

Table 27.4 Currently available antiretroviral drugs[9]

Nucleoside RT* inhibitors (NRTIs)	Non-nucleoside RT inhibitors (NNRTIs)	Protease inhibitors (HIV PIs)	Fusion (entry) inhibitors	Integrase inhibitors
• abacavir (ABC) • zidovudine (ZDV) • didanosine (DDI) • emtricitabine (FTC) • stavudine (D4T) • lamivudine (3TC) • AZT + 3TC (Combivir) • AZT + 3TC + abacavir (Trizivir) • tenofovir (TFV)**	• nevirapine (NEV) • delavirdine (DLV) • efavirenz (EFV) • etravirine (ETR) • rilpivirine (RPV)	• saquinavir (SQV) • indinavir (IDV) • ritonavir (RTV) • fosamprenavir (FAPV) • lopinavir/ritonavir (LPV) • atazanavir (ATZ) • tipranavir (TPV) • darunavir (DRV)	• enfuvirtide (T20) • maraviroc (MVC)≠	• raltegravir (RAL) • dolutegavir • elvitegavir **Combination of classes e.g.** • Atripla (TFV, EFV, FTC) • Eviplera (TFV, FTC, RPV)

* RT = reverse transcriptase
** a nucleotide analogue RTI
≠ a CCR5 antagonist

use of antiretroviral therapy are constantly changing. Updated guidelines can be found on the internet at www.hivatis.org, www.bhiva.org, www.ashm.org.au or www.aidsinfo.nih.gov/guidelines. Viral resistance is the limiting factor, no matter how potent an individual drug may be at reducing viral load initially. The trials of combined zidovudine and lamivudine demonstrated both a more sustained decrease in plasma viral load than either drug did alone, and a more delayed development of viral resistance. There are now many antiretroviral drugs available for use in Australia (see TABLE 27.4) and clinicians have a much wider scope of treatments available. However, many questions remain about combination therapy and further trials using viral load as a clinical endpoint should provide pointers for treatment. Currently the use of three drugs, referred to as highly active antiretroviral therapy (HAART), is favoured. There are many possible combinations. Side effects, which are often severe—including cardiovascular disease—and affect the quality of life, remain a problem. Resistance to HAART is now a problem. Effective (90%) results have been achieved with TRIO (etravirine, darunavir and raltegravir) therapy.[11] Investigators are evaluating the benefits of dual therapy through the SWORD-1 and SWORD-2 studies. Long-term treatment with fewer agents would be popular if of proven efficacy. Subcutaneous injections of interleukin-2 have been shown to boost immunity.

When to start[12,13]

This is a controversial issue. CD_4 cell count guidelines:

- <350/μL—treat with ART
- 350–500/μL—strongly consider, offer or closely monitor

Current thinking favours early treatment. Refer to current international guidelines (see Australasian Society for HIV, Viral Hepatitis and Sexual Health Medicine: www.ashm.org.au). The most widely used and preferred regimen consists of 2 NTIs plus either an NNRI or a protease inhibitor,[9] e.g. emtricitabine + tenofovir + efavirenz or rilpivirine.

Be aware of:

- drug interactions (www.hiv-druginteractions.org)
- contraindicated drug combinations[9]
- adverse effects[9]
- opportunistic infections

HAART (highly active antiretroviral therapy)

This is a combination of three (or more) agents with one or more penetrating the blood–brain barrier.

Pneumocystis jiroveci[9]

This is an important cause of pneumonia and not usually seen until the CD_4^+ cell count is <200/μL. It is usually treated with trimethoprim + sulfamethoxazole (cotrimoxazole) oral or IV for 21 days depending on severity, which is also given orally as prophylaxis when the cell count reaches <200. Alternative agents are IV pentamidine or oral dapsone, clindamycin and atovaquone.

Acute HIV Infection

Treatment of seroconversion illness is not of proven clinical benefit (to date) but is optional and some clinics offer it.

Pre-exposure prophylaxis (PrEP)

This can be considered for those at risk. Selected tablets such as tenofovir or Truvada are taken around time of sex.[14] Refer to your local sexual health clinic.

Post-exposure prophylaxis (PEP)

Undertake a risk assessment—PEP is not recommended for low-risk cases but those with significant high risk should be considered for PEP. It should be commenced within 72 hours of exposure and usually involves 2–3 antiretroviral agents taken daily for 28 days.[15] Refer to 'Needle-stick and sharps injuries' for protocol (see CHAPTER 132).

The HIV test: the role of the family doctor[13]

The astute GP will use the opportunity of a request for an HIV test to explore preventive and sexual health issues. A full sexual history and drug history must incorporate the 'three Cs' of counselling, confidentiality and consent in the pre-test interview.

Many HIV-positive patients have described how the results left them bewildered and devastated, especially with an unexpected positive result. Part of the reason given was the lack of any form of pre-test counselling. Ideally, management involves shared care with an expert consultant, with whom close liaison is essential.

Initial consultation

- First establish why the patient is presenting 'now' for the test.
- Explore the 'hidden component' of the patient's consultation.
- Take a full sexual, medical and drug-taking history. It is recognised that this can be embarrassing for both the doctor and the patient, but those experienced in this process advise the following approach:
  - Establish a supportive, non-judgmental atmosphere. Encourage disclosure of history and patterns of partners and sexual practices in a gender-neutral situation. Make no assumptions about sexual preferences; they will be indicated by the patient as the history evolves, provided you allow this to happen; this will take time.
- Non-judgmental, matter-of-fact questions such as 'Have you injected yourself with drugs?' and 'Do you have sex with men or women or both?' may permit honest disclosure.
- Stress the importance of disclosure of prior, known infections with STIs. Assess the patient's risk for an STI.
- Assess the patient's coping strategies and social network.

Pre-test counselling

- Give information on the test (what it tells and does not tell).
- Explain about the false negative and 'window period'.
- Give appropriate information about HIV disease and other STIs.
- Dispel any myths about transmission of infection.
- Give preventive advice on safer practices (sex and IV drugs).
- Assess the possible coping mechanisms of the patient.
- Assess the patient's social support networks and interpersonal bonds.
- Reassure about confidentiality. This is a legal requirement.
- Discuss who to tell: informing sexual contacts.
- Offer tests other than STIs.

Finally:

- Discuss how the patient will cope with the test result.
- Discuss legal requirements (check with state laws).
- Advise of need for informed consent (not only for HIV test but other STIs).
- Make arrangements to discuss the test results face to face.

Consider the useful question: 'How would your behaviour change, if at all, as a result of having this test today?'

Test result (about 2 weeks later)

This must be given in consultation (whether positive or negative): avoid the telephone.

The negative test result

- Provide reassurance.
- Emphasise the safe sex information.
- Counter any suggestion that current risk-taking behaviour is safe.
- Retest if in high-risk category or known HIV contact or in a 'window period' of 12 weeks.
- A test in 3 months helps rule out recent acquisition.
- Maintain confidentiality.

The positive test result

This is a very traumatic experience and good communication skills are essential. The result should be stated clearly. Good pretest history taking, risk assessment and counselling will make the task of informing the patient of a positive test result a lot easier. Being able to inform the patient of a greatly improved prognosis due to combination drug therapy is also of assistance in breaking the news. Be warm and open. Many patients want to be touched for reassurance. The words 'you are not dying' can be firmly stated a few times. Educate the patient about the difference between HIV infection and the acquired immunodeficiency syndrome. Discuss with the patient to whom he or she is going to tell the result and help the patient decide on the most supportive friend. Ask the patient what he or she is going to do after the consultation and make an appointment for the next day. Give the patient an HIV support line number for overnight telephone support if required. Discuss the issue of contact tracing briefly and in more depth at the next consultation, because sexual contacts should be notified. However, avoid an information overload.

Start immediate post-test counselling and education. Emphasise that an HIV-positive status does not equal AIDS and need not lead to it in the short term. Organise a consultant's appointment and provide sound patient education material.

Interview and full clinical assessment

- Assessment of general health. Assess risk factors for cardiovascular disease and diabetes since ART can increase the overall risk at least two-fold.[16]
- Particular assessment of prior psychiatric history and confirm prior STIs and drugs
- Evidence of EBV (glandular fever), hepatitis B, HIV illness (acute seroconversion illness)
- Further counselling and discussion of specific problems
- Assessment of bonds and relationships with regard to support

Examination—to set a base level

- Full examination, skin, CNS—especially fundi, chest, abdomen and genitals; urine and lung function test
- Monitor temperature and weight

Blood tests—to set a base level and check immune status

- Repeat HIV antibody test (if any possibility of error)
- CD_4 cells with FBE and a differential WCC
- Viral load test
- G-6-PD screen for enzyme deficiency
- Serology for syphilis (RPR), hepatitis A, B and C (very important), toxoplasmosis, CMV
- Test for gonorrhoea and *Chlamydia*, herpes and thrush (if indicated)
- Mantoux test for tuberculosis

Encourage a holistic approach to health maintenance and enhancement. Explore the patient's feelings, anxieties, fears and confidentiality concerns. Reinforce safer practices.

The second post-positive result consultation

- Give results of repeat HIV test and baseline tests.
- Explore patient's understanding, feelings, coping abilities and spiritual issues (if appropriate).
- Some of the common questions that patients with HIV infection ask are:
  - Am I going to get sick?
  - How long will I live for?
  - Are there any treatments available?
  - Is there a cure?
  - What is going to happen to me?
  - Should I tell my friends?
  - Should I tell my family?
  - What are the social and legal issues?

It is worth pre-empting these questions and having ready appropriate answers for that particular patient.

- Give appropriate reassurance: prognosis is now much better, in respect of long remission, than appreciated.
- Discuss support systems.
- Check personal prophylaxis (safer sex and needle-sharing habits).
- Reinforce lifestyle strategies and suggest how patients can help themselves: give case examples.
- Recommend meditation, mindfulness and appropriate literature.
- Provide appropriate referrals (if needed): specialist counsellors, self-help and support groups, meditation classes.
- Advise patients about their legal and ethical responsibilities not to pass on the infection to others.
- Organise contact tracing.

- Address the difficult issue of telling sexual partners.
- If the patient is unwilling to inform sexual partners or is uncertain of who they may be, then contact-tracing organisations run through state government offices are of assistance in tracing sexual partners who may be at risk.
- If a patient refuses to inform a sexual partner of the risk, then the doctor may disclose this information to the patient's partner in the following circumstances: if there is a clear risk of transmission; if the patient has been given education and counselling and this has been ignored; or if the doctor in the case has sought advice from colleagues and institutional ethics committee and before disclosure discussed it with the medical defence organisation. The doctor then should provide the patient with written advice that the patient must notify the partner, and if the patient still refuses to do so then the doctor has the right to do so.
- Discuss 'safer sex' guidelines. Condom usage is essential to prevent further viral loading and this needs to be explained, as well as the reason of protecting others.
- Advise on the importance of compliance with medication. There is rapid rebound of the virus when ART is stopped.
- Different criteria are used to guide treatment of children.

Continuing maintenance consultations

- Provide appropriate support, encouragement and counselling.
- Frequency depends on CD_4 cell count (e.g. 3–6 monthly).
- Examination:
  - Check general condition, temperature and weight.
  - Look for unusual lung infection, diarrhoea, skin lesions, tongue and oropharynx, fevers, wasting and neurological signs.
  - Examine for signs of CMV retinitis (at risk if CD_4 count <100 cells/μL).
  - Monitor for depressive illness.
  - Look for early signs of AIDS-related dementia.
- Tests: CD_4 cell count and syphilis serology; viral load test; chest X-ray and induced sputum (if cough, shortness of breath), faeces microculture if diarrhoea persists, *Candida* mouth swabs and herpes swabs appropriately.
- Treat intercurrent illness.
- Prophylaxis—this is managed according to immune status: if CD_4 count <200 cells/μL use cotrimoxazole to prevent opportunistic infections, particularly PJP.

Contact tracing

Contacts of HIV-positive patients should be traced and offered testing with counselling.[5] Patients with HIV infection must be advised of the risk they pose to seronegative sexual partners. A person who has HIV or is at risk of HIV infection must not make any blood, semen or tissue donation. Because of the probable association between genital ulcerative disease and HIV transmission, the effective management of STIs is part of the general strategy for HIV control.

Table 27.5 Red flags for HIV infection

Persistent
Fever
Headache
Weight loss
Diarrhoea
Dry cough
Dyspnoea on exertion
Visual disturbance
Neurological
• seizures
• peripheral neuropathy
• others
Psychiatric
• depression/mania
• sleep disturbance
• signs of dementia
Laboratory
Viral count >10 000 copies/mm
Cell count 200–250/μL or less

Prevention of HIV infection

Counselling the person at risk regarding 'safer practices'

No effective vaccine has been developed. Modification of behaviour is the only valid strategy for prevention of HIV infection. Education programs to encourage sexual practices that reduce the exchange of genital secretions (safe sex) may achieve risk reduction for sexually active individuals. Condoms provide a barrier if used properly and consistently but may be too easily damaged to offer reliable protection during anal

27

intercourse. A water-based lubricant such as K-Y gel or Lubafax should be used: oil-based lubricants such as Vaseline weaken condoms.

Discuss alternative sex practices, including touching, cuddling, body-to-body rubbing and mutual masturbation.

Emphasise the importance of being in control with drug taking, IV usage, safe sex practices and the needle-exchange program.

Of special importance is the finding that the most important biological risk factor for HIV transmission is the presence of other active STIs in either partner. This includes chlamydia, gonorrhoea, syphilis and genital herpes. Herpes is also likely to increase the risk of HIV transmission during both homosexual and heterosexual intercourse, even in the presence of condoms.[13,14,15]

Health professionals

Care should be exercised whenever blood samples are taken or sharps have been used. Advise safe disposal of sharps and other disposables and appropriate sterilisation of material. Gloves should be worn for all invasive procedures. Management of needle-stick injuries and other at-risk exposures is described in CHAPTER 132. Blood donors need to be carefully screened.

Community education

Educating the community in a non-emotional, responsible way about AIDS should be a priority. While the personal, community and global benefits of effective AIDS education are generally acknowledged, the fear of addressing such a sensitive issue sometimes results in failure to act.[16,17] AIDS education in schools in particular can be an important strategy. People with HIV infection would be appropriate resource educators and the use of videos would be a most appropriate medium for education.

When to refer[18]

Most patients with HIV disease need referral to a specialist or clinic that can manage the patient expertly and sympathetically.

Referral should take place at the time of:

- onset of a life-threatening opportunistic infection
- the need to initiate antiretroviral drug therapy
- administration of prophylactic pentamidine therapy
- serious psychological problems related to HIV-positive status

Acknowledgment

Part of this text, including clinical manifestations, prevention and contact tracing is reproduced from the *Handbook on Sexually Transmitted Diseases*[5] (copyright Commonwealth of Australia, reproduced by permission).

Patient education resources

Hand-out sheets from *Murtagh's Patient Education* 7th edition:

- HIV infection and AIDS
- HIV post-exposure prophylaxis

Other resources

Australasian Society for HIV, Viral Hepatitis and Sexual Health Medicine (ASHM). Patient fact sheets. <www.ashm.org.au>

HIV drug interactions. <www.hiv.druginteractions.org>

References

1. Baker D, Pell C, Donovan B. HIV infection as a chronic disease: optimising outcomes. Medicine Today, February 2014; 15 (2): 16–26.
2. Stewart GJ. The challenge: the clinical diagnosis of HIV. Med J Aust, 1993; 158: 31–4.
3. Kumar P, Clark M. *Clinical Medicine* (7th edn). London: Elsevier Saunders, 2009: 184.
4. Pohl M. Managing HIV patients in general practice. Patient Management, 1989; June: 49–61.
5. NHMRC. *Handbook on Sexually Transmitted Diseases.* Canberra: Department of Community Services & Health, 1995: 1–55.
6. McCoy R. Alarm bells. When to worry about your patient with HIV. Aust Fam Physician, 1997; 26: 803–9.
7. Available from: www.cdc.gov (US Centers for Disease Control and Prevention update on HIV/AIDS developments).
8. Bradford D. Update on issues for HIV management. Aust Fam Physician, 1997; 26: 812–17.
9. Expert group for Antibiotic guidelines. HIV infection. In: eTG complete. Melbourne: Therapeutic Guidelines Ltd. Available from: <www.tg.org.au>, accessed January 2018.
10. Kidd M, McCoy R. Managing HIV/AIDS. Part 2—Treatment. Medical Observer, March 2002: 36–7.
11. Yazdanpanah Y, Fagard C, Descamps D et al. High rate of virologic success with raltegravir plus etravirine and darunavir/ritonavir in treatment-experienced patients with multidrug-resistant virus: results of the ANRS 139 TRIO trial. XVII International AIDS Conference (AIDS 2008). August 3–8, 2008. Mexico City. Abstract THAB0406.
12. Buckley N (Chair). *Australian Medicines Handbook.* Adelaide: Australian Medicines Handbook Pty Ltd, 2013: 187–9.
13. Clinical and Translational Science Institute. Strategic Timing on Antiretroviral Treatment (START). University of Minnesota. Available from: <https://clinicaltrials.gov/ct2/show/NCT00867048>, accessed February 2018.

14 Nikolopoulos GK et al. Pre exposure Prophylaxis for HIV: Evidence and Perspectives. Curr Pharm Des, 29 March 2017. Available from: <www.readbyqxmd.com/read/28356043/pre-exposure-prophylaxis-for-hiv-evidence-and-perspectives>, accessed February 2018.
15 HIV/AIDS: 'Let's talk about it'. ASHM, 2005. Available from: <www.ashm.org.au>.
16 World Health Organization report. *AIDS Prevention through Health Promotion.* Geneva: WHO, 203.
17 Rogers G. How to treat: HIV care and prevention—Part 1. Australian Doctor, 2006; 3 February: 25–32.
18 Bradford DL. Acquired immune deficiency syndrome. In: *MIMS Disease Index* (2nd edn). Sydney: IMS Publishing, 1996: 1–5.

28 Baffling viral and protozoal infections

It is certainly a one-sided opinion—even though generally adopted at the moment—that all infectious agents which are still unknown must be bacteria. Why should not other microorganisms just as well be able to exist as parasites in the body of animals?

Robert Koch (1843–1910), *Zur Untersuchung von Pathogenen Organismen* (1881)

Almost any infection, especially if subacute or insidious in its onset, can be baffling and can belong to the 'fever of undetermined origin' group of infections. Syphilis and tuberculosis were the great mimics of the past. Now malaria and Epstein–Barr mononucleosis (EBM) can be regarded as important mimics. EBM (Epstein–Barr mononucleosis, infectious mononucleosis, glandular fever) can be a perennial baffler and can be confused with HIV infection in its primary clinical phase. Any of the febrile diseases can be confusing before declaring themselves with classic symptoms such as the jaundice of hepatitis or the rash of dengue fever, or before serological tests become positive.

Viral and protozoal infections that can present as masquerades include:

- HIV infection (especially primary)
- EBV
- TORCH organisms: toxoplasmosis, rubella, CMV, HSV
- hepatitis A, B, C, D, E
- mosquito-borne infections: malaria, dengue fever, yellow fever/other haemorrhagic fevers, Japanese encephalitis, Ross River fever, West Nile fever

The TORCH organisms (TORCH being an acronym for toxoplasmosis, rubella, CMV and herpes) are well known for their adverse intra-uterine effects on the fetus. Three are viral (toxoplasmosis is a protozoan) and the first three of these fetal pathogens are acquired by passage across the placenta. Most of these organisms are noted for being opportunistic infections in immunocompromised patients, especially in later stage HIV infection.

The mosquito-borne infections causing encephalitis and haemorrhagic fevers are mainly viral, apart from the protozoan causing malaria, and are of particular significance in travellers returning from endemic areas (refer to CHAPTER 15).

The major protozoal diseases of humans are:

- blood: malaria, trypanosomiasis
- GIT: giardiasis, amoebiasis, cryptosporidium
- tissues: toxoplasmosis, leishmaniasis, babesiosis

Most of the world's serious protozoal infections—malaria, African trypanosomiasis, leishmaniasis, amoebiasis—occur in tropical areas and are listed and explained in CHAPTER 15.

Four similar clinical presentations

Four infections—EBV, primary HIV, CMV and toxoplasmosis—produce almost identical clinical presentations and tend to be diagnosed as glandular fever or pseudoglandular fever. It is important for the first contact practitioner to consider all four possibilities, especially keeping in mind the possibility of HIV infection.

A worthwhile approach is to make a provisional diagnosis based on the clinical variations as presented in TABLE 28.1.

Screening tests are:

- FBE, especially WCC
- EBV-specific antibodies
- serological test for CMV (specific antibodies)
- serological test for toxoplasmosis (specific antibodies—acute and convalescent)
- HIV antibody test (ELISA)
- NAAT (PCR) testing

Epstein–Barr mononucleosis

EBM is a febrile illness caused by the human herpes virus 4 (Epstein–Barr) virus, one of the eight known herpes viruses. It can mimic diseases such as HIV primary infection, streptococcal tonsillitis, viral hepatitis and acute lymphatic leukaemia. There are three forms: the febrile, the anginose (with sore throat, see FIG. 28.1) and the glandular (with lymphadenopathy).

It may occur at any age but usually between 10 and 35 years; it is commonest in the 15–25 years age group.

Table 28.1 Clinical features differentiating HIV, EBV, CMV and toxoplasmosis infections (all can present with a similar illness)

Feature	EBV infection	HIV infection	CMV infection	Toxoplasmosis
Onset	Insidious	Acute	Insidious	Insidious or acute
Fever	A feature Intermittent	A feature	Quotidian (afternoon spikes)	Low grade
Fatigue/malaise	Common	Common, severe	Common	Common
Tonsillar hypertrophy	Common	Mild enlargement	Uncommon	Uncommon
Exudative pharyngitis	Common	Rare	Rare	Occurs
Mucocutaneous ulcers	Rare	Common	Unknown	Unknown
Skin rash	About 5%	Common	About 5%	About 10%
Jaundice	About 8%	Rare	Uncommon	Uncommon
Diarrhoea	Unknown	Occurs	Unknown	Unknown
Cervical lymphadenopathy	Common	Common	Uncommon	Common (a feature)
Hepatomegaly	About 8%	Rare	Common	Occasional
Splenomegaly	About 50%	Rare	About 50%	Up to 30%
Atypical lymphocytes	In 80–90%	In <50%	Common	Uncommon

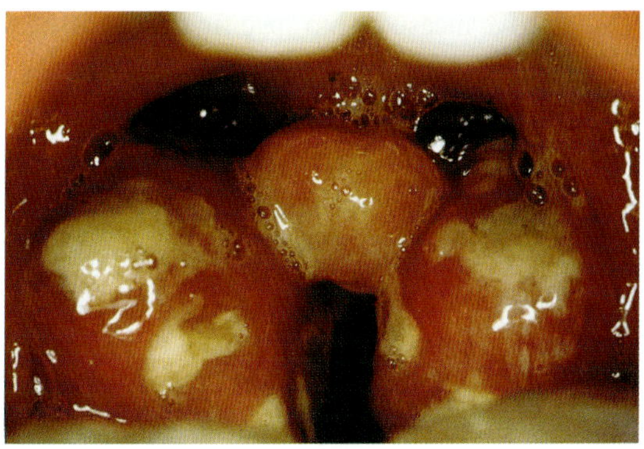

FIGURE 28.1 Tonsillitis of Epstein–Barr mononucleosis. This is often confused with bacterial tonsillitis.

In most young children primary EBV infection is asymptomatic.

Occurrence and transmission

EBM has an annual incidence of 4–5 new cases in a population of 2500.[1] It usually affects people in their late teenage years or early 20s. It is endemic in most countries, affecting over 95% of the adult population worldwide. Subclinical infection is common in young children. The incubation period is at least 1 month but data are insufficient to define it accurately.

EBV is excreted in oropharyngeal secretions during the illness and for some months (sometimes years) after the clinical infection. EBM has a low infectivity and isolation is not necessary. It is apparently transmitted only by close contact, such as kissing and sharing drinking vessels.

Progress of the primary infection is checked partly by specific antibodies (which might prevent cell-to-cell spread of the virus) and partly by a cellular immune response, involving cytotoxic T-cells, which eliminates the infected cells. This response accounts for the clinical picture. The virus is never eliminated from the body. The nature of EBV is not yet fully understood.

Second attacks and fatalities do occur and there is a possible association between EBM and lymphoma.[3]

Clinical features

The typical clinical features are presented in TABLE 28.2 and FIGURE 28.2.

DxT sore throat + fever + lymphadenopathy → EBM

The rash

The rash of EBM is almost always related to antibiotics given for tonsillitis. The primary rash, most often non-specific, pinkish and maculopapular (similar to that of rubella), occurs in about 5% of cases only.

The secondary rash is most often precipitated by one of the penicillins, especially ampicillin or amoxycillin. About 90–100% of patients prescribed ampicillin or amoxycillin will be affected; up to 50% of those given penicillin will develop the rash. It can be extensive and sometimes has a purplish tinge (see FIG. 28.3).

Table 28.2 Clinical features of EBM[1,2,4]

Symptoms
Slow onset malaise 1–6 weeks
Fever
Myalgia
Headaches, anorexia
Blocked nose—mouth breathing
Nasal quality to voice
Sore throat (85%)
Anorexia, nausea ± vomiting
Rash—primary 5%
Dyspepsia
Clinical findings
Exudative pharyngitis (84%)
Petechiae of palate (not pathognomonic) (11%)
Lymphadenopathy, especially posterior cervical
Rash—maculopapular
Splenomegaly (50%)
Jaundice ± hepatomegaly (5–10%)
Clinical or biochemical evidence of hepatitis

The complications of EBM are presented in TABLE 28.3 and the differential diagnoses in TABLE 28.4.

Diagnosis

The following laboratory tests confirm the diagnosis of EBM:

- WCC shows absolute lymphocytosis.
- Blood film shows atypical lymphocytes.

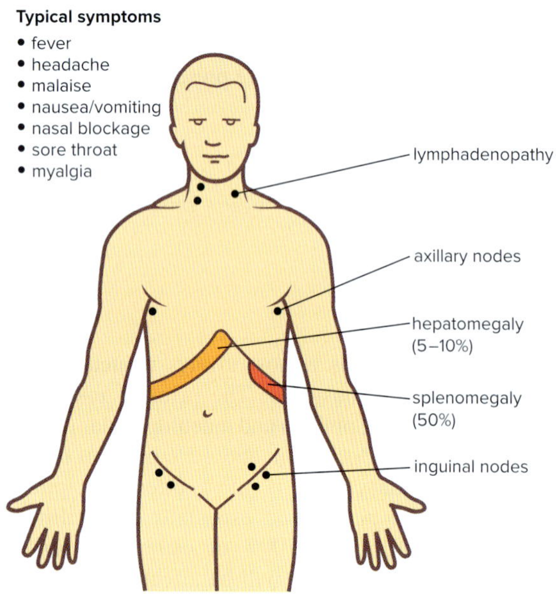

FIGURE 28.2 Clinical features of Epstein–Barr mononucleosis

- Paul–Bunnell or Monospot test for heterophil antibody is positive (although positivity can be delayed or absent in 10% of cases).
- Diagnosis confirmed (if necessary) by EBV-specific antibodies, viral capsid antigen (VCA) antibodies—IgM, IgG and EB nuclear antigen (EBN-A).

Culture for EBV and tests for specific viral antibodies are not performed routinely.

False positives for the Paul–Bunnell test are:

- hepatitis
- Hodgkin lymphoma
- acute leukaemia

Prognosis

EBM usually runs an uncomplicated course over 6–8 weeks. Major symptoms subside within 2–3 weeks. Patients should be advised to take about 4 weeks off work.

Treatment

- Supportive measures (no specific treatment)
- Rest (the best treatment) during the acute stage, preferably at home and indoors
- NSAIDs or paracetamol to relieve discomfort

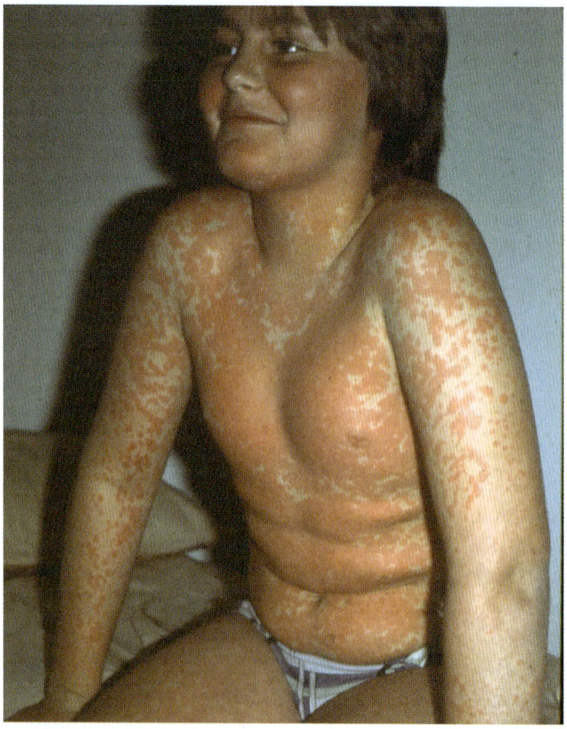

FIGURE 28.3 Typical purplish maculopapular rash of EBM precipitated by ampicillin prescribed for the acute tonsillitis of EBM

Table 28.3	Complications of EBM[1]
Common	
Antibiotic-induced skin rash Prolonged debility Hepatitis Depression	
Rare	
Cardiac: • myocarditis • pericarditis Haematological: • agranulocytosis • haemolytic anaemia • thrombocytopenia Respiratory tract: • upper airway obstruction (lymphoid hypertrophy) Miscellaneous: • ruptured spleen Neurological: • cranial nerve palsies, especially facial palsy • Guillain–Barré syndrome • meningoencephalitis • transverse myelitis	

- Gargle soluble aspirin or 30% glucose to soothe the throat
- Advise against alcohol, fatty foods, continued activity, especially contact sports (risk of splenic rupture)
- Ensure adequate hydration
- Corticosteroids reserved for: neurological involvement, thrombocytopenia, threatened airway obstruction (not recommended for uncomplicated cases)

Post-EBM malaise

Some young adults remain debilitated and depressed for some months. Lassitude and malaise may extend up to a year or so.

Cytomegalovirus infection

CMV has a worldwide distribution and causes infections that are generally asymptomatic. The virus (human herpes virus 5) may be cultured from various sites of healthy individuals. It has its most severe effects in the immunocompromised, especially those with AIDS, and also in recipients of solid organ transplants and bone marrow grafts; 90% of AIDS patients are infected with CMV and 95% have disseminated CMV at autopsy. CMV infection can be an important development following massive blood transfusion, including those given to infants or from organ transplantation. The incubation period of CMV ranges from 20 to 60 days and the illness generally lasts about 2 to 6 weeks.[2]

Table 28.4	Differential diagnoses of EBM[1]
Other agents that cause typical EBM syndrome	
• HIV infection (acute initial illness) • CMV • toxoplasmosis	
Exudative tonsillitis resembling EBM	
• acute streptococcal pharyngitis • adenovirus infection • diphtheria (unlikely in Australia)	
Hepatitis A, B, C, D, E	
Lymphadenopathy, fever and splenomegaly	
• lymphoma • leukaemia	
Complications of EBM without other manifestations	
• encephalitis	
Others	
• drug reaction • influenza	

Clinical features

Three important clinical manifestations are described.

1. *Perinatal disease*
   Intrauterine infection may cause serious abnormalities in the fetus, including CNS involvement (microcephaly, hearing defects, motor disturbances), jaundice, hepatosplenomegaly, haemolytic anaemia and thrombocytopenia. Up to 30% of CMV-affected infants have mental retardation[3] (see CHAPTER 109).
2. *Acquired CMV infection*
   In healthy adults, CMV produces an illness similar to EBM with fever, malaise, arthralgia and myalgia, generalised lymphadenopathy and hepatomegaly. However, cervical lymphadenopathy and exudative pharyngitis are rare.
   The infection may be spread by blood transfusion, and CMV should be suspected on clinical grounds in a patient with a febrile illness resembling EBM following major surgery, such as open heart surgery or kidney transplantation, and where extensive transfusion has been necessary.

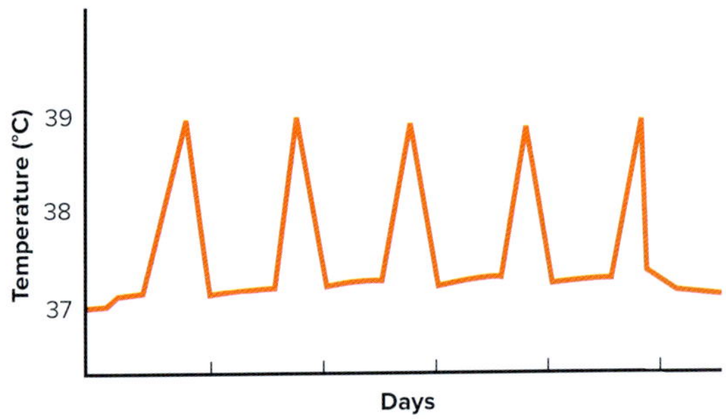

FIGURE 28.4 Cytomegalovirus infection: typical quotidian intermittent fever pattern

The fever often manifests as quotidian intermittent fever spiking to a maximum in the mid-afternoon and falling to normal each day (see FIG. 28.4). There is often a relative lymphocytosis with atypical lymphocytes but the heterophil antibody test is negative. Liver function tests are often abnormal.

Diagnosis: Specific diagnosis can be made by demonstrating rising antibody titres from acute and convalescent (2 weeks) sera. A four-fold increase indicates recent infection. PCR testing can be used. The virus can be isolated from the urine and blood.

3 *CMV disease in the immunocompromised host* Disseminated CMV infection occurs in the immune-deficient person, notably HIV infection causing opportunistic severe pneumonia, retinitis (a feature of AIDS), encephalitis and diffuse involvement of the gastrointestinal tract.

Treatment

In the patient with normal immunity no treatment apart from supportive measures is required, as the infection is usually self-limiting. In immunosuppressed patients various antiviral drugs, such as ganciclovir, foscarnet and fomivirsen (intraocular) have been used with some benefit.[5]

Toxoplasmosis

Toxoplasmosis, which is caused by *Toxoplasma gondii,* an obligate intracellular protozoan, is a worldwide, albeit rare, infection. The definitive host in its life cycle is the cat (or pig or sheep) and the human is an intermediate host. However, clinical toxoplasmosis is very uncommon. Infection in humans usually occurs through eating foodstuffs contaminated by infected cat faeces. Its main clinical importance is an opportunistic infection.

The five major clinical forms of toxoplasmosis are:[5]

1. asymptomatic lymphadenopathy (the commonest)
2. lymphadenopathy with a febrile illness, similar to EBM
3. acute primary infection: a febrile illness similar to acute leukaemia or EBM; a rash, myocarditis, pneumonitis, chorioretinitis and hepatosplenomegaly can occur
4. neurological abnormalities—includes headache and neck stiffness, sore throat and myalgia
5. congenital toxoplasmosis—this is a rare problem but if it occurs it typically causes CNS involvement and has a poor prognosis

In the immunocompromised, clinical forms 3 and 4 are typical features with meningoencephalitis being a serious development.

Diagnosis

Diagnosis is by serological tests (to show a four-fold rise in antibodies), which are sensitive and reliable.

Treatment

Patients with a mild illness or with asymptomatic infection require no treatment. Children under 5 years may be treated to avoid the possible occurrence of chorioretinitis. Symptomatic patients are treated with pyrimethamine plus sulphadiazine. Clindamycin is usually used in pregnant patients.

Viral respiratory infections

Life-threatening viral respiratory infections include the virulent influenza viruses such as avian (bird) influenza and swine influenza and severe acute respiratory distress syndrome (SARS). These conditions are presented in CHAPTER 49.

Ross River fever

Mosquito-borne infections have devastating consequences in tropical regions (see CHAPTER 15), while others cause less morbidity and include Ross River fever.

Epidemic polyarthritis of Ross River virus (RRV), which is an alpha virus, occurs in all states of Australia. It is most prevalent in mosquito-prone areas (especially during the summer) and in tropical and temperate coastal regions and inland riverine areas.[7] Subclinical infection is common with variable clinical manifestations.

Clinical features

- All age groups, especially 20–30 years
- Incubation period 3–21 days (usually 7–11)

Symptoms (major)

- Polyarthritis (75% of patients)—mainly fingers, wrists, feet, ankles and knees
- Maculopapular rash—widespread, often 'subtle', mainly trunk and limbs
- Myalgia

DxT polyarthritis + fever + rash → Ross River fever

Other symptoms

- Pyrexia (mild)
- Headache
- Nausea
- Fatigue with excercise

Signs (which may be present) include joint swelling (mainly hands and feet), tenosynovitis around the wrists and ankles (poor prognostic sign), the rash and mild lymphadenopathy.

Outcome

In many patients the illness resolves within 2 to 6 weeks and most feel normal within 3 months, but some with a more severe arthritis can enter a chronic phase lasting 18 months or more. Depression is a common sequela.

Diagnosis

Diagnosis is by antibody testing of serum. The differential diagnosis includes other viral infections that cause arthritis, such as hepatitis B, rubella, Barmah Forest virus (a mosquito-borne virus) and dengue, and early rheumatiod arthritis and rheumatic fever.

Barmah Forest virus, which is common in Australia, has a similar clinical presentation but is less severe.[8]

Treatment

Treatment is symptomatic with bed rest and simple analgesics such as aspirin. NSAIDs are used for more severe cases. Oral corticosteroids are effective but should be avoided if possible. An inactivated RRV vaccine is being developed.[9]

Deadly infections (worldwide)

The WHO, in its 1996 and 2011 reports,[10] estimated that the leading cause of approximately 50 million deaths in the world was infectious diseases, which accounted for about one-third or 17 million deaths. Other figures included diseases of the circulatory system (15 million deaths, including ischaemic heart disease—7.7 million—and stroke—6.2 million) and cancer (6 million deaths, approximately 12%).

The reports indicated that nearly 50 000 people are dying every day from infectious diseases such as cholera, hepatitis B, malaria, tuberculosis and HIV (see TABLE 28.5). Tuberculosis tends to occur in people with HIV. At least 30 new infections have emerged in the past 20 years, and for many of them there is no treatment, cure or vaccine. These include some infections causing infant diarrhoea, *Legionella pneumophila*, *Lyme borreliosis* (Lyme disease), the Hantaan virus (which can cause a fatal haemorrhagic fever), HIV and hepatitis E and C.

The reports also said that until recently the struggle for control over infectious diseases had seemed almost over, with smallpox eradicated and six other diseases, including polio, leprosy and guinea-worm disease, singled out for eradication within a few years. A pleasing improvement occurred in measles and neonatal tetanus. However, half the world's 6 billion people were at risk of many infectious diseases, since many that seemed under control such as tuberculosis and malaria were becoming more prevalent. Some, such as yellow fever and cholera, were striking in new regions. Other infections were resistant to drugs and virtually untreatable. The previously almost forgotten infections such as *Yersinia* (the plague) had re-emerged.

The deadly haemorrhagic fevers that have broken out in isolated epidemics include the zoonotic African

Table 28.5 The world's deadliest infectious diseases

	Infectious disease	Cause	Annual deaths
1	Acute lower respiratory infections (mostly pneumonia)	Bacterial or viral	3 400 000 (approx. 3.1 million children)
2	Diarrhoeal diseases	Bacterial or viral	1 900 000
3	HIV/AIDS	Viral	1 100 000
4	Tuberculosis	Bacterial	1 800 000
5	Malaria	Protozoal	438 000
Other significant infections			
6	Hepatitis B	Viral	
7	Measles	Viral	
8	Neonatal tetanus	Bacterial	
9	Pertussis	Bacterial	
10	Intestinal worm disease		

Source: World Health Organization, 2011 and 2015 figures

diseases—Ebola haemorrhagic fever, Marburg haemorrhagic fever and Lassa fever. These are caused by filoviruses and for most no specific treatment is available.

Other deadly viruses include rabies (a rhabdo virus; see CHAPTER 15); the paramyxoviruses—Hanta (RNA) virus, which causes haemorrhagic and pulmonary complications; the henipavirus family, which are naturally harboured in fruit bats and include Hendra virus, Nipah virus and Cedar virus.

Another serious infection that emerged sporadically was the so-called 'flesh eating' *Streptococcus A* infection, which was a particularly virulent strain causing localised destruction of soft tissue.

West Nile encephalitis caused by a mosquito-transmitted virus and carried by birds has surfaced in the US and beyond, causing thousands of cases and hundreds of deaths.

The lessons to be learned include careful surveillance, attention to prevention, especially with effective immunisation programs, rational antibiotic prescribing and care with travelling to developing tropical countries.

Patient education resources

Hand-out sheets from *Murtagh's Patient Education* 7th edition:

- Glandular fever
- Hepatitis B
- Hepatitis C
- Influenza
- Malaria
- Pertussis

References

1 Charles PGP. Infectious mononucleosis. Aus Fam Physician, 2003; 32 (10): 755–8.

2 Fauci AS, Braunwald E et al. *Harrison's Principles of Internal Medicine* (17th edn). New York: McGraw-Hill, 2008: 1106–9.

3 Papadakis MA, McPhee SJ. *Current Medical Diagnosis and Treatment* (52nd edn). New York: Lange, 2013: 1263–5.

4 Maeda E et al. Spectrum of Epstein-Barr virus related diseases: a pictorial review. Jpn J Radiology, January 2009; 27(1): 4–19. [PMID19373526]

5 Rawlinson W, Scott G. Cytomegalovirus. Aust Fam Physician, 2003; 32 (10): 789–93.

6 Kumar PJ, Clark ML. *Clinical Medicine* (7th edn). London: Elsevier Saunders, 2009: 160.

7 Whitby M. Ross River fever. In: *MIMS Disease Index* (2nd edn). Sydney: IMS Publishing, 1996: 452–3.

8 Russell RC, Doggett SL. *Ross River and Barmah Forest Virus.* University of Sydney, Department of Medical Entomology, 2014. <http://medent.usyd.edu.au/fact/>, see Ross River and Barmah Forest.

9 Wressnigg N et al. An inactivated Ross River virus vaccine is well tolerated and immunogenic in an adult population in a randomized phase 3 trial. Clinical and Vaccine Immunology, 2015; 22(3): 267–73.

10 World Health Organization. *Annual Report.* Geneva: WHO, May 2011 and 2015.

Baffling bacterial infections 29

In its beginning the malady is easier to cure but difficult to detect, but later it becomes easy to detect but difficult to cure.

NICCOLÒ MACHIAVELLI (1469–1527), *ON TUBERCULOSIS*

Bacterial infections can present diagnostic brainteasers, and a high index of suspicion is needed to pinpoint the diagnosis. Many are rarely encountered, thus making diagnosis more difficult yet demanding vigilance and clinical flexibility.

The list includes:

- tuberculosis
- infective endocarditis
- syphilis
- septicaemia
- the zoonoses (e.g. brucellosis, Lyme disease)
- clostridial infections: tetanus, gas gangrene, puerperal infection, botulism, pseudomembranous colitis
- hidden suppuration: abscess, osteomyelitis
- mycoplasma infections: atypical pneumonia
- *Chlamydia* infections: psittacosis, non-specific arthritis, pelvic inflammatory disease, trachoma, atypical pneumonia
- legionnaire disease
- Hansen disease

Chlamydia and rickettsial organisms have been confirmed as being small bacterial organisms.

Tuberculosis

Tuberculosis (TB), caused by *Mycobacterium tuberculosis,* still has a worldwide distribution with a very high prevalence in Asian countries where 60–80% of children below the age of 14 years are affected.[1] This has special implication in Australia, where large numbers of Asian migrants are settling. The WHO estimates that one-third of the world's population is infected by the tubercle bacillus. It remains a deadly disease with about 2 million people worldwide dying of TB every year and 8 million new cases a year.

Clinical features

TB can be a mimic of other diseases and a high level of suspicion is necessary to consider the diagnosis, especially if there are only extrapulmonary manifestations. There may be no symptoms or signs, even in advanced disease. Ideally patients should be referred early for specialist management.

High risk people/situations

- newborn and infants
- adults over 60 years
- patients with HIV/AIDS
- chronic disease, e.g. diabetes
- crowded or unsanitary living conditions
- people affected by alcohol and drugs
- immigrants and refugees from endemic countries (especially Indian sub-continent, Papua New guinea, South East Asia, Sub Sahara and South Africa)

DxT malaise + cough + weight loss ± fever/night sweats + haemoptysis ➔ pulmonary TB

Primary infection

The primary infection usually involves the lungs. Transmission is by droplet infection. The focus is usually subpleural in the upper to mid zones and is almost always accompanied by lymph node involvement.

Erythema nodosum may accompany the primary infection (see FIG. 29.1). Primary TB is symptomless in most cases although there may be a vague, 'not feeling well' illness associated with a cough. In most people this pulmonary focus heals but leaves some surviving tubercle bacilli, even if it becomes calcified (the Ghon focus).

Progressive primary tuberculosis

If the immune response is inadequate, progressive primary TB develops, with constitutional and pulmonary symptoms. Rarely, haematogenous spread can occur to the lungs ('miliary tuberculosis'), to the pleural space (tuberculosis pleural effusion) or to extrapulmonary sites such as the meninges and bone.

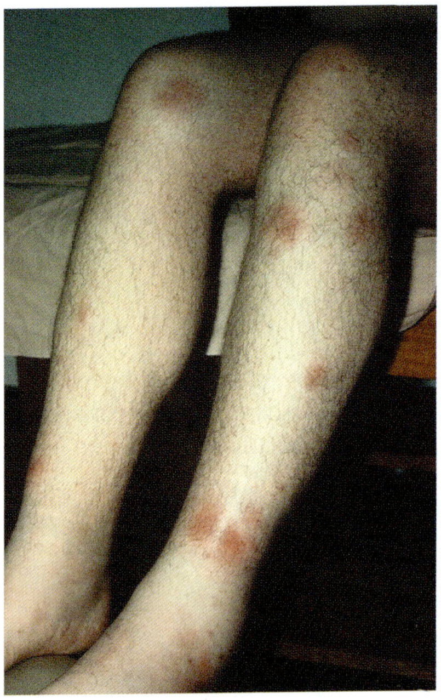

FIGURE 29.1 Classic erythema nodosum involving the legs of a patient with pulmonary tuberculosis

Latent TB infection (LTBI)

LTBI is the presence of infection without evidence of active disease (contained by the immune system) and inability to transmit the infection. However, reactivation may occur if the host's immune defences are impaired (occurs in about 10%). LTBI is very common in children in and from developing countries. Consider HIV in these people. The tubercular skin test is primarily intended to identify these people with a view to prophylaxis therapy. The standard preferred regimen is isoniazid (10 mg/kg up to 300 mg (o) daily for 6–9 months). This decision should be made by a consultant.

Post-primary or adult-type pulmonary TB

Most cases of TB in adults are due to reactivation of disease some years later and not to re-infection. Symptoms of active TB include persistent cough, sputum production, haemoptysis, fever, sweating, malaise, weight loss and anorexia. The factors causing this include poor social living conditions with malnutrition, diabetes and other factors lowering natural immunity, such as immunosuppressant drugs, corticosteroids, lymphoma and HIV infection (later stage). The chest X-ray is usually abnormal—classic apical disease with infiltration and cavitation with fibrotic changes.

> **Practice tip**
>
> TB! – Think HIV.

Reactivated pulmonary TB

This usually presents with constitutional symptoms of poor health and night sweats, and a cough that is initially dry but may become productive and be bloodstained (see CHAPTER 42). Sometimes the infection will be asymptomatic. The natural history of TB is illustrated in FIGURE 29.2.

Extrapulmonary TB

The main sites of extrapulmonary disease (in order of frequency in Australia) are the lymph nodes (the commonest, especially in young adults and children), genitourinary tract (kidney, epididymis, Fallopian tubes), pleura and pericardium, the skeletal system (arthritis and osteomyelitis with cold abscess formation), CNS (meningitis and tuberculomas), the eye (choroiditis, iridocyclitis), the skin (lupus vulgaris), the adrenal glands (Addison disease—see CHAPTER 23) and the GIT (ileocaecal area and peritoneum). This is increasing, especially in HIV patients.

These sites are illustrated in FIGURE 29.3.

Miliary tuberculosis

This disorder follows diffuse dissemination of tubercle bacilli via the bloodstream especially in those with chronic disease and immunosuppression. It can occur within 3 years of the primary infection or much later because of reactivation.

The symptoms, which are insidious, include weight loss, fever and malaise. Choroidal tubercules are pathognomonic. The classic chest X-ray is multiple 1–2 mm nodules in lung fields. It is fatal without treatment.

TB in children[3]

Children living in close contact with people with smear-positive pulmonary TB are highly vulnerable to acquiring the primary infection. A possible complication is miliary TB. The lifetime risk of TB disease in children with LTBI is in the order of 5–15%.[4] Children with LTBI should be considered for prophylaxis with a course of isoniazid.

Primary disease is the more common form in young children. Reactivation is more common in adolescents.

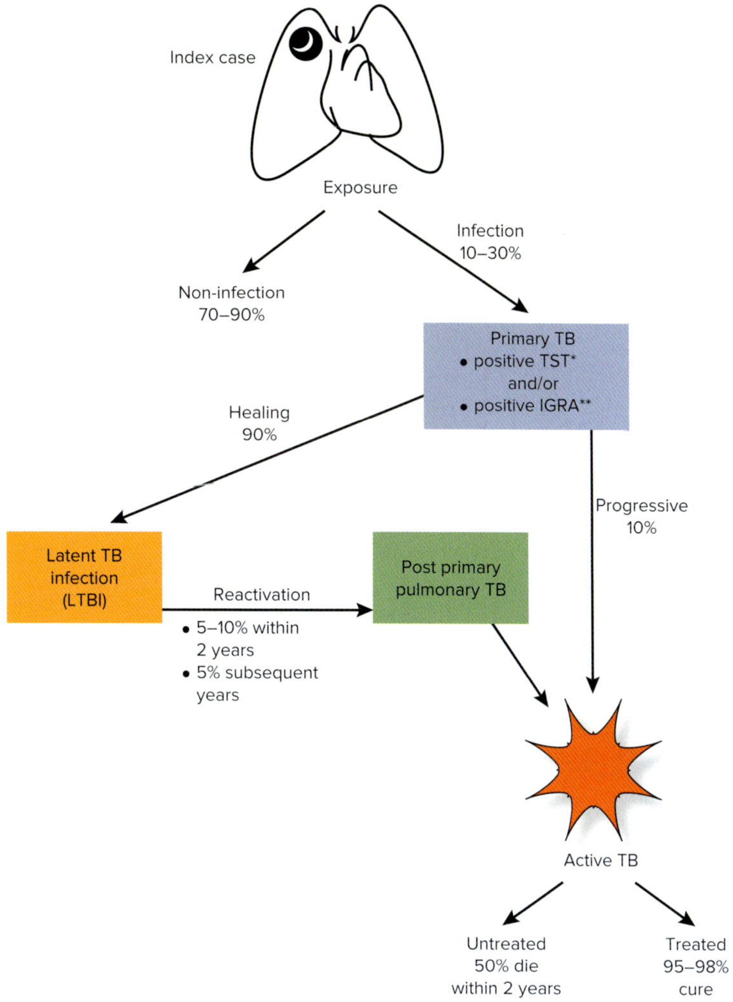

FIGURE 29.2 Natural history of TB infection

* TST = tuberculin skin test

** IGRA = interferon gamma release assay

Based on WHO algorithm and Dr Grant Jenkin (personal communication)

Diagnosis[2]

A high index of suspicion is critical for the diagnosis of TB. Tests include:

- Mantoux tuberculin test (TST) (a guide only)
- chest X-ray; CT scan if doubtful
- sputum or bronchial excrction or gastric aspirates for stain (acid-fast bacilli) and culture (takes about 6–8 weeks but important). Ideally requires 3 specimens over 3 days including one early morning
- immunochromatographic finger-prick test (new and promising)
- interferon gamma release assay (IGRA)
- NAAT/PCR test—less sensitive than culture
- biopsies on lesions/lymph nodes may be necessary. The hallmark is caseating granulomata
- fibrc-optic bronchoscopy to obtain sputum may be necessary
- consider HIV studies

Tuberculin (Mantoux) testing and BCG vaccination

A tuberculin (Mantoux) test should be performed prior to BCG vaccination in all individuals over 6 months

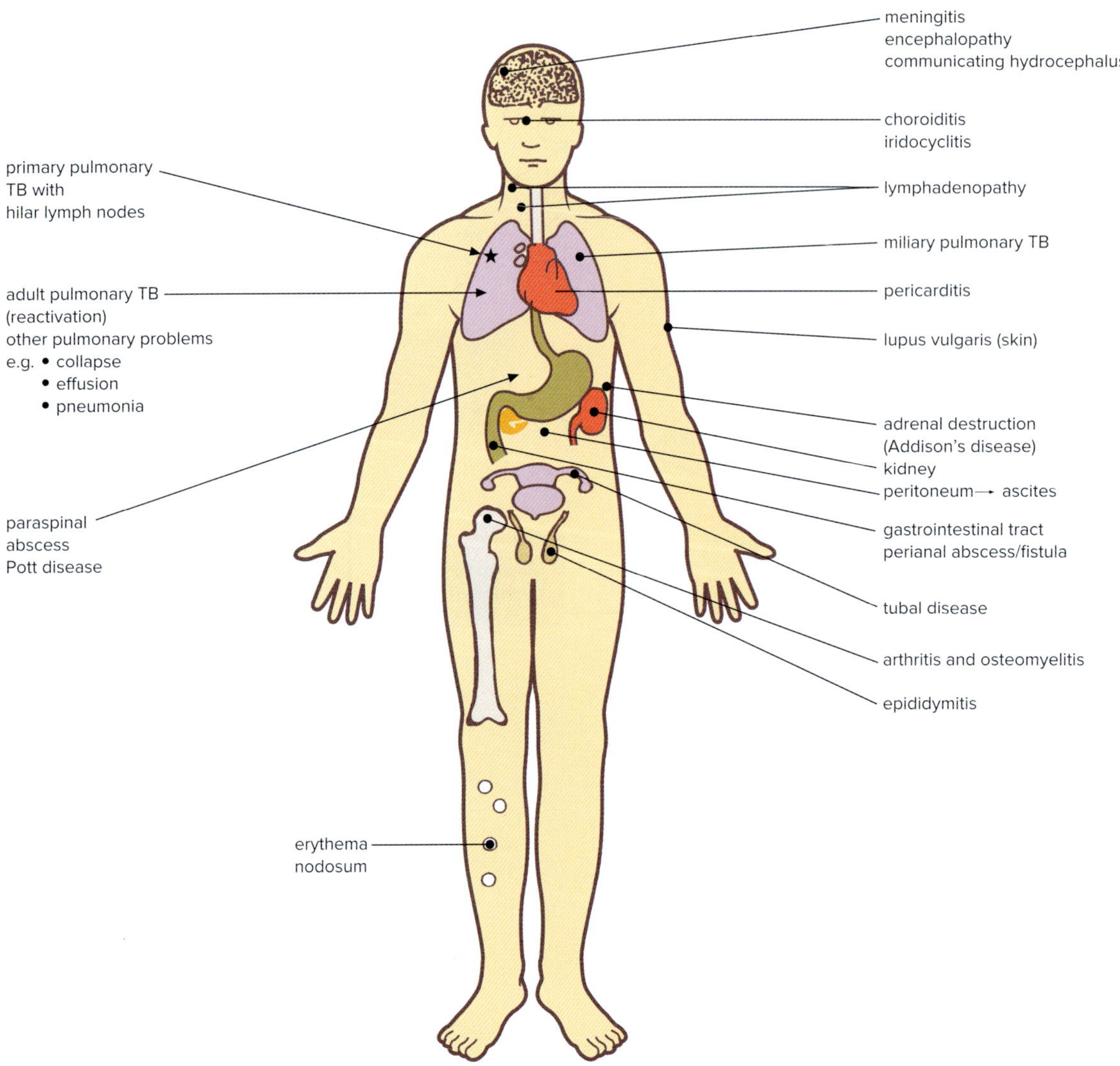

FIGURE 29.3 Pulmonary and extrapulmonary distribution of tuberculosis: the primary infection starts in the lung and then spread throughout the body, especially to the lymph nodes

of age. (It is read at 48–72 hours.) It is not a good test to diagnose TB.

If area of induration:

- <5 mm—negative (*note:* may be negative in presence of very active pulmonary infection)
- 5–10 mm—typical of past BCG vaccination
- >5 mm—significant in immunocompromised, close contacts and HIV infection
- >10 mm—positive = tuberculosis infection (active or inactive)
- >15 mm—highly significant for 'normal' people

The BCG vaccination should be given if the reaction is <5 mm induration. Do not give it for a reaction >5 mm.

BCG vaccination is recommended for:

- ATSI neonates in regions of high incidence
- neonates born to patients with leprosy or family history of leprosy
- children <5 years travelling for long periods to countries of high TB prevalence

BCG vaccination should be considered for:

- neonates in household with immigrants or visitors recently arrived from countries of high prevalence (e.g. South-East Asia) (*note:* tuberculin test not necessary for neonates <14 days)
- children and adolescents <16 years with continued exposure to active TB patient and where isoniazid therapy is contraindicated

- others at increased risk (and where value of BCG vaccine uncertain), such as health care workers, travellers >5 years with significant exposure

BCG vaccination is contraindicated for:

- tuberculin reactions >5 mm
- immunocompromised or malignancies involving bone marrow lymphatics (can disseminate infection)
- high-risk HIV infection
- significant fever or intercurrent illness
- generalised skin diseases, including keloid tendency
- pregnancy
- previous infection

Areas of concern

Drug resistance

This includes the increasing emergence of forms resistant to two or more front-line drugs—multidrug-resistant TB (MDR-TB). TB is much more aggressive in the immunocompromised and if not adequately treated can be fatal in 2 months, especially if they have MDR-TB. Treatment compliance is a huge issue and so the directly observed therapy (DOT) strategy for isoniazid in children is a WHO priority, as is 'DOTS plus' to control MDR-TB. TB is a more pressing problem in children requiring early treatment.

Management and treatment[5,6]

Referral to experienced specialist care is appropriate. The current antimicrobial treatment is to use four antituberculous drugs initially (rifampicin + isoniazid + pyrazinamide + ethambutol) daily for 2 months, then rifampicin + isoniazid daily for a further 4 months. The usual precautions with adverse reactions are required. Pyridoxine 25 mg daily is recommended for adults taking isoniazid. A 3-times-weekly regimen is also an option if DOT is employed. Corticosteroids may be prescribed. Notify appropriate jurisdictional public health authorities. Promote healthy lifestyle advice.

Syphilis

Although syphilis is uncommon, it is increasing in the general population. It is extremely common in certain Indigenous groups and is frequently acquired from sexual contacts overseas.[5,8]

It presents either as a primary lesion or through the chance finding of positive syphilis serology. Family physicians should be alert to the various manifestations of secondary syphilis, which can cause difficulties in diagnosis. Congenital syphilis is rare where there is general serological screening of antenatal patients. Early syphilis—less than 2 years duration and based on positive serology—includes primary, secondary and latent syphilis.

Clinical features[7,8]

Primary syphilis

The primary lesion or chancre usually develops at the point of inoculation after an incubation period averaging 21 days. The chancre is typically firm, painless, punched out and clean (see FIG 29.4). The adjacent lymph nodes are discretely enlarged, firm and non-suppurating. Any anorectal ulcer or sore should be considered as syphilis until proved otherwise.

Untreated, early clinical syphilis usually resolves spontaneously within 4 weeks, leading to latent disease, which may proceed to late destructive lesions.

Secondary syphilis

The interval between the appearance of the primary chancre and the onset of secondary manifestations varies from 6 to 12 weeks after infection. Constitutional symptoms, including fever, headache, malaise and general aches and pains, may precede or accompany the signs of secondary syphilis.

The most common feature of the secondary stage of infection is a rash, which is present in about 80% of cases. The rash is typically a symmetrical, generalised, coppery-red maculopapular eruption on the face, trunk, palms and soles and is neither itchy nor tender. It can resemble any skin disease except those characterised by vesicles.

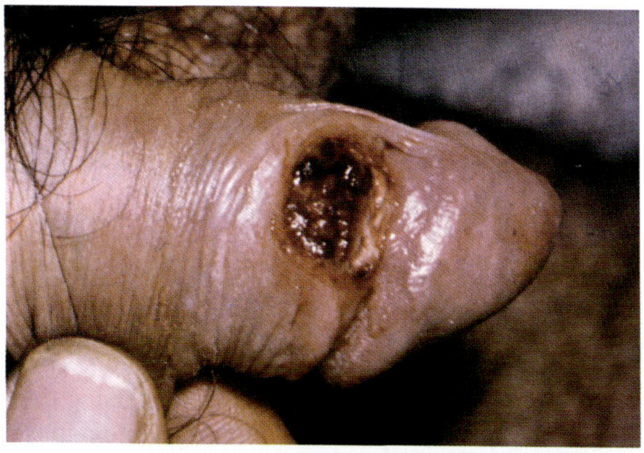

FIGURE 29.4 Chancre of primary syphilis in adolescent. This painless, innocuous-looking lesion was associated with a firm, enlarged linguinal lymph node. Dark field examination revealed many motile treponema.

Latent syphilis

Positive serology in a patient without symptoms or signs of disease is referred to as latent syphilis and is the commonest presentation of syphilis in Australia today. Possibly because of the widespread use of antibiotics, the infection often proceeds to the latent stage without a recognised primary or secondary stage.

Late (tertiary) syphilis

Tertiary manifestation of syphilis (follows >2 years latency), which is very rare, may be 'benign' with development of gummas (granulomatous lesions) in almost any organ, or more serious with cardiovascular or CNS involvement. Benign gummatous disease is rare but cardiovascular disease and neurosyphilis occasionally occur. Careful management and follow-up of patients with early or latent disease is essential to prevent late sequelae. It can only be detected by blood tests.

Neurosyphilis includes:

- meningovascular (e.g. cranial nerve palsies)
- tabes dorsalis (e.g. sensory ataxia, lightning pains, Charcot joints)
- general paresis of the insane (e.g. dementia, psychosis)

Think of syphilis

Syphilis should not be overlooked as a cause of oral, ocular or anorectal lesions. The diagnosis of syphilis depends on a detailed history, careful clinical examination and specific examinations.

Underlying these approaches is the need to think of the possibility of syphilis with concurrent STIs.

Syphilis and HIV infection[8]

HIV and syphilis are commonly associated. In patients with AIDS and syphilis, standard regimens for syphilis are not always curative. Seronegative syphilis has been reported in patients with HIV infection. Lymphadenopathy in a patient with HIV infection may be due to coexisting secondary syphilis.

Diagnosis

Dark field examination[7]

Spirochaetes can be demonstrated by microscopic examination of smears from early lesions using dark field techniques and provide an immediate diagnosis in symptomatic syphilis. The direct fluorescent antibody techniques (FTAABS) can be used on this smear.

Serology

Serological tests provide indirect evidence of infection, and the diagnosis of asymptomatic syphilis relies heavily on these tests. The main types of tests are:

- reagin tests (VDRL and RPR)—not specific for syphilis but useful for screening
- treponemal tests (TPPA, TPI, EIA, FTA-abs)—specific tests, with the latter being sensitive and widely used
- PCR (blood or CSF)—very sensitive

Treatment

Refer to CHAPTER 117.

Infective endocarditis

Infective endocarditis, although uncommon, has high morbidity and mortality. It can be a difficult problem to diagnose but must be considered in the differential diagnosis of fever, especially in patients with a history of cardiac valvular disorders. It is caused by microbial infection of the cardiac valves or endocardium. Previously referred to as bacterial endocarditis, the term *infective endocarditis* is preferred because not all the infecting organisms are bacteria.

It may present as a fulminating or acute infection but more commonly runs an insidious course and is referred to as subacute (bacterial) endocarditis. Its incidence is increasing, probably due to the increasing number of elderly people with degenerative valve disease, more invasive procedures, IV drug use and increased cardiac catheterisation.[9]

DxT FUO + cardiac murmur + embolism → endocarditis

Risk factors

- Past history of endocarditis
- Rheumatically abnormal valves, especially ASTIP
- Congenitally abnormal valves
- Mitral valve prolapse
- Calcified aortic valve
- Congenital cardiac defects (e.g. VSD, PDA)
- Prosthetic valves, shunts, conduits
- IV drug use
- Central venous catheters
- Temporary pacemaker electrode catheters

Note: Only about 50% of patients with infective endocarditis have previously known heart disease.[7]

Responsible organisms[10]

- *Streptococcus viridans* (50% of cases) most susceptible to penicillin
- *Streptococcus bovis*
- *Enterococcus faecalis*
- *Staphylococcus aureus* (causes 50% of acute form)
- *Candida albicans/Aspergillus* (IV drug users)
- *Staphylococcus epidermidis*
- *Coxiella burnetii* (Q fever)
- HACEK group (Gram –ve bacilli) (5–10% of cases)

Presentations

- Acute endocarditis
- Subacute endocarditis
- Prosthetic endocarditis

Infective endocarditis without cardiac murmur is frequently seen in IV drug users who develop infection on the tricuspid valve.

Warning signs for development of endocarditis

- Change in character of heart murmur
- Development of a new murmur
- Unexplained fever and cardiac murmur = infective endocarditis (until proved otherwise)
- A febrile illness developing after instrumentation (e.g. urethral dilatation) or minor and major surgical procedures (e.g. dental extraction, tonsillectomy, abortion)

The 'classic tetrad' of clinical features:[9] signs of infection, signs of heart disease, signs of embolism, immunological phenomena

There is a significant high mortality and morbidity from infective endocarditis, which is often related to a delay in diagnosis.

A golden rule

Culture the blood of every patient who has a fever and a heart murmur.

Clinical features

The classic clinical features are summarised in FIGURE 29.5.

The patients are often elderly, appear pale and ill, with intermittent fever, and complain of vague aches and pains. The full clinical presentation takes time to develop. A febrile illness of 1 to 2 weeks duration is a common presentation.

Investigation

This includes:

- FBE and ESR: ESR ↑, anaemia and leukocytosis
- urine: proteinuria and microscopic haematuria
- blood culture: positive in about 75%[7] (at least 3 sets of samples—aerobic and anaerobic culture)
- echocardiography—to visualise vegetations (TOE more sensitive than TTE)
- chest X-ray
- ECG

Consider kidney function tests and C-reactive protein.

Management

The patient should be referred because optimal management requires close cooperation between physician, microbiologist and cardiac surgeon.

Any underlying infection should be treated (e.g. drainage of dental abscess). Bactericidal antibiotics are chosen on the basis of the results of the blood culture and antibiotic sensitivities. Four blood cultures should be sent to the laboratory within the first hour of admission and treatment should seldom be delayed longer than 24 hours.

Antimicrobial treatment[10,11]

Consultation with an infectious diseases physician or clinical microbiologist should be sought.

Empirical treatment[11]

Once cultures have been taken, prompt empirical antimicrobial treatment should be commenced, especially in fulminating infection suspected to be endocarditis (usually due to *Staphylococcus aureus*). Benzylpenicillin, gentamicin and flucloxacillin/dicloxacillin are recommended, for example (adults):

- benzylpenicillin 1.8 g IV, 4 hourly
  plus
  flucloxacillin/dicloxacillin 2 g IV, 4 hourly
  plus
  gentamicin 4–6 mg/kg IV, daily
- Vancomycin is indicated in certain circumstances

For specific organisms isolated on culture and prosthetic valve endocarditis confer with a consultant.

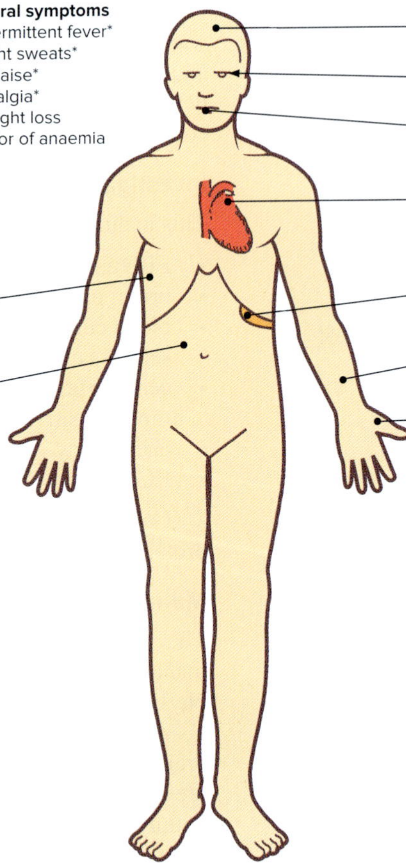

FIGURE 29.5 Infective endocarditis: possible clinical features

Prevention

Antibiotic prophylaxis[10,11]

The evidence for prophylaxis of endocarditis is not clear, and current international practice is not to treat low-risk cardiac abnormalities having procedures with a low incidence of bacteraemia.

It is advisable to discuss the relative risks with patients.

If in doubt, discuss the issue with the patient's cardiologist or an infectious diseases specialist.[8,10]

References for specific conditions: see References[5,12] and see also http://circ.ahajournals.org (Paediatrics).

Low-risk patients

These include patients with murmurs not due to valve disorders, isolated secundum ASD, pacemakers, implanted defibrillators, previous rheumatic fever without valve dysfunction, previous CABGS, mitral valve prolapse without regurgitation, complete surgical or device closures of congenital heart defects.

No prophylaxis is recommended in these patients.

High risk of adverse outcomes[11]

These include past history of endocarditis, prosthetic heart valves, most congenital heart disease especially cyanotic types and those with repaired defects, hypertrophic cardiomyopathy, cardiac transplantation recipients who develop cardiac valvulopathy, rheumatic heart disease in Indigenous patients, all acquired valvular heart disease, mitral valve prolapse with regurgitation and surgically fashioned systemic-pulmonary shunts.

Procedures requiring prophylaxis[11]

- Dental: invasive dental surgery—any procedure causing bleeding from gingiva, bone or mucosa, for example, dental extractions, drainage of abscess, osteotomies, dental implants, replanting avulsed teeth, periodontal procedures including probing, endodontic surgery, intraligamentary local anaesthetic injections, root canal work

- Other procedures—examples are:
  - genitourinary procedures in the presence of infection, for example, D&C, IUCD, urethral dilatation, circumcision, prostatic surgery, vaginal delivery in presence of infection or prolonged labour
  - gastrointestinal tract procedures in presence of infection
  - respiratory tract procedures—tonsillectomy/adenoidectomy, rigid bronchoscopy, nasal and sinus surgery
  - incision and drainage of local abscess, for example, boils, perirectal, dacryocystitis

Recommended antibiotics

Dental procedures and URT interventions (*S. viridans* and *Streptococcus* cover):[11]

- phenoxymethylpenicillin 2 g (child 40 mg/kg up to 2 g) orally 1 hour before procedure
  or
- amoxycillin 2 g (child 50 mg/kg up to adult dose) orally 30 minutes beforehand (if not on long-term penicillin)
  or
- amoxy/ampicillin 2 g (50 mg/kg up to adult dose) IV just before procedure commences or IM 30 minutes before if having a general anaesthetic
  or
- if hypersensitive to penicillin: clindamycin or lincomycin

Genitourinary and gastrointestinal procedures[11]

Enterococci prophylaxis

- amoxy/ampicillin (child: 50 mg/kg up to 2 g) IV (just before procedure)
  or
- amoxy/ampicillin 2 g (child 50 mg/kg up to 2 g) IM 30 minutes beforehand

If hypersensitive to penicillin: vancomycin or teicoplanin plus gentamicin.

Zoonoses

Zoonoses are those diseases and infections that are naturally transmitted between vertebrate animals and humans (see TABLE 29.1). Zoonotic diseases (which are not restricted to farming communities) can present as a mild illness but are prolonged in duration and can have debilitating sequelae.[14] There is a long list of diseases, which vary from country to country, and includes plague, rabies, scrub typhus, Lyme disease, tularaemia, hydatid disease, orf, anthrax, erysipeloid, listeriosis, campylobacteriosis and ornithosis (psittacosis).

Diagnosis[15]

If a zoonosis is overlooked in the differential diagnosis, many will remain undiagnosed and untreated.

Table 29.1 Major zoonoses in Australia

Zoonosis	Organism(s)	Animal host	Mode of transmission	Main presenting features
Q fever	*Coxiella burnetii*	Various wild and domestic animals	Inhaled dust Animal contact Unpasteurised milk	Fever, rigors, myalgia, headache, dry cough
Leptospirosis	*Leptospira interrogans or pomona*	Various domestic animals	Infected urine contaminating cuts or sores	Fever, myalgia, severe headache, macular rash
Brucellosis	*Brucella abortus*	Cattle	Contamination of cuts or sores by animal tissues Unpasteurised milk	Fever (undulant), sweats, myalgia, headache, lymphadenopathy
Lyme disease	*Borrelia burgdorferi*	Marsupials (probable)	Tick bites	Fever, myalgia, arthritis, backache, doughnut-shaped rash
Psittacosis	*Chlamydia psittaci*	Birds: parrots, pigeons, ducks, etc.	Inhaled dust	Fever, myalgia, headache, dry cough
Bovine tuberculosis	*Mycobacterium bovis*	Cattle	Unpasteurised milk	Fever, sweats, weight loss, cough (as for human pulmonary TB)
Listeriosis	*Listeria monocytogenes*	Various wild and domestic animals	Unpasteurised milk or cheese Contaminated vegetables Person to person	Mild febrile illness (in most) Meningoencephalitis in those susceptible (neonates, pregnancy, elderly, etc.)

29

> **Practice tip**
>
> Think of a zoonosis in patients presenting with a flu-like illness and features of atypical pneumonia.

Fever and sweats (flu-like illness)

Any patient with undiagnosed fever should be questioned about exposure to animals, recent travel both in and out of Australia, animal bites, cat scratches, consumption of raw milk, mosquito and tick bites, pets and occupation.

Rash

- Consider rickettsial illness such as leptospirosis, Q fever, Lyme disease

Cough or atypical pneumonia

- Consider Q fever, psittacosis, bovine TB

Arthralgia/arthritis

- Consider Lyme-like disease, Ross River fever

Meat workers

- Consider Q fever, leptospirosis, orf, anthrax

Papular/pustular lesions

- Consider orf, anthrax (black)

Brucellosis

Brucellosis (undulant fever, Malta fever) has diminished in prevalence since the campaign to eradicate it from cattle. Entry is mainly by the mouth, or abraded or cut skin.

Clinical features (acute brucellosis)

- Incubation period 1–3 weeks
- Insidious onset: malaise, headache, weakness
- A prolonged febrile illness
- The classic fever pattern is undulant (refer to CHAPTER 53)

Possible:

- arthralgia
- lymphadenopathy
- hepatomegaly
- spinal tenderness
- splenomegaly (if severe)

Complications such as epididymo-orchitis, osteomyelitis and endocarditis can occur. Localised infections in sites such as bones, joints, lungs, CSF, testes and cardiac valves are possible but uncommon.

Symptoms of chronic brucellosis are virtually indistinguishable from chronic fatigue syndrome and can present with FUO.

> **DxT** malaise + headache + undulant fever → brucellosis

Diagnosis

- Blood cultures if febrile (positive in 50% during acute phase)[10,13]
- *Brucella* agglutination test (rising titre)—acute and convalescent (3–4 weeks) samples
- *Brucella* PCR testing—sensitive and rapid

Treatment[3]

- Adults: doxycycline 100 mg (o) bd for 6 weeks + rifampicin 600 mg (o) daily for 6 weeks
  or
  gentamicin 4–6 mg/kg/day IV statim then daily for 2 weeks (monitor)
- Children: cotrimoxazole + rifampicin
  or
  gentamicin
- Relapses do occur (10%)—prolonged therapy

Prevention and control

Involves eradication of brucellosis in cattle, care handling infected animals and pasteurisation of milk. No vaccine is currently available for use in humans.

Q fever

Q fever is a zoonosis due to *Coxiella burnetii.* It is the most common abattoir-associated infection in Australia and can also occur in farmers and hunters. It usually resolves spontaneously within 2 weeks. Rash is not a major feature but can occur if the infection persists without treatment.

Clinical features

- Incubation period 1–3 weeks
- Sudden onset fever, rigors and myalgia
- Dry cough (may be pneumonia in 20%)[13]
- Petechial rash (if persisting infection)
- ± Abdominal pain

Persistent infection may cause pneumonia or endocarditis so patients with valvular disease are at risk of endocarditis (culture is negative). It is a rare cause of hepatitis. The acute illness may resolve spontaneously but a chronic relapsing disease may follow. Untreated chronic infection is usually fatal.

> **DxT** fever + headache + prostration → Q fever

Diagnosis

- Serodiagnosis is by antibody levels in acute phase and 2–3 weeks later (4-fold increase)
- *Coxiella burnetii* PCR

Treatment[3]

- Doxycycline 100 mg (o) bd for 14 days
- For endocarditis or chronic disease: prolonged course of doxycycline plus clindamycin or rifampicin
- Children: >8 same antibiotics according to weight; <8 cotrimoxazole (instead of doxycycline)

Prevention

The disease can be prevented in abattoir workers by using Q fever vaccine.

Leptospirosis

Leptospirosis follows contamination of abraded or cut skin or mucous membranes with *Leptospira*-infected urine of many animals including pigs, cattle, horses, rats and dogs. In Australia it is almost exclusively an occupational infection[14] of farmers (especially with flooded farmland in tropics) and workers in the meat industry. There is a risk to dairy farmers splashed with urine during milking. Early diagnosis is important to prevent it passing into the immune phase.

Clinical features

- Incubation period 3–20 days (average 10)
- Fever, chills, myalgia
- Severe headache
- Chest pain (possibly haemoptysis)
- Macular rash
- Light-sensitive conjunctivitis (marked suffusion)

Some may develop the immune phase (after an asymptomatic period of 1–3 days) with aseptic meningitis or jaundice and nephritis (icterohaemorrhagic fever, Weil syndrome) with a significant mortality.

> **DxT** abrupt fever + headache + conjunctivitis → leptospirosis

Diagnosis

- High or rising titre of antibodies: can be cultured

Treatment[5]

Mild cases may not require treatment (adult doses shown).

- Doxycycline 100 mg (o) bd for 7 days
  or
- benzylpenicillin 1200 mg IV, 6 hourly for 7 days
  or
- ceftriaxone 1 g IV daily for 7 days

Lyme and lyme-like disease

Lyme disease (known as Lyme borreliosis) was first described in 1975 and named after the town Lyme in Connecticut (US). It is widespread in the US and is now appearing in other countries but is not endemic in Australia. Sporadic cases are seen in visitors or travellers. The illness encountered here and in other countries is described as debilitating symptom complexes attributed to ticks. Traditional Lyme disease, which is highly infective, is caused by a spirochaete, *Borrelia burgdorferi,* and transmitted by *Ixodes* ticks, so that people living and working in the bush are susceptible. It has been reported in deer farmers. Lyme disease presents in three stages. If suspected refer to an infectious disease physician for expert advice.

The pathognomic sign is erythema migrans—a characteristic pathognomonic rash, usually a doughnut-shaped, well-defined rash about 6 cm in diameter at the bite site.

Stage 1: erythema migrans, flu-like illness
Stage 2: neurological problems such as limb weakness and cardiac problems
Stage 3: arthritis

Diagnosis

- Clinical pattern especially rash of erythema migrans + serology and PCR

Treatment

- Remove tick
- A typical regimen for adults is doxycycline 100 mg bd for 21 days or amoxycillin

Psittacosis ('bird fanciers disease')

Most patients are bird fanciers. Psittacosis accounts for 1–5% of hospital admissions for pneumonia. The disease may follow a low-grade course over several months but can have a dramatically acute presentation of flu-like illness. It is indistinguishable from other atypical pneumonias except for history of contact with birds.

Clinical features

- Incubation period 1–2 weeks
- Fever, malaise, myalgia
- Headache
- Cough (usually dry)
- Minimal chest signs
- Splenomegaly (sometimes)

Mortality can be as high as 20% if untreated.

Diagnosis

- Serology—rising antibody and PCR
- Chest X-ray

Treatment[3]

- Doxycycline 200 mg (o) or clarithromycin 250 mg, 12 hourly for 14 days (o)

Listeriosis[15]

Listeriosis is caused by *Listeria monocytogenes*, a bacterium widespread in nature that can contaminate food and has been found in many fresh (e.g. fruit and vegetables) and processed foods (e.g. dairy products, especially unpasteurised milk, soft cheese, processed meats and smoked seafood). Its significance lies in the mortality rate in high-risk groups such as pregnant women, the immunocompromised, frail aged, and very young but especially neonates and fetuses. Babies may be stillborn or aborted.

Clinical features

It may be subclinical but possible presentations include:

- influenza-like illness (usually mild)
- food poisoning, gastroenteritis (atypical)
- meningitis, especially infants, elderly
- septicaemia (in susceptible)
- pneumonia (in susceptible)

Diagnosis

- Microscopy, culture or isolation of organism from infected site or blood
- Serological tests available

Treatment

- Amoxycillin 1 g (o) 8 hourly or IV for 10–14 days[5,13]

Other zoonoses

- Mosquito-transmitted infections: Murray Valley encephalitis, Ross River virus, Barmah Forest virus
- Infections from bites and scratches: cat-scratch disorder, rat bite fever
- Hydatid disease, orf, milker's nodules
- Toxoplasmosis, histoplasmosis, hookworm

CLOSTRIDIAL INFECTIONS

Tetanus

This sometimes misdiagnosed bacterial infection (*Clostridium tetani*) can appear from one day to several months after the injury, which may have been forgotten. A total of 10–20% of patients with tetanus have no identifiable wound of entry.[16] Neonatal tetanus can occur from contamination of the umbilical stump. It is a significant cause of postpartum maternal mortality worldwide.

Clinical features

- Prodrome: fever, malaise, headache
- Trismus (patient cannot open mouth)
- Risus sardonicus (a grin-like effect from hypertonic facial muscles)
- Opisthotonos (arched trunk with hyperextended neck)
- Spasms, precipitated by minimal stimuli

Differential diagnosis: phenothiazine toxicity, strychnine poisoning, rabies, dental abscess

Management

- Give tetanus antitoxin and human tetanus immunoglobin
- Refer immediately to expert centre
- Intubate and ventilate if necessary

Gangrene/Gas gangrene[5]

Gangrene (necrotising soft tissue infection) can involve skin and subcutaneous fat, fascia and muscle.

Gas gangrene (clostridial myonecrosis) is caused by entry of one of several clostridia organisms, for example, *Clostridium perfringens*, into devitalised tissue, such as exists following severe trauma to a leg.

Clinical features

- Sudden onset of pain and swelling in the contaminated wound
- Brownish serous exudate
- Gas in the tissue on palpation or X-ray
- Prostration and systemic toxicity
- Circulatory failure ('shock')

Management

- Refer immediately to surgical centre for debridement

- Start benzylpenicillin 2.4 g IV, 4 hourly + clindamycin
- Hyperbaric oxygen if available

Botulism[5]

Botulism is food poisoning caused by the neurotoxin of *Clostridium botulinum.* It can be infant botulism, of wound origin or food borne. From 12 to 36 hours after ingesting the toxin from canned, smoked or vacuum-packed food (e.g. home-canned vegetables or meat) visual problems such as diplopia suddenly appear. Suspect botulism if cranial nerve weakness with normal sensation. General muscle paralysis and prostration quickly develop. Refer immediately for antitoxin and intensive care.

PNEUMONIA

Surprisingly the initial presentation of pneumonia can be misleading, especially when the patient presents with constitutional symptoms such as fever, malaise and headache rather than respiratory symptoms. A cough, although usually present, can be relatively insignificant in the total clinical picture. This problem applies particularly to atypical pneumonia but can occur with bacterial pneumonia, especially lobar pneumonia (refer to CHAPTER 42).

The atypical pneumonias[5,12]

Refer to CHAPTER 42.

Clinical features

- Fever, malaise
- Headache
- Minimal respiratory symptoms, non-productive cough
- Signs of consolidation absent
- Chest X-ray (diffuse infiltration) incompatible with chest signs

> **DxT** 'flu' + headache + dry cough → atypical pneumonia

Serology tests and treatment

Blood tests and PCR tests are available for all the following causative organisms:

Mycoplasma pneumoniae (the commonest)

- Adolescents and young adults: treat with doxycycline (first line) 200 mg statim then 100 mg daily for 14 days

  or

  with roxithromycin 300 mg (o) daily for 14 days

Legionella pneumophila (legionnaire disease)

- Related to cooling systems in large buildings
- Incubation 2–10 days
- Diagnostic criteria include: prodromal-like illness; a dry cough, influenza-like illness, confusion or diarrhoea; lymphopenia with marked leukocytosis; hyponatraemia; PCR test and urinary antigen assay
- Treatment for mild disease: azithromycin 500 mg (o) daily for 5 days or doxycycline 100 mg (o) 12 hourly for 10–14 days
- Patients can become very prostrate with complications—treat with azithromycin (o or IV) or erythromycin (IV or o) plus (if very severe) add ciprofloxacin or rifampicin for 14–21 days

Chlamydia psittaci (psittacosis)

- Treat with doxycycline 100 mg bd for 14 days

Coxiella burnetii (see Q fever section)

Acknowledgment

Part of this text, on the clinical manifestations of syphilis, is reproduced from the *Handbook on Sexually Transmitted Diseases*[8] (copyright Commonwealth of Australia, reproduced by permission).

Resources

World Health Organization. *Guidelines for national tuberculosis programmes on the management of tuberculosis in children* (2nd edn). Geneva: WHO, 2014. Available from: <http://apps.who.int/medicinedocs/documents/s21535en/s21535en.pdf>, accessed February 2018.

National Heart Foundation of New Zealand. Guidelines for prophylaxis of infective endocarditis associated with dental and other medical interventions.

Royal Children's Hospital Melbourne. Guidelines for prophylaxis against infection in asplenic children. Melbourne: RCH, 2010.

References

1 Kumar PJ, Clark ML. *Clinical Medicine* (7th edn). London: Elsevier Saunders, 2009: 863.

2 National Institute for Health Care Excellence (NICE). Tuberculosis: clinical diagnosis and management of tuberculosis, and measures for its prevention and control (CG117). London: NICE, 2011.

3 World Health Organization. *Guidelines for national tuberculosis programmes on the management of tuberculosis in children* (2nd edn). Geneva: WHO, 2014. Available

29

from: <http://apps.who.int/medicinedocs/documents/s21535en/s21535en.pdf>, accessed February 2018.

4 Thompson K et al. *Paediatric Handbook* (8th edn). Oxford: Wiley-Blackwell, 2009: 131–2.

5 Expert group for Antibiotic guidelines. Tuberculosis. In: eTG complete. Melbourne: Therapeutic Guidelines Ltd. Available from: <www.tg.org.au>, accessed January 2018.

6 Soto-Martinez M, Ranganathan S. Tuberculosis (Part 2). Medical Observer, 11 March 2011: 25–7.

7 Hart G. Syphilis. In: *MIMS Disease Index* (2nd edn). Sydney: IMS Publishing, 1996: 493–6.

8 NHMRC. *Handbook on Sexually Transmitted Diseases.* Canberra: Department of Community Services & Health, 1990: 23–9.

9 Oakley C. Infective endocarditis. Med Int, 1986; 21: 872–8.

10 Speed B. Endocarditis, infective. In: *MIMS Disease Index* (2nd edn). Sydney: IMS Publishing, 1996: 167–9.

11 Expert group for Antibiotic guidelines. Prophylaxis of infection. In: eTG complete. Melbourne: Therapeutic Guidelines Ltd. Available from: <www.tg.org.au>, accessed January 2018.

12 Zhu F. *Australian Anti-infection Handbook* (2nd edn). Sydney: Palmer Higgs Books Online, 2010.

13 Scott J. Zoonoses. Current Therapeutics, 1995; April: 42–5.

14 Benn R. Australian zoonoses. Current Therapeutics, 1990; July: 31–40.

15 NHMRC Statement. Listeria, advice to medical practitioners. Canberra: NHMRC, 1992.

16 Fauci AS et al. *Harrison's Principles of Internal Medicine* (17th edn). New York: McGraw-Hill Medical, 2008: 898.

Infections of the central nervous system

30

Bacterial meningitis is a medical emergency especially meningococcus meningitis which can cause rapid deterioration of the patient. Consider it if a sudden onset of the classical triad is accompanied by high fever and the signs of a very sick child. Meningococcal meningitis may be accompanied by a petechial rash and septic shock (Waterhouse–Friderichsen syndrome).

ANISHA BAHRA & KATIA CIKUREL, *NEUROLOGY,* 1999[1]

Infections of the central nervous system cover general conditions such as meningitis and encephalitis and specific organisms such as syphilis and polio. This section is highlighted because the conditions that are difficult to diagnose can have morbid outcomes, especially if the conditions are misdiagnosed. They are representative of classic 'not-to-be-missed' conditions.

Key symptoms suggestive of cerebral infection are headache, seizures and altered conscious level.

Meningitis

Meningitis is inflammation of the meninges (pia and arachnoid) and the cerebrospinal fluid (CSF).

The classic triad is:

- headache
- photophobia
- neck stiffness

Other symptoms include malaise, vomiting, fever and drowsiness.

Causes (organisms)[1,2]

Bacteria

- *Streptococcus pneumoniae*, *Haemophilus influenzae* (especially children), *Neisseria meningitides* (the big three)
- *Listeria monocytogenes*, *Mycobacterium tuberculosis*, Group B *Streptococcus*, *Strep. agalactiae* (common in newborn), *Staphylococcus* spp., Gram −ve bacilli, such as *Escherichia coli*, *Borrelia burgdorferi*, *Treponema pallidum*

Viruses

- Enteroviruses (Coxsackie, echovirus, poliovirus) mumps, herpes simplex HSV type 1, 2 or 6, varicella zoster virus, EBV, HIV (primary infection)

Fungi

- *Cryptococcus neoformans* or *C. gattii*
- *Histoplasma capsulatum*

Investigations

- Lumbar puncture (see TABLE 30.1)
- CT scan
- Blood culture—all patients with suspected meningitis
- CSF microculture/PCR (PCR useful even if antibiotics given)
- Specific serology, e.g. HIV, EBV

Note: If significant delay with these, do not withhold treatment.

Bacterial meningitis[2]

Bacterial meningitis is basically a childhood infection. Neonates and children aged 6–12 months are at greatest risk. Meningococcal disease can take the form of either meningitis or septicaemia (meningococcaemia) or both. Most cases begin as septicaemia, usually via the nasopharynx. The onset is usually sudden (see CHAPTER 96).

Clinical features (typical)

Infancy

- Fever, pallor, vomiting ± altered conscious and mental state
- Lethargy
- Increasing irritability with drowsiness
- Refusal to feed, indifference to mother
- Neck stiffness (not always present)
- Cold extremities (a reliable sign)
- May be bulging fontanelle
- Kernig sign (see FIG. 30.1): unreliable
- Brudzinski sign (see FIG. 30.2): more reliable sign of meningeal irritation
- Opisthotonos (see FIG. 30.3): rare

Table 30.1 CSF findings in meningitis

	Bacterial (pyogenic)	Tuberculosis	Viral (aseptic)
CSF appearance	Cloudy/pus	Opalescent	Usually clear
CSF pressure	↑↑↑	↑↑ or N	↑ or N
Predominant cell	Neutrophils	Lymphocytes	Lymphocytes
Cell count/mm^3	100–1000 +	50–1000	10–1000
Glucose	↓↓↓	↓↓	Normal

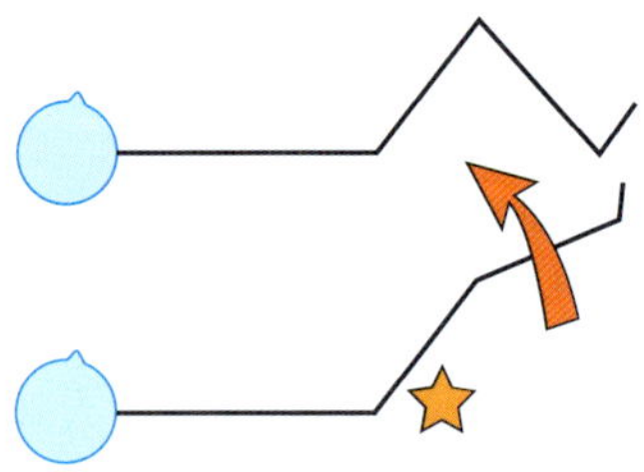

FIGURE 30.1 Kernig sign: pain in hamstrings with inability to straighten leg on passive knee extension with hip flexed at 90°

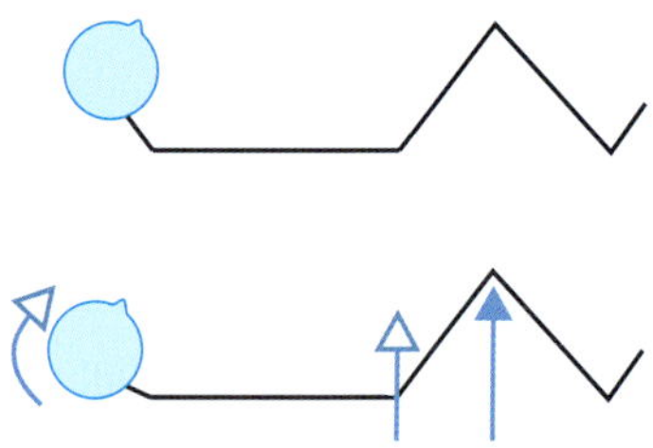

FIGURE 30.2 Brudzinski sign: neck flexion causes involuntary flexion of hip and knee

Children over 3 years, adolescents, adults

- Meningeal irritation more obvious (e.g. headache, fever, vomiting, neck stiffness)
- Later: delirium, altered conscious state

Note: Antibiotics may mask symptoms. Suspect meningitis if fever >3 days in reasonably well child on antibiotics.[3]

Fulminating

- Dramatic sudden-onset shock, purpura (does not blanch on pressure) ± coma
- Usually due to meningococcal septicaemia, also *H. influenzae* type B, *Streptococcus pneumoniae*, *Listeria monocytogenes*

Note: septic shock may ensue without signs of meningitis.

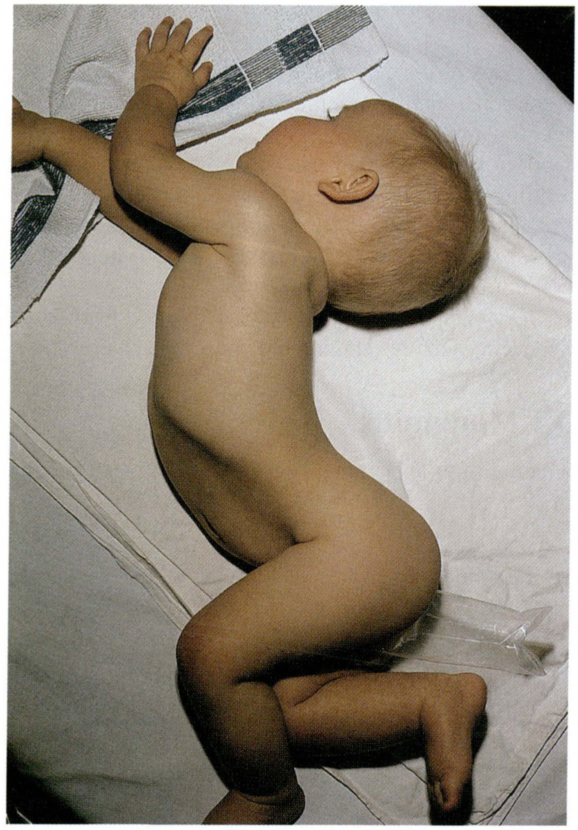

FIGURE 30.3 Opisthotonos caused by advanced meningitis

Treatment (suspected meningitis)[4]

First: oxygen + IV access and consult

- Take blood for culture (within 30 minutes of assessment)—ideally prior to hospitalisation
- For child give bolus of 10–20 mL/kg of N saline with added bolus up to total 60 ml/kg if signs of hypoperfusion
- Admit to hospital for lumbar puncture (preliminary CT scan to assess safety of LP in adults)
- Dexamethasone 0.15 mg/kg up to 10 mg IV (start at same time as antibiotics—shown to improve outcome)[5]

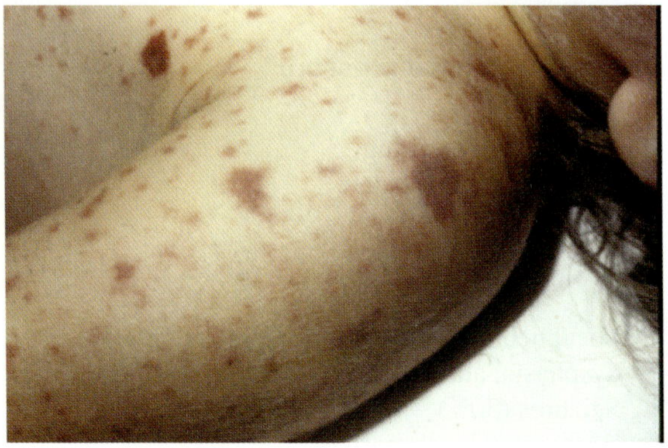

FIGURE 30.4 Meningococcaemia with typical early purpuric rash in a 2-year-old child

- Ceftriaxone 2 g (child >1 month: 50 mg/kg up to 2 g) IV statim then 12 hourly for 4 days
  or
  cefotaxime 2 g (child: 50 mg/kg up to 2 g) IV 6 hourly for 3–5 days (note that IM injection is painful)

Note: IV preferable but IM or interosseous better than nothing.

Antibiotics of proven effectiveness are cefotaxime, ceftriaxone, meropenem and penicillin.

Treatment (meningococcaemia—all ages)

Treatment is extremely urgent once suspected (e.g. petechial or purpuric rash on trunk and limbs) (see FIG. 30.4). It should be given before reaching hospital. Empirical treatment is:

- benzylpenicillin 2.4 g (child: 60 mg/kg IV up to 2.4g) statim (continue for 5 days)
- if IV access not possible give IM
  or
- ceftriaxone 2 g (child >1 month 50 mg/kg up to 2 g) IV or IM 12 hourly for 5 days

Note: Penicillin dose guide for suspected meningitis in child: <1 year 300 mg, 1–9 years 600 mg, 10+ years 1.2 g.

Specific organisms—*streptococcus pneumoniae:* benzyl penicillin or cephalosporin; Group B *streptococcus:* benzyl penicillin; *H influenza:* cephalosporin.

Prevention

- meningococcal vaccines—B and ACWY given separately

Viral meningitis[1,6]

This is basically a childhood infection. The most common causes are human herpes virus 6 (the cause of roseola infantum) and enteroviruses (Coxsackie and echovirus).

Most cases are benign and self-limiting, but the clinical presentation can mimic bacterial meningitis although there are fewer obvious signs of meningeal irritation. Lumbar puncture is important for diagnosis and also PCR for enterovirus. If positive it can allow early cessation of antibiotics if commenced empirically.[2] Treatment which is symptomatic includes rehydration and analgesics. Acyclovir is given for herpes meningitis. The immunocompromised require special management.

> **Practice tip**
>
> Very cold hands? Think meningitis.

Encephalitis[1,6]

Encephalitis is inflammation of the brain parenchyma. It is mainly caused by viruses although other organisms including some bacteria, *Mycoplasma*, *Rickettsia* and *Histoplasma* can cause encephalitis. Suspect it when a viral prodrome is followed by irrational behaviour, altered conscious state and possibly cranial nerve lesions.

> **Practice tip**
>
> Consider the possibility of (non-infective) autoimmune encephalitis.

Clinical features

These can vary from mild to severe.

- Constitutional: fever (not inevitable), malaise, myalgia
- Meningeal features: headache, photophobia, neck stiffness
- Cerebral dysfunction: altered consciousness—confusion, drowsiness, personality changes, irrational behaviour, seizures, coma
- Focal neurological deficit

Causes (viral organisms)

- Herpes simplex type 1 or 2, enteroviruses, mumps, CMV, EBV, HIV, measles, influenza, arboviruses, for example, Japanese B, West Nile, Murray Valley encephalitis, Ross River
- Consider cerebral malaria in the differential diagnosis

There are three forms of mediated viral encephalitis: direct, delayed (latent) and immune mediated (postinfectious encephalomyelitis).

Toxoplasma gondii

A protozoal infection seen in immunocompromised patients, especially HIV. Refer for specialist advice.

Investigations

- Lumbar puncture: CSF (usually aseptic meningitis)
- CSF PCR for viral studies, esp. HSV, toxoplasma
- CT scan—often shows cerebral oedema
- Gadolinium enhanced MRI
- EEG—characteristic waves

Treatment

Organise hospitalisation where treatment will be supportive. Suspected herpes simplex encephalitis should be treated with IV aciclovir immediately.

Note: Meningoencephalitis is meningitis plus some parenchymal involvement of brain substance.

Autoimmune encephalitis

This is a recently identified group of neuropsychiatric disorders seen typically in young people.[7] There is a prodrome of fever and headache followed by days or weeks of psychiatric behavioural problems with bizarre symptoms and movements. It may be related to a paraneoplastic manifestation, e.g. ovarian cancer. Diagnosis is confirmed by blood and CSF antibody testing (anti-NMDA receptor). Specialist referral for diagnosis and specific immunotherapy is appropriate.

Brain abscess and subdural empyema[4,8]

A brain (cerebral) abscess is a focal area of infection in the cerebrum or cerebellum. It presents as a space-occupying intracerebral lesion. Suspect in any patient with a raised intracranial pressure. The infection can reach the brain by local spread or via the bloodstream, for example, endocarditis or bronchiectasis. There may be no clue to a focus of infection elsewhere but it can follow ear, sinus, dental, periodontal or other infection and also a skull fracture. The organisms are polymicrobial, especially microaerophilic cocci and anaerobic bacteria in the non-immunosuppressed. In the immunosuppressed, *Toxoplasma*, *Nocardia* sp. and fungi.

Clinical features

Raised intracranial pressure

- Headache
- Nausea and vomiting
- Altered conscious state
- Papilloedema

Other

- Focal neurological signs such as hemiplegia, dysphasia, ataxia
- Seizures (30%)
- Fever (may be absent)
- Signs of sepsis elsewhere, e.g. teeth, endocarditis

Investigations

- MRI (if available) or CT scan
- FBE, ESR/CRP, blood culture
  Note: lumbar puncture is contraindicated.
- Consider endocarditis

Management

Management is urgent neurosurgical referral. Aspiration or biopsy is essential to guide antimicrobial treatment which may (empirically) include metronidazole IV and a cephalosporin, e.g. ceftriaxone IV. Nocardiosis is treated with other antibiotics.

Spinal subdural or epidural abscess[9]

These uncommon focal infections can be extremely difficult to diagnose so an index of suspicion is required to consider such an abscess. The usual organism is *Staphylococcus aureus.*

Clinical features[6]

- Back pain (increasing) ± radiculopathy
- Percussion tenderness over spine
- Evolving neurological deficit, e.g. gradual leg weakness and sensory loss ± fever (may be absent)

Causes

- Associated infection: furuncle, decubitus ulcer, adjacent osteomyelitis, discitis, other
- Back trauma with haematoma
- Post-subdural or epidural anaesthetic block
- One-third is spontaneous

Investigations

- Blood culture
- MRI scan to localise abscess and spinal cord pressure

Management

Urgent neurosurgical referral. Empirical therapy while awaiting culture results may include di/flucloxacillin IV, + gentamicin IV or vancomycin IV.

Prion-transmitted diseases[10,11]

Prions are proteinaceous infected particles devoid of nucleic acid that can present with a wide spectrum of neurological presentations. The feature is transmissible spongiform encephalopathy (TSE), with Creutzfeldt–Jakob disease being the classic example. Other examples of TSE forms affecting humans are variant CJD, kuru (New Guinea) and fatal familial insomnia.

Creutzfeldt–Jakob disease

There are three distinct forms of CJD: sporadic (80–85%), familial (15%) and iatrogenic (1%). The annual incidence is one per million people. Usual transmission is from contaminated human tissue (e.g. corneal graft), cadaver pituitary human gonadotrophin or eating contaminated beef. There is no specific treatment for the disease.

DxT fatigue + psychiatric symptoms + myoclonus → CJD

Clinical features

- Progressive dementia (starts with personality change and memory loss—eventual loss of speech)
- Myoclonus/muscle spasms
- Fatigue and somnolence
- Variable neurological features (e.g. ataxia, chorea)

Diagnosis

- MRI: high signal intensity in thalami
- CSF: positive 14-3-3 protein immunoassay
- EEG
- Brain biopsy after death (ultimate confirmation)

Management

- Supportive: no proven specific treatment

Poliomyelitis[11]

Polio is a highly contagious enterovirus (picornavirus) transmitted through the faeco-oral route and is a specific spinal cord anterior horn cell enterovirus. It remains endemic in the tropics. Most infections (95%) are asymptomatic. *Note:* myelitis means inflammation of the spinal cord.

Clinical features

- Flu-like syndrome, with fever and sore throat, then
- 'Pre-paralytic' stage: nausea and vomiting, headache, stiff neck (meningeal irritation)
- Paralytic (0.1%): LMN lesion (flaccid paralysis)—may include spinal polio especially of lower limbs and/or bulbar polio ± respiratory failure. No sensory loss.

There are 2 levels of polio: minor (recovery in a few days) and major.

Diagnosis

- Viral studies of throat and faeces—culture and PCR
- Serology
- CSF: leucocytosis, esp. lymphocytes

Management

Symptomatic paralytic patients should be referred to hospital. Prevention is through vaccination.

Post-polio syndrome

Many years after the primary infection (usually 20–40 years) this may present with new muscle weakness and pain as dysfunction of surviving motor neurones develops. Refer to specialist unit.

Non-viral causes of flaccid paralysis[12,13]

- *Borrelia burgdorferi* (Lyme disease), *Mycoplasma*, diphtheria, botulism, transverse myelitis, syphilis

Syphilis

Neurosyphilis can present at any stage of syphilis. The main syphilitic syndromes affecting the CNS are:

- Asymptomatic syphilis: present during the interval between the secondary and tertiary stages of syphilis.
- Meningitis including acute basal meningitis and meningovascular syphilis. The latter can present with a cerebrovascular accident.
- Tabes dorsalis causing meningoradiculitis with degeneration of the parenchyma of the spinal columns of the spinal cord and involvement of the pupils. Features include lightning pains, Charcot joints, ataxia and neurotrophic ulcers, Argyll Robertson pupils.
- General paralysis of the insane with marked personality change, dementia, dysarthria and seizures.

OTHER INFECTIONS THAT CAN INVOLVE THE CNS

30

Tuberculosis

Neurological TB may include tuberculosis meningitis, tuberculoma (presenting as a cerebral abscess), spinal arachnoiditis and spinal involvement (Pott disease). Treatment with multiple antimicrobial agents is usually complex and prolonged.

Human immunodeficiency virus

HIV involvement may be direct with primary infection causing encephalopathy ('AIDS' dementia), myelopathy or acute atypical meningitis in addition to secondary opportunistic infection. The latter include CNS toxoplasmosis, cytomegalovirus, herpes simplex myelitis, varicella zoster and others (see CHAPTER 27).

Helminthic infections

Worm infestations that can (rarely) cause intracerebral lesions through the formation of cysts or granulomas include cysticercosis (tapeworms), *Echinococcus* (hydatid) and *Schistosoma.*

Other infections may present with seizures. These include:

- Botulism (see CHAPTER 29)
- Tetanus (see CHAPTER 29)
- Rabies (see CHAPTER 15)
- Hansen disease (leprosy) (see CHAPTER 15)

Patient education resources

Hand-out sheets from *Murtagh's Patient Education* 7th edition:

- Bacterial meningitis and meningococcus

References

1 Bahra A, Cikurel K. *Neurology.* London: Mosby, 1999: 195–7.
2 Thomson K, Tey D, Marks M. *Paediatric Handbook* (8th edn). Oxford: Wiley-Blackwell, 2009: 407–13.
3 Hewsen P, Oberklaid F. Recognition of serious illness in babies. Journal of Paediatrics and Child Health, 2000; 36: 221–5.
4 Expert group for Antibiotic guidelines. Central nervous system infections. In: eTG complete. Melbourne: Therapeutic Guidelines Ltd. Available from: <www.tg.org.au>, accessed January 2018.
5 Brower MC et al. Corticosteroids for acute bacterial meningitis. Cochrane Database Syst Rev. 2013; (6): CD004405.
6 Venkatesan A et al. Case definition, diagnostic algorithm and priorities in encephalitis: consensus statement of the international encephalitis consortium. Clin Infect Dis, 2013; 57(8): 1114–28.
7 Lancaster E. The diagnosis and treatment of autoimmune encephalitis. J Clin Neurol, 2016; 12(1): 1–13.
8 Helweg-Larsen J et al. Pyogenic brain abscess, a 15 year survey. BMC Infect Dis, 2012; 12: 332.
9 Beers MD, Porter RS et al. *The Merck Manual* (18th edn). Whitehouse Station: Merck Research Laboratories, 2006: 1850–1.
10 Beers MD, Porter RS et al. *The Merck Manual* (18th edn). Whitehouse Station: Merck Research Laboratories, 2006: 1914–5.
11 Beers MD, Porter RS et al. *The Merck Manual* (18th edn). Whitehouse Station: Merck Research Laboratories, 2006: 1853.
12 Bahra A, Cikurel K. *Neurology.* London: Mosby, 1999: 204–5.
13 Longmore M, Wilkinson I et al. *Oxford Handbook of Clinical Medicine.* Oxford: Oxford University Press, 2007: 420.

Chronic kidney failure 31

I have never yet examined the body of a patient dying with dropsy attended by albuminous urine, in whom some obvious derangement was not discovered in the kidneys.

RICHARD BRIGHT 1827

Chronic kidney failure

In the diagnostic model the problem of chronic kidney failure (CKF) as a masquerade has been highlighted. The reason for this is that the dysfunction associated with progressive chronic kidney disease (CKD) can be difficult to diagnose as there may be no or minimal symptoms. The underlying cause needs to be identified. In fact the patient may present with a subtle terminal illness. It is important that all general practitioners are aware of the seriousness of the problem and keep it in mind when the patient presents with apparent minor problems such as fatigue or weakness. Sometimes the kidneys can develop acute failure, which may recover or progress to chronicity.

> If CKD is detected early and managed appropriately then the otherwise inevitable deterioration in kidney function can be reduced by as much as 50% and may even be reversible.[1]

Table 31.1 Significant causes of chronic kidney failure (approximate order of prevalence)

Diabetes mellitus
Glomerulonephritis • IgA nephropathy (commonest)
Hypertension
Vascular • atherosclerosis, including kidney artery stenosis
Polycystic kidneys
Obstructive nephropathy/reflux • bilateral ureteric obstruction • bladder outflow obstruction: prostatic enlargement,
Drugs, including analgesic nephropathy
Lupus and other connective tissue disorders
Vasculitides, e.g. polyasteritis nodosa (PAN)
Gout
Amyloidosis
Multiple myeloma
Hypercalcaemia

Key facts and checkpoints

- 10% of people attending general practice[1] have CKD but most do not know it.
- At least 95 people per million of the population are treated for end-stage kidney disease/kidney failure (ESKF) each year.
- Two-thirds of these are under 60 years of age.
- Important causes are glomerulonephritis (25%), diabetes mellitus (35%), polycystic kidney disease (8%), reflux nephropathy (8%) and hypertension (13%) (see TABLE 31.1).[2]
- The commonest cause of ESKF in Australia is diabetes mellitus.
- The commonest cause of nephritis leading to kidney failure in Australia is IgA nephropathy.
- In children the incidence of chronic kidney failure is quite low (1 to 2 per million of the population).[2]
- Warmer climates, poorer living conditions and certain genetic predispositions are associated with a higher prevalence of kidney failure.
- Kidney failure should be considered in the diagnosis of patients with unexplained anaemia, unexplained poor health and unusually high analgesic intake.[2]
- CKD is an important risk factor for cardiovascular disease.
- Uraemic symptoms are non-specific and usually are not recognised until the creatinine clearance is less than 20% of normal.
- CKF is characterised by the accumulation of uraemic toxins and a deficiency of kidney hormones that cause dysfunction of organs other than kidneys.
- This interaction can cause phosphate retention, secondary hyperparathyroidism and bone disorders such as osteomalacia.
- Age is an issue—we lose 1% of renal function per year
- It is possible to identify stages of kidney failure (see TABLE 31.2).

Table 31.2 Classification of chronic kidney disease stages[1,3]

CKD stage	GFR (mL/min)	Description	Clinical action plan
1	>90	Evidence of kidney damage (e.g. scarring on ultrasound, proteinuria/haematuria)	
2	60–89	Evidence of kidney damage Mild kidney failure	Further investigation for those at risk: • Assess proteinuria • Urinalysis • BP Cardiovascular risk reduction: • BP, cholesterol, blood glucose, smoking, obesity
3 3a 3b	30–59 44–59 30–44	Moderate kidney failure	As above. • Avoid nephrotoxic drugs • Monitor eGFR 3 monthly • Prescribe antiproteinuric drugs, ACE inhibitors or ARBs if appropriate • Address anaemia, acidosis, hyperparathyroidism • Ensure drug dosages are appropriate for level of kidney function Consider referral to nephrologist
4	15–29	Severe kidney failure	As above. • Referral to nephrologist • Prepare for dialysis or transplantation (if appropriate)
5	<15	End-stage kidney failure	As above. • Institute dialysis or transplantation (if appropriate)

Acute kidney failure

Acute kidney failure (AKF, a forerunner of CKF) is defined as a sudden (days to weeks) decrease in kidney function (azotaemia) with or without oliguria. It results in dysfunctional fluid and electrolyte balance and nitrogenous waste excretion with a sudden increase in blood urea and creatinine levels.

AKF is usually classified into:

- prerenal (e.g. acute circulatory failure → kidney hypoperfusion)
- postrenal (e.g. obstruction)
- kidney (intrinsic) (e.g. acute glomerulonephritis)

Early diagnosis with hospital admission is important and this is achieved by being aware of the patient at risk and the early detection of hypovolaemia, hypertension or hypotension, oliguria or urine abnormalities.

Treatment options include renal dialysis, blood filtration and fluid and electrolyte restriction.

DxT malaise (extreme) + a/n/v + confusion (± oliguria) ➔ AKF

Chronic kidney disease and failure

Chronic kidney disease (CKD) is diagnosed as:[1]

- an estimated or measured glomerular filtration rate (GFR)[1] <60 mL/min/1.73m^2 that is present for ≥3 months with or without evidence of kidney damage

  or
- evidence of kidney damage with or without decreased GFR that is present for ≥3 months as evidenced by the following, irrespective of the underlying cause:
  - albuminuria
  - haematuria after exclusion of urological causes
  - structural abnormalities (e.g. on kidney imaging tests)
  - pathological abnormalities (e.g. renal biopsy)

Chronic kidney (or renal) failure (CKF) is defined as a severe reduction in nephron mass over an extended period of time, resulting in uraemia. It can present surreptitiously and be a real master of disguise in clinical practice. Asymptomatic CKF may be discovered on routine health screening, as a chance finding in hospitalised or hypertensive patients, or during follow-up of patients with known kidney disease.[4] Symptoms only manifest when stage 4 is reached.

Important clinical associations[5]

The possibility of CKF should be monitored in patients with:

- diabetes mellitus
- hypertension
- established cardiovascular disease
- severe gout
- a history of urinary tract abnormality (e.g. vesicoureteric reflux, bladder outflow obstruction) or kidney failure

The possibility of CKF should be considered and investigated in patients presenting with:

- unexplained poor health
- hypertension
- anaemia
- pruritus
- hyperparathyroidism
- pericarditis
- urinary tract symptoms or signs: proteinuria, haematuria, oedema, nocturia, loin pain, prostatic obstruction
- neurological disturbances: confusion, coma, peripheral neuropathy, seizures

Patients with CKF may present with features of acute kidney failure with the intervention of complicating factors such as:

- drug toxicity
- infection
- fluid imbalance

Urgent treatment of the following conditions, which can lead to rapid kidney failure, is essential:

- progressive nephritis
- systemic lupus erythematosus
- vasculitides (see CHAPTER 32), for example, polyarteritis nodosa, Wegener granulomatosis

Risk factors for chronic kidney disease[5]

Non-modifiable	Modifiable
Age >60	Diabetes mellitus
Family history	Hypertension
Aboriginal or Torres Strait Islander origin >30 years	Smoking
History of acute injury	Obesity—BMI ≥30

The clinical approach

History

A hallmark of early-stage CKF is a non-specific history and examination, and the diagnosis is very difficult in the absence of a known past history of kidney disease. Inquire about drugs, UTIs, LUTs, systemic disease and family history. The diagnosis can be established only by kidney function tests. Symptoms from CKF are rare unless the creatinine clearance is less than 20% of normal and only become common when less than 10% of normal.

In patients with chronic kidney disease, symptomatic uraemia may be precipitated by prerenal factors, such as fluid loss from vomiting or diarrhoea, infection, antibiotic therapy especially tetracyclines, or increasing hypertension.

Symptoms and signs

The symptoms and signs of CKF are summarised in FIGURE 31.1.

The common early presenting symptoms are generally non-specific and referable to the GIT, presumably due to the formation of ammonia in the upper GIT. However, anaemia is the main cause of symptoms.

Such symptoms, which indicate uraemia, include:

- malaise
- anorexia, nausea, vomiting
- tiredness/lethargy
- nocturia
- restless legs (esp. if eGFR <15)
- pruritus
- dyspnoea

If a patient presents with these symptoms and has a sallow 'lemon' tinge appearance due to a combination of anaemia and brownish pigmentation, then CKF should be highly suspected.

DxT fatigue + a/n/v + sallow skin → CKF

Physical examination[6]

General inspection of the patient with CKF will usually reveal a sallow complexion with yellow-brown pigmentation in the skin, which is often dry and pruritic. The patient's mental state should be noted. The respiratory and pulse rates are usually rapid because of anaemia and metabolic acidosis. Other findings may include bruising, uraemic fetor, reduced mental status, pericarditis and peripheral neuropathy. The abdomen should be carefully palpated, especially in the kidney areas. A rectal examination is indicated to detect

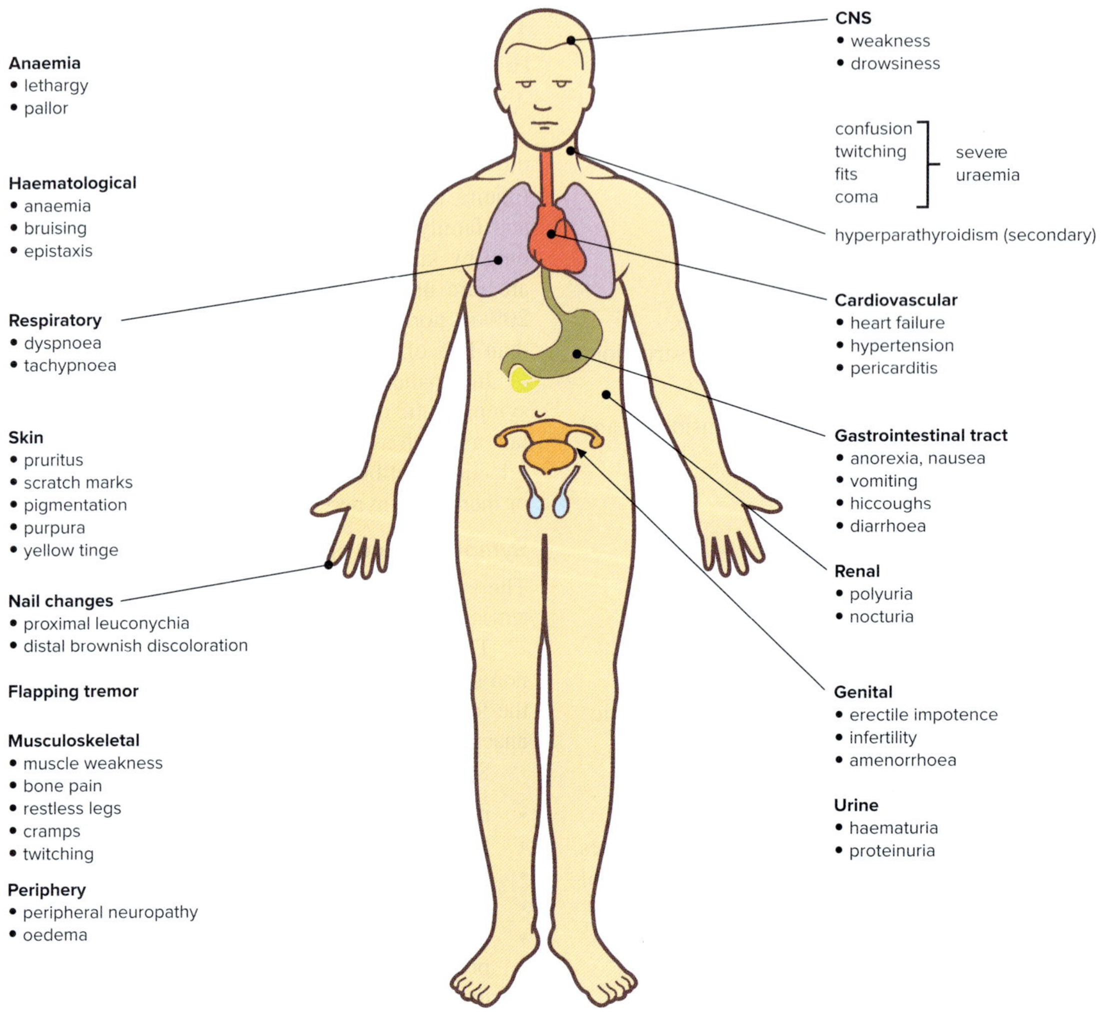

FIGURE 31.1 Clinical features of chronic kidney failure

prostatomegaly or other rectal or pelvic pathology. Ophthalmoscopic examination may show hypertensive or diabetic retinopathy. Urinalysis should test glucose, blood and protein. This involves a dipstick testing on the first morning specimen. Proteinuria should be confirmed with a 24-hour urine protein estimation or (preferably) an albumin creatinine ratio (ACR). Two out of these three positive results are required.

ACR guidelines

Normoalbuminuria

Men:	<2.5 mg/mmol
Women:	<3.5 mg/mmol

Microalbuminuria

Men:	2.5–25 mg/mmol
Women:	3.5–35 mg/mmol

Macroalbuminuria (if persistent, indicates moderate to severe CKF)

Men:	>25 mg/mmol
Women:	>35 mg/mmol

Investigations

- Urine dipstick (poor sensitivity and specificity)[1]
- 24-hour urine protein
- Albumin creatinine ratio
- Microculture of urine
- ESR and FBE (? anaemia)
- Kidney function tests (most appropriate for the GP):
  - plasma urea
  - plasma creatinine
  - creatinine clearance (more precise)
  - eGFR (the new standard)

- Plasma electrolytes:
  - sodium, potassium, chloride, bicarbonate
  - calcium and phosphate
- Consider:
  - magnesium, urate, glucose
  - lipids
  - prescribed drug level
  - cardiac studies
  - protein electrophoresis (? myeloma)
  - ANA for lupus
  - ANCA for vasculitis
- Determination of underlying cause:
  - imaging of urinary tract—ultrasound
  - immunological tests
  - kidney biopsy
- Biochemical changes—elevation of:
  - potassium
  - phosphate
  - creatinine and urea
  - urinary protein
  - hydrogen ions → acidosis; anion group
- Consider renal biopsy

Monitoring CKD

The traditional test in identifying and monitoring CKD is the serum creatinine level.[7] The normal range is about 40–120 μmol/L (0.04–0.12 mmol/L) but the laboratory will indicate their appropriate reference level. However, serum creatinine is an unreliable and insensitive marker of CKD. To improve detection and management guidelines laboratories now report on estimated glomerular filtration rate (eGFR) using the CKP-EPI (chronic kidney disease epidemiology collaboration) formula with every request for serum creatinine concentration, which is required to calculate to GFR.[8]

Although common in older people, an eGFR <60 is associated with increased risks of adverse clinical outcomes, especially renal and cardiovascular.

Guiding rule

eGFR = 140 − age

Drug prescribing in CKD[3,9]

Drugs that can damage the kidneys include:

- classic nephrotoxic drugs, e.g. gentamicin, vancomycin
- NSAIDs, COX-2 inhibitors
- ACE inhibitors and AIIR blockers (ARBs)
- aminoglycosides
- cephalosporins (various)
- tetracyclines
- lithium
- colchicine

Beware of the 'triple whammy'

- NSAIDs/COX-2 inhibitors
- ACE inhibitors
- diuretics

These three agents individually or in combination are implicated in over 50% of cases of iatrogenic acute kidney failure.[10]

Diuretics should be used with care.

Drugs causing hyperkalaemia

- NSAIDs/COX-2
- ACE inhibitors
- ARBs
- Aldactone
- Moduretic
- Trimethoprim
- Digoxin

Increased risk of adverse reaction

- Allopurinol:
  - vasculitis
  - liver dysfunction
- Statins:
  - liver dysfunction
  - myopathy
  - rhabdomyolysis
- Gemfibrozil: rhabdomyolysis

  Do not use statins and gemfibrozil together.

- Beta lactams: interstitial nephritis
- LMW heparin: bleeding
- Aspirin/NSAID: GIT bleeding
- Omeprazole and related agents: interstitial nephritis

Dangerous drug accumulation is presented in TABLE 31.3.

Management

The basic object is to slow progression of disease. The patient should be referred to an appropriate specialist as early as possible. The underlying disease and any abnormalities causing progressive kidney damage must be corrected where possible. The management of CKF is based on the team approach involving specialists and paramedical personnel, including a

31

Table 31.3 Dangerous drug accumulation in kidney impairment[7]

Drug	Problem
Aciclovir	Confusion, encephalopathy
Cotrimoxazole	Steven Johnson syndrome
Flagyl (long term)	Peripheral neuropathy
Penicillin (high dose IV)	Seizures
Quinalones: • ciprofloxacin • norfloxacin	Seizures
Metformin	Lactic acidosis
Sulfonylureas	Prolonged hypoglycaemia
Insulin	Hypoglycaemia
Atenolol	Bradycardia/heart block
Digoxin	Nausea, bradycardia
Sotalol	Ventricular tachycardia (Mg required before conversion)
Codeine	Confusion, acute brain syndrome
Methotrexate	Liver dysfunction Bone marrow depression
Lithium	Tremor—confusion Thyroid dysfunction

dietitian. Attention to lifestyle, especially nutrition and fluid control, is fundamental. The patient is usually faced with years of ongoing care so that an empathic support team based around the patient's GP is very important to the patient, who will require considerable psychosocial support. The common problem of depression necessitates surveillance.

Optimum treatment includes:

- regular review
- good blood pressure control (the most effective way to slow progression)
- keeping plasma phosphate levels in normal range
- maintaining effective fluid and electrolyte balance
- prompt treatment of intercurrent illness
- judicious use of drugs
- avoiding treatment errors, especially with drugs
  - avoid potassium-sparing diuretics
  - avoid nephrotoxic medications
  - other drugs that may cause problems include digoxin, tetracyclines, gentamicin, NSAIDs, nitrofurantoin and ACE inhibitors (ACEIs)
- rapid treatment of complications, especially salt and water depletion and acute urinary tract infection
- diet: low protein, sodium and potassium
- avoid toxins: nicotine, alcohol, caffeine
- treating anaemia with human recombinant erythropoietin and iron (iron infusions)
- attention to an advanced care plan

Targets: goals of management[1,5]

The following are optimal targets for patients with chronic kidney disease:

• blood pressure	$<$140/90 mm Hg if proteinuria $\leq$130/80 mm Hg if albuminuria, diabetes
• cholesterol	total $<$4.0 mmol/L LDL $<$2.5 mmol/L
• blood sugar	pre-prandial 4.4–6.8 mmol/L
• HbA1c	$\leq$7%
• haemoglobin	100–115 g/L
• serum potassium	$\leq$6 mmol/L
• BMI	25 kg/m^2
• serum albumin	$>$35 g/L
• albuminuria	$\geq$50% reduction of baseline value
• acidosis	HCO^{-}_3 $>$22 mmol/L
• phosphate	PO^{-}_4 $\leq$1.75 mmol/L
• no smoking	
• alcohol	$\leq$2 standard drinks/day

The main goal is to treat blood pressure, achieve resolution of proteinuria and reduce CVD risk. Recommend an advanced care plan.

Blood pressure control

- No added salt diet (with care)
- Drug control: none of the antihypertensive agents is specifically contraindicated but those eliminated mainly by the kidney (e.g. ACE inhibitors, atenolol, sotalol) should be given in lower dosage. ACE inhibitors should not be used in the presence of kidney artery stenosis; loop diuretics (e.g. frusemide) are effective in larger doses.[2] The first-line agents are ACEIs or ARBs, which should not be used together. They should be ceased if the creatinine levels exceed 30% above baseline or if the serum K exceeds 6 mmol/L (despite dose

reduction).[4] The non-dihydropyridine calcium channel blockers are next choice. Beta blockers can be used. Diuretics have a vital role in the patient with diastolic heart failure (see CHAPTER 88).[9] Control the blood pressure to the lowest tolerable level since a lower level is associated with a slower decline in GFR.

Anaemia

- Exclude chronic infection and iron deficiency.
- Give iron for iron deficiency and also erythropoietin especially for Hb <100 g/L initiated in a renal unit.
- Avoid transfusions where possible.

Hyperphosphataemia control

- Balanced nutrition to reduce dietary phosphate
- Protein restriction
- Calcium carbonate tablets (to bind phosphate)

Hyperkalaemia treatment

(A concern if >6.5 mmol/L.)

- Low potassium diet
- Cease ACEI/ARB/spironolactone (if applicable)
- Nebulised salbutamol
- IV insulin and dextrose
- IV calcium gluconate
- Oral resonium A
- Then dialysis

Dialysis

Dialysis is indicated when all other methods fail. About two-thirds of patients receive haemodialysis and about 22% are on continuous ambulatory peritoneal dialysis and automated overnight peritoneal dialysis (nocturnal dialysis).

The preferred access is via an AV fistula usually between the radial artery and a cephalic vein.

Transplantation

Transplantation is the treatment of choice for kidney failure except where contraindicated, such as with active malignancy or tuberculosis and perhaps the elderly. However, a critical shortage of donors remains a problem. Rejection and infection are problems, occurring especially in the first 6 months. As a rule, never stop the immunosuppressants. With time there is a high rate of malignancy especially of skin, lymphoma × 5–10 and solid organs × 2–3 (except breast and prostate).

Chronic kidney failure in children

The incidence of CKF in children is about two per million of the total population per year. The commonest causes include chronic glomerulonephritis, obstructive nephropathy and reflux nephropathy. Identification of structural kidney abnormalities by obstetric ultrasound and early investigation of urinary tract infections may decrease the incidence of CKF. Dialysis and transplantation are normally considered for children over 2 years of age with end-stage CKF. For children under 2 years there are complex ethical, psychological and technical problems.[7] Nevertheless the prognosis for such treatment is poor.

Chronic kidney failure in elderly

An eGFR <60 is common but still predictive of significant increased risk of adverse clinical outcomes. Do not regard as physiological. Individualise management.

When to refer[4]

- (Glomerular) haematuria
- eGFR <30 (stage 4 or 5 CKD)
- Rapidly declining kidney function
- Significant proteinuria >1 g/24 hours or ACR >30
- Glomerular haematuria with macroalbuminuria
- Kidney impairment + hypertension (poor control)
- Diabetes with kidney impairment: eGFR <60 or albuminuria/proteinuria

Any person with rapidly declining eGFR and/or signs of acute nephritis (oliguria, haematuria, oedema and acute hypertension) should be regarded as a medical emergency.

Patient education resources

Hand-out sheets from *Murtagh's Patient Education* 7th edition:

- Kidney disease

References

1 Kidney Health Australia. *Chronic Kidney Disease: Management in General Practice* (3rd edn). Melbourne: 2015 e-version. Available from: <www.kidney.org.au>, accessed January 2018.

2 Fox CH et al. A quick guide to evidence-based chronic kidney disease care for the primary care physician. Postgrad Med, 2008; 120(2): E01–6.

31

3 Johnson DW, Usherwood T. Chronic kidney disease. Aust Fam Physician, 2005; 34(11): 915–21.

4 Kumar PJ, Clark M. *Clinical Medicine* (7th edn). London: Elsevier Saunders, 2009: 625–42.

5 RACGP. *Royal Australian College of General Practitioners Guidelines for Preventive Activities in General Practice* (9th edn). East Melbourne: RACGP, 2016: 96–7.

6 Tally N, O'Connor S. *Clinical Examinations* (5th edn). Sydney: Maclennan & Petty, 2006: 186–7.

7 Robinson MJ, Roberton DM. *Practical Paediatrics* (5th edn). Melbourne: Churchill Livingstone, 2003: 610–1.

8 Johnson DW, Usherwood T. Automated reporting of GFR: coming to a laboratory near you. Aust Fam Physician, 2005; 34(11): 925–8.

9 Cunninghan M. Drug therapy in the renally challenged. Monash University Update for GPs. Seminar proceedings November, 2005: 1–8.

10 Thomas MC. Diuretics, ACE inhibitors and NSAIDs—'the triple whammy'. Med J Aust, 21 Feb 2000: 172.

Resources

Kidney Health Australia, <www.kidney.org.au>

Renal Drug Reference Guide, <www.renaldrugreference.com.au>

ATSIP, <www.naccho.org.au>

Australian absolute cardiovascular disease risk calculator, <www.cvdcheck.org.au>

NICE guidelines, chronic kidney disease, <www.nice.org.uk>

Connective tissue disease and the systemic vasculitides

32

In its more aggravated forms diffuse scleroderma is one of the most terrible of all human ills. Like Tithonus to 'wither slowly' and like him to be 'beaten down and marred and wasted', until one is literally a mummy, encased in an ever shrinking, slow contracting skin of steel, is a fate not pictured in any tragedy.

Sir William Osler 1898

The inflammatory connective tissue diseases and the related vasculitides are groups of disorders that are difficult to classify because their causation is generally unknown. They all cause joint and soft tissue inflammation and multiple other possible manifestations that create diagnostic difficulties.

Autoimmune diseases[1]

These are disorders in which the body's immune system damages its own specific organs or systems. The connective tissue diseases are a classic subgroup of autoimmune disease. Rheumatoid arthritis is the most common autoimmune disease. Organ-specific autoimmune diseases include diabetes type 1, Hashimoto thyroiditis, pernicious anaemia, IgA glomerulonephritis, Graves disease, autoimmune hepatitis and myasthenia gravis.

It is convenient to consider a working classification of joint pain (see TABLE 32.1) that includes apparent joint pain (arthralgia), as some of the inflammatory disorders cause problems in the soft tissues around joints (e.g. giant cell arteritis and hydroxyapatite crystallopathy of the tendons around the shoulder joint).

Vasculitis is, in fact, a condition common to the connective tissue disorders and to the so-called vasculitides (see TABLE 32.2).

A major concern to all is that the diagnosis of these conditions is elusive and often delayed.

Table 32.1 A classification of rheumatological pain

Hyperacute (red hot) joints	Crystals	Urate: gout
		Calcium pyrophosphate; hydroxyapatite
	Pus	Example: staphylococcal septic arthritis
Inflammation of joints	Symmetrical	Example: rheumatoid arthritis
	Asymmetrical	Example: spondyloarthropathies
Non-inflammatory joint disorder	Typical	Primary osteoarthritis (e.g. in hands)
	Atypical	Example: post-trauma, haemochromatosis
Joint and soft tissue inflammation	Connective tissue disorders	SLE
		Scleroderma
		Polymyositis/dermatomyositis
		Polyarteritis nodosa
	Vasculitides	Giant cell arteritis
		Polymyalgia rheumatica
Non-articular (soft tissue) inflammation	Generalised	Examples: fibrositis, fibromyalgia, polymyalgia
	Localised	Examples: plantar fasciitis, epicondylitis

Source: After Dr Stephen Hall, personal communication

Table 32.2 List of connective tissue disorders and systemic vasculitides

Connective tissue disorders
Rheumatoid arthritis
SLE
Systemic sclerosis/limited scleroderma
Polymyositis/dermatomyositis
Mixed connective tissue disease
Sjögren syndrome
Raynaud phenomenon (including Raynaud syndrome)
Systemic vasculitides
Large vessel predominantly: • giant cell arteritis/temporal arteritis/polymyalgia rheumatica • Takayasu arteritis • Behçet syndrome
Medium vessel (mainly affects visceral vessels): • polyarteritis nodosa • Kawasaki disease
Small vessel (mainly): • immunoglobulin A vasculitis (Henoch–Schönlein purpura) • hypersensitivity vasculitis • essential cryoglobulinaemia
Antineutrophil cytoplasmic antibody (ANCA) associated: • granulomatosis with polyangiitis (Wegener granulomatosis) • eosinophilic granulomatosis polyangiitis (Churg–Strauss vasculitis) • microscopic polyangiitis

Inflammatory connective tissue disease

The term 'connective tissue disease' (CTD) is a generic label applied to a group of disorders characterised by systemic inflammation, presumed initiated by an autoimmune response to an autoantigen and perpetuated by unknown factors.[2] The vasculitides are a variety of CTD.

The CTDs comprise three classic conditions, namely systemic lupus erythematosus (SLE), systemic sclerosis (scleroderma) and polymyositis/dermatomyositis (see FIG. 32.1).[1]

Mixed connective tissue disorder includes features of all three disorders and is sometimes referred to as 'overlap' syndrome. Other related disorders classified as CTDs include sicca syndromes such as Sjögren syndrome and Raynaud syndrome.

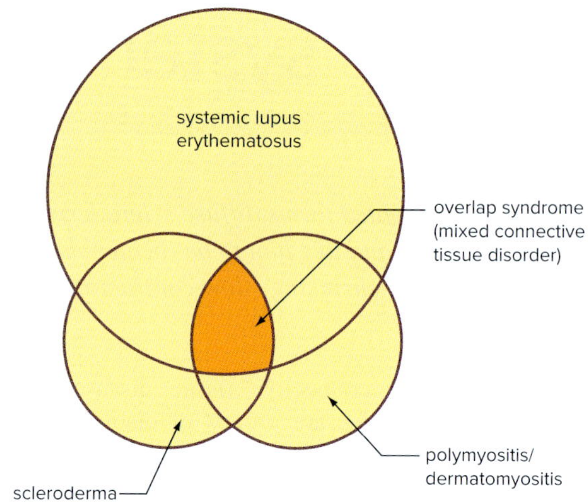

FIGURE 32.1 The classic connective tissue disorders

Common features include:

- fatigue
- arthralgia or arthritis
- multisystem involvement
- vasculitis
- immunological abnormalities
- sicca (dry skin and mucous membranes)
- Raynaud phenomenon

Investigations in connective tissue disease

The rapidly growing list of investigations, particularly those of auto-antibodies, can be confusing. Baseline investigations to consider are FBE, ESR, C-reactive protein and rheumatoid factor. The rheumatoid factor can be positive in a great range of disorders, including rheumatoid arthritis, SLE, systemic sclerosis, Sjögren syndrome, chronic liver disease and various viral (e.g. hepatitis), bacterial (e.g. tuberculosis) and parasitic (e.g. malaria) infections. There is usually a low titre, except in rheumatoid arthritis. X-rays and HLA-B_{27} tests are not recommended.

TABLE 32.3 summarises the majority of autoantibodies that can be tested. The antinuclear antibody (ANA) test is a generic term for auto-antibodies to several different cellular antigens. It is very sensitive for SLE, but not absolutely specific (false positives occur with viral arthritis and others, e.g. Sjögren). It is especially useful in the young female presenting with fatigue, small joint arthralgia and dermatological features of SLE.

The more specific antibodies for SLE, namely to double-stranded DNA (dsDNA) and extractable

Table 32.3 Auto-antibodies in connective tissue disease[2]

Antibody	Feature
Antinuclear antibody (ANA)	High sensitivity 95%, low specificity for SLE
Anti-dsDNA	High sensitivity and specificity for SLE (60%): found in rheumatoid arthritis
Antibodies to extractable nuclear antigens (ENA)	
Smith (Sm)	Highly specific for SLE
U1 RNP	Common in mixed connective tissue disease, SLE
Ro (SSA)	Common in Sjögren syndrome, SLE and some other connective tissue diseases
La (SSB)	Common in Sjögren syndrome, SLE (15%)
Scl-70 (antitopoisomerase)	Common in 20–30% of patients with scleroderma
Jo1	Common in 30% of patients with polymyositis
Anticentromere lc	High sensitivity and specificity for CREST syndrome
Antineutrophil cytoplasm (ANCA)	High sensitivity and specificity for Wegener granulomatosis
Antiphospholipids	Diagnostic in antiphospholipid syndrome
Anti-cardiolipin	
Anti-β_2-GP1 antibodies	
Lupus anticoagulants 1gM × 1gG aPL	Present in 5–10% of SLE

nuclear antigens (ENA), should only be ordered if there is a significantly positive ANA.

Antiphospholipid antibody syndrome

This syndrome may occur with SLE or in isolation and is responsible for recurrent arterial and/or venous thromboembolism, recurrent spontaneous abortions or thrombocytopenia in the presence of antiphospholipid antibodies but without features of SLE. Livedo reticularis, skin ulcers and neuropsychiatric disturbances have also been noted. If suspected, commence aspirin 150–300 mg (o) daily and refer to a consultant.

Systemic lupus erythematosus

SLE (lupus), which is the commonest of the connective tissue disorders, is described as the 'great pretender'.[3] It is a multisystem autoimmune disorder with a wide variety of clinical features that are due to vasculitis (see FIG. 32.2). Arthritis is the commonest feature of SLE (90% of cases). Milder manifestations outnumber more severe forms.

Clinical features[4]

- Prevalence about 1 in 1000 of population
- Mainly affects women in 'high oestrogen' period (90% of cases)
- Peak onset between 15 and 45 years
- Fever, malaise, tiredness common
- Multiple drug allergies, e.g. sulfonamides
- Problems with oral contraceptive pill and pregnancy
- Course of remission and flares

DxT polyarthritis + fatigue + skin lesions → SLE

Classification criteria

(SLE = four or more of these 11 criteria)

- Malar (butterfly) rash
- Discoid rash
- Photosensitivity
- Arthritis (non-erosive arthritis in ≥2 peripheral joints)
- Oral ulcers (usually painless)
- Serositis (pleurisy or pericarditis)
- Kidney features (proteinuria or cellular casts)
- Neurological features (intractable headache, seizures or psychosis)
- Haematological features (haemolytic anaemia, leucopenia, lymphopenia or thrombocytopenia)
- Immunological features (positive anti-DNA, antiphospholipid antibodies or anti-Sm tests and false positive syphilis serology)
- Positive antinuclear antibody (ANA) test

Note: Drugs that can cause a lupus-like syndrome are discussed in CHAPTER 35).

Diagnosis

- ESR/CRP—elevated in proportion to disease activity
- ANA test—positive in 95% (perform first) (key test)

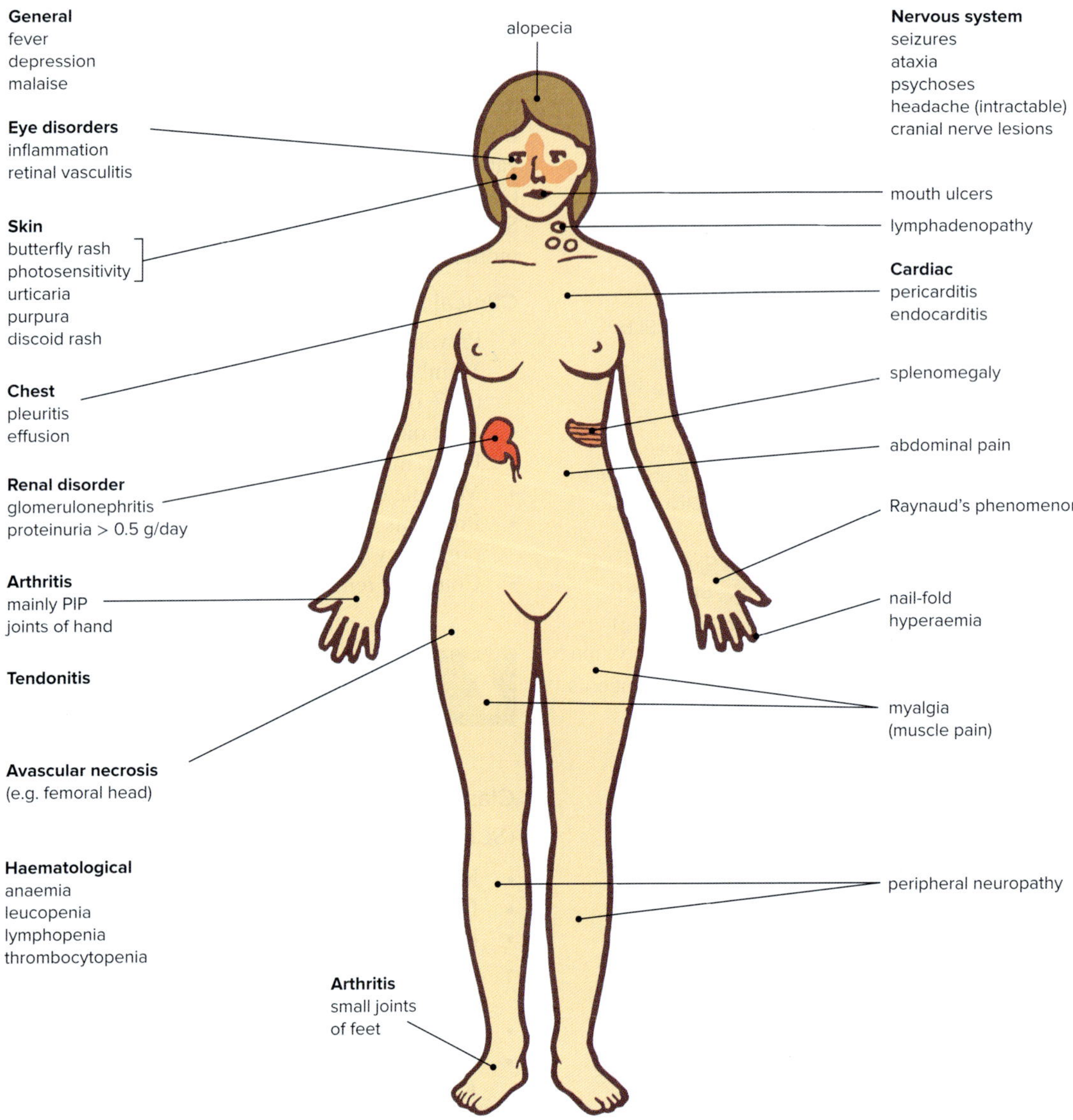

FIGURE 32.2 Clinical features of SLE

- dsDNA antibodies—90% specific for SLE but present in only 60% (key test)
- ENA antibodies, especially Sm—highly specific
- Rheumatoid factor—positive in 50%
- LE cell test—inefficient and not used

The diagnosis cannot be made on blood tests alone. Supportive clinical evidence is necessary.

For suspected SLE, the recommended approach is to perform an ANA test. If positive then order dsDNA and ENA antibodies.

Management[5]

- Appropriate explanation, support and reassurance, use of sunscreens (refer to CHAPTER 121)
- Refer to consultant rheumatologist for shared care in a multidisciplinary team: urgent if severe organ damage

Treatment[2]

Based on severity and organ involved.

- Mild: NSAIDs (for arthralgia)
- Moderate (especially skin, joint serosa involved): low-dose antimalarials (e.g. hydroxychloroquine

up to 6 mg/kg once daily) (e.g. 400 mg (o) daily for 3 months, then 200 mg daily long term)

- Severe: corticosteroids are the mainstay (e.g. prednisolone initially 25-60 mg (o) daily then 7.5–15 mg (o) daily): immunosuppressive drugs (e.g. azathioprine, methotrexate with folic acid, bDMARDs (e.g. rituximab, belimumab) may be used for severe arthralgia
- Avoid drugs in those in clinical remission and with normal complement levels.
- Avoid excessive sunlight.
- Other treatments, such as plasma exchange and immunosuppressive regimens, are available for severe disease.
- Keep in mind antiphospholipid antibody syndrome, especially with recurrent fetal loss and thrombotic episodes.

Systemic sclerosis (scleroderma)

This can present as a polyarthritis affecting the fingers in 25% of patients, especially in the early stages. Soft tissue swelling produces a 'sausage finger' pattern. Scleroderma mainly affects the skin with fibrotic thickening. It presents with Raynaud phenomenon in over 85% of patients (see FIG. 32.3).

There are three clinical variants:

1 limited cutaneous disease, e.g. morphea
2 cutaneous with limited organ involvement (CREST)
3 diffuse systemic disease (systemic sclerosis)

Clinical features[2,6]

- Female to male ratio = 3:1
- A progressive disease of multiple organs
- Raynaud phenomenon
- Stiffness of fingers and other skin areas (see FIG. 32.4)
- 'Bird-like' facies (mouth puckered)
- Dysphagia and diarrhoea (malabsorption)
- Oesophageal dysmotility
- Respiratory symptoms: pulmonary fibrosis
- Cardiac symptoms: pericarditis, pulmonary arterial hypertension, etc.
- Look for tight skin on chest (Roman breastplate)

DxT finger discomfort + arthralgia + GORD (± skin tightness) → scleroderma

Diagnosis[2,6]

- ESR may be raised
- Normocytic normochromic anaemia may be present
- ANA test—up to 90% positive (relatively specific)
- Rheumatoid factor—positive in 30%

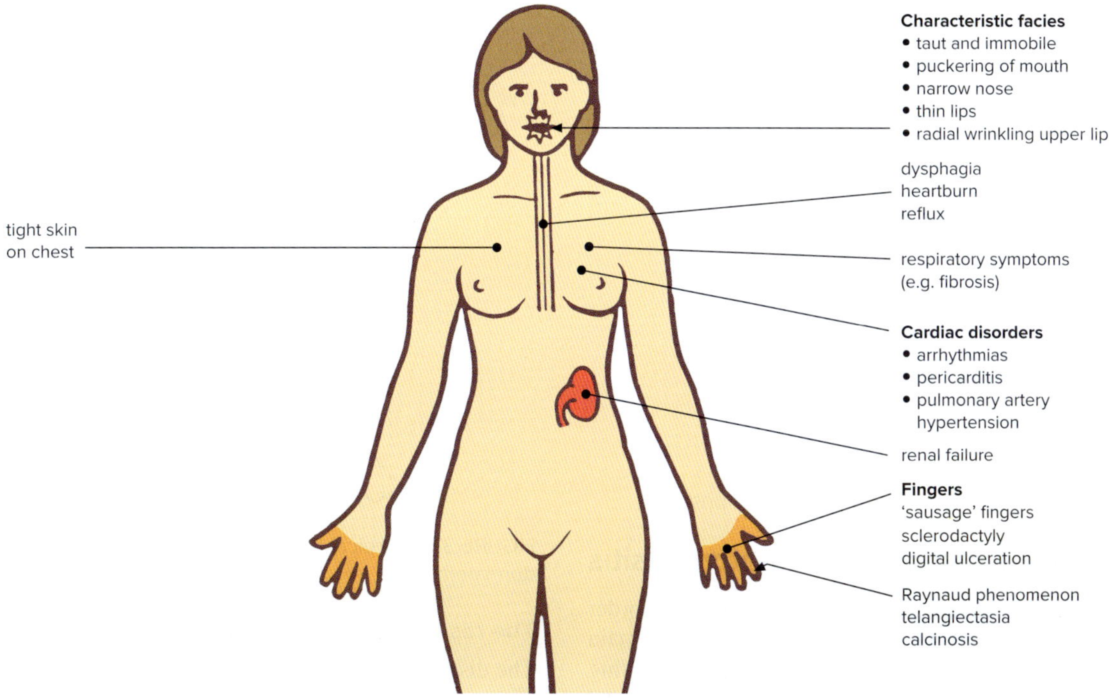

FIGURE 32.3 Clinical features of scleroderma

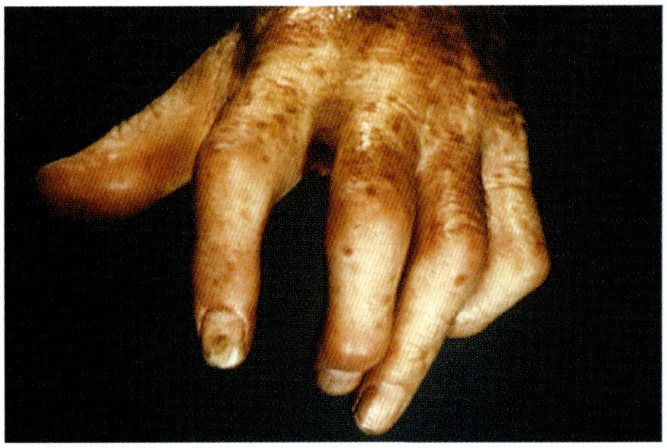

FIGURE 32.4 Scleroderma showing stiff, taut skin of fingers

- Anticentromere antibodies—specific (positive in 90% with limited disease and 5% with diffuse)
- Antitopoisomerase I (anti-Scl-70) antibody is specific but only positive in 20–30%
- Skin biopsy—increase in dermal collagen

Management

- Refer to consultant for shared care
- Empathic explanation, patient education
- Analgesics and NSAIDs for pain
- Avoid vasospasm (no smoking, beta blockers, ergotamine); calcium channel blockers such as nifedipine may help Raynaud
- Treat malabsorption if present; skin emollients
- D-penicillamine can help if there is significant systemic or cutaneous involvement[8]

Localised scleroderma

- Morphea—plaques of erythema with violaceous periphery, feels hard; mainly on trunk
- Linear—may be 'en coup de sabre' (a sabre stroke)

CREST syndrome

Clinical features

- Calcinosis
- Raynaud phenomenon
- Oesophageal dysmotility
- Sclerodactyly
- Telangiectasia
- Anticentromere antibody (invariably positive)

Polymyositis and dermatomyositis

Polymyositis is an uncommon systemic disorder with inflammation of skin and muscle whose main feature is symmetrical muscle weakness and wasting involving the proximal muscles of the shoulder and pelvic girdles.

Clinical features

- Any age group
- Peak incidence 40–60 years
- Female to male ratio = 2:1
- Muscle weakness and wasting proximal limb muscles
- Main complaint is weakness
- Muscle pain and tenderness in about 50%
- Arthralgia or arthritis in about 50% (resembles distribution of rheumatoid arthritis)
- Dysphagia in about 50% due to oesophageal involvement
- Raynaud phenomenon
- Consider associated malignancy: lung and ovary

DxT weakness + joint and muscle pain + violaceous facial rash → dermatomyositis

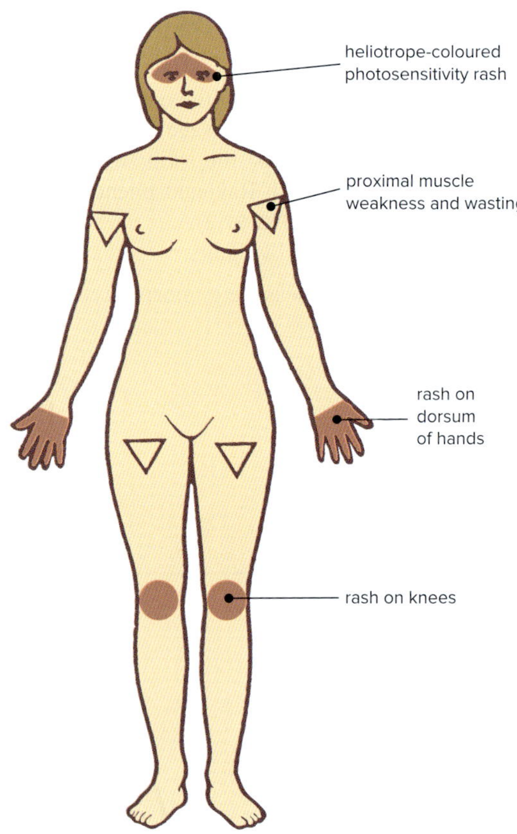

FIGURE 32.5 Clinical features of polymyositis/dermatomyositis

The rash

The distinctive rash shows features of photosensitivity. There is heliotrope (violet) discolouration of the eyelids (see FIG. 32.6), forehead and cheeks, and possible

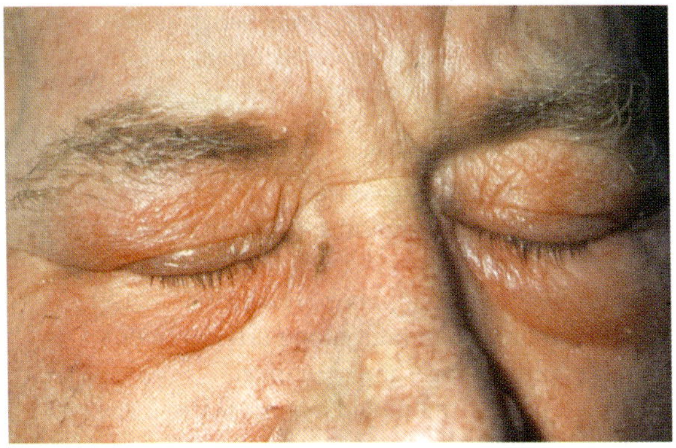

FIGURE 32.6 Heliotrope discolouration of eyelids in dermatomyositis

erythema resembling sunburn and peri-orbital oedema. There is a characteristic rash on the hands, especially the fingers and nail folds. The knees and elbows are commonly involved.

Differential diagnosis: statin-induced necrotising myositis (↑ CK levels).

Diagnosis

- Muscle enzyme studies (serum creatine kinase and aldolase)
- Biopsies—skin and muscle
- EMG studies—show characteristic pattern

Treatment includes corticosteroids and cytotoxic drugs. Early referral is appropriate.

Sjögren syndrome

The under-diagnosed syndrome of dry eyes (keratoconjunctivitis sicca) in the absence of rheumatoid arthritis or any other autoimmune disease is known as primary Sjögren syndrome (SS). There is lymphoid infiltration of the exocrine glands:

- primary SS—limited or multisystem
- secondary SS—occurs in association with other CTDs including rheumatoid arthritis (accounts for 50%) or systemic sclerosis

Clinical features

- Fatigue
- Sicca (xerostomia, dry eyes, dry vagina)
- Difficulty swallowing food
- Increased dental caries; denture dysfunction
- Salivary gland enlargement; reduced salivation
- Xerotrachea → chronic dry cough; hoarseness
- Dyspareunia
- Arthralgia ± non-erosive arthritis

Although considered benign, it can transform into non-Hodgkin lymphoma (approx. 1 in 44 cases).

DxT dry eyes + dry mouth + arthritis ➜ Sjögren syndrome

Diagnosis

- Autoantibody tests—positive ANA (ENA), Ro (SSA), La (SS-B)
- Elevated ESR, +ve RA factor, possibly anaemia
- Schirmer's tear test (measures conjunctival dryness)

Management

- Referral to rheumatologist
- Treatment is symptomatic for dry eyes, mouth and vagina; arthralgia
- NSAIDs, hydroxychloroquine or steroids for arthritis

Raynaud phenomenon[2]

(Refer also to CHAPTER 64.)

It is classified as either primary (without associated disease) or secondary (when associated with any CTD).

Patients with primary Raynaud may progress to a CTD but the likelihood is low (5–15%) and the delay to diagnosis is long (average of 10 years).[2] The more severe the Raynaud, the more likely it is to progress to systemic disease.

Raynaud is a clinical syndrome of episodic arteriolar vasospasm usually involving the fingers and toes (one or two at a time). It may also involve the nose, ear or nipple.

The vasculitides[2]

The vasculitides or vasculitis syndromes are a heterogeneous group of disorders involving inflammation and necrosis of blood vessels, the clinical effects and classification depending on the size of the vessels involved (see TABLE 32.2). They are a variety of CTD.

Small vessel vasculitis is the common type encountered in practice. Medium vessel vasculitis includes polyarteritis nodosa and large vessel vasculitis includes giant cell arteritis.

Symptoms suggestive of vasculitis include systemic (malaise, fever, weight loss, arthralgia), skin lesions (e.g. purpura, ulcers, infarction), respiratory (wheeze, cough, dyspnoea), ENT (epistaxis, sinusitis, nasal crusting), chest pain (angina), kidney (haematuria, proteinuria, CKF) and neurological (various, e.g. sensorimotor).

Small vessel vasculitis

This is associated with many important disorders, such as rheumatoid arthritis, SLE, bacterial endocarditis, Henoch–Schönlein purpura and hepatitis B. Skin lesions are usually associated with these disorders and the most common presentation is painless, palpable purpura, such as occurs with Henoch–Schönlein purpura.

> **Practice tip**
>
> Consider vasculitis in any unidentified multisystem disorder.

Rarer but deadly causes

The major vasculitides called systemic vasculitides are polyarteritis nodosa (PN), polymyalgia rheumatica (PR), giant cell arteritis (GCA), Takayasu arteritis, Behçet syndrome, Churg–Strauss vasculitis and Wegener granulomatosis (WG). Unfortunately, many patients die or become terminally ill before the diagnosis is suspected.

> **Practice tip**
>
> If a serious ANCA-associated disease is suspected, early diagnosis is life-saving because of sinister kidney damage. Perform a urine examination for haematuria and proteinuria. If positive, order an ANCA test. If positive, refer urgently.

Henoch–Schönlein purpura

More details are presented about this vasculitis disorder in CHAPTER 39.

Takayasu arteritis[2]

Known as 'pulseless disease' or 'aortic arch syndrome', this vasculitis involves the aortic arch and other major arteries. It typically affects young Japanese female adults. Features include absence of peripheral pulses and hypertension.

Polyarteritis nodosa

The hallmark of PN is necrotising vasculitis of the small and medium arteries leading to skin nodules, infarctive ulcers and other serious manifestations. The cause is unknown but associations are found with drug abusers (especially adulterated drugs), B-cell lymphomas, other drugs and hepatitis B surface antigen. It should be suspected in any multisystemic disease of obscure aetiology.

Clinical features

- Young to middle-aged men
- Constitutional symptoms: fever, malaise, myalgia, weight loss
- Migratory arthralgia or polyarthritis
- Subcutaneous nodules along arterial lines
- Livedo reticularis and skin ulcers
- Kidney impairment and hypertension
- Cardiac disorders: arrhythmia, failure, infarction
- Diagnosis confirmed by biopsy or angiogram
- ESR raised
- Treatment is with corticosteroids and immunosuppressants. Refer for specialist care. Meticulous control of blood pressure is essential.
- Death is usually from kidney disease

> **DxT** arthralgia + weight loss + fever (± skin lesions) → polyarteritis nodosa

Giant cell arteritis and polymyalgia rheumatica

The basic pathology of this very important disease complex is GCA (synonyms: temporal arteritis, cranial arteritis). The clinical syndromes are polymyalgia rheumatica and temporal arteritis. The clinical manifestations of polymyalgia rheumatica invariably precede those of temporal arteritis, of which there is about a 50% association. The diagnosis is based on clinical grounds. No definite cause has been found.

Urgently refer any patient with giant cell arteritis.

Clinical features (polymyalgia rheumatica)

- Pain and stiffness in proximal muscles of shoulder and pelvic girdle, cervical spine (refer FIG. 32.7)
- Symmetrical distribution
- Typical ages 60–70 years (rare <50)
- Both sexes: more common in women
- Early morning stiffness lasting >45 minutes
- May be systemic symptoms: weight loss, malaise, anorexia
- Painful restriction of movement of shoulders and hips (other joints not usually involved)
- Signs may be absent later in day
- ESR typically >40 but may be normal

Differential diagnosis: polymyalgic onset rheumatoid arthritis.

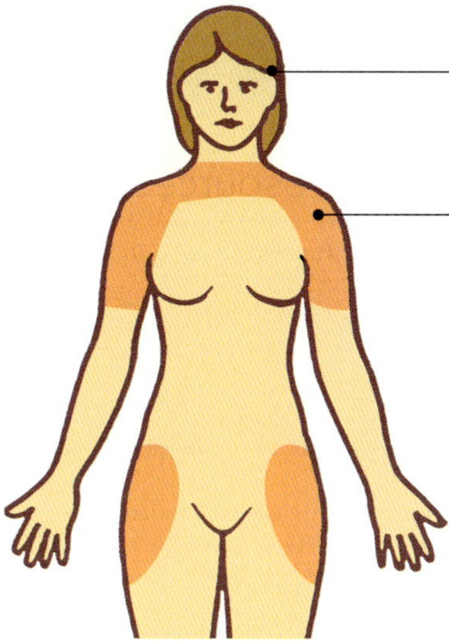

FIGURE 32.7 Polymyalgia rheumatica: typical sites of areas of pain and stiffness

> **DxT** /malaise + painful shoulder girdle + morning stiffness (>50 years) ➔ polymyalgia rheumatica

Clinical features (temporal arteritis)

- Headache—unilateral, throbbing (CHAPTER 56)
- Visual symptoms, e.g. diplopia
- Temporal tenderness
- Polymyalgia rheumatica
- Loss of pulsation of temporal artery
- Jaw claudication
- Biopsy of temporal artery (5 cm) is diagnostic

> **DxT** fatigue/malaise + headache + jaw claudication ➔ temporal arteritis

Investigation

- No specific test for polymyalgia rheumatica
- ESR—extremely high, around 100
- C-reactive protein—elevated
- Mild anaemia (normochromic, normocytic)

Treatment for uncomplicated disease[9]

Refer any patient with GCA urgently.

Prednisolone

- Starting dose
  - temporal (giant cell) arteritis: 40–60 mg (o) daily initially for 2–4 weeks (+ aspirin 100 mg/day) then gradual reduction according to ESR/CRP
  - polymyalgia rheumatica: 15 mg (o) daily for 2–4 weeks, then taper
- Taper down gradually to the minimum effective dose (often <5 mg daily) according to the clinical response and the ESR and CRP. Aim for treatment for 2 years. Relapses are common.
- If complicated (e.g. evolving visual loss) give IV methylprednisolone for 3 days prior to oral agents.

Other drugs

- Azathioprine or methotrexate can be used as steroid-sparing agents.

> **Practice tip**
>
> In giant cell arteritis, a delay in diagnosis after presenting with amaurosis fugax and non-specific symptoms can have tragic consequences, in the form of ischaemic events such as blindness and strokes.

Behçet syndrome[2]

Behçet syndrome is a systemic (multiorgan) vasculitis of unknown aetiology, affecting veins and arteries of all sizes. The main feature is painful oral ulceration and the hallmark is the 'pathergy' reaction whereby simple trauma such as a pinprick can cause a papule or pustule to form within a few hours at the site.

Clinical features

- Male to female ratio = 2:1
- Recurrent oral and/or genital ulceration
- Arthritis (usually knees)
- Skin changes, e.g. erythema nodosum
- Ocular symptoms—pain, reduced vision, floaters (ocular inflammation)

There is no specific diagnostic test.

Associated problems/complications: repeated uveitis and retinitis → blindness, colitis, venous thrombosis, meningoencephalitis.

Treatment: high-dose steroids and specific ulcer treatment. DMARDs or bDMARDs may be required.

> **Practice tip**
>
> Patients with Behçet eye disease should be referred promptly for an ophthalmological opinion, which may be sight-saving.[2]

32

Wegener granulomatosis[2]

Now called 'granulomatosis with polyangiitis', this rare vasculitis of unknown cause has a classic triad: upper respiratory tract (URT) granuloma, fleeting pulmonary shadows (nodules) and glomerulonephritis. Without treatment it is invariably fatal and sometimes the initial diagnosis is that made at autopsy. It is difficult to diagnose, especially as the patient (usually young to middle-aged) presents with a febrile illness and respiratory symptoms, but early diagnosis is essential. It usually gets confused with benign nasal conditions.

Clinical features

- Adolescence to elderly, mean age 40–45 years
- Constitutional symptoms (as for PN)
- Lower respiratory tract (LRT) symptoms (e.g. cough, dyspnoea)
- Oral ulcers
- Upper respiratory symptoms: rhinorrhoea, epistaxis, sinus pain, nasal septum loss, ear dysfunction
- Eye involvement—orbital mass
- Polyarthritis
- Kidney involvement—usually not clinically apparent (about 75% get glomerulonephritis)
- Chest X-ray points to diagnosis—multiple nodes, cavitations
- Antineutrophil antibodies (c-ANCA) are a useful diagnostic marker (not specific)
- Diagnosis confirmed by biopsy, usually an open lung biopsy
- Better prognosis with early diagnosis and treatment with appropriate DMARD

DxT malaise + URTs (e.g. rhinitis, sinusitis) + LRTs (e.g. wheeze, cough) ➜ granulomatosis with polyangiitis

DxT asthma + rhinitis + vasculitis + hypereosinophilia ➜ Churg–Strauss vasculitis

Patient education resources

Hand-out sheets from *Murtagh's Patient Education* 7th edition:

- Rheumatoid arthritis
- Systemic lupus erythematosus

References

1. Kumar PJ, Clark ML. *Clinical Medicine* (7th edn). London: Elsevier Saunders, 2009: 73–7.
2. Expert group for Rheumatology guidelines. Inflammatory connective tissue disease. In: eTG complete. Melbourne: Therapeutic Guidelines Ltd. Available from: <www.tg.org.au>, accessed January 2018.
3. Hanrahan P. The great pretender: SLEs. Aust Fam Physician, 2001; 30(7): 636–40.
4. Nikpour M et al. A systematic review of prevalence, disease characteristics and management of systemic lupus erythematosus in Australia: Inter Med J, 2014; 44(12a): 1170–9.
5. Gill JM, Quisel AM et al. Diagnosis of systemic lupus erythematosus. AM Fam Physician, 2003; 68(11): 2179–86.
6. Randell P. Scleroderma. In: *MIMS Disease Index* (2nd edn). Sydney: IMS Publishing, 1996: 458–60.
7. Chaisson NF, Hassoun PM. Systemic sclerosis-associated pulmonary hypertension. Chest, 2013; 144(4): 1346–56.
8. Steen VD et al. D-penicillamine therapy in progressive systemic sclerosis. Ann Intern Med, 1982; 97: 652–9.
9. Hernandez-Rodriguez J et al. Treatment of polymyalgia rheumatica: a systematic review. Arch Intern Med, 2009; 169(20): 1839–50.

Neurological dilemmas 33

The disease is of long duration; to connect, therefore, the symptoms which occur in its later stages with those which mark its commencement, requires a continuance of observation of the same case, or at least a correct history of its symptoms, even for several years.

JAMES PARKINSON (1755–1824), *AN ESSAY ON THE SHAKING PALSY*

In general practice there are many neurological problems that present a diagnostic dilemma, with some being true masquerades for the non-neurologist. This applies particularly to various seizure disorders, space-occupying lesions in the cerebrum and the cerebellum, demyelinating disorders, motor neurone disorders and peripheral neuropathies.

The most common pitfall that occurs with neurological disorders is misdiagnosis, and the most common reason for misdiagnosis is an inadequate history. Failure to appreciate the neurological meaning of points elicited during the history is another reason for misdiagnosis.

Some very important neurological disorders are presented in this section: Parkinson disease, which is common and can be easily misdiagnosed, especially when the classic 'pill rolling' tremor is absent or mild; multiple sclerosis (MS), because it is difficult to diagnose initially; and acute idiopathic demyelinating polyneuropathy (Guillain–Barré syndrome), because it can be rapidly fatal if misdiagnosed. MS can masquerade as almost anything—'If you don't know what it is, think of MS.'

Another brain teaser for the family doctor is to diagnose accurately the various types of epilepsy. The most commonly misdiagnosed seizure disorders are complex partial seizures or atypical generalised tonic–clonic seizures (see CHAPTER 54).[1] Even more difficult is the differentiation of real seizures from pseudo- or non-epileptic seizures. As a rule neurological conditions should be referred early for specialist management.

Diplopia

The onset of diplopia (double vision) in adults is often acute, very distressing and invariably easy to diagnose. It is invariably binocular, which usually results from extraocular muscular imbalance or weakness. The type of binocular diplopia—vertical, horizontal or oblique—provides clues in identifying the affected muscle. Monocular diplopia is double vision that occurs in one eye when the other is covered. It arises from the eye itself.

The diagnostic strategy model is outlined in TABLE 33.1.

Table 33.1 Diplopia: diagnostic strategy model

Probability diagnosis
Binocular:
Ocular nerve palsy (3, 4, 6)—various causes
CVA/TIA
Opthalmoplegic migraine
Physiological (disparateness)
Drug effect, e.g. alcohol, benzodiazepines
Monocular:
Eye disorder, e.g. cataract, refractive error, cornea
Serious disorders not to be missed
Vascular:
CVA/TIA
Infection:
Intraocular abscess
Sinusitis
Botulism
HIV/AIDS
Tumour/cancer:
Involving 3, 4 or 6 cranial nerves
Other
Facial bone trauma/head injury
Guillain–Barré syndrome
Pitfalls (often missed)
Any orbital infiltration
Rarities:
Multiple sclerosis
Myasthenia gravis
Orbital myositis
Cavernous sinus thrombosis
Wernicke's encephalopathy
Seven masquerades checklist
Diabetes: mononeuritis
Drugs, e.g. sedatives, opioids, alcohol
Thyroid/other endocrine—hyperthyroid?
Is the patient trying to tell me something?
A consideration if nil findings
Some cases are idiopathic

Diagnosis

Diplopia should be differentiated from blurred vision, which is like 'ghosting' on a TV screen.

Office tests

Test for double vision with each eye occluded. If diplopia persists, it is uniocular. If, however, double vision disappears when either eye is covered, there is a defect of one of the muscles moving the eyeball. Determine whether diplopia occurs in any particular direction of gaze. It is most marked when moved in the direction of action of the weak muscle. Ask patient to follow your finger, red pin or penlight with both eyes and move it in an H pattern.

- 3rd nerve—eye turned out: divergent squint
- 6th nerve—failure to abduct: convergent squint (see FIG. 33.1).

33

Key investigations

- Nil for most cases
- First line: urinalysis, blood sugar, FBE, ESR/CRP (? arteritis)
- Consider: TFTs, imaging if indicated (refer)
- ESR (consider arteritis)

  Note:
- Exclude 3rd and 6th nerve palsies as they may be secondary to life-threatening conditions.
- Refer urgently if diplopia is binocular, of recent onset and persistent

Motor weakness

Muscle weakness is a common feature of many disorders ranging from neurogenic and myogenic disorders to metabolic and psychiatric. It is very important clinically to be able to differentiate upper motor neurone (UMN) signs from lower motor neurone (LMN) signs (see TABLE 33.2).

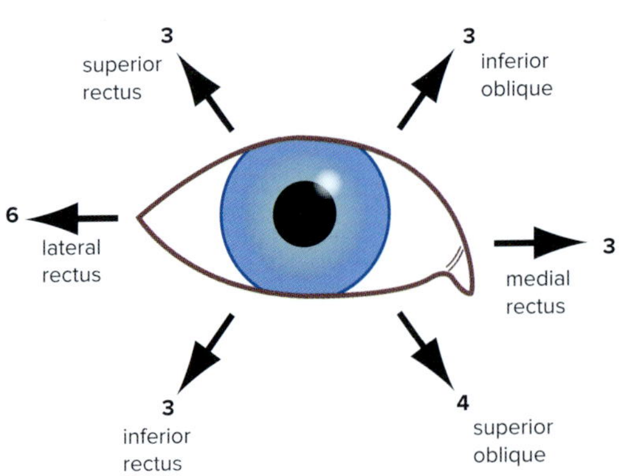

FIGURE 33.1 Direction of movement of the right eye indicating the responsible extra-ocular muscles and cranial nerves (3 = oculomotor, 4 = trochlear, 6 = abducens)

Table 33.2 Clinical differences between a lower motor neurone lesion and an upper motor neurone lesion

Manifestation	UMN	LMN
Weakness	Present	Present
Wasting	Absent or mild	Marked
Power	Reduced	Reduced
Tone	Usually increased (spastic paralysis) ± clonus	Absent or decreased (flaccid paralysis)
Fasciculations	Absent	May be present
Reflexes	Brisk tendon reflexes Abdominal absent Extensor plantar response	Absent or diminished Downgoing plantar response

Upper motor neurone lesions

UMN signs occur when a lesion has interrupted a neural pathway at a level above the anterior horn cell.[2] Examples include lesions in motor pathways in the cerebral cortex, internal capsule, brain stem or spinal cord.

Clinical examples include stroke (thrombosis, embolism or haemorrhage in the brain), tumours of the various pathways, demyelinating disease (e.g. multiple sclerosis) and infection (e.g. HIV).

Lower motor neurone lesions

LMN signs occur when a lesion interrupts peripheral neural pathways from the anterior horn cell, that is, the spinal reflex arc.

Clinical examples include peripheral neuropathy, Guillain–Barré syndrome, poliomyelitis and a thickened peripheral nerve (e.g. leprosy).

Note: A spinal cord lesion causes LMN signs at the level of the lesion and UMN signs below that level.

Neurogenic and myogenic muscle weakness

It is also important to distinguish between weakness caused by neurological conditions, especially those causing LMN lesions and muscular disorders. The features are compared in TABLE 33.3. Myotonia is muscle stiffness with difficulty in relaxation after voluntary contraction, e.g. dystrophia myotonica (myotonic dystrophy) (see TABLE 33.7).

Table 33.3 Muscle weakness: main clinical differences between neurogenic and myogenic lesions

Myogenic weakness	Neurogenic weakness
Reflexes often present despite severe weakness	Reflexes often absent despite minimal weakness
Weakness out of proportion to wasting	Wasting out of proportion to weakness
Sensation normal	± Sensory changes
No fasciculation (polymyositis may cause fasciculation)	Fasciculation a feature

Motor neurone disease (MND)

MND is a progressive neuromuscular disorder resulting in muscular limb and bulbar weakness due to death of motor neurones in the brain, brain stem and spinal cord. The sensory system is not involved, nor the cranial nerves to the eye muscles. Five to 10% of MND is inherited with an autosomal dominant pattern; the rest is sporadic. The three main patterns are:

1. amyotrophic lateral sclerosis (Lou Gehrig disease)—combined LMN muscle atrophy plus UMN hyper-reflexia, leading to progressive spasticity. This is the most common type.
2. progressive muscle atrophy—wasting beginning in the distal muscles; widespread fasciculation
3. progressive bulbar (LMN) palsy and pseudobulbar palsy (LMN lesions in the brainstem motor nuclei). Results in wasted fibrillating tongue, weakness of chewing and swallowing, and of facial muscles.

Symptoms and signs

- Weakness or muscle wasting—first noticed in hands (weak grip) or feet
- Stumbling (spastic gait, foot drop)
- Difficulty with swallowing
- Difficulty with speech, for example, slurring, hoarseness
- Fasciculation (twitching) of skeletal muscles and fibrillating tongue
- Cramps
- Emotional instability, depression
- ± Muscle pain

The diagnosis is clinical. There are no diagnostic tests, but neurophysiological tests and MRI of the brain and cord help differentiate from other conditions.

MND is incurable and progresses to death usually within 3–5 years from ventilatory failure/aspiration pneumonia.

No treatment is proven to influence outcome although riluzole, a sodium channel blocker, appears to slow progression slightly. Baclofen 10 mg bd may help symptoms of cramp. Botulinum toxin may help spasticity and propantheline or amitriptyline for drooling. Multidisciplinary care is essential.

Tremor

Tremor is an important symptom to evaluate correctly. The diagnostic model, including causes is presented in TABLE 33.4. A common pitfall in patients presenting with tremor is for Parkinson disease (PD) to be diagnosed as benign essential tremor and for benign essential tremor to be diagnosed as PD, but the clinical distinction is not always easy and it must be remembered that as many as 20% will experience both concurrently.

Resting tremor—Parkinsonian

The tremor of PD is present at rest. The hand tremor is most marked with the arms supported on the lap and during walking. The characteristic movement is 'pill-rolling' where movement of the fingers at the metacarpophalangeal joints is combined with movements of the thumb. The resting tremor decreases on finger–nose testing. The best way to evoke the tremor is to distract the patient, such as focusing attention on the left hand with a view to 'examining' the right hand or by asking the patient to turn the head from side to side.

Action or postural tremor

This fine tremor is noted by examining the patient with the arms outstretched and the fingers apart. The tremor may be rendered more obvious if a sheet of paper is placed over the dorsum of the hands. The tremor is present throughout movement, being accentuated by voluntary contraction.

Causes

- Essential tremor (also called familial tremor or benign essential tremor)
- Senile tremor
- Physiological
- Anxiety/emotional
- Hyperthyroidism
- Alcohol
- Drugs, for example, drug withdrawal (e.g. heroin, cocaine, alcohol), amphetamines, lithium, sympathomimetics (bronchodilators), sodium valproate, heavy metals (e.g. mercury), caffeine, amiodarone
- Phaeochromocytoma

33

Table 33.4 Tremor: diagnostic strategy model

Probability diagnosis Benign essential (familial) tremor Senility Physiological Parkinson disease (including drug-induced PD) Anxiety/emotional Alcohol	**Key history** • Nature of the tremor: resting, intention, pill-rolling, flapping (asterixis) • Family history of tremor • Evidence of cognitive changes or other neurological problems • Systems review: respiratory, cardiac, liver, kidneys
Serious disorders not to be missed *Vascular:* cerebral infarction → Parkinsonism *Infection* meningoencephalitis tertiary syphilis *Cancer/tumour:* cerebral tumour (frontal lobe) *Other:* toxicity from organ failure (kidney, liver, lungs)	**Key examination** • General appearance and vital signs • Respiratory, cardiac, abdominal (esp. liver) and neurological examination **Key investigations** According to above: • FBE and ESR • thyroid functions tests (hyperthyroidism), LFTs, pulse oximetry/blood gases • drug screen • MRI
Pitfalls often missed Cerebellar disease Multiple sclerosis Fragile X sydrome Alzheimer dementia Uraemia of kidney failure CO_2 retention of respiratory failure Hepatic failure *Rarities:* hepatolenticular degeneration (Wilson disease) lesion of midbrain (red nucleus)	**Diagnostic tips** • Essential tremor eased by a small quantity of alcohol • Triad of essential tremor: postural or action tremor, head tremor, positive family history • Look for Parkinson tetrad: resting tremor, bradykinesia, rigidity, postural instability • Look for cerebellar tetrad: intention tremor, dysarthria, nystagmus, ataxic gait • Typical drugs that induce Parkinsonism are phenothiazine, butyrophenones, reserpine
Seven masquerades checklist Drugs (withdrawal, e.g. opioids, stimulants, illicit agents, benzodiazepines, caffeine, alcohol; adverse reactions, e.g. sympathomimetics, β agonists, lithium, phenthiazines, valproate, amiodarone, alcohol) Thyroid/other endocrine (hyperthyroidism, hypoglycaemia, phaeochromocytoma)	
Is the patient trying to tell me something? Anxiety (esp. hyperventilation)	

Intention tremor (cerebellar disease)

This coarse oscillating tremor is absent at rest but exacerbated by action and increases as the target is approached. It is tested by 'finger–nose–finger' touching or running the heel down the opposite shin, and past pointing of the nose is a feature. It occurs in cerebellar lobe disease and with lesions of cerebellar connections.

Flapping (metabolic tremor)

A flapping or 'wing-beating' tremor is observed when the arms are extended with hyperextension of the wrists. It involves slow, coarse and jerky movements of flexion and extension at the wrists.

Note: Flapping (asterixis) is not strictly a tremor.

Causes

- Wilson syndrome
- Hepatic encephalopathy

- Uraemia
- Respiratory failure
- Lesions of the red nucleus of the midbrain (the classic cause of a flap)

Essential tremor

Essential tremor, which is probably the most common movement disorder (2–5% prevalence), has been variously called benign, familial, senile or juvenile tremor.

Clinical features

- Autosomal dominant disorder (variable penetrance)
- Often begins in early adult life, even adolescence
- Usually begins with a slight tremor in both hands
- May involve head (titubation), chin and tongue and rarely trunk and legs
- Interferes with writing (not micrographic), handling cups of tea and spoons, etc.
- Tremor most marked when arms held out (postural tremor); less evident at rest
- Tremor exacerbated by anxiety
- May affect speech if it involves bulbar musculature
- Relieved by alcohol
- Can swing arm and gait normal

Triad of features

- Positive family history
- Tremor with little disability
- Normal gait

Distinguishing essential tremor from Parkinson disease

This is not always easy as a postural tremor can be present in PD although the hand tremor is most marked at rest with the arms supported on the lap. Parkinsonian tremor is slower at 4–6 Hz while essential tremor is much faster at around 8–13 Hz. Imaging is unnecessary.

A most useful way to differentiate the two causes is to observe the gait. It is normal in essential tremor but in PD there may be loss of arm swing and the step is usually shortened with stooped posture and shuffling gait.

Management

Most patients do not need treatment and all that is required is an appropriate explanation.[1] If necessary, use propranolol (first choice) or primidone 62.5 mg nocte (up to 250 mg).[3] A typical starting dose of propranolol is 10–20 mg bd; many require 120–240 mg/day.[3] If the tremor is only intrusive at times of increased emotional stress, intermittent use of benzodiazepines (e.g. lorazepam 1 mg) 30 minutes before exposure to the stress may be all that is required. Modest alcohol intake (e.g. a glass of whisky) is very effective. A standard drink of alcohol often alleviates the tremor. Larger doses of alcohol have no additional effect. If drugs fail, deep brain stimulation to the thalamus can be used.

Parkinson disease

Parkinson disease (PD) is a disorder of the automatic processor of the brain which relies on dopamine to maintain movements at a selected size and speed. Loss of dopamine causes movements to become smaller and slower. The pathological features are loss of dopamine-producing neurones from the substantia nigra in the brain stem together with Lewy bodies in the neurones.[4] Genetic factors occur in 5% of individuals.

One of the most important clinical aspects of PD, which has a slow and insidious onset, is the ability to make an early diagnosis. Sometimes this can be very difficult, especially when the tremor is absent or mild, as occurs with the atherosclerotic degenerative type of Parkinsonism. The lack of any specific abnormality on special investigation leaves the responsibility for a diagnosis based on the history and examination. As a general rule of thumb the diagnosis of PD is restricted to those who respond to levodopa (L-dopa)—the rest are termed Parkinsonism or 'Parkinson plus'.

The classic quintet of PD

1. tremor (at rest)
2. rigidity
3. bradykinesia
4. postural instability
5. gait freezing

$\geq$2 signs = Parkinson disease

Key facts and checkpoints

- PD is a most common and disabling chronic neurological disorder. About 90% are idiopathic.
- The prevalence in Australia is 120–150 per 100 000.[5] Lifetime risk is 1 in 40.
- The mean age of onset is between 58 and 62 years.[5]
- The incidence rises sharply over 70 years of age (peak 65 years).[5]
- The diagnosis is based on the history and examination.
- Always think of PD in an older person presenting with falls.
- A reduced sense of smell is one of the first symptoms. Others that may precede PD include

constipation, REM sleep disorders and orthostatic hypotension.
- Non-motor automatic dysfunctions: cognition, behaviour, mood.
- Hemi-Parkinsonism can occur; all the signs are confined to one side and thus must be differentiated from hemiparesis. In fact, most cases of PD start unilaterally.
- Always consider drug-induced Parkinsonism. The usual drugs are phenothiazines, butyrophenones and reserpine. Tremor is uncommon but rigidity and bradykinesia may be severe.
- Other causes include vascular (atherosclerosis) and normal pressure hydrocephalus.

Refer to TABLE 33.5.

Signs

- Power, reflexes and sensation are usually normal.
- The earliest abnormal physical signs to appear are loss of dexterity of rapid alternating movements and absence of arm swing, in addition to increased tone with distraction.

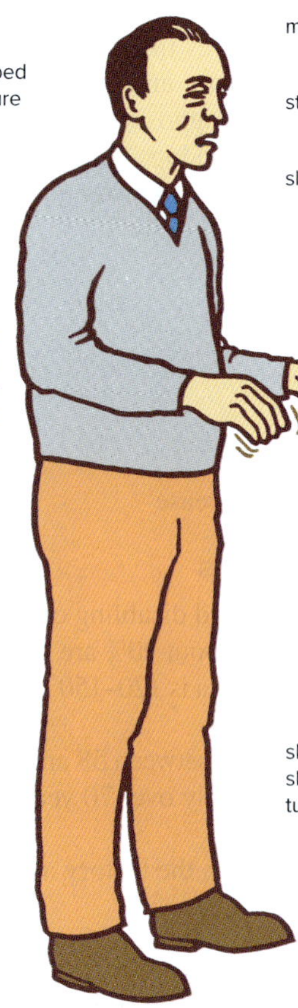
masked facies
stooped posture
staring expression
slow, monotonous speech
failure to swing arm or arms
pill-rolling tremor at rest
slow and shuffling gait
short steps
turning by 'numbers'

FIGURE 33.2 Basic clinical features of Parkinson disease[6]

- Positive frontal lobe signs, such as grasp and glabellar taps (only allow three blinks), are more common with Parkinsonism.

Note: There is no laboratory test for PD—it is a clinical diagnosis. Hypothyroidism and depression, which also cause slowness of movement, may cause confusion with diagnosis.

Note: The Steele–Richardson–Olszewksi syndrome (also known as progressive supranuclear palsy—PSP parkinsonism, mild dementia and vertical gaze dysfunction) is worth considering.

Three major traps in missing early diagnosis:[5]

- Age: 10–15% are <50 years at onset
- Belief that it is a disease of men: M = F
- Absence of resting tremor (only 50% have it at onset)

Principles of management

- Provide appropriate explanation and education.
- Explain that PD is slowly progressive and is improved but not cured by treatment. It is associated with increased mortality (RR death compared with general population ranges 1.6 to 3). The question of whether treatment reduces mortality remains controversial.[7]
- Refer to a specialist for shared care—from outset.
- Support systems are necessary for advanced PD.
- Walking sticks (which spread the centre of gravity) with appropriate education into their use may be necessary to help prevent falls, and constant care is required, so that admission to a nursing home for end-stage disease may be appropriate.
- Correct dopamine deficiency and/or block cholinergic excess in the brain.

Management (pharmacological)[8,9]

Avoid postponing treatment. It should be commenced as soon as symptoms interfere with working capacity or the patient's enjoyment of life. This will be apparent only if the correct questions are asked as the patient may accept impaired enjoyment without appreciating that it is due to PD. Start low—L-dopa 100/25 (½ tab bd) and go slow. There is usually no difference between the L-dopa preparations. The dosage should be tailored so that the patient neither develops side effects nor is on an inadequate dose of medication without significant therapeutic benefit (see TABLE 33.6). The dose usually progresses to 1 tab bd, then consider add-on therapy.

The older drugs, such as anticholinergics and amantadine, still have a place in modern management but

Table 33.5 Parkinson disease: symptoms and signs (a checklist)

General	Tiredness Lethargy Restlessness Trouble getting out of chair or car and turning over in bed
Tremor	Present at rest Slow rate—4 to 6 cycles per second Alternating, especially arms Pill-rolling (severe cases) *Note:* may be absent or unilateral
Rigidity	'Cogwheel'—'juddering' on passive extension of the forearm—feels like going through cogs Lead pipe—limbs resist passive extension through movement (constant resistance)
Motor: bradykinesia/hypokinesia	Slowness of initiating a movement Difficulty with fine finger tasks Micrographia (see FIG. 33.3) Masked facies Relative lack of blinking Impaired convergence of eyes Excessive salivation (late) Swallowing problems (can aspirate) Difficulty turning over in bed and rising from a chair Slow, soft monotonous speech/dysarthria
Gait disorder	No arm swing on one or both sides Start hesitation Slow, shuffling and narrow based Short steps (petit pas) Slow turning circle ('turn by numbers') 'Freezing' when approaching an obstacle Festination
Disequilibrium	Poor balance Impaired righting reflexes Falls—may be first thing that leads to presentation
Posture	Progressive forward flexion of trunk (stooped) Flexion of elbow at affected side
Autonomic symptoms	Constipation (common) Postural hypotension—may be induced by treatment
Neuropsychiatric	Depression (early), anxiety, sleep disorder Progressive dementia in 30–40% usually after 10 years[6] Hallucinations—either with Lewy body dementia or treatment

L-dopa, which basically counters bradykinesia, is the best drug and the baseline of treatment. With the onset of disability (motor disturbances) L-dopa in combination with a decarboxylase inhibitor (carbidopa or benserazide) in a 4:1 ratio should be introduced. L-dopa therapy does not significantly improve tremor but improves

Table 33.6 Anti-Parkinson drugs[8,9]

Agent	Main adverse effects
Dopaminergic (standard and slow release)	
• L-dopa + benserazide	Nausea and vomiting (initially) Orthostatic hypotension
• L-dopa + carbidopa	Involuntary dyskinetic movements Psychiatric disturbances Compulsive behaviour (as below) On–off phenomena End-of-dose failure Constipation
Dopamine agonists	
Ergot derivatives (not recommended): • bromocriptine • cabergoline • pergolide	Nausea and vomiting Dizziness, fatigue, somnolence Compulsive behaviours (gambling, punding, hypersexuality) Orthostatic hypotension
Non-ergot derivatives: • pramipexole • ropinirole • rotigotine	
• apomorphine	Nausea, psychosis, dyskinesia
Anticholinergics	
• benzhexol	Dryness of mouth GIT upset Constipation
• benztropine	Confusion in elderly
• biperiden	Contraindicated in glaucoma and prostatism
COMT inhibitors	
• entacapone	Diarrhoea, discoloured urine
• combination entacapone/ L-dopa-carbidopa (Stalevo)	Sleep problems
MAO-B inhibitors	
• selegiline	Dry mouth
• rasagiline	Neuropsychiatric disturbances Nausea Dizziness, fatigue Insomnia
Others	
• amantadine	Nausea and vomiting Insomnia Nightmares Neuropsychiatric disturbances Ankle oedema Livedo reticularis

rigidity, dyskinesia and gait disorder. Consider benzhexol or benztropine if tremor is the feature, especially in young patients.

The new non-ergot derivative dopamine agonists can be used in treatment, especially with the L-dopa 'on–off' phenomenon (fluctuations throughout the day). They are preferred to the ergot derivatives because of a superior adverse effect profile. They appear to be most effective when used in combination. The ergot derivatives can have serious adverse effects,

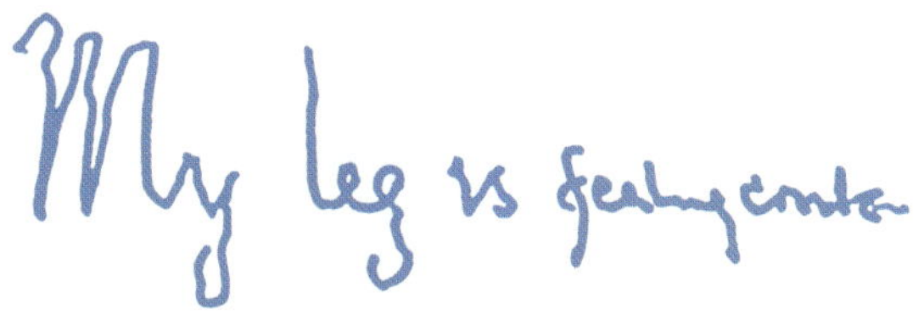

FIGURE 33.3 Micrographia, one of the signs of Parkinson disease

including cardiac valve damage, and are no longer recommended. Selegiline is an effective second-line drug, especially in combination with Sinemet. If there is associated pain, depression or insomnia, the tricyclic agents (e.g. amitriptyline) can be effective.

Entacapone has the potential to increase 'on time' and reduce motor fluctuations in L-dopa treated patients who are beginning to experience end-of-dose failure. The initial dose is 200 mg and best used when combined with L-dopa.

Treatment strategy[8,9]

Mild (minimal disability):

- L-dopa preparation (low dose), e.g. L-dopa 100 mg + carbidopa 25 mg (½ tab bd—increase gradually as necessary to 1 tab (o) tds)

  or

- amantadine 100 mg (o) daily may help the young or the elderly for up to 12 months—if inadequate response
- selegiline up to 5 mg bd can be added to L-dopa if necessary

Moderate (independent but disabled, e.g. writing, movements, gait):

- L-dopa preparation
- selegiline 1 mg bd

  and/or

- Add if necessary—non-ergot dopamine agent
  - pramipexole start with 0.25 mg transdermally daily
  - rotigotine start with 2 mg daily

Severe (disabled, dependent on others):

- L-dopa (to maximum tolerated dose) + non-ergot dopamine agent
- Add entacapone 200 mg (o) with each dose of L-dopa, e.g. Stalevo
- Consider antidepressants

An example of a practical treatment algorithm is presented in FIGURE 33.4.

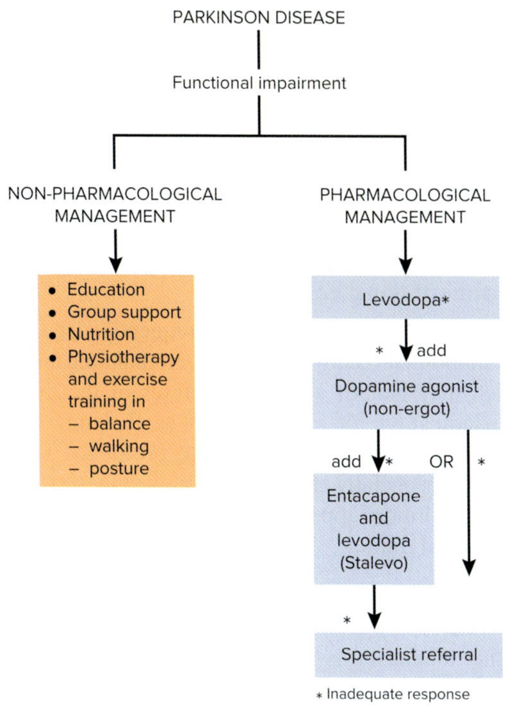

FIGURE 33.4 Management of early Parkinson disease: one possible pathway

Long-term problems

After 3–5 years of L-dopa treatment, side effects may appear in about one-half of patients:[5]

- involuntary movements—dyskinesia
- end-of-dose failure (reduced duration of effect to 2–3 hours only)—consider entacapone
- 'on–off' phenomenon (sudden inability to move, with recovery in 30–90 minutes)
- early morning dystonia, such as clawing of toes (due to disease—not a side effect)

  Specialist advice is appropriate.

Advanced disease[8]

Under consultant and good home/nursing care:

- Apomorphine can be used for severe akinesia not responsive to L-dopa
- For nausea and vomiting side effects: domperidone 20 mg (o) tds 24 hours prior to apomorphine
- Better control may also be achieved with: amantadine 100 mg (o) bd
- Duodopa—levodopa into jejunum

Contraindicated drugs

- Phenothiazines and other older antipsychotics
- Butyrophenones

Multidisciplinary care

This important strategy includes physiotherapy, occupational therapy, physical therapy, e.g. tai chi, and psychiatry/psychology, e.g. CBT, mindfulness.

Treatment (surgical)

The preferred method is high-frequency deep brain stimulation via electrodes into the subthalamic nucleus, which may benefit all major features of the disease. The indication for surgery such as thalamotomy is erratic and disabling responses to prolonged L-dopa therapy, especially for annoying dyskinesias. It is considered more appropriate for younger patients with a unilateral tremor.[8]

When to refer

If the diagnosis is unclear at the time of initial presentation, it is appropriate either to review the patient at a later date or to refer the patient for more neurological assessment.

Once diagnosed or highly suspected it is best to refer to establish the diagnosis and to seek advice on initiation of treatment. Patients and families usually prefer this approach. In the initial years before motor fluctuations develop, management could be performed by the GP according to an overall plan developed in liaison with a neurological colleague. When fluctuations develop and end-stage diseases manifest (e.g. gait disorders), specialist supervision is appropriate.[1]

Red flags in Parkinson disease and differential diagnosis[10]

Bilateral onset (PSP)
Poor response to L-dopa
Dysautonomia—bladder, orthostatic hypotension (MSA)
Dystonia (PSP)
Anterocollis (head flexed) (MSA)
Retrocollis (head extended) (PSP)
Myoclonus (CBD, CJD)
Early onset dementia (LBD)

CBD = corticobasal degeneration, CJD = Creutzfeldt–Jakob disease, LBD = Lewy body dementia, MSA = multiple system atrophy, PSP = progressive supranuclear palsy

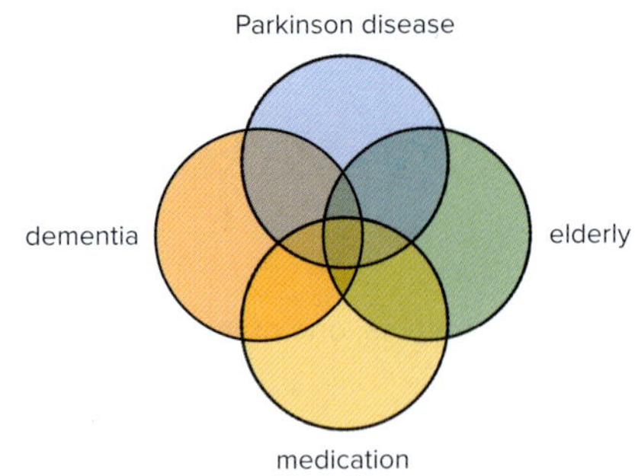

FIGURE 33.5 Factors contributing to psychosis

Cognitive impairment with Parkinson disease[4,11]

This may be due to multiple factors including Parkinson associated dementia, Lewy body dementia, Alzheimer disease and medication, all of which can induce psychosis, but L-dopa is the least likely. Neuropsychiatric symptoms, which can be varied and bizarre and usually worse in the evening, can occur. Factors contributing to psychosis are illustrated in FIGURE 33.5. Management is based on monotherapy with gradual build-up of L-dopa to maximum tolerated dose, for example, 450–600 mg/day.

Practice tips for Parkinson disease

- One of the simplest diagnostic tools for PD, as compared with Parkinsonism, is a trial of therapy with L-dopa. The response is excellent while that for Parkinsonism is poor.
- L-dopa is the gold standard for therapy.
- Ensure that a distinction is made between drug-induced involuntary movements and the tremor of PD.
- Keep the dose of L-dopa as low as possible to avoid these drug-induced involuntary movements.
- In the elderly with a fractured hip always consider PD (a manifestation of disequilibrium).
- Remember the balance of psychosis and PD in treatment.
- Keep in mind the 'sundown' effect—patients often go psychotic as the sun goes down.
- Don't fail to attend to the needs of the family, who often suffer in silence.
- If drugs are to be withdrawn they should be withdrawn slowly.

Management (psychotic problems)

- Treat as an inpatient
- Exclude and treat comorbidities, e.g. UTI
- Eliminate and wean off worst drugs
- Increase L-dopa slowly to 150 mg tds or qid
- Give quetiapine or olanzapine at night-time

Paraesthesia and numbness

The diagnostic strategy model for paraesthesia and numbness is presented in TABLE 33.7.

Table 33.7 Paraesthesia and numbness: diagnostic strategy model

Probability diagnosis
Diabetic peripheral neuropathy
Nutritional peripheral neuropathy, esp. alcohol, B12, folate
Hyperventilation with anxiety
Nerve root pressure, e.g. sciatica, cervical spondylosis
Nerve entrapment, esp. carpal tunnel syndrome
Serious disorders not to be missed
Vascular:
CVA/TIA
Peripheral vascular disease
Infection:
AIDs
Lyme disease/suspected tick-borne disease
Leprosy
Some viral infections
Tumour/cancer:
Disseminated malignancy
Cerebral/spinal cord tumours
Other:
Uremia
Guillain–Barré syndrome
Trauma to spinal cord
Marine fish toxins, e.g. toadfish, ciguatera
Pitfalls (often missed)
Migraine variant with focal signs
Multiple sclerosis/transverse myelitis
Hypocalcaemia
Rarities:
Chronic inflammatory polyneuropathy
Amyloidosis
Heavy metal toxicity, e.g. lead
Seven masquerades checklist
Diabetes
Drugs, e.g. cytotoxic agents, interferon (see list)
Anaemia—pernicious anaemia
Thyroid/other endocrine—hypothyroid?
Spinal dysfunction
Is the patient trying to tell me something?
Consider conversion reaction (hysteria), severe anxiety disorder
Some cases may be idiopathic

Multiple sclerosis

Multiple sclerosis (MS) is the most common cause of progressive neurological disability in the 20–50 year age group.[10] It is generally accepted that MS is an autoimmune disorder. Genetic and environmental factors are believed to play a role.[12] Early diagnosis is difficult because MS is characterised by widespread neurologic lesions that cannot be explained by a single anatomical lesion, and the various symptoms and signs are subject to irregular exacerbations and remissions. The lesions are 'separated in time and space'. The most important issue in diagnosis is the need for a high index of suspicion. The use of MRI has revolutionised the diagnosis of MS.

MS is a primary demyelinating disorder with demyelination occurring in plaques throughout the white and grey matter of the brain, brain stem, spinal cord and optic nerves. The clinical features depend on their location. There is a loss of brain volume.

There is a variety of types of MS—relapsing remitting (most common), secondary progressive, progressive relapsing and primary progressive—together with 'benign' and 'malignant' forms.

Clinical features

See FIGURE 33.6.

- More common in females (3:1)
- Peak age of onset is in the fourth decade
- Transient motor and sensory disturbances
- UMN signs
- Symptoms develop over several days but can be sudden
- Monosymptomatic initially in about 80%
- Only 20% have a benign disease
- Multiple symptoms initially in about 20%
- Common initial symptoms include:
  - visual disturbances of optic neuritis (blurred vision or loss of vision in one eye—sometimes both); central scotoma with pain on eye movement (looks like unilateral papilloedema)
  - diplopia (brain-stem lesion)
  - weakness in one or both legs, paraparesis or monoparesis
  - sensory impairment in the lower limbs and trunk: numbness, paraesthesia; band-like sensations; clumsiness of limb (loss of position sense); feeling as though walking on cotton wool
  - vertigo (brain-stem lesion)
- Subsequent remissions and exacerbations that vary from one individual to another

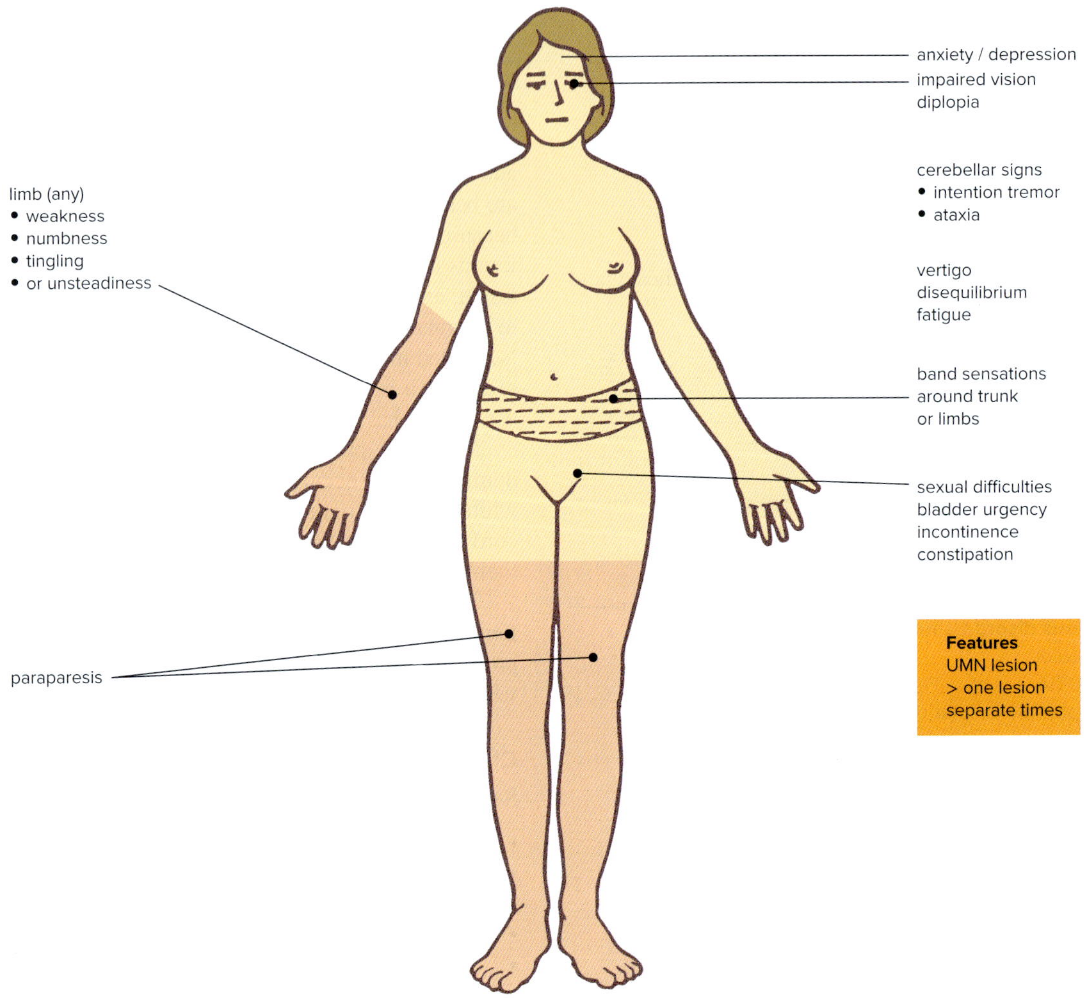

FIGURE 33.6 Basic clinical signs in multiple sclerosis

- 80% have a relapsing remitting disease
- There is a progressive form, esp. in women around 50 years
- Anxiety, depression and other mood disorders are common

Symptoms causing diagnostic confusion

- Bladder disturbances, including retention of urine and urgency
- 'Useless hand' due to loss of position sense
- Facial palsy
- Trigeminal neuralgia
- Psychiatric symptoms

In established disease, common symptoms are fatigue, impotence and bladder disturbances.

Examination (neurological)

The findings depend on the site of the lesion or lesions and include optic atrophy, weakness, hyper-reflexia, extensor plantar responses, nystagmus (two types—cerebellar or ataxic), ataxia, incoordination and regional impairment of sensation.

Diagnosis

The diagnosis is clinical along with the MRI and depends on the following determinants:

- Lesions are invariably UMN.
- >1 part of CNS is involved, although not necessarily at time of presentation.
- Episodes are separated in time and space.
- Practically MS can only be diagnosed after a second relapse or when the MRI shows new lesions.[10]

- An early diagnosis requires evidence of contrast-enhancing lesions or new T2 lesions on the MRI indicating dissemination in time.
- The diagnostic criteria is based on the internationally accepted 2010 McDonald criteria (refer to www.nice.org.uk).[12,13]

Other neurological disorders such as infections (e.g. encephalitis), malignancies, spinal cord compression, spinocerebellar degeneration and others must be excluded.

Investigation

- Lumbar puncture: oligoclonal IgG detected in CSF in 90% of cases[14] (only if necessary)
- Visual evoked potentials: abnormal in about 90% of cases
- MRI scan: usually abnormal, demonstrating MS lesions in about 90% of cases[14]

Course and prognosis

- The course is variable and difficult to predict. An early onset (<30 years) is usually 'benign' while a late onset (≥50 years) is often 'malignant'.
- MS follows a classic history of relapses and remissions in 80–85% of patients.[14]
- The rate of relapse is about once in 2 years.
- About 20% have a progressive course from the onset with a progressive spastic paraparesis (applies mainly to late-age onset).
- The average duration of MS is about 40 years from diagnosis to death.[14]
- A 'benign' course occurs in about 30% of patients with 10–20% never suffering major disability.
- The median time to needing a walking aid is 15 years.[8]
- The likelihood of developing MS after a single episode of optic neuritis is about 60%.

Management principles

- All patients should be referred to a neurologist for confirmation of the diagnosis, which must be accurate.
- Explanation about the disorder and its natural history should be given.
- Acute relapses require treatment if causing significant disability.
- Depression and anxiety, which are common, require early treatment, e.g. paroxetine.
- CBT or mindfulness-based interventions.

Treatment (relapses)

Mild relapses

Mild symptoms, such as numbness and tingling, require only confirmation, rest and reassurance.

Moderate relapses

- Prednisolone—in outpatient setting

Severe relapses or attacks[8,15]

These attacks include optic neuritis, paraplegia or brain-stem signs. Admit to hospital for IV therapy:

- methylprednisolone 1 g in 200 mL saline by slow IV infusion (1 hour) daily for 3 days

  Plasma exchange may be used.

  Observe carefully for cardiac arrhythmias.

Drugs to prevent relapses[16]

Currently first-line immunomodulators are the interferons, glatiramer acetate and the monoclonal antibodies natalizumab and alemtuzumab.

Interferon beta-1b (SC injection) and beta-1a (IM injection) appear to be effective (but expensive) for those with frequent and severe attacks.

New agents being evaluated include teriflunamide, daclizumab, ocrelizumab and Biotin.

Treatment (symptoms)[7,16]

Spasticity

- Physiotherapy
- Baclofen 10–25 mg (o) nocte
- For continuous drug therapy: baclofen 5 mg (o) tds, increasing to 25 mg (o) tds + diazepam 2–10 mg (o) tds
- An alternative is dantrolene

Paroxysmal (e.g. neuralgias)

- Carbamazepine or gabapentin

Cannabis

The reported efficacy of the cannabis-based medicine Stativex for relaxation, pain and bladder function is still being debated. One RCT showed a positive effect on detrusor activity.[18]

See references 8 and 16 for treatment of other symptoms.

Peripheral neuropathy

Peripheral neuropathy (PN) refers to all conditions causing nerve damage outside the central nervous system. It can be a mononeuropathy, such as carpal tunnel syndrome; mononeuropathy multiplex involving multiple single nerves in an asymmetric pattern (as in vasculitides); or a polyneuropathy, which is a diffuse symmetric disorder best referred to as PN. It can be classified according to clinical progression as acute, subacute or chronic. The manifestations can be sensory, motor, autonomic or mixed (sensorimotor).

- Sensory symptoms: tingling, burning, numbness in extremities, unsteady gait (loss of position sense)
- Motor symptoms (LMN): weakness or clumsiness in hands, foot/wrist drop
- Signs: may be classic 'glove and stocking' sensory loss, sensory ataxia, LMN signs—distal muscle wasting, muscle weakness, reflexes absent or depressed, fasciculations

Causes

- Mostly sensory: diabetes mellitus, vitamin deficiency (folate, B1, B6, B12), alcohol, various neurotoxic drugs, leprosy, uraemia (CKF), amyloidosis, malignancy
- Mostly motor: lead poisoning, porphyria, various neurotoxic drugs, Charcot–Marie–Tooth syndrome (peroneal muscle atrophy), acquired inflammatory polyneuropathies—acute (Guillain–Barré syndrome) and chronic (chronic inflammatory demyelinating polyneuropathy)

Note: In many instances no cause is found despite a full history and examination.

Management

Refer to a suitably qualified consultant for diagnosis particularly via electrophysiology.

Acute inflammatory polyradiculoneuropathy (Guillain–Barré syndrome)

Guillain–Barré syndrome, which is a rapidly progressive and treatable cause of PN or ascending radiculopathy, is potentially fatal. Early diagnosis of this serious disease by the family doctor is crucial as respiratory paralysis may lead to death. The underlying pathology is segmental demyelination of the peripheral nerves and nerve roots.

Clinical features

- Weakness in the limbs (usually symmetrical)
- Paraesthesia or pain in the limbs (less common)
- Both proximal and distal muscles affected, usually starts peripherally and moves proximally
- Facial and bulbar paralysis (rare)
- Weakness of extraocular muscles (rarely)
- Reflexes depressed or absent
- Variable sensory loss but rare

Within 3–4 weeks the motor neuropathy, which is the main feature, progresses to a maximum disability, possibly with complete quadriparesis and respiratory paralysis.[19]

Investigation

- CSF protein is elevated; cells are usually normal.
- Motor nerve conduction studies are abnormal.

Management

- Admit to hospital.
- Respiratory function (vital capacity) should be measured regularly (2–4 hours at first).
- Tracheostomy and artificial ventilation may be necessary.
- Physiotherapy to prevent foot and wrist drop and other general care should be provided.
- Treatment is with plasma exchange or IV immunoglobulin (0.4 g/kg/day for 5 days), which may need to be continued monthly.[8]
- Corticosteroids are not generally recommended.

Outcome

About 80% of patients recover without significant disability. Approximately 5% relapse.[19]

Chronic inflammatory demyelinating polyneuropathy[8,20]

This acquired immunological disorder is similar to Guillain–Barré syndrome except that it has a slower and more protracted course. Diagnosis is by nerve studies and treatment is with corticosteroids, plasmapheresis or IV immunoglobin.

Charcot–Marie–Tooth syndrome

This is an inherited autosomal dominant polyneuropathy with an insidious onset from puberty. Clinical features include weakness in the legs, variable distal sensory loss and muscle atrophy giving the 'inverted champagne bottle' appearance of the legs. The features vary according to the various subgroups. Refer for electrodiagnostic studies and specific genetic testing.

Familial periodic paralysis

An autosomal dominant skeletal muscle disorder. Clinical features:

- young patient (usually adolescent)
- day after vigorous exercise awakens with weakness in limbs (for 4–24 hours)
- flaccid paralysis/loss of deep tendon reflexes

Related to potassium levels—measure during symptoms. Classify as high, low or normal.

Table 33.8	Clinical classification of acquired myasthenia gravis
Group I	Ocular MG
Group IIA	Mild generalised MG
Group IIB	Moderate to severe MG
Group III	Acute severe (fulminating) MG with respiratory muscle weakness
Group IV	Late (chronic) severe MG

Myasthenia gravis

Myasthenia gravis (MG) is an acquired autoimmune disorder that usually affects muscle strength. Patients have fluctuating symptoms and variable distribution of muscle weakness. All degrees of severity, ranging from occasional mild ptosis to fulminant quadriplegia and respiratory arrest, can occur[21] (see TABLE 33.8). It is associated with thymic tumour and other autoimmune diseases, for example, RA, SLE, thyroid and pernicious anaemia.

Clinical features

- Painless fatigue with exercise
- Weakness also precipitated by emotional stress, pregnancy, infection, surgery
- Variable distribution of weakness:
  - ocular: ptosis (60%) and diplopia (see FIG. 33.7); ocular myasthenia only remains in about 10%
  - bulbar: weakness of chewing, swallowing, speech (ask to count to 100), whistling and head lolling
  - limbs (proximal and distal)
  - generalised
  - respiratory: breathlessness, ventilatory failure

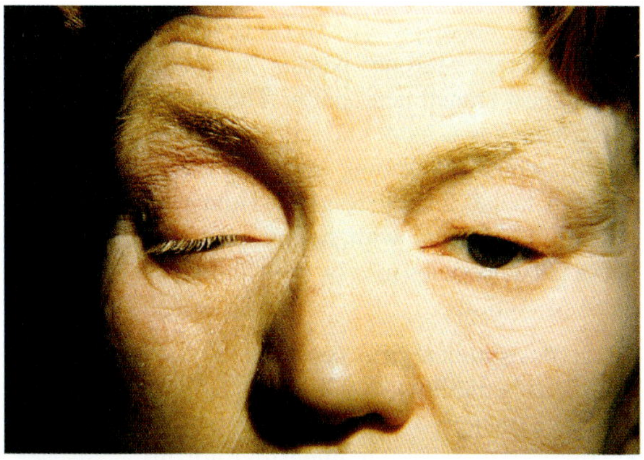

FIGURE 33.7 Myasthenia gravis in a 40-year-old woman with a 12-month history of increasing muscular weakness including drooping of the eyelids. Ptosis, especially on the right side, is apparent.

Note: The classic MG image is 'the thinker'—the hand used to hold the mouth closed and the head up.

Diagnosis

- Serum anti-acetylcholine receptor antibodies
- Electrophysiological tests if antibody test negative
- CT scan to detect thymoma
- Edrophonium test still useful but potentially dangerous (atropine is the antidote)

Management principles[8,21]

- Refer for consultant management.
- Detect possible presence of thymoma with CT or MR scan of thorax. If present, removal is recommended.
- Thymectomy is recommended early for generalised myasthenia, especially in all younger patients with hyperplasia of the thymus, even if not confirmed preoperatively.
- Plasmapheresis is useful for acute crisis or where temporary improvement is required or patients are resistant to treatment.
- Avoid drugs that are relatively contraindicated.
- Pharmacological agents:
  - anticholinesterase inhibitor drugs (e.g. pyridostigmine, neostigmine or distigmine) should be used only for mild-to-moderate symptoms
  - corticosteroids are useful for all grades of MG (should be introduced slowly).

Practice tips for myasthenia gravis

- The combination of ocular and facial weakness should alert the family doctor to the possibility of a neuromuscular disorder, especially MG or mitochondrial myopathy.[20] Look for weakness and fatigue.
- Beware of facioscapulohumeral dystrophy.
- Ptosis may develop only after looking upwards for a minute or longer.
- Smiling may have a characteristic snarling quality.

Ptosis

It is worth remembering that the four major causes of ptosis are:

1. 3rd cranial nerve palsy—ptosis, eye facing 'down and out', dilated pupil, sluggish light reflex
2. Horner syndrome—ptosis, miosis (constricted pupil), ipsilateral loss of sweating

3 Mitochondrial myopathy—progressive external ophthalmoplegia or limb weakness, induced by activity—no pupil involvement
4 Myasthenia gravis—ptosis and diplopia, no pupil involvement

Dystonia

Dystonias are sustained or intermittent abnormal repetitive movements or postures resulting from alterations in muscle tone. The dystonic spasms may affect one (focal) or more (segmental) parts of the body or the whole body (generalised).

Key facts and checkpoints

- Misdiagnosis is common as transient symptoms may be mistaken for an emotional or psychiatric disorder. Many cases take years to diagnose.
- Dystonias are often regarded as nervous tics.
- The cause is thought to be disorders of the basal ganglia of the brain, but mainly there is no known specific cause.
- Neuroleptic and dopamine receptor blocking agents (e.g. L-dopa, metoclopramide) can induce a severe generalised dystonia (e.g. oculogyric crisis) which is treated with benztropine 1–2 mg IM or IV.[8] However, L-dopa is the drug of choice in some L-dopa responsive dystonias.

Focal dystonias

- *Blepharospasm* is a focal dystonia of the muscles around the eye resulting in uncontrolled blinking, especially in bright light. This is best treated with botulinum toxin, type A.
- *Oromandibular dystonia* affects the jaw, tongue and mouth, resulting in jaw grinding movements and grimacing. Proper speech and swallowing may be disrupted.
- *Meige syndrome* is a combination of blepharospasm and oromandibular dystonia.

Note: It must be differentiated from the buccal-lingual-facial movements of tardive dyskinesia.

- *Hemifacial spasm* involves involuntary, irregular muscle contractions and spasms affecting one side of the face. It usually starts with twitching around the eye and then spreads to involve all the facial muscles on one side. It is usually due to irritation of the facial nerve in its intracranial course and surgical intervention may alleviate this problem.
- *Writer's cramp, typist's cramp, pianist's cramp, golfer's cramp* are all occupational focal dystonias of the hand and/or forearm initiated by performing these skilled acts.
- *Cervical dystonia* or *spasmodic torticollis* is a focal dystonia of the unilateral cervical muscles. It usually begins with a pulling sensation followed by twisting or jerking of the head, leading to deviation of the head and neck to one side. In early stages patients can voluntarily overcome the dystonia.
- *Laryngeal* or *spastic dystonia* is a focal dystonia of the laryngeal muscles resulting in a strained, hoarse or creaking voice. It may lead to inability to speak in more than a whisper.

Treatment

The current treatment for focal or segmental (spread to an adjacent body region) dystonias is localised injection of purified botulinum A toxin into the affected muscle groups. The dosage is highly individualised and needs to be repeated at intervals of 3 and 6 months. The injections have to be given with great caution, ideally by a registered injector.

Tics

Motor and vocal tics are a feature of Tourette disorder. If socially disabling treat with:

- haloperidol 0.25 mg (o) nocte, very gradually increasing to 2 g (max.) daily[7]

  or

- clonidine 25 mcg (o) bd for 2 weeks, then 50–75 mcg bd

Facial nerve (Bell) palsy[15]

Facial (7th nerve palsy), which is an acute unilateral lower motor neurone paresis or paralysis, is the commonest cranial neuropathy. The classic type is Bell palsy, which is usually idiopathic although attributed to an inflammatory swelling involving the facial nerve in the bony facial canal. In Ramsay–Hunt syndrome, which is due to infection with herpes zoster causing facial nerve palsy, vesicles may be seen on the ipsilateral ear.

Associations:

- herpes simplex virus (postulated)
- diabetes mellitus
- hypertension
- thyroid disorder, e.g. hyperthyroidism

Clinical features

- Abrupt onset (can worsen over 2–5 days)
- Weakness in the face (complete or incomplete)

- Preceding pain in or behind the ear
- Impaired blinking
- Bell phenomenon—when closing the eye it turns up under the half-closed lid

Less common:

- Difficulty eating
- Loss of taste—anterior two-thirds of tongue
- Hyperacusis

Management

- prednisolone 1 mg/kg (o) (usually 60 mg) daily in the morning for 5 days (start within 48 hours of onset)

Note: This is controversial, but recent randomised trials and a Cochrane review support the use of prednis(ol)one. No good evidence for antiviral drugs.

- Patient education and reassurance
- Adhesive patch or tape over eye if corneal exposure (e.g. windy or dusty conditions, during sleep)
- Artificial tears if eye is dry and at bedtime
- Massage and facial exercises during recovery

Note:

- At least 70–80% achieve full spontaneous recovery; higher if mild.
- Electromyography and nerve excitability or conduction studies are a prognostic guide only.
- No evidence that nucleoside analogue, for example, aciclovir, is useful but should be used for Ramsay–Hunt syndrome.
- No evidence that surgical procedures to decompress the nerve are beneficial.[15]

Patient education resources

Hand-out sheets from *Murtagh's Patient Education* 7th edition:

- Bell palsy
- Tremor: essential tremor
- Parkinson disease

References

1 Iansek R. *Pitfalls in Neurology.* Melbourne: Proceedings of Monash University Medical School Update Course, 1999: 40–4.

2 Talley NJ, O'Connor S. *Clinical Examination* (5th edn). Sydney: Churchill Livingstone, 2005: 345–6.

3 Wolfe N et al. Tremor: how to treat. Australian Doctor, 29 June 2007: 29.

4 Silver D. Impact of functional age on the use of dopamine agonists in patients with Parkinson disease. Neurologist, 2006; 12: 214–23.

5 Selby G, Herkes G. Parkinson's disease. In: *MIMS Disease Index* (2nd edn). Sydney: IMS Publishing, 1996: 395–8.

6 Beran R. Parkinson disease: Part 1. Update. Medical Observer, 26 September 2008.

7 Barton S et al. *Clinical Evidence* (Issue 5). London: BMJ Publishing Group, 2001: 906–13.

8 Expert group for Neurology guidelines. Parkinson disease. In: eTG complete. Melbourne: Therapeutic Guidelines Ltd. Available from: <www.tg.org.au>, accessed January 2018.

9 Beran R. Parkinson disease: Part 2. Update. Medical Observer, 3 October 2008.

10 Butler E. *Neurology Update 2016.* Melbourne: Proceedings of Monash University Medical School Update Course, 2016 (available on request).

11 Buckley N (Chair). *Australian Medicines Handbook.* Adelaide: Australian Medicines Handbook Ltd, 2016: 739–40.

12 Beran R. Multiple sclerosis: Part 1. Update. Medical Observer, 30 October 2009.

13 Polman CH et al. Diagnostic criteria for multiple sclerosis: 2005 revisions to the 'McDonald Criteria'. Ann Neural, 2005; 58: 840–6.

14 McLeod JR. Multiple sclerosis. In: *MIMS Disease Index* (2nd edn). Sydney: IMS Publishing, 1996: 321–3.

15 Barton S et al. *Clinical Evidence* (Issue 5). London: BMJ Publishing Group, 2001: 894–904.

16 Beran R. Multiple sclerosis: Part 2. Update. Medical Observer, 6 November 2009.

17 Milanese C et al. A double blind study on azathioprine in the treatment of multiple sclerosis. J Neurology, 1993; 240: 295–8.

18 Kavia R et al. Randomised controlled trial of cannabis based medicine (CBM, Stativex®) to treat detrusor overactivity in multiple sclerosis. Neurourol Urodyn, 2004; 23(5/6): 607.

19 Pollard J. Neuropathy, peripheral. In: *MIMS Disease Index* (2nd edn). Sydney: IMS Publishing, 1996: 346.

20 Beran R. Peripheral neuropathy: Part 2. Update. Medical Observer, 26 June 2009.

21 Darveniza P. Myasthenia gravis. In: *MIMS Disease Index* (2nd edn). Sydney: IMS Publishing, 1996: 324–6.

Resources

Parkinson disease <www.parkinsons.org.au>
Multiple sclerosis <www.msaustralia.org.au>
Amyotrophic lateral sclerosis <www.mnd.aust.asn.au>

Diagnostic triads of neurological dilemmas

All triads show a chronic onset unless indicated by an asterisk (acute onset).

If you see this combination of signs:	Consider:
Charcot's triad:	
• dysarthria + intention tremor + nystagmus	→ cerebellar disease (typical of MS)
• visual disturbance (blurred or transient loss) + weakness in limbs ± paraesthesia in limbs	→ multiple sclerosis
Note: There are many combinations of MS (Charcot's has historical interest).	
• rigidity + bradykinesia + resting tremor	→ Parkinson disease
• tremor (postural or action) + head tremor + absence of Parkinsonian features	→ essential tremor
• fatiguable and weakness of eyelids and eye movements + limbs + bulbar muscles (speech and swallowing)	→ myasthenia gravis
• ascending weakness of limbs + of face + areflexia*	→ Guillain–Barré syndrome (GBS)
• (episodic) vertigo + tinnitus + hearing loss*	→ Ménière syndrome
• dementia + myoclonus + ataxia	→ Creutzfeldt–Jakob disease
• drowsiness + vomiting + headache (waking)	→ ↑ intracerebral pressure
• enophthalmos + meiosis + ptosis ± anhydrosis	→ Horner syndrome
• blank spell + lip-smacking (or similar automation) + olfactory/gustatory hallucination	→ complex partial seizure
• gradual spread (Jacksonian march) of focal jerking (mouth, arm or leg) or sensory disturbance or (rarely) visual field disturbance	→ simple partial seizure
• ↑ intracranial pressure +/or focal signs +/or epilepsy	→ cerebral tumour
• dysphagia + dysphonia/dysarthria + spastic tongue	→ pseudobulbar palsy
• recurrent: headache (often unilateral) + nausea (± vomiting) + visual aura*	→ migraine with aura (formerly 'classical migraine')
• recurrent: severe retro-orbital headache + rhinorrhoea + lacrimation*	→ cluster headache
• instantaneous: headache ± vomiting ± neck stiffness	→ subarachnoid haemorrhage until disproven
• headache + visual obscurations + papilloedema (often in obese young female)	→ benign intracranial hypertension
• acute and transient: amaurosis fugax or dysphasia or hemiplegia*	→ TIA (carotid)
• typical facies (temporalis atropy and frontal balding) + muscle weakness esp. hands (± myotonia) + cataracts	→ dystrophia myotonica (myotonic dystrophy)
• ataxias + ophthalmoplegia + areflexia*	→ Miller–Fisher variant of GBS
• vertigo + provoked by movement (especially rolling in bed) + Hallpike test +ve	→ BPPV
• UMN signs + LMN signs + fasciculations	→ motor neurone disease
• leg weakness + ataxic gait + clumsiness (appears about 12 years)	→ Friedreich ataxia
• limb weakness + flaccid paralysis (day after exercise in a young person)	→ familial periodic paralysis

Part 3

Problem solving in general practice

34 Abdominal pain

A great fit of the stone in my left kidney: all day I could do but three or four drops of water, but I drunk a draught of white wine and salet oyle, and after that, crabs' eyes in powder with the bone in the carp's head and then drunk two great draughts of ale with buttered cake; and I voyded with an hour much water and a stone as big as an Alexander seed. God be thanked!

JOHN DEE 1594

Abdominal pain represents one of the top 15 presenting symptoms in primary care[1] and varies from a self-limiting problem to a life-threatening illness requiring immediate surgical intervention. Abdominal pain can be considered to be acute, subacute, chronic or recurrent. It can embrace all specialties, including surgery, medicine, gynaecology, geriatrics and psychiatry. For acute abdominal conditions it is important to make a rapid diagnosis in order to reduce morbidity and mortality. Most cases require surgical referral (see TABLE 34.1). Lower abdominal pain in women adds another dimension to the problem and will be presented in a separate chapter (CHAPTER 103).

Table 34.1 Surgical causes of the acute abdomen

Process	Organ involved	Disorder
Inflammation	Bowel	Inflammatory bowel disease
	Appendix	Appendicitis
	Gall bladder	Cholecystitis
	Liver	Hepatitis
	Pancreas	Pancreatitis
	Fallopian tube	Salpingitis
	Colonic diverticulae	Diverticulitis
Perforation	Duodenum	Perforated duodenal ulcer
	Stomach	Perforated gastric ulcer
	Colon (diverticula or cancer)	Faecal peritonitis
	Gall bladder	Biliary peritonitis
	Appendix	Appendicitis
Obstruction	Gall bladder	Biliary colic
	Small intestine	Acute small bowel obstruction
	Large bowel	Acute large bowel obstruction
	Ureter	Ureteric colic
	Urethra	Acute urinary retention
	Mesenteric artery occlusion	Intestinal infarction
Haemorrhage	Fallopian tube	Ruptured ectopic pregnancy
	Spleen or liver	Ruptured spleen or liver (haemoperitoneum)
	Ovary	Ruptured ovarian cyst
	Abdominal aorta	Ruptured abdominal aortic aneurysm (AAA)
Torsion (ischaemia)	Sigmoid colon	Sigmoid volvulus
	Ovary	Torsion ovarian cyst
	Testes	Torsion of testes

Key facts and checkpoints

- The commonest causes of the acute abdomen in two general practice series were:
  Series 1—acute appendicitis (31%) and the colics (29%);[2]
  Series 2—acute appendicitis (21%), the colics (16%), mesenteric adenitis (16%).[3] The latter study included children.
- An international study involving referral to 26 surgical departments in 17 countries revealed non-specific abdominal pain (34%), acute appendicitis (28%) and cholecystitis (10%) as the most common conditions.[1]
- As a general rule, upper abdominal pain is caused by lesions of the upper GIT and lower abdominal pain by lesions of the lower GIT.
- Colicky midline umbilical abdominal pain (severe) → vomiting → distension = small bowel obstruction (SBO).
- Midline lower abdominal pain → distension → vomiting = large bowel obstruction (LBO).
- If cases of acute abdomen have a surgical cause, the pain nearly always precedes the vomiting.
- Mesenteric artery occlusion must be considered in an elderly person with arteriosclerotic disease or in patients with atrial fibrillation presenting with severe abdominal pain or following myocardial infarction.
- Up to one-third of presentations of abdominal pain are considered to be non-specific, whereby no specific cause is found.

A diagnostic approach

A summary of the separate diagnostic models for acute abdominal pain and chronic abdominal pain are presented in TABLES 34.2 and 34.3.

Probability diagnosis

The most common causes of acute abdomen are acute appendicitis, acute gastroenteritis, an irritable bowel syndrome, the various 'colics' and ovulation pain (mittelschmerz). Mesenteric adenitis is common in children. The various causes of chronic or recurrent abdominal pain are presented in TABLE 34.3. A study on chronic abdominal pain[4] showed that the commonest reasons (approximate percentages) were no discoverable causes (50%), minor causes including muscle strains (16%), irritable bowel syndrome (12%), gynaecological causes (8%), peptic ulcers and hiatus hernia (8%).

Table 34.2 Acute abdominal pain (adults): diagnostic strategy model (excluding trauma)

Probability diagnosis
Acute gastroenteritis
Acute appendicitis
Mittelschmerz/dysmenorrhoea
Irritable bowel syndrome
Biliary colic/renal colic
Serious disorders not to be missed
Cardiovascular:
• myocardial infarction (usually inferior)
• ruptured AAA
• dissecting aneurysm aorta
• mesenteric artery occlusion/ischaemia
Neoplasia:
• large or small bowel obstruction
Severe infections:
• acute salpingitis
• peritonitis/spontaneous bacterial peritonitis
• ascending cholangitis
• intra-abdominal abscess
Pancreatitis
Ectopic pregnancy
Small bowel obstruction/strangulated hernia
Sigmoid volvulus
Perforated viscus
Pitfalls (often missed)
Acute appendicitis
Myofascial tear
Pulmonary causes:
• pneumonia
• pulmonary embolism
Faecal impaction (elderly)
Herpes zoster
Rarities:
Porphyria
Lead poisoning
Henoch–Schönlein purpura
Haemochromatosis
Haemoglobinuria
Addison disease
Seven masquerades checklist
Depression
Diabetes (ketoacidosis)
Drugs (especially narcotics)
Anaemia (sickle cell)
Endocrine disorder (thyroid storm, Addison)
Spinal dysfunction
UTI (including urosepsis)
Is the patient trying to tell me something?
May be very significant.
Consider Munchausen syndrome, sexual dysfunction and abnormal stress.

34

Table 34.3 Chronic or recurrent abdominal pain (adult): diagnostic strategy model

Probability diagnosis

Irritable bowel syndrome
Diverticular disease
Mittelschmerz/dysmenorrhoea
Peptic ulcer/gastritis

Serious disorders not to be missed

Cardiovascular:
- mesenteric artery ischaemia
- AAA

Neoplasia:
- bowel/stomach cancer
- pancreatic cancer
- ovarian tumours

Severe infections:
- hepatitis
- recurrent PID

Pitfalls (often missed)

Adhesions
Appendicitis
Food allergies
Lactase deficiency
Constipation/faecal impaction
Chronic pancreatitis
Crohn disease
Endometriosis
Diverticulitis
Rarities:
Tropical infections (e.g. hydatids, melioidosis, malaria, strongyloides)
Uraemia
Lead poisoning
Porphyria
Sickle cell anaemia
Hypercalcaemia
Addison disease

Seven masquerades checklist

Depression
Drugs
Endocrine disorder (Addison disease)
Spinal dysfunction
UTI

Is the patient trying to tell me something?

A strong possibility: consider hypochondriasis, anxiety, sexual dysfunction, Munchausen syndrome.

Serious disorders not to be missed

Most of the causes of the acute abdomen are serious and early diagnosis is mandatory to reduce mortality and morbidity.

It is vital not to misdiagnose a ruptured ectopic pregnancy, which causes lower abdominal or suprapubic pain of sudden onset, or the life-threatening vascular causes, such as a ruptured or dissecting aortic aneurysm, mesenteric artery occlusion and myocardial infarction (which can present as epigastric pain).

Perforated ulcers (now uncommon) and strangulated bowel, such as volvulus of the sigmoid and entrapment of the small bowel in a hernial orifice or around adhesions, also demand an early diagnosis.

There are some important 'red flag' symptoms and signs[1] of abdominal emergencies demanding urgent attention (see box):

Red flag pointers for acute abdominal pain

History	Signs
Collapse at toilet	Pallor and sweating
Lightheadedness	Hypotension
Ischaemic heart disease	Atrial fibrillation or tachycardia
Progressive-vomiting pain, distension	Fever
Menstrual abnormalities	Prostration
Malignancy	Rebound tenderness and guarding
Lack of flatus	Decreased urine output

Note: collapsing at toilet (points to intra-abdominal bleeding)

Dangers of misdiagnosis

- Ectopic pregnancy → rapid hypovolaemic shock
- Ruptured AAA → rapid hypovolaemic shock
- Gangrenous appendix → peritonitis/pelvic abscess
- Perforated ulcer → peritonitis
- Obstructed bowel → gangrene

Pitfalls

A very common pitfall is misdiagnosing acute appendicitis, especially in the elderly, in children, in pregnancy and in those taking steroids, where the presentation may be atypical. Early appendicitis presents typically with central abdominal pain that shifts to the right iliac fossa (RIF) some 4–6 hours later. This causes confusion early on. It can cause diarrhoea with abdominal pain, especially if a pelvic appendix, and can be misdiagnosed as acute gastroenteritis.

Disaccharidase deficiencies, such as lactase deficiency, are associated with cramping abdominal pain, which may be severe. The pain follows some time, maybe hours, after the ingestion of milk and is accompanied by the passage of watery stool. The association with milk may be unrecognised by the patient.

Herpes zoster, especially in the elderly patient with unilateral abdominal pain in the dermatomal distribution, is a trap. Referred pain from conditions above the diaphragm, such as myocardial infarction, pulmonary embolism and pneumonia, can be misleading. The rare general medical causes, such as diabetes ketoacidosis, acute porphyria, Addison disease, lead poisoning, tabes dorsalis, sickle cell anaemia, haemochromatosis and uraemia often create a diagnostic dilemma and should be kept in mind.

Specific pitfalls

- Misdiagnosing a ruptured ectopic pregnancy in the patient on contraception or with a history of normal menstruation or where the brownish vaginal discharge is mistaken for a normal period.
- Failing to examine hernial orifices in a patient with intestinal obstruction.
- Misleading temporary improvement (easing of pain) in perforation of gangrenous appendix or perforated peptic ulcer.
- Overlooking acute mesenteric artery obstruction in an elderly patient with colicky central abdominal pain.
- Attributing abdominal pain, frequency and dysuria to a urinary infection when the cause could be diverticulitis, pelvic appendicitis, salpingitis or a ruptured ectopic pregnancy.
- Failing to examine testes.

Seven masquerades checklist

Depression, diabetes, drugs, spinal dysfunction and UTI can all cause abdominal pain although the pain may be more subacute or chronic. Abdominal pain and even tenderness can accompany diabetic ketoacidosis. Drugs that can cause abdominal pain are listed in TABLE 34.4.

Spinal dysfunction of the lower thoracic spine and thoracolumbar junction can cause referred pain to the abdomen. The pain is invariably unilateral, radicular in distribution, and related to activity. It can be confused with intra-abdominal problems such as biliary disease (right-sided), appendicitis and Crohn disease (right side), diverticular disorder (left-sided) and pyelonephritis.

Psychogenic considerations

Psychogenic factors can be most relevant, especially in recurrent or chronic abdominal pain where no specific cause can be identified in most cases.[5] Bain and Spaulding found that 40% of cases of adult abdominal pain had non-structural causes with 28% having psychiatric diagnoses and 6% spastic colon. They noted that 'psychological disturbances are often fairly easy to identify if care is taken to obtain the personal history and to assess the patient's personality, but the diagnostic terms used to describe psychological disturbances lack precision'.

Munchausen syndrome is hospital admission by deception, often with severe abdominal pain without convincing clinical signs or abnormal investigation. Diagnosis requires a high level of suspicion.

Table 34.4 Drugs to consider as a cause of abdominal pain (other than illicit drugs)

Drugs
Alcohol
Antibiotics (e.g. erythromycin)
Aspirin
Corticosteroids
Cytotoxic agents
Tricyclic antidepressants (e.g. imipramine)
Iron preparations
Nicotine
NSAIDs/COX-2 inhibitors
Sodium valproate
Phenytoin

The clinical approach

History

The urgency of the history will depend on the manner of presentation, whether acute or chronic. Pain has to be analysed according to its quality, quantity, site and radiation, onset, duration and offset, aggravating and relieving factors and associated symptoms and signs.

Special attention has to be paid to:

- anorexia, nausea or vomiting
- micturition
- bowel function
- menstruation/contraception
- drug intake

Key questions

Point to where the pain is and where it travels to.

Questions to ask:

- What type of pain is it: is it constant or does it come and go?
- How severe would you rate it from 1 to 10?

34

- Have you ever had previous attacks of similar pain?
- What else do you notice when you have the pain?
- Do you know of anything that will bring on the pain? Or relieve it?
- What effect does milk, food or antacids have on the pain?
- Have you noticed any sweats or chills or burning of urine?
- Are your bowels behaving normally? Have you been constipated or had diarrhoea or blood in your motions?
- Have you noticed anything different about your urine?
- What medications do you take?
- How much aspirin do you take?
- Are you smoking heavily or taking heroin or cocaine?
- How much alcohol do you drink?
- How much milk do you drink?
- Have you travelled recently?
- What is happening with your periods? Is it mid-cycle or are your periods overdue?
- Does anyone in your family have bouts of abdominal pain?
- Do you have a hernia?
- What operations have you had for your abdomen?
- Have you had your appendix removed?

Examination

A useful checklist for conducting the examination is:

- general appearance
- oral cavity
- vital parameters: temperature, pulse, BP, respiratory rate (record these in the notes)
- chest: check heart and lungs for upper abdominal pain (especially if absent abdominal signs)
- abdomen: inspection, auscultation, palpation and percussion (in that order)

The abdominal examination should be performed with the patient lying flat with one pillow under the head and the abdomen uncovered from xiphisternum to groin. Ask the patient to breathe through the mouth during the examination. Consider the following:

- inguinal region (including hernial orifices) and femoral arteries
- rectal examination: mandatory
- vaginal examination (females): for suspected problems of the fallopian tubes, uterus or ovaries
- thoracolumbar spine (if referred spinal pain suspected)
- urine analysis: white cells, red cells, glucose and ketones, porphyrins
- special clinical tests: Murphy sign (a sign of peritoneal tenderness with acute cholecystitis); psoas and obturator signs
- look for hernias: Spigelian hernias occur through defects in transversus abdominal muscle lateral to the rectus sheath—usually below the level of the umbilicus

Guidelines

- *Palpation:* start away from the painful side, palpate with gentleness—note any guarding or rebound tenderness: guarding indicates peritonitis; rebound tenderness indicates peritoneal irritation (bacterial peritonitis, blood). Feel for maximum site that corresponds to focus of the problem
- *Patient pain indicator:* the finger pointing sign indicates focal peritoneal irritation; the spread palm sign indicates visceral pain
- *Atrial fibrillation:* consider mesenteric artery obstruction
- *Tachycardia:* sepsis and volume depletion
- *Tachypnoea:* sepsis, pneumonia, acidosis
- *Pallor and 'shock':* acute blood loss
- *Auscultation:* note bowel activity or a succussion splash (best before palpation and percussion)

Causes of a 'silent abdomen': diffuse sepsis, ileus, mechanical obstruction (advanced).

If distension, consider the six F's: fat, fluid, flatus, faeces, fetus, frightening growths.

Hypertympany indicates mechanical obstruction.

Physical signs may be reduced in the elderly, grossly obese, severely ill and patients taking corticosteroid therapy.

Investigations

The following investigations may be selected:

- haemoglobin—anaemia with chronic blood loss (e.g. peptic ulcer, cancer, oesophagitis)
- blood film—abnormal red cells with sickle cell disease
- WCC—leucocytosis with appendicitis (75%),[2] acute pancreatitis, mesenteric adenitis (first day only), cholecystitis (especially with empyema), pyelonephritis
- ESR—raised with cancer, Crohn disease, abscess, but non-specific
- C-reactive protein (CRP)—use in diagnosing and monitoring infection, inflammation (e.g. pancreatic). Preferable to ESR
- liver function tests—hepatobiliary disorder

- serum amylase and/or lipase (preferable)—if raised to greater than three times normal upper level acute pancreatitis is most likely; also raised partially with most intra-abdominal disasters (e.g. ruptured ectopic pregnancy, perforated peptic ulcers, ruptured empyema of gall bladder, ruptured aortic aneurysm)
- faecal elastase—chronic pancreatitis
- pregnancy tests—urine and serum β-HCG: for suspected ectopic
- *Helicobacter pylori* testing
- urine:
  - blood: ureteric colic (stone or blood clot), urinary infection
  - white cells: urinary infection, appendicitis (bladder irritation)
  - bile pigments: gall bladder disease
  - porphobilinogen: porphyria (add Ehrlich aldehyde reagent)
  - ketones: diabetic ketoacidosis
  - air (pneumaturia): fistula (e.g. diverticulitis, other pelvic abscess, pelvic cancer)
- faecal blood—mesenteric artery occlusion, intussusception ('redcurrant jelly'), colon cancer, diverticulitis, Crohn disease and ulcerative colitis

Radiology

The two main screening tests are plain abdominal X-ray and CT scan. The following tests can be considered according to the clinical presentation:

- plain X-ray abdomen (erect and supine): look for (see FIG. 34.1):
  - kidney/ureteric stones—70% opaque[2]
  - biliary stones—only 10–30% opaque

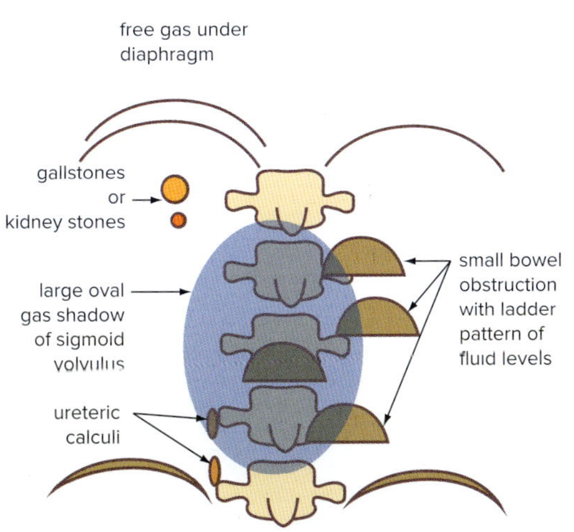

FIGURE 34.1 The acute abdomen: signs to watch for on plain abdominal X-ray

  - air in biliary tree
  - calcified aortic aneurysm
  - marked distension sigmoid → sigmoid volvulus
  - distended bowel with fluid level → bowel obstruction
  - enlarged caecum with large bowel obstruction
  - blurred right psoas shadow → appendicitis
  - 'coffee bean' sign → volvulus
  - a sentinel loop of gas in left upper quadrant (LUQ) → acute pancreatitis
- chest X-ray: air under diaphragm → perforated ulcer
- ultrasound: good for hepatobiliary system, kidneys and female pelvis: look for:
  - gallstones
  - ectopic pregnancy
  - pancreatic pseudocyst
  - aneurysm aorta/dissecting aneurysm
  - hepatic metastases and abdominal tumours
  - thickened appendix
  - paracolic collection

  Note: can be affected by gas shadows
- IVP
- contrast-enhanced X-rays (e.g. Gastrografin meal): diagnosis of bowel leakage
- barium enema
- HIDA or DIDA nuclear scan—diagnosis of acute cholecystitis (good when US unhelpful)
- CT scan: gives excellent survey of abdominal organs including masses and fluid collection:
  - pancreatitis (acute and chronic)
  - undiagnosed peritoneal inflammation (best)
  - trauma
  - diverticulitis
  - leaking aortic aneurysm
  - retroperitoneal pathology
  - appendicitis (especially with oral contrast)
- ERCP: shows bile duct obstruction and pancreatic disease
- MRI scan (especially useful with contrast)

Other tests:

- ECG
- endoscopy upper GIT
- sigmoidoscopy and colonoscopy

Diagnostic guidelines

General rules

- Upper abdominal pain is caused by lesions of the upper GIT.

- Lower abdominal pain is caused by lesions of the lower GIT or pelvic organs.
- Early severe vomiting indicates a high obstruction of the GIT.
- Acute appendicitis features a characteristic 'march' of symptoms: pain → anorexia, nausea → vomiting.

Pain patterns

The pain patterns are presented in FIGURE 34.2. Colicky pain is a rhythmic pain with regular spasms of recurring pain building to a climax and fading. It is virtually pathognomonic of intestinal obstruction. Ureteric colic is a true colicky abdominal pain, but so-called biliary colic and kidney colic are not true colics at all.

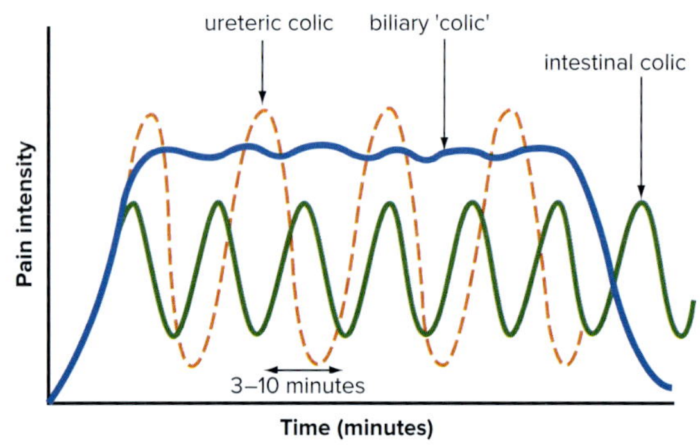

FIGURE 34.2 Characteristic pain patterns for various causes of 'colicky' acute abdominal pain

Site of pain

Typical pain sites of abdominal pain (general guidelines only) are presented in FIGURE 34.3. Epigastric pain usually arises from disorders of the embryologic foregut, such as the oesophagus, stomach and duodenum, hepatobiliary structures, pancreas and spleen. However, as some disorders progress the pain tends to shift from the midline to the right (gall bladder and liver) or left (spleen). Periumbilical pain usually arises from disorders of structures of the embryologic midgut, while structures from the hindgut tend to refer pain to the lower abdomen or suprapubic region.

The intra-abdominal sensory receptors can be considered as innervating visceral or parietal peritoneum. Visceral mechanoreceptors are triggered by intestinal distension or tension on mesentery or blood vessels while nociceptors are triggered by mechanical, thermal and chemical stimuli. The pain from viscera is felt as diffuse and poorly localised while stimulation of parietal peritoneal nociceptors gives a pain that is experienced directly at the site of insult.

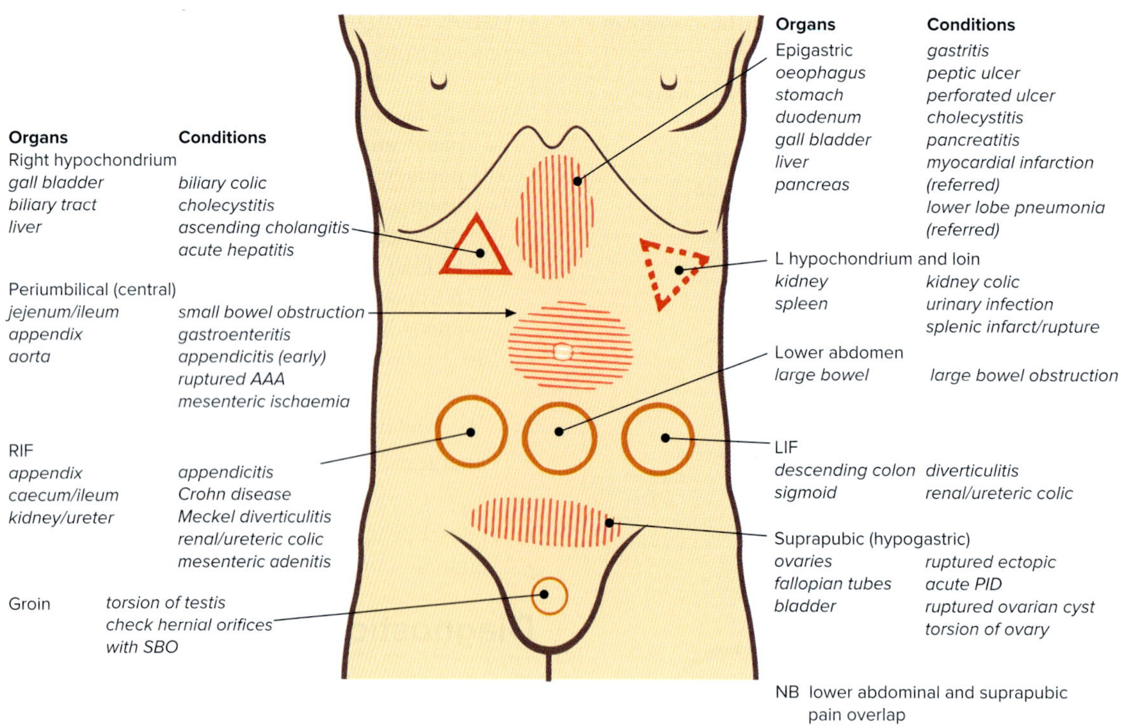

FIGURE 34.3 Typical sites of various causes of acute abdominal pain

Abdominal pain in children

Abdominal pain is a common complaint in children, especially recurrent abdominal pain, which is one of the most common complaints in childhood. The problem causes considerable anxiety in parents and it is important to differentiate the severe problems demanding surgery from non-surgical problems. About one in 15 will have a surgical cause for pain.[6] A good rule is to rule out a urinary infection with urinalysis.

Table 34.5 Acute abdominal pain in children

The causes of abdominal pain can be considered in the diagnostic model category.

1 Common causes/probability diagnosis:
- infant 'colic'
- gastroenteritis (all ages)
- mesenteric adenitis

2 Serious causes, not to be missed:
- intussusception (peaks at 6–9 months)
- acute appendicitis (mainly 5–15 years)
- bowel obstruction/strangulated hernia

3 Pitfalls:
- child abuse
- constipation/faecal impaction
- torsion of testes
- lactose intolerance
- peptic ulcer
- infections: mumps, tonsillitis, pneumonia (especially right lower lobe), EBM, UTI
- adnexal disorders in females (e.g. ovarian)

4 Rarities:
- Meckel diverticulitis
- Henoch–Schönlein purpura
- sickle crisis
- lead poisoning

5 Seven masquerades checklist:
- diabetes mellitus
- drugs
- UTI

6 Psychogenic consideration:
- important cause

Infant 'colic' (period of infant distress)

This is the occurrence in a well baby of regular, unexplained periods of inconsolable crying and fretfulness, usually in the late afternoon and evening, especially between 2 weeks and 16 weeks of age. No cause for the apparent abdominal pain can be found and it lasts for a period of at least 3 weeks. It is very common and occurs in about one-third of infants.

Clinical features

- Baby between 2 and 16 weeks old
- Prolonged crying—at least 3 hours
- Occurrence at least 3 days a week
- Crying worst at around 10 weeks of age
- Crying during late afternoon and early evening
- Child flexing legs and clenching fists as if severe 'stomach ache'
- Normal physical examination

Management

Reassure and explain to the parents. Advise the parents:

- Use gentleness (such as subdued lighting where the baby is handled, soft music, speaking softly, quiet feeding times).
- Avoid quick movements that may startle the baby.
- Make sure the baby is not hungry—underfeeding can make the baby hungry.
- If the baby is breastfed, express the watery foremilk before putting the baby to the breast.
- Provide demand feeding (in time and amount).
- Make sure the baby is burped, and give posture feeding.
- Provide comfort from a dummy or pacifier.
- Provide plenty of gentle physical contact.
- Cuddle and carry the baby around (e.g. take a walk around the block).
- A carrying device such as 'snuggly' or 'Mei Tai Sling' allows the baby to be carried around at the time of crying.
- Make sure the mother gets plenty of rest during this difficult period.
- Do not worry about leaving a crying child for 10 minutes or so after 15 minutes of trying consolation.

Medication

Drugs are not generally recommended, but for very severe problems some preparations can be helpful (e.g. simethicone [Infacol wind drops]).

Intussusception

Intussusception is the diagnosis that should be foremost in one's mind with a child aged between 3 months and 2 years presenting with sudden onset of severe colicky abdominal pain, coming at intervals of about 15 minutes and lasting for 2–3 minutes. Early diagnosis, within 24 hours of the onset, is essential, for after this time there is a significant rise in morbidity and mortality. It is due to the telescoping of a segment of bowel into the adjoining distal segment (e.g. ileocaecal segment), resulting in intestinal obstruction. It is usually idiopathic but can have a pathological lead point (4–12 years) (e.g. polyp, Meckel diverticulum).

Typical clinical features[7]

See FIGURE 34.4.

- Male babies > female
- Range: birth to school age, usually 5–24 months
- Sudden-onset acute pain with shrill cry
- Vomiting
- Lethargy
- Pallor with attacks
- Intestinal bleeding: redcurrant jelly (60%)[7]

DxT pale child + severe 'colic' + vomiting → acute intussusception

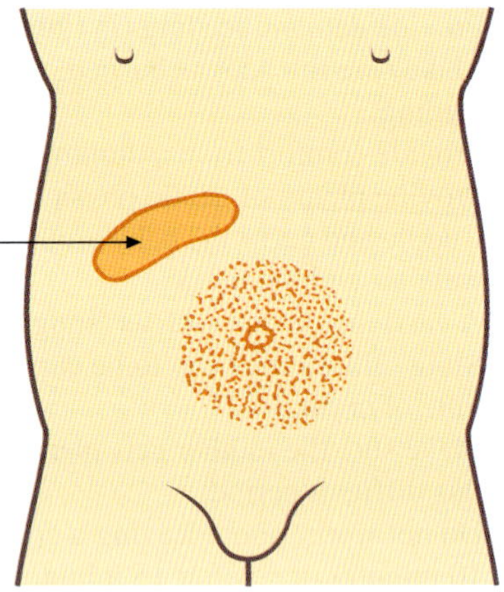

FIGURE 34.4 Typical features with pain distribution of acute intussusception

Signs

- Pale, anxious and unwell
- Sausage-shaped mass in right upper quadrant (RUQ) anywhere between the line of colon and umbilicus, especially during attacks (difficult to feel)
- Signe de dance (i.e. emptiness in RIF to palpation)
- Alternating high-pitched active bowel sounds with absent sounds
- Rectal examination: ± blood ± hard lump

Diagnosis

- Ultrasound
- Oxygen or barium enema (with caution) also used for diagnosis and treatment

Treatment[7]

- Hydrostatic reduction by air or oxygen from the 'wall' supply (preferred) or barium enema
- Surgical intervention may be necessary

Differential diagnosis

- Acute gastroenteritis: can be difficult in those cases where there is some loose stool with intussusception and with blood and mucus without much watery stool in gastroenteritis. However, usually attacks of pain are of shorter duration, and there is loose watery stool, fever and no abdominal mass. If doubtful refer as possible intussusception.
- Impacted faeces can lead to spasms of colicky abdominal pain—usually an older child with a history of constipation.
- Other causes of intestinal obstruction (e.g. irreducible inguinal hernia, volvulus, intra-abdominal band).

Drugs

In any child complaining of acute abdominal pain, enquiry should be made into drug ingestion. A common cause of colicky abdominal pain in children is cigarette smoking (nicotine); consider other drugs such as marijuana, cocaine and heroin.

Acute appendicitis in children

This may occur at any age, being more common in children of school age (10–12 years) and in adolescence, and uncommon in children under 3 years of age. Special problems of early diagnosis occur with the very young (younger than 3 years) and in intellectually disabled children, many of whom present with peritonitis.

Vomiting occurs in at least 80% of children with appendicitis and diarrhoea in about 20%. The temperature is usually only slightly elevated but in about 5% of cases it exceeds 39°C.[2]

In children the physical examination, especially eliciting abdominal (including rebound) tenderness, and the rectal examination demand considerable tact, patience and gentleness. Jumping or hopping induces pain.

A serious point of confusion can occur between pelvic appendicitis, causing diarrhoea and vomiting, and acute gastroenteritis. A high CRP level >50 mg/L is a feature of appendicitis.[6] A particularly severe case of apparent gastroenteritis, especially if persistent, should be regarded as pelvic appendicitis until proved otherwise. Ultrasound is the preferred imaging.

Mesenteric adenitis

This presents a difficult problem in differential diagnosis with acute appendicitis because the history can be very similar. At times the distinction may be almost impossible. In general, with mesenteric adenitis localisation of pain and tenderness is not as definite, rigidity is less of a feature, the temperature is higher, and anorexia, nausea and vomiting are also lesser features. The illness lasts about five days followed by a rapid recovery. Comparisons between the two are presented in TABLE 34.6, but if in any doubt it is advisable to consider the problem as acute appendicitis, admit for observation and be prepared for laparoscopy/laparotomy.

Mesenteric adenitis can sometimes present an anaesthetic risk and patients are usually quite ill in the immediate postoperative period. Treatment is symptomatic and includes ample fluids and paracetamol.

Table 34.6 Comparison of the features of acute appendicitis and mesenteric adenitis in children (guidelines only)

	Acute appendicitis	Mesenteric adenitis
Typical child	Older	Younger
Site of onset of pain	Midline Shifting to right	RIF Can be midline
Preceding respiratory illness	Uncommon	Invariable: URTI or tonsillitis
Anorexia, nausea, vomiting	++	±
Colour	Usually pale	Flushed: malar flush
Temperature	N or ↑	↑↑ → ↑↑↑
Abdominal palpation	Tender in RIF Guarding ± Rigidity	Tender in RIF Minimal guarding Usually no rigidity
Rectal examination	Invariably tender	Often tender but lesser degree
Psoas and obturator tests	Usually positive	Usually negative
Full blood examination	Leucocytosis	Lymphocytosis

RIF = right iliac fossa

Recurrent abdominal pain

Recurrent abdominal pain (RAP)—three distinct episodes of abdominal pain over 3 or more months—occurs in 10% of school-aged children. In only 5–10% of children will an organic cause be found so that in most cases the cause remains obscure.[8]

Causes (organic)

An organic cause, however, must be considered and excluded. Organic disease is more likely if:

- the pain is other than periumbilical
- the pain radiates rather than remains localised
- the pain wakes the child from sleep
- the pain is accompanied by nausea and vomiting
- the child is not completely well between attacks
- there is associated weight loss
- there is failure to thrive

Possible causes

- Constipation
- Childhood migraine equivalent (pain with extreme pallor)
- Lactose intolerance (symptoms related to milk ingestion)
- Intestinal parasites (may disturb child about 60 minutes after falling asleep)

Investigations

- Urine analysis and MSU
- FBE and ESR
- Plain X-ray (assesses faecal retention)

Non-organic RAP

Clinical features

Typical clinical features include:

- acute and frequent colicky abdominal pain
- pain localised to or just above umbilicus
- no radiation of pain
- pain lasts less than 60 minutes
- nausea frequent and vomiting rare
- diurnal (never wakes the child at night)
- minimal umbilical tenderness
- anxious child
- obsessive or perfectionist personality
- one or both parents intense about child's health and progress

Psychogenic factors

Although psychogenic factors are very relevant in individual cases there is scant hard evidence to support the widely held hypothesis[8] that such factors account for the vast majority of RAP. Some children will have obvious psychological problems or even be school avoidant, a common factor being family disruption.

Management[8]

- Give explanation, reassurance and support (ensure that the patient is involved in the discussion).
- Reassurance can only be given following a careful examination and thoughtfully chosen investigations.
- Avoid investigations, especially radiological if possible (FBE and MCU are okay).
- Acknowledge that the child has pain.
- Emphasise that the disorder is common, and usually traverses childhood without ill effects.
- Recommend simple measures (e.g. local warmth, brief rest for painful episodes).
- Advise review if episodes change in nature, pain persists for hours or there are new symptoms.
- Identify any life stresses and provide insight therapy.
- Enquire about family structures and function, and school performance.
- Discourage identification with the sick role.
- Refer for psychological assessment and counselling if necessary.

34

Abdominal pain in the elderly

The elderly can suffer from a wide spectrum of disorders. Ischaemic events, emboli, cancer (in particular) and diverticulae of the colon are more common in old age; duodenal ulcer is less so. Those causes of abdominal pain that occur with more frequency include:

- vascular catastrophies: ruptured AAA, mesenteric artery occlusion
- perforated peptic ulcer
- biliary disorders: biliary pain and acute cholecystitis
- diverticulitis
- sigmoid volvulus
- strangulated hernia
- intestinal obstruction
- cancer, especially of the large bowel
- herpes zoster, causing unilateral root pain
- constipation and faecal impaction

Problems arise with management because the pain threshold is raised (colic in particular is less severe) and there is an attenuated response to infection so that fever and leucocytosis can be absent. Non-specific signs, such as confusion, anorexia and tachycardia, might be the only systemic evidence of infection.

Abdominal aortic aneurysm

An AAA may be asymptomatic until it ruptures or may present with abdominal discomfort and a pulsatile mass noted by the patient. There tends to be a family history and thus screening is appropriate in such families. Ultrasound screening is advisable in first-degree relatives over 50 years.

The risk of rupture is related to the diameter of the AAA and the rate of increase in diameter. The normal diameter of the abdominal aorta, which is palpated just above the umbilicus, is 10–30 mm, being 20 mm on average in the adult; an aneurysm is greater than 30 mm in diameter.[9] Refer if $\geq$ 40 mm. Greater than 50 mm is significantly enlarged and is chosen as the arbitrary reference point to operate because of the exponential rise in risk of rupture with an increasing diameter. Refer all cases. The patency of a Dacron graft after 5 years is approximately 95% (see FIG. 34.5). Newer techniques include endovascular aneurysm repair.

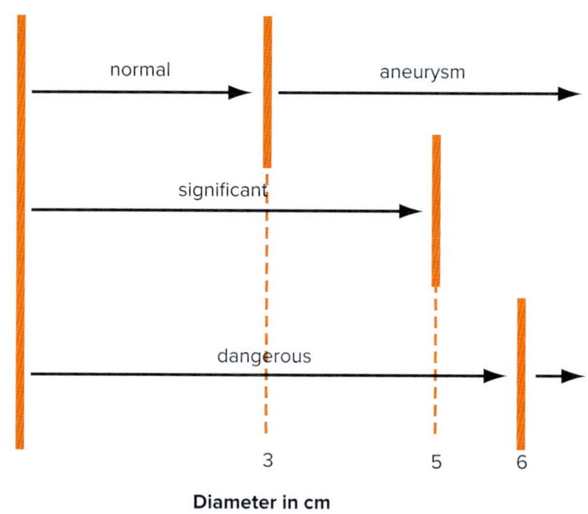

FIGURE 34.5 Guidelines for normal and abnormal widths of the abdominal aorta in adults (to exact scale)

Investigations

- Ultrasound (good for screening) in relatives >50 years (obesity a problem)
- CT scan (clearer imaging). Helical/spiral scan is investigation of choice.
- MRI scan (best definition)

Rupture of aneurysm

This is a real surgical emergency in an elderly person who presents with acute abdominal and perhaps back pain with associated circulatory collapse (see FIG. 34.6). The patient often collapses at toilet because

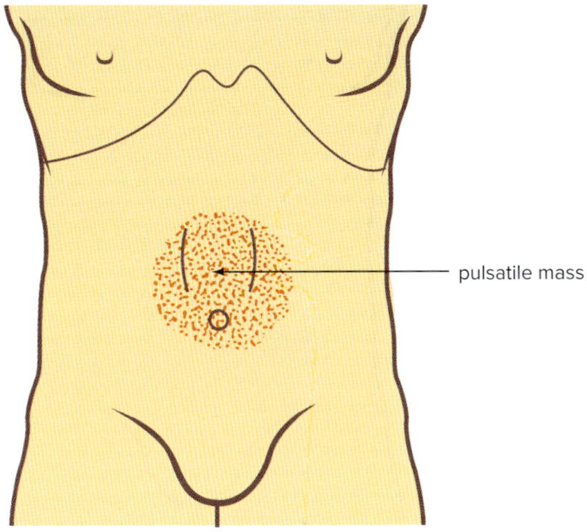

FIGURE 34.6 Typical pain distribution of a ruptured abdominal aortic aneurysm

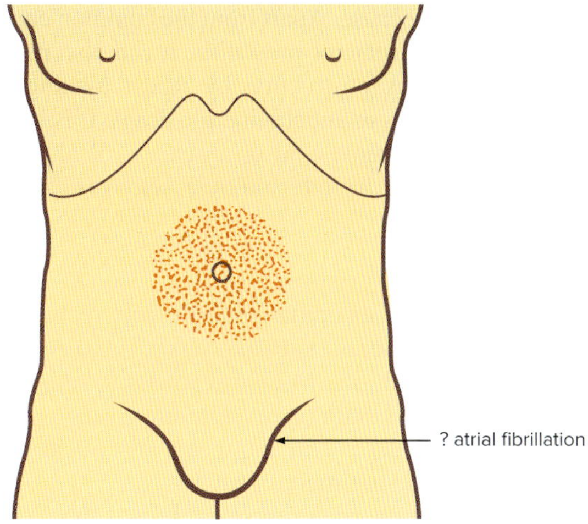

FIGURE 34.7 Typical pain distribution of mesenteric arterial occlusion

they feel the need to defecate and the resultant Valsalva manoeuvre causes circulatory embarrassment.

The patient should be transferred immediately to a vascular surgical unit, which should be notified in advance. Two important emergency measures for the 'shocked' patient are intravenous access for plasma expanding fluid (a central venous line is best if possible) and swift action.

> **DxT** intense abdominal pain + pale and 'shocked ± back pain ➔ ruptured AAA

Mesenteric artery occlusion

Acute intestinal ischaemia arises from superior mesenteric artery occlusion from either an embolus or a thrombosis in an atherosclerotic artery. Another cause is an embolus from atrial fibrillation. Necrosis of the intestine soon follows if intervention is delayed.

Clinical features

- Abdominal pain—gradually becomes intense (see FIG. 34.7). Patients develop a 'fear of eating'
- Profuse vomiting
- Watery diarrhoea—blood in one-third of patients (later) (refer CHAPTER 44)
- Patient becomes confused

> **DxT** anxiety and prostration + intense central pain + profuse vomiting ± bloody diarrhoea ➔ mesenteric arterial occlusion

Signs

- Localised tenderness, rigidity and rebound over infarcted bowel (later finding)
- Absent bowel sounds (later)
- Shock develops later
- Tachycardia (may be atrial fibrillation and other signs of atheroma)

Investigations

- CRP may be elevated intestinal alkaline phosphatase.
- X-ray (plain) shows 'thumb printing' due to mucosal oedema on gas-filled bowel.
  CT scanning gives the best definition while mesenteric arteriography is performed if embolus is suspected. However, it is commonly only diagnosed at laparotomy.

Management

Early surgery may prevent gut necrosis but massive resection of necrosed gut may be required as a life-saving procedure. Early diagnosis (within a few hours) is essential.

Note:

- Mesenteric venous thrombosis can occur but usually in patients with circulatory failure.
- Inferior mesenteric artery occlusion is less severe and survival more likely.

Acute retention of urine

Acute retention of urine with a volume of 600+ mL usually causes severe lower abdominal pain, which may not be apparent in a senile or dementing person.

Find and treat the cause. Apart from the common cause of an enlarged prostate or prostatitis, it can also result from bladder neck obstruction by faecal loading or other pelvic masses or anticholinergic drugs. It is often precipitated by extreme cold or an excess of alcohol. Neurogenic causes include multiple sclerosis, spinal injury and diabetes.

Management

- Perform a rectal examination and empty rectum of any impacted faecal material.
- Catheterise with size 14 Foley catheter to relieve obstruction and drain (give antibiotic cover).
- Have the catheter in situ and seek a urological opinion. Send specimen for MCU.
- If there is any chance of recovery (e.g. if the problem is drug-induced), withdraw drug, leave catheter in for 48 hours, remove and give trial of prazosin 0.5 mg bd or terazosin.
- In some instances, it may be worth giving analgesics, ambulating the patient and attempting voiding by standing up to the sound of running water. A hot bath may also provide a simple solution.
- Check for prostate cancer and renal impairment.
- Perform neurological examination of lower limbs and perianal area.

34

Chronic retention of urine

May be painless, of insidious onset and present with overflow of urine. Bladder capacity may be >1.5 L.

Faecal impaction

Faecal impaction is encountered typically in the aged, bedridden, debilitated patient. It may closely resemble malignant obstruction in its clinical presentation.[10] Spurious diarrhoea can occur, which is known as 'faecal incontinence' (see CHAPTER 36).

Acute appendicitis

Acute appendicitis is mainly a condition of young adults but it affects all ages (although uncommon under 3 years). It is the commonest surgical emergency and special care has to be taken with the very young and the very old. The symptoms can vary because of the different positions of the appendix. It is basically a clinical diagnosis.

Clinical features

See FIGURE 34.8. Typical clinical features are:

- maximum incidence 20–30 years
- initial pain is central abdominal (sometimes colicky)
- increasing severity and then continuous

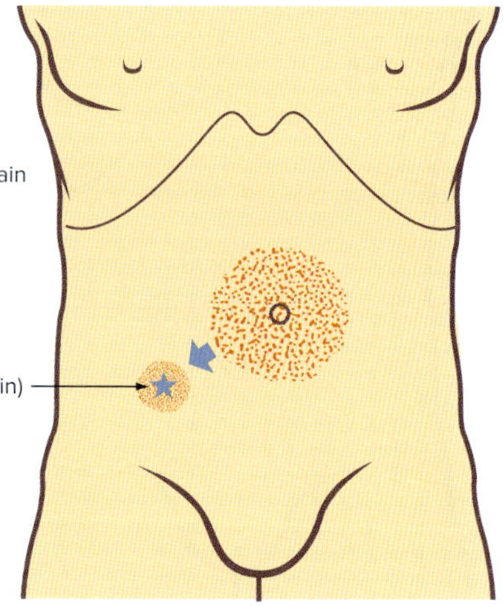

FIGURE 34.8 Typical pain distribution of acute appendicitis

- shifts and localises to RIF within 6 hours
- may be aggravated by walking (causing a limp) or coughing
- sudden anorexia
- nausea and vomiting a few hours after the pain starts
- ± diarrhoea and constipation

DxT localised RIF pain + a/n/v + guarding → acute appendicitis

Signs

- Patient looks unwell
- Flushed at first, then pale
- Furred tongue and halitosis
- May be febrile
- Tenderness in RIF, usually at McBurney point
- Local rigidity and rebound tenderness
- Guarding
- ± Superficial hyperaesthesia
- ± Psoas sign: pain on resisted flexion of right leg, on hip extension or on elevating right leg (due to irritation of psoas especially with retrocaecal appendix)
- ± Obturator sign: pain on flexing patient's right thigh at the hip with the knee bent and then internally rotating the hip (due to irritation of internal obturator muscle)
- Rovsing sign: rebound tenderness in RIF while palpating in LIF
- PR: anterior tenderness to right, especially if pelvic appendix or pelvic peritonitis

Variations and cautions

- Abscess formation → localised mass and tenderness
- Retrocaecal appendix: pain and rigidity less and may be no rebound tenderness; loin tenderness; positive psoas test
- Pelvic appendix: no abdominal rigidity; urinary frequency; diarrhoea and tenesmus; very tender PR; obturator tests usually positive
- Elderly patients: pain often minimal and eventually manifests as peritonitis; can simulate intestinal obstruction
- Pregnancy (occurs mainly during second trimester): pain is higher and more lateral; harder to diagnose; peritonitis more common
- Perforation more likely in the very young, the aged and the diabetic

Investigations

Few investigations including imaging are of value:

- blood cell count shows a leucocytosis (75%) with a left shift
- urea and electrolytes—to assess hydration prior to surgery
- CRP—elevated
- plain X-ray may show local distension, blurred psoas shadow and fluid level in caecum
- ultrasound shows a thickened appendix (86% sensitivity, 81% specificity);[11] affected by gas shadow
- CT scan also accurate (94% sensitivity, 98% specificity) and allows other causes, especially in the female pelvis, to be evaluated[12]
- laparoscopy
- β-HCG

Management

Immediate referral for surgical removal—the gold standard. If perforated, cover with cefotaxime and metronidazole. It is reasonable to offer a conservative approach with careful monitoring and antibiotics in selected patients. One detailed study showed that surgery was the safest option.[13]

Small bowel obstruction

The symptoms depend on the level of the obstruction (see TABLE 34.7). The more proximal the obstruction, the more severe the pain.

Main causes

- Outside obstruction (e.g. adhesions—commonest cause, previous laparotomy), strangulation in hernia or pockets of abdominal cavity (see FIG. 34.9)—this may lead to a 'closed loop' obstruction.[14]
- Lumen obstructions (e.g. foreign body, trichobezoar, gallstones, intussusception, malignancy).

Table 34.7 Small bowel obstruction: difference between a high and a low obstruction

	High	Low
Frequency of spasms	3–5 minutes	6–10 minutes
Intensity of pain	+ + +	+
Vomiting	Early, frequent Violent	Later Less severe
Content:	Gastric juices, then green	Faeculent (later)
Dehydration and degree of illness	Marked	Less prominent
Distension	Minimal	Marked

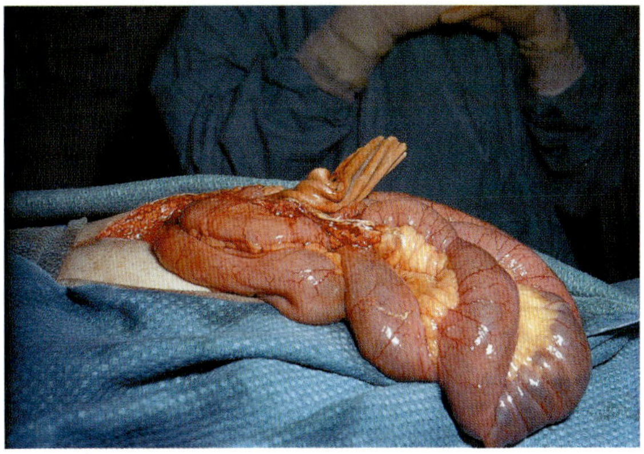

FIGURE 34.9 Operative findings (corrugated drainage material) in a 65-year-old man with subacute bowel obstruction after a 21-year history of nagging abdominal pain following a cholecystectomy

Clinical features

- Severe colicky epigastric and periumbilical (mainly) pain (see FIG. 34.10)
- Spasms last about 1 minute
- Spasms every 3–10 minutes (according to level)
- Vomiting
- Absolute constipation (nil after bowel emptied)
- No flatus
- Abdominal distension (especially if lower SBO)

DxT colicky central pain + vomiting + distension → SBO

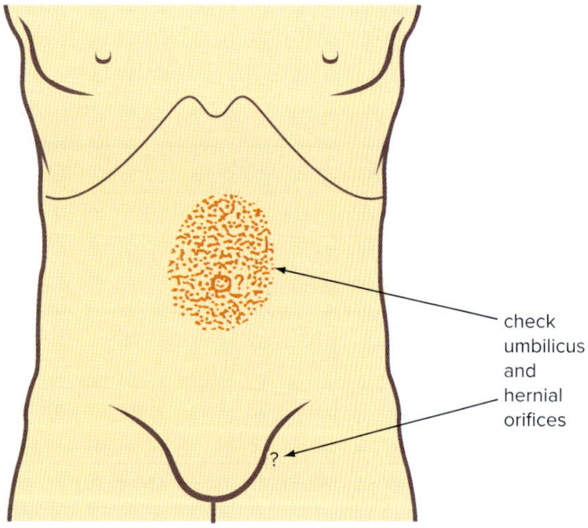

FIGURE 34.10 Typical pain distribution of small bowel obstruction

34

Signs and tests

- Patient weak and sitting forward in distress
- Visible peristalsis, loud borborygmi
- Abdomen soft (except with strangulation)
- Tender when distended
- Increased sharp, tinkling bowel sounds
- Dehydration rapidly follows, especially in children and elderly
- PR: empty rectum, may be tender
  Note: check all hernial orifices, including umbilicus
- X-ray: plain erect film confirms diagnosis—'stepladder' fluid levels (4–5 for diagnosis) in 3–4 hours
  - Gastrografin follow-through for precise diagnosis with caution. It can cause severe diarrhoea and may be therapeutic in adhesive obstruction.
- ± CT scan (especially if extrinsic causation)

Management

- IV fluids and bowel decompression with nasogastric tube
- Laparotomy or hernia repair

Large bowel obstruction

The cause is commonly colon cancer (75% of cases), especially on the left side, but it can occur in diverticulitis or in volvulus of the sigmoid colon (10% of cases) and caecum.[10] Sigmoid volvulus is more common in older men and has a sudden and severe onset. The pain is less severe than in SBO. Be wary of the non-surgical causes, simple constipation or acute pseudo-obstruction of the colon (Ogilvie syndrome). Consider ileus.

Clinical features

- Sudden-onset colicky pain (even with cancer)
- Each spasm lasts less than 1 minute
- Usually hypogastric midline pain (see FIG. 34.11)
- Vomiting may be absent (or late)
- Absolute constipation (obstipation), no flatus

DxT colicky pain + distension ± vomiting → LBO

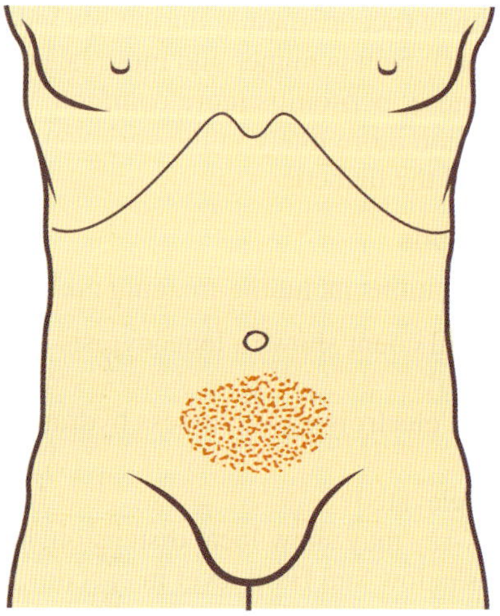

FIGURE 34.11 Typical pain distribution of large bowel obstruction

Signs and tests

- Increased bowel sounds, especially during pain
- Distension early and marked
- Local tenderness and rigidity
- PR: empty rectum; may be rectosigmoid cancer or blood. Check for faecal impaction
- X-ray: distension of large bowel with separation of haustral markings, especially caecal distension
  - sigmoid volvulus shows a distended loop and 'coffee bean' sign
  - Gastrografin enema confirms diagnosis

Management

- Drip and suction
- Surgical referral

Perforated peptic ulcer

Perforation of a peptic ulcer can cause acute abdominal pain both with and without a prior history of peptic ulcer. It is an acute surgical emergency requiring immediate diagnosis. Consider a history of drugs, especially NSAIDs and H_2-receptor antagonists. Perforated ulcers may follow a heavy meal. There is usually no back pain. May be painless with steroids.

The maximal incidence is 45–55 years, most common in males, and a perforated duodenal ulcer is more common than a gastric ulcer.

Consider the clinical syndrome in three stages:

1 prostration
2 reaction (after 4 hours)—symptoms may improve
3 peritonitis (after 4 hours)—severe pain

Clinical features

See FIGURE 34.12. Typical clinical features are:

- sudden-onset severe epigastric pain
- continuous pain but lessens for a few hours
- epigastric pain at first, and then generalised to whole abdomen
- pain may radiate to one or both shoulders (uncommon) or right lower quadrant
- nausea and vomiting (delayed)
- hiccough is a common late symptom

DxT sudden severe pain + anxious, still, 'grey', sweaty + deceptive improvement ➔ perforated peptic ulcer

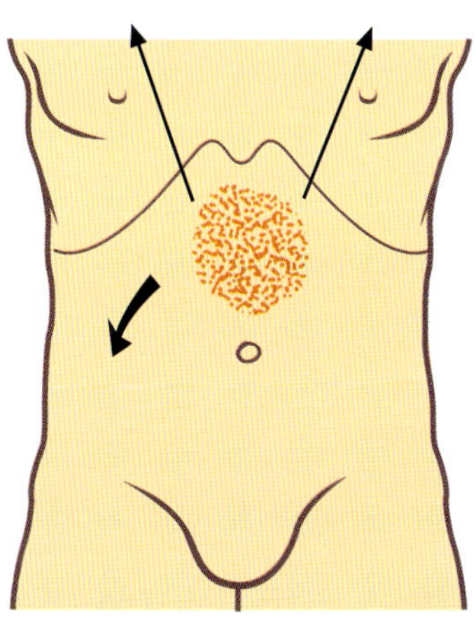

FIGURE 34.12 Typical features of perforated peptic ulcer with typical pain radiation

Signs and tests (typical of peritonitis)

- Patient lies quietly (pain aggravated by movement and coughing)
- Pale, sweating or ashen at first
- Board-like rigidity
- Guarding
- Maximum signs at point of perforation
- No abdominal distension
- Contraction of abdomen (forms a 'shelf' over lower chest)
- Bowel sounds reduced (silent abdomen)
- Shifting dullness may be present
- Pulse, temperature and BP usually normal at first
- Tachycardia (later) and shock later (3–4 hours)
- Breathing is shallow and inhibited by pain
- PR: pelvic tenderness
- X-ray: chest X-ray may show free air under diaphragm (in 75%)—need to sit upright for prior 15 minutes
  - limited Gastrografin meal can confirm diagnosis
  - CT scan is accurate

Management

- Pain relief
- Drip and suction (immediate nasogastric tube)
- Broad-spectrum antibiotics
- Immediate laparotomy after resuscitation
- Conservative treatment may be possible (e.g. later presentation and Gastrografin swallow indicates sealing of perforation)

Ureteric colic

Kidney (renal) colic is not a true colic but a constant pain due to blood clots or a stone lodged at the pelvic–ureteric junction; ureteric colic, however, presents as severe true colicky pain due to stone movement, dilatation and ureteric spasm. Fortunately, the majority of urinary calculi are small and will pass spontaneously.

Guidelines:

- loin pain—stone in kidney
- kidney/ureteric colic—ureteric stone
- strangury—stone in bladder

Clinical features

- Maximum incidence 30–50 years (M > F)
- Intense colicky pain: in waves, each lasting 30 seconds with 1–2 minutes respite
- Begins in loin and radiates around the flank to the groin, thigh, testicle or labia (see FIG. 34.13)
- Usually lasts <8 hours
- ± Vomiting

DxT intense pain (loin) ➔ groin + microscopic haematuria ➔ ureteric colic

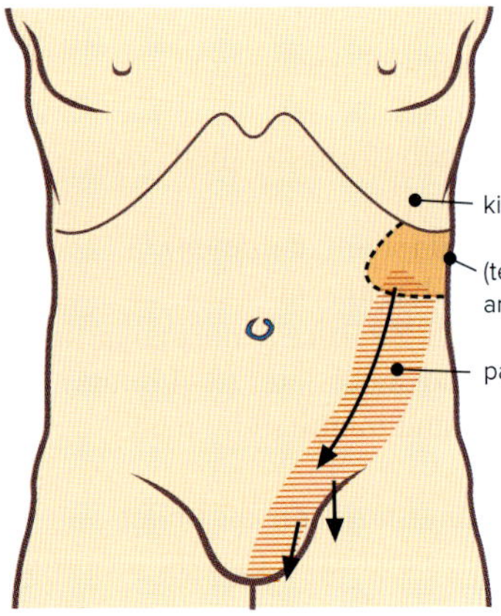

FIGURE 34.13 Ureteric colic: typical radiation of pain in left ureteric colic

34

Signs

- Patient restless: may be writhing in pain
- Pale, cold and clammy
- Tenderness at costovertebral angle
- ± Abdominal and back muscle spasm
- Smoky urine due to haematuria

Diagnosis

- Urine: microscopy; blood testing strip (negative does not exclude calculus)
- Plain X-ray: most stones—kidney, ureter, bladder (75%)—are radio-opaque (calcium oxalate and phosphate)
- IVP: confirms opacity, level of obstruction, kidney function and any anatomical abnormalities
- Ultrasound: may locate calculus but will exclude obstruction
- Non-contrast spiral KUB-CT is the 'gold standard' (sensitivity 97%, specificity 96%) (will show easily missed radiolucent[11] uric acid stones)

Management

If the diagnosis is in doubt (especially if narcotic addiction is suspected) get the patient to pass urine in the presence of an examiner and test for haematuria. While awaiting passage of urine, an indomethacin suppository may be tried for pain relief.

Routine treatment (average size adult)

- morphine 2.5 to 5 mg IV[15] statim then titrate to effect
  or
  fentanyl 50–100 mcg IV then titrate to effect
- Avoid high fluid intake, especially IV fluids—provokes distension of ureter and aggravates pain.
- Most cases settle and the patient can go home when pain relief is obtained and an IVP arranged for the next day.
- Further pain can be alleviated by indomethacin suppositories but should be limited to two a day.
- An effective alternative treatment is diclofenac 75 mg IM injection then 50 mg (o) tds for 1 week. Several clinical trials have shown that NSAIDs by IM injection, including ketorolac (10–30 mg IM [or IV] 4–6 hourly), are effective and at least as efficacious as opioids.[15,16,17] Consider an anti-emetic.

Outcome and follow-up

- The calculus is likely to pass spontaneously if <5 mm (90% <4 mm pass spontaneously).[16]
- If >5 mm intervention will usually be required by extracorporeal shock wave lithotripsy or surgery.
- If the patient passes the calculus, he or she should retrieve it and present it for analysis.
- A repeat IVP may be necessary if there is evidence of obstruction for more than 3 weeks.
- Persistent obstruction causes sepsis.
- The cause of the 'stone' should be considered. Search for causes such as hyperparathyroidism, hypercalcaemia, hyperoxaluria and UTI.
- Fever with ureteric colic indicates an obstructed infected kidney.

When to refer[16]

Any of the following:

- stone >5 mm in diameter
- high-grade obstruction
- gross hydronephrosis
- fever/UTI
- unremitting pain
- stone fails to progress
- type 2 diabetes
- staghorn calculus
- presence of solitary kidney

Facts about urinary tract calculi

- The prevalence is 1 to 3 per 1000 population per year[16]
- The lifelong incidence is 10%
- The recurrence is up to 75% (most within 2 years)
- The typical age range is 20–50 years (peaks at 28 years)
- Pregnancy is a risk factor
- Male to female ratio = 3:1

- The incidence is inversely proportional to fibre intake and proportional to ingestion of animal protein and persistently low urinary volume
- Formed from urinary supersaturation with calcium (calcium oxalate, 75–80%), uric acid (7%) and cysteine (rare): also infected calculi (struvite)—Mg^+, NH_4^+, PO_4^- (5%)

'Phony' colic

Some patients who present with typical colic may be feigning their pain mainly because they are opioid dependent and seeking drugs by deception. As ureteric colic can affect young people (peak age 28 years) this can be a very difficult management issue, even for the experienced.

The use of CT scanning would help in locating calculi in such patients. If in doubt an appropriate agent would be ketorolac (Toradol) 10–30 mg IM.

It is advisable to obtain a specimen of urine passed in the presence of an examiner and then tested for microscopic blood. While awaiting passage of urine an indomethacin suppository may be tried for pain relief.

Recurrent urinary calculi

Investigations

- Serum electrolytes, urea, creatinine
- Serum calcium, phosphate, uric acid, magnesium
- Serum alkaline phosphatase
- Urine sample—microbiology and culture
- At least two consecutive 24-hour urine samples
- Stone analysis
- IVP

Dietary advice is given in CHAPTER 10.

Biliary pain

Abdominal pain can be produced by contraction of the biliary tree upon an obstructing stone or inspissated bile. Although the stereotyped patient is female, 40, fat, fair and fertile it can occur from adolescence to old age and in both sexes.

Clinical features

See FIGURE 34.14.

Typical clinical features are:

- acute onset severe pain
- post-prandial or at night (often wakes 2–3 am)
- constant pain (not colicky)
- lasts 20 minutes to 2–6 hours
- maximal RUQ or epigastrium
- may radiate to tip of right shoulder or scapula
- painful episode builds to a crescendo for about 20 minutes; may recede or last for hours
- some relief by assuming flexed posture
- ± nausea and vomiting with considerable retching
- often a history of biliary pain (may be mild) or jaundice
- often precipitated by a fatty meal

DxT severe pain + vomiting + pain radiation → biliary colic

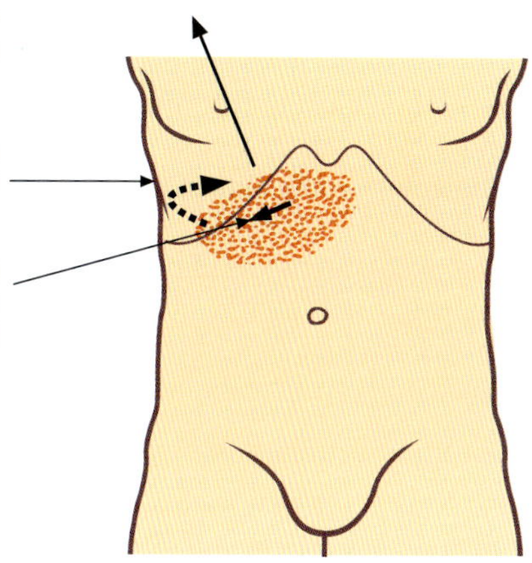

FIGURE 34.14 Typical site of pain of biliary colic and acute cholecystitis

Signs

- Patient anxious and restless, usually in a flexed position or rolling in agony
- Localised tenderness (Murphy sign) over fundus of gall bladder (on transpyloric plane)
- Slight rigidity

Diagnosis

- Abdominal ultrasound (to diagnose gallstones)/ DIDA
- Helical CT
- Intravenous cholangiography if previous cholecystectomy
- LFTs may show elevated bilirubin and alkaline phosphatase

Management

- Pain relief:[18]
  morphine 2.5–5 mg IV statim then titrate to effect (age-dependent)
  or
  fentanyl 50–100 mcg IV statim then titrate to effect

34

or
ketorolac 10–30 mg IM 4–6 hourly (max 90 mg daily)
- Gallstone dissolution with ursodeoxycholic acid or lithotripsy (in those unable to have surgery)
- Cholecystectomy (main procedure)

Gallstone facts[18]

- Gallstones form from bile in the gall bladder and sometimes in the bile duct (especially post-cholecystectomy)
- Two main types—cholesterol and pigment (bilirubin)
- Lifetime risk in first world countries is 12–20%
- 70% of people with gall bladder stones are asymptomatic, but risk of developing symptoms is about 15% over 20 years
- Cholecystectomy almost never indicated for such stones
- Complications: acute cholecystitis (may lead to empyema, perforation, cholecystoenteric fistula), obstructive jaundice, cholangitis and acute pancreatitis (pancreatic duct obstruction)

34

Microlithiasis (biliary 'sludge')

This condition, which causes biliary 'colic' due to spasm of the sphincter of Oddi, often follows prolonged fasting. Cholecystectomy may be necessary.

Acute cholecystitis

Cholecystitis is associated with gallstones in over 90% of cases[18] and there is usually a past history of biliary pain. It occurs when a calculus becomes impacted in the cystic duct and inflammation develops. It is very common in the elderly. The acute attack is often precipitated by a large or fatty meal. The causative organisms are usually aerobic bowel flora (e.g. *E. coli, Klebsiella* species and *Enterococcus faecalis).*

Clinical features

- Steady severe pain and tenderness
- Localised to right hypochondrium or epigastrium
- Nausea and vomiting (bile) in about 75%
- Aggravated by deep inspiration

Signs

- Patient tends to lie still
- Localised tenderness over gall bladder (positive Murphy sign)
- Muscle guarding
- Rebound tenderness
- Palpable gall bladder (approximately 15%)
- Jaundice (approximately 15%)
- ± Fever

Diagnosis

- Ultrasound: gallstones but not specific for cholecystitis
- HIDA scan: demonstrates obstructed cystic duct—the usual cause
- WCC and CRP: can be elevated

Treatment

- Bed rest
- IV fluids
- Nil orally
- Analgesics
- Antibiotics
- Cholecystectomy

If evidence of sepsis, use amoxy/ampicillin 1 g IV, 6 hourly plus gentamicin 4–6 mg/kg IV daily.[20]

Change to amoxycillin + clavulanate 875 + 125 mg (o) 12 hourly when afebrile.

Acute pancreatitis

With acute pancreatitis there may be a past history of previous attacks or a past history of alcoholism (35%) or gallstone disease (40–50%). It is commonly precipitated by fatty foods and alcohol, mumps, hypertriglyceridaemia and some antidiabetic medications, e.g. gliptins.

Clinical features

See FIGURE 34.15.

Typical clinical features are:

- sudden onset of severe constant deep epigastric pain but onset can be steady
- lasts hours or a day or so
- pain may radiate to back
- pain may be relieved by sitting forwards
- nausea and vomiting
- sweating and weakness

DxT severe pain + nausea and vomiting + relative lack of abdominal signs → acute pancreatitis

Signs

- Patient is weak, pale, sweating and anxious
- Tender in epigastrium
- Lack of guarding, rigidity or rebound
- Reduced bowel sounds (may be absent if ileus)
- ± Abdominal distension
- Fever, tachycardia ± shock

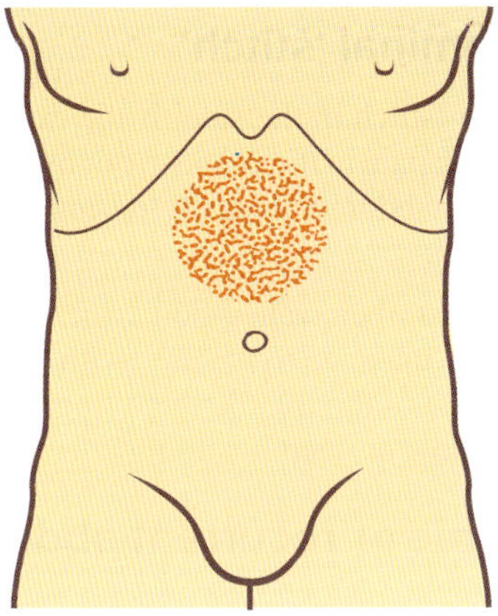

FIGURE 34.15 Typical pain distribution of acute pancreatitis

Diagnosis

- WCC—leucocytosis
- Serum lipase (preferred as more sensitive and specific) or serum amylase
- CRP—elevated
- Serum glucose ↑, calcium ↓
- Blood gases: P_aO_2 (? pulmonary complications)
- LFTs: ? obstructive pattern
- Plain X-ray, may be sentinel loop
- CT scan (especially for complications)
- Ultrasound better for detecting cysts and unsuspected gallstones

Management[20]

- Arrange admission to hospital.
- Basic treatment is bed rest, nil orally, nasogastric suction (if vomiting), IV fluids and analgesics (morphine).
- Use morphine 2.5–5 mg IV or fentanyl 50–100 mcg IV statim then titrate to effect.
- May require ERCP if obstructive LFTs.

Chronic pancreatitis

In comparison to acute pancreatitis, the pain of chronic pancreatitis is milder but more persistent. There may be epigastric pain boring through to the back. Symptoms may relapse and worsen. Investigate with CT scan and ultrasound and faecal elastase (N > 200 μg/g stool: pancreastic exocrine insufficiency < 200 μg/g stool). MRCP is the most sensitive imaging study. The patient with this problem is often labelled as 'gastritis', 'ulcer' or 'neurotic' because of the indeterminate nature of the pain. Malabsorption and diabetes may result from pancreatitis and weight loss and steatorrhoea become prominent features.

Pain associated with pancreatic cancer is indistinguishable from that of chronic pancreatitis but generally tends to be more severe and more prominent in the back. Use paracetamol for pain. Give pancreatic enzyme supplements (e.g. pancrelipase) for steatorrhoea.

Acute diverticulitis

The patient with acute diverticulitis is usually over 40 years of age, with long-standing, grumbling, left-sided abdominal pain and constipation, but can have irregular bowel habit. It occurs in less than 10% of patients with diverticular disorder.[2] (Refer CHAPTER 44.)

Clinical features

See FIGURE 34.16.

Typical clinical features are:

- acute onset of pain in the left iliac fossa
- pain increased with walking and change of position
- usually associated with constipation

DxT acute pain + left–sided radiation + fever → acute diverticulitis

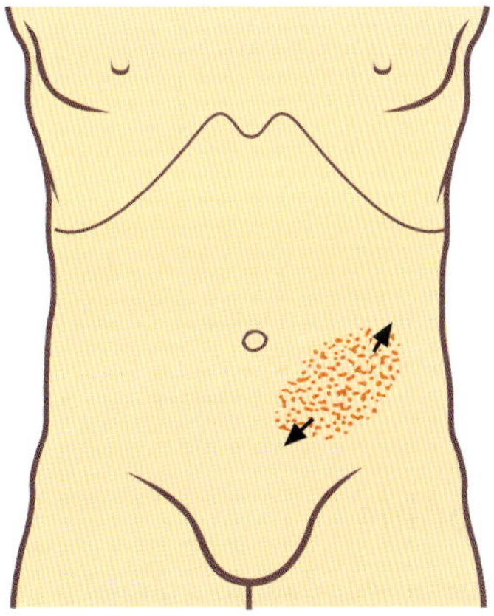

FIGURE 34.16 Typical pain distribution of acute diverticulitis

Signs

- Tenderness, guarding and rigidity in LIF
- Fever
- May be inflammatory mass in LIF

34

Investigations

- FBE: leucocytosis
- Elevated ESR
- Pus and blood in stools
- Abdominal ultrasound/CT scan (especially—can detect fistula, abscess, or perforation)
- Erect chest X-ray
- Erect and supine abdominal X-ray

Complications

- Bleeding (can be profuse, especially in elderly)
- Perforation (high mortality)
- Abscess
- Peritonitis
- Fistula (bladder, vagina, small bowel)
- Intestinal obstruction

Treatment[20]

- Hospital admission
- Rest the GIT: nil orally, drip and suction
- One landmark study showed that a 'wait and see' approach without antibiotics can be considered appropriate in patients with an uncomplicated initial attack of diverticulitis[21]
- Analgesics
- Antibiotics:
  mild cases: amoxycillin + clavulanate 875/125 mg (o) 12 hourly for 5 days
  or
  metronidazole + cephalexin
  severe cases: (amoxy) ampicillin 1 g IV 6 hourly
  +
  gentamicin 5–7 mg/kg IV/day
  +
  metronidazole 500 mg IV 12 hourly
  or
  metronidazole + ceftriaxone 1 g IV/day
- Surgery for complications
- Screening colonoscopy after acute episode

Peritonitis

Can be generalised due to intra-abdominal sepsis following perforation of a viscus, e.g. peptic ulcer, appendix, diverticulum. Typical signs are as for perforated peptic ulcer. Key investigations are peritoneal fluid culture and CT scan. Surgical intervention is usually required. Usual antibiotic treatment is IV cephalosporins or amoxy/ampicillin + gentamicin + ss metronidazole.[19] Spontaneous bacterial peritonitis can occur in any patient with ascites.

Abdominal 'stitch'

The common 'stitch in the side' is the experience of a sharp, stabbing pain in the epigastric or hypochondrium regions of the abdomen, usually during running. The sufferer should:

- stop and rest, then walk—don't run
- apply deep massage to the area with the palps (fleshy tips) of the middle three fingers
- perform slow or deep breathing

Chronic or recurrent abdominal pain

Advances in technology, particularly the use of ultrasound, CT scanning and endoscopy, have increased the opportunities for diagnosing chronic or recurrent abdominal pain in adults.

If the patient has 'red flag' symptoms (see below) and the above investigations are unavailable, consider the possibility of conditions such as pancreatic cancer, ovarian cancer, small bowel tumours, mesenteric ischaemia, Crohn disease, metabolic disorders such as lactase deficiency, and rarer conditions as outlined in TABLE 34.3.

Other investigations that may help:

- MRI
- laparoscopy—this may allow the identification of chronic adhesive obstruction, small bowel tumours or inflammation, or intra-abdominal malignancy

Red flags for organic disease[12]

- Older patient
- Nocturnal pain or diarrhoea
- Progressive symptoms
- Rectal bleeding
- Fever
- Anaemia
- Weight loss
- Abdominal mass
- Faecal incontinence or urgency (recent onset)

Chronic appendicitis

It is possible to have recurrent episodes of subacute inflammation of the appendix. If suspected, laparoscopy performed during or soon after an attack is diagnostic.

Adhesions

There is no firm evidence that intra-abdominal adhesions are painful apart from complications such as bowel obstruction. Sometimes patients are 'cured' by laparoscopic divisions of adhesions.

Peptic ulcer (gastric or duodenal)

See CHAPTER 47.

Clinical features

- Usually central epigastric pain
- Burning pain
- Relieved by antacids or food or milk
- DU: usually 2–3 hours after meals or wakes from sleep
- GU: may occur after meals but inconsistent relationship to eating

When to refer

- All cases of acute abdominal pain where urgent surgical intervention is required
- Special urgency and early diagnosis is important with: ruptured ectopic pregnancy, ruptured AAA, mesenteric artery occlusion, ruptured viscus, perforated peptic ulcer, strangulated obstructed bowel, intussusception
- All cases where the diagnosis is not apparent
- All cases where surgery is necessary
- Medical causes, such as diabetic ketoacidosis and porphyria

Practice tips

- Special caution is required at the extremes of age when the symptoms and signs do not often reflect the seriousness of the underlying pathology.
- If an elderly patient presents with intense acute abdominal pain, inadequately relieved by strong parenteral injections, likely causes include mesenteric artery occlusion, acute pancreatitis and ruptured or dissecting aortic aneurysm.
- When an inflamed appendix ruptures, the abdominal pain improves for a significant period of time.
- Consider gallstones and duodenal ulcer if the patient is woken (e.g. at 2–3 am) with abdominal pain.
- Pus cells and red cells may be present in the urine with appendicitis when a pelvic appendix involves the bladder and a retrocaecal appendix involves the ureter.
- Consider diabetic ketoacidosis in a patient with abdominal pain, tenderness and rigidity and deep sighing respiration.

Patient education resources

Hand-out sheets from *Murtagh's Patient Education* 7th edition:
- Appendicitis
- Diverticular disease
- Gallstones
- Infant colic
- Irritable bowel
- Kidney stones

References

1. De Wit NJ. Acute abdominal pain. In: Jones R et al., eds. *Oxford Textbook of Primary Care.* Vol. 2. Oxford: Oxford University Press, 2004: 738–40.
2. Sandler G, Fry J. Acute abdominal pain. In: *Early Clinical Diagnosis.* Lancaster: MTP Press, 1986: 137–76.
3. Murtagh J. *The Anatomy of a Rural Practice.* Melbourne: Monash University Monograph, 1980: 34.
4. Sandler G, Fry J. Chronic abdominal pain. In: *Early Clinical Diagnosis.* Lancaster: MTP Press, 1986: 177–86.
5. Bain ST, Spaulding WB. The importance of coding presenting symptoms. CMAJ, 1967; 97 (16): 953–9.
6. Holland AJ. Acute abdominal pain in children. Australian Doctor, 2009; 7 August: 25–32.
7. Hutson JM, Woodward AA, Beasley SW. *Jones Clinical Paediatric Surgery.* Oxford: Blackwell Publishing, 2003: 139–45.
8. Dilley A. Abdominal surgical problems in children. Medical Observer, 23 April 2004: 31–4.
9. Appleberg M. Abdominal aortic aneurysms: how to treat. Australian Doctor, 2001; 22 June: iii–iv.
10. Hunt P, Marshall V. *Clinical Problems in General Surgery.* Sydney: Butterworths, 1991: 193–243.
11. Humes DJ. Acute appendicitis. BMJ, 2006; 333: 530–4.
12. Rao P, Boland G. Imaging of acute right lower abdominal quadrant pain. Clin Radiol, 1998; 53: 639–49.
13. Ashrafizadeh A, Koneru S, Thomas JH et al. Non-operative treatment of acute appendicitis: is this possible?. Medicine Today, August 2017; 18: 8.
14. Crawford J, Jarvis T, Hugh T. Acute abdominal pain: how to treat. Australian Doctor, 2008; 2 August: 27–34.
15. Expert group for Analgesic. Acute pain. In: eTG complete [Internet]. Melbourne: Therapeutic Guidelines Ltd. Available from: <www.tg.org.au>, accessed January 2018.
16. Laerum E, Murtagh J. Kidney coli and recurrent urinary calculi. Aust Fam Physician, 2001; 30 (1): 36–41.

17 Laerum E et al. Oral diclofenac in the treatment of recurrent kidney colic. A double-blind comparison with placebo. Eur Urol, 1995; 28: 108–11.

18 Expert group for Gastrointestinal. Biliary and pancreatic disorders. In: eTG complete [Internet]. Melbourne: Therapeutic Guidelines Ltd. Available from: <www.tg.org.au>, accessed January 2018.

19 Tooceli J, Wright T. Gallstones. Med J Aust, 1998; 169: 166–71.

20 Expert group for Antibiotic. Intra-abdominal infection. In: eTG complete [Internet}. Melbourne: Therapeutic Guidelines Ltd. Available from: <www.tg.org.au>, accessed January 2018.

21 Daniels L, Unlu C, de Korte N et al. Randomized clinical trial of observational versus antibiotic treatment for the first episode of CT-proven uncomplicated acute diverticulitis. Br J Surg, 2017; 104 (1): 52–61.

Arthritis 35

Rheumatic disorders are common in old age: much of rheumatology is geriatric and much of geriatrics is rheumatology.

DR FRANK DUDLEY HART[1] 1983

The clinical evaluation of the patient presenting with the complaint of arthralgia (painful joints) or arthritis (inflammation of the joints) can be a difficult and challenging exercise because it can be a presentation of many systemic disorders, some of which are rare. Important considerations are sex, age, the pattern of joint involvement (monoarticular or polyarticular), immediate and more remote history, family history and drug use—all of which may provide important diagnostic clues. Polyarthritis, which implies the active inflammation of five or more joints, presents a more challenging diagnostic problem.

Key facts and checkpoints

- In a UK National Morbidity Survey, rheumatic disease composed just over 7% of all morbidity presenting to the family doctor.[2]
- The commonest cause was osteoarthritis (OA), which affects 5–10% of the population.
- The same study indicated an episode rate for arthritis/arthralgia of 38.6 per 1000 population.
- The population incidence of rheumatoid arthritis (RA) is 1–2%.
- There should be no systemic manifestations with OA.
- One-quarter of disability in elderly people is due to severe joint disease.
- Systemic diseases that may predispose to, or present with, an arthropathy include the connective tissue disorders, diabetes mellitus, a bleeding disorder, previous tuberculosis, the spondyloarthropathies such as psoriasis, SBE, hepatitis B, rheumatic fever, the various vasculitic or arteritic syndromes (the vasculitides) such as Wegener granulomatosis, HIV infection, lung cancer, haemochromatosis, sarcoidosis, hyperparathyroidism, Whipple disease and Paget disease.
- The pain of inflammatory disease is worse at rest (e.g. on waking in the morning) and improved by activity.
- Early diagnosis and management of RA results in considerably better outcomes.
- Causes of monoarthritis include crystal deposition disease, sepsis, osteoarthritis, trauma and spondyloarthritis.
- Gout and septic arthritis have a recognised cause and cure.
- Acute gout is almost exclusive to males: in women, it is usually seen only in those who are postmenopausal or taking thiazide diuretics.

A diagnostic approach

A summary of the diagnostic strategy model is presented in TABLE 35.1.

Probability diagnosis

The probability diagnoses for the patient presenting with arthritis are:

- osteoarthritis (mono- or polyarthritis)
- viral arthritis (if acute and polyarthritis)

OA is very common in general practice. It may be primary, which is usually symmetrical, and can affect many joints. This clinical pattern is different from secondary OA, which follows injury and other wear-and-tear causes.

Viral polyarthritis is more common than realised. It presents usually within 10 days of the infection, and is usually mild.

Clinical features (viral arthritis)

- Acute onset
- A polyarthritis
- Symmetric inflammation
- Mainly of hands and feet
- Rash—persists for 24 hours minimum
- Terminates rapidly—over days
- FBE: lymphopaenia, lymphocytosis, ± atypical lymphocytes

It tends to terminate quickly and spontaneously without permanent damage to joints. It is caused by many viruses, including those causing influenza,

35

Table 35.1 Arthralgia: diagnostic strategy model

Probability diagnosis
Osteoarthritis
Viral polyarthritis (e.g. parvovirus)

Serious disorders not to be missed
Infection:
- rheumatic fever
- endocarditis
- tuberculosis
- brucellosis
- pyogenic (septic) arthritis: e.g. gonococcus, *Staphylococcus, Kingella kingae*
- HIV arthropathy
- dengue fever

Cancer:
- bronchogenic carcinoma
- leukaemia/lymphoma
- secondary malignancy

Other:
- rheumatoid arthritis (RA)
- connective tissue disorders: SLE, scleroderma, polymyositis and dermatomyositis, psoriasis, other

Pitfalls (often missed)
Fibromyalgia syndrome
Polymyalgia rheumatica
Crystal deposition:
- gout
- pyrophosphate (pseudogout)

Haemarthrosis
Dengue fever
Lyme disease
Ross River virus
Avascular necrosis
Rarities:
Other vasculitides (e.g. polyarteritis nodosa)
Haemochromatosis
Sarcoidosis
Whipple disease
Hyperparathyroidism
Familial Mediterranean fever
Amyloidosis
Pigmented villonodular synovitis

Seven masquerades checklist
Depression (unlikely)
Diabetes (? arthropathy)
Drugs (especially narcotics)
Endocrine disorder (thyroid storm, Addison disease)
Spinal dysfunction (possible spondyloarthropathies)

Is the patient trying to tell me something?
Always a consideration with pain. Psychogenic factors aggravate chronic arthritic conditions.

mumps, rubella, varicella, hepatitis B and C, infectious mononucleosis (more muscle aching), cytomegalovirus, parvovirus, Australian epidemic polyarthritis due to the alphaviruses, Ross River virus (see CHAPTER 28) and Barmah Forest virus. Adenovirus is common in children.

Serious disorders not to be missed

These include rheumatoid arthritis (RA), which can start as a monoarthritis; pyogenic arthritis, including gonococcus, *Staphylococcus, Kingella* sp. and *Streptococcus* infections; tuberculosis; rheumatic fever; and bacterial endocarditis. Early diagnosis of septic arthritis is very important as it can destroy a hip in 24 hours.

It is important to be forever watchful for rheumatic fever (RF). It presents typically as a migratory polyarthritis involving large joints sequentially, one becoming hot, red, swollen and very painful as the other subsides. It rarely lasts more than 5 days in any one joint.

A flitting polyarthritis can also occur with endocarditis in addition to a systemic upset and a cardiac murmur. Gonococcal infection may present in a single joint or as flitting polyarthritis, often accompanied by a rash. Brucellosis can cause arthritis and sacroiliitis and can be confused with the spondyloarthropathies.

HIV infection is becoming a great mimicker. It can present as a chronic oligoarticular asymmetrical arthritis.[3] It can also present as a rash very similar to psoriasis.

With the large influx of migrants from South-East Asia the possibility of tuberculosis presenting as arthritis should be kept in mind.

Connective tissue disorders may be involved. They include SLE, progressive systemic sclerosis (scleroderma), and dermatomyositis. It is most inappropriate to settle with a general diagnosis such as 'rheumatism' or 'arthritis' and where doubtful it is important to find the specific entity causing the problem.

In respect to malignant disease, arthralgia is associated with acute leukaemia, lymphoma and neuroblastoma in children and with bronchial carcinoma, which may cause hypertrophic osteoarthropathy, especially of the wrist and ankle (not a true arthritis but simulates it). Occasionally polyarthritis may be the first feature of an occult neoplasm. Monoarticular metastatic disease may involve the knee (usually from lung or breast).

Red flag pointers for polyarthritis

- Fever
- Weight loss
- Profuse rash
- Lymphadenopathy
- Cardiac murmur
- Severe pain and disability
- Malaise and fatigue
- Vasculitic signs
- Two or more systems involved

Pitfalls

There are several pitfalls, most of which are rare. A common pitfall is gout. This applies particularly to older women taking diuretics, whose osteoarthritic joints, especially of the hand, can be affected. The condition is often referred to as nodular gout and does not usually present as acute arthritis.

Fibromyalgia syndrome is a real puzzle (see CHAPTER 37) as it can mimic the connective tissue disorders in its early presentation—typically a woman in the third or fourth decade.

Another 'trap' is haemarthrosis in a patient with a bleeding disorder.

Infective causes that may be overlooked are dengue fever, especially in travellers returning from a tropical or subtropical area, and Lyme disease, which is now surfacing in many countries, especially where ticks are found.

There are many rare causes of arthritis. Sarcoidosis causes two forms: an acute benign form, usually in the ankles and knees, and a chronic form with long-standing sarcoidosis that involves joints (large or small) adjacent to underlying bone disease.

Then there are the uncommon vasculitides, which can cause confusion in diagnosis. This group includes polyarteritis nodosa, hypersensitive vasculitis, polymyalgia rheumatica/giant cell arteritis, Wegener granulomatosis, Henoch–Schönlein purpura and Behçet syndrome.

Haemochromatosis can present with a degenerative arthropathy that characteristically affects the second or third metacarpophalangeal joints.[3]

Other rare causes of arthritis are erythema nodosum, serum sickness and Sjögren syndrome.

General pitfalls

- Not searching beyond RA when an RA pattern polyarthritis may be part of another systemic disease
- Failing to search for some cause of arthritis other than OA in a patient, especially an elderly patient (i.e. underdiagnosing); an important example of this is polymyalgia rheumatica
- Failing to consider the various drug interactions between NSAIDs, over-the-counter medications and other drugs used by the elderly
- Underdiagnosing and misdiagnosing through lack of appreciation of the many causes of arthritis, especially those presenting as part of a systemic disease

Seven masquerades

Drug-induced arthritis usually affects the hands and is generally symmetrical. The drugs may induce autoantibodies (e.g. ANA, ANCA). Those that include a lupus syndrome include the anti-epileptics, chlorpromazine and some cardiac drugs. Various antibiotics have been associated with arthralgia, e.g. minocycline, while diuretics, especially frusemide and thiazides, can precipitate gout. The problem usually resolves promptly after withdrawal of the agent.[4]

Intravenous drug abuse may be associated with septic arthritis, hepatitis B and C, HIV-associated arthropathy, SBE with arthritis and serum sickness reactions.

Hyperthyroidism can uncommonly cause acropathy (clubbing and swelling of the fingers) and may present as pseudogout, while hypothyroidism can present with an arthropathy or cause proximal muscle pain, stiffness and weakness. Diabetes mellitus may cause an arthropathy that can be painless or mild to moderately painful.

The spondyloarthropathies may be a causative factor. They often present with an acute monoarthritis, particularly in teenagers, some time before causing sacroiliitis and spondylitis.

Psychogenic considerations

Although 'arthralgia' is an uncommon complaint in psychoneurotic disorders, any pain syndrome can be a significant manifestation. The usual cause of arthralgia is inflammation in the joint—that is, arthritis—but a functional cause is encountered from time to time.

Furthermore, some patients who are unfortunate enough to acquire arthritis, especially the more serious disorders, certainly develop ongoing emotional and psychological problems that appear to aggravate their total problem.

So-called 'growing pains' of the lower limb are common in children, and the physical examination and investigations are normal. Parents need to be reassured that it is a benign condition, while recognising that emotional factors may be quite significant. As Apley pointed out, 'physical growth is not painful, but emotional growth can hurt like hell'.[5]

The clinical approach

A priority is to determine whether or not the arthritis is caused by a primary rheumatic disorder or whether it is part of an underlying systemic disorder.

History

Very careful enquiry about the exact onset of the arthritis is important. This includes whether it was acute or insidious, and confined to specific joints or flitting as in rheumatic fever and sometimes in infective endocarditis. Is it a true polyarthritis or monoarthritis? Symmetrical or asymmetrical? It is also important to differentiate between arthralgia (pains in or around the joints) and arthritis (inflammation of the joints). Not all arthralgia is arthritis.

A family history is important because a positive family history is associated with conditions such as RA (rarely), ankylosing spondylitis, connective tissue disorders (rarely), psoriasis, gout, pseudogout and haemophilia.

A very hot, red, swollen joint suggests either infection or crystal arthritis.

Key questions

- Can you carefully point out exactly where you feel the pain?
- Does the pain move from joint to joint or stay in the same joint?
- Are you aware of anything that brought on the pain?
- Does the pain disturb you at night?
- Do your joints feel very sore or stiff when you wake up in the morning?
- What effect does exercise or activity have on the pain or stiffness?
- Have you had an injury in the past to your painful joint(s)?
- Do you get pain over both your shoulders and upper arms?
- Have you got a skin rash? Is it new?
- Have you had a fever, sweats or chills?
- Do you get very tired, weak or out of sorts?
- Have you noticed any change in the colour of your urine?
- Have you had a sore throat?
- Have you had sinus trouble?
- Have you had acute pain in your big toe or in other joints before?
- Do you have a history of psoriasis?
- Do you have a history of rheumatic fever?
- Do you have pain in your neck or lower back or in other joints?
- Have you had any diarrhoea?
- Have you had a discharge from your penis?
- Have you had any problems with your eyes?
- What drugs are you taking? Are you taking fluid tablets (diuretics)?
- How much alcohol would you drink a day?
- Have you been visiting the countryside or exposed to ticks or have you been to a deer farm?
- Have you travelled overseas recently?
- Have you been at risk of getting an STI?
- Have you been drinking untreated milk recently?
- Have you had cats as pets, especially as a child (associated with RA)?

Examination

A systematic examination of the affected joint or joints should be performed, looking for signs of inflammation, deformity, swelling and limitation of movement. Tenderness and warmth indicates inflammatory activity. Erythema indicates gouty arthritis or other crystallopathy, rheumatic fever or septic arthritis.

Joint swelling:

- acute (1–4 hours) with intense pain = blood infection or crystals (e.g. gout)
- subacute (1–2 days) and soft = fluid (synovial effusion)
- chronic and bony = osteoarthritis
- chronic and soft/boggy = synovial proliferation

A coarse crepitus suggests OA. Each joint should be examined specifically. Inspection should note the presence of lumps or bumps such as Heberden nodes on the osteoarthritic DIP joints of the hands, Bouchard nodes on the osteoarthritic PIP joints of the hands, and rheumatoid nodules, which are the only pathognomonic finding of RA and gouty tophi. Signs that may be of diagnostic help are presented in FIGURE 35.1.

The specific inflamed joint or joints may give an indication of the disease process. Typical joints affected by various arthropathies are illustrated in FIGURE 35.2.

Investigations

TABLE 35.2 lists the many investigations that are used to reach a diagnosis. Clinical acumen permits a judicious selection of specific tests rather than ordering an expensive battery.

It is important to keep in mind the many specific serological tests to detect infective causes of arthralgia. These include Australian epidemic polyarthritis, Lyme disease, rubella, *Brucella*, hepatitis B, gonococcus, mycoplasma, HIV tests, parvovirus and Barmah Forest virus.

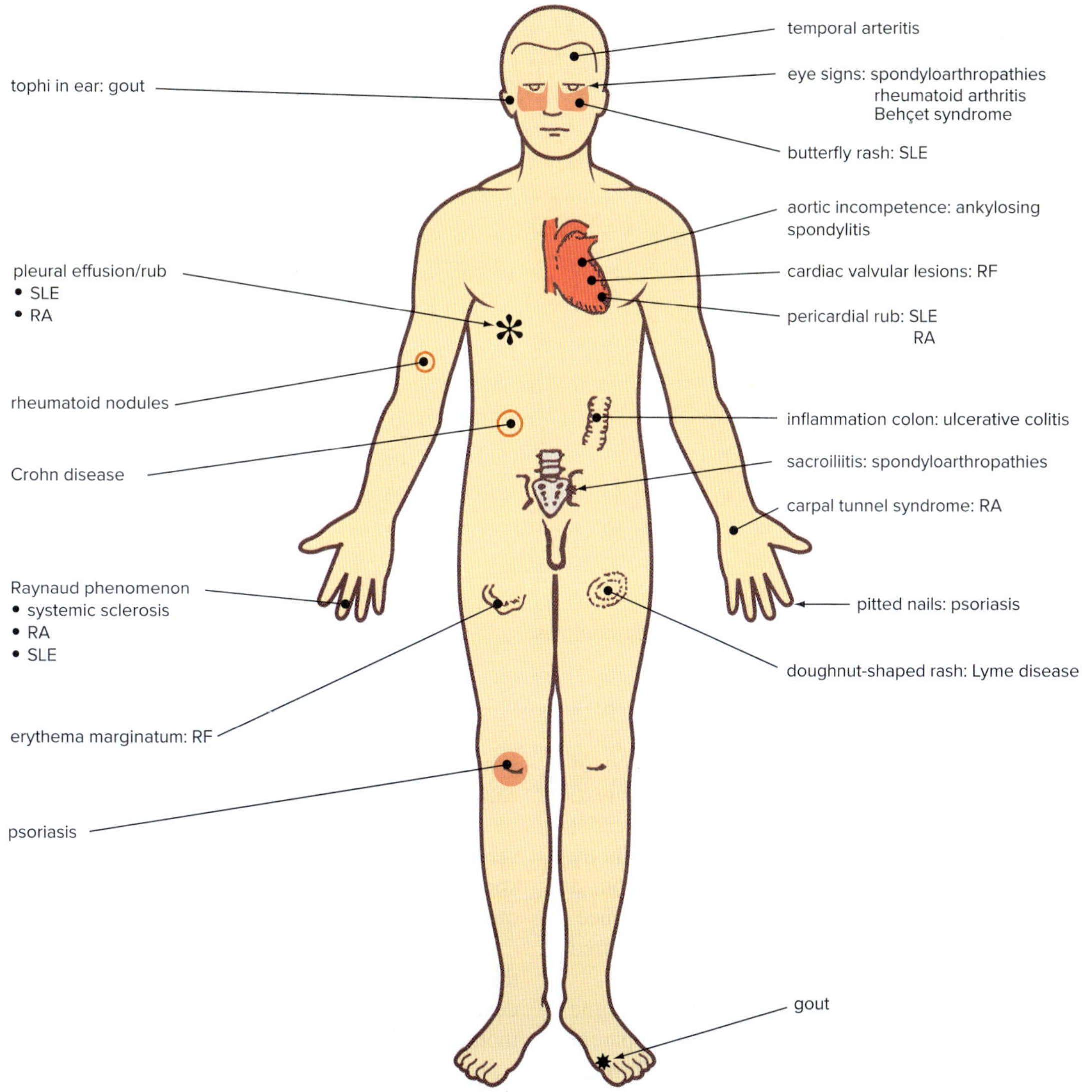

FIGURE 35.1 Physical examination: possible findings to consider in diagnosis

35

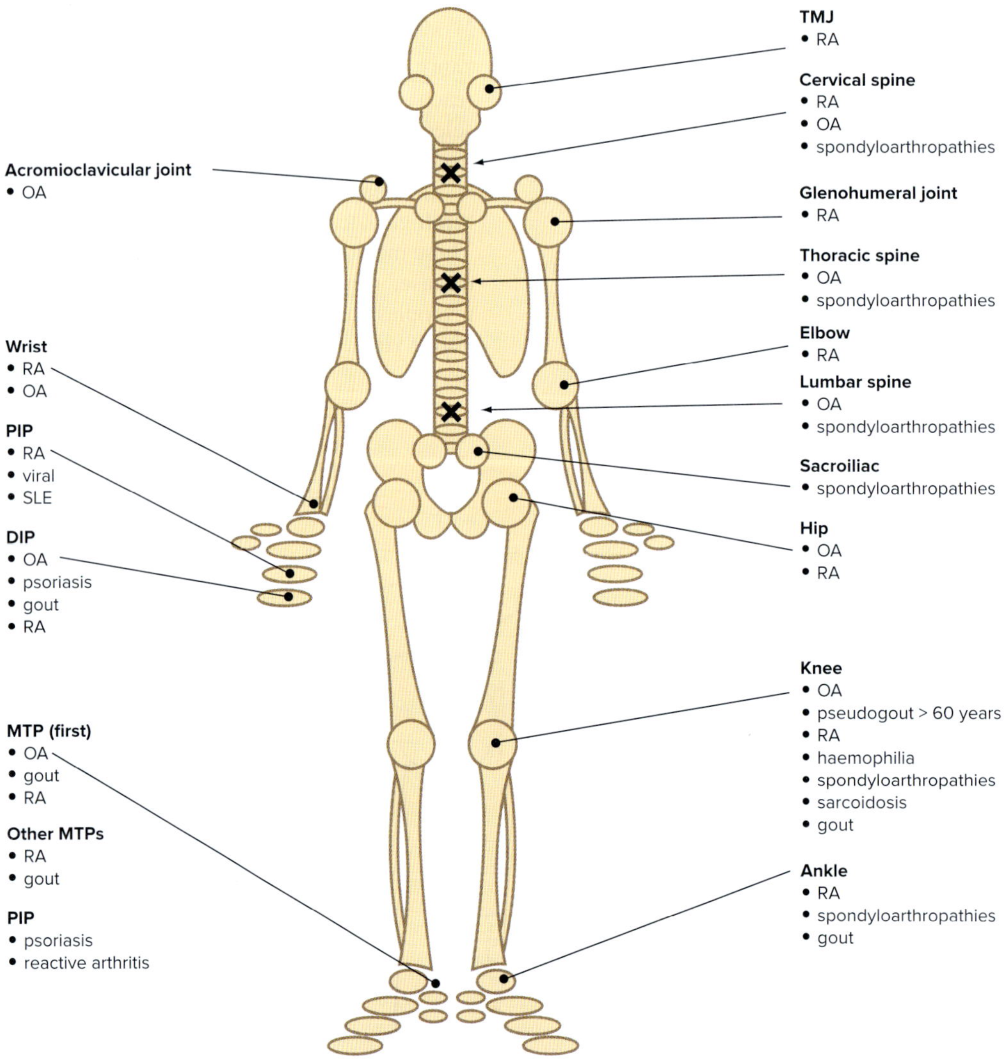

FIGURE 35.2 Joints typically affected by various arthropathies

In reference to viral serology, a positive immunoglobulin M (IgM) antibody test is presumptive evidence of recent infection and is likely to be of diagnostic significance in this clinical context. However, sometimes IgM antibodies can persist for months or years.[6] A positive IgG antibody result indicates previous exposure to the virus but a single positive titre is of no diagnostic significance. Seroconversion or at least a fourfold rise on paired sera confirms recent infection (see FIG. 35.3).

Plain X-ray is invaluable, although in some conditions radiological changes may be apparent only when the disease is well established. Typical X-ray changes for common conditions are presented in FIGURE 35.4. Arthrography has limited value in the diagnosis of polyarthritis but is very useful for specific joints such as the shoulder and the knee. Ultrasound examination for joints such as the shoulder and the hip can be very useful.

HLA-B_{27} should not be used for arthritis screening. It has a high sensitivity for ankylosing spondylitis, but low specificity, and should rarely be ordered.[6]

The various immunological tests for diagnosis of the connective tissue disorders are outlined with the description of each condition. Such screening tests include:

- rheumatoid factor and anti-CCP
- antinuclear antibodies
- dsDNA antibodies

Table 35.2 Investigations for arthritis

Appropriate tests can be selected from the following:

- urine analysis: blood, protein, sugar
- synovial fluid: analysis, culture
- radiology—plain X-ray*
- blood and other cultures
- haemoglobin and differential WCC
- ESR*
- C-reactive protein
- serum uric acid, creatinine*
- 24-hour urinary uric acid
- rheumatoid factor
- anti-CCP (cyclic citrullinated peptide) antibody*
- antinuclear antibody (screening test for SLE)*
- dsDNA antibodies
- extractable nuclear antigen (ENA) antibodies
- HLA-B_{27} (poor predictive value)
- various specific serological tests (e.g. Australian epidemic polyarthritis, rubella, Lyme disease, hepatitis B, Barmah Forest virus, parvovirus)
- HIV serology
- antistreptolysin O titre
- streptococcal anti-DNase B
- arthroscopy and biopsy
- bone scan

**Key tests*

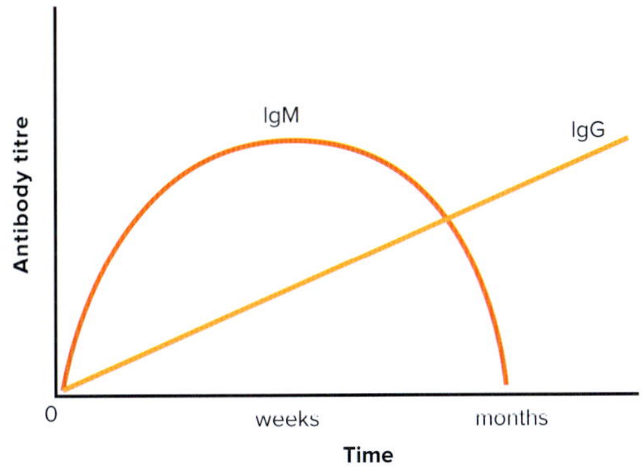

FIGURE 35.3 Time course of IgG and IgM antibodies in viral arthritis

The LE cell test has been superseded by the antinuclear, dsDNA and ENA (especially Sm) antibody tests but the latter should only be performed if there is an elevated ANA test.[6]

Arthritis in children

Arthralgia (joint pain) is a common problem in childhood and, although arthritis is rare, the complaint demands considerable respect because of the many

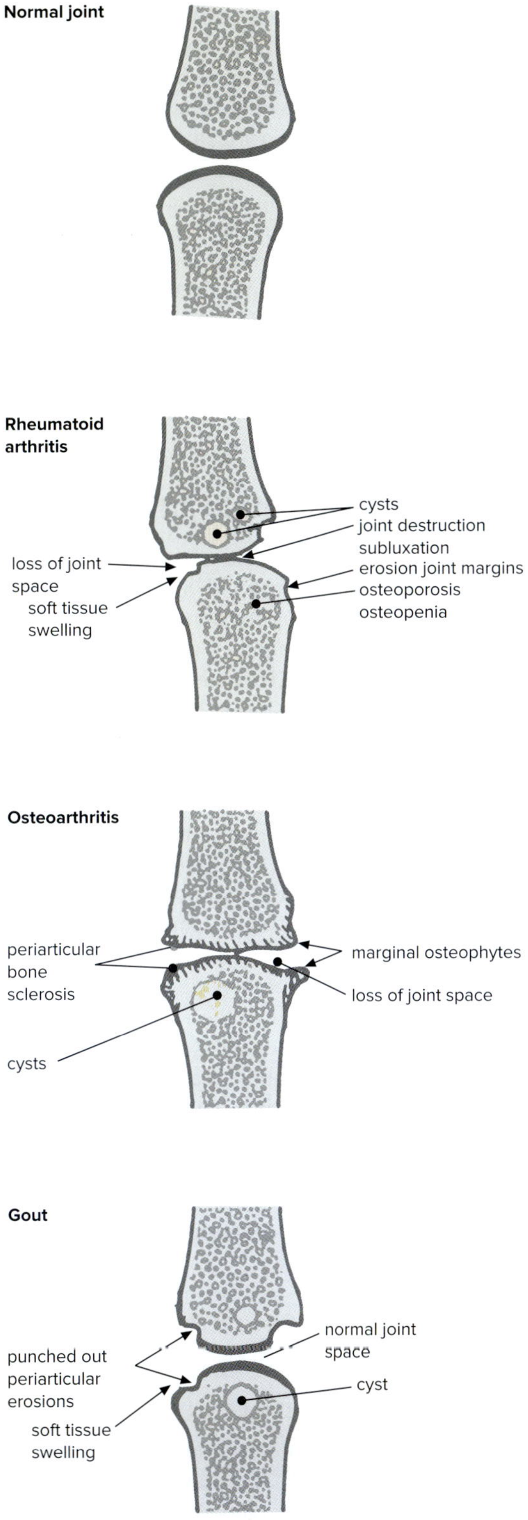

FIGURE 35.4 X-rays for common arthritic conditions: typical changes

35

serious problems causing it. Particular consideration should be given to rheumatic fever, septic arthritis, osteomyelitis and meningoccaemia. Arthritis may be part of an infectious disease such as rheumatic fever, rubella, mumps, varicella, cytomegalovirus infection, erythema infectiosum (human parvovirus), influenza or other viral infection, and is occasionally encountered with Henoch–Schönlein purpura. Actually, viral arthritis is very common in children. An FBE is helpful as it may show lymphopaenia, lymphocytosis or atypical lymphocytes.[1] It is worth noting that underlying bone tumours can present as joint pain if the tumour is adjacent to the joint.

Note: Acute-onset monoarticular arthritis associated with fever is septic until proven otherwise.

Juvenile idiopathic arthritis

JIA, also known as juvenile chronic arthritis and juvenile rheumatoid arthritis (US), is defined as a chronic arthritis persisting for a minimum of 6 weeks (some criteria suggest 3 months) in one or more joints in a child younger than 16 years of age.[5] It is rare, affecting only about 1 in 1000 children, but produces profound medical and psychosocial problems.

35

The commonest types of JIA are oligoarticular (pauciarticular) arthritis, affecting four or fewer joints (about 50%), and polyarticular arthritis, affecting five or more joints (about 40%). Systemic onset arthritis, previously known as Still syndrome, accounts for about 10% of cases. It is usually seen in children under the age of 5 but can occur throughout childhood. The child can present with a high remittent fever and coppery red rash, plus other features, including lymphadenopathy, splenomegaly and pericarditis. Arthritis is not an initial feature but develops ultimately, usually involving the small joints of the hands, wrists, knees, ankles and metatarsophalangeal joints.

These children should be referred once the problem is suspected or recognised. JIA is not a benign disease—50% have persistent active disease as adults.

Rheumatic fever typically occurs in children and young adults, the first attack usually occurring between 5 and 15 years of age.

Arthritis in perspective

Five per cent of all children complain of recurrent lower limb pain, which often awakens them from their sleep. There may be emotional factors involved and parents need appropriate reassurance. A careful history and physical examination are essential, and perhaps simple basic investigations may be appropriate. As Rudge[5] points out, we have to be vigilant against underdiagnosis, misdiagnosis and overdiagnosis. Refer to growing pains (see CHAPTER 91) and post-activity musculoskeletal pain (see CHAPTER 66).

Rheumatic fever

RF is an inflammatory disorder that typically occurs in children and young adults following a group A *Streptococcus pyogenes* infection. It is common in developing countries and among Indigenous Australians (see CHAPTER 134) but uncommon in first world countries.[8]

Clinical features

- Young person 5–15 years (can be older)
- Acute-onset fever, joint pains, malaise
- Flitting arthralgia mainly in leg (knees, ankles) and arm (elbows and wrists)
- One joint settles as the other is affected
- May follow a sore throat

However, the symptoms depend on the organs affected and arthritis may be absent.

Diagnosis

Based on clinical criteria:

2 or more major criteria
or
1 major + 2 or more minor criteria

in the presence of supporting evidence of preceding Group A streptococcal infection.

Major criteria

- Carditis
- Polyarthritis
- Chorea (involuntary abnormal movements)
- Subcutaneous nodules
- Erythema marginatum

Minor criteria

- Fever (≥38°C)
- Previous RF or rheumatic heart disease
- Monoarthralgia
- Raised ESR >30 mm/hr or CRP >30 mg/L
- ECG—prolonged PR interval

Investigations

A selective combination of:

- FBC
- throat swab
- ESR

- streptococcal ASOT
- streptococcal anti-DNase B (repeat in 10–14 days)
- C-reactive protein
- plus ECG and echocardiogram (if ↑ PR) and CXR.

Treatment

- Rest in bed until CRP normal for 2 weeks
- Benzathine penicillin 900 mg IM (450 mg in child <20 kg) statim or phenoxymethylpenicillin 500 mg (o) bd, 10 days
- Paracetamol 15 mg/kg (o) 4 hourly (max. 60 mg/kg/day); aspirin or naproxen for arthritis
- Diuretics for carditis (may be ACE inhibitor and corticosteroids)
- Prophylactic long-term penicillin

Septic arthritis

Acute sepsis (see FIG. 35.5) can affect any joint at any age, although it is more common in children. It evolves over hours or days and can rapidly destroy a joint structure. It is an emergency in the hip joint of children. Check for IV drug use. The commonest organisms are *S. aureus, Kingella kingae* and *N. gonorrhoea*. Diagnosis is by blood culture and synovial fluid analysis and culture. Treatment is with drainage and washout of the joint and IV followed by oral antibiotics, e.g. di/flucloxacillin.

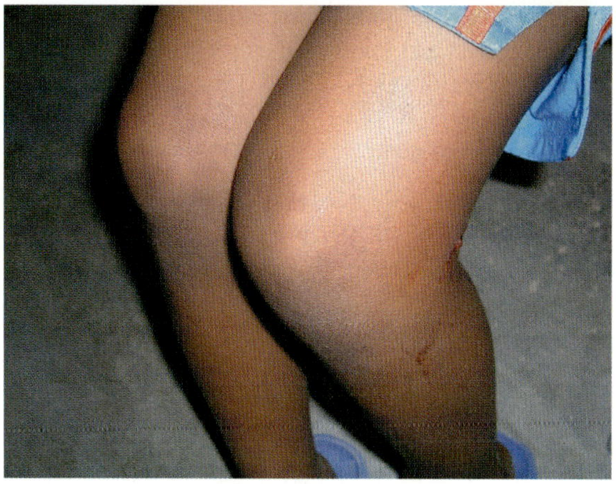

FIGURE 35.5 Septic arthritis in a young girl who presented with a painful swollen left knee and difficulty walking. A knee aspiration revealed turbid fluid with elevated leukocytes. The joint fluid culture grew *Staphylococcus aureus*.

Arthritis in the elderly

OA is very common with advancing age and for this reason care has to be taken not to simply attribute other causes of arthritis to OA. Other musculoskeletal conditions that become more prevalent with increasing age are:

- polymyalgia rheumatica
- Paget disease of bone
- avascular necrosis
- gout
- pseudogout (pyrophosphate arthropathy)
- malignancy (e.g. bronchial carcinoma)

Pseudogout

This crystal deposition arthropathy (chondrocalcinosis) is noted by its occurrence in people over 60 years. It usually affects the knee joint but can involve other joints.

Rheumatoid arthritis

Although it usually begins between the ages of 30 and 40 it can occur in elderly patients, when it occasionally begins suddenly and dramatically. This is called ‘explosive’ RA and fortunately tends to respond to small doses of prednisolone and has a good prognosis.[7] RA in the elderly can present as a polymyalgia rheumatica syndrome.

35

Osteoarthritis

OA is the most common type of arthritis, occurring in about 10% of the adult population and in 50% of those aged over 60.[8] It is a degenerative disease of cartilage and may be primary or secondary to causes such as trauma and mechanical problems, septic arthritis, crystallopathy or previous inflammatory disorders, or structural disorders such as SCFE and Perthes disorder.

The arthritis

Primary OA is usually symmetrical and can affect many joints. Unlike other inflammatory disease the pain is worse on initiating movement and loading the joint, and eased by rest. OA is usually associated with stiffness, especially after activity, in contrast to RA.

Joints involved

In primary OA all the synovial joints may be involved, but the main ones are:

- first carpometacarpal (CMC) joint of thumb
- first metatarsophalangeal (MTP) joint of great toe
- distal interphalangeal (DIP) joints of hands

Other joints that are affected significantly are the proximal interphalangeal joints, the knees, hips, acromioclavicular joints and joints of the spine, especially the facet joints of the cervical (C5–6, C6–7) and lumbar regions (L3–4, L4–5, L5–S1) (see FIG. 35.6).

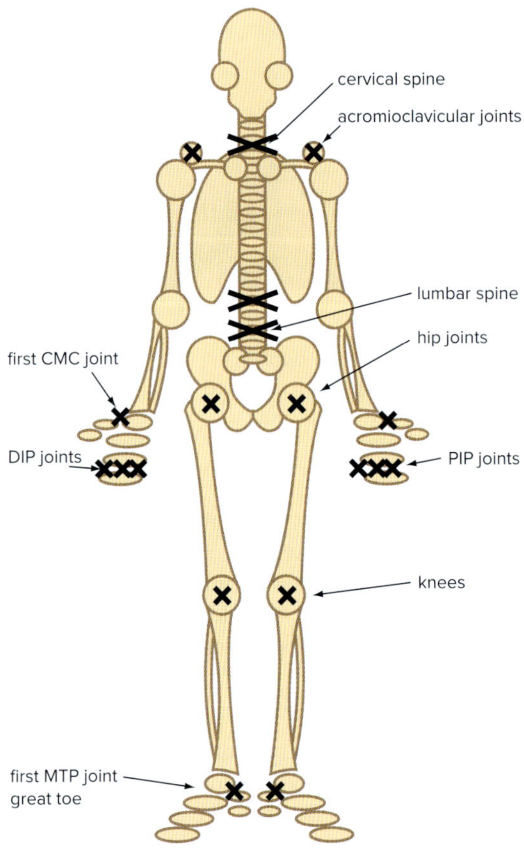

FIGURE 35.6 Osteoarthritis: typical joint distribution

Clinical features

- Pain: worse by the end of the day, aggravated by use, relieved by rest, worse in cold and damp
- Variable morning stiffness
- Variable disability

Signs

(See FIG. 35.7.)

- Hard and bony swelling
- Crepitus
- Signs of inflammation (mild)
- Restricted movements
- Joint deformity

Note: There should be no systemic manifestations.

Crystal arthropathy can complicate OA, especially in the fingers of people taking diuretics (e.g. nodular gout).

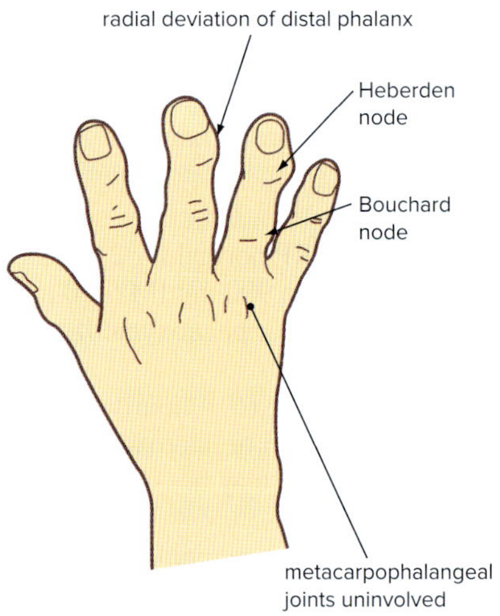

FIGURE 35.7 Typical clinical features of osteoarthritis of the hand

Differentiation from an inflammatory arthropathy

OA does not exhibit the typical inflammatory pattern. The clinical diagnosis is based on:

- gradual onset of pain after activity (worse towards the end of the day)
- the pattern of joint involvement
- the lack of soft tissue swelling
- the transient nature of the joint stiffness or gelling
- takes <30 minutes to settle after rest while inflammatory arthritis takes at least 30 minutes

Diagnosis

The diagnosis is clinical and radiological but the degree of changes on X-ray do not always parallel levels of symptoms.[8]

X-ray findings

- Joint space narrowing with sclerosis of subchondral bone
- Formation of osteophytes on the joint margins or in ligamentous attachments
- Cystic areas in the subchondral bone
- Altered shape of bone ends

Principles of management

- Provide explanation and reassurance including patient education hand-outs.
- Correct modifiable risk factors: obesity, injury, overuse.
- Control pain and maintain function with appropriate drugs.

- Suggest judicious activity, exercise and physical therapy.
- Consider factors lowering the coping threshold (e.g. stress, depression, anxiety, overactivity).
- Refer for surgical intervention for debilitating and intractable pain or disability. Examples include OA of hip, knee, shoulder, first CMC joint of thumb, and first MTP joint, where surgery is now very successful. Osteotomies still have a limited place for a varus or valgus deformity of the knee.

Treatment (optimal)

- *Explanation.* Provide patient education and reassurance that arthritis is not the crippling disease perceived by most patients.
- *Exercise.* A graduated exercise program is essential to maintain joint function. Aim for a good balance of relative rest with sensible exercise. It is necessary to stop or modify any exercise or activity that increases the pain. Systematic reviews have found that both exercise and education may help reduce the pain and disability in people with OA of the hip or knee.[9]
- *Rest.* Rest during an active bout of inflammatory activity only; prolonged bed rest contraindicated.
- *Heat.* Recommended is a hot-water bottle, warm bath or electric blanket to soothe pain and stiffness. Advise against getting too cold.
- *Diet.* If overweight it is important to reduce weight to ideal level. Obesity increases the risk of OA of the knee approximately fourfold and weight loss may slow progression;[10] otherwise, no specific diet has been proven to cause or improve OA. Some people claim that their arthritis is improved by having a nutritious balanced diet consisting of fish, rice and vegetables and avoiding meat, dairy produce, alcohol, pepper and spices.
- *Correction of predisposing factors and aids.* Apart from weight reduction the following may help: walking stick, heel raise for leg length disparity, back brace, elastic or hinged joint support (e.g. knee).
- *Physiotherapy.* Referral should be made for specific purposes such as:
  - correct posture and/or leg length disparity
  - supervision of a hydrotherapy program
  - heat therapy and advice on simple home heat measures
  - teaching and supervision of isometric strengthening
  - exercises (e.g. for the neck, back, quadriceps muscle)
- *Occupational therapy.* Refer for advice on aids in the home, more efficient performance of daily living activities, protection of joints, and on the wide range of inexpensive equipment and tools.
- *Simple analgesics* (regularly for pain). Use paracetamol/acetaminophen (avoid codeine or dextropropoxyphene preparations, and aspirin if recent history of dyspepsia or peptic ulceration). Take before activity. Systematic reviews found that NSAIDs and simple analgesics reduce the pain of OA but there is no good evidence that NSAIDs are superior to simple analgesics (e.g. paracetamol) or that any one of the many NSAIDs is more effective than others.[9]
- *NSAIDs and aspirin.* These are the first-line drugs for more persistent pain not relieved by paracetamol or where there is evidence of inflammation, such as pain worse with resting and nocturnal pain. The risk versus benefit equation always has to be weighed carefully. As a rule, NSAIDs should be avoided if possible. Significant risks of NSAIDs are:
  - gastric erosion with bleeding
  - gastric ulceration
  - depression of kidney function (check kidney function beforehand)
  - hepatotoxicity

  Note: Change to a suppository form will not necessarily render the upper GIT safe from irritation.

- *COX-2 specific inhibitors (CSIs).* Refer to CHAPTER 12. These new generation agents, represented mainly by celecoxib and etoricoxib, should be considered where there is an indication for an NSAID but when the risk of NSAID-induced ulceration and bleeding is high.[11] Evidence shows that they have a similar efficacy to other NSAIDs and a modest absolute reduction in GIT complications.[11] The usual precautions need monitoring.
- *Intra-articular (IA) corticosteroids.* As a rule IA corticosteroids are not recommended but occasionally can be very effective for an inflammatory episode of distressing pain and disability on a background of tolerant pain (e.g. a flare-up in an osteoarthritic knee).
- *Viscosupplementation.* Intra-articular hylans, e.g. hyaluronan weekly for 3–5 weeks especially for OA of knee. Supported by level I evidence.
- *Complementary therapy.* Glucosamine, a natural amine sugar, derived from chitin in shellfish shells, has had anecdotal claims of efficacy for

the treatment of OA. Level II evidence has shown a modest benefit for the knees.[13] Further studies indicate inadequate evidence to support its general use.[8] The dose is 1500–2000 mg (o) daily in divided doses, with food. It is well tolerated (it is contraindicated in those with a significant seafood allergy). A 3–4 month trial may be worthwhile.[8]
- *Epidemiological studies* (level III evidence) suggest that OA patients whose diet is rich in antioxidants, such as vitamin C, vitamin D and green tea, have slower progression of joint space narrowing on X-ray over long-term follow-up.[14]
- *Contraindicated drugs.* For OA these include the immunosuppressive and disease-modifying drugs such as oral corticosteroids, gold, anti-malarials and cytotoxic agents.
- *Surgery.* Refer for surgical intervention if debilitating and intractable pain or disability. Examples include OA of the hip, knee, shoulder, first CMC joint of thumb and first MTP joint.

Rheumatoid arthritis

35

RA, which is an autoimmune polyarticular systemic disease of unknown aetiology, is the commonest chronic inflammatory polyarthritis and affects about 1–2% of the population. The disorder can vary from a mild to a most severe debilitating expression. About 10–20% of patients have a relentless progression and require aggressive drug therapy.[14]

Genetic factors may represent a risk of 15–70% of developing RA.

The arthritis

RA generally presents with the insidious onset of pain and stiffness of the small joints of the hands and feet. The pain is persistent rather than fleeting and mainly affects the fingers where symmetrical involvement of the PIP joints produces spindling while the metacarpophalangeal joints develop diffuse thickening as does the wrist (see FIG. 35.8). In 25% of cases RA presents as arthritis of a single joint such as the knee,[7] a situation leading to confusion with Lyme disease or a spondyloarthropathy. Differential diagnosis is polyarticular gout.

Joints involved

- Hands: MCP and PIP joints, DIP joints (30%)
- Wrist and elbows
- Feet: MTP joints, tarsal joints (not IP joints), ankle
- Knees (common) and hip (delayed—up to 50%)
- Shoulder (glenohumeral) joints

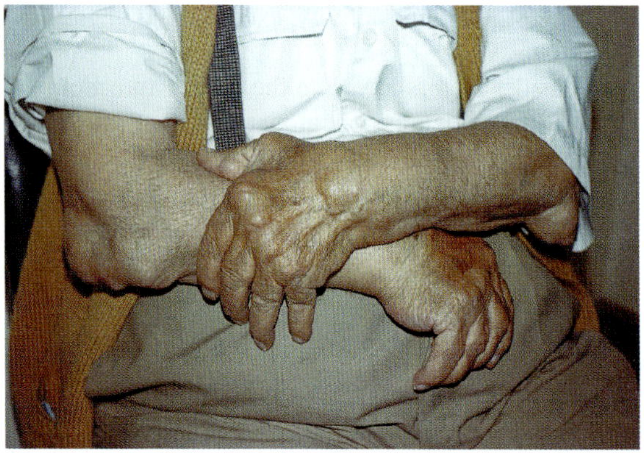

FIGURE 35.8 Chronic rheumatoid arthritis showing classic features of deformities including subluxation of joints and rheumatoid nodules

- Temporomandibular joints
- Cervical spine (not lumbar spine)

Refer to FIGURE 35.9.

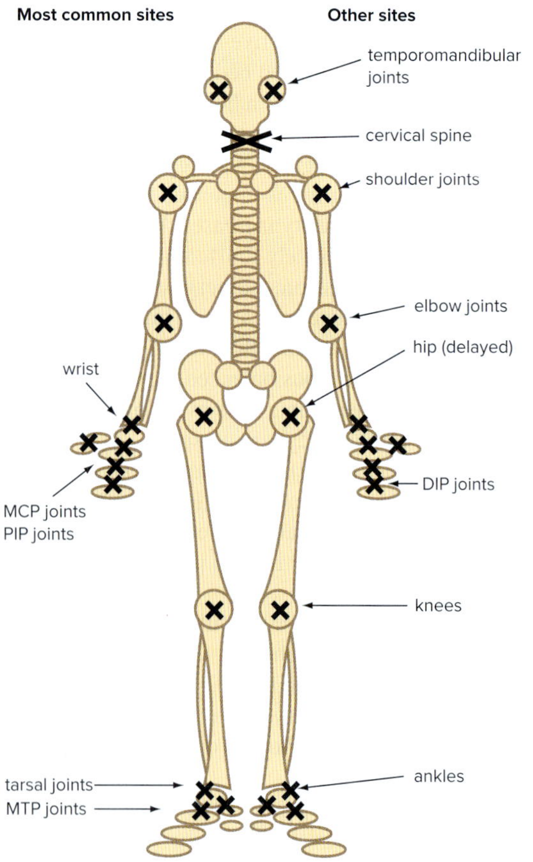

FIGURE 35.9 Rheumatoid arthritis: typical joint distribution

Clinical features

- Insidious onset but can begin acutely (explosive RA)
- Any age 10–75 years: peak 30–50 years but bimodal 25–50 (peak age) and 65–75
- Female to male ratio = 3:1
- Joint pain: worse on waking, nocturnal pain, disturbed sleep; relieved with activity
- Morning stiffness—can last hours
- Rest stiffness (e.g. after sitting)
- General: malaise, weakness, weight loss, fatigue
- Disability according to involvement

Signs

- Soft swelling (effusion and synovial swelling), especially of wrist, MCP and PIP joints
- Warmth
- Tenderness on pressure or movement
- Limitation of movement
- Muscle wasting
- Later stages: deformity, subluxation, instability or ankylosing
- Look for swan necking, boutonnière and z deformities, ulnar deviation (see FIG. 35.10)
- Check for a number of everyday functions, for example:
  - power grip (lifting a jug of water)
  - precision grip (using a key or pen), undoing buttons
  - hook grip (carrying a bag)

The various possible extra-articular manifestations are summarised in FIGURE 35.11.

Investigations

- ESR/CRP usually raised according to activity of disease
- Anaemia (normochromic and normocytic) may be present
- Rheumatoid factor
  - positive in about 70–80% (less frequent in early disease)
  - 15–25% of RA patients will remain negative[14]
- Anti-cyclic citrullinated peptide (anti-CCP) antibodies: more specific for RA (96% specificity)
- X-ray changes:
  - erosion of joint margin
  - loss of joint space (may be destruction)
  - juxta-articular osteoporosis
  - cysts
  - advanced: subluxation or ankylosing
- MRI—helpful for early diagnosis

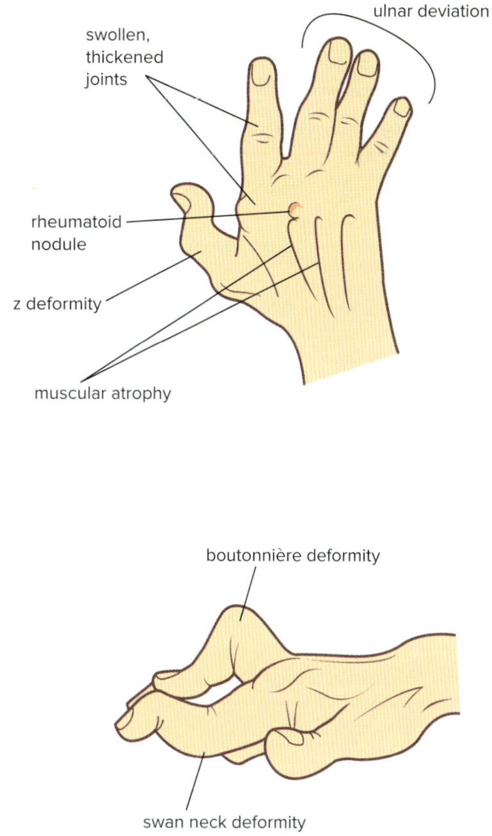

FIGURE 35.10 Chronic rheumatoid arthritis: typical signs

Criteria for the diagnosis of RA are presented in TABLE 35.3.

Principles of management[8,15]

- Give patient education support and appropriate reassurance. The diagnosis generally has distressful implications, and so the patient and family require careful explanation and support. Some patients have little or no long-term problems but even in mild cases, continuing care and medical supervision is important.
- There has been a radical shift from palliation to early induction of disease remission, to prevent joint damage and reduce morbidity from malignancy (especially lymphoma) and cardiovascular disease.
- Since many studies show disease progression in the first 2 years, relative aggressive treatment with disease-modifying antirheumatic drugs (DMARDs) from the outset is advisable, rather than to start stepwise with analgesics and NSAIDs only.[16]

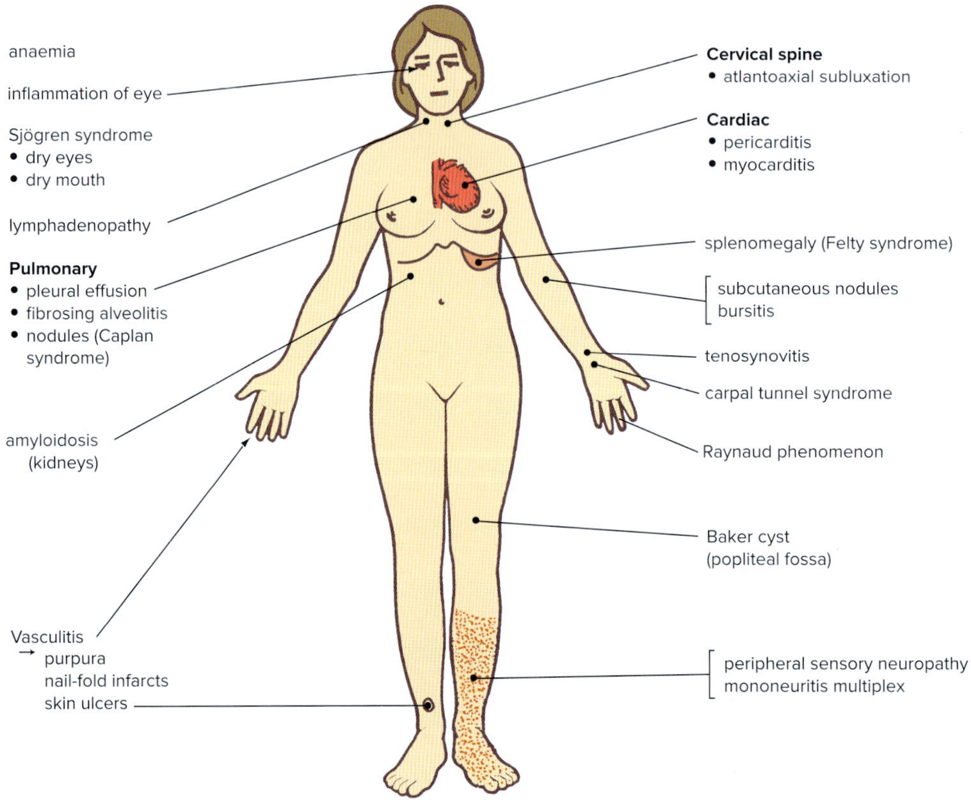

FIGURE 35.11 Rheumatoid arthritis: significant non-articular clinical manifestations

Table 35.3 Revised criteria for features suggestive of rheumatoid arthritis[8]

Family history of inflammatory arthritis
Symptom duration of >6 weeks
Early-morning stiffness of >1 hour
Arthritis in three or more regions
Swelling in five or more joints
Bilateral compression tenderness of the metatarsophalangeal joints
Symmetry of the areas affected
Presence of rheumatoid nodules
Rheumatoid factor positivity
Raised inflammatory markers (ESR/CRP) in absence of infection
Anti-cyclic citrullinated peptide antibody positivity
Bony erosions evident on radiographs of the hands or feet, although these are uncommon in early disease

Key points

- If the RA factor is positive, it is non-specific—order the anti-CCP antibody to confirm the diagnosis.
- RA has a strong cardiovascular risk factor.

- Use a team approach where appropriate, including an early consultant referral for obvious or suspected RA or positive anti-CCP for diagnosis and collaborative support.
- Fully assess the patient's functional impairment and impact on home life, work and social activity. Involve the family in decision making.
- Make judicious use of pharmaceutical agents. For serious cases consultant collaboration is essential.
- Review the patient regularly, continually assessing progress and drug tolerance. The disease activity can be monitored with plain X-rays, ultrasound of hands (especially if hands are thick), CRP ± ESR.

Specific advice

- *Rest and splinting.* This is necessary where practical for any acute flare-up of arthritis.
- *Exercise.* It is important to have regular exercise, especially walking and swimming. Have hydrotherapy in heated pools.
- *Smoking cessation.* This is strongly recommended.
- *Referral.* Referring to physiotherapists and occupational therapists for expertise in exercise supervision, physical therapy and advice regarding coping in the home and work is important.

- *Joint movement.* Each affected joint should be put daily through a full range of motion to keep it mobile and reduce stiffness.
- *Diet.* Although there is no special diet that seems to cause or cure RA, there is evidence that avoiding animal fats (dairy products and some meats) and using fish oils is beneficial.[18] A nourishing, well-balanced diet is common sense and obesity must be avoided.

Therapies used in the management of rheumatoid arthritis are presented in TABLE 35.4.

Table 35.4 Therapies used in the management of rheumatoid arthritis[15,17]

Therapies
Education (rest, literature, weight loss, joint protection advice)
NSAIDs
Simple analgesics
DMARDs: Conventional synthetic DMARDs • Immunosuppressants: – azathioprine – cyclosporin – leflunomide – methotrexate Biological DMARDs • Cytokine inhibitors – anti-TNF α agents: abatacept, adalimumab, certolizumab, etanercept, infliximab, golimumab, rituximab – anti-Interleukin-1 agents; anakinra, tocilizumab
Gold salts
Quinolones: • hydroxychloroquine • chloroquine
Others: • D-penicillamine • sulfasalazine
Glucocorticoids: • oral prednisolone • intra-articular • intravenous (steroid 'pulses')
Fish body oil
Physical therapy (hydrotherapy, isometric exercises)
Occupational therapy (splints, aids and appliances)
Orthopaedic surgery (synovectomy, joint replacement, arthrodesis, plastic hand surgery)
Chiropody, footwear, insoles

Source: After Reilly and Littlejohn[15,17]

Management (pharmacological)[18]

Best under consultant direction.

- NSAIDs are effective and still have a place, but the adverse effects are a problem.
- The use of DMARDs and biological DMARDs improves long-term outcomes.
- Methotrexate is the 'backbone' of treatment.
- It should be continued when starting other DMARDs.
- Supplementation with folic acid can improve gastrointestinal symptoms and reduce the risk of liver dysfunction.
- Beware of the increased risk of infection in patients on combination DMARD regimes.
- When indicated, vaccination for pneumococcus, influenza, hepatitis A and B and HPV is recommended for all DMARDs.
- Any pain can be managed with paracetamol or NSAIDs. Avoid opioid analgesics if possible.
- Glucocorticoids are appropriate for flares of RA.

Fish oil

Fish oil in doses to deliver 4 g of omega-3 long-chain polyunsaturated fatty acids daily (typically 0.2 g/kg) over several months has been shown to reduce symptoms and the need for NSAIDS through its anti-inflammatory activity.[8,18]

35

Glucocorticoids

Oral use should be considered in patients with severe disease as a temporary adjunct to DMARD therapy and where other treatments have failed or are contraindicated.

The dose is prednisolone 5–10 mg (o) daily. Avoid doses higher than 15 mg daily if possible.

Intra-articular injections of depot preparations are effective in larger joints.

Disease-modifying antirheumatic drugs (DMARDs)

These agents target synovial inflammation and prevent joint damage. The choice depends on several factors, but is best left to the specialist coordinating care. In most patients with recently diagnosed RA, methotrexate is the cornerstone of management and should be commenced as early as possible.

Initial dose: methotrexate 5–10 mg (o) once weekly, increasing to maximum of 25 mg weekly (o) SC depending on clinical response and toxicity. Add folic acid 5–10 mg twice weekly (not on the day methotrexate is given).[8]

Biological DMARDs (bDMARDs) are the newer agents, which should be considered if remission is not achieved with appropriate methotrexate monotherapy, 'triple therapy' or other combinations. All bDMARDs are more effective when combined with methotrexate.

Warning: All practitioners should be aware of the increased risk of infectious diseases such as the atypical pneumonias, tuberculosis and listeriosis while taking bDMARDs. All patients should report unusual or unexpected fever or symptoms. Injection site reactions are common.

Standard initial drug therapy

Monotherapy with methotrexate (or occasionally another DMARD) is standard. Less than 20% will reach disease remission and, if not achieved, increase the dose or consider combination therapy. Many patients are managed on conventional DMARDs.

Combination therapy

35

Consider standard triple therapy: methotrexate + sulfasalazine + hydroxychloroquine.

Triple therapy can be used if methotrexate monotherapy has failed or initially on diagnosis, depending on the severity of the disease. Monitoring for FBE, LFTs and annual eye checks is necessary.

Several other double combinations may be used (e.g. methotrexate with cyclosporin, leflunomide or a bDMARD).

CONNECTIVE TISSUE DISEASES

The connective tissue disorders have the common feature of arthritis or arthralgia. Refer to CHAPTER 32.

Arthritis is the commonest clinical feature of SLE (over 90%).[7] It is a symmetrical polyarthritis involving mainly small and medium joints, especially the proximal interphalangeal and carpal joints of the hand. It is usually non-erosive and non-deforming, although deformities of fingers and thumbs can occur due to laxity of ligaments, tendons and capsules, causing joint instability.

The initial presentation is similar to RA.

Scleroderma can present as a polyarthritis affecting the fingers of the hand in 25% of patients, especially in the early stages. Soft tissue swelling produces a 'sausage finger' pattern.

Arthralgia and arthritis occur in about 50% of patients with polymyositis/dermatomyositis and may be the presenting feature before the major feature of muscle weakness and wasting of the proximal muscles of the shoulder and pelvic girdles appear. The small joints of the hand are usually affected and it may resemble RA.

Crystal arthritis

Arthritis, which can be acute, chronic or asymptomatic, is caused by a variety of crystal deposits in joints. The three main types of crystal arthritis are monosodium urate (gout), calcium pyrophosphate dihydrate (CPPD) and calcium phosphate (usually hydroxyapatite).[19] Refer to TABLE 35.5.

Table 35.5 Crystal-induced disorders

Crystals	Associated disease/ syndrome	Typical joints or region affected
Monosodium urate	Acute gout Tophaceous gout Asymptomatic Chronic gouty arthritis	Metatarsophalangeal joint of big toe Also: other foot joints, ankle, knee and patellar bursa, wrist, fingers
Calcium pyrophosphate dihydrate (CPPD)	Acute pseudogout Destructive arthropathy (like RA) Asymptomatic (most common)	Knee, wrist In older people >60 years (average age 72) F >M (2.7:1)
Basic calcium phosphate	Acute calcific periarthritis Destructive arthropathy Acute arthritis	Shoulder (supraspinatus)

Gout (monosodium urate crystal disorder)

Gout is an abnormality of uric acid metabolism resulting in hyperuricaemia and urate crystal deposition. Urate crystals deposit in:

- joints—acute gouty arthritis
- soft tissue—tophi and tenosynovitis
- urinary tract—urate stones

Four typical stages of gout are recognised:

- *Stage 1*—asymptomatic hyperuricaemia
- *Stage 2*—acute gouty arthritis
- *Stage 3*—intercritical gout (intervals between attacks)
- *Stage 4*—chronic tophaceous gout and chronic gouty arthritis

Asymptomatic hyperuricaemia:

- 10 times more common than gout[7]
- Elevated serum uric acid (>0.42 mmol/L in men, > 0.36 mmol/L in women)
- Absence of clinical manifestations
- Usually does not warrant treatment

Clinical features

Typical clinical features of gout include:[8]

- mainly a disorder of men (5–8% prevalence)
- onset earlier in men (40–50) than women (60+)
- acute attack: excruciating pain in great toe (see FIG. 35.12), early hours of morning

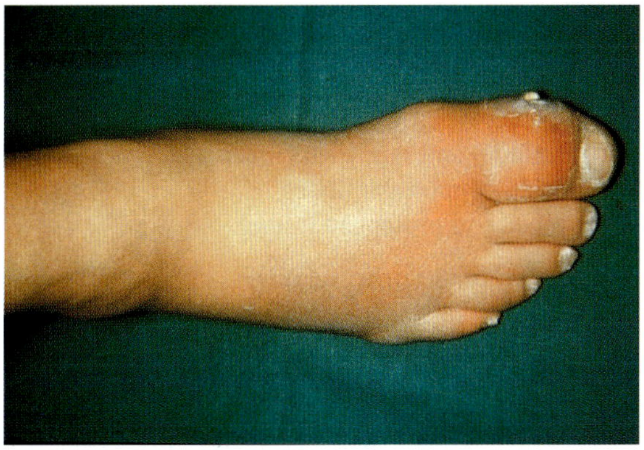

FIGURE 35.12 Gout showing typical red, shiny, swollen arthritis of the first MTP joint with desquamation of the skin

- skin over joint—red, shiny, swollen and hot
- exquisitely tender to touch
- relief with colchicine, NSAIDs, corticosteroids
- can subside spontaneously (3–10 days) without treatment

Causes/precipitating factors

- Alcohol excess (e.g. binge drinking)
- Surgical operation
- Starvation
- Drugs (e.g. frusemide, thiazide diuretics)
- Chronic kidney disease
- Myeloproliferative disorders
- Lymphoproliferative disorders (e.g. leukaemia)
- Sugary soft drinks[21]
- Cytotoxic agents (tumour lysis)
- Hypothyroidism
- Low-dose aspirin
- Others

The arthritis

Monoarthritis in 90% of attacks:

- MTP joint great toe—75%
- other joints—usually lower limbs: other toes, ankles, knees

Polyarticular onset is more common in old men and may occur in DIP and PIP joints of fingers. No synovial joint is immune.

Refer to FIGURE 35.13.

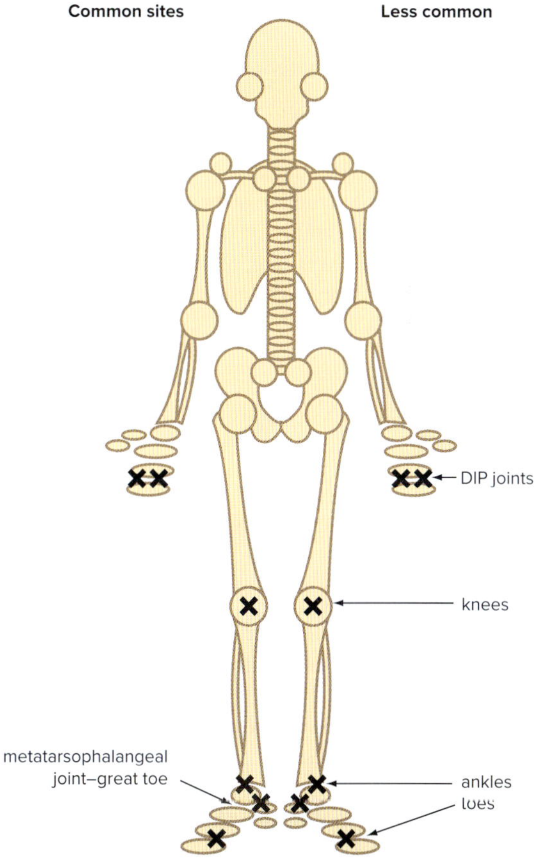

FIGURE 35.13 Gout: possible joint distribution

Other features

- Prone to recurrence
- Tophi in ears, elbows (olecranon bursa), big toes, fingers, Achilles tendon (can take many years)

35

- Can cause patellar bursitis
- Can get cellulitis (does not respond to antibiotics)

Nodular gout

Develops in postmenopausal women with kidney impairment taking diuretic therapy who develop pain and tophaceous deposits around osteoarthritic interphalangeal (especially DIP) joints of fingers.

Diagnosis

- Synovial fluid aspirate of affected joint, bursa or tophus → typical uric acid crystals using compensated polarised microscopy; this should be tried first (if possible) as it is the only real diagnostic feature
- Elevated serum uric acid (up to 30% can be within normal limits with a true acute attack)[19]
- X-ray: punched out erosions at joint margins

Management

Management of gout includes these principles:

- good advice and patient education information
- provision of rapid pain relief
- preventing further attacks
- prevention of destructive arthritis and tophi
- dealing with precipitating factors and comorbid conditions (e.g. alcohol dependence, obesity, CKD, polycythaemia vera, diabetes, hypertension)

35

The acute attack[8,20,21]

NSAIDs (except aspirin), in full dosage, are first-line and effective.

give orally until symptoms abate (up to 4–5 days) then continue for one week

or

Corticosteroids:

prednisolone 15–30 mg (o) daily until symptoms abate,[22,23] then decrease gradually

or

local corticosteroid injection up to a maximum of two affected sites[23]

or

intramuscular (in difficult cases) e.g. tetracosactrin 1 mg

or

Colchicine:

colchicine 0.5 mg (o) statim, then 0.5 mg every 6 or 8 hours until pain relief (usually 24–28 hours) or diarrhoea develops (max. 6 mg/24 hours)[21]

Note:

- Must be given early
- Avoid if kidney impairment
- Avoid use with macrolide antibiotics, e.g. clarithromycin, especially in CKD
- Avoid long-term use

Note:

- Avoid aspirin and urate pool lowering drugs (probenecid, allopurinol, sulphinpyrazone)[22]
- Monitor kidney function and electrolytes

Long-term therapy

When acute attack subsides, preventive measures with the aim of treating through diet include:

- weight reduction
- a normal, well-balanced diet
- avoidance of purine-rich food, such as organ meats (liver, brain, kidneys, sweetbread), tinned fish (sardines, anchovies, herrings), shellfish and game
- reducing red and processed meats, french fries and sweet treats
- reduced intake of alcohol
- reduced intake of sugary soft drinks (fructose)[24]
- good fluid intake (e.g. water—2 litres a day)
- avoidance of drugs such as diuretics (thiazides, frusemide) and salicylates/low-dose aspirin
- wearing comfortable shoes
- avoidance of prolonged fasting

Prevention (drug prophylaxis)

Allopurinol (a xanthine oxidase inhibitor) is the first-line drug of choice: dose 100–300 mg daily.

Indications:

- frequent acute attacks > 1 attack in 12 months
- tophi or chronic gouty arthritis
- kidney stones or uric acid nephropathy
- hyperuricaemia

Adverse effects:

- rash (2%)
- severe allergic reaction (rare)

Precautions:

- beware of kidney insufficiency and elderly patients—use lower doses
- beware of drug interactions:
  - azathioprine and 6 mercaptopurine—potentially lethal
  - amoxycillin—prone to rashes
- avoid initiating or changing allopurinol during an acute attack

Method: treatment of intercritical and chronic gout

- Commence allopurinol 6–8 weeks after last acute attack.
- Start with 50 mg daily for the first week and increase by 50 mg weekly to maximum 300 mg.
- Check uric acid level after 4 weeks: aim for level <0.38 mmol/L.
- Add colchicine 0.5 mg bd for 6 months (to avoid precipitation of gout) or indomethacin 25 mg bd or other NSAIDs.

Febuxostat (an alternative xanthine oxidase inhibitor): dose is 40 mg (o) initially, increasing to 80 mg

Probenecid (uricosuric agent)—a second-line agent

Good for hyperexcretion of uric acid by blocking renal tubular reabsorption. Dose: 500 mg/day (up to 2 g)

Note: Aspirin antagonises effect.

Prophylaxis of a flare of gout[8]

colchicine 0.5 mg (o) daily or bd
or
prednisolone 5mg (o) daily
or
an NSAID, e.g. diclofenac 25–50 mg (o) up to 200 mg/day

Calcium pyrophosphate crystal disorder (pseudogout)[8]

The finding of calcification of articular cartilage on X-ray examination is usually termed chondrocalcinosis. This is mainly a disorder of the elderly superimposed on an osteoarthritic joint. The acute attack is similar to an acute attack of gout but it affects the following joints (in order):

- knee
- 2nd and 3rd MCP joints
- wrist
- shoulder
- ankle
- elbow

It can affect tendons, especially the Achilles tendon, and cause a fever resembling septic arthritis.

The crystals in synovial fluid are readily identified by phase-contrast microscopy. X-rays are helpful in showing calcification of the articular cartilage.

Management is based on aspiration and installation of a depot glucocorticosteroid by injection into the joint (if joint infection excluded) plus analgesia. Be cautious of using NSAIDs in the elderly—paracetamol is preferred. Colchicine can be used.

Treatment includes:[8]

indomethacin 50 mg (o) tds (if tolerated) until symptoms abate
and/or
colchicine 0.5 mg (o) tds until attack subsides
and
paracetamol 500–1000 mg (o) four times daily, if necessary

THE SPONDYLOARTHRITIDES

The spondyloarthritides are a group of related inflammatory arthropathies with common characteristics affecting the spondyles (vertebrae) of the spine. It is appropriate to regard them as synonymous with the seronegative spondyloarthropathies in contradistinction to RA, which is seropositive and affects the cervical spine only. Apart from back pain, this group tends to present with oligoarthropathy in younger patients. The arthritis is characteristically peripheral, asymmetrical, affects the lower limbs and can exhibit dactylitis (e.g. 'sausage' digits).

Features[25]

- Sacroiliitis with or without spondylitis
- Enthesopathy (enthesitis), especially plantar fasciitis, Achilles tendonitis, costochondritis
- Peripheral arthritis, especially larger lower limb joints
- Extra-articular features (e.g. iritis/anterior uveitis, mucocutaneous lesions, psoriasiform skin and nail lesions, chronic GIT and GU inflammation)
- Absent rheumatoid factor
- Association with HLA-B_{27} antigen
- Familial predisposition

The group of disorders

1. Axial spondyloarthritis, including ankylosing spondylitis
2. Reactive arthritis
3. Inflammatory bowel disease (enteropathic arthritis)
4. Psoriatic arthritis
5. Juvenile onset ankylosing spondylitis
6. Unclassified spondyloarthritis—partial features only

Ankylosing spondylitis

This usually presents with an insidious onset of inflammatory back and buttock pain (sacroiliac joints and spine) and stiffness in young adults (age

<40 years), and 20% present with peripheral joint involvement before the onset of back pain. It usually affects the girdle joints (hips and shoulders), knees or ankles. At some stage, over 35% have joints other than the spine affected. The symptoms are responsive to NSAIDs (see CHAPTER 38).

Key clinical criteria[8]

- Low back pain persisting for >3 months
- Associated morning stiffness >30 minutes
- Awoken with pain during second half of night
- Improvement with exercise and not relieved by rest
- Limitation of lumbar spine motion in sagittal and frontal planes
- Chest expansion ↓ relative to normal values
- Unilateral sacroiliitis (grade 3 to 4)
- Bilateral sacroiliitis (grade 2 to 4)

Reactive arthritis

Reactive arthritis is a form of arthropathy in which non-septic arthritis and often sacroiliitis develop after an acute urogenital infection (usually *Chlamydia trachomatis*) or an enteric infection (e.g. *Salmonella, Shigella*).

35

> **DxT** urethritis + conjunctivitis ± iritis + arthritis → reactive arthritis

The arthritis (Reiter's syndrome), which commences 1–3 weeks post infection, tends to affect the larger peripheral joints, especially the ankle (talocrural) and knees, but the fingers and toes can be affected in a patchy polyarthritic fashion. Mucocutaneous lesions, including keratoderma blennorrhagica and circinate balanitis, may occur, although the majority develop peripheral arthritis only (see FIG. 35.14).

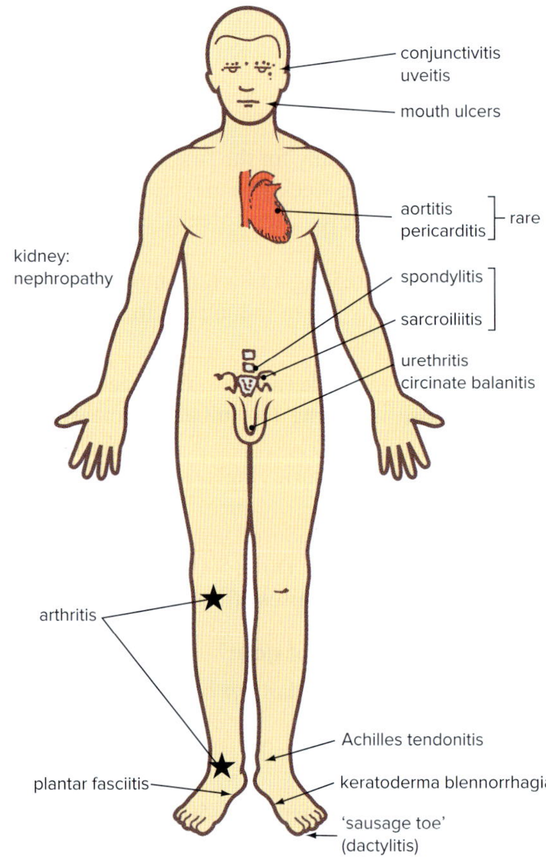

FIGURE 35.14 Possible clinical features of reactive arthritis

Enteropathic spondyloarthritidy

Inflammatory bowel disease (ulcerative colitis, Crohn disease and Whipple disease) may rarely be associated with peripheral arthritis and sacroiliitis.

Psoriatic arthritis

Like reactive arthritis, this can develop a condition indistinguishable from ankylosing spondylitis. It is therefore important to look beyond the skin condition of psoriasis, for about 5% will develop psoriatic arthropathy. It can have several manifestations:

1 mainly DIP joints
2 identical RA pattern but RA factor negative
3 identical ankylosing spondylosis pattern with sacroiliitis and spondylitis
4 monoarthritis, especially knees
5 severe deformity or 'mutilans' arthritis

Unclassified spondyloarthritides

Patients in this category seem to be the most frequently encountered in family practice. They clearly have a spondyloarthropathy but fail to meet the criteria for any one of the individual entities within the group. A typical patient is a young male in his third decade with a painful knee or other joint, unilateral (or bilateral) back pain with one of the entheseal problems (e.g. plantar fasciitis).

Investigations for spondyloarthritides

- X-rays:
  - radiological sacroiliitis is central to the diagnosis

- changes include narrowing of SIJs, margin irregularity, sclerosis of peri-articular bone and eventually bony fusion. Spondylitis usually follows
- ESR and CRP: most patients have an elevated ESR and CRP at some stage of their disease
- HLA-B_{27}: this test has low specificity and has limited value except that it predicts risk to offspring if positive
- Microbiology: in patients with a history of reactive arthritis, cultures should be obtained from the urethra, faeces, urine and blood[24]

Principles of management

- Identify the most active elements of the disease and treat accordingly.
- Provide patient and family education with appropriate reassurance: this is vital. Stress that, although the disease is non-curable, treatment is effective and long-term prognosis generally good.
- Provide regular assessment and support.
- Give genetic counselling—in cases of ankylosing spondylitis with positive HLA-B_{27}, the risk to offspring is significant.
- Give advice regarding work, especially with posture.
- Acute anterior uveitis requires prompt treatment and monitoring by an ophthalmologist.
- Refer for physiotherapy for exercises, stretching program, postural exercises and hydrotherapy. Appropriate physiotherapy slows deterioration in spinal function.[25]
- Consider referral for occupational therapy.
- Pharmacological agents:[8]
  - NSAIDs (e.g. indomethacin 75–200 mg (o) daily or 100 mg rectally nocte daily or ketoprofen 100 mg rectally nocte to control pain, stiffness and synovitis)
  - sulphasalazine (if NSAIDs ineffective)
  - intra-articular corticosteroids for severe monoarthritis and intralesional corticosteroids for enthesopathy

Refer for advice on above and especially for DMARD and bDMARD therapy.

Cautions

- Careful monitoring is required with NSAIDs and sulphasalazine.
- Systemic corticosteroids are not indicated.
- Immunosuppressants (low-dose weekly methotrexate) and bDMARDs may be needed for severe intractable problems with psoriasis and reactive arthritis.
- These conditions should be managed in collaboration with a consultant.

When to refer

- Consider referring most severe true inflammatory disorders for diagnosis and initiation of treatment (e.g. RA, spondyloarthropathy, connective tissue disorders and suspicion of a vasculitide)
- Osteoarthritis:
  - generalised joint pain
  - associated systemic symptoms
  - deteriorating joint function
  - intractable pain (especially at rest)
  - if surgical procedure is contemplated[8]
- Rheumatoid arthritis:
  - all patients initially
  - persistent inflammation of a joint or joints
  - patient ill and corticosteroids contemplated
  - if a surgical procedure is contemplated
- Spondyloarthropathies:
  - initial referral for confirmation of diagnosis and initiation of treatment
  - disease unresponsive to conventional treatment
  - sudden deterioration in symptoms, especially pain
  - onset of uveitis or other ocular complications
  - adverse drug reactions
- Undiagnosed arthritis in presence of constitutional symptoms
- Suspicion of a suppurative or serious infective condition (e.g. septic arthritis, endocarditis, brucellosis)
- Children with evidence of juvenile idiopathic arthritis (e.g. Still syndrome)

Practice tips

- Morning stiffness and pain, improving with exercise = RA.
- Flitting polyarthritis and fever = rheumatic fever; ?endocarditis; ?SLE.
- Polyarthritis (usually PIPs) and rash = viral arthritis or drug reaction.
- If rheumatoid arthritis involves the neck, beware of atlantoaxial subluxation and spinal cord compression.
- If the patient is young—think of SLE.

continued

continued

- If a patient returns from overseas with arthralgia, think of drug reactions, hepatitis, Lyme disease, but if the pain is intense consider dengue fever.
- Consider the possibility of Lyme disease in people with a fever, rash and arthritis who have been exposed to tick bites in rural areas.
- If a patient presents with Raynaud phenomenon and arthritis, especially of the hands, consider foremost RA, SLE and systemic sclerosis.
- Avoid the temptation to apply on doubtful grounds a broad label such as arthritis or rheumatoid, or a precise diagnosis such as RA, and introduce drugs.[27]

Patient education resources

Hand-out sheets from *Murtagh's Patient Education* 7th edition:

- Gout
- Osteoarthritis
- Rheumatoid arthritis

References

1 Hart FD. *Practical Problems in Rheumatology.* London: Dunitz, 1985: 77.
2 Cormack J, Marinker M, Morrel D. *Practice: A Handbook of Primary Health Care.* London: Kluwer-Harrop Handbooks, 1980; 3 (61): 1–12.
3 Lassere M, McGuigan L. Systemic disease presenting as arthritis: a diagnostic approach. Aust Fam Physician, 1991; 20: 1683–714.
4 Carroll GJ, Taylor AL. Drug-induced musculoskeletal syndromes. Current Therapeutics, 2000; Feb: 47–50.
5 Rudge S. Joint pain in children: assessing the serious causes. Modern Medicine Australia, 1990; May: 113–21.
6 Barraclough D. Rheumatology symptoms: will investigation make a difference? Aust Fam Physician, 2001; 30 (4): 322–6.
7 Kumar PJ, Clarke ML. *Clinical Medicine* (7th edn). London: Saunders, 2009: 523–9.
8 Expert group for Rheumatology. In: eTG complete [Internet]. Melbourne: Therapeutic Guidelines Ltd. Available from: <www.tg.org.au>, accessed Sept 2017.
9 Barton S (ed.). *Clinical Evidence.* London: BMJ Publishing Group, 2001: 808–18.
10 Felson DT. Weight and osteoarthritis. J Rheumatol Suppl, 1995; 43: 7–9.
11 Day R. COX-2 specific inhibitors: should I prescribe them? Current Therapeutics, 2000; Feb: 9–11.
12 Reginster JY et al. A controlled trial of glucosamine for osteoarthritis of the knee. Lancet, 2001; 357: 251–6.
13 McAlindon J, Felson DT. Nutrition: risk factors for osteoarthritis. Ann Rheum Dis, 1997; 56: 397–442.
14 Shmerling RH, Delbanco TL. How useful is the rheumatoid factor? An analysis of sensitivity, specificity and predictive value. Arch Intern Med, 1992; 152: 2417–20.
15 Wilson TD, Hill CL. Managing the drug treatment of rheumatoid arthritis. Aust Pres, 2017; 40: 51–8
16 Ostor A, McColl G. What's new in rheumatoid arthritis. Aust Fam Physician, 2001; 30 (4): 314–20.
17 Reilly P, Littlejohn G. Current treatment concepts in arthritis. Aust Fam Physician, 1989; 18: 1499–1509
18 Cleland LG, James MJ, Proudman SM. Fish oil: what the prescriber needs to know. Arthritis Research and Therapy, 2006; 8 (1): 202–11.
19 Hall S. Crystal arthritis: a clinician's view. Aust Fam Physician, 1991; 20: 1717–24.
20 Buckley N (Chair). *Australian Medicines Handbook.* Adelaide: Australian Medicines Handbook Pty Ltd, 2016; 699–701
21 Graf SW, Whittle SL, Wechalekar MD et al. Australian and New Zealand recommendations for the diagnosis and management of gout: integrating systematic literature review and expert opinion in the 3e Initiative. Int J Rheum Dis, 2015; 18 (3): 341–51.
22 Wechalekar MD, Vinik O, Moi JH et al. The efficacy and safety of treatments for acute gout: results from a series of systematic literature reviews including Cochrane reviews on intraarticular glucocorticoids, colchicine, nonsteroidal antiinflammatory drugs, and interleukin-1 inhibitors. J Rheumatol Suppl, Sept 2014; 92: 15–25.
23 Janssens H, Janssen M et al. Use of oral prednisolone or naproxen for treatment of gout arthritis: a double blind randomised equivalence trial. Lancet, 2008; 371 (9627): 1854–60.
24 Choi HK, Curham G. Soft drinks, fructose consumption and the risk of gout in men: prospective cohort study. BMJ online, 31 January 2008: 39449.819271 BE.
25 Edmonds JP. Spondyloarthropathies. Med J Aust, 1997; 166: 214–18.
26 Vilitanen JV et al. Fifteen months follow up of intensive inpatient physiotherapy and exercise in ankylosing spondylitis. Clin Rheumatol, 1995; 14: 413–19.
27 Hart FD. Early clinical diagnosis of 12 forms of arthritis. Modern Medicine Australia, 1989; March: 34–40.
28 Kincaid-Smith P, Larkins R, Whelan G (eds). *Problems in Clinical Medicine.* Sydney: MacLennan and Petty, 1989: 391.

Anorectal disorders 36

Duncan ill with very bad piles—operated on last night, or, since that sounds alarming, lanced. Can't really sympathise with that particular disease, though the pain is terrible. Must laugh.

VIRGINIA WOOLF 1934, *DIARY ENTRY*

Anorectal problems are common in family practice and tend to cause anxiety in the patient that is often related to the fear of cancer. This fear may be well founded for many instances of rectal bleeding and lumps. It is important to keep in mind the association between haemorrhoids and large bowel cancer.

Anorectal problems include:

- pain
- lumps
- discharge
- bleeding
- pruritus

Common anorectal conditions are illustrated in FIGURE 36.1.

ANORECTAL PAIN (PROCTALGIA)

The patient may complain that defecation is painful or almost impossible because of anorectal pain.

Causes

Pain without swelling:

- anal fissure
- anal herpes
- ulcerative proctitis

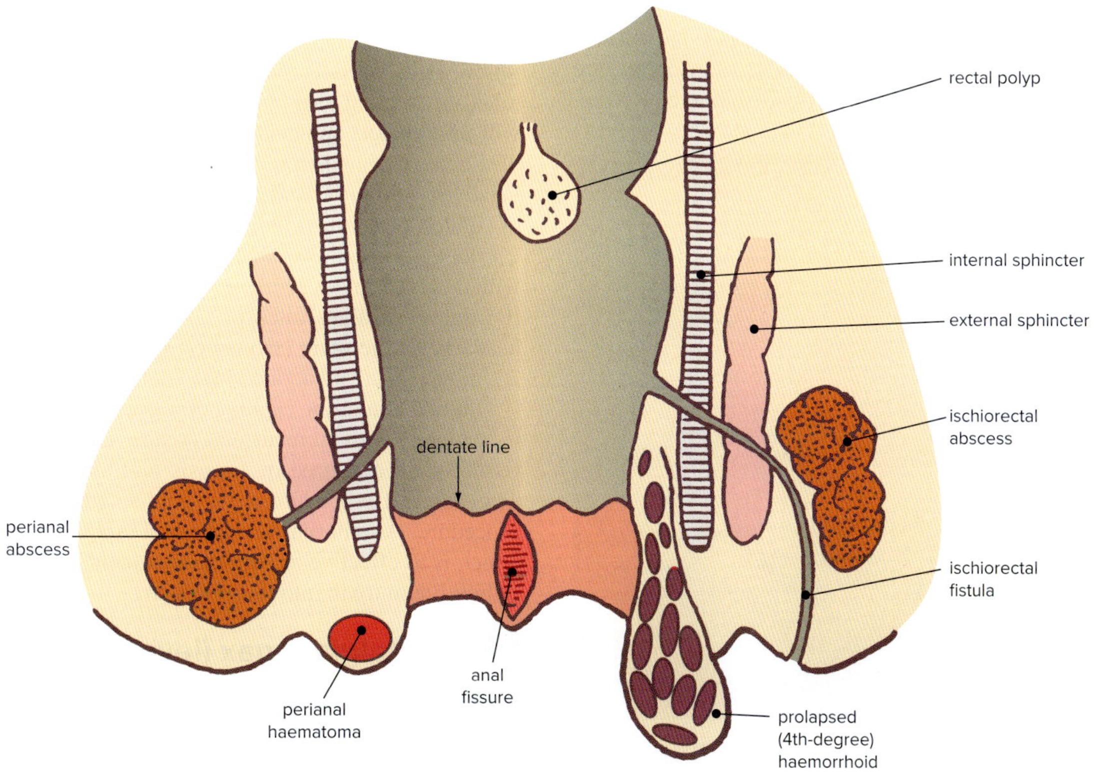

FIGURE 36.1 Common anorectal conditions

- proctalgia fugax
- solitary rectal ulcer
- tenesmus

Painful swelling:

- perianal haematoma
- strangulated internal haemorrhoids
- abscess: perianal, ischiorectal
- pilonidal sinus
- fistula-in-ano (intermittent)
- anal carcinoma

Anal fissure

Anal fissures cause pain on defecation and usually develop after a period of constipation (may be a brief period) and tenesmus. Other associations are childbirth and opioid analgesics.[1] Sometimes the pain can be excruciating, persisting for hours and radiating down the back of both legs. Anal fissures, especially if chronic, can cause minor anorectal bleeding (bright blood) noted as spotting on the toilet paper.

Examination

On inspection the anal fissure is usually seen in the anal margin, situated in the midline posteriorly (6 o'clock)—90% of fissures. The fissure appears as an elliptical ulcer involving the lower third of the anus from the dentate line to the anal verge (see FIG. 36.2).[1]

Digital examination and sigmoidoscopy are difficult because of painful anal sphincter spasm.

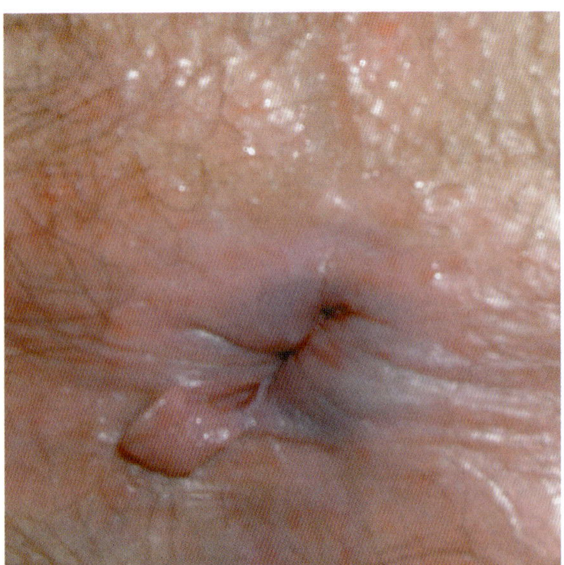

FIGURE 36.2 Anal fissure with prominent skin tag situated in the mid posterior position of the anal verge: the 6 o'clock position

If there are multiple fissures, Crohn disease should be suspected. These fissures look different, being indurated, oedematous and bluish in colour.

In chronic anal fissures a sentinel pile is common and in long-standing cases, a subcutaneous fistula is seen at the anal margin, with fibrosis and anal stenosis.[1]

Red flag pointers for anorectal pain

- Weight loss
- Change in bowel habits
- Fever >38°C
- Recurrent (consider Crohn disease)
- Exquisitely painful PR (consider abscess)

Treatment

The aim is to disrupt the cycle of anal sphincter spasm, allowing improved blood flow to assist healing. Management is conservative, with avoidance of hard stools and warm salt (sitz) baths after bowel movements. A high-residue diet and avoidance of constipation (aim for soft bulky stools) may lead to resolution and long-term prevention. A combined local anaesthetic and corticosteroid ointment applied to the fissure can provide relief but may not promote healing. Topical local anaesthetic applied before passing a stool may relieve pain but does not promote healing. Hot baths relax the internal anal sphincter. An acute anal fissure will usually heal spontaneously or within a few weeks of a treatment involving a high-fibre diet, sitz baths or laxatives.[2] A conservative treatment is the application of diluted glyceryl trinitrate ointment (e.g. Rectogesic 2% three times daily for 6 weeks to the lower anal canal) with a gloved finger gently inserted into the anal canal. It achieves healing rates of about 50%.[3,4] Transient headache is the main adverse effect. An alternative is 2% diltiazem cream applied twice daily for 6–8 weeks.

Lateral internal sphincterotomy is indicated in patients with a recurrent fissure and a chronic fissure with a degree of fibrosis and anal stenosis.[5] This surgical procedure is the gold-standard surgical procedure. An alternative 'chemical' sphincterotomy, which is as effective as surgical treatment, is injection of botulinum toxin into the sphincter.

Proctalgia fugax (levator ani spasm)

Clinical features

- Episodic fleeting rectal pain
- Varies from mild discomfort to severe spasm

- Last 3–30 minutes
- Often wakes patient from sound sleep
- Can occur any time of day
- A functional bowel disorder of unknown aetiology
- Affects adults, being more common in women

Management[6]

- Explanation and reassurance re self-healing
- An immediate drink (preferably hot) and local warmth with firm flannel pressure to the perineum
- Salbutamol inhaler (2 puffs statim) worth a trial but anecdotal evidence only

Alternatives include glyceryl trinitrate spray for the symptom or possibly antispasmodics, calcium channel blockers and clonidine.

Solitary rectal ulcer syndrome

These ulcers occur in young adults; they can present with pain but usually present as the sensation of a rectal lump causing obstructed defecation and bleeding with mucus. The ulcer, which is usually seen on sigmoidoscopy about 10 cm from the anal margin on the anterior rectal wall, can resemble cancer. Management is difficult and a chronic course is common. Treatment includes a high-residue diet and the avoidance of constipation.

Tenesmus

Tenesmus is an unpleasant sensation of incomplete evacuation of the rectum. It causes the patient to attempt defecation at frequent intervals. The most common cause is irritable bowel syndrome. Another common cause is an abnormal mass in the rectum or anal canal, such as cancer (e.g. prostate, anorectal), haemorrhoids or a hard faecal mass. In some cases, despite intensive investigation, no cause is found and it appears to be a functional problem.

Perianal haematoma

A perianal haematoma (thrombosed external haemorrhoid) is a purple tender swelling at the anal margin caused by rupture of an external haemorrhoidal vein following straining at toilet or some other effort involving a Valsalva manoeuvre. The degree of pain varies from a minor discomfort to severe pain. It has been described as the 'five day, painful, self-curing pile', which may lead to a skin tag. Spontaneous rupture with relief of symptoms can occur.

Management

Surgical intervention is recommended, especially in the presence of severe discomfort. The treatment depends on the time of presentation after the appearance of the haematoma.

1. *Within 24 hours of onset.* Perform simple aspiration without local anaesthetic using a 19 gauge needle while the haematoma is still fluid.
2. *From 24 hours to 5 days of onset.* The blood has clotted and a simple incision under local anaesthetic over the haematoma with deroofing with scissors (like taking the top off a boiled egg) to remove the thrombosis by squeezing is recommended. Removal of the haematoma reduces the chances of the development of a skin tag, which can be a source of anal irritation.
3. *Day 6 onwards.* The haematoma is best left alone unless it is very painful or (rarely) infected. Resolution is evidenced by the appearance of wrinkles in the previously stretched skin.

Follow-up

The patient should be reviewed in 4 weeks for rectal examination and proctoscopy, to examine for any underlying internal haemorrhoid that may predispose to further recurrence. Prevention includes an increased intake of dietary fibre and avoidance of straining at stool.

Strangulated haemorrhoids

A marked oedematous circumferential swelling will appear if all the haemorrhoids are involved. If only one haemorrhoid is strangulated, proctoscopy will help to distinguish it from a perianal haematoma. Initial treatment is with rest and ice packs and then haemorrhoidectomy at the earliest possible time. It is best to refer for urgent surgery.

Perianal cellulitis[6]

This occurs mainly in pre-school and school-aged children. It is usually caused by *Streptococcus pyogenes*. Check for a fissure.

Perianal anorectal abscess

This is caused by infection by polymicrobial organisms of one of the anal glands that drain the anal canal.

Clinical features

- Severe, constant, throbbing pain
- Fever and toxicity
- Hot, red, tender swelling adjacent to anal margin
- Non-fluctuant swelling

Careful examination is essential to make the diagnosis. Look for evidence of a fistula, Crohn disease and anorectal cancer.

Treatment

Drain via a cruciate incision, which may need to be deep (with trimming of the corners) over the point of maximal induration. A drain tube can be inserted for 7–10 days. Packing is not necessary.

Antibiotics

If a perianal or perirectal abscess is recalcitrant or spreading with cellulitis, use:

- metronidazole 400 mg (o) 12 hourly for 5–7 days plus
- cephalexin 500 mg (o) 6 hourly for 5–7 days[7]

Ischiorectal abscess

An ischiorectal abscess presents as a larger, more diffuse, tender, dusky red swelling in the buttock. The presence of an abscess is usually very obvious but the precise focus is not always obvious on inspection. Antibiotics are of little help and surgical incision and drainage as soon as possible is necessary. A deep general anaesthetic is necessary.

Pilonidal sinus and abscess

Recurrent abscesses and discharge in the sacral region (at the upper end of the natal cleft about 6 cm from the anus) can be caused by a midline pilonidal sinus, which often presents as a painful abscess. Once the infection has settled it is important to excise the pits, allow free drainage of the midline cavity and lateral tracks and remove all ingrown hair. Antibiotics, which should be guided by culture (e.g. cephalexin and metronidazole), are given to complement surgical drainage only if there is severe surrounding cellulitis. Pilonidal means 'a nest of hairs' and the problem is particularly common in hirsute young men (see FIG. 36.3). Refer for excision of the sinus network if necessary, possibly marsupialisation.

Fistula-in-ano[5]

An anal fistula is a tract that communicates between the perianal skin (visible opening) and the anal canal, usually at the level of the dentate line. It usually arises from chronic perianal infection, especially following discharge of an abscess. It is common in patients with Crohn disease. Symptoms include recurrent abscesses, discharge of blood, pus or serous fluid, swelling and anal pain. A surgical opinion is necessary to determine the appropriate surgical procedures, which may be complex if it traverses sphincter musculature.

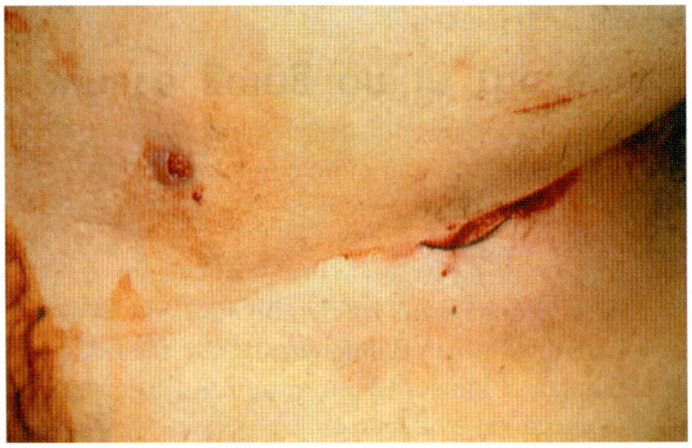

FIGURE 36.3 Pilonidal sinus revealing a pilonidal sinus and a lateral sinus opening after shaving. It shows the characteristic tuft of hairs protruding from the midline sinus.

ANORECTAL LUMPS

Anorectal lumps are relatively common and patients are often concerned because of the fear of cancer. A lump arising from the anal canal or rectum, such as an internal haemorrhoid, tends to appear intermittently upon defecation, and reduce afterwards.[1] Common prolapsing lesions include second- and third-degree haemorrhoids, hypertrophied anal papilla, polyps and rectal prolapse. Common presenting lumps include skin tags, fourth-degree piles and perianal warts (see TABLE 36.1).

Table 36.1 Common anal lumps
Prolapsing lumps
Second- and third-degree haemorrhoids
Rectal prolapse
Rectal polyp
Hypertrophied anal papilla
Persistent lumps
Skin tag
Perianal warts (condylomata accuminata)
Anal cancer
Fourth-degree haemorrhoids
Perianal haematoma
Perianal abscess

Skin tags

The skin tag is usually the legacy of an untreated perianal haematoma. It may require excision for aesthetic reasons, for hygiene or because it is a source of pruritus ani or irritation. A tag may be associated with a chronic fissure.

Treatment (method of excision)

A simple elliptical excision at the base of the skin tag is made under local anaesthetic. Suturing of the defect is usually not necessary.

Perianal warts

It is important to distinguish the common viral warts from the condylomata lata of secondary syphilis. Local therapy includes the application of podophyllin every 2 or 3 days by the practitioner or imiquimod.

Rectal prolapse

This is protrusion from the anus to a variable degree of the rectal mucosa (partial) or the full thickness of the rectal wall. It appears to be associated with constipation and chronic straining, leading to a lax sphincter. Features can include mucus discharge, bleeding, tenesmus, a solitary rectal ulcer and faecal incontinence (75%).

Visualisation of the prolapse is an important part of the diagnosis. Surgery such as rectopexy (fixing the rectum to the sacrum) is the only effective treatment for a complete prolapse.[5]

Temporary shrinking of a visible prolapse in an emergency situation can be achieved by a liberal sprinkling of fine crystalline sugar.

Internal haemorrhoids

Haemorrhoids or piles are common and tend to develop between the ages of 20 and 50 years. Roughly one out of two Westerners suffers from them by the time they reach the age of 50.[3] Internal haemorrhoids are a complex of dilated arteries, branches of the superior haemorrhoidal artery and veins of the internal haemorrhoidal venous plexus (see FIG. 36.4). The commonest cause is chronic constipation related to a lack of dietary fibre and inappropriate habit.

Anatomically there are three classical sites, namely 3, 7 and 11 o'clock (see FIG. 36.5).

Clinical stages and pathology[3]

- *Stage 1:* First-degree internal haemorrhoids: three bulges form above the dentate line. Bright bleeding is common.
- *Stage 2:* Second-degree internal haemorrhoids: the bulges increase in size and slide downwards so that the patient is aware of lumps when straining at stool, but they disappear upon relaxing. Bleeding is a feature.

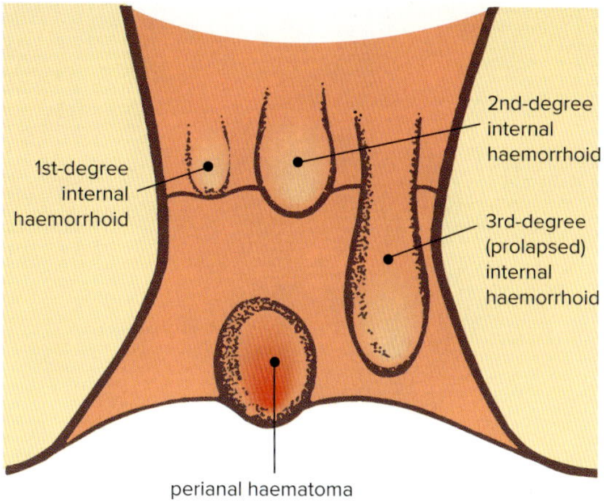

FIGURE 36.4 Classification of haemorrhoids

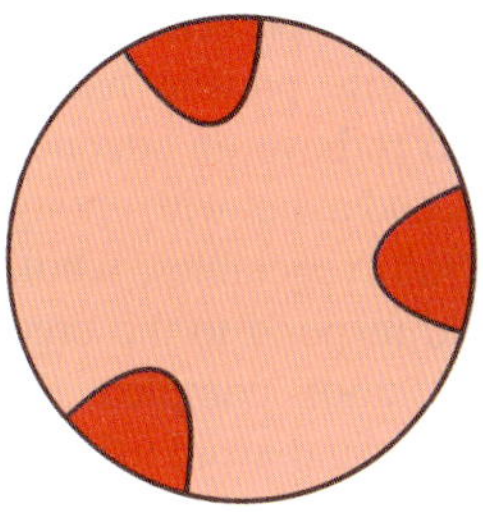

FIGURE 36.5 Three sites of primary haemorrhoids, looking into the anus from below

- *Stage 3:* Third-degree internal haemorrhoids: the pile continues to enlarge and slide downwards, requiring manual replacement to alleviate discomfort. Bleeding is also a feature.
- *Stage 4:* Fourth-degree internal haemorrhoids: prolapse has occurred and replacement of the prolapsed pile into the anal canal is impossible.

Symptoms

Bleeding is the main and, in many people, the only symptom. The word 'haemorrhoid' means flow of blood. Other symptoms include prolapse, mucoid discharge, irritation/itching, tenesmus, incomplete bowel evacuation and pain (see FIG. 36.6).

Treatment

Invasive treatment of haemorrhoids is based on three main procedures: rubber band ligation, cryotherapy and sphincterotomy. Injection is now not so favoured, while a meta-analysis concluded that rubber band ligation was the most effective non-surgical therapy.[8] Surgery is generally reserved for large strangulated piles. The best

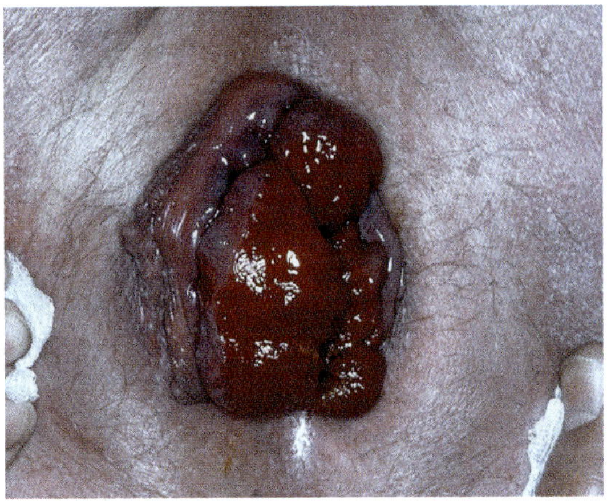

FIGURE 36.6 Severely prolapsed haemorrhoids requiring surgery

treatment, however, is prevention, and softish bulky faeces that pass easily prevent haemorrhoids. People should be advised to have an adequate intake of non-caffeinated fluids and a diet with enough fibre by eating plenty of fresh fruit, vegetables, wholegrain cereals or bran. They should respond to the urge to defecate and avoid straining at stool, complete their bowel action within a few minutes and avoid using laxatives.

ANAL DISCHARGE

Anal discharge refers to the involuntary escape of fluid from or near the anus. The causes may be considered as follows.[5]

1. *Continent*
   - Anal fistula
   - Pilonidal sinus
   - STIs: anal warts, gonococcal ulcers, genital herpes
   - Solitary rectal ulcer syndrome
   - Cancer of anal margin
2. *Incontinent*
   - Minor incontinence—weakness of internal sphincter
   - Severe incontinence—weakness of levator ani and puborectalis
3. *Partially continent*
   - Faecal impaction
   - Rectal prolapse

Anal (faecal) incontinence

Studies have revealed that up to 1 in 10 people suffer some degree of faecal incontinence, which is a common reason for institutionalisation of the elderly.[9] Patients may be reluctant to seek medical advice and doctors often do not ask specifically about the condition. The problem is as common in men as in women.

Apart from ageing, risk factors include perianal injury, such as childbirth injury, anal surgery, irritable bowel syndrome and neurological disorders.

If there are symptoms of anal incontinence postnatally, early referral to a physiotherapist, continence nurse adviser or colorectal surgeon is advisable.[10]

Among the various possible treatments there are surgical possibilities, which vary from direct sphincter repair, directed injections such as collagen and silicone into the anal sphincter, and an artificial anal sphincter (e.g. Acticon Neosphincter). A colostomy may be the last resort. It is worth keeping in mind asking patients about the possibility of this problem and knowing 'to whom to refer'.

Rectal bleeding

Patients present with any degree of bleeding from a smear on the toilet tissue to severe haemorrhage. Various causes are presented in FIGURE 36.7. Common causes are polyps, colon and rectal cancer, ischaemic colitis, diverticular disease and haemorrhoids.

Local causes of bleeding include excoriated skin, anal fissure, a burst perianal haematoma and anal cancer. A characteristic pattern of bright bleeding

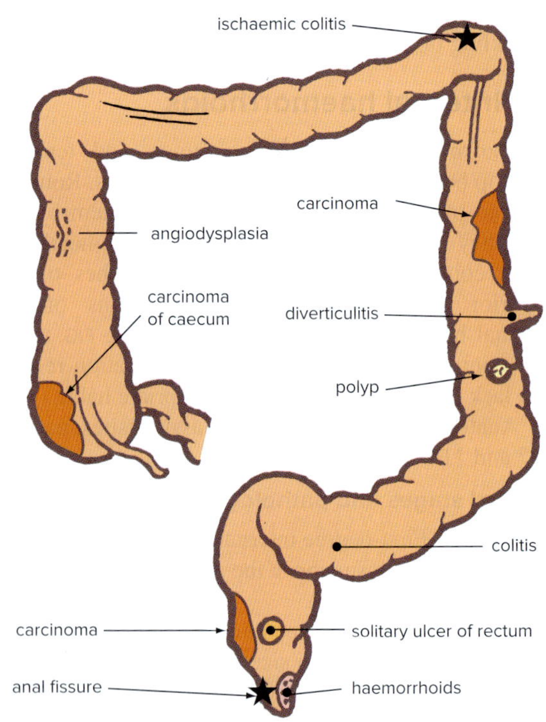

FIGURE 36.7 Various causes of rectal bleeding

is found with haemorrhoids. It is usually small non-prolapsing haemorrhoids that bleed.

The nature of the blood (e.g. bright red, dark red or black) and the nature of the bleeding (e.g. smear, streaked on stool, mixed with stool, massive) gives an indication of the source of the bleeding (see TABLE 36.2). Black tarry (melaena) stool indicates bleeding from the upper gastrointestinal tract and is rare distal to the lower ileum. Patients with melaena should be admitted to hospital.

Table 36.1 Presentation and causes of rectal bleeding[6]

Presentation	Causes
Bright red blood in toilet separate from faeces	Internal haemorrhoids
Bright red blood on toilet paper	Internal haemorrhoids Fissure Anal cancer Pruritus Anal warts and condylomata
Blood and mucus on underwear	Third-degree haemorrhoids Fourth-degree haemorrhoids Prolapsed rectum Mucosal prolapse Prolapsed mucosal polyp
Blood on underwear (no mucus)	Ulcerated perianal haematoma Anal cancer
Blood and mucus mixed with faeces	Colorectal cancer Proctitis Colitis, ulcerative colitis Large mucosal polyp Ischaemic colitis
Blood mixed with faeces (no mucus)	Small colorectal polyps Small colorectal cancer
Melaena (black tarry stools)	Gastrointestinal bleeding (usually upper) with long transit time to the anus
Torrential haemorrhage (rare)	Diverticular disorder Angiodysplasia
Large volumes of mucus in faeces (little blood)	Villous papilloma of rectum Villous papilloma of colon
Blood in faeces with menstruation (rare)	Rectal endometriosis

Source: Orlay, G. *Office Proctology*, page 11.[11] © Copyright 1987 George Orlay—reproduced with permission

Frequent passage of blood and mucus indicates a rectal tumour or proctitis, whereas more proximal tumours or extensive colitis present different patterns.

Substantial haemorrhage, which is rare, can be caused by diverticular disorder, angiodysplasia or more proximal lesions such as Meckel diverticulum and even duodenal ulcers. Angiodysplasias are 5 mm collections of dilated mucosal capillaries and thick-walled submucosal veins, found usually in the ascending colon of elderly patients who have no other bowel symptoms. The bleeding is persistent and recurrent. The site is identified by technetium-labelled red cell scan or colonoscopy.

The history should also include an analysis of any associated symptoms such as pain, diarrhoea or constipation, presence of lumps and a sensation of urgency or unsatisfied defecation. The latter symptoms point to a rectal cause. Associated change of bowel habit suggests a diagnosis of cancer of the rectum or left colon. Bleeding from right colon cancer is often occult, presenting as anaemia.

The examination includes a general assessment, anal inspection, digital rectal examination and proctosigmoidoscopy. Even if there is an anal lesion, proximal bleeding must be excluded in all cases by sigmoidoscopy[3] and by colonoscopy if there are any bowel symptoms or no obvious anal cause or a doubt about a lesion causing the symptoms.

Red flag pointers for rectal bleeding

- Age >50 years
- Change of bowel habit
- Weight loss
- Weakness, fatigue
- Brisk bleeding
- Constipation
- Haemorrhoids (may be sinister)
- Family history of cancer

Pruritus ani

Pruritus ani, which is itching of the anus, can be a distressing symptom that is worse at night, during hot weather and during exercise. It is seen typically in adult males with considerable inner drive, often at times of stress and in hot weather when sweating is excessive. In children, threadworm infestation should be suspected. It may be part of general itching, such as with a skin disorder, or localised whereby various anorectal disorders have to be excluded. Seborrhoeic dermatitis is a particularly common underlying factor. Consider also the more uncomfortable lichen sclerosus with its ivory white sclerotic plaques, which may also be present in the genital region.

Signs

The skin changes can vary from minimal signs to marked pathology that can show linear ulceration, maceration or lichenification (see FIG. 36.8). Superficial skin changes can be moist and macerated or dry and scaly. Full anorectal examination is necessary.

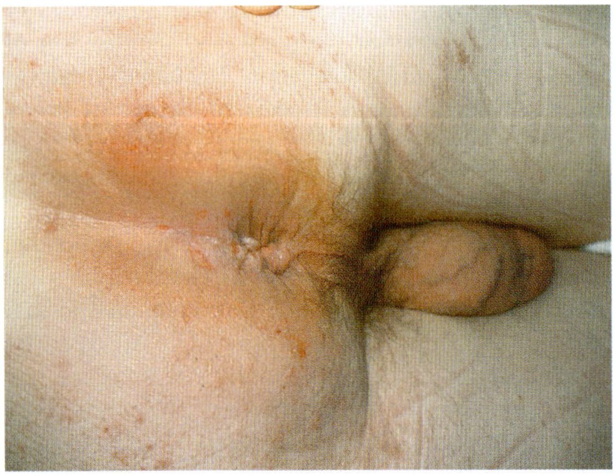

FIGURE 36.8 Lichen chronicus simplex. Lichenification from scratching with longstanding pruritus (see CHAPTER 122)

Causes and aggravating factors

- Psychological factors:
  - stress and anxiety
  - fear of cancer
- Generalised systemic or skin disorders:
  - seborrhoeic dermatitis
  - eczema
  - lichen sclerosus
  - diabetes mellitus
  - candidiasis
  - psoriasis (look for fissures in natal cleft)
  - antibiotic treatment
  - worms: pinworm (threadworm)
  - diarrhoea causing excoriation
  - Crohn disease
- Local anorectal conditions:
  - haemorrhoids, skin tags
  - fissures/fistula
  - faecal incontinence
  - warts
- Zealous hygiene to lack of hygiene
- Contact dermatitis:
  - dyed or perfumed toilet tissue, soap, powder
  - clothing
- Excessive sweating (e.g. tight pantyhose in summer)

Diagnosis

- Urinalysis (? diabetes)
- Anorectal examination
- Scrapings and microscopy to detect organisms
- Stool examination for intestinal parasites

Treatment

- Treat the cause (if known) and break the scratch cycle.
- Avoid local anaesthetics, antiseptics.
- Advise aqueous cream or a soap substitute to wash anus (instead of soap).
- Most effective preparations (for short[12] courses):

  methylprednisolone aceponate 0.1% in a fatty ointment; once daily until symptoms settle (up to 4 weeks)
  or
  hydrocortisone 1% cream/ointment
  or
  hydrocortisone 1% cream with clioquinol 3% or clotrimazole 1% (especially if dermatosis and *Candida* suspected)

If an isolated area and resistant, infiltrate 0.5 mL of triamcinolone intradermally. Fractionated X-ray therapy can be used if very severe. For a lichenified perianal area, use a potent corticosteroid ointment, e.g. betamethasone dipropionate 0.05% daily until clear.

Patient education about anal hygiene is essential.

Practice tips for pruritus ani

- Most cases of uncomplicated pruritus ani resolve with simple measures, including explanation and reassurance.
- Avoid perfumed soaps and powders. Use bland aqueous cream or a mild soap substitute.
- Otherwise prescribe a corticosteroid, especially methylprednisolone aceponate 0.1%. Once symptoms are controlled, use hydrocortisone 1%.[12]
- Lifestyle stress and anxiety underlie most cases.
- In obese patients with intertrigo and excessive sweating, strap the buttocks apart with adhesive tape.
- Consider perianal lichen simplex and lichen sclerosus in patients presenting with 'a sore bottom'.

Patient education resources

Hand-out sheets from *Murtagh's Patient Education* 7th edition:

- Anal fissure
- Haemorrhoids
- Pruritus ani

References

1. Gold D. Benign anal conditions: how to treat. Australian Doctor, 20 January 2012: 19–25.
2. Utzig MJ, Kroesen AJ, Buhr HJ. Conservative treatment of anal fissure. Am J Gastroenterol, 2003; 98: 968–74.
3. Lund JN, Scholefield JH. A randomised, prospective, double-blind, placebo-controlled trial of glyceryl trinitrate ointment in the treatment of anal fissure. Lancet, 1997; Jan 4: 11–13.
4. Nelson R. Nonsurgical therapy for anal fissure. Cochrane Database Syst Rev. 2006, Issue 4. Art No. CD003431.
5. Schnitzler M. Benign perianal conditions. Update. Medical Observer, 23 March 2007: 31–4.
6. Expert group for Gastroenterology. Perianal disorders. In: eTG complete [Internet]. Melbourne: Therapeutic Guidelines Ltd. Available from:<www.tg.org.au>, accessed Sept 2017.
7. Expert group for Antibiotics. Abscess. In: eTG complete [Internet]. Melbourne: Therapeutic Guidelines Ltd. Available from: <www.tg.org.au>, accessed Sept 2017.
8. MacRae HM, McLeod RS. Comparison of haemorrhoidal treatments: a meta-analysis. Can J Surg, 1997; 40 (1): 14–7.
9. Kalantar JS, Howell S, Talley NJ. Prevalence of faecal incontinence and associated risk factors. Med J Aust, 2002; 176: 54–7.
10. Rieger N. Faecal incontinence: how to treat. Australian Doctor, 15 February 2008: 21–6.
11. Orlay G. *Office Proctology*. Sydney: Australasian Medical Publishing Company, 1987: 11–52.
12. Expert group for Dermatology. Pruritus ani. In: eTG complete [Internet]. Melbourne:Therapeutic Guidelines Ltd. Available from: <www.tg.org.au>, accessed Sept 2017.

37 Thoracic back pain

The maladies that afflict the clerks aforesaid arise from three causes; first constant sitting, secondly the incessant movement of the hand and always in the same direction, and thirdly the strain on the midline from the effort not to disfigure the books by error or cause loss to their employers.

THE PHYSICIAN RAMAZZINI 1713

Thoracic (dorsal) or upper back pain, which is defined as pain localised between the neck and above the costal margin, is common in people of all ages. It accounts for 10–15% of all spinal pain and has a 1-year prevalence in 20% of adults. Dysfunction of the joints of the thoracic spine, with its unique costovertebral joints (which are an important source of back pain), is very commonly encountered in medical practice, especially in people whose lifestyle creates stresses and strains through poor posture and heavy lifting. It is also referred to as non-specific thoracic spinal pain. Muscular and ligamentous strains may be common, but they rarely come to light in practice because they are self-limiting and not severe.

This dysfunction can cause referred pain to various parts of the chest wall and can mimic the symptoms of various visceral diseases, such as angina, biliary colic and oesophageal spasm. In similar fashion, heart and gall bladder pain can mimic spinal pain.

Key facts and checkpoints

- The commonest site of pain in the spine is the costovertebral articulations especially the costotransverse articulation (see FIG. 37.1).
- Pain of thoracic spinal origin may be referred anywhere to the chest wall, but the commonest sites are the scapular region, the paravertebral region 2–5 cm from midline and, anteriorly, over the costochondral region.
- Thoracic (also known as dorsal) pain is more common in patients with abnormalities such as kyphosis and Scheuermann disease.
- Trauma to the chest wall (including falls on the chest such as those experienced in body contact sport) commonly lead to disorders of the thoracic spine.
- Unlike the lumbar spine, the joints are quite superficial and it is relatively easy to find the affected (painful) segment.
- Intervertebral disc prolapse is very uncommon in the thoracic spine.
- The older patient presenting with chest pain should be regarded as having a cardiac cause until proved otherwise.
- If the chest pain is non-cardiac, then the possibility of referral from the thoracic spine should be considered.
- The thoracic spine is the commonest site in the vertebral column for metastatic disease.
- Scheuermann disease, which affects the lower thoracic spine in adolescents, is often associated with kyphosis and recurrent thoracic back pain. Always inspect the thoracic spine of the younger patient for kyphosis and scoliosis, ideally at 9 years of age.
- Palpation is the most important component of the physical examination.

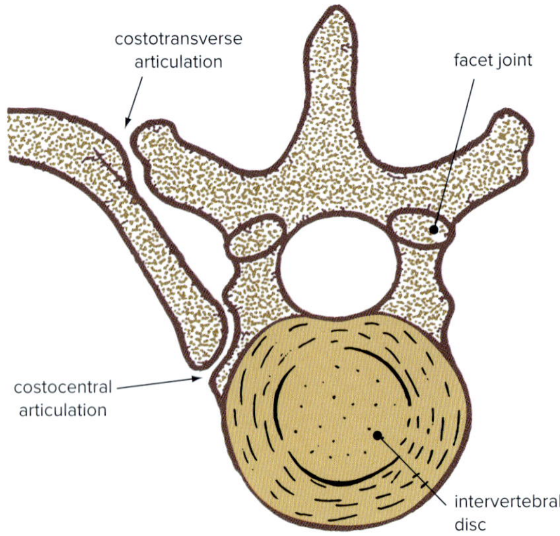

FIGURE 37.1 The functional unit of the thoracic spine

A diagnostic approach

A summary of the diagnostic strategy model is presented in TABLE 37.1.

Table 37.1 Thoracic back pain: diagnostic strategy model

Probability diagnosis
Musculoligamentous strains (mainly postural) Vertebral dysfunction (non-specific back pain)
Serious disorders not to be missed
Cardiovascular: • acute coronary syndromes, esp. myocardial infarction • dissecting aneurysm • pulmonary infarction • epidural haematoma (blood-thinning agents) Neoplasia: • myeloma • lung (with infiltration) • metastatic disease Severe infections: • epidural abscess • pleurisy • infectious endocarditis • osteomyelitis Pneumothorax Osteoporosis
Pitfalls (often missed)
Angina Gastrointestinal disorders • oesophageal dysfunction • peptic ulcer (penetrating) • hepatobiliary • pancreatic Herpes zoster Spondyloarthropathies Costochondritis: • Tietze syndrome Fibromyalgia syndrome Polymyalgia rheumatica Notalgia paraesthetica Chronic infection: • tuberculosis • brucellosis
Seven masquerades checklist
Depression Diabetic radiculopathy Spinal dysfunction UTI
Is the patient trying to tell me something?
Yes, quite possible with many cases of back pain.

Probability diagnosis

The commonest cause of thoracic back pain is musculoskeletal, due usually to musculoligamentous strains caused by poor posture. However, these pains are usually transitory and present rarely to the practitioner. The problems that commonly present are those caused by dysfunction of the lower cervical and thoracic spinal joints, especially those of the mid-thoracic (interscapular) area.

Arthritic conditions of the thoracic spine are not relatively common although degenerative osteoarthritis is encountered at times; the inflammatory spondyloarthropathies are uncommon.

The various systemic infectious diseases such as influenza and Epstein–Barr mononucleosis can certainly cause diffuse backache but should be assessed in context.

Not to be missed

A special problem with the thoracic spine is its relationship with the many thoracic and upper abdominal structures that can refer pain to the back. These structures are listed in TABLE 37.2 but, in particular, myocardial infarction and dissecting aneurysm must be considered. A complex problem described by neurosurgeons is the patient presenting with severe sudden thoracic back pain caused by an epidural haematoma related to aspirin or warfarin therapy.

Table 37.2 Non-musculoskeletal causes of thoracic back pain

Heart	Myocardial infarction Angina Pericarditis
Great vessels	Dissecting aneurysm Pulmonary embolism (rare) Pulmonary infarction Pneumothorax Pneumonia/pleurisy
Oesophagus	Oesophageal rupture Oesophageal spasm Oesophagitis Oesophageal cancer
Subdiaphragmatic disorders of:	Gall bladder Stomach Duodenum Pancreas Subphrenic collection
Miscellaneous infections	Herpes zoster Bornholm disease Infective endocarditis
Psychogenic	

Cardiopulmonary problems

The acute onset of pain can have sinister implications in the thoracic spine where various life-threatening cardiopulmonary and vascular events have to be kept in mind. The pulmonary causes of acute pain include spontaneous pneumothorax, pleurisy and pulmonary infarction. Thoracic back pain may be associated with infective endocarditis due to embolic phenomena. The ubiquitous myocardial infarction or acute coronary occlusion may, uncommonly, cause interscapular back pain, while the very painful dissecting or ruptured aortic aneurysm may cause back pain with hypotension.

Osteoporosis

Osteoporosis, especially in people over 60 years, including both men and women, must always be considered in such people presenting with acute pain, which can be caused by a pathological fracture. The association with pain following inappropriate physical therapy such as spinal manipulation should also be considered.

Acute infections

Infective conditions that can involve the spine include osteomyelitis, tuberculosis, brucellosis, syphilis and *Salmonella* infections. Such conditions should be suspected in young patients (osteomyelitis), farm workers (brucellosis) and migrants from South-East Asia and third world countries (tuberculosis). The presence of poor general health and fever necessitates investigations for these infections.

37

Neoplasia

Fortunately, tumours of the spine are uncommon. Nevertheless, they occur frequently enough for the full-time practitioner in back disorders to encounter some each year, especially metastatic disease.

The three common primary malignancies that metastasise to the spine are those originating in the lung, breast and the prostate (all paired structures). The less common primaries to consider are the thyroid, the kidney and adrenals and malignant melanoma.

Reticuloses such as Hodgkin lymphoma can involve the spine. Primary malignancies that develop in the vertebrae include multiple myeloma and sarcoma.

Benign tumours to consider are often neurological in origin. An interesting tumour is the osteoid osteoma, which is aggravated by consuming alcohol and relieved by aspirin.

The tumours of the spine are summarised in TABLE 37.3.

Table 37.3 Significant tumours affecting the thoracic and lumbar spine

	Benign	Malignant
Of bone	Osteoid osteoma Haemangioma Osteoblastoma Aneurysmal bone cyst Eosinophilic granuloma	Primary: • multiple myeloma • lymphomas (e.g. Hodgkin) • sarcoma
Spinal	Extradural: • lipoma • neuroma • fibroma Intradural: • neuroma • ependymoma • chordoma • meningioma	Secondary: • breast • lung • prostate • adrenals/kidney • thyroid • melanoma Direct spread: • stomach • large bowel • pancreas • uterus/cervix/ovary

Source: After Kenna and Murtagh[2]

The symptoms and signs that should alert the clinician to malignant disease are:

- back pain occurring in an older person
- unrelenting back pain, unrelieved by rest (this includes night pain)
- rapidly increasing back pain
- constitutional symptoms (e.g. unexplained weight loss, fever, malaise)
- a history of treatment for cancer (e.g. excision of skin melanoma)

Red flag pointers for thoracic back pain[1]

The red flag pointers are similar to those for low back pain (see CHAPTER 38).

Fracture pointer
Major trauma
Minor trauma:
- osteoporosis
- female >50 years
- male >60 years

Malignancy pointer
Age >50
Past history malignancy

Unexplained weight loss
Pain at rest
Constant pain
Night pain
Pain at multiple sites
Unresponsive to treatment

Infection pointer
Fever
Night sweats
Risk factors for infection

Other serious conditions
Chest pain/heaviness
Shortness of breath, cough

FBE, ESR, CRP and a plain X-ray of the thoracic spine should be the initial screening test in the presence of these pointers.

A common trap for the thoracic spine is lung cancer, such as mesothelioma, which can invade parietal pleura or structures adjacent to the vertebral column.

Pitfalls

Pitfalls include ischaemic heart disease presenting with interscapular pain, herpes zoster at the pre-eruption stage and the various gastrointestinal disorders. Two commonly misdiagnosed problems are a penetrating duodenal ulcer presenting with lower thoracic pain and oesophageal spasm, which can cause thoracic back pain.

Inflammatory rheumatological problems are not common in the thoracic spine but occasionally a spondyloarthropathy such as ankylosing spondylitis manifests here, although it follows some time after the onset of sacroiliitis.

Seven masquerades checklist

Spinal dysfunction is the outstanding cause in this checklist, but urinary tract infection may occasionally cause lower thoracic pain. Depression always warrants consideration in any pain syndrome, especially back pain. It can certainly cause exaggeration of pre-existing pain from vertebral dysfunction or some other chronic problem.

Psychogenic considerations

Psychogenic or non-organic causes of back pain can present a complex dilemma in diagnosis and management. The causes may be apparent from the incongruous behaviour and personality of the patient, but often the diagnosis is reached by a process of exclusion. There is obviously some functional overlay in everyone with acute or chronic pain, hence the importance of appropriate reassurance to these patients that their problem invariably subsides with time and that they do not have cancer.

Anatomical and clinical features

The functional unit of the thoracic spine is illustrated in FIGURE 37.1. Although there is scant literature and evidence about the origins of pain in the thoracic spine,[3] the strongest evidence indicates that pain from the thoracic spine originates mainly from the apophyseal joints and rib articulations. Any one thoracic vertebra has 10 separate articulations, so the potential for dysfunction and the difficulty in clinically pinpointing the precise joint at a particular level are apparent.

The costovertebral joints are synovial joints unique to the thoracic spine and have two articulations—costotransverse and costocentral. Together with the apophyseal joints, they are capable of presenting with well-localised pain close to the midline or as referred pain, often quite distal to the spine, with the major symptoms not appearing to have any relationship to the thoracic spine.

Generalised referral patterns are presented in FIGURE 24.2 (see CHAPTER 24), while the dermatome pattern is outlined in FIGURE 37.2.

The pain pattern acts as a guide only because there is considerable dermatomal overlap within the individual and variation from one person to another. It has been demonstrated that up to five nerve roots may contribute to the innervation of any one point in the anterior segments of the trunk dermatomes, a fact emphasised by the clinical distribution of herpes zoster.

Upper thoracic pain[1]

Dysfunction of the joints of the upper thoracic spine usually gives rise to localised pain and stiffness posteriorly but also can cause distal symptoms, probably via the autonomic nervous system.

A specific syndrome called the T4 syndrome[4] has been shown to cause vague pain and paraesthesia in the upper limbs and diffuse, vague head and posterior neck pain. Examination may reveal hypomobility of the upper thoracic segments. It has been proven to respond to spinal manipulation, which restores full mobility.

However, most of the pain, stiffness and discomfort arise from dysfunction of the upper and middle thoracic segments with patients presenting with the complaint of pain between 'my shoulder blades'.

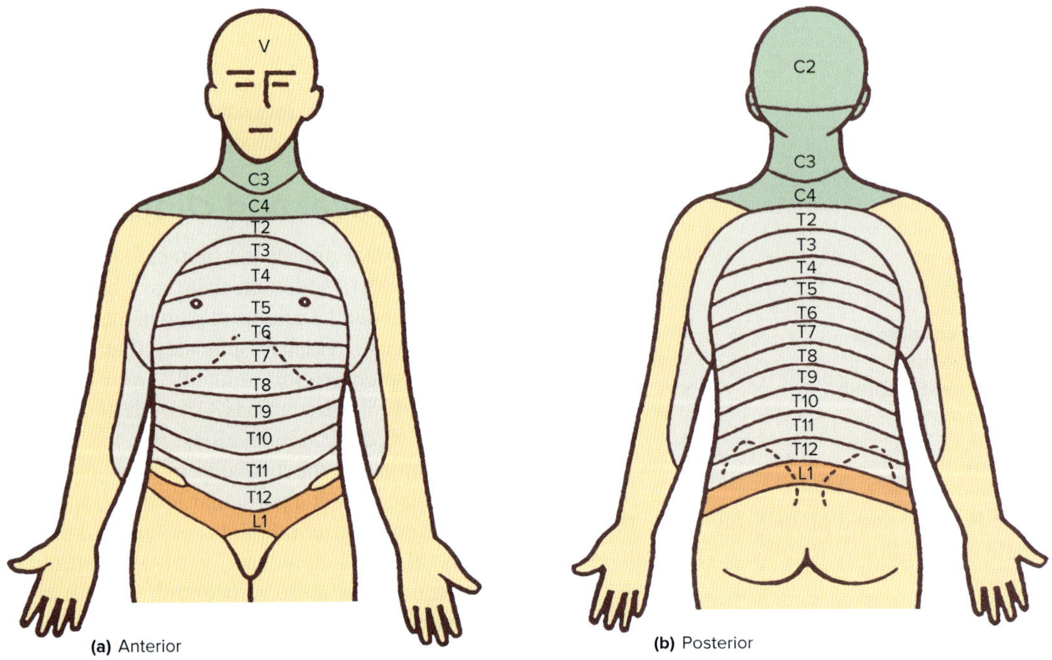

FIGURE 37.2 Dermatomes for the thoracic nerve roots, indicating possible referral areas.

Source: Reproduced with permission from C Kenna and J Murtagh. *Back Pain and Spinal Manipulation* (2nd edn), Oxford: Butterworth-Heinemann, 1997

37

Costovertebral joint dysfunction[1]

The unique feature of the thoracic spine is the costovertebral joint. Dysfunction of this joint commonly causes localised pain approximately 3–4 cm from the midline where the rib articulates with the transverse process and the vertebral body. In addition, it is frequently responsible for referred pain ranging from the midline, posterior to the lateral chest wall, and even anterior chest pain.

When the symptoms radiate laterally, the diagnosis is confirmed only when movement of the rib provokes pain at the costovertebral joint. This examination will simultaneously reproduce the referred pain.

FIGURE 37.3 presents the pattern of referred pain from these joints and highlights the capacity of the thoracic spine to refer pain centrally to the anterior chest and upper abdomen. Confusion arises for the clinician when the patient's history focuses on the anterior chest pain and fails to mention the presence of posterior pain, should it be present. The shaded areas on FIGURE 37.3 represent those areas where the patient experiences pain following the injection of hypertonic saline into the posterior elements of the spine.

The clinical approach

History

The history of a patient presenting with thoracic back pain should include a routine pain analysis, which usually provides important clues for the diagnosis. The age, sex and occupation of the patient are relevant. Pain in the thoracic area is very common in people who sit bent over for long periods, especially working at desks. Students, secretaries and stenographers are therefore at risk, as are nursing mothers, who have to lift their babies.

People who are kyphotic or scoliotic or who have 'hunchbacks' secondary to disease such as tuberculosis and poliomyelitis also suffer from recurrent pain in this area.

Older people are more likely to present with a neoplastic problem in the thoracic spine and with osteoporosis. Senile osteoporosis is usually a trap because it is symptomless until the intervention of a compression fracture. Symptoms following such a fracture can persist for 3 months.

Pain that is present day and night indicates a sinister cause.

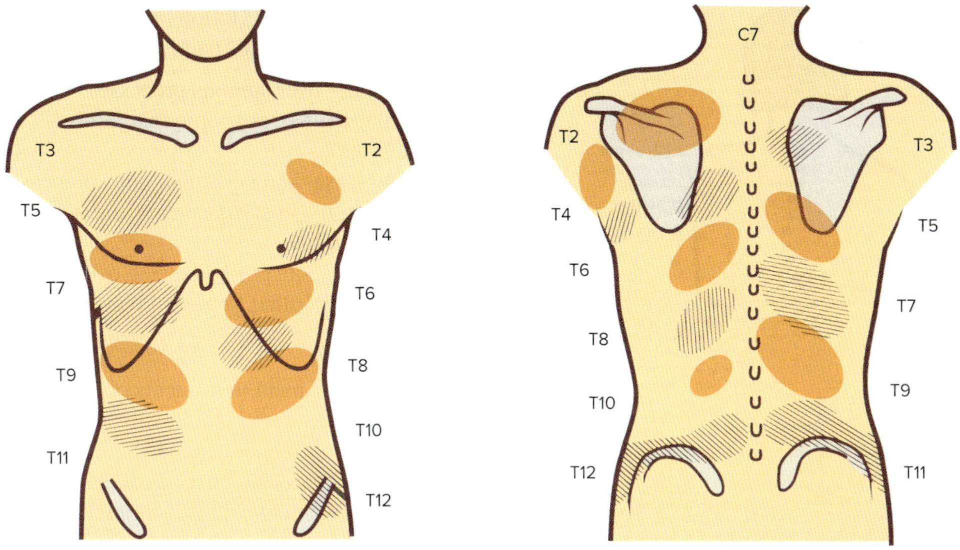

FIGURE 37.3 Kellegren's (1939) pain referral patterns after stimulation of deep joints of the thoracic spine

Features of the history that give an indication that the pain is arising from dysfunction of the thoracic spine include:

- *Aggravation and relief of pain on trunk rotation.* The patient's pain may be increased by rotating (twisting) towards the side of the pain but eased by rotating in the opposite direction.
- *Aggravation of pain by coughing, sneezing or deep inspiration.* This can produce a sharp catching pain which, if severe, tends to implicate the costovertebral joint. Care must be taken to rule out pneumonia and pleurisy.
- *Relief of pain by firm pressure.* Patients may state that their back pain is eased by firm pressure such as leaning against the corner of a wall.

It is very important to be able to differentiate between chest pain due to vertebral dysfunction and that caused by myocardial ischaemia.

Key questions

- Can you recall injuring your back, such as by lifting something heavy?
- Did you have a fall onto your chest or back?
- Is the pain present during the night?
- Do you have low back pain or neck pain?
- Does the pain come on after walking or any strenuous effort?
- Does the pain come on after eating or soon after going to bed at night?
- Have you noticed a fever or sweating at any time, especially at night?
- Have you noticed a rash near where you have the pain?
- What drugs are you taking? Do you take drugs for arthritis or pain? Cortisone?
- What happens when you take a deep breath, cough or sneeze?

Examination

The examination of the thoracic spine is straightforward with the emphasis on palpation of the spine—central and laterally. This achieves the basic objective of reproducing the patient's symptoms and finding the level of pain. The 'LOOK, FEEL, MOVE, X-RAY' clinical approach is most appropriate for the thoracic spine.

Inspection

Careful inspection, especially of posture, is important since it may be possible to observe at a glance why the patient has thoracic pain. Note the symmetry, any scars, skin creases and deformities, 'flat spots' in the spine, the nature of the scapulae or evidence of muscle spasm. Look for kyphosis and scoliosis.

Kyphosis may be generalised, with the back having a smooth uniform contour, or localised where it is due to a collapsed vertebra, such as occurs in an older person with osteoporosis. Generalised kyphosis is common in the elderly, especially those with degenerative spinal disease. In the young it may reflect the important Scheuermann disease.

The younger person in particular should be screened for scoliosis (see FIG. 37.4), which becomes

37

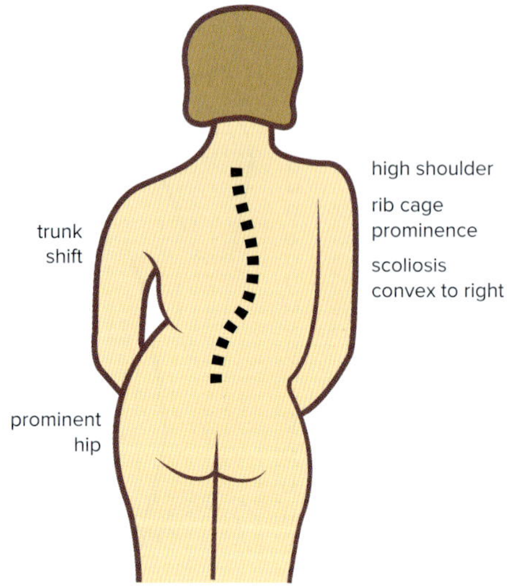

FIGURE 37.4 Adolescent idiopathic scoliosis: typical configuration of the trunk and thoracic spine

more prominent on forward flexion (see FIG. 37.6). Look for any asymmetry of the chest wall, inequality of the scapulae and differences in the levels of the shoulders. A useful sign of scoliosis is unequal shoulder levels and apparent 'winging' of scapula. When viewed anteriorly a difference in the levels of the nipples indicates the presence of scoliosis, or other problems causing one shoulder to drop. Inspection should therefore take place with posterior, lateral (side) and anterior views. For acute pain, check the skin for evidence of herpes zoster (rash or scars).

Palpation[2]

The best position is to have the patient prone on the examination table with the thoracic spine preferably in slight flexion. This is achieved by lowering the top of the table.

Test passive extension of each joint with firm pressure from the pad of the thumbs or the bony hand (either the pisiform prominence or the lateral border of the fifth metacarpal). Spring up and down with a few firm oscillations, keeping the elbows straight, but being well above the patient. Ask the patient if the pressure reproduces the pain.

Apart from asking the patient 'Is that the pain?' note:

- the distribution of pain and its change with movement
- the range of movement
- the type of resistance in the joint
- any muscle spasm

Palpation must follow a set plan in order to reproduce the patient's pain. The sequence is as follows:

1 central—over spinous processes
2 unilateral—over apophyseal joints (2–3 cm from midline)
3 transverse—on side of spinous processes
4 unilateral—costotransverse junctions (4–5 cm from midline)
5 unilateral—over ribs (spring over posterior rib curve with ulnar border of hand, along axis of rib)

Movements

There are four main movements of the thoracic spine to assess, the most important of which is rotation, as this is the movement that so frequently reproduces the patient's pain where it is facet joint or costovertebral in origin.

The movements of the thoracic spine and their normal ranges are:

1 Extension	30°
2 Lateral flexion L and R	30°
3 Flexion	90°
4 Rotation L and R	60°

Ask the patient to sit on the table with hands placed behind the neck and then perform the movements. Check these four active movements, noting any hypomobility, the range of movement, reproduction of symptoms and function and muscle spasm.

Neurological examination

This includes sensory testing for altered sensation in a dermatomal distribution.

Investigations

The plain X-ray and MRI scan is of no utility in patients with non-specific back pain but has a place in the presence of red flags, where the MRI is most appropriate to investigate suspected serious pathology. A plain X-ray may exclude basic bony abnormalities and diseases, such as osteoporosis and malignancy. CT scanning has a minimal role in the evaluation of thoracic spinal pain.

Other investigations to consider are:

- FBE and ESR/CRP
- serum alkaline phosphatase
- serum electrophoresis for multiple myeloma
- Bence–Jones protein analysis
- *Brucella* agglutination test
- blood culture for pyogenic infection and bacterial endocarditis
- tuberculosis studies
- HLA-B_{27} antigen for spondyloarthropathies
- ECG or ECG stress tests (suspected angina)

- gastroscopy or barium studies (peptic ulcer)
- MRI scanning if myelopathy is suspected
- radionuclide bone scan if neoplastic or metabolic disease is suspected

Thoracic back pain in children

The most common cause of thoracic back pain in children is 'postural backache', also known as 'TV backache', which is usually found in adolescent schoolgirls and is a diagnosis of exclusion.

Important, although rare, problems in children include infections (tuberculosis, discitis and osteomyelitis) and tumours such as osteoid osteoma and malignant osteogenic sarcoma.

Dysfunction of the joints of the thoracic spine in children and particularly in adolescents is very common and often related to trauma such as a heavy fall in sporting activities or falling from a height (e.g. off a horse). Fractures, of course, have to be excluded.

Inflammatory disorders to consider are juvenile ankylosing spondylitis and spinal osteochondrosis (Scheuermann disease), which may affect adolescent males in the lower thoracic spine (around T9) and thoracolumbar spine. The latter condition may be asymptomatic, but can be associated with back pain, especially as the patient grows older. It is the commonest cause of kyphosis.

It is important to screen adolescent children for idiopathic scoliosis, which may be without associated backache.

Kyphosis[5]

Kyphosis is the normal curve of the thoracic spine when viewed from the side. The normal range is 20–45° (see FIG. 37.5). An excessive angle (>45–50°) occurs with a kyphotic deformity. In children a congenital cause is likely (present from infancy); in adolescents it is usually due to Scheuermann disease or is postural; in adults consider ankylosing spondylitis—and osteoporosis in the elderly. Tuberculosis of the spine can cause a gross deformity. Children with significant kyphosis should be referred for management which includes exercises, bracing or surgery.

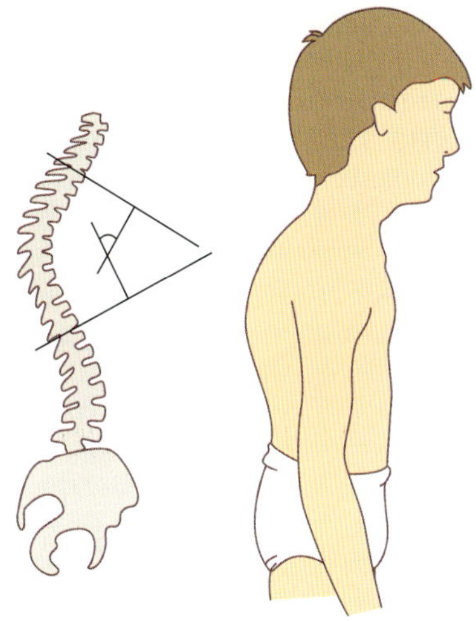

FIGURE 37.5 Illustration of kyphosis, which is measured by the angle between the uppermost and lowermost inclined vertebrae on the lateral X-ray

Scheuermann disease

This is a structural saggital plane deformity of unknown cause affecting the T7, 8, 9 or T11, 12 areas.

Clinical features

- Age 11–17 years
- Males > females
- Lower thoracic spine
- Thoracic pain or asymptomatic
- Increasing thoracic kyphosis over 1–2 months
- Wedging of the vertebrae
- Pain in the wedge, especially on bending (only 20% present with pain)
- Short hamstrings
- Cannot touch toes
- Diagnosis confirmed by X-ray (lateral standing)—shows Schmorl node and anterior vertebral body wedging

Treatment

- Explanation and support
- Extension exercises, avoid forward flexion
- Postural correction
- Avoidance of sports involving lifting and bending
- Consider bracing or surgery if serious deformity
- If detected early hyperextension body casts followed by a Milwaukee brace can prevent deformity

37

Adolescent idiopathic scoliosis

A degree of scoliosis is detectable in 5% of the adolescent population.[6] The vast majority of curves, occurring equally in boys and girls, are mild and of no consequence. Eighty-five per cent of significant curves in adolescent scoliosis occur in girls.[6] Inheritance is a factor. The highest incidence is in first-degree female relatives (12%). The scoliotic deformity develops at 10 years of age. Such curves appear during the peripubertal period, usually coinciding with the growth spurt. The screening test (usually in 12–14 year olds but ideally as early as 9) is to note the contour of the back on forward flexion (see FIG. 37.6). The routine physical screening check of an adolescent should include this area.

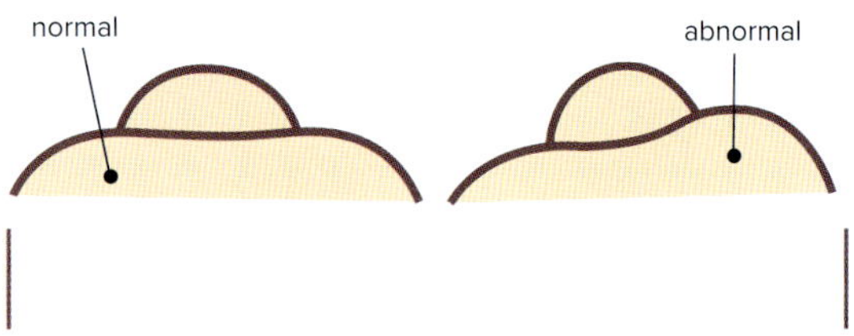

FIGURE 37.6 Screening for adolescent idiopathic scoliosis: testing asymmetry by forward flexion

The test

The subject stands with the feet parallel and together, and bends forward as far as possible with outstretched hands, palms facing each other, pointed between the great toes.

Investigation

A single erect PA spinal X-ray is sufficient;[7] the Cobb angle (see FIG. 37.7) is the usual measurement yardstick.

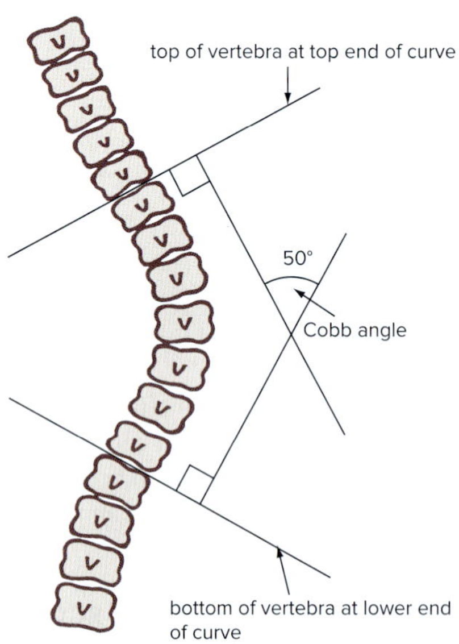

FIGURE 37.7 Scoliosis: the Cobb angle method of curve measurement

Management

Aims

- To preserve good appearance—level shoulders and no trunk shift
- Prevent increasing curve in adult life: less than 45°
- *Not* to produce a straight spine on X-ray

Methods

- Braces:
  - Milwaukee brace (rarely used)
  - high-density polyethylene underarm orthosis
  - to be worn for 20–22 hours each day until skeletal maturity is reached.
- Surgical correction: depends on curve and skeletal maturity

Guidelines for treatment

- Still growing:

<20°	observe (repeat examination + X-ray)
20–30°	observe, brace if progressive
30–45°	brace
≥45–50°	operate

- Growth complete:

<45°	leave alone
>45°	operate

Referral to consultant: >20°

Thoracic back pain in adults

Elderly patients: thoracic back pain due to mechanical causes is not such a feature in the elderly, although vertebral dysfunction still occurs quite regularly. However, when the elderly person presents with thoracic pain, a very careful search for organic disease is necessary. Special problems to consider are:

- malignant disease (e.g. multiple myeloma, lung, prostate)
- osteoporosis
- vertebral pathological fractures
- polymyalgia rheumatica
- Paget disease (may be asymptomatic)
- herpes zoster
- visceral disorders: ischaemic heart disease, penetrating peptic ulcer, oesophageal disorders, biliary disorders

Dysfunction of the thoracic spine

Also referred to as non-specific thoracic back pain, this is the outstanding cause of pain in adulthood presenting to the practitioner and is relatively easy to diagnose. It is often referred to as the thoracic hypomobility syndrome with the disorder arising in the facet joints, costovertebral joints and thoracic musculoligamentous structure, singularly or in combination. The most efficacious treatment for painful dysfunctional problems varies according to practitioners with a special interest in this area. There is a paucity of studies and evidence supporting the multiplicity of therapies, especially focal injections and physical therapy. Many claim and bear testimony that appropriate skilled mobilisation and manipulation therapy provides effective short-term, sometimes immediate, relief.[8]

Typical profile:[2]

Age	Any age, especially between 20 and 40 years.
History of injury	Sometimes slow or sudden onset
Site and radiation	Spinal and paraspinal—interscapular, arms, lateral chest, anterior chest, substernal, iliac crest
Type of pain	Dull, aching, occasionally sharp; severity related to activity, site and posture
Aggravation	Deep inspiration, postural movement of thorax, slumping or bending, walking upstairs, activities (e.g. lifting children, making beds), beds too hard or soft, sleeping or sitting for long periods
Association	Chronic poor posture
Diagnosis confirmation	Examination of spine, therapeutic response to manipulation

Management

First-line management

- Explanation with printed information
- Reassurance, including spontaneous recovery likely
- Continued activity according to pain level
- Back education program
- Analgesics, if required (e.g. paracetamol 1 g (o) qid or 1.33g (o) 8-hourly), is first line
- Posture education and specific mobilising exercise program, esp. extension and rotation exercises to overcome stiffness
- Physical therapy: a short course of spinal mobilisation and manipulation (if appropriate) to help with pain and mobility

Spinal mobilisation and manipulation

Spinal mobilisation is helpful but the more forceful manipulative therapy (with extreme care) produces better and quicker results. There are many techniques that can be employed, the choice depending on which part of the back is affected.[7] The sternal thrust (Nelson hold) technique is widely used for upper thoracic segments and the crossed pisiform technique (patient prone) or posteroanterior indirect thrust (patient supine—see FIG. 37.8) is claimed to be the most—effective for the mid-thoracic spine. There is level II evidence that spinal manipulation is effective compared with placebo.[8]

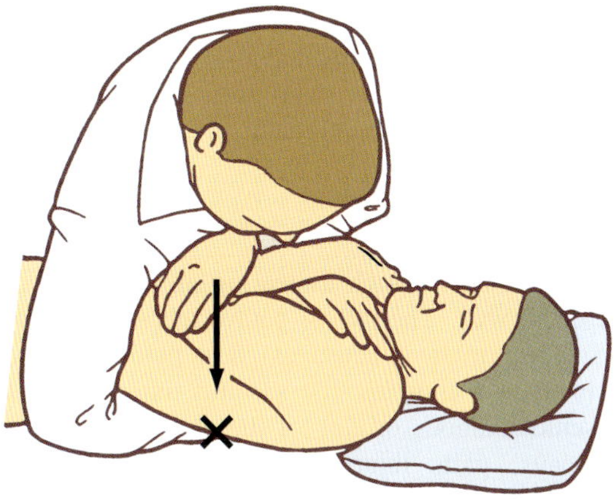

FIGURE 37.8 Manipulation of the mid-thoracic spine by the posteroanterior indirect thrust technique in a patient with no spinal disease or red flags

Source: Reproduced with permission from C Kenna and J Murtagh. *Back Pain and Spinal Manipulation* (2nd edn). Oxford: Butterworth-Heinemann, 1997

37

Thoracic disc protrusion

Fortunately, a disc protrusion in the thoracic spine is uncommon. This reduced incidence is related to the firm splintage action of the ribcage. Most disc protrusions occur below T9, with the commonest site, as expected, being T11–12.

The common presentation is back pain and radicular pain that follows the appropriate dermatome so disc protrusion should be considered in patients with neurological signs at thoracic levels. This may include a flaccid area of the lower abdominal musculature.

However, disc lesions in the thoracic spine are prone to produce spinal cord compression, manifesting as sensory loss, bladder incontinence and signs of upper motor neurone lesion. The disc is relatively inaccessible to surgical intervention, but over the past decade there has been a significant improvement in the surgical treatment of thoracic disc protrusions, due to the transthoracic lateral approach.

Syrinx

A syrinx usually comes to notice as a radiological finding in the presence of thoracic back pain when it may in fact be asymptomatic. It is a rare, fluid-filled neurological cavity within the spinal cord. It is usually a congenital anomaly, but a neoplasm needs to be excluded. An MRI of the spinal cord defines the problem. Any symptoms usually appear between adolescence and age 50, due to a central cord syndrome (see CHAPTER 62). A syrinx usually begins at the cervical level and extends down. Treat conservatively, but refer to an expert, who may consider surgical intervention if it is symptomatic.

Muscle injury

Muscular injuries such as tearing are uncommon in the chest wall. The strong paravertebral muscles do not appear to be a cause of chest pain, but strains of intercostal muscles, the serratus anterior and the musculotendinous origins of the abdominal muscles can cause pain. Injuries to these muscles can be provoked by attacks of violent sneezing or coughing or overstrain, e.g. lifting a heavy suitcase down from an overhead luggage rack.

SCAPULOTHORACIC JOINT DISORDERS[9]

37

The gliding plane between the scapula and thoracic wall permits a considerable range of scapular movement, which contributes significantly to movement of the shoulder. Several muscles, including the rhomboids, serratus anterior and levator scapulae, help stabilise scapular movement and may be a source of pain in the scapular region.

Snapping scapula

The patient complains of a loud cracking or snapping sound upon abduction of the scapula. There is often associated crepitus. Pain is felt along the medial scapular border. The patient may develop a habit ('tic') of neurotically clicking the shoulder back and forth.

On examination, there is usually generalised hypermobility of the scapula, abnormal movement and tenderness to palpation along the medial edge on full abduction.

The cause (uncommon) may be an underlying bony abnormality such as a bony spur on the superior border of the scapula or an osteoma. X-rays should include a lateral view of the scapula to search for this possibility.

Treatment

- Explanation and reassurance (if X-rays normal)—otherwise resect any bone abnormality.
- Avoid repeated scapular movement and 'trick' movements.
- Appropriate exercises under physiotherapy supervision.
- Infiltrate any very tender area in the muscle (with care) with local anaesthetic and steroid.
- Deep massage to the tender focus.

Scapulocostal syndrome

This condition causes localised pain and tenderness, often severe, along the upper part of the medial scapular border, with radiation around the chest wall and shoulder girdle to the neck. Pain is usually worse with prolonged shoulder use towards the end of the day. It is commonly seen in typists, gymnasts and other sportspeople. It is related to poor posture. The cause may include friction between the scapula and the thoracic wall, scoliosis, trauma and myofascial strain due to poor posture.

Treatment

- Avoid the movements producing the pain.
- Posture and re-education exercises and scapula stretching.
- Deep friction massage.
- Local injections of local anaesthetic and corticosteroid into the tender area.

Winging of the scapula

The asymmetry may not be apparent until the patient tries to contract the serratus anterior against resistance by pushing the outstretched arm against the wall. There may be parascapular discomfort. The common cause is neurogenic paralysis of the serratus anterior muscle. Paralysis may result from injury to the long thoracic nerve (from C5, 6, 7 nerve roots) such as a neck injury or a direct blow to the suprascapular area and from injury to the brachial plexus such as excessive carrying of heavy packs, severe traction on the arm or forceful cervical manipulation. Most cases settle spontaneously, although it may take 1–2 years.

FIBROMYALGIA, FIBROSITIS AND MYOFASCIAL TRIGGER POINTS

Fibromyalgia is relatively uncommon, but when encountered it presents an enormous management problem. It is not to be confused with so-called fibrositis or tender trigger points. Referral to a specialist with expertise in this condition or to a multidisciplinary pain clinic for the definitive diagnosis is recommended.

Fibrositis is not a diagnosis but a symptom, indicating a localised area of tenderness or pain in the soft tissues, especially of the upper thoracic spine. It is probably almost always secondary to upper thoracic or lower cervical spinal dysfunction.

Myofascial trigger points

As described by Travell and Rinzler,[10] a trigger point is characterised by:

- circumscribed local tenderness
- localised twitching with stimulation of juxtaposed muscle
- pain referred elsewhere when subjected to pressure

Trigger spots also tend to correspond to the acupuncture points for pain relief.

Treatment[11]

Local injection is relatively easy and may give excellent results. Identify the maximal point of pain and inject 5–8 mL of local anaesthetic (LA; e.g. lignocaine/lidocaine 1%) into the painful point (see FIG. 37.9). Post-injection massage or exercises should be performed.

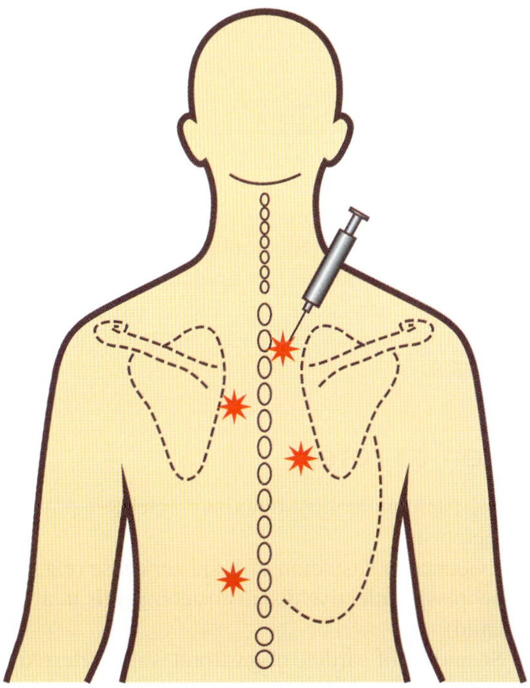

FIGURE 37.9 Injection for myofascial trigger points

Don't:

- use large volumes of LA
- use corticosteroids
- cause bleeding

Do:

- use a moderate amount of LA (only)

Fibromyalgia syndrome[12]

AKA chronic diffuse non-inflammatory pain. Its pathophysiology is poorly understood.

Clinical features

The main diagnostic features are:

1 a history of widespread pain (neck to low back)
2 pain in 11 of 18 tender points on digital palpation

These points must be painful, not tender. Smythe and Moldofsky have recommended 14 of these points on a map as a guide for management[12] (see FIG. 37.10). No consistent measurable investigations have been identified.

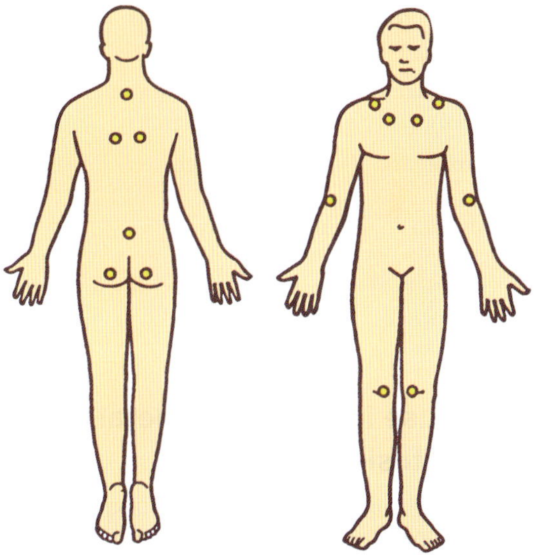

FIGURE 37.10 Fibromyalgia syndrome: typical tender points (the tender point map represents the 14 points recommended for use as a standard for diagnostic or therapeutic studies)

Other features

- Female to male ratio = 4:1
- Usual age onset 29–37 years: diagnosis 44–53 years
- Poor sleep pattern
- Dermatographia

- Fatigue (similar to chronic fatigue syndrome)
- Psychological disorders (e.g. anxiety, depression, tension headache, irritable digestive system)

This disorder is very difficult to treat and is usually unresponsive in the long term to passive physical therapy or injections.[13] Patients require considerable explanation, support and reassurance, including screening with ESR/CRP. Best evidence to date supports the value of educational programs and regular aerobic exercise.[14] Consider referral to a specialist or fibromyalgia clinic.

Treatment

- Explanation, patient education, reassurance and counselling
- Attention to sleep disorders, stress factors and physical factors[14]
- Relaxation program
- Rehabilitation: graduated exercise program (e.g. walking, water exercises, swimming or cycling)
- Use paracetamol for first-line analgesia
- Carefully assess any change in the nature or pattern of symptoms

Medication (often disappointing but worth a trial)

Antidepressants (of proven short-term value);[15,16] start low then monthly increments as tolerated:

amitriptyline 10–50 mg (o) nocte

or

dothiepin 25–75 mg (o) nocte

or

37 duloxetine 30 mg (o) mane, increasing to 60 mg over 2 weeks[17]

Note: NSAIDs are of no proven benefit.

Diffuse idiopathic skeletal hyperostosis (DISH)

DISH is ligamentous ossification of the spine leading to progressive stiffness and possible pain in some parts. Possible associated metabolic disorder e.g. diabetes. Ankylosing spondylitis is a differential diagnosis.

There is no specific treatment. Manage as for spinal dysfunction.

Serious pitfalls

The following points regarding serious vertebral organic disease are worth repeating in more detail.

Metastatic disease[18]

Secondary deposits in the thoracolumbar spine may be the first presenting symptoms of malignant disease. Any patient of any age presenting with progressive severe night pain of the back should be regarded as having a tumour and investigated with a technetium bone scan as part of the primary investigations.

Secondary deposits in the spine can lead to rapid onset paralysis due to spinal cord infarction. Many such metastases can be controlled in the early stages with radiotherapy.

Multiple myeloma

Osteoporotic vertebral body collapse should be diagnosed only when multiple myeloma has been excluded. Investigations should include an ESR, Bence–Jones protein analysis, and immunoglobulin electrophoresis.

Early treatment of multiple myeloma can hold this disease in remission for many years and prevent crippling vertebral fractures (see CHAPTER 26).

Infective discitis, vertebral osteomyelitis and epidural/subdural abscess

Severe back pain in an unwell patient with fluctuating temperature (fever) should be considered as infective until proved otherwise. Investigations should include blood cultures, serial X-rays and nuclear bone scanning. Biphasic bone scans using technetium with either indium or gallium scanning for white cell collections usually clinch this diagnosis.

Strict bed rest with high-dose antibiotic therapy is usually curative. If left untreated, vertebral end plate and disc space collapse is common and extremely disabling. Consider tuberculosis osteomyelitis in people at risk. Suspect an epidural abscess in the presence of persistent and increased back pain. Percuss the spine for localised tenderness (see CHAPTER 30).

When to refer

- Persistent pain or dysfunction—refer to a physical therapist.
- Evidence or suspicion of a sinister cause (e.g. neoplasia, infective discitis/osteomyelitis in a child).
- Suspicion of cardiac or gastrointestinal referred (persistent) pain.
- Significant idiopathic adolescent scoliosis or kyphosis (e.g. Scheuermann disease).

Patient education resources

Hand-out sheets from *Murtagh's Patient Education* 7th edition:

- Exercises for your thoracic spine
- Fibromyalgia
- Scoliosis

Practice tips

- Feelings of anaesthesia or paraesthesia associated with thoracic spinal dysfunction are rare.
- Thoracic back pain is frequently associated with cervical lesions.
- Upper thoracic pain and stiffness is common after 'whiplash'.
- The T4 syndrome of upper to mid-thoracic pain with radiation (and associated paraesthesia) to the arms is well documented.
- Symptoms due to a fractured vertebra usually last 3 months and to a fractured rib 6 weeks.
- The pain of myocardial ischaemia, from either angina or myocardial infarction, can cause referred pain to the interscapular region of the thoracic spine.
- Beware of the old trap of herpes zoster in the thoracic spine, especially in the older person.
- Consider multiple myeloma as a cause of an osteoporotic collapsed vertebra.
- Examine movements with the patient sitting on the couch and hands clasped behind the neck.
- Spinal disease of special significance in the thoracic spine includes osteoporosis and neoplasia, while disc lesions, inflammatory diseases and degenerative diseases (spondylosis) are encountered less frequently than with the cervical and lumbar spines.
- It is imperative to differentiate between spinal and cardiac causes of chest pain: either cause is likely to mimic the other. A working rule is to consider the cause as cardiac until the examination and investigations establish the true cause.
- Always X-ray the thoracic spine following trauma, especially after motor vehicle accidents, as wedge compression fractures (typically between T4 and T8) are often overlooked.
- Plain X-ray, CT scan or MRI are of no utility in patients with non-specific thoracic back pain.
- MRI is the most appropriate imaging to investigate suspected serious pathology.

References

1. Australian Acute Musculoskeletal Pain Guidelines Group. *Evidence-Based Management of Acute Musculoskeletal Pain—A Guide for Clinicians.* Bowen Hills, QLD: Australian Academic Press, 2004.
2. Kenna C, Murtagh J. *Back Pain and Spinal Manipulation* (2nd edn). Oxford: Butterworth-Heinemann, 1997: 165–74.
3. Johansson MS et al. Incidence and prognosis of mid-back pain in the general population: a systemic review. Eur J Pain, 2017; 21 (1): 20–8.
4. McGuckin N. The T4 syndrome. In: Grieve GD (ed.), *Modern Manual Therapy of the Vertebral Column.* London: Churchill Livingstone, 1986: 370–6.
5. Sponseller P. *The 5-minute Orthopaedic Consult.* Philadelphia: Lippincott, Williams and Wilkins, 2001: 184–5.
6. Stephens J. Idiopathic adolescent scoliosis. Aust Fam Physician, 1984; 13: 180–4.
7. Anonymous. *The Easter Seal Guide to Children's Orthopaedics.* Toronto: The Easter Seal Society, 1982: 64–7.
8. Schiller L. Effectiveness of spinal manipulation therapy in the treatment of mechanical thoracic back pain. J Manip Physiol Ther, 2001; 24: 394–401.
9. Corrigan B, Maitland G. *Practical Orthopaedic Medicine.* Sydney: Butterworths, 1986: 384–5.
10. Travell J, Rinzler SH. The myofascial genesis of pain. Postgrad Med, 1952; 11: 425–34.
11. Simons D. Understanding effective treatments of myofascial trigger points. J Bodyw Mov Ther, 2002; 6: 81–5.
12. Smythe HA, Moldofsky H. Two contributions to understanding of the 'fibrositis' syndrome. Bull Rheum Dis, 1977; 28: 928–31.
13. Clauw DJ. Fibromyalgia: a clinical review. JAMA, 2014; 311 (15): 1,547–55.
14. Theadom A, Cropley M et al. Mind and body therapy for fibromyalgia. Cochrane Database Syst Rev. 2015, Issue 4. Art No. CD001980.
15. Jaeschke R, Adachi J, Guyatt G et al. Clinical usefulness of amitriptyline in fibromyalgia: the results of 23 N-of-I randomised controlled trials. J Rheumatol, 1991; 18: 447–51.
16. Expert group for Rheumatology. Fibromyalgia. In: eTG complete [Internet]. Melbourne: Therapeutic Guidelines Ltd. Available from: <www.tg.org.au>, accessed January 2018.
17. Chappell AS, Littlejohn G et al. A 1-year safety and efficacy study of duloxetine in patients with fibromyalgia. Clin J Pain, 2009; 25 (5): 365–75.
18. Young D, Murtagh J. Pitfalls in orthopaedics. Aust Fam Physician, 1989; 18: 653–4.

38 Low back pain

Last Wednesday night while carrying a bucket of water from the well, Hannah Williams slipped upon the icy path and fell heavily upon her back. We fear her spine was injured for though she suffers acute pain in her legs she cannot move them. The poor wild beautiful girl is stopped in her wildness at last.

FRANCIS KILVERT 1874

Low back pain accounts for at least 5% of general practice presentations. It is a massive problem worldwide. The most common cause is minor soft tissue injury, but patients with this do not usually seek medical help because the problem settles within a few days.

Most back pain in patients presenting to GPs is postulated to be due to dysfunction of elements of the mobile segment, namely the facet joint, the intervertebral joint (with its disc) and the ligamentous and muscular attachments. This problem, often referred to as mechanical back pain, will be described as vertebral dysfunction—a general term that, while covering radicular and non-radicular pain, includes dysfunction of the joints of the spine, although the specific origin in most instances cannot be determined. It is therefore appropriate to refer to this as 'non-specific back pain'.[1]

Key facts and checkpoints

- Back pain accounts for at least 5% of all presenting problems in general practice in Australia and 6.5% in Britain.[2]
- In the US it is the commonest cause of limitation of activity in those under the age of 45.[2]
- Approximately 85–90% of the population will experience back pain at some stage of their lives, while 70% of the world's population will have at least one disabling episode of low back pain in their lives.[2]
- At least 50% of these people will recover within 2 weeks and 90% within 6 weeks, but recurrences are frequent and have been reported in 40–70% of patients; 2–7% develop chronic pain.[3]
- The most common age groups are the 30s, 40s and 50s, the average age being 45 years.[4]
- The most common cause of back pain is a minor strain to muscles and/or ligaments, but people suffering from this type of back pain usually do not seek medical treatment as most of these soft-tissue problems resolve rapidly.
- The main cause of back pain presenting to the doctor is dysfunction of the intervertebral joints of the spine due to injury, also referred to as mechanical back pain (at least 70%).
- The second most common cause of back pain is spondylosis (synonymous with osteoarthritis and degenerative back disease). It accounts for about 10% of cases of low back pain.
- L5 and S1 nerve root lesions represent most of the cases of sciatica presenting in general practice. They tend to present separately but can occur together with a massive disc protrusion.
- An intervertebral disc prolapse has been proven in only 6–8% of cases of back pain.[2]

Causes of low back pain

To develop a comprehensive diagnostic approach, the practitioner should have a clear understanding of the possible causes of low back and leg pain and of the relative frequency of their clinical presentations. The major causes of low back pain in several hundred patients presenting to the author's general practice are summarised in TABLE 38.1.

Relevant causes are illustrated in FIGURE 38.1.

Table 38.1 Major causes of low back ± leg pain presenting in the author's general practice

Patients	%
Vertebral dysfunction (non-specific back pain)	71.8
Lumbar spondylosis	10.1
Depression	3.0
Urinary tract infection	2.2
Spondylolisthesis	2.0
Spondyloarthropathies	1.9
Musculoligamentous strains/tears	1.2
Malignant disease	0.8
Arterial occlusive disease	0.6
Other	6.4
Total	100.0

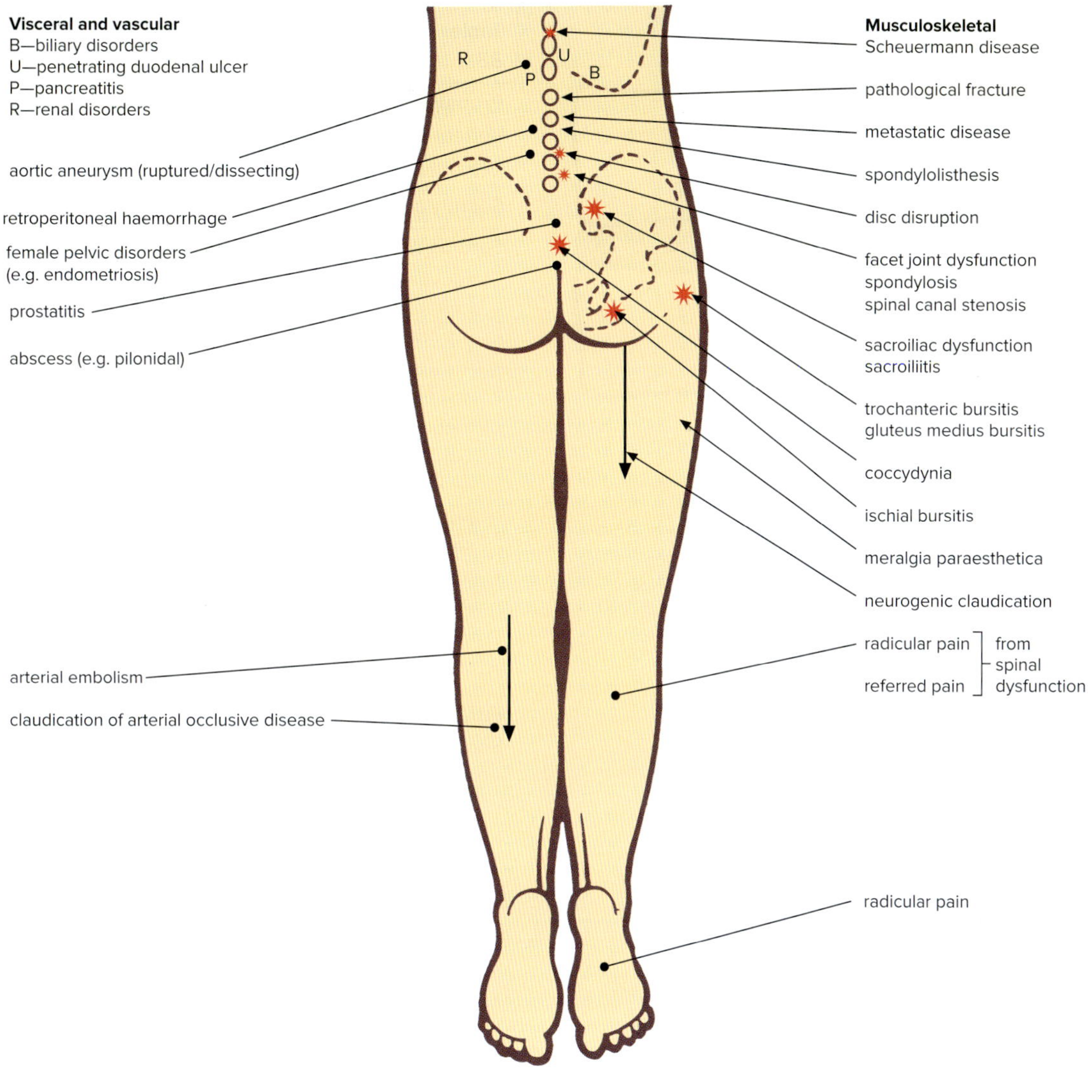

FIGURE 38.1 Relevant causes of back pain with associated buttock and leg pain

Anatomical and pathophysiological concepts

Recent studies have focused on the importance of disruption of the intervertebral disc in the cause of back pain. A very plausible theory has been advanced by Maigne[3] who proposes the existence, in the involved mobile segment, of a minor intervertebral derangement (MID). He defines it as 'isolated pain in one intervertebral segment, of a mild character, and due to minor mechanical cause'.

The MID always involves one of the two apophyseal joints in the mobile segment, thus initiating nociceptive activity in the posterior primary dermatome and myotome.

Maigne points out that the functional ability of the mobile segment depends intimately upon the condition of the intervertebral disc. Thus, if the disc is injured, other elements of the segment will be affected. Even a minimal disc lesion can produce apophyseal joint dysfunction, which is a reflex cause of protective muscle spasm and pain in the corresponding segment, with loss of function (see FIG. 38.2).

In theory, any structure with a nociceptive nerve supply may be a source of pain. Such structures include the ligaments, fascia and muscles of the lumbosacral spine, intervertebral joints, facet joints, dura mater and sacroiliac joints.[5]

Actually, pain can theoretically arise from any innervated structure in the region of the spine. It can be

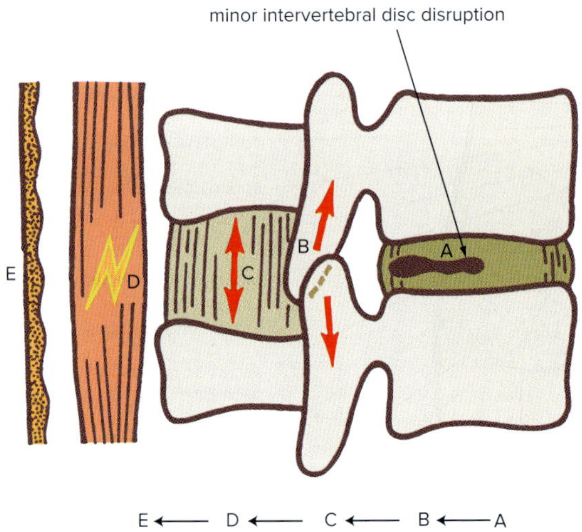

FIGURE 38.2 Reflex activity from a MID in the intervertebral motion segment. Apart from the local effect caused by the disruption of the disc (A), interference can occur in the facet joint (B) and interspinous ligament (C) leading possibly to muscle spasm (D) and skin changes (E) via the posterior rami.

Source: Reproduced with permission from C Kenna and J Murtagh. *Back Pain and Spinal Manipulation.* Sydney: Butterworths, 1989

neurogenic, spondylogenic, viscerogenic, vasculogenic or rarely psychogenic.

A diagnostic approach

A summary of the diagnostic strategy model is presented in TABLE 38.2.

38

Probability diagnosis

The commonest cause of low back pain is vertebral dysfunction or mechanical pain, which then has to be further analysed. The term can embrace musculoskeletal strain, discogenic and posterior ligament pain, and facetogenic dysfunction/pain.

Degenerative changes in the lumbar spine (lumbar spondylosis) are commonly found in the older age group. This problem, and one of its complications, spinal canal stenosis, is steadily increasing along with the ageing population.

Serious disorders not to be missed

It is important to consider malignant disease, especially in an older person. It is also essential to consider infection such as acute osteomyelitis and tuberculosis, which is often encountered in recent immigrants, especially those from Asia and central Africa. The uncommon epidural or subdural abscess should also be kept in mind, especially if any fever (see CHAPTER 30). These conditions are considered in more detail under infections of the central nervous

Table 38.2 Low back pain: diagnostic strategy model
Probability diagnosis
Vertebral dysfunction (non-specific low back pain)
Musculoligamentous strain/sprain
Spondylosis (degenerative OA)
Serious disorders not to be missed
Cardiovascular:
• ruptured aortic aneurysm
• retroperitoneal haemorrhage (anticoagulants)
Neoplasia:
• myeloma
• metastases
Severe infections:
• vertebral osteomyelitis
• epidural abscess
• septic discitis
• tuberculosis
• pelvic abscess/PID
Osteoporotic compression fracture/other fracture
Cauda equina compression
Pitfalls (often missed)
Spondyloarthropathies:
• ankylosing spondylitis
• reactive arthritis
• psoriasis
• bowel inflammation
Sacroiliac dysfunction
Spondylolisthesis
Claudication:
• vascular
• neurogenic/spinal canal stenosis
Paget disease
Prostatitis
Endometriosis
Seven masquerades checklist
Depression
Spinal dysfunction
UTI
Is the patient trying to tell me something?
Quite likely. Consider lifestyle, stress, work problems, malingering, conversion reaction

Note: Associated buttock and leg pain included.

system. For pain or anaesthesia of sudden onset, especially when accompanied by neurological changes in the legs, consider cauda equina compression due to a massive disc prolapse and also retroperitoneal haemorrhage. It is important to ask patients if they are taking anticoagulants. See TABLE 38.3.

Table 38.3 'Red flag' pointers to serious low back pain conditions[6]

Age >50 years or <20 years
History of cancer
Temperature >37.8°C
Constant pain—day and night esp. severe night pain
Unexplained weight loss
Symptoms in other systems, e.g. cough, breast mass
Significant trauma
Features of spondyloarthropathy, e.g. peripheral arthritis (e.g. age <40 years, night-time waking)
Neurological deficit
Drug or alcohol abuse especially IV drug use
Use of anticoagulants
Use of corticosteroids
No improvement over 1 month
Possible cauda equina syndrome:

- saddle anaesthesia
- recent onset bladder dysfunction/overflow incontinence
- bilateral or progressive neurological deficit

Pitfalls

The inflammatory disorders must be kept in mind, especially the spondyloarthropathies, which include psoriatic arthropathy, ankylosing spondylitis, reactive arthritis, inflammatory bowel disorders such as ulcerative colitis and Crohn disease, and reactive arthritis. The spondyloarthropathies are more common than appreciated and must be considered in the younger person presenting with features of inflammatory back pain (i.e. pain at rest, relieved by activity). The old trap of confusing claudication in the buttocks and legs, due to a high arterial obstruction, with sciatica must be avoided.

General pitfalls

- Being unaware of the characteristic symptoms of inflammation and thus misdiagnosing one of the spondyloarthropathies.
- Overlooking the early development of malignant disease or osteomyelitis; if suspected, and an X-ray is normal, a radionuclide scan should detect the problem.
- Failing to realise that mechanical dysfunction and osteoarthritis can develop simultaneously, producing a combined pattern.
- Overlooking anticoagulants as a cause of a severe bleed around the nerve roots and corticosteroids leading to osteoporosis.
- Not recognising back pain as a presenting feature of the drug addict.

Red flag pointers for low back pain

There are several so-called 'red flag' or precautionary pointers to a serious underlying cause of back pain (see TABLE 38.3). Such symptoms and signs should alert the practitioner to a serious health problem and thus guide selection of investigations, particularly appropriate imaging of the lumbar spine.

Seven masquerades checklist

Of these conditions, depression and urinary tract infection have to be seriously considered. For the young woman with upper lumbar pain, especially if she is pregnant, the possibility of a urinary tract infection must be considered. These patients may not have urinary symptoms, such as dysuria and frequency.

Depressive illness has to be considered in any patient with a chronic pain complaint. This common psychiatric disorder can continue to aggravate or maintain the pain even though the provoking problem has disappeared.

This is more likely to occur in people who have become anxious about their problem or who are under excessive stress. Many doctors treat such patients with a therapeutic trial of antidepressant medication, for example, amitriptyline or doxepin.

Psychogenic considerations

The patient may be unduly stressed, not coping with life or malingering. It may be necessary to probe beneath the surface of the presenting problem.

A patient with low back pain following lifting at work poses a problem that causes considerable anguish to doctors, especially when the pain becomes chronic and complex. Chronic pain may be the last straw for patients who have been struggling to cope with personal problems; their fragile equilibrium is upset by the back pain. Many patients who have been dismissed as malingerers turn out to have a genuine problem. The importance of a caring, competent practitioner with an insight into all facets of his or her patient's suffering, organic and functional, becomes obvious. The tests for non-organic back pain are very useful in this context.

Yellow flag pointers

This term has been introduced to identify psychosocial and occupational factors that may increase the risk of chronicity in people presenting with acute back pain. Consider psychological issues if:

- abnormal illness behaviour
- 'fear avoidance': concern re pain on activity
- compensation issues
- unsatisfactory restoration of activities
- failure to return to work
- unsatisfactory response to treatment
- treatment refused
- atypical presenting physical signs

Nature of the pain

The nature of the pain may reveal its likely origin. Establish where the pain is worst—whether it is central (proximal) or peripheral. The following are general characteristics and guides to diagnosis:

- aching throbbing pain = inflammation (e.g. sacroiliitis)
- deep aching diffuse pain = referred pain (e.g. dysmenorrhoea)
- superficial steady diffuse pain = local pain (e.g. muscular strain)
- boring deep pain = bone disease (e.g. neoplasia, Paget disease)
- intense sharp or stabbing (superimposed on a dull ache) = radicular pain (e.g. sciatica)

A comparison of the significant features of the two most common types of pain—mechanical and inflammatory—is presented in TABLE 38.4.

38

The clinical approach

History

Analysing the history invariably guides the clinician to the diagnosis. The pain patterns have to be carefully evaluated and it is helpful to map the diurnal variations of pain to facilitate the diagnosis (see FIG. 38.3).

It is especially important to note the intensity of the pain and its relation to rest and activity. In particular, ask whether the pain is present during the night, whether it wakes the patient, is present on rising or whether it is associated with stiffness.

Continuous pain, present day and night, is suggestive of neoplasia or infection. Pain on waking also suggests inflammation or depressive illness. Pain provoked by activity and relieved by rest suggests mechanical dysfunction while pain worse at rest and relieved by moderate activity is typical of inflammation. In some patients the coexistence of mechanical and inflammatory causes complicates the pattern.

Pain aggravated by standing or walking that is relieved by sitting is suggestive of spondylolisthesis.

Table 38.4 Comparison of the patterns of pain for inflammatory and mechanical causes of low back pain[8]

Feature	Inflammation	Mechanical
History	Insidious onset	Precipitating injury/ previous episodes
Nature	Aching, throbbing	Deep dull ache, sharp if root compression
Stiffness	Severe, prolonged Morning stiffness	Moderate, transient
Effect of rest	Exacerbates	Relieves
Effect of activity	Relieves	Exacerbates
Radiation	More localised, bilateral or alternating	Tends to be diffuse, unilateral
Intensity	Night, early morning	End of day, following activity

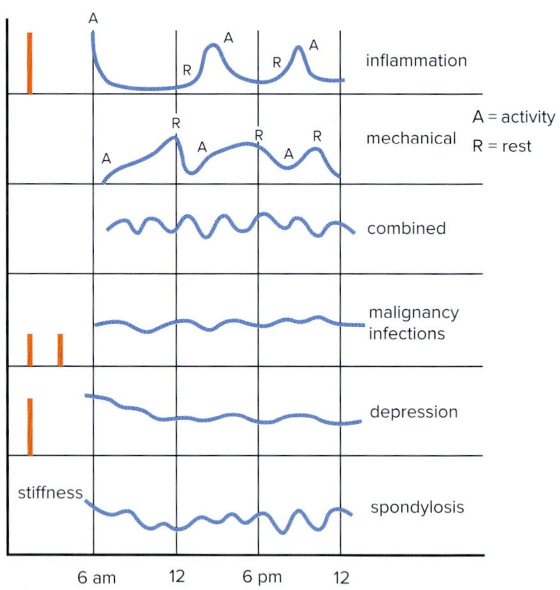

FIGURE 38.3 Typical daily patterns of pain for conditions causing back pain. Note conditions that can wake patients from sleep and also the combined mechanical and inflammatory patterns.

Pain aggravated by sitting (usually) and improved with standing indicates a discogenic problem.

Pain of the calf that travels proximally with walking indicates vascular claudication; pain in the buttock that descends with walking indicates neurogenic claudication. This latter problem is encountered more frequently in older people who have a tendency to spinal canal stenosis associated with spondylosis.

Key questions

- What is your general health like?
- Can you describe the nature of your back pain?
- Was your pain brought on by an injury?
- Is it worse when you wake in the morning or later in the day?
- How do you sleep during the night?
- What effect does rest have on the pain?
- What effect does activity have on the pain?
- Is the pain worse when sitting or standing?
- What effect does coughing or sneezing or straining at the toilet have?
- What happens to the pain in your back or leg if you go for a long walk?
- Do you have a history of psoriasis, diarrhoea, penile discharge, eye trouble or severe pain in your joints?
- Do you have any urinary symptoms?
- What medication are you taking? Are you on anticoagulants?
- Are you under any extra stress at work or home?
- Do you feel tense or depressed or irritable?

Examination

Physical examination

The basic objectives of the physical examination are to reproduce the patient's symptoms, detect the level of the lesion and determine the cause (if possible) by provocation of the affected joints or tissues. This is done using the time-honoured method of joint examination—look, feel, move and test function. The patient should be stripped to a minimum of clothing so that careful examination of the back can be made. A neurological examination of the lower limb should be performed if symptoms extend below the buttocks. It is important to perform a rectal examination to check for flaccidity in a patient with suspected cauda equina syndrome.

A useful screening test for a disc lesion and dural tethering is the slump test.[7]

The main components of the physical examination are:

1 inspection
2 active movements:
   - forward flexion (to reproduce the patient's symptoms)
   - extension (to reproduce the patient's symptoms)
   - lateral flexion (R & L) (to reproduce the patient's symptoms)
3 provocative tests (to reproduce the patient's symptoms)
4 palpation (to detect level of pain)
5 neurological testing of lower limbs (if appropriate)
6 testing of related joints (hip, sacroiliac)
7 assessment of pelvis and lower limbs for any deformity (e.g. leg shortening)
8 general medical examination, including rectal examination

Important landmarks

The surface anatomy of the lumbar region is the basis for determining the vertebral level. Key anatomical landmarks include the iliac crest, spinous processes, the sacrum and the posterior superior iliac spines (PSISs).

- The tops of the iliac crest lie at the level of the L3–4 interspace (or the L4 spinous process).
- The PSISs lie opposite S2.

Inspection

Inspection begins from the moment the patient is sighted in the waiting room. A patient who is noted to be standing is likely to have a significant disc lesion. Considerable information can be obtained from the manner in which the patient arises from a chair, moves to the consulting room, removes the shoes and clothes, gets onto the examination couch and moves when unaware of being watched.

The spine must be adequately exposed and inspected in good light. Patients should undress to their underpants; women may retain their brassiere and it is proper to provide them with a gown that opens down the back. Note the general contour and symmetry of the back and legs, including the buttock folds, and look for muscle wasting. Note the lumbar lordosis and any abnormalities, such as lateral deviation. If lateral deviation (scoliosis) is present it is usually away from the painful side.

Note the presence of midline moles, tufts of hair or haemangioma that might indicate an underlying congenital anomaly, such as spina bifida occulta.

Movements of the lumbar spine

There are three main movements of the lumbar spine. As there is minimal rotation, which mainly occurs at the thoracic spine, rotation is not so important. The movements that should be tested, and their normal ranges, are as follows:

- extension (20–30°) (see FIG. 38.4a)
- lateral flexion, left and right (30°) (see FIG. 38.4b)
- flexion (75–90°: average 80°) (see FIG. 38.4a)

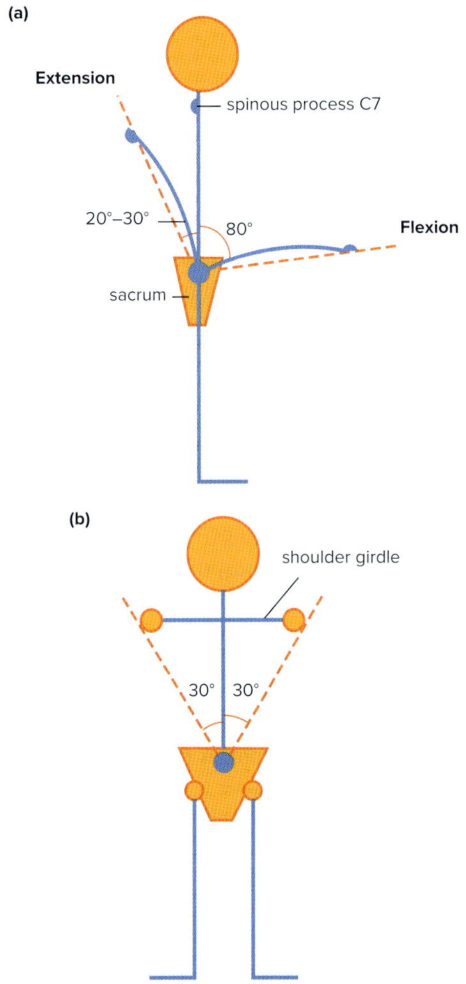

FIGURE 38.4 **(a)** Degrees of movement of the lumbar spine: flexion and extension, **(b)** degree of lateral flexion of the lumbar spine

Source: Reproduced with permission from C Kenna and J Murtagh. *Back Pain and Spinal Manipulation.* Sydney: Butterworths, 1989

Measurement of the angle of movement can be made by using a line drawn between the sacrum and large prominence of the C7 spinous process.

Palpation

Have the patient relaxed, lying prone, with the head to one side and the arms by the sides. The levels of the spinous processes are identified by standing behind the patient and using your hands to identify the L4 and L5 spinous processes in relation to the top of the iliac crests. Mark the important reference points.

Palpation, which is performed with the tips of the thumbs opposed, can commence at the spinous process of L1 and then systematically proceed distally to L5 and then over the sacrum and coccyx. Include the interspinous spaces as well as the spinous processes. When the thumbs (or other part of the hand such as the pisiforms) are applied to the spinous processes, a firm pressure is transmitted to the vertebrae by a rocking movement for three or four 'springs'. Significant reproduction of pain is noted.

Palpation occurs at three main sites:

- centrally (spinous processes to coccyx)
- unilateral—right and left sides (1.5 cm from midline)
- transverse pressure to the sides of the spinous processes (R and L)

Straight leg raising (SLR) test (Lasègue test)

This test is a passive test by the practitioner. The patient lies supine with both knees extended and the ankle dorsiflexed. The affected leg is raised slowly, keeping the knee extended. If sciatica with dural irritation is present, 20° to 60° of elevation causes reproduction of pain.

Slump test

The slump test is an excellent provocation test for lumbosacral pain and is more sensitive than the SLR test. It is a screening test for a disc lesion and dural tethering. It should be performed on patients who have low back pain with pain extending into the leg, and especially for posterior thigh pain.

A positive result is reproduction of the patient's pain, and may appear at an early stage of the test (when it is ceased).

Method:

1. The patient sits on the couch in a relaxed manner with knees at the edge of the table.
2. The patient then slumps forward (without excessive trunk flexion), and then places the chin on the chest.
3. The unaffected leg is straightened.
4. The affected leg only is then straightened (see FIG. 38.5).
5. Both legs are straightened together.
6. The foot of the affected straightened leg is dorsiflexed.

Note: Take care to distinguish from hamstring pain. Deflexing the neck relieves the pain of spinal origin, not hamstring pain.

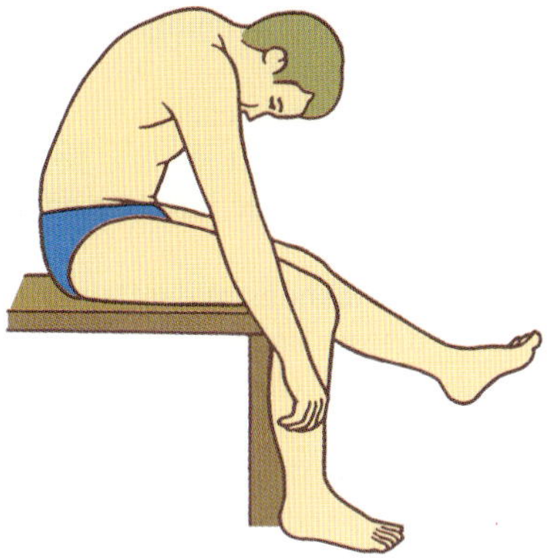

FIGURE 38.5 The slump test: one of the stages

Significance of the slump test

- It is positive if the back or leg pain is reproduced.
- If positive, it suggests disc disruption.
- If negative, it may indicate lack of serious disc pathology.
- If positive, one should approach manual therapy with caution.

Neurological examination[7]

A neurological examination is performed only when the patient's symptoms, such as pain, paraesthesia, anaesthesia and weakness, extend into the leg.

The importance of the neurological examination is to ensure that there is no compression of the spinal nerves from a prolapsed disc or from a tumour. This is normally tested by examining those functions that the respective spinal nerves serve, namely skin sensation, muscle power and reflex activity.

The examination is not daunting but can be performed quickly and efficiently in 2 to 3 minutes by a methodical technique that improves with continued use. The neurological examination consists of:

1 quick tests: walking on heels (L5), walking on toes (S1)
2 dural stretch tests: slump test, straight leg raising
3 specific nerve root tests (L4, L5, S1): sensation, power, reflexes

Main nerve roots

Refer to FIGURE 38.6 and to TABLE 66.3.

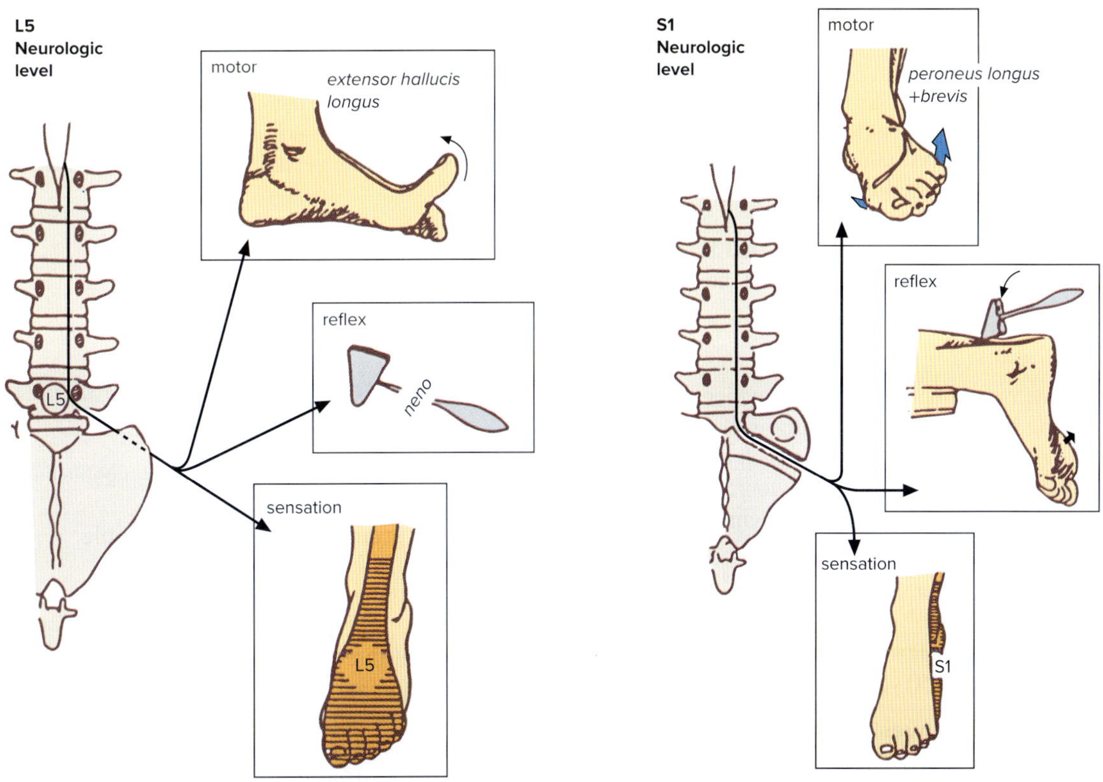

FIGURE 38.6 The main motor, sensory and reflex features of the nerve roots L5 and S1

Source: Reproduced with permission of Pearson Education Inc. Upper Saddle River, New Jersey. S Hoppenfeld. *Physical Examination of the Spine and Extremities.* 1st © 1976

L3:

- femoral stretch test (prone, flex knee, extend hip)
- motor—extension of knee
- sensation—anterior thigh
- reflex—knee jerk (L3, L4)

L4:

- motor—resisted inversion foot
- sensation—inner border of foot to great toe
- reflex—knee jerk

L5:

- motor: walking on heels, resisted extension great toe
- sensation—middle three toes (dorsum)
- reflex—nil

S1:

- motor: walking on toes, resisted eversion foot
- sensation—little toe, most of sole
- reflex—ankle jerk (S1, S2)

Other examination

The method of examining the sacroiliac and hip joints is outlined in CHAPTER 65.

Investigations

Investigations for back pain can be classified into three broad groups: front-line screening tests; specific disease investigations; and procedural and preprocedural tests.

Plain X-rays of the lumbar spine are not routinely recommended in acute non-specific low back pain (pain <6 weeks) in the absence of 'red flags' as they are of limited diagnostic value and no benefits in physical function are observed.[1]

38

Screening tests

These are most important for the patient presenting with chronic back pain, especially in the presence of 'red flags', when serious disease such as malignancy, osteoporosis, infection or spondyloarthropathy must be excluded. The screening tests for chronic pain are:

- plain X-ray
- urine examination (office dipstick)
- FBE; ESR/CRP
- serum alkaline phosphatase
- PSA in males >50 years

Specific disease investigation

Such tests include:

- peripheral arterial studies
- HLA-B_{27} antigen test for ankylosing spondylitis and reactive arthritis
- serum electrophoresis for multiple myeloma (paraprotein)
- PSA for possible prostate cancer
- *Brucella* agglutination test
- blood culture for pyogenic infection and bacterial endocarditis
- bone scanning to demonstrate inflammatory or neoplastic disease and infections (e.g. osteomyelitis) before changes are apparent on plain X-ray
- tuberculosis studies
- X-rays of shoulder and hip joint
- electromyographic (EMG) studies to screen leg pain and differentiate neurological diseases from nerve compression syndromes
- radioisotope scanning
- technetium pyrophosphate scan of SIJ for ankylosing spondylitis
- selective anaesthetic block of facet joint under image intensification
- selective anaesthetic block of medial branches of posterior primary rami and other nerve roots

Procedural and preprocedural diagnostic tests

These tests should be kept in reserve for red flag pointers to chronic disorders, especially mechanical disorders, that remain undiagnosed and unabated, and where surgical intervention is planned for a disc prolapse requiring removal.

Depending on availability and merit, such tests include:

- CT scan
- myelography or radiculography
- discography
- MRI

Summary of diagnostic guidelines for spinal pain

- Continuous pain (day and night) = neoplasia, especially malignancy or infection.
- The big primary malignancy is multiple myeloma.
- The big three metastases are from lung, breast and prostate.
- The other three metastases are from thyroid, kidney/adrenal and melanoma.
- Pain with standing/walking (relief with sitting) = spondylolisthesis.
- Pain (and stiffness) at rest, relief with activity = inflammation.
- In a young person with inflammation think of ankylosing spondylitis.

- Stiffness at rest, pain with or after activity, relief with rest = osteoarthritis.
- Pain provoked by activity, relief with rest = mechanical dysfunction.
- Pain in bed at early morning = inflammation, depression or malignancy/infection.
- Pain in periphery of limb = discogenic → radicular or vascular → claudication or spinal canal stenosis → claudication.
- Pain in calf (ascending) with walking = vascular claudication.
- Pain in buttock (descending) with walking = neurogenic claudication.
- One disc lesion = one nerve root (exception is L5–S1 disc).
- One nerve root = one disc (usually).
- Two or more nerve roots—consider neoplasm.
- The rule of thumb for the lumbar nerve root lesions is L3 from L2–3 disc, L4 from L3–4, L5 from L4–5 and S1 from L5–S1.
- A large disc protrusion can cause bladder symptoms, either incontinence or retention.
- A retroperitoneal bleed from anticoagulation therapy can give intense nerve root symptoms and signs.

Back pain in children

The common mechanical disorders of the intervertebral joints can cause non-specific back pain in children, which must always be taken seriously. Like abdominal pain and leg pain, it can be related to psychogenic factors, so this possibility should be considered by diplomatically evaluating problems at home, at school or with sport. It is helpful to remember that tight hamstrings are associated with non-specific back discomfort with poor forward flexion.

Especially in children under the age of 10, it is very important to exclude organic disease. Infections such as osteomyelitis and tuberculosis are rare possibilities, and 'discitis' has to be considered. This painful condition can be idiopathic, but can also be caused by the spread of infection from a vertebral body. It has characteristic radiological changes.

Tumours causing back pain include the benign osteoid osteoma and the malignant osteogenic sarcoma. Osteoid osteoma is a very small tumour with a radiolucent nucleus that is sharply demarcated from the surrounding area of sclerotic bone. Although more common in the long bones of the leg, it can occur in the spine.

In older children and adolescents (in whom back pain is common) the organic causes of back pain are more likely to be inflammatory, congenital or from developmental anomalies and trauma.

A prolapsed intervertebral disc, which can occur in adolescents, can be very unusual in its presentation. There is often marked spasm, with a stiff spine and lateral deviation, which may be out of proportion to the relatively lower degree of pain.

Other important conditions to consider are Scheuermann disease (which largely affects thoracic spine) and early onset ankylosing spondylitis.

Spondylolisthesis can occur in older children, usually due to a slip of L5 or S1, because the articular facets are congenitally absent or because of a stress fracture in the pars interarticularis. It is necessary to request standing lateral and oblique X-rays.

Consider a lumbar stress fracture in the adolescent, which can be caused by activity involving rotation and extension of the spine such as cricket fast bowling. It has an insidious onset and requires a high index of suspicion.

Back pain in the elderly

Traumatic spinal dysfunction is still the most common cause of back pain in the elderly and may represent a recurrence of earlier dysfunction. It is amazing how commonly disc prolapse and facet joint injury can present in the aged. However, degenerative joint disease is very common and, if advanced, can present as spinal stenosis with claudication and nerve root irritation due to narrowed intervertebral foraminae.

Special problems to consider are malignant disease, degenerative spondylolisthesis, vertebral pathological fractures and occlusive vascular disease.

ACUTE BACK AND LEG PAIN DUE TO VERTEBRAL DYSFUNCTION

Mechanical disruption of the vertebral segment or segments is the foremost cause to consider, while the main serious clinical syndromes are secondary to disruption with or without prolapse of the intervertebral disc, usually L4–5 or L5–S1.

TABLE 38.5 presents the general clinical features and diagnosis in acute back pain (fractures excluded) following vertebral dysfunction: the symptoms and signs can occur singly or in combination.

Fortunately, syndromes A and B are extremely rare, but, if encountered, urgent referral to a surgeon is mandatory. Clinical features of the cauda equina syndrome are presented in FIGURE 38.7. Syndrome B can follow a bleed in patients taking anticoagulant therapy or be caused by a disc sequestration after inappropriate spinal manipulation.

Table 38.5 Clinical features and diagnosis of vertebral dysfunction leading to low back and leg pain[7]

Clinical features	Frequency	Diagnosis
Syndrome A (surgical emergency) Saddle anaesthesia (around anus, scrotum or vagina) Distal anaesthesia Evidence of UMN or LMN lesion Loss of sphincter control or urinary retention Progressive weakness of legs peripherally and areflexia (often bilateral)	Very rare	Spinal cord (UMN) or cauda equina (LMN) compression (FIGURE 38.7)
Syndrome B (probable surgical emergency) Anaesthesia or paraesthesia of the leg Foot drop Motor weakness Absence of reflexes	Uncommon	Large disc protrusion, paralysing nerve root
Syndrome C Distal pain with or without paraesthesia Radicular pain (sciatica) Positive dural stretch tests	Common	Posterolateral disc protrusion on nerve root or disc disruption
Syndrome D Non-specific lumbar pain (unilateral, central or bilateral) ± buttock and posterior thigh pain	Very common	Disc disruption or facet dysfunction or unknown (non-specific) causation

Vertebral dysfunction with non-radicular pain (non-specific back pain)

This outstanding common cause of low back pain is considered to be due mainly to dysfunction of the pain-sensitive facet joint. The precise pathophysiology is difficult to pinpoint.

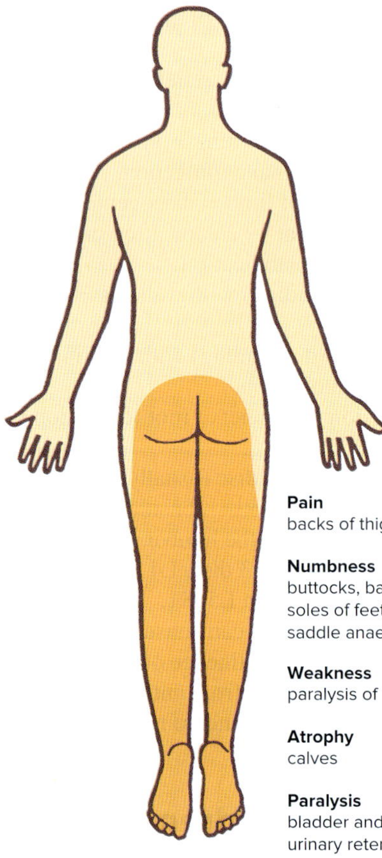

FIGURE 38.7 Cauda equina syndrome due to massive prolapsed intervertebral disc

Typical profile[8]

Age	Any age—late teens to old age, usually 22–55 years
History of injury	Yes, lifting or twisting
Site and radiation	Unilateral lumbar (may be central) Refers over sacrum, SIJ areas, buttocks
Type of pain	Deep aching pain, episodic
Aggravation	Activity, lifting, gardening, housework (vacuuming, making beds, etc.)
Relief	Rest, warmth
Associations	May be stiffness, usually good health
Physical examination (significant)	Localised tenderness—unilateral or central L4, L5 or S1 levels, may be restricted flexion, extension, lateral flexion
Diagnosis confirmation	Investigation, which is usually inappropriate, invariably normal

Note: diagnosis made clinically

38

Management[1,6,8]

- Activity directed by degree of pain but normal activity encouraged from outset
- Reassure that it is rarely serious and usually settles in time
- Back education program
- Analgesics—paracetamol (as for thoracic back pain)
- Consider short-term oral NSAIDs (particularly if inflammatory pattern)
- Exercise program and swimming (as tolerated)—conflicting evidence re efficacy
- Physical therapy—mobilisation, manipulation (for persistent problems, but conflicting evidence) (see later in this chapter)

Current evidence for acute low back pain can be summarised as follows:[3,6,7]

- beneficial—advice to stay active and reassurance, NSAIDs
- likely to be beneficial—analgesics, spinal mobilisation/manipulation and stretching (reduces period of morbidity)
- unknown—back exercises, trigger point injections, acupuncture

For chronic low back pain (pain >12 weeks):

- beneficial—back exercises, multidisciplinary treatment program
- likely benefit—analgesics, NSAIDs, trigger point injections, spinal mobilisation/manipulation

Radiculopathy

Radicular pain, caused by nerve root compression from a disc protrusion (most common cause) or tumour or a narrowed intervertebral foramina, typically produces pain in the leg related to the dermatome and myotome innervated by that nerve root. Leg pain may occur alone without back pain and vary considerably in intensity.

The two nerve roots that account for most of these problems are L5 and S1 and the commonest disc lesion is L4–5, closely followed by L5–S1. A disc can be confined, extruded or sequestrated. Most settle with time (6–12 weeks). The management is outlined at the end of this chapter and under 'Sciatica' (see CHAPTER 66).

Spondylolisthesis

About 5% of the population have spondylolisthesis but not all are symptomatic. The pain is caused by extreme stretching of the interspinous ligaments or of the nerve roots. The onset of back pain in many of these patients is due to concurrent disc degeneration rather than a mechanical problem. The pain is typically aggravated by prolonged standing, walking and exercise. The physical examination is quite diagnostic.

- Physical examination (significant): stiff waddling gait, increased lumbar lordosis, flexed knee stance, tender prominent spinous process of 'slipped' vertebrae, limited flexion, hamstring tightness or spasm
- Diagnosis confirmation: lateral X-ray (standing) (see FIG. 38.8)

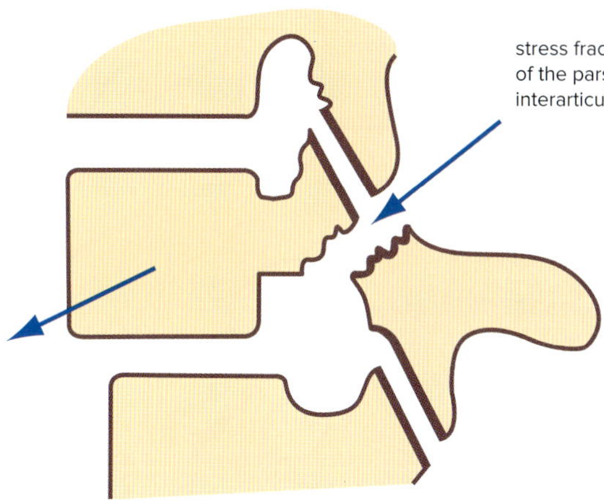

FIGURE 38.8 Spondylolisthesis: illustrating a forward shift of one vertebra on another

Management

This instability problem can be alleviated with relief of symptoms by getting patients to follow a strict flexion exercise program for at least 3 months. The objective is for patients to 'splint' their own spine by strengthening the abdominal and spinal muscles.

Extension of the spine should be avoided, especially hyperextension. Gravity traction might help. Recourse to lumbar corsets or surgery (for spinal fusion) should be resisted, although it is appropriate in a few severe intractable cases.

Lumbar spondylosis

Lumbar spondylosis, also known as degenerative osteoarthritis or osteoarthrosis, is a common problem of wear and tear that may follow vertebral dysfunction, especially after severe disc disruption and degeneration.

38

Stiffness of the low back is the main feature of lumbar spondylosis. Although most people live with and cope with the problem, progressive deterioration can occur, leading to subluxation of the facet joints. Subsequent narrowing of the spinal and intervertebral foramen leads to spinal canal stenosis (see FIG. 38.9).

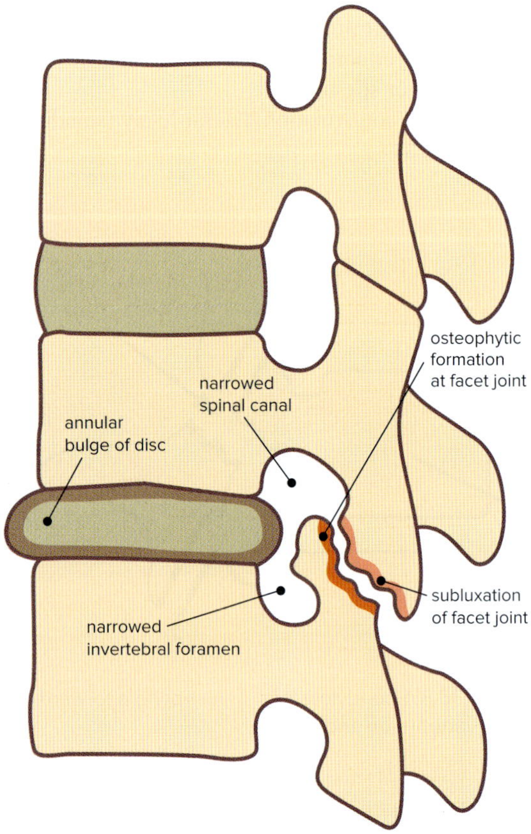

FIGURE 38.9 Lumbar spondylosis with degeneration of the disc and facet joint, leading to narrowing of the spinal canal and intervertebral foramen (spinal canal stenosis)

Management

- Basic analgesics (depending on patient response and tolerance)
- NSAIDs (judicious use)
- Appropriate balance between light activity and rest
- Exercise program and hydrotherapy (if available)—physiotherapy supervision
- Regular mobilisation therapy may help
- Consider trials of electrotherapy, such as TENS and acupuncture
- Consider decompressive surgery for spinal canal stenosis (see CHAPTER 66)

THE SPONDYLOARTHRITIDES

The seronegative spondyloarthropathies are a group of disorders characterised by involvement of the sacroiliac joints with an ascending spondylitis and extraspinal manifestations, such as oligoarthritis and enthesopathies (see FIG. 38.10; refer to CHAPTER 35). The pain and stiffness that are the characteristic findings of spinal involvement are typical of inflammatory disease: namely, worse in the morning, may occur at night and improves rather than worsens with exercise.

The main disorders in this group are ankylosing spondylitis, psoriatic arthritis, reactive spondyloarthropathies and the inflammatory bowel diseases. Hence the importance of searching for a history of psoriasis, diarrhoea, urethral discharge, eye disorders and episodes of arthritis in other joints.

Treatment

The earlier the treatment the better the outlook for the patient; the prognosis is usually good (see earlier in chapter). Refer to consultant for shared care. The basic objectives of treatment are:

- prevention of spinal fusion in a poor position
- relief of pain and stiffness
- maintenance of optimum spinal mobility

Malignant disease

It is important to identify malignant disease and other space-occupying lesions as early as possible because of the prognosis and the effect of a delayed diagnosis on treatment.

With respect to the neurological features, more than one nerve root may be involved and major neurological signs may be present without severe root pain. The neurological signs will be progressive.

If malignant disease is proved and myeloma is excluded, a search should be made for the six main primary malignancies that metastasise to the spine

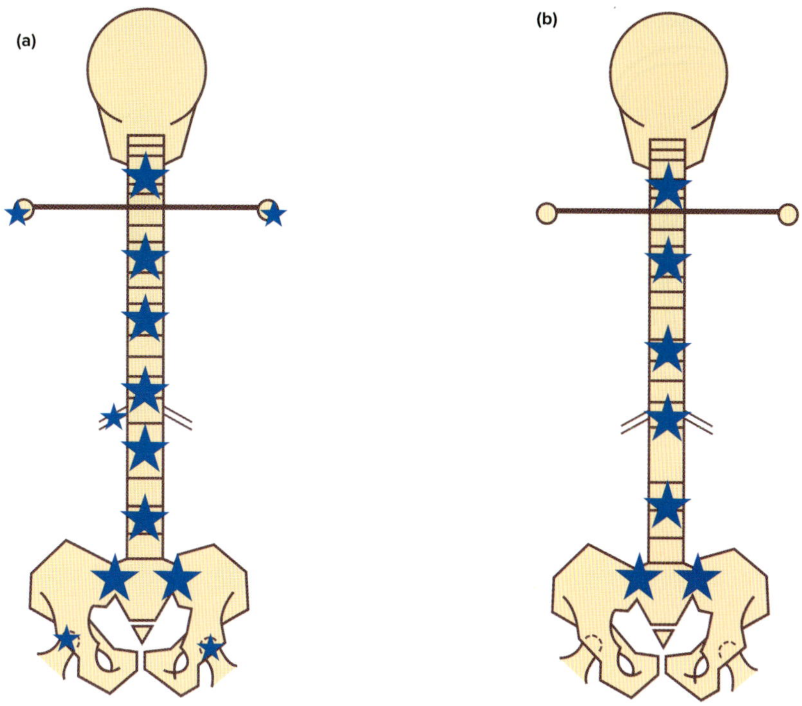

FIGURE 38.10 **(a)** Ankylosing spondylitis and psoriasis: main target areas on vertebral column and girdle joints **(b)** Crohn disease and ulcerative colitis: main target areas of enteropathies. Reactive arthritis targets the lumbar spine and sacroiliac joints only

(see FIG. 38.11). If the bone is sclerotic consider prostatic secondaries, some breast secondaries or Paget disease.

Non-organic back pain

Like headache, back pain is a symptom of an underlying functional, organic or psychological disorder. Pre-occupation with organic causation of symptoms may lead to serious errors in the assessment of patients with back pain. Any vulnerable aching area of the body is subject to aggravation by emotional factors.

Depressed patients are generally less demonstrative than patients with extreme anxiety and conversion disorders and malingerers, and it is easier to overlook the non-organic basis for their problem.

A trial of antidepressants for a minimum of 3 weeks is recommended and quite often a positive response with relief of backache eventuates.

Failure to consider psychological factors in the assessment of low back pain may lead to serious errors in diagnosis and management. Each instance of back pain poses a stimulating exercise in differential diagnosis. A comparison of organic and non-organic features is presented in TABLE 38.6.

Assessment of the pain demands a full understanding of the patient. One must be aware of his or her type of work, recreation, successes and failures; and one must relate this information to the degree of incapacity attributed to the back pain.

Patients with psychogenic back pain, especially the very anxious, tend to overemphasise their problem. They are usually demonstrative, the hands being used to point out various painful areas almost without prompting. There is diffuse tenderness even to the slightest touch and the physical disability is out of proportion to the alleged symptoms. The pain distribution is often atypical of any dermatome and the reflexes are almost always hyperactive. It must be remembered that patients with psychogenic back pain—for example, depression and conversion disorders—do certainly experience back pain and do not fall for the traps set for the malingerer.

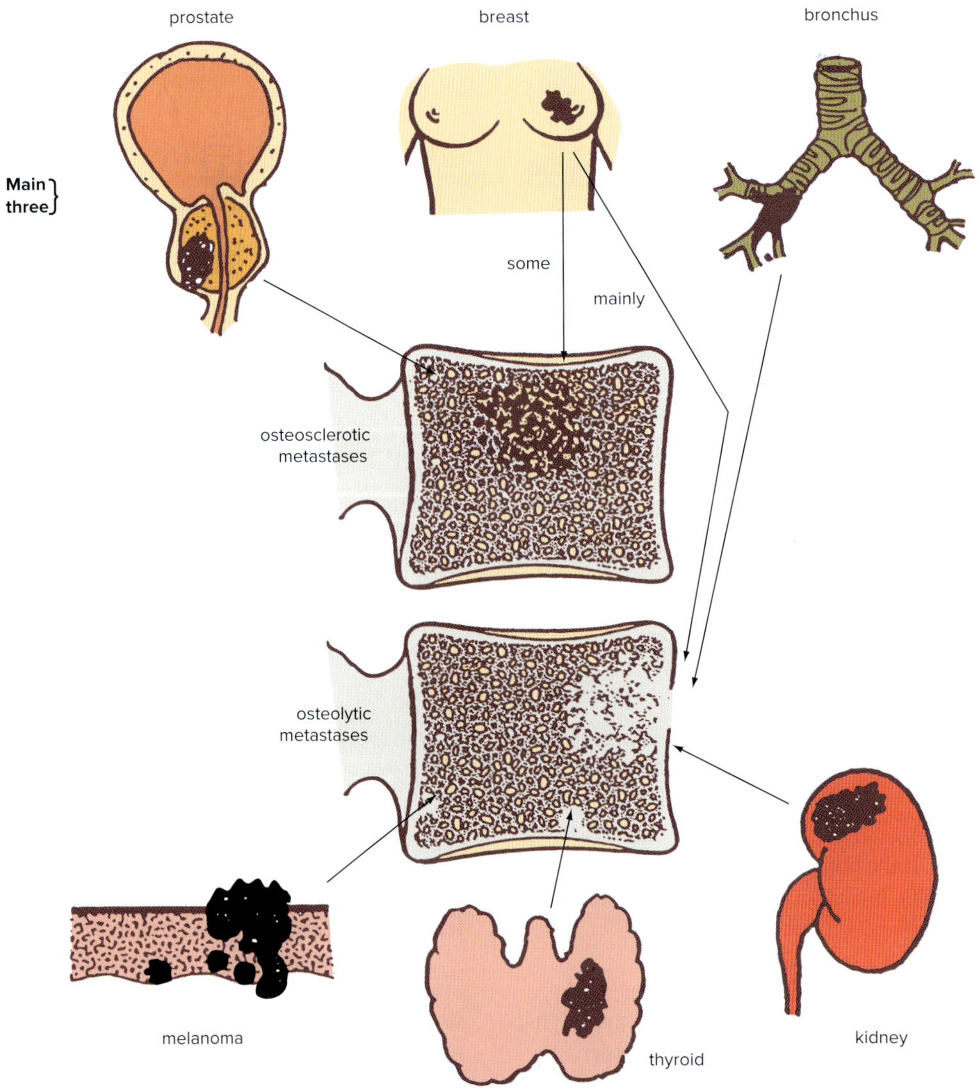

FIGURE 38.11 Important primary malignancies metastasising to the spine. Note the difference between sclerotic and osteoporotic metastases; multiple myeloma also causes osteoporotic lesions

Treatment options for back pain

General aspects of management[1,6]

The aim of treatment is to reduce pain, maintain function and minimise disability and work absenteeism and importantly the risk of chronicity.

Advice to stay active. Evidence from randomised controlled trials confirms that, in people with acute low back pain, advice to stay active speeds symptomatic recovery, reduces chronic disability and results in less time off work compared with bed rest or usual care.[6] Encourage the patient to stay at work or return early if possible. Keep moving despite discomfort.[7]

The caring knowledgeable therapist. Evidence supports the positive value of education and reassurance from a confident, supportive and knowledgeable therapist.

Relative rest. For acutely painful debilitating back problems, 2 days of strict rest lying on a firm surface is optimal treatment.[9] Resting for longer than 3 days does not produce any significant healing, and patients should be encouraged to return to activities of daily living as soon as possible.

Patient education. Appropriate educational material leads to a clear insight into the causes and aggravation of the back disorder plus coping strategies. This can

Table 38.6 Comparison of general clinical features of organic and non-organic based low back pain[8]

Symptoms	Organic disorders	Non-organic disorders
Presentation	Appropriate	Often dramatic
Pain	Localised	Bilateral/diffuse Sacrococcygeal
Pain radiation	Appropriate Buttock, specific sites	Inappropriate Front of leg/whole leg
Time pattern	Pain-free times	Constant, acute or chronic
Paraesthesia/anaesthesia	Dermatomal Points with finger	May be whole leg Shows with hands
Response to treatment	Variable Delayed benefit	Patient often refuses treatment Initial improvement (often dramatic) then deterioration (usually within 24 hours)
Signs		
Observation	Appropriate Guarded	Overreactive under scrutiny Inconsistent
Tenderness	Localised to appropriate level	Often inappropriate level Withdraws from probing finger
Spatial tenderness (Magnuson)	Consistent	Inconsistent
Active movements	Specific movements affected	Often all movements affected
Axial loading test	No back pain (usually)	Back pain
SLR 'distraction' test	Consistent	Inconsistent
Sensation	Dermatomal	Non-anatomical 'sock' or 'stocking'
Motor	Appropriate myotome	Muscle groups (e.g. leg 'collapses')
Reflexes	Appropriate May be depressed	Brisk hyperactive

be a component of cognitive behaviour therapy (if considered appropriate)

Heat. Thermography (hot or cold) is beneficial. Heat in the form of heat bags, hot flannels and similar methods can be of benefit, especially in the first 2–4 weeks of acute low back pain. Evidence shows that heat is more effective than placebo for pain relief.[6]

Exercises. An early graduated exercise program as soon as the acute phase settles has been shown to promote healing and prevent relapses.[10] All forms of exercise (extension, flexion and isometric) appear to be equally effective (see FIG. 38.12). Supervised swimming is an excellent activity for back disorders. Physiotherapist supervision is optimal.

Studies support the use of exercises for chronic back pain rather than acute pain.[3]

Pharmacological agents

Basic analgesics[11]

Paracetamol is recommended as the first-line analgesic but evidence is not clear cut. Evidence indicates that short-term NSAIDs (used cautiously) may benefit individual patients where paracetamol is ineffective.

NSAIDs[11]

These are second-line and particularly useful where there is clinical evidence of inflammation, especially with the spondyloarthropathies, severe spondylosis and in acute radicular pain, to counter irritation on the nerve root. NSAIDs have been shown to be more effective than placebo in acute back pain for pain relief and overall improvement. There is no evidence to distinguish different NSAIDs.[3]

Opioids[6,11]

The role of opioids is limited because any pain-control benefits are outweighed by the potential risks. They are not recommended but may be considered when paracetamol and NSAIDs are not recommended or are unable to provide pain control.

Injection techniques

Trigger point injection

This may be effective for relatively isolated points using 5–8 mL of local anaesthetic. Studies indicate that it is likely to be more beneficial for chronic back pain.[3]

38

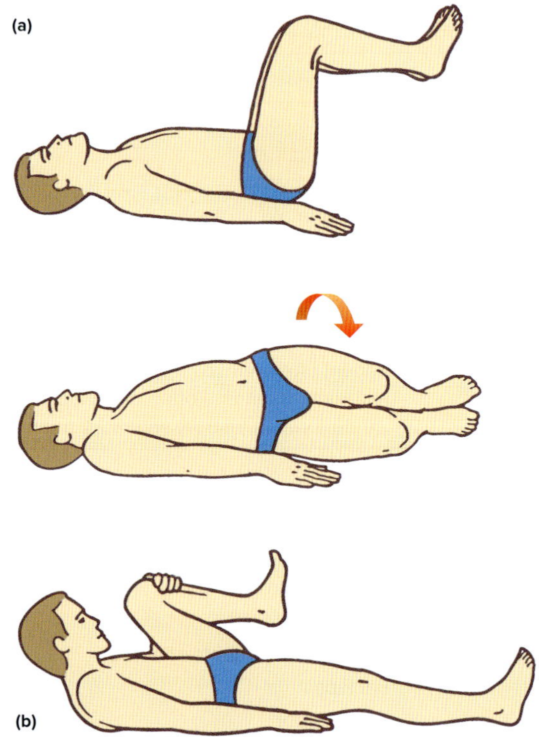

FIGURE 38.12 Examples of exercises for low back pain: **(a)** rotation exercise; **(b)** flexion exercise

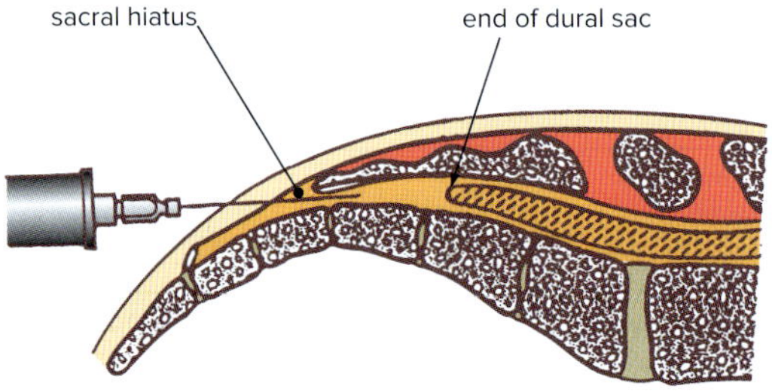

FIGURE 38.13 Caudal epidural injection: the needle should lie free in the space and be well clear of the dural sac

Physical therapy

Active exercises are the best form of physical therapy (see FIG.38.12a, b).

Passive spinal stretching at the end range is a safe, effective method (see FIG. 38.14). Spinal mobilisation is a gentle, repetitive, rhythmic movement within the range of movement of the joint. It is safe and quite effective and a variation of stretching.

Spinal manipulation is a high-velocity thrust at the end range of the joint. It is generally more effective and produces a faster response, but requires accurate diagnosis and greater skill. It is more effective for uncomplicated dysfunctional low back

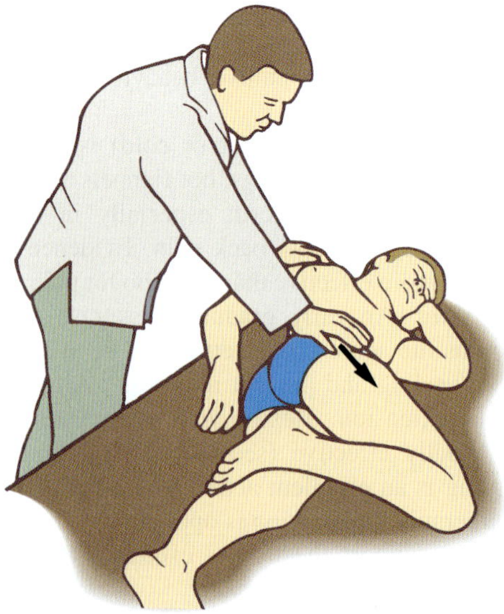

FIGURE 38.14 Lumbosacral spinal stretching technique (for right-sided pain): a traditional technique. Illustration shows direction of line of force

Source: Reproduced with permission from C Kenna and J Murtagh. *Back Pain and Spinal Manipulation.* Sydney: Butterworths, 1989[7]

Chymopapain

This enzyme has been advocated for the treatment of acute nuclear herniation that is still intact. The indications are similar for surgical discectomy. However, studies show that although it is more effective than placebo, it is less effective than surgical discectomy.[12]

Facet joint injection

Corticosteroid injection under radio-image intensification is widely used in some clinics. The procedure is delicate and expertise is required. Best evidence to date does not support the use of these injections.

Epidural injections

Injections of local anaesthetic with or without corticosteroids are used for chronic pain, especially for nerve root pain. The author favours the caudal (trans-sacral) epidural injection for persistent sciatica using 15 mL of half-strength local anaesthetic only (e.g. 0.25% bupivacaine) (see FIG. 38.13).

Others favour the use of steroids and the lumbar epidural approach. The evidence regarding effectiveness is conflicting.[5]

pain (without radicular pain), especially acute pain (see FIG. 38.15).[3,6,13,14] However, the evidence from controlled trials is conflicting. Adverse effects are uncommon, but can be serious.

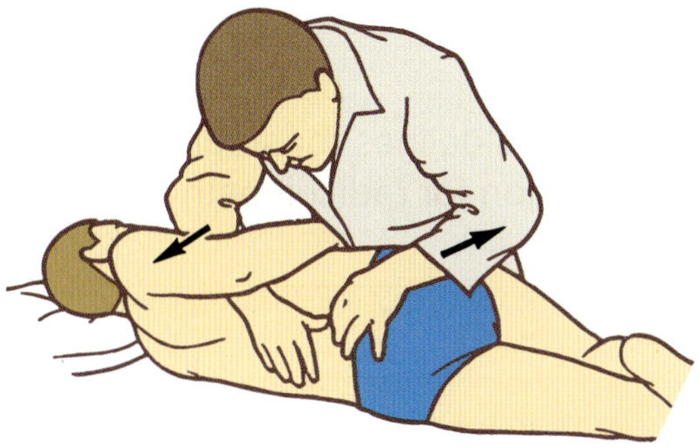

FIGURE 38.15 Lumbar spinal stretching manipulation: illustration of the specific technique for the L4–5 level with arrows indicating the direction of applied force

Source: Reproduced with permission from C Kenna and J Murtagh. *Back Pain and Spinal Manipulation.* Sydney: Butterworths, 1989[7]

Other treatments

The following treatments have advocates for the management of back pain, although clear-cut evidence for the efficacy of these modalities is still lacking:

- hydrotherapy
- traction
- TENS
- therapeutic ultrasound
- facet joint injection
- posterior nerve root (medial branch) blocks with or without denervation (by cryotherapy or radiofrequency)
- percutaneous vertebroplasty (injection of bone cement into fractured vertebra of osteoporosis)
- deep friction massage (in conjunction with mobilisation and manipulation)
- acupuncture (evidence for short-term benefit)
- biofeedback
- gravitational methods (home therapy)
- lumbar supports

MANAGEMENT GUIDELINES FOR LUMBOSACRAL DISORDERS (SUMMARY)

The management of 'mechanical' back pain depends on the cause. Since most of the problems are mechanical and there is a tendency to natural resolution, conservative management is quite appropriate. The rule is: 'if patients with uncomplicated back pain receive no treatment, one-third will get better within 1 week and by 3 weeks almost all the rest of the other two-thirds are better'.[14,15] Practitioners should have a clear-cut management plan with a firm, precise, reassuring and conservative clinical approach.

The problems can be categorised into general conditions for which the summarised treatment protocols are outlined.

- Acute pain = pain less than 6 weeks
- Subacute pain = pain 6–12 weeks
- Chronic pain = pain greater than 12 weeks

Acute low back pain[6]

The common problem of low back pain caused by facet joint dysfunction and/or limited disc disruption usually responds well to the following treatment (see box). The typical patient is aged 20–55 years, is well and has no radiation of pain below the knee.[15,16]

Most of these patients can expect to be relatively pain-free in 14 days and can return to work early (some may not miss work and this should be encouraged). The evidence concerning spinal manipulation is that it reduces the period of disability.

Management of non-specific acute low back pain (summary)[17]

- Explanation and reassurance? cognitive behaviour therapy
- Back education program
- Encouragement of normal daily activities, including work, according to degree of comfort
- Regular non-opioid analgesics (paracetamol or NSAIDs)
- Prescribe exercises (provided non-aggravating)
- Physical therapy: stretching of affected segment, muscle energy therapy, spinal mobilisation or manipulation (if no contraindication)[6,11,13,15]
- Review in about 5 days (probably best time for consideration of physical therapy)
- No investigation needed initially

Sciatica with or without low back pain

Sciatica is a more complex and protracted problem to treat, but most cases will gradually settle within 12 weeks (refer to CHAPTER 66). Conservative management is usually recommended in the first 6–8 weeks.

38

Acute[6]

- Explanation and reassurance
- Back education program
- Resume normal activities as soon as possible
- Regular non-opioid analgesics with review as the patient mobilises
- NSAIDs for 10–14 days, then cease and review
- If severe pain unrelieved, add an opioid that works well for the patient, such as tapentadol SR 50 mg (o) bd as necessary, for short-term use[17]
- Walking and swimming
- Weekly or 2-weekly follow-up
- Consider: a course of corticosteroids for very severe pain,[6] e.g. prednisolone 50 mg for 5 days, then 25 mg for 5 days, gradually tapering to 3 weeks in total.
  or
  30 mg daily mane for 3 weeks, tapering to 0 over next 2 weeks (efficacy not clearly established)

Chronic

- Reassurance that problem will subside (assuming no severe neurological defects)
- Consider epidural anaesthesia (if slow response)
- Consider amitriptyline 10–25 mg (o) nocte increasing to maximum 75–100 mg or duloxetine

Note: An important controlled prospective study comparing surgical and conservative treatment in patients with sciatica over 10 years showed that there was significant relief of sciatica in the surgical group for 1–2 years but not beyond that time. At 10 years, both groups had the same outcome, including neurological deficits.[18]

38

Sacroiliac dysfunction

See CHAPTER 66.

Chronic back pain

The basic management of the patient with uncomplicated chronic back pain should follow the following guidelines:

- back education program and ongoing support
- encouragement of normal activity
- exercise program
- mindfulness-based stress reduction (evidence based)
- analgesics (e.g. paracetamol 665 mg (o) 8-hourly)
- NSAIDs for 14–21 days (especially if inflammation, i.e. pain at rest—relieved by activity and poor response to non-pharmacological treatment) and review
- duloxetine or amitriptyline (second-line therapy)[1,7]
- trial of mobilisation or manipulation (at least three treatments)—if no contraindications[12,13] (low-quality evidence)
- consider trigger point injection
- a multidisciplinary rehabilitation team approach is recommended/back schools

General guidelines for surgical intervention for radiculopathy

Absolute

- Bladder/bowel control disturbance; perineal sensory change
- Progressive motor disturbance (e.g. significant foot drop, weakness in quadriceps)

Relative

- Severe prolonged pain or disabling pain
- Failure of conservative treatment with persistent pain (problem of permanent nerve damage)
- If all four of the following criteria are met:[6]
  — leg pain equal to or worse than back pain
  — positive straight leg raise test
  — no response to conservative therapy after 4–6 weeks
  — imaging shows a lesion corresponding to symptoms

Prevention of further back pain

Patients should be informed that an ongoing back care program should give them an excellent outlook. Prevention includes:

- education about back care, including a good layperson's reference
- golden rules to live by: how to lift, sit, bend, play sport and so on
- an exercise program: a tailor-made program for the patient
- posture and movement training, such as the Alexander technique[19] or the Feldenkrais technique[20]

When to refer

Urgent referral

- Myelopathy, especially acute cauda equina compression syndrome
- Severe radiculopathy with progressive neurologic deficit
- Spinal fractures

Other referrals

- Recalcitrant spinal canal stenosis
- Neoplasia or infection
- Undiagnosed back pain
- Paget disease
- Continuing pain of 3 months' duration without a clearly definable cause

Practice tips

- Back pain that is related to posture, aggravated by movement and sitting, and relieved by lying down is due to vertebral dysfunction, especially a disc disruption.
- The pain from most disc lesions is generally relieved by rest.
- Plain X-rays are of limited use, especially in younger patients, and may appear normal in disc prolapse.
- Remember the possibility of depression as a cause of back pain; if suspected, consider a trial of antidepressants.
- If back pain persists, possibly worse during bed rest at night, consider malignant disease, depressive illness or other systemic diseases.
- Pain that is worse on standing and walking, but relieved by sitting, is probably caused by spondylolisthesis.
- If pain and stiffness is present on waking and lasts longer than 30 minutes upon activity, consider inflammation.
- Avoid using strong analgesics (especially opioids) in any chronic non-malignant pain state.
- Bilateral back pain is more typical of systemic diseases, while unilateral pain typifies mechanical causes.
- Back pain at rest and morning stiffness in a young person demand careful investigation: consider inflammation such as ankylosing spondylitis and reactive arthritis.
- A disc lesion of L5–S1 can involve both L5 and S1 roots. However, combined L5 and S1 root lesions should still be regarded with suspicion (e.g. consider malignancy).
- A large central disc protrusion can cause bladder symptoms, either incontinence or retention.
- Low back pain of very sudden onset with localised spasm and protective lateral deviation may indicate a facet joint syndrome.
- The T12–L1 and L1–2 discs are the groin pain discs.
- The L4–5 disc is the back pain disc.
- The L5–S1 disc is the leg pain disc.
- Severe limitation of SLR (especially to less than 30°) indicates lumbar disc prolapse.
- A preventive program for dysfunctional back pain based on back care awareness and exercises is mandatory advice.
- Remember that most back problems resolve within a few weeks, so avoid overtreatment.

Patient education resources

Hand-out sheets from *Murtagh's Patient Education* 7th edition:

- Backache
- Exercises for your lower back
- Sciatica
- Spondylosis

References

1 Australian Acute Musculoskeletal Pain Guidelines Group. *Evidence-Based Management of Acute Musculoskeletal Pain: A Guide for Clinicians.* Bowen Hills: Australian Academic Press, 2004. <https://www.nhmrc.gov.au/_files_nhmrc/file/publications/synopses/cp95.pdf> (accessed 23/5/2018).

2 Sloane P, Slatt M, Baker R. *Essentials of Family Medicine.* Baltimore: Williams & Wilkins, 1988: 228–35.

3 Barton S (ed.). *Clinical Evidence.* London: BMJ Publishing Group, 2001: 772–87.

4 Maigne R. Manipulation of the spine. In: Basmajian JV (ed.). *Manipulation, Traction and Massage.* Paris: RML, 1986: 71–96.

5 Bogduk N. The sources of low back pain. In: Jaysom M (ed.). *The Lumbar Spine and Back Pain* (4th edn). Edinburgh: Churchill Livingstone, 1992: 61–88.

6 Expert group for Rheumatology. Low back pain. In: eTG complete [Internet]. Melbourne: Therapeutic Guidelines Ltd. Available from: <www.tg.org.au>, accessed Sept 2017.

7 Kenna C, Murtagh J. *Back Pain and Spinal Manipulation* (2nd edn). Oxford: Butterworth Heinemann, 1997: 70–164.

8 Kamper SJ, Maher CG, Buchbinder R. Non-specific low back pain: manage initially with reassurance, activity and analgesia. Modern Medicine, June 2013: 19–35.

9 Deyo RA, Diehl AK, Rosenthal M. How many days of bed rest for acute low back pain? A randomised clinical trial. N Engl J Med, 1986; 315: 1064–70.

10 Kendall PH, Jenkins SM. Exercises for backache: a double blind controlled study. Physiotherapy, 1968; 54: 154–7.

11 Chou R, Deyo R, Friedly J et al. Non-invasive treatments for low back pain. Agency for Healthcare Research and Quality 2016. <www.effectivehealthcare.ahrq.gov> (accessed 23/5/2018).

12 Gibson JNA et al. Surgery for lumbar disc prolapse. Cochrane Database Syst Rev. 2002, Issue 2. Art No. CD001350.

13 Blomberg S, Svardsudd K, Mildenberger F. A controlled, multicentre trial of manual therapy in low back pain. Scand J Prim Health Care, 1992; 10: 170–8.

14 Royal College of General Practitioners et al. *Clinical Guidelines for the Management of Acute Low Back Pain.* London: RCGP, 1996.

15 Kuritzky L. Low back pain. Family Practice, Audio-Digest California Medical Association: 1996; 44: 14.

16 Deyo RA. Acute low back pain: a new paradigm for management. Br Med J, 1996; 313: 1343–4.

17 Qaseem A, Wilt TJ et al. Noninvasive treatments for acute, subacute, and chronic low back pain: a clinical practice guideline from the American College of Physicians. Ann Intern Med, 2017; 166 (7): 514–30.

18 Weber et al. A controlled prospective study with 10 years observation of patients with sciatica. Spine, 1983; 8: 131–40.

19 Hodgkinson L. *The Alexander Technique.* London: Piatkus, 1988: 1–97.

20 Feldenkrais M. *Awareness Through Movement.* New York: Harper & Row, 1972.

Bruising and bleeding 39

My pa is one mask of brooses both blue and green.

Charles Dickens (1812–70), *Nicholas Nickleby*

Many patients present with the complaint that they bruise easily but only a minority turn out to have an underlying blood disorder. Purpura is bleeding into the skin or mucous membranes, appearing as multiple small haemorrhages that do not blanch on pressure. Smaller purpuric lesions that are 2 mm or less in diameter (pinhead size) are termed petechiae, while larger purpuric lesions are called ecchymoses (see FIG. 39.1).

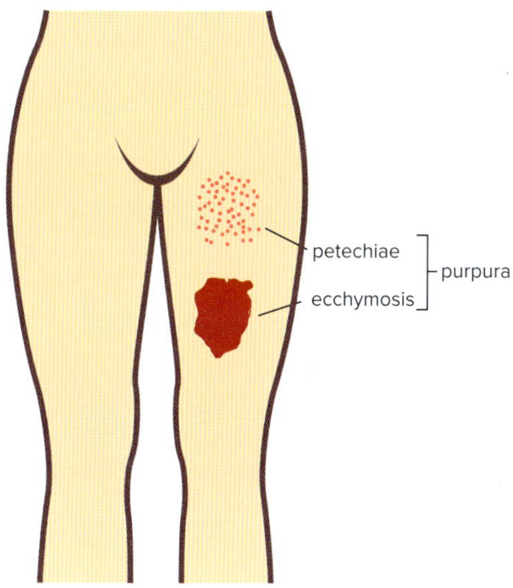

FIGURE 39.1 Purpuric rash (petechiae and ecchymoses)

Bruises are large areas of bleeding that are a result of subcutaneous bleeding. If bruising is abnormal and out of proportion to the offending trauma, then a disturbance of coagulation is suggested (see FIG. 39.2). The three spontaneous pathways that arrest bleeding following injury are vasoconstriction, platelet plugging of gaps and the coagulation cascade (intrinsic and extrinsic pathways).

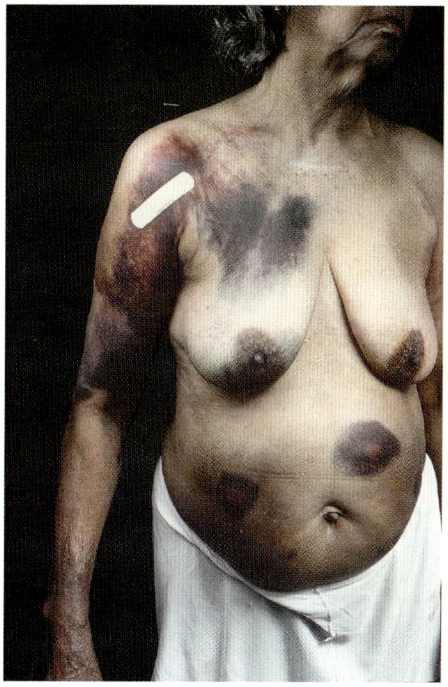

FIGURE 39.2 Severe bleeding in a diabetic patient with systemic fibrinolysis. Note the bleeding following insulin injections into the abdominal wall and an injection into the shoulder joint.

Source: Photo courtesy Hatem Salem

The decision to investigate is difficult because decisions have to be made about which patients warrant investigation and whether the haemostatic defect is due to local or systemic pathology.[1] The ability to identify a bleeding disorder is important because of implications for surgery, pregnancy, medication and genetic counselling.

Differential diagnosis

'Palpable purpura' due to an underlying systemic vasculitis is an important differential problem. The petechiae are raised so finger palpation is important. The cause is an underlying vasculitis affecting small vessels (e.g. polyarteritis nodosa).

Key facts and checkpoints

- Purpura = petechiae + ecchymoses.
- Abnormal bleeding is basically the result of disorders of (1) the platelet, (2) the coagulation mechanism or (3) the blood vessel.

continued

continued

- There is no substitute for a good history in the assessment of patients with bleeding disorders.
- An assessment of personal and family histories is the first step in the identification of a bleeding disorder.
- When a patient complains of 'bruising easily' it is important to exclude thrombocytopenia due to bone marrow disease and clotting factor deficiencies such as haemophilia.
- The commonest cause of an acquired bleeding disorder is drug therapy (e.g. aspirin, NSAIDs, cytotoxics and oral anticoagulants).
- In general, bleeding secondary to platelet defects is spontaneous, associated with a petechial rash and occurs immediately after trauma or a cut wound.[1] The bleeding is usually mucosal (e.g. bleeding from gingiva, menorrhagia, epistaxis and petechiae).
- Laboratory assessment should be guided by the clinical impression.
- Bleeding caused by coagulation factor deficiency is usually traumatic and delayed (e.g. haemorrhage occurring 24 hours after a dental extraction in a haemophiliac).
- The routine screening tests for the investigation of patients with bleeding disorders can occasionally be normal despite the presence of an undeniable bleeding disorder and even a severe haemorrhagic state. Second-line investigations will need to be undertaken.

Causes of clinical disorders

The three major mechanisms of systemic bleeding disorders are (the Virchow triad):

1 coagulation deficiencies (reduction or inhibition of circulatory coagulation factors)
2 platelet abnormalities: of platelet number or function
3 vascular defects: of vascular endothelium

39

Bleeding disorders can also be divided into impaired primary or secondary haemostasis. Primary haemostatic disorders which are the most common include von Willebrand disease (vWD), thrombocytopenia and platelet function disorders. Examples of disorders of secondary haemostasis are disorders of fibrin formation and the haemophilias.[2]

A list of differential diagnoses of systemic bleeding disorders is presented in TABLE 39.1.[1]

Table 39.1 Differential diagnoses of systemic bleeding disorders

Vascular disorders

(a) Inherited:
- hereditary haemorrhagic telangiectasia
- Marfan syndrome; other connective tissue disorders

(b) Acquired:
- infection (e.g. meningococcus, measles, dengue)
- purpura simplex
- senile purpura
- Henoch–Schönlein purpura
- steroid purpura
- vitamin C deficiency (scurvy)

Coagulation factor deficiency or inhibitor

(a) Inherited:
- haemophilia A
- haemophilia B
- vWD

(b) Acquired:
- disseminated intravascular coagulation (DIC)
- liver disease
- vitamin K deficiency
- oral anticoagulant therapy or overdosage

Thrombocytopenia

(a) Inherited:
- Fanconi syndrome
- amegakaryocytic thrombocytopenia

(b) Acquired:
(Immune)
- immune thrombocytopenic purpura
- drug-induced thrombocytopenia (e.g. heparin)
- thrombotic thrombocytopenic purpura
- post-transfusion purpura

(Non-immune)
- disseminated intravascular coagulation
- bone marrow replacement (e.g. leukaemia) or failure
- splenic pooling

Functional platelet disorders

(a) Inherited:
- Glanzmann thrombasthenia
- Bernard–Soulier syndrome
- storage pool deficiency

(b) Acquired:
- drug-induced (e.g. aspirin, NSAIDs)
- uraemia /kidney failure
- myeloproliferative disorders
- dysproteinaemias

Source: After Mitchell et al.[1] Adapted from Bleeding disorders, *MIMS Disease Index* (2nd edn) 1996 with permission of MIMS Australia, a division of MediMedia Australia Pty Ltd

The clinical approach

Differentiation of coagulation factor deficiencies and platelet disorders as the cause of a bleeding problem can usually be determined by a careful evaluation of the history and physical examination.

History

Factors that suggest the presence of a systemic bleeding defect include:

- spontaneous haemorrhage
- severe or recurrent haemorrhagic episodes, e.g. epistaxis
- bleeding from multiple sites
- bleeding out of proportion to the degree of trauma
- cutaneous bleeding
- gastrointestinal bleeding
- postpartum haemorrhage
- bleeding from tooth extraction/oral cavity
- menorrhagia
- muscle haematomas or haemarthrosis

If a bleeding diathesis is suspected it is essential to determine whether local pathology is contributing to the blood loss (e.g. postoperative bleeding, postpartum bleeding, gastrointestinal haemorrhage).

Diagnostic tips

- Platelet abnormalities present as early bleeding following trauma.
- Coagulation factor deficiencies present with delayed bleeding after initial haemostasis is achieved by normal platelets.
- A normal response to previous coagulation stresses (e.g. dental extraction, circumcision or pregnancy) indicates an acquired problem.
- If acquired, look for evidence of MILD: Malignancy, Infection, Liver disease, Drugs.
- A diagnostic strategy is outlined in TABLE 39.2.

Family history

A positive family history can be a positive pointer to the diagnosis:

- sex-linked recessive pattern: haemophilia A or B
- autosomal dominant pattern: vWD, dysfibrinogenaemias
- autosomal recessive pattern: deficiency of coagulation factors V, VII and X

Enquire whether the patient has noticed blood in the urine or stools and whether menorrhagia is present in women. A checklist for a bleeding history is

Table 39.2	Purpura: diagnostic strategy model
Probability diagnosis	
Simple purpura (easy bruising syndrome) Senile purpura Corticosteroid-induced purpura Immune thrombocytopenic purpura Henoch–Schönlein purpura Liver disease, especially alcoholic cirrhosis Increased intravascular pressure, e.g. coughing, vomiting	
Serious disorders not to be missed	
Malignant disease: • leukaemia • myeloma Aplastic anaemia Myelofibrosis Severe infections: • septicaemia • meningococcal infection • measles • typhoid • dengue/chikungunya Disseminated intravascular coagulation Thrombotic thrombocytopenic purpura Fat embolism	
Pitfalls (often missed)	
Haemophilia A, B vWD Post-transfusion purpura Trauma (e.g. domestic violence, child abuse) *Rarities:* • hereditary telangiectasia (Osler–Weber–Rendu syndrome) • Ehlers–Danlos syndrome • scurvy • Fanconi syndrome	
Seven masquerades checklist	
Drugs: examples (see 'Medication Record') • sodium valproate • various antibiotics • quinine/quinidine • thiazide diuretics • NSAIDs/salicylates • cytotoxics • oral anticoagulants/heparin Anaemia: • aplastic anaemia	
Psychogenic factors	
Factitial purpura	

presented in TABLE 39.3. The actual size and frequency of the bruises should be recorded where possible and if none are present at the time of the consultation the patient should return if any bruises reappear.

Table 39.3 Checklist for a bleeding history

Skin bruising	Tonsillectomy
Epistaxis	Other operations
Injury	Childbirth
Domestic violence	Haematuria
Menorrhagia	Rectal bleeding
Haemarthrosis	Drugs
Tooth extraction	Family history
Unusual haematomas	Comorbidities (e.g. liver disease, kidney disease)

Key questions

- How long has the problem been apparent to you?
- Do you remember any bumps or falls that might have caused the bruising?
- What sort of injuries cause you to bruise easily?
- Have you noticed bleeding from other areas such as your nose or gums?
- Has anyone in your family had a history of bruising or bleeding?
- What is your general health like?
- Do you have any tiredness, weight loss, fever or night sweats?
- Did you notice a viral illness or sore throat beforehand?
- How much alcohol do you drink?
- What happened in the past when you had a tooth extracted?
- Have you ever had painful swelling in your joints?

39

Medication record

It is mandatory to obtain a complete drug history. Examples of drugs and their responses are:

- vascular purpura:
  - prednisolone/other steroids
- thrombocytopenia:
  - cytotoxic drugs
  - carbamazepine
  - gold
  - sodium valproate
  - heparin
  - ranitidine
  - sulphonamides
  - quinine, quinidine
  - thiazide diuretics
  - penicillins, vancomycin
  - chloramphenicol
- functional platelet abnormalities:
  - aspirin
  - NSAIDs
- coagulation factor deficiency:
  - warfarin

Examination

Careful examination of the skin is important. Note the nature of the bleeding and the distribution of any rash, which is characteristic in Henoch–Schönlein purpura. Senile purpura in the elderly is usually seen over the dorsum of the hands, extensor surface of the forearms and the shins. Purpura on the legs indicates platelet disorders, meningococcal septicaemia and paraproteinaemias; on the fingers and toes indicates vasculitis.

Note the lips and oral mucosa for evidence of hereditary telangiectasia. Gum hypertrophy occurs in monocytic leukaemia. Search for evidence of malignancy, such as sternal tenderness, lymphadenopathy and splenomegaly. Examine the ocular fundi for evidence of retinal haemorrhages. Urinalysis, searching for blood (microscopic or macroscopic), is important.

Investigations

The initial choice of investigations depends upon the bleeding pattern.

If coagulation defect suspected:

- prothrombin time (PT), i.e. INR
- activated partial thromboplastin time (APTT)
- fibrinogen level
- thrombin time (TT)

If platelet pathology suspected:

- platelet count
- skin bleeding time (of doubtful value)
- platelet function analyser (PFA-100)

If inherited disorders suspected:

- factor VIII
- vW factor activity
- vW factor antigen

The full blood examination and blood film is useful in pinpointing the aetiology. Platelet morphology gives a diagnostic guide to inherited platelet disorders. The skin-bleeding time as a screening test of haemostasis has been shown recently to be severely limited by its lack of specificity and sensitivity and its routine use cannot be recommended. It is not a useful predictor of surgical risk of haemorrhage.[1,3] Other sophisticated tests, such as von Willebrand's screen and platelet aggregation (e.g. PFA-100), can be advised by the consulting haematologist. One of considerable value is the bone marrow examination, which is useful to exclude the secondary causes of thrombocytopenia, such as leukaemia, other marrow infiltrations and aplastic anaemia.

Other tests to consider: ESR/CRP, autoimmune screening, kidney function tests, LFTs, plasma electrophoresis, skin biopsy. Be cautious of pseudo-thrombocytopenia due to laboratory error—exclude on a blood film and consider a repeat collection.

A summary of appropriate tests is presented in TABLE 39.4 and of blood changes for some coagulation factor deficiencies in TABLE 39.5.

Table 39.4 Laboratory investigation checklist for the easy bruiser

Full blood count
Platelet count
Prothrombin time (INR)
Thrombin time (TT)
Activated partial thromboplastin time

Table 39.5 Blood changes for specific coagulation factor disorders

	Haemophilia A	vWD	Vitamin K deficiency
PT	Normal	Normal	↑
APTT	↑	↑	↑
TT	Normal	Normal	Normal

Abnormal bleeding in children

Abnormal bleeding in children is not uncommon and once again the clinical history, particularly the past and family history, provides the most valuable information. It is important to keep non-accidental injury, such as child abuse, in mind in the child presenting with 'easy bruising'. However, it is appropriate to exclude a bleeding disorder, especially a platelet disorder. Vigorous coughing or vomiting in a child can cause petechiae on or around the eyelids.

Coagulation disorders, including haemophilia and vWD, are usually suspected on clinical grounds because of widespread bruising or because of prolonged bleeding following procedures such as circumcision and tonsillectomy.

A common condition is haemorrhagic disease of the newborn, which is a self-limiting disease usually presenting on the second or third day of life because of a deficiency of coagulation factors dependent on vitamin K. The routine use of prophylactic vitamin K in the newborn infant has virtually eliminated this problem.

Idiopathic (immune) thrombocytopenic purpura (ITP) is the commonest of the primary platelet disorders in children. Both acute and chronic forms have an immunological basis. The diagnosis is based on the peripheral blood film and platelet count. The platelet count is commonly below 50 000/mm^3 (50 × 10^9/L). Spontaneous remission within 4 to 6 weeks occurs with acute ITP in childhood.[3]

The commonest vascular defects in childhood are:

- anaphylactoid (Henoch–Schönlein) purpura
- infective states
- nutritional deficiency (usually inadequate dietary vitamin C)

Henoch–Schönlein purpura

HSP, which is a type of IgA vasculitis, is the commonest vasculitis of children. It affects the small vessels, producing a leucocytoclastic vasculitis with a classic triad of non-thrombocytopenic purpura, large joint arthritis and abdominal pain. It is diagnosed clinically by the characteristic distribution of the rash (which is a palpable purpura) over the lower limbs, extending onto the buttocks (see FIG. 39.3), but it can also involve the upper limbs, trunk and even the face.

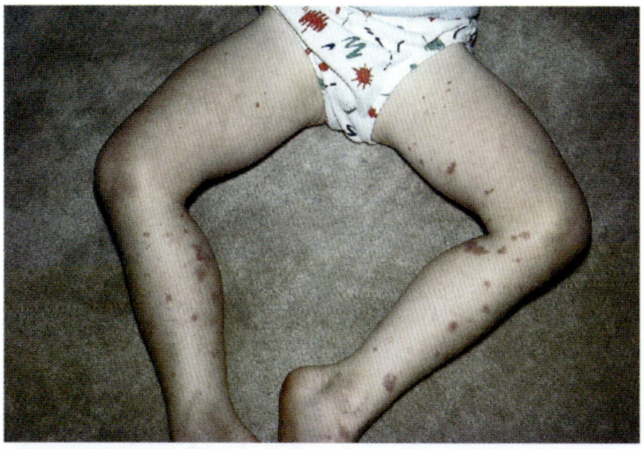

FIGURE 39.3 Henoch–Schönlein purpura in a 5-year-old boy showing the typical distribution of the rash on the lower limbs

39

The onset of HSP typically follows an upper respiratory tract infection including a group A streptococcal tonsillopharyngitis.

The bleeding time, coagulation time and platelet counts are normal. The prognosis is good; most recover fully in a few months.

Clinical features

- All ages, mainly in children
- Rash, mainly on buttocks and legs (see FIG. 39.4)[4]
- Rash can occur on hands, arms and trunk
- Arthritis: mainly ankles and knees
- Abdominal pain—colicky (vasculitis of GIT)
- Haematuria (reflects nephritis)

Associations

- Kidney involvement—deposition of IgA immune complex (a serious complication)
- Melaena
- Intussusception
- Scrotal involvement

Investigations

- FBE
- Urine: protein and blood; spun specimen, micro for casts

Management

- Largely symptomatic—analgesics
- No specific therapy
- Short course of steroids for abdominal pain (if intussusception excluded)
- If haematuria: follow-up urine microscopy and kidney function especially if no resolution

DxT arthralgia + purpuric rash ± abdominal pain → Henoch–Schönlein purpura

Practice tip

Beware of CKF in HSP.

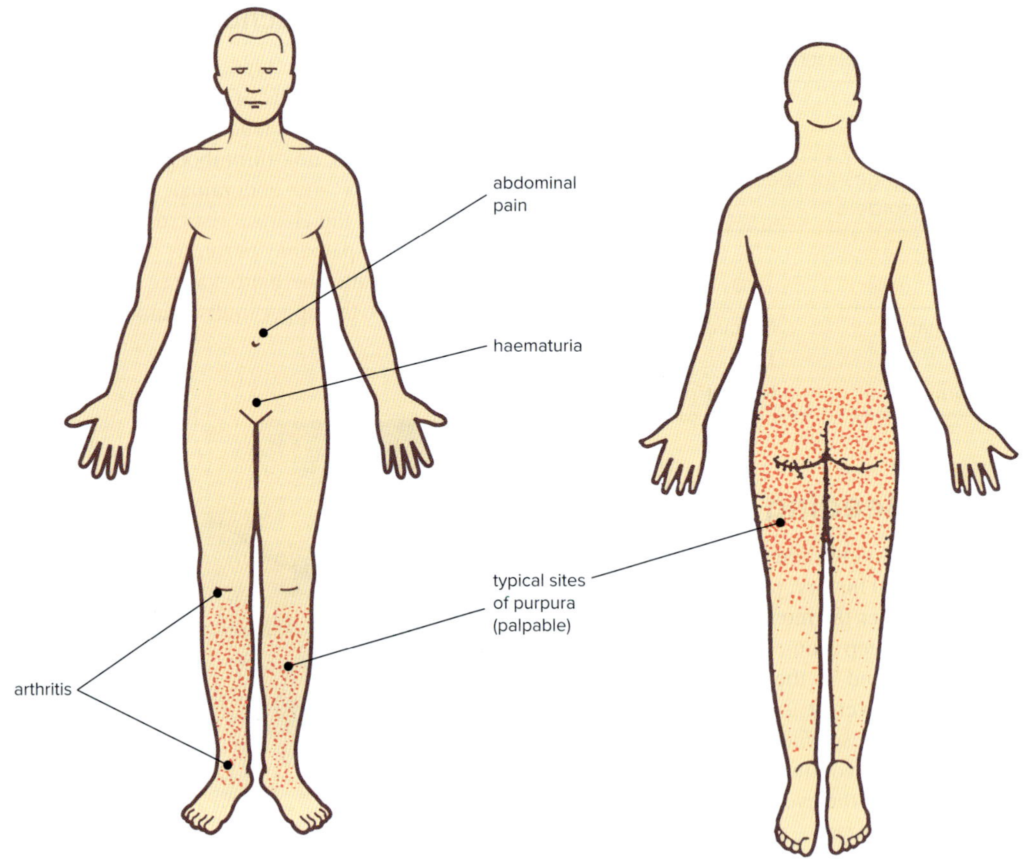

FIGURE 39.4 Henoch–Schönlein purpura: typical distribution

Infective states

The purpura associated with severe infections, such as meningococcaemia and other septicaemias, is due primarily to a severe angiitis. Disseminated intravascular coagulation usually follows.[3]

Abnormal bleeding in the elderly

The outstanding causes are senile purpura and purpura due to steroids.[5] The cause in both instances is atrophy of the vascular supporting tissue.

VASCULAR DISORDERS

The features are:

- easy bruising and bleeding into skin
- ± mucous membrane bleeding
- investigations normal

Simple purpura (easy bruising syndrome)

This is a benign disorder occurring in otherwise healthy women usually in their 20s or 30s. The feature is bruising on the arms, leg and trunk with minor trauma. The patient may complain of heavy periods. Major challenges to the haemostatic mechanism, such as dental extraction, childbirth and surgery, have not been complicated by excessive blood loss.

Factitial purpura

Unexplained bruising or bleeding may represent self-inflicted abuse or abuse by others. In self-inflicted abuse, the bruising is commonly on the legs or areas within easy reach of the patient.

PLATELET DISORDERS

The features are:

- petechiae ± ecchymoses
- bleeding from mucous membranes
- platelet counts <50 000/mm^3 (50 × 10^9/L)

Immune (idiopathic) thrombocytopenic purpura

Clinical features[5]

- Acute onset in children
- Easy bruising and petechiae
- Epistaxis, bleeding gums and menorrhagia common
- No systemic illness
- Splenomegaly rare
- Isolated thrombocytopenia: platelets may be <20 000/mm^3
- Other blood cells normal
- Otherwise normal physical examination
- Normal bone marrow with normal or increased megakaryocytes (acute leukaemia and aplastic anaemia should be excluded)

DxT bruising + oral bleeding + epistaxis → ITP

The two distinct types caused by immune destruction of the platelets are:

- acute thrombocytopenia of childhood—usually in children, usually postviral
- chronic ITP—autoimmune disorder, usually in adult women; all cases should be referred to a specialist unit

Acute thrombocytopenia of childhood

This is caused by a reaction to a virus infection resulting in the production of cross-reacting antibodies against platelets.

There is an early risk of spontaneous haemorrhage, so refer/admit to hospital especially if the platelet count is <30 × 10^9/L or there is active bleeding.

The prognosis is good, invariably self-limiting—90% resolve in 6 months. It may recur with further viral infections. The rest pass into chronic ITP.

Bleeding is treated with immunoglobulin or steroids.

Chronic idiopathic (immune) thrombocytopenic purpura

Chronic ITP is a relapsing illness that rarely undergoes spontaneous remission and may require treatment with prednisolone or biological agents, e.g. rituximab. Ask about drug history. Some require splenectomy, but this operation is avoided where possible, especially in young children, because of the subsequent risk of severe infection, particularly with *Streptococcus pneumoniae*.[5] (Refer later in this chapter.)

Thrombotic thrombocytopenic purpura

This is an uncommon life-threatening syndrome of haemolytic anaemia, thrombocytopenia and extremely high LDH. Clinical features include fever (non-infectious), neurologic and kidney abnormalities. The defect is in the absence of a specific protease in the plasma.

COAGULATION DISORDERS

The features are:

- ecchymoses
- haemarthrosis and muscle haematomas
- usually traumatic and delayed

The inherited disorders such as haemophilia A and B are uncommon and involve deficiency of one factor only. The acquired disorders, such as disseminated intravascular coagulation (DIC), occur more commonly and invariably affect several anticoagulation factors (see TABLE 39.6).

Table 39.6 International nomenclature of clotting factors

Factor	Common synonyms
I	Fibrinogen*
II	Prothrombin*
III	No longer used
IV	Calcium
V	Proaccelerin
VI	No longer used
VII	Proconvertin (tissue factor)
VIII	Antihaemophilic factor A Antihaemophilic globulin
IX	Antihaemophilic factor B (Christmas factor)
X	Stuart–Prower factor
XI	Plasma thromboplastin antecedent
XII	Hageman factor, contact factor
XIII	Fibrin stabilising factor

Inherited coagulation disorders

A list of the inherited bleeding disorders is included in TABLE 39.1. The better-known disorders are vWD, haemophilia A and haemophilia B (Christmas disease).

von Willebrand disease

This is the most common disorder of haemostasis (incidence 1% of population) and is usually a mild problem with an excellent prognosis.[6] There are about 22 types.

Clinical features

- Autosomal dominant inheritance (common types)
- Equal sex incidence
- Prolonged bleeding time
- Bleeding tendency exacerbated by aspirin
- Platelets normal
- Defective platelet adhesion at site of trauma combined with factor VIII deficiency[6]
- APTT prolonged
- Positive vW factor antigen
- Menorrhagia and epistaxis common
- Haemarthroses rare

DxT menorrhagia + bruising + increased bleeding—1. incisions 2. dental 3. mucosal → vWD

Treatment

- No specific treatment
- Avoid aspirin (including Alka-Seltzer), NSAIDs, IM injections
- Be cautious of surgical and dental procedures
- Preparations that help include desmopressin acetate (DDAVP), factor VIII concentrates and tranexamic acid

Haemophilia A

Clinical features

- Spontaneous haemarthroses, especially knees, ankles and elbows, are almost pathognomonic
- X-linked recessive pattern of inheritance
- Invariably only males affected (1 in 5000)
- Females theoretically affected if haemophiliac father and carrier mother
- The human factor gene has long been identified
- Severity levels:
  - severe—bleed spontaneously
  - moderate—bleed with mild trauma or surgery
  - mild—bleed after major trauma or surgery
- Deficiency of factor VIII
- APTT prolonged
- Normal prothrombin time and fibrinogen
- Many seropositive for HIV, hepatitis B or C (factor VIII concentrate transmission)
- Low platelet count should suspect HIV-associated ITP[6]

DxT spontaneous haemarthrosis + muscle bleeds + delayed bleeding → haemophilia A

Treatment

- Infusion of recombinant factor VIII concentrates[7]
- Avoid aspirin

Haemophilia B (Christmas disease)

- Identical clinical features to haemophilia A
- Also an X-linked recessive hereditary disorder
- Incidence of 1 in 30 000
- Deficiency of coagulation factor IX
- Same laboratory findings as haemophilia A apart from specific factor assays
- Treatment is with recombinant factor IX concentrates

Splenectomy

Main indications:

- immune thrombocytopenic purpura
- haemolytic anaemias esp. hereditary spherocytosis
- hypersplenism
- trauma
- Hodgkin/non-Hodgkin lymphoma

Post-splenectomy management[8]

Immediate problem is thrombocytosis (↑ platelets to 600–1000 × 10^9/L) for 2–3 weeks with risk of thromboembolism.

Long-term risk is overwhelming infection (pneumococcus [especially] *Haemophilus influenzae* and meningococcus), especially in young children in the first 2 years post-splenectomy. For elective surgery give immunisation at least 2 weeks before surgery. Lifelong prophylaxis should be considered in select patients such as those severely immunocompromised.

Prophylaxis

- Education about risks and early recognition of infection (special care with malaria)
- Pneumococcal immunisation—give 2–3 weeks preoperative, repeat 5-yearly; avoid in pregnancy
- Haemophilus type B vaccine—once only if not immunised
- Meningococcus vaccine—every 5 years
- Influenza vaccine—annual
- Long-term penicillin: amoxycillin daily or phenoxymethylpenicillin bd
- Urgent hospital admission if infection develops

Management principles for bleeding[1]

- Make the correct diagnosis.
- Stop or avoid drugs affecting the haemostatic system.
- Control bleeding episodes with appropriate drugs, blood products and local measures, such as simple compression or topical haemostatic agents.
- Infuse appropriate blood components for the treatment of coagulation factor deficiencies and some platelet disorders (e.g. factor VIII for haemophilia A, fresh frozen plasma for multiple factor deficiency).
- Refer patients with identified defects to a consultant haematologist or haemophilia centre.
- Supervise advanced planning in patients intending pregnancy, surgery or dental extraction.

When to refer[1]

- Management of haemorrhage is not amenable to simple measures such as local therapy with simple compression and other measures.
- Elective surgery or pregnancy is being planned.
- Platelet count <30 × 10^9/L.

Practice tips

- A careful history and physical examination will usually pinpoint the cause of the bleeding disorder.
- Drug therapy can lead to unmasking of pre-existing haemostatic disorders (e.g. platelet dysfunction induced by aspirin may cause spontaneous bleeding in patients with underlying vWD).
- Think of disseminated intravascular coagulation (DIC) in any acutely ill patient with abnormal bleeding from sites such as the mouth or nose, venepuncture or with widespread ecchymoses. The clinical situations are numerous, such as septicaemia, obstetric emergencies, disseminated malignant disease, falciparum malaria and snake bites.
- Be cautious of non-prescription therapies affecting oral anticoagulants or causing platelet dysfunction (e.g. gingko biloba).

39

References

1 Mitchell CA, Dear A, Salem H. Bleeding disorders. In: *MIMS Disease Index* (2nd edn). Sydney: IMS Publishing, 1996: 69–71.

2 Tran HAM. Bleeding disorders: does this patient have an increased risk of bleeding? Common sense pathology. Australian Doctor, 2008, March.

3 McPherson J, Street A. Tests of haemostasis: detection of the patient at risk of bleeding. Australian Prescriber, 1995; 18 (2): 38–40.

4 Thomson K, Tey D, Marks M et al. *Paediatric Handbook* (8th edn). Oxford: Wiley-Blackwell, 2009: 280–1.

5 Proven D et al. International consensus report on the investigation and management of primary immune thrombocytopenia. Blood, 2010; 115 (2): 168–86.

6 Kumar PJ, Clark ML. *Clinical Medicine* (7th edn). London: Saunders, 2009: 423.

7 Papadakis M, McPhee SJ. *Current Medical Diagnosis and Treatment* (52nd edn). New York: The McGraw-Hill Companies, 2013: 551–2.

8 Expert group for Antibiotic. Prophylaxis-medical. In: eTG complete [Internet]. Melbourne: Therapeutic Guidelines Ltd. Available from: <www.tg.org.au>, accessed January 2018.

Resources

Post surgical management—splenectomy. Spleen Australia.

Coagulation cascade. https://en.wikipedia.org/wiki/coagulation

Chest pain

There is a disorder of the breast marked with strong and peculiar symptoms, considerable for the kind of danger belonging to it. The seat of it, and sense of strangling, and anxiety with which it is attended, may make it not improperly be called angina pectoris.

WILLIAM HEBERDEN (1710–1801)

The presenting problem of chest pain is common yet very threatening to both patient and doctor because the underlying cause in many instances is potentially lethal, especially with chest pain of sudden onset. The causes of acute chest pain are summarised and presented in FIGURE 40.1.

Key facts and checkpoints

- Chest pain represents an acute coronary event until proved otherwise.
- Immediate life-threatening causes of spontaneous chest pain are:
  - myocardial infarction (MI) and unstable angina (acute coronary syndromes: ACS)
  - pulmonary embolism
  - aortic dissection
  - tension pneumothorax
- The main differential diagnoses of ACS include aortic dissection, pericarditis, oesophageal reflux and spasm, biliary colic and hyperventilation with anxiety.
- The history remains the most important clinical factor in the diagnosis of ischaemic heart disease. With angina a vital clue is the reproducibility of the symptom.
- Consider unstable angina = pre-myocardial infarction.
- Unrecognised MI may be atypical (50%) or silent (50%). More common with diabetes, hypertension, elderly and females.

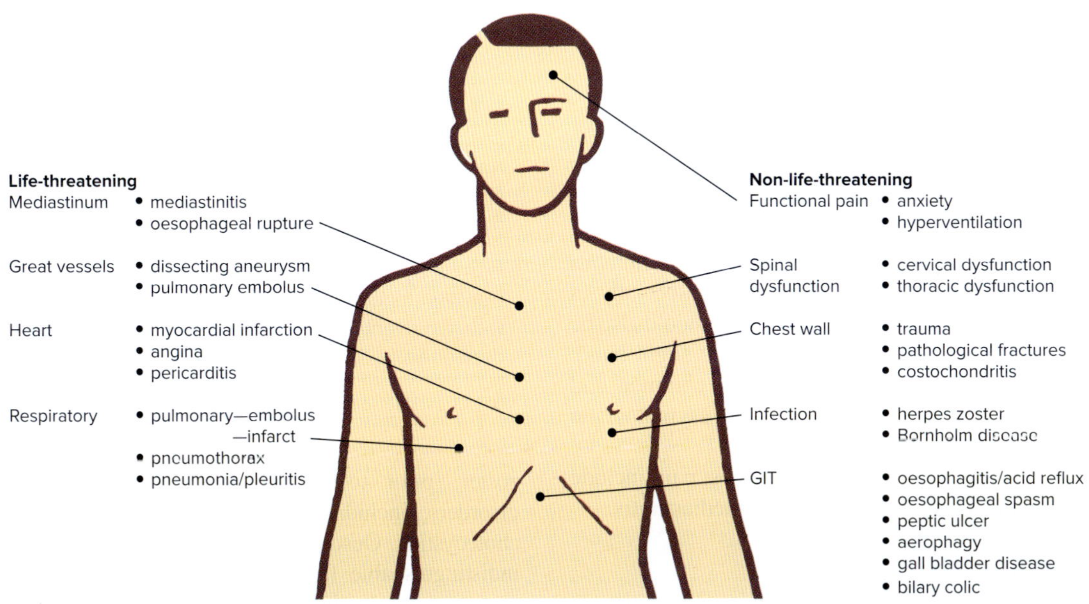

FIGURE 40.1 Causes of acute chest pain

A diagnostic approach

The diagnostic strategy model (see TABLE 40.1) can be used to analyse chest pain according to the five self-posed questions.

Probability diagnosis

The commonest causes encountered in general practice are musculoskeletal or chest wall pain and psychogenic disorders. The former is a very important yet often overlooked cause and sometimes inappropriately referred to as fibrositis or neuralgia. Causes include costochondritis, muscular strains, dysfunction of the sternocostal joints and dysfunction of the lower cervical spine or upper thoracic spine, which can cause referred pain to various areas of the chest wall. Angina is common and must always be considered. If angina-like pain lasts longer than 15 minutes myocardial infarction must be excluded. The best predictor of coronary pain is chest pain with pain in both arms.

Red flag pointers for acute chest pain

- Dizziness/syncope
- Pain in arms L>R, jaw
- Thoracic back pain
- Sweating
- Palpitations
- Syncope
- Haemoptysis
- Dyspnoea
- Pain on inspiration
- Pallor
- Past history: ischaemia, diabetes, hypertension

Serious disorders not to be missed

The usual triad of malignancy, myocardial ischaemia and severe infections (see TABLE 40.1) must be considered. In addition, other cardiovascular catastrophes, such as a dissecting aortic aneurysm and pulmonary embolus, must be excluded, although uncommon, especially in those at risk. Spontaneous pneumothorax should also be considered, especially in a young male of slight build. Malignancies of the lung are relatively common and may present as pain when the previously asymptomatic tumour invades nerves or the spine.

The severe infections that cause chest pain include pneumonia/pleurisy, pericarditis and mediastinitis.

Pitfalls

Unfortunately, myocardial infarction and angina are often missed. Referred pain from spinal dysfunction, especially if referred anteriorly, is commonly overlooked. Other pitfalls include a cough fracture of a rib, herpes zoster (prior to the eruption) and gastrointestinal disorders, including oesophageal spasm, reflux and cholecystitis. Oesophageal problems may be clinically indistinguishable from angina. Mitral valve prolapse can cause chest pain although the mechanism is unclear: think of it in an unwell female prone to palpitations and chest pain. The pain tends to be sharp, fleeting, non-exertional and located near the cardiac apex.

Table 40.1 Chest pain: diagnostic strategy model

Probability diagnosis
Musculoskeletal (chest wall)
Psychogenic
Angina

Serious disorders not to be missed
Cardiovascular:
- acute coronary syndromes
- aortic dissection
- pulmonary embolism/infarction

Neoplasia:
- lung cancer
- tumours of spinal cord and meninges

Severe infections:
- pneumonia/pleuritis (pleurisy)
- mediastinitis
- pericarditis

Pneumothorax, esp. tension
Oesophageal rupture

Pitfalls (often missed)
Mitral valve prolapse
Oesophageal spasm
Gastro-oesophageal reflux disease
Biliary colic/acute cholecystitis
Herpes zoster
Fractured rib (e.g. cough fracture)
Spinal dysfunction
Muscular tear
Rarities:
- pancreatitis
- Bornholm disease (pleurodynia)
- cocaine inhalation (can ↑ ischaemia)
- hypertrophic cardiomyopathy

Seven masquerades checklist
Depression (possible)
Anaemia (indirect)
Drugs (e.g. cocaine)
Spinal dysfunction

Is the patient trying to tell me something?
Consider functional causes, especially anxiety or panic with hyperventilation (e.g. takotsubo syndrome), opioid dependency.

Note: Chest pain is myocardial ischaemia until proved otherwise.

General pitfalls

General pitfalls include:

- not being 'coronary aware' in patients presenting with chest pain
- referred pain from spinal disorders, especially of the lower cervical spine—one of the great pitfalls in medical practice
- labelling chest pain as psychological in an anxious patient presenting with acute chest pain
- assuming that pain radiating down the inside of the left arm is always cardiac in origin
- being unaware that up to 20% of myocardial infarctions are silent, especially in elderly patients, and that pulmonary embolism is often painless if the main pulmonary veins are involved

Seven masquerades checklist

Of this group spinal dysfunction is possible. Disc lesions from the lower cervical spine are unlikely to cause chest wall pain, but dysfunction of the facet joints of this area of the spine and the upper thoracic spine are common causes of referred pain to the chest wall. Nerve root pain from spinal problems is rarely found in the chest wall. Pathological fractures secondary to osteoporosis or malignancy in the vertebrae cause posterior wall pain. Cocaine users can present with chest pain.

Psychogenic considerations

With psychogenic causes the pain can occur anywhere in the chest, and tends to be continuous and sharp or stabbing rather than constricting. Associated symptoms include palpitations, deep breathing, fatigue, tremor, agitation and anxiety. Abnormal stress, tension, anxiety or depression may precipitate the pain, which often lasts hours or days.

The clinical approach

History

A meticulous history of the behaviour of the pain is the key to diagnosis. The pain should be analysed into its usual characteristics with the SOCRATES system. Association with serious medical problems such as diabetes, Marfan syndrome, anaemia and connective tissue disorders (e.g. SLE, RA) should be kept in mind. Consider coronary risk factors. The ability to take a detailed history will obviously be limited with severe acute pain.

Associated symptoms

- *Syncope.* Consider myocardial infarction, pulmonary embolus and dissecting aneurysm.
- *Pain on inspiration.* Consider pleuritis, pericarditis, mediastinitis, pneumothorax and musculoskeletal (chest wall pain).
- *Thoracic back pain.* Consider spinal dysfunction, acute coronary syndromes, angina, aortic dissection, pericarditis and gastrointestinal disorders such as a peptic ulcer, biliary colic/cholecystitis and oesophageal spasm.

Key questions

- Where exactly do you get the pain? Can you pinpoint it?
- Does the pain travel anywhere?
- Can you give me a careful description of the pain?
- How long did the pain last and could you do anything to relieve it?
- Is the pain brought on by exertion and relieved by rest?
- Do cold conditions bring it on?
- Do you have any other symptoms, such as breathlessness, faintness, fever, nausea or vomiting, dizziness, weight loss, sweating or back pain?
- Is the pain made worse by breathing or coughing, or by movement or pressing on that area?
- Is there any blood in any sputum you bring up?
- Is your pain associated with what you eat and drink? Or with a bitter taste in your mouth?
- Do you get the pain on stooping over and after lying in bed at night?
- Do antacids relieve your pain?
- Have you noticed a rash where you get the pain?
- Have you had a blow to your chest or an injury to your back?

Examination

The examination should focus on the following areas:

- general appearance—evidence of atherosclerosis (senile arcus, thickened vessels), pale and sweating (myocardial infarction, dissecting aneurysm or pulmonary embolus), hemiparesis (? aortic dissection)
- pulses—both radial and femoral—check for nature of pulse and absence of femoral pulses
- blood pressure
- temperature
- palpation of chest wall, lower cervical spine and thoracic spine—look for evidence of localised tenderness, pathological fracture, spinal dysfunction, herpes zoster
- palpation of legs—check for evidence of deep venous thrombosis
- examination of chest—check for evidence of pneumothorax

- auscultation of chest:
  - reduced breath sounds, hyper-resonant percussion note and vocal fremitus → pneumothorax
  - friction rub → pericarditis or pleurisy
  - basal crackles → cardiac failure
  - apical systole murmur → mitral valve prolapse
  - aortic diastolic murmur → proximal dissection (aortic regurgitation)

Note: In the presence of a myocardial infarction, the examination may be normal but the patient, apart from being cold, clammy or shocked, may have muffled heart sounds, a gallop rhythm, a systolic murmur. With an aortic dissection the patient may also appear cold, clammy and shocked, but may show absent femoral pulses, hemiparesis and a diastolic murmur of aortic regurgitation.

- upper abdominal palpation—check for tenderness suggestive of gall bladder disease or peptic ulceration

Possible findings on examination of a patient with chest pain are presented in FIGURE 40.2.[1]

Investigations[1]

The following investigations to aid diagnosis are available, although the majority are sophisticated and confined to hospitals with high-technology imaging departments. The fundamental tests that are readily available to the GP—ECG, chest X-ray and cardiac enzymes—should help confirm the diagnosis in most

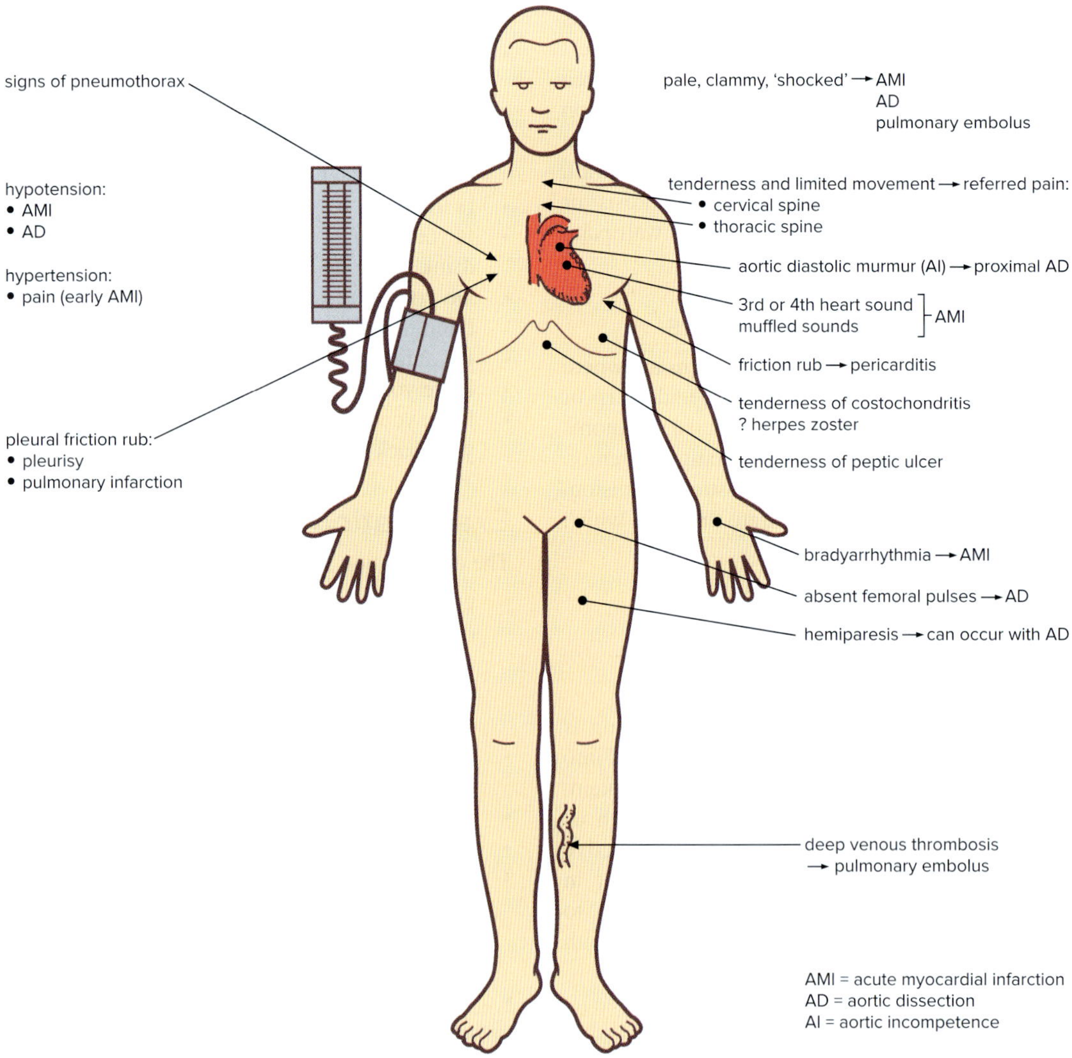

FIGURE 40.2 Possible examination findings in a patient with chest pain

instances. All patients with undifferentiated chest pain should have a 12-lead ECG.

Electrocardiogram (ECG)

This may be diagnostic for ischaemia and myocardial infarction, although it is important to bear in mind that it may be normal with both, including the early minutes to hours of an acute infarction.

It can be helpful to differentiate between myocardial infarction, pulmonary embolism and pericarditis. The ECG in pulmonary embolism may be normal but if massive may show right axis deviation, right BBB and right ventricular strain. Pericarditis is characterised by low voltages and saddle-shaped ST segment elevation.

Exercise stress test

This is the key test for defining chest pain as cardiac in origin. Physical stress, such as the motor-driven treadmill or a bicycle ergometer, is used to elicit changes in the ECG to diagnose myocardial ischaemia.

Exercise thallium scan

This radionuclide myocardial perfusion scan using thallium can complement the exercise ECG.

Ambulatory ECG Holter monitor

This monitor is especially useful for silent ischaemia, variant angina and arrhythmias.

Chest X-ray

The routine CXR is taken in full inspiration. Ask for an expiration film if pneumothorax is suspected.

Blood glucose

Tests association with diabetes.

Haemoglobin and blood film

Anaemia is a possible associated factor.

Serum enzymes

Damaged necrosed myocardial tissue releases cellular enzymes, which are markers of this damage:

- troponin I and troponin T (the key marker)–on arrival and 2 hours later (ADAPT trial protocol)
- creatinine kinase (CK) and creatinine kinase–myocardial bound fraction (CK–MB)[2]
- myoglobin

Transthoracic echocardiography

This can be used in the early stages of myocardial infarction to detect abnormalities in heart wall motion, when ECGs and enzymes are not diagnostic. Stress echocardiography is a new technique that is useful where standard exercise testing has been unhelpful.

Transoesophageal echocardiography (TOE)

More sensitive and is the investigation for dissecting aneurysm (immediate diagnosis), prosthetic valves and embolisation.

Isotope scanning

1. Technetium-99m pyrophosphate studies:
   - myocardium—to diagnose posterolateral myocardial infarction in the presence of bundle branch block
   - pulmonary—to diagnose pulmonary embolism
2. Gated blood pool nuclear scan (radionuclide ventriculography)—this scan tests left ventricular function at rest and exercise in patients with myocardial ischaemia.

Angiography (arteriography)

Angiography, including CT angiogram, should be selective:

1. coronary—to evaluate coronary arteries
2. pulmonary—to diagnose pulmonary thromboembolism
3. coronary computed tomograph
4. MRI

Oesophageal studies

- Endoscopy
- Barium swallow
- Oesophageal manometry
- Radionucleide transit studies

Spine—X-ray

- Cervical spine
- Thoracic spine

Site, radiation and features of chest pain syndromes

Myocardial ischaemia[1]

Coronary artery disease includes the acute coronary syndromes (unstable angina and myocardial infarction), stable angina and other variants of angina.

The typical retrosternal distribution of myocardial ischaemia is shown in FIGURE 40.3. Retrosternal pain or pain situated across the chest anteriorly should be regarded as cardiac until proved otherwise.

The wide variation of sites of pain, umbilicus to jaw, including neck, inside of arms, epigastrium and interscapular, should always be kept in mind (see FIG. 40.4). Pain is referred into the left arm more commonly than into the right arm. The best predictor of AMI is pain in both arms.

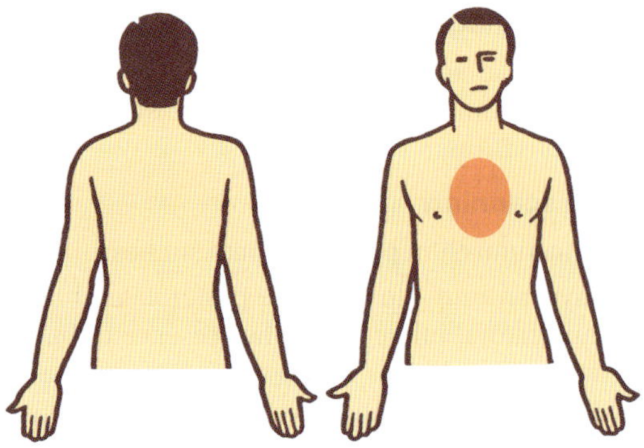

FIGURE 40.3 Pain of myocardial ischaemia: typical site

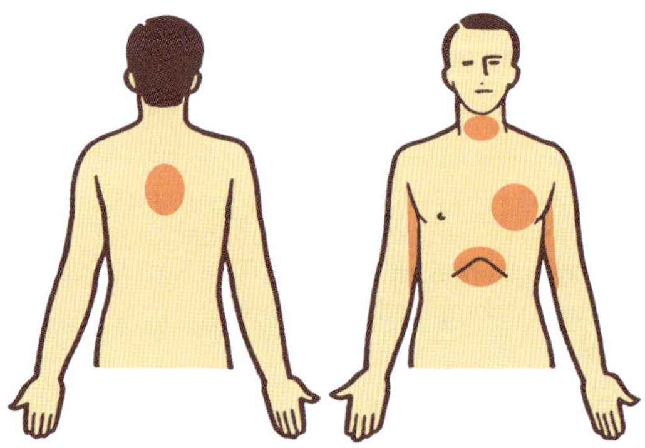

FIGURE 40.4 Pain of myocardial ischaemia: other sites

The quality of the pain is usually described as pressure, heaviness or tightness. The patient often uses the clenched fist sign to illustrate a sense of constriction.

The radiation of pain will assist in differentiating ischaemic pain from that caused by pericarditis. Enquiry about precipitating and relieving factors will enable a differentiation to be made between ischaemic pain and the almost identical pain caused by reference from the spine. Associated symptoms include dyspnoea, dizziness, nausea and vomiting and sweating (diaphoresis).

If a retrosternal pain almost identical with that of myocardial ischaemia is precipitated not by exertion but by bending, lifting, straining or lying down, oesophageal reflux and spasm is a possible diagnosis. This is frequently confused with ischaemic heart disease and can cause radiation into the left arm.

Stable angina. The pain of angina tends to last a few minutes only (average 3–5 minutes) and is relieved by rest and glyceryl trinitrate (nitroglycerine). The pain may be precipitated by an arrhythmia.

The types of acute coronary syndromes are summarised in TABLE 40.2.[3]

Table 40.2 Types of acute coronary syndromes

	Serum markers		
	Creatinine kinase	Troponin	ECG at evaluation
Unstable angina			
Low risk	Normal	Non-detectable	Normal
High risk	Normal	Detectable	ST depression
Myocardial infarction			
Non-ST elevation (NSTEMI)	Elevated	Detectable	ST depression, no Q wave
ST elevation (STEMI)	Elevated	Detectable	± Q wave or new LBBB

STEMI = ST elevation myocardial infarction

Myocardial infarction. Ischaemic pain lasting longer than 15–20 minutes is usually infarction. However, it can resolve in a few minutes or within 24 hours. The pain is typically heavy and crushing, and can vary from mild to intense. Occasionally the attack is painless, typically in diabetics. Pallor, sweating and vomiting may accompany the attack.

Unstable angina. This term includes rest angina, new onset effort angina, post infarct angina and post coronary procedure angina. Severe ischaemic chest pain can last 15–20 minutes or more. It is classified as low risk or high risk 'minor myocardial damage'.

For management purposes it is best to classify the clinical presentation of acute ischaemic chest pain as an ST elevation myocardial infarction (STEMI) or a non-ST elevation acute coronary syndrome (NSTEACS), which includes NSTEMI and unstable angina.

Aortic dissection

Chest pain is present in 75% of dissections. The pain, which is usually sudden, severe and midline, has a tearing or ripping sensation and is usually situated retrosternally and between the scapulae (see FIG. 40.5). It radiates to the abdomen, flank and legs. An important diagnostic feature is the inequality in the pulses (e.g. carotid, radial and femoral). There may also be occlusion of the coronary or kidney arteries with appropriate symptoms and signs. Hemiplegia, aortic incompetence or cardiac tamponade can occur. Consider a CT angiogram.

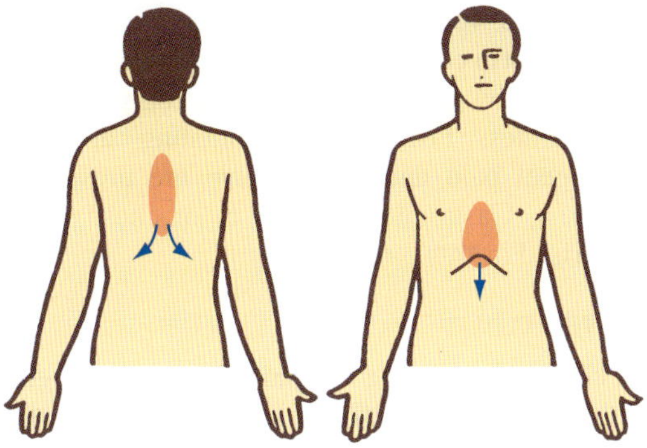

FIGURE 40.5 Pain of aortic dissection

Pulmonary embolism[3]

This may have a dramatic onset following occlusion of the pulmonary artery or a major branch, especially if more than 50% of the cross-sectional area of the pulmonary trunk is occluded. There are three general types: massive (obstructive shock or BP< 90 mmHg), submassive (acute without hypotension but right ventricular dysfunction) and non-massive (low risk).

The diagnosis can present clinical difficulties, especially when dyspnoea is present without pain. It can be asymptomatic. Embolism usually presents with retrosternal chest pain (see FIG. 40.6) and may be associated with syncope and breathlessness. In addition, hypotension, acute right heart failure or cardiac arrest occurs with a massive embolus. The physical examination can be deceptively normal. Pulmonary infarction is generally less dramatic than embolism and it is usually accompanied by pleuritic chest pain and haemoptysis. It complicates embolism in about 10% of patients. The diagnosis is usually confirmed by a CT pulmonary angiogram (best) and/or V/Q scan (see later in chapter) and ECG (look for T wave inversion V1–V4). The D-dimer test may be useful.

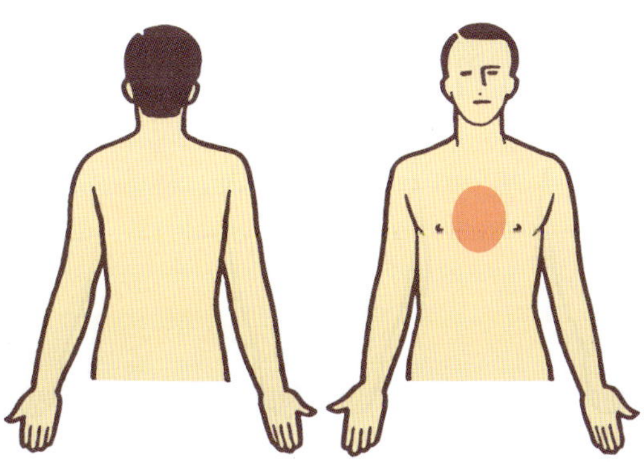

FIGURE 40.6 Pain of pulmonary embolism

Pleuritis[4]

Inflammation of the pleura is due to underlying pneumonia (viral or bacterial), pulmonary infarction, tumour infiltration or connective tissue disease (e.g. SLE).

Clinical features

- Often sudden onset
- Pain usually localised without radiation
- Sharp knife-like pain
- Continuous pain with sharp exacerbations
- Aggravated by inspiration, sneezing and coughing
- May be associated dyspnoea, cough, haemoptysis

Epidemic pleurodynia (Bornholm disease)

Unilateral severe knife-like intermittent chest pain and adjacent upper abdominal pain ('the devil's grip') following an URTI—affecting any age. Other symptoms include fever, malaise, headache, malaise and tender truncal muscles. It is caused by a Coxsackie B virus. CXR is normal; diagnosis is by exclusion. It usually settles within a week with simple analgesics. Recurrences may follow.

Acute pericarditis[5]

The clinical presentation depends on the cause, whether viral (commonest), a connective tissue disorder, bacterial, uraemia or post-AMI. There may be fever, malaise, fatigue and anxiety.[4]

- Signs: friction rub, tachycardia, paradoxical pulse
- Investigations: ECG, CXR, echocardiography

Pericarditis causes three distinct types of pain:

1. pleuritic (the commonest), aggravated by cough and deep inspiration, sometimes brought on by swallowing; worse with lying flat, relieved by sitting up and leaning forward
2. steady, crushing, retrosternal pain that mimics myocardial infarction
3. pain synchronous with the heartbeat and felt over the praecordium and left shoulder

Occasionally, two and rarely all three types of pain may be present simultaneously (see FIG. 40.7).

The cardinal sign is a pericardial friction rub (often transient). Treatment depends on the cause—may be NSAIDs ± colchicine or corticosteroids.

Spontaneous pneumothorax

The acute onset of pleuritic pain and dyspnoea in a patient with a history of asthma or emphysema is the hallmark of a pneumothorax. It is due to a rupture of a subpleural 'bleb' or a small air-containing cyst. It often occurs in young, slender males without a history of lung disorders. The pain varies from mild to severe and can be felt anywhere in the chest, sometimes being retrosternal. Typical pain distribution is shown in FIGURE 40.8. The diagnosis is made on expiration film.

If a tension pneumothorax becomes painful and dyspnoea becomes rapidly more intense, urgent decompression of air is essential (see later in chapter). A comparison of the serious causes of acute chest pain is summarised in TABLE 40.3.

Oesophageal pain

Gastro-oesophageal reflux can cause oesophagitis characterised by a burning epigastric or retrosternal pain that may radiate to the jaw. The pain is aggravated or precipitated by lying flat or bending over, especially after meals, and is more frequent at night. The pain is worse if oesophageal spasm is present. Oesophageal motor disorders, including spasm, may occur in isolation. The pain may radiate uncommonly to the back (see FIG. 40.9). It may be precipitated by eating, especially hot or cold food and drink, and may be relieved by eating or by glyceryl trinitrate (nitroglycerine) and other nitrates. Features differentiating angina-like oesophageal pain and cardiac pain are presented in TABLE 40.4. Gastrointestinal causes of chest pain are summarised in TABLE 40.5.[1]

Spinal pain

The commonest cause of pain of spinal origin is vertebral dysfunction of the lower cervical or upper dorsal region (see CHAPTER 37). The spinal problem may be a disc prolapse (relatively common in the lower cervical spine, but rare in the upper thoracic spine) or dysfunction of the facet joints or costovertebral joints causing referred pain. This referred pain can be present anywhere in the chest wall, including anterior chest, which causes confusion with cardiac pain (see FIG. 40.10). The pain is dull and aching. It may be aggravated by exertion, certain body movements or deep inspiration. The old trap for unilateral nerve root pain is herpes zoster.

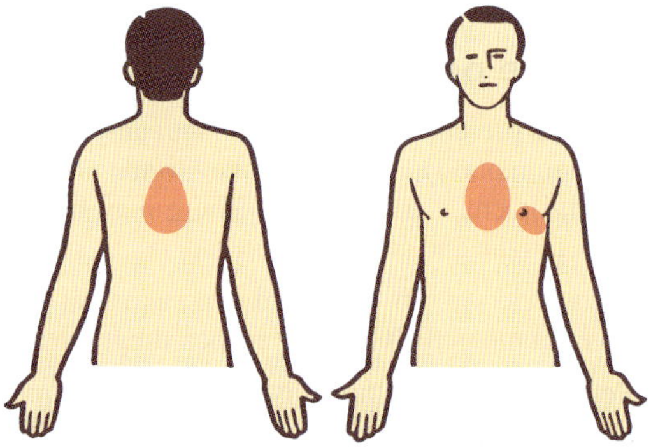

FIGURE 40.7 Pain of pericarditis

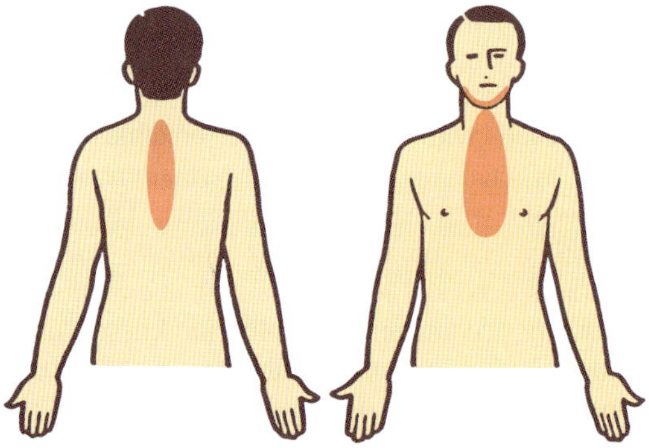

FIGURE 40.9 Oesophageal pain

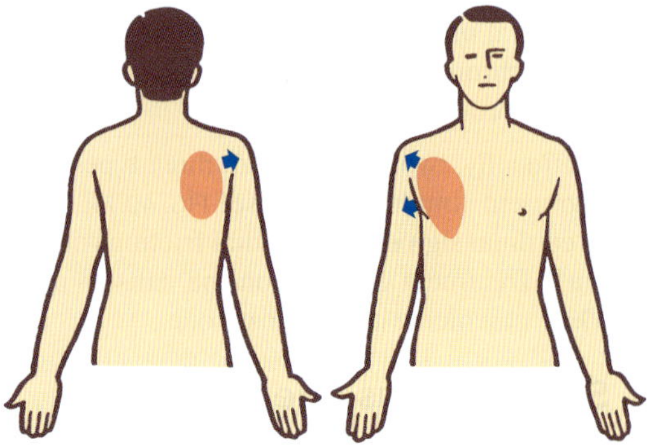

FIGURE 40.8 Pain of pneumothorax (right side)

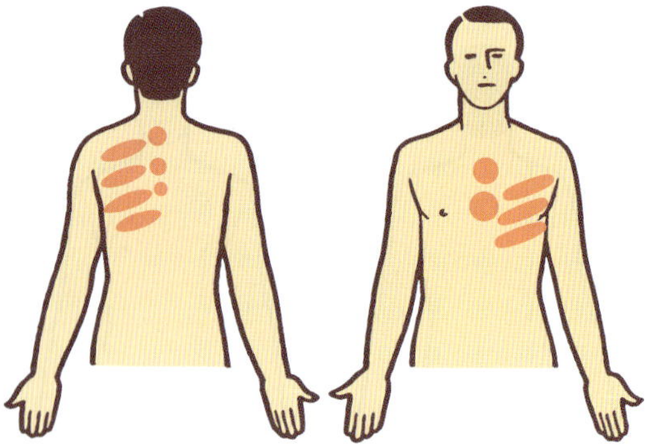

FIGURE 40.10 Possible pain sites for thoracic spinal dysfunction (left side)

40

Table 40.3 A comparison of the serious causes of acute chest pain

	Myocardial infarction	Angina	Pulmonary embolus	Aortic dissection	Pericarditis	Pneumothorax
Pain intensity	+ → + + + +	+	+ → + + +	+ + + + +	+ → + + +	+ → + + +
Pain quality	Heavy Crushing Vice-like Burning	Heavy Aching Tightness Burning	Dull Heavy	Tearing Searing	Heavy Aching ± sharp	Tightness Sharp Stabbing
Pain site	Deep retrosternal	Deep retrosternal	Retrosternal	Anterior chest	Substernal	Lateral chest
Pain radiation	Throat/lower jaw Left arm (often) Right arm (uncommon) Back (uncommon)	As for infarction	Lateral chest (pleuritic)	Front to back of chest Down back to abdomen Arms	Left arm (uncommon) Right arm (rare) Throat (rare) Back	Lateral chest
History	Family, risk factors	Family, risk factors	Phlebitis Calf pain Immobility Surgery Malignancy	Atherosclerosis Hypertension ? Marfan	Viral infection MI	Asthma COAD Old TB
Associated symptoms	Pallor, nausea, sweating, vomiting, dyspnoea, syncope	Strangling in throat	Dyspnoea, syncope, sweating, vomiting, cyanosis, agitation, haemoptysis	Syncope, pallor, cyanosis, Neurological: • hemiparesis • paraplegia	Fever, malaise ± pleuritic pain	Dyspnoea, cough, ? cyanosis
Pulse	Variable ? arrhythmias	Variable ? arrhythmias	Tachycardia	Unequal some ? absent	Weak if effusion	Tachycardia
Cardiac auscultation	± Gallop rhythm murmur of MI	S_3 during attack	↓ pulmonary S_2, S_3 or S_4	± Murmur of AI	± Pericardial friction rub	
Chest auscultation	Basal crackles		± Adventitious sounds			↓ Breath sounds
Chest X-ray			± Localised oligaemia or infarction	Widening of mediastinum	↑ Cardiac silhouette if effusion	Diagnostic—expiration film
ECG	Q waves ST elevation T inversion (variable)	Normal or ST depression	R axis deviation S_1, Q_3, T_3 sign	May show myocardial infarction	Saddle-shaped elevated ST segments	
Special definitive diagnostic tests	Serum enzymes: troponin I or T Cardiac scanning	Stress ECG Coronary angiography Technetium scanning Enzymes	Lung scanning CT pulmonary angiography V/Q scan	TOE Ultrasound Aortic angiography CT scan	Echocardiography (if effusion)	

Table 40.4 Features differentiating angina-like oesophageal pain and cardiac pain

	Favour oesophageal	Favour cardiac	Non-discriminating
Precipitating factors	Meals, posture	Consistently with exercise	Emotion
Relieving factors	Antacids		Rest, nitrates
Radiation	Epigastrium	Arm	Back
Associated symptoms	Heartburn, regurgitation, dysphagia	Dyspnoea	Sweating

Table 40.5 A comparison of gastrointestinal causes of chest pain

	Acid reflux	Oesophageal spasm	Peptic ulcer	Gall bladder disease
Site	Epigastric	Deep retrosternal	Deep retrosternal	Right hypochondrium
Radiation	Retrosternal Throat	Back	To back (DU)	Below right scapula Tip right shoulder
Quality	Burning	Constricting	Gnawing	Deep ache
Precipitation	Heavy meals Wine/coffee Lying Bending	Eating hot/cold food and drinks	Eating: • GU: 30 min • DU: 2–3 hours	Fatty food
Relief	Standing Antacids	Antispasmodics Nitroglycerine	Antacids	Getting onto hands and knees
Associated symptoms	Water brash	Dysphagia	Dyspepsia	Flatulence Dyspepsia

GU = gastric ulcer; DU = duodenal ulcer

Costochondritis[4]

This causes mild to moderate anterior chest wall pain that may radiate to the chest, back or abdomen. It is usually unilateral, sharp in nature and exaggerated by breathing, physical activity or a specific position. It may be preceded by exercise or a URTI and can persist for several months. It is diagnosed by eliciting tenderness at the costochondral junction of the affected ribs and needs to be differentiated from Tietze syndrome, where there is a tender, fusiform swelling at the costochondral junction (refer to CHAPTER 100).

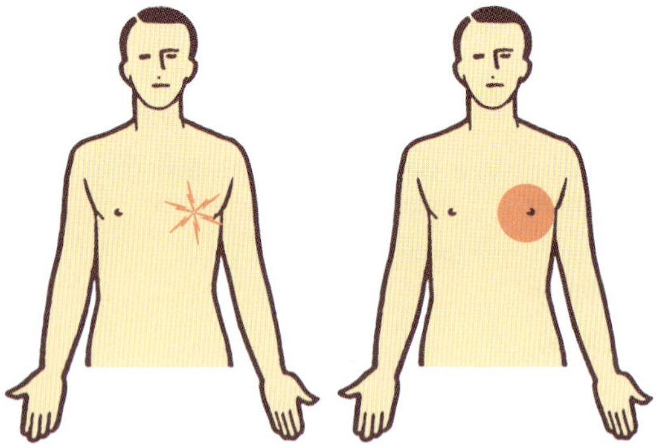

FIGURE 40.11 Typical sites of psychogenic pain

Psychogenic pain

Psychogenic chest pain can occur anywhere in the chest, but often it is located in the left submammary region, usually without radiation (see FIG. 40.11). It tends to be continuous and sharp or stabbing. It may mimic angina but tends to last for hours or days. It is usually aggravated by tiredness or emotional tension and may be associated with shortness of breath, fatigue and palpitations.

Da Costa syndrome (effort syndrome) is recurrent attacks of stabbing left-sided submammary pain, usually associated with anxiety ± depression.

Takotsubo cardiomyopathy or 'broken heart syndrome' presents with acute chest pain and shortness of breath. It mimics an acute anterior myocardial infarction. It is caused by a major catecholamine discharge following an emotionally stressful event, resulting in apical left ventricular ballooning. Treatment is usually with aspirin, beta blockers and ACE inhibitors. Most patients recover completely.

Chest pain in children

Chest pain in children is rarely the result of serious pathology but is an important complaint, especially in adolescents. A US study has shown that the mean age for childhood chest pain is 11.9 years.[5] Most cases are of unknown aetiology (probably psychogenic), while common causes include musculoskeletal disorders, cough-induced pain, costochondritis, psychogenic disturbance (includes hyperventilation) and asthma.[6] See TABLE 40.6.

Table 40.6 Causes of chest pain in children: diagnostic model

Probability diagnosis
Musculoskeletal (chest wall pain)
• cough strain (10%)
• injury
• muscle strain
• costochondritis
• precordial catch syndrome (stitch in side)
• asthma
Note: Most cases are unknown (21%)
Serious disorders not to be missed
Vascular
• ischaemic pain: structural cardiac conditions
• arrhythmias (e.g. PSVT)
Infection
• pericarditis
• myocarditis
• pneumonia
• herpes zoster
Other:
• pneumothorax
• POTS syndrome
Pitfalls (often missed)
Kawasaki syndrome
Breast disorders
Cocaine inhalation
Rarities:
• Bornholm disease
• oesophagitis or gastric pain
Is the patient trying to tell me something?
Psychogenic: stress, anxiety, depression (10%)

Source: Adapted from Selbst[4]

Chest pain in children younger than 12 years old is more likely to have a cardiorespiratory cause, such as cough, asthma, pneumonia or heart disease, while chest pain in adolescents is more likely to be associated with a psychogenic disturbance.

Causes of musculoskeletal pain include strains to pectoral, shoulder or back muscles after excessive exercise, and minor trauma from sports such as football or wrestling.

Breast problems can present as chest pain.

Cardiac causes

Myocardial ischaemia is very rare in children but should be considered in any child with exercise-induced chest pain, adolescents with long-standing diabetes and children with sickle-cell anaemia.

Precordial catch (Texidor twinge or stitch in the side)[5]

This complaint, which is common in children and adolescents, presents as a unilateral low chest pain that lasts usually 30 seconds to 3 minutes, typically with exercise, such as long-distance running. The pain is relieved by straightening up and taking very slow deep breaths followed by shallow breaths.

Chest pain in the elderly

Chest pain is a very important symptom in the elderly as the life-threatening cardiovascular conditions—myocardial infarction and angina, dissecting aneurysm and ruptured aorta—are an increasing manifestation with age. In a community survey in Glasgow, 20% of men and 12% of women over 65 years were found to have ischaemic heart disease.[8] The elderly patient presenting with chest pain is most likely to have angina or myocardial infarction. Other important disorders to consider are herpes zoster, cough fracture of the rib, malignancy, pleurisy, pulmonary embolus and gastro-oesophageal reflux.

Chest pain in adults

Angina pectoris

Main features

- There is a 2–3% incidence between 25 and 64 years.[9]
- The history is the basis of diagnosis.
- Angina is an oppressive discomfort rather than a pain, typically transient and lasting <10 mins.
- It is mainly retrosternal: radiates to arms, jaw, throat, back.
- It may be associated with shortness of breath, nausea, faintness and sweating.
- It occurs during exercise, emotion, after meals or in cold.
- It is relieved within a few minutes with rest.
- Physical examination is usually not helpful, except during an attack.
- Mitral valve prolapse, oesophageal spasm and dissecting aneurysm are important differential diagnoses.
- The causes of angina are summarised in TABLE 40.7.

Note: Ensure that the patient is not anaemic or thyrotoxic. Fever and tachycardia also have to be excluded.

Table 40.7 Causes of angina

Coronary artery atheroma
Valvular lesions (e.g. aortic stenosis)
Rapid arrhythmias
Anaemia
Rarities:
• vasculitis
• trauma
• collagen disease

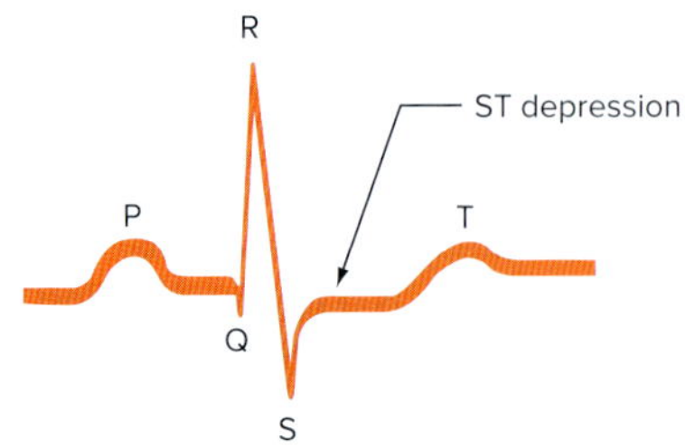

FIGURE 40.12 Typical ECG pattern for angina pectoris: this tracing is usually observed during an attack

Note: there is no specific ECG of angina; the most that can be said is that an ECG is consistent with angina

Variants[1,9]

- *Stable angina.* Pain occurs with exertion and is usually predictable with no symptom change during the past month.
- *Unstable angina* (also referred to as crescendo angina, pre-infarct angina and acute coronary insufficiency). It is increasing angina (severity and duration) over a short period of time, precipitated by less effort and may come on at rest, especially at night. It may eventually lead to complete infarction, often with relief of symptoms. It is due to unstable plaque.
  - *Nocturnal angina.* Pain occurs during the night. It is related to unstable angina.
  - *Decubitus angina.* The pain occurs when lying flat and is relieved by sitting up.
  - *Variant angina or Prinzmetal angina or spasm angina.*[7] The pain occurs at rest and without apparent cause. It is associated with typical transient ECG changes of ST elevation (as compared with the classic changes of ST depression during effort angina). It can lead to infarction and cause arrhythmias. It is caused by coronary artery spasm.

Aids to diagnosis

ECG

This may be normal or show ischaemia or evidence of earlier infarction. During an attack it may be normal or show well-marked depression of the ST segment, symmetrical T-wave inversion (see FIG. 40.12) or tall upright T waves.

Exercise ECG

This is positive in about 75% of patients with severe coronary artery disease and should be performed if the diagnosis is in doubt, for prognostic reasons or to aid in the timing of additional investigations (e.g. coronary angiography). A normal stress test does not rule out coronary artery disease.

Exercise thallium-201 scan

This test is helpful in some difficult circumstances such as in the presence of left branch bundle block (LBBB), old infarction and Wolff–Parkinson–White (WPW) syndrome (when exercise test is of little use) and with mitral valve prolapse, which gives high false positive tests. It helps determine the presence and extent of reversible myocardial ischaemia since thallium is only taken up by perfused tissue.

Ambulatory ECG Holter monitoring

This may be useful in some patients.

Gated blood pool nuclear scan

This test assesses the ejection fraction, which is a reliable index of ventricular function and thus aids assessment of patients for coronary artery bypass surgery.

Echocardiography

This assesses global and regional wall motion abnormalities and assesses valvular dysfunction and pericardium status.

Coronary angiography

This test accurately outlines the extent and severity of coronary artery disease. It is usually used to determine the precise coronary artery anatomy prior to surgery.

The relationship between the degree of angina and coronary artery disease is not clear-cut. Some people with severe angina have normal coronary arteries.

Indications for coronary angiography are presented in TABLE 40.8.

'Ultrafast CT' may replace traditional angiography.

Table 40.8 Indications for coronary angiography

Strong positive exercise stress test
Suspected left main coronary artery disease
Angina resistant to medical treatment
Suspected but not otherwise proven angina
Acute coronary syndromes
Angina after myocardial infarction
Patients over 30 years with aortic and mitral valve disease being considered for valve surgery

40

Management of stable angina

Preventions

This is especially important for those with a positive family history and an unsatisfactory lifestyle. Modification of risk factors:

- no smoking
- weight reduction
- healthy eating/optimal low-fat diet
- exercise
- control of hypertension
- control of diabetes
- control of blood lipids

General advice for the stable angina patient

- Reassure patient that angina has a reasonably good prognosis: 30% survive more than 10 years;[10] spontaneous remission can occur.
- Attend to any risk factors.
- If inactive, take on an activity such as walking for 20 minutes a day.
- Take regular exercise to the threshold of angina.
- If tense and stressed, cultivate a more relaxed attitude to life—consider a stress management/relaxation course.
- Avoid precipitating factors.
- Don't excessively restrict lifestyle.

Medical treatment[5]

The acute attack and episodic angina

- Nitrates:
  glyceryl trinitrate 300–600 mcg tab sublingually, max 1800 mcg
  or
  glyceryl trinitrate SL 400 mcg metered dose spray: 1 spray; repeat after 5 minutes if pain persists (maximum three doses)
  or
  isosorbide dinitrate 5 mg sublingually; repeat every 5 minutes if pain persists (maximum 3 tablets)
  or
  nifedipine 5 mg capsule (suck or chew) if intolerant of nitrates
- Aspirin 150 mg (o)

Tips about glyceryl trinitrate tablets:

- if pain persists for longer than 10 minutes despite two doses of nitrates, take a third dose and call for an ambulance
- warn patient about headache and other side effects
- sit down to take the tablet
- take ½ (initially) or 1 tablet every 5 minutes
- take a maximum of 3 tablets in 15 minutes
- tablets must be fresh
- discard the bottle after being opened for 3 months or after 2 days if carried on the person
- keep tablets out of light and heat
- if pain relieved quickly, spit out residual tablet
- advise patient to get medical advice if no relief after 3 tablets

Note: avoid nitrates if patient has taken sildenafil or vardenafil in the previous 24 hours or tadalafil in the previous 5 days.

Prevention of angina

Moderate stable angina

Regular predictable attacks precipitated by moderate exertion. For prevention:

add to aspirin (if not contraindicated)
beta blocker, e.g. atenolol 25–100 mg (o) once daily
or
metoprolol 25–100 mg (o) twice daily
plus nitrates
glyceryl trinitrate (transdermal: ointment or patches) daily (use for 14 hours only)
or
isosorbide mononitrate 30 mg (o) SR tablet mane, increasing to 120 mg if required

Note: Aim for a daily nitrate-free interval.

Persistent angina

Not prevented by beta blocker:

add
a dihydropyridine calcium-channel blocker (CCB)
nifedipine CR 30–60 mg (o) once daily
or
amlodipine 2.5–10 mg (o) once daily
plus nitrates

If beta blocker contraindicated (use a non-dihydropyridine calcium-channel blocker):

diltiazem 30–90 mg (o) tds or CR 180–360 mg (o) daily
or
verapamil (according to directions)

Refractory stable angina

Consider adding nicorandil 5 mg (o) bd, increasing after a week to 10–20 mg bd or replacing the CCB with perhexiline
or
ivabradine and seeking specialist advice

Unstable angina

Includes onset of angina at rest, abrupt worsening of angina and angina following acute myocardial infarction.

- Should be hospitalised for stabilisation and further evaluation. May need IV nitrate therapy.
- The objectives are to optimise therapy and consider coronary angiography with a view to a corrective procedure.

Rules of practice

- For variant angina (spasm) use nitrates and calcium antagonist (avoid beta blockers).
- As a rule, avoid the combination of verapamil and a beta blocker (risk of tachycardia and heart block).
- Do not combine a dihydropyridine CCB with a non-dihydropyridine CCB.
- Tolerance to nitrate use is a problem, so 24-hour coverage with long-acting preparations is not recommended.
- Consider using the potassium channel opening vasodilator nicorandil 5 mg (o) bd to 10–20 mg (o) bd (after 1 week). Can use as alternative to long-acting nitrates. The new agent ivabradine can be considered.
- Nitrates can be used prophylactically prior to any exertion that is likely to provoke angina (e.g. glyceryl trinitrate spray or tablet *or* isosorbide dinitrate 5 mg tablet)
- Avoid nitrates if the patient has used a 5 phosphodiesterase inhibitor in the past 1–5 days.

Non-medical treatment[5]

Percutaneous intervention (PCI) and coronary angioplasty (the gold standard)

One current technique is dilating coronary atheromatous obstructions by inflating a balloon against the obstruction—percutaneous transluminal coronary angioplasty (PTCA) (see FIG. 40.13) and maintaining patency with intracoronary stent devices.

Two complications of the balloon inflation angioplasty are acute coronary occlusion (2–4%) and restenosis, which occurs in 30% in the first 6 months after angioplasty.[10]

Intra-coronary stents

PTCA followed by stenting is now the most favoured procedure to maintain patency of the obstructed coronary vessel (see FIG. 40.14). Modern drug eluting stents, which include drugs such as primolimus, sirolimus or paclitaxel, can be used as well as the bare metal stent. Stent patients require long-term antiplatelet agents (e.g. aspirin plus clopidogrel) (specialist advice is required).

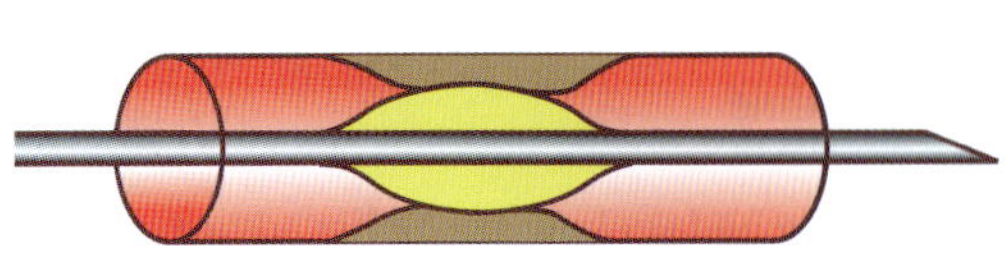

FIGURE 40.13 Percutaneous transluminal angioplasty (PTCA) with an inflatable balloon

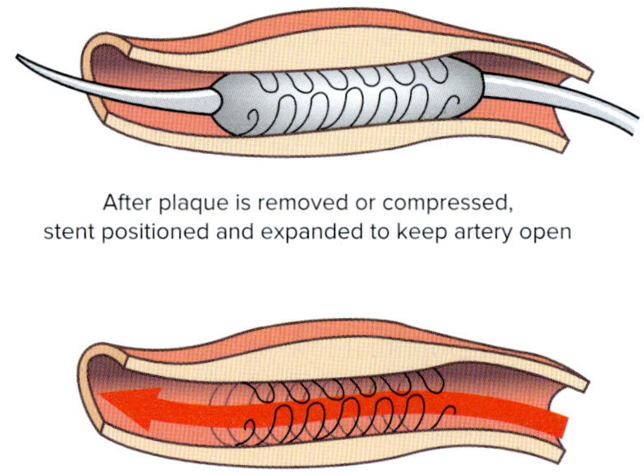

FIGURE 40.14 Illustration of stenting a coronary artery

Coronary artery surgery

The main surgical techniques in current use are coronary artery bypass grafting (CABG) using either a vein (usually the saphenous) (see FIG. 40.15) or internal mammary arterial implantation (see FIG. 40.16) or both and endarterectomy.

Symptomatic patients with significant left main coronary obstruction should undergo bypass surgery, and those with two or three vessel obstruction and

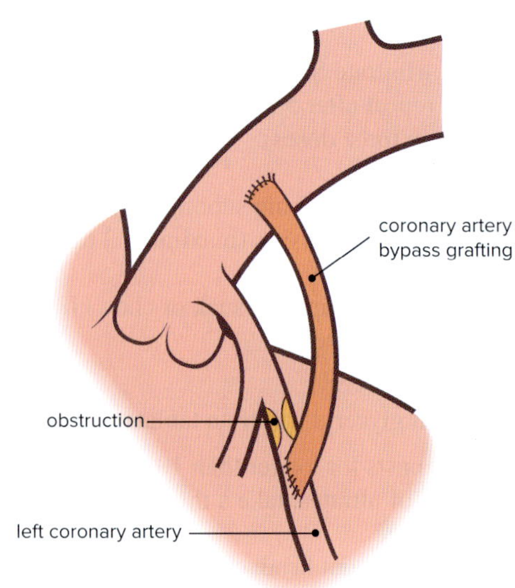

FIGURE 40.15 Coronary artery bypass grafting to relieve coronary obstruction

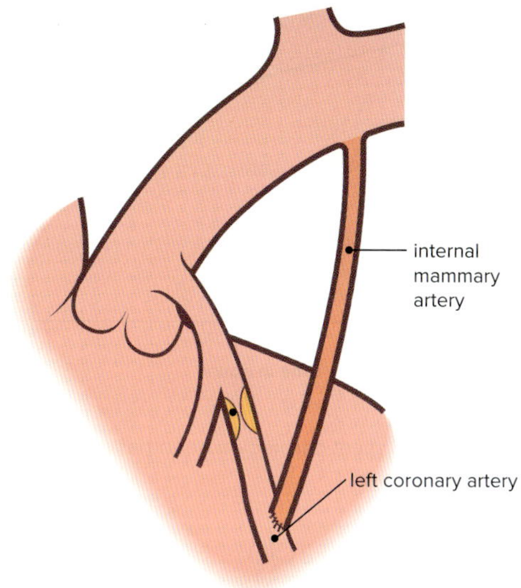

FIGURE 40.16 Internal mammary arterial transplantation to relieve obstruction

good ventricular function are often considered for angioplasty or surgery. A significant improvement in the quantity and quality of life can be expected.

Myocardial infarction

Clinical guidelines[11]

- Variable pain; may be mistaken for indigestion
- Similar to angina but more oppressive
- So severe, patient may fear imminent death—*angor animi*
- About 20% have no pain. These have a high mortality rate
- 'Silent infarcts' in diabetics, hypertensives, females and elderly; one report (*European Heart Journal,* 14 February 2006, online) reported that 40% of infarcts were silent and undetected in older patients
- 60% of those who die do so before reaching hospital, within 2 hours of the onset of symptoms
- Hospital mortality is 8–10%[10]
- Like CVA, seems to peak at 6–10 am

Diagnosis is based on 2 out of 3 criteria: history of prolonged ischaemic pain, typical ECG appearance, and rise and fall of cardiac enzymes.

Aetiology

- Thrombosis with occlusion
- Haemorrhage under a plaque
- Rupture of a plaque
- Coronary artery spasm

Signs

These may be:

- no abnormal signs
- pale/grey, clammy, dyspnoeic
- restless and apprehensive
- variable BP with pain ↓ heart pump failure
- variable pulse: watch for bradyarrhythmias
- mild cardiac failure: third or fourth heart sound, basal crackles

Investigations

1 *ECG.* The ECG is valuable with characteristic changes in a full thickness infarction. The typical features (see FIG. 40.17) are:
  - the Q wave: broad (>1 mm) and deep >25% length R wave
    - occurs normally in leads AVR and V1; III (sometimes)
    - abnormal if in other leads
    - occurs also with WPW and ventricular tachycardia (VT)
    - usually permanent feature after full thickness AMI
  - T wave and ST segment:
    - transient changes (inversion and elevation respectively)

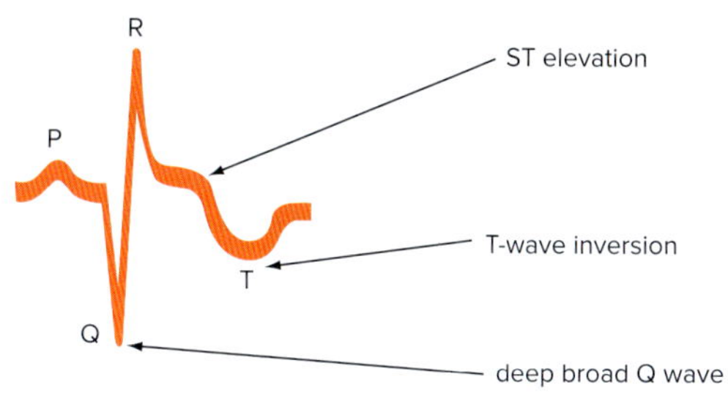

FIGURE 40.17 Typical ECG features of myocardial infarction, illustrating a Q wave, ST elevation and T-wave inversion

The typical progression is shown in FIGURE 40.18.

Note:

- Q waves do not develop in subendocardial infarction.
- The strategies for management of AMI are based on the distinction between Q wave (transmural) or non-Q wave (subendocardial) infarction.
- Q wave infarction has been proved to benefit from thrombolytic therapy, but non-Q wave infarction has not.
- If new LBBB think AMI (in LBBB no Q wave).
- A normal ECG, especially early, does not exclude AMI. Q waves may take days to develop.

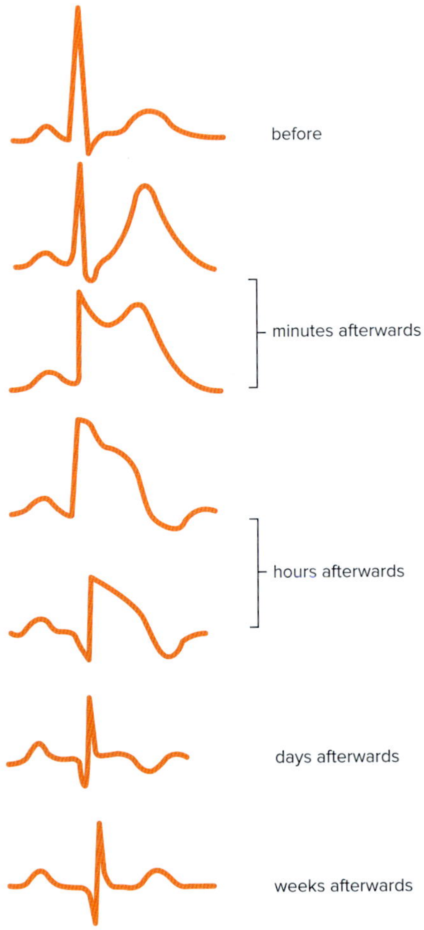

FIGURE 40.18 Typical evolution of ECG changes with myocardial infarction

2 *Cardiac enzymes.* The typical enzyme patterns are presented in FIGURE 40.19. As a rule, large infarcts tend to produce high serum enzyme levels. The elevated enzymes can help time the infarct:
   - troponin I or T:
     - starts rising at 3–12 hours, peaks at 24 hours and persists for about 5–14 days
     - now the preferred test
     - positive in unstable angina
     - raised in aortic dissection and kidney impairment
     - may have to wait until 10 hours before recording a negative result
     - not useful for repeat MI
     - both proteins, I and T, provide same information
     - reference interval <0.1 μg/L

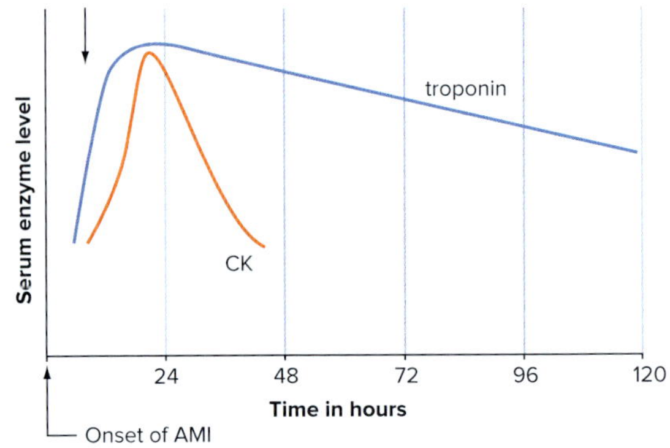

FIGURE 40.19 Typical cardiac enzyme patterns following myocardial infarction

   - creatinine kinase (CK):
     - after delay of 6–8 hours from the onset of pain it peaks at 20–24 hours and usually returns to normal by 48 hours
     - CK–MB: myocardial necrosis is present if >15% of total CK; unlike CK, it is not affected by intramuscular injections

3 *Technetium pyrophosphate scanning*
   - It is performed from 24 hours to 14 days after onset.
   - It scans for 'hot spots', especially when a posterolateral AMI is suspected and ECG is unhelpful because of pre-existing LBBB.

4 *Echocardiography.* This is used to assist diagnosis when other tests are not diagnostic.

Note: The clinical diagnosis may be the most reliable, as the ECG and enzymes may be negative.

Management of acute coronary syndromes

General principles[11,12]

- Aim for immediate attendance if suspected.
- Pre-hospital: make diagnosis, assess risk, ensure stability. A 12-lead ECG should be arranged ASAP.
- Call a mobile coronary care unit.
- Achieve coronary perfusion and minimise infarct size.
- Prevent and treat cardiac arrest; have a defibrillator available to treat ventricular fibrillation.
- Optimal treatment is in a modern coronary care unit (if possible) with continuous ECG monitoring (first 48 hours) and a peripheral IV line (consider intranasal oxygen only if hypoxaemic <94% saturation).

- Pay careful attention to relief of pain and apprehension.
- Establish a caring empathy with the patient.
- Give aspirin as early as possible (if no contraindications): 300 mg chewed or dissolved sublingually.
- Prescribe a beta blocker and an ACE inhibitor early (if no contraindications).

Note: For a STEMI it is important to re-establish flow as soon as possible, usually by either thrombolytic therapy or primary angioplasty (preferably with stenting). Rescue angioplasty is usually used when large infarcts have not perfused at 60–90 minutes.[5]

Hospital management[5,11]

- As for first-line management.
- Confirm ECG diagnosis: STEMI or NSTEACS.
- Take blood for cardiac enzymes, particularly troponin levels, urea and electrolytes.
- Organise an urgent cardiology consultation for risk stratification and a decision whether to proceed to coronary angiography and coronary reperfusion with PCI (or CABG) or with thrombolysis.

Management of STEMI[12]

The optimal first-line treatment for the patient with a STEMI is urgent referral to a coronary catheter laboratory ideally within 60 minutes (the golden hour) of the onset of pain for assessment after coronary angiography for percutaneous transluminal coronary angioplasty (PTCA). If available and performed by an interventional cardiologist it has the best outcomes (level I evidence).

The principle is to achieve rapid reperfusion via primary angioplasty with a stent (optimal stent status currently under evaluation).

Adjunct therapy will include dual antiplatelet therapy—aspirin and a $P2Y_{12}$ inhibitor (clopidogrel, ticagrelor or prasugrel) and anticoagulation with low molecular weight heparin or unfractionated heparin, a statin and an ACE inhibitor.

Urgent reperfusion guidelines

- Within 60 minutes of symptom onset STEMI: PCI (optimal)
- Within 90 minutes of onset STEMI: PCI (acceptable)
- If these targets are not reached: fibrinolysis within 30 minutes of arrival

First-line management (e.g. outside hospital)

- Perform an ECG and classify ACS into STEMI or NSTEACS, and notify the medical facility that will receive the patient (discuss over the telephone). The ECG is the sole test required to select patients for emergency perfusion
- Oxygen 4–6 L/min only if hypoxaemic (aim to keep P_aO_2 >90%)
- Secure an IV line (withdraw blood for tests especially troponin levels)
- Glyceryl trinitrate (nitroglycerine) 300 mcg (½ tab) SL or spray 400 mcg (every 5 minutes as necessary to maximum of three doses). Beware of sildenafil (Viagra) and related drugs use and bradycardia—correct with atropine
- Aspirin 300 mg
- Morphine 2.5 mg IV statim bolus: then 1 mg/min every 5–10 mins until pain relief (up to 15 mg) (If feasible, it is preferable to give IV morphine 1 mg/min until relief of pain; this titration is easier in hospital.)

Management of NSTEACS

NSTEACS can progress to a STEMI; therefore all patients with NSTEACS should have ongoing monitoring in hospital and their risk stratified to direct management decisions.

Reperfusion therapy[13,14]

All patients with acute myocardial infarction should be considered for admission to a coronary care unit for monitoring and expert care. The decision of reperfusion therapy by PCI or fibrinolytic therapy will be determined by unit policy based on availability of PCI.

Fibrinolytic therapy

If angioplasty is unachievable either through timing or the unavailability of the service (such as in rural locations), thrombolysis is an indication for STEMI and the sooner the better, but preferably within 12 hours of the commencement of chest pain.[5,12] The decision should be made by an experienced consultant, especially as PCI is not usually possible once fibrinolytic therapy has been given.

Second-generation fibrin-specific agents (reteplase, alteplase or tenecteplase) are the agents of choice. Streptokinase can be used but it is inappropriate for use in Indigenous people and those who have received it on a previous occasion. There are several other contraindications for the use of fibrinolytic agents.

Further management strategies include:

- Full heparinisation for 24–36 hours (after rt-PA—not after streptokinase), especially for large anterior transmural infarction with risk of embolisation, supplemented by warfarin.
- Use LMW heparin (e.g. enoxaparin 1 mg/kg SC bd or unfractionated heparin 5000–7500 units SC 12-hourly).

Further management of STEMI (? myocardial infarction)

- Antiplatelet therapy: aspirin + clopidogrel
- Beta blocker (if no thrombolytic therapy or contraindications) as soon as possible:
  atenolol 25–100 mg (o) daily
  or
  metoprolol 25–100 mg (o) twice daily
- Consider glyceryl trinitrate IV infusion if pain recurs
- Start early introduction of ACE inhibitors (within 24–48 hours) in those with significant left ventricular (LV) dysfunction (and other indications)
- Statin therapy to lower cholesterol
- Treat hypokalaemia
- Consider magnesium sulphate (after thrombolysis)
- Consider frusemide

Post-AMI drug management

Proven:[1,12,13]

- beta blockers—within 12 hours
- ACE inhibitors—within 24 hours
- aspirin 75–150 mg and clopidogrel 75 mg (o) daily or both (alternatives to clopidogrel: ticagrelor or prasugrel)
- lipid-lowering drugs (e.g. statins)
- warfarin
  Targets:
- BP <140/90; TC <4 mmol/L; LDLC <2 mmol/L; TG <2 mmol/L

Ongoing management

- Education and counselling
- Bed rest 24–48 hours
- Continuing ECG monitoring
- Check serum potassium and magnesium
- Early mobilisation to full activity over 7–12 days
- Light diet
- Sedation
- Beta blocker (o): atenolol or metoprolol
- Anticoagulation where indicated (certainly if evidence of thrombus with echocardiography)
- ACE inhibitors for left ventricular failure and to prevent remodelling
- monitor psychological issues (e.g. anxiety)

On discharge

- Rehabilitation program
- Continued education and counselling
- No smoking
- Reduce weight
- Encourage consumption of omega-3 fatty acids
- Regular exercise, especially walking
- Exercise test (to be considered)
- Continue beta blockers for 2 years
- Continue ACE inhibitors
- Aspirin 100–300 mg daily and clopidogrel 75 mg daily
- Anticoagulation where indicated (at least 3 months)
- Statin therapy

Special management issues

Indications for coronary angiography

- Development of angina
- Strongly positive exercise test
- Consider after use of streptokinase

Management of the extensive infarction

- ACE inhibitors (even if no CCF)
- Radionuclide studies (to assess left ventricular function)
- Beta blockers (proven value in severe infarction) if no contraindications or LV dysfunction
- Anticoagulation

Treating and recognising complications of STEMI

Acute left ventricular failure

- Signs: basal crackles, extra (third or fourth) heart sounds, X-ray changes
- Treatment (according to severity) (refer to CHAPTER 88):
  - oxygen
  - diuretic (e.g. frusemide)
  - morphine IV
  - glyceryl trinitrate: IV, SL, (o) or topical
  - ACE inhibitors

Cardiogenic shock (a major hospital management procedure)

Requires early specialist intervention which may include:

- adrenaline—titrated to BP
- treat hypotension with inotropes
- intra-aortic balloon pump
- urgent angiography ± angioplasty/surgery

Pericarditis

This occurs in first few days after AMI (usually anterior AMI), with onset of sharp pain.

- Signs: pericardial friction rub
- Treatment:[9] anti-inflammatory medication (e.g. aspirin, indomethacin or ibuprofen for pain) with caution

  Note: Avoid anticoagulants.

Post-AMI syndrome (Dressler syndrome)

This occurs weeks or months later, usually around 6 weeks.

- Features: pericarditis, fever, pericardial effusion (an autoimmune response)
- Treatment: as for pericarditis

Left ventricular aneurysm

This is a late complication.

- Clinical: cardiac failure
- Features: arrhythmias, embolisation
- Signs: double ventricular impulse, fourth heart sound, visible bulge on X-ray
- Diagnosis: 2D electrocardiography
- Treatment:
  - antiarrhythmic drugs
  - anticoagulants
  - medication for cardiac failure
  - possible aneurysmectomy

Right ventricular infarction

This may accompany inferior MI and is life-threatening.

Ventricular septal rupture and mitral valve papillary rupture

This presents with severe cardiac failure and a loud pansystolic murmur. Both have a poor prognosis and early surgical intervention may be appropriate.

Cardiac arrhythmias

All types are common with STEMI and require treatment according to guidelines in CHAPTER 70. Methods may include defibrillation, cardioversion and pacemaking. Past infarct prophylaxis with IV lignocaine is not indicated.[5,15]

Anxiety and depression

Patients require anticipatory guidance and support including education, reassurance and counselling. If necessary, anxiolytic agents and antidepressants may help recovery.

Management of other serious spontaneous causes of chest pain

Aortic dissection

- Early definitive diagnosis is necessary: best achieved by transoesophageal echocardiography.
- 50% of patients are hypertensive; so need pharmacological control of hypertension with IV nitroprusside and beta blockers.
- Emergency surgery needed for many, especially for type A (ascending aorta involved).

Note: There is an increased incidence during pregnancy.

Pulmonary embolus

Investigations to diagnose suspected pulmonary embolus (choose from):[4,17,18]

- chest X-ray and ECG
- CT pulmonary angiography (first-line study)
- radionucleide imaging—the ventilation/perfusion (V/Q) study
- digital subtraction angiography
- D-dimer assay—useful but not specific
- Doppler sonography of lower limbs
- arterial blood gases
- Wells score: if >3, highly probable; if >6, diagnostic

Management (specialist care)

Needs supportive medical care and anticoagulation:

heparin IV: 5000 U as immediate bolus, continuous infusion 30 000 U over 24 hours or 12 500 U (sc) bd
or
low molecular weight heparin

Note: The dose of heparin should then be adjusted daily to maintain the APTT at between 1.5 and 2 times control, or INR >2.

- Continue heparin 5–10 days.
- Warfarin (o) after 3–4 days or immediate; then continue heparin for 3 days after international normalised ratio (INR) at desired level.

Note: Thrombolytic therapy either IV or into the pulmonary artery can be used for major embolism. Surgical embolectomy is rarely necessary but needed if very extensive.

Pneumothorax

- Most episodes resolve spontaneously without drainage (at least 20% lung collapse).
- Drainage of the pleural space indicated for a large pneumothorax >25% pleural area, with persistent dyspnoea.
- Guidelines:
  - <25% collapse, no symptoms: observe
  - <25% collapse + persisting symptoms: drain
  - >25% collapse: usually drain
- For recurrent attacks, excision of cysts or pleurodesis may be necessary.
- Statistics indicate a 30–50% recurrence rate of spontaneous pneumothorax (most within 12 months), 35% on the same side, 10–15% on the opposite side. Recurrence should not recur after a pleurodesis where the lung surface has been rendered adherent to the chest wall.

Acute tension pneumothorax

For urgent cases insert a 12–16 gauge needle into the pleural space through the second intercostal space on the affected side. Replace with a formal intercostal catheter connected to underwater seal drainage.

Treatment of oesophageal disorders

Gastro-oesophageal reflux

- Achieve normal weight if overweight.
- Avoid coffee, alcohol and spicy foods.
- Avoid large meals and overeating (keep to small meals).
- Use antacids or alginate compounds (e.g. Gaviscon, Mylanta Plus).
- If persistent:

  acid suppression—H_2-receptor blockers (e.g. cimetidine, ranitidine)

  or

  proton-pump inhibitors (e.g. omeprazole)

40

Oesophageal spasm[19]

Long-acting nitrates (e.g. isosorbide dinitrate 10 mg tds)

or

Calcium-channel blockers (e.g. nifedipine CR 20–30 mg once daily)

Note: Attend to lifestyle and dietary factors, as for reflux.

Musculoskeletal causes of chest wall pain

There are many musculoskeletal causes, most of which can be eliminated by the history and physical examination. Some of the causes listed in TABLE 40.9 are very uncommon and often part of a general disorder, such as ankylosing spondylitis. Muscular tears or strains of the chest wall are quite common. A differential diagnosis is a fractured rib including a cough fracture.

Table 40.9 Musculoskeletal causes/origins of chest wall pain (front and back)

Injury to thoracic spine → dysfunction
Vertebral fracture:
- trauma
- pathological:
  - osteoporosis
  - metastatic disease
  - multiple myeloma

Intercostal muscle strains/tears
Rib disorders:
- fractures
- slipping rib

Costochondritis
Tietze syndrome
Fibromyalgia

Musculoskeletal chest pain is typically aggravated or provoked by movements such as stretching, deep inspiration, sneezing and coughing. The pain tends to be sharp and stabbing in quality but can have a constant aching quality.

Costochondritis is a common cause of anterior pain, which is generally well localised to the costochondral junction and may also be a component of an inflammatory disorder, such as one of the spondyloarthropathies.

Management is generally conservative with analgesics, gentle massage with analgesic creams and NSAIDs if there is an inflammatory component. Other measures that can help for very painful chest wall problems are localised injections of local anaesthetic with or without corticosteroids (with care not to penetrate the parietal pleura) and a modified support (especially for rib injuries) in the form of a special elasticised rib belt (called a universal rib belt) that gives excellent support and symptom relief while permitting adequate lung expansion.

Posterior chest (thoracic back) pain

Disorders of the musculoskeletal system represent the most common cause of thoracic (dorsal) back pain, especially dysfunction of the joints of the thoracic spine. Refer to CHAPTER 37 for more detail. Probably the commonest cause is costovertebral dysfunction caused by overstress of rib articulations with vertebrae (the costovertebral joints). This fact is clearly demonstrated with the midline thoracic back pain following cardiac surgery when these joints are compressed during sternotomy and splaying of the chest walls.

The back pain may be associated with simultaneous referred anterior chest pain or abdominal pain (see FIG. 37.3 in CHAPTER 37).

Acute thoracic back pain

Although posterior pain is invariably caused by vertebral dysfunction, there are several other important causes, including serious bone disease (leading to compression fractures) and life-threatening visceral and vascular causes. Refer to red flag pointers and TABLE 37.3 and management guidelines in CHAPTER 37.

Note:

- Intervertebral disc protrusions are rare in the thoracic spine.
- Rarely, a penetrating peptic ulcer can present with mid to lower thoracic back pain.

When to refer

- Obvious or suspected myocardial infarction, especially with extensive infarction
- Transfer to major centre with complications of AMI:
  - rupture of septum or papillary muscle
  - aneurysm
  - refractory arrhythmias
  - cardiogenic shock
- Patients with persistent post-infarction angina
- Angina:
  - patient with angina not responding to drug treatment
  - patient with unstable angina
  - angina lasting for longer than 15 minutes (unresponsive to sublingual nitrate) needs urgent hospital admission
- Suspected or proven pulmonary embolus or dissecting aneurysm or other serious life-threatening problem (after initial first-line measures, e.g. decompression of tension pneumothorax)
- Suspected oesophageal or other gastrointestinal disorder (e.g. duodenal ulcer), for endoscopy or appropriate gastroenterological evaluation

Practice tips

- All sudden acute chest pain is cardiac (and potentially fatal) until proven otherwise.
- A careful history is the basis of the diagnosis.
- Mitral valve prolapse is often an undiagnosed cause of chest pain: keep it in mind, especially if pain is recurrent and intermittent (proved by echocardiography).
- Calcium antagonists can cause peripheral oedema, so be careful not to attribute this to heart failure.
- The pain of oesophageal spasm can be very severe and mimic myocardial infarction.
- Oesophageal spasm responds to glyceryl trinitrate: do not confuse with angina.
- Intervertebral disc protrusions are a very rare cause of severe sudden thoracic pain (T2–9).
- Infective endocarditis can cause pleuritic posterior chest pain.
- Family doctors need to monitor carefully patients who are taking anticoagulants. The INR ratio, which needs to be kept between 2 and 3, should be tested at least monthly.
- The sudden onset of dyspnoea without chest pain can occur frequently with (painless) myocardial infarction and pulmonary embolism.
- If a patient recovering from an AMI suddenly develops shortness of breath, consider ventricular septal rupture, mitral valve papillary rupture (with mitral regurgitation), pulmonary embolus and other serious complications.
- Treat (indefinitely) all post-MI patients with ACE inhibitors, and all post-MI and acute ischaemic syndrome patients with beta blockers.[15,16]
- Use antiplatelet agents indefinitely—100–300 mg aspirin daily or, if contraindicated, clopidogrel 75 mg daily or warfarin. Some studies favour combining aspirin and clopidogrel.

Patient education resources

Hand-out sheets from *Murtagh's Patient Education* 7th edition:

- Angina
- Cardiovascular (including coronary) risk factors

References

1. Juergens C. Chest pain: how to treat. Australian Doctor, 2005; 2 September: 27–34.
2. Than M, Cullen L et al. 2-hour accelerated diagnostic protocol to assess patients with chest pain symptoms using contemporary troponins as the only biomarker: the ADAPT trial. J Am Coll Cardiol, 2012; 59 (23): 2091–8.
3. Management of unstable angina guidelines 2000. Med J Aust, 2000; 173 (8): Suppl.
4. Worsnop C, Pierce R. Pleuritic chest pain. Medicine Today, 2005; 6 (3): 53–60.
5. Expert group for Cardiovascular. Acute chest pain. In: eTG complete [Internet]. Melbourne: Therapeutic Guidelines Ltd. Available from: <www.tg.org.au>, accessed May 2017.
6. Selbst S, Ruddy R, Clark B et al. Paediatric chest pain: a prospective study. Paediatrics, 1988; 82: 319–23.
7. Reynolds JL. Precordial catch syndrome in children. Southern Medical Journal, 1989; 82 (10): 1228–30.
8. Kennedy RD, Andrews GR, Mitchell JRA. Ischaemic heart disease in the elderly. British Heart Journal, 1977; 39: 1121–7.
9. Caspari P. Angina pectoris. In: *MIMS Disease Index* (2nd edn). Sydney: IMS Publishing, 1996: 35–8.
10. Kumar P, Clark M. *Clinical Medicine.* London: Saunders, 2003: 769–74.
11. Psaltis P. Management of acute coronary syndrome. In: Monash University: update course notes, 2013: 2–20.
12. Aroney C, Aylward P (Co-chairs). Guidelines for the management of acute coronary syndromes 2006. Med J Aust, 2006; 184 (8): Suppl.
13. Acute Coronary Syndromes Working Group. Guidelines for the management of acute coronary syndromes. MJA, 2006; 184 (8): S1–S30. © 2006. The Medical Journal of Australia—reproduced with permission.
14. Chew DP, Aroney C, Aylward P et al. 2011 Addendum to the National Heart Foundation of Australia/Cardiac Society of Australia and New Zealand Guidelines for the management of acute coronary syndromes (ACS) 2006. Heart Lung Circ, 2011; 20 (8): 487–502.
15. Barton S (ed.). *Clinical Evidence.* London. BMJ Publishing Group, 2001: 8–23.
16. American Heart Association guidelines for myocardial ischaemia. Circulation, 2001; 104: 1577–9.
17. Rashford S. Acute pleuritic chest pain. Aust Fam Physician, 2001; 30 (9): 841–5.
18. Lau L. *Imaging Guidelines* (4th edn). Melbourne: RANZC Radiologists, 2001: 70.
19. Expert group for Gastrointestinal. Oesophageal disorder. In: eTG complete [Internet]. Melbourne: Therapeutic Guidelines Ltd. Available from: <www.tg.org.au>, accessed Sept 2017.

Constipation

41

I have finally kum to the konklusion, that a good reliable set of bowels iz wurth more tu a man, than enny quantity of brains.

HENRY SHAW (1818–85), *JOSH BILLINGS*

Constipation is the difficult passage of small hard stools. The Rome III criteria define it has having two or more of the following, for at least 12 weeks:

- infrequent passage of stools <3/week
- passage of lumpy or hard stools at least 25% of time
- straining >25% of time
- sensation of incomplete evacuation >25% of time
- use of manual manoeuvres >25% of time
- sensation of anorectal obstruction/blockage >25% of time

Accordingly it affects more than 1 in 5 in the population.[1]

However, the emphasis should be on the consistency of the stool rather than on the frequency of defecation; for example, a person passing a hard stool with difficulty once or twice a day is regarded as constipated, but the person who passes a soft stool comfortably every two or three days is not constipated. Various causes of chronic constipation are summarised in FIGURE 41.1.

Key facts and checkpoints

- The survey showed 10% of adults and 6% of children reported constipation in the preceding 2 weeks.[1]
- Up to 20% of British adults take regular laxatives.[2]
- Constipation from infancy may be due to Hirschsprung disorder.
- Diet is the single most important factor in preventing constipation.
- Beware of the recent onset of constipation in the middle-aged and the elderly.
- Bleeding suggests cancer, haemorrhoids, diverticular disorder and inflammatory bowel disease.
- Unusually shaped stools (small pellets or ribbon-like) suggest irritable bowel syndrome.
- Always examine the abdomen and rectum.
- Plain abdominal X-rays are generally not useful in the diagnosis of chronic constipation.
- The flexible sigmoidoscope is far superior to the rigid sigmoidoscope in investigation of the lower bowel.
- Intractable constipation (obstipation) is a challenge at both ends of the age spectrum but improved agents have helped with management.

A diagnostic approach

Using the diagnostic strategy model (see TABLE 41.1), the five self-posed questions can be answered as follows.

Probability diagnosis

The commonest is 'idiopathic' constipation where there is no structural or systemic disease. This is also referred to as 'functional' constipation.

Probably the most frequent single factor causing constipation in Western society is deficiency in dietary fibre, including fruit, green leafy vegetables and wholemeal products. The amount of fibre in our diet is directly related to stool weight and to colonic transit time. The average colonic transit time in the large bowel for Westerners is 60 hours; for a rural African on a very high-fibre diet it is 30 hours. Other compounding factors are dehydration, lack of physical activity and inappropriate bowel habits. Constipation is also a common problem in pregnancy.

Serious disorders not to be missed

Neoplasia

It is obvious that colonic or anorectal neoplasms must not be missed in a patient, especially middle-aged or elderly, presenting with constipation or other change in bowel habit. Most cases present with either complete or incomplete bowel obstruction.

Extrinsic malignancy, such as lymphoma or ovarian cancer, compressing or invading the rectum, also has to be considered. Cancer of the large bowel is most prevalent in our society and appropriate

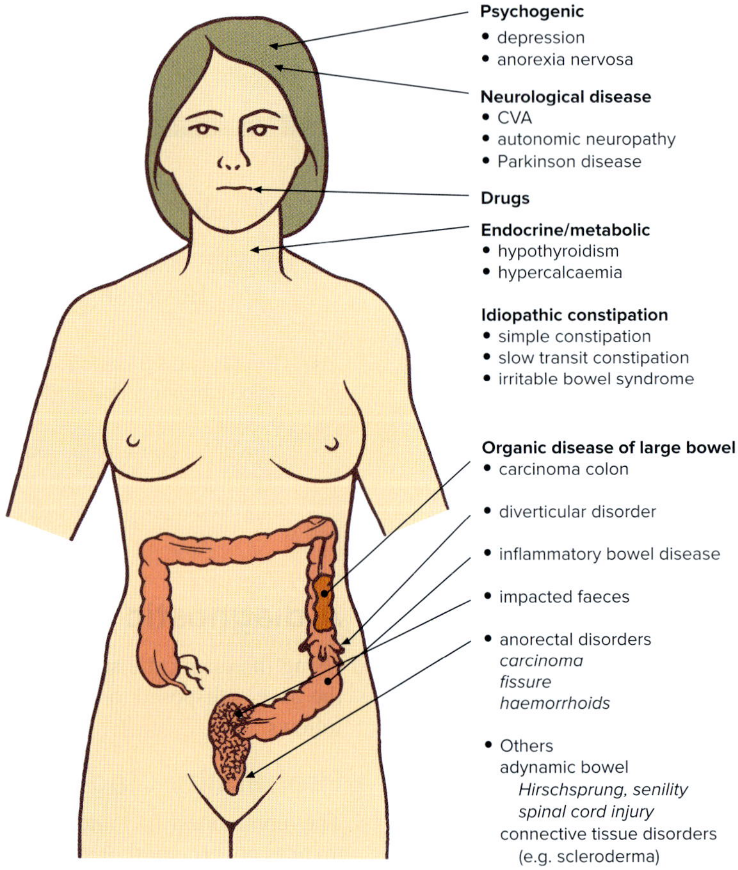

FIGURE 41.1 Causes of chronic constipation

screening examinations, including rectal examination, sigmoidoscopy and colonoscopy, must be considered where appropriate.

Megacolon

In children it is important to detect the presence of megacolon, for example megacolon secondary to Hirschsprung disorder. Symptoms dating from birth suggest Hirschsprung disorder, which occasionally may present for the first time in adult life.

Neurological disorders

Constipation, often with faecal impaction, is a common accompaniment to paraplegia, multiple sclerosis, cerebral palsy and autonomic neuropathy.

Alarm symptoms

- Recent constipation in >40 years of age
- Rectal bleeding
- Family history of cancer

Pitfalls

The pitfalls can be summarised as follows:

- impacted faeces
- depressive illness
- purgative abuse
- local anal lesions
- drugs

Although patients with impacted faeces usually present with spurious diarrhoea, it is a form of idiopathic constipation and is very commonly encountered in general practice, especially in bedridden elderly people.

Anal pain or stenosis, such as fissure-in-ano, thrombosed haemorrhoids, perianal haematoma or ischiorectal abscess, leads to constipation when the patient is hesitant to defecate.

General pitfalls and tips

- Ensure the patient is truly constipated, and not having unreal expectations of regularity.
- Ensure that the anthraquinone group of laxatives, including 'Ford pills', is never used long term

because they cause melanosis coli and associated megacolon.

- Be very wary of alternating constipation and diarrhoea (e.g. colon cancer).
- In a busy practice be careful not to let 'familiarity breed contempt' (e.g. onset of hyperparathyroidism, cancer).
- Avoid relying solely on the rectal examination to exclude cancer.

Seven masquerades checklist

Three of the primary masquerades (see TABLE 41.1) are important causes of constipation, namely drugs, depression and hypothyroidism. Many drugs (see TABLE 41.2) may be associated with constipation, especially codeine and its derivatives, antidepressants, aluminium and calcium antacids. A careful drug history is thus mandatory. Fortunately the constipation is usually relieved once the drug is withdrawn. Constipation can be a significant symptom in all types of depressive illness and may be aggravated by treatment with antidepressants.

The metabolic causes of constipation include hypothyroidism, hypercalcaemia and porphyria. We occasionally encounter the patient with hypercalcaemia, for example, hyperparathyroidism, but thyroid dysfunction is relatively common in general practice.

Table 41.1 Chronic constipation: diagnostic strategy model
Probability diagnosis
Functional constipation[3] • primary—slow transit, dyssynergic defecation • lifestyle—diet, low fluids, bad habits
Serious disorders not to be missed
Intrinsic neoplasia: colon, rectum or anus, especially colon cancer Extrinsic malignancy (e.g. lymphoma, ovary) Hirschsprung (children)
Pitfalls (often missed)
Impacted faeces Local anal lesions, e.g. fissure, haemorrhoids Drug/purgative abuse Hypokalaemia Depressive illness Acquired megacolon Diverticular disease Stricture, e.g. Crohn disease *Rarities:* • lead poisoning • hypercalcaemia • hyperparathyroidism • dolichocolon (large colon)/megarectum • Chagas disease • neuromuscular, e.g. systemic sclerosis
Seven masquerades checklist
Depression Diabetes (autonomic neuropathy) Drugs (TABLE 41.2) Thyroid disorder (hypo); hyperparathyroidism Spinal dysfunction (severe only)
Is the patient trying to tell me something?
May be functional (e.g. depression, anorexia nervosa).

Table 41.2 Drugs associated with constipation
Analgesics (inhibitors of prostaglandin synthesis)
Antacids (containing calcium carbonate or aluminium hydroxide)
Anticholinergic agents, antispasmodics
Antidiarrhoeal agents
Antiepileptics
Antihistamines (H_1-receptor blockers)*
Antiparkinson drugs*
Antipsychotic drugs,* e.g. clozapine, risperidone
Barbiturates
Barium sulphate
Benzodiazepines
Calcium-channel blockers (verapamil)
Calcium supplements
Cholestyramine
Clonidine
Cough mixtures
Cytotoxic drugs
Diuretics that cause hypokalaemia
Gabapentin
Ganglionic blocking agents
Heavy metal (especially lead)
5-HT_3 receptor antagonists e.g. ondansetron
Iron supplements
Laxatives (chronic use)
Monoamine oxidase inhibitors
Muscle relaxants
Opioid analgesics (e.g. codeine)
SSRIs
Tricyclic antidepressants*

* Denotes anticholinergic effect.

41

Diabetes rarely can be associated with constipation when an autonomic neuropathy can lead to alternating bouts of constipation and diarrhoea.

Psychogenic considerations

Constipation may be a manifestation of an underlying functional problem and psychiatric disorder, such as depression, anorexia nervosa, schizophrenia or drug abuse. Drug abuse must always be considered, keeping in mind that narcotics and laxatives present with rebound constipation. More commonly, it may reflect the inactive lifestyle of the patient and provide a good opportunity for appropriate counselling.

The clinical approach

History

It is important to ask patients to define exactly what they mean by constipation. Somc people believe that just as the earth rotates on its axis once a day, so should their bowels open daily to ensure good health. As always, a careful history is appropriate, including stool consistency, frequency, ease of evacuation, pain on defecation and the presence of blood or mucus. A dietary history is very relevant in the context of constipation.

Key questions

- How often do you go to the toilet?
- What are your bowel motions like?
- Are they bulky, hard, like rabbit pellets or soft?
- Is there pain on opening your bowels?
- Have you noticed any blood?
- Have you noticed any lumps?
- Do you have any soiling on your underwear?
- How do you feel in yourself?
- What medications are you taking?

Diary

Ask the patient to keep a 10-day diary recording frequency and nature of stools, and whether any difficulty was experienced when passing stool.

Examination

41

The important aspects are abdominal palpation and rectal examination. Palpation may reveal the craggy mass of a neoplasm, faecal retention (especially in the thin patient) or a tender spastic colon. The perianal region should be examined for localised disease. The patient should be asked to bear down to demonstrate perianal descent, haemorrhoids or mucosal prolapse. Perianal sensation and the anal reflex should be tested. Digital rectal examination is mandatory, and may reveal a rectal tumour and faecal impaction, as well as testing for rectal size and tone. If there is a history from infancy, a normal or narrow rectum suggests congenital megacolon (Hirschsprung disorder) but, if dilated, acquired megacolon.

General signs that may be significant in the diagnosis of constipation are summarised in FIGURE 41.2.

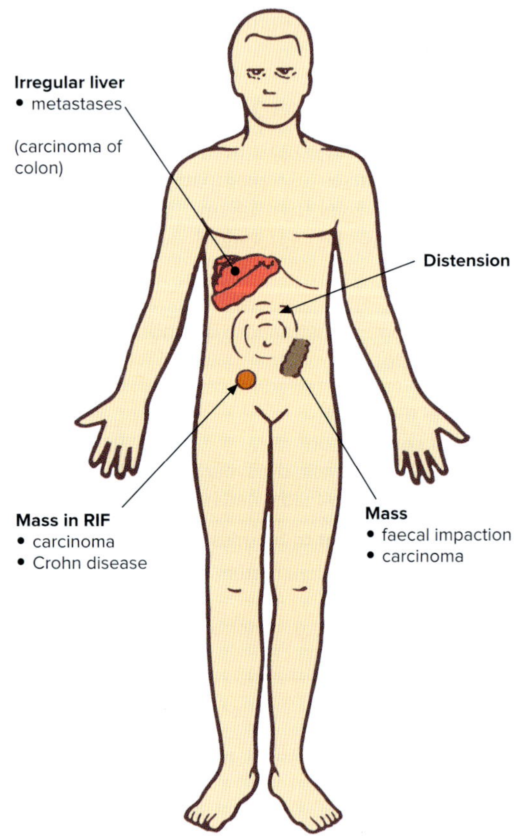

FIGURE 41.2 Possible significant abdominal signs in the patient with constipation

Rectal examination

The most important first step is to *do* the examination.

Method

- Explain to the patient what will happen.
- After inspection with the patient in the left lateral position and with knees drawn up, a lubricated gloved index finger is placed over the anus.
- Part the buttocks.
- Ask the patient to concentrate on slow deep breathing.
- With gentle backwards pressure the finger is then inserted slowly into the anal canal and then into the rectum (it helps patient comfort if they push down or squeeze to accommodate the finger).

- Rotate the finger anteriorly to feel the prostate in males and the cervix in females.
- The finger will reach to about 7–8 cm with gentle thrusting into the perineum.
- Gently withdraw the finger and examine the whole circumference of the rectum by sweeping the finger from posterior on both sides.

Points to note

- Any pain: fissure, proctitis, excoriation from diarrhoea (a rectal examination will not be possible in the presence of a fissure)
- Induration from a chronic fissure or fistula in the anal canal
- The sphincter tone
- The nature of the faeces (? impaction)
- The rectal wall: cancer is usually indurated, elevated and ulcerated; a villous adenoma has a soft velvety feel
- Posteriorly: the sacrum and coccyx
- Laterally: the side walls of the pelvis
- Anteriorly: cervix and pouch of Douglas in the female; prostate and rectovesical pouch in the male

Prostate examination

- It feels larger if the patient has a full bladder.
- The normal prostate is a firm smooth rubbery bilobed structure (with a central sulcus) about 3 cm in diameter.
- A craggy hard mass suggests cancer.
- An enlarged smooth mass suggests benign hypertrophy.
- A tender, nodular or boggy mass suggests prostatitis.

Practice tip on treatment

A suitable method of doing a rectal examination on a home visit (in the absence of gloves in the doctor's bag) is to apply moist soap around the finger and caked under the nail (in case of breakage), then plastic wrap and finally petroleum jelly (e.g. Vaseline).

Before resorting to a good old-fashioned '3H' enema (hot water, high and a hell of a lot), use a sorbitol compound (e.g. Microlax 5 mL enema). It can be carried in the doctor's bag, is very easy to insert and is most effective.

A common pitfall

In the female, the cervix or a vaginal tampon can be mistaken for a mobile extrarectal tumour.

Endoscopy

Sigmoidoscopy—in particular, flexible sigmoidoscopy with examination of the rectosigmoid—is important in excluding local disease; search for abnormalities such as blood, mucus or neoplasia. The insufflation of air sometimes reproduces the pain of the irritable bowel syndrome.

It is worth noting that 60% of polyps and cancers will occur in the first 60 cm of the bowel[4] and diverticular disorder should be evident with the flexible sigmoidoscope.

The presence of melanosis coli is an important sign—it may give a pointer to the duration of the constipation and the consequent chronic intake (perhaps denied) of anthraquinone laxatives.

Investigations

These can be summarised as follows:

- Haematological:
  - haemoglobin
  - ESR
- Stools for occult blood
- Biochemistry (where suspected):
  - thyroid function tests
  - serum calcium
  - serum potassium
  - carcinoembryonic antigen (a tumour marker)
- Radiological:
  - CT colonography (virtual colonography)
  - double contrast barium enema (especially for primary colonic disease, e.g. megacolon)
  - bowel transit studies, using radio-opaque shapes taken orally and checking progress by abdominal X-ray or stool collection
- Physiological tests:
  - anal manometry—test anal tone
  - rectal sensation and compliance, using an inflatable rectal balloon
  - dynamic proctography, to determine disorders of defecation
  - Rectal biopsy, to determine aganglionia

Idiopathic constipation

It is best to classify idiopathic constipation into three subgroups:

1. simple constipation
2. slow transit constipation
3. normal transit constipation (irritable bowel syndrome)

Of these, the commonest is simple constipation, which is essentially related to a faulty diet and bad habit.

Avery Jones,[7] who defined the disorder, describes it as being due to one or more of the following causes:

- faulty diet—inadequate dietary fibre
- neglect of the call to stool
- unfavourable living and working conditions
- lack of exercise
- travel

Dyschezia, or lazy bowel, is the term used to describe a rectum that has become unresponsive to faecal content, and this usually follows repeated ignoring of calls to defecate.

Slow transit constipation occurs primarily in women with an apparently normal colon, despite a high-fibre intake and lack of the other causes described by Avery Jones. Many are young, with a history dating from early childhood or, more commonly, adolescence. Constipation may follow childbirth, uncomplicated abdominal surgery or a period of severe dieting. However, in the majority no precipitating cause is evident.

A *defecatory disorder* is where there is a paradoxical contraction rather than normal relaxation of the anal sphincter and associated muscles responsible for evacuation. Also known as dyssynergic dysfunction.

Management

Most patients have simple constipation and require reassurance and education once an organic cause has been excluded. Encourage modification of lifestyle.

Advice to patients

- Adequate exercise, especially walking, is important.
- Develop good habit: answer the call to defecate as soon as possible. Develop the 'after breakfast habit'. Allow time for a good relaxed breakfast and then sit on the toilet. Don't miss meals—food stimulates motility.
- Avoid laxatives and codeine compounds (tablets or mixture).
- Take plenty of fluids, especially water and fruit juices (e.g. prune juice).
- Eat an optimal bulk diet. Eat foods that provide bulk and roughage, such as vegetables and salads, cereals (especially wheat fibre), fresh and dried fruits, and wholemeal bread. Enough fibre should be taken to convert stools that sink to stools that float.

Examples of food with good bulk properties are presented in TABLE 41.3.[8] Fruit has good fibre, especially in the skin, and some have natural laxatives (e.g. prunes, figs, rhubarb, apricots).

41

Table 41.3 Foods with bulk-forming properties (from least to most)

Potato
Banana
Cauliflower
Peas
Cabbage
Lettuce
Apple
Carrot
Bran

Treatment (pharmaceutical preparations)

Some patients may not tolerate unprocessed bran but tolerate pharmaceutical preparations better (see TABLE 41.4). An appropriate choice would be one of the hydrophilic bulk-forming agents such as ispaghula or psyllium. Avoid stimulant laxatives except for short sharp treatments.

First-line therapy[6]

Use a general bulking agent e.g. psyllium or ispaghula granules 1–2 teaspoonsful (o) once or twice daily, or Benefiber® 2 teaspoonsful (o) twice daily.

Second-line therapy

Use an osmotic laxative or a fibre-based stimulant preparation e.g. macrogol 3350 + 1–2 sachets, each dissolved in 125 mL water once daily

or

lactulose syrup, 15–30 mL (o) daily until response, then 10–20 mL daily

or

dried fruits with senna leaf (Nu-Lax) 10 g nocte

or

docusate + senna (50–80 mg), 1–2 tabs nocte

Third-line therapy

(Recheck cause.)

Magnesium sulphate 1–2 teaspoons (15 g) in water once or twice daily (if normal kidney function)

or

as capsules (Colocap Balance) 15 caps over 15 minutes

or

combined bulking/stimulating agent (e.g. frangula/sterculia [Normacol plus])

or

glycerin suppository (retain for 15–20 minutes)

or
sodium citrate or phosphate enema (e.g. Fleet Enema)
or
Microlax enema

Constipation in children

Constipation is quite common in children but no cause has been discovered in up to 95%. The most common factor is diet. Constipation often begins after weaning or with the introduction of cow's milk. It is rare with breastfeeding. Low fibre intake and a family history of constipation may be associated factors.[5] Most children develop normal bowel control by 4 years of age (excluding any physical abnormality). It is normal to have a bowel movement every 2–3 days, providing it is of normal consistency and is not painful.

It is important to differentiate between encopresis and constipation:

Constipation usually appears between 2 and 4 years of age, and up to a third of primary school-aged children will report constipation over a 12-month period. In toddlers, the gender distribution is equal, but by age 5, boys are more likely to get constipation than girls, with the frequency of faecal incontinence three times higher in boys.

Constipation in children is defined as having two or more of the following over the previous 2 months:

- <3 bowel motions per week
- >1 episode of faecal incontinence per week (previously referred to as encopresis)
- large stools in rectum or palpable on abdominal examination
- retentive posturing (e.g. 'stiff as a board' standing/lying, tip toes, crossed legs, braces against furniture) and withholding behaviour (e.g. refuses, hides, requests nappy, denies need to go)
- painful defecation

Faecal incontinence, which is a consequence of chronic constipation, is the passage of stool in an inappropriate place in children who have been toilet trained. It can present as soiling, due to faecal retention with overflow of liquid faeces (spurious diarrhoea) aka encopresis.

Constipation is nearly always functional (>95%),[6] though the GP should check for any red flags for a pathological cause (see below). The key feature in functional constipation is chronic faecal retention leading to rectal dilatation and insensitivity to the normal defecation reflex.

Table 41.4 Therapeutic agents (laxatives) to treat constipation (with examples)

Hydrophilic bulk-forming agents
Psyllium mucilloid (Agiofibe, Metamucil)
Sterculia (Granocol, Normacol)
Ispaghula (Agiolax, Fybogel)
Methylcellulose
Wheat bran/dextrin (Benefiber)
Crude fibre (Fibyrax Extra)
Stimulant (irritant) laxatives
Sodium picosulfate
Anthraquinones: senna (Senokot/Sennetabs), senna with dried fruits (Nu-Lax), sennosides A and B; cascara
Frangula bark (in Normacol Plus)
Castor oil
Triphenylmethanes: bisacodyl (e.g. Dulcolax); picsulfate
Osmotic laxatives
Macrogol 3350 with electrolytes (e.g. Movicol)
Magnesium sulphate (Epsom salts/Colocap Balance)
Magnesium hydroxide (milk of magnesia)
Lactulose (several agents)
Mannitol
Sodium phosphate mixture
Sorbitol (Sorbilax)
Saline laxatives
Stool-softening/lubricating agents
Liquid paraffin (Agarol)
Docusate—poor evidence of efficacy
Poloxamer
Glycerin suppositories
Sorbital/sodium compounds (Microlax)
Laxatives in suppository form
Glycerin/glycerol suppository
Sorbitol sodium compounds (e.g. Fleet Enema)
Sodium phosphate enema (e.g. Fleet)
Stimulant microenema or suppository (e.g. Bisa-lax)
Stool-softener microenema (e.g. Enamax)
Prokinetic agent
Prucalopride

Note: ColonLYTELY used for colonoscopy preparation contains macrogol, sodium sulphate and other mineral salts

Red flag pointers for organic causes

- Blood in stools
- Perianal disease
- Fever
- Weight loss/delayed growth
- Delayed meconium/thin strip-like stools
- Vomiting
- Urinary symptoms
- Abnormal neurological findings in legs
- Medications used for children with behavioural/developmental issues

Normally the rectum is empty just prior to defecation; with faecal retention, the rectum is stretched, weak and numb and it can leak.

Other important conditions

Hirschsprung disorder:

- consider if delay in passing first meconium stool and subsequent constipation

Anal fissure in infants:

- consider if stool hard and associated with pain or bleeding
- the mainstay of treatment is dietary manipulation

Principles of treatment of functional constipation[5,6]

- Encourage relaxed child–parent interaction with toilet training, such as appropriate encouragement, 'after breakfast habit' training, regular toileting (where possible), three times/day for 3–5 minutes, reinforce desired behaviour with stickers on an age-appropriate chart.
- Introduce psychotherapy or behaviour modification program, especially where 'fear of the toilet' exists.
- Establish an empty bowel: remove any severely impacted faeces with microenemas (e.g. Microlax), and even disimpaction under anaesthesia if necessary. A good guide if faecal 'rocks' are visible on X-ray.
- Advice for parents of children over 18 months:
  - Drink ample non-milk fluids each day—several glasses of water, unsweetened fruit juice (be cautious of cow's milk).
  - Use prune juice, which contains sorbitol.
  - Get regular exercise—walking, running, outside games or sport.
  - Provide high-fibre foods—high-fibre cereals, wholegrain bread, brown rice, wholemeal pasta, fresh fruit with skins left on where possible, dried fruits such as sultanas, apricots or prunes, fresh vegetables.
- Advice on correct posture and position—'how to do a poo':[5]
  - Feet supported (e.g. with a foot stool)
  - Knees higher than bottom and apart
  - Leaning forward with elbows on knees
  - Encourage child to push out stomach
  - Ensure privacy (including at preschool/school)
- Laxatives—if constipation has been brief in duration, treat for 3 months, but for chronic constipation, treat for 6 months minimum.
- Can use macrogol 3350 (Movicol), paraffin oil or lactulose.
- For acute faecal impaction, high-dose laxatives can be used until liquid stools are achieved, and then revert back to maintenance treatment. Enemas are suitable only for children with acute severe rectal pain or distress and are rarely required.
- Use a pharmaceutical preparation as a last resort to achieve regularity.

First line:[6]

- paraffin oil (e.g. Parachoc): RCT evidence indicates suitable and better than stimulant laxative

  or

  osmotic laxative (e.g. lactulose): 1–3 mg/kg
  - 1–5 years: 10 mL per day
  - >5 years: 15 mL per day

  or

  macrogol 3350 with electrolytes:
  - 2–12 years: 1 sachet Movicol-Half in 60 mL water once daily
  - >12 years: 1 sachet Movicol (or 2 Movicol-Half) daily

Severe constipation/faecal impaction:

- consider admission to hospital
- abdominal X-ray
- macrogol 3350 with electrolytes (double above doses and water)
- Microlax enema

If unsuccessful, add ColonLYTELY via nasogastric tube *or* sodium phosphate enema (Fleet Enema) (not <2 years).

Constipation in the elderly

Constipation is a common problem in the elderly, with a tendency for idiopathic constipation to increase with age. In addition, the chances of organic disease increase with age, especially colorectal cancer, so this problem requires attention in the older patient. Faecal impaction is a special problem in the aged confined largely to bed. Constipation is often associated with Parkinson disease. In the elderly, an osmotic laxative such as sorbitol or lactulose may be required for long-standing refractory constipation, but stimulant and other non-osmotic laxatives should be avoided.

Faecal impaction

This is a difficult problem, especially in the older person who may not be aware of the problem especially if they have spurious diarrhoea. Symptoms include malaise, anorexia and nausea, confusion, headache,

41

abdominal discomfort ± colic and bloating, a sense of inadequate defecation and frequent amounts of small stool. Complications include spurious diarrhoea, faecal incontinence, bowel obstruction, urinary incontinence or retention. It often follows opioid medication. Confirm with rectal examination ± plain X-ray of abdomen. Treat with oral or osmotic laxatives (e.g. 8 sachets of macrogol 3350 for 3 days with or without rectal suppositories) or enema, e.g. Fleet Enema, Microlax.

Manual disimpaction

If manual disimpaction should be necessary, the unpleasant procedure can be rendered virtually odourless if the products are 'milked' or scooped directly into a container of water. A large plastic cover helps restrict the permeation of the smell.

Discomfort and embarrassment are reduced by this method and by adequate premedication (e.g. IV midazolam and IV fentanyl) if large faecaliths are present.

Colorectal cancer

General features

- Commonest GIT malignancy
- Second most common cause of death from cancer in Western society
- Generally men over 50 years (90% of all cases)
- Mortality rate about 60%
- Good prognosis if diagnosed early
- Two-thirds in descending colon and rectum

Refer to section on genetics of colorectal cancer (see CHAPTER 18).

Predisposing factors

- Ulcerative colitis (long-standing)
- Familial: familial adenomatous polyposis (FAP), hereditary non-polyposis colorectal cancer
- Colonic adenomata
- Decreased dietary fibre
- Age >50 years

Lifetime risk

This is determined by the family history (see TABLE 41.5).

Consider referral to a familial cancer clinic for assessment.

Table 41.5 Family history and lifetime risk of colorectal cancer[5]

Family history	Lifetime risk
None: population risk	1:50
One first-degree relative >45 years	1:17
One first-degree relative and one second-degree relative	1:12
One first-degree relative <45 years	1:10
Two first-degree relatives (any age)	1:6
Hereditary non-polyposis colon cancer	1:2
Familial adenomatous polyposis	1:1

Symptoms

- Blood in the stools
- Mucus discharge
- Recent change in bowel habits (constipation more common than diarrhoea)
- Alternating constipation with spurious diarrhoea
- Bowel leakage when flatus passed
- Unsatisfactory defecation (the mass is interpreted as faeces)
- Abdominal pain (colicky) or discomfort (if obstructing)
- Rectal discomfort
- Symptoms of anaemia
- Rectal examination—this is appropriate because many cancers are found in the lowest 12 cm and most can be reached by the examining finger

Obstruction (distension with ↑ pain)

If obstructing, there is a risk of rupture of the caecum.

Surgery is needed to circumvent the closed loop obstruction.

Spread

- Lymphatics → epigastric and para-aortic nodes
- Direct → peritoneum
- Blood → portal circulation

Various forms of presentation of large bowel cancers are shown in FIGURE 41.3.

Investigations

- FOBT: immunochemical tests (e.g. Inform and InSure) do not require dietary or medication restriction
- CT colonography (investigation of choice)
- Serum CEA level is not useful for diagnosis but is useful for monitoring response to treatment
- Sigmoidoscopy, especially flexible sigmoidoscopy
- Double contrast, barium enema may miss tumours and is being superseded by other imaging
- Ultrasonography and CT scanning not useful in primary diagnosis; valuable in detecting spread especially hepatic metastases
- PET scanning (if available) is useful for follow-up

If FOBT is positive—investigate by colonoscopy or by flexible sigmoidoscopy.

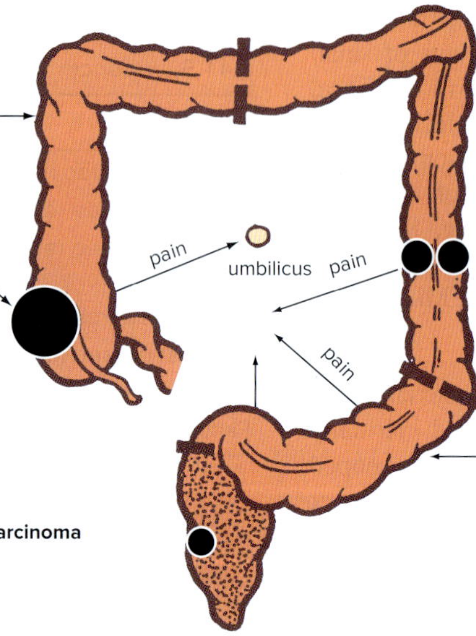

FIGURE 41.3 Various forms of presentation of large bowel cancer

Screening[10]

An FOBT every 2 years is now recommended for all people from 50 years (see guidelines in CHAPTER 9).

Colonoscopy is recommended as follows:

- Moderate risk: every five years from 50 years or 10 years younger than when a family member presented
- High risk: guided by clinical genetics team but as a rule yearly or 2 yearly commencing at 25 years, and every 12 months from 12–15 years of age if a strong family history of FAP.[11]

In addition, flexible sigmoidoscopy and rectal biopsy for those with ulcerative colitis. Refer to a bowel cancer specialist to plan appropriate surveillance.

Management

Early surgical excision is the treatment, with the method depending on the site and extent of the cancer. Dukes' classification gives a guide to prognosis (see TABLE 41.6). The survival rates for Dukes C cancer have improved with more effective chemotherapy.

There are other classifications for staging of colorectal cancer, including the 0, I, II, III, IV and TNM systems.

Follow-up includes:

- CEA antigen
- colonoscopy
- abdominal imaging: ultrasound or CT scan of liver

Table 41.6 Modified Dukes' classification of colorectal cancer

Stage	Pathologic description	Approx. treated 5-year survival %*
A	Cancer limited to mucosa and submucosa	92
B	Cancer extends into muscularis or serosa	75
C	Cancer involves regional lymph nodes	46
D	Distant metastases (e.g. liver)	7

* percentage ranges cover several studies

Source: Cancer Council Australia, 2008

Overall survival over 50%[11]

Congenital megacolon

Hirschsprung disorder (aganglionosis)

Clinical features

- Congenital
- Constipation from infancy
- Abdominal distension from infancy
- Possible anorexia and vomiting
- Male to female ratio = 8:1

- Rectal examination—narrow or normal rectum
- Abdominal X-ray/barium enema—distended colon full of faeces to narrow rectum
- Diagnosis, confirmed by full thickness biopsy, shows absence of ganglion cells
- Absent rectoanal reflex on anal manometry

Treatment

Resect narrow segment after preliminary colostomy.

Acquired megacolon

Clinical features

- In older children and adults
- Mainly due to bad habit
- Can be caused by:
  - chronic laxative abuse
  - milder form of Hirschsprung disorder
  - Chagas disease (Latin America)[2]
  - hypothyroidism (cretinism)
  - systemic sclerosis
- Marked abdominal distension
- Rectal examination—dilate loaded rectum, lax sphincter
- Abdominal X-ray/barium enema—distended colon full of faeces but no narrowed segment

Treatment

Re-education of bowel habit is required.

When to refer[4]

Patients with constipation or change in bowel habit of recent onset without obvious cause need further investigation.

- Patients with chronic symptoms who do not respond to simple measures should be referred.

Practice tips

- The objectives of treatment should be to exclude organic disease and then reassure and re-educate the patient about normal bowel function.
- Discourage long-term use of laxatives, suppositories and microenemas.
- The laxatives to discourage should include anthraquinone derivatives, bisacodyl, phenolphthalein, magnesium salts, castor oil and mineral oils.
- First-line treatment of functional constipation (unresponsive to simple measures) is a bulking agent. An osmotic laxative is good second-line therapy.
- Bleeding with constipation indicates associated organic illness—exclude bowel cancer. Bright red blood usually means haemorrhoids.
- Beware of hypokalaemia causing constipation in the elderly patient on diuretic treatment.
- If cancer can be felt on rectal examination, an abdominal perineal procedure with colostomy usually follows; if not, an anterior resection is generally the rule.

Patient education resources

Hand-out sheets from *Murtagh's Patient Education* 7th edition:

- Bowel cancer
- Constipation

References

1 Rome Foundation. Rome III diagnostic criteria for functional gastroenterological disorders. J Gastrointestinal Liver Disease, 2006; 15 (3): 307–12.

2 Arce DA, Ermocilla MD et al. Evaluation of constipation. American Family Physician, 2002; 65: 2283–90.

3 Gibson P. Constipation. In: Monash University, 2012 update course proceedings.

4 Bolin T. Constipation. In: *MIMS Disease Index* (2nd edn). Sydney: IMS Publishing, 1996: 127–9.

5 Guree A, Rimer R, Marks M. In: *Paediatric Handbook* (9th edn). Oxford: Wiley Blackwell, 2015: 98–101.

6 Tabber MM, DiLorenzo et al. Evaluation and treatment of functional constipation in infants and children: evidence-based recommendations from ESPGHAN and NASPGHAN. J Paediatr Gastroenterol Nutr. 2014; 58 (2): 258–70.

7 Barton S (ed.). *Clinical Evidence*. London: BMJ Publishing Group, 2001: 231–5.

8 Expert group in Gastrointestinal. Functional gastrointestinal disorders. In: eTG complete [Internet]. Melbourne: Therapeutic Guidelines Ltd. Available from: www.tg.org.au, accessed September 2017.

9 Avery Jones F, Godding FW. *Management of Constipation*. Oxford: Blackwell Scientific Publications, 1972: 16.

10 Sali A. Preventive initiatives in medicine and surgery. Aust Fam Physician, 1985; 14: 1314.

11 Houlston RS, Murday V. Screening and genetic counselling for relatives of patients with colorectal cancer in a family cancer clinical. BMJ, 1990; 301: 366–8.

12 Royal Australian College of General Practitioners. *Guidelines for Preventive Activities in General Practice* (9th edn). East Melbourne: RACGP, 2016: 105–9.

13 Colorectal Cancer. In: *Guidelines* (4th edn). Sydney: Gastroenterological Society of Australia, 2013: 10–18.

42 Cough

I bounded into bed. The bound made me cough—I spat—it tasted strange—it was bright red blood—I don't want to find this is real consumption—I shan't have my work written. That's what matters. How unbearable it would be to die—nothing real finished.

KATHERINE MANSFIELD (1888–1923), DIARY ENTRY 1918

Cough is one of the five most common symptoms presenting in family practice. There is a wide range of causes (see TABLE 42.1) with the great majority being minor and self-limiting, although the possibility of serious causes such as bronchial carcinoma should always be kept in mind.

It is a feature of smokers, who often have a morning cough with little sputum. Coughing can also be initiated by pleural irritation. It is a reflex that provides an essential protective service. It serves to remove substances that may have been accidentally inhaled and removes excess secretions or exudates that may accumulate in the airway.

Table 42.1 Significant causes of cough

Non-productive (dry cough)
Upper respiratory tract infection
Lower respiratory tract infection:
• viral
• mycoplasma
Inhaled irritants:
• smoke
• dust
• fumes
Drugs
Inhaled foreign body
Bronchial neoplasm
Pleurisy
Interstitial lung disorders:
• fibrosing alveolitis
• extrinsic allergic alveolitis
• pneumoconiosis
• sarcoidosis
Tuberculosis
Left ventricular failure (esp. nocturnal cough)
Whooping cough (pertussis)
Gastro-oesophageal reflux and hiatus hernia
Postnasal drip
Productive cough
Chronic bronchitis
Bronchiectasis
Pneumonia
Asthma
Foreign body (later response)
Bronchial carcinoma (dry or loose)
Lung abscess
Tuberculosis (when cavitating)

Key facts and checkpoints

- Cough is the commonest manifestation of lower respiratory tract infection.
- Cough is the cardinal feature of chronic bronchitis.
- Cough is a feature of asthma with sputum production, especially at night.
- Cough can have a psychogenic basis.
- Cough may persist for many weeks following an acute upper respiratory tract infection (URTI) as a result of persisting bronchial inflammation and increased airway responsiveness.[1]
- Postnasal drip is the commonest cause of a persistent or chronic cough, especially causing nocturnal cough due to secretions (mainly from chronic sinusitis) tracking down the larynx and trachea during sleep.
- The commonest causes of haemoptysis are URTI (24%), acute or chronic bronchitis (17%), bronchiectasis (13%), TB (10%). Unknown causes totalled 22% and cancer 4% (figures from a UK study).[2]

A diagnostic approach

A summary of the diagnostic strategy model is presented in TABLE 42.2.

Probability diagnosis

The most common cause of cough is an acute respiratory infection, whether a URTI or acute bronchitis.[3] Persistent

Table 42.2 Cough: diagnostic strategy model
Probability diagnosis
Upper respiratory infection
Postnasal drip/rhinitis/sinusitis
Smoking
Acute bronchitis
Chronic bronchitis/COPD
Serious disorders not to be missed
Cardiovascular:
• left ventricular failure
Neoplasia:
• lung cancer
Severe infections:
• tuberculosis
• pneumonia
• influenza
• lung abscess
• HIV infection
• SARS (coronavirus)
Asthma
Cystic fibrosis
Inhaled foreign body
Pneumothorax
Pitfalls (often missed)
Atypical pneumonias
Gastro-oesophageal reflux (nocturnal)
Smoking (children/adolescents)
Bronchiectasis
Whooping cough (pertussis)
Interstitial lung disorders
Sarcoidosis
Seven masquerades checklist
Drugs (several)
Is the patient trying to tell me something?
Anxiety and habit.

coughing with a URTI is usually due to the development of sinusitis with a postnasal drip.

Chronic bronchitis is also a common cause of cough.

Serious disorders not to be missed

Bronchial carcinoma must not be overlooked. A worsening cough is the commonest presenting problem. A bovine cough is suggestive of cancer: the explosive nature of a normal cough is lost when laryngeal paralysis is present, usually resulting from bronchial carcinoma infiltrating the left recurrent laryngeal nerve.

Chronic cough may be the first presentation of *Pneumocystis jiroveci* pneumonia in an HIV-infected patient. Careful but tactful questioning of the patient in relation to IV drug use, sexual practice and previous blood transfusions is important. Important causes of a chronic cough are summarised in TABLE 42.3.

Table 42.3 Some causes of chronic cough[2,4,5]
Normal chest X-ray (includes most causes)
Chronic postnasal drip*
Asthma*
Asthma + postnasal drip
Postinfective bronchial hyper-responsiveness
Gastro-oesophageal reflux:*
• symptomatic
• asymptomatic
Chronic bronchitis
Chronic heart failure
Drugs (e.g. ACE inhibitors, inhaled steroids, salazopyrin)
Snoring and obstructive sleep apnoea
Irritants: occupational and household
Smoker's cough
Whooping cough (pertussis)
Habit
Functional
Idiopathic
Abnormal chest X-ray
Bronchiectasis
Cancer: bronchial, larynx
Cardiac failure
COPD
Cystic fibrosis
Inhaled foreign body
Interstitial lung disorders (e.g. sarcoidosis)
Tuberculosis

* top three

The possibility of a foreign body should always be kept in mind, especially in children, and severe infections such as TB and pulmonary abscess must not be misdiagnosed.

Red flag pointers for cough

- Age >50 years
- Smoking history
- Asbestos history exposure
- Persistent cough
- Overseas travel
- TB exposure
- Haemoptysis
- Unexplained weight loss
- Dyspnoea
- Fever

It is also important not to overlook asthma in which a nocturnal cough, without wheezing, is a feature in children.

Pitfalls

Causes that tend to be overlooked, especially in the presence of a normal X-ray, are gastro-oesophageal reflux, postnasal drip and asthma. Gastro-oesophageal reflux is more common as a cause of reflex coughing, especially at night, than appreciated. Whooping cough, especially immunisation-modified, can be difficult to diagnose, particularly if the characteristic whoop is absent.

General pitfalls

- Attributing cough due to bronchial carcinoma in a smoker to 'smoker's cough'
- Overlooking TB, especially in the elderly, by equating symptoms to old age, bronchitis or even smoking
- Overlooking the fact that bronchial carcinoma can develop in a patient with other pulmonary conditions, such as chronic bronchitis
- Being slow to order a chest X-ray
- Failing to recognise that pertussis presents in adults

Seven masquerades checklist

The applicable masquerade is drugs, many of which can produce a wide variety of disorders of the respiratory tract that cause a cough. Pulmonary infiltration with fibrosis may result from some cytotoxic drugs, especially bleomycin. Over 20 different drugs are known to produce an SLE-like syndrome, sometimes complicated by pulmonary infiltrates and fibrosis. Cough can be a feature of some of the ACE inhibitors and beta blockers, inhaled steroids and sulfasalazine.

Psychogenic considerations

A cough can occur for psychosocial reasons. Coughing is under cerebral control and a slight cough before commencing a speech is normal and presumably assists in clearing mucus from around the vocal cords.[6] This can readily become a nervous habit or mannerism. A typical 'psychogenic' cough is barking in quality—the 'Cape Barren goose' cough. It does not occur during sleep.

The clinical approach

History

42

The nature of the cough may provide important diagnostic clues, but it is the associated symptoms, such as the nature of the sputum, breathlessness, wheezing and constitutional symptoms, that provide the most helpful diagnostic value. A diagnosis of asthma should not be made if the predominant symptom is cough without airflow limitation such as wheeze. A history of smoking habits, past and present, is essential and an occupational and hobby history requires investigation. Significant occupations (past or present) include mining (pneumoconiosis), aircraft manufacturing (asbestosis and mesothelioma), farming ('farmer's lung'—allergic pneumonitis from mouldy hay) and bird handling ('bird fancier's lung'—allergic alveolitis or psittacosis from pigeons or budgerigars). A past history of recurrent lung infections from childhood is suggestive of cystic fibrosis and bronchiectasis, a history of hay fever and eczema suggests asthma, while a family history involves asthma, cystic fibrosis, emphysema (α_1-antitrypsin deficiency) and tuberculosis.

Key questions[7]

- How would you describe the cough?
- How long has the cough been present?
- Do you cough up sputum?
- Describe the sputum, especially its colour.
- Is there any blood in the sputum?
- How much sputum do you produce—a teaspoonful, an eggcupful or more?
- Is there a burning sensation in your throat or chest when you cough?
- Have you noticed any other symptoms?
- What about chest pain or fever, shivers or sweats?
- Do you have a wheeze?
- Have you had previous attacks of wheezing or hay fever?
- Is there a history of asthma in your family?
- Have you lost weight?
- Has anyone in the family had TB or a persistent cough?
- How much do you smoke?
- Are you exposed to any smoke or fumes?
- What kind of work do you do?
- Where have you worked in the past?
- Is there a chance you have been exposed to asbestos?
- Do you keep birds or pets at home?
- Do you have any birds nesting outside your bedroom?
- Is there a possibility of a foreign body such as a peanut 'having gone down the wrong way'?
- Have you had an operation recently or been confined to bed?
- Have you noticed any swelling of your legs?
- Have you been exposed to birds such as pigeons?

Examination

Physical examination includes a general examination with a search for features such as enlarged cervical or axillary glands, which may indicate bronchial carcinoma, as would Horner syndrome (constricted pupil, ptosis). A careful examination of the lungs and cardiovascular system is also appropriate. Fine crackles on auscultation indicate pulmonary oedema of heart failure, interstitial pulmonary fibrosis and early lobar pneumonia, while coarse crackles indicate resolving pneumonia, bronchiectasis and TB. Careful inspection of the sputum forms an important part of the physical examination of the lungs. This should include its colour and consistency, presence of particulate matter and a 24-hour sputum watch.

Investigations

This applies particularly to patients with haemoptysis. Investigations include:[8]

- haemoglobin, blood film and white cell count
- sputum cytology and culture
- ESR (elevated with bacterial infection, bronchiectasis, TB, lung abscess and bronchial carcinoma), CRP
- pulmonary function tests/spirometry
- radiology:
  - plain chest X-ray (shows many problems)
  - tomography: helps more precise localisation of lesion, may show cavitation
  - bronchography: shows bronchiectasis (a very unpleasant procedure)
  - CT scanning (more sensitive than plain X-ray)
  - CT pulmonary angiogram
  - ventilation/perfusion isotope scan: for pulmonary infarction
  - echocardiogram (pulmonary hypertension)
- skin tests
- lung biopsy
- bronchoscopy (best at time of haemoptysis)

However, all that is needed initially is a plain chest X-ray.

Diagnostic characteristics

There are important characteristics of cough that may point to the causation. TABLE 42.1 compares typical causes of dry and productive cough.

Character of the cough

- Brassy → tracheitis and bronchitis (major bronchi); extrinsic pressure on trachea (e.g. tumour)
- Barking → laryngeal disorders (e.g. laryngitis)
- Croupy (with stridor) → laryngeal disorders (e.g. laryngitis, croup)
- Hollow 'bovine' (no power) → vocal cord paralysis (left-recurrent laryngeal nerve)
- Weak cough → indicates bronchial carcinoma
- Paroxysmal with whoops → whooping cough
- Painful → tracheitis; left ventricular failure
- Dry chronic → GORD, drugs (e.g. ACE)

Timing

- Nocturnal cough →
  - asthma
  - left ventricular failure
  - postnasal drip
  - chronic bronchitis
  - whooping cough
- Waking cough →
  - bronchiectasis, asthma
  - chronic bronchitis
  - GORD

Associations

- Changing posture →
  - bronchiectasis
  - lung abscess
- Meals →
  - hiatus hernia (possible)
  - oesophageal diverticulum
  - tracheo-oesophageal fistula
- Wheezing →
  - asthma
- Breathlessness →
  - asthma
  - left ventricular failure
  - COPD

Sputum

A healthy, non-smoking individual produces approximately 100–150 mL of mucus a day. This normal bronchial secretion is swept up the airways towards the trachea by the mucociliary clearance mechanism and is usually swallowed. The removal from the trachea is assisted also by occasional coughing although this is carried out almost subconsciously.[6]

Excess mucus is expectorated as sputum. The commonest cause of excess mucus production is cigarette smoking. Mucoid sputum is clear and white.

Character of sputum

- Clear white (mucoid) → normal or uninfected bronchitis
- Yellow or green (purulent) → due to cellular material (neutrophils or eosinophil granulocytes)

  - ± infection (not necessarily bacterial infection)
  - asthma due to eosinophils
  - bronchiectasis (copious quantities)
- Rusty → lobar pneumonia (*S. pneumoniae*): due to blood
- Thick and sticky → asthma
- Profuse, watery → alveolar cell carcinoma
- Thin, clear mucoid → viral infection
- Redcurrant jelly → bronchial carcinoma
- Profuse and offensive → bronchiectasis; lung abscess
- Thick plugs (cast-like) → allergic bronchopulmonary *Aspergillus;* bronchial carcinoma
- Pink frothy sputum → pulmonary oedema

Haemoptysis

Blood-stained sputum (haemoptysis), which varies from small flecks of blood to massive bleeding, requires thorough investigation. Always consider malignancy or TB. Often the diagnosis can be made by chest X-ray. Causes are presented in TABLE 42.4. Haemoptysis must be distinguished from blood-stained saliva caused by nasopharyngeal bleeding or sinusitis and also from haematemesis.[6] Acute bronchitis produces streaky haemoptysis.

Productive cough

- Chronic bronchitis: mucoid or purulent; rarely exceeds 250 mL per day[6]
- Bronchiectasis: purulent sputum; up to 500 mL/day
- Asthma: mucoid or purulent; tenacious sputum
- Lung abscess: purulent and foul-smelling
- Foreign body: can follow impaction

Cough in children[3]

Cough in children is a very common symptom, but troublesome persistent cough is a great cause of anxiety among parents and probably the commonest symptom for which the family doctor is consulted. Age-related causes of chronic cough (present at least 4 weeks) are presented in TABLE 42.5. Most children with chronic cough do NOT have asthma. A chest X-ray is advisable for a persistent cough.

Common causes of cough generally are:

- asthma
- recurrent viral bronchitis
- acute URTIs
- allergic rhinitis
- croup

Table 42.4 Haemoptysis (adults): diagnostic strategy model

Haemoptysis (adults): diagnostic strategy model
Probability diagnosis
Acute chest infection
• URTI (24%)
• bronchitis
Chronic bronchitis
Trauma: Chest contusion, prolonged coughing
Cause often unknown (22%)
Serious disorders not to be missed
Vascular:
• pulmonary infarction/embolus
• LHF → pulmonary oedema
• mitral stenosis
• pulmonary hypertension
• AV malformation
Infection:
• lobar pneumonia (rusty sputum)
• tuberculosis
• lung abscess
Cancer/tumour (4%):
• bronchogenic carcinoma
• tumour of the larynx or trachea
Other:
• blood disorders including anticoagulants
• cystic fibrosis
Pitfalls (often missed)
Foreign body
Bronchiectasis (13%)
Latrogenic (e.g. endotracheal intubation)
Spurious haemoptysis (blood from nose or throat)
Factitious (e.g. Munchausen syndrome)

Note: Haemoptysis must be distinguished from blood-stained saliva caused by nasopharyngeal bleeding or sinusitis, also haematemesis.[6] Copious haemoptysis is due to bronchiectasis or TB.

Disorders not to be missed are:

- asthma
- cystic fibrosis
- inhaled foreign body
- tracheo-oesophageal fistula
- pneumonia
- whooping cough

Several clinicians describe the catarrhal child syndrome as the commonest cause of cough.[3] This refers to children who develop a postnasal drip following acute respiratory infection and allergic rhinitis. Recurrent cough in children can usually be

Table 42.5 Chronic cough in children: age-related causes to consider

Early months of life
Milk inhalation/reflux
Asthma
Toddler/preschool child
Asthma
Bronchitis
Whooping cough
Cystic fibrosis
Croup
Foreign body inhalation
Tuberculosis
Bronchiectasis
Early school years
Asthma
Bronchitis
Mycoplasma pneumonia
Adolescence
Asthma
Psychogenic
Smoking

Source: After Selecki and Helman[9]

explained by recurrent viral respiratory infections which commonly occur when first exposed to other children. Their airways tend to be overactive. There is a slight predisposition to asthma.

If asthma is suspected, a therapeutic trial of salbutamol 200 mcg 4 hourly via a spacer may be worthwhile.

Psychogenic causes

Habit cough can occur in children, especially those with a history of school phobia. The cough does not occur during sleep and remains unchanged with exertion or infection.

Croup (laryngotracheobronchitis)

Clinical features

- Characteristic harsh barking inspiratory cough with stridor
- Prodrome of URTI for 2 days
- Sounds like a dog barking or a seal
- Children 6 months to 6 years
- Fever variable (rarely >39°)
- Usually 11 pm to 2 am
- Auscultation confirms inspiratory stridor
- Occurs in small local epidemics

Management—refer to CHAPTER 96.

Cough in the elderly

Important causes of cough to consider in the elderly include chronic bronchitis, lung cancer, pulmonary infarct (check calves), bronchiectasis and left ventricular failure, in addition to the acute upper and lower respiratory infections to which they are prone. It is important to be surveillant for bronchial carcinoma in an older person presenting with cough, bearing in mind that the incidence rises with age. One study found the causes of chronic cough in the elderly to be postnasal drip syndrome 48%, gastro-oesophageal reflux 20% and asthma 17%.[10]

COMMON RESPIRATORY INFECTIONS

Respiratory infections, especially those of the upper respiratory tract, are usually regarded as trivial, but they account for an estimated one-fifth of all time lost from work and three-fifths of time lost from school, and are thus of great importance to the community.[11] The majority of respiratory infections are viral in origin and antibiotics are therefore not indicated.

URTIs are those involving the nasal airways to the larynx, while lower respiratory tract infections (LRTIs) affect the trachea downwards.

Combined URTIs and LRTIs include influenza, measles, whooping cough and laryngotracheobronchitis.

The common cold (acute coryza)

This highly infectious URTI, which is often mistakenly referred to as 'the flu', produces a mild systemic upset and prominent nasal symptoms (see FIG. 42.1).

Clinical features

- 24–48 hours of weakness
- Malaise and tiredness
- Sore, runny nose
- Sneezing
- Sore throat
- Slight fever

Other possible symptoms:

- headache
- hoarseness
- cough

The watery nasal discharge becomes thick and purulent in about 24 hours and persists for up to a week. Secondary bacterial infection is uncommon.

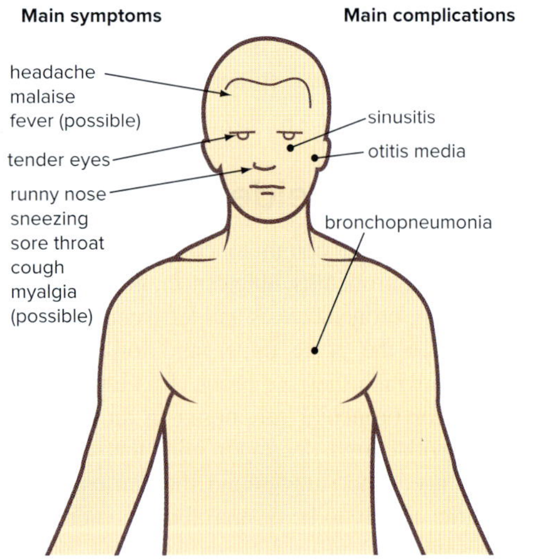

FIGURE 42.1 The main symptoms and complications of the common cold

Management

Advice to the patient includes:

- rest—adequate sleep and rest
- drink copious fluids
- stop smoking (if applicable)
- analgesics—paracetamol (acetaminophen) or aspirin (max. 8 tablets a day in adults)
- steam inhalations for a blocked nose
- cough mixture for a dry cough
- gargling aspirin in water or lemon juice for a sore throat (avoid aspirin in children <16 years)
- vitamin C powder or tablets (e.g. 2 g daily) may aid recovery; however, clinical trials are inconclusive
- clinical trials of vitamin C, zinc lozenges and echinacea give contradictory results to date[11]

Influenza

Influenza causes a relatively debilitating illness and should not be confused with the common cold. The differences are presented in TABLE 42.6. The incubation period is usually 1–3 days and the illness commences abruptly with a fever, headache, shivering and generalised muscle aching (see FIG. 42.2).

Clinical criteria[12]

During an influenza epidemic:

- fever >38°C plus at least one respiratory symptom and one systemic symptom
- cough (dry)
- sore throat
- coryza
- prostration or weakness
- myalgia
- headache
- rigors or chills

Table 42.6 Comparison of common cold and influenza

	Common cold	Influenza
Incubation period	12 hours to 5 days	1–3 days
Fever	±	+ +
Cough	(later)	+
Sore throat	+ +	±
Rhinitis sneezing rhinorrhoea	+	± late symptom
Muscle aches	–	+
Toxaemia	–	±
Causes	Rhinoviruses Parainfluenza Influenza B, C Coronavirus RSV	Influenza A Influenza B Novel strains influenza A e.g. H5N1

Diagnosis: Nasal/throat swabs for viral PCR (rapid and best); viral antigen detection or culture.

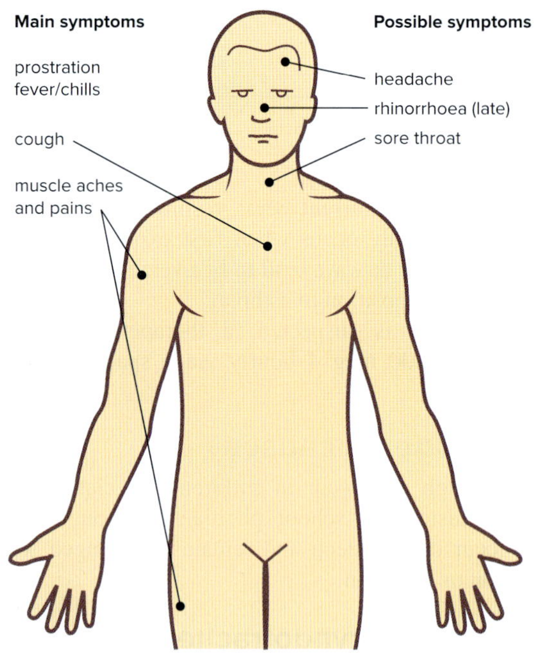

FIGURE 42.2 The main features of influenza

Complications

- Tracheitis, bronchitis, bronchiolitis
- Secondary bacterial infection
- Pneumonia due to *Staphylococcus aureus* (mortality up to 20%)[1]
- Toxic cardiomyopathy with sudden death (rare)
- Encephalomyelitis (rare)
- Depression (a common sequela)

Management

Advice to the patient includes:

- rest in bed until the fever subsides and patient feels better
- analgesics: paracetamol and aspirin or ibuprofen are effective, especially for fever
- fluids: maintain high fluid intake (water and fruit juice)
- freshly squeezed lemon juice and honey preparation

Antiviral agents[12]

- Neuraminidase inhibitors (cover influenza A and B):
  zanamivir (Relenza) 10 mg by inhalation bd for 5 days
  oseltamivir (Tamiflu) 75 mg (o) bd (child 2 mg/kg) for 5 days

Both should be commenced within 36 hours of onset and given for 5 days.

Note: These antiviral agents have questionable benefit in a low-risk population, but treatment for vulnerable patients is appropriate.

Prevention

Influenza vaccination offers some protection for up to 70% of the population for about 12 months.[1] (See CHAPTER 9.)

Swine origin flu

(The swine variety of H1N1 influenza A.)

This strain presents with typical influenza symptoms commonly accompanied by gastrointestinal symptoms (especially diarrhoea). Like avian flu, it tends to occur in a pandemic and affects the young in particular.

The treatment is the same as for influenza in general, with neuraminidase inhibitors. A vaccine is now available.

Avian (bird) flu due to H5N1 strain: refer to CHAPTER 28.

Middle East respiratory syndrome (MERS–CoV)

This is a viral respiratory disease of varying severity caused by a novel coronavirus. Symptoms include cough, fever and dyspnoea. Endemic to the Middle East, especially Saudi Arabia. No specific treatment but supportive. Significant mortality rate.

BRONCHITIS

Acute bronchitis

This is acute inflammation of the tracheobronchial tree that usually follows an upper respiratory infection. Although generally mild and self-limiting, it may be serious in debilitated patients.

Clinical features

Features of acute infectious bronchitis are:

- cough and sputum (main symptoms)
- wheeze and dyspnoea
- usually viral infection
- can complicate chronic bronchitis—often due to *Haemophilus influenzae* and *Streptococcus pneumoniae*
- scattered wheeze on auscultation
- fever or haemoptysis (uncommon)

Outcome

- It improves spontaneously in 4–8 days in healthy patients.

Treatment[12,14,15]

- Symptomatic treatment
- Inhaled bronchodilators for airflow limitation
- Antibiotics usually not needed in previously healthy adult or child
- Use antibiotics only if evidence of acute bacterial infection with fever, increased sputum volume and sputum purulence:

  amoxycillin 500 mg (o) 8-hourly for 5 days
  or
  especially if mycoplasma suspected, doxycycline 200 mg (o) statim, 100 mg, daily for 5 days.

Chronic bronchitis

This is a chronic productive cough for at least 3 successive months in 2 successive years:

- wheeze, progressive dyspnoea
- recurrent exacerbations with acute bronchitis
- occurs mainly in smokers

Refer to COPD (in CHAPTER 83).

PNEUMONIA[16]

This is inflammation of lung tissue. It usually presents as an acute illness with cough, fever and purulent sputum plus physical signs and X-ray changes of consolidation.

However, the initial presentation of pneumonia can be misleading, especially when the patient presents with constitutional symptoms (fever, malaise and headache) rather than respiratory symptoms. A cough, although usually present, can be relatively insignificant in the total clinical picture. This diagnostic problem applies particularly to atypical pneumonia but can occur with bacterial pneumonia, especially lobar pneumonia.

Community-acquired pneumonia[12,14]

CAP occurs in people who are not or have not been in hospital recently, and who are not institutionalised or immunocompromised. The choice of antibiotic is initially empirical. CAP is usually caused by a single organism, especially *Streptococcus pneumoniae,* which is now becoming resistant to antibiotics.[15] Treatment is usually for 5–10 days for most bacterial causes, 2 weeks for *Mycoplasma* or *Chlamydia* infection and 2–3 weeks for *Legionella.*

Typical pneumonia

The commonest community-acquired infection is with *Streptococcus pneumoniae* (majority), now becoming resistant to antibiotics, *Haemophilus influenzae*[15] (mainly in COPD), *M. pneumoniae* (young adults), *Klebsiella pneumoniae.*

Clinical features

- Often history of viral respiratory infection
- Rapidly ill with high temperature, dry cough, pleuritic pain, rigors or night sweats
- 1–2 days later may be rusty-coloured sputum
- Rapid and shallow breathing follows
- Examination: focal chest signs, consolidation
- Investigations: CXR, sputum M&C, oxygen saturation, specific tests/serology, PCR
- Complications: pleural effusion, empyema, lung abscess, respiratory failure

The atypical pneumonias

Refer to CHAPTER 29.

42

Clinical features

- Fever, malaise
- Headache
- Minimal respiratory symptoms, non-productive cough
- Signs of consolidation absent
- Chest X-ray (diffuse infiltration) incompatible with chest signs

Causes

- Virus, e.g. influenza
- *Mycoplasma pneumoniae*—the commonest:
  - adolescents and young adults
  - treat with:

  roxithromycin 300 mg (o) daily
  or
  doxycycline 100 mg bd for 14 days
- *Legionella pneumophila* (legionnaire disease):
  - related to cooling systems in large buildings
  - incubation 2–10 days

  Diagnostic criteria include:

- prodromal influenza-like illness
- a dry cough, confusion or diarrhoea
- very high fever (may be relative bradycardia)
- lymphopaenia with moderate leucocytosis
- hyponatraemia

Patients can become prostrate with complications. Treat with:

azithromycin IV (first line) or erythromycin (IV or oral)
plus (if very severe)
ciprofloxacin or rifampicin

- *Chlamydia pneumoniae:*
  - similar to *Mycoplasma*
- *Chlamydia psittaci* (psittacosis):
  - treat with doxycycline, roxithromycin or erythromycin
- *Coxiella burnetti* (Q fever):
  - treat with doxycycline 200 mg (o) statim then 100 mg daily for 14 days

Antibiotic treatment according to severity[11,12]

This is usually empirical.

Mild pneumonia

This does not require hospitalisation.

amoxycillin/clavulanate 875/125 mg (o) 12-hourly for 5–7 days or amoxycillin 1 g 8-hourly especially if *S. pneumoniae* isolated or suspected
plus (especially if atypical pneumonia suspected)
roxithromycin 300 mg (o) daily for 5 days or
doxycycline 100 mg bd for 5 days

Moderately severe pneumonia

This requires hospitalisation (see Guidelines box for severe pneumonia and hospital admission). Monitor with CXR; oximeter (keep $P_aO_2 \geq 94\%$).

- Neonates
- Age over 65 years
- Coexisting illness
- High temperature: >38°C
- Clinical features of severe pneumonia
- Involvement of more than one lobe
- Inability to tolerate oral therapy

  benzylpenicillin 1.2 g IV 4–6 hourly for 7 days
  or
  procaine penicillin 1.5 g IM daily (drugs of choice for *S. pneumoniae*) plus doxycycline
  or
  ceftriaxone 1 g IV daily for 7 days (in penicillin-allergic patient)
- If not so severe and oral medication tolerated, can use amoxycillin/clavulanate or cefaclor or doxycycline
- In tropical regions use a different regimen (refer to eTG)
- If atypical pneumonia, use doxycycline, erythromycin or roxithromycin

Severe pneumonia

The criteria for severity (with increased risk of death) are presented in the box on Guidelines for severe pneumonia and hospital admission.[14,15,16] The CURB-65 score indicates severity (Confusion, Urea > 7 mmol/L, Respiratory rate ≥30/min, BP <90/60 mmHg, Age ≥65).[17]

azithromycin 500 mg IV daily (covers *Mycoplasma, Chlamydia* and *Legionella*)
plus
cefotaxime 1 g IV 8-hourly
or
ceftriaxone 1 g IV daily
add
flucloxacillin for *Staphylococcus aureus*

Guidelines for severe pneumonia and hospital admission: the red flags

- Altered mental state/acute onset confusion
- Rapidly deteriorating course
- Respiratory rate >30 per minute
- Pulse rate >100 per minute
- BP <90/60 mmHg
- CURB-65 ≥2
- Hypoxia P_aO_2 <60 mm Hg or O_2 saturation <92%
- Leucocytes $<4 \times 10^8$L or $>20 \times 10^9$/L
- Multilobular involvement on CXR

Pneumonia in children

Clinical features

- Tachypnoea, expiratory grunt
- Possible focal chest signs
- Diagnosis often only made by chest X-ray

Pathogens

- Viruses are the most common cause in infants.
- *Mycoplasma* is common in children over 5 years.
- *S. pneumoniae* is a cause in all age groups.
- Pathogens are difficult to isolate—may need blood culture.

Treatment

Depends on age and tropical vs non-tropical. Almost all those under 48 months should be admitted to hospital. Indicators for hospital admission are shown in the box.

- Minimal handling
- Careful observations including pulse oximetry
- Attend to hydration
- Antibiotics indicated in all cases. Refer to guidelines for 5 years and older[12]

  Mild (general guidelines only):[16]

  amoxycillin (o) or roxithromycin (o)

  Moderate:

  benzylpenicillin IV + roxithromycin (o) or doxycycline (o)

  Severe:[15]

  ceftriaxone IV or cefotaxamine IV ± azithromycin (o)

  Note: Refer to eTG for various age groups and tropical regions.

Pneumonia in children: guidelines for hospitalisation[14]

Infants:
- RR>70
- Intermittent apnoea
- Not feeding

Older children:
- RR>50
- Grunting
- Signs of dehydration

Both groups:
- $S_aO_2 \leq 92\%$
- Cyanosis
- Difficulty breathing
- Family/social issues

CHRONIC PERSISTENT COUGH

A cough associated with a viral respiratory infection should last no more than 2 weeks. If it does, it is termed *persistent*. A cough lasting 2 months or more is defined as a chronic cough. A cough that lasts longer than 3–4 weeks requires scrutiny. TABLE 42.3 includes some causes of chronic cough.

A chronic cough can be divided into productive and non-productive. If productive, the presence of pus is significant, as purulent sputum usually means bacterial infection in the bronchi and/or sinuses.[4] The main organisms are *Haemophilus influenzae* (the most common), *S. pneumoniae* and *Moraxella*. Such infections are most susceptible to amoxycillin or amoxycillin/clavulanate or parenteral cephalosporins.

Non-productive cough

Some of the many causes of a non-productive cough are included in TABLE 42.1 and more than one may be operative in a patient simultaneously; for example, an allergic snorer with oesophageal reflux taking an ACE inhibitor for hypertension may have a viral respiratory infection.[4] It has been shown that a non-productive or irritating cough is usually caused by persistent stimulation of irritant receptors in the trachea and major bronchi, and may result in the production of small amounts of mucoid sputum.

Investigations to be considered in intractable chronic cough include a chest X-ray, spirometry, CT scan of the thorax (searching in particular for a tumour) and ambulatory oesophageal pH monitoring.

If bronchial hyper-responsiveness is proven, a trial of inhaled or oral corticosteroids can be used in these patients.[5]

Gastro-oesophageal reflux

This common condition is the most likely cause of a persistent, non-productive cough in an apparently well patient with a history of reflux. Recent studies utilising 24-hour ambulatory oesophageal pH monitoring have demonstrated that in patients with persistent unexplained cough the predominant cause is asymptomatic gastro-oesophageal reflux.[4,5] In the absence of evidence of aspiration, the cough is considered to be due to stimulation of a distal oesophageal-tracheobronchial reflex. Other studies have established a relationship between bronchial asthma and reflux or swallowing disorders whereby microaspiration can initiate an inflammatory response in the airways.

Indications for 24-hour ambulatory oesophageal pH monitoring in chronic cough include:

- unexplained chronic cough after clinical assessment
- symptomatic gastro-oesophageal reflux
- chronic cough with known aetiology unresponsive to therapy

If reflux is proven or suspected, treat with routine conservative anti-reflux measures and at least a 4-week trial of histamine H_2-receptor antagonists. If cough persists, refer for further evaluation.[5]

If all investigations and treatment trials (including anti-reflux and corticosteroids) prove unrewarding, a trial of ipratropium bromide both nebulised (500 mcg, qid) and to a lesser degree metered dose inhaler (4 × 20 μg puffs qid) has been found to be effective.[5,17]

However, for patients with idiopathic chronic cough it is important to provide ongoing interest and support, and not eventually to dismiss them as 'just a cough'.

Bronchial carcinoma

Lung cancer accounts for 25% of cancer deaths in men and 24% of cancer deaths in women (rapidly rising), with cigarette smoking being the most common cause of lung cancer in both sexes.[11] It is also the most common lethal cancer in both sexes in Australia. Bronchial carcinoma accounts for over 95% of primary lung malignancies. The prognosis is poor—the 5-year overall survival is 12–14%.[18] The mesothelioma incidence continues to rise.

Clinical features

- Most present between 50 and 70 years (mean 67 years)
- Only 10–25% asymptomatic at time of diagnosis[9]
- If symptomatic—usually advanced and not resectable

Local symptoms

- Cough (42%)
- Chest pain (22%)
- Wheezing (15%)
- Haemoptysis (7%)
- Dyspnoea (5%)

General

- Anorexia, malaise
- Weight loss—unexplained

Others

- Unresolved chest infection
- Hoarseness
- Symptoms from metastases

The possible physical findings are summarised in FIGURE 42.3.

Investigations

- Chest X-ray
- Sputum cytology
- CT scanning
- Fibre-optic bronchoscopy
- PET scanning
- Fluorescence bronchoscopy (helps early detection)
- Tissue diagnosis where possible

Note: Based on a 2003 Cochrane review, no proven effect of any screening for asymptomatic patients.

Causes of a solitary pulmonary nodule on X-ray are presented in TABLE 42.7.

Management

Refer to a respiratory physician to determine the type of cancer. They are usually classified as small

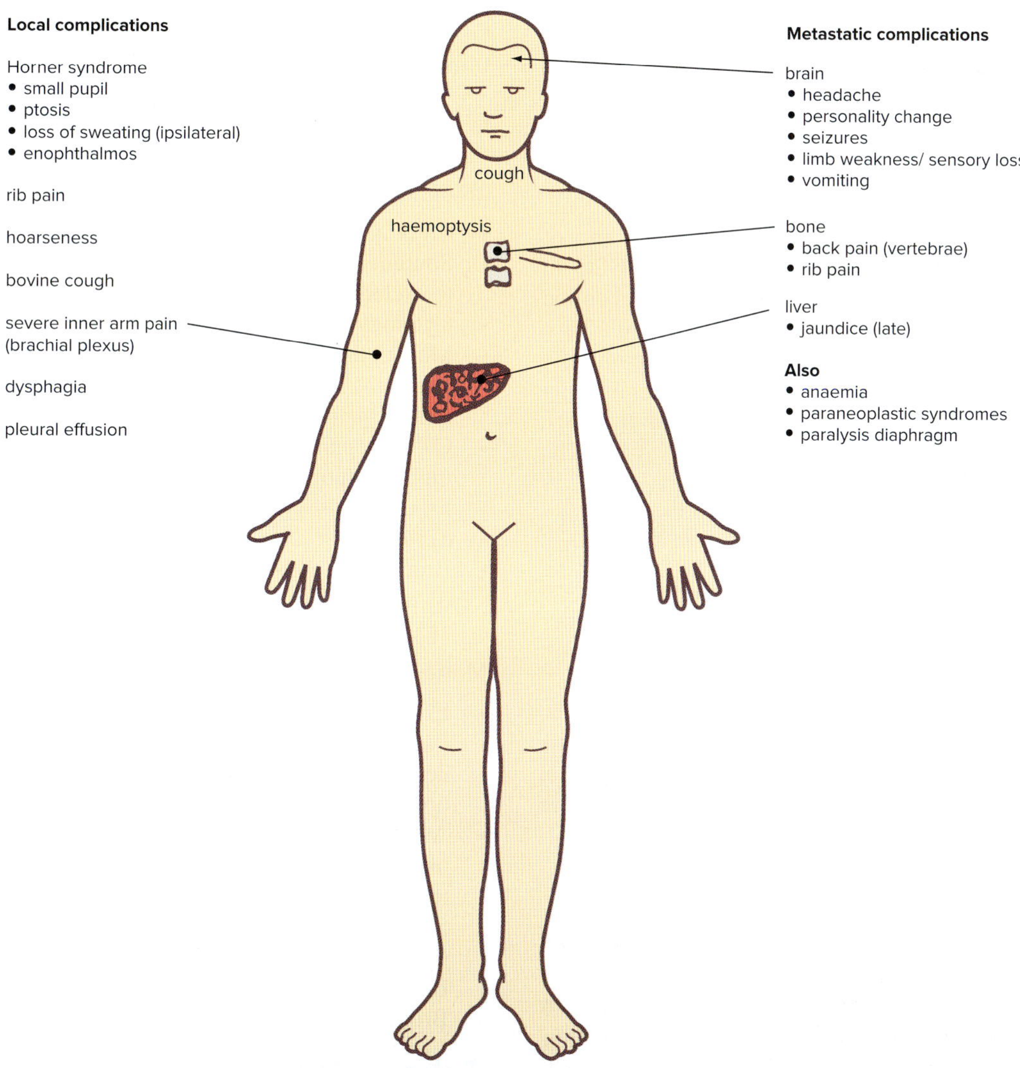

FIGURE 42.3 Possible physical findings of bronchial carcinoma

Table 42.7 Causes of a solitary pulmonary nodule (on X-ray)[19]

Common
Bronchial carcinoma
Secondary tumour
Solitary metastasis
Granuloma (e.g. TB)
Hamartoma
Less common
Bronchial adenoma
Foreign body
AVM
Hydatid
Others (e.g. haematoma, cyst, carotid tumour)

cell lung (oat cell) poorly differentiated cancer (15–20% incidence) (SCLC) and non-small cell lung cancer (NSCLC), which includes squamous cell carcinoma, adenocarcinoma and large cell carcinoma (approximately 20–30% of each). The main aim of management is a curative resection of NSCLC in those who can benefit from it. Surgery is not an option for SCLC since it metastasises so rapidly (80% have metastasised at the time of diagnosis).[14] Chemotherapy is suitable for the deadly SCLC but currently only extends life expectancy from 3–20 months (at best). It also has an important place in treating NSCLC. The main role of radiotherapy is palliative.

Mesothelioma

Mesothelioma is a malignant tumour of mesothelial cells usually at the pleura. It is associated with prior asbestos exposure, possibly decades earlier (90% report exposure).

Clinical features include chest pain, dyspnoea, weight loss and recurrent pleural effusions. Diagnosis is based on imaging and on histology after pleural biopsy. Prognosis is poor and treatment is palliative support.

Bronchiectasis

Bronchiectasis is dilatation of the bronchi when their walls become inflamed, thickened and irreversibly damaged, usually after obstruction followed by infection. Predisposing causes include whooping cough, measles, TB, inhaled foreign body (e.g. peanuts in children), bronchial carcinoma, cystic fibrosis and congenital ciliary dysfunction (Kartagener syndrome). The left lower lobe and lingula are the commonest sites for localised disease.

Clinical features

- Chronic cough—worse on waking
- Mild cases: yellow or green sputum only after infection
- Advanced:
  - profuse purulent offensive sputum
  - persistent halitosis
  - recurrent febrile episodes
  - malaise, weight loss
- Episodes of pneumonia
- Sputum production related to posture
- Haemoptysis (blood-stained sputum or massive) possible

Examination

- Clubbing
- Coarse crackles over infected areas (usually lung base)
- Other respiratory signs are given in TABLE 49.6 (see CHAPTER 49).

Investigations

- Chest X-ray (normal or bronchial changes)
- Sputum examination: for resistant pathogens and to exclude TB
- Cytology: to rule out neoplasia
- Main pathogens: *Streptococcus pneumoniae, Pseudomonas aeruginosa, Haemophilus influenzae* (commonest), *Staphylococcus aureus*
- CT scan: can show bronchial wall thickening—high-resolution CT scan is the new gold standard for diagnosis
- Spirometry
- Bronchograms: very unpleasant and used only if diagnosis in doubt or possible localised disease amenable to surgery (rare)

Management[20]

- Explanation and preventive advice.
- Postural drainage (e.g. lie over side of bed with head and thorax down for 10–20 minutes three times a day).
- Antibiotics for acute exacerbations according to organism—it is important to eradicate infection to halt the progress of the disease. Amoxycillin 500 mg (o) tds for 14 days or doxycyclin 200 mg (o) daily (if child ≥8 years) is recommended for first presentation.[20] Avoid long-term use.
- Bronchodilators, if evidence of bronchospasm.[21]

Tuberculosis

Although cough is a feature, pulmonary TB may be symptomless and detected by X-ray screenings.[8] (Refer to CHAPTER 29.)

Symptomatic treatment of cough

Symptomatic treatment of cough should be reserved for patients who have acute self-limiting causes of cough, especially an acute viral infection. There are many cough mixtures available and the major constituents of these mixtures are shown in TABLE 42.8.[8] The recommended mixture should be tailored to the patient's individual requirements. These mixtures should be used only in the short term.[20] Cough medicines are generally not recommended in children. The Therapeutic Guidelines Ltd recommend that cough and cold medicines, especially cough suppressants, antihistamines and related products, should not be given under 6 years. Consider sucrose and glycerol syrup (a demulcent).[21]

Strategies recommended to manage chronic cough in adults include:[21]

- sedating antihistamine at night
- PPIs because recurrent coughing causes acid reflex and vice versa
- low-dose inhaled corticosteroid

Short term: codeine phosphate 25–30 mg (o) every 3–6 hours.

If intractable: 2 mL lignocaine 2% via nebuliser, for 5–10 minutes up to 4 times daily for up to 7 days.

Table 42.8 Cough mixtures: major constituents

Cough mixtures: major constituents
Cough suppressants
Opioid (use with caution):
Codeine
Dihydrocodeine
Hydrocodone
Pholcodine
Ethylmorphine
Normethadone
Others:
Carbetapentane
Dextromethorphan
Oxolamine
Expectorants/mucolytics
Senega
Ammonia
Guaiphenesin
Bromhexine
Analgesics/antipyretics
Paracetamol (acetaminophen)
Salicylates (e.g. aspirin)
Decongestants
Sympathomimetic:
Ephedrine
Pseudoephedrine
Phenylephrine
Phenylpropanolamine
Methoxyphenamine
Antihistamine:
Promethazine
Pheniramine
Chlorpheniramine
Diphenhydramine
Dexchlorpheniramine
Brompheniramine
Triprolidine
Anticholinergic:
Atropine
Isopropamide

Source: After Williams and Bowes[8]

When to refer

- Patients in whom bronchoscopy is necessary to exclude bronchial carcinoma
- Persistent hoarseness in a patient who requires expert laryngeal examination
- Evidence of pulmonary TB

Practice tips

- Unexplained cough over the age of 50 is bronchial carcinoma until proved otherwise (especially if there is a history of smoking).
- Consider TB in the presence of an unusual cough ± wheezing.
- Bronchoscopy is essential to exclude adequately a suspicion of bronchial carcinoma when the chest X-ray is normal.
- Bright red haemoptysis in a young person may be the initial symptom of pulmonary TB.
- Avoid settling for a diagnosis of bronchitis as an explanation of haemoptysis until bronchial carcinoma has been excluded.
- Coughing may be so severe that it terminates in vomiting or loss of consciousness (post-tussive syncope).
- Large haemoptyses are usually due to bronchiectasis or TB.
- The presence of white cells in the sputum renders it yellow or green (purulent) but does not necessarily imply infection.

Patient education resources

Hand-out sheets from *Murtagh's Patient Education* 7th edition:

- Common cold
- Croup
- Influenza
- Pneumonia

References

1 Kumar PJ, Clarke ML. *Clinical Medicine* (7th edn). London: Elsevier, 2009: 819.

2 Walsh TD. *Symptom Control.* Oxford: Blackwell Scientific Publications, 1989; 81: 81–8, 235–9.

3 Fitzgerald D. Children with chronic or recurrent cough. Medical Observer, 22 November 2002: 32–3.

4 Burns M. Chronic cough. Aust Fam Physician, 1996; 25: 161–7.

5 Ing A. Intractable cough. In: *MIMS Disease Index* (2nd edn). Sydney: IMS Publishing, 1996: 130–3.

6 Kincaid-Smith P, Larkins R, Whelan G. *Problems in Clinical Medicine.* Sydney: MacLennan & Petty, 1990: 105–8.

7 Davis A, Bolin T, Ham J. *Symptom Analysis and Physical Diagnosis* (2nd edn). Sydney: Pergamon Press, 1990: 56–60.

8 Williams TJ, Bowes G. Cough as a symptom in adult life. Modern Medicine Australia, 1992; June: 84–92.

9 Selecki Y, Helman A. Chronic cough in children. Australian Doctor, 1989; 18 September: i–iv.

10 Smyrinos NA et al. From a prospective study of chronic cough: diagnostic and therapeutic aspects in older adults. Arch Intern Med, 1988; 158: 1222–8.

11 McPhee SJ, Papadakis MA. *Current Medical Diagnosis and Treatment* (56th edn). New York: McGraw-Hill Education, 2017: 214.

12 Expert group for Antibiotic. Respiratory. In: eTG complete [Internet]. Melbourne: Therapeutic Guidelines Ltd. Available from: <www.tg.org.au>, accessed September 2017.

13 Barton S (ed.). *Clinical Evidence.* London: BMJ Publishing Group, 2001: 319–22.

14 Stocks N, Melbye H. Community acquired pneumonia: how to treat. Australian Doctor, 16 March 2007: 25–32.

15 Charles PG et al. The etiology of community-acquired pneumonia in Australia: why penicillin plus doxycycline or a macrolide is the most appropriate therapy. Clin Infect Dis, 2008; 46 (10): 1513–21.

16 Thompson K, Tey D, Marks M. *Paediatric Handbook* (8th edn). Melbourne: Blackwell Science, 2009: 514, 606.

17 Chalmers JD et al. Severity assessment tools for predicting mortality in hospitalised patients with community-acquired pneumonia. Systematic review and meta-analysis. Thorax, 2010; 65 (10): 878–83.

18 National Health and Medical Research Council. *Assessment and Management of Lung Cancer. Evidence-Based Guidelines. A Guide for GPs.* NH&MRC, 2005.

19 Lau L (ed.). *Imaging Guidelines* (4th edn). Melbourne: RANZC Radiologists, 2001: 64.

20 Schroeder K, Fahey T. Systematic review of randomised controlled trials of over the counter cough medicines for acute cough. BMJ, 2002; 324: 329–31.

21 Buckley N (Chair). *Australian Medicines Handbook.* Adelaide: Australian Medicines Handbook Pty Ltd, 2016: 891–2.

Deafness and hearing loss 43

There are two kinds of deafness. One is due to wax and is curable; the other is not due to wax and is not curable.

Sir William Wilde (1815–76)

Deafness is defined as impairment of hearing, regardless of its severity.[1] It is a major community health problem requiring a high index of suspicion for diagnosis, especially in children. Deafness may be conductive, sensorineural or a combination of both (mixed).

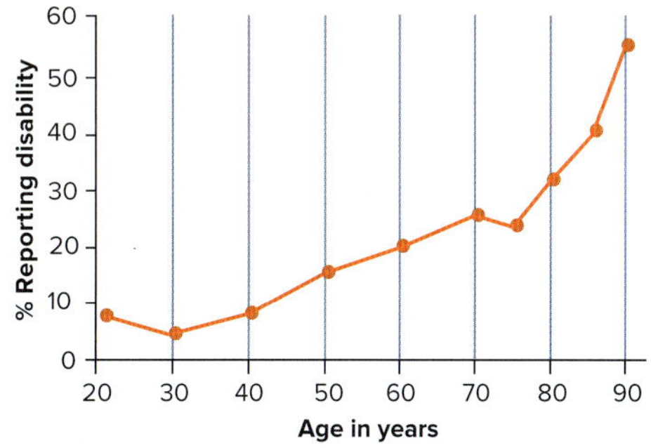

FIGURE 43.1 Prevalence of hearing problems with increasing age

Key facts and checkpoints

- Deafness occurs at all ages but is more common in the elderly (see FIG. 43.1). Fifty per cent of people over 80 years have deafness severe enough to be helped by a hearing aid.
- The threshold of normal hearing is from 0–20 decibels (dB), about the loudness of a soft whisper.
- One in seven of the adult population suffers from some degree of significant hearing impairment (over 20 dB in the better-hearing ear).[2]
- One child in every 1000 is born with a significant hearing loss. The earlier it is detected and treated the better.
- Degrees of hearing impairment with vocal equivalent:[2,3]
  - mild = loss of 20–40 dB (soft-spoken voice is 20dB)
  - moderate = loss of 40–60 dB (normal-spoken voice is 40dB)
  - severe = loss of 70–90 dB (loud spoken voice)
  - profound = loss of over 90 dB (shout is 90–120dB)
- More women than men have a hearing loss.
- People who have worked with high noise levels (>85 dB) are more than twice as likely to be deaf.
- There is a related incidence of tinnitus with deafness.

A diagnostic approach

It is useful to consider the causes of deafness in terms of pathophysiology (conductive or sensorineural hearing loss) and anatomical sites (see FIG. 43.2).

Conductive hearing loss is caused by an abnormality in the pathway conducting sound waves from the outer ear to the inner ear,[1] as far as the footplate of the stapes.

Sensorineural hearing loss (SNHL) is a defect central to the oval window involving the cochlea (sensor), cochlear nerve (neural) or, more rarely, central neural pathways.[1]

Congenital deafness is an important consideration in children, while presbyacusis is very common in the aged. The commonest acquired causes of deafness are impacted cerumen (wax), serous otitis media and otitis externa. Noise-induced deafness is also a common problem.

It is important not to misdiagnose an acoustic neuroma, which can present as acute deafness, although slow progressive loss is more typical. A summary of the diagnostic strategy model, which includes several important causes of deafness, is presented in TABLE 43.1 and a checklist of ototoxic drugs in TABLE 43.2.

Symptoms

The symptoms vary so that some barely notice a problem while others are severely disabled.

Common symptoms include inability to:

- hear speech and other sounds loudly enough
- hear speech and music clearly, even when loud enough
- understand speech even when loud enough—a problem of language reception

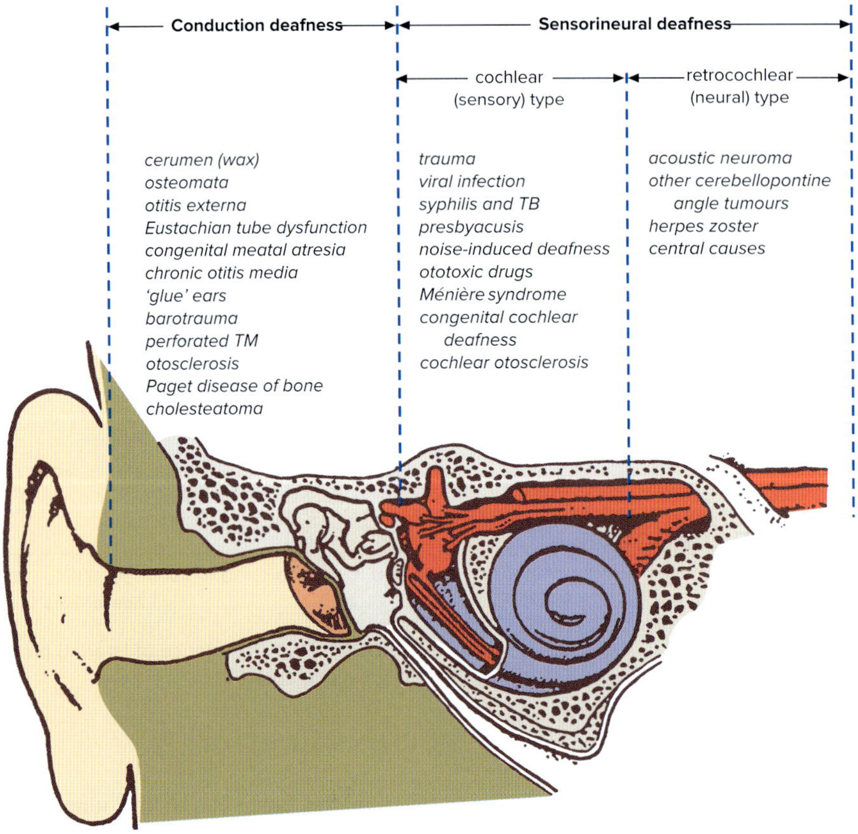

FIGURE 43.2 Causes of deafness according to anatomical site

People with mild hearing loss notice only subtle differences and may have trouble hearing certain high-frequency sounds, such as 's', 'f' or 'th'. They may also have trouble hearing in certain situations, such as at a party or in a crowd where there is a lot of background noise. Those with moderate hearing loss have trouble hearing in many situations.

The clinical approach

History

The history should include an account of the onset and progression of any deafness, noise exposure, drug history, a history of swimming or diving, air travel and head injury and family history. A recent or past episode of a generalised infection would be relevant and the presence of associated aural symptoms, such as ear pain, discharge, tinnitus and vertigo. Vertigo may be a symptom of Ménière syndrome, multiple sclerosis, acoustic neuroma or syphilis.

Several important clues can be obtained from the history. The often sudden onset of hearing loss in an ear following swimming or showering is suggestive of wax, which swells to block the ear canal completely.

Patients with conductive loss may hear better in noisy conditions (paracusis) because we raise our voices when there is background noise. Conversely, people with sensorineural deafness (SND) usually have more difficulty hearing in noise as voices become unintelligible.

Examination

Inspect the facial structures, skull and ears. The ears are inspected with an otoscope to visualise the external meatus and the tympanic membrane (TM) and the presence of obstructions such as wax, inflammation or osteomata.

The examination requires a clean external auditory canal. Gentle suction is useful for cleaning pus debris. Syringing is reserved for wax in people with an intact TM and a known healthy middle ear.

It is an advantage to have a pneumatic attachment to test drum mobility. Reduction of TM mobility is an important sign in secretory otitis media.

Table 43.1 Deafness and hearing loss: diagnostic strategy model

Probability diagnosis
Impacted cerumen
Serous otitis media
Otitis externa
Congenital (children)
Presbyacusis
Serious disorders not to be missed
Neoplasia:
• acoustic neuroma
• temporal lobe tumours (bilateral)
• otic tumours
• nasopharyngeal carcinoma
Infection:
• generalised infections (e.g. mumps, measles)
• meningitis
• syphilis
Perforated tympanic membrane
Cholesteatoma
Perilymphatic fistula (post-stapedectomy)
Ménière syndrome
Pitfalls (often missed)
Foreign body
Temporal bone fracture
Otosclerosis
Barotrauma
Noise-induced deafness
Rarities:
• Paget disease of bone
• multiple sclerosis
• osteogenesis imperfecta
Seven masquerades checklist
Diabetes
Drugs
Thyroid disorder (hypo)
Is the patient trying to tell me something?
Unlikely.

There are several simple hearing tests. The distance at which a ticking watch can be heard can be used but the advent of the digital watch has affected this traditional method.

Whisper test

Occlude far ear. Have the patient cover near eye with one hand to prevent lip reading. Place your mouth at the near side. Strongly whisper '68' then '100' from a distance of 50 cm. Ask the patient to repeat the words. Then repeat using a normal speaking voice.

Table 43.2 Known ototoxic drugs

Alcohol
Aminoglycosides:
• amikacin
• gentamicin
• kanamycin
• neomycin
• streptomycin
• tobramycin
Diuretics:
• ethacrynic acid
• frusemide
Chemotherapeutic agents
Quinine and related drugs
Salicylates/aspirin excess

Hair-rubbing method

In children and in adults with a reasonable amount of hair grab several hairs close to the external auditory canal between the thumb and index finger. Rub the hairs lightly together at 5 cm (high sensitivity) to produce a relatively high-pitched 'crackling' sound (see FIG. 43.3). If this sound cannot be heard, a moderate hearing loss is likely (usually about 40 dB or greater). Like the whisper test, this test is a rough guide only.

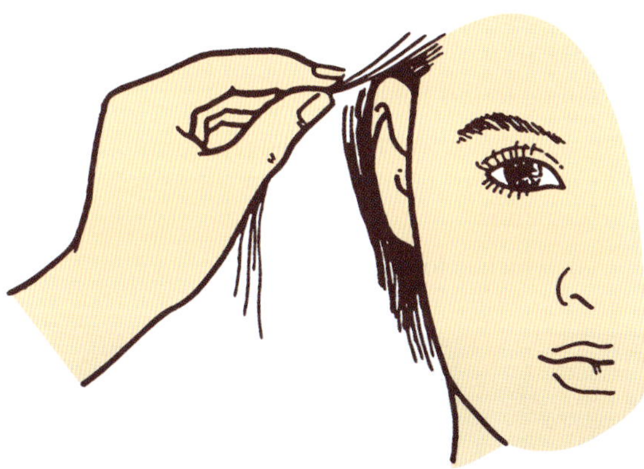

FIGURE 43.3 Simple hair-rubbing method of testing possible deafness

Tuning fork tests

If deafness is present, its type (conduction or sensorineural) should be determined by tuning fork testing. The most suitable tuning fork for preliminary testing is the C_2 (512 cps) fork. The fork is best activated by striking it firmly on the bent elbow.

43

Weber test

The vibrating tuning fork is applied firmly to the midpoint of the skull or to the central forehead or to the teeth.

This test is of value only if the deafness is unilateral or bilateral and unequal (see FIG. 43.4). Normally the sound is heard equally in both ears in the centre of the forehead. With sensorineural deafness the sound is transmitted to the normal ear, while with conduction deafness it is heard better in the abnormal ear.

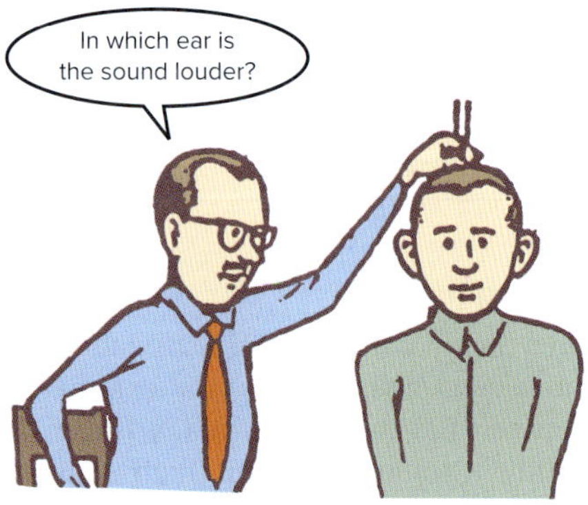

FIGURE 43.4 Weber test

Lateralisation of the sound to one ear indicates a conductive loss on that side, or a sensorineural loss on the other side.

Rinne test

The tuning fork is held:

- outside the ear (tests air conduction) and
- firmly against the mastoid bone (tests bone conduction)

Ask which is louder.

It therefore compares air and bone conduction in the same ear (see FIG. 43.5). A variation of the test includes placing the tuning fork on the mastoid process and the patient indicates when it can no longer be heard. The fork is then placed at the external auditory meatus and the patient indicates whether the sound is now audible. Normally air conduction is better than bone conduction and the sound will again be heard.

A comparison of the interpretation of these tests is summarised in TABLE 43.3.

Table 43.3 A comparison of the Rinne and Weber tests

State of the hearing	Rinne test	Weber test
Normal	Positive: AC >BC	Equal in both ears
Conduction deafness	Negative: BC >AC	Louder in the deaf ear
Very severe conduction deafness	Negative: BC >AC May hear BC only	Louder in the deaf ear
Sensorineural deafness	Positive: AC >BC	Louder in the better ear
Very severe sensorineural deafness	'False' negative (without masking)	Louder in the better ear

AC = air conduction; BC = bone conduction

Audiometric assessment

Audiometric assessment includes the following:

- pure tone audiometry
- impedance tympanometry
- electric response audiometry
- oto-acoustic emission testing

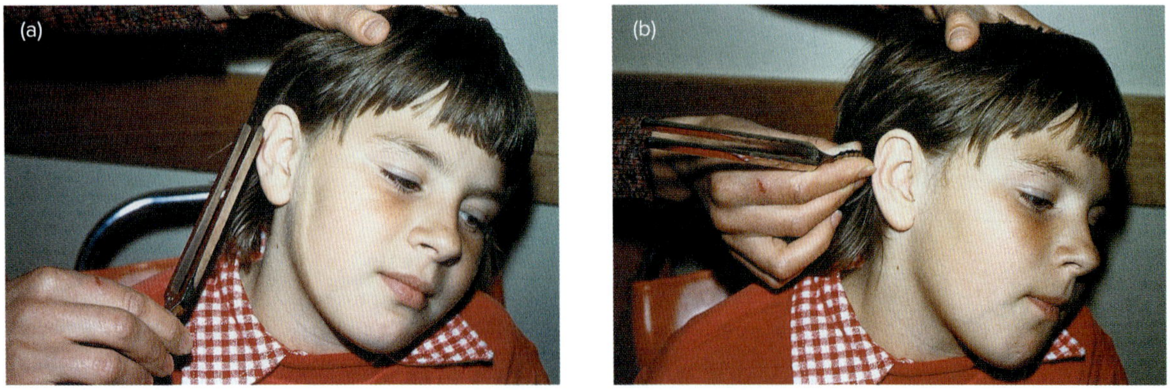

FIGURE 43.5 Rinne test comparing air conduction **(a)** with bone conduction **(b)**

Pure tone audiometry[4,5]

Pure tone audiometry is a graph of frequency expressed in hertz versus loudness expressed in decibels. The tone is presented either through the ear canal (a test of the conduction and the cochlear function of the ear) or through the bone (a test of cochlear function).

FIGURES 43.6 and 43.7 are typical examples of pure tone audiograms.

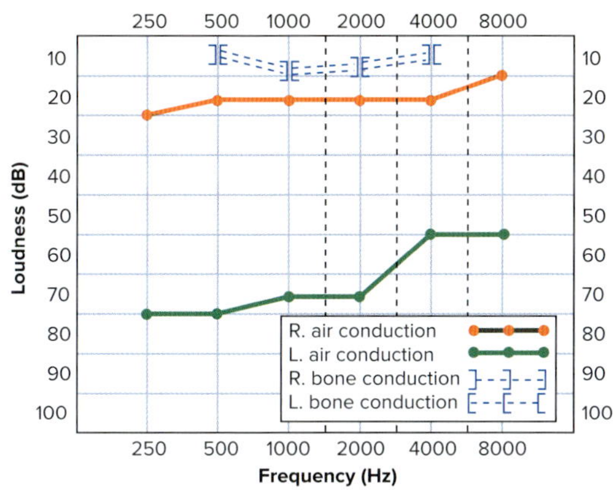

FIGURE 43.6 Pure tone audiogram for severe conductive deafness in left ear

Source: After Black[4]

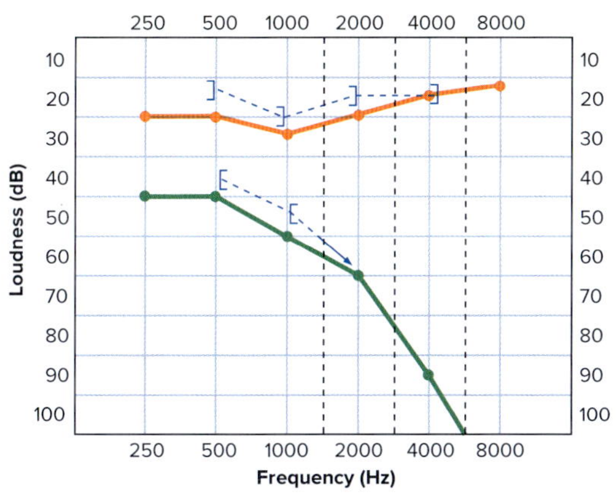

FIGURE 43.7 Pure tone audiogram for unilateral (left) sensorineural deafness. Suspect a viral or congenital origin in children; check adults for acoustic neuroma.

The difference between the two is a measure of conductance. If the two ears have different thresholds, a white noise masking sound is applied to the better ear to prevent it hearing sound presented to the test ear. The normal speech range occurs between 0 and 20 dB in soundproof conditions across the frequency spectrum.

Tympanometry

Tympanometry measures the mobility of the tympanic membrane, the dynamics of the ossicular chain and the middle-ear air cushion. The test consists of a sound applied at the external auditory meatus, otherwise sealed by the soft probe tip.

Deafness in children

Deafness in childhood is relatively common and often goes unrecognised. One to two of every 1000 newborn infants suffer from SND.[1] Congenital deafness may be due to inherited defects, to prenatal factors such as maternal intrauterine infection or drug ingestion during pregnancy, or to perinatal factors such as birth trauma, and haemolytic disease of the newborn.

Deafness may be associated with Down syndrome and Waardenburg syndrome. Waardenburg syndrome, which is dominantly inherited, is diagnosed in a patient with a white forelock of hair and different coloured eyes.

Acquired deafness accounts for approximately half of all childhood cases. Purulent otitis media and secretory otitis media are common causes of temporary conductive deafness. However, one in 10 children will have persistent middle-ear effusions and mild to moderate hearing loss in the 15–40 dB range.[6]

Permanent deafness in the first few years of life may be due to virus infections, such as mumps or meningitis, ototoxic antibiotics and several other causes.

Screening[1]

The aim of screening should be to recognise every deaf child by the age of 8 months to 1 year—before the vital time for learning speech is wasted. High-risk groups should be identified and screened, for example, a family history of deafness, maternal problems of pregnancy, perinatal problems, survivors of intensive care, very low birthweight and gestation <33 weeks, cerebral palsy and those with delayed or faulty speech. The guidelines for early signs of normal hearing are presented in TABLE 43.4.

Optimal screening times:

- 8–9 months (or earlier)
- school entry

There has been a proposition from the National Universal Hearing Screening Committee to introduce testing of newborn hearing following results[7] supporting this strategy after the finding of a higher incidence than appreciated. The average age at which these deaf children were diagnosed was 26 months.

Table 43.4 Early signs of normal hearing

Age	Typical response
1 month	Should notice sudden constant sounds (e.g. car motor, vacuum cleaner) by pausing and listening.
3 months	Should respond to loud noise (e.g. will stop crying when hands are clapped).
4 months	Should turn head to look for source of sound, such as mother speaking behind the child.
7 months	Should turn instantly to voices or even to quiet noises made across the room.
10 months	Should listen out for familiar everyday sounds.
12 months	Should show some response to familiar words and commands, including his or her name.

Early signs of hearing loss

A high index of suspicion is essential in detecting hearing loss in children and any parental concern should be taken seriously. The presentation of hearing loss will depend on whether it is bilateral or unilateral, its severity and age of onset.

Typical presentations include:

- malformation of skull, ears or face
- failure to respond in an expected way to sounds, especially one's voice
- preference for, or response only to, loud sounds
- no response to normal conversation or to television
- speech abnormality or delay
- absence of 'babbling' by 12 months
- no single words or comprehension of simple words by 18 months
- learning problems at school
- disobedience
- other behavioural problems
- inability to detect sound direction (unilateral loss)
- inability to follow simple commands or less than 20 spoken words by 2 years

Screening methods

Hearing can be tested at any age. No child is too young to be tested and this includes the newborn. Informal office assessments, such as whispering in the child's ear or rattling car keys, are totally inadequate for excluding deafness and may be potentially harmful if they lead to false reassurance.

Pneumatic otoscopy is essential to exclude middle-ear effusions.

Pure tone audiometry is unreliable in children under 4 years of age, so special techniques such as tympanometry are required. Tympanometry assesses TM compliance, and is highly sensitive and specific for detecting middle-ear pathology in children beyond early infancy.

Auditory brain stem response testing is used to evaluate children (particularly young infants) for whom information on behavioural hearing tests is either unobtainable or unreliable.[6]

Management

Children with middle-ear pathology and hearing loss should be referred to a specialist. All children with SNHL (even those with profound deafness), as well as children with conductive losses not correctable by surgery, benefit from amplification. All children need referral to a specialist centre skilled in educational and language remediation.

Deafness in the elderly[8]

The prevalence of hearing loss increases exponentially with age. The commonest reason for bilateral progressive SND is presbyacusis, which is the high-frequency hearing loss of advancing age (see FIG. 43.8). There appears to be a genetic predisposition to presbyacusis.[8]

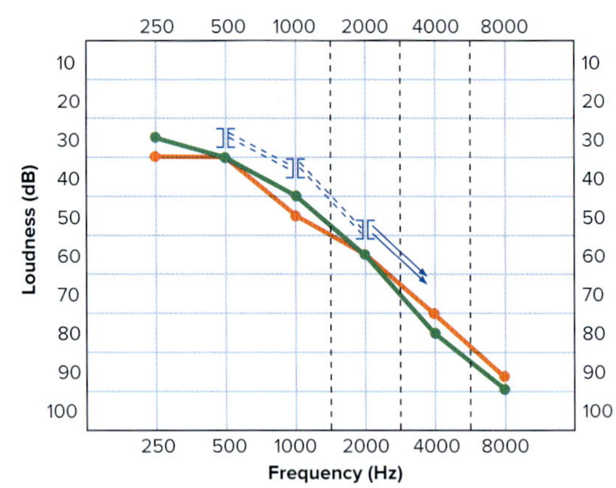

FIGURE 43.8 Presbyacusis: bilateral high-frequency sensorineural deafness

Some features include:

- loss of high-frequency sounds
- usually associated with tinnitus
- intolerance to very loud sounds
- difficulty picking up high-frequency consonants, e.g. 'f', 's'—these sounds are often distorted or unheard, and there is confusion with words such as 'fit' and 'sit', 'fun' and 'sun'

Deafness is associated with various types of mental illness in the aged, including anxiety, depression, paranoid delusions, agitation and confusion because of sensory deprivation. The possibility of deafness should be kept in mind when assessing these problems.

Signs indicating referral for hearing test

Possible indications for referring the older person:

- speaking too loudly
- difficulty understanding speech
- social withdrawal
- lack of interest in attending parties and other functions
- complaints about people mumbling
- requests to have speech repeated
- complaints of tinnitus
- setting television and radio on high volume

Sudden deafness

Sudden deafness refers to sudden SNHL of greater than 30–35 dB with an onset period of between 12 hours and 3 days.[9] It specially excludes gradual progressive causes of SND, such as cumulative noise trauma or presbyacusis, and also excludes causes of sudden deafness that may be related to pathology in the external auditory canal, TM or middle ear.

The main causes are given in TABLE 43.5.

Table 43.5 Causes of sudden deafness

Trauma:

- head injury
- diving
- flying
- acoustic blast

Postoperative:

- previous stapedectomy

Viral infections (e.g. mumps, measles, herpes zoster)
Ototoxic drugs (e.g. aminoglycosides, gentamicin)
Cerebellopontine angle tumours (e.g. acoustic neuroma)

Vascular disease:

- polycythaemia
- diabetes
- stroke
- vasculitis

Ménière syndrome
Cochlear otosclerosis

In several instances, despite a careful clinical examination and investigation, an explanation for sudden SND cannot be found. The cause of deafness in these cases is thought to be either vascular obstruction of the end artery system or viral cochleitis.[7,8] Fortunately, spontaneous recovery usually results.

Patients with sudden SND require immediate referral. It is a difficult problem both in diagnosis and management. Early diagnosis and a high index of suspicion are fundamental.[8] Two important conditions that deserve special reference are perilymphatic fistula, which occurs after stapedectomy, and an acoustic neuroma presumably causing compression of the internal auditory artery by the tumour in the internal auditory meatus.

Investigations: FBE, ESR, ANCA; TB ELISPOT; viral titres; evoked response audiometry; MRI.

Otosclerosis

Otosclerosis is a disease of the bone surrounding the inner ear and is the most common cause of conductive hearing loss in the adult with a normal tympanic membrane. The normal middle ear bone is replaced by vascular, spongy bone that becomes sclerotic.

Clinical features[3]

Usually:

- a progressive disease
- develops in the 20s and 30s
- family history (autosomal dominant)
- bilateral or unilateral
- female preponderance
- affects the footplate of the stapes
- may progress rapidly during pregnancy
- conductive hearing loss
- begins in lower frequencies, then progresses
- SND may be present
- impedance audiometry shows characteristic features of conductive loss with a mild sensorineural loss
- may be associated with Ménière syndrome

Management

- Referral to an ENT consultant
- Stapedectomy (approximately 90% effective)
- Hearing aid (less effective alternative)

Cholesteatoma[7]

A cholesteatoma is a sac of keratinising squamous epithelium that arises from a perforation involving the periphery of the TM. In other words, it is a ‘big sac of skin' (refer to CHAPTER 50). It is dangerous to the ear because it tends to expand and destroy adjacent structures, including the TM, ossicular chain and cochlear. Destruction of the first two may result in conductive hearing loss of up to 60 dB. Irreversible SND caused by otic capsule erosion may also occur. Surgical correction is mandatory.

Wax impaction[10]

Ear wax impaction occurs in about 5% of the normal population but is more prevalent in older people especially with the use of hearing aids. It is also common in those who use cotton buds (which should be avoided), where cerumen is packed onto the TM leading to a conductive hearing loss. The average wax production is 2.81 mg/week. Most ear wax clears spontaneously without treatment.

Methods of removal include:

- gentle syringing with warm (body temperature) water or normal saline solution—by trained practitioner (avoid syringing if infection or perforated TM)
- consider cerumenolytic drops for several days before syringing
  - carbamide peroxide (Ear Clear)
  - docusate sodium (Waxsol)
  - hydrogen peroxide
  - sodium bicarbonate
  - oil based (e.g. olive oil, almond oil)

Keratosis obturans is an accumulation of keratin to form a pearly-white plug that requires removal.

Noise-induced hearing loss

Clinical features

- Onset of tinnitus after work in excessive noise
- Speech seems muffled soon after work
- Temporary loss initially but becomes permanent if noise exposure continues
- High-frequency loss on audiogram

Sounds exceeding 85 dB are potentially injurious to the cochlea, especially with prolonged exposures. Common sources of injurious noise are industrial machinery, weapons and loud music.

Tinnitus

The diagnostic strategy is presented in TABLE 43.6.

Tinnitus is defined as a sound perceived by the ear that arises from an internal source. When pathology in the inner ear is the cause, the tinnitus is non-pulsating, continuous and may have variable frequencies and intensity.

A thorough history and examination should be conducted so that tinnitus can be classified as objective (e.g. heard with stethoscope) or non-objective and pulsatile, or non-pulsatile.

Precautions:

- exclude wax, drugs including marijuana, NSAIDs, salicylates, quinine and aminoglycosides,[9] vascular disease, depression, anaemia, aneurysm, vascular tumours (e.g. glomus tumour), venous hum (jugular vein), acoustic neuroma (progressive and unilateral), Ménière syndrome and infections (e.g. viral cochleitis)
- if pulsatile, consider carotid artery lesions, including a caroticocavernous fistula and an AV fistula

Table 43.6 Diagnostic strategy for tinnitus

Probability diagnosis
Ear wax or debris
Sensorineural hearing loss (esp. noise-induced)
Otosclerosis
Ageing
Ear infection (e.g. viral cochleitis)
Ménière syndrome
Serious disorders not to be missed
Vascular:
• arteriovenous malformation
• arterial bruits (esp. carotid)
• venous hum (jugular)
Infection:
• suppurative otitis media
Cancer/tumour:
• acoustic neuroma (unilateral)
Other:
• head injury
Pitfalls (often missed)
Impacted wisdom tooth
Temporomandibular injury
Alcoholism
Rarities:
• superior canal dehiscence
• glomus jugulare tumour
• syphilis
Seven masquerades checklist
Anaemia (severe)
Depression
Drugs (aspirin, NSAIDs, loop diuretics, marijuana, quinine, aminoglycosides)
Spinal dysfunction
Is the patient trying to tell me something?
Consider if subjective tinnitus

- beware of lonely elderly people living alone (suicide risk)

Note: Otosclerosis in young adults causes deafness and tinnitus.

Investigations

- Audiological examination by audiologist
- Tympanometry and speech discrimination
- MRI or CT scan (if serious cause suspected or head injury)

Management

- Treat any underlying cause and aggravating factors. Otherwise, minimise symptoms.
- Educate and reassure the patient (tinnitus is nearly always amenable to treatment).
- Encourage a patient support group.

Holistic approach (options)

Mainly based on acoustic desensitisation:

- Relaxation techniques, address any anxiety
- Tinnitus retraining therapy (clinical psychologist)
- Cognitive behaviour therapy techniques
- Background 'noise' (e.g. music played during night for masking)
- Tinnitus maskers
- Hearing aids (based on audiologist assessment)
- Consider hypnotherapy

Medical (trials of options)

- Clonazepam 0.5 mg nocte (with care)
- Minerals (e.g. zinc and magnesium)
- Betahistine (Serc) 8–16 mg daily (max. 32 mg)
- Carbamazepine or sodium valproate
- Antidepressants if depressed

Acute severe tinnitus

- Lignocaine 1% IV slowly (up to 5 mL)

Hearing aids

Hearing aids are most useful in conductive deafness. This is due to the relative lack of distortion, making amplification simple. In SND the dual problem of recruitment and the hearing loss for higher frequencies may make hearing aids less satisfactory. Modern aids selectively amplify higher frequencies and 'cut out' excessive volume peaks that would cause discomfort. A trial of such aids should be made by a reliable hearing-aid consultant following full medical assessment.

Cochlear implants[8,11]

The cochlear implant or 'bionic ear' is used in adults and children with severe hearing loss unresponsive to powerful hearing aids. The implant consists of an array of 22 electrodes inserted into the cochlea following mastoidectomy, attached to a receiver implanted in the skull next to the ear. External sounds are detected by an external processor worn behind the ear and connected to the implanted receiver with an external induction coil. Near normal speech and hearing may be achieved in children with congenital or acquired deafness with early implantation. The device is most suitable for children over 2 years and adults with severe deafness.

Advice for families

Relatives and close friends need considerable advice about coping with deaf family members. They should be told that the deaf person may hear in a quiet room but not in a crowd, and advised of the range of aids and services available and the importance of proper maintenance of any hearing aids (especially with aged people).

Do

- Face the light when speaking to them.
- Speak directly to them.
- Speak clearly and naturally.
- Speak at a uniform pitch: avoid lowering your voice during or at the end of a sentence.
- Speak within 2 metres.
- Be tolerant and relaxed.
- Be patient with mistakes.
- Write key words on a paper pad when necessary.

Don't

- Speak with your back to them.
- Mumble your words.
- Use exaggerated lip movements.
- Shout.
- Put your hand or fingers over your mouth when talking.
- Repeat one word over and over.

Red flags for priority referral[8]

- Asymmetrical sensorineural hearing loss
- Cranial nerve defects
- Ear canal or middle-ear mass
- Deep ear pain
- Discharging ear

When to refer

- See 'Red flags' above.
- Sudden deafness.
- Any child with suspected deafness, including poor speech and learning problems, should be referred to an audiology centre.
- Any child with middle-ear pathology and hearing loss should be referred to a specialist.
- Unexplained deafness.

Practice tips

- A mother who believes her child may be deaf is rarely wrong in this suspicion.
- Suspect deafness in an infant with delayed development and in children with speech defects or behavioural problems.
- Audiological assessment should be performed on children born to mothers with evidence of intrauterine infection by any of the TORCH organisms (toxoplasmosis, rubella, cytomegalovirus and herpes virus).
- No child is too young for audiological assessment. Informal office tests are inadequate for excluding hearing loss.
- Sounds tend to be softer in conductive hearing loss and distorted with sensorineural loss.
- People with conductive deafness tend to speak softly, hear better in a noisy environment, hear well on the telephone and have good speech discrimination.
- People with SND tend to speak loudly, hear poorly in a noisy environment, have poor speech discrimination and hear poorly on the telephone.

Patient education resources

Hand-out sheets from *Murtagh's Patient Education* 7th edition:

- Hearing problems in children
- Hearing impairment in older people
- Tinnitus

References

1 Lasak JM et al. Hearing loss: diagnosis and management. Prim Care, 2014; 41 (1): 19–31.

2 Fagan P. Assessing hearing in clinical practice. Medical Observer, 10 March 2006: 23–5.

3 Papadakis MA, McPhee SJ. *Current Medical Diagnosis and Treatment* (56th edn). New York: McGraw-Hill Education, 2017: 209–10.

4 Black B. Pure tone audiograms. Aust Fam Physician, 1988; 17: 906–7.

5 Cootes H. Interpret audiograms: therapy update. Australian Doctor, 25 May 2007: 41–6.

6 Jarman R. Hearing impairment. Australian Paediatric Review, 1991; 4: 2.

7 Fortnum HM et al. Prevalence of permanent childhood hearing impairment in the United Kingdom and implications for universal neonatal hearing screening: questionnaire-based ascertainment study. BMJ, 2001; 323: 536–40.

8 Sale P, Patel N. Hearing loss in the ageing patient: how to treat. Australian Doctor, 15 April 2011: 27–34.

9 Pohl DV. Sudden deafness. Modern Medicine Australia, 1990; June: 72–8.

10 Buckley N (Chair). *Australian Medicines Handbook*. Adelaide: Australian Medicines Handbook Pty Ltd, 2016: 422.

11 Black B, Harvey L. Tinnitus: update. Medical Observer, 13 August 2004: 31–3.

12 Atlas M, Lowinger D. The GP's essential guide to hearing loss. Medicine Today, 2000; June: 48–59.

Diarrhoea

44

A dirty cook gives diarrhoea quicker than rhubarb.

TUNG-SU PAI (TIME UNCERTAIN)

Diarrhoea is defined as an intestinal disorder characterised by abnormal frequency and liquidity of faecal evacuations.

Acute self-limiting diarrhoea, which is very common and frequently not seen by the medical practitioner, is usually infective and mild, and resolves within days. In Australia most infective cases are viral. The causes of diarrhoea are numerous, thus making a detailed history and examination very important in leading to the diagnosis. 'Chronic' diarrhoea is that lasting at least 4–6 weeks. Important causes are presented in FIGURE 44.1.

The terminology for acute infective diarrhoea can be confusing. A simple classification is:

- vomiting and diarrhoea = gastroenteritis
- diarrhoea (only) = enteritis

Key facts and checkpoints

- The characteristics of the stool provide a useful guide to the site of the bowel disorder.
- Disorders of the upper GIT tend to produce diarrhoea stools that are copious, watery or fatty, pale yellow or green.
- Colonic disorder tends to produce stools that are small, of variable consistency, brown and may contain blood or mucus.
- Acute gastroenteritis should be regarded as a diagnosis of exclusion.
- Chronic diarrhoea is more likely to be due to protozoal infection (e.g. amoebiasis, giardiasis or *Cryptosporidium*) than bacillary dysentery.
- A history of travel, especially to countries at risk of endemic bowel infections, is essential.
- Certain antibiotics can cause an overgrowth of *Clostridium difficile*, which produces pseudomembranous colitis.
- Coeliac disease, although a cause of failure to thrive in children, can present at any age.
- In disorders of the colon, the patient experiences frequency and urgency but passes only small amounts of faeces.
- Diarrhoea can be classified broadly into four types:
  - acute watery diarrhoea
  - bloody diarrhoea (acute or chronic)
  - chronic watery diarrhoea
  - steatorrhoea

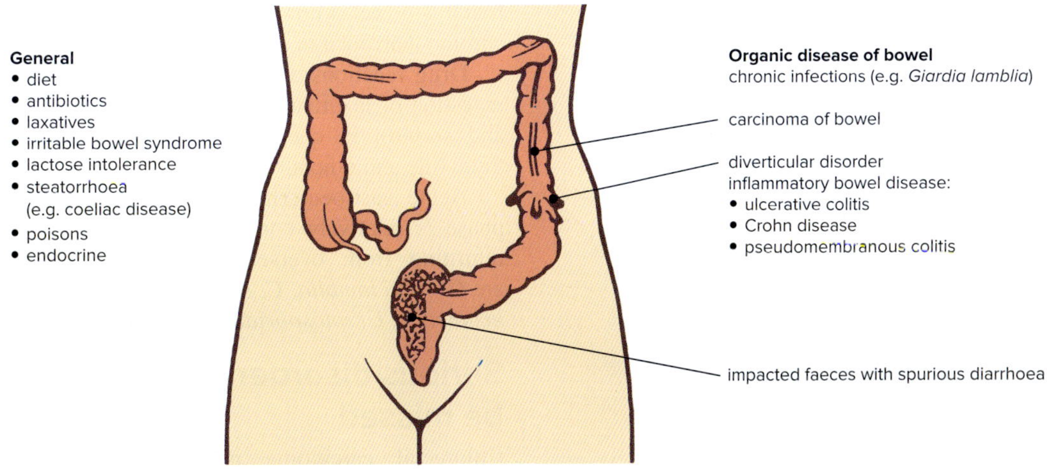

FIGURE 44.1 Important causes of chronic diarrhoea

44

A diagnostic approach

A summary of the diagnostic strategy model is presented in TABLE 44.1.

Table 44.1 Diarrhoea: diagnostic strategy model

Probability diagnosis

Acute:
- Gastroenteritis/infective enteritis (viral/bacterial)
- Dietary indiscretion
- Antibiotic reaction

Chronic:
- Irritable bowel syndrome
- Drug reactions (e.g. laxatives)
- Chronic infections

Serious disorders not to be missed

Neoplasia:
- colorectal cancer
- ovarian cancer
- peritoneal cancer

HIV infection (AIDS)

Infections:
- cholera
- typhoid/paratyphoid
- amoebiasis
- malaria
- enterohaemorrhagic *E. coli* enteritis

Inflammatory bowel disease:
- Crohn/ulcerative colitis
- pseudomembranous colitis

Non-microbial food poisoning e.g. death cap mushroom
Intussusception
Pelvic appendicitis/pelvic abscess

Pitfalls (often missed)

Coeliac disease
Faecal impaction with spurious diarrhoea
Lactase deficiency
Giardia lamblia infection
Cryptosporidium infection
Cytomegalovirus in immunocompromised
Malabsorption states (e.g. coeliac disease)
Vitamin C and other oral drugs
Nematode infections:
- strongyloides (threadworm)
- whipworm

Radiotherapy
Diverticulitis
Post-GIT surgery
Ischaemic colitis (elderly)

Rarities:
- Addison disease (see CHAPTER 23)
- carcinoid tumours
- zinc deficiency in children
- short bowel syndrome
- amyloidosis
- toxic shock
- Zollinger–Ellison syndrome

Seven masquerades checklist

Diabetes
Drugs (e.g. metformin)
Thyroid disorder (hyper)

Is the patient trying to tell me something?

Yes, diarrhoea may be a manifestation of anxiety state or irritable bowel syndrome.

Probability diagnosis

Acute diarrhoea

Common causes are:

- gastroenteritis/enteritis:
  - bacterial: *Salmonella* sp., *Campylobacter jejuni, Shigella* sp., enteropathic *Escherichia coli, Staphylococcus aureus* (food poisoning)
  - viral: rotavirus (50% of children hospital admissions[1]), norovirus, astrovirus, adenovirus
- dietary indiscretions (e.g. binge eating)
- antibiotic reactions

Red flag pointers for diarrhoea

- Unexpected weight loss
- Persistent/unresolved
- Blood in stool
- Fever
- Overseas travel
- Severe abdominal pain
- Family history: bowel cancer, Crohn disease

Chronic diarrhoea

Irritable bowel syndrome was the commonest cause of chronic diarrhoea in a UK study.[1]

Drug reactions are also important. These include ingestion of laxatives, osmotic agents such as lactose and sorbitol in chewing gum, alcohol, antibiotics, thyroxine and others.

Acute gastroenteritis that persists into a chronic phase is relatively common, especially in travellers returning from overseas. Important considerations are *Giardia lamblia, C. difficile, Yersinia, Entamoeba histolytica, Cryptosporidium* and HIV infection.

Serious disorders not to be missed

Colorectal carcinoma must be considered with persistent diarrhoea, especially if of insidious onset.

AIDS due to symptomatic HIV infection needs consideration, especially in those at risk. The serious infectious disorders that can affect international travellers, such as cholera, typhoid, paratyphoid and amoebiasis, should also be kept in mind.

In children, coeliac disease and cystic fibrosis can present as chronic diarrhoea, while intussusception, although not causing true diarrhoea, can present as loose, redcurrant jelly-like stools and should not be misdiagnosed (as gastroenteritis). Appendicitis must also be considered in the onset of acute diarrhoea and vomiting.

Infection with enterohaemorrhagic strains of *E. coli* (e.g. O157:H7, O111:H8) may lead to the haemolytic uraemic syndrome or thrombotic thrombocytopenic purpura, particularly in children. What appears to be simple enteritis can eventuate to be fatal. If suspected, avoid giving antibiotics.

Clue: Think of it with atypical gastroenteritis and bloody diarrhoea. Avoid antibiotics.

Death cap mushroom (the world's most lethal)—*Amanita phalloides* (FIGURE 44.2)—causes severe gastroenteritis followed by delayed hepatic failure and AKF.

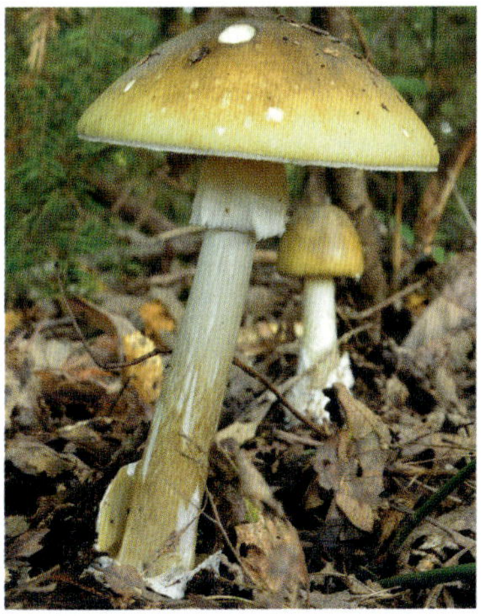

FIGURE 44.2 *Amanita phalloides* (death cap mushroom)
Source: Shutterstock.com

Pitfalls

There are many traps in evaluating the patient with diarrhoea, including drug ingestion, especially vitamin C (sodium ascorbate powder), which causes diarrhoea. Faecal impaction with spurious diarrhoea is an age-old pitfall, as is lactase deficiency, which may go undiagnosed for many years. In recent times infection with *G. lamblia* may smoulder on for months with watery, offensive stools before diagnosis.

General pitfalls

- Not considering acute appendicitis in acute diarrhoea—can be retrocaecal or pelvic appendicitis
- Missing faecal impaction with spurious diarrhoea
- Failing to perform a rectal examination
- Failing to consider acute ischaemic colitis in an elderly patient with the acute onset of bloody diarrhoea stools (following sudden abdominal pain in preceding 24 hours)

Seven masquerades checklist

The significant masquerades include diabetes, when an autonomic neuropathy may cause alternating bouts of constipation and diarrhoea, thyrotoxicosis and drugs. Drugs that can cause diarrhoea are summarised in TABLE 44.2.

Pseudomembranous colitis (antibiotic-associated diarrhoea)[2]

This potentially fatal colitis can be caused by the use of any antibiotic, especially clindamycin, lincomycin, ampicillin and the cephalosporins (an exception is vancomycin).

Table 44.2 Drugs that can cause diarrhoea
Alcohol, esp. chronic abuse (often overlooked!)
Antibiotics, esp. penicillin derivatives
Antihypertensives, selected (e.g. methyldopa)
Acarbose
Cardiac agents (e.g. digoxin, quinidine)
Chenodeoxycholic acid
Cisapride
Colchicine
Cytotoxic agents (e.g. methotrexate)
Food and drug additives: sorbitol, mannitol, fructose, lactose
Heavy metals
H_2-receptor antagonists
Iron-containing compounds
Laxatives
Magnesium-containing antacids/magnesium supplements
Metformin
Misoprostol
NSAIDs
Orlistat
Prostaglandins
Quinidine
Salicylates
Sildenafil
Statins
Theophylline
Thyroxine

It is usually due to an overgrowth of *C. difficile*, which produces a toxin that causes specific inflammatory lesions, sometimes with a pseudomembrane. It may occur, uncommonly, without antibiotic usage.

Clinical features

- Profuse, watery diarrhoea
- Abdominal cramping and tenesmus ± fever
- Within 2 days of taking antibiotic (can start up to 4 to 6 weeks after usage)
- Persists 2 weeks (up to 6) after ceasing antibiotic

Diagnosed by characteristic lesions on sigmoidoscopy and a tissue culture assay and/or PCR for *C. difficile* toxin.

Treatment[2]

- Cease antibiotic
- Need hygiene measures to prevent spread
- Mild to moderate: metronidazole 400 mg (o) tds for 10 days
- Severe: vancomycin 125 mg (o) qid for 10 days (in consultation with specialist). Beware of toxic megacolon.

Psychogenic considerations

Anxiety and stress can cause looseness of the bowel. The irritable bowel syndrome, which is a very common condition, may reflect underlying psychological factors and most patients find that the symptoms are exacerbated by stress. Look for evidence of depression.

In children chronic diarrhoea can occur with the so-called 'maternal deprivation syndrome', characterised by growth and developmental retardation due to adverse psychosocial factors.

The clinical approach

History

As always, the history is the key to the diagnosis. First establish what the patient means by the term 'diarrhoea', his or her normal pattern and how the presenting problem varies from normal.

It is important to analyse the nature of the stools, the frequency of diarrhoea, associated symptoms, including abdominal pain, and constitutional symptoms, such as fever. Food intake in the past 72 hours and recent travel abroad may give a clue to acute gastroenteritis or food poisoning (an acute, self-limiting illness of diarrhoea and vomiting). The difference between food poisoning and infective gastroenteritis is presented in TABLE 44.3. However, there can be an overlap of features from a specific organism and the exercise may be semantic, but it may provide a clue to food-borne causation. A summary of non-microbial food poisoning is presented in TABLE 44.4.

Table 44.3 Comparison of acute diarrhoea due to bacterial food poisoning and infective gastroenteritis

	Food poisoning	Infective gastroenteritis
Responsible organisms	Toxins from: *Staphylococcus aureus* *Salmonella* sp. *Clostridium perfringens* *Clostridium difficile* *Vibrio parahaemolyticus* *Aeromonas hydrophilia* *Bacillus cereus*	Viral Bacterial, e.g. *Campylobacter jejuni* *Escherichia coli* *Shigella* sp. *Salmonella* sp.
Incubation period (onset from contact)	Short—within 24 hours Average—12 hours *S. aureus*—2–4 hours	3–5 days
Diarrhoea	Watery	Diarrhoea ± blood
Other features	Abdominal cramps (milder) Dehydration Headache Vomiting	Abdominal cramps
Typical foods	Chicken Meat Seafood Rice Custards and cream (*S. aureus*)	Milk Water Chicken

A drug history is relevant, as is a family history of diarrhoea, which may be significant for coeliac disease, Crohn disease and cystic fibrosis.

Enquire sensitively about sexual activity. Patients at risk from HIV infection should be discreetly evaluated.

Table 44.4 Non-microbial food poisoning[3]

Food (specific types)	Toxin	Onset	Features (symptoms)
Mushrooms	Muscarine	Minutes to hours	N, V, D, P: CNS symptoms
Toadstools	Amatoxin	Hours	N, V, D, P: hepatic failure
Immature or sprouting potatoes	Solanine	Within hours	N, V, D, P Throat constriction
Fish	Ichthysarcotoxin Various (e.g. ciguatera, scombrotoxin)	10–60 minutes (occasionally longer)	N, V, D, P Circumoral tingling CNS symptoms Collapse
Mussels	Mytilotoxism	5–30 minutes	N, V, P CNS: paralysis
Grain, esp. rye	Ergot fungus Alphatoxin	Minutes to 24 hours	N, V, P Circulatory and CNS
Fava beans (favism)	Enzyme deficiency	Rapid	V, D Acute haemolysis

N = nausea; V = vomiting; D = diarrhoea; P = abdominal pain

Key questions

Acute diarrhoea

- Where did you eat in the 24 hours before the diarrhoea started?
- What food did you eat during this time?
- Did you have chicken or seafood recently? (Chicken may be contaminated with *Salmonella* or *Campylobacter* and seafood with *Vibrio parahaemolyticus.*)
- Did any other people get the same problem?
- Have you travelled overseas recently? Where?
- Have you noticed any blood or mucus in your motions?
- Have you had any previous attacks?
- Have you noticed fever, weakness or other symptoms?

Chronic diarrhoea

- Have you noticed any blood or mucus in the motion?
- Have you travelled overseas recently? Where?
- Do you have pain and is it relieved by opening your bowels or passing wind?
- Does anyone else in your family have diarrhoea?
- Have you had any operations on your abdomen recently?
- What medications are you taking?
- Are you taking antibiotics?
- Do you take vitamin C for your health?
- Do you take laxatives?
- How much alcohol do you drink? Fruit juice?
- How much milk do you drink?
- What about thick shakes, ice-cream and yoghurt?
- Do you get clammy or shaky, or have you lost weight?
- Have you had trouble with pain in your joints, back pain, eye trouble or mouth ulceration?
- Do you have trouble flushing your motions down the toilet?
- Do you get diarrhoea during the night?
- Are you under a lot of stress?

Significance of symptoms

Abdominal pain

Central colicky abdominal pain indicates involvement of the small bowel, while lower abdominal pain points to the large bowel.

Nature of stools

If small volume, consider inflammation or carcinoma of colon; if large volume, consider laxative abuse and malabsorption.

If there is profuse bright red bleeding, consider diverticulitis or carcinoma of colon, and if small amounts with mucus or mucopus consider inflammatory bowel disorder. The presence of blood in the stools excludes functional bowel disorder. Diarrhoea at night suggests organic disease. In steatorrhoea the stools are distinctively pale, greasy, offensive, floating and difficult to flush. It is exacerbated by fatty foods.

'Rice water' stool is characteristic of cholera and 'pea soup' stool of typhoid fever.

Examination

The extent of the examination depends on the nature of the presenting problem. If it is acute, profuse and associated with vomiting, especially in a child, the examination needs to be general to assess the effects of fluid, electrolyte and nutritional loss. An infant's life is in danger from severe gastroenteritis and this assessment is a priority. The general nutritional and electrolyte assessment is also relevant in chronic diarrhoea with malabsorption, and this includes looking for evidence of muscle weakness (e.g. hypokalaemia, hypomagnesaemia, tetany [hypocalcaemia], bruising [vitamin K loss]).

The examination should also focus on the abdomen (systematic palpation), the rectum and the skin. Possible helpful signs are included in FIGURE 44.3.

The stool

Ideally the stool should be examined. The consistency of the stool as an aid to diagnosis[2,4] is summarised in TABLE 44.5, the features of the stool in TABLE 44.6, and the characteristics that distinguish between small and large bowel diarrhoea[1] are presented in TABLE 44.7. Note the presence of blood or mucus or steatorrhoea.

Bloody diarrhoea

Consider: inflammatory bowel disease, colonic polyps, carcinoma, infective especially *Shigella, Salmonella, Campylobacter, E. coli,* amoebiasis, colitis (pseudomembranous, ischaemic).

Investigations[3]

The following list includes a range of tests that may be required. Appropriate tests should be judiciously selected and in some instances, such as acute self-limiting diarrhoea, no investigations are necessary.

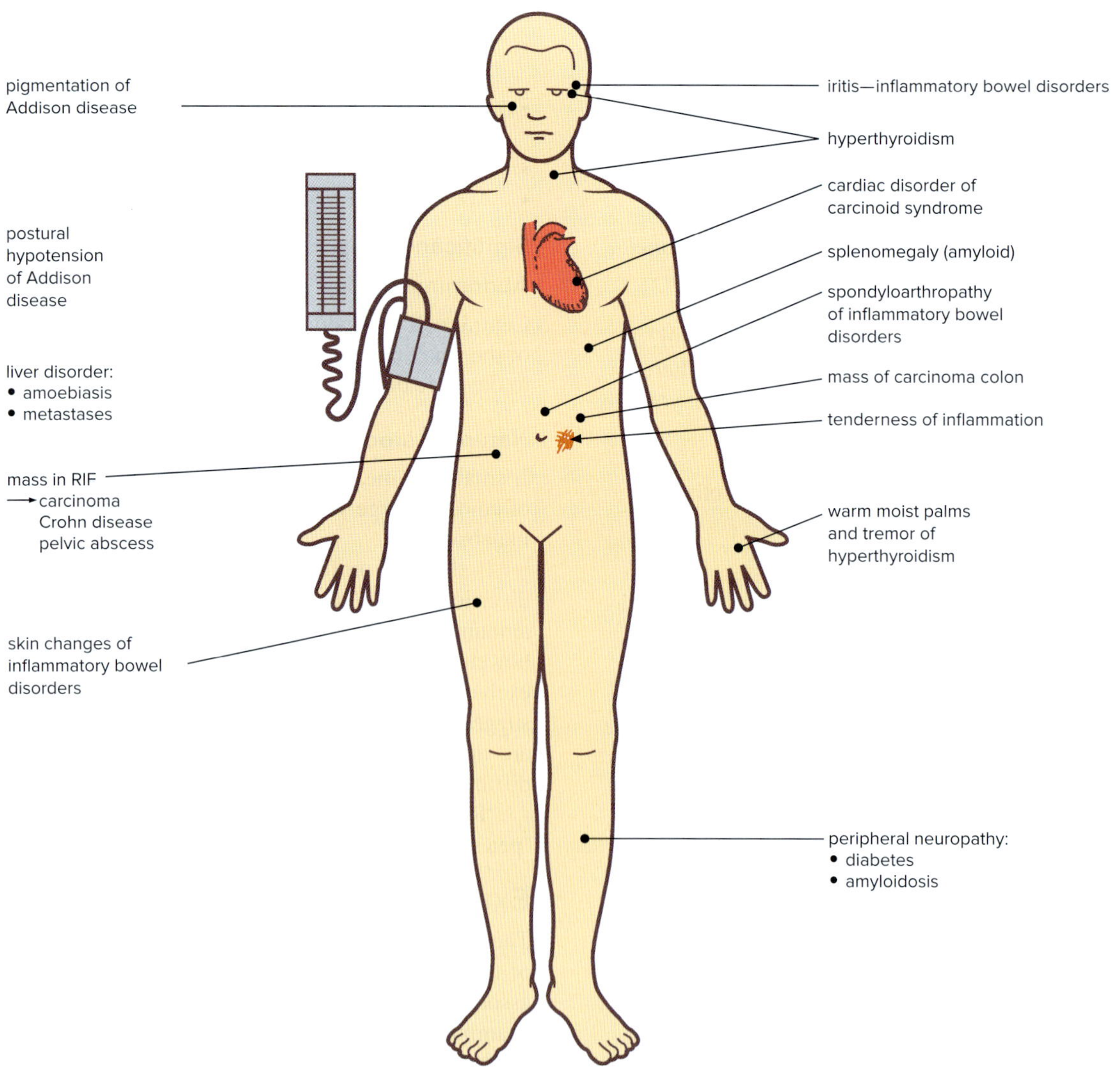

FIGURE 44.3 Possible significant signs in the patient with diarrhoea

Table 44.5 Stool consistency as an aid to diagnosis

Consistency	Probable cause
Liquid and uniform	Small bowel disorder (e.g. gastroenteritis)
Loose with bits of faeces	Colonic disorder
Watery, offensive, bubbly	*Giardia lamblia* infection
Liquid or semiformed, mucus ± blood	*Entamoeba histolytica*
Bulky, pale, offensive	Malabsorption
Pellets or ribbons	Irritable bowel syndrome

Table 44.6 Stool features as an aid to diagnosis

Stool appearance	Cause to consider
China clay	Obstructive jaundice
Black stool	Melaena (blood) in faeces
Pea soup	Typhoid fever
Rabbit pellets	Irritable bowel syndrome
Redcurrant jelly	Intussusception
Rice water	Cholera
Silver stool	Carcinoma of ampulla of Vater
Toothpaste	Hirschsprung disease

Table 44.7 Distinction between small and large bowel diarrhoea

	Small bowel	Large bowel
Volume	Large	Small
Pain	Central	Lower/LIF
Borborygmi	+ +	–
Undigested food	+	–
Steatorrhoea	+/–	–
Blood	–	+
Mucus	–	+
Urgency	–	+
Tenesmus	–	+

- Stool tests:
  - microscopy for parasites and red and white cells (warm specimen for amoebiasis)
  - cultures: may need special requests for *Campylobacter* sp., *C. difficile* and toxin, *Yersinia* sp., *Cryptosporidium* sp., *Aeromonas* sp. (stools must be collected fresh on three occasions)
- Blood tests: haemoglobin; MCV, WCC, ESR, iron, ferritin, folate, vitamin B12, calcium, electrolytes, thyroid function, HIV tests
- Antibody tests, total IgA (e.g. IgA anti-endomysial, IgA transglutaminase for coeliac disease); PCR tests (where applicable)
- Haemagglutination tests for amoebiasis
- *C. difficile* tissue culture assay
- Malabsorption studies
- Endoscopy:
  - proctosigmoidoscopy
  - flexible sigmoidoscopy/colonoscopy (with biopsy)
  - small bowel biopsy (coeliac disease)
- Radiology:
  - plain X-ray abdomen—of limited value
  - small bowel enema
  - barium enema, especially double contrast

Note: HIV patients should be investigated in specialist centres.

Principles of treatment[3]

When an underlying cause of diarrhoea can be identified, apart from some common infections, management should be directed at that cause. There are a few situations in which the causative bacterial or parasitic pathogen requires specific treatment, for example, giardiasis. The management is determined by the nature of the pathogen and the severity of the illness.

However, in Australia most infective cases are viral. The basic principle therefore is to achieve and maintain adequate hydration until the illness resolves. In adults and children oral rehydration is indicated unless there is evidence of impending circulatory 'shock' demanding intravenous therapy. Oral rehydration solution containing sodium, potassium and glucose should be considered for patients with mild to moderate dehydration. Adults should drink 2 to 3 L of the solution in 24 hours. Normal food intake may start after rehydration.

In general, treatment should not be directed specifically at altering the frequency and consistency of the stools. The antimotility drugs (loperamide, diphenoxylate and codeine) have a role restricted to short-term control of symptoms in adults during periods of significant social inconvenience, such as travel. It must be emphasised that antimotility drugs are never indicated for management of acute diarrhoea in infants and children.[5]

The traditional absorbent agents, such as kaolin/pectin mixtures, activated charcoal and other mineral clays, have not been shown to be of value and may interfere with absorption of other drugs. They should not be used.

44

Specific antibiotics are reserved for the treatment of giardiasis, amoebiasis, antibiotic-associated diarrhoea, cholera and typhoid. Although antibiotics are usually unnecessary, in most cases they may be indicated for severe cases of *Campylobacter* enteritis, *Salmonella* enteritis, shigellosis and traveller's diarrhoea. Lactobacillus has been shown to reduce the duration of diarrhoea in rotavirus-related enteritis and antibiotic-associated diarrhoea.

Diagnostic triads for diarrhoea

DxT Acute diarrhoea + colicky abdominal pain ± vomiting ➜ gastroenteritis

DxT (Young adult) diarrhoea ± blood and mucus + abdominal cramps ➜ inflammatory bowel disease (UC/Crohn)

DxT As above + constitutional symptoms ± eyes/joints ➜ Crohn disease

DxT Pale bulky offensive stools, difficult to flush, weight loss ➜ malabsorption

DxT Fatigue + weight loss + iron deficiency ➜ coeliac disease

DxT Failure to thrive (child) + recurrent chest infections ➜ cystic fibrosis

DxT Altered bowel habit: diarrhoea ± constipation ± rectal bleeding ± abdominal discomfort ➜ colorectal carcinoma

DxT Diarrhoea (fluid/incontinent) + constipation +++ abdominal discomfort + anorexia/nausea ➜ faecal impaction

DxT Profuse watery diarrhoea + abdominal cramps and increasing distension (on antibiotics) ➜ pseudomembranous colitis (Girotra's triad)

DxT Variable diarrhoea/constipation + abdominal discomfort + mucus PR + flatulence ++ ➜ irritable bowel syndrome

MALABSORPTION

It is important to distinguish the steatorrhoea of various malabsorption syndromes from diarrhoea. Important causes are presented in TABLE 44.8.

The common causes are coeliac disease, chronic pancreatitis and postgastrectomy.

Clinical features

- Bulky, pale, offensive, frothy, greasy stools
- Stools difficult to flush down toilet
- Weight loss
- Prominent abdomen

Table 44.8 Important causes of malabsorption

Primary mucosal disorders
Gluten-sensitive enteropathy (coeliac disease)
Tropical sprue
Lactose intolerance (lactase deficiency)
Crohn disease (regional enteritis)
Whipple disease
Parasite infections (e.g. *Giardia lamblia*)
Lymphoma
Maldigestion states
Lumenal abnormalities:
• postsurgery (e.g. gastrectomy, ileal resection)
• systemic sclerosis
Pancreatic disorders
Chronic pancreatitis
Cystic fibrosis
Pancreatic tumours (e.g. Zollinger–Ellison)

- Failure to thrive (in infants)
- Increased faecal fat
- Signs of multiple vitamin deficiencies (e.g. A, D, E, K)
- Sore tongue (glossitis)
- Hypochromic or megaloblastic anaemia (possible)

Refer for specific investigations (e.g. FBE, barium studies, small bowel biopsy, faecal fat [>21 g/3 days]).

Coeliac disease[2]

Synonyms: coeliac sprue, gluten-sensitive enteropathy.

Note: It can appear at *any* age; refer to coeliac disease in children (see later in chapter).

It is widely underdiagnosed because most patients present with non-GIT symptoms, such as tiredness.

There is a genetic factor in this autoimmune disorder with a 1 in 10 chance if a first-degree relative is affected. Consider screening under 2 years if there is such an association.

Clinical features

- Classic tetrad: diarrhoea, weight loss, iron/folate deficiency, abdominal bloating
- Malaise, lethargy
- Flatulence
- Mouth ulceration
- Diarrhoea with constipation (alternating)
- Pale and thin patient
- No subcutaneous fat

Diagnosis

- Elevated faecal fat
- Characteristic duodenal biopsy: villous atrophy (key test)

- Total IgA level
- IgA antigliadin antibodies (screening—limited)
- IgA anti-endomysial antibodies (>90% sensitivity and specificity)
- IgA transglutaminase antibodies (>90% sensitivity and specificity)

Associations

- Iron-deficiency anaemia
- Type 1 diabetes
- Pernicious anaemia
- Primary biliary cirrhosis
- Subfertility
- Malignancy, especially lymphoma
- Dermatitis herpetiformis
- IgA deficiency
- Autoimmune thyroid disease
- Osteoporosis
- Neurological (e.g. seizures, ataxia, peripheral neuropathy)
- Down syndrome

Management

- Diet control: high complex carbohydrate and protein, low fat, gluten-free (no wheat, barley, rye and oats)
- Treat specific vitamin and mineral deficiencies
- Give pneumococcal vaccination (increased risk of pneumococcus sepsis)

Gluten-free diet

Avoid foods containing gluten either as an obvious component (e.g. flour, bread, oatmeal), or as a hidden ingredient (e.g. dessert mix, stock cube).

Forbidden foods include:

- standard bread, pasta, crispbreads, flour
- standard biscuits and cakes
- breakfast cereals made with wheat or oats
- oatmeal, wheat bran, barley/barley water
- 'battered' or breadcrumbed fish, etc.
- meat and fruit pies
- most stock cubes and gravy mixes

Whipple disease

This is a rare malabsorption disorder usually affecting white males. It is caused by the bacillus *Tropheryma whipplei*. It may involve the heart, lungs and CNS.

Clinical features

- Males >40 years
- Chronic diarrhoea (steatorrhoea)
- Arthralgia (migratory seronegative arthropathy mainly of peripheral joints)
- Weight loss
- Lymphadenopathy
- ± Fever

Diagnosis

- PCR for *T. whipplei*
- Jejunal biopsy—stunted villi

Treatment

IV ceftriaxone for 2 weeks then cotrimoxazole or tetracycline for up to 12 months

This produces a dramatic improvement.

Diarrhoea in the elderly

The older the patient, the more likely a late onset of symptoms that reflect serious underlying organic disease, especially malignancy. Colorectal cancer needs special consideration. The older the patient, especially the bedridden elderly patient, the more likely the presentation of faecal impaction with spurious diarrhoea. The possibility of drug interactions, including digoxin, should also be considered. Ischaemic colitis must be considered in an elderly patient.

Ischaemic colitis

This is due to atheromatous occlusion of mesenteric vessels (low blood flow) (see CHAPTER 34).

Clinical features

Clinical features include:

- sharp abdominal pain in an elderly patient with bloody diarrhoea (low blood flow)
  or
- periumbilical pain and diarrhoea about 15–30 minutes after eating
- maybe loud bruits over central abdomen
- other evidence of generalised atherosclerosis
- barium enema shows 'thumb printing' sign due to submucosal oedema
- the definitive test is aortography and selective angiography of mesenteric vessels
- most episodes resolve—may be followed by a stricture

Diarrhoea in children

The commonest cause of diarrhoea in children is acute infective gastroenteritis, but there are certain conditions that develop in childhood and infancy and require special attention. The presentation of small amounts of redcurrant jelly-like stool with intussusception should also be kept in mind. Of the many causes only a few are commonly seen. The two

44

commonest causes are infective gastroenteritis and antibiotic-induced diarrhoea.

Important causes of diarrhoea in children are:

- infective gastroenteritis
- antibiotics
- overfeeding (loose stools in newborn)
- dietary indiscretions
- toddler's diarrhoea
- sugar (carbohydrate) intolerance
- food allergies (e.g. milk, soy bean, wheat, eggs)
- maternal deprivation
- malabsorption states: cystic fibrosis, coeliac disease

Note: Exclude surgical emergencies (e.g. acute appendicitis), infections (e.g. pneumonia), septicaemia, otitis media <5 years.

Acute gastroenteritis

Note: Dehydration from gastroenteritis is an important cause of death, particularly in obese infants (especially if vomiting accompanies the diarrhoea).

Definition

It is an illness of acute onset, of less than 10 days' duration associated with fever, diarrhoea and/or vomiting, where there is no other evident cause for the symptoms.[5]

Causes

- Mainly rotavirus (developed countries) and adenovirus: viruses account for about 80%
- Bacterial: *C. jejuni* and *Salmonella* sp. (two commonest), *E. coli* and *Shigella* sp.
- Protozoal: *G. lamblia, E. histolytica, Cryptosporidium*
- Food poisoning—staphylococcal toxin

Differential diagnoses. These include septicaemia, urinary tract infection, intussusception, appendicitis, pelvic abscess, partial bowel obstruction, diabetes mellitus and antibiotic reaction[4] (see TABLE 44.9).

Table 44.9 Differential diagnosis of acute diarrhoea and vomiting in children

Bowel infection:

- viruses
- bacteria
- protozoal
- food poisoning—staphylococcal toxin

Systemic infection

Abdominal disorders:

- appendicitis
- pelvic abscess
- intussusception
- malrotation

Urinary tract infection

Antibiotic reaction

Diabetes mellitus

Note: Exclude acute appendicitis and intussusception in the very young.

Symptoms

- Anorexia, nausea, poor feeding, vomiting, fever, diarrhoea (fever and vomiting may be absent)
- Fluid stools (often watery) 10–20 per day
- Crying—due to pain, hunger, thirst or nausea
- Bleeding—uncommon (usually bacterial)
- Anal soreness

Viral indication: large volume, watery, typically lasts 2–3 days, systemic symptoms uncommon.

Bacterial indication: small motions, blood, mucus, abdominal pain and tenesmus.

Dehydration: must be assessed (see TABLE 44.10).

Complications:

- febrile convulsions
- sugar (lactose) intolerance (common)
- septicaemia, especially *Salmonella*

Management

Management is based on the assessment and correction of fluid and electrolyte loss.[5,6] Since dehydration is usually isotonic with equivalent loss of fluid and electrolytes, serum electrolytes will be normal.

Note: The most accurate way to monitor dehydration is to weigh the child, preferably without clothes, on the same scale each time. However, the easiest is clinical assessment (e.g. vomiting, no urine, lethargy and thirst).

Avoid

- Drugs: antidiarrhoeals, anti-emetics and antibiotics
- Lemonade or similar sugary soft drink: osmotic load too high, can use if diluted 1 part to 4 parts water but sugar may be poorly tolerated

To treat or not to treat at home

- Treat at home—if family can cope, vomiting is not a problem and no dehydration.
- Admit to hospital—if dehydration or persisting vomiting or family cannot cope; also infants <6 months and high-risk patients.

Advice to parents (for mild-to-moderate diarrhoea)

If applicable, remove child from day care or school and keep away from food preparation areas. Advise about

Table 44.10 Assessment of hydration[2]

	Mild	Moderate	Severe
Body weight loss	4–5%	6–9%	≥9%
Symptoms/general observations	Thirsty Alert Restless	Thirsty Restless Lethargic Irritable	Infants: drowsy, limp, cold, sweaty, cyanotic limbs, comatose Older: apprehensive, cold and sweaty, cyanotic limbs
Signs	Normal	Dry mucous membranes, absent tears Tachycardia Mildly sunken eyes	Rapid feeble pulse Hypotensive Sunken eyes and fontanelles Very dry mucous membranes
Pinched skin test	Normal (<2 seconds)	Retracts slowly (1–2 seconds)	Retracts very slowly (>2 seconds)
Urine output	Normal	Decreased	Nil
Treatment	Oral rehydration: • small amounts of fluids often • continue breast-feeding • solids after 24 hours • provide maintenance fluid and loss	Oral rehydration: • consider nasogastric tube for steady fluid infusion *or* • IV infusion	Admit to hospital Urgent IV infusion: isotonic fluid (0.9% saline) Start with bolus 20 mL/kg

hygiene, including handwashing and napkin disposal. If children are not dehydrated, encourage eating and drinking as tolerated.

General rules[6,7]

- Give small amounts of fluids often
- Start solids after 24 hours
- Continue breastfeeding (should be increased in frequency, e.g. hourly)
  or
- Continue formula feeding if tolerated or resume it after 24 hours.
- Consider stool culture and test for rotavirus for symptoms that persist and worsen

Day 1

Give fluids, a little at a time and often (e.g. 5 mL every 1–2 minutes by spoon or syringe or 50 mL every 15 minutes if vomiting a lot). A good method is to give 200 mL (about 1 cup) of fluid every time a watery stool is passed or a big vomit occurs.

The ideal fluid is Gastrolyte or Repalyte (new formulation). Other suitable oral rehydration preparations are WHO-recommended solutions Electrolade and Glucolyte.

A new product is Hydralyte paediatric rehydration, which is a solution as an 'ice-block' formulation:

- children 1–2 years—one 'ice-block' per hour
- older children—as often as desired.

Warning: Do *not* use straight lemonade or mix up Gastrolyte with lemonade or fluids other than water.

Alternatives are:	
• lemonade (not low-calorie)	1 part to 6 parts water
• sucrose (table sugar)	1 teaspoon to 120 mL water
• glucose	1 teaspoon to 120 mL water
• cordials (not low-calorie)	1 part to 16 parts water
• fruit juice	1 part to 4 parts water

Method of assessing fluid requirements[3]

- Fluid loss (mL) = % dehydration × body weight (kg) × 10
- Maintenance (mL/kg/24 h): 1–3 mo: 120 mL; 4–12 mo: 100 mL; >12 mo: 80 mL
- Allow for continuing loss.

Example: 8 month 10 kg child with 5% dehydration:
Fluid loss = 5 × 10 × 10 = 500 mL
Maintenance = 100 × 10 = 1000 mL
Total 24-hour requirement (min.) = 1500 mL
Approximate average hourly requirement = 60 mL

- Aim to give more (replace fluid loss) in the first 6 hours.
- Rule of thumb: give 100 mL/kg (infants) and 50 mL/kg (older children) in first 6 hours.

Days 2 and 3

Reintroduce your baby's milk or formula diluted to half strength (i.e. mix equal quantities of milk or formula and water). Their normal food can be continued but do not worry that your child is not eating food. Solids can be commenced after 24 hours. Best to start with bread, plain biscuits, jelly, stewed apple, rice, porridge or non-fat potato chips. Avoid fatty foods, fried foods, raw vegetables and fruit, and wholegrain bread.

Day 4

Increase milk to normal strength and gradually continue reintroduction to usual diet.

Breastfeeding. If your baby is not vomiting, continue breastfeeding but offer extra fluids (preferably Gastrolyte) between feeds. If vomiting is a problem, express breast milk for the time being while you follow the oral fluid program.

Note: Watch for lactose intolerance as a sequela—explosive diarrhoea after introducing formula. Replace with a lactose-free formula.

If acute invasive or persistent *Salmonella* are present, give antibiotics (ciprofloxacin or azithromycin).

CHRONIC DIARRHOEA IN CHILDREN[6]

Sugar intolerance

Synonyms: carbohydrate intolerance, lactose intolerance.

The commonest offending sugar is lactose.

Diarrhoea often follows acute gastroenteritis when milk is reintroduced into the diet (some recommend waiting for 2 weeks). Stools may be watery, frothy, smell like vinegar and tend to excoriate the buttocks. They contain sugar. Exclude giardiasis.

A simple test follows.

- Line the napkin with thin plastic and collect fluid stool.
- Mix 5 drops of liquid stool with 10 drops of water and add a Clinitest tablet (detects lactose and glucose but not sucrose).
- A positive result indicates sugar intolerance.

Diagnosis: lactose breath hydrogen test.

Treatment

- Remove the offending sugar from the diet.
- Use milk preparations in which the lactose has been split to glucose and galactose by enzymes, or use soy protein.

Note: Most milk allergies improve with age.

Toddler's diarrhoea ('cradle crap')

A clinical syndrome of loose, bulky, non-offensive stools with fragments of undigested food in a well, thriving child. The onset is usually between 8 and 20 months. Associated with high fructose intake (fruit juice diarrhoea).

Diagnosis by exclusion; treatment by dietary adjustment.

Cow's milk protein intolerance[7]

This is not as common as lactose intolerance. Diarrhoea is related to taking a cow's milk formula and relieved when it is withdrawn.

Allergic responses to cow's milk protein may result in a rapid or delayed onset of symptoms. Delayed onset may be more difficult to diagnose, presenting with diarrhoea, malabsorption or failure to thrive.

It is diagnosed by unequivocal reproducible reactions to elimination and challenge. If diagnosed, remove cow's milk from the diet and replace with either soy milk, a hydrolysed or an elemental formula (see CHAPTER 80).

Inflammatory bowel disorders

These disorders, which include Crohn disease and ulcerative colitis, can occur in childhood. A high index of suspicion is necessary to make an early diagnosis. Approximately 5% of cases of chronic ulcerative colitis have their onset in childhood.[5]

Chronic enteric infection

Responsible organisms include *Salmonella* sp., *Campylobacter, Yersinia, G. lamblia* and *E. histolytica.* With persistent diarrhoea, it is important to obtain microscopy of faeces and aerobic and anaerobic stool cultures. *G. lamblia* infestation is not an uncommon finding and may be associated with malabsorption, especially of carbohydrate and fat. Giardiasis can mimic coeliac disease.

Coeliac disease

(See earlier in chapter.)

Clinical features in childhood:

- usually presents at 9–18 months, but any age
- previously thriving infant

- anorexia, lethargy, irritability
- failure to thrive
- malabsorption—abdominal distension
- offensive frequent stools

  Diagnosis: duodenal biopsy (definitive).
  Treatment: remove gluten from diet.

Cystic fibrosis

Cystic fibrosis, which presents in infancy, is the commonest of all inherited disorders (1 per 2500 live births). Refer to CHAPTER 18.

ACUTE GASTROENTERITIS IN ADULTS

Features

- Invariably a self-limiting problem (1–3 days)
- Abdominal cramps
- Possible constitutional symptoms (e.g. fever, malaise, nausea, vomiting)
- Other meal-sharers affected → food poisoning
- Consider dehydration, especially in the elderly
- Consider possibility of enteric fever

Traveller's diarrhoea

The symptoms are usually as above, but very severe diarrhoea, especially if associated with blood or mucus, may be a feature of a more serious bowel infection such as amoebiasis. Possible causes of diarrhoeal illness are presented in TABLE 14.1, in CHAPTER 14. Most traveller's diarrhoea is caused by *E. coli,* which produces a watery diarrhoea within 14 days of arrival in a foreign country. (For specific treatment refer to the section on Traveller's diarrhoea in CHAPTER 14.)

Persistent traveller's diarrhoea

Any traveller with persistent diarrhoea after visiting less developed countries, especially India and China, may have a protozoal infection such as amoebiasis or giardiasis.

If there is a fever and blood or mucus in the stools, suspect amoebiasis. Giardiasis is characterised by abdominal cramps, flatulence and bubbly, foul-smelling diarrhoea.

Principles of treatment of diarrheoa

Acute diarrhoea

- Maintenance of hydration:

  Antiemetic injection (for severe vomiting)
  prochlorperazine IM, statim
  or
  metoclopramide IV, statim
- Antidiarrhoeal preparations:
  (avoid if possible: loperamide preferred)

  loperamide (Imodium) 2 caps statim then 1 after each unformed stool (max: 8 caps/day)
  or
  diphenoxylate with atropine (Lomotil) 2 tabs statim then 1–2 (o) 8-hourly

General advice to patient

Rest

Your bowel needs a rest and so do you. It is best to reduce your normal activities until the diarrhoea has stopped.

Diet

Eat as normally as possible but drink small amounts of clear fluids such as water, tea, lemonade and yeast extract (e.g. Marmite). Then eat low-fat foods such as stewed apples, rice (boiled in water), soups, poultry, boiled potatoes, mashed vegetables, dry toast or bread, biscuits, most canned fruits, jam, honey, jelly, dried skim milk or condensed milk (reconstituted with water).

At first, avoid alcohol, coffee, strong tea, fatty foods, fried foods, spicy foods, raw vegetables, raw fruit (especially with hard skins), Chinese food, wholegrain cereals and cigarette smoking.

On the third day introduce dairy produce, such as a small amount of milk in tea or coffee and a little butter or margarine on toast. Add also lean meat and fish (either grilled or steamed).

Treatment (antimicrobial drugs)[2,8]

Bacterial diarrhoea in adults and older children is usually self-limiting and does not require antibiotic treatment (they may be used to shorten the course of a persistent infection). *Campylobacter, Salmonella, Shigella* and *E. coli* are the most common causes. As a rule, use oral rehydration solution 2–3 L orally over 24 hours if mild to moderate dehydration. If severe, intravenous rehydration with N saline is recommended.

It is advisable not to use antimicrobials except where the following specific organisms are identified. The drugs should be selected initially from the list below or modified according to the results of culture and sensitivity tests.[3] Only treat if symptoms have persisted for more than 48 hours. Adult doses are shown for the following specific enteric infections based on faecal culture. Recommended empirical therapy is ciprofloxacin or norfloxacin.

Shigella dysentery (moderate to severe)

cotrimoxazole (double strength) 1 tab (o) 12-hourly for 5 days: use in children (children's doses)
or
norfloxacin 400 mg (o) 12-hourly for 5 days (preferred for adults)
or
ciprofloxacin 500 mg (o) bd for 5 days

Giardiasis

This protozoal infestation is often misdiagnosed. It should be considered for a persistent profuse, watery, bubbly, offensive diarrhoea (see CHAPTER 15).

tinidazole 2 g (o), single dose (may need repeat)
or
metronidazole 400 mg (o) tds for 7 days
(in children: 30 mg/kg/day [to max. 1.2 g/day] as single daily dose for 3 days)

Salmonella enteritis

Antibiotics are not generally advisable, but if severe or prolonged use:

ciprofloxacin 500 mg (o) bd for 5–7 days
or
azithromycin 1 g (o) day, then 500 mg for 6 days
or
ceftriaxone IV or ciprofloxacin IV if oral therapy not tolerated

Note: Salmonella is a notifiable disease; infants under 15 months are at risk of invasive *Salmonella* infection.

Campylobacter

A zoonosis that is usually self-limiting.

Antibiotic therapy indicated in severe or prolonged cases:

azithromycin 500 mg (o) 12-hourly for 3 days
or
ciprofloxacin 500 mg (o) 12-hourly for 3 days
or
norfloxacin 400 mg (o) 12-hourly for 5 days

Cryptosporidium species

Usually self-limiting, may need fluid and electrolytes and anti-motility agents.

If severe, nitazoxanide (shared care).

Amoebiasis (intestinal)

See CHAPTER 15.

metronidazole 600–800 mg (o) tds for 6–10 days
plus
diloxanide furoate 500 mg (o) tds for 10 days

Blastocystitis hominis (a parasitic infection)

Pathogenicity is disputed: give therapy only if severe. Associated with poor hygiene (travel, pets, dam/tank water, oysters).

metronidazole for 7 days
Specialist advice should be sought.

Treatment for special enteric infections

Typhoid/paratyphoid fever

See CHAPTER 15.

azithromycin 1 g (o) daily for 7 days
or
(if not acquired in the Indian subcontinent or SE Asia)

ciprofloxacin 500 mg (o) 12-hourly for 7–10 days (use IV if oral therapy not tolerated)

If ciprofloxacin is contraindicated (e.g. in children) or not tolerated, then use:

ceftriaxone 3 g IV daily until culture and sensitivities available, then choose oral regimens

If severe: administer same drug and dosage IV for first 4–5 days.

Cholera

Antibiotic therapy reduces the volume and duration of diarrhoea. Rehydration is the key.

azithromycin 1 g (child 20 mg/kg up to 1 g) (o) as a single dose
or
ciprofloxacin 1 g (o) as a single dose

For pregnant women and children:

amoxycillin (child: 10 mg/kg up to) 250 mg (o) 6-hourly for 4 days

INFLAMMATORY BOWEL DISEASE[3]

Inflammatory bowel disease (IBD) should be considered when a young person presents with:

- bloody diarrhoea and mucus
- colonic pain and fever
- urgency to visit toilet and feeling of incomplete defecation
- constitutional symptoms including weight loss and malaise
- extra-abdominal manifestations such as arthralgia, low back pain (spondyloarthropathy), eye problems (iridocyclitis), liver disease and skin lesions (pyoderma gangrenosum, erythema nodosum)

Investigations include FBE, vitamin B12 and folate, LFTs (abnormal enzymes), HLA B_{27}, faecal calprotectin (if normal, no intestinal inflammation; if abnormal, needs colonoscopy) and lactoferrin.

Two important disorders are ulcerative colitis (UC) and Crohn disease, which have equal sex incidence and can occur at any age, but onset peaks between 20 and 40 years.

Ulcerative colitis

Clinical features

- Mainly a disease of Western societies
- Mainly in young adults (15–40 years)
- High-risk factors—family history, previous attacks, low-fibre diet
- Recurrent attacks of loose stools
- Blood, or blood and pus, or mucus in stools
- Abdominal pain slight or absent
- Fever, malaise and weight loss uncommon
- Begins in rectum (continues proximally)—affects only the colon: it usually does not spread beyond the ileocaecal valve
- An increased risk of carcinoma after 7–10 years

Main symptom

- Bloody diarrhoea

Diagnosis

- Faecal calprotectin: a sensitive test
- Proctosigmoidoscopy: a granular red proctitis with contact bleeding
- Barium enema: characteristic changes

Prognosis

- 5% mortality in an acute attack
- Recurrent attacks common

Crohn disease

Synonyms: regional enteritis, granulomatous colitis.

The cause is unknown but there is a genetic link.

Clinical features

- Recurrent diarrhoea in a young person (15–40 years)
- Blood and mucus in stools (less than UC)
- Colicky abdominal pain (small bowel colic)
- Right iliac fossa pain (confused with appendicitis)
- Constitutional symptoms (e.g. fever, weight loss, malaise, anorexia, nausea)
- Signs include perianal disorders (e.g. anal fissure, fistula, ischiorectal abscess), mouth ulcers
- Skip areas in bowel: ½ ileocolic, ¼ confined to small bowel, ¼ confined to colon, 4% in upper GIT

Main symptom

- Colicky abdominal pain

Diagnosis

- Sigmoidoscopy: 'cobblestone' appearance (patchy mucosal oedema)
- Colonoscopy: useful to differentiate from UC
- Biopsy with endoscopy

Prognosis

Less favourable than UC with both medical and surgical treatment.

Management principles of both

- Education and support, including support groups
- Treat under consultant supervision
- Treatment of acute attacks depends on severity of the attack and the extent of the disorder:
  - mild attacks: manage out of hospital
  - severe attacks: hospital, to attend to fluid and electrolyte balance
- Role of diet controversial: consider a high-fibre diet but maintain adequate nutrition
- Pharmaceutical agents (the following can be considered):
  - 5-aminosalicylic acid derivatives (mainly UC): sulfasalazine (mainstay), olsalazine, mesalazine. Usually start with these agents
  - corticosteroids (mainly for acute flares): oral, parenteral, topical (rectal foam, suppositories or enemas)
  - for severe disease, immunomodifying drugs (e.g. azathioprine, cyclosporin, methotrexate) and biological agents (e.g. infliximab)
- Surgical treatment: reserve for complications; avoid surgery if possible

ALTERNATING DIARRHOEA AND CONSTIPATION

Alternating diarrhoea and constipation are well-known symptoms of incomplete bowel obstruction (cancer of colon and diverticular disease) and irritable bowel syndrome.

Irritable bowel syndrome (IBS)[3,8,10]

Clinical features

- Typically in younger women (21–40 years)
- Any age or sex can be affected
- May follow attack of gastroenteritis/traveller's diarrhoea
- Cramping abdominal pain (central or iliac fossa)—see FIGURE 44.4
- Pain usually relieved by passing flatus or by defecation
- Variable bowel habit (constipation more common)
- Diarrhoea usually worse in morning—several loose, explosive bowel actions with urgency

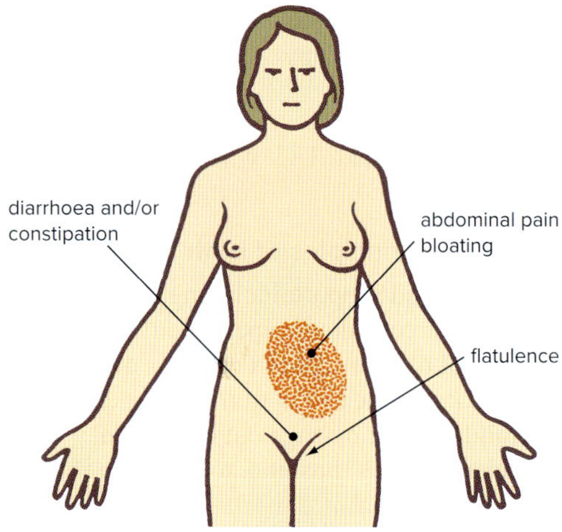

FIGURE 44.4 Classic symptoms of irritable bowel syndrome

- The Bristol stool chart was devised to assist with the subclassification of stool types and bowel habits <www.continence.org.au/pages/bristol-stool-chart.html>
- Often precipitated by eating
- Faeces sometimes like small, hard pellets or ribbon-like
- Anorexia and nausea (sometimes)
- Bloating, abdominal distension, borborygmi
- Tiredness common

The Rome III diagnostic criteria for IBS are presented in TABLE 44.11.

Table 44.11 Rome III diagnostic criteria for irritable bowel syndrome*[11]

In the preceding 3 months, the patient has had abdominal discomfort for at least 3 days per month with two of the following three features:

- relieved by defecation
- onset associated with a change in stool frequency
- onset associated with a change in form (appearance) of stool (loose, watery or pellet-like)

Symptoms that cumulatively support the diagnosis of irritable bowel syndrome:

- abnormal stool frequency (for research purposes may be defined as more than three bowel movements per day and fewer than three bowel movements per week)
- abnormal stool form (lumpy/hard or watery/mushy)
- abnormal stool passage (straining, urgency or feeling of incomplete evacuation)
- passage of mucus
- bloating or feeling of abdominal distension

Note: Red flags must be excluded

* in absence of structural or metabolic abnormalities to explain symptoms

IBS is a diagnosis of exclusion. A thorough physical examination, investigations (FBE, ESR and stool microscopy or culture) and colonoscopy are necessary. Insufflation of air at colonoscopy may reproduce the abdominal pain of IBS.

Possible related causes

Bowel infection, food irritation (e.g. spicy foods), lactose (milk) intolerance, excess-fibre wheat products, high fatty foods, carbonated drinks, laxative overuse, use of antibiotics and codeine-containing analgesics, psychological factors.

Management

The patient must be reassured and educated with advice that the problem will not cause malignancy or inflammatory bowel disease and will not shorten life expectancy. The basis of initial treatment is simple dietary modification (FODMAPs), exercise, fluids (2–3 L water daily) and non-fermentable fibre.

Red flag pointers for non-IBS disease[9]

- Age of onset >50 years
- Fever
- Unexplained weight loss
- Rectal bleeding
- Pain waking at night
- Persistent daily diarrhoea/steatorrhoea
- Recurrent vomiting
- Major change in symptoms
- Mouth ulcers
- ↑ CRP, ESR
- Anaemia
- Family history bowel cancer or IBD

Self-help advice to the patient

Anyone with IBS should try to work on the things that make the symptoms worse. If you recognise stresses and strains in your life, try to develop a more relaxed lifestyle. You may have to be less of a perfectionist in your approach to life.

Focus on establishing a regular eating pattern. Try to avoid any foods that you can identify as causing the problem. You may have to cut out smoking and alcohol and avoid laxatives and codeine (in painkillers). A high-fibre (non-fermentable) and low-carbohydrate diet and 2–3 L of water a day may be the answer to your problem.

A low-FODMAP diet can produce good benefits.[11] FODMAP refers to fermentable oligosaccharides, disaccharides, monosaccharides and polyols, which are poorly absorbed. All of these carbohydrates need to be eliminated (under a dietitian's guidance) then reintroduced one at a time.

See <www.med.monash.edu/cecs/gastro/fodmap>, available as an app—the Monash University Low-FODMAP Diet.

Diverticular disorder

Diverticular disorder is a problem of the colon (90% in descending colon) and is related to lack of fibre in the diet. It is usually symptomless.

Clinical features

- Typical in middle-aged or elderly—over 40 years
- Increases with age
- Present in one in three people over 60 years (Western world)
- Diverticulosis—symptomless
- Diverticulitis—infected diverticula and symptomatic (refer CHAPTER 34)
- Constipation or alternating constipation/diarrhoea
- Intermittent cramping lower abdominal pain in LIF
- Tenderness in LIF
- Rectal bleeding—may be profuse (± faeces)
- May present as acute abdomen or subacute obstruction
- Usually settles in 2–3 days

Complications (of diverticulitis)

- Abscess
- Perforation
- Peritonitis
- Obstruction (refer CHAPTER 34)
- Fistula—bladder, vagina

Investigations

- WBC and ESR—to determine inflammation
- Sigmoidoscopy
- Barium enema

Management

- It usually responds to a high-fibre diet.
- Avoidance of constipation.

Advice to the patient

The gradual introduction of fibre with plenty of fluids (especially water) will improve any symptoms you may have and reduce the risk of complications. Your diet should include:

1 cereals, such as bran, shredded wheat, muesli or porridge
2 wholemeal and multigrain breads
3 fresh or stewed fruits and vegetables

Bran can be added to your cereal or stewed fruit, starting with 1 tablespoon and gradually increasing to 3 tablespoons a day. Fibre can make you feel uncomfortable for the first few weeks, but the bowel soon settles with your improved diet.

When to refer

Children with diarrhoea

- Infant under 3 months
- Moderate to severe dehydration
- Diagnosis of diarrhoea and vomiting in doubt (e.g. blood in vomitus or stool, bile-stained vomiting, high fever or toxaemia, abdominal signs suggestive of appendicitis or obstruction)
- Failure to improve or deterioration
- A pre-existing chronic illness

Adults with diarrhoea

- Patient with chronic or bloody diarrhoea
- Any problem requiring colonoscopic investigation
- Patients with anaemia
- Patients with weight loss, abdominal mass or suspicion of neoplasia
- Patients with anal fistulae
- Patients not responding to treatment for giardiasis
- Infection with *E. histolytica*
- Long-term asymptomatic carrier of typhoid or paratyphoid fever
- Patient with persistent undiagnosed nocturnal diarrhoea
- Patients with IBS with a significant change in symptoms
- Patients with inflammatory bowel diseases with severe exacerbations, possibly requiring immunosuppressive therapy and with complications
- Patients with ulcerative colitis of more than 7 years' duration (screening by colonoscopy for carcinoma)

Practice tips

- Oral antidiarrhoeal drugs are contraindicated in children; besides being ineffective they may prolong intestinal recovery.
- Anti-emetics can readily provoke dystonic reactions in children, especially if young and dehydrated.
- Acute diarrhoea is invariably self-limiting (lasts 2–5 days). If it lasts longer than 7 days, investigate with culture and microscopy of the stools.
- If diarrhoea is associated with episodes of facial flushing or wheezing, consider carcinoid syndrome.

continued

44

continued

- Recurrent pain in the right hypochondrium is usually a feature of IBS (not gall bladder disease).
- Recurrent pain in the right iliac fossa is more likely to be IBS than appendicitis.
- Beware of false correlations or premature conclusions (e.g. attributing the finding of diverticular disorder on barium meal to the cause of the symptoms).
- Undercooked chicken is a common source of enteropathic bacterial infection.
- Consider alcohol abuse if a patient's diarrhoea resolves spontaneously on hospital admission.

Patient education resources

Hand-out sheets from *Murtagh's Patient Education* 7th edition:

- Coeliac disease in adults
- Coeliac disease in children
- Diarrhoea—acute diarrhoea in adults
- Gastroenteritis in children

References

1 Bolin T, Riordan SM. Acute and persistent diarrhoea. Current Therapeutics, 2001; May: 47–57.

2 Cheng AC et al. Australasian Society for Infectious Diseases guidelines for the diagnosis and treatment of *Clostridium difficile* infection. Med J Aust, 2011; 194 (7): 353–8.

3 Expert group for Gastrointestinal. Supportive measures of gastroenteritis. In: eTG complete [Internet}. Melbourne: Therapeutic Guidelines Ltd. Available from: www.tg.org.au, accessed September 2017.

4 Dalton C. Foodborne illness: how to treat. Australian Doctor, 15 April: 2005; 39–46.

5 Robinson MJ, Roberton DM. *Practical Paediatrics* (5th edn). Edinburgh: Churchill Livingstone, 2003: 675–90.

6 Oberklaid F. Management of gastroenteritis in children. In: *The Australian Paediatric Review.* Melbourne: Royal Children's Hospital, 1990: 1–2.

7 Gwee A, Rimer R, Marks M. *Paediatric Handbook* (9th edn). Oxford: Wiley-Blackwell, 2015: 90–5.

8 Onwuezobe IA et al. Antimicrobials for treating symptomatic non-typhoidal *Salmonella* infection (Cochrane Review). Cochrane Database Syst Rev. 2012, Issue 11. Art No. CD001167.

9 Ellard K, Malcolm A. Irritable bowel syndrome. Medical Observer, 30 March 2007: 29–32.

10 NICE. Irritable bowel syndrome in adults: diagnosis and management of irritable bowel syndrome in primary care, 2008. <www.nice.org.uk> (accessed 25/5/2018).

11 Rome Foundation. Rome III diagnostic criteria for functional gastrointestinal disorders. J Gastrointestin Liver Dis, 2006; 15 (3): 307–12.

12 Gibson PR. Irritable bowel syndrome. Australian Doctor, 13 April 2012: 17–34.

13 Gibson PR, Shepherd SJ. Evidence-based dietary management of functional gastrointestinal symptoms: the FODMAP approach. J Gastroenterol Hepatology, 2010; Feb 25 (2): 2528.

The disturbed patient

45

There is not a sight in nature so mortifying as that of a Distracted Person, when his imagination is troubled, and his whole soul is disordered and confused.

JOSEPH ADDISON (1672–1719)

The disturbed and confused patient is a complex management problem in general practice. The cause may be a single one or a combination of several abnormal mental states (see TABLE 45.1).[1] The cause may be an organic mental disorder, which may be a long-term insidious problem such as dementia, or an acute disorder (delirium), often dramatic in onset. On the other hand, the cause of the disturbance may be a psychiatric disorder such as panic disorder, mania, major depression or schizophrenia.

The manifestations of the disturbance are many and include perceptual changes and hallucinations, disorientation, changes in consciousness, changes in mood from abnormally elevated to gross depression, agitation and disturbed thinking, including delusions.

Table 45.1 A general classification of psychiatric disorders[1]

Organic mental disorders:
- acute organic brain syndrome (delirium)
- chronic organic brain syndrome (dementia)

Psychoactive and substance use disorders:
- toxic states
- drug dependency
- withdrawal states

Schizophrenic disorders

Mood disorders:
- major depression
- bipolar (manic depressive) disorder
- adjustment disorders with depressed mood
- dysthymia

Anxiety disorders:
- generalised anxiety disorder
- panic disorder
- obsessive–compulsive disorder
- phobic disorders
- post-traumatic stress disorder

Disorders specific to children

Other disorders:
- postpartum psychiatric illness
- eating disorders
- personality disorders
- body dysmorphic disorder

Key facts and checkpoints

- Depression affects 15% of people over 65 and can mimic or complicate any other illness, including delirium and dementia.[1]
- Elderly patients with depression are at a high risk of suicide.
- Always search vigorously for the cause or causes of delirium.
- Seeing patients in their home is the best way to evaluate their problem and support systems. It allows opportunities for a history from close contacts and for checking medication, alcohol intake and other factors.
- The diagnosis of dementia can be overlooked: a Scottish study showed that 80% of demented patients were not diagnosed by their GP.[2]
- Patients with a chronic brain syndrome (dementia) are at special risk of an acute brain syndrome (delirium) in the presence of infections and many prescribed drugs.[1]
- Consider prescribed and illicit substances, including the severe anticholinergic delirium syndrome.
- The key feature of dementia is impaired memory.
- The two key features of delirium are disorganised thought and attention.
- Hallucination guidelines:
  - auditory: psychoses, e.g. schizophrenia
  - visual: almost always organic disorder
  - olfactory: temporal lobe epilepsy
  - tactile: cocaine abuse, alcohol withdrawal

A diagnostic approach

A summary of the diagnostic strategy model for the disturbed or confused patient is presented in TABLE 45.2.

Table 45.2 The disturbed mind: diagnostic strategy model

Probability diagnosis
The 4 Ds:
- dementia
- delirium (look for cause)
- depression
- drugs: toxicity, withdrawal

Serious disorders not to be missed
Cardiovascular:
- CVAs
- cardiac failure
- arrhythmia
- acute coronary syndromes

Neoplasia:
- cerebral
- cancer (e.g. lung)

Severe infections:
- septicaemia
- HIV infection
- infective endocarditis

Hypoglycaemia
Bipolar disorder/mania
Schizophrenia states
Anxiety/panic
Subdural haematoma

Pitfalls (often missed)
Illicit drug withdrawal
Fluid and electrolyte disturbances
Faecal impaction (elderly)
Urinary retention (elderly)
Hypoxia
Pain syndromes (elderly)
Rarities:
- autoimmune encephalitis
- hypocalcaemia/hypercalcaemia
- kidney failure
- hepatic failure
- prion diseases (e.g. Creutzfeldt–Jakob disease)

Seven masquerades checklist (all possible)
Depression
Diabetes
Drugs
Anaemia
Thyroid disorder
Spinal dysfunction (severe pain in elderly)
UTI

Is the patient trying to tell me something?
Consider anxiety, depression, emotional deprivation or upset, change in environment, serious personal loss.

Glossary of terms

Alzheimer disease A term used for both senile and presenile dementia, which has characteristic pathological degenerative changes in the brain.

Cognition The mental functions of perception, thinking and memory. It is the process of 'knowing'.

Compulsions Repeated, stereotyped and seemingly purposeful actions that the person feels compelled to carry out but resists, realising they are irrational (most are associated with obsessions).

Confusion Disorientation in time, place and person. It may be accompanied by a disturbed conscious state (see TABLE 75.1, CHAPTER 75).

Conversion The process by which thoughts or experiences unacceptable to the mind are repressed and converted into physical symptoms.

Delirium (also termed 'toxic confusional state') A relatively acute disorder in which impaired consciousness is associated with abnormalities of perception or mood.

Delusions Abnormal, illogical or false beliefs that are held with absolute conviction despite evidence to the contrary.

Dementia An acquired, chronic and gradually progressive deterioration of memory, intellect and personality. Presenile dementia or early onset dementia is dementia under 65 years of age. Senile dementia refers to older patients (usually over 80 years).

Dissociation A psychological disorder in which unpleasant memories or emotions are split off from consciousness and the personality and buried into the unconsciousness.

Depersonalisation An alteration in the awareness of the self—the person feels unreal.

Hallucinations Disorders of perception quite divorced from reality. Features:
- mostly auditory or visual
- a false perception—not a distortion
- perceived as normal perceptions
- independent of the person's will

Illusions False interpretations of sensory stimuli such as mistaking people or familiar things.

Obsessions Recurrent or persistent thoughts, images or impulses that enter the mind despite efforts to exclude them.

Somatisation The conversion of mental experiences or states into bodily symptoms, with no physical causation.

Probability diagnosis

The diagnosis depends on the age and presentation of the patient. In a teenager the probable causes of acute confusion or irrational behaviour include drug toxicity or withdrawal, schizophrenia, severe depression or a behavioural disorder.

It is the elderly who commonly present with confusion. The questions that must be asked are:

- Is the problem one of the 4 Ds—dementia, delirium, depression, drugs or something else?
- If delirium is the problem, what is the cause?

Depression affects 15% of people over 65 and can mimic other causes of confusion and behavioural disturbance.

Significant prescribed drugs include hypnotics, sedatives, oral hypoglycaemics, antihypertensives, digoxin, antihistamines, anticholinergic drugs and antipsychotics.

Serious disorders not to be missed

There are many serious underlying disorders that must be considered, especially with delirium (see TABLE 45.3). Cerebral organic lesions, including space-occupying lesions (e.g. cerebral tumour, subdural haematoma), severe infection (systemic or intracerebral) and cancer at any site, especially lung, breast, bowel, or lymphoma, must be ruled out.

The sudden onset of delirium may suggest angina, myocardial infarction or a cerebrovascular accident. Twenty per cent of patients with delirium also have underlying heart failure.[3]

Pitfalls

There are many pitfalls, especially with drug toxicity or withdrawal from the so-called illicit drugs. In the elderly in particular, fluid and electrolyte disturbances, such as dehydration, hypokalaemia, hyponatraemia and hypocalcaemia, can cause delirium. Bowel disturbances such as faecal impaction or constipation can cause delirium and incontinence of both faeces and urine.

Seven masquerades checklist

All the following disorders can cause disturbed or confused behaviour, particularly in the elderly:

- depression: a very important cause of 'pseudodementia'
- drugs: toxicity or withdrawal (see TABLE 45.4)

Table 45.3 Important causes of delirium (typical examples of each group)

Drug intoxication and drug sensitivity	
Anticholinergics	
Antidepressants	
Sedatives	
Alcohol, opioids etc.	
Withdrawal from substances of abuse and prescribed drugs	
Alcohol	
Opioids	
Amphetamines	
Cannabis	
Sedatives and anxiolytics	
Infections	
Specific:	Urinary tract
	Lower respiratory (e.g. pneumonia)
	Otitis media
	Cellulitis
Intracranial:	Meningitis
	Encephalitis
Systemic:	Infective endocarditis
	Septicaemia
	HIV virus
	Other viral infections
	Malaria
Metabolic disturbances	
Uraemia, hepatic failure	
Electrolyte disturbances	
Dehydration	
Endocrine disturbances	
Diabetic ketoacidosis, hypoglycaemia	
Hypothyroidism/hyperthyroidism	
Nutritional and vitamin deficits	
Vitamin B complex deficiency (esp. B6, B12)	
Wernicke encephalopathy	
Hypoxia	
Respiratory failure, cardiac failure, anaemia	
Vascular	
CVA	
Acute coronary syndromes	
Head injury and other intracranial problems	
Seizures	
Complex partial seizures	
'Subtle' causes	
Pain (e.g. herpes zoster)	
Emotional upset	
Environmental change	
Peri-operative	
Faecal impaction	
Urinary retention	

Table 45.4 Prescribed drugs that can cause delirium

Anticholinergic:
- antiparkinsonian (e.g. benztropine)
- tricyclic antidepressants

Tranquillisers and hypnotics:
- major tranquillisers (e.g. chlorpromazine)
- minor tranquillisers (e.g. diazepam)
- hypnotics
- lithium

Anti-epileptics
Antihistamines 1 and 2
Antihypertensives
Corticosteroids
Cardiac drugs:
- digoxin
- diuretics
- beta blockers

Opioids
Sympathomimetics

- diabetes: especially hypoglycaemia, which can occur with type 2
- anaemia: often from self-neglect or chronic blood loss
- thyroid disorders: both hyperthyroidism and hypothyroidism can present with disturbed behaviour; 'myxoedemic madness' may be precipitated by atropine compounds
- urinary tract infection: causes or contributes to 20% of cases of hallucinations or illusions[2]
- spinal dysfunction: with its many severe pain syndromes, such as sciatica, can be a significant factor

Psychogenic factors

Apart from the primary psychiatric disorders of anxiety, depression, mania and schizophrenia, relatively simple and subtle social problems, such as loneliness, boredom, a domestic upset, financial problem or similar issues, can trigger a confusional state.

The clinical approach

History

Developing rapport with the disturbed or confused patient is essential and can be helped by a warm handshake or a reassuring pat on the shoulder. The basis of the history is a careful account from relatives or witnesses about the patient's behaviour.

When communicating with the patient, speak slowly and simply (avoid shouting), face the patient and maintain eye contact. Important features are the past history and recent psychosocial history, including recent bereavement, family upsets and changes in environment. Search for evidence of depression and note any organic symptoms such as cough, constipation and so on.

Mental status examination

The most practical bedside screening test of mental function is the Mental Status Questionnaire of Kahn and colleagues,[4] which includes 10 simple questions.

1. What is the name of this place?
2. What city are you in now?
3. What year is it?
4. What month is it?
5. What is the date today?
6. What year were you born?
7. When is your birthday?
8. How old are you?
9. Who is the prime minister/president?
10. Who was the prime minister/president before him?

(Interpretation: normal 9–10; mildly impaired 8–9; confused/demented 7 or less.)

Other MMSEs are presented in CHAPTER 8.

Examination

The patient's general demeanour, dress and physical characteristics should be noted at all times. Assess the patient's ability to hear, see, speak, reason, obey commands, stand and walk. Any problems related to the special senses can cause confusion.

Look for features of alcohol abuse, Parkinson disease and hypothyroidism.

Examine the neurological system and keep in mind the possibility of a subdural haematoma, which may have followed a forgotten fall.

Don't omit the rectal examination to exclude faecal impaction, melaena, cancer and prostatomegaly (in males), and also check the bladder for evidence of chronic retention.

Investigations

Investigations to consider for delirious or demented patients (unknown cause):

- urinalysis and microscopy
- cultures of blood and urine
- total and differential blood count; ESR
- blood glucose
- urea and creatinine and electrolytes

- calcium and phosphate
- vitamin D
- thyroid function tests
- liver function tests
- serum vitamin B12 and folate levels
- ECG/troponin (? acute coronary syndrome)
- chest X-ray
- cerebral CT scan, especially non-contrast CT
- syphilis serology
- HIV
- arterial blood gases

Behavioural emergencies: management of the acutely disturbed patient[1]

Delirious or psychotic patients can be paranoid and respond defensively to the world around them. This behaviour can include aggressive and violent behaviour resulting in danger to themselves, their friends and family and to their medical attendants.

Dangerousness should be assessed from features such as the patient's past history (especially previous dangerous behaviour), age and sex, recent stress, victim behaviour, muscle bulk, presence of weapons, degree of overactivity and the manner of handling of the present distress by others. The patient may be in a state of acute panic and trying to flee a situation or in an agitated psychotic state prepared to confront the situation. It should be emphasised that most violent individuals are not mentally ill.

Most cases require an injection (the ideal intravenous administration can be extremely difficult and hazardous), which is often interpreted as a physical attack. It may not be possible to diagnose the cause of the problem before giving the injection.

Approach to management

- Assess the environment and don't move into the patient's space until in a position of control.
- React calmly. Communicate calmly and simply.
- State your task firmly and simply.
- Try to control the disturbed patient gently.
- Ensure the safety of all staff and make certain that heroics are not attempted in dangerous circumstances.
- An adequate number of staff to accompany the doctor is essential—six is ideal (one for immobilisation of each limb, one for the head and one to assist with drugs).[1]
- Patients should be placed on the floor in the prone position.

Principles of sedative administration[1]

- Use the safest possible route of administration whenever possible (i.e. oral in preference to parenteral but often impractical). Intravenous administration has the lowest margin of safety.
- Parenteral administration should be restricted to severely disturbed patients.
- Closely monitor vital signs during and after sedative administration.
- Avoid intramuscular diazepam because of poor absorption.
- Be cautious of intravenous midazolam (Hypnovel) in such patients because of the risk of respiratory depression.
- Avoid benzodiazepines in patients with respiratory insufficiency. Haloperidol is an alternative.
- Patients have died from cardiopulmonary arrest after repeated sedative administration (especially benzodiazepines), so intensive monitoring is essential.

Monitor the following adverse effects:

- respiratory depression
- hypotension
- dystonic reactions, including choking
- neuroleptic malignant syndrome

Treatment options[1]

The treatment in acute medical and psychiatric settings depends on the appropriate mode of administration. Benzodiazepines are generally the drugs of first choice over antipsychotics in tranquillisation.[5] However, the IV route allows titration to the desired degree of sedation and has a more immediate effect.

Intravenous medication

diazepam or midazolam 5 mg IV initially

then

2.5–5 mg increments IV, repeated every 3–4 minutes until required level of sedation (rousable drowsiness) is reached—up to a maximum of 20–30 mg, when specialist advice is needed especially if further boluses are necessary

and/or droperidol 5–10 mg IV

Intramuscular medication

If this route considered appropriate:

midazolam 5–10 mg IM

or (if history of benzodiazepine tolerance)

droperidol 5–10 mg IM
or
olanzapine 5–10 mg repeated every 2–4 hours
or
combination midazolam/droperidol

(These first two injections can be repeated in 20 minutes if required. Droperidol is similar to haloperidol but more sedating. Keep in mind the rare but potentially fatal laryngeal dystonia with high doses—cover with benztropine 2 mg IM.)

Oral medication (if considered appropriate)

diazepam 5–20 mg (o), repeated every 2–6 hours (max: 120 mg/24 hours)
or
lorazepam 1–2 mg (o), repeated every 2–6 hours (max: 10 mg/24 hours)

If sedation is not achieved, add an antipsychotic medications e.g. olanzapine 5–10 mg initially or risperidone 0.5–1 mg initially.

Postdisturbance evaluation

Determine the likely cause, such as:

- acute organic brain syndrome: toxic causes, infection
- alcohol or drugs (illicit or prescribed): intoxication, withdrawal
- manic illness
- severe depression
- schizophrenic syndrome
- severe panic

Acute organic brain syndrome (delirium)

The many labels of acute organic brain syndrome include:

- delirium
- acute confusional state
- toxic confusional state
- confusional episode
- acute brain syndrome

Main clinical features

- Clouding of conscious state
- Disorientation
- Impaired attention
- Impaired memory
- Global cognitive defect—onset over days/hours

Refer to the box.

DSM-5 criteria for delirium[5]

Diagnosis of delirium requires evidence of:

A Disturbance of consciousness, attention and awareness
B Clinical features appearing over a short period
C A change in cognition:
- perceptual disturbance
- incoherent speech
- disorientation
- memory impairment/deficit

D A & C not better explained by another disorder
E Evidence of a cause

Other clinical features[1]

- The patients are usually elderly.
- Anxiety and agitation can be severe but in hypoactive deliria (usually due to metabolic disturbance) the conscious state can vary from drowsiness to coma.
- Odd behaviour with mood swings can occur.
- Psychotic symptoms can occur.
- Delusions are usually fleeting.
- The disturbance is usually worse at night and may be aggravated by sedation.
- Visual hallucinations are a feature of alcohol withdrawal.
- Attacks on bystanders may result (uncommon).

Always seek a cause.[1] A list of causes is presented in TABLE 45.3. The most important causes are:

- infections (usually in urinary tract, lungs or ear, or systemic in young or elderly)
- prescribed drugs

Anticholinergic delirium

Consider this cause (from drugs with anticholinergic properties or illicit substances). Features include hyperactivity, marked thought disorder, vivid visual hallucinations and very disturbed behaviour.

Differential diagnosis of delirium

In the earlier stages it may mimic the various psychiatric disorders, including anxiety, depression, various hallucinatory states, particularly agitated schizophrenia (rarely), extreme manic states, complex partial seizures, dementia. Consider deafness. Delirium is common in the hospital setting.

Investigations

Investigations are those listed under 'The clinical approach' earlier in the chapter.

Treatment

Principles:

- Acute delirium is a medical emergency.
- Establish normal hydration, electrolyte balance and nutrition.
- Consider alcohol withdrawal and give a trial of thiamine when the cause of delirium is unknown.
- Attend to helpful environmental factors (e.g. calm atmosphere, a night-light, orientation clues, presence of friends and relatives).
- Give oxygen if hypoxic, e.g. respiratory distress

Medication

Medication[1] may not be needed, but it will be if there are symptoms of anxiety, aggression or psychosis (doses for a fit adult).

For anxiety and depression:
midazolam 1.25–5 mg IM
For psychotic behaviour:
haloperidol 0.5 mg (o) as a single dose
or
olanzapine 2.5–10 mg (o) daily in 1 or 2 doses

If oral administration is not possible or when parenteral medication is required (cover with benztropine 2 mg (o) or IM):

haloperidol 0.5 mg IM as single dose
or
olanzapine 2.5 mg IM as single dose
For anticholinergic delirium:
tacrine hydrochloride 15–30 mg with caution by slow IV injection (an antidote)
Note:

- For hypoxia, give oxygen.
- Avoid benzodiazepines, especially in children and in patients with respiratory insufficiency.
- Consider necessity for pain relief.
- Use lower doses of parenteral medications in the very old and frail.

Dementia (chronic organic brain syndrome)

Dementia or neurocognitive disorder is an important diagnosis to consider in the elderly patient. The DSM criteria for dementia are presented in CHAPTER 8.

The main feature of dementia is impairment of memory, especially recent memory, when the person cannot remember what has happened a few hours (or even moments) earlier but may clearly remember the events of the past.

The more serious behavioural changes encountered with dementia tend to occur in the advanced stages. However, these disturbances may be precipitated by illness such as infections, emotional upset and drugs. These serious disturbances include:

- uninhibited behaviour
- hallucinations (generally uncommon)
- paranoid delusions

If a stable patient becomes acutely disturbed, delirium should be suspected.

Presenile dementia—Alzheimer type

The main features are:

- onset in late 50s and early 60s
- insidious onset
- early loss of short-term memory
- progressive decline in intellect
- death in 5–10 years
- more common in Down syndrome

Differential diagnosis of dementia

There are two approaches to the differential diagnosis, including consideration of the classic causes of disturbed behaviour as summarised in the mnemonic in TABLE 45.5.[6]

However, the foremost differential diagnosis should be 'pseudodementia' caused by severe depression.

Table 45.5 Differential diagnosis of dementias

D = **D**elirium
drugs (see toxic)

E = **E**motional disorder = depression
endocrine = thyroid

M = **M**emory = benign forgetfulness

E = **E**lective = anxiety disorders/neuroses

N = **N**eurological:
- CVA
- head trauma

T = **T**oxic:
- drugs/medication
- metabolic disease

I = **I**ntellect—low or retarded

A = **A**mnesic disorders—Korsakov syndrome

S = **S**chizophrenia (chronic)

Source: McLean[6]

45

Table 45.6 Comparison of schizophrenia and dementia

	Dementia	Schizophrenia
Onset	Middle-aged or elderly	Young
Memory	Always impaired	Usually unaffected
Delusions	Rare	Frequent
Hallucinations	Uncommon	Frequent
Thought broadcasting	Never	Frequent

A simple comparison between schizophrenia and dementia is shown in TABLE 45.6.

A vigorous search for a possible cause of dementia is warranted since there are a significant number of reversible causes. In particular, it is important to exclude the psychiatric conditions that may mimic dementia.

Treatment[1]

- To control psychotic symptoms or disturbed behaviour:
  risperidone 0.5–2 mg (o) daily
  or
  olanzapine 2.5–10 mg (o) daily in 1 or 2 doses
- To control symptoms of anxiety and agitation: oxazepam 15 mg (o) 1 to 4 times daily. Avoid benzodiazepines for more than 2 weeks
- For depression—administer antidepressants

The acute psychotic patient

Acute psychosis is the presence of the mental state where appreciation of reality is impaired as evidenced by the presence of typical psychotic symptoms such as delusions, hallucinations, mood disturbance and bizarre behaviour.[7] Refer to the diagnostic strategy for hallucinations in TABLE 45.7.

The differential diagnoses of patients presenting with psychoses is presented in TABLE 45.8.

Table 45.7 Hallucinations: diagnostic strategy model

Probability diagnosis
Drugs (illicit or prescribed)
Alcohol (acute or chronic)
Schizophrenia
Febrile delirium
Affective (mood) disorders
Drug withdrawal (incl. alcohol, hypnotics)
Dementias (esp. Lewy body)

Serious disorders not to be missed
Vascular:
- cerebrovascular disease
- migraine (luminous)

Infections:
- encephalitis/meningitis
- septicaemia
- any serious febrile illness

Tumours:
- cerebral tumours
- cancer treatment

Other:
- hypoxia
- liver failure
- metabolic/electrolyte imbalance
- dehydration

Pitfalls (often missed)
Major depression
Extreme fatigue
Vitamin deficiency (esp. B group)
Seizure disorders (esp. complex partial)
Rarities:
- narcolepsy
- post-concussion
- bereavement
- multiple sclerosis

Seven masquerades checklist
Depression
Diabetes
Drugs (iatrogenic/social, illicit)
Thyroid/other endocrine (hypothyroid)
Urinary tract infection (esp. elderly)

Is the patient trying to tell me something?
Consider conversion disorder (hysteria); fabrication.

Early diagnosis

Early recognition of a psychosis, particularly schizophrenia, is extremely important, as early intervention leads to improved outcomes. Early or prodromal symptoms include the following:

- social withdrawal
- reduced attention and concentration
- reduced drive and motivation
- depressed mood
- anxiety
- irritability/agitation
- suspiciousness
- sleep disturbance
- deterioration in role functioning

Table 45.8	Causes of psychoses[7]

Functional psychoses:
- schizophrenia
- schizophreniform disorder (shorter duration of symptoms)
- schizoaffective disorder (core symptoms of schizophrenia + mood symptoms)
- bipolar mood disease (depressed or manic phase)

Drug-induced psychoses
Organic-based psychoses
Other:
- delusional disorder (paranoid psychoses)
- brief psychotic disorder (rapid resolution)
- folie à deux (psychosis occurring simultaneously in two close associates)

It is appropriate to ask the correct questions in order to elicit psychotic symptoms. These are presented in TABLE 45.9.

DSM-5 key diagnostic criteria[5]—schizophrenia

A Two or more of following, each present for a significant portion of time during a 1-month period
  1. delusions
  2. hallucinations
  3. disorganised speech
  (at least one of these: 1–3)
  4. grossly disorganised or catatonic behaviour
  5. negative symptoms, e.g. flat affect (avolition)

B Social, learning or occupational dysfunction
C Continuous signs of disturbance for at least 6 months
D No evidence of other psychoses, e.g. bipolar
E Not attributable to effects of substance abuse or other medical condition

Schizophrenia and associated disorders

The term 'schizophrenia' (Bleuler 1911) refers to a group of severe psychiatric illnesses characterised by severe disturbances of emotion, language, perception, thought processes, volition and motor activity. The causes of schizophrenia disorders are unknown, but genetic factors and drug abuse are implicated.

Table 45.9 Questions for eliciting psychotic symptoms

Anxiety	Have you been feeling especially nervous or fearful? Have you felt tense and shaky, or experienced palpitations?
Depressed mood	Have you been feeling sad or 'down in the dumps' recently, not enjoying activities as much as before?
Elevated mood	Have you been feeling especially good in yourself, more cheerful than usual and full of life?
Auditory hallucinations	Do you hear voices of people talking to you even when there is no-one nearby?
Thought insertion	Have you felt that thoughts are being put into your mind? Do you experience telepathy?
Thought withdrawal	Have you experienced thoughts being taken out of your mind?
Thought broadcasting	Have you felt that other people are aware of your thoughts?
Thought echo	Have you experienced voices or people echoing your thoughts?
Delusion of control	Have you felt under the control or influence of an outside force?
Delusions of reference	Do programs on the television or radio hold special meaning for you?
Delusions of persecution	Do you feel that you are being singled out for special treatment? Is there a conspiracy against you?
Delusions of grandeur	Do you feel special, with unusual abilities or power?
Delusions of guilt	Do you believe that you have sinned or have done something deserving punishment?

Reproduced with permission

Source: Moulds[5]

Signs and symptoms of schizophrenia

- Positive
  - delusions
  - hallucinations
  - thought disorder
  - disorganised speech and behaviour
- Negative
  - flat affect
  - poverty of thought
  - lack of motivation
  - social withdrawal
  - reduced speech output

- Cognitive
  - distractibility
  - impaired working memory
  - impaired executive function (e.g. planning)
  - impaired insight
- Mood
  - mania (elevation)
  - depression

Other features include:

- bizarre behaviour
- subject to tension, anxiety or depression
- deterioration in work and study performance
- peak incidence 15–25 years[8] —smaller peak at 40 years
- lifetime prevalence 1 in 100
- equal sex incidence
- high risk of suicide

Differential diagnosis

Organic factors need to be excluded, especially drugs:

- amphetamines
- hallucinogens (e.g. LSD)
- marijuana

Also consider complex partial seizures and a personality disorder. Other psychoses are presented in TABLE 45.8.

A comparison of delirium, dementia and functional psychosis is presented in TABLE 45.10.

Management

Drug treatment is only a part of total management. Explanation and appropriate reassurance to the family with patient and family supportive care is obviously essential. Supportive psychotherapy is important in all phases. A team approach is necessary to cope with the disorder, which usually has a devastating effect on the family. Referral for specialist care is appropriate.

Acute phase

- Hospitalisation usually necessary
- Drug treatment for the psychosis[1]

Drug treatment may include the first-generation (typical or conventional) antipsychotics such as haloperidol and chlorpromazine, which are effective for managing the 'positive' symptoms, or the second generation (atypical) antipsychotics such as risperidone, olanzapine, quetiapine, clozapine, amisulpride and aripiprazole, which in addition are more effective at treating the 'negative' and other symptoms of schizophrenia.[9]

The usual practice rule is to start with a second-generation antipsychotic at a low dose and titrate upwards at a rate and to a level that is optimal for the patient. Patients with a first psychotic episode may respond to lower than usual doses.[5]

1 When oral medication is possible, first-line treatment (for the first episode) is one of (with starting doses):[1,10,11]
amisulpride 100 mg nocte
asenapine 5 mg sublingual bd
aripiprazole 10 mg once daily
lurasidone 40 mg once daily
olanzapine 5 mg nocte
paliperidone 3 mg nocte
quetiapine 50 mg bd → 200 mg bd (by day 5)

Table 45.10 Comparison of the clinical features of delirium, dementia and acute functional psychoses[8]

Feature	Delirium	Dementia	Acute psychosis
Onset	Rapid	Slow—insidious	Rapid
Duration	Hours to weeks	Months to years	Depends on response to treatment
Course over 24 hours	Fluctuates—worse at night	Minimal variation	Minimal variation
Consciousness	Reduced	Alert	Alert
Perception	Misperceptions common, especially visual	Misperceptions rare	May be misperceptions
Hallucinations	Common, visual (usually) or auditory	Uncommon	Common, mainly auditory
Attention	Distractable	Normal to impaired	Variable—may be impaired
Speech	Variable, may be incoherent	Difficulty finding correct words	Variable: normal, rapid or slow
Organic illness or drug toxicity	One or both present	Often absent	Usually absent

risperidone 0.5–1 mg nocte → 2 mg nocte
zipraside 40 mg bd → 80 mg bd (risk of ↑ QT)
zuclopenthixol 20 mg nocte

> ## Practice tips
>
> Typical initial oral therapy:
>
> olanzapine 5 mg
>
> *or*
>
> risperidone 0.5 mg

If response is inadequate in 3 weeks increase the dose according to prescribing guidelines.

If no response after 4–6 weeks consider a change to:[12]

- an alternative second-generation agent (above)
  or
- a first-generation antipsychotic such as:
  chlorpromazine 200 mg once daily → 500 mg
  haloperidol 1.5 mg once daily → 7.5 mg
  trifluoperazine 2 mg bd

2 Parenteral medication should be avoided if possible in acute care, but if required:[1,11]
  haloperidol 2.5–10 mg IM, initially, up to 20 mg in 24 hours, depending on the response
  or
  olanzapine 5–10 mg IM initially (do not use with benzodiapines concurrently)
  add
  benztropine 1–2 mg (o) bd (to avoid dystonic reaction)
  or
  zuclopenthixol acetate 50–150 mg IM as a single dose

If dystonic reaction:
  benztropine 1–2 mg IV or IM
If very agitated use:
  diazepam 5–10 mg (o) up to 40 mg/day or 5–10 mg IV

Chronic phase

Long-term antipsychotic medication is recommended to prevent relapse.[1]

- Examples of oral medication regimens:[11,12]
  olanzapine 5–10 mg (o) nocte
  or
  risperidone 0.5–1 mg (o) bd up to 2–4 mg
  or
  quetiapine 150 mg (o) bd
- Aim for lowest possible dose to maintain control.
- Chlorpromazine is not recommended for long-term use because of photosensitivity reactions.
- Use depot preparations if compliance is a problem (usually test dose first):[1,10]
  fluphenazine decanoate 12.5 mg IM, initially then 12.5–50 mg every 2–4 weeks
  or
  haloperidol decanoate 50 mg IM, initially then 50–200 mg every 4 weeks
  or
  flupenthixol decanoate 10 mg IM, initially then 20–40 mg every 2–4 weeks
  or
  risperidone 25–25 mg IM initially then every 2 weeks, titrated to clinical response
  or
  zuclopenthixol 100 mg IM, initially then titrated to 200–400 mg every 2–4 weeks

  Tips with depot preparations:
- Start with IM test doses and then titrate to recommended controlling levels (half or full starting dose).
- May take 2–4 months to produce a stable response, so oral supplements may be necessary.
- Not as effective as oral therapy.
- Give as deep IM injection with 21 gauge needle in buttock.
- Use lowest possible dose to avoid tardive dyskinesia.
- Reassess at least every 3 months.
- Closely monitor patient for movement disorders.

Drug-resistant schizophrenia[13,14]

Consider other causes (e.g. substances abuse). ECT may help the agitated patient, especially if catatonic. Consider a trial of clozapine (12.5 mg (o) bd initially increasing to 200–600 mg daily), with strict monitoring for blood dyscrasias and cardiotoxicity, or olanzapine (5–20 mg daily). A trial of adjunctive ECT should be considered in patients who fail to respond to clozapine.

Movement disorders from antipsychotic medication[1]

Acute dystonias

- Usually bizarre muscle spasms affect face, neck, tongue and trunk
- Oculogyric crises, opisthotonos and laryngeal spasm

  Treatment:
  benztropine 1–2 mg IV or IM

Akathisia

- Subjective or objective motor restlessness of feet and legs
- Generally later onset in course of treatment

45

Treatment:

- reduce dosage until akathisia less troublesome or substitute thioridazine
- can use oral propranolol, diazepam or benztropine as a short-term measure

Parkinsonian

- Seen relatively early in treatment
- The akinesia can be confused with drug-induced depression

Treatment:

- use lower dose or substitute a phenothiazine in low dosage
- alternatively, use benztropine or benzhexol

Tardive dyskinesia[1]

Tardive dyskinesia is a syndrome of abnormal involuntary movements of the face, mouth, tongue, trunk and limbs. This is a major problem with the use of long-term antipsychotic drugs and may occur months or years (usually) after starting treatment and with drug withdrawal. Avoid prolonged use of metoclopramide.

Differential diagnosis:

- spontaneous orofacial dyskinesia
- senile dyskinesia
- ill-fitting dentures
- neurological disorders causing tremor and chorea

If drug withdrawal is ineffective, use tetrabenazine 12.5 mg (o) daily, increasing as necessary.[12] The risks and benefits of continuing therapy have to be weighed.

Note: Because of the difficulty with managing tardive dyskinesia, prevention in the form of using the lowest possible dosage of antipsychotic medication is essential. This involves regular review and adjustment if necessary.

Neuroleptic (antipsychotic) malignant syndrome

This is a potentially fatal adverse effect that can develop at any time. It develops in hours to days.

Syndrome: high temperature, muscle rigidity, altered consciousness. Milder variants can occur (refer to CHAPTER 53).

Treatment:

- discontinue medication
- ensure adequate hydration with IV fluids
- if life-threatening:

  bromocriptine 2.5 mg (o) bd, gradually increasing to 5 mg (o) tds
  and
  dantrolene 50 mg IV every 12 hours for up to 7 doses
- consultant referral

Cardiac dysfunction

Various psychotrophic agents, particularly the phenothiazines, are prone to cause the adverse effect of prolongation of the QT interval with potential severe outcomes.

Bipolar disorder

The mood disorders are divided into depressive disorders and bipolar disorders. Bipolar is a broad term to describe a recurrent illness with episodes of either mania or depression with return to normal function in between. The swing in moods in bipolar disorders (manic depressive disorders) is illustrated in FIGURE 45.1. It affects 1%–2% of the population.

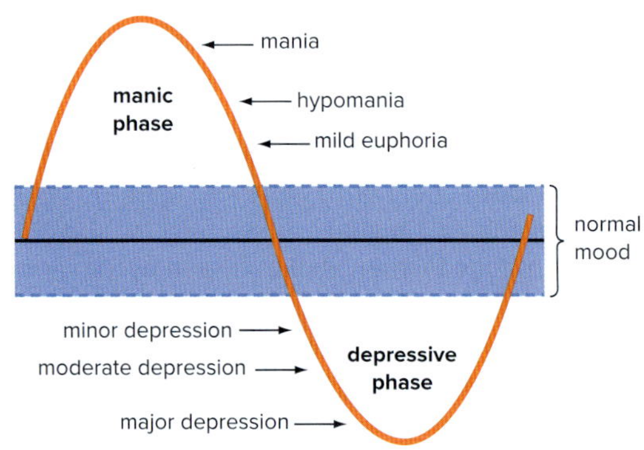

FIGURE 45.1 Bipolar disorder (manic depression): possible mood swings

DSM-5 criteria for a manic episode[5]

A Distinct period for at least 1 week of abnormal and persistent elevated, expansive or irritable mood

B Three or more of these unusual features:
1. inflated self-esteem or grandiosity
2. decreased need for sleep
3. talkative/accelerated speech
4. racing thoughts or flights of ideas
5. distractability as reported or observed
6. increased goal-directed activity or psychomotor agitation
7. excessive activity with 'painful' consequences

C Marked impaired social or occupational functioning or need for hospitalisation or psychotic features

D Episode not due to substance abuse or other medical condition

A–D = a manic episode: at least one in a lifetime for diagnosis

Bipolar I disorder has one fully fledged manic or mixed episode and usually depressive episodes.

Bipolar II disorder is defined as a major depressive episode with at least one hypomanic episode lasting a minimum of 4 days but no classic manic episodes.

The symptoms of mania may appear abruptly, usually in the teens or young adulthood.

Typical inherent features, in addition to the above, include:

- reckless behaviour, overspending
- hasty decisions (e.g. job resignation, hasty marriages)
- impaired judgment
- increased sexual drive, energy and activity
- poor insight into the problem
- variable psychotic symptoms—paranoia, delusions, auditory hallucinations

Note: The peak onset is in early adult life. The exact cause is unknown, but there is a strong hereditary basis. Episodes may be precipitated by stress.

'Hypomania' is the term used to describe the symptoms of mania that are similar to but less severe (without criterion C) and of shorter duration.

The subsequent major depressive phase is associated with a high risk of suicide.

Good questions to ask the patient with suspected 'bipolar' disorder:

- How have you been feeling in yourself?
- Have you felt especially good about yourself?
- Do you feel that you are special or have special powers?
- Have you been spending more than usual?
- Have you been needing less sleep than usual?

Management of acute mania[1,15]

This is a medical emergency requiring hospitalisation for protection of both family and patient. Involuntary admission is usually necessary. It may be a first episode or a relapse due to poor treatment compliance or substance abuse. A recent meta-analysis indicates that antipsychotics are the most efficacious drugs.

Treatment

First line:[1]

olanzapine 5 mg (o) nocte initially then increasing to 10 mg
or
risperidone 1 mg (o) nocte initially then increasing to 2 mg

Second line:

haloperidol or a second-generation antipsychotic e.g. aripiprazole[16]
or
lithium carbonate 750–1000 mg (o) daily in 2 or 3 divided doses increasing according to serum levels
or (a mood stabilising agent)
sodium valproate 200–400 mg (o) bd initially
or
carbamazepine 100–200 mg (o) bd initially

If a parenteral antipsychotic drug is required:

haloperidol 5–10 mg IM or IV
Repeat in 15–30 minutes if necessary
(risk of tardive dyskinesia)
Change to oral medication as soon as possible

Failure to respond to treatment:[17,18,19]

- ensure maximum concentration of first drug
- switch to a different drug e.g. olanzapine to lithium
- combine drugs, e.g. second-degree antipsychotic + lithium
- ECT is of proven benefit for recalcitrant problems

Remember to provide supportive psychotherapy with appropriate psychosocial interventions.

Prophylaxis for recurrent bipolar disorder

(Over 90% will have a recurrence at some time: consider medication if two or more episodes of either mania or depression in the previous 4 years.)

Recommended prophylactic agents[5]

lithium carbonate125–500 mg (o) bd then adjusted
or
second-generation antipsychotic agent
or (if depression prominent)
lamotrigine or carbamazine or sodium valproate

Use long-term lithium (e.g. 3–5 years). Target plasma level for maintenance is usually 0.6–0.8 mmol/L. A US study recommended lithium as the prime mood stabiliser.[16]

- If poor response, use another agent.
- Unwanted side effects of lithium include:
  - a fine tremor
  - muscle weakness
  - weight gain
  - gastrointestinal symptoms
  - hypothyroidism
  - nephrotoxicity
- With anti-epileptics, adjust dosage according to clinical response and toxicity.

45

Management of bipolar depression[10,17]

This is a difficult component to treat and antidepressants should not be used alone.[11] Many mood-stabilising agents appear to have a bimodal (antidepressant and antimania) effect and can be useful in the absence of classical antidepressants.[15]

A recommended regimen is:

an antidepressant (e.g. SSRI, SNRI or MAOI)
plus
lithium, valproate, carbamazepine, quetiapine, lamotrigine or olanzapine (one of these used for prophylaxis)

Antidepressants are usually withdrawn within 1–2 months because of a propensity to precipitate mania.

ECT is an effective treatment for bipolar depression while psychological therapies such as CBT and psychoeducation have proven efficacy.

Bipolar I patients usually recover but proceed to have further episodes of depression or mania.[11]

Liaison with family and carers

Promote a caring support and pyschoeducation program for patient and family. Educate about the patient's 'relapse signature' for a manic or depressive episode.

Body dysmorphic disorder[5]

Body dysmorphic disorder is characterised by a preoccupation with the belief that some aspect of physical appearance is abnormal, unattractive or diseased. The person's concern and distress is out of proportion to any imagined or actual defect and usually not amenable to reassurance. This preoccupation causes significant functional impairment. The condition rarely presents directly and may be over-represented in the area of dermatology or plastic surgery. It begins in late childhood or early adolescence. The person's focus is on the face, head or secondary sexual characteristics.

Patients may be helped by counselling and psychotherapy including CBT. There is clinical evidence that SSRIs help if the symptoms suggest an obsessive–compulsive disorder. An antipsychotic agent may help where beliefs are delusional or in the context of a psychotic disorder.

Depression

Depression is very common and presents in a great range of severity. In the context of 'the disturbed patient' depression can be confused with dementia or a psychosis, particularly if the following are present:

- psychomotor agitation
- psychomotor retardation
- delusions
- hallucinations

Assessment[1]

The following questions need to be addressed:

- Is the depression primary (i.e. not secondary to another psychiatric condition such as schizophrenia or anxiety disorder)?
- Is it part of a bipolar disorder? Has there been a previous manic or hypomanic episode? If so, a different approach to treatment is required.
- Is the depression caused by another illness or physical factor (e.g. hypothyroidism, cerebrovascular disease or medication)?
- Is the patient psychotic?
- Is the patient a suicide risk?

The treatment of depression is presented in CHAPTER 19.

Psychoactive substance use disorders

It is important for the GP to be aware of the effects of self-administration of psychoactive substances, especially their toxic or withdrawal effects. They form a significant consideration for the differential diagnosis of disturbed patient behaviour. The following substances can cause these effects.

Alcohol

Toxic and withdrawal effects, including delirium tremens, are outlined in CHAPTER 21. Abrupt withdrawal can cause symptoms ranging from tremors, agitation and dysphoria (feeling thoroughly miserable) to fully developed delirium tremens. Epileptic seizures may also occur.

Barbiturate dependence

Tolerance and symptoms on withdrawal are the main features. Barbiturate withdrawal is a very serious, life-threatening problem and may be encountered in elderly people undergoing longstanding hypnotic withdrawal. Symptoms include anxiety, tremor, extreme irritability, twitching, seizures and delirium.

Management[1]

Undertake withdrawal with medical supervision as an inpatient.

Transfer the patient to phenobarbitone or diazepam.
phenobarbitone 120 mg (o) hourly until sedation
or
phenobarbitone 30 mg for each 100 mg of shorter-acting barbiturate

reduce the dose gradually over 10–14 days
or
diazepam 20–40 mg orally, daily
reduce the dose gradually over 10–14 days

Benzodiazepine dependence

Withdrawal symptoms in the dependent patient include anxiety, restlessness, irritability, palpitation and muscle aches and pains, but delirium and seizures are uncommon except with very high doses. The shorter the half-life, the greater the dependence.

Withdrawal is best achieved by supervising a gradual reduction in dosage aided by relaxation techniques and behavioural strategies to help patients cope with insomnia and anxiety.

Refer to CHAPTER 21 for the effects of opioid dependence, stimulant substance abuse, hallucinogen abuse and cannabis use and dependence.

Psychiatric disorders of childhood and adolescence[1]

The following disturbance problems do occur and must be taken seriously, especially the potential for suicide in the second decade. Many of these disorders are presented in more detail in CHAPTER 94.

Attention deficit hyperactivity disorder

Clinical features:

- short attention span
- distractibility
- overactivity
- impulsiveness
- antisocial behaviour

Depression

Major depression follows the same criteria as for adults. Suicidal ideation has to be considered and taken very seriously if present. Imipramine is probably the drug of choice.

Bipolar disorders

Mania is seldom diagnosed before puberty. Adolescents may present (uncommonly) with symptoms of mania or hypomania.

Schizophrenia and related disorders

Schizophrenia is rare before puberty. The criteria for diagnosis are similar to adults:

- delusion
- thought disorder
- hallucinations
- 6 months or more of deterioration in functioning

Autism

Aggression and irritability can be a feature, especially during adolescence.

Tourette syndrome

Behavioural problems can be part of this syndrome, which requires the attention of an experienced consultant.

Obsessive–compulsive disorders

In about one-third of cases the onset is between 5 and 15 years of age.

VIOLENCE AND DANGEROUSNESS

Dangerousness has been defined as a 'propensity to cause serious physical injury or lasting psychological harm to others' and, in the context of people with mental illness, 'the relative probability of their committing a violent crime'.[20]

Dangerousness is not related only to mental illness and, interestingly, most offenders have no psychiatric diagnosis. It is not an inherited, immutable characteristic of an individual but tends to surface on impulse in a particular context given a whole range of situational factors. Prediction of the risk of violence is not straightforward.

Various groups have been identified as contributing risk factors for violent conduct.[20]

- Schizophrenic psychoses, including: older male paranoid schizophrenics; younger males prone to act violently and impulsively, presumably due to hallucinatory commands
- Morbid jealousy: associated with delusions of infidelity
- Antisocial personality disorder
- Mood disorder: violence, usually associated with depression (rarely mania); parents with severe depression; history of suicide attempts in depression
- Episodic discontrol syndrome (similar to intermittent explosive disorder)
- Intellectual disability combined with personality disorder and behavioural disturbances
- Alcohol abuse or dependency
- Amphetamine or benzodiazepine abuse or dependency

From a management viewpoint, homicidal threats must be taken very seriously.

The diagnostic strategy model for antisocial behaviour in adults is presented in TABLE 45.11.

45

45

Table 45.11 Antisocial behaviour in adults: diagnostic strategy model

Probability diagnosis
Functional (no medical or mental component)
Drugs (alcohol, illicit or prescribed)
Alcohol (acute or chronic)
Antisocial personality disorder (esp. cluster B)
Affective (mood) disorders
Drug withdrawal (incl. alcohol, hypnotics)
Mental impairment

Serious disorders not to be missed
Vascular:
- cerebrovascular disease (incl. SAH)
- acute coronary syndromes

Infections:
- encephalitis/meningitis
- HIV/AIDS
- septicaemia

Tumours:
- cerebral tumours

Other:
- post-ictal (epilepsy)
- delirium
- subdural haematoma
- psychosis (schizophrenia, bipolar, paraphrenia)
- schizotypal personality disorder

Pitfalls (often missed)
Head injury
Fluid and electrolyte imbalance
Dementia (esp. early)
Rarities:
- neurosyphilis
- prion disease (e.g. CJD)
- premenstrual dysphoria syndrome

Seven masquerades checklist
Depression (major)
Diabetes (hypoglycaemia)
Drugs (iatrogenic/social, illicit)
Thyroid/other endocrine (hyper/hypothyroid)

Is the patient trying to tell me something?
Consider conversion disorder (hysterical fugue)
Malingering/fabrication
Severe anxiety/panic

SUICIDE AND PARASUICIDE

The haunting issue of suicide and parasuicide is presented in CHAPTER 19. The disturbed patient is always a suicide risk rather than a homicide risk. The importance of recognising depression with an associated suicide risk in the elderly patient has been emphasised heavily in this chapter.

Facts and figures[21]

- More than 90% of suicides occur without underlying chronic conditions but most people are significantly depressed at the time.
- In Australia, suicide is the second most common cause of death between the ages of 11 and 25 years. Children as young as 5 years of age have committed suicide.
- Those who talk about suicide may attempt it later.
- About half of those committing suicide have seen a doctor within their last month of life.
- Around 80–90% of suicides have given clear or subtle warnings to family, friends or doctors.
- There is no evidence that asking patients about suicidal ideation provokes suicidal acts.
- Doctors in Australia and other Western countries have a high suicide rate.

Suicide risk

Blumenthal's[22] overlapping model lists five groups of risk factors (see FIG. 45.2):

1 Psychiatric disorders:
  - affective disorder and alcohol abuse in adults
  - schizophrenia
  - depression and conduct disorder in young people
  - anorexia nervosa

2 Personality traits:
  - impulsiveness and aggression

3 Environmental and psychosocial factors:
  - poor social supports
  - chronic medical illness (e.g. AIDS)
  - significant loss

4 Family history and genetics (both nature and nurture):
  - emulation of relatives
  - specific ethnic groups in custody

5 Biological factors:
  - possible serotonin deficiency

Parasuicide

Parasuicide is attempted suicide; in many cases, patients are drawing attention to themselves as a 'plea for help'. It is important for the GP to take an active role in the support of the patient and family after discharge from hospital, but preferably in conjunction with a psychiatric or counselling service. Arrange frequent consultations at first and ensure adequate follow-up, especially for missed appointments.

PERSONALITY DISORDERS

People with personality disorders may become very distressed and acutely disturbed under stress or provocation, and this may involve dramatic scenes,

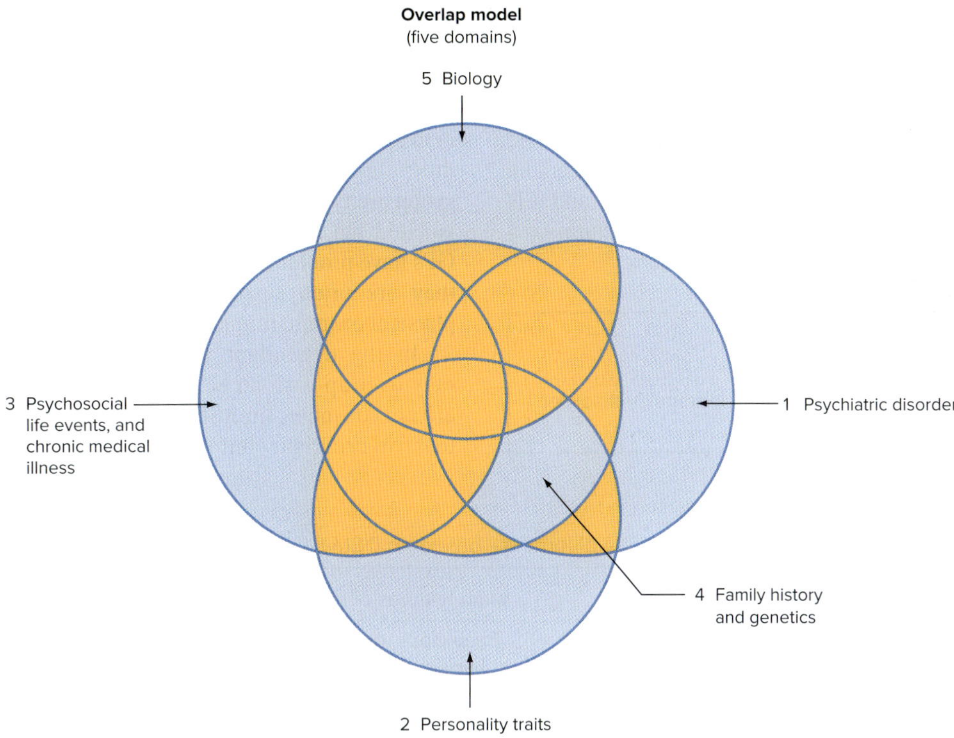

FIGURE 45.2 Overlap model for understanding suicidal behaviour.

Source: After Blumenthal SJ, Kupfer DJ, Generalised treatable strategies for suicidal behaviour, *Annals New York Academy of Science,* 1986; 487: 327–40.

including public suicide threats. It is important to recognise personality disorders because they usually cause considerable distress to the patients, their family, society and GPs. The prevalence is estimated as 11–12%.[1]

In practice, the personality disorders of most concern are those that present with hostility, either verbal or physical, particularly if a suicide or homicide threat is involved. It is a mistake to assume that those patients who manifest violent or psychopathic behaviour have a personality disorder or, conversely, that the meek and mild are free from personality disorder.

The diagnosis of personality disorder can be difficult. As practitioners we tend to have a 'gut feeling' about the diagnosis but often find it difficult to classify the personality of the patient and then to manage it appropriately.

The main characteristics of a personality disorder are:[1]

- lack of confidence and low self-esteem
- long history from childhood
- difficulties with interpersonal relationships and society
- recurrent maladaptive behaviour
- relatively fixed, inflexible and stylised reaction to stress
- minimal insight
- perception of difficulties as external to themselves

The medical/psychiatric significance:

- maladaptive relationships with GPs and society
- problem of sexually dysfunctional lives
- risk of substance abuse and self-destructive behaviour
- prone to depression and anxiety (usually low grade)
- susceptible to 'breakdown' under stress

Personality is the result of a genetic template and the continuing interaction of the person with outside influences (peer pressures, family interactions, influential events) and personal drives in seeking an identity. The outcome is a unique behaviour pattern manifesting as a personality trait or character reflective of the individual's self-image and fundamental to his or her sense of personal identity.[24]

Although personality is unique, it is possible to make a hypothesis that one is normal or abnormal.

If abnormal, it is possible to stereotype it according to the predominant symptoms or behaviours.

Using the International Classification of Disease (ICD-10) and the DSM-5 classification, various subtypes are readily identifiable (see TABLE 45.12),[5] which can be considered in three main groups. There is a considerable overlap between the subtypes within a group[25] and it is more important to understand the specific features of a person's personality than to categorise them.[26]

> **Practice tip**
>
> The cardinal feature of antisocial personality disorder is lack of empathy.

The antisocial personality disorders (ASPD) group (1–2% of population) tend to come to the attention of GPs more frequently, with some individuals representing 'heart-sink' patients because of demanding, angry or aggressive behaviour. They are more common among people in prison. The withdrawn group are typically withdrawn, suspicious and socially isolated but fall short of a true psychotic syndrome. GPs have problems communicating with them because they are often suspicious, which can make proper physical examination and management difficult.

In the dependent and inhibited groups, which may overlap with an anxiety state, the main features are nervousness, timidity, emotional dependence and fear of criticism and rejection. They are frequent

Table 45.12 Summary of main personality disorders—based on DSM-5

Main cluster group	Subtypes	Main features of disorder
Cluster A Withdrawn *Synonyms:* • odd • eccentric	Paranoid	Suspicious, oversensitive, argumentative, defensive, hyperalert, cold and humourless
	Schizoid	Shy, emotionally cold, introverted, detached, avoids close relationships
	Schizotypal	Odd and eccentric, sensitive, suspicious and superstitious, socially isolated, odd speech, thinking and behaviour. Falls short of criteria for schizophrenia
Cluster B Antisocial *Synonyms:* • dramatic • emotional • sociopathic • flamboyant • erratic	Antisocial (sociopathic, psychopathic)	Impulsive, insensitive, selfish, callous, superficial charm, lack of guilt, low frustration level, doesn't learn from experience, relationship problems (e.g. promiscuous), reckless disregard for safety of self and others, lack of self-control
	Histrionic (hysterical)	Self-dramatic, egocentric, immature, vain, dependent, manipulative, easily bored, emotional scenes, inconsiderate, seductive, craves attention and excitement
	Narcissistic ('prima donna')	Morbid self-admiration, exhibitionist, insensitive, craves and demands attention, exploits others, preoccupied with power, lacks interest in and empathy with others, bullying, insightless; 'charming, disarming, alarming', prone to fits of destructive anger and revenge
	Borderline ('hell-raiser')	Confused self-image/identity, impulsive, reckless, emptiness, 'all or nothing' relationships—emotionally unstable and intense, damaging reckless behaviour, full of anger and guilt, lacks self-control, uncontrolled gambling, spending etc. *Note:* High incidence of suicide and parasuicide; drug abuse
Cluster C Dependent *Synonyms:* • anxious • fearful • inhibited	Avoidant (anxious)	Anxious, self-conscious, fears rejection, timid and cautious, low self-esteem, overreacts to rejection and failure
	Dependent	Passive, weak-willed, lacks vigour, lacks self-reliance and confidence, overaccepting, avoids responsibility, seeks support, excessive need to be cared for
	Obsessional (obsessive–compulsive, anankastic)	Rigid, perfectionist, pedantic, indecisive, egocentric, preoccupied with orderliness and control, cautious

Note: The 'dark antisocial triad': narcissism, psychopathy (seeks control) and Machiavellianism (the end justifies the means).[23]

attenders (the 'fat file' syndrome) and are often accompanied by friends and relatives because of their insecurity.

Management

The best treatment is a supportive, 'therapeutic' community and an understanding and supportive GP. Psychotherapies are the key to long-term treatment. It is vital to understand that people with personality disorders perceive the world from a fundamentally different perspective. Problematic patients, if agreeable, may respond well to psychological intervention and behavioural techniques, especially operant conditioning (reinforcing acceptable behaviour) and averse conditioning (correcting inappropriate behaviour).[1,24] CBT has the most to offer.

The borderline and narcissistic disorders in particular respond well to specific types of psychotherapeutic intervention. Patients' self-esteem needs careful support while maladaptive modes of behaviour are confronted. Hospitalisation is rarely required except for those at risk of suicide (e.g. antisocial patients).

Medication has limitations but may be useful to treat those individuals who temporarily decompensate into a psychosis, an anxiety state or depression. One study has shown that antipsychotic medication in low dosage (e.g. haloperidol 5 mg daily) is effective in treating the problematic behaviours in paranoid and some antisocial personality disorders.[27]

There are dangers to the therapist and it is important not to 'buy into' a particular psychopathy, especially with seductive, manipulative or paranoid patients.[22]

When to refer[21]

Indications for referral to a psychiatrist:

- severe depression
- high suicide risk
- actual suicide attempt: recent or in the past
- suspected psychiatric disorders in the elderly: ?depression or schizophrenia; ?depression or dementia
- failure to improve with treatment
- poor family and social supports

Patient education resources

Hand-out sheets from *Murtagh's Patient Education* 7th edition:

- Bipolar disorder
- Personality disorders
- Schizophrenia

References

1 Expert group for Psychotropic. In: eTG complete [Internet]. Melbourne: Therapeutic Guidelines Ltd. Available from: <www.tg.org.au>, accessed September 2017.

2 Biro G. Dementia. Australian Doctor Weekly, 1990; 16 February: I–VIII.

3 Biro G. Delirium in the elderly. Australian Doctor Weekly, 1989; 1 December: I–VIII.

4 Kahn RL et al. Brief objective measures of the determination of mental status in the aged. Am J Psychiatry, 1960; 117: 326–9.

5 Kupfer DJ (Chair). *Diagnostic and Statistical Manual of Mental Disorder* (5th edn). Washington DC: American Psychiatric Publishing, 2013.

6 McLean S. Is it dementia? Aust Fam Physician, 1992; 21: 1762–6.

7 Keks N, Blashki G. The acutely psychotic patient: assessment and initial management. Aust Fam Physician, 2006; 35 (3): 90–4.

8 Norman T, Judd F. Schizophrenia. In: *MIMS Disease Index* (2nd edn). Sydney: IMS Publishing, 1996: 455–7.

9 Lovric K. Schizophrenia: update. Medical Observer, 17 September; 2004: 31–2.

10 Blashki G, Judd F, Piterman L. *General Practice Psychiatry.* Sydney: McGraw-Hill, 2007: 189–90.

11 Buckley N (Chair). *Australian Medicines Handbook.* Adelaide. Australian Medicines Handbook Pty Ltd, 2016: 831–6.

12 Hartling L et al. Antipsychotics in adults with schizophrenia: comparative effectiveness of first-generation versus second-generation medications: a systematic review and meta-analysis. Ann Intern Med, 2012; 157 (7): 498–511.

13 McEvoy JP et al. Effectiveness of clozapine versus olanzapine, quetiapine, and risperidone in patients with chronic schizophrenia who did not respond to prior atypical antipsychotic treatment. Am J Psychiatry, 2006; 163 (4): 600–10.

14 Leucht S et al. Antipsychotic drugs versus placebo for relapse prevention in schizophrenia: a systematic review and meta-analysis. Lancet, 2012; 379 (9831): 2063–71.

15 Smith LA, Cornelius V et al. Pharmacological intervention for acute bipolar mania: a systematic review of randomised placebo controlled trials. Bipolar Disorders, 2007; 9 (6): 551–60.

16 Sachs GS. A 25-year-old woman with bipolar disorder. JAMA, 2001; 285: 454–62.

17 Lovic K. Bipolar affective disorder: update. Medical Observer, 25 November 2005: 25–8.

18 Cipriani A et al. Comparative efficacy and acceptability of antimanic drugs in acute mania: a multiple-treatments meta-analysis. Lancet, 2011; 378 (9799): 1306–15.

19 Geddes JP et al. Lithium plus valproate combination therapy versus monotherapy for relapse prevention in bipolar I disorder (BALANCE): a randomised open-label trial. Lancet, 2010; 375 (9712): 385–95

20 Beaumont PJV, Hampshire RB. *Textbook of Psychiatry.* Melbourne: Blackwell Scientific Publications, 1989: 283–4.

21 Biro G. Suicide. Australian Doctor Weekly, 1991; 26 April: I–VIII.

22 Blumenthal S. Suicide—a guide to risk factors, assessment and treatment of suicidal patients. Med Clin North Am, 1988; 72: 937–63.

23 Jonason PK, Webster GD. The dirty dozen: a concise measure of the dark triad. Psychol Assess, 2010; 22 (2): 420–32.

24 Papadakis MA, McPhee SJ et al. *Current Medical Diagnosis and Treatment* (52nd edn). New York: The McGraw-Hill Companies, 2013: 1051–2.

25 Pullen I, Wilkinson G et al. *Psychiatry and General Practice Today*. London: RC Psych & RCGP, 1994: 180–3.

26 Kaplan R. Personality disorders: diagnoses and treatment. Medical Observer, 24 August 2001: 32–3.

27 Soloff PH et al. Progress in pharmacotherapy of borderline disorders: a double blind study of amitriptyline, haloperidol and placebo. Arch Gen Psychiatry, 1986; 43: 691–7.

Resources

NICE Pathways: Personality disorders. National Institute for Health and Care Excellence (NICE) <https://pathways.nice.org.uk/pathways/personality-disorders>

Dizziness/vertigo

46

I got my giddiness in 1690 (at the age of 23) by eating 100 golden pippins at a time at Richmond. Four years later at a place 20 miles further on in Surrey I got my deafness; and these two 'friends' have visited me one or other year since, and being old acquaintances have often sought fit to come together.

JONATHAN SWIFT (1667–1745), DESCRIBING HIS MÉNIÈRE SYNDROME

When patients complain of 'dizziness', they can be using this term to describe many different phenomena, and hence a careful history is required to unravel the problem. Other patients may use different terms to explain the same sensation, for example, 'giddiness', 'swimming in the head', 'my brain spinning', 'whirling' and 'swinging'.

'Dizzy' comes from an old English word, *dysig*, meaning foolish or stupid. Strictly speaking, it means unsteadiness or lightheadedness—without movement or motion or spatial disorientation.

'Vertigo', on the other hand, comes from the Latin *vertere* (to turn) and *-igo* for a condition. It should describe a hallucination of rotation of self or the surroundings in a horizontal or vertical direction.[1]

The term 'dizziness', however, is generally used collectively to describe all types of equilibrium disorders and, for convenience, can be classified as shown in FIGURE 46.1.

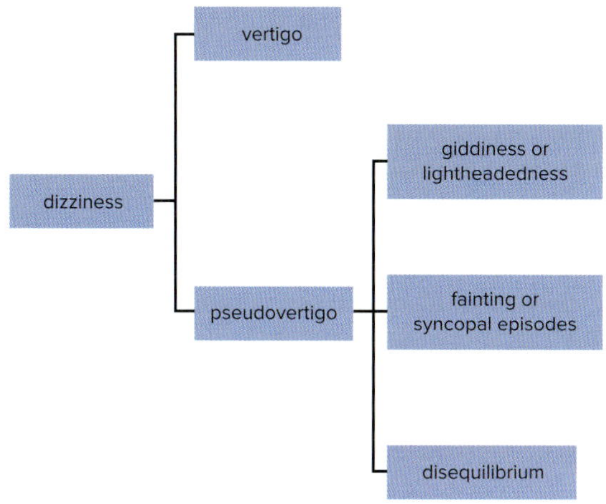

FIGURE 46.1 Classification of dizziness

Key facts and checkpoints

- Approximately one-third of the population will have suffered from significant dizziness by age 65 and about a half by age 80.[2]
- The commonest causes in family practice are postural hypotension and hyperventilation.
- The ability to examine and interpret the sign of nystagmus accurately is important in the diagnostic process.
- A drug history is very important, including prescribed drugs and others such as alcohol, cocaine, marijuana and illicit drugs.
- Ménière syndrome is overdiagnosed. It has the classic triad: vertigo–tinnitus–deafness (sensorineural).
- Vertebrobasilar insufficiency is also overdiagnosed as a cause of vertigo. It is a rare cause but may result in dizziness and sometimes vertigo but rarely in isolation.

Defined terminology

Vertigo

Vertigo is defined as an episodic sudden sensation of circular motion of the body or of its surroundings or an illusion of motion, usually a rotatory sensation. Other terms used by the patient to describe this symptom include 'everything spins', 'my head spins', 'the room spins', 'whirling', 'reeling', 'swaying', 'pitching' and 'rocking'. It is frequently accompanied by autonomic symptoms such as nausea, retching, vomiting, pallor and sweating.

Vertigo is characteristically precipitated by standing or turning the head or by movement. Patients have to walk carefully and may become nervous about descending stairs or crossing the road and usually seek support. Therefore the vertiginous patient is usually very frightened and tends to remain immobile during an attack.

Patients may feel as though they are being impelled by some outside force that tends to pull them to one side, especially while walking.

True vertigo is a symptom of disturbed function involving the vestibular system or its central connections. It invariably has an organic cause. Important causes are presented in TABLE 46.1, while FIGURE 46.2 illustrates central neurological centres that can cause vertigo.

Nystagmus is often seen with vertigo and, since 80–85% of causes are due to an ear problem, tinnitus and hearing disorders are also associated. In acute cases there is usually a reflex autonomic discharge producing sweating, pallor, nausea and vomiting.

Giddiness

Giddiness is a sensation of uncertainty or ill-defined lightheadedness. Other terms used by patients include 'a swimming sensation', 'walking on air' and 'ground going beneath me'. It usually contains no elements of rotation, impulsion, tinnitus, deafness, nausea or vomiting.

The patient with giddiness, although fearful of falling or swooning, can nonetheless walk without difficulty if forced to do so.

Giddiness is a typical psychoneurotic symptom.

Syncopal episodes

Syncope may present as a variety of dizziness or lightheadedness in which there is a sensation of

Table 46.1 Causes of vertigo

Peripheral disorders
Labyrinth: • labyrinthitis: viral or suppurative • Ménière syndrome • benign paroxysmal positional vertigo (BPPV) • drugs • trauma • chronic suppurative otitis media
Eight nerve: • vestibular neuronitis • acoustic neuroma • drugs
Cervical vertigo
Central disorders
Brain stem (TIA or stroke): • vertebrobasilar insufficiency • infarction
Cerebellum: • degeneration • tumours
Migraine
Multiple sclerosis

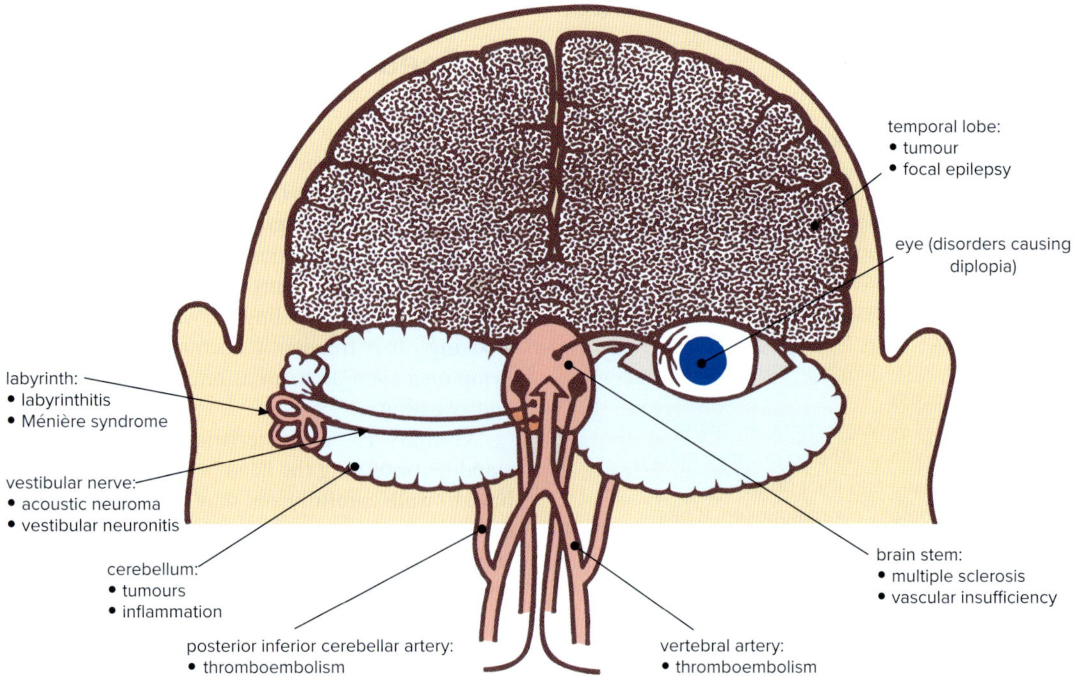

FIGURE 46.2 Diagrammatic illustration of central centres that can cause vertigo

impending fainting or loss of consciousness. Common causes are cardiogenic disorders and postural hypotension, which are usually drug-induced.

Disequilibrium

Disequilibrium implies a condition in which there is a loss of balance or instability while walking, without any associated sensations of spinning. Other terms used to describe this include 'unsteadiness on feet', 'the staggers', 'swaying feeling' and 'dizzy in the feet'.

Disequilibrium is usually of neurogenic origin.

A diagnostic approach

A summary of the diagnostic strategy model is presented in TABLE 46.2.

Probability diagnosis

In medical school we gain the wrong impression that the common causes of dizziness or vertigo are the relatively uncommon causes, such as Ménière syndrome, aortic stenosis, Stokes–Adams attacks, cerebellar disorders, vertebrobasilar disease and hypertension. In the real world of medicine, one is impressed by how often dizziness is caused by relatively common benign conditions, such as hyperventilation associated with anxiety, simple syncope, postural hypotension due to drugs and old age, inner ear infections, wax in the ears, post head injury, motion sickness and alcohol intoxication. In most instances making the correct diagnosis (which, as ever, is based on a careful history) is straightforward, but finding the underlying cause of true vertigo can be very difficult.

The common causes of vertigo seen in general practice are benign paroxysmal positional vertigo (BPPV, so often related to cervical vertebral dysfunction), accounting for about 25% of cases, acute vestibulopathy (vestibular neuronitis) and vestibular migraine.

Viral labyrinthitis is basically the same as vestibular neuronitis, except that the whole of the inner ear is involved so that deafness and tinnitus arise simultaneously with severe vertigo. The most common causes of recurrent spontaneous vertigo are Ménière syndrome and vestibular migraine.

Serious disorders not to be missed

Neoplasia

The important serious disorders to keep in mind are space-occupying tumours, such as acoustic neuroma, medulloblastoma and other tumours (especially

Table 46.2 Dizziness/vertigo: diagnostic strategy model

Probability diagnosis
Anxiety-hyperventilation (G)
Postural hypotension (G/S)
Simple faint—vasovagal (S)
Acute vestibulopathy (V)
Benign paroxysmal positional vertigo (V)
Motion sickness (V)
Vestibular migraine (V)
Cervical dysfunction/spondylosis
Serious disorders not to be missed
Neoplasia:
• acoustic neuroma
• posterior fossa tumour
• other brain tumours, primary or secondary
Intracerebral infection (e.g. abscess)
Cardiovascular:
• arrhythmias
• myocardial infarction
• aortic stenosis
Cerebrovascular:
• vertebrobasilar insufficiency
• brain stem infarct (e.g. PICA thrombosis)
Multiple sclerosis
Carbon monoxide poisoning
Pitfalls (often missed)
Ear wax—otosclerosis
Arrhythmias
Hyperventilation
Alcohol and other drugs
Cough or micturition syncope
Vestibular migraine/migrainous vertigo
Parkinson disease
Ménière syndrome (overdiagnosed)
Rarities:
• Addison disease (CHAPTER 23)
• neurosyphilis
• autonomic neuropathy
• hypertension
• subclavian steal
• perilymphatic fistula
• Shy–Drager syndrome
Seven masquerades checklist
Depression
Diabetes (possible: hypo/hyper)
Drugs
Anaemia
Thyroid disorder (possible)
Spinal dysfunction
UTI (possible)
Is the patient trying to tell me something?
Very likely. Consider anxiety and/or depression.

Note: G = giddiness; S = syncope; V = vertigo

posterior fossa tumours) capable of causing vertigo, intracerebral infections and cardiovascular abnormalities.

It is important to bear in mind that the commonest brain tumour is a metastatic deposit from lung cancer.[3]

Red flags for dizziness/vertigo

- neurological signs
- ataxia out of proportion to vertigo
- nystagmus out of proportion to vertigo
- central nystagmus
- central eye movement abnormalities

46

Acoustic neuroma

This uncommon tumour should be suspected in the patient presenting with the symptoms shown in the diagnostic triad below. Headache may occasionally be present.

DxT (unilateral) tinnitus + hearing loss + unsteady gait → acoustic neuroma

Diagnosis is best clinched by high-resolution MRI. Audiometry and auditory evoked responses are also relevant investigations.

Cardiac disorders

Cardiac disorders that must be excluded for giddiness or syncope are the various arrhythmias, such as Stokes–Adams attacks caused by complete heart block, aortic stenosis and myocardial infarction.

Cerebrovascular causes

The outstanding cerebrovascular causes of severe vertigo are vertebrobasilar insufficiency and brain stem infarction. Vertigo is the commonest symptom of transient cerebral ischaemic attacks in the vertebrobasilar distribution.[1]

Severe vertigo, often in association with hiccoughs and dysphagia, is a feature of the variety of brain stem infarctions known as the lateral medullary syndrome due to posterior inferior cerebellar artery (PICA) thrombosis. There is a dramatic onset of vertigo with cerebellar signs, including ataxia and vomiting. There are ipsilateral cranial nerve (brain stem) signs with contralateral spinothalamic sensory loss of the face and body. Diagnosis is by CT or MRI scanning.

Neurological causes

Important neurological causes of dizziness are multiple sclerosis and complex partial seizures.

The lesions of multiple sclerosis may occur in the brain stem or cerebellum. Young patients who present with a sudden onset of vertigo with 'jiggly' vision but without auditory symptoms should be considered as having multiple sclerosis. Five per cent of cases of multiple sclerosis present with vertigo.

Pitfalls

A list of conditions causing dizziness that may be misdiagnosed is presented in TABLE 46.2. Wax in the ear certainly causes dizziness, though its mechanism of action is controversial. Cough and micturition syncope do occur, although they are uncommon.

Ménière syndrome is a pitfall in the sense that it tends to be overdiagnosed.

Seven masquerades checklist

Of these conditions, drugs and vertebral dysfunction (of the cervical spine) stand out as important causes. Depression demands attention because of the possible association of anxiety and hyperventilation.

Diabetes mellitus has an association through the possible mechanisms of hypoglycaemia from therapy or from an autonomic neuropathy.

Drugs

Drugs usually affect the vestibular nerve rather than the labyrinth. Drugs commonly associated with dizziness are presented in TABLE 46.3.

Table 46.3 Drugs that can cause dizziness

Alcohol
Antibiotics: streptomycin, gentamicin, kanamycin, tetracyclines
Antidepressants
Anti-epileptics: phenytoin
Antihistamines
Antihypertensives
Aspirin and salicylates
Cocaine
Diuretics in large doses: intravenous frusemide, ethacrynic acid
Glyceryl trinitrate
Quinine–quinidine
Tranquillisers: phenothiazines, phenobarbitone, benzodiazepines

Cervical spine dysfunction

It is not uncommon to observe vertigo in patients with cervical spondylosis or post cervical spinal injury. It has been postulated[4] that this may be caused by the generation of abnormal impulses from proprioceptors in the upper cervical spine, or by osteophytes compressing the vertebral arteries in the vertebral canal. Some instances of BPPV are associated with disorders of the cervical spine.

Psychogenic considerations

This may be an important aspect to consider in the patient presenting with dizziness, especially if the complaint is giddiness or lightheadedness. An underlying anxiety, particularly agoraphobia and panic disorder, may be the commonest cause of this symptom in family practice and clinical investigation of hyperventilation may confirm the diagnosis. The possibility of depression must also be kept in mind.[5] Many of these patients harbour the fear that they may be suffering from a serious disorder, such as a brain tumour or multiple sclerosis, or face an impending stroke or insanity. Appropriate reassurance to the contrary is often positively therapeutic for that patient.

The clinical approach

The essentials of the diagnostic approach include careful attention to the history and physical examination, and judicious selection of specific office tests and special investigations.

History

It is important to get patients to explain the precise nature of the symptoms, even asking their opinion as to the cause of their dizziness.

Key questions

The following questions should be addressed:

- Is it vertigo or pseudovertigo?
- Symptom pattern:
  - paroxysmal or continuous?
  - effect of position and change of posture?
- Any aural symptoms? Tinnitus? Deafness?
- Any visual symptoms?
- Any neurological symptoms?
- Any nausea or vomiting?
- Any symptoms of psychoneurosis?
- Any recent colds?
- Any recent head injury (even trivial)?
- Any drugs being taken?
  - alcohol?
  - marijuana?
  - hypotensives?
  - psychotropics?
  - other drugs?

Examination

A full general examination is appropriate with particular attention being paid to the cardiovascular and central nervous systems and the auditory and vestibular mechanisms.

46

Guidelines

Examination guidelines are:

1. ear disease:
   - auroscopic examination: ? wax ? drum
   - hearing tests
   - Weber and Rinne tests
2. the eyes:
   - visual acuity
   - test movements for nystagmus
3. cardiovascular system:
   - evidence of atherosclerosis
   - blood pressure: supine, standing, sitting
   - cardiac arrhythmias
4. cranial nerves:
   - 2nd, 3rd, 4th, 6th and 7th
   - corneal response for 5th
   - 8th—auditory nerve
5. the cerebellum or its connections:
   - gait
   - coordination
   - reflexes
   - Romberg test
   - finger nose test: ? past pointing
6. the neck, including cervical spine
7. general search for evidence of:
   - anaemia
   - polycythaemia
   - alcohol dependence

Office tests for dizziness

- Ask the patient to perform any manoeuvre that may provoke the symptom.
- Carry out head positional testing to induce vertigo and/or nystagmus (e.g. Hallpike manoeuvre in FIG. 46.3 or head impulse test/head thrust). Avoid if prominent spontaneous vertigo and nystagmus.
- Take blood pressure measurements in three positions.

- Perform forced hyperventilation (20–25 breaths per minute) for 2 minutes.
- Carry out palpation of carotid arteries and carotid sinus (with care).

Investigations

Appropriate laboratory tests should be selected from TABLE 46.4.

46

Table 46.4 Investigations

Haemoglobin
Blood glucose
ECG: ? Holter monitor
Audiometry
Brain-stem evoked audiometry
Caloric test
Visual evoked potentials (MS)
Electrocochleography
Electro-oculography (electronystagmography)
Rotational tests
Radiology:

- chest X-ray (? bronchial carcinoma)
- cervical spine X-ray
- CT scan
- MRI (the choice to locate acoustic neuroma or other tumour—may detect MS and vascular infarction)

Diagnostic guidelines

- A sudden attack of vertigo in a young person following a recent URTI is suggestive of vestibular neuronitis.
- Dizziness is a common symptom in menopausal women and is often associated with other features of vasomotor instability.
- Phenytoin therapy can cause cerebellar dysfunction.
- Postural and exercise hypotension are relatively common in the older atherosclerotic patient.
- Acute otitis media does not cause vertigo but chronic otitis media can, particularly if the patient develops a cholesteatoma, which then erodes into the internal ear causing a perilymphatic fistula.

Dizziness in children

Dizziness is not a common symptom in children. Vertigo can have sinister causes and requires referral because of the possibility of tumours, such as a medulloblastoma. A study by Eviatar and Eviatar[6] of vertigo in children found that the commonest cause was a seizure focus particularly affecting the temporal lobe. Other causes included psychosomatic vertigo, vestibular migraine and vestibular neuritis.

Apart from the above causes it is important to consider:

- infection (e.g. meningitis, meningoencephalitis, cerebral abscess)
- trauma, especially to the temporal area
- middle-ear infection
- labyrinthitis (e.g. mumps, measles, influenza)
- BPPV (short-lived attacks of vertigo in young children between 1 and 4 years of age: tends to precede adulthood migraine)[7]
- hyperventilation
- drugs—prescribed
- illicit drugs (e.g. cocaine, marijuana)
- cardiac arrhythmias
- alcohol toxicity

A common trap is the acute effect of alcohol in curious children who can present with the sudden onset of dizziness.

Dizzy turns in girls in late teens

- These are commonly due to blood pressure fluctuations.
- Give advice related to reducing stress, lack of sleep and excessive exercise.
- Reassure that it settles with age (rare after 25 years).

Dizziness in the elderly

Dizziness is a relatively common complaint of the elderly. Common causes include postural hypotension related mainly to drugs prescribed for hypertension or other cardiovascular problems. Cerebrovascular disease, especially in the areas of the brain stem, is also relevant in this age group. True vertigo can be produced simply by an accumulation of wax in the external auditory meatus, being more frequent than generally appreciated.

Middle-ear disorder is also sometimes the cause of vertigo in an older person but disorder of the auditory nerve, inner ear, cerebellum, brain stem and cervical spine are common underlying factors.

Malignancy, primary and secondary, is a possibility in the elderly. The possibility of cardiac arrhythmias as a cause of syncopal symptoms increases with age.

Dizzy turns in elderly women

If no cause such as hypertension is found, advise them to get up slowly from sitting or lying, and to wear firm elastic stockings.

Acute vestibulopathy (vestibular failure)

Causes:

- vestibular neuritis
- stroke—AICA or PICA

Vestibular neuritis covers both vestibular neuronitis and labyrinthitis, which are considered to be a viral infection of the vestibular nerve and labyrinth respectively, causing a prolonged attack of vertigo that can last for several days and be severe enough to require admission to hospital.[8]

It is analogous to a viral infection of the 7th nerve causing Bell palsy. The attack is similar to Ménière syndrome except that there is no hearing disturbance.

> **DxT** acute vertigo + nausea + vomiting → vestibular neuronitis

> **DxT** same symptoms + hearing loss ± tinnitus → acute labyrinthitis

Characteristic features

- single attack of vertigo without tinnitus or deafness
- usually preceding 'flu-like' illness
- mainly in young adults and middle age
- abrupt onset with vertigo, ataxia, nausea and vomiting
- generally lasts days to weeks
- examination shows lateral or unidirectional nystagmus—rapid component away from side of lesion (no hearing loss)
- caloric stimulation confirms impaired vestibular function

It is basically a diagnosis of exclusion.

Treatment

- Rest in bed, lying very still
- Gaze in the direction that eases symptoms

The following drugs can be used (see TABLE 46.5):

prochlorperazine (Stemetil) 12.5 mg IM (if severe vomiting), but may slow recovery, or 5–10 mg (o) tds
or
promethazine 10–25 mg IM or slow IV then 10–25 mg (o) for 48 hrs
or
(recommended as best)
diazepam (which decreases brain-stem response to vestibular stimuli)[2] 5–10 mg IM for the acute attack, then 5 mg (o) tds for 2–3 days

A short course of corticosteroids often promotes recovery (e.g. prednisolone 1 mg/kg (up to 100 mg) (o) daily in morning for 5 days, then taper over 15 days and cease).[1,10]

46

Table 46.5 Symptomatic relief of acute vertigo: pharmaceutical options[9]

Anti-emetics:

- prochlorperazine
- metoclopramide

Antihistamines:

- promethazine
- betahistine

Benzodiazepines (short period use for vertigo):

- diazepam
- lorazepam

Outcome

Both are self-limiting disorders and usually settle over 5–7 days or several weeks. Labyrinthitis usually lasts longer and during recovery rapid head movements may bring on transient vertigo.

Benign paroxysmal positional vertigo

BPPV is a common type of acute vertigo that is induced by changing head position—particularly tilting the head backwards, changing from a recumbent to a sitting position or turning to the affected side.

Features

- Affects all ages, especially the elderly
- The female to male ratio is 2:1
- Recurs periodically for several days
- Each attack is brief, usually lasts 10–60 seconds, and subsides rapidly
- Severe vertigo on getting out of bed
- Can occur on head extension and turning head in bed
- Attacks are not accompanied by vomiting, tinnitus or deafness (nausea may occur)

46

- In one large series 17% were associated with trauma, 15% with viral labyrinthitis, while about 50% had no clear predisposing factor other than age. One accepted theory of causation is that fine pieces of floating crystalline calcium carbonate deposits (otoconia) that are loose in the labyrinth settle in the posterior semicircular canal and generate endolymphatic movement.[11] It may also be a variation of cervical dysfunction.
- Diagnosis is confirmed by head position testing: head impulse (head thrust) test or Hallpike manoeuvre (refer to YouTube for these manoeuvres).[12] In the latter, from a sitting position, the patient's head is rapidly taken to a head-hanging position 30° below the level of the couch—do three times, with the head (1) straight, (2) rotated to the right, (3) rotated to the left. Hold on for 30 seconds and observe the patient carefully for vertigo and nystagmus. There is a latent period of a few seconds before the onset of the symptoms—see FIGURE 46.3.
- Tests of hearing and vestibular function are normal
- There is usually spontaneous recovery in weeks (most return to regular activity after 1 week)
- Recurrences are common: attacks occur in clusters

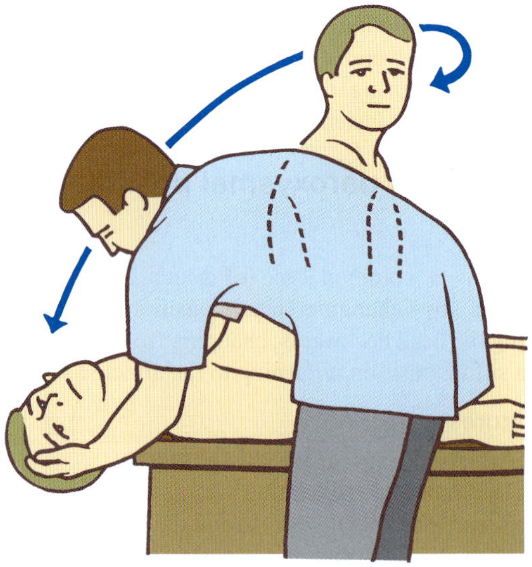

FIGURE 46.3 Hallpike manoeuvre: positional testing for benign paroxysmal positional vertigo (head rotated to 45° then taken rapidly from a sitting position to a hanging position). Repeat with head turned to the opposite side. A positive response is the onset of symptoms ± nystagmus with the affected ear lowermost.

Management

- Give appropriate explanation and reassurance
- Avoidance measures: encourage the patient to move in ways that avoid the attack
- Drugs are not recommended
- Special exercises
- Cervical traction may help

Particle repositioning manoeuvres

Patient-performed exercises. Most patients appear to benefit from exercise, such as the Brandt–Daroff procedure[13] or the Cawthorne–Cooksey exercises[9] that consist essentially of repeatedly inducing the symptoms of vertigo. Rather than resorting to avoidance measures, the patient is instructed to perform positional exercises to induce vertigo, hold this position until it subsides, and repeat this many times until the manoeuvre does not precipitate vertigo. The attacks then usually subside in a few days.

Therapist-performed exercises. Physical manoeuvres performed as an office procedure include the Epley and Semont manoeuvres.

Surgical treatment

Rarely surgical treatment is required; it involves occlusion of the posterior semicircular canal rather than selective neurectomy.

Ménière syndrome

This is caused by a build-up of endolymph.

- It is commonest in the 30–50 years age group.
- It is characterised by paroxysmal attacks of vertigo, tinnitus, nausea and vomiting, sweating and pallor, deafness (progressive).
- Onset is abrupt—patient may fall and then be bedridden for 1–2 hours. Patient doesn't like moving head.
- Attacks last 30 minutes to several hours.
- There is a variable interval between attacks (twice a month to twice a year).
- Nystagmus is observed only during an attack (often to side opposite affected inner ear).
- Examination:
  - sensorineural deafness (low tones)
  - caloric test: impaired vestibular function
  - audiometry: sensorineural deafness, loudness recruitment
  - special tests
- There are characteristic changes in electrocochleography.

> **DxT** vertigo + vomiting + tinnitus + sensorineural deafness → Ménière syndrome

Treatment

The aim is to reduce endolymphatic pressure by reducing the sodium and water content of the endolymph.

Acute attack[14]

Anticipation of attack (fullness, tinnitus):

prochlorperazine 25 mg suppository

or

30 g urea crystals in orange juice (preferably 30 minutes before in prodromal phase)

Treatment:

diazepam 5 mg IV ± prochlorperazine 12.5 mg IM. Consider betahistine 8 mg (o) tds if persistent or episodic or a diuretic e.g. hydrochlorothiazide 25 mg (o) daily

Long term

- Reassurance with a careful explanation of this condition to the patient, who often associates it with malignant disease
- Excess intake of salt, tobacco and coffee to be avoided
- A low-salt diet is the mainstay of treatment (<3 g per day)
- Alleviate abnormal anxiety by using stress management, meditation or possibly long-term sedation (fluid builds up with stress)
- Referral for neurological assessment
- Diuretic (e.g. hydrochlorothiazide/amiloride daily)—check electrolytes regularly

Surgery may be an option for intractable cases.

Vestibular migraine (migrainous vertigo)

Migraine is a relatively common cause of vertigo and often unrecognised because of its many guises. It should be strongly suspected if there is a past and/or family history of migraine and also where there is a history of recurrent bouts of spontaneous vertigo or ataxia that persist for hours or days in the absence of aural symptoms.[15] Vertigo, which is usually not violent, may take the place of the aura that precedes the headache or may be a migraine equivalent whereby the vertigo replaces the symptoms of headache, which may be an inconspicuous feature in some cases. Nausea and vomiting may be present. Pizotifen or propranolol are recommended for prophylaxis.

When to refer

- Vertigo of uncertain diagnosis, especially in children
- Possibility of tumour, or bacterial infection
- Vertigo in presence of suppurative otitis media despite antibiotic therapy
- Presumed viral labyrinthitis not abating after 3 months
- Vertigo following trauma
- Presumed Ménière syndrome, not responding to conservative medical management
- Evidence of vertebrobasilar insufficiency
- BPPV persisting for more than 12 months despite treatment with particle repositioning exercises

46

Practice tips

- A careful drug history often pinpoints the diagnosis.
- Always consider cardiac arrhythmias as a cause of acute dizziness.
- Consider phenytoin therapy as a cause of dizziness in an epileptic patient.
- If an intracerebral metastatic lesion is suspected, consider the possibility of carcinoma of the lung as the primary source.
- Three important office investigations to perform in the evaluation are blood pressure measurement (lying, sitting and standing), hyperventilation and head positional testing.
- Cervical vertigo is very common and appropriate cervical mobilisation methods, with care, should be considered.
- BPPV is also common and prescribing a set of exercises to desensitise the labyrinth is recommended. Use either the Brandt–Daroff procedure or the Cawthorne–Cooksey program.[11]
- Think of migraine particularly in a younger patient presenting with unexplained recurrent vertigo.

Patient education resources

Hand-out sheets from *Murtagh's Patient Education* 7th edition:

- Labyrinthitis
- Ménière syndrome
- Vertigo: benign positional vertigo
- Vertigo: exercises for benign positional vertigo

References

1 Expert group for Neurology. Vestibular neuritis. In: eTG complete [Internet]. Melbourne: Therapeutic Guidelines Ltd. Available from: <www.tg.org.au>, accessed September 2017.

2 Sloane PD, Slatt LM, Baker RM. *Essentials of Family Medicine*. Baltimore: Williams & Wilkins, 1988.

3 Kuo C-H, Pang L, Chang R. Vertigo: assessment in general practice. Aust Fam Physician, 2008; 37: 341–7.

4 Lance JW. *A Physiological Approach to Clinical Neurology*. London: Butterworths, 1970: 162–79.

5 Paine M. Dealing with dizziness. Australian Prescriber, 2005; 28: 94–7.

6 Eviatar L, Eviatar A. Vertigo in children: differential diagnosis and treatment. Paediatrics, 1977; 59: 833–7.

7 Tunnessen WW Jr. *Signs and Symptoms in Paediatrics*. Philadelphia: Lippincott, 1988: 591–4.

8 Waterson J. Dizziness: how to treat. Australian Doctor, 7 March; 2003: 1–8.

9 Hain TC, Yacovino D. Pharmacologic treatment of persons with dizziness. Neurol Clin, 2005; 23: 831–53.

10 Strupp M, Zingler VC, Arbuson V et al. Methylprednisolone, valacyclovir or the combination for vestibular neuritis. N Engl J Med, 2004; 351: 354–61.

11 Brandt T, Daroff DB. Physical therapy for BPPV. Arch Otolaryngol, 1980; 106: 484–5.

12 Kuo CH, Pang L, Chang R. Vertigo—part 1—assessment in general practice. Aust Fam Physician, 2008; 37 (5): 341–7.

13 Froehling IA, Bowen JM, Mohr DN et al. The canalith repositioning procedure for BPPV: a randomised controlled trial. Mayo Clin Proc, 2000; 75: 695–700.

14 Tonkin JP. Meniere's disease. Current Therapeutics, 1995; 36: 39–43.

15 Pohl D. Vertigo. In: *MIMS Disease Index* (2nd edn). Sydney: IMS Publishing, 1996: 568–71.

Dyspepsia (indigestion) 47

Half the patients who get you up in the middle of the night and think they are dying are suffering from wind!

Francis Young (1884–1954), Advice to a younger doctor

Dyspepsia or indigestion is a difficult, sometimes vague, symptom to define or evaluate and requires very careful questioning to clarify the exact nature of the complaint.

Dyspepsia embraces the following:

- nausea
- heartburn/regurgitation
- upper abdominal discomfort
- lower chest discomfort
- acidity
- epigastric fullness, bloating or unease
- abdominal distension

The discomfort can sometimes amount to pain. Diagnoses to consider in dyspeptic patients are summarised in TABLE 47.1.

Glossary of terms

Dyspepsia Pain or discomfort centred at the upper abdomen that is chronic or recurrent in nature.

Flatulence Excessive wind. It includes belching, abdominal bloating or passing excessive flatus.

Heartburn A central retrosternal or epigastric burning sensation that spreads upwards to the throat.

Table 47.1 Diagnoses to consider in dyspeptic patients[1]

Gastrointestinal disorders
Gastro-oesophageal reflux, including hiatus hernia
Functional (non-ulcer) dyspepsia
Oesophageal motility disorders (dysmotility)
Peptic ulcer
Upper GIT malignancies (e.g. oesophagus, stomach, pancreas)
Hepatobiliary disease (e.g. hepatitis, biliary dyskinesia, cholelithiasis)
Pancreatitis
Upper GIT inflammation: • oesophagitis • gastritis • duodenitis
Irritable bowel syndrome
Non-gastrointestinal disorders
Myocardial ischaemia
Drug reaction
Alcohol effect
Somatisation
Anxiety/stress
Depression

Flatulence

Excessive belching

- Usually functional
- Organic disease uncommon
- Due to air swallowing (aerophagy)
- Common in anxious people who gulp food and drink
- Associated hypersalivation

Management tips

- Make patient aware of excessive swallowing
- Avoid fizzy (carbonated) soft drinks
- Avoid chewing gum
- Don't drink with meals
- Don't mix proteins and starches
- Eat slowly and chew food thoroughly before swallowing
- Eat and chew with the mouth closed

If persistent: simethicone preparation (e.g. Mylanta II, Phazyme).

If desperate: place one small cork between the back teeth after meals for 30 minutes.

Excessive flatus

Flatus arises from two main sources:

- swallowed air
- bacterial fermentation of undigested carbohydrate

Exclude:

- malabsorption
- irritable bowel syndrome
- anxiety → aerophagy
- drugs, especially lipid-lowering agents
- lactose intolerance

Management

- Assess diet (e.g. high fibre, beans and legumes, cabbage, onions, grapes and raisins)
- Avoid drinking with eating, especially with leafy vegetables
- Cook vegetables thoroughly
- Trial a lactose-free diet
- Consider simethicone preparations (e.g. No Gas)

Key facts and checkpoints

- Dyspepsia or indigestion is a common complaint; 80% of the population will have experienced it at some time.
- Consider heartburn as ischaemic heart disease until proved otherwise.
- The presence of oesophagitis is suggested by pain on swallowing hot or cold liquids (odynophagia).
- All reflux is not due to hiatus hernia.
- Many patients with hiatus hernia do not experience heartburn.
- All patients with dysphagia must be investigated to rule out malignancy.
- Ten per cent of people in the community develop peptic ulcer (PU) disease.
- The major feature of PU disease is epigastric pain.
- The pain of duodenal ulcer (DU) classically occurs at night.
- At any time, 10–20% of chronic NSAIDs users have peptic ulceration (greater than non-users).[2]
- NSAIDs and *Helicobacter pylori* infection are the most important risk factors for upper GIT disease.
- NSAIDs mainly cause gastric ulcers (GU, gastric antrum and prepyloric region), with the duodenum affected to a lesser extent.
- Dyspeptic symptoms correlate poorly with NSAID-associated ulcer.

A diagnostic approach

A summary of the diagnostic strategy model is presented in TABLE 47.2.

It is best to consider dyspepsia as:

- ulcer-like—localised pain
- dysmotility-like—diffuse discomfort, feeling full after meals (early satiety), nausea, bloating
- acid-reflux-like—indigestion or heartburn with acid reflux or regurgitation

The ulcer-like category may be due to an ulcer and if not is termed functional (non-ulcer) dyspepsia.

Table 47.2 Dyspepsia: diagnostic strategy model

Probability diagnosis
Irritable upper GIT (functional dyspepsia)
Gastro-oesophageal reflux
Drugs
Oesophageal motility disorder (e.g. gastroparesis)
Serious disorders not to be missed
Neoplasia:
• cancer: stomach, pancreas, oesophagus
Cardiovascular
• ischaemic heart disease
• congestive cardiac failure
Pancreatitis
Peptic ulcer (PU) disease
Pitfalls (often missed)
Myocardial ischaemia
Food allergy (e.g. lactose intolerance)
Pregnancy (early)
Hepatobiliary disease
Other gall bladder disease
Post vagotomy
Achalasia
Duodenitis
Autoimmune gastritis
Rarities:
• hyperparathyroidism
• mesenteric ischaemia
• Zollinger–Ellison syndrome
• kidney failure
• scleroderma
Seven masquerades checklist
Depression
Diabetes (rarely)
Drugs
Is this patient trying to tell me something?
Anxiety and stress are common associations of which patients are often unaware. Consider irritable bowel syndrome; somatisation.

Pitfalls

Perhaps the commonest mistake is to attribute the discomfort of myocardial ischaemia to a disorder of the GIT. A sense of fullness or pressure in the epigastrium can certainly accompany ischaemia.

General pitfalls

- Reflux oesophagitis and PU can mimic ischaemic heart disease.
- Overlooking gastric cancer as a cause of dyspepsia.
- Failing to stress that weight reduction to ideal level will generally alleviate gastro-oesophageal reflux.
- Overlooking drugs as a cause (see TABLE 47.3).

Table 47.3 Drugs that may cause dyspepsia
Alcohol
Anticholinergics
Aspirin
Bisphosphonates, esp. alendronate
Calcium-channel blockers
Corticosteroids
Digitalis
Lipid-lowering agents
Narcotics
Nicotine
NSAIDs
Potassium supplements (slow release)
Tetracycline; erythromycin
Theophylline
Tricyclic antidepressants

The clinical approach

History

It is worthwhile spending some time clarifying the exact nature of the presenting complaint: what the patient means by 'indigestion' or 'heartburn'.[1] The relationship of the symptom to eating is very important, and whether it occurs after each meal or after specific meals.

In particular, care should be taken to consider and perhaps exclude ischaemic heart disease.

Key questions

- How would you describe the discomfort?
- Can you show me exactly where it is and where it radiates?
- What makes your discomfort worse?
- What relieves your discomfort?
- What effect do food, milk and antacids have?
- What effect do coffee, onions or garlic have?
- What effect does a big meal have?
- What about drinking alcohol? Wine?
- What effect does exercise have?
- Do fried or fatty foods make it worse?
- Do hot spicy foods affect it?
- Does the problem come on at night soon after you go to bed?
- Does it wake you up at night?
- Does bending over (e.g. gardening) make it worse?
- Do you have periods of freedom from the problem?
- Are you under a lot of stress or have a lot of worry?
- Do you go flat out all day?
- Do you rush your meals?
- Do you chew your food properly?
- What drugs or medicines do you take?
- How much alcohol do you have? Do you smoke?
- Have you noticed anything else when you have the problem?
- Do you get constipated or have diarrhoea?
- Have you lost weight recently?
- Do you feel the discomfort between your shoulder blades, or in your shoulders or throat?
- Do you experience shortness of breath, syncope or dizziness?

Symptoms analysis

Site and radiation

The site and radiation of pain or discomfort can provide a lead to the diagnosis. Refer to FIGURE 40.9 in CHAPTER 40. If it is felt in the interscapular area, consider oesophageal spasm, gall bladder disease or a DU. Retrosternal discomfort indicates oesophageal disorders or angina, while epigastric discomfort suggests disorders of the biliary system, stomach and duodenum.

Character of the pain

There tends to be considerable overlap in the character of the pain from the various disorders but some general characteristics apply:

- burning pain → gastro-oesophageal reflux (GORD)
- constricting pain → ischaemic heart disease or oesophageal spasm
- deep gnawing pain → PU
- heavy ache or 'killing' pain → psychogenic pain

Aggravating and relieving factors

Examples of these factors include:

- eating food may aggravate a GU but relieve a DU

- eating fried or fatty foods will aggravate biliary disease, functional dyspepsia and oesophageal disorders
- bending will aggravate GORD
- alcohol may aggravate GORD, oesophagitis, gastritis, PU, pancreatitis

Associated symptoms

Relevant examples:

- difficulty in swallowing → oesophageal disorders
- lump or constriction in throat → psychogenic
- acid regurgitation → GORD, oesophagitis
- anorexia, weight loss → stomach cancer
- water brash → GORD, hiatus hernia, PU
- symptoms of anaemia → chronic oesophagitis or gastritis, PU, cancer (stomach, colon)
- flatulence, belching, abnormal bowel habits → irritable bowel syndrome
- diarrhoea 30 minutes after meal → mesenteric ischaemia

Examination

The physical examination does not often provide the key to the diagnosis but it is important to perform very careful palpation and inspection. Look for evidence of clinical anaemia and jaundice. Diffuse mild abdominal tenderness and a pulsatable abdominal aorta are common findings but do not necessarily discriminate between organic and functional problems. Specific epigastric tenderness suggests peptic ulceration while tenderness over the gall bladder area (Murphy sign) indicates gall bladder disease. An epigastric mass indicates stomach cancer.

Investigations

Do not overinvestigate. Investigations tend to be unrewarding in most instances of dyspepsia and could be postponed if the history is suggestive of a functional cause and the symptoms are not severe.[1] A trial of treatment such as changing adverse lifestyle factors, dietary modification and antacids could be the initial approach. Age is important in determining the extent of investigations, which are more relevant in those over 40 years.

The investigation of choice is endoscopy, which is superior to barium studies in investigation of the upper GIT. Gastroscopy is indicated for the *alarm* symptoms:

- abnormal symptoms of reflux/dyspepsia
- change of symptoms
- dysphagia
- unexplained weight loss
- GIT bleeding
- pain radiating to back
- pain waking at night
- abnormal signs on examination
- other tests: fasting serum gastrin (? hypersecretion)

Helicobacter pylori tests[3]

Helicobacter pylori has been proved to cause ulcers. Most DUs and about two-thirds of GUs have been attributed to *H. pylori* infection.

Non-invasive tests:

- serological—IgG antibodies (sensitivity 85–90%, specificity 90–99%); excellent for diagnosis, not for follow-up
- urea breath test (high sensitivity 97% and specificity 96%), good for follow-up
- stool antigen test (sensitivity 96%, specificity 97%)

Invasive tests:

- gastric mucosal biopsy during endoscopy can detect *H. pylori* through histology or rapid urease testing or *H. pylori* culture

Dyspepsia in the elderly

An organic disorder is more likely in the older patient, in whom it is important to consider stomach cancer. Symptoms such as anorexia, vomiting and weight loss point to such a problem.

Other conditions causing dyspepsia that are more prevalent in this age group are:

- constipation
- mesenteric artery ischaemia
- congestive cardiac failure

Dyspepsia in children

Dyspepsia is an uncommon problem in children but can be caused by drugs, oesophageal disorders and gastro-oesophageal reflux in particular.[4] Reflux can be considered to be physiological or pathological.

Gastro-oesophageal reflux

Regurgitation of feeds because of gastro-oesophageal reflux is a common physiological event in newborn infants. A mild degree of reflux is normal in babies, especially after they burp; this condition is called *posseting*.

Symptoms

Milk will flow freely from the mouth soon after feeding, even after the baby has been put down for a sleep. Sometimes the flow will be forceful and may even be out of the nose.

Despite this vomiting or regurgitation, the babies are usually comfortable and thrive. Some infants will cry, presumably because of heartburn.[4]

In a small number the reflux may be severe enough (pathological) to cause serious problems such as oesophagitis with haematemesis or anaemia, stricture formation, failure to thrive, apnoea and aspiration.

Prognosis

Reflux gradually improves with time and usually ceases soon after solids are introduced into the diet. Most cases clear up completely by the age of 9 or 10 months, when the baby is sitting. Severe cases tend to persist until 18 months of age.

Investigations

These are not necessary in most cases but in those with persistent problems or complications referral to a paediatrician is recommended. The specialist investigations include barium meal with cine scanning, oesophageal pH monitoring or endoscopy and biopsy.

Management

Appropriate reassurance with parental education is important. It should be pointed out that changes in feeding practice and positioning will control most reflux.

The infant should be placed on the left side for sleeping with the head of the cot elevated about 20–30 degrees. The old bucket method, in which the child is placed in a bucket, is not necessary.

Smaller, more frequent feeds and thickening agents are appropriate.

Thickening of feeds

Giving the baby thicker feeds usually helps those with more severe reflux. The old-fashioned remedy of using cornflour blended in bottles is still useful.

Bottle-fed babies (powdered milk formula):

Carobel: Add slightly less than 1 full scoop per bottle.

Gaviscon: Mix slightly less than ½ teaspoon of Infant Gaviscon Powder with 120 mL of formula in the bottle.

Cornflour (maize based): Mix 1 teaspoon with each 120 mL of formula. Check with your doctor or nurse for the proper method.

Prethickened formulas include Karicare and S26 AR: Very simple to use but more expensive.

Breastfed babies:

Carobel: Add slightly less than 1 full scoop to 20 mL cool boiled water or 20 mL expressed breast milk and give just before the feed.

Gaviscon: Mix slightly less than ½ teaspoon of Infant Gaviscon Powder with 20 mL cool boiled water or expressed breast milk and give just after the feed.

For persistent or complicated reflux, including painful oesophagitis, specialist-monitored treatment will include the use of antacids and H_2-receptor blocking agents (e.g. ranitidine).[5]

Gastro-oesophageal reflux disease (GORD)[6,7] in adults

47

Clinical features

- Nausea
- Bloating and belching
- Heartburn
- Acid regurgitation, especially lying down at night
- Water brash (mouth fills with saliva)
- Nocturnal cough with possible asthma-like symptoms
- Diagnosis usually made on history
- Investigation usually not needed (reserve for alarm features as described in the red flag box and non-responsive treatment)

Red flag pointers for upper GIT endoscopy

- Anaemia (new onset)
- Dysphagia
- Odynophagia (painful swallowing)
- Haematemesis or melaena
- Unexplained weight loss >10%
- Vomiting
- Older age >50 years
- Chronic NSAID use
- Severe frequent symptoms
- Family history of upper GIT or colorectal cancer
- Short history of symptoms
- Unresponsive *H. pylori* treatment

Complications

- Oesophagitis ± oesophageal ulcer
- Iron-deficiency anaemia
- Oesophageal stricture
- Respiratory: chronic cough, asthma, hoarseness
- Barrett oesophagus (from prolonged reflux)

Barrett oesophagus

- Usually a metaplastic response to prolonged reflux
- A premalignant condition (adenocarcinoma)
- Lower oesophagus lined with gastric mucosa (at least 3 cm) of metaplastic columnar epithelium
- Prone to ulceration
- Needs careful management, which includes PPIs for symptoms of oesophagitis + reflux
- Consider 2 yearly endoscopies with biopsies
- Diagnosed by endoscopy and biopsy

Investigations[6]

- Endoscopy (see Red flag pointers)—perform prior to empirical therapy. Limited role—about one third negative
- Barium swallow and meal
- 24-hour ambulatory oesophageal pH monitoring

47

Management of GORD[6,7,8,9]

Stage 1

- Patient education/appropriate reassurance
- Consider acid suppression or neutralisation
- Attend to lifestyle:
  - reduce weight if overweight (this alone may abolish symptoms)
  - reduce or cease smoking
  - reduce or cease alcohol (especially with dinner)
  - avoid fatty foods (e.g. pastries, french fries)
  - reduce or cease coffee, tea and chocolate
  - avoid coffee and alcohol late at night
  - avoid gaseous drinks
  - leave at least 3 hours between the evening meal and retiring
  - increase fibre intake (e.g. high fibre cereals, fruit and vegetables)
  - small regular meals and snacks
  - eat slowly and chew food well
  - sleep on the left side
  - main meal at midday; light evening meal
  - avoid spicy foods and tomato products
- Drugs to avoid: anticholinergics, theophylline, nitrates, calcium-channel blockers, doxycycline. Pill-induced oesophagitis occurs, especially with tetracyclines, slow-release potassium, iron sulphate, corticosteroids, NSAIDs—avoid taking dry; use ample fluids
- Elevation of head of bed or wedge pillow: if GORD occurs in bed, sleep with head of bed elevated 10–20 cm on wooden blocks or use a wedge pillow (preferable)
- Antacids (see TABLES 47.4 and 47.5): best is liquid alginate/antacid mixture, e.g. Gaviscon/Mylanta plus 20 mL on demand or 1–2 hours after meals and at bedtime

Table 47.4 Antacids in common use

Antacids	
Water soluble:	Calcium carbonate
	Sodium: • bicarbonate • citrotartrate
	Note: Excess is prone to cause alkalosis—apathy, mental changes, stupor, kidney dysfunction, tetany
Water insoluble:	Aluminium: • hydroxide • glycinate • phosphate
	Magnesium: • alginate • carbonate • hydroxide • trisilicate
Combination antacids	
Antacid + alginic acid	
Antacid + oxethazaine	
Antacid + simethicone	

Table 47.5 Side effects of common antacids

Aluminium hydroxide	Constipation
Magnesium trisilicate	Diarrhoea
Sodium bicarbonate	Alkalosis
	Milk alkali syndrome
	Aggravation of hypertension
Calcium carbonate	Alkalosis
	Constipation
	Milk alkali syndrome
	Hypercalcaemia

Antacids are appropriate for rapid relief of mild intermittent or occasional breakthrough symptoms but are ineffective for long-term management.

Stage 2[6]

If no relief after several weeks, the following approaches are recommended by the Gastroenterological Society of Australia (GESA).[6]

Reduce acid secretion. Select from:

- Proton-pump inhibitor (PPI) for 4 weeks (preferred agent) 30–60 minutes before food
  lansoprazole 30 mg mane
  or
  omeprazole 20 mg mane
  or
  pantoprazole 40 mg mane
  or
  esomeprazole 20 mg mane
  or
  rabeprazole 20 mg mane
- H_2-receptor antagonists (oral use for 8 weeks)
  famotidine 20 mg bd
  or
  nizatadine 150 mg bd or 300 mg nocte
  or
  ranitidine 150 mg bd pc or 300 mg nocte
- Antacids are useful for daytime symptoms

Although the more traditional step-up approach of 1. Antacids → 2. H_2-receptor antagonists → 3. PPI can be used, there has been a change to favour a high level (more potent) initial therapy with PPIs at standard dose (a step-down approach; see FIG. 47.1). This is based on the grounds of outcomes, speed of response and total cost. May need to eradicate *H. pylori* if present.

Surgery is usually for young patients with severe reflux. The gold standard is a short, loose 360-degree fundoplication.

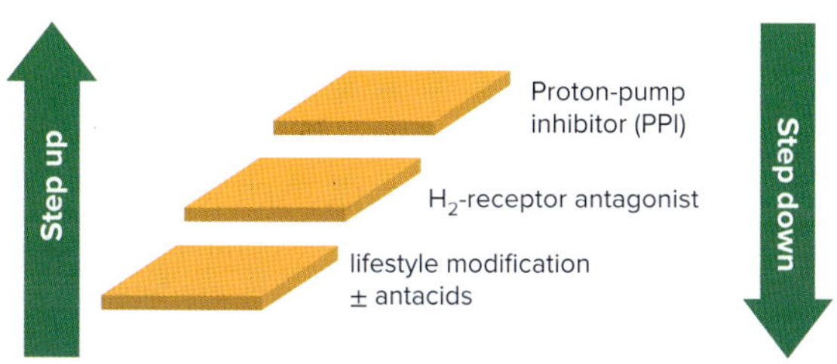

FIGURE 47.1 The stepwise approach to the management of dyspeptic symptoms[7]

Functional (non-ulcer) dyspepsia[7, 10]

This term applies to the 60% of patients presenting with dyspepsia in which there is discomfort on eating in the absence of demonstrable organic disease. This can be considered in two categories (although there is overlap):

- ulcer-like dyspepsia
  or
- dysmotility-like dyspepsia

Ulcer-like dyspepsia

Treat as for GORD. A practical approach is to commence with a 4-week trial of a PPI or an H_2-receptor antagonist and cease if symptoms resolve.[7]

Dysmotility-like dyspepsia

Clinical features

- Discomfort with early sense of fullness on eating
- Nausea
- Overweight
- Emotional stress
- Poor diet (e.g. fatty foods)
- Similar lifestyle guidelines to GORD

Management

- Treat as for GORD (stage 1).
- Include antacids.
- If not responsive:
  - Step 1: H_2-receptor antagonists
  - Step 2: prokinetic agents

  domperidone 10 mg tds
  or
  metoclopramide 10 mg tds

Peptic ulcer disease[10,11]

Features (general)

- Common: 10–20% incidence over a lifetime
- Point prevalence of ulcer disease: 3–5%
- DU:GU = 4:1
- DUs common in men 3:1
- Cumulative mortality of 10%
- Risk factors:
  - male sex
  - family history
  - smoking (cause and delayed healing)
  - stress
  - common in blood group O
  - NSAIDs 2–4 times increase in GU and ulcer complications
  - *H. pylori:* if absent and no NSAIDS, no ulcer
- Unproven risk factors:
  - corticosteroids
  - alcohol (except for gastric erosion)
  - diet (does reduce recurrence of PU)
- Types of ulcers:
  - lower oesophageal
  - gastric
  - stomal (postgastric surgery)
  - duodenal

Note: If NSAIDs and *H. pylori* are not implicated, it is referred to as idiopathic (affects a small population group).

47

Clinical features

- Episodic burning epigastric pain related to meals (1–2 hours after)
- Relieved by food or antacids (generally)
- Dyspepsia common
- May be 'silent' in elderly on NSAIDs
- Physical examination often unhelpful

Investigations

- Endoscopy (investigation of choice):[12] 92% predictive value
- Barium studies: 54% predictive value
- Serum gastrin (consider if multiple ulcers)
- *H. pylori* test: serology or urea breath test; diagnosis usually based on urease test performed at endoscopy

Complications

- Perforation
- Bleeding → haematemesis and melaena
- Obstruction—pyloric stenosis
- Anaemia (blood loss)
- Cancer (in GU)
- Oesophageal stenosis

Bleeding peptic ulcer

This can be treated with endoscopic haemostasis with heater probe or injection of adrenaline or both. Also IV omeprazole 80 mg bolus, then 8 mg/hr IV infusion for 3 days. Surgery is an option. IV esomeprazole or pantoprazole can also be used.

Management of peptic ulcer disease

Aims of treatment:

- relieve symptoms
- accelerate ulcer healing
- prevent complications
- minimise risk of relapse

The treatment of a GU is similar to that for a DU except that GUs take about 2 weeks longer to heal and the increased risk of malignancy has to be considered.

Stage 1[7]

General measures: (lifestyle and symptom relief)

- same principles as for GORD
- stop smoking
- avoid irritant drugs: NSAIDs, aspirin
- normal diet but avoid foods that upset
- antacids

If *H. pylori* positive—eradicate with combined therapy. Confirm eradication with a urea breath test (DU) or repeat gastroscopy (GU) and repeat if still present.[8]

If *H. pylori* negative—treat with full-dose PPI.

Proton-pump inhibitors (PPIs) provide more potent acid suppression and heal GUs and DUs more rapidly than H_2-receptor antagonists.

- 4–8-week oral course

Use with caution in:

- the elderly
- those on drugs, especially warfarin, anticonvulsants, beta blockers
- liver disease

Therapy to eradicate *Helicobacter pylori*[13,14]

This organism has a proven link with PU disease (both DU and benign non-drug induced GU), gastric cancer and maltoma (a gastric lymphoma) because of mucosal infection. This hypothesis is supported by a very low relapse of DU in subjects eradicated of *H. pylori*. Most infected people are asymptomatic but infection leads to a lifetime risk of peptic ulcer disease in 15–20% and of gastric cancer in up to 2%.[10] Twenty per cent of people have a variety of symptoms including those from gastritis and duodenitis. Treatment is based on combination triple or quadruple therapy, which can achieve a successful eradication rate of 85–90%.

Drug treatment regimens (examples)[7]

First-line therapy:

PPI (e.g. omeprazole or esomeprazole 20 mg)
plus
clarithromycin 500 mg
plus
amoxycillin 1 g
All orally twice daily for 7 days; this is the preferred regimen (available as a combination pack)
Note: a 10–14-day course improves eradication rate by approx. 5%.[1]
or
PPI + clarithromycin + metronidazole 400 mg (twice daily for 7 days)—if hypersensitive to penicillin
or
PPI + amoxycillin + levofloxacin (for salvage therapy)
or
other combinations: quadruple therapy e.g. bismuth + PPI + tetracycline + metronidazole (for failed triple combination)

Note: Resistance to metronidazole is common (>50%) and to clarithromycin is increasing (about 5% plus), but uncommon with tetracycline and amoxycillin.[6]

Antacids are good for daytime relief.

Maintenance anti-secretory therapy is usually unnecessary for *H. pylori* ulcers after successful eradication.[7]

For children with confirmed *H. pylori:*

PPI + amoxycillin + clarithromycin

Surgical treatment

Indications (now uncommon) include:

- failed medical treatment after 1 year
- complications:
  - uncontrollable bleeding
  - perforation
  - pyloric stenosis
- suspicion of malignancy in GU
- recurrent ulcer after previous surgery

NSAIDs and peptic ulcers[7,15]

1. *Ulcer identified in NSAID user:*
   - stop NSAID (if possible)
   - check smoking and alcohol use
   - try alternative anti-inflammatory analgesic:
     - paracetamol
     - COX-2 selective drug
     - enteric-coated, slow-release aspirin
     - corticosteroids intra-articular or oral
   - PPI for 4 weeks (gives best results)

   Note: Healing time is doubled if NSAID continued.[2] About 90% heal within 12 weeks. Check healing by endoscopy at 12 weeks. Do *H. pylori* test.

2 *Prevention of ulcers in NSAID user:*[15]

Primary prophylaxis is usually reserved for those at significantly increased risk, e.g. older persons (>75 years) and past history PU.

Use one of the following PPIs:[7]

esomeprazole 20 mg bd for 7 days

or

omeprazole 20 mg daily

or

pantoprazole 40 mg daily

Increased dietary fibre assists DU healing and prevention.

Note: Do *H. pylori* test and, if present, it should be eradicated with combination therapy after the ulcer has healed, especially in people who continue to take NSAIDs.[1]

Autoimmune gastritis[7]

This is an inflammatory condition with antibodies to parietal cells and intrinsic factor. It is asymptomatic and may lead to pernicious anaemia. Diagnosis is confirmed by histology or endoscopy. *H. pylori* is absent.

Treat with iron and vitamin B12 if they are low.

Stomach cancer

Clinical features

- Male to female ratio = 3:1
- Usually asymptomatic early
- Consider if upper GIT symptoms in patients over 40 years, especially weight loss
- Recent-onset dyspepsia in middle age
- Dyspepsia unresponsive to treatment
- Vague fullness or epigastric distension
- Anorexia, nausea, ± vomiting
- Dysphagia—a late sign
- Onset of anaemia
- Changing dyspepsia in GU
- Changing symptoms in pernicious anaemia
- *H. pylori* is implicated as a cause and its treatment reduces the risk[1]

Risk factors: ↑ age, blood group A, smoking, sugar, atrophic gastritis

Limited physical findings

- Palpable abdominal mass (20%)
- Signs (see FIG. 47.2) in advanced cases

DxT malaise + anorexia + dyspepsia + weight loss → stomach cancer

DxT triple loss of appetite + weight + colour → stomach cancer

Investigations

- Endoscopy and biopsy is optimal test
- Barium meal—false negatives

Treatment

- Surgical excision: may be curative if diagnosed early but overall survival is poor (22% at 5 years)

When to refer

- Infants with persistent gastro-oesophageal reflux not responding to simple measures
- Failure to respond to stage 1 therapy for heartburn, when endoscopy is required
- Patients with persistent or recurrent ulcers
- Any patient with a PU complication, such as haemorrhage, obstruction or perforation

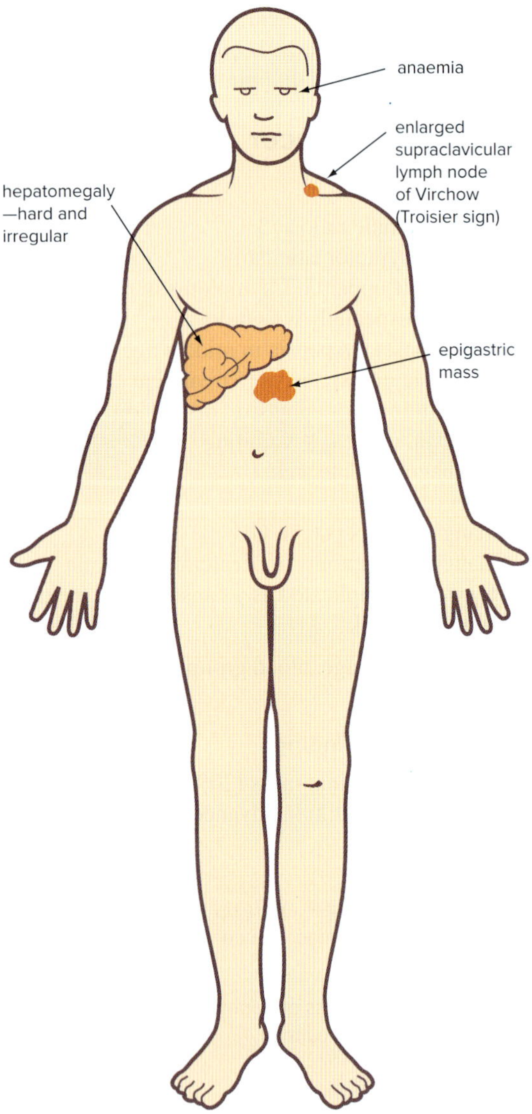

FIGURE 47.2 Late signs of stomach cancer

Practice tips

- Scleroderma is a rare but important cause of oesophagitis.
- Advise patients never to 'dry swallow' medications.
- Dysphagia always warrants investigation, not observation.
- Beware of attributing anaemia to oesophagitis.
- Epigastric pain aggravated by any food, relieved by antacids = chronic GU.
- Epigastric pain before meals, relieved by food = chronic DU.
- Keep in mind the malignant potential of a GU.
- A change in the nature of symptoms with a GU suggests the possibility of malignant change.
- Avoid the long-term use of water-soluble antacids.
- Investigate the alarm symptoms—dysphagia, bleeding, anaemia, weight loss, waking at night, pain radiating to the back.

Patient education resources

Hand-out sheets from *Murtagh's Patient Education* 7th edition:

- Heartburn
- Hiatus hernia
- Peptic ulcer
- Reflux disease
- Reflux in infants

References

1 Buckley N (Chair). *Australian Medicines Handbook*. Adelaide: Australian Medicines Handbook Pty Ltd, 2016: 513–22.
2 Pritchard P. The management of upper gastrointestinal problems in patients taking NSAIDs. Aust Fam Physician, 1991; 20: 1739–41.
3 McGarity B, Morgia M. Peptic ulcer disease: an update on diagnosis and treatment. Medicine Today, 2001; December: 33–7.
4 Sewell J. Gastro-oesophageal reflux. Australian Paediatric Review, 1991; 3: 2.
5 Gwee A, Rimer R, Marks M. *Paediatric Handbook* (9th edn). Oxford: Wiley-Blackwell, 2015: 96–7.
6 *Gastro-oesophageal Reflux Disease in Adults: Guidelines* (5th edn). Sydney: Gastroenterological Society of Australia, 2011.
7 Expert group for Gastrointestinal. Gastric disorders. In: eTG complete [Internet]. Melbourne: Therapeutic Guidelines Ltd. Available from: <www.tg.org.au>, accessed October 2017.
8 *GORD and Non-ulcer Dyspepsia*. NPS News, 2001; PPR review No. 11.
9 Fock KM et al. Asia-Pacific consensus on the management of gastroesophageal reflux disease: update. J Gastroenterol Hepatol, 2008; 23: 8–22.
10 Katelaris P. Dyspepsia: update. Australian Doctor, 2005; 7 October; 2005: 23–5.
11 Madge S, Yeomans N. Stomach and duodenal ulcers. Current Therapeutics, 2001; September: 69–72.
12 Korman M, Sievert W. Peptic ulcers. In: *MIMS Disease Index* (2nd edn). Sydney: IMS Publishing, 1996: 400–2.
13 Ford A, Delaney B et al. Eradication therapy for peptic ulcer disease in *Helicobacter* positive patients (Cochrane Review). Cochrane Database. Syst Rev. 2004, Issue 4. Art No. CD003840.
14 Sugano K et al. Kyoto global consensus report on Helicobacter pylori gastritis. Gut, 2015; 64 (9): 1353–67.
15 Chan FK, To KF, Wu JC. Eradication of *Helicobacter pylori* and risk of peptic ulcers in patients starting long term treatment with NSAIDs: a randomised trial. Lancet, 2002; 359 (9300): 9–13.

Dysphagia

48

We swallow approximately 1200 times daily, largely subconsciously. While we take the fundamental function for granted, disordered swallowing can be a devastating condition, with substantial morbidity for those affected.

IAN COOK 1996

Dysphagia is difficulty in swallowing. It is a common problem affecting up to 22% of patients in the general practice setting.[1] It is usually associated with a sensation of hold-up of the swallowed bolus and is sometimes accompanied by pain.

Its origin is considered as either oropharyngeal or oesophageal. Oropharyngeal dysphagia is usually related to neuromuscular dysfunction and is commonly caused by stroke. Oesophageal dysphagia is usually due to motor disorders, such as achalasia or diffuse oesophageal spasm, and to peptic oesophageal strictures often secondary to reflux. In this type of dysphagia there is a sensation of a hold-up, which may be experienced in either the cervical or retrosternal region.[1] Causes are usually classified as functional, mechanical and neurological (see TABLE 48.1).

Table 48.1 Causes of dysphagia

Functional	Examples: muscle tension, 'express swallowing'
Neurological	Examples: stroke, myasthenia, MND
Mechanical	
• luminal	Example: foreign body
• mural	Example: stricture, tumour
• extramural	Example: extrinsic compression (i.e. goitre)

Dysphagia must not be confused with globus sensation, which is the sensation of the constant 'lump in the throat' although there is no actual difficulty swallowing food. If dysphagia is progressive or prolonged then urgent attention is necessary.

There are only a few common causes of dysphagia and these are usually readily diagnosed on the history and two or three investigations. A careful history is very important, including a drug history and psychosocial factors.

Diagnostic guidelines

- Any disease or abnormality affecting the tongue, pharynx or oesophagus can cause dysphagia.
- Patients experience a sensation of obstruction at a definite level with swallowing food or water; hence, it is convenient to subdivide dysphagia into oropharyngeal and oesophageal.
- Pain from the oropharynx is localised to the neck.
- Pain from the oesophagus is usually felt over the T2–6 area of the chest.
- Oropharyngeal causes: difficulty initiating swallowing; food sticks at the suprasternal notch level; regurgitation; aspiration.
- Oesophageal causes: food sticks to mid to lower sternal level; pain on swallowing solid foods, especially meat, potatoes and bread, and then eventually liquids.
- A pharyngeal pouch usually causes regurgitation of undigested food and gurgling may be audible over the side of the neck.
- Neurological disorders typically result in difficulty swallowing or coughing or choking due to food spillover, especially with liquids.
- Dysphagia for solids only indicates a structural lesion, such as a stricture or tumour.
- Dysphagia for liquids and solids is typical of an oesophageal motility disorder, namely achalasia.[2]
- GORD tends to exclude achalasia.

Red flag pointers for dysphagia

- Age >50 years
- Recent or sudden onset
- Unexplained weight loss
- Painful swallowing
- Progressive dysphagia
- Dysphagia for solids
- Hiccoughs
- Hoarseness
- Neurological symptoms/signs

- Gastroenterologists claim that the big three common causes referred to them are benign peptic stricture, cancer and achalasia.[3]
- Intermittent dysphagia for both liquids and solids is characteristic of a motility disorder such as oesophageal achalasia.
- Malignant oesophageal obstruction is usually evident when there is a short history of rapidly progressive dysphagia and significant weight loss.[4]

A summary of the diagnostic strategy model is presented in TABLE 48.2.

Examination

It is worthwhile focusing on the following features:

- general examination including hands and skin ? scleroderma
- assess nutritional status including BMI
- mouth, pharynx, larynx (look for paralysis) ? dentition
- neck, especially for lymph nodes and thyroid
- neurological, especially cranial nerve function and muscle weakness disorders or evidence of stroke
- special oesophageal obstruction test:
  - hand the patient a glass of water and place a stethoscope over the left upper quadrant of abdomen
  - measure time between swallowing and murmur produced by bolus passing the cardia (normal: 7–10 seconds)
- assess aspiration risk, e.g. through having a sip of water[1]

Investigations

- Full blood examination: ? anaemia
- Neurological cause: oesophageal motility study (manometry)
- Mechanical:
  - extrinsic compression (e.g. barium swallow, CT scan, chest X-ray)
  - intrinsic (e.g. endoscopy ± barium swallow)
  - PET scan: good for identifying oesophageal cancer and gastro-oesophageal function

The primary investigation in suspected pharyngeal dysphagia is a video barium swallow[5] while endoscopy is generally the first investigation in cases of suspected oesophageal dysphagia. Barium swallow should precede endoscopy in the latter when there is a suspected oesophageal 'ring' and suspected oesophageal dysmotility. If endoscopy and radiology are negative, consider oesophageal motility studies to look specifically for achalasia or other less common motility disorders.

Table 48.2 Dysphagia: diagnostic strategy model (excluding oropharyngeal infections and strokes)

Probability diagnosis
Functional (e.g. 'express' swallowing, psychogenic)
Tablet-induced irritation
Pharyngotonsillitis
GORD/reflux oesophagitis
Serious disorders not to be missed
Neoplasia:
• cancer of the pharynx, oesophagus, stomach
• extrinsic tumour
AIDS (opportunistic oesophageal infection in immunocompromised, also candidiasis, herpes and viral oesophagitis)
Stricture, usually benign peptic stricture
Oesophageal food bolus obstruction
Scleroderma
Neurological causes:
• pseudobulbar palsy
• multiple sclerosis/myasthenia gravis
• motor neurone disease (amyotrophic sclerosis)
• Parkinson disease
Pitfalls (often missed)
Foreign body
Drugs (e.g. phenothiazines, bisphosphanates)
Subacute thyroiditis
Extrinsic lesions (e.g. lymph nodes, goitre)
Upper oesophageal web (e.g. Plummer–Vinson syndrome)
Diffuse oesophageal spasm
Eosinophilic oesophagitis
Radiotherapy
Achalasia
Upper oesophageal spasm (mimics angina)
Rarities (some):
• Sjögren syndrome
• aortic aneurysm
• aberrant right subclavian artery
• lead poisoning
• cervical osteoarthritis (large osteophytes)
• other neurological causes
• other mechanical causes
Seven masquerades checklist
Depression
Drugs
Thyroid disorder
Is the patient trying to tell me something?
Yes. Could be functional ? globus sensation.

SPECIFIC CONDITIONS

Benign peptic stricture

- Fibrous stricture of lower third oesophagus (can be higher)
- Follows years of reflux oesophagitis
- Usually older patients
- Dysphagia with solid food
- Diagnosis confirmed by endoscopy and barium swallow

Treatment

- Dilate the stricture
- Treat reflux vigorously

Oesophageal cancer

- Dysphagia at beginning of meal
- Progressive dysphagia for solid food steadily progressive over weeks
- Can remain silent and tends to be invasive when diagnosed
- Hiccoughs may be an early sign
- Hoarseness and cough (upper third)
- Discomfort or pain—throat, retrosternal, interscapular
- Weight loss can be striking
- Associations: GORD, tobacco, Barrett oesophagus
- Diagnosis confirmed by barium swallow and endoscopy
- Both SCC upper third (commonest) and adenocarcinoma, distal third
- Adenocarcinoma associated with Barrett mucosa
- Treatment is usually palliative surgery
- Plummer–Vinson syndrome

DxT fatigue + progressive dysphagia + weight loss → oesophageal cancer

Barrett oesophagus

See CHAPTER 47.

Achalasia

- A disorder of oesophageal motility
- Widely dilated oesophagus
- Empties poorly through a smoothly tapered lower end
- Gradual onset of dysphagia for both liquids and solids
- Fluctuating symptoms—dysphagia, regurgitation
- Chest discomfort
- Diagnosis confirmed by barium swallow or manometry
- Manometry is the only way to diagnose with certainty[1]

Treatment

- Conservative in the elderly (e.g. nifedipine/or endoscopic botulinum toxin injection into the sphincter)[6]
- Pneumatic dilatation of lower oesophageal sphincter or surgical myotomy

  Note: Prokinetic drugs have no place in treatment.

Drug-induced oesophageal injury[3]

- Tetracycline, especially doxycycline, can cause painful ulceration in all age groups.
- Delayed passage of some drugs (due to pre-existing disorders) can cause local ulceration, even perforation (especially in the elderly) (e.g. iron tablets, slow-release potassium, aspirin, NSAIDs, bisphosphonates, zidovudine, antibiotics).
- The elderly are prone to the problem if they ingest drugs upon retiring to bed with insufficient liquid washdown.

Management

- Stop drugs or swallow them upright with a glass of water
- Take antacids

Globus sensation (cricopharyngeal spasm)

Also referred to as 'globus hystericus' or 'lump in the throat', it is the subjective sensation of a lump in the throat. It appears to be associated with psychological stress (e.g. unresolved hurt, grief, non-achievement). Suppression of sadness is most often implicated.[6] No specific aetiology or physiological mechanism has been established. The symptom can be associated with GORD, from frequent swallowing or emotionally based dry throat.

Clinical features

- Sensation of being 'choked up' or 'something stuck' or lump—a very real sensation
- Not affected by swallowing
- Eating and drinking may provide relief
- Normal investigations

48

Approach to patient

- Careful history and examination
- Exclude organic cause (refer TABLE 48.2)
- May require investigations if doubtful diagnosis

Management

- Usually settles with education, reassuring support and time (up to several months)
- Avoid swallowing very hot drinks
- No drug of proven value
- Treat any underlying psychological disorder

Odynophagia

Pain on swallowing is basically caused by irritation of an inflamed or ulcerated (in particular) mucosa by the swallowed food bolus, usually meat, which may impact.

Important causes include:

- GORD (the commonest cause) with associated oesophagitis
- oesophageal spasm, especially distal oesophagus
- oesophageal candidiasis, especially in the immunosuppressed
- herpes simplex oesophagitis, in the immunosuppressed
- cytomegalovirus oesophagitis, in the immunosuppressed
- pill-induced oesophagitis/ulceration
- oesophageal cancer
- achalasia

Eosinophilic oesophagitis[7, 8]

Eosinophilic oesophagitis is increasingly being recognised as a cause of dysphagia, gastro-oesophageal reflux and acute food bolus obstruction in both children (particularly) and adults. It may present as infant colic.[8] It should be considered in those who regularly experience food getting stuck in their throat. It is associated with allergic disorders such as hay fever, cow's milk allergy and asthma. The IgE is elevated. Refer to gastroscopy, which may show eosinophilic infiltrates in the oesophagus on mucosal biopsies. However, symptoms usually resolve within 72 hours of eliminating the offending food. A six-food elimination diet (cow's milk protein, wheat, soy, eggs, seafood and peanuts) has been shown to reduce symptoms in up to 90%.[1] Treatment of the acute attack includes IM buscopan and a swallowed topical corticosteroid aerosol, e.g. fluticasone twice daily for 8 weeks.[9]

Practice tips

- Although dysphagia is a common psychogenic symptom, it must always be taken seriously and investigated.
- Mechanical dysphagia represents cancer until proved otherwise.
- Progressive dysphagia and weight loss in an elderly patient is oesophageal cancer until proved otherwise.
- Oesophageal cancer usually causes pain, wasting and regurgitation.
- Globus sensation or hystericus, an anxiety disorder, should not be confused with dysphagia. It is the subjective sensation of a lump or mass in the throat. Usually seen in young women.
- Cancer-induced achalasia occurs with tumours at the gastro-oesophageal junction usually due to adenocarcinoma of the stomach.
- Severe oesophageal reflux predisposes to adenocarcinoma.
- Oesophageal strictures can be benign, usually secondary to chronic reflux oesophagitis, or due to malignancy.
- Be careful of a change of symptoms in the presence of long-standing reflux. Consider stricture or cancer.
- A prominent hard lymph node in the left supraclavicular fossa (Troisier sign) is suggestive of cancer of the stomach.
- Dysphagia can be caused by a tight fundoplication and can be diagnosed by manometry or barium swallow.[1]

Dietary adjustments (dysphagia diets)

1 Thin liquids, e.g. fruit juice, coffee, tea
2 Nectar-thick liquids, e.g. creamy soup, tomato juice
3 Honey-consistency diet (honey-thick liquids)
4 Pudding-thick foods, e.g. mashed bananas, cooked cereals, purees
5 Mechanical soft foods, e.g. meat loaf, baked beans, casseroles
6 Chewy foods, e.g. pizza, cheese, bagels
7 Foods that fall apart, e.g. bread, rice, muffins

Consider nutritional methods such as nasogastric feeding and gastrostomy.

References

1 Kuo P, Holloway R. Dysphagia: how to treat. Australian Doctor, 8 February 2013: 21–8.
2 Trate DM, Parkman HP, Fisher RS. Dysphagia: evaluation, diagnosis and treatment. Primary Care, 1996; 23: 417–32.
3 Breen K. A practical approach to patients with dysphagia or pain on swallowing. Modern Medicine Australia, 1992; 3: 50–6.
4 Abeygunasekera S. Difficult and painful swallowing: a guide for GPs. Medicine Today, 2003; 4 (10): 33–40.
5 Roman S, Kahrilas PJ. Management of spastic disorders of the esophagus. Gastroenterol Clin North Am, 2013; 42 (1): 27–43.
6 Porter RS, Kaplan JL (eds). *The Merck Manual* (19th edn). NJ: Merck Sharp & Dohme Corp., 2011: 78.
7 Kakakios A, Heine R. Eosinophilic oesophagitis. Med J Aust, 2006; 185 (7): 401.
8 Thomson K, Tey D, Marks M. *Paediatric Handbook* (8th edn). Oxford: Wiley-Blackwell, 2009: 232.
9 Expert group for Gastrointestinal. Disorders of the oesophagus. In: eTG complete [Internet]. Melbourne: Therapeutic Guidelines Ltd. Available from: www.tg.org.au, accessed September 2017.

49 Dyspnoea

When man grows old . . . there is much gas within his thorax, resulting in panting and troubled breathing.

HUANG TI (2697–2597 BCE), *THE YELLOW EMPEROR'S CLASSIC OF INTERNAL MEDICINE*

Dyspnoea is the subjective sensation of breathlessness that is excessive for any given level of physical activity. It is a cardinal symptom affecting the cardiopulmonary system and can be very difficult to evaluate. Appropriate breathlessness following activities such as running to catch a bus or climbing several flights of stairs is not abnormal but may be excessive due to obesity or lack of fitness.

Key facts and checkpoints

- Determination of the underlying cause of dyspnoea in a given patient is absolutely essential for effective management.
- The main causes of dyspnoea are lung disease, heart disease, obesity and functional hyperventilation.[1]
- The most common cause of dyspnoea encountered in family practice is airflow obstruction, which is the basic abnormality seen in chronic asthma and chronic obstructive pulmonary disease (COPD).[2]
- Wheezing, which is a continuous musical or whistling noise, is an indication of airflow obstruction.
- Some patients with asthma do not wheeze and some patients who wheeze do not have asthma.
- Other important pulmonary causes include restrictive disease, such as fibrosis, collapse and pleural effusion.
- Dyspnoea is not inevitable in lung cancer but occurs in about 60% of cases.[3]
- Normal respiratory rate is 12–16 breaths/minute.

Terminology

It is important to emphasise that dyspnoea or breathlessness is a subjective sensation of the desire for increased respiratory effort and must be considered in relation to the patient's lifestyle and individual tolerance of discomfort. It also depends on the age, physical fitness and physical expectations of the person. Patients may complain of tightness in the chest and this must be differentiated from angina.

The American Thoracic Society guide for grades of dyspnoea is:

Grade 0	No breathlessness except with strenuous exercise
Grade 1	Breathlessness when hurrying on the level or walking up a slight hill
Grade 2	Walks slower than people of the same age on the level because of breathlessness or has to stop for breath when walking at own pace on level
Grade 3	Stops for breath after walking about 100 yards (91 metres) or a few minutes on the level
Grade 4	Too breathless to leave the house or breathless when dressing or undressing

Glossary of terms

Hyperpnoea An increased level of ventilation (e.g. during exertion).

Hyperventilation Overbreathing.

Orthopnoea Breathlessness lying down flat.

Paroxysmal nocturnal dyspnoea Inappropriate breathlessness causing waking from sleep.

Tachypnoea An increased rate of breathing.

Difference between heart and lung causes

The distinguishing features between dyspnoea due to heart disease and to lung disease are presented in TABLE 49.1.

The history is a good indication and a useful guideline is that dyspnoea at rest is typical of lung disease, especially asthma, while it tends to be present on effort with heart disease as well as with COPD.

Wheezing

Wheezing is any continuous musical expiratory noise heard with the stethoscope or otherwise. Wheeze includes stridor, which is an inspiratory wheeze.

Table 49.1 Comparison of distinguishing features between dyspnoea due to heart disease and lung disease

Lung disease	Heart disease
History of respiratory disease	History of hypertension, cardiac ischaemia or valvular heart disease
Slow development	Rapid development
Present at rest	Mainly on exertion
Productive cough common	Cough uncommon and then 'dry'
Aggravated by respiratory infection	Usually unaffected by respiratory infection

Source: After Sandler[1]

Common causes of wheezing

Localised:

- partial bronchial obstruction:
  - impacted foreign body
  - impacted mucus plugs
  - extrinsic compression

Generalised:

- asthma
- obstructive bronchitis
- bronchiolitis

'Cardiac asthma' and bronchial asthma

The term 'cardiac asthma' is used to describe a wheezing sensation such as that experienced with paroxysmal nocturnal dyspnoea. Differentiating features are presented in TABLE 49.2.

Table 49.2 Comparison of distinguishing features between 'cardiac asthma' and bronchial asthma

	Cardiac	Bronchial
Dyspnoea	Mainly inspiratory	Mainly expiratory
Cough	Follows dyspnoea	Precedes dyspnoea
Sputum	Pink and frothy	Thick and gelatinous
Relief	Standing up (by an open window) Intravenous diuretic/CPAP, morphine	Coughing up sputum Bronchodilator
Lung signs	Mainly crackles	Mainly wheezes

Is it asthma or COPD?

This question is often asked, especially in the middle-aged or elderly person with dyspnoea. Differentiating features are presented in TABLE 49.3.

Table 49.3 Comparison of asthma and COPD

	Asthma	COPD
Symptoms <35 years	Common	Unusual
Smoking history	Possible	Invariable
Chronic cough	Uncommon	Common
Dyspnoea	Diurnal and variable	Constant and progressive
Response to inhaled bronchodilator	Good	Poor
Nocturnal waking with symptoms	Common	Uncommon
Airflow obstruction	Reversible	Non-reversible

A diagnostic approach

A summary of the diagnostic strategy model is presented in TABLE 49.4.

49

Table 49.4 Dyspnoea: diagnostic strategy model

Probability diagnosis

Bronchial asthma
Bronchiolitis (children)
COPD
Ageing; lack of fitness/physical deconditioning
Left heart failure
Obesity

Serious disorders not to be missed

Cardiovascular:

- acute heart failure (e.g. AMI)
- arrhythmia
- pulmonary embolism
- fat embolism
- pulmonary hypertension
- dissecting aneurysm
- cardiomyopathy
- pericardial tamponade
- anaphylaxis

Neoplasia:

- bronchial carcinoma, other malignancy

Severe infections:

- SARS
- avian influenza
- pneumonia
- acute epiglottitis (children)

Respiratory disorders:

- inhaled foreign body

continued

Table 49.4 *continued*

• upper airways obstruction • pneumothorax • atelectasis • pleural effusion • tuberculosis • Acute respiratory distress syndrome (ARDS) Neuromuscular disease: • infective polyneuritis • poliomyelitis
Pitfalls (often missed) Interstitial lung disease: • idiopathic pulmonary fibrosis • hypersensitivity pneumonitis • sarcoidosis (others) Chemical pneumonitis Metabolic acidosis Radiotherapy Kidney failure (uraemia) Multiple small pulmonary emboli
Seven masquerades checklist Depression Diabetes (incl. ketoacidosis) Drugs Anaemia Thyroid disorder (thyrotoxicosis) Spinal dysfunction (ankylosing spondylitis)
Is the patient trying to tell me something? Consider functional hyperventilation (anxiety and panic attacks).

49

Probability diagnosis

The common causes of dyspnoea are lung disease, heart disease, obesity, anaemia (tissue hypoxia) and functional hyperventilation. More specifically, bronchial asthma, COPD, acute pulmonary infections and left heart failure (often insidious) are common individual causes.

Serious disorders not to be missed

Severe cardiovascular events such as acute heart failure, which may be precipitated by myocardial infarction (may be silent, especially in diabetics), a life-threatening arrhythmia, pulmonary embolism, dissecting aneurysm or a cardiomyopathy (such as viral myocarditis) require early diagnosis and corrective action. Recurrent pulmonary embolism may present a diagnostic problem. There may be a history of deep venous thrombosis, pregnancy, malignancy or taking the contraceptive pill.[4]

Severe infections such as lobar pneumonia, tuberculosis and myocarditis must be considered. In children acute epiglottitis, croup, bronchiolitis, pneumonia and bronchitis are serious infections responsible for respiratory distress.

Primary carcinoma is an important consideration, especially in dyspnoea of gradual onset. Other malignant conditions to consider are metastases, lymphangitis carcinomatosis, lymphomas and pleural mesothelioma. Pleural effusion may be the mode of presentation of some of these serious disorders.

Pitfalls

Interstitial pulmonary disease can be a diagnostic dilemma because the physical signs and X-ray appearances can be minimal in the early stages despite the presence of significant dyspnoea. Allergic alveolitis, such as that caused by birds (e.g. hypersensitivity to their droppings) can be a pitfall. The diagnosis is easier if a known disease associated with pulmonary infiltration, such as sarcoidosis, is present. Measuring the diffusing capacity will help with diagnosis.

Pericardial tamponade may cause difficulty in diagnosis either with an acute onset, such as malignancy involving pericardium, or insidiously. The patient usually has a weak pulse with pulsus paradoxus, hypotension and a raised jugular venous pressure.

It is important to be careful not to attribute dyspnoea simply to obesity or lack of fitness when it could have a true organic disorder such as heart failure.

Seven masquerades checklist

Most of the masquerades have to be considered as underlying causes. Depression can be associated with dyspnoea, anaemia is an important cause of dyspnoea, thyrotoxicosis can rarely present with dyspnoea, and diabetic ketoacidosis can cause rapid deep breathing.

Drugs must also be considered, especially as a cause of interstitial pulmonary fibrosis that presents with dyspnoea, cough and fever. Drugs that cause this disorder include several cytotoxic agents (especially bleomycin, cyclophosphamide, methotrexate), amiodarone, sulphasalazine, penicillamine, nitrofurantoin, gold salts and adrenergic nasal sprays.[3] Poisons that may cause hyperventilation are salicylate, methyl alcohol, theophylline overdosage and ethylene glycol. Anaemia must be considered especially in those at risk. Dyspnoea is unlikely to be caused solely by chronic anaemia unless the haemoglobin level is less than 8 g/dL.[4] It is more likely to occur if another predisposing cause, such as ischaemic heart disease, is present.

Psychogenic considerations

Functional dyspnoea or hyperventilation is common. However, it is important to exclude organic causation such as asthma, drugs and thyrotoxicosis before settling with the psychogenic label and to reassure

Red flag pointers for dyspnoea

History	Examination
Increased age	Pallor/cyanosis
Sudden onset	Dyspnoea at rest
Ischaemic heart disease	Fever
Migrant: Africa, Asia	Hypotension
Recent travel	Tachycardia
Asthma/allergy	Tachypnoea
Unexplained weight loss	Calf tenderness
Haemoptysis	Chest wall signs
Significant trauma	Altered conscious state
HIV	Elevated JVP
Drugs: social, biologicals	Wheezing

the patient strongly if there is no organic cause. Any uncomfortable sensation in the chest may be interpreted as dyspnoea by anxious patients. Depression, anxiety and panic attacks may be underlying the problem. Characteristic associated features of hyperventilation with anxiety include dizziness, faintness, palpitations, yawning, paraesthesia of the hands and legs, inability to take a deep breath or a sensation of smothering. These patients may exhibit sighing and irregular breathing on examination. In true psychogenic dyspnoea, chest X-rays and pulmonary function tests are normal but symptoms are often reproduced after 15–30 seconds of voluntary hyperventilation. It is important to remember that it may be present in a patient who has organic disease of a mild degree such as asthma.

Table 49.5 Typical causes of dyspnoea related to time of onset

Sudden
Lung collapse
Inhaled foreign body/other choking
Spontaneous pneumothorax
Arrhythmia
Anaphylaxis
Myocardial infarction
Pulmonary embolism
Rapid (over a few hours)
Asthma
Hyperventilation (can be sudden)
Acute exacerbations of COPD
Pneumonia
Diabetic ketoacidosis
Extrinsic allergic alveolitis
High altitude
Left heart failure (acute pulmonary oedema)
Pericardial tamponade
Poisons
Over days or weeks
Congestive heart failure
Pleural effusion
Carcinoma of the bronchus/trachea
Over months or years
COPD
Tuberculosis
Fibrosing alveolitis
Pneumoconiosis
Non-respiratory causes
Anaemia
Hyperthyroidism
Obesity

The clinical approach

History

Special attention should be paid to evaluating exactly what the patient means by breathlessness or restriction of breathing. The analysis should then include provoking factors and associated symptoms with a view to differentiating between pulmonary causes such as asthma and COPD. Wheeze is often (but not always) present in asthma and chronic airflow obstruction. Most respiratory causes of dyspnoea also produce cough. The rate of development of dyspnoea gives an indication of the possible cause (see TABLE 49.5).[5] The sudden onset of dyspnoea at rest is suggestive of pulmonary embolism or pneumothorax. Severe dyspnoea developing over 1 or 2 hours is most likely due to left heart failure or bronchial asthma. Bronchial asthma is usually easily distinguished from left heart failure by the history of previous attacks, by the absence of chest pain and the absence of cardiac murmurs. 'My breathing feels tight' indicates asthma. A complaint of 'suffocation or feeling smothered' or 'just not getting enough air' may be a pointer to functional dyspnoea.

The dyspnoea of asthma tends to occur at rest and at night, while that with chronic airflow obstruction occurs with exertion.

Examination

The routine findings from inspection, percussion and auscultation will determine whether the underlying lung disease is localised or generalised. The generalised findings for various disorders of the lungs are summarised in TABLE 49.6.

Careful inspection is mandatory. The patient should be stripped to the waist and observed for factors such as

Table 49.6 Comparison of examination findings for various lung disorders

	Trachea	Chest wall movement	Percussion note	Breath sounds	Vocal fremitus	Adventitious sounds
Normal	Midline	Equal expansion	Resonant	Vesicular	Normal	Nil: ± few transient inspiratory basal crackles
Asthma	Midline	Decreased (bilateral)	Resonant	Vesicular—prolonged expiration	Normal or decreased	Expiratory wheezes
Emphysema	Midline	Decreased (bilateral)	Resonant to hyper-resonant	Vesicular—decreased	Decreased	Nil or the crackles and wheezes of chronic bronchitis
Consolidation (e.g. lobar pneumonia)	Midline	Decreased on affected side	Dull	Bronchial	Increased	Fine late inspiratory crackles
Collapse: major bronchus	Towards affected side	Decreased (unilateral)	Dull	Absent or decreased	Absent or decreased	Nil
Collapse: peripheral bronchus	Towards affected side	Decreased (unilateral)	Dull	Bronchial	Increased	Coarse crackles
Pleural effusion (>500 mL)	Towards opposite side (if massive)	Decreased (unilateral)	Stony dull	Absent or decreased	Absent or decreased	None
Pneumothorax (large)	Towards opposite side (if tension)	Decreased (unilateral)	Hyper-resonant	Absent or decreased	Absent or decreased	None
Fibrosis (generalised)	Midline	Decreased (bilateral)	Normal	Vesicular	Increased	Fine crackles
Bronchiectasis	Midline	Slight decrease	Resonant to dull	Bronchial	Normal or decreased	Coarse crackles ± localised wheeze

49

cyanosis, clubbing, pallor, mental alertness, dyspnoea at rest, use of accessory muscles, rib retraction and any other abnormalities of the chest wall. A coarse tremor or flap of the outstretched hands indicates carbon dioxide intoxication.[6] To obtain maximum value from auscultation, request the patient to open his or her mouth and take deep breaths. Adventitious sounds that are not audible during tidal breathing may then be heard. Wheezes are high-pitched continuous sounds heard either in expiration or inspiration, being more pronounced in expiration.

Crackles are short interrupted sounds heard mainly at the end of inspiration, resembling the crackling sound of hair being rubbed between the fingers near the ear. Fine crackles, previously referred to as crepitations, occur typically in lobar pneumonia and diffuse interstitial fibrosis, and are not cleared by coughing. Medium crackles are typical of congestive cardiac failure, and coarse crackles indicate airway mucus and usually clear on coughing.

Causes of pulmonary crackles

- Left ventricular failure
- Idiopathic pulmonary fibrosis
- Extrinsic allergic alveolitis
- Pneumonia
- Bronchiectasis
- Chronic bronchitis
- Asbestosis
- Pulmonary fibrosis

Investigations

The two most important initial investigations for respiratory disease are chest X-ray and pulmonary function tests.

Pulmonary function tests (PFTs)

These relatively simple tests provide considerable information.

Peak expiratory flow rate

The most practical instrument for office use to detect chronic airway obstruction due to asthma or chronic bronchitis is the mini peak flow meter, which measures peak expiratory flow rate (PEFR).

The interpretation of the tests, which vary according to sex, age and height, requires charts of predicted normal values. A chart for PEFR in normal adult subjects is presented in Appendix V. The value for a particular patient should be the best of three results.

Spirometry

Spirometry is the gold standard test. The measurement of the forced vital capacity (FVC) and the forced expiratory volume in one second (FEV_1) provide a very useful guide to the type of ventilatory deficit. Both the FVC and the FEV_1 are related to sex, age and height.

The FEV_1 expressed as a percentage of the FVC is an excellent measure of airflow limitation. In normal subjects it is approximately 70%. A normal spirometry pattern is shown in FIGURE 49.1 and abnormal patterns in FIGURE 49.2. FIGURE 49.3 summarises the relative values for these conditions.

Lung volume

Tidal volume (TV) and vital capacity (VC) can be measured by a simple spirometer but the total lung

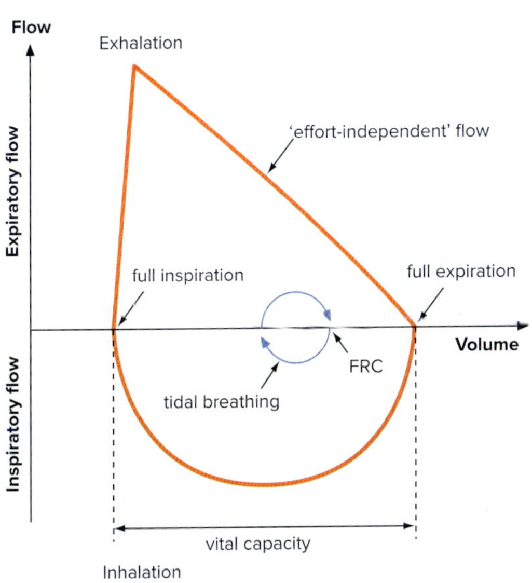

FIGURE 49.1 Spirometry patterns showing normal flow volume loop.

Source: Reprinted with permission

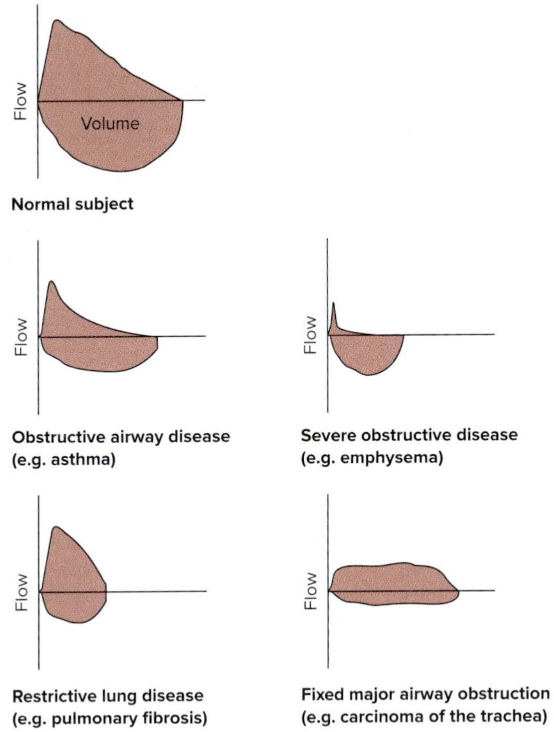

FIGURE 49.2 Maximum expiratory and inspiratory flow volume curves with examples of relative changes of patterns.

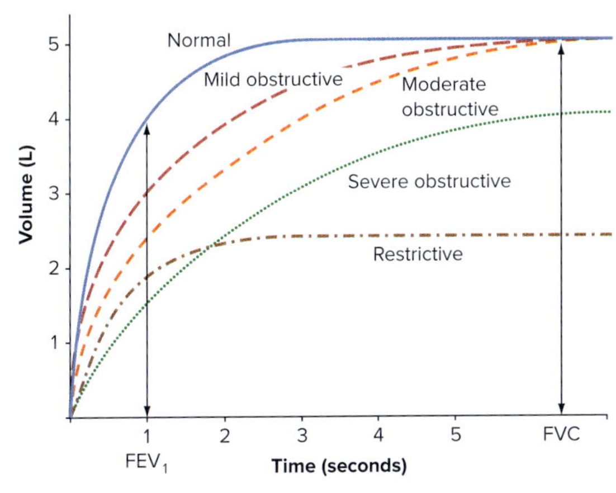

FIGURE 49.3 Spirograms

capacity and the residual volume are measured by the helium dilution method in a respiratory laboratory.

Diffusing capacity (gas transfer factor)

This test measures the carbon monoxide uptake by a single breath analysis for whole lungs. In normal lungs the transfer factor is a true measure of the diffusing capacity of the lungs for oxygen and depends on the thickness of the alveolar-capillary membrane.[5] Gas transfer is usually reduced in patients with severe degrees of emphysema and fibrosis, anaemia and congestive cardiac failure. Useful for COPD and interstitial lung disease. Normal in asthma.

Pulse oximetry

The outstanding monitoring aid, transcutaneous pulse oximetry, estimates oxygen saturation (SpO_2) of capillary blood. The estimates are generally very accurate and correlate to within 5% of measured arterial O_2 saturation (SaO_2).[7] The ideal level is 97–100%; median levels—neonates 97%, children 98%, adults 98%. <92% is very serious.

Histamine challenge test

This test indicates the presence of airway or bronchial hyper-reactivity, which is a fundamental feature with asthma. The test should not be performed on those with poor lung function and only performed by a respiratory technician under medical supervision. The test is potentially dangerous.

Other investigations (to select from)

- Haemoglobin, red cell indices and PCV
- White blood cell count (e.g. eosinophilia of asthma)
- Sputum, culture and cytology
- Tuberculosis tests
- ESR/CRP
- Arterial blood gas analysis
- Cardiological investigations:
  - ECG, including exercise
  - echocardiography (technically difficult in emphysema)
  - nuclear gated blood pool scan to assess heart function
  - cardiac enzymes
- Other medical imaging:
  - high-resolution CT
  - MRI
  - ventilation and perfusion radionuclide scan (pulmonary embolism)
- Bronchoscopy, especially fibre-optic bronchoscopy
- Thoracocentesis and pleural biopsy
- Open lung biopsy
- $Alpha_1$-antitrypsin measurement (normal range 1.1–2.2 g/L)

Pleural effusion

Key points

- Normal pleural space has 10–20 mL fluid
- Can be detected on X-ray if >300 mL fluid in pleural space
- Can be detected clinically if >500 mL fluid
- Can be subpulmonary—simulates a raised diaphragm
- May be asymptomatic
- Dyspnoea common with large effusion
- Chest pain in setting of pleuritis, infection or trauma
- Signs: refer TABLE 49.6
- The fluid may be transudate or exudate (diagnosed by aspirate)
- If blood stained—malignancy, pulmonary infarction, TB

Transudate

Protein content <25 g/L; lactic dehydrogenase <200 IU/L.

Causes

- Heart failure (90% of cases)
- Hypoproteinaemia, e.g. nephrotic syndrome
- Liver failure with ascites
- Constrictive pericarditis
- Hypothyroidism
- Ovarian tumour—right-sided effusion (Meigs syndrome)

Exudate

Protein content >35 g/L; lactic dehydrogenase >200 IU/L

Causes

- Infection—bacterial pneumonia, pleurisy, empyema, TB, viral
- Malignancy—bronchial carcinoma, mesothelioma, metastatic
- Pulmonary infarction
- Connective tissue diseases (e.g. SLE, RA)
- Acute pancreatitis
- Lymphoma
- Sarcoidosis
- HIV with parasitic pneumonia

Management

Aspiration if symptomatic: may require repeats and pleurodesis. Treat the underlying cause.

Dyspnoea in children

There are numerous causes of dyspnoea in children but the common causes are asthma, bronchiolitis and pulmonary infections. The important infections that can be fatal—croup, epiglottitis and myocarditis—must be kept in mind and intensively managed.

Bronchiolitis is an important cause of respiratory distress in infants under 6–12 months. It should not be confused with asthma (refer to CHAPTER 96).

Sudden breathlessness or stridor may be due to an inhaled foreign body. Signs of lobar collapse may be present but physical examination may be of little help and a chest X-ray is essential.

Cardiovascular disorders, including congenital heart disease, can cause dyspnoea. Extra respiratory causes include anaemia, acidosis, aspiration, poisoning and hyperventilation.

Dyspnoea in the elderly

Dyspnoea in the elderly is common and is caused usually by heart failure and COPD. The other associations with ageing, such as lung cancer, pulmonary fibrosis and drugs, are relevant. The classic problem of the aged is acute heart failure that develops typically in the early morning hours. The acute brain syndrome is a common presentation of all these disorders.

Respiratory disease in the elderly

The respiratory system, like most other bodily systems, matures until about the age of 25 years and subsequently slowly loses efficiency due to a variety of factors such as disease, smoking, pollution and ageing. There is a decline in lung function and gas exchange and decreased ventilatory responses to hypoxia and hypercapnia.

Heart failure

Heart failure occurs when the heart is unable to maintain sufficient cardiac output to meet the demands of the body. Dyspnoea is a common early symptom as pulmonary congestion causes hypoxia (increased ventilation) and decreased compliance (increased work). The incidence of congestive cardiac failure (CCF) has been increasing steeply, partly due to the ageing population.

Symptoms

- Increasing dyspnoea progressing to (in order):
  - fatigue, especially exertional fatigue
  - paroxysmal nocturnal dyspnoea
  - weight change: gain or loss

It is convenient to divide heart failure into left and right heart failure but they rarely occur in isolation and often occur simultaneously. Right failure is invariably secondary to left failure. Furthermore, some cardiologists stress the importance of differentiating between systolic and diastolic dysfunction. Both present in the same way clinically and hence referral for cardiac studies to obtain measurement of the left ventricular function is required. This permits an accurate diagnosis and guide to treatment and an accurate prognosis.

Refer to Chronic heart failure (CHAPTER 88).

Chronic obstructive pulmonary disease

Chronic bronchitis and emphysema should be considered together as both these conditions usually coexist to some degree in each patient. An alternative, and preferable, term—chronic obstructive pulmonary disease (COPD)—is used to cover chronic bronchitis and emphysema with chronic airflow limitation.[6]

For more detail on the management of COPD refer to CHAPTER 83.

Interstitial Lung Diseases

Interstitial lung diseases comprise a group of disorders that have the common features of inflammation (pneumonitis) and fibrosis of the interalveolar septum, representing a non-specific reaction of the lung to injury of various causes.[8,9]

In many there is a hypersensitivity reaction to various unusual antigens. The fibrosis may be localised as following unresolved pneumonia, bilateral as with tuberculosis or widespread.

Consider the possibility of fibrosis of the lungs in chronic dyspnoea and a dry cough with normal resonance.

Causes of widespread interstitial pulmonary fibrosis include:

- idiopathic pulmonary fibrosis
- hypersensitivity pneumonitis (extrinsic allergic alveolitis)
- drug-induced
- lymphangitis carcinomatosis
- various occupational lung disorders
- rheumatoid arthritis
- sarcoidosis
- acute pulmonary oedema
- immunological/multisystemic disease (e.g. connective tissue disorders, RA, vasculitis, inflammatory bowel disease)

Common clinical features:

- dyspnoea and dry cough (insidious onset)
- fine inspiratory crackles at lung base with faint breath sounds
- cyanosis and finger clubbing may be present
- PFTs:
  - restrictive ventilatory deficit
  - decrease in gas transfer factor
- characteristic X-ray changes

High-resolution CT scanning has been a major advance in diagnosis. May show ‘honeycomb lung’.

Idiopathic pulmonary fibrosis

Idiopathic pulmonary fibrosis, also known as idiopathic fibrosing interstitial pneumonia and cryptogenic fibrosing alveolitis, is the most common diagnosis among patients presenting with interstitial lung disease.

Patients usually present in the fifth to seventh decade with the clinical features as outlined under interstitial lung diseases such as slowly progressive dyspnoea over months to years. Chest X-ray abnormalities are variable but include bilateral diffuse nodular or reticulonodular shadowing favouring the lung bases. High-resolution CT scans are effective for diagnosis. Open lung biopsy may be needed for diagnosis and staging. The usual prognosis is poor, with death occurring about 3.5–5 years after diagnosis. The usual treatment is high doses of oral corticosteroids with azathioprine and no smoking.[9,10]

If refractory, refer to a palliative care service.[11]

Pulmonary sarcoidosis

Sarcoidosis is a multisystemic disorder of unknown aetiology, which is characterised by non-caseating granulomatous inflammation that involves the lung in about 90% of affected patients. A characteristic feature is bilateral hilar lymphadenopathy, which is often symptomless and detected on routine chest X-ray (CXR). Radiological lung involvement can be associated with or occur independently of hilar lymphadenopathy.

49

Clinical features[8,9]

- May be asymptomatic (one-third)
- Onset usually third or fourth decade (but any age)
- Bilateral hilar lymphadenopathy (on CXR)
- Cough
- Fever, malaise, arthralgia
- Skin lesions: erythema nodosum, lupus pernio
- Ocular lesions (e.g. anterior uveitis)
- Other multiple organ lesions (uncommon)
- Overall mortality 2–5%

Erythema nodosum with an acute swinging fever, malaise and arthralgia in a young adult female is diagnostic of sarcoidosis.

Diagnosis

Histological evidence from biopsy specimen, usually transbronchial biopsy (essential if an alternative diagnosis, e.g. lymphoma, cannot be excluded) or skin biopsy in cases of erythema nodosum. A better modern diagnostic method is biopsy via video-assisted thoracoscopy.

Supporting evidence:

- elevated serum ACE (non-specific)
- PFTs: restrictive pattern; impaired gas transfer in advanced cases
- ±ve Kveim test (not recommended these days)
- serum calcium

Treatment

Sarcoidosis may resolve spontaneously (hilar lymphadenopathy without lung involvement does not require treatment).

Indications for treatment with corticosteroids:

- no spontaneous improvement or worsening after 3–6 months
- symptomatic pulmonary lesions
- eye, CNS and other systems involvement
- hypercalcaemia, hypercalciuria
- erythema nodosum with arthralgia
- persistent cough

Corticosteroid treatment[9]

- Prednisolone 0.5 mg/kg (up to 50 mg) (o) daily for 4–6 weeks, then reduce to lowest dose that maintains improvement.[9] If there is a response, taper the dose to 10–15 mg (o) daily as a maintenance dose for 6–12 months.[9]
- Prednisolone 20–30 mg for 2 weeks for erythema nodosum of sarcoidosis.

Glossary of terms

Chronic airflow limitation A physiological process measured as impairment of forced expiratory flow, which is the major cause of dyspnoea in these patients.

Chronic bronchitis A clinical condition characterised by a productive cough on most days for at least 3 months of the year for at least 2 consecutive years in the absence of any other respiratory disease that could be responsible for such excessive sputum production (such as tuberculosis or bronchiectasis).

COPD A chronic, slowly progressive disorder characterised by the presence of airway obstruction, which may (or may not) be partially reversible by bronchodilator therapy.[8]

Emphysema This is defined in pathological rather than clinical terms, as permanent dilatation and destruction of lung tissue distal to the terminal bronchioles.

Hypersensitivity pneumonitis

Hypersensitivity pneumonitis (extrinsic allergic alveolitis) is characterised by a widespread diffuse inflammatory reaction in both the small airways of the lung and the alveoli, due to the inhalation of allergens, which are usually spores of micro-organisms such as thermophilic actinomycetes in 'farmer's lung' or (more commonly) avian protein from droppings or feathers in 'bird fancier's lung'. Occupational causes of extrinsic alveolitis have been described by Molina[12] (see TABLE 49.7).

Table 49.7 Various causes of hypersensitivity pneumonitis (extrinsic allergic alveolitis)

Occupation/disease	Source of antigen
Farmer's lung	Mouldy hay, grain and straw
Bagassosis	Mouldy sugar cane fibre (bagasse)
Bird fancier's lung	Avian proteins: dropping dust (e.g. from pigeons); 'bloom' on budgerigar feathers
Mushroom worker's lung	Mushroom compost
Cheese washer's lung	Moulds or mites on cheese
Wheat weevil lung	Infested wheat flour (insect)
Ventilator pneumonitis	Humidified hot air system Air-conditioning system
Wood pulp worker's disorder	Contaminated wood dust
Detergent worker's disorder	Proteolytic enzymes
Suberosis	Mouldy cork bark
Rat handler's lung	Rat urine and serum
Malt worker's lung	Mouldy barley
Coffee worker's lung	Coffee dust
Sisal worker's lung	Sisal dust
Sericultural workers	Silkworms
Furrier's lung	Fur dust
Sausage workers	Dust
Prawn workers	Prawn fumes

Illness may present as acute or subacute episodes of pyrexia, chills and malaise with dyspnoea and a peripheral neutrophil several hours after exposure.[12] Management is based on prevention, namely avoiding exposure to allergens or wearing protective, fine-mesh masks. Prednisolone can be used (with caution) to control acute symptoms. It should be pointed out that this allergic disorder is different from the infection psittacosis.

Drug-induced interstitial lung disease[9]

Drugs are an important cause of this disorder and have three main effects:

1. *Alveolitis with or without pulmonary fibrosis.* This is mainly due to cytotoxic drugs, nitrofurantoin and amiodarone. The drug should be removed and consideration given to prescribing prednisolone 50 mg (o) daily for several weeks, depending on response.
2. *Eosinophilic reactions.* This is presumably an immunological reaction, which may present as wheezing, dyspnoea, a maculopapular rash and pyrexia. The many implicated drugs include various antibiotics, NSAIDs, cytotoxic agents, major tranquillisers and antidepressants, and anti-epileptics. Treatment is drug removal and a short course of prednisolone 20–40 mg (o) daily for 2 weeks.
3. *Non-cardiogenic acute pulmonary oedema.* This is rare and has been reported to occur with opioids, aspirin, hydrochlorothiazide, β2-adrenoceptor agonists (given IV to suppress premature labour), cytotoxics, interleukin-2, heroin.

OCCUPATIONAL PULMONARY DISEASE

Various types of acute and chronic pulmonary diseases are related to exposure to noxious substances such as dusts, gases and vapours in the workplace. Common chemical causes include formaldehyde used in processed woods, e.g. chipboard and medium-density fibre. GPs have a crucial role in the identification of the possible work-relatedness of lung disease.

Disorders due to chemical agents include:

- obstructive airways disorders, such as occupational asthma, acute bronchitis, (chronic) industrial bronchitis, byssinosis (asthma-like condition due to cotton dust)
- hypersensitivity pneumonitis
- pulmonary fibrosis (pneumoconiosis) due to mineral dust
- lung cancer due to industrial agents such as asbestos, various hydrocarbons
- pleural disorders, usually associated with asbestosis

Pneumoconiosis

The term 'pneumoconiosis' refers to the accumulation of dust in the lungs and the reaction of tissue to its presence, namely chronic fibrosis. The main cause worldwide is inhalation of coal dust, a specific severe variety being progressive massive fibrosis (complicated coal worker's pneumoconiosis) in which the patient suffers severe dyspnoea of effort and a cough often productive of black sputum. TABLE 49.8 summarises the important causes.

Table 49.8 Selected pneumoconioses

Fibrotic lung disease	Agent	Typical occupations
Coal dust		
Coal worker's pneumoconiosis	Coal dust	Coal mining
Metal dust		
Siderosis	Metallic iron or iron oxide	Mining
		Welding
		Foundry work
Inorganic dusts		
Silicosis	Silica (silicon dioxide)	Quarrying
		Rock mining
		Stone cutting
		Sandblasting
Silicate dusts		
Asbestosis	Asbestos	Mining
		Shipbuilding
		Insulation
		Power stations
		Wharf labouring

49

Of particular concern are diseases caused by inhalation of fibres of asbestos, which is a mixture of silicates of iron, magnesium, cadmium, nickel and aluminium. These diseases include asbestosis, diffuse pleural thickening, pleural plaques, mesothelioma and increased bronchial carcinoma in smokers. Pulmonary asbestosis has classic X-ray changes but high-resolution CT scans may be required to confirm the presence of calcified pleural plaques. It usually takes 10–20 years from exposure for asbestosis to develop and 20–40 years for mesothelioma to develop,[8] while bronchial carcinoma is caused by the synergistic effects of asbestosis and cigarette smoking.

Acute respiratory distress syndrome (ARDS)

ARDS, also known as acute lung injury and formerly called 'adult respiratory distress syndrome', refers to acute hypoxaemic respiratory failure following a pulmonary or systemic insult with no apparent cardiogenic cause of pulmonary oedema. This occurs about 12–48 hours after the event.[13] The most common cause is sepsis, which accounts for about one-third of ARDS patients. The mortality rate is 30–40%, increasing if accompanied by sepsis. Management is based on early diagnosis, early referral, identification and treatment of the underlying condition and then optimal intensive care.[14]

Clinical features

- Sudden onset of respiratory distress
- Stiff lungs—reduced lung compliance
- Refractory hypoxaemia
- Bilateral pulmonary infiltrates on X-ray
- No apparent evidence of congestive heart failure
- Absence of elevated left atrial pressure
- Specific gas exchange abnormalities
- Signs: tachypnoea, laboured breathing, rib retraction, central cyanosis, fine crackles on auscultation

The differential diagnoses are pneumonia and acute heart failure. Common risk factors/associations for ARDS include (indirectly—systemic)—sepsis, shock, trauma, burns, drug overdose (e.g. heroin), multiple transfusions, obstetric complications (e.g. eclampsia, amniotic fluid embolism), and many direct causes such as pulmonary aspiration, toxic gas inhalation, blast injury and pneumonia (e.g. SARS). Admit patient to an intensive care unit.

Severe acute respiratory syndrome (SARS)[7]

SARS is a respiratory illness of varying severity (mild to severe) with a known mortality rate of about 10% of clinically established cases. All cases to date exhibit a high fever of >38°C. It is considered to be an atypical pneumonia caused by a quite unique coronavirus (SARS–CoV). Cases have acquired SARS following exposure to endemic areas of South-East Asia. Severe cases (up to 10% mortality) can progress to ARDS.

Suspected case = fever >38°C + cough, breathing difficulty or dyspnoea + contact with SARS person/area. Plain X-rays may show pulmonary infiltrates while high-resolution CT scans may show typical patterns.

Key features

- Symptoms of atypical pneumonia: fever, cough, dyspnoea
- Associated may be myalgia, diarrhoea, headache, sore throat, rhinorrhoea, confusion, malaise, rash

- Virulent virus—droplet spread by close contact
- Incubation period 2–7 days
- Crackles and wheezes may be present on auscultation but no hallmark sign
- Non-specific X-ray signs
- Prime CT scans may show typical changes
- Diagnosis confirmed by PCR studies or isolation of the virus on culture
- Complications appear to be confined to the lung

Optimal treatment for SARS by drugs is still being evaluated. Management is supportive; supplemental oxygen is required. Preventive measures, including wearing of face masks (NIOSH standard mask best) and appropriate infection control procedures, are important. Wear a mask, gloves, goggles and gown for clinical assessment of suspected cases and switch off air-conditioning (refer to CHAPTER 28).

Practice tips

- Remember to order a chest X-ray and pulmonary function tests in all doubtful cases of dyspnoea.
- All heart diseases have dyspnoea as a common early symptom.
- Increasing dyspnoea on exertion may be the earliest symptom of incipient heart failure.
- Several drugs can produce a wide variety of respiratory disorders, particularly pulmonary fibrosis and pulmonary eosinophilia. Amiodarone and cytotoxic drugs, especially bleomycin, are the main causes.
- Dyspnoea in the presence of lung cancer may be caused by many factors, such as pleural effusion, lobar collapse, upper airway obstruction and lymphangitis carcinomatosis.
- The abrupt onset of severe dyspnoea suggests pneumothorax or pulmonary embolism.
- If a patient develops a relapse of dyspnoea while on digoxin therapy, consider the real possibility of digoxin toxicity and/or electrolyte abnormalities leading to left heart failure.
- Recurrent attacks of sudden dyspnoea, especially waking the patient at night, are suggestive of asthma or left heart failure.
- Causes of hyperventilation include drugs, asthma, thyrotoxicosis and panic attacks/anxiety.

Bronchial carcinoma

Dyspnoea is associated with about 60% of cases of lung cancer[3] (see CHAPTER 42). It is not a common early symptom unless bronchial occlusion causes extrinsic collapse. In advanced cancer, whether primary or secondary, direct spread or metastases may cause dyspnoea. Other factors include pleural effusion, lobar collapse, metastatic infiltration, upper airway obstruction due to superior vena cava (SVC) obstruction and lymphangitis carcinomatosis. A special problem arises with coexisting chronic bronchitis and emphysema.

When to refer

- Patients with acute onset of severe dyspnoea
- All patients with heart failure resistant to initial therapy or where the diagnosis is in doubt
- Patients with pulmonary disease of uncertain aetiology, especially those requiring respiratory function tests
- Those in whom lung cancer is suspected

Patient education resources

Hand-out sheets from *Murtagh's Patient Education* 7th edition:

- Asthma
- Asthma in children
- Chronic obstructive pulmonary disease
- Asthma: dangerous asthma
- Heart failure

49

References

1. Stenton C. The MRC breathlessness scale. Occup Med (Lond), 2008; 58 (3): 226–7.
2. Cormack J, Marinker M, Morrell D. *Practice: A Handbook of Primary Health Care*. London: Kluwer-Harrap Handbooks, 1980; 3 (29): 3.
3. Walsh TD. *Symptom Control*. Boston: Blackwell Scientific Publications, 1989: 157–64.
4. Beck ER, Francis JL, Souhami RL. *Tutorials in Differential Diagnosis* (3rd edn). Edinburgh: Churchill Livingstone, 1993: 37.
5. Kelly DT. Cardiac failure. In: *MIMS Disease Index* (2nd edn). Sydney: IMS Publishing, 1996: 97–9.
6. Kumar PJ, Clark ML. *Clinical Medicine* (7th edn). London: Elsevier, 2009: 819–28.
7. Porter RS, Kaplan JL. *The Merck Manual of Diagnosis and Therapy* (19th edn). NJ: Merck Sharp & Dohme Corp., 2011: 1856.
8. Papadakis MA, McPhee SP. *Current Medical Diagnosis and Treatment* (52nd edn). New York: The McGraw-Hill Companies, 2013: 1602.
9. Expert group for Respiratory. Interstitial lung disease. In: eTG complete [Internet]. Melbourne: Therapeutic Guidelines Ltd. Available from: <www.tg.org.au>, accessed September 2017.
10. National Institute for Health and Care Excellence (NICE). Idiopathic pulmonary fibrosis [CG163]. London: NICE, 2013. <www.nice.org.uk> (accessed 29/5/2018).

11 Raghu G et al. An official ATS/ERS/JRS/ALAT statement: idiopathic pulmonary fibrosis: evidence-based guidelines for diagnosis and management. Am J Respir Crit Care Med, 2011; 183 (6): 788–824.

12 Molina C. Occupational extrinsic allergic alveolitis. In: Pepys J, ed., *Clinics in Immunology and Allergy*. London: WB Saunders, 1984: 173–90.

13 Papadakis MA, McPhee SP. *Current Medical Diagnosis and Treatment* (56th edn). New York: McGraw-Hill Education, 2017; 319–21.

14 Ware LB et al. The acute respiratory distress syndrome. N Engl J Med, 2000; 342: 1334.

The painful ear

50

The ears should be kept perfectly clean; but it must never be done in company. It should never be done with a pin, and still less with the fingers, but always with an ear picker.

St Jean Baptiste de la Salle (1651–1719)

Pain in the ear (otalgia) is a common symptom in general practice. It affects all ages, but is most prevalent in children, where otitis media is the commonest cause. Ear pain may be caused by disorders of the ear or may arise from other structures, and in many instances the precise diagnosis is difficult to make. Important causes of ear pain are summarised in TABLE 50.1.[1]

A patient with a painful ear often requests urgent attention, and calls in the middle of the night from anxious parents of a screaming child are commonplace. Infants may present with nothing except malaise, vomiting or screaming attacks.

Key facts and checkpoints

- Of patients presenting with earache, 77% can be expected to have acute otitis media and 12% otitis externa.
- Approximately 1 in every 25 patients in general practice will present with an earache.
- Two-thirds of children will sustain at least one episode of otitis media by their second birthday; 1 in 7 children will have had more than 6 episodes by this age.[2]
- Otitis media is unlikely to be present if the tympanic membrane (TM) is mobile. Pneumatic otoscopy greatly assists diagnosis since the most valuable sign of otitis media is absent or diminished motility of the TM.
- Bullous myringitis, which causes haemorrhagic blistering of the eardrum or external ear canal, is an uncommon cause of severe pain. It is caused by a virus, probably influenza.[3] Consider herpes zoster.
- The antibiotic of first choice for acute otitis media (children and adults) is amoxycillin.
- Otitis externa can be distinguished from otitis media by pain on movement of the pinna.

Table 50.1 Causes of ear pain

1 Ear

External ear:

- Perichondritis
- Otitis externa:
  - *Candida albicans*
  - *Aspergillus nigra*
  - *Pseudomonas* spp.
  - *Staphylococcus aureus*
- Furunculosis
- Trauma
- Neoplasia
- Herpes zoster (Ramsay–Hunt syndrome)
- Viral myringitis
- Wax-impacted

Middle ear:

- Eustachian insufficiency
- Eustachian tube dysfunction
- Barotrauma
- Acute otitis media
- Chronic otitis media and cholesteatoma
- Acute mastoiditis

2 Periotic cause

Dental disorders e.g. dental abscess; malocclusion

Upper cervical spinal dysfunction

TMJ arthralgia

Parotitis

Temporal arteritis

Lymph node inflammation

Other referred causes

Pharyngeal disorders

Tonsillitis

Glossopharyngeal neuralgia

A diagnostic approach

The five self-posed questions can be answered using the diagnostic strategy model (see TABLE 50.2).

Probability diagnosis

The commonest cause of ear pain is acute otitis media. Chronic otitis media and otitis externa are also common. In the tropics, 'tropical ear' due to acute bacterial otitis is a particular problem. Temporomandibular joint

Table 50.2	The painful ear: diagnostic strategy model
Probability diagnosis	
Otitis media (viral or bacterial)	
Otitis externa (fungal, viral or bacterial)	
TMJ arthralgia	
Eustachian tube dysfunction	
Serious disorders not to be missed	
Neoplasia of external ear	
Cancer of other sites (e.g. tongue, nasopharynx)	
Herpes zoster (Ramsay–Hunt syndrome)	
Acute mastoiditis	
Cholesteatoma	
Necrotising otitis externa	
Pitfalls (often missed)	
Foreign bodies in ear	
Hard ear wax	
Barotrauma	
Dental causes (e.g. abscess)	
Referred pain: neck, throat	
Unerupted wisdom tooth and other dental causes	
TMJ arthralgia	
Facial neuralgias, esp. glossopharyngeal	
Chondromalacia nodularis helicies	
Furuncles of canal or pinna	
Post tonsillectomy:	
• from the wound	
• from TMJ due to mouth gag	
Seven masquerades checklist	
Depression	
Spinal dysfunction (cervical)	
Is the patient trying to tell me something?	
Unlikely, but always possible with pain. More likely in children. Consider factitious pain.	

50

(TMJ) arthralgia, which may be acute or chronic, is also common and must be considered, especially when otitis media and otitis externa are excluded.

Serious disorders not to be missed

As always, it is important not to overlook malignant diseases, especially the obscure ones, such as cancer of the tongue, palate or tonsils, which cause referred pain.

Locally destructive cholesteatoma associated with chronic otitis media must be searched for. It signifies the 'unsafe' ear (see FIG. 50.1) that must be distinguished from the so-called 'safe' ear (see FIG. 50.2).

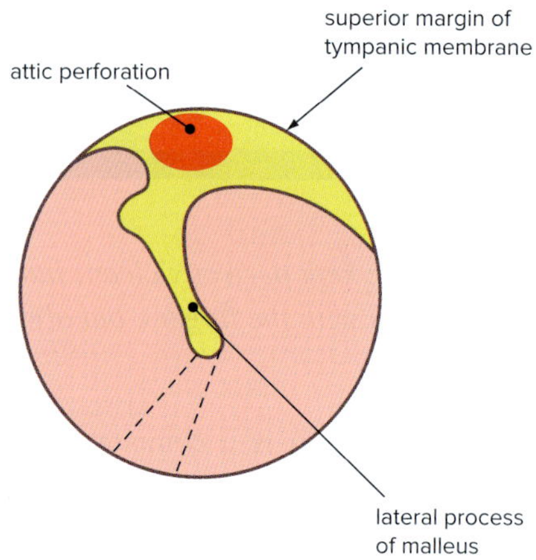

FIGURE 50.1 Infected ear: unsafe perforation

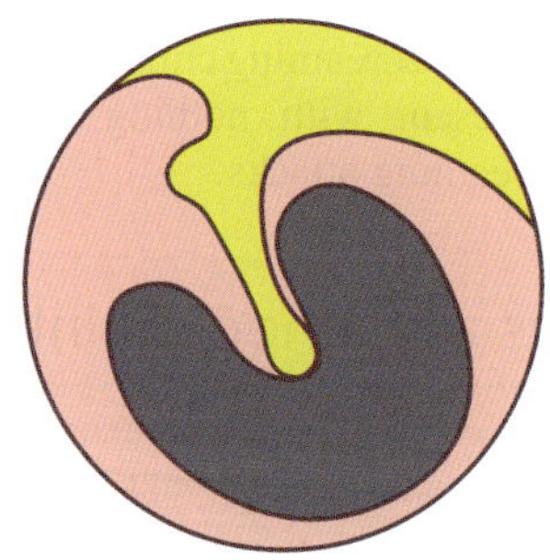

FIGURE 50.2 Infected ear: safe perforation

Herpes zoster should be considered, especially if it does not erupt on the pinna and is confined to the ear canal (usually the posterior wall), and especially in the older person.

Pitfalls

The medical aphorism 'more things are missed by not looking than by not knowing' applies particularly to the painful ear—good illumination and focusing the auroscope are mandatory. Particular attention should be paid to the external canal—look for hard wax, otitis externa, furuncles and foreign objects such as insects.

It may not be possible to visualise the TMs so it is important to clean the canal to permit this (if possible, on the first visit). Otitis media may coexist with otitis externa. Barotrauma should be considered, especially if pain follows air travel or diving.

General pitfalls

- Failing to visualise the TM before diagnosis and treatment
- Not checking out possible referral sites such as the oropharynx and teeth
- Overlooking common musculoskeletal causes such as TMJ arthralgia and cervical spondylosis
- Failing to recognise the unsafe ear

Red flag pointers for painful ear

- Offensive discharge >9 days
- Downward displacement of pinna
- Swelling behind ear
- Neurological symptoms (e.g. headaches, drowsiness)
- Older person: unexplained, intractable ear pain
- Persistent fever

Seven masquerades checklist

Of the conditions in the checklist, depression and dysfunction of the upper cervical spine have to be considered. Depressive illnesses should be considered in any patient complaining of chronic pain.

Disorders of the upper cervical spine are a commonly overlooked cause of periotic pain. Pain from the C2 and C3 levels is referred to the posterior region of the ear.

Psychogenic considerations

Such factors are unlikely, unless the pain causes discomfort in the periotic region, which is likely to be magnified by a depressive state.

The clinical approach

History

In assessing the painful ear the relevant features are:

- site of pain and radiation
- details of the onset of pain
- nature of the pain
- aggravating or relieving factors, especially swimming
- associated features such as deafness, discharge, vertigo, tinnitus and irritation of the external ear, sore throat

Agonising pain may be caused by perichondritis or furunculosis of the external ear and by the rare problem of herpes zoster (Ramsay–Hunt syndrome).[3] Movement of the pinna markedly increases the pain of acute otitis externa and perichondritis, and movement of the jaw usually causes an exacerbation of TMJ arthralgia or severe otitis externa.

Key questions (especially children)

- Where is the pain?
- Is it in the ear, behind or below it?
- Is it in one ear or both ears?
- Have you noticed any other symptoms such as sore throat, fever or vomiting?
- Has anyone hit you over the ear?
- Has there been a discharge from the ear?
- Have you noticed any deafness?
- Are you allergic to penicillin?
- Have you been swimming in a spa, and where?
- Have you been in an aeroplane?

Examination

The patient's general state and behaviour is observed during the history taking. Sudden, jabbing pain may indicate neuralgia, particularly glossopharyngeal neuralgia or a severe infection. The external ear is carefully inspected and the pinna manipulated to determine any tenderness.

Palpate the face and neck and include the parotid glands, regional lymph nodes, the mastoid process and the skin. Inspect the TMJs—tenderness from dysfunction typically lies immediately in front of the external auditory meatus. Palpate the TMJ over the lateral aspect at the joint disc. Ask the patient to open the mouth fully when tenderness is maximal. The TMJ can be palpated posteriorly by inserting the little finger into the external canal.

Inspect both ear canals and TMs with the auroscope, using the largest earpiece that comfortably fits into the canal. Better visualisation of the TM can be achieved by pulling the pinna back and downwards in young children and up and back in older children—see FIGURE 50.3 for normal appearance. Impacted wax may not explain the otalgia. If herpes zoster involves the facial nerve, vesicles may be noted in and around the external auditory meatus (notably the posterior wall).

If the diagnosis is still doubtful look for causes of referred pain; inspect the cervical spine, the nose and postnasal space and the mouth, including the teeth, pharynx and larynx.

Pharyngeal and mandibular causes of periotic pain are summarised in FIGURES 50.4 and 50.5.

Inspect sites supplied by the nerves V2, IX, X, XI, C1, C2 and C3 to exclude other causes of referred pain.

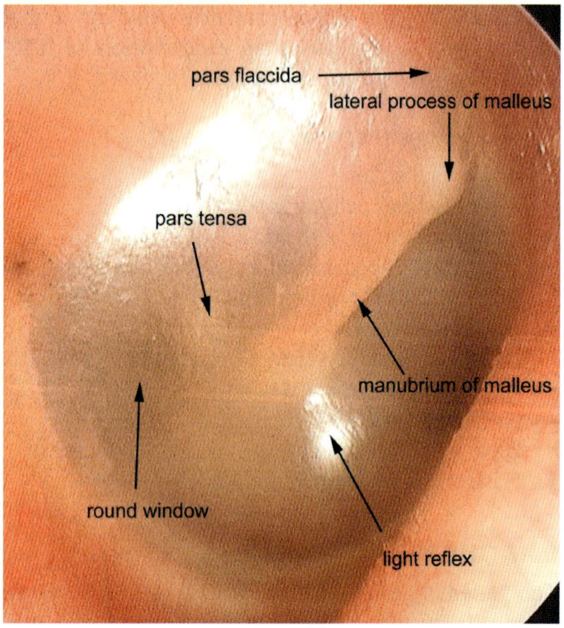

FIGURE 50.3 Normal right tympanic membrane

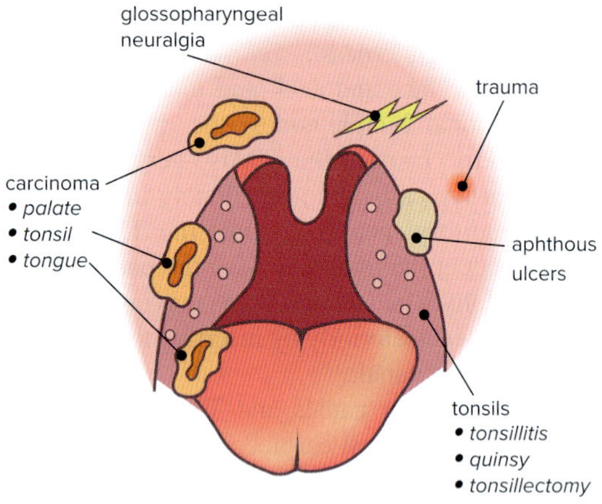

FIGURE 50.4 Pharyngeal causes of otalgia

Source: Courtesy of Bruce Black

Investigations

Investigations are seldom necessary. Hearing tests are essential, especially for children. Simple tests such as speech discrimination, hair rubbing and tuning fork tests can be used. Otherwise audiometry can be used. Audiometry combined with tympanometry and physical measurement of the volume of the ear canal can be performed in children, irrespective of age.

Swabs from discharge, especially to determine bacterial causes, such as *Staphylococcus aureus* or *Pseudomonas* spp. infection, may be necessary. However, swabs are of no value if the TM is intact.

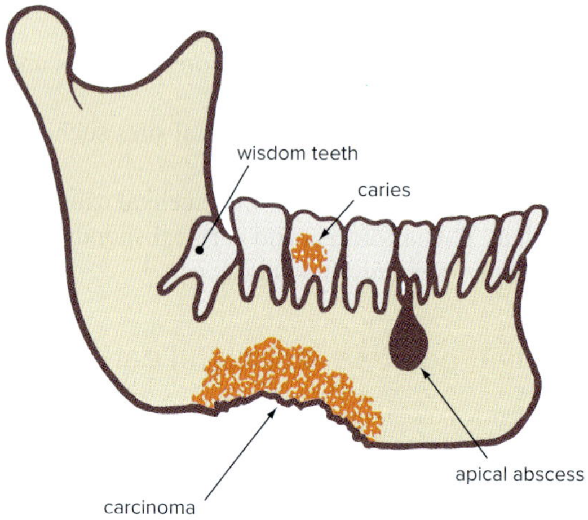

FIGURE 50.5 Mandibular causes of otalgia

Source: Courtesy of Bruce Black

Radiology and CT/MRI scanning may be indicated for special conditions such as a suspected extraotic malignancy.

Ear pain in children

Important causes of primary otalgia in children include otitis media, otitis externa, external canal furuncle or abscess, chronic eczema with fissuring of the auricle, impacted wax, foreign body, barotrauma, perichondritis, mastoiditis and bullous myringitis. Secondary otalgia includes pharyngeal lesions, dental problems, gingivostomatitis, mumps and postauricular lymphadenopathy. Peritonsillar abscess (quinsy) may cause ear pain.

Foreign bodies

Foreign bodies (FBs) are frequently inserted into the ear canal (see FIG. 50.6). They can usually be syringed out or lifted with thin forceps. Various improvised methods can be used to remove FBs in cooperative children. These include a probe to roll out the FB or a rubber catheter used as a form of suction or otherwise a fine sucker.[6]

Probe method

This requires good vision using a head mirror or head light and a thin probe. The probe is inserted under and just beyond the FB. Lever it in such a way that the tip of the probe 'rolls' the foreign body out of the obstructed passage.

Rubber catheter suction method

The only equipment required for this relatively simple and painless method is a straight rubber catheter (large type) and perhaps a suction pump. The end of the

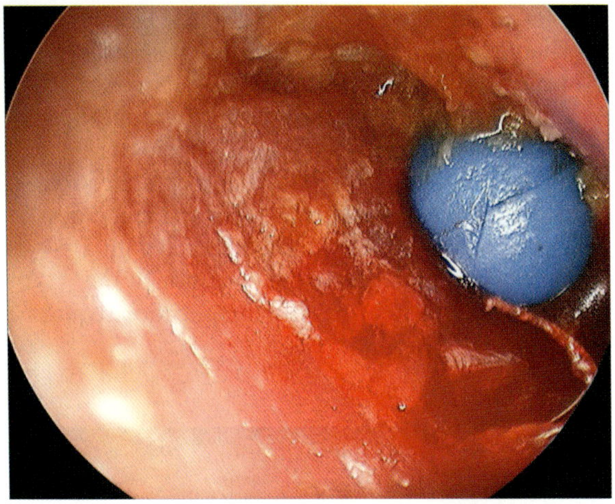

FIGURE 50.6 Foreign body (bead) in ear canal of a 3-year-old child, showing reactive tissue in ear canal

catheter is cut at right angles, a thin smear of petroleum jelly is applied to the rim and this end is applied to the FB. Suction is applied either orally or by a pump. Gentle pump suction is preferred but it is advisable to pinch closed the suction catheter until close to the FB as the hissing noise may frighten the child.

Insects in the ear

Live insects should be immobilised by first instilling Aquaear drops or olive oil, and then syringing the ear with warm water.

Dead flies that have originally been attracted to pus are best removed by suction.

Note: If simple methods such as syringing fail to dislodge the FB it is important to refer for examination and removal under microscopic vision. Syringing should not be performed if there is a possibility of the FB perforating the TM.

Otitis media in children

Otitis media is very common in children and is the most common reason a child is brought in for medical attention. Persistent middle ear effusions may follow and affect the language and cognitive development of young children.

Clinical features

- Two peaks of incidence: 6–12 months of age and school entry
- Seasonal incidence coincides with URTIs
- Bacteria cause two-thirds of cases[5]
- The commonest organisms are *Streptococcus pneumoniae, Haemophilus influenzae* and *Moraxella catarrhalis*
- Fever, irritability, otalgia and otorrhoea may be present
- The main symptoms in older children are increasing earache and hearing loss
- Pulling at the ears is a common sign in infants
- Removal of wax is necessary in about 30% to visualise the TM

Visualisation of the tympanic membrane

Use the largest ear speculum that will comfortably fit in the child's ear. A good technique to enable the examination of the ears (also nose and throat) in a reluctant child is where the child is held against the parent's chest while the parent's arm embraces the child's arm and trunk.

Note the following features of the TM: translucency, colour, position and motility.

Treatment

Many children with viral URTIs have mild reddening or dullness of the eardrum and antibiotics are not warranted, particularly in the absence of systemic features (fever and vomiting).[5] Best practice at this stage is symptomatic relief with analgesics and either watchful waiting, especially in healthy children over 6 months, or antibiotics.[6] In contrast, where the eardrum is red or yellow and bulging, with loss of anatomical landmarks, antibiotic therapy is indicated.[7]

The debate about the role of antibiotics in acute otitis media is controversial. An Australian study revealed that antibiotics provided only modest benefit: up to 20 children must be treated to prevent one child from experiencing pain by 2–7 days after presentation.[6,8,9] A North American survey concluded: 'treat children who are very ill (approximately 15%) with antibiotics immediately. Treat all others for pain and pain only and follow up according to age. Treat with antibiotics if more serious symptoms develop, or the fever, pain and other symptoms do not resolve within the time frame'.[9]

50

Possible clinical indications for antibiotics in children with painful otitis media[5,6]

Consider immediate treatment:

- acute OM in the only hearing ear
- risk of complications in those at risk, e.g. cochlear implant (usually IV antibiotics) or Indigenous children

Other considerations:

- sick child with fever
- vomiting
- red–yellow bulging TM
- loss of TM landmarks or perforation
- persistent fever and pain after 48 hours' conservative approach

The antibiotic of choice for children with systemic features is:[5]

amoxycillin 15 mg/kg 8-hourly up to 500 mg (o) for 5 days
or
amoxycillin 30 mg/kg 12-hourly (o) for 5 days

Amoxycillin is also the preferred choice in the US and UK.[10]

If β-lactamase-producing bacteria are suspected or documented, or initial treatment fails, use:

(if resistance to amoxycillin is suspected or proven) amoxycillin/potassium clavulanate
or
cefaclor 12.5 mg/kg/day (max. 750 mg/day) orally in three divided doses for 5–7 days (if penicillin hypersensitive) or cefuroxamine

With appropriate treatment most children with acute otitis media are significantly improved within 48 hours. Parents should be encouraged to contact their doctor if no improvement occurs within 72 hours. This problem is usually due to a resistant organism or suppuration. The patient should be re-evaluated at 10 days.[10]

It is of interest that some practitioners refer to the 'Pollyanna' phenomenon when treating otitis media; that is, all antibiotics seem to work!

Antibiotic drops

A randomised trial has found that antibiotic eardrops are superior to oral antibiotics for the treatment of acute otorrhoea in children with grommets.[11] This method has advocates among specialists who recommend ciprofloxacin drops following aural toilet.

Symptomatic treatment

Rest the patient in a warm room with adequate humidity. Use analgesics such as paracetamol (acetaminophen) or ibuprofen in high dosage. Although the use of antihistamines and decongestants has not been verified scientifically, the author has found nasal decongestants (as oxymetazoline nasal drops or sprays) effective in distressed children with an associated URTI. Otherwise, avoid antihistamines and decongestants.

Follow-up: adequate follow-up with hearing assessment is mandatory.

Complications[5,6]

- *Middle ear effusion.* 70% of children will have an effusion present 2 weeks from the time of diagnosis, 40% at 4 weeks, with 10% having persistent effusions for 3 months or more. If the effusion is still present at 6–8 weeks, a second course of antibiotics should be prescribed.[2] If the effusion persists beyond 3 months, refer for an ENT opinion or earlier if an associated speech delay or educational difficulty (especially a 20 dB hearing loss).
- *Acute mastoiditis.* This is a major complication that presents with pain, swelling and tenderness developing behind the ear associated with a general deterioration in the condition of the child (see FIG 50.7). Such a complication requires immediate referral.

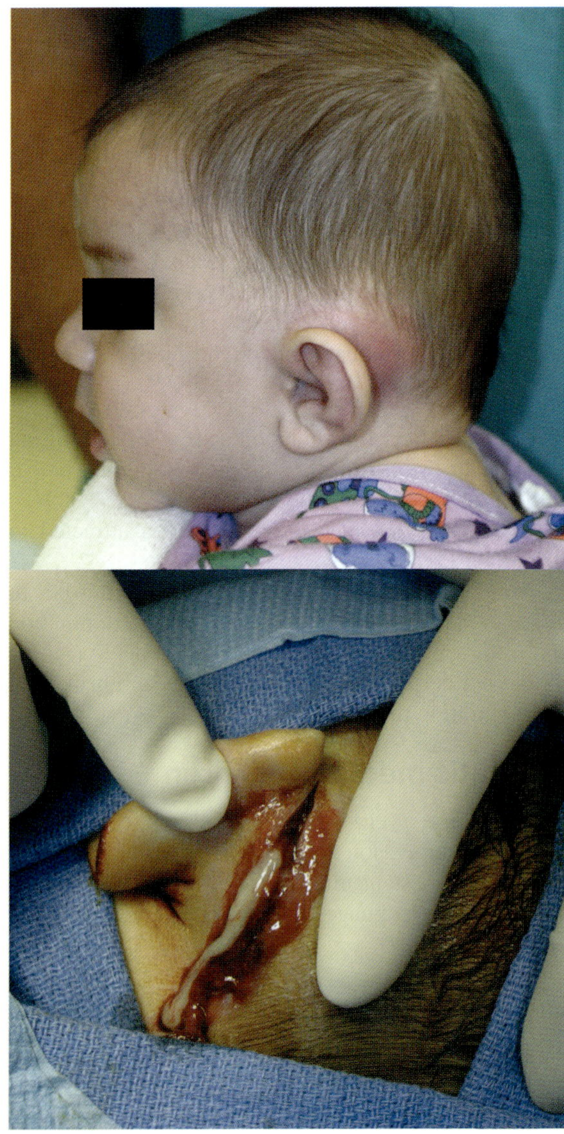

FIGURE 50.7 Mastoiditis in a child with recurrent otitis media showing erythema and swelling behind the ear. Surgical drainage was performed

- *Chronic suppurative otitis media.* Discharge through a perforation of the TM >6 weeks.
- *Rare complications.* These include labyrinthitis, petrositis, facial paresis and intracranial abscess.
- *Serous otitis media (glue ear).* This represents incomplete resolution of suppurative otitis media. Signs include loss of drum mobility, hearing loss and abnormal impedance confirmed by pneumatic otoscopy or tympanometry. Most resolve spontaneously but any necessary treatment includes medications such as bromhexine elixir and Demazin syrup, auto-inflations and Otovent assisted nasal inflation.

If an effusion lasts for >3 months, arrange for a hearing assessment and consider referral to an ENT surgeon for possible tympanostomy tubes (grommets).[13]

Note: a proposed *S. pneumoniae* and *H. influenzae* conjugate vaccine may be an effective preventive measure for childhood otitis media.

Recurrent acute otitis media

Antibiotic prevention of acute otitis media is indicated (arguably) if it occurs more often than every other month or for three or more episodes in 6 months or >4 in 12 months:[14]

chemoprophylaxis (for about 4 months)

amoxycillin twice daily (first choice)

or

cefaclor twice daily

Consider *Pneumococcus* vaccine in children over 18 months of age (if not already given) in combination with the antibiotic. Avoid smoke exposure (cigarettes and wood fires) and group child care.

Consider review by ENT consultant.

Viral infections

Most children with viral URTIs have mild–moderate reddening or dullness of the eardrum and antibiotics are not warranted. If painful bullous otitis media is present, either prick the bulla with a sterile needle for pain relief, or instil dehydrating eardrops such as anhydrous glycerol.

Ear pain in adults and the elderly

Causes of otalgia that mainly afflict the elderly include herpes zoster (Ramsay–Hunt syndrome), TMJ arthralgia, temporal arteritis and neoplasia. It is especially important to search for evidence of malignancy.

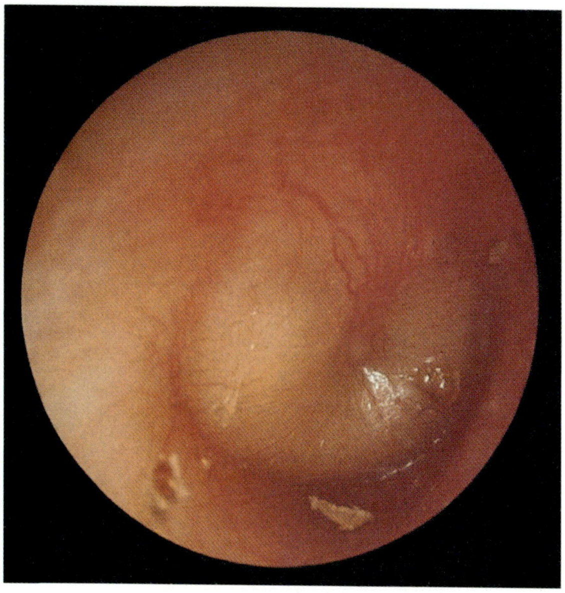

FIGURE 50.8 Acute otitis media causing true otalgia. The ear drum bulges laterally due to pus in the middle ear. Perforation and otorrhoea imminent.

Acute otitis media

Acute otitis media causes deep-seated ear pain, deafness and often systemic illness (see FIG. 50.8). The sequence of symptoms is a blocked ear feeling, pain and fever. Discharge may follow if the TM perforates, with relief of pain and fever.

The commonest organisms are viruses (adenovirus and enterovirus), and the bacteria *H. influenzae, S. pneumoniae, Moraxella* (previously *Neisseria catarrhalis*) and β-haemolytic streptococci.

The two cardinal features of diagnosis are inflammation and middle ear effusion.

Appearance of the tympanic membrane (all ages)

Translucency. If the middle ear structures are clearly visible through the drum, otitis media is unlikely.

Colour. The normal TM is a shiny pale-grey to brown: a yellow colour is suggestive of an effusion.

Diagnosis

The main diagnostic feature is the redness of the TM. The inflammatory process usually begins in the upper posterior quadrant and spreads peripherally and down the handle of the malleus (see FIG. 50.9). The TM will be seen to be reddened and inflamed with engorgement of the vessels, particularly along the handle of the malleus. The loss of light reflex follows and anatomical features

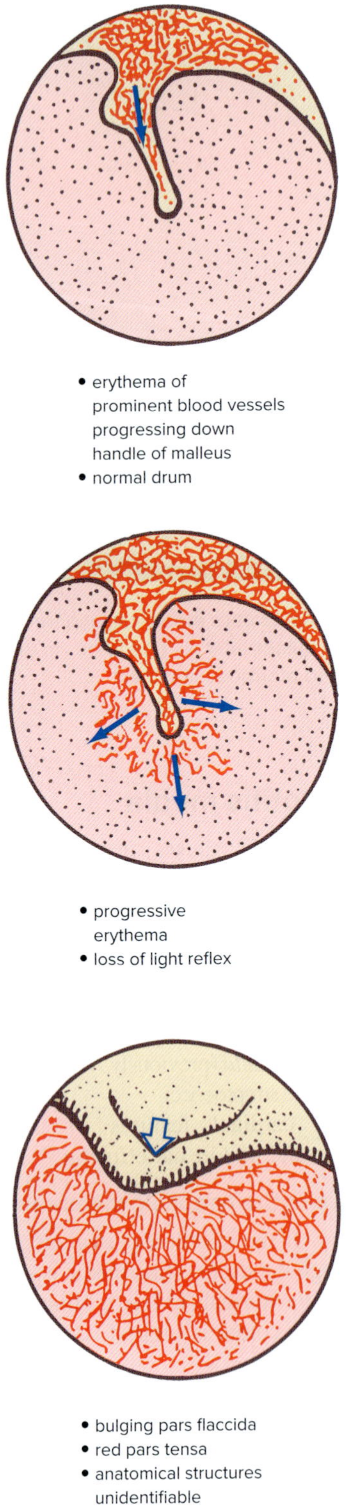

FIGURE 50.9 The appearances of the left tympanic membrane in the progressive development of acute otitis media

then become difficult to recognise as the TM becomes oedematous. Bulging of the drum is a late sign. Blisters are often seen on the TM and this is thought to be due to a viral infection in the epidermal layers of the drum.

Treatment of acute otitis media (adults)

- Analgesics to relieve pain
- Adequate rest in a warm room
- Nasal decongestants for nasal congestion
- Antibiotics until resolution of all signs of infection
- Treat associated conditions (e.g. adenoid hypertrophy)
- Follow-up: review and test hearing audiometrically

Antibiotic treatment[5]

First choice:

amoxycillin 750 mg (o) bd for 5 days[5]
or
500 mg (o) tds for 5 days

A longer course (up to 10 days) may be required depending on severity and response to 5-day course.

Alternatives:

doxycycline 100 mg (o) bd for 5–7 days (daily for milder infections)
or
cefaclor 250 mg (o) tds for 5–7 days
or
(if resistance to amoxycillin is suspected or proven) amoxycillin/potassium clavulanate 500/125 mg (o) tds for 5 days (the most effective antibiotic)

Consider surgical intervention for failed therapy.

CHRONIC OTITIS MEDIA

There are two types of chronic suppurative otitis media and they both present with deafness and discharge without pain. The discharge occurs through a perforation in the TM: one is safe (see FIG. 50.10a), the other unsafe (see FIG. 50.10b).

Chronic discharging otitis media (safe)[5,13]

If aural discharge persists for >6 weeks after a course of antibiotics, treatment can be with topical steroid and antibiotic combination drops, following ear toilet. The toileting can be done at home by dry mopping with rolled tissue spear. If persistent, referral to exclude cholesteatoma or chronic osteitis is advisable.

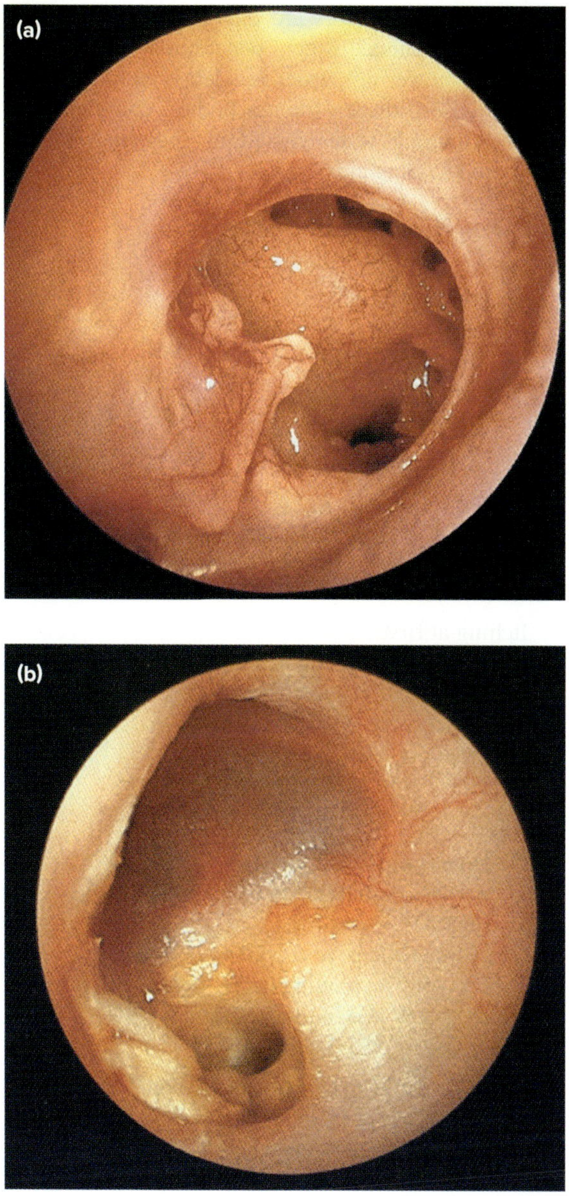

FIGURE 50.10 **(a)** Chronic otitis media with loss of the tympanic membrane; this is 'safe ear' **(b)** Unsafe ear: chronic otitis media with attic cholesteatoma.

Recognising the unsafe ear

Examination of an infected ear should include inspection of the attic region, the small area of drum between the lateral process of the malleus, and the roof of the external auditory canal immediately above it. A perforation here renders the ear 'unsafe' (see FIG. 50.1); other perforations, not involving the drum margin (see FIG. 50.2), are regarded as 'safe'.[13]

Cholesteatoma[12]

Refer CHAPTER 43.

The status of a perforation depends on the presence of accumulated squamous epithelium (termed cholesteatoma) in the middle ear, because this erodes bone. An attic perforation contains such material; safe perforations do not.

Red flags for cholesteatoma include meningitis-type features, cranial nerve deficits, sensorineural hearing loss and persistent deep ear pain.

Cholesteatoma is visible through the hole as white flakes, unless it is obscured by discharge or a persistent overlying scab. Either type of perforation can lead to chronic infective discharge, the nature of which varies with its origin. Mucus admixture is recognised by its stretch and recoil when this discharge is being cleaned from the external auditory canal. The types of discharge are compared in TABLE 50.3.

Table 50.3 Comparison of types of discharge

	Unsafe	Safe
Source	Cholesteatoma	Mucosa
Odour	Foul	Inoffensive
Amount	Usually scant, never profuse	Can be profuse
Nature	Purulent	Mucopurulent

Management

If an attic perforation is recognised or suspected, specialist referral is essential. Cholesteatoma cannot be eradicated by medical means: surgical removal is necessary to prevent a serious infratemporal or intracranial complication. Adjunct suction with care may be necessary to decompress the mass.

DIAGNOSTIC STRATEGY FOR EAR DISCHARGE (OTORRHOEA) MASS

Otitis externa[13]

Otitis externa (see FIG. 50.11), also known as 'swimmer's ear', 'surfer's ear' and 'tropical ear', is common in a country whose climate and coastal living leads to extensive water sports. It is more prevalent in hot humid conditions and therefore in the tropics.

Table 50.4	Ear discharge: diagnostic strategy model
Probability diagnosis Acute otitis media with perforation Chronic suppurative otitis media Furuncle (boil) of ear canal Infected otitis externa Reactive skin conditions (e.g. eczema) Liquefied wax	
Serious disorders not to be missed Infections: • *Pseudomonas pyocyanae* • cholesteatoma • herpes zoster oticus • mastoiditis Cancer: • malignancy with discharge (e.g. SCC) Other: • cerebrospinal fluid otorrhoea (fractured temporal bone) • necrotising otitis media	
Pitfalls (often missed) Foreign body with infection/liquidisation (e.g. insects) Trauma ± blood Rarities: • keratitis obliterans • branchial or salivary fistula • Wegener granulomatosis	
Is the patient trying to tell me something? Factitious ? Excessive manipulation of ear canal	
Diagnostic tip Acute ear discharge is most likely due to otitis externa or perforated ear drum with otitis media	

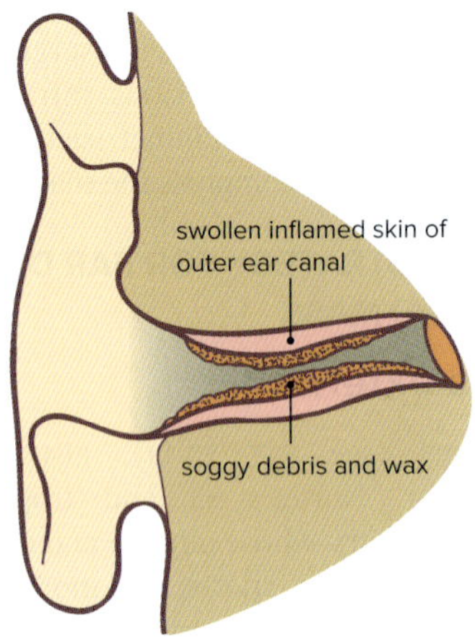

FIGURE 50.11 Otitis externa

50

Predisposing factors are allergic skin conditions, ear canal trauma, water penetration (swimming, humidity, showering), water and debris retention (wax, dermatitis, exostoses), foreign bodies, contamination from swimming water including spas, and use of Q tips and hearing aids.

Common responsible organisms

- Bacteria:
  - *Pseudomonas* sp.
  - *Escherichia coli*
  - *S. aureus*
  - *Proteus* sp.
  - *Klebsiella* sp.
- Fungi:
  - *Candida albicans*
  - *Aspergillus* sp.

Clinical features

- Itching at first
- Otalgia/pain (mild to intense) in 70%
- Fullness in ear canal
- Scant discharge
- Hearing loss

Signs

- Oedema (mild to extensive)
- Tenderness on moving auricle or jaw
- Erythema
- Discharge (offensive if coliform)
- Pale cream 'wet blotting paper' debris—*C. albicans*
- Black spores of *Aspergillus nigra*
- TM granular or dull red

Obtain culture, especially if resistant *Pseudomonas* sp. suspected, by using small ear swab.

Note: 'Malignant' otitis externa occurs in diabetics due to *Pseudomonas* infection at base of skull.

Management

Aural toilet

Meticulous aural toilet by gentle suction and dry mopping with a wisp of cotton wool on a fine brooch under good lighting is the keystone of management. This enables topical medication to be applied directly to the skin.

Syringing

This is appropriate in some cases but the canal must be dried meticulously afterwards. For most cases it is not recommended.

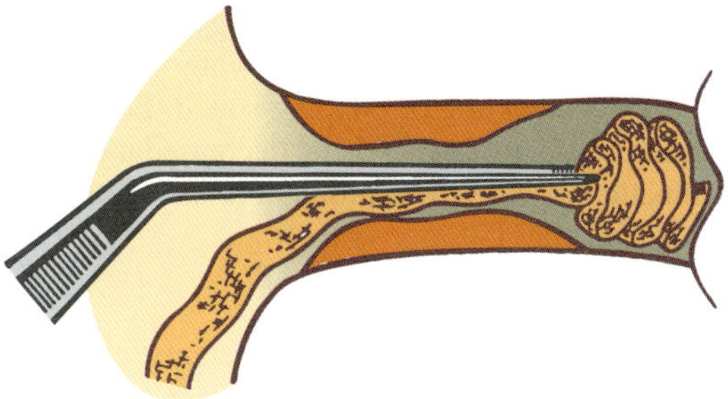

FIGURE 50.12 Insertion of a wick; it is packed gradually by short back-and-forth movements of the forceps.
Source: Courtesy of Bruce Black

Dressings

Dressings are essential in all but the mildest forms. After cleaning and drying, insert 10–20 cm of 4 mm Nufold gauze impregnated with a steroid and antibiotic cream.

For severe otitis externa, a wick is important and will reduce the oedema and pain in 12–24 hours (see FIG. 50.12). The wick can be soaked in an astringent (e.g. aluminium acetate 4% solution or glycerin and 10% ichthammol). The wick needs replacement daily until the swelling has subsided.

Topical antimicrobials for acute diffuse otitis externa[5]

Most effective, especially when the canal is open, is an antibacterial, antifungal and corticosteroid preparation such as Kenacomb or Sofradex drops (2–3 drops tds), Locacorten-Vioform drops (2–3 drops bd) or Ciproxin HC (3 drops bd). Be cautious of ear drops with neomycin (hypersensitivity). The tragus should be pumped for 30 seconds after instillation by pressing on it repeatedly, within the limitation of any pain.

Other measures[13]

- Strong analgesics are essential
- Antibiotics have a minimal place in treatment unless a spreading cellulitis has developed (refer if in doubt)
- Prevent scratching and entry of water
- Use a wick soaked in combination steroid and antibiotic ointment for more severe cases

> **Practice tip for severe 'tropical ear'**
>
> Prednisolone (o) 15 mg statim then 10 mg 8-hourly for six doses followed by:
>
> - Merocel ear wick
> - topical Kenacomb or Sofradex drops

Prevention

- Keep the ear dry, especially those involved in water sports
- Protect the ear with various waterproofing methods:
  - cotton wool coated with petroleum jelly
  - an antiseptic drying agent (e.g. ethanol) after swimming and showering
  - tailor-made ear plugs (e.g. EAR foam plugs)
  - silicone putty or Blu-Tack
  - a bathing cap pulled well forward allows these plugs to stay *in situ*
- Avoid poking objects such as hairpins and cotton buds in the ear to clean the canal
- If water enters, shake it out or use Aquaear (acetic acid) drops (spirit drops to help dry the canal)

Necrotising otitis externa

This severe complication, usually due to *Pseudomonas aeruginosa*, can occur in the immunocompromised, diabetic or elderly patient. It involves cartilage and bone and should be considered with treatment failure, severe persistent pain, fever and visible granulation tissue. Urgent referral is advisable.

Ear exostoses ('surfer's ear')

These periosteal bony overgrowths are usually caused by water retention in the ear. They are often multiple. They tend to trap keratin, wax and water, leading to infection.

50

Prevention

- Use plugs or Blu-Tack to waterproof ear.
- Dry thoroughly with hair dryer after swimming.

They may require surgical removal.

Acute localised otitis externa (furunculosis)

Furunculosis is a staphylococcal infection of the hair follicle in the outer cartilaginous part of the ear canal. It is usually intensely painful. Fever occurs only when the infection spreads in front of the ear as cellulitis. The pinna is tender on movement—a sign that is not a feature of acute otitis media. The furuncle (boil) may be seen in the external auditory meatus (see FIG. 50.13).

Management

- If pointing, it can be incised after a local anaesthetic or freezing spray
- Warmth (e.g. use hot washcloth, hot water bottle)
- If fever with cellulitis—flu/dicloxacillin or cephalexin

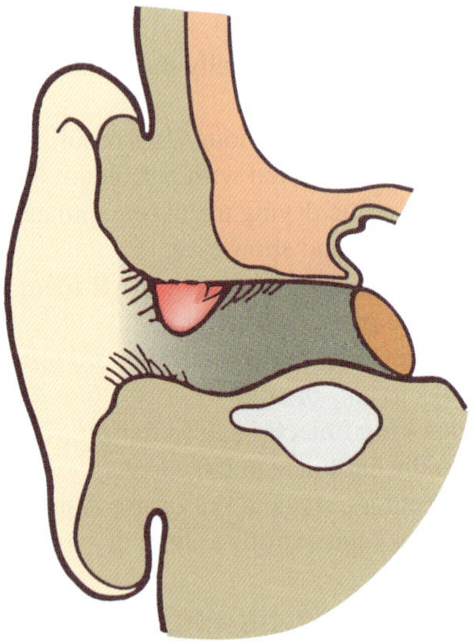

FIGURE 50.13 Furuncle (boil) in hair-bearing area at opening of the ear canal

Perichondritis

Perichondritis is infection of the cartilage of the ear characterised by severe pain of the pinna, which is red, swollen and exquisitely tender. It is rare and follows trauma or surgery to the ear. As the organism is frequently *P. pyocyaneus,* the appropriate antibiotics must be carefully chosen (e.g. ciprofloxacin).

Infected ear lobe

The cause is most likely a contact allergy to nickel in an earring, complicated by a *S. aureus* infection.

Management

- Discard the earrings
- Clean the site to eliminate residual traces of nickel
- Swab the site and then commence antibiotics (e.g. flucloxacillin or erythromycin)
- Instruct the patient to clean the site daily, and then apply the appropriate ointment
- Use a 'noble metal' stud to keep the tract patent
- Advise the use of only gold, silver or platinum studs in future

Eustachian tube dysfunction

This is a common cause of discomfort.[15] Symptoms include fullness in the ear, pain of various levels and impairment of hearing. The most common causes of dysfunction are disorders causing oedema of the tubal lining, such as viral URTI and allergy when the tube is only partially blocked; swallowing and yawning may elicit a crackling or popping sound. Examination reveals retraction of the TM and decreased mobility on pneumatic otoscopy. The problem is usually transient after a viral URTI.

Treatment

- Systemic and intranasal decongestants (e.g. pseudoephedrine or corticosteroids in allergic patients)
- Autoinflation by forced exhalation against closed nostrils (avoid in active intranasal infection)
- Avoid air travel, rapid altitude change and underwater diving

Otic barotrauma

Barotrauma is damage caused by undergoing rapid changes in atmospheric pressure in the presence of an occluded Eustachian tube (see FIG. 50.14). It affects scuba divers and aircraft travellers.

The symptoms include temporary or persistent pain or pressure in both ears, deafness, vertigo, tinnitus and perhaps discharge.

Inspection of the TM may reveal (in order of seriousness): retraction; erythema; haemorrhage (due to extravasation of blood into the layers of the TM); fluid or blood in the middle ear; perforation. Perform conductive hearing loss tests with tuning fork.

Treatment

Most cases are mild and resolve spontaneously in a few days, so treat with analgesics and reassurance. Menthol inhalations are soothing and effective. Refer

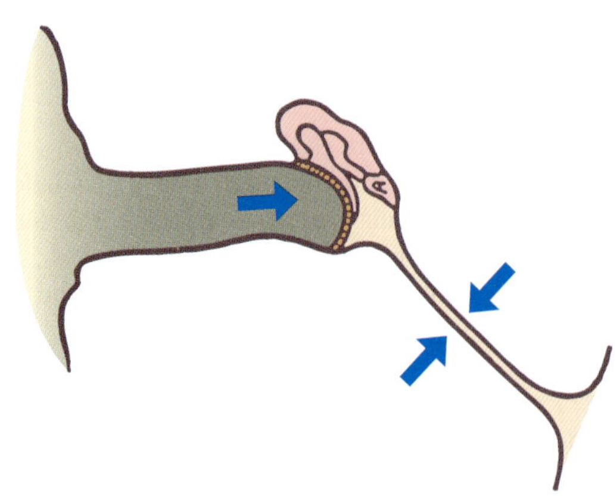

FIGURE 50.14 Mechanism of barotrauma, with blocking of the Eustachian tube due to increased pressure at the sites indicated.

Source: Courtesy of Bruce Black

if any persistent problems for consideration of the Politzer bag inflation or myringotomy.

Prevention

Flying. Perform repeated Valsalva manoeuvres during descent. Use decongestant drops or sprays before boarding the aircraft, and then 2 hours before descent.

Diving. Those with nasal problems, otitis media or chronic tubal dysfunction should not dive.

Penetrating injury to tympanic membrane

A penetrating injury to the TM can occur in children and adults from various causes such as pencils and slivers of wood or glass. Bleeding invariably follows and infection is the danger.

Management

- Remove blood clot by suction toilet or gentle dry mopping
- Ensure no FB is present
- Check hearing
- Prescribe a course of broad-spectrum antibiotics (e.g. cotrimoxazole)
- Prescribe analgesics
- Instruct patient not to let water enter ear
- Review in 2 days and then regularly
- At review in 1 month, the drum should be virtually healed
- Check hearing 2 months after injury

Complete healing can be expected within 8 weeks in 90–95% of such cases.[16]

Temporomandibular joint arthralgia

If rheumatoid arthritis is excluded, a set of special exercises, which may include 'chewing' a piece of soft wood over the molars, invariably solves this problem (see CHAPTER 52). If an obvious dental malocclusion is present, referral is necessary.

When to refer

Otitis media

- Incomplete resolution of acute otitis media
- Persistent middle ear effusion for 3 months after an attack of acute otitis media
- Persistent apparent or proved deafness
- Evidence or suspicion of acute mastoiditis or other severe complications
- Frequent recurrences (e.g. four attacks a year)
- Presence of craniofacial abnormalities

Other ear problems

- Attic perforation/cholesteatoma
- FBs in ear not removed by simple measures such as syringing
- No response to treatment after 2 weeks for otitis externa
- Suspicion of carcinoma of the ear canal
- Acute TM perforation that has not healed in 6 weeks
- Chronic TM perforation (involving lower two-thirds of TM)

Practice tips

- The pain of acute otitis media may be masked by fever in babies and young children.
- A red TM is not always caused by otitis media. The blood vessels of the drum head may be engorged from crying, sneezing or nose blowing. In crying babies, the TM as well as the face may be red.
- In otitis externa, most cases will resolve rapidly if the ear canal is expanded and then cleaned meticulously.
- If an adult presents with ear pain but normal auroscopy, examine possible referral sites, namely TMJ, mouth, throat, teeth and cervical spine.
- Consider mastoiditis if foul-smelling discharge is present over 7+ days.
- Antibiotics have no place in the treatment of otic barotrauma.
- It is good practice to make relief of distressing ear pain a priority. Adequate analgesics must be given. There is a tendency to give too low a dose of paracetamol in children. The installation of nasal drops in infants with a snuffy nose and acute otitis media can indirectly provide amazing pain relief.
- Spirit ear drops APF are a cheap and simple agent to use for recurrent otitis externa where wetness of the ear canal is a persistent problem.

Patient education resources

Hand-out sheets from *Murtagh's Patient Education* 7th edition:

- Earache in children
- Ear infection (otitis media)
- Ear: otitis externa
- Ear: wax in your ear

References

1 Black B. Otalgia. Aust Fam Physician, 1987; 16: 292–6.

2 Lieberthal AS et al. The diagnosis and management of acute otitis media. Pediatrics, 2013; 131 (3): e964–99.

3 Ludman H. *ABC of Otolaryngology* (3rd edn). London: BMJ, 1993.

4 Murtagh J. *Practice Tips* (6th edn). Sydney: McGraw-Hill, 2013: 134–6.

5 Expert group for Antibiotic. Ear, nose and throat infections. In: eTG complete [Internet]. Melbourne: Therapeutic Guidelines Ltd. Available from: <www.tg.org.au>, accessed September 2017.

6 Morris PS, Leach AJ. Managing otitis media: an evidence-based approach. Australian Prescriber, 2009; 32 (6): 155–9.

7 Del Mar C, Glasziou P, Hayem M. Are antibiotics indicated for the initial treatment of acute otitis media in children? A meta analysis. BMJ, 1997; 314: 1526–9.

8 Venekamp RP et al. Antibiotics for acute otitis media in children (Cochrane Review). Cochrane Database. Syst Rev. 2013, Issue 1. Art No. CD000219.

9 Rosser W, Shafir M. *Evidence-Based Family Medicine.* Hamilton: BC Decker, 1998: 111–13.

10 Gunasekera H. Otitis media in children: how to treat. Australian Doctor, 18 July 2008: 33–40.

11 Van Dongen TM, van der Heijden GJ et al. Treatment of otitis media in children under 2 years of age. N Eng J Med, 2014; 370: 723–33.

12 Black B. Otitis media: how to treat. Australian Doctor, 29 November 2002: I–VIII.

13 Kaushik V, Malik T, Saeed SR. Intervention for acute otitis externa (Cochrane Review). Cochrane Database. Syst Rev. 2010, Issue 1. Art No. CD004740.

14 Buckley N (Chair). *Australian Medicines Handbook.* Adelaide: Australian Medicines Handbook Pty Ltd, 2013: 386–7.

15 Papadakis MD, McPhee SJ. *Current Medical Diagnosis and Treatment* (52nd edn). New York: The McGraw-Hill Companies, 2013; 201–2.

16 Kruger R, Black B. Penetrating injury eardrum. Aust Fam Physician, 1986; 15: 735.

Resources

National Health and Medical Research Council (NHMRC). Australian Clinical Practice Guidelines. <https://www.clinicalguidelines.gov.au>

National Institute for Health and Care Excellence (NICE). Respiratory tract infection: Antibiotic prescribing. London: NICE, 2008. <https://www.nice.org.uk/guidance/cg69/evidence/full-guideline-196853293>

The Royal Children's Hospital Melbourne. Australian clinical practice guidelines for managing acute otitis media. Melbourne: RCH, last updated April 2018. <https://www.rch.org.au/clinicalguide/guideline_index/Acute_otitis_media/>

The red and tender eye 51

Those with sore eyes . . . find the light painful, while the darkness, which permits them to see nothing, is restful and agreeable.

DIO CHRYSOSTOM (40–115 CE)

A red eye accounts for at least 80% of patients with eye problems encountered in general practice.[1] An accurate history combined with a thorough examination will permit the diagnosis to be made in most cases without recourse to specialist ophthalmic equipment. A summary of the diagnostic strategy model is presented in TABLE 51.1.

Table 51.1 The red and tender eye: diagnostic strategy model

Probability diagnosis Conjunctivitis: • bacterial • adenovirus • allergic
Serious disorders not to be missed Acute glaucoma Uveitis: • acute iritis • choroiditis Corneal ulcer Herpes simplex keratitis Microbial keratitis (e.g. fungal, amoebic, bacterial) Herpes zoster ophthalmicus Penetrating injury Endophthalmitis Orbital cellulitis Trachoma
Pitfalls (often missed) Scleritis/episcleritis Foreign body Trauma—contusion, penetrating injury Ultraviolet light 'keratitis' Blepharitis Cavernous sinus arteriovenous fistula
Seven masquerades checklist Drugs (hypersensitivity) Thyroid disorder (hyperthyroidism)
Is the patient trying to tell me something? Unlikely.

Key facts and checkpoints

- Acute conjunctivitis accounts for over 25% of all eye complaints seen in general practice.[2]
- A purulent discharge indicates bacterial conjunctivitis.[3]
- A clear or mucous discharge indicates viral or allergic conjunctivitis.
- Viral conjunctivitis can be slow to resolve and may last for weeks.
- Pain and visual loss suggest a serious condition such as glaucoma, uveitis (including acute iritis) or corneal ulceration.
- Beware of the unilateral red eye—think beyond bacterial or allergic conjunctivitis. It is rarely conjunctivitis and may be a corneal ulcer, keratitis, foreign body, trauma, uveitis or acute glaucoma.[4]
- Keratitis (inflammation of the cornea) is one of the most common causes of an uncomfortable red eye. Apart from the well-known viral causes (herpes simplex, herpes zoster, adenovirus and measles), it can be caused by fungal infection (usually on a damaged cornea), bacterial infection or inflammatory disorder such as ankylosing spondylitis.[5]
- Herpes simplex keratitis (dendritic ulcer) often presents painlessly as the neurotrophic effect grossly diminishes sensation.

The clinical approach

The five essentials of the history are:

- history of trauma, especially as indicator of intraocular foreign body (IOFB)
- vision
- the degree and type of discomfort
- presence of discharge
- presence of photophobia

The social and occupational history is also very important. This includes a history of exposure to a 'red eye' at school, work or home; incidents at work such as injury, welding, foreign bodies or chemicals; and genitourinary symptoms.

When examining the unilateral red eye keep the following diagnoses in mind:

- trauma
- foreign body, including IOFB
- corneal ulcer
- iritis (uveitis)
- viral conjunctivitis (commonest type)
- acute glaucoma

The manner of onset of the irritation often gives an indication of the cause. Conjunctivitis or uveitis generally has a gradual onset of redness, while a small foreign body will produce a very rapid hyperaemia. Photophobia occurs usually with uveitis and keratitis. It is vital to elicit careful information about visual acuity. The wearing of contact lenses is very important as these are prone to cause infection or the 'overwear syndrome', which resembles an acute ultraviolet (UV) burn.

The key eye symptoms

The key eye symptoms are:

- itch
- irritation
- pain (with pus or watering)
- loss of vision (red or white eye)
  - red = front of eye
  - white = back of eye

Key questions

- Have you noticed blurring of your vision?
- Have you been in close contact with others with the same condition?
- Have you had a cold or running nose recently?
- Do you wear contact lenses?
- Can you recall scratching or injuring your eye?
- What were you doing at the time you noticed trouble?
- Have you been putting any drops, ointments or cosmetics in or around your eye?
- Do you suffer from hay fever?
- Do you have any problems with your eyelids?
- Had your eyes been watering for some time beforehand?
- Have you had any other problems?
- Have you been exposed to arc welding?

Red eye red flags (urgent ophthalmic referral)[3,6]

- Severe ocular pain
- Severe orbital pain
- Reduction of vision
- Loss of vision
- Diplopia
- Dilated pupil
- Abnormal corneal signs
- Globe displacement
- Endophthalmitis
- Microbial keratitis ± contact lens use

Loss of vision in the red eye

Consider:

- iritis (uveitis)
- scleritis
- acute glaucoma (pain; nausea and vomiting)
- chemical burns

The painful red eye

Causes to consider:

- keratitis
- uveitis (iritis)
- episcleritis
- scleritis
- acute glaucoma
- hypopyon (pus in the anterior chamber)
- endophthalmitis (inflammation of internal structures—may follow surgery)
- corneal abrasion/ulceration

Pain with discharge:

- keratitis

Pain with photophobia:

- uveitis
- episcleritis

Examination

The basic equipment:

- eye testing charts at 45 cm (18 in) and 300 cm (10 ft)
- multiple pinholes
- torch (e.g. Cobalt blue)
- magnifying aid (e.g. binocular loupe)
- glass rod or cotton bud to aid eyelid eversion
- fluorescein sterile paper strips
- anaesthetic drops
- Schiotz tonometer
- ophthalmoscope
- Ishihara colour vision test

The four essentials of the examination are:

- testing and recording vision
- meticulous inspection under magnification
- testing the pupils
- testing ocular tension[4]

Also:

- local anaesthetic test
- fluorescein staining
- subtarsal examination

Inspection

A thorough inspection is essential, noting the nature of the inflammatory injection, whether it is localised (episcleritis) or diffuse, viewing the iris for any irregularity, observing the cornea, and searching for foreign bodies, especially under the eyelids, and for any evidence of penetrating injury. No ocular examination is complete until the eyelid is everted and closely inspected. Both eyes must be examined since many patients presenting with conjunctivitis in one eye will have early signs of conjunctivitis in the other. Use fluorescein to help identify corneal ulceration. Local anaesthetic drops instilled prior to the examination of a painful lesion are recommended. The local anaesthetic test is a sensitive measure of a surface problem—if the pain is unrelieved a deeper problem must be suspected.

Palpate for enlarged pre-auricular lymph nodes, which are characteristic of viral conjunctivitis.

The nature of the injection is important. In conjunctivitis the vessels are clearly delineated and branch from the corners of the eye towards the cornea, since it involves mainly the tarsal plate. Episcleral and scleral vessels are larger than conjunctival vessels and are concentrated towards the cornea (see FIG. 51.1).

Ciliary injection appears as a red ring around the limbus of the cornea (the ciliary flush), and the individual vessels, which form a parallel arrangement, are not clearly visible. Ciliary injection may indicate a more serious deep-seated inflammatory condition such as anterior uveitis or a deep corneal infection. The presence of fine follicles on the tarsal conjunctivae indicates viral infection while a cobblestone appearance indicates allergic conjunctivitis.

Note: Slit lamp examination is ideal for the examination of the eye.

Investigations

These include:

- swab of discharge for micro and culture or for viral studies
- ESR/CRP

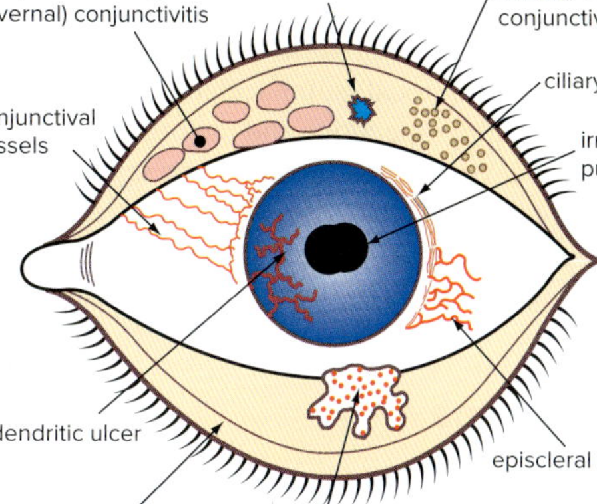

FIGURE 51.1 Physical signs to search for in a patient with a red eye (eyelids everted)

- HLA B27 antigen
- imaging

Red eye in children

Children can suffer from the various types of conjunctivitis (commonly), uveitis and trauma. Of particular concern is orbital cellulitis, which may present as a unilateral swollen lid and can rapidly lead to blindness if untreated. Bacterial, viral and allergic conjunctivitis are common in all children. Conjunctivitis in infants is a serious disorder because of the immaturity of tissues and defence mechanisms. Serious corneal damage and blindness can result.

51

Neonatal conjunctivitis (ophthalmia neonatorum)

This is conjunctivitis in an infant less than 1 month old and is a notifiable disease. Chlamydial and gonococcal infections are uncommon but must be considered if a purulent discharge is found in the first few days of life.[7] In both conditions the parents must be investigated for associated venereal infection and treated accordingly (this includes contact tracing) (see CHAPTER 134).

Chlamydia trachomatis accounts for 50% or more of cases. Its presentation in neonates is acute, usually 1–2 weeks after delivery, with moderate mucopurulent discharge. It is a systemic disease and may be associated with pneumonia. The diagnosis is confirmed by PCR tests on the conjunctival secretions.

Treatment is with azithromycin 20 mg/kg orally, daily for 3 days. Regular face washing and the treatment of all household contacts is recommended.[7]

Neisseria gonorrhoeae conjunctivitis, which usually occurs within 1–2 days of delivery, requires vigorous treatment with intravenous cephalosporins or penicillin and local sulphacetamide drops. The discharge is highly infectious and the organism has the potential for severe corneal infection or septicaemia.[7]

Other common bacterial organisms can cause neonatal conjunctivitis, and herpes simplex virus type II can cause conjunctivitis and/or eyelid vesicles or keratitis.[2]

Trachoma

More than 6 million people worldwide have trachoma-caused blindness.

Trachoma is a chlamydial conjunctivitis that is prevalent in outback areas and in the Indigenous population. *C. trachomatis* is usually transmitted by human contact between children and parents and also by flies, especially where hygiene is inadequate. It is the most common cause of blindness in the world. Recurrent and untreated disease leads to lid scarring and inturned lashes (entropion) with corneal ulceration and visual loss. It is important to commence control of the infection in childhood.

Treatment

- Prevention/community education
- Antibiotics—azithromycin
- Surgical correction (where relevant)

Blocked nasolacrimal duct

Delayed development of the nasolacrimal duct occurs in about 6% of infants,[7] resulting in blocked lacrimal drainage; the lacrimal sac becomes infected, causing a persistent discharge from one or both eyes. In the majority of infants, spontaneous resolution of the problem occurs by the age of 6 months.

Management

- Local antibiotics for infective episodes
- Bathing with normal saline
- Frequent massage over the lacrimal sac
- Referral for probing of the lacrimal passage before 6 months if the discharge is profuse and irritating or between 6 and 12 months if the problem has not self-corrected (refer CHAPTER 91)

Red eye in the elderly

In an elderly patient there is an increased possibility of acute glaucoma, uveitis and herpes zoster. Acute angle closure glaucoma should be considered in any patient over the age of 50 presenting with an acutely painful red eye.

Eyelid conditions such as blepharitis, trichiasis, entropion and ectropion are more common in the elderly.

ACUTE CONJUNCTIVITIS

Acute conjunctivitis is defined as an episode of conjunctival inflammation lasting less than 3 weeks.[2] The two major causes are infection (either bacterial or viral) and acute allergic or toxic reactions of the conjunctiva (see TABLE 51.2).

> **Practice tips**
>
> Be cautious of loss of vision, pain or photophobia—refer if appropriate.

Clinical features

- Diffuse hyperaemia of tarsal or bulbar conjunctivae
- Absence of ocular pain, good vision, clear cornea
- Infectious conjunctivitis is bilateral (usually) or unilateral (depending on the cause), with a discharge, and a gritty or sandy sensation

Bacterial conjunctivitis

Bacterial infection may be primary, secondary to a viral infection or secondary to blepharitis.

History

Purulent discharge with sticking together of eyelashes in the morning is typical. It usually starts in one eye and spreads to the other. There may be a history of contact with a person with similar symptoms. The organisms are usually picked up from contaminated fingers, face cloths or towels.

Clinical features

- Gritty red eye
- Purulent discharge
- Clear cornea

Examination

There is usually a bilateral mucopurulent discharge with uniform engorgement of all the conjunctival blood vessels and a non-specific papillary response (see FIG. 51.2). Fluorescein staining is negative.

Causative organisms

These include:

- *Streptococcus pneumoniae*
- *Haemophilus influenzae*
- *Staphylococcus aureus*
- *Streptococcus pyogenes*
- *N. gonorrhoeae* (a hyperacute onset)
- *Pseudomonas aeruginosa*

Table 51.2 Major causes of a red eye

	Site of inflammation	Pain	Discharge	Vision	Photophobia	Pupil	Cornea	Ocular tension
Bacterial conjunctivitis	Conjunctiva, including lining of lids (usually bilateral)	Irritation—gritty	Purulent, lids stuck in the morning	Normal	No	Normal	Normal	Normal
Viral conjunctivitis	Conjunctiva, lining of lids often follicular (uni or bilateral)	Gritty	Watery	Normal	No	Normal	Normal	Normal
Allergic (vernal) conjunctivitis	Conjunctiva, papillary swellings on lid linings (bilateral)	Gritty—itching	Watery	Normal	No	Normal	Normal	Normal
Contact hypersensitivity (dermato-conjunctivitis)	Conjunctiva and eyelids Oedema	Itching	Watery	Normal—may be blurred	No	Normal	Normal	Normal
Subconjunctival haemorrhage	Beefy red area fading at edge (unilateral)	No	No	Normal	No	Normal	Normal	Normal
Herpes simplex keratitis	Unilateral—circumcorneal Dendritic ulcer	Yes—gritty	No, reflex lacrimation	Blurred, but variable, depends on site	Yes	Normal	Abnormal	Normal
Corneal ulcer	Unilateral—circumcorneal (exclude foreign body)	Yes	No, reflex lacrimation	Blurred, but variable, depends on site	Yes	Normal	Abnormal	Normal
Scleritis/episcleritis	Localised deep redness Tender area	Yes	No	Normal	Yes	Normal	Normal	Normal
Acute uveitis/iritis	Maximum around cornea	Yes—radiates to brow, temple, nose	No, reflex lacrimation	Blurred	Yes	Constricted, may be irregular	Normal	Normal or low
Acute glaucoma	Diffuse but maximum circumcorneal	Yes, severe with nausea and vomiting	No, reflex lacrimation	Haloes around lights	Yes	Dilated Absent light reflex	Hazy	Hard, elevated

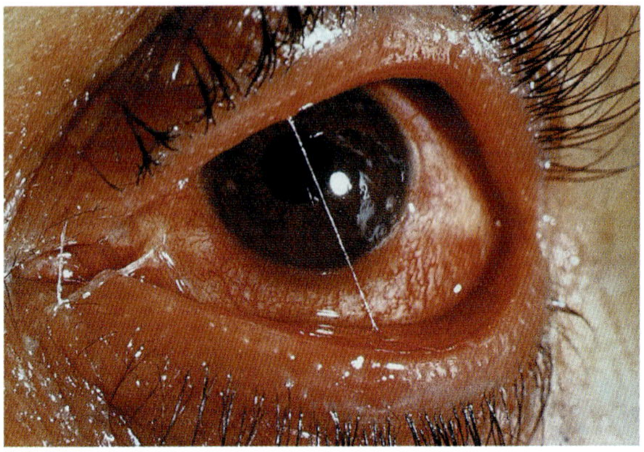

FIGURE 51.2 Acute bacterial conjunctivitis with mucopurulent discharge, no corneal stain

Diagnosis is usually clinical, but a swab should be taken for smear and culture with:[2]

- hyperacute or severe purulent conjunctivitis
- prolonged infection
- neonates

Management[7]

Limit the spread by avoiding close contact with others, use of separate towels and good ocular hygiene. Clear away debris and mucus with saline solution before topical treatment. Exclude serious causes.

Mild cases

51

Mild cases may resolve with saline irrigation of the eyelids and conjunctiva but may last up to 14 days if untreated.[8] An antiseptic eye drop such as propamidine isethionate 0.1% (Brolene) 1–2 drops, 6–8-hourly for 5–7 days can be used. Cooled black tea is reportedly widely used in Middle Eastern countries with good effect.

More severe cases

Chloramphenicol 0.5% eye drops, one drop 1–2 hourly for 24 hours,[1] decrease to 4 times a day for another 7 days (max. 10 days—cases of aplastic anaemia have been reported with long-term use).

Also use chloramphenicol 1% eye ointment each night or framycetin 0.5% eye drops, 1–2 drops every 1–2 hours for the first 24 hours, decreasing to 8-hourly until discharge resolves for up to 7 days.

Note: Never pad a discharging eye.

> **Practice tip**
>
> Brick-red eye—think of chlamydia.

Specific organisms

- *Pseudomonas* and other coliforms: use topical gentamicin and tobramycin.
- *N. gonorrhoeae:* use appropriate systemic antibiotics depending on sensitivity. Use ceftriaxone 1 g IM or IV as a single dose.[7]
- *Chlamydia trachomatis*—may be sexually transmitted (a full STI screen is advisable). Shows a brick-red follicular conjunctivitis with a stringy mucus discharge. Treatment is with azithromycin.

Viral conjunctivitis

The most common cause of this very contagious condition is adenovirus.

History

It is commonly associated with URTIs and is the type of conjunctivitis that occurs in epidemics (pink eye).[1] The conjunctivitis usually has a 2–3 week course; it is initially one-sided but with cross-infection occurring days later in the other eye. It can be a severe problem with a very irritable, watering eye.

Examination

The examination should be conducted with gloves. It is usually bilateral with diffuse conjunctival infection and productive of a scant watery discharge. Viral infections typically but not always produce a follicular response in the conjunctivae (tiny, pale lymphoid follicles) and an associated pre-auricular lymph node (see FIG. 51.3). Subconjunctival haemorrhages may occur with adenovirus infection. High magnification, ideally a slit lamp, may be necessary to visualise some of the changes, such as small corneal opacities, follicles and keratitis.

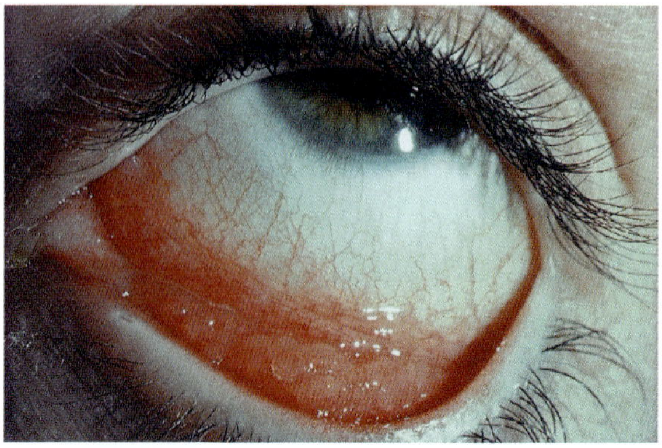

FIGURE 51.3 Viral conjunctivitis: watery eye, lid swelling, typical eyelid follicles, associated local lymphadenopathy

Diagnosis is based on clinical grounds and a history of infected contacts. Viral culture and serology can be performed to identify epidemics.

Treatment

- Limit cross-infection by appropriate rules of hygiene and patient education.
- Treatment is symptomatic—cool compress and topical lubricants (artificial tear preparations), naphazoline (e.g. Albalon), vasoconstrictors (e.g. phenylephrine) or saline bathing.
- Do not pad; avoid bright light.
- Watch for secondary bacterial infection. Avoid corticosteroids, which reduce viral shedding and prolong the problem.

Primary herpes simplex infection

This viral infection produces follicular conjunctivitis. About 50% of patients have associated lid or corneal ulcers/vesicles, which are diagnostic.[2] Only a minority (less than 15%) develop corneal involvement with the primary infection.

Dendritic ulceration highlighted by fluorescein staining is diagnostic (see FIG. 51.4). Antigen detection or culture may allow confirmation.

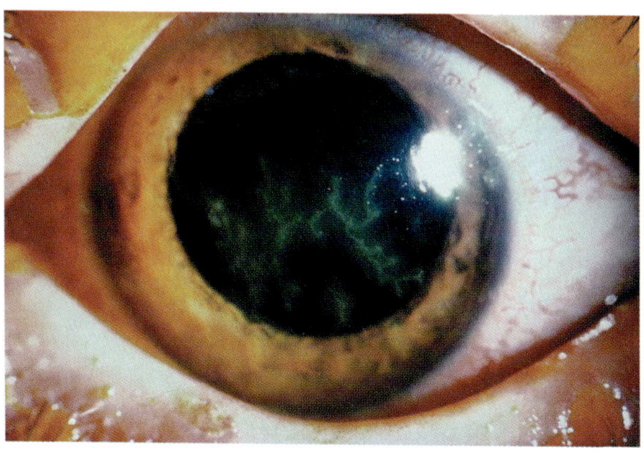

FIGURE 51.4 Herpes simplex keratitis—gritty, watery eye with typical dendritic ulcer, stained with fluorescein

Treatment (herpes simplex keratitis)

- Attend to eye hygiene
- Aciclovir 3% ointment, five times a day for 14 days or for at least 3 days after healing[7]
- Atropine 1% 1 drop, 12-hourly, for the duration of treatment will prevent reflex spasm of the pupil (specialist supervision)
- Debridement by a consultant

Never use corticosteroids and refer all new cases early to a consultant.

Chlamydial conjunctivitis

Chlamydial conjunctivitis is encountered in three common situations:

- neonatal infection (first 1–2 weeks)
- young patient with associated venereal infection
- isolated Aboriginal people with trachoma

Take swabs for culture and PCR testing.
Systemic antibiotic treatment:[8]

neonates: azithromycin 20 mg/kg orally, daily for 3 days[7]
children over 6 kg and adults: azithromycin 1 g (o) as single dose

Note: Partner must be treated in cases of STI.

ALLERGIC CONJUNCTIVITIS

Allergic conjunctivitis results from a local response to an allergen. It includes:

- vernal (hay fever) conjunctivitis
- contact hypersensitivity reactions, e.g. reaction to preservatives in drops

Vernal (hay fever) conjunctivitis

This is usually seasonal and related to pollen exposure. There is usually associated rhinitis (see CHAPTER 80).

Treatment

Tailor treatment to the degree of symptoms. Antihistamines may be required but symptomatic measures usually suffice. 51

Treatment options:

1 Topical antihistamines/vasoconstrictors
2 Mast cell stabilisers, e.g. sodium cromoglycate 2% drops, 1–2 drops per eye four times daily or ketotifen
3 Combination of 1 and 2
4 Topical steroids (severe cases)

Artificial tear preparations may give adequate symptomatic relief.

Contact hypersensitivity

Common topical allergens and toxins include topical ophthalmic medications, especially antibiotics, contact lens solutions (often the contained preservative) and a wide range of cosmetics, soaps, detergents and chemicals. Clinical features include burning, itching and watering with hyperaemia and oedema of the conjunctiva and eyelids. A skin reaction of the lids usually occurs.

Treatment

- Withdraw the causative agent.
- Apply normal saline compresses.
- Treat with naphazoline or phenylephrine.
- If not responding, refer for possible corticosteroid therapy.

Subconjunctival haemorrhage

Subconjunctival haemorrhage, which appears spontaneously, is a beefy red localised haemorrhage with a definite posterior margin (see FIG. 51.5). If it follows trauma and extends backwards, it may indicate an orbital fracture. It is usually caused by a sudden increase in intrathoracic pressure such as coughing and sneezing. It is not related to hypertension but it is worthwhile measuring the blood pressure to help reassure the patient.

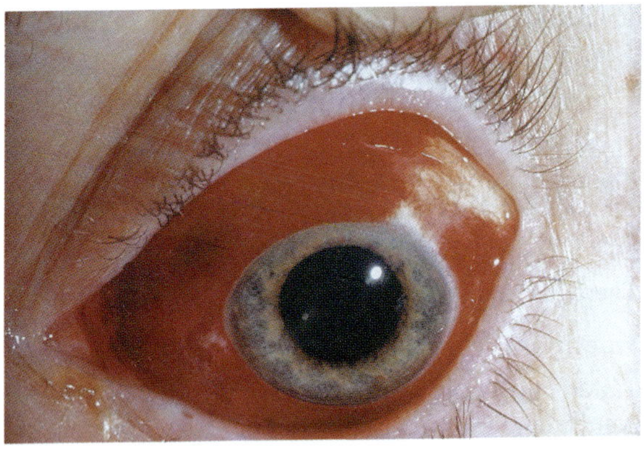

FIGURE 51.5 Subconjunctival haemorrhage: usually a localised haemorrhage that appears spontaneously. It is pain free. If traumatic and extends posteriorly, it may indicate an orbital fracture

Management

No local therapy is necessary. The haemorrhage absorbs over 2 weeks. Patient explanation and reassurance is necessary. If haemorrhages are recurrent, a bleeding tendency should be excluded.

Episcleritis and scleritis

Episcleritis and scleritis present as a localised area of inflammation (see FIGS 51.1 and 51.6). The episclera is a vascular layer that lies just beneath the conjunctiva and adjacent to the sclera. Both may become inflamed, but episcleritis (which is more localised) is essentially self-limiting, while scleritis (which is rare) is more serious as the eye may perforate.[3] Both conditions may be confused with inflammation associated with a foreign body, pterygium or pinguecula. There are no significant associations with episcleritis, which is usually idiopathic, but scleritis may be associated with connective tissue disease, especially rheumatoid arthritis and herpes zoster and rarely sarcoidosis and tuberculosis.

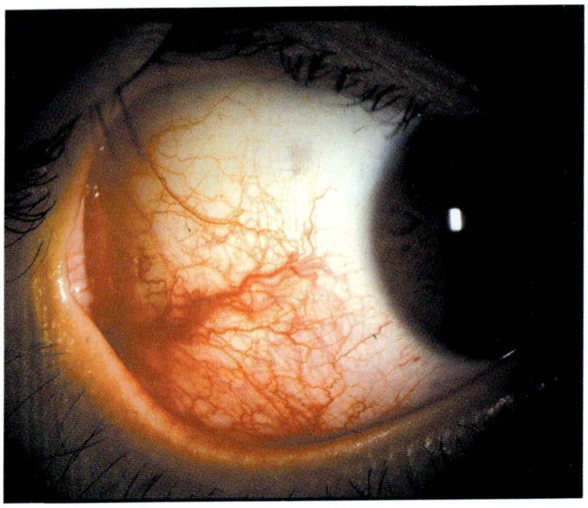

FIGURE 51.6 Episcleritis showing inflammation of the conjunctival and episclerical tissue only. Note the absence of violaceous colour that is seen in scleritis

Clinical features

Episcleritis:

- no discharge
- no watering
- vision normal (usually)
- often sectorial
- usually self-limiting

Treat with topical or oral steroids.

Scleritis:

- painful loss of vision
- urgent referral

History

A red and sore eye is the presenting complaint. There is usually no discharge but there may be reflex lacrimation. Scleritis is much more painful than episcleritis[3] and the eye becomes intensely red.

Examination

With scleritis, there is a localised area of inflammation that is tender to touch (FIG. 51.6), and which is more extensive than with episcleritis, being uniform across the eye. The inflamed vessels are larger than the conjunctival vessels.

Management

An underlying cause such as an autoimmune condition should be identified. Refer the patient, especially for scleritis. Corticosteroids or NSAIDs may be prescribed.

Uveitis (iritis)

The iris, ciliary body and the choroid form the uveal tract, which is the vascular coat of the eyeball.[7]

Anterior uveitis (acute iritis or iridocyclitis) is inflammation of the iris and ciliary body and this is usually referred to as acute iritis (see FIG. 51.7). The iris is sticky and sticks to the lens. The pupil may become small because of adhesions, and the vision is blurred.

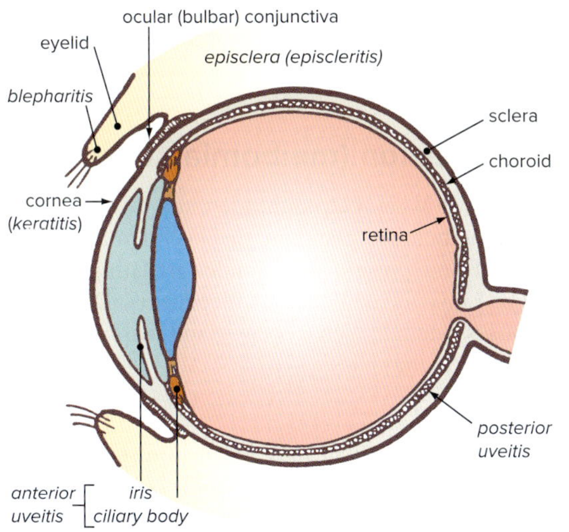

FIGURE 51.7 Diagrammatic representation of eye structures involved in inflammatory disorders

Causes include autoimmune-related diseases such as the seronegative arthropathies (e.g. ankylosing spondylitis), SLE, IBD, sarcoidosis and some infections (e.g. toxoplasmosis and syphilis).

Clinical features

- Eye redness, esp. around the edge of the iris
- Eye discomfort or pain
- Increased tearing
- Blurred vision
- Sensitivity to light
- Floaters in the field of vision
- Small pupil

The examination findings are summarised in TABLE 51.2. The affected eye is red, with the infection being particularly pronounced over the area covering the inflamed ciliary body (ciliary flush). However, the whole bulbar conjunctivae can be infected. The patient should be referred to a consultant. Slit lamp examination aids diagnosis.

Management involves finding the underlying cause. Treatment includes pupil dilatation with atropine drops and topical steroids to suppress inflammation. Systemic corticosteroids may be necessary. The prognosis of anterior uveitis is good if treatment and follow-up are maintained, but recurrence is likely.

Posterior uveitis (choroiditis) may involve the retina and vitreous membrane. Blurred vision and floating opacities in the visual field may be the only symptoms. Pain is not a feature. Referral to detect the causation and for treatment is essential.

Acute glaucoma

Acute glaucoma should always be considered in a patient over 50 years presenting with an acutely painful red eye. Permanent damage will result from misdiagnosis. The attack characteristically strikes in the evening or early morning when the pupil becomes semidilated.[3]

Clinical features

- Patient >50 years
- Pain in one eye
- ± Nausea and vomiting
- Impaired vision
- Haloes around lights
- Hazy cornea
- Fixed semidilated pupil
- Eye feels hard

51

Management

Urgent ophthalmic referral is essential since emergency treatment is necessary to preserve the eyesight. If immediate specialist attention is unavailable, treatment can be initiated with acetazolamide (Diamox) 500 mg IV and pilocarpine 4% drops to constrict the pupil or pressure-lowering drops.

Keratoconjunctivitis sicca

Dry eyes are a common problem, especially in elderly women. Lack of lacrimal secretion can be functional (e.g. ageing), or due to systemic disease (e.g. rheumatoid arthritis, SLE, Sjögren syndrome), drugs (e.g. β-blockers) or other factors, including the menopause. Up to 50% of patients with severe dry eye have Sjögren syndrome.

Clinical features

- A variety of symptoms
- Dryness, grittiness, stinging and redness

- Sensation of foreign body (e.g. sand)
- Photophobia if severe
- Slit light examination diagnostic with special stains

Treatment

- Treat the cause.
- Bathe eyes with clean water.
- Use artificial tears: hypromellose (e.g. Tears Naturale), polyvinyl alcohol (e.g. Tears Plus).
- Be cautious of adverse topical reactions.
- Refer severe cases.

EYELID AND LACRIMAL DISORDERS

There are several inflammatory disorders of the eyelid and lacrimal system that present as a 'red and tender' eye without involving the conjunctiva. Any suspicious lesion should be referred.

Stye (external hordeolum)

A stye is an acute abscess of a lash follicle or associated glands of the anterior lid margin, caused usually by *S. aureus*. The patient complains of a red tender swelling of the lid margin, usually on the medial side (see FIG. 51.8). A stye may be confused with a chalazion, orbital cellulitis or dacryocystitis.

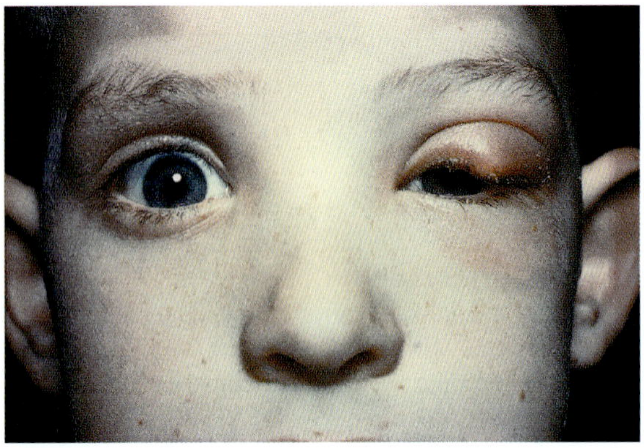

FIGURE 51.8 Hordeolum—a stye. This is a focal staphylococcal infection of the root of an eyelash

Management

- Use heat to help it discharge by using direct steam from a thermos (see FIG. 51.9) onto the enclosed eye or by hot compresses.
- Perform lash epilation to allow drainage of pus (incise with a size 11 blade if epilation does not work).
- Use chloramphenicol ointment if the infection is spreading locally.[3]

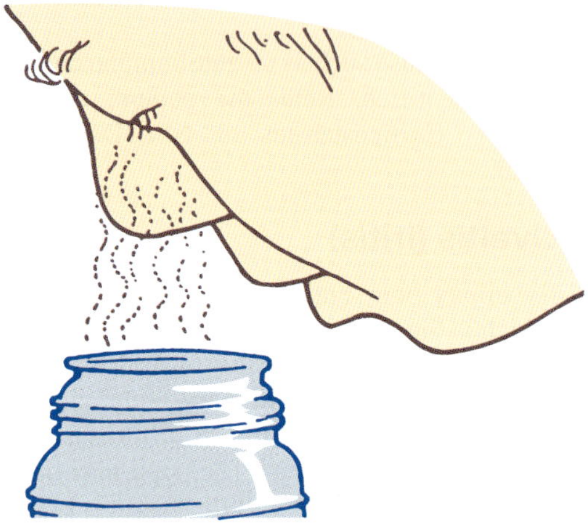

FIGURE 51.9 Steaming the painful eye: allow steam to rise from a thermos onto the closed eye for 10–15 minutes

Chalazion (meibomian cyst)

Also known as an internal hordeolum, this granuloma of the meibomian gland in the eyelid may become inflamed and present as a tender irritating lump in the lid. Look for evidence of blepharitis. Differential diagnoses include sebaceous gland carcinoma and basal cell carcinoma.

Management

Conservative treatment may result in resolution. This involves heat either as steam from a thermos or by applying a hot compress (a hand towel soaked in hot water) followed by light massage and the application of chloramphenicol ointment for 5 days. If the chalazion is very large, persistent or uncomfortable, or is affecting vision, it can be incised and curetted under local anaesthesia. This is best performed through the inner conjunctival surface using a chalazion clamp (blepharostat) (see FIG. 51.10).

Meibomianitis is usually a staphylococcal micro-abscess of the gland, and oral antistaphylococcal antibiotics (not topical) are recommended (e.g. di/flucloxacillin 500 mg (o) 6-hourly for adults). Surgical incision and curettage may also be necessary.

Blepharitis

This common chronic condition is characterised by inflammation of the lid margins (anterior blepharitis) and is commonly associated with secondary ocular effects such as styes, chalazia and conjunctival or corneal ulceration (see FIG. 51.11). Posterior blepharitis, which involves abnormalities of the

51

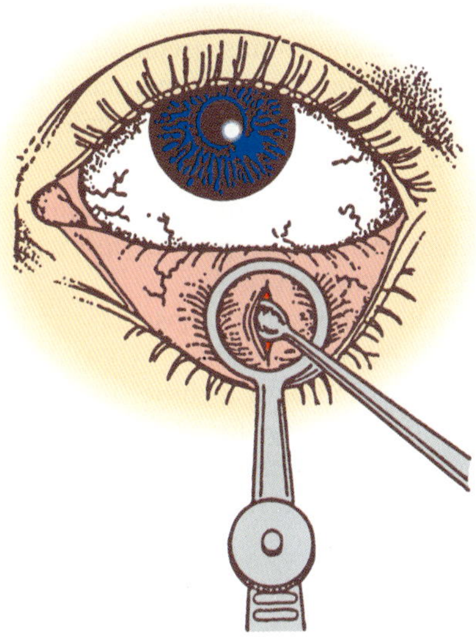

FIGURE 51.10 Excision of a meibomian cyst, using a chalazion clamp and curette

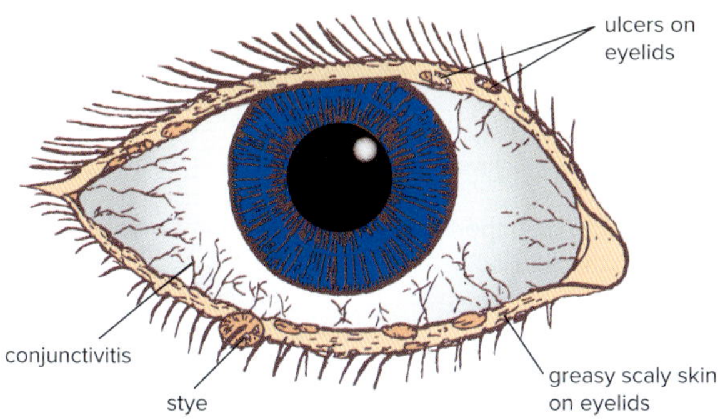

FIGURE 51.11 Blepharitis: common complicating features

submucus meibomian glands at the rim of the eyelids, is frequently associated with seborrhoeic dermatitis (especially) and atopic dermatitis, and less so with rosacea.[8] There is a tendency to colonisation of the lid margin with *S. aureus,* which causes an ulcerative infection.

The two types are:

- anterior blepharitis—staphylococcal
- posterior blepharitis—seborrhoeic and rosacea

Clinical features[9]

- Persistent sore eyes or eyelids
- Irritation, grittiness, burning, dryness and 'something in the eye' sensation
- Lid or conjunctival swelling and redness
- Crusts or scales around the base of the eyelids
- Discharge or stickiness, especially in morning
- Inflammation and crusting of the lid margins

Management

Anterior blepharitis

- Eyelid hygiene is the mainstay of therapy. The crusts and other debris should be gently cleaned with a cotton wool bud dipped in a 1:10 dilution of baby shampoo or a solution of sodium bicarbonate, once or twice daily. Application of a warm water or saline soak with gauze for 20 minutes is also effective. Proprietary lid solutions or wipes can also be used. If not controlled, apply chloromycetin 1% ointment once or twice daily for 4 weeks and review.

Posterior blepharitis

- Follow the same hygiene methods as above but with firm eye massage towards the lid margins.
- Ocular lubricants such as artificial tear preparations may greatly relieve symptoms of keratoconjunctivitis sicca (dry eyes).
- Control scalp seborrhoea with regular medicated shampoos.
- If persistent, short-term use of a mild topical corticosteroid ointment (e.g. hydrocortisone 0.5%) can be effective.
- Treat infection with an antibiotic ointment smeared on the lid margin (this may be necessary for several months) (e.g. tetracycline hydrochloride 1% or framycetin 0.5% or chloramphenicol 1% ointment to lid margins 3–6-hourly).[8]
- If not controlled by topical measures, use systemic antibiotics such as doxycycline 50 mg daily for at least 8 weeks (erythromycin for children <8 years), or flucloxacillin may be required for lid abscess.
- Avoid wearing make-up and contact lenses if inflammation is present.

51

Dacryocystitis

Acute dacryocystitis is infection of the lacrimal sac secondary to obstruction of the nasolacrimal duct at the junction of the lacrimal sac (see FIG. 51.12). Inflammation is localised over the medial canthus. There is usually a history of a watery eye for months beforehand. The problem may vary from being mild (as in infants) to severe with abscess formation.

Management

- Use local heat: steam or a hot moist compress.
- Use analgesics.
- In mild cases, massage the sac and duct with warm compresses, and instil astringent drops (e.g. zinc sulphate + phenylephrine) or chloromycetin 1% eye drops if inflammation.

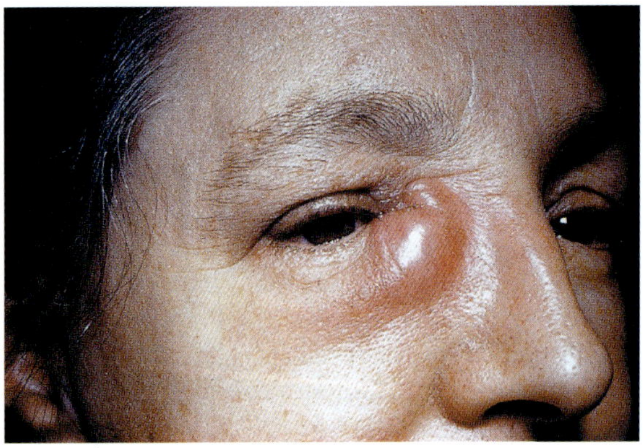

FIGURE 51.12 Acute dacryocystitis with abscess formation. Associated obstruction of the nasolacrimal duct at the junction of the lacrimal sac, which has become infected

- For acute cases, systemic antibiotics are best guided by results of Gram's stain and culture but initially use di/flucloxacillin or cephalexin.
- Measures to establish drainage are required eventually. Recurrent attacks or symptomatic watering of the eye are indications for surgery such as dacryocystorhinostomy.

Dacroadenitis

Dacroadenitis is infection of the lacrimal gland presenting as a tender swelling on the outer upper margin of the eyelid. It may be acute or chronic and has many causes. It is usually caused by a viral infection (e.g. mumps), which is treated conservatively with warm compresses. Bacterial infection is treated with appropriate antibiotics.

Orbital cellulitis

Orbital cellulitis includes two basic types—peri-orbital (or preseptal), which is soft tissue infection of the eyelids, and orbital (or postseptal) cellulitis. The latter, which arises from infection of the paranasal sinus or orbital trauma, is a potentially blinding and life-threatening condition. It is especially important in children in whom blindness may develop in hours. The patient, often a child, presents with unilateral swollen eyelids that may be red. Ask about a history of sinusitis, peri-ocular trauma, surgery, bites and immunocompromise issues.

Features to look for in orbital cellulitis include:[3]

- a systemically unwell patient
- proptosis
- peri-ocular swelling and erythema
- tenderness over the sinuses
- ocular nerve compromise (reduced vision, impaired colour vision or abnormal pupils)
- restricted and painful eye movements (see FIG. 51.13)

In peri-orbital cellulitis, which usually follows an abrasion, there is no pain or restriction of eye movement (see FIG. 51.14).

Immediate referral to hospital for specialist treatment is essential for both types. Treatment is with IV cefotaxime until afebrile, then amoxycillin/clavulanate for 7–10 days for peri-orbital cellulitis and for orbital cellulitis, IV cefotaxime + di(flu) cloxacillin together followed by amoxycillin/clavulanate (o) 10 days.[7]

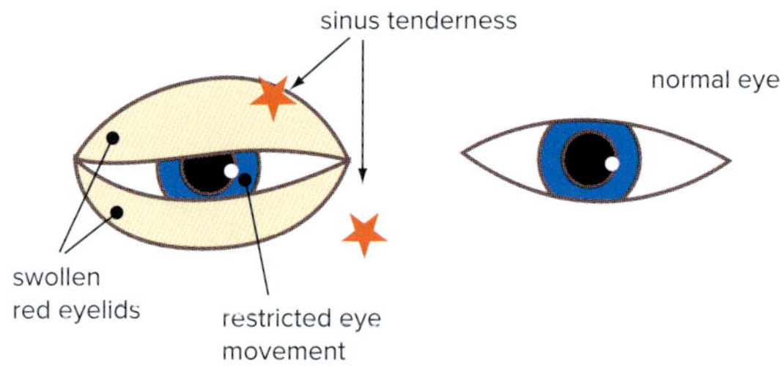

FIGURE 51.13 Important signs in the patient presenting with orbital cellulitis

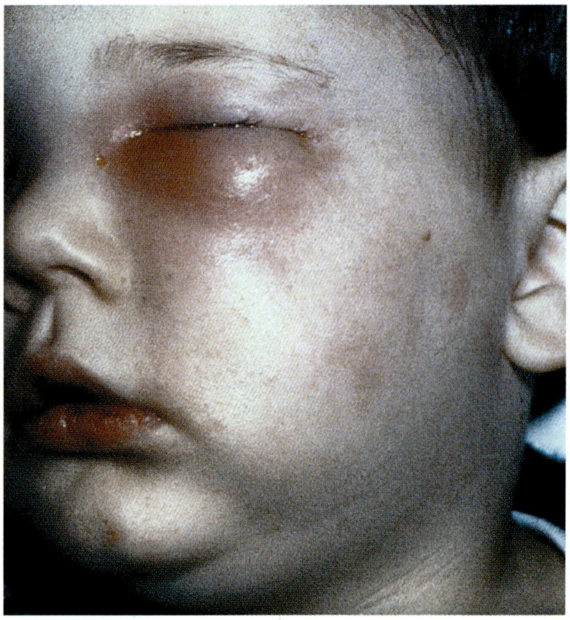

FIGURE 51.14 Peri-orbital cellulitis following an abrasion to the eye. Treat this as an urgent condition

Herpes zoster ophthalmicus

Herpes zoster ophthalmicus (shingles) affects the skin supplied by the ophthalmic division of the trigeminal nerve. The eye may be affected if the nasociliary branch is involved. The rash usually appears on the tip of the nose. Ocular problems include conjunctivitis, uveitis, keratitis and glaucoma.

Immediate referral is necessary if the eye is red, vision is blurred or the cornea cannot be examined. Apart from general eye hygiene, treatment usually includes one of the oral anti-herpes virus agents such as oral aciclovir 800 mg, five times daily for 10 days or (if sight is threatened) aciclovir 10 mg/kg IV slowly 8-hourly for 10 days (provided this is commenced within 3 days of the rash appearing)[5,8] and topical aciclovir ointment 4-hourly (see CHAPTER 122).

Pinguecula and pterygium[10]

Pinguecula is a yellowish elevated nodular growth on either side of the cornea in the area of the palpebral fissure. It is common in people over 35 years. The growth tends to remain static but can become inflamed—pingueculitis. Usually no treatment is necessary unless they are large, craggy and uncomfortable, when excision is indicated. If irritating, topical astringent drops such as naphazoline compound drops (e.g. Albalon) can give relief.

Pterygium is a fleshy overgrowth of the conjunctiva onto the nasal side of the cornea and usually occurs in adults living in dry, dusty, windy areas. Excision of a pterygium by a specialist is indicated if it is likely to interfere with vision by encroaching on the visual axis, or if it becomes red and uncomfortable or disfiguring.

CORNEAL DISORDERS[11]

Patients with corneal conditions typically suffer from ocular pain or discomfort and reduced vision. The common condition of dry eye may involve the cornea while contact lens disorders, abrasions/ulcers and infection are common serious problems that threaten eyesight. Inflammation of the cornea—keratitis—is caused by factors such as UV light, e.g. 'arc eye', herpes simplex, herpes zoster ophthalmicus and the dangerous microbial keratitis. Bacterial keratitis is an ophthalmological emergency that should be considered in the contact lens wearer presenting with pain and reduced vision.

Topical corticosteroids should be avoided in the undiagnosed red eye.

Corneal abrasion and ulceration

There are many causes of abrasions, particularly trauma from a foreign body embedded on the corneal surface or 'cul-de-sac' FB, contact lenses, fingernails including 'french nails', and UV burns. The abrasion may be associated with an ulcer, which is a defect in the epithelial cell layer of the cornea. Common causes of a corneal ulcer are listed in TABLE 51.3.

Table 51.3 Corneal ulceration: common causes

Trauma
Contact lens wear/injury
Infection—microbial keratitis:
- bacterial (e.g. *Pseudomonas* [contact lens])
- viral (e.g. herpes simplex [dendritic ulcer], herpes zoster ophthalmicus)
- fungal
- protozoal (e.g. *Acanthamoeba*)

Neurotrophic (e.g. trigeminal nerve defect)
Immune-related (e.g. rheumatoid arthritis)
Spontaneous corneal erosion
Chronic blepharitis
Overexposure (e.g. eyelid defects)

Symptoms

- Ocular pain
- Foreign body sensation
- Watering of the eye (epiphora)
- Blepharospasm
- Blurred vision

Diagnosis is best performed with a slit lamp using a cobalt blue filter and flourescein staining.

Management (corneal ulcer)

- Stain with fluorescein.
- Check for a foreign body.
- Treat with chloramphenicol 1% ointment ± homatropine 2% (if pain due to ciliary spasm).
- Double eye pad (if not infected).
- Review in 24 hours.
- A 6 mm defect heals in 48 hours.
- Consider early specialist referral.

Superficial punctate keratitis

Punctate keratopathy presents as scattered small lesions on the cornea that stain with fluorescein if they are deep enough. It is a non-specific finding and may be associated with blepharitis, viral conjunctivitis, trachoma, keratitis sicca (dry eyes), UV light exposure (e.g. welding lamps, sunlamps), contact lenses and topical ocular agents. Management involves treating the cause and careful follow-up.

Practice tips

- Think corneal abrasion if the eye is 'watering' and painful (e.g. caused by a large insect such as a grasshopper or other foreign body).
- If a slit lamp is unavailable, the direct ophthalmoscope can be used to provide illumination as well as blue light for corneal examination. Magnifying loupes can then be used for viewing the illuminated cornea.

Microbial keratitis

This is responsible for at least 1.5 million new cases of blindness every year in the developing world and for significant morbidity in developed countries.

Risk factors

- Contact lens wear
- Corneal trauma, especially agriculture trauma
- Corneal surgery
- Post-herpetic corneal lesion
- Dry eye
- Corneal anaesthetic
- Corneal exposure (e.g. VII nerve lesion)
- Ocular surface disease, including ulceration

Pseudomonas aeruginosa is the most common causative organism in contact lens wearers.

Acanthamoeba is associated with bathing or washing in contaminated water.

51

Urgent referral to an ophthalmologist or eye clinic is needed to avoid rapid corneal destruction with perforation, especially with bacterial keratitis. An appropriate 'covering' topical antibiotic is ciprofloxacin 0.3% ointment.

Problems with contact lenses

Because a contact lens is a foreign body, various complications can develop and a history of the use of contact lenses is important in the management of a red eye.

Infection

Infection is more likely to occur with soft rather than hard lenses. They should not be worn when sleeping since this increases the risk of infection 10-fold.[12] One cause is *Acanthamoeba* keratitis acquired from contaminated water that may be used for cleaning the lenses.

Hard lens trauma

This may cause corneal abrasions with irreversible endothelial changes or ptosis, especially with the older polymethyl-methacrylate-based lenses. Patients should change to modern gas-permeable hard lenses.

Lost lenses

Patients should be reassured that lenses cannot go behind the eye. The edge of the lens can usually be seen by everting the upper lid.

Preventive measures[13]

- Wash hands before handling lenses.
- Do not use tap water or saline.
- Clean lenses with disinfecting solution.
- Store overnight in a clean airtight case with fresh disinfectant.
- Change the lens container solution daily.
- Discard disposable lenses after 2 weeks.
- Do not wear lenses while sleeping.
- Do not wear lenses while swimming in lakes, rivers or swimming pools.

Refer to an ophthalmologist if a painful red eye develops, especially if a discharge is present.

Flash burns

A common problem, usually presenting at night, is bilateral painful eyes caused by UV 'flash burns' to both corneas some 5–10 hours previously. The mechanism of injury is UV rays from a welding machine causing superficial punctate keratitis. Other sources of UV light such as sunlamps and snow reflection can cause a reaction.

Management

- Local anaesthetic (long-acting) drops: once-only application (do not allow the patient to take home more drops).
- Instil homatropine 2% drops statim or other short-acting ocular dilating agent (be careful of glaucoma).
- Use analgesics (e.g. codeine plus paracetamol) for 24 hours.
- Use broad-spectrum antibiotic eye ointment in lower fornix (to prevent infection).
- Use firm eye padding for 24 hours, when eyes reviewed (avoid light).

The eye usually heals completely in 48 hours. If not, check for a foreign body.

Note: Contact lens 'overwear syndrome' gives the same symptoms.

Cavernous sinus arteriovenous fistula

Such a fistula produces conjunctival hyperaemia but no inflammation or discharge. The lesion causes raised orbital venous pressure. The fistula may be secondary to head injuries or may arise spontaneously, particularly in postmenopausal women. It needs radiological investigation.

The classic symptom is a 'whooshing' sound synchronous with the pulse behind the eye, and the sign is a bruit audible with the stethoscope placed over the orbit.

Penetrating eye injuries

These require urgent referral to an ophthalmologist.

Consider:

- X-ray
- tetanus prophylaxis
- transport by land
- injection of anti-emetic (e.g. metoclopramide)

Use no ointment or eye drops, including local anaesthetic.

If significant delay is involved, give one dose (in adults) of:[8]

gentamicin 1.5 mg/kg IV plus
cefotaxime 1 g or ceftriaxone 1 g IV (can give ceftriaxone IM but with lignocaine 1%)
or
vancomycin IV + oral ciprofloxacin

Hyphaema

With hyphaema, a common blunt sporting injury, bleeding from the iris collects in the anterior chamber of the eye (see FIG. 51.15). The danger is that, with exertion, a secondary bleed from the ruptured vessel could fill the anterior chamber with blood, blocking the escape of aqueous humour and causing a severe secondary glaucoma. Loss of the eye can occur with a severe haemorrhage. It is likely to happen between the second and fourth days after the injury.

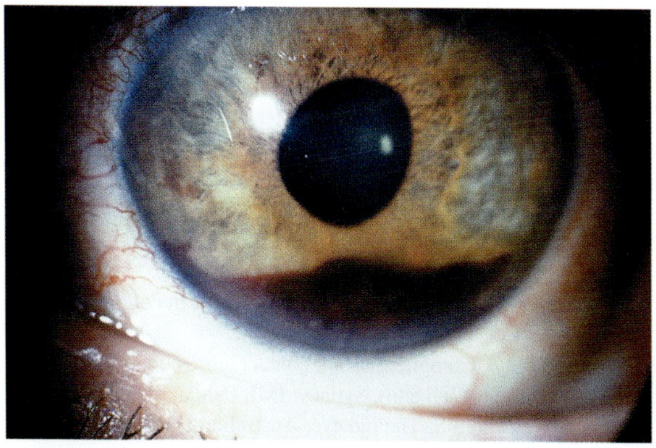

FIGURE 51.15 Hyphaemia of the eye showing blood in the anterior chamber; this occurred in a 29-year-old man who was struck in the eye by a squash ball

Management

- First, exclude a penetrating injury.
- Avoid unnecessary movement: vibration will aggravate bleeding. (For this reason, do not use a helicopter if evacuation is necessary.)
- Avoid smoking and drinking alcohol.
- Do not give aspirin (can induce bleeding).
- Prescribe complete bed rest for 5 days and review the patient daily.
- Apply padding over the injured eye for 4 days.
- Administer sedatives as required.
- Beware of 'floaters', 'flashes' and field defects.

Arrange ophthalmic consultation after 1 month to exclude glaucoma and retinal detachment. No sport before this time.

Endophthalmitis[14]

This is an intra-ocular bacterial infection that may complicate any penetrating injury, including intra-ocular surgery. It should be considered in patients with such a history presenting with a red painful eye. Pus may be seen in the anterior chamber (hypopyon).

Urgent referral is mandatory. If significant delay, use ciprofloxacin (o) + vancomycin IV as single doses.[7]

Epiphora (watering eyes)

This has many causes and is more common in older people.

The main causes are drainage obstruction and excessive tear production, which includes physical and chemical irritants, blepharitis and entropion. Management depends on the person's age. Remove any mucoid discharge and massage the nasolacrimal sac.

Antibiotics are indicated only for conjunctivitis, blepharitis or dacryocystitis. Probing of the ducts or even surgery may be required.

When to refer

- Uncertainty about the diagnosis
- Patients with uveitis, acute glaucoma, episcleritis/scleritis or corneal ulceration
- Deep central corneal and intra-ocular foreign bodies
- Prolonged infections, with a poor or absent response to treatment or where therapy may be complicating management

- Infections or severe allergies with possible ocular complications
- Sudden swelling of an eyelid in a child with evidence of infection suggestive of orbital cellulitis—this is an emergency
- Emergency referral is also necessary for hyphaema, hypopyon, penetrating eye injury, acute glaucoma, severe chemical burn
- Herpes zoster ophthalmicus: if the external nose is involved then the internal eye may be involved
- Summary for urgent referral:
  - trauma (significant)/penetrating injury
  - hyphaema >3 mm
  - corneal ulcer
  - severe conjunctivitis
  - uveitis/acute iritis
  - Behçet syndrome
  - acute glaucoma
  - giant cell arteritis
  - orbital cellulitis (pre- and post-)
  - acute dacryocystitis
  - keratitis
  - episcleritis/scleritis
  - endophthalmitis
  - herpes zoster ophthalmicus

Note: As a general rule never use corticosteroids or atropine in the eye before referral to an ophthalmologist.

51

Practice tips

- Avoid long-term use of any medication, especially antibiotics (e.g. chloramphenicol: course for a maximum of 10 days).[2]
  Note: Beware of allergy or toxicity to topical medications, especially antibiotics, as a cause of persistent symptoms.
- As a general rule, avoid using topical corticosteroids or combined corticosteroid/antibiotic preparations.
- Never use corticosteroids in the presence of a dendritic ulcer.
- To achieve effective results from eye ointment or drops, remove debris such as mucopurulent exudate with bacterial conjunctivitis or blepharitis by using a warm solution of saline (dissolve a teaspoon of kitchen salt in 500 mL of boiled water) to bathe away any discharge from conjunctiva, eyelashes and lids.
- A gritty sensation is common in conjunctivitis but the presence of a foreign body must be excluded.[3]
- Beware of the contact lens 'overwear syndrome', which is treated in a similar way to flash burns.

Red eye golden rules

- Always test and record vision
- Beware of the unilateral red eye
- Conjunctivitis is almost always bilateral
- Irritated eyes are often dry
- Never use steroids if herpes simplex is suspected
- A penetrating eye injury is an emergency
- Consider an intra-ocular foreign body
- Beware of herpes zoster ophthalmicus if the nose is involved
- Irregular pupils: think iritis, injury and surgery
- Never pad a discharging eye
- Refer patients with eyelid ulcers
- If there is a corneal abrasion look for a foreign body

Source: Based on J Colvin and J Reich[4]

Patient education resources

Hand-out sheets from *Murtagh's Patient Education* 7th edition:

- Blepharitis
- Bloodshot eye
- Chalazion (meibomian cyst)
- Conjunctivitis
- Foreign body in the eye
- Stye

References

1. McDonnell P. Red eye: an illustrated guide to eight common causes. Modern Medicine Australia, 1989; October: 37–9.
2. Della NG. Acute conjunctivitis. In: *MIMS Disease Index*. Sydney: IMS Publishing, 1991–92: 113–15.
3. Kuzniarz M. Red eye. Medical Observer, 11 May 2012: 27–30.
4. Colvin J, Reich J. Systematic examination of the red eye. Aust Fam Physician, 1976; 5: 153–65.
5. Maclean H. Keratitis (viral and fungal). In: *MIMS Disease Index*. Sydney: IMS Publishing, 1991–92: 301–3.
6. Robinson MJ, Roberton DM. *Practical Paediatrics* (5th edn). Melbourne: Churchill Livingstone, 2003: 759.
7. Expert group for Antibiotic. Eye infections. In: eTG complete [Internet]. Melbourne: Therapeutic Guidelines Ltd. Available from: <www.tg.org.au>, accessed September 2017.
8. Lindsley K, Matsumura S et al. Interventions for chronic blepharitis (Cochrane Review). Cochrane Database. Syst Rev. 2012, Issue 5. Art No. CD005556.
9. Colvin J. Painful eye: an emergency call. Aust Fam Physician, 1985; 14: 1258.
10. Watson SL. Common corneal conditions. Medicine Today, 2005; 6 (5): 22–30.
11. Schein OD, Poggio EC. Ulcerative keratitis in contact lens wearers. Cornea, 1990; 9 (1): 55–8.
12. Lazarus MG. Complications of contact lenses. In: *MIMS Disease Index* (2nd edn). Sydney: IMS Publishing, 1996: 121–3.
13. Sehu W, Zagora S. The red eye. Australian Doctor. 12 October 2012: 23–30.
14. Barry P, Cordovés L, Gardner S. European Society of Cataract Refractive Surgeons (ESCRS). Guidelines for prevention and treatment of endophthalmitis following cataract surgery. Dublin, Ireland, 2013.

Pain in the face

52

It's as though the devil suddenly thrust red hot electric needles through my right cheek towards my ear.

PATIENT (ANONYMOUS), DESCRIBING 'TIC DOULOUREUX'

When a patient complains of pain in the face rather than the head, the physician has to consider foremost the possibilities of dental disorders, sinus disease, especially of the maxillary sinuses, temporomandibular joint (TMJ) dysfunction, eye disorders, lesions of the oropharynx or posterior third of the tongue, trigeminal neuralgia and chronic paroxysmal hemicrania.

The key to the diagnosis is the clinical examination because even the most sophisticated investigation may provide no additional information.

A basic list of causes of facial pain is presented in TABLE 52.1.[1] The causes can vary from the simple, such as aphthous ulcers, herpes simplex and dental caries, to serious causes, such as carcinoma of the tongue, sinuses and nasopharynx or osteomyelitis of the mandible or maxilla.

Key facts and checkpoints

- Dental disorders are the commonest cause of facial pain, accounting for up to 90% of pain in and about the face.[2]
- The most common dental disorders are dental caries and periodontal diseases.
- The mean age of onset of trigeminal neuralgia is 50–52 years.
- There is a similarity in the 'occult' causes of pain in the ear and in the face (refer to FIGS 50.4 and 50.5).
- Sinusitis occurs mainly as part of a generalised upper respiratory infection. Swimming is another common predisposing factor.
- Dental root infection must be sought in all cases of maxillary sinusitis.

A diagnostic approach

A summary of the diagnostic strategy model is presented in TABLE 52.2.

Table 52.1 Diagnoses to consider in orofacial pain

Positive physical signs
Cervical spinal dysfunction
Dental pathology
Erysipelas
Eye disorders
Herpes zoster
Nasopharyngeal cancer
Oropharyngeal disorders: • ulceration (aphthous, infective, traumatic, others) • cancer • gingivitis/stomatitis • tonsillitis • erosive lichen planus
Paranasal sinus disorders
Parotid gland: • mumps • sialectasis • cancer • pleomorphic adenoma
TMJ dysfunction
Temporal arteritis
Absent physical signs
Atypical facial pain
Chronic paroxysmal hemicrania
Depression-associated facial pain
Facial migraine (lower half headache)
Glossopharyngeal neuralgia
Migrainous neuralgia (cluster headache)
Trigeminal neuralgia (tic douloureux)

Probability diagnosis

The commonest cause of facial pain is dental disorders, especially dental caries. Another common cause is sinusitis, particularly maxillary sinusitis.

TMJ dysfunction causing TMJ arthralgia is a very common problem encountered in general practice and

52

Table 52.2 Pain in the face: diagnostic strategy model

Probability diagnosis

Dental pain:
- caries
- periapical abscess
- fractured tooth

Maxillary/frontal sinusitis
TMJ dysfunction

Serious disorders not to be missed

Cardiovascular:
- myocardial ischaemia
- aneurysm of cavernous sinus
- internal carotid aneurysm
- ischaemia of posterior inferior cerebellar artery

Neoplasia:
- cancer: mouth, sinuses, nasopharynx, tonsils, tongue, larynx, salivary gland
- metastases: orbital, base of brain, bone

Severe infections:
- herpes zoster
- erysipelas
- periapical abscess → osteomyelitis
- acute sinusitis → spreading infection

Temporal arteritis

Pitfalls (often missed)

TMJ dysfunction
Migraine variants:
- facial migraine
- chronic paroxysmal hemicrania

Atypical facial pain
Eye disorders:
- glaucoma
- iritis
- optic neuritis

Chronic dental neuralgia (odontalgia)
Salivary gland:
- infection, mumps, suppuration, calculus, obstruction, cancer

Acute glaucoma (upper face)
Cranial nerve neuralgias:
- trigeminal neuralgia
- glossopharyngeal neuralgia

Seven masquerades checklist

Depression
Spinal dysfunction (cervical spondylosis)

Is the patient trying to tell me something?

Quite probably. Atypical facial pain has underlying psychogenic elements.

it is important to have some simple basic strategies to give the patient.

Red flag pointers for pain in the face

- Persistent pain: no obvious cause
- Unexplained weight loss
- Trigeminal neuralgia: possible serious cause
- Herpes zoster involving nose
- Person >60 years: consider temporal arteritis, malignancy

Serious disorders not to be missed

It is important not to overlook cancer of various structures, such as the mouth, sinuses, nasopharynx, tonsils, tongue, larynx and parotid gland, which can present with atypical chronic facial pain.

It is important therefore to inspect these areas, especially in the elderly, but lesions in the relatively inaccessible nasopharynx can be easily missed. Nasopharynx cancer spreads upwards to the base of the skull early and patients can present with multiple cranial nerve palsies before either pain or bloody nasal discharge.[1]

Tumours may arise in the bones of the orbit, for example, lymphoma or secondary cancer, and may cause facial pain and proptosis. Similarly, any space-occupying lesion or malignancy arising from the region of the orbit or base of the brain can cause facial pain by involvement (often destruction) of trigeminal sensory fibres. This will lead to a depressed ipsilateral corneal reflex.

Also, aneurysms developing in the cavernous sinus[1] can cause pain via pressure on any of the divisions of the trigeminal nerve, while aneurysms from the internal carotid arising from the origin of the posterior communicating artery can cause pressure on the oculomotor nerve.

Temporal arteritis typically causes pain over the temporal area but can cause ischaemic pain in the jaws when chewing.

Pitfalls

Commonly overlooked causes of facial pain include TMJ arthralgia and dental disorders, especially of the teeth, which are tender to percussion, and oral ulceration. Diagnosing the uncommon migraine variants, particularly facial migraine and chronic paroxysmal hemicrania, often presents difficulties, including differentiating between the neuralgias.

Glossopharyngeal neuralgia, which is rare, causes pain in the back of the throat, around the tonsils and adjacent fauces. The lightning quality of the pain of neuralgia gives the clue to diagnosis.

Common pitfalls

- Failing to refer unusual or undiagnosed causes of facial pain
- Overlooking infective dental causes, which can cause complications
- Failing to consider the possibility of malignant disease of 'hidden' structures in the older patient
- Unaware that facial pain never crosses the midline

Seven masquerades checklist

Of these, depression and cervical spinal dysfunction must be considered. The upper cervical spine can cause facial pain from lesions of C2 or C3 via the lesser occipital or greater auricular (see FIG. 52.1) nerves, which may give pain around the ear. It is important to remember that the C2 and C3 nerves share a common pathway with the trigeminal nerve (see CHAPTER 62).

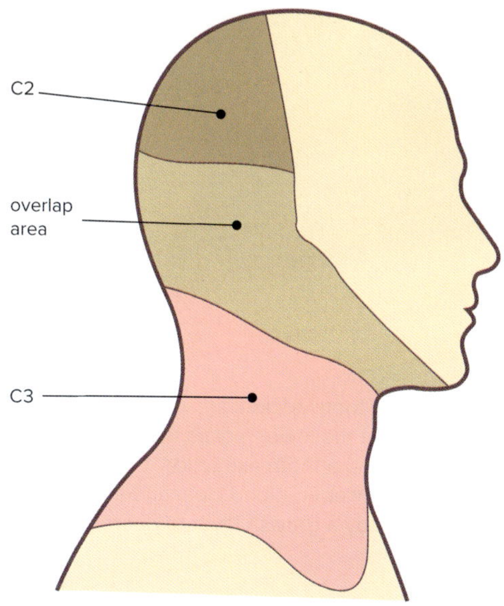

FIGURE 52.1 Dermatomes of C2 and C3, with the overlap area indicated

Depressive illness can present with a variety of painful syndromes and facial pain is no exception. The features of depression may be apparent and thus antidepressants should be prescribed. Usually the facial pain and the depression subside concomitantly.

Psychogenic considerations

Psychogenic factors have to be considered in every painful condition. They are considered to be high in patients with atypical facial pain.

The clinical approach

History

Diagnosis of nearly all types of facial pain must be based almost entirely on the history. It is often difficult to delineate the exact nature and distribution of the pain. The history should include the typical analysis of pain, especially noting the site and radiation of the pain.

Examination

The patient's general state and behaviour should be noted. Any sudden jabbing pain in the face causing the characteristic 'tic' may indicate neuralgia.

Palpate the face and neck to include the parotid glands, eyes, regional lymph nodes and the skin. Inspect the TMJs and cervical spine. Carefully inspect the nose, mouth, pharynx and postnasal space. In particular inspect the teeth, percussing each tooth if dental disorder is suspected. Bimanual palpation of the floor of the mouth is performed to detect induration or submandibular and submental lymph node enlargement.

The sinuses, especially the maxillary sinuses, should be inspected and a torch light should be placed inside the mouth to test transillumination of the maxillary sinuses. It works best when one symptomatic side can be compared with an asymptomatic side.

Perform a neurological examination on the cranial nerves with special emphasis on the trigeminal, oculomotor and glossopharyngeal nerves.

Investigations

If investigations are being contemplated referral may be appropriate. The association of multiple sclerosis and tumours with neuralgias may have to be investigated. Radiological investigations include plain X-rays of the paranasal sinuses, CT scans, MRI and orthopantomograms.

Facial pain in children

Apart from trauma, facial pain in children is almost invariably due to dental problems, rarely migraine variants and occasionally childhood infections such as mumps and gingivostomatitis. A serious problem sometimes seen in children is orbital cellulitis secondary to ethmoiditis.

52

Sinusitis occurs in children, especially older children, and it should be suspected with persistent bilateral mucopurulent rhinorrhoea (beyond 10 days).

Facial pain in the elderly

Many of the causes of facial pain have an increased incidence with age, in particular trigeminal neuralgia, herpes zoster, cancer, glaucoma, TMJ dysfunction and cervical spondylosis. Glossopharyngeal neuralgia does not seem to have a particular predilection for the elderly. Xerostomia due to decreased secretions of salivary glands may cause abrasion with minor trauma. It may aggravate the pain of glossitis, which is common in the elderly.

DENTAL DISORDERS

Dental caries

Dental caries, impacted teeth, infected tooth sockets and dental roots can cause pain in the maxillary and mandibular regions. Caries with periapical and apical abscess formation produces pain from infection extending around the apex of the tooth into the alveolar bone. Retention of a fractured root may cause unilateral paroxysmal pain. Impacted third molars (wisdom teeth) may be associated with surrounding soft tissue inflammation (pericoronitis), causing pain that may be localised to the mandible or radiate via the auriculotemporal nerve to the ear. *Candida albicans*, which is an oral commensal, may colonise dentures causing hyperaemia and painful superficial ulceration of the denture-bearing mucosa. Antibiotics are of no proven use.

Features of dental caries

- Pain is usually confined to the affected tooth but it may be diffuse.
- Pain is almost always aggravated by thermal changes in the mouth:
  - cold—if dental pulp vital
  - hot—if dental pulp is necrotic
- Pain may be felt in more than one tooth.
- Dental pain will not cross the midline.
- Antibiotics are not indicated.

Treatment of dental pain

- Arrange urgent dental consultation
- Pain relief:[3]

  aspirin 600 mg (o), 4–6 hourly
  or
  ibuprofen 400 mg (o), 4–6 hourly
  or
  paracetamol 0.5–1 g (o), 4–6 hourly

Tooth abscess, inflamed wisdom tooth, spreading dental infection or root canal infection[4]

Dental treatment will usually alleviate the problem; however, if severe:

amoxycillin 500 mg (o) tds for 5 days
If unresponsive:
amoxycillin/clavulanate 875/125 mg (o) bd (adjust to children's dose)
add metronidazole 400 mg (o) 12-hourly for 5 days
For patients hypersensitive to penicillin:
clindamycin 300–450 mg (o) 8-hourly for 5 days

Gingivitis and periodontitis

Refer to CHAPTER 72

Alveolar osteitis (dry socket)

Refer urgently for specialised toileting and insertion of dressing. This usually heals naturally in 14 days. Antibiotics are of no proven use (see FIG. 52.2).[3,4]

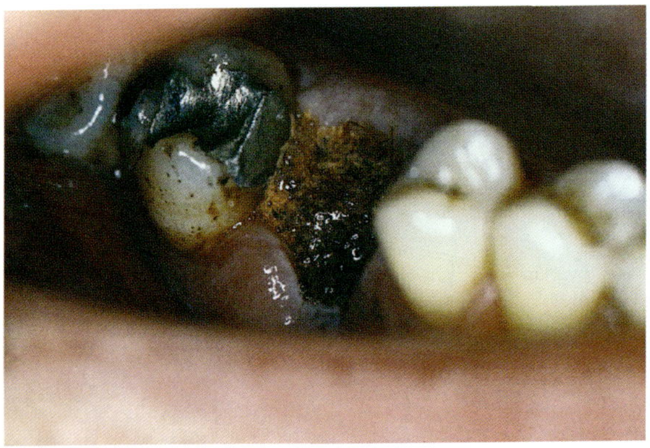

FIGURE 52.2 Dry tooth socket: this is a very painful condition mainly in the lower molars unrelieved by analgesics following a tooth extraction 1–3 days earlier. The socket has few or no blood clots and sensitive bone surfaces covered by a greyish layer of necrotic tissue

KNOCKED-OUT OR BROKEN TEETH

If a permanent (second) tooth is knocked out, it can be saved by immediate proper care. Likewise, a broken tooth should be saved and urgent dental attention sought.

The knocked-out tooth

- Place the tooth in its original position, preferably immediately (see FIG. 52.3); if dirty, put it in milk before replacement or, better still, place it under

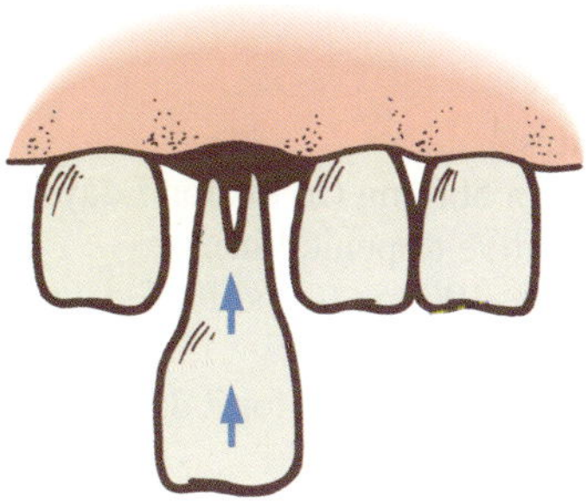

FIGURE 52.3 Replacement of a knocked-out tooth

the tongue and 'wash it' in saliva. Do not use water, and do not wipe or touch the root.
- Fix the tooth by moulding strong silver foil (e.g. cooking foil) over it and the adjacent teeth.
- Refer the patient to his or her dentist or dental hospital as soon as possible.

Note: Teeth replaced within half an hour have a 90% chance of successful re-implantation.

Ludwig angina[4]

This is a rapidly swelling cellulitis occurring in both the sublingual and submaxillary spaces without abscess formation, often arising from a root canal infection. It resembles an abscess and should be treated as one. It is potentially life-threatening as it can compromise the airway.

Management

- Culture and sensitivity testing
- Specialist consultation
- Empirical treatment:

  amoxycillin 2 g IV, 6-hourly
  plus
  metronidazole 500 mg IV, 12-hourly

Pain from paranasal sinuses

Infection of the paranasal sinuses may cause localised pain. Localised tenderness and pain may be apparent with frontal or maxillary sinusitis. Sphenoidal or ethmoidal sinusitis causes a constant pain behind the eye or behind the nose, often accompanied by nasal blockage. Chronic infection of the sinuses may be extremely difficult to detect. The commonest organisms are *Streptococcus pneumoniae, Haemophilus influenzae* and *Moraxella catarrhalis.*

Expanding lesions of the sinuses, such as mucocoeles and tumours, cause local swelling and displace the contents of the orbit—upwards for maxillary, laterally for the ethmoids and downwards for the frontal.

Maxillary sinusitis

The maxillary sinus is the one most commonly infected.[5] It is important to determine whether the sinusitis is caused by stasis following a URTI or acute rhinitis, or due to dental root infection. Most episodes are of viral origin.

Clinical features (acute sinusitis)

- Facial pain and tenderness (over sinuses)
- Toothache
- Headache
- Purulent postnasal drip
- Nasal discharge
- Nasal obstruction
- Rhinorrhoea
- Cough (worse at night)
- Prolonged fever
- Epistaxis

Suspect bacterial cause if high fever and purulent nasal discharge.

Clinical features (chronic sinusitis)

- Vague facial pain
- Offensive postnasal drip
- Nasal obstruction
- Toothache
- Malaise
- Halitosis

Some simple office tests

Diagnosing sinus tenderness[6]

To differentiate sinus tenderness from non-sinus bone tenderness palpation is useful. This is best done by palpating a non-sinus area first and last (see FIG. 52.4), systematically exerting pressure over the temporal bones (T), then the frontal (F), ethmoid (E) and maxillary (M) sinuses, and finally zygomas (Z), or vice versa.

Differential tenderness both identifies and localises the main sites of infection (see FIG. 52.4).

Diagnosing unilateral sinusitis

A simple way to assess the presence or absence of fluid in the frontal sinus, and in the maxillary sinus (in particular), is the use of transillumination. It works best when one symptomatic side can be compared with an asymptomatic side.

It is necessary to have the patient in a darkened room and to use a small, narrow-beam torch. For the maxillary sinuses remove dentures (if any). Shine the

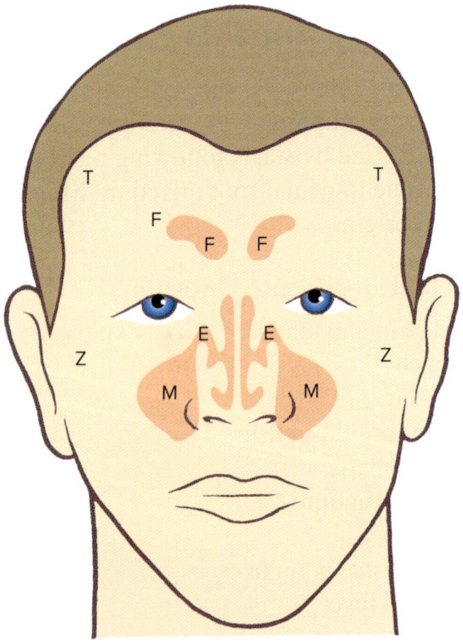

FIGURE 52.4 Diagnosing sinus tenderness: T (temporal) and Z (zygoma) represent no sinus bony tenderness, for purposes of comparison

light inside the mouth (with lips sealed), on either side of the hard palate, pointed at the base of the orbit. A dull glow seen below the orbit indicates that the antrum is air-filled. Diminished illumination on the symptomatic side indicates sinusitis.

A CT scan may show mucosal thickening without fluid levels. Plain films are not indicated.

Management (acute bacterial sinusitis)

52

Principles

- Exclude dental root infection.
- Control predisposing factors.
- Use appropriate antibiotic therapy.
- Establish drainage by stimulation of mucociliary flow and relief of obstruction.

Guidelines for antibiotic therapy

Consider therapy for severe cases displaying at least three of the following:

- persistent mucopurulent nasal discharge (>7–10 days)
- facial pain
- poor response to decongestants
- tenderness over the sinuses especially maxillary
- tenderness on percussion of maxillary molar and premolar teeth that cannot be attributed to by a single tooth

Measures

- Analgesics
- Antibiotics:[4]
  amoxycillin 500 mg (o) tds for 7 days
  or (if sensitive to penicillin)
  doxycycline 100 mg (o) bd for 7 days
  or
  cefaclor 500 mg (o) tds for 7 days
  or
  amoxycillin + clavulanate 875/125 mg (o) tds for 7–14 days if poor response to above (indicates resistant *H. influenzae*)
- In complicated or severe disease, use intravenous cephalosporins or flucloxacillin
- Nasal decongestants (oxymetazoline-containing nasal drops or sprays)[5] for 5 days (only if congestion)
- Inhalations (a very important adjunct)
- Nasal saline irrigation

Antihistamines and mucolytics are of no proven value.

Invasive methods

Surgical drainage may be necessary by atrial lavage or frontal sinus trephine.

Inhalations for sinusitis

The old method of towel over the head and inhalation bowl can be used, but it is better to direct the vapour at the nose. Equipment needed is a container, which can be an old disposable bowl, a wide-mouthed bottle or tin, or a plastic container.

For the inhalant, several household over-the-counter preparations are suitable such as Friar's Balsam (5 mL), Vicks VapoRub (1 teaspoon), or menthol (5 mL).

The cover can be made from a paper bag (with its base cut out), a cone of paper or a small cardboard carton (with the corner cut away).

Method

1 Add 5 mL or 1 teaspoon of the inhalant to 0.5 L (or 1 pint) of boiled water in the container.
2 Place the paper or carton over the container.
3 Get the patient to apply nose and mouth to the opening and breathe in the vapour deeply and slowly through the nose, and then out slowly through the mouth.
4 This should be performed for 5–10 minutes, three times a day, especially before retiring.

After inhalation, upper airway congestion can be relieved by autoinsufflation.

Chronic sinusitis

Chronic sinusitis or recurrent sinusitis may arise from chronic infection or allergy. It may be associated with nasal polyps and vasomotor rhinitis, but is frequently associated with a structural abnormality of the upper airways. Refer to CHAPTER 59.

It does not usually cause pain unless an acute infection intervenes. The acute or chronic attack is treated as for the acute attack but with 14 days of antibiotics. Those with an allergic mucous membrane may respond to intranasal corticosteroids. Surgical intervention will benefit chronic recurrence with mechanical blockage.

TMJ dysfunction

This condition is due to abnormal movement of the mandible, especially during chewing. The basic causes are dental malocclusion and masticatory muscle dysfunction. Check for bruxism. The pain is felt over the joint and tends to be localised to the region of the ear and mandibular condyle, but it may radiate forwards to the cheek and even the neck.

Examination

- Check for pain and limitation of mandibular movements, especially on opening the mouth.
- Palpate about the joint bilaterally for tenderness, which typically lies immediately in front of the external auditory meatus; palpate the temporalis and masseter muscles.
- Palpate the TMJ over the lateral aspect of the joint disc.
- Ask the patient to open the mouth fully when tenderness is maximal. The TMJ can be palpated posteriorly by inserting the little finger into the external canal.
- Check for crepitus in mandibular movement.

Management

If organic disease such as rheumatoid arthritis and obvious dental malocclusion is excluded, a special set of instructions or exercises can alleviate the annoying problem of TMJ arthralgia in about 3 weeks. Warm packs may help. Provide patient education advice and self-care.

Method 1: 'Chewing' the piece of soft wood

- Obtain a rod of soft wood approximately 15 cm long and 1.5 cm wide. An ideal object is a large carpenter's pencil.
- Instruct the patient to position this at the back of the mouth so that the molars grasp the object with the mandible thrust forward.
- The patient then rhythmically bites on the object with a grinding movement for 2–3 minutes at least 3 times a day.

Method 2: The 'six by six' program

This is a specific program recommended by some dental surgeons. The six exercises should be carried out six times on each occasion, six times a day, taking about 1–2 minutes.

Instruct the patient as follows:

1. Hold the front one-third of your tongue to the roof of your mouth and take six deep breaths.
2. Hold the tongue to the roof of your mouth and open your mouth six times. Your jaw should not click.
3. Hold your chin with both hands keeping the chin still. Without letting your chin move, push up, down and to each side. Remember, do not let your chin move.
4. Hold both hands behind your neck and pull chin in.
5. Push on upper lip so as to push head straight back.
6. Pull shoulders back as if to touch shoulder blades together.

These exercises should be pain-free. If they hurt, do not push them to the limit until pain eases.

Treatments

Injection into the TMJ[7]

- Indications: painful rheumatoid arthritis, osteoarthritis or TMJ dysfunction not responding to conservative measures. Inject a 1 mL solution of local anaesthetic and corticosteroid in equal parts.
- Dental management that may be required for malfunction of the bite includes dental occlusal splinting.
- NSAIDs: A trial of NSAIDs, e.g. ibuprofen 400 mg (o) tds for 10 days, for TMJ inflammation may need consideration. Cease if no response after 10 days.

52

Inflammatory or ulcerative oropharyngeal lesions

A variety of ulcerative conditions and infections of structures such as gingivae, tongue, tonsils, larynx and pharynx can cause facial pain (refer to CHAPTER 72). Gingivostomatitis, herpes labialis (cold sores) and aphthous ulceration are common examples. Lesions of the posterior third of the tongue, the oropharynx, tonsils and larynx may radiate to the region of the ear via the tympanic branch of the ninth nerve or the auricular branch of the tenth nerve.

Trigeminal neuralgia

Trigeminal neuralgia (tic douloureux) is a condition of often unknown cause that typically occurs in patients over the age of 50, affecting the second and third divisions of the trigeminal nerve and on the same side of the face. Brief paroxysms of pain, often with associated trigger points, are a feature.

Clinical features

- Site: sensory branches of the trigeminal nerve (see FIG. 52.5) almost always unilateral (often right side)
- Radiation: tends to commence in the mandibular division and spreads to the maxillary division and (rarely) to the ophthalmic division
- Quality: excruciating, searing jabs of pain like a burning knife or electric shock
- Frequency: variable and no regular pattern
- Duration: seconds to 1–2 minutes (up to 15 minutes)
- Onset: spontaneous or trigger point stimulus
- Offset: spontaneous
- Precipitating factors: talking, chewing, touching trigger areas on face (e.g. washing, shaving, eating), cold weather or wind, turning onto pillow
- Aggravating factors: trigger points usually in the upper and lower lip, nasolabial fold or lower eyelid (see FIG. 52.6)
- Relieving factors: nil
- Associated features: rarely occurs at night; spontaneous remissions for months or years
- Signs: there are no signs, normal corneal reflex

Causes

- Unknown
- Local pressure on the nerve root entry zone by tortuous pulsatile dilated small vessels (probably up to 75%)
- Multiple sclerosis
- Neurosyphilis
- Tumours of the posterior fossa

Note: Precise diagnosis is essential. MRI may be helpful.

Treatment

- Patient education, reassurance and empathic support is very important in these patients.

Medical therapy

carbamazepine (from onset of the attack to resolution)[8] 50 mg (elderly patient) or 100 mg (o) bd initially; gradually increase the dose to avoid drowsiness every 7 days to 200 mg bd (maintenance); higher dosage to maximum 600 mg bd may be necessary

Alternative drugs if carbamazepine not tolerated or ineffective (but question the diagnosis if lack of response):

gabapentin 300 mg daily initially, then increase
lamotrigine 400 mg (o) daily

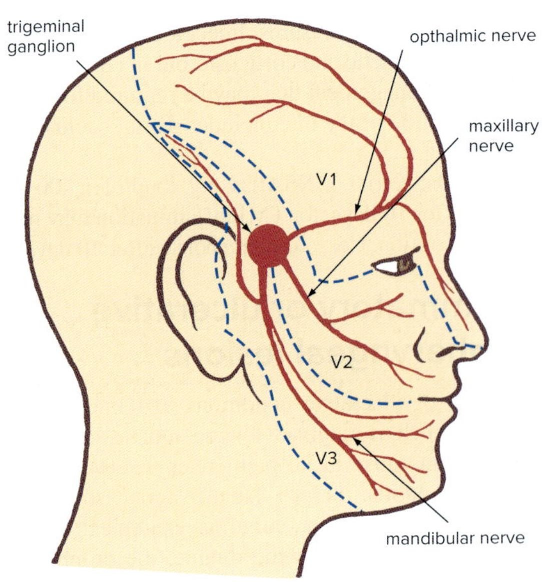

FIGURE 52.5 Typical cutaneous sensory distribution of the trigeminal nerve and its branches

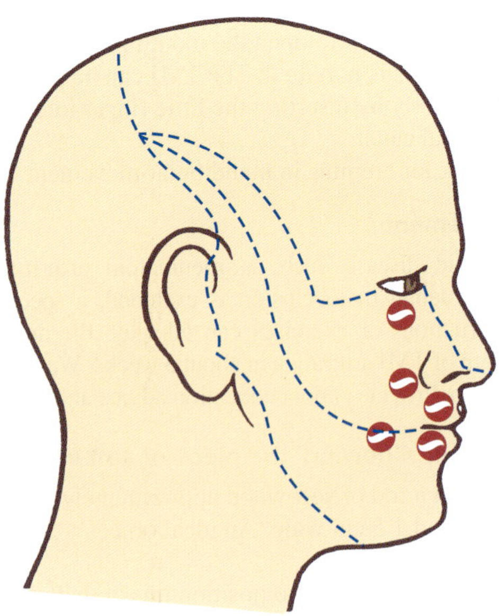

FIGURE 52.6 Trigeminal neuralgia: typical trigger points

phenytoin 300–500 mg daily
clonazepam
baclofen
sodium valproate

Surgery

- Refer to a neurosurgeon if medication ineffective
- Possible procedures include:
  - decompression of the trigeminal nerve root (e.g. gel foam packing between the nerve and blood vessels)
  - if severe, refer for neuroablative treatment, e.g. thermocoagulation/radiofrequency neurolysis
  - surgical division of peripheral branches

Glossopharyngeal neuralgia[8,9,10]

This is an uncommon condition of the ninth cranial nerve and branches of the vagus nerve with similar clinical features of severe, lancinating pains, particularly felt in one ear, the base of the tongue or beneath the angle of the jaw. The pain usually lasts 30–60 seconds.

- Sites: back of throat around tonsillar fossa and adjacent fauces deep in ear, back of tongue
- Radiation: ear canal, neck
- Triggers: swallowing, coughing, talking, yawning, laughing
- Treatment: as for trigeminal neuralgia

Migrainous neuralgia (cluster headache)

As described in CHAPTER 56, the pain is unilateral and centred around the eye with associated lacrimation and stuffiness of the nose.

Facial migraine (lower half headache)[8]

Migraine may rarely affect the face below the level of the eyes, causing pain in the area of the cheek and upper jaw. It may spread over the nostril and lower jaw. The pain is dull and throbbing, and nausea and vomiting are commonly present. The treatment is as for other varieties of migraine with simple analgesics or ergotamine for infrequent attacks.

Chronic paroxysmal hemicrania

In the rare condition of chronic or episodic paroxysmal hemicrania there is a unilateral facial pain that can resemble chronic cluster headache but the duration is briefer, about 15 minutes, and it may recur many times a day even for years. It responds dramatically to indomethacin.[11]

Herpes zoster and postherpetic neuralgia

Refer to CHAPTER 121. Herpes zoster may present as hyperaesthesia or a burning sensation in any division of the fifth nerve, especially the ophthalmic division.

Atypical facial pain

This is mainly a diagnosis of exclusion whereby patients, usually middle-aged to elderly women, complain of diffuse pain in the cheek (unilateral or bilateral) without demonstrable organic disease. The pain does not usually conform to a specific nerve distribution (although in the maxillary area), varies in intensity and duration and is not lancinating as in trigeminal neuralgia. It is usually described as deep-seated and 'boring', severe, continuous and throbbing in nature. It is a very confusing and difficult problem to treat. These patients tend to show psychoneurotic tendencies but caution is needed in labelling them as functional.

Treatment

Trial of an antidepressant[8], e.g.:

amitriptyline 10–75 mg nocte (first line)
or
dothiepin 25–150 mg nocte

Temporal arteritis

This may produce mild or severe unilateral or bilateral headache. There may be ischaemic pain in the jaws when chewing. There may be marked scalp tenderness over the affected arteries. See CHAPTER 32 for management.

52

Erysipelas

Classical erysipelas is a superficial form of cellulitis involving the face. It usually presents with the sudden onset of butterfly erythema with a well-defined edge (see FIG. 52.7). It often starts around the nose and there may be underlying sinus or dental infection which should be investigated. There is an associated 'flu-like' illness and fever. It is invariably caused by *Streptococcus pyogenes*. Treatment is by phenoxymethylpenicillin or di/flucloxacillin for 7–10 days.

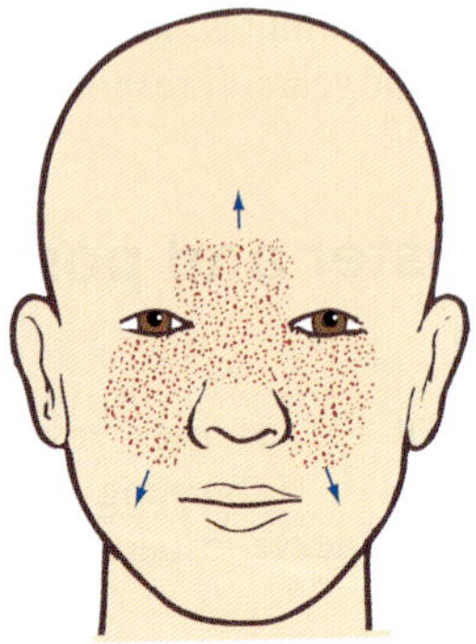

FIGURE 52.7 Erysipelas: typical spreading distribution of the infection

When to refer

- Severe trigeminal or glossopharyngeal neuralgia
- Unusual facial pain, especially with a suspicion of malignancy
- Continuing pain of uncertain cause
- Positive neurological signs, such as impaired corneal reflex, impaired sensation in a trigeminal dermatome, slight facial weakness, hearing loss on the side of the neuralgia
- Possible need for surgical drainage of sinusitis—indications for surgery include failure of appropriate medical treatment, anatomical deformity, polyps, uncontrolled sinus pain[5]
- Dental root infection causing maxillary sinusitis
- Other dental disorders

Practice tips

- Malignancy must be excluded in the elderly with facial pain.
- Problems from the molar teeth, especially the third (wisdom), commonly present with peri-auricular pain without aural disease and pain in the posterior cheek.
- Facial pain never crosses the midline; bilateral pain means bilateral lesions.[12]
- If no obvious cause of persistent pain, refer to exclude sinister cause: don't overdiagnosis sinusitis.

Patient education resources

Hand-out sheets from *Murtagh's Patient Education* 7th edition:

- Sinusitis
- Temporomandibular joint dysfunction

References

1 Beck ER, Francis JL, Souhami RL. *Tutorials in Differential Diagnosis.* Edinburgh: Longman Cheshire, 1987: 161–4.

2 Gerschman JA, Reade PC. Orofacial pain. Aust Fam Physician, 1984; 13: 14–24.

3 Expert group for Analgesic. Oral and dental. In: eTG complete [Internet]. Melbourne: Therapeutic Guidelines Ltd. Available from: <www.tg.org.au>, accessed September 2017.

4 Kumar R, Sambrook P, Goss AW. Mismanagement of dental infection. Aust Prescr, 2011; 34: 40–1.

5 Stevens M. The diagnosis and management of acute and chronic sinusitis. Modern Medicine Australia, 1991; April: 16–26.

6 Bridges-Webb C. Diagnosing sinus tenderness: practice tip. Aust Fam Physician, 1981; 10: 742.

7 Murtagh J. *Practice Tips* (7th edn). Sydney: McGraw-Hill, 2017: 48–9.

8 Expert group for Neurology. Facial pain. In: eTG complete [Internet]. Melbourne: Therapeutic Guidelines Ltd. Available from: <www.tg.org.au>, accessed September 2017.

9 Mendelsohn M, Lance J, Wheatley D. Facial pain: how to treat. Australian Doctor, 7 November; 2003: 31–6.

10 Wiffen PJ et al. Carbamazepine for acute and chronic pain in adults (Cochrane Review). Cochrane Database. Syst Rev. 2011, Issue 19. Art No. CD005451.

11 Burns R. Pitfalls in headache management. Aust Fam Physician, 1990; 19: 1825.

12 Quail G. Diagnosing facial pain: non oro-dental causes. New Zeal Dent J, 2017; 113: 17–21.

Fever and chills

53

Why! the fever itself is nature's instrument.

THOMAS SYDENHAM (1624–89), *MEDICAL OBSERVATIONS*

Although fever is a sign of disease and usually occurs in response to infection (mainly viral), its presence is recognised as playing an important role in the individual's defence against infection. The infecting pathogen triggers hypothalamic receptors, causing the thermostatic mechanisms to be reset to maintain core temperature at a higher level. The elevation in temperature results from increased heat production (e.g. shivering) or decreased loss (e.g. peripheral vasoconstriction). The elevation in body temperature activates T-cell production, increases the effectiveness of interferons and limits the replication of some common viruses.[1]

Key facts and checkpoints

- Fever plays an important physiological role in the defence against infection.
- Normal body temperature (measured orally mid-morning) is 36–37.2°C (average 36.8°C).
- Fever can be defined as an early-morning oral temperature >37.2°C or a temperature >37.8°C at other times of the day.[2]
- Oral temperature is about 0.4°C lower than core body temperature.
- Axillary temperature is 0.5°C lower than oral temperature.
- Rectal, vaginal and ear drum temperatures are 0.5°C higher than oral and reflect core body temperature.
- There can be a normal diurnal variation of 0.5–1°C (lowest in early morning and highest in late afternoon).
- Fevers due to infections have an upper limit of 40.5–41.1°C.
- Hyperthermia (temperature above 41.1°C) and hyperpyrexia appear to have no upper limit.
- Infection remains the most important cause of acute fever.[3]
- Symptoms associated with fever include sweats, chills, rigors and headache.
- General causes of fever include infections, malignant disease, mechanical trauma (e.g. crush injury), vascular accidents (e.g. infarction, cerebral haemorrhage), immunogenic disorders (e.g. drug reactions, SLE), acute metabolic disorders (e.g. gout), and haemopoietic disorders (e.g. acute haemolytic anaemia).[3]
- Drugs can cause fever, presumably because of hypersensitivity.[3] Important examples are allopurinol, antihistamines, barbiturates, cephalosporins, cimetidine, methyldopa, penicillins, isoniazid, quinidine, phenolphthalein (including laxatives), phenytoin, procainamide, salicylates and sulphonamides.
- Drug fever should abate by 48 hours after discontinuation of the drug.[4]
- Infectious diseases at the extremes of age (very young and aged)[3] often present with atypical symptoms and signs. Their condition may deteriorate rapidly.
- Overseas travellers or visitors may have special, even exotic infections and require special evaluation (refer to CHAPTER 15).
- Immunologically compromised patients (e.g. AIDS patients) pose a special risk for infections, including opportunistic infections.
- A febrile illness is characteristic of the acute infection of HIV: at least 50% have an illness like glandular fever. Think of it!

Chills/rigors[2]

The abrupt onset of fever with a chill or rigor is a feature of some diseases. Examples include:

- bacteraemia/septicaemia
- pneumococcal pneumonia
- pyogenic infection with bacteraemia
- lymphoma
- pyelonephritis
- visceral abscesses (e.g. perinephric, lung)
- malaria
- biliary sepsis (Charcot triad—jaundice, right hypochondrial pain, fever/rigors)

Features of a true chill are teeth chattering and bed shaking, which is quite different from the chilly sensations that occur in almost all fevers, particularly those in viral infections. The event lasts 10–20 minutes.

Other features:

- shaking cannot be stopped voluntarily
- absence of sweating
- cold extremities and pallor (peripheral vascular shutdown)
- dry mouth and pilo-erection: lasts 10–20 minutes

Hyperthermia

Hyperthermia or hyperpyrexia is a temperature greater than 41.1°C. A more accurate definition is a state when the body's metabolic heat production or environmental heat load exceeds normal heat loss capacity. Hyperthermia may be observed particularly in the tropics, in malaria and heatstroke. It can occur with CNS tumours, infections or haemorrhages because of its effect on the hypothalamus.

Heatstroke (sunstroke, thermic fever)[5]

This is the sudden onset of hot, dry, flushed skin with a rapid pulse, temperature above 40°C, and confusion or altered conscious state in a person exposed to a very hot environment. The BP is usually not affected initially but circulatory collapse may precede death. It is a life-threatening emergency. The diagnosis is clinical. Differential diagnoses include severe acute infection, toxic shock, food, chemical and drug poisoning. The elderly and debilitated are susceptible as are children left in cars.

Treatment

- Immediate effective cooling water applied to skin
- Icepacks at critical points (e.g. axillae, neck, head)
- Ice water bath if possible
- Aim to bring down temperature by 1°C every 10 minutes

53

Malignant hyperthermia

This is a rare hereditary disorder characterised by rapidly developing hyperpyrexia, muscular rigidity and acidosis in patients undergoing major surgery.

Sweats

Sweating is a heat loss mechanism, and diffuse sweating that may soak clothing and bedclothing permits rapid release of heat by evaporation. In febrile patients the skin is usually hot and dry—sweating occurs in most when the temperature falls. It is characteristic of only some fevers (e.g. septic infections and rheumatic fever).

Factitious fever

Factitious fever is usually encountered in hospitalised patients attempting to malinger. The situation is usually suspected when:

- a series of high temperatures is recorded to form an atypical pattern of fluctuation
- there is excessively high temperature (41.1°C) and above
- a recorded high temperature is unaccompanied by warm skin, tachycardia and other signs of fever such as a flushed face and sweating
- there is an absence of diurnal variation

The patient may have surreptitiously dipped the thermometer in warm water, placed it in contact with a heat source or heated the bulb by friction with bedclothes or even mucous membranes of the mouth.

Neuroleptic malignant syndrome

This is often confused with 'malignant' hyperthermia and heat stroke. The syndrome includes high temperature, muscle rigidity, autonomic dysfunction and altered consciousness. It is a rare and potentially lethal reaction in patients taking antipsychotic drugs, particularly occurring with haloperidol alone or with other drugs especially lithium carbonate. Refer to CHAPTER 45.

Measurement of temperature

Temperature can be measured by several methods, including the mercury thermometer, the liquid crystal thermometer and the electronic probe thermometer. The mercury thermometer is a most widely used and effective temperature-measuring instrument. However, it is less popular now and not favoured for infant use by the American Academy of Paediatricians.

Basic rules of usage for the mercury thermometer

1. Before use, shake down to 35–36°C.
2. After use:
   - shake down and store in antiseptic
   - do not run under hot water
   - wipe rectal thermometer with alcohol and store separately
3. Recording time is 3 minutes orally and 1–2 minutes rectally.

Accidental breakage in the mouth

If a child bites off the end of a mercury thermometer there is no need for alarm, as the small amount of mercury is non-toxic and the piece of glass will usually pass in the stool.

Oral use

1 Place under the tongue at the junction of the base of the tongue and the floor of the mouth to one side of the frenulum—the 'heat' pocket.
2 Ensure that the mouth is kept shut.
3 Remove dentures.

Note: This is unsuitable for children 4 years and under, especially if irritable.

Rectal use

This is an appropriate route for babies and young children under the age of 4 years but should be used with care. The rule is '2–3 cm in for 2–3 minutes' and some authorities claim that this method is the gold standard, especially in infants.

Method

1 Lubricate the stub with petroleum or KY jelly.
2 Insert for 2–3 cm past anal verge.
3 Keep the thermometer between the flexed fingers with the hand resting on the buttocks (see FIG. 53.1).

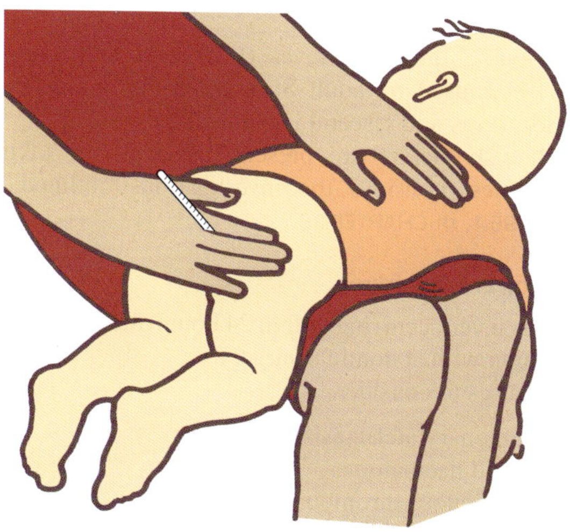

FIGURE 53.1 Rectal temperature measurement in infants

Don't:

- dig thermometer in too hard
- hold it too rigidly
- allow the child to move around

Axillary use

This is unreliable with poor sensitivity and generally should be avoided but may be practical in young children.[6]

If used, place high in the axilla for 3 minutes. Fever is present if the temperature is above 37.2°C.

Groin use

This route is not ideal but is more reliable than the axilla. It closely approximates oral temperature. In infants, the thigh should be flexed against the abdomen.

Vaginal use

This is mainly used as an adjunct to the assessment of ovulation during the menstrual cycle. It should be placed deeply in the vagina for 5 minutes before leaving bed in the morning.

Digital peak hold thermometer

Infrared aural (eardrum) use

Otic thermography is now accepted standard practice. The temperature can be measured in 3 seconds, with the infrared device (e–2 therm) placed in the ear canal. First, hold the child's head firmly to avoid any movement, then take temperature. Wait 2 minutes before taking the temperature in the same ear. The tympanic membrane (TM) accurately reflects hypothalamic temperature, which in turn reflects core body temperature. The TM is also immune from the effects of eating, drinking and smoking. A systematic review in the Cochrane study questions its reliability. It is poor in small infants but useful over the age of 6 months.[7] However, some Australian authorities believe that in general practice the benefits of convenience outweigh the lack of accuracy.[8] The normal range is the same as for rectal temperature.

Digital electronic pacifier (dummy) thermometer

This is a popular method for infants and younger children, favoured by many paediatricians in the US.

Skin use

Plastic strip thermometers placed on the forehead are very inaccurate and should not be used.

The clinical approach

The initial approach is to evaluate the severity of the problem and the nature of the illness. Some infections, particularly bacterial infections, are life-threatening and this requires urgent diagnosis and hospital admission.

According to Yung and Stanley[3] it is helpful to consider fever in three categories: less than 3 days duration; between 4 and 14 days duration; and protracted fever (more than 14 days).

Fever of less than 3 days duration

This is very commonly encountered in family practice, often due to a self-limiting viral infection of the respiratory tract. It is important, however, to be vigilant for other infections, so evidence of an infectious disease, urinary tract infection, pneumonia or other infection should be sought. A routine urine examination, especially in females, is an important screening investigation. The majority of patients can be managed conservatively.

Fever present for 4–14 days

If fever persists beyond 4–5 days a less common infection should be suspected since most common viral infections will have resolved by about 4 days.[3] A careful history is mandatory, as outlined later in the chapter for fever of unknown origin (FUO). The basic examination and investigations are along similar lines.

Temperature chart

Charting the patterns of fever may be a diagnostic help because some febrile conditions follow a predictable temperature pattern.[9] Examples are presented in FIGURE 53.2.

Intermittent fever

This is a fever in which the temperature rises for a few hours each day and then returns to normal (see FIG. 53.2a). Examples include various pyogenic infections, cytomegalovirus and lymphoma.

53

Relapsing fever

The fever returns to normal for days before rising again. Malaria is the classic example of periodic relapsing fever: in quartan fever, caused by *Plasmodium malariae* (see FIG. 53.2a), the attacks occur every 72 hours (the term *quartan* means every 4th day by inclusive counting). This compares with tertian fever from *Plasmodium vivax* in which paroxysms of malaria occur every 48 hours, that is, every 3rd day.

Remittent fever

This is a fever in which the temperature returns towards normal for a variable period but is always elevated (see FIG. 53.2d). Common examples are collections of pus (e.g. pelvic abscess, wound infection, empyema and carcinoma). It is a common feature of empyema.

Undulant fever

Undulant fever is characterised by bouts of continuous or remittent fever for several days, followed by afebrile remissions lasting a variable number of days. It is commonly a feature of brucellosis infection but is also seen in the lymphomas, especially Hodgkin lymphoma (see FIG. 53.2b). The latter is referred to as Pel–Ebstein fever with fevers lasting 3–10 days followed by afebrile periods of 3–10 days.

Continuous fever pattern

This is common with viral infections such as influenza (see FIG. 53.2c).

Quotidian fever

In this pattern the fever recurs daily (see FIG. 53.2d). Daily fever spikes in the morning are characteristic of *Pseudomonas* infection (e.g. pulmonary superinfection); afternoon spikes are indicative of cytomegalovirus infection; and evening spikes suggest localised collection of pus (e.g. empyema of the gall bladder).

Double quotidian fever (two fever spikes in a day) is caused by adult Still syndrome, gonococcal endocarditis and visceral leishmaniasis.

If risk factors are present, especially if taking antibiotics, consider the investigations outlined in TABLE 96.1, in CHAPTER 96.

Postoperative fever

This is fever occurring within 24 hours after surgery—common with abdominal surgery.

Causes to consider:

- pulmonary atelectasis (common)
- wound haematoma
- deep venous thrombosis
- myocardial infarction
- allergic drug reaction
- transfusion reaction

Septic problems related to the operation usually develop after several days.

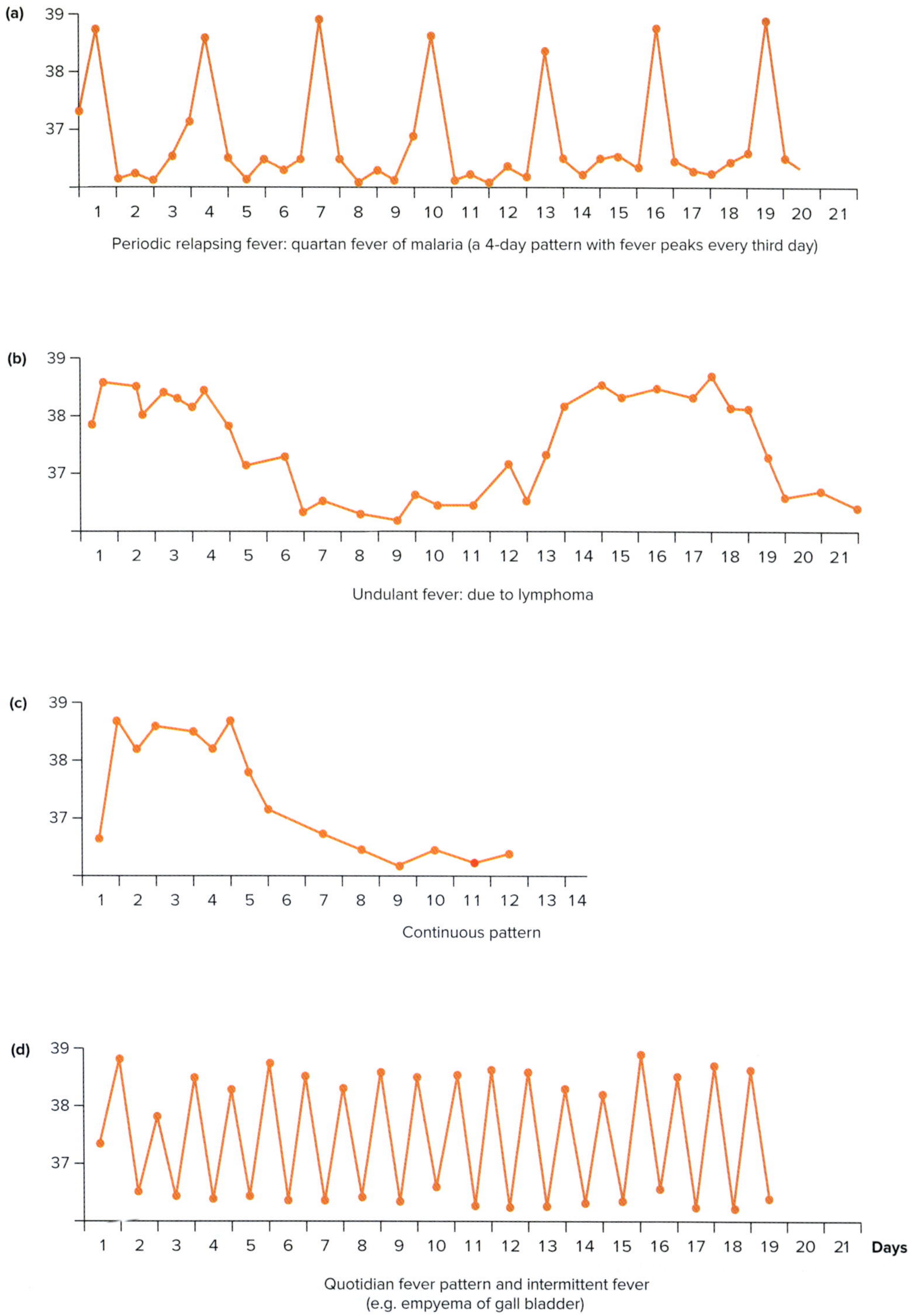

FIGURE 53.2 Examples of fever patterns from temperature charts

Fever in children

In children, most authorities would consider a fever of 38.5°C and above to be significant and warrant close scrutiny.[10] If it is below this, it is not caused by teething or swaddling.

Important causes not to be missed:

- urinary infection
- meningitis/encephalitis
- pneumonia
- septicaemia/bacteraemia
- osteomyelitis
- septic arthritis
- pertussis
- abscess

The fever is usually a response to a viral infection. Fever itself is not harmful until it reaches a level of 41.5°C.[1] Hyperthermia is uncommon in children. Temperatures above 41°C are usually due to CNS infection or the result of human error, for example:

- shutting a child in a car on a hot day
- overwrapping a febrile child

Complications include dehydration (usually mild) and febrile convulsions, which occur in 5% of febrile children between 6 months and 5 years. Febrile convulsions are triggered by a rapid rise in temperature rather than its absolute level.

Note: Teething does *not* cause fever.

Approach to the febrile infant

It is important to decide whether the child looks well or seriously ill. Identification of the very ill child is presented in CHAPTER 96.

If the child is well and has no risk factors (e.g. unreliable caregiver, poor access to treatment, medical risk factors, taking antibiotics) treat expectantly. The only test required is urine microscopy and culture. Educate the caregiver about review if serious signs develop. Treat the fever as outlined in TABLE 96.1, in CHAPTER 96.

Management

- Treatment of low-grade fevers should be discouraged.
- Treatment of high-grade fevers includes:
  - treatment of the causes of the fever (if appropriate)
  - adequate fluid intake/increased fluids
  - paracetamol (acetaminophen) is the preferred antipyretic since aspirin is potentially dangerous in young children (use paracetamol if temperature >38.5°C). The usual dose of 10–15 mg/kg every 4–6 hours may represent undertreatment. Use 20 mg/kg as a loading dose and then 15 mg/kg maintenance
  - evidence favours tepid sponging for first 30 minutes combined with paracetamol[11]
  - ibuprofen 5–10 mg/kg every 6 hours is a suitable antipyretic

Advice to parents

- Dress the child in light clothing (stripping off is unnecessary).
- Do not overheat with too many clothes, rugs or blankets.
- Give frequent small drinks of light fluids, especially water.
- Sponging with cool water and using fans is not effective.

Febrile convulsions

Refer to CHAPTER 96.

Fever in the elderly

The elderly tend to have a problem with impaired thermoregulation and so they may not develop a fever in response to suppurative infection compared with younger people. This can be misleading in the diagnostic process.

Important facts

- Any fever in the elderly is significant.
- Viral infection is a less common cause of fever in the elderly.
- Fever in the elderly is sepsis until proven otherwise (common sites are the lungs and urinary tract).

The elderly are more vulnerable to hyperthermia and hypothermia. Heatstroke classically occurs in epidemic form during a heatwave. The syndrome consists of hyperpyrexia, decreased sweating, delirium and coma. The core temperature is usually over 41°C.

'Alarm bell' signs

In many patients the existence of a life-threatening infective illness is obvious and prompt action is essential. In others the diagnosis is not clear-cut but there are certain warning signs (see Red flags box).

These 'red flag' symptoms and signs are obviously super 'sensitive'. Patients with some of these features may have potentially life-threatening diseases, but this list would include many with viral infections.

Fever of undetermined origin

Fever of undetermined origin (FUO), also referred to as pyrexia of unknown origin (PUO), has the following (Petersdorf–Beeson modified) criteria:[12]

- illness for at least 3 weeks
- fevers >38.3°C (100.9°F) on several occasions
- undiagnosed after 1 week of intensive study

Red flag pointers for fever

- High fever
- Repeated rigors
- Drenching night sweats
- Severe myalgia (? sepsis)
- Severe pain anywhere (? sepsis)
- Severe sore throat or dysphagia (? *Haemophilus influenzae* epiglottitis)
- Altered mental state
- Incessant vomiting
- Unexplained rash
- Jaundice
- Marked pallor
- Tachycardia
- Tachypnoea

Most cases represent unusual manifestations of common diseases and not rare or exotic diseases. Examples are tuberculosis, bacterial endocarditis, hepatobiliary disease and lung cancer.[13]

Keep in mind that the longer the duration of fever, the less likely the diagnosis is to be infectious—fevers that last greater than 6 months are rarely infectious (only 6%). One study showed that 9% are factitious.[14]

Patients with FUO in definite need of further investigation are:

- babies <3 months of age
- children with fever >40°C
- adults >50 years
- diabetics
- the immunocompromised
- travellers

A diagnostic approach

A knowledge of the more common causes of FUO is helpful in planning a diagnostic approach (refer to TABLE 53.1).

History

The history should include consideration of past history, occupation, travel history, sexual history, IV drug use (leads to endocarditis and abscesses), animal contact, medication and other relevant factors. Symptoms such as pruritus, a skin rash and fever patterns may provide clues for the diagnosis. The average patient with a difficult FUO needs to have a careful history taken on at least three separate occasions.[15]

Examination

A common mistake is the tendency to examine the patient only once and not re-examine. The patient

Table 53.1 Diagnostic strategy for fever that is prolonged (FUO)

Probability diagnosis

Pyogenic abscess (anywhere, e.g. liver, pelvis
Pneumonia (viral, bacterial, atypical)
Epstein–Barr mononucleosis
Viral upper respiratory tract infection
Urinary infection (incl. chronic pyelonephritis)

Serious disorders not to be missed

Vascular:

- vasculitides (polyarteritis nodosa, giant cell arteritis/polymyalgia)

Infection:

- HIV/AIDS
- malaria and other tropical diseases
- zoonoses (e.g. leptospirosis, Q fever, listeriosis)
- typhoid/paratyphoid fever
- tuberculosis
- osteomyelitis
- chronic septicaemia/bacteraemia
- infective endocarditis
- Lyme disease
- syphilis (secondary)

Cancer (up to 30%):

- lymphoma and leukaemia
- solid cancers (e.g. lung, kidney)
- disseminated

Other:

- inflammatory bowel disease (e.g. Crohn)

Pitfalls (often missed)

Connective tissue disorder (e.g. rheumatoid arthritis, systemic lupus erythematosus)
Sarcoidosis
Drug idiosyncrasies

Rarities:

- factitious fever

Note: Up to 20% remain unknown.

should be examined regularly (as for history taking) as physical signs can develop eventually. HIV infection must be excluded. Special attention should be paid to the following (see FIG. 53.3):

- skin—look for rashes, vesicles and nodules
- the eyes and ocular fundi
- temporal arteries
- sinuses and ears (canal and TM)
- teeth and oral cavity—? dental abscess, other signs
- heart—murmurs, pericardial rubs
- lungs—abnormalities including consolidation, pleuritic rub
- abdomen—enlarged/tender liver, spleen or kidney
- rectal and pelvic examination (note genitalia)
- lymph nodes, especially cervical (supraclavicular)
- blood vessels, especially of the legs—? thrombosis
- urine (analysis)

Investigations[16]

Basic investigations include:

- haemoglobin, red cell indices and blood film
- white cell count
- ESR/C-reactive protein
- chest X-ray and sinus films
- urine examination (analysis and culture)
- routine blood chemistry
- blood cultures

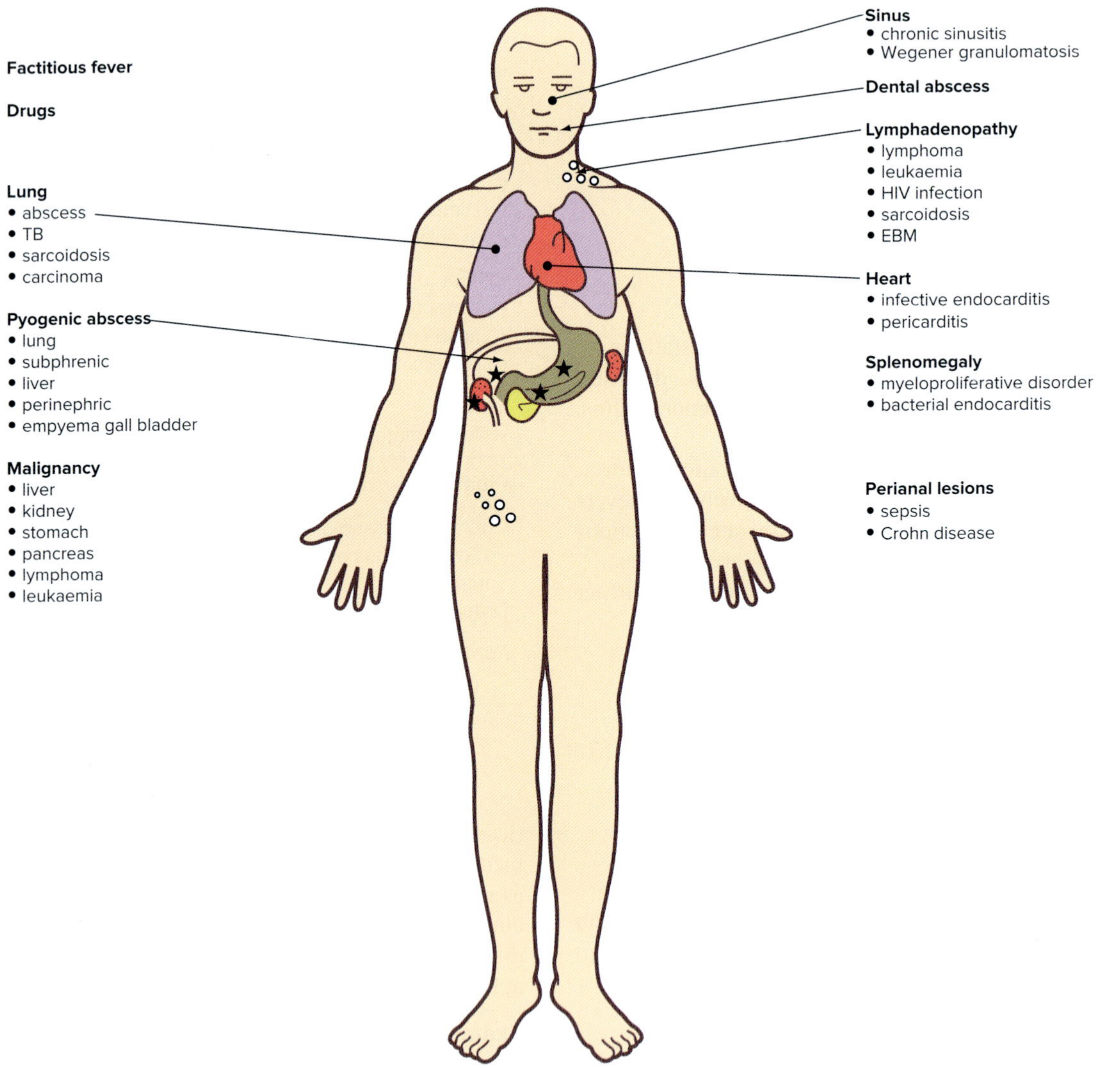

FIGURE 53.3 Sites to consider in FUO (malignancy is indicated by a star)

53

Further possible investigations (depending on clinical features):

- stool microscopy and culture
- culture of sputum (if any)
- specific tests for malaria, typhoid, EBM, Q fever, brucellosis, psittacosis, cytomegalovirus, toxoplasmosis, syphilis, various tropical diseases and others
- NAAT (e.g. PCR) tests
- HIV screening
- tests for rheumatic fever
- tuberculin test
- tests for connective tissue disorders (e.g. DNA antibodies, C-reactive protein)
- upper GIT series with small bowel follow-through
- CT and ultrasound scanning for primary and secondary neoplasia
- gall bladder functioning
- occult abscesses
- MRI—best for detecting lesions of the nervous system
- echocardiography—for suspected endocarditis
- isotope scanning for specific causes
- aspiration or needle biopsy
- laparoscopy for suspected pelvic infection
- tissue biopsies (e.g. lymph nodes, skin, liver, bone marrow) as indicated

FUO in children

Fever in children is usually a transient phenomenon and subsides within 4–5 days. At least 70% of all infections are viral. Occasionally a child will present with FUO which may be masked from antibiotic administration. Common causes of prolonged fever in children differ from those in adults. Most cases are not due to unusual or esoteric disorders,[17] the majority representing atypical manifestation of common diseases.

A summary of the common causes (with the most common ranked first) is as follows.[17]

Infectious causes (40%)

- Viral syndrome
- Urinary tract infection
- Pneumonia
- Pharyngitis
- Sinusitis
- Meningitis

Collagen–vascular disorders (15%)

- Rheumatic arthritis
- Systemic lupus erythematosus
- Rheumatic fever
- Henoch–Schönlein syndrome

Neoplastic disorders (7%)

- Leukaemia
- Reticulum cell sarcoma
- Lymphoma

Inflammatory diseases of the bowel (4%)

Septicaemia

The diagnosis of septicaemia can be easily missed, especially in small children, the elderly and the immunocompromised, and in the absence of classic signs, which are:

- fever
- rash (suggestive of meningococcus)
- tachycardia
- tachypnoea
- cool extremities

Patients with septicaemia require urgent referral as it has a very high mortality rate.[18] Investigations should include two sets of blood cultures and other appropriate cultures (e.g. urine, wound, sputum). Empirical initial treatment in adults (after blood cultures) is di/flucloxacillin IV and gentamicin IV.[19]

Glossary of terms

Bacteraemia The transient presence of bacteria in the blood (usually asymptomatic) caused by local infection or trauma.

Septicaemia (sepsis) The multiplication of bacteria or fungi in the blood, usually causing a systemic inflammatory response (SIRS). SIRS is defined as two or more of (in adults):

- temperature >38°C or <36°C
- respiratory rate >20/min
- heart rate >90/min
- WCC >12 × 10^9/L or <4 × 10^9/L

Severe sepsis Sepsis associated with organ dysfunction, hypoperfusion or hypotension with two or more of: fever, tachycardia, tachypnoea and elevated WCC.

Septic shock Sepsis with critical tissue perfusion causing acute circulatory failure including hypotension and peripheral shutdown—cool extremities, mottled skin, cyanosis. Consider *S. aureus* (food poisoning, tampon use) and *S. pyogenes.*

Pyaemia A serious manifestation of septicaemia whereby organisms and neutrophils undergo

continued

continued

embolisation to many sites, causing abscesses, especially in the lungs, liver and brain.

Primary septicaemia Septicaemia where the focus of infection is not apparent, while in secondary septicaemia a primary focus can be identified. Examples of secondary septicaemia in adults are:

- urinary tract (e.g. *Escherichia coli*)
- respiratory tract (e.g. *Streptococcus pneumoniae*)
- pelvic organs (e.g. *Neisseria gonorrhoeae*)
- skin (e.g. *Staphylococcus aureus*)
- gall bladder (e.g. *E. coli, Streptococcus faecalis*)

Patients with septicaemia require urgent referral.

Patient education resources

Hand-out sheets from *Murtagh's Patient Education* 7th edition:

- Febrile convulsions
- Fever

References

1. Sewell J. Fever in childhood. Problems in clinical medicine. Australian Paediatric Review, 1990; 2: 2.
2. Yung AP, McDonald MI, Spelman DW et al. *Infectious Diseases: A Clinical Approach.* Melbourne: Self-published, 2001: 13–16.
3. Yung A, Stanley P. Problems in infectious diseases. In: Kincaid Smith P et al. *Problems in Clinical Medicine.* Sydney: MacLennan & Petty, 1990: 326–35.
4. Lipsky BA, Hirshmann JV. Drug fever. JAMA, 1981; 245: 851–4.
5. McPhee S, Papadakis S. *Current Medical Diagnosis and Treatment* (52nd edn). New York: The McGraw-Hill Companies, 2013: 1548.
6. Craig JV et al. Temperature measurement at the axilla compared with rectum in children and young people: systematic review. BMJ, 2000; 320: 1174–8.
7. Duce SJ. A systematic review of the literature to determine optimal methods of temperature measurement in neonates, infants and children (Cochrane Review). In: The Cochrane Library, 1996: 1–124.
8. Nogrady B. Ear temperature readings get green light. Australian Doctor, 30 August, 2002: 3.
9. Beck ER, Francis JL, Souhami RL. *Tutorials in Differential Diagnosis* (3rd edn). Edinburgh: Churchill Livingstone, 1995: 209–13.
10. Fitzgerald D. Assessing fever in children. Medical Observer, 23 May 2003: 36–7.
11. Bernath VF, Anderson JN, Silagy CA. Tepid sponging and paracetamol for reduction of body temperature in children. Med J Aust, 2002; 176: 30.
12. Roth AR, Basello GM. Approach to the adult patient with fever of unknown origin. Am Fam Physician, 2003; 68: 2223–8.
13. Papadakis S, McPhee S. *Current Medical Diagnosis and Treatment* (52nd edn). New York: The McGraw-Hill Companies, 2013: 1276–8.
14. Gelfand JR. Fever of unknown origin. In: Braunwald E et al. *Harrison's Principles of Internal Medicine* (15th edn, Vol. 1). New York: McGraw-Hill, 2001: 805–6.
15. Braunwald E et al. *Harrison's Principles of Internal Medicine* (15th edn). New York: McGraw-Hill, 2001: 90–106.
16. Naito T, Mizooka M et al. Diagnostic workup for fever of unknown origin: a multicenter collaborative retrospective study. BMJ Open, 2013; 3.
17. Tunnessen WW Jr. *Signs and Symptoms in Paediatrics* (2nd edn). Philadelphia: JB Lippincott, 1988: 3–6.
18. Burrell AR, McLaws ML et al. Sepsis kills: early intervention saves lives. Med J Aust, 2016; 204: 73.
19. Expert group for Antibiotic. Severe sepsis and septic shock. In: eTG complete [Internet]. Melbourne: Therapeutic Guidelines Ltd. Available from: <www.tg.org.au>, accessed October 2017.

Faints, fits and funny turns 54

Persons who have had frequent and severe attacks of swooning, without any manifest cause, die suddenly.

HIPPOCRATES (?460–377 BCE), *APHORISMS, 11, 41*

When patients present with the complaint of a 'funny turn' it is usually possible to determine that they have one of the more recognisable presenting problems, such as fainting, 'blackouts', lightheadedness, weakness, palpitations, vertigo or migraine. However, there are patients who do present with confusing problems that warrant the label of 'funny turn'. The most common problem with funny turns is that of misdiagnosis, so a proper and adequate history-taking is of great importance.

It is important to remember that seemingly 'funny turns' may be the subjective interpretation of cultural and linguistic communication barriers, especially in an emotional and frustrated patient.[1] Various causes of faints, fits and funny turns are presented in TABLE 54.1. A useful simple classification is to consider them as:

- syncope
- seizures
- sleep disorders—sleep apnoea/narcolepsy/cataplexy
- labyrinthine

Key facts and checkpoints

- The commonest cause of 'funny turns' presenting in general practice is lightheadedness, often related to psychogenic factors such as anxiety, panic and hyperventilation.[2] Patients usually call this 'dizziness'.
- Absence attacks occur with minor forms of epilepsy and with partial seizures such as complex partial seizures.
- The psychomotor attack of complex partial seizure presents as a diagnostic difficulty. The most commonly misdiagnosed seizure disorder is that of complex partial seizures or variants of generalised tonic–clonic seizures (tonic or clonic or atonic).
- The diagnosis of epilepsy is made on the history (or video electroencephalogram/EEG), rather than on the standard EEG, although a sleep-deprived EEG is more effective.
- The triad—angina + dyspnoea + blackout or lightheadedness—indicates aortic stenosis.
- Severe cervical spondylosis can cause vertebrobasilar ischaemia by causing pressure on the vertebral arteries that pass through the intervertebral foramina, especially with head turning or looking up.

A diagnostic approach

A summary of the diagnostic strategy model is presented in TABLE 54.2.

Red flag pointers for faints, fits and funny turns

- Onset in older person
- Neurological symptoms and signs
- Headache
- Tachycardia
- Irregular pulse
- Fever
- Rash
- Drugs: social or prescribed
- Cognitive impairment
- Confusion: gradual onset

The clinical approach

History

The clinical history is of paramount importance in unravelling the problem. A reliable eye-witness account of the 'turn' is invaluable, as is the setting or circumstances in which the 'episode' occurred.

It is essential at first to determine exactly what the patient means by 'funny turn'. In the process of questioning it is appropriate to evaluate the mental state and personal and social factors of the patient. It may be appropriate to confront the patient about feelings of depression, anxiety or detachment from reality.

Table 54.1 Faints, fits and funny turns: checklist of causes (excluding tonic–clonic seizure and stroke)

Psychogenic/communication problems

Breath-holding attack
Conversion reactions (hysteria)
Culture/language conflicts
Fugue states
Hyperventilation
Malingering
Personality disorders
Phobia/anxiety states
Psychoses/severe depression

Other conditions

Transient ischaemic attacks
Complex partial seizure (temporal lobe epilepsy)
Tonic, clonic or atonic seizures
Primary absence seizure
Migraine variants or equivalents, e.g. acute confusional migraine
Familial periodic paralysis
Cardiovascular disorders:

- arrhythmias
- Stokes–Adams attacks
- postural hypotension
- long QT syndrome
- aortic stenosis

Vertigo
Drug reaction
Alcohol and other substance abuse
Hypoglycaemia
Anaemia
Head injury
Amnesic episodes
Metabolic/electrolyte disturbances
Vasovagal/syncope
Carotid sinus sensitivity
Cervical spondylosis
Sleep disorders:

- sleep apnoea
- narcolepsy/cataplexy

Autonomic failure

Table 54.2 Faints, fits and funny turns: diagnostic strategy model

Probability diagnosis
Anxiety related/hyperventilation
Vasovagal syncope
Postural hypotension
Breath-holding attacks/febrile convulsions (children)

Serious disorders not to be missed
Cardiovascular:

- arrhythmias
- aortic stenosis
- postural orthostatic tachycardia syndrome (POTS)

Cerebrovascular:

- TIAs

Neoplasia:

- space-occupying lesions

Subdural/extradural haematomas
Severe infections:

- infective endocarditis

Hypoglycaemia

Pitfalls (often missed)
Atypical migraine
Cardiac arrhythmias/long QT syndrome
Simple partial seizures
Complex partial seizures
Atypical tonic–clonic seizures
Acute confusional state/delirium
Drugs/alcohol/marijuana
Electrolyte disturbances (e.g. hypokalaemia)
Sleep disorders
Transient global amnesia
Rarities:

- atrial myxoma

Seven masquerades checklist
Depression
Diabetes (hypoglycaemia)
Drugs
Anaemia
Spinal dysfunction (cervical spondylosis)

Is the patient trying to tell me something?
Highly likely. Pseudo-seizures, psychogenic and 'communication' disorders quite significant.

It is important to break up the history into three components. First is the lead-up to the episode; second is an adequate description of what took place during the episode; third are the events that took place after the episode.

Apart from the events, note the patient's feelings, symptoms, circumstances and provocative factors. Search for possible secondary gain.

Onset

A sudden onset may be due to cardiovascular causes, especially arrhythmias, which may include the more common supraventricular tachycardias in addition to the less common but more dramatic arrhythmias that may cause unconsciousness. Other causes of a sudden onset include the various epilepsies, vasovagal attacks and TIAs.

Precipitating factors[2]

Enquire about precipitating factors such as emotion, stress, pain, heat, fright, exertion, suddenly standing up, coughing, head movement or hypersomnolence:

- emotion and stress suggest hyperventilation
- fright, pain → vasovagal attack
- standing up → postural hypotension
- exertion → aortic stenosis
- head movement → cervical spondylosis with vertebrobasilar insufficiency
- hypersomnolence → narcolepsy

Associated symptoms[2]

Certain associated symptoms give an indication of the underlying disorder:

- breathing problems and hyperventilation suggest an anxiety state
- tingling in extremities or tightening of the hand → anxiety/hyperventilation
- visual problems → migraine or TIA
- fear or panic → anxiety or complex partial seizure
- hallucinations (taste/smell/visual) → complex partial seizure
- speech problems → TIA or anxiety
- sweating, hunger feelings → hypoglycaemia
- related to food → migraine
- first thing in morning → consider 'hangover'

Drug history

This requires careful analysis and includes alcohol intake and illicit drugs such as marijuana, cocaine and amphetamines. Prescribed drugs that can cause lightheadedness or unconsciousness are listed in TABLE 54.3 and those causing seizures in TABLE 54.4.

Table 54.3 Typical drugs that may cause lightheadedness or blackouts

Alcohol
Antiepileptics
Antihypertensives
Barbiturates
Benzodiazepines
Opioids
OTC anticholinergic compounds
Peripheral vasodilators:
- ACE/ARB inhibitors
- glyceryl trinitrate
- hydralazine
- prazosin

Phenoxybenzamine
SSRI antidepressants
Tricyclic antidepressants

Table 54.4 Important causes of convulsive seizures

Epilepsy:
- first presentation
- known patient with recurrence

Cerebral hypoxia
Hypoglycaemia
Poor cerebral perfusion:
- oedema of eclampsia

Neurotrauma
Cerebrovascular accident
CNS infections:
- meningitis
- encephalitis
- septicaemia
- septic emboli
- cerebral abscess

Toxins
Alcohol excess
Hyperthermia
Metabolic disorders
Drugs:
- antidepressants
- theophylline
- amphetamine
- antibiotics, e.g. norfloxacin, ciprofloxacin
- cocaine
- local anaesthetics

Anaphylaxis
Expanding brain lesion:
- neoplasm
- haematoma

Sudden cessation of certain drugs such as phenothiazines can also be responsible for 'funny turns'.

Past history

The past history may give an indication of the cause of the 'turn'. Such conditions include hypertension, migraine, epilepsy, rheumatic heart disease, diabetes, atherosclerosis (e.g. angina, vascular claudication), alcohol or other substance abuse and psychiatric disorders.

Diary of events

If the diagnosis is elusive it may help to get the patient to keep a diary of circumstances in which events take place, keeping in mind the importance of the time period prior, during and post episode.

Examination

Important focal points of the physical examination include:

- evaluation of the mental state, especially for anxiety
- looking for evidence of anaemia, alcohol abuse and infection
- cerebrovascular examination: carotid arteries, ocular fundi, bruits
- cardiovascular examination: pulses, BP, heart (the BP should be taken lying, sitting and standing)
- the cervical spine

Various manoeuvres

Subject the patient to a number of manoeuvres to try to induce various sensations in order to identify the one that affects them. These should include sudden assumption of the erect posture from a squat, spinning the patient and then a sudden stop, head positioning with either ear down (see FIG. 46.3, CHAPTER 46), Valsalva manoeuvre, and hyperventilation for 60 seconds. Children can spin a showbag 'windmill' while hyperventilating (blowing). Ask 'Which one mimics your complaint?'

Investigations

Depending on the clinical findings, investigations can be selected from the following tests:

- full blood count: ? anaemia ? polycythaemia
- blood sugar: ? diabetes ? hypoglycaemia
- metabolic studies: urea and electrolytes, calcium, magnesium
- ECG: ? ischaemia ? arrhythmia
- 24-hour ambulatory cardiac (Holter) monitor: ? arrhythmia
- radiology/imaging and neuroimaging:
  - cervical X-ray
  - chest X-ray
  - carotid duplex Doppler scan: ? carotid artery stenosis
  - CT scan
  - MRI scan
- EEG or video EEG; include those recorded with sleep deprivation, hyperventilation or photic stimulation
- positron emission tomography (PET) or single photon emission computerised tomography (SPECT) may show localised brain dysfunction when others are negative

In neonates and children

The various forms of seizures are also encountered in childhood, when most patients with epilepsy are diagnosed. They can be categorised as subtle (staring, eye deviation, abnormal sucking or lip smacking) or tonic and clonic. Benign sleep myoclonus occurs in infants normally only during sleep and usually resolves by 2 months of age. There is a concern, supported by evidence, that children are being misdiagnosed. It is appropriate to take a visual recording of the attack.[3]

Neonatal seizures are dangerous and require specialised care to identify the cause and quickly stop the seizure. Pyridoxine may be used.

EPILEPSY SYNDROMES

The following are special age-related epilepsy syndromes seen in children.[4,5] (See CHAPTER 84.)

Febrile seizures

Tonic–clonic seizures occur in 2–5% of children usually aged 3 months to 6 years who have a high fever generally caused by a viral infection. The long-term prognosis is good. For seizures lasting more than 5 minutes, use midazolam or diazepam.

Salaam attacks or infantile spasms

Also known as West syndrome, these are generalised tonic seizures with sudden flexion of the arms, forward flexion of the trunk and extension of the legs, lasting only a few seconds, with the usual age of onset between 4 and 12 months. They are usually restricted to the first 3 years of life and are replaced by other forms of attacks. ECG shows typical hypsarrhythmias. Prognosis for cognitive development is also unfavourable. The most effective therapy is corticotrophin (ACTH), e.g. tetracosactin IM injection. Otherwise, oral prednisolone, vigabatrin, benzodiazepines or sodium valproate can be used.

Lennox–Gastaut syndrome (myoclonic epilepsy of infancy)

This uncommon syndrome refers to a triad of severe difficult-to-control seizures (usually tonic with drop attack), mental retardation and characteristic EEG. The seizures usually begin between the ages of 1 and 6 years, with a peak onset at 3–5 years. Prognosis is poor. Sodium valproate is the therapy of choice.

Benign focal childhood epilepsy with centrotemporal spikes

This disorder usually begins in children aged 2–13 years, with a peak age of 5–8 years. It is the most common form of childhood focal epilepsy, and there is a strong family history of epilepsy. The main feature is a simple partial motor or somatosensory seizure involving the face and mouth during sleep, producing a typical 'glugging' sound. The child usually wakes from sleep, goes to the parents and is unable to speak and has hemifacial contortions. It may progress to a tonic–clonic seizure. There is a characteristic EEG pattern. The prognosis is excellent as remission usually occurs around puberty. Carbamazepine is the therapy of choice.

Childhood and juvenile absence epilepsy

These children present with frequent absence seizures (formerly 'petit mal'), often over a hundred daily. Peak age of onset is 4–9 years. The absence seizures can be very subtle. Signs include alteration of awareness (usually in the classroom), sudden onset, facial and other automatisms. Juvenile absence epilepsy presents later (10–15 years). First-line treatment is ethosuximide (best tolerated) or sodium valproate.

Juvenile myoclonic epilepsy (myoclonic epilepsy of Janz)

This is a triad of seizures: myoclonic jerks, tonic–clonic seizures and absences. Onset is around puberty but may occur earlier. The myoclonic jerks and tonic–clonic seizures usually occur in the early morning after waking. Mental development is usually as normal, but the disorder is generally lifelong and is well controlled with sodium valproate.

Medial temporal lobe epilepsy

This syndrome of complex partial seizures, which usually last 1–3 minutes, is seen in childhood. Transient postictal confusion and speech dysfunction is common. Those with medically intractable seizures respond well to surgery.

Dravet syndrome

Known as severe myoclonic epilepsy of infancy, it is a catastrophic form with a very poor prognosis. It is largely inherited. Early diagnosis and treatment are essential.

NON-EPILEPTIC EVENTS RESEMBLING EPILEPTIC SEIZURES[4]

Many normal and abnormal behaviours seen in children resemble seizures but are unrelated to epilepsy. A careful history is very important. The following are examples:

- *Postures of spasticity and movement disorders.* These occur in children with neurological disorders such as cerebral palsy.
- *Syncope.* The child may describe a 'sinking feeling', or 'everything getting louder' prior to the loss of consciousness.
- *Breath-holding.* This often occurs after a crying spell and clonic movements may be seen at the end of the event.
- *Masturbation.* This behaviour leads to a tonic-like posture of the legs and preoccupation, especially in young girls.[6]
- *Munchausen-by-proxy.*[7] This syndrome of fictitious epilepsy described by a parent is becoming more recognised.
- *Psychogenic seizures (pseudo seizures).* A diagnostic dilemma exists when these coexist with genuine seizures. These should be suspected when they occur in particular circumstances and the description of the 'seizure' is bizarre.
- *Shuddering.* Shuddering or shivering spells can resemble myoclonic jerks.
- *Night terrors.*[8] These episodes, which usually affect children aged 2–4 and 6–9, generally develop within 2 hours of sleep onset and last 1–2 minutes (sometimes longer). They are alarming and the child usually cannot be reassured or settled. A 6-week trial of phenytoin or imipramine can be used for severe problems.
- *Tics.* Motor tics can be quite complex but are usually brief involuntary movements involving the face and upper limbs.
- *Cardiac causes.* For example, long QT syndrome.

Blackouts

The important causes of blackout include the various syncopes that are listed in TABLE 75.4 (see CHAPTER 75) and the various forms of epilepsy. The classic tonic–clonic seizure is described in CHAPTER 74, while descriptions of other seizures producing blackouts or funny turns now follow.

Important causes of convulsions (tonic–clonic seizures) are listed in TABLE 54.4. Refer also to CHAPTER 84.

Complex partial seizures

In complex partial seizures (known also as temporal lobe epilepsy) the symptomatology varies considerably from patient to patient and is often a diagnostic problem. It is the commonest type of focal epilepsy and the attacks vary in time from momentary to several minutes (usually 1–3 minutes).

Possible manifestations[2]

- Commonest: slight disturbance of perception and consciousness
- Hallucinations: visual, taste, smell, sounds
- Absence attacks or vertigo
- Illusions—objects/people shrink or expand
- Affective feelings—fear, anxiety, anger
- Dyscognitive effects: *déjà vu* (familiarity), *jamais vu* (unreality), waves emanating from epigastrium
- Objective signs: lip-smacking, swallowing/chewing/sucking, unresponsive to commands or questions, pacing around a room
- Postictal drowsiness

Unreal or detached feelings are common in complex partial seizures. There can be permanent short-term memory loss. The sensation of strange smells or tastes is more common than auditory or visual hallucinations.[1] They can progress to tonic–clonic seizures.

Diagnosis

- EEG is diagnostic in 50–60% of cases; a repeat EEG will increase rate to 60–80%
- EEG/video telemetry helpful with frequent attacks
- CT or MRI scan—to exclude tumour when diagnosis confirmed

Medication (see CHAPTER 84)

carbamazepine (first choice):[5,9] children and adults
or
sodium valproate (second choice): not <2 years
or (others)
vigabatrin, phenytoin, phenobarbitone, tiagabine, benzodiazepines, ethosuximide, levetiracetam

54

Tonic–clonic seizures

The classic seizure sequence: aura—cry—fall—fit (clonic then tonic-incontinence).

Variants of tonic–clonic seizures are more common than realised. Some patients may simply stiffen or drop to the ground while others may have one or two jerks or shakes only:

- stiffen and fall = tonic
- floppy and fall = atonic
- shaking only = clonic

Refer to CHAPTER 75 and CHAPTER 84.

Simple partial seizures

In simple partial seizures (Jacksonian epilepsy) there is no loss of consciousness. These include focal seizures, which may proceed to a generalised tonic–clonic seizure or to motor seizures.

Jacksonian (motor seizure)

Typically, jerking movements begin at the angle of the mouth or in the thumb and index finger and 'march' to involve the rest of the body (e.g. thumb → hand → limb → face ± leg on one side and then on to the contralateral side). A tonic–clonic or complex partial seizure may follow.

Medication

carbamazepine (first choice)[5]: children and adults
or
sodium valproate (second choice) not <2 years
or (others)
phenytoin, vigabatrin, gabapentin

Absence seizure

This type of generalised epilepsy typically affects children from 4 years up to puberty:[2] (see CHAPTER 84).

- child ceases activity and stares suddenly
- child is motionless (may blink or nod)
- no warning
- sometimes clonic (jerky) movement of eyelids, face, fingers
- may be lip-smacking or chewing (called complex absence)
- only lasts few seconds—usually 5–10 seconds
- child then carries on as though nothing happened
- usually several per day (not just one or two)
- may lead to generalised seizures in adulthood
- two types—childhood and juvenile

Diagnosis

Best evoked in the consulting room by hyperventilation and 'windmill'.

EEG:

- classic 3 Hz wave and spike
- may be normal

- always include hyperventilation
- easier with sleep deprivation

Medication

ethosuximide (first choice)[5,10]
or
sodium valproate (second choice)
or (others) e.g. clonazepam, gabapentin
childhood absence may not need pharmacotherapy

Note: Beware of hepatoxicity with sodium valproate, especially in those under 2 years.

The first seizure

The decision to treat the first seizure with medication is based on several factors. Since 50% of patients will never have another seizure, treatment is not usually recommended. However, if two or more seizures occur over more than 24 hours, patients are likely to experience more and require treatment. The risk is increased in specific types, such as partial (focal) seizures, those with ECG abnormalities and a lesion on neuroimaging.[5,12]

Narcolepsy

Narcolepsy is characterised by brief spells of irresistible sleep during daytime hours, usually in inappropriate circumstances, even during activity. Its cause is unknown. Although patients are usually aware of their disorder, some may have no insight into the problem and present with the complaint of unusual turns. Narcolepsy can present as 'attacks' in which the patient may crumple and fall without losing consciousness. It can be part of a tetrad syndrome (daytime hypersomnolence, cataplexy, hypnogogic and hypnopompic hallucinations, sleep paralysis).

Other features:

- onset in teens or 20s
- can have several attacks per day

Refer to CHAPTER 71.

Diagnosis

- A clinical diagnosis

If doubtful:

- EEG monitoring
- sleep laboratory studies (sleep latency test)—rapid eye movement is a hallmark

Medication[11]

dexamphetamine (in slowly increasing doses to 60 mg daily)
or
methylphenidate (immediate release) up to 60 mg daily
or
modafinil 200–400 mg (o) daily
or
tricyclic antidepressants (e.g. clomipramine, imipramine, fluoxetine), for associated cataplexy

AMNESIC EPISODES

Amnesic episodes in which people cannot recall events or their own identity can be psychogenic (commonly), such as fugue states, conversion disorder, severe depression and factitious states. They may be related to an organic problem such as epilepsy, sleep apnoea, cerebrovascular disorder, post-trauma, Wernicke–Korsakoff syndromes and drugs (e.g. alcohol, cannabis and anaesthetic agents).

Transient global amnesia[5,13,14]

This is a benign, self-limited profound amnesic episode of unknown aetiology tending to occur in middle-aged or elderly people. Proposed causation includes transient ischaemia or dysfunction of the temporal lobes, similar to temporal lobe epilepsy or a migraine variant.

Clinical features

- Typically last 4–8 hours (up to 24 hours)
- Identity and conscious state preserved
- Agitated, perplexed, anxious patient
- State of bewilderment (e.g. 'where am I?')
- Anterograde and retrograde amnesia
- Frequent repetition of questions
- Able to perform complex motor skills (e.g. driving)
- Usually single episode (20% recurrence)
- Complete resolution: good prognosis
- No abnormal neurological signs
- All investigations unhelpful

Four diagnostic criteria (after Caplan)[12]

- Witnessed onset of attack (essential for diagnosis)
- Dysfunction during attack limited to amnesia and repetitive queries
- No other neurological features
- Memory loss should be transient, lasting no longer than 24 hours

54

Management

- Reassuring explanation/education
- Special investigations, including angiography, not needed if conform to above criteria
- No active treatment usually needed

Cerebrovascular disorders

Cerebrovascular disease is one of the major causes of mortality and morbidity in developed countries and can cause recurrent attacks of ischaemia in the carotid and vertebrobasilar systems (particularly vertebrobasilar insufficiency), which may present as 'funny turns'. In particular, brain-stem ischaemia causes 'funny turns' such as impaired consciousness, including transient global amnesia, drop attacks and the 'locked-in' syndrome.

Orthostatic intolerance and syncope

There are three main syndromes of autonomic instability with orthostatic intolerance leading to syncope

1 *Reflex (vasovagal) syncope.* This affects 30% of the population, has a strong family history and an onset in the young. There is a hypotensive response. The multiple precipitants include coughing, micturition, fright, standing, heat and defecation (straining). Although consciousness quickly returns, recovery can be delayed (e.g. malaise for 12–24 hours). See CHAPTER 75.
2 *Postural orthostatic tachycardia syndrome (POTS).*[15] This is orthostatic intolerance with dysautonomia upon changing from the supine to the upright position or head up tilt. Tachycardia with decreased ventricular filling is a feature with hypotension and possibly syncope. There are myriad symptoms including dizziness, fatigue, blurred vision, chest pain and cognitive impairment. Some consider it a variety of chronic fatigue syndrome. It has an adolescent onset and a familial history. Referral to a 'syncope' unit is recommended for this complex and debilitating condition. One treatment option is fludrocortisone acetate. Another is the vasopressor/hypertensive agent midodrine to treat dysautonomia and orthostatic hypotension.
3 *Autonomic failure.* This is age related and can be primary (e.g. multiple system atrophy) or secondary (e.g. diabetes, amyloid). It leads to hypoperfusion syncope. Precipitants include orthostasis, meals and alcohol. Recovery from syncope is rapid.

Psychogenic or communication disorders

Psychogenic causes have to be considered. 'Hysterical fugue' is one such manifestation. The problem can be a communication disorder, such as an emotional person trying to communicate a problem in a language foreign to them.

Patients with psychiatric disorders such as schizophrenia or depression may experience feelings of depersonalisation or unreality, which can be interpreted as a 'turn' or even temporal lobe epilepsy.

Patients who complain of vague and bizarre symptoms, such as 'queer feelings in the head', 'swimming sensation', 'unreal feelings' and 'walking on air' are likely to have an anxiety state.

Severe anxiety or panic attacks typically cause lightheadedness that presents as a 'funny turn'. Other somatic symptoms include palpitations, sweating, inability to swallow, headache, breathlessness and manifestations of hyperventilation.

Pitfalls in management[2]

- The main pitfall associated with seizure disorders and epilepsy is misdiagnosis (not all seizures are generalised tonic–clonic in nature).
- Failing to place appropriate emphasis on the history in making the diagnosis.
- Misdiagnosing syncope with some involuntary movements for epilepsy.
- Overlooking cardiac arrhythmias as a cause of funny turns, including recurrent dizziness.
- Failing to consider the possibility of aortic stenosis with syncopal attacks.
- Misdiagnosing vertigo and syncope for TIA.
- Mistaking visual or sensory migraine equivalents in young adults for TIA.
- Overlooking drugs (including self-administered drugs) as a cause of lightheadedness.

When to refer

- Transient ischaemic attacks, especially if the diagnosis is in doubt
- Clinical suspicion of or proven cardiac arrhythmias
- Evidence of aortic stenosis
- Seizures
- General uncertainty of the diagnosis

Practice tips

- A detailed clinical analysis is more important in the first instance than laboratory tests. The key to accurate diagnosis is a very careful history, taking the patient second by second through the attack and events preceding the turn.
- Talk to as many eyewitnesses as possible in unravelling the cause.
- For 'undiagnosed turns', ask the patient to keep a diary with an accurate record of the attack, including preceding events.
- Remember that migraine is a great mimic and can cause confusion in diagnosis.
- Remember that the EEG can be normal in the confirmed epileptic.
- The more bizarre the description of a 'funny turn', the more likely a functional problem is the cause.
- Transient hypoglycaemia can mimic a TIA.

Patient education resources

Hand-out sheets from *Murtagh's Patient Education* 7th edition:

- Fainting (syncope)

References

1 Kincaid-Smith P, Larkins R, Whelan G. *Problems in Clinical Medicine.* Sydney: MacLennan & Petty, 1990: 159–64.

2 Porter RS, Kaplan JL. *The Merck Manual of Diagnosis and Therapy* (19th edn). Whitehouse Station, N.J.: Merck Sharp & Dohme Corp., 2011: 2041–8.

3 Hindley D, Ali A, Robson C. Diagnoses made in a secondary care 'fits, faints and funny turns' clinic. Arch Dis Child, 2006; 91 (3): 214–8.

4 Stewart I, Bye A. The diagnosis of childhood fits and funny turns. Modern Medicine Australia, 1994; 37 (8): 65–72.

5 Expert group for Neurology. Epilepsy and seizures. In: eTG complete [Internet]. Melbourne: Therapeutic Guidelines Ltd. Available from: <www.tg.org.au>, accessed October 2017.

6 Fleisher DR, Morrison A. Masturbation mimicking abdominal pain or seizures in young girls. J Paediatr, 1990; 116: 810–14.

7 Meadow R. Fictitious epilepsy. Lancet, 1984; 2: 25–8.

8 Rothner AD. Not everything that shakes is epilepsy: the differential diagnosis of paroxysmal nonepileptiform disorders. Cleve Clin J Med, 1989; 56 (Suppl, part 2): 206S–213S.

9 Scott AK. Management of epilepsy. In: *Central Nervous System.* London: British Medical Association, 1995: 1–2.

10 Levine M et al. *Drugs of Choice: A Formulary for General Practice.* Ottawa: Canadian Medical Association, 1995: 98–9.

11 Sofou K, Kristjansdottir et al. Management of prolonged seizures and status epilepticus in childhood: a systematic review. J Child Neurol, 2009; 24 (8): 918–26.

12 Bonnett LJ et al. Risk of recurrence after a first seizure and implications for driving: further analysis of the Multicentre study of early Epilepsy and Single Seizures. BMJ, 2010; 341.

13 Caplan LR. Transient global amnesia: criteria and classification. Neurology, 1986; 36: 441.

14 Horne M. Neurology quiz. Aust Fam Physician, 1994; 23: 935.

15 Thieben MJ, Sandroni P et al. Postural orthostatic tachycardia syndrome: the Mayo Clinic experience. Mayo Clin Proc, March 2007; 82 (3): 308–13.

55 Haematemesis and melaena

The 'once smelt never forgotten' sickly smell of melaena can be diagnosed from a distance of 20 metres without trying.

EMERGENCY ROOM SUPERVISOR, BRISBANE 1985

Acute severe upper GI haemorrhage is an important medical emergency. The dramatic symptom of haematemesis follows bleeding from the oesophagus, stomach and duodenum. More than half the patients are over 60 years of age.[1]

Haematemesis is the vomiting of blood appearing as fresh blood or 'coffee grounds'. Melaena is the passage of black tarry stools, with 50 mL or more of blood required to produce melaena stool (Greek *melas* = black). Melaena occurs in most patients with upper GI haemorrhage and haematemesis occurs in over 50%.[1]

Although the incidence is declining, the mortality rate of upper GI haemorrhage remains high at approximately 6–8%.[2]

Key facts and checkpoints

- Chronic peptic ulceration accounts for most cases of upper GI haemorrhage.
- Haematemesis is almost always associated with some degree of blood in the stools, although melaena may not necessarily accompany it, especially if bleeding occurs from the oesophagus.
- Black stool caused by oral iron therapy or bismuth-containing antacid tablets can cause confusion.
- Always check for a history of drug intake, especially aspirin and NSAIDs.
- Corticosteroids in conventional therapeutic doses are thought to have no influence on GI haemorrhage.
- The volume of bleeding is best assessed by its haemodynamic effects rather than relying on the patient's estimation, which tends to be excessive.
- Melaena is generally less life-threatening than haematemesis.
- Resuscitation of the patient is the first task.
- A sudden loss of 20% or more of circulatory blood volume usually produces signs of shock such as tachycardia, hypotension, faintness and sweating. Younger patients can compensate better and tolerate a larger loss prior to the development of shock.[1] A useful guide is that shock in a previously well 70 kg man indicates an acute blood loss of at least 1000–1500 mL.

Causes of upper GI bleeding

The major cause of bleeding is chronic peptic ulceration of the duodenum and stomach, accounting for about half of all cases.[3,4] The other major cause is acute gastric ulcers and erosions, which account for at least 20% of cases. Aspirin and NSAIDs are responsible for many of these bleeds. Causes are summarised in TABLE 55.1 and illustrated in FIGURE 55.1.

Table 55.1 Diagnostic strategy model for upper gastrointestinal bleeding (haematemesis)[5,6]

Probability diagnosis

Chronic peptic ulcer (stomach and duodenum)
Acute gastric ulcers/erosions
Oesophagitis (incl. GORD)
Mallory–Weiss (emetogenic) syndrome
Drugs: aspirin, NSAIDs, anticoagulants, clopidogrel

Serious disorders not to be missed

Vascular:
- oesophageal varices
- blood dyscrasias
- vascular malformation/angiodysplasia
- hereditary coagulopathy

Cancer:
- gastric or oesophageal

Other:
- chronic liver disease

Pitfalls (often missed)

Stomach ulcer
Swallowed blood (e.g. epistaxis)
Collagen diseases (e.g. scleroderma)
Rarities:
- ruptured oesophagus
- hereditary haemorrhagic telangiectasia
- scurvy
- ingested poisons (e.g. acid, alkali, arsenic)
- gastric antral vascular ectasia

Mallory–Weiss syndrome

In this condition a tear occurs at the lower end of the oesophageal mucosa (at the oesophagogastric

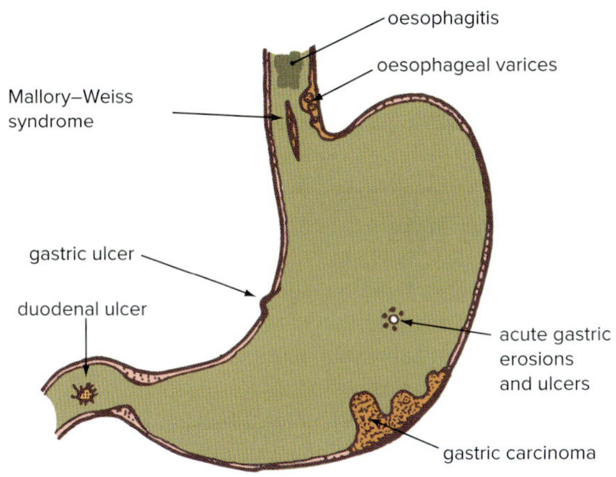

FIGURE 55.1 Important causes of haematemesis and melaena

junction) because of an episode of severe or protracted vomiting or coughing. Blood appears in the vomitus after a bout of heavy vomiting or dry retching. It is usually seen in alcoholic patients. It is usually a self-limiting lesion. A definite diagnosis can only be made by oesophagoscopy.

Gastro-oesophageal varices

Such varices are caused by portal hypertension, which in turn is usually due to cirrhosis of the liver. There is a raised incidence of peptic ulcer in those with liver cirrhosis, especially in biliary and alcohol-induced cirrhosis, so this should be kept in mind as a possible source of bleeding. Mortality is about 30%, despite advances, and 70% for untreated patients.[6]

Primary prevention of bleeding from varices is with the use of beta blockers such as propranolol if no contraindications.[7]

Management includes injection sclerotherapy, and then intravenous octreotide or terlipressin if it fails. Passage of a Sengstaken–Blakemore or Minnesota tube into the oesophagus and stomach to provide tamponade and the radiological procedure of using a transjugular intrahepatic portosystemic stent are possible options.

The clinical approach

History

It is important to establish the nature of the vomitus and the possibility of bleeding arising from the mouth, nose or pharynx. A coffee grounds vomitus indicates that the blood has been in contact with gastric acid. Oesophageal bleeding tends to lead to vomiting of fresh blood. Questions to help pinpoint the possible aetiology should be asked. Patients may confuse vomiting up and coughing up blood.

Table 55.2	Drugs associated with gastrointestinal haemorrhage[2]
Aspirin	
Clopidogrel	
Other antiplatelet drugs	
Heparin/new oral anticoagulants	
NSAIDs/COX-2 inhibitors	
Prednisolone	
SSRI antidepressants	
Warfarin	

Key questions

- What drugs have you been taking? (see TABLE 55.2)
- Have you been taking aspirin or tablets for arthritis or back pain?
- How much have you vomited?
- What did the vomit look like?
- Did you notice black dots like coffee grounds or any blood clots?
- Have you had any indigestion, heartburn or stomach pains recently?
- Have you lost any weight unexpectedly?
- Have you opened your bowels and if so what was the colour?
- Have you noticed whether your bowel motions were black or unusual in any way?
- How much alcohol do you drink?
- Have you had any previous operations on your stomach for a peptic ulcer?
- Were you vomiting normal vomit before the blood appeared?
- Have you been eating beetroot or other bright red foodstuffs?

Examination

The patient's general state, particularly the circulation, should be assessed immediately on presentation. It is critical to assess the patient's haemodynamic status with vital signs of heart rate, blood pressure and postural changes.[2] A careful abdominal examination should be performed including a digital rectal examination. As a rule abdominal findings are not remarkable except when a mass, hepatomegaly or splenomegaly, is found. Other evidence of liver disease should be sought. 55

Investigations

Investigations to determine the source of the bleeding should be carried out in a specialist unit. Upper gastrointestinal endoscopy is the single most useful test and will detect the cause of the bleeding in at least 80% of cases.[3]

The haemoglobin level will not be an appropriate guide to blood loss or the need for transfusion during the early stages, because haemodilution occurs gradually over the 24 hours following a severe bleed. However, a level below 90 g/L during this period is usually regarded as an indication for transfusion.

Other tests to consider include FBE, *H. pylori*, LFTs, plain abdominal X-ray, coagulation profile.

Management

The immediate objectives are:

1 restore an effective blood volume (if necessary)
2 establish a diagnosis to allow definitive treatment

All patients with a significant bleed should be admitted to hospital and referred to a specialist unit. Urgent resuscitation is required where there has been a large bleed and there are clinical signs of shock. Such patients require insertion of intravenous lines and rapid infusion of isotonic saline followed by a plasma expander (e.g. Haemaccel) followed by transfusion with blood commenced as soon as possible.

Proton pump inhibitors should be commenced in most cases especially as 50% of bleeding is from peptic ulceration. Oral administration may be possible in most cases but intravenous PPI (e.g. omeprazole 80 mg over 15–30 minutes followed by IV infusion for up to 3 days)[7,8] is appropriate for the seriously ill.[4] Eventually switch to oral PPIs.

In many patients bleeding is insufficient to decompensate the circulatory system and they settle spontaneously. Approximately 85% of patients stop bleeding within 48 hours.[3]

In some instances intervention via upper endoscopy to achieve haemostasis of bleeding point with a heater probe (e.g. Gold Probe) or injection with adrenaline or both or application of clips will be employed. Occasionally surgery will be necessary to arrest bleeding but should be avoided if possible in patients with acute gastric erosion.

Practice tips

- Ask the patient not to dispose of the evidence of vomitus, if possible.
- Patients with haematemesis should be assessed in the emergency department.
- Peptic ulcer disease remains the most common cause of upper gastrointestinal bleeding (UGIB).
- Upper endoscopy is the gold standard for diagnosis and therapy for acute UGIB.

References

1 Papadakis MA, McPhee SJ. *Current Medical Diagnoses and Treatment* (56th edn). New York: The McGraw-Hill Companies, 2017: 504–7.
2 Worthley DL, Fraser RJ. Management of acute bleeding in the upper gastrointestinal tract. Australian Prescriber, 2005; 28: 62–6.
3 Kumar PJ, Clark ML. *Clinical Medicine* (7th edn). London: Elsevier Saunders, 2009: 291–3.
4 Fulde GW. *Emergency Medicine* (4th edn). Marrickville: Elsevier, 2007: 299–301.
5 Beck ER, Francis JL, Souhami RL. *Tutorials in Differential Diagnosis* (3rd edn). Edinburgh: Churchill Livingstone, 1995: 75–9.
6 Norton I, Chan C. Upper gastrointestinal bleeding: clinical review. Medical Observer, 9 April 2010: 1–3.
7 Expert group for Gastrointestinal. Bleeding peptic ulcers. In: eTG complete [Internet]. Melbourne: Therapeutic Guidelines Ltd. Available from: <www.tg.org.au>, accessed October 2017.
8 Sachar H, Vaidya K, Laine L. Intermittent vs continuous proton pump inhibitor therapy for high-risk bleeding ulcers: a systematic review and meta-analysis. JAMA Intern Med, 2014: 174 (11): 1755–62.

Headache

56

When the head aches, all the body is out of tune.

MIGUEL DE CERVANTES (1547–1616)

Headache, one of the cardinal symptoms known to human beings, is a very common complaint in general practice. When a patient presents with 'headache' we need to have a sound diagnostic and management strategy as the problem can be confusing. The key to analysing the symptom of headache is to know and understand the cause, for 'one only sees what they know'.

The patient's manner of presentation can confuse us because many tend to influence us with preconceived ideas that they will verbalise—'I think I need my blood pressure checked' or 'My eyes need testing'—or they may not mention their anxiety about a cerebral tumour or an impending stroke.

Hypertension is such a rare cause of headache that one is tempted to stress the adage 'hypertension does not cause headache', but we do encounter the occasional patient whose headache appears to be caused by hypertension and it is mandatory to measure the blood pressure of patients presenting with headache. Patients expect this routine and reassurance is difficult without the appropriate physical examination. Where headaches and hypertension coexist, assume that the headaches are not due to hypertension.

The diagnosis of serious causes of headache depends on a careful history, a high index of suspicion of the 'different' presentations and the judicious use of CT scanning.

Key facts and checkpoints

- Eighty-five per cent of the population will have experienced headache within 1 year and 38% of adults will have had a headache within 2 weeks.[1]
- Forty per cent of children will have experienced one or more headaches by the age of 7 and 75% by the age of 15.[2]
- Headache can be classified as primary or secondary, e.g. intracranial pathology, TMJ, cervical spine.
- Migraine affects at least 10% of the adult population and one-quarter of these patients require medical attention for their attacks at some stage.[3] It is under-recognised and poorly managed in the community.[4]
- Five per cent of children suffer from migraine by the age of 11 years.[3]
- Seventy per cent of sufferers have a positive family history of migraine.
- Many headaches previously considered to be tension related are secondary to disorders of the neck, eyes, teeth, temporomandibular joints or other structures.[3]
- Drug-induced headaches are common and must be considered in the history.
- In children the triad of symptoms—dizziness, headache and vomiting—indicates medulloblastoma of the posterior fossa until proved otherwise.
- A typical triad of symptoms in an adult with a cerebral tumour (advanced) is headache, vomiting and convulsions.
- Eye strain is not a common cause.
- Secondary bronchogenic bronchial carcinoma is the commonest cause of intracerebral malignancy.
- Primary headaches must be differentiated from secondary headaches.[5]

A diagnostic approach

A summary of the diagnostic strategy model is presented in TABLE 56.1.

Probability diagnosis

The commonest cause of headache presenting in general practice is respiratory infection.[1] The most common causes of chronic recurrent headache are so-called transformed migraine, tension-type headache and combination headaches. Combination headaches, typified by relatively constant pain lasting for many days, have a mix of components such as tension, depression, cervical dysfunction, vascular headache and drug dependence. Neurologists may refer to these headaches as 'tension-vascular headache'. Tension headache is less common than previously promulgated.[3]

Table 56.1 Headache: diagnostic strategy model

Probability diagnosis Acute: respiratory infection Chronic: • tension-type headache • combination headache • migraine • transformed migraine
Serious disorders not to be missed Cerebrovascular: • subarachnoid haemorrhage • stroke/TIA • intracranial haemorrhage • carotid or vertebral artery dissection • temporal arteritis • cerebral venous thrombosis, e.g. venous sinus Neoplasia: • cerebral tumour • pituitary tumour Severe infections: • meningitis, esp. fungal • encephalitis • intracranial abscess Haematoma: extradural/subdural Glaucoma (acute) Benign intracranial hypertension
Pitfalls (often missed) Cervical spondylosis/dysfunction Dental disorders Refractive errors of eye Sinusitis Ophthalmic herpes zoster (pre-eruption) Exertional headache Paroxysmal hemicrania Hypoglycaemia Post-traumatic headache Post-spinal procedure (e.g. epidural, lumbar puncture) Sleep apnoea *Rarities:* • Paget disease • post-sexual intercourse • Cushing syndrome • Conn syndrome • Addison disease • dysautonomic cephalgia
Seven masquerades checklist Depression Diabetes Drugs Anaemia Thyroid/endocrine disorder Spinal dysfunction (cervicogenic/occipital neuralgia UTI
Is the patient trying to tell me something? Quite likely if there is an underlying psychogenic disorder.

Transformed migraine[6]

This describes the progressive increase in frequency of migraine attacks until the headache recurs daily. The typical migraine features become modified so that the pattern resembles that of tension headache but with the unilateral situation of migraine. Analgesic abuse can transform episodic migraine into chronic daily headache.

Serious disorders not to be missed

For the acute onset of headache it is vital not to miss subarachnoid haemorrhage (SAH) or meningitis. Intracranial haemorrhage, especially involving cerebellar, intraventricular and frontal lobe areas, needs to be considered.

Acute 'thunderclap' headache[6]

This is a sudden severe headache that can be caused by the following:

- enlarging aneurysm—an enlarging aneurysm or vascular malformation can cause acute headache
- SAH—the pain is typically occipital, localised at first then generalised and may vary in intensity
- meningitis—must be considered if the headache is generalised, especially in the presence of malaise, fever and neck stiffness: the ache, which is constant and severe, may begin abruptly

For chronic headache, space-occupying lesions including subdural haematomas must be considered. Since headaches tend to decrease with age, headaches developing in the elderly should be viewed with suspicion and this includes considering temporal arteritis (TA). Benign intracranial hypertension should be considered, especially in young obese women. The dangerous cryptococcal meningitis can be difficult as the CT scan may be normal.

Tips on sinister causes of headache[4]

- The most important indicator is time course: beware of acute or subacute tempo.
- Be suspicious of any focal symptoms or signs (except for typical migraine aura).
- Beware of fever, confusion, altered mental state or neck stiffness.

Pitfalls

The list (see TABLE 56.1) contains some controversial causes of headache, although some should be obvious if a careful history is elucidated. These include post-traumatic headache, post-procedural headache (e.g. lumbar puncture and spinal anaesthesia) and exertional headache. Sinusitis can be overlooked in the absence of respiratory signs. Refractive errors of the eye, although an uncommon cause of headache, do warrant consideration.

General pitfalls

- Overinvestigating the patient with headache, especially as a substitute for a careful history and examination
- Failing to appreciate that a combination of factors and cervical dysfunction are common causes of headache
- Omitting to measure the blood pressure in the patient complaining of headache
- Rushing in with antibiotics for a patient (especially children) with fever and headache—bacterial meningitis may be masked
- Attributing the early headache of a space-occupying lesion to tension or hypertension

Seven masquerades checklist

Of the masquerades, depression and drugs are important causes of headache. Cervical dysfunction is certainly an important cause and tends to be ignored by some doctors. Australian figures are misleading because many of these patients tend to gravitate to alternative health professionals.

A UK study placed headache from cervical spondylosis on almost equal terms with migraine.[1]

The explanation for referral of pain from disorders of the upper cervical spine to the head and eye is that some afferent fibres from the upper three cervical nerve roots converge on cells in the posterior horn of the spinal cord (which can also be excited by trigeminal afferent fibres), thus conveying to the patient the impression of head pain through this shared pathway (see FIG. 56.1).

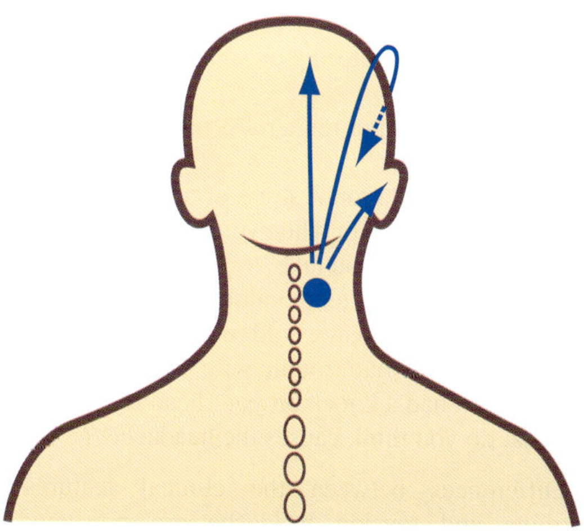

FIGURE 56.1 Typical headache referral patterns for dysfunction of the upper cervical spinal segments

Question the possibility of the effect of any drug the patient is taking: important examples are alcohol, analgesics (rebound), antihypertensives (several), caffeine, COCP, corticosteroids, NSAIDs (especially indomethacin), vasodilators, e.g. CCBs, nitrates, PDE inhibitors (e.g. sildenafil). Anaemia can cause headache, usually if the haemoglobin level falls below 100 g/L.[6] Hypo- and hyperthyroidism may also cause headache, and in diabetics hypoglycaemia is often responsible.

Psychogenic considerations

Headache, like tiredness, is one of those symptoms that may reflect a 'hidden agenda'. Of course, the patient may be depressed (overt or masked) or may have a true anxiety state. The most characteristic feature of psychogenic headache is that the headache is present virtually every minute of the day for weeks or months on end. However, it is common for patients to deny that they are anxious, depressed or unduly stressed. For this reason a detailed history is important to identify lifestyle factors and historical events that can be associated with headache.

Some patients are fearful of their headache lest it represents a cerebral tumour, stroke or hypertension and need appropriate reassurance.

Conversion reactions and other aspects of compensation rewards, especially following an accident (e.g. rear-end collision), may make the symptom of headache difficult to manage. Headache, like backache, is one of the prime symptoms perpetuated or exaggerated for secondary gain.

Severe headaches, especially simulated migraine, are common 'tickets of entry' for drug addicts seeking narcotics from empathic practitioners. Such patients require very skilled management.

Timelines for causes of headache/ facial pain

Acute severe headache, e.g.:

- subarachnoid haemorrhage
- benign sex or exertional headache
- migraine/cluster headache

Subacute headache (recent onset, increasing):

- expanding intracranial lesion
- temporal arteritis

Recurrent episodes, e.g.:

- migraine/cluster headache
- benign sex or exertional headache
- neuralgias, e.g. trigeminal

Chronic headache, e.g.:

- tension-type headache
- transformed migraine/rebound headache
- cervicogenic/post-traumatic
- atypical facial pain

Diurnal patterns of pain

Plotting the fluctuation of headache during the day provides vital clues to the diagnosis (see FIG. 56.2). The patient who wakes up with headache could have vascular headache (migraine), cervical spondylosis, depressive illness, hypertension or a space-occupying lesion. It is usual for migraine to last hours, not days, which is more characteristic of tension headache. The pain of frontal sinusitis follows a typical pattern, namely onset around 9 am, building to a maximum by about 1 pm, and then subsiding over the next few hours. In the absence of respiratory symptoms it is likely to be misdiagnosed as tension headache. The pain from combination headache tends to follow a most constant pattern throughout the day and does not usually interrupt sleep.

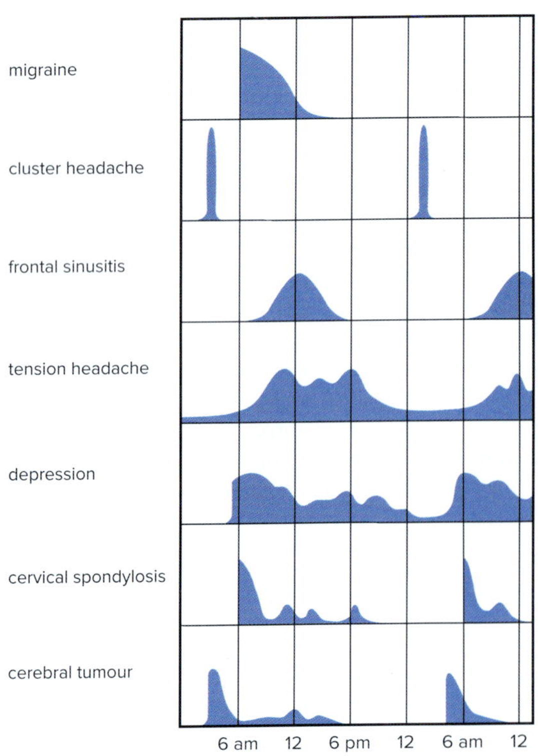

FIGURE 56.2 Typical diurnal patterns of various causes of headache; the relative intensity of pain is plotted on the vertical axis

The clinical approach

History

A full description of the pain including a pain analysis should be obtained using one of the mnemonics (see CHAPTER 12) with an emphasis on relieving factors and associations.

It is useful to get the patient to plot on a prepared grid the relative intensity of the pain and the times of day (and night) that the pain is present. The history, especially of the tempo of the condition, should help diagnose headaches secondary to specific pathology.

Key questions[7]

- Can you describe your headaches?
- How often do you get them?
- Can you point to exactly where in the head you get them?
- Do you have any pain in the back of your head or neck?
- What time of the day do you get the pain?
- Do you notice any other symptoms when you have the headache?
- Do you feel nauseated and do you vomit?
- Do you experience any unusual sensations in your eyes, such as flashing lights?
- Do you get dizzy, weak or have any strange sensations?
- Does light hurt your eyes?
- Do you get any blurred vision?
- Do you notice watering or redness of one or both of your eyes?
- Do you get pain or tenderness on combing your hair?
- Are you under a lot of stress or tension?
- Does your nose run when you get the headache?
- What tablets do you take?
- Do you get a high temperature, sweats or shivers?
- Have you had a heavy cold recently?
- Have you ever had trouble with your sinuses?
- Have you had a knock on your head recently?
- What do you think causes the headaches?

Differences between the clinical features of migraine and tension headache are presented in TABLE 56.2. 'Red flag' indicators of a serious cause of headache are outlined in the box.

Table 56.2 A comparison of typical clinical features of migraine and tension headache[5]

	Migraine	Tension headache
Family history	✓	
Onset before age 20	✓	
Prodromata	✓	
Bilateral		✓
Unilateral	✓	
Throbbing	✓	
Constant		✓
Less than one per week	✓	
Continuous daily		✓
Lasts less than 24 hours	✓	
Vomiting	✓	
Aggravated by the pill	✓	
Aggravated by alcohol	✓	
Relieved by alcohol		✓

Examination

For the physical examination it is appropriate to use the basic tools of trade, namely the thermometer, sphygmomanometer, pen torch, and diagnostic set, including the ophthalmoscope and the stethoscope. Inspect the head, temporal arteries and eyes. Areas to palpate include the temporal arteries, the facial and neck muscles, the cervical spine and sinuses, the teeth and temporomandibular joints. Search especially for signs of meningeal irritation and papilloedema.

Red flag indicators for headache

- Sudden onset especially if no previous history
- Severe and debilitating pain
- Progressive
- Fever
- Vomiting
- Disturbed consciousness/confusion, drowsiness
- Personality change
- Worse with bending, coughing or sneezing
- Maximum in morning
- Wakes patient at night
- Neurological and visual symptoms/signs
- Seizure
- Young obese female: ? on medication
- 'New' in elderly, especially >50 years
- Post-head injury

A mental state examination is mandatory and includes looking for altered consciousness or cognition and assessment of mood, anxiety–tension–depression, and any mental changes. Neurological examination includes assessment of visual fields and acuity, reactions of the pupils and eye movements in addition to sensation and motor power in the face and limbs and reflexes, including the plantar response. 'Red flag' pointers from physical examination are given in the box.

Red flag pointers: from physical examination

- Altered consciousness or cognition
- Meningism
- Abnormal vital signs: BP, temperature, respiration
- Focal neurological signs, including pupils, fundi, eye movement
- Tender, poorly pulsatile temporal arteries

Special signs

- *Upper cervical pain sign.* Palpate over the C2 and C3 areas of the cervical spine, especially two finger breadths out from the spinous process of C2. If this is very tender and even provokes the headache it indicates headache of cervical origin.
- *Ewing sign for frontal sinusitis.* Press your finger gently upwards and inwards against the orbital roof medial to the supra-orbital nerve. Pain on pressure is a positive finding and indicates frontal sinusitis.
- *The invisible pillow sign.* The patient lies on the examination table with head on a pillow. The examiner then supports the head with his or her hands as the pillow is removed. The patient is instructed to relax the neck muscles and the examiner removes the supporting hands. A positive test indicating tension from contracting neck muscles is when the patient's head does not readily change position. This is uncommon.

Investigations

Investigations can be selected from:

- haemoglobin ? anaemia
- WCC: leucocytosis with bacterial infection
- ESR/CRP: ? temporal arteritis
- radiography:
  - chest X-ray, if suspected intracerebral malignancy
  - cervical spine
  - skull X-ray, if suspected brain tumour, Paget disease, deposits in skull
  - sinus X-ray, if suspected sinusitis
  - CT scan: detection of brain tumour (most effective), cerebrovascular accidents (valuable), SAH

- radioisotope scan (technetium-99m) to localise specific tumours and haematoma
- MRI: very effective for intracerebral pathology but expensive; produces better definition of intracerebral structures than CT scanning but not as sensitive for detecting bleeding; detects intracranial vasculitis in temporal arteries
- lumbar puncture: diagnosis of meningitis, suspected SAH (only if CT scan normal)
  Note: Dangerous if raised intracranial pressure.

Headache in children

Respiratory infections and febrile illnesses are common causes of headache in children but there are other causes that reflect the common causes in adults. Many childhood headaches are isolated but are chronic in a significant number. Migraine is relatively common before adolescence, while tension or muscle contraction headache is more common after adolescence.

Consider often overlooked causes such as hair traction, eye strain (measure and record vision) and hypoglycaemia. Children who have long periods without regular eating are prone to headache including exacerbations of migraine. They should not skip breakfast.[8]

Young children rarely experience sinus headache and this should not really be considered until the sinuses develop, around 5 years for the frontal sinuses.

From 1% of children aged 7 years to 5% or more of children aged 15 years suffer from migraine, with girls developing it at a higher rate[2] with increasing age. There is a strong family history. As a rule the prognosis is good as the majority will have no migraines in the long term. The type is mainly common migraine with symptoms such as malaise or nausea: classic migraine with the typical aura is not a feature of childhood migraine. The rather dramatic migraine, such as vertebrobasilar migraine, is frequent in adolescent girls and hemiplegia occurs in infants and children, especially with their first migraine attack.[9] Vomiting is not necessarily an associated symptom in children.

The possibility of cerebral space-occupying lesions requires due consideration, especially if the headaches are progressive. These are present typically in the morning and are associated with symptoms such as vomiting, dizziness, diplopia, ataxia, personality changes and deterioration of school performance. Symptoms that indicate a cerebral tumour or other serious problem are outlined in TABLE 56.3.

Neonates and children aged 6–12 months are at the greatest risk from meningitis and it is important to keep this in mind.

56

Table 56.3 Pointers to serious causes of headache in children

Headache features
Persistent or recurrent
Present first thing in morning
Wakes child at night
No past history
No family history
Associated poor health
Associated neurological symptoms
Unilateral localisation

Source: After Wright[2]

Management of the non-serious causes of headache includes reassurance (especially of parents), discouragement of excessive emphasis on the symptom and simple medications, such as paracetamol for the younger child and aspirin for the adolescent. Patients with undiagnosed and/or problematic headache should be referred.

Pharmacological treatment in children[9]

Tension headache and migraine:

paracetamol 20 mg/kg (o) statim then 15 mg/kg 4–6-hourly up to 90 mg/kg/day (max. 4 g daily)
or
ibuprofen 5–10 mg/kg (o) statim up to 40 mg/kg/day (not for children <6 months)

Headache in the elderly

A recent onset of headache in the elderly has to be treated with caution because it could herald a serious problem, such as a space-occupying lesion (e.g. neoplasm, subdural haematoma), TIA, trigeminal neuralgia or vertebrobasilar insufficiency. Cervical spondylosis is age-related and may be an important factor in the ageing patient. Age-related headaches are summarised in TABLE 56.4.

Late-life migraine can be mistaken for cerebrovascular disease, especially in the presence of preceding neurological symptoms. It is the sequence of the visual and sensory symptoms with the spread from face to tongue to hand over some minutes, with clearing in one area as it appears that helps distinguish migraine from transient ischaemic attacks (TIAs). Although some patients experience headache with TIAs it is not a distinguishing feature. Vomiting is suggestive of migraine rather than cerebrovascular disease.[10]

Table 56.4 Age-related causes of headache	
Children	Intercurrent infections Psychogenic Migraine Meningitis Post-traumatic
Adults, including middle age	Migraine Cluster headache Tension Cervical dysfunction Subarachnoid haemorrhage Combination
Elderly	Cervical dysfunction Cerebral tumour Temporal arteritis Neuralgias Paget disease Glaucoma Cervical spondylosis Subdural haemorrhage

Tension-type headache

Tension or muscle contraction headaches are typically a symmetrical (bilateral) tightness. They tend to last for hours and recur each day. They are often associated with cervical dysfunction and stress or tension, although the patient usually does not realise the headaches are associated with tension until it is pointed out. Seventy-five per cent of patients are females.[3]

IHS criteria for tension-type headache[11]

The International Headache Society (IHS3) criteria for episodic tension-type headaches involve the following:

A The patient should have had at least 10 of these headaches.

B The headaches last from 30 minutes to 7 days.

C The headaches must have at least two of the following four:
1 non-pulsating quality
2 mild or moderate intensity
3 bilateral location
4 no aggravation with routine physical activity

D The headaches must have both of the following:
1 no nausea or vomiting
2 photophobia and phonophobia are absent, or one but not the other is present

E Not attributable to another disorder.

IHS = International Headache Society

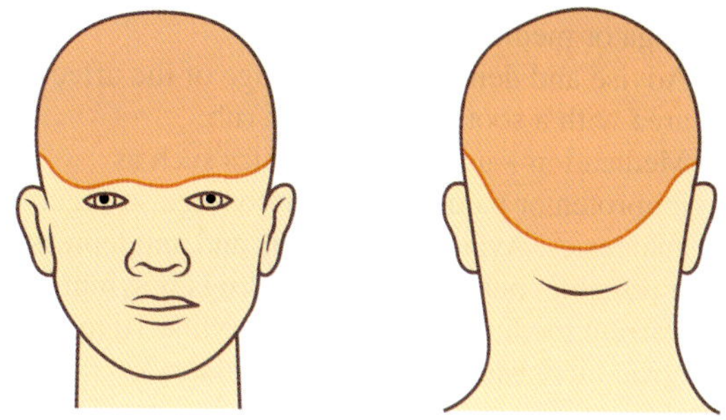

FIGURE 56.3 Typical distribution of pain in tension-type headache

Clinical features (tension headache)

Site:	frontal, over forehead and temples (see FIG. 56.3)
Radiation:	occiput
Quality:	dull ache, like a 'tight pressure feeling', 'heavy weight on top of head', 'tight band around head'; may be tightness or vice-like feeling rather than pain
Frequency:	almost daily
Duration:	hours (can last days)
Onset:	after rising, gets worse during day
Aggravating factors:	stress, overwork with skipping meals
Relieving factors:	alcohol
Associated features:	lightheadedness, fatigue, neck ache or stiffness (occiput to shoulders), perfectionist personality, anxiety/depression
Physical examination:	muscle tension (e.g. frowning), scalp often tender to touch, 'invisible pillow' sign may be positive

Management[9]

- Careful patient education: explain that the scalp muscles get tight like the calf muscles when climbing up stairs.
- Counselling and relevant advice; CBT is as effective as any drug in all ages
  - Learn to relax your mind and body.
  - During an attack, relax by lying down in a hot bath and practise meditation.
  - Be less of a perfectionist: do not be a slave to the clock.
  - Don't bottle things up, stop feeling guilty, approve of yourself, express yourself and your anger.

- Advise stress reduction, relaxation therapy and yoga or meditation classes.
- Advise and demonstrate massage of the affected area with a soothing analgesic rub.
- Medication—use mild analgesics such as ibuprofen or paracetamol. Discourage stronger analgesics. Avoid tranquillisers and antidepressants if possible, but consider these drugs if symptoms warrant medication (e.g. amitriptyline 10 mg (o) nocte increasing to 75 mg if necessary).

Special notes:

- The general aim is to direct patients to modify their lifestyle and avoid tranquillisers and analgesics.
- It is unusual to be awoken from sleep.
- Beware of depression.
- Consider muscle energy therapy and/or mobilisation of the neck followed by exercises if there is evidence of cervical dysfunction.
- Recommend a meditation program.

Migraine

Migraine, or the 'sick headache', is derived from the Greek word meaning 'pain involving half the head'. It affects at least 1 person in 10, is more common in females (18% of women, 6% men) and peaks between 20 and 50 years. There are various types of migraine (see TABLE 56.5), with classic migraine (headache, vomiting and aura) and common migraine (without the aura) being the best known. The most common trigger factor is stress.[3]

Table 56.5 Types of vascular headache

Common migraine (aura is vague or absent)
Classic migraine
Complicated migraine
Unusual forms of migraine:
- hemiplegic
- basilar
- retinal
- migrainous (vestibular) vertigo
- migrainous stupor
- ophthalmoplegic
- migraine equivalents
- status migrainosus

Cluster headache
Chronic paroxysmal hemicrania
Menstrual migraine
Lower half headache
Benign exertional-sex headache (beware of SAH)
Miscellaneous (e.g. icepick pains, 'ice-cream' headache)

Source: After Day[12]

DxT headache + vomiting + visual aura → migraine with aura (classic)

IHS3 criteria for common migraine[11]

The IHS3 criteria for migraine without aura involve the checklist following.

A The patient should have had at least five attacks fulfilling criteria B and D.
B The headaches last 4–72 hours.
C The headache must have at least two of the following:
  1 unilateral location
  2 pulsing quality
  3 moderate or severe intensity, inhibiting or prohibiting daily activities
  4 headache worsened by routine physical activity
D The headache must have at least two of the following:
  1 nausea and/or vomiting
  2 photophobia and phonophobia
E Not attributable to another disorder.

IHS3 criteria for migraine with typical aura (classic)[11]

A At least two attacks fulfilling criteria B and C.
B One or more of the following fully reversible aura symptoms: visual, sensory, speech and/or language, motor, brainstem, retinal.
C At least two of:
  1 at least one aura symptom spreads gradually over at least 5 minutes
  2 each aura symptom lasts 5–60 minutes
  3 at least one symptom is unilateral
  4 headache follows aura within 60 minutes
D Not attributable to another disorder including TIA.

Management

Patient education: provide explanation and reassurance, especially if bizarre visual and neurological symptoms are present. Patients should be reassured about the benign nature of their migraine. For each migraine sufferer, an individual treatment plan including a migraine action plan should be devised.

Counselling and advice

- Tailor the advice to the individual patient.
- Avoid known trigger factors, especially tension, fatigue, hunger and constant physical and mental stress.

- Advise keeping a diary of foodstuffs or drinks that can be identified as trigger factors. Consider a low amine diet: eliminate chocolate, cheese, red wine, coffee, walnuts, tuna, Vegemite, spinach and liver.
- Practise a healthy lifestyle, relaxation programs, meditation techniques and biofeedback training.
- Be open to non-drug therapies (e.g. trial of acupuncture, hypnotherapy).

Clinical features (classic migraine)

Site:	temporofrontal region (unilateral) (see FIG. 56.4); can be bilateral
Radiation:	retro-orbital and occipital
Quality:	intense and throbbing
Frequency:	1 or 2 per month
Duration:	4–72 hours (average 6–8 hours)
Onset:	paroxysmal, often wakes with it
Offset:	spontaneous (often after sleep)
Precipitating factors:	tension and stress (commonest); others in TABLE 56.6
Aggravating factors:	tension, activity
Relieving factors:	sleep, vomiting
Associated factors:	nausea, vomiting (90%) irritability aura — visual 25% (scintillation, scotoma, hemianopia, fortification) — sensory (unilateral paraesthesia)
Other pointers:	abdominal pain in childhood; family history of migraine, asthma and eczema

Treatment of the acute attack

- Commence treatment at earliest impending sign.
- Mild headaches may require no more than conventional treatment with 'two aspirin (or paracetamol) and a good lie down in a quiet dark room'.[5,9]
- Rest in a quiet, darkened, cool room.
- Place cold packs on the forehead or neck.
- Drink copious water but avoid drinking coffee, tea or orange juice.
- Avoid moving around too much.
- Do not read or watch television.
- For patients who find relief from simply 'sleeping off' an attack, consider prescribing temazepam 10 mg or diazepam 10 mg in addition to the following measures.[3]
- For moderate attacks use oral ergotamine or sumatriptan and for severe attacks use injection therapy.
- Avoid pethidine and other opioids.

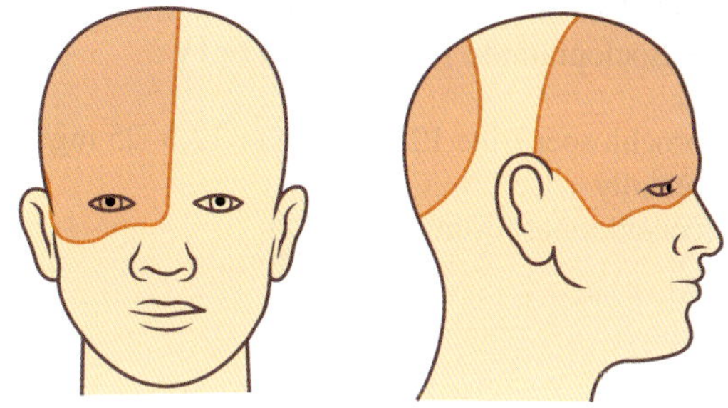

FIGURE 56.4 Typical distribution of pain in migraine (right side)

Table 56.6 Migrainous trigger factors

Exogenous
Foodstuffs—chocolate, oranges, tomatoes, citrus fruits, cheeses, gluten sensitivity (possible)
Alcohol—especially red wine
Drugs—vasodilators, oestrogens, monosodium glutamate, nitrites ('hot dog' headache), indomethacin, OCP, codeine
Glare or bright light* (32%)
Emotional stress* (63%)
Head trauma (often minor) (e.g. jarring—'footballer's migraine')
Allergen
Climatic change
Excessive noise
Strong perfume
Endogenous
Tiredness, physical exhaustion, oversleeping
Lack of sleep
Stress, relaxation after stress—'weekend migraine'
Exercise/physical stress
Hormonal changes
— puberty
— menstruation*
— climacteric
— pregnancy
Hunger
Familial tendency
?Personality factors

*Most common

Medication (if necessary)[9,13,14]

First-line medication acute migraine:

- aspirin or paracetamol + anti-emetic: e.g. soluble aspirin (Disprin Direct) 600–900 mg (o) *and* metoclopramide 10 mg (o)
- paracetamol or ibuprofen (for children)
- consider NSAIDs (e.g. ibuprofen, naproxen, diclofenac rapid)

If nausea and vomiting is a feature:

- metoclopramide 10–20 mg IM or IV
  or
- prochlorperazine 12.5 mg IM or 12.5–25 mg rectally
- consider nasal sumatriptan

Alternatives:
Choose a triptan preparation.
Triptans

- sumatriptan (a serotonin receptor agonist)[9]
  50–100 mg (o) at the time of prodrome, repeat in 2 hours if necessary to maximum dose 300 mg/24 hours
  or
  nasal spray 10–20 mg per nostril (up to 40 mg/24 hours)
  or
  6 mg, SC injection, repeat in 1 or more hours to maximum dose 12 mg/24 hours
  or
- zolmitriptan 2.5–5 mg (o), repeat in 2 hours if necessary (max. 10 mg/24 hours)
  or
- naratriptan 2.5 mg (o), repeat in 4 hours (max. 5 mg/24 hours)
  or
- rizatriptan 10 mg wafer, repeat in >2 hours (max. 30 mg/24 hours)
  or
- eletriptan 40–80 mg (o) up to 160 mg/24 hours

Avoid triptans in patients with coronary artery disease, Prinzmetal angina, uncontrolled hypertension or during pregnancy. Do not use with ergotamine simultaneously and cease if chest pain develops, albeit transient in a young patient. Use with caution in patients taking SSRIs, MAOIs and lithium.

Treatment of the severe attack

(If other preparations ineffective.)

> **Practice tip for early migraine attack**
>
> A triptan + a NSAID, e.g. naproxen or ibuprofen[15]

Caution: Consider the possibility of underlying cerebral vascular malformation, SAH or opioid addiction.

- If at home:[12]
  sumatriptan 6 mg (SC)
- If in surgery or emergency room:
  metoclopramide 10 mg (IV) slowly over 2 minutes + oral analgesics
  or
  metoclopramide 10 mg (IV) + dihydroergotamine 0.5 mg IV slowly
  or
  sumatriptan 6 mg (SC)
  or
  chlorpromazine 0.1 mg/kg IV infusion over 30 mins

Caution: Do not use ergotamine preparations if sumatriptan used in previous 6 hours, and do not use sumatriptan if ergotamine preparations used in previous 24 hours.

> **Practice tips for severe classic migraine:**
>
> - IV metoclopramide + 1 litre N saline IV in 30 minutes + oral aspirin or paracetamol
> - Continue high fluid intake

Prophylaxis

Non-drug self-management with avoidance of any known trigger factors is the key. Acupuncture has a place in management.[16]

Consider prophylactic therapy for frequent attacks that cause disruption to the patient's lifestyle and well-being, a rule of thumb being two or more severe migraine attacks per month; certainly consider it for weekly attacks and a poor response to therapy for the acute attack. Do not give ergotamine.[10]

The most commonly used drugs include:

- beta blockers—propranolol 40 mg (o) bd or tds (max. 320 mg/day), metoprolol, atenolol*
- tricyclic antidepressants—amitriptyline*
- sodium valproate*
- pizotifen 0.5–2.0 mg at night
- cyproheptadine (ideal for children)
- clonidine
- methysergide (reserve for unresponsive severe migraine) 1 mg tds after food—up to 4 months only (discontinued in Australia)
- calcium-channel blockers—nifedipine, verapamil
- NSAIDs—naproxen, indomethacin, ibuprofen
- MAOIs—phenelzine, moclobemide
- sumatriptan
- gabapentin
- topiramate
- botulinum toxin into muscles of the face, scalp or neck

* first line

For consideration:

- melatonin
- anti-CGRP monoclonal antibodies

Menstrual migraine[9]

Naproxen 550 mg (o) bd, 48 hours before expected attack for 4–10 days, oestradiol gel 1.5 mg transdermally, once daily for 7 days or mefenamic acid.

Guidelines[9,13]

Select the initial drug according to the patient's medical profile:

- if low or normal weight—pizotifen
- if hypertensive—a beta blocker
- if depressed or anxious—amitriptyline
- if tension—a beta blocker
- if cervical spondylosis—naproxen
- food-sensitive migraine—pizotifen
- menstrual migraine—naproxen or mefenamic acid or ibuprofen or oestradiol transdermal gel

Commonly prescribed first-line drugs are propranolol or pizotifen:[10]

propranolol 40 mg (o) bd or tds (at first) increasing to 320 mg daily (if necessary)
pizotifen 0.5–1 mg (o) nocte (at first) increasing to 3 mg a day (if necessary)

Each drug should be tried for 2 months before it is judged to be ineffective. Amitriptyline 50 mg nocte can be added to propranolol, pizotifen (beware of weight gain) or methysergide and may convert a relatively poor response to very good control.[3]

Cluster headache

Cluster headache is also known as migrainous neuralgia. It occurs in paroxysmal clusters of unilateral headache that typically occur nightly, usually in the early hours of the morning, although patients may have headaches that occur at other times. A hallmark is the pronounced cyclical nature of the attacks and at least five attacks. It occurs typically in males (6:1 ratio) and is rare in childhood. There are no visual disturbances or vomiting.

DxT retro-orbital headache + rhinorrhoea + lacrimation ➜ cluster headache

Management

Acute attack (brief treatment seldom effective):

- consider 100% oxygen 10 L/min for 15 min (usually good response)
- sumatriptan 6 mg SC injection (or 20 mg intranasal) *or*
- metoclopramide 10 mg IV + dihydroergotamine 0.5 mg IV slowly or 1 mg IM
- consider local anaesthetic—greater occipital nerve block

Avoid alcohol during cluster.

Prophylaxis (once a cluster starts)

Consider the following:

- methysergide 1 mg (o) once daily up to 3 mg bd
- prednisolone 50 mg/day for 10 days then taper over 3 weeks (as a bridging treatment)
- lithium 250 mg (o) bd
- verapamil SR 160 mg (o) daily up to 320 mg
- pizotifen
- indomethacin (helps confirm diagnosis)
- sodium valproate

Note: Some of the above can be used long term for frequent clusters. Prevention of further attacks is the main focus of cluster headache treatment.[5]

Clinical features

Site:	over or about one eye (see FIG. 56.5); always same side
Radiation:	frontal and temporal regions
Quality:	severe
Frequency:	one every other day and 8 per day for more than half the time
Duration:	15–180 minutes (average 30 minutes); the clusters last 4–6 weeks (can last months)
Onset:	suddenly during night (usually), same time about 2–3 hours after falling asleep; the 'alarm clock' headache (e.g. 2–4 am)
Offset:	spontaneous
Aggravating factors:	alcohol (during cluster)
Relieving factors:	drugs
Associated features:	family history; rhinorrhoea and/or congestion, ipsilateral nose; lacrimation; flushing and/or sweating of forehead and cheek; redness of ipsilateral eye; eyelid oedema; miosis and/or ptosis; sensation of fullness in ear; a sense of restlessness or agitation (see FIG. 56.6)

Cervicogenic headache

Headache from neck disorders (cervical dysfunction or spondylosis), referred to as cervicogenic, is far more common than realised and is very rewarding

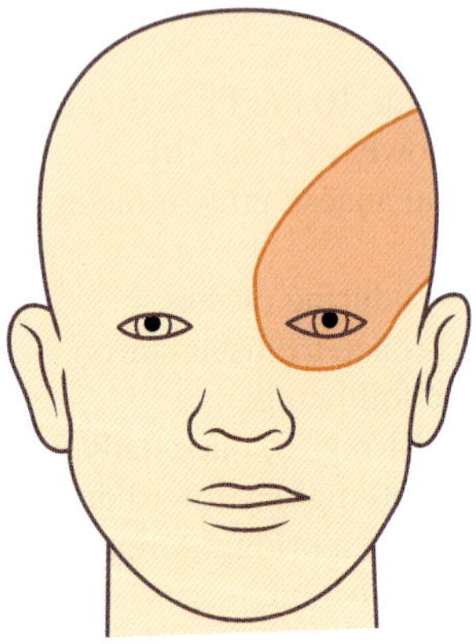

FIGURE 56.5 Typical distribution of pain in cluster headache

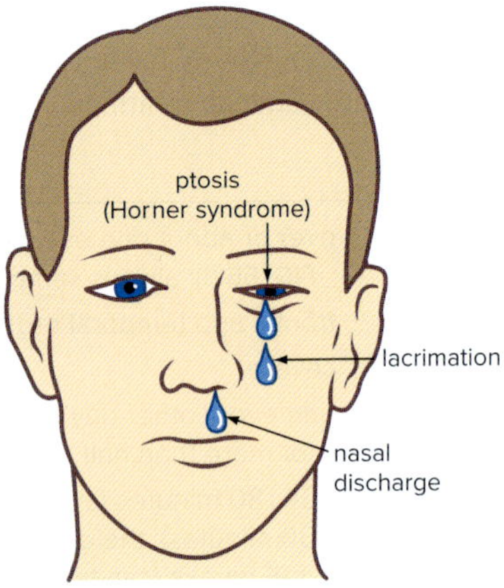

FIGURE 56.6 Features of an attack of cluster headache: ptosis, lacrimation and a discharge from the nostril on the side of pain

to treat by physical therapy, including mobilisation and manipulation and exercises in particular. See CHAPTERS 24 and 62.

Headache can be caused by abnormalities in any structure innervated by the upper two cervical nerves C2, C3 (usually the C1–2, C2–3 facet joints). Pain from cervical structures can be referred retro-orbitally and over one-half of the head. The headache is often incorrectly diagnosed as migraine but clinical examination of the neck helps differentiation.[17] The neck may be responsible for so-called 'tension' headache but clinical differentiation can be more difficult.

Occipital neuralgia, which is uncommon, causes intermittent neuralgia or lancinating pain in the C2 distribution and may radiate to the front-orbital area (see FIG. 56.7).

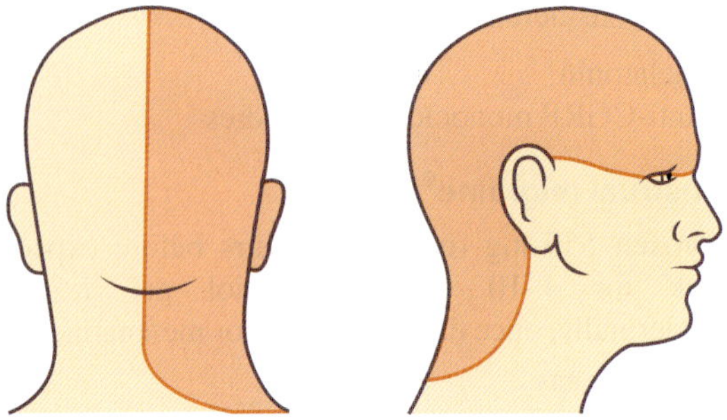

FIGURE 56.7 Typical distribution of pain in cervical dysfunction (right side)

Clinical features

The pain is usually sited in the occipital region with possible radiation to the parietal region, vertex of skull and behind the eye (see FIG. 56.7). It is usually present on waking and settles during the day. There is usually a history of trauma including an MVA or blow to the head. Associated features include stiffness and grating of the neck. On examination there is usually tenderness to palpation over the C1, C2 and/or C3 levels of the cervical spine, especially on the side of the headache.

Treatment

- Physiotherapy modalities: hydrotherapy, muscle energy therapy, mobilisation, manipulation (from experts) and neck exercises (very important)
- Supportive neck pillow
- Heat pack, especially for acute pain
- NSAIDs for cervical spondylosis
- For intractable cases consider mobilisation under general anaesthesia, injections of corticosteroids around, or surgical section of the greater occipital nerve for occipital neuralgia.[17]

Combination headache

Combined (also known as mixed) headaches are common and often diagnosed as psychogenic headache or atypical migraine. They have a combination of various degrees of:

- tension and/or depression
- cervical dysfunction
- vasospasm (migraine)
- drugs: analgesics (rebound), alcohol, nicotine, caffeine, NSAIDs

The headache, which has many of the features of tension headache, is usually described as a heavy deep ache 'as though my head is ready to burst'. It tends to be constant, being present throughout every waking moment. It tends to last for days (average 3–7) but can last for weeks or months. It is often related to stress and adverse working conditions, and sometimes follows an accident.

Management

An important strategy is to evaluate each possible component of the headache as a stepwise trial by an elimination process:

- drug evaluation and modification
- cervical dysfunction—physical therapy if present
- depression
- tension and stress
- other psychogenic factors (e.g. conversion reaction)
- vasospasm

Treatment includes cognitive therapy, reassurance that the patient does not have a cerebral tumour, and lifestyle modification. The most effective medication is amitriptyline or other antidepressant. Propranolol and the antiepileptics can be considered.

Temporal arteritis

TA is also known as giant cell arteritis or cranial arteritis. There is usually a persistent unilateral throbbing headache in the temporal region and scalp sensitivity with localised thickening, with or without loss of pulsation of the temporal artery. It is related to polymyalgia rheumatica—20% of sufferers will develop TA. See CHAPTER 32.

TA is a type of collagen disease causing inflammation of extracranial vessels, especially the superficial temporal artery. It usually presents as a unilateral intermittent headache in a person over 50 years.

Clinical features

Age:	over 50 years (mean age 70 years)
Site:	forehead and temporal region (unilateral) (see FIG. 56.8)
Radiation:	down side of head towards occiput
Quality:	severe burning pain
Frequency:	daily, a constant ache
Duration:	usually constant (getting worse)
Onset:	non-specific, tends to be worse in morning
Offset:	nil
Aggravating factors:	stress and anxiety
Relieving factors:	nil
Associated features:	malaise, vague aches and pains in muscles (especially of neck), weight loss
Other pointers:	intermittent blurred vision
	tenderness on brushing hair
	jaw claudication on eating
	polymyalgia rheumatica
	hypertension
	abnormal emotional behaviour

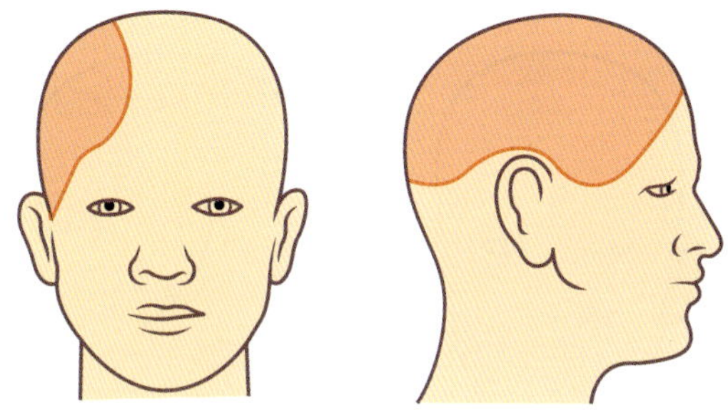

FIGURE 56.8 Typical distribution of pain in temporal arteritis (right side)

TA may also involve the intracranial vessels, especially the ophthalmic artery or posterior ciliary arteries, causing optic atrophy and blindness. Vision is impaired in about one-half of patients at some stage. Once the patient goes blind it is usually irreversible.

Diagnosis

Diagnosis is by biopsy and histological examination of the superficial temporal artery. The ESR is usually markedly elevated but may be normal. The biopsy may be normal as TA has a focal nature. MRI has a high sensitivity and specificity.

Note: Consider it with any 'new' headache.

Treatment

TA is very responsive to corticosteroids; start treatment immediately to prevent permanent blindness. Initial medication is prednisolone 40–60 mg orally daily in two divided doses initially for 2–4 weeks. Dose reduction and progress is monitored by the clinical state and ESR and CRP levels.[10] Concomitant use of H2-receptor antagonists may be appropriate initially. Temporal arteritis may take 1–2 years to resolve.

Frontal sinusitis

The headache of frontal sinusitis can be a diagnostic problem especially in the absence of, or a lapse in time since, an obvious upper respiratory infection or vasomotor rhinitis. Some patients do not have a history of a preceding respiratory infection, nor any signs of nasal obstruction or fever. Contrary to popular belief, sinusitis is a relatively uncommon source of headache.

Clinical features

It presents typically as a frontal or retro-orbital headache (see FIG. 56.9). A characteristic is its diurnal variation, developing in the morning around 9 am, being most intense in the middle of the day, then subsiding to offset around 6 pm.

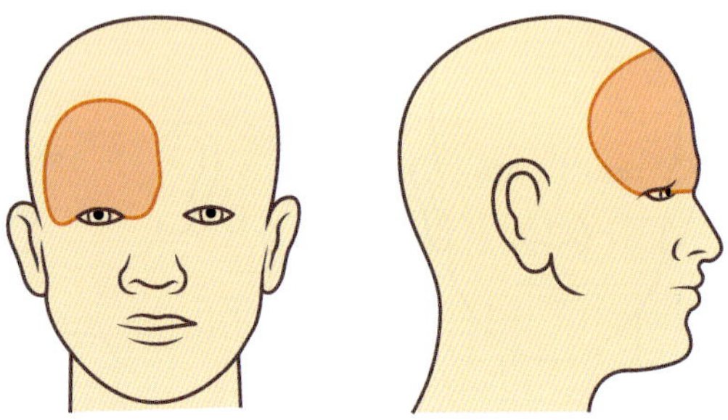

FIGURE 56.9 Typical distribution of pain of frontal sinusitis (right side)

Examination

There is tenderness over the frontal sinus and pain on percussion over the sinus. Ewing sign may be elicited. Fever and oedema of the upper eyelid may be present.

Management

Principles of treatment

- Drain the sinus conservatively using steam inhalations
- Antibiotics: amoxycillin or amoxycillin/clavulanate or cefaclor or doxycycline
- Analgesics

Referral

If resolution cannot be accomplished by conservative means then referral to an ENT specialist is advisable. Acute purulent sinusitis can be treacherous if it persist and spreads, causing collections of pus in the extradural or subdural space, cerebral abscess or blood-borne spread of infection.

Complications

- Orbital cellulitis
- Subdural abscess
- Osteomyelitis
- Cavernous sinus thrombosis

Symptoms indicating spread of infection:

- increase in fever and chills
- vomiting
- oedema of the eyelids and forehead
- visual disturbances
- dulling of the sensorium
- convulsions

Raised intracranial pressure

Important causes of a space-occupying lesion include a cerebral tumour and subdural haematoma. Sometimes it is not possible to differentiate between a subdural and an extradural haematoma, although the latter classically follows an acute injury (see CHAPTER 75). Typical features are generalised headache, usually worse in the morning, aggravated by abrupt changes in intracranial pressure and later associated with vomiting and drowsiness. Headache is an uncommon presenting symptom of a cerebral tumour.

> **DxT** drowsiness + vomiting + seizure → raised intracranial pressure

Clinical features

Site:	generalised, often occipital
Radiation:	retro-orbital
Quality:	dull, deep steady ache
Frequency:	daily
Duration:	may be hours in morning
Onset:	worse in mornings, usually intermittent, can awaken from sleep
Offset:	later in day (if at all)
Aggravating factors:	coughing, sneezing, straining at toilet
Relieving factors:	analgesics (e.g. aspirin), sitting, standing
Associated features:	vomiting (without preceding nausea); vertigo/dizziness; drowsiness; seizures; confusion (later); neurological signs (depending on side)

Examination

- Focal CNS signs
- Papilloedema (see FIG. 56.10) (but may be absent)

Intracerebral tumours

- Incidence is 5–10 per 100 000 population
- Two peaks of incidence: children <10 years[3] and 35–60 years

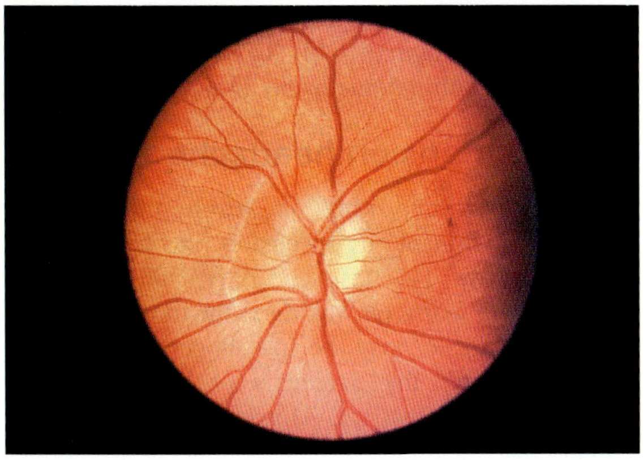

FIGURE 56.10 Papilloedema with swollen optic disc of the ocular fundus due to raised intracranial pressure

- Main types of tumour:
  - children: medulloblastoma, astrocytoma (posterior fossa), ependymoma, glioma (brain stem)
  - adults: cerebral glioma, meningioma, pituitary adenoma, cerebral metastases (e.g. lung)

Investigations

- CT scan and MRI

Subarachnoid haemorrhage

SAH is a life-threatening event that should not be overlooked at the primary care level. The incidence is 12 per 100 000 population per annum. About 40% of patients die before treatment, while about one-third have a good response to treatment.

Approximately 75% will present with an acute severe headache and the remainder with loss of consciousness.

Clinical features

- Sudden severe 'thunderclap' headache
- Occipital location
- Localised at first, then generalised
- Pain and stiffness of the neck follows
- Vomiting and loss of consciousness often follow
- Confusion or a lowered consciousness level
- ± seizures
- Kernig sign positive (see CHAPTER 30)
- Neurological deficit may include: hemiplegia (if intracerebral bleed), third nerve palsy (partial or complete) (see FIG. 56.11)

About one-third of patients experience a 'sentinel' headache.

DxT occipital headache + vomiting + neck stiffness → SAH

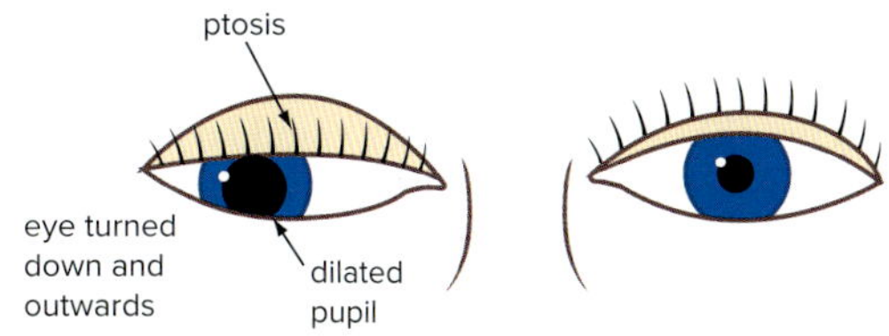

FIGURE 56.11 Third nerve palsy (right side)

Diagnosis

CT scanning is the investigation of choice and should be performed in the first few hours (blood has dispersed by 6 hours). Lumbar puncture is not necessary if the diagnosis can be made by CT, but is used if the CT scan is negative (usually 10–20% of cases). It may be falsely negative after 7 days. Even blood staining of CSF and xanthochromia is a positive feature on lumbar puncture.

Special notes

- Less severe headaches can cause diagnostic difficulties.
- Consider an angioma rather than an aneurysm as the cause of SAH if previous episodes.

Management

Immediate referral for possible surgical intervention is required. If there is lingering doubt, review the patient within 12–24 hours.

Meningitis

The headache of meningitis is usually generalised and radiates to the neck. It is constant and severe and occasionally may begin abruptly. It is aggravated by flexion of the neck. Brudzinski sign (neck flexion) and Kernig sign are positive. Fever and neck stiffness are usually present. Urgent referral to hospital is necessary. If meningitis is suspected or if a child or adult has headache with fever and neck stiffness, antibiotics must not be given until a lumbar puncture has been performed.

Drug rebound headache

Rebound headaches are usually associated with analgesic and ergotamine dependence. A long list of over-the-counter and prescription medications can cause rebound, for example, aspirin, paracetamol, ibuprofen, opioids and caffeine. The headache is present on waking and typically persists throughout the day but fluctuates in intensity. It is a mild to moderate, dull, bilateral ache with a distribution similar to tension headache. Drug rebound headaches should be suspected in any patient who complains of headache 'all day every day'. A careful drug history should be taken. Treatment includes gradual withdrawal of the drugs and the substitution of antiemetics and amitriptyline or beta blocker over about 14 days.

Chronic paroxysmal hemicrania

This is a rare headache syndrome that overlaps with cluster headache and facial pain. The unilateral pain, which can be excruciating, is located in the area of the temple, forehead, eye and upper face. It can radiate to the ear, neck and shoulder. It differs from cluster headaches in that the patients are invariably female, the paroxysms are short (average 20–30 minutes) and more frequent, with attacks occurring up to 14 times a day. The disorder resembles cluster headaches in nature and distribution and associated autonomic features, such as ipsilateral nasal stuffiness or rhinorrhoea, lacrimation, conjunctival injection and ptosis. The aetiology is unknown but the headache often responds dramatically to indomethacin (25 mg (o) tds).[10]

Post-traumatic headache

This is a continuous, diffuse type of headache with associated psychological symptoms such as dizziness, irritability and depression. It can persist for 6–12 months and is best treated with aspirin or paracetamol. If unresponsive and persistent, amitriptyline or sodium valproate can be tried.[9]

Post-lumbar-puncture headache[9]

This is common and is usually present when standing or sitting and rapidly improves with lying flat. It is a form of low-pressure headache, possibly due to CSF leakage. It can be severe with nausea and vomiting. In most resolution occurs within 2–7 days. Treatment includes bed rest until resolution. If persistent, referral for an epidural blood patch is recommended.

Trigeminal neuralgia

The pain of trigeminal neuralgia comes in excruciating paroxysms, which last for seconds to minutes only and usually affect the face rather than the head (see CHAPTER 52). The lightning-like jabs of searing or burning pain usually last 1 to 2 minutes but can last as long as 15 minutes.

Icepick headache

Icepick headaches are similar sudden stabbing pains lasting a few seconds usually at the temple (often bilateral) and are more common in migraine sufferers. They can occur unpredictably 30 or more times a day. Treatment is with indomethacin 25 mg tds.[9]

Hypertension headache

It tends to occur only in severe hypertension such as malignant hypertension or hypertensive encephalopathy. The headache is typically occipital, throbbing and worse on waking in the morning.

The headache may be psychogenic in origin, developing after the diagnosis of hypertension is disclosed to the patient. However, the occasional patient has genuine headache related to milder hypertension and this serves as an accurate indicator of their blood pressure level.

Benign intracranial hypertension (pseudotumour cerebri)

This is a rare but important sinister headache condition that typically occurs in young obese women mainly in the second to fifth decades but can occur at any age. Key features are headache, visual blurring and obscurations, nausea and papilloedema. It is considered to be due to a disturbance in the CSF circulation. The CT and MRI scans are normal but lumbar puncture reveals increased CSF pressure and normal CSF analysis.

It is sometimes linked to drugs, including tetracyclines (most common), nitrofurantoin, oral contraceptive pill, steroids and vitamin A preparations. The main concern is visual deficits from the high intracranial pressure. Urgent referral is essential. Medical treatment includes weight reduction, corticosteroids and diuretics. The treatment of choice to alleviate symptoms is repeated lumbar puncture. Surgery, which involves decompression of the optic nerves or lumbo-peritoneal shunting, is sometimes required for failed medical therapy.

> **DxT** headache + visual obscurations + nausea → benign intracranial hypertension

HEADACHES RELATED TO SPECIFIC ACTIVITIES

Sex headache

This can manifest as a dull or explosive headache, provoked by sexual arousal and activity, especially with orgasm. Some are clearly a form of exertional headache. Sometimes sex headache is mistaken for

SAH, but if the severe headache coincided with orgasm, was not associated with vomiting or neck stiffness, or settled within hours, SAH is unlikely. Treatment is with prophylactic beta blockers or ergotamine 1 mg (o) 1–2 hours before activity.

Cough and exertional headache

Some people experience a severe transient pain with factors such as coughing, sneezing, stooping, straining, lifting and various sporting activities. It is usually benign and examination is normal. A CT scan is indicated if there are focal signs or if the symptoms do not settle.

Treatment is indomethacin 25 mg (o) 2–3 times daily for cough headache and 1–2 hours before exertional activity.

Gravitational headache

Occipital headache, coming on when standing upright and relieved by lying down, is characteristic of a post-lumbar puncture, an epidural block or low-pressure headache. It can last for several weeks after the procedure.

'Ice-cream' headache

Frontal or global headache can be provoked by the rapid ingestion of very cold food and drink. It is a form of vascular headache.

When to refer

- Evidence or suspicion of SAH or intracerebral haematoma
- Complicated migraine
- Uncertain diagnosis
- Positive neurological signs despite typical headaches

Practice tips

- A patient >55 years presenting with unaccustomed headache has an organic disorder such as TA, intracerebral tumour or subdural haematoma until proved otherwise.
- The ESR is an excellent screening test to diagnose TA but occasionally can be normal in the presence of active TA.
- If a patient presents twice within 24 hours to the same practice or hospital with headache and vomiting, consider other causes apart from migraine before discharging the patient.[8]
- If migraine attacks are severe and unusual (e.g. always on the same side) consider the possibility of cerebral vascular malformation.
- CT scans and MRI have superseded other investigations in the diagnosis of cerebral tumours and intracranial haemorrhage but should be ordered sparingly and judiciously.
- If a headache is occipital in origin or accompanied by neck pain, consider the likely possibility of cervical dysfunction and refer to the appropriate therapist once the diagnosis is established.
- For recurrent migraine sufferers emphasise the importance of trigger factor avoidance and of taking aspirin and metoclopramide medication at the earliest warning of an attack.
- A severe headache of sudden onset is SAH until proved otherwise. It is overlooked sometimes.
- SAH is overlooked sometimes, mainly because it is not considered in the differential diagnosis. Suspect with very severe and protracted headache, drowsiness and neck stiffness.
- Medical evidence indicates that most headaches are related to fatigue, stress or migraine triggers and respond to application of heat or cold, exercise and common analgesics, including aspirin and ibuprofen.[18]
- If women with migraine demand the oral contraceptive, use a low-dose oestrogen preparation and monitor progress.
- The use of narcotics for migraine treatment (such as pethidine and codeine) is to be avoided whenever possible—the frequent use of ergotamine, analgesics or narcotics can transform episodic migraine into chronic daily headache.[4]

Patient education resources

Hand-out sheets from *Murtagh's Patient Education* 7th edition:

- Migraine
- Tension headache

References

1 Cormack J, Marinker M, Morrell D. The patient complaining of headache. In: *Practice*. London: Kluwer Medical, 1982: 3–12.
2 Wright M. Recurrent headaches in children. Australian Paediatric Review, 1991; 1 (6): 1–2.
3 Anthony M. Migraine and tension headache. In: *MIMS Disease Index* (2nd edn). Sydney: IMS Publishing, 1996: 313–16.
4 Stark R. Management of headache. Proceedings of 25th update course for GPs. Monash University, 2003.
5 Beran R. *Headache in Neurology for General Practitioners*. Sydney: Elsevier, 2012: 46–55.

6 Lance JW. Headache and facial pain. Med J Aust, 2000; 172: 450–5.
7 Davis A, Bolin T, Ham J. *Symptom Analysis and Physical Diagnosis.* Sydney: Pergamon, 1990.
8 Smith L. Childhood headache. In: Australian Doctor Education, GP Paediatrics, 2005.
9 Expert group for Neurology. Headache. In: eTG complete [Internet]. Melbourne: Therapeutic Guidelines Ltd. Available from: <www.tg.org.au>, accessed October 2017.
10 Burns R. Pitfalls in headache management. Aust Fam Physician, 1990; 19: 1821–6.
11 IHS Classification ICHD-3: 2013. Refer <www.ihs-classification.org/en/> or <www.sagepub.co.uk>.
12 Day TJ. Migraine and other vascular headaches. Aust Fam Physician, 1990; 19: 1797–804.
13 Heywood J, Zagami A. Treating acute migraine attack. Current Therapeutics, 1997; 37 (12): 33–7.
14 Buckley N (Chair). *Australian Medicines Handbook.* Adelaide: Australian Medicines Handbook Pty Ltd, 2016: 750–2.
15 Mannix LK, Martin VT et al. Combination treatment for menstrual migraine and dysmenorrhea using sumatriptan-naproxen: two randomized controlled trials. Obstet Gynecol, 2009; 114 (1):106–13.
16 Linde K, Allais G et al. Acupuncture for migraine prophylaxis. Cochrane Database. Syst Rev. 2009. Art No. CD001218.
17 Anthony M. The treatment of migraine—old methods, new ideas. Aust Fam Physician, 1993; 22: 1401–05.
18 Rosser W, Shafir MS. *Evidence-Based Family Medicine.* Hamilton: BC Decker Inc., 1998: 164–6.

Hoarseness

57

Hoarseness results from imperfect phonation due to impairment of normal vocal cord mobility or vibration. It is an important symptom as it may signal a serious cause such as malignancy or a disease with potential for airway obstruction.[1]

RAYMOND L CARROLL 1996

Hoarseness (dysphonia) is defined as an altered voice due to a laryngeal disorder.[2] It is an important symptom of laryngeal disease presenting in general practice, and ranges from the very common, trivial, self-limiting condition of viral upper respiratory tract infection to a life-threatening disorder (see TABLE 57.1). It may be of sudden presentation lasting only a few days or develop gradually and persist for weeks or months. The cut-off point between acute and chronic hoarseness is three weeks duration, by which time most self-limiting conditions have resolved. Hoarseness pertains to harsh, raspy, gravelly or rough tones of voice rather than pitch or volume. Rarely, hoarseness can be a functional or deliberate symptom referred to as 'hysterical aphonia'.[3] In this condition, patients purposely hold the cords apart while speaking.

Table 57.1 Hoarseness: diagnostic strategy model

Probability diagnosis
Viral URTI: acute laryngitis
Non-specific irritative laryngitis (Reinke oedema)
Vocal abuse (shouting, screaming, etc.)
Nodules and polyps of cords
Presbyphonia in elderly: 'tired' voice
Acute tonsillitis

Serious disorders not to be missed
Cancer: larynx, lung, including recurrent laryngeal nerve palsy, oesophagus, thyroid
Imminent airway obstruction (e.g. acute epiglottitis, croup)
Other rare severe infections (e.g. TB, diphtheria)
Foreign body
Motor neurone disease
Aortic arch aneurysm
Myasthenia gravis

Pitfalls (often missed)
Toxic fumes
Vocal abuse
Benign tumours of vocal cords (e.g. polyps, 'singer's nodules', papillomas)
Gastro-oesophageal reflux → pharyngolaryngitis
Goitre
Vocal cord palsy
Dystonia
Physical trauma (e.g. post-intubation), haematoma
Fungal infections (e.g. *Candida* with steroid inhalation, immunocompromised)
Allergy (e.g. angioedema)
Leucoplakia
Vocal cord dysfunction
'Floppy trachea' syndrome
Systemic autoimmune disorders (e.g. SLE, Wegener granulomatosis)

Seven masquerades checklist
Consider:
- drugs: antipsychotics, anabolic steroids, opium users
- smoking → non-specific laryngitis
- hypothyroidism, acromegaly

Is the patient trying to tell me something?
Consider:
- functional aphonia
- functional stridor

Key facts and checkpoints

- In acute hoarseness, the diagnosis is usually obvious from the history alone. Examples include acute upper respiratory tract infection (URTI) or vocal overuse.
- Think 'hypothyroidism' if unusual hoarseness develops.
- Laryngeal cancer must be excluded if hoarseness persists for longer than 3 weeks in an adult. It can arise intrinsic or extrinsic to the vocal cords.

continued

continued

- Intermittent hoarseness is invariably secondary to a benign disorder. Constant or progressive hoarseness suggests malignancy.
- Non-malignant vocal cord lesions, which include polyps, vocal nodules, contact ulcers, granulomas, other benign tumours and leucoplakia, account for about half of all voice disorders.
- In cases of chronic hoarseness the larynx must be visualised for diagnosis but the following are common:
  - children—'screamer's nodules'
  - adults—non-specific irritant laryngitis
- Acute laryngeal oedema may develop as a component of the life-threatening acute angioedemic allergic response.
- Elderly or debilitated patients may exhibit a shaky or soft 'pseudohoarse' voice due to a weakened respiratory effort. This is termed phonaesthenia or presbyphonia.
- Contact ulcers of the larynx occur on the posterior third of the vocal cords where the mucosa is thin. The resultant weak hoarse voice may be accompanied by painful phonation. The ulcers may develop into granulomas. Apart from intubation, the condition is usually found in forceful orators who misuse their larynx when attempting to lower the pitch of their voice.[3]

The clinical approach

History

Note the nature and duration of the voice change. Inquire about corticosteroid inhalations, excessive or unaccustomed voice straining (especially singing), recent surgery, possible reflux, smoking or exposure to environmental pollutants. Elicit associated respiratory or general symptoms such as cough and weight loss. Consider symptoms of hypothyroidism.

Examination

Palpate the neck for enlargement of the thyroid gland or cervical nodes. Perform a simple oropharyngeal examination except if epiglottitis is suspected. Check for signs of hypothyroidism, such as coarse dry hair and skin, slow pulse and mental slowing. Perform indirect laryngoscopy if skilled in the procedure.

Investigations

The following need to be considered:

- Thyroid function tests.
- Chest X-ray if it is possibly due to lung cancer with recurrent laryngeal nerve palsy.
- Indirect laryngoscopy (the gag reflex may preclude this).
- Direct laryngoscopy with a flexible fibre-optic endoscope with possible biopsy (the most sensitive investigation).
- The choice of imaging to detect suspected neoplasia or laryngeal trauma is special CT scan.

Management principles

Acute hoarseness

- Treat according to cause.
- Advise vocal rest or minimal usage at normal conversational level.
- Avoid irritants (e.g. dust, tobacco, alcohol).
- Consider inhalations and cough suppressants in cases of acute URTI and coughing paroxysms.

Chronic hoarseness

- Establish the diagnosis.
- Consider referral to ENT specialist.

Hoarseness in children

- It is worth bearing in mind that stridor in infants can be caused by a congenital abnormality of the larynx, including laryngomalacia (congenital laryngeal stridor), which is particularly noticeable when the child is asleep; laryngeal stenosis (congenital laryngeal narrowing); and laryngeal paralysis due to birth trauma of the vagus nerve. Vocal cord paralysis/palsy is the most common laryngeal abnormality in children (20% of cases) after laryngomalacia.[3]
- In children exclude the acute infections—laryngotracheobronchitis (croup), tonsillitis and epiglottitis.
- Persistent hoarseness in children is due commonly to vocal cord nodules related to vocal abuse, such as screaming and yelling, often due to noisy children's games.
- It is important to exclude a juvenile papilloma in a hoarse child.[4]

SPECIFIC CONDITIONS

Acute laryngitis

Most cases are caused by the respiratory viruses—rhinovirus, influenza, para-influenza, Coxsackie, adenovirus and respiratory syncytial virus, resulting in vocal cord oedema (be cautious of group A *Streptococcus*). The main symptom is hoarseness, which usually persists for 3–14 days and leads to loss of voice. Even speaking can be painful. Aggravating factors include smoking, excessive alcohol drinking, and exposure to irritants and pollutants, air-conditioning systems and very cold weather.

Management

- Rest at home, including voice rest (the best treatment).
- Use the voice sparingly, avoid whispering.
- Use a warm sialagogue (e.g. hot lemon drinks).
- Drink ample fluids, especially water.
- Avoid smoking, passive smoke and alcohol.
- Have hot, steamy showers as humidity helps.
- Use steam inhalations (e.g. 5 minutes, three times a day).
- Use cough suppressants, especially mucolytic agents.
- Use simple analgesics, such as paracetamol or aspirin, for discomfort.
- Antibiotics are of no proven use unless there is evidence of bacterial infection. Corticosteroids are rarely indicated.

Chronic laryngitis: 'barmaid syndrome'

This typically occurs in a heavy smoker who works in a heavy smoking environment, who is a heavy drinker and continually talks or sings. It is a combination of vocal abuse and chemical irritation. Hoarseness often comes and goes. Treatment involves modification of these factors and screening for vocal cord tumours.

Chronic laryngitis due to laryngopharyngeal reflux is treated with an 8–12 week empirical course of proton-pump inhibitors as well as dietary and lifestyle modification.[2]

Benign tumours of the vocal cords

These include nodules (most common) (see FIG. 57.1), polyps (second most common), cysts and papules. Vocal cord nodules, including 'singer's nodules', may respond well to conservative measures such as voice rest and vocal therapy. If not, they can be removed by microlaryngeal surgery or laser therapy. Dependent polyps and papillomas are removed by microsurgery.

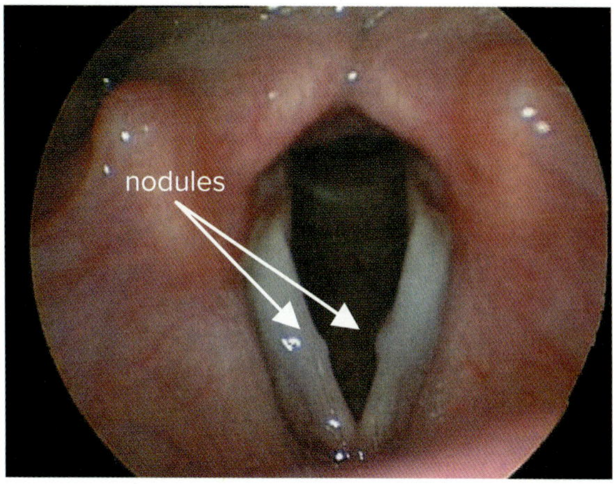

FIGURE 57.1 Vocal cord nodules

Laryngeal cancer

Squamous cell carcinoma usually occurs in patients with a history of chronic laryngitis, smoking and alcohol use. Symptoms include hoarseness, stridor, haemoptysis and dysphagia. It may be preceded by leucoplakia, which is treated by vocal cord stripping under microsurgery. The diagnosis based on persistent hoarseness is made after fibre-optic laryngoscopy and biopsy by a specialist. The patient may present with an unexplained cervical lymph node. The condition is curable if detected early. Small local tumours can be treated by radiotherapy or laser therapy. Larger tumours usually require laryngectomy and perhaps dissection of the cervical lymph nodes (commando operation). Such radical surgery demands considerable patient support, including education about speech, eating and tracheostomy care.

Vocal cord dysfunction[6]

This condition is paradoxical vocal (or fold) adduction on inspiration and abduction on expiration, causing inspiratory airway obstruction and stridor. It tends to be misdiagnosed as asthma. Apart from dyspnoea and stridor (usually inspiratory) and wheezing, symptoms may include intermittent hoarseness, chest and/or throat tightness, a noisy rasping sound and a choking or suffocating sensation. Patients may complain about a feeling 'like breathing through a straw'. Diagnosis is by observing inspiratory closure of the vocal cords with direct laryngoscopy. The mainstay of treatment is speech therapy.

57

Excessive dynamic airways collapse ('floppy trachea')[7]

Also known as adult tracheobronchomalacia, this is defined as pathological collapse and narrowing of the airway lumen by ≥50%. It is due to laxity of the posterior membrane into the airway lumen (in the presence of structurally intact cartilage) during forced expiration. Symptoms include breathing difficulty, coughing, difficulty clearing secretions, dyspnoea and stridor. Respiratory failure and death can occur. Diagnosis is with CT scanning and fibre-optic bronchoscopy. Treatment varies from conservative to surgery (minimal to radical). Refer to a respiratory physician.

When to refer[1]

- Acute cases that are unexplained, fail to respond by 3–4 weeks or recur.
- All chronic cases.
- Any case with stridor or non-tender cervical lymphadenopathy.
- Patients requiring voice therapy when vocal abuse is identified.

Practice tips

- Consider intubation as a possible cause of transient hoarseness, especially in these times of day surgery.[5]
- Consider gastro-oesophageal reflux disease in the elderly but avoid such a diagnosis without specialist investigation for other causes.
- If stridor is present with acute hoarseness, the airway is compromised. Be on stand-by for possible emergency intervention.
- Prevention is the best treatment for laryngeal cancer (i.e. quit smoking).
- Recurrent laryngeal nerve palsy may be associated with cancer of the lung and mediastinum, or diabetes, or may be idiopathic.

References

1 Carroll RL. Hoarseness. In: *MIMS Disease Index* (2nd edn). Sydney: IMS Publishing, 1996: 239–40.
2 Bova R, McGuinness J. Hoarseness: a guide to voice disorders. Medicine Today, 2007; 8 (2): 38–44.
3 Priestly J, Havas TE. Benign vocal fold lesions. Medical Observer, 19 November 2012: 1–3.
4 Birman C, Fitzsimons, Quayle S. Little voices: therapy update. Australian Doctor, 7 May 2004: 49–50.
5 Hopcroft K, Forte V. *Symptom Sorter* (4th edn). Oxford: Radcliffe Publishing, 2011; 316–8.
6 Indrees M et al. Vocal cord dysfunction in bronchial asthma. A review article. J Asthma, 2015; 52 (4): 327–35.
7 Murgu S, Colt H. Tracheobronchomalacia and excessive dynamic airway collapse. Clin Chest Med, 2013; 34 (3): 527–55.

Jaundice

58

The disease is produced by black bile when it flows into the liver. The symptoms are these: 'an acute pain in the liver, also below the breast, a feeling of suffocation is strong during these days and becomes less strong later'. The liver is tender to palpation and the complexion of the patient is somewhat livid. These are symptoms that occur in the beginning but as the disease progresses, the fever diminishes in strength and the patient feels sated after ingesting a little amount of food. He must drink melikration [a mixture of water and honey].

HIPPOCRATES ON HEPATITIS

Jaundice is a yellow discolouration of the skin and mucosal surfaces caused by the accumulation of excessive bilirubin.[1] It is a cardinal symptom of hepatobiliary disease and haemolysis. Important common causes include gallstones, hepatitis A, hepatitis B, hepatitis C, drugs, alcohol and Gilbert syndrome. The commonest clinical encounter with jaundice, especially physiological jaundice, is in the newborn. As for all patients, the history and examination are paramount, but investigations are essential to clinch the diagnosis of jaundice.

The three major categories of jaundice are (see FIG. 58.1):

- obstructive:
  - extrahepatic
  - intrahepatic
- hepatocellular
- haemolytic

Key facts and checkpoints

- Jaundice is defined as a serum bilirubin level exceeding 19 μmol/L.[2]
- Clinical jaundice manifests only when the bilirubin level exceeds 50 μmol/L.[1]
- However, jaundice is difficult to detect visually below 85 μmol/L if lighting is poor.
- It can be distinguished from yellow skin due to hypercarotenaemia (due to dietary excess of carrots, pumpkin, mangoes or pawpaw) and hypothyroidism by involving the sclera.
- The most common causes of jaundice recorded in a general practice population are (in order) viral hepatitis, gallstones, pancreatic cancer, cirrhosis, pancreatitis and drugs.[3]
- Always take a full travel, drug and hepatitis contact history in any patient presenting with jaundice.
- Acute hepatitis is usually self-limiting in patients with hepatitis A and in adults with hepatitis B but progresses to chronic infections with hepatitis C and children with hepatitis B.[4]
- A fatty liver (steatosis) can occur not only with alcohol excess but also with obesity, diabetes and starvation. There is usually no liver damage and thus no jaundice.
- Almost all patients with chronic hepatitis C will be cured with a course of oral direct-acting antiviral agents, but only if they are diagnosed, assessed, treated and monitored appropriately.

Table 58.1 Abbreviations used in this chapter

Hepatitis A virus	HAV
Hepatitis A antibody	anti-HAV
Immunoglobulin M	IgM
Immunoglobulin G	IgG
Hepatitis B virus	HBV
Hepatitis B surface antigen	HBsAg
Hepatitis B surface antibody	anti-HBs
Hepatitis B core antibody	anti-HBc
Hepatitis Be antigen	HBeAg
Hepatitis C virus	HCV
Hepatitis C virus antibody	anti-HCV
Hepatitis D (Delta) virus	HDV
Hepatitis E virus	HEV
Hepatitis F virus	HFV
Hepatitis G virus	HGV

58

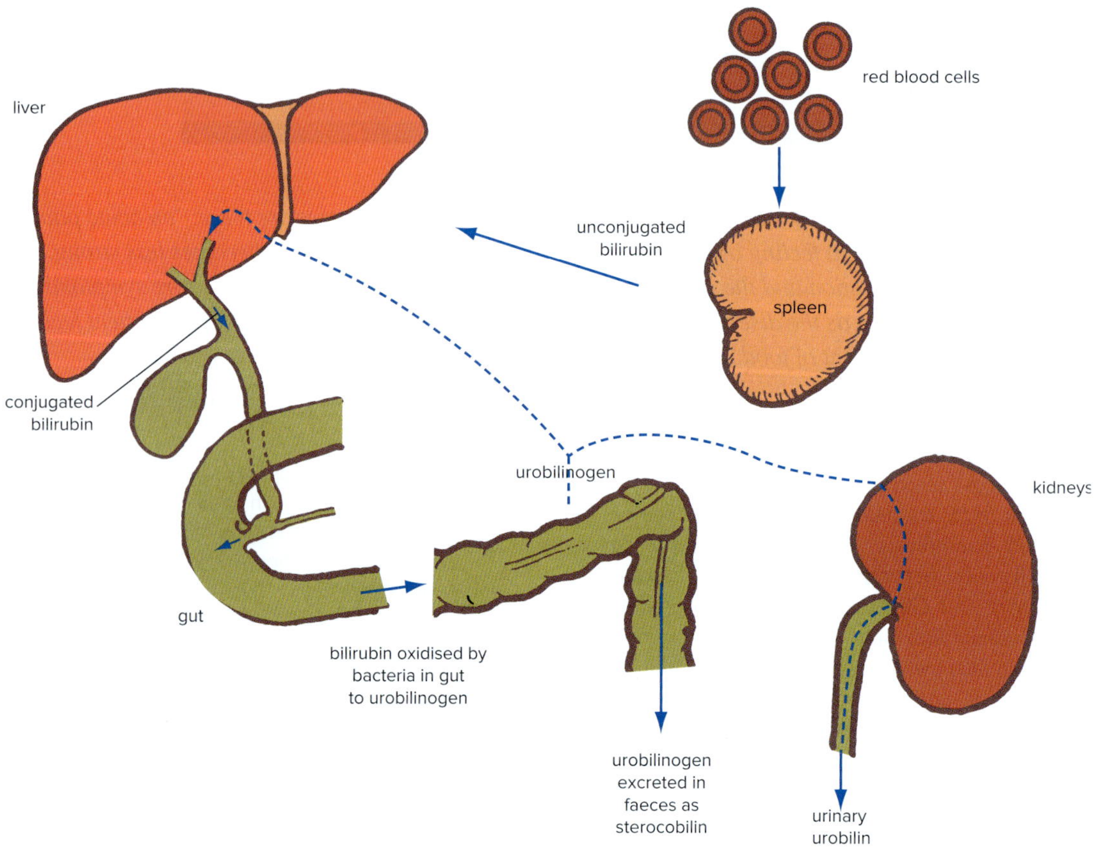

FIGURE 58.1 The jaundice pathway

A diagnostic approach

A summary of the diagnostic strategy model is presented in TABLE 58.2.

Probability diagnosis

The answer depends on the age and social grouping of the patient, especially if the patient indulges in risk-taking behaviour or has travelled overseas.

Viral hepatitis A, B or C account for the majority of cases of jaundice.

In the middle-aged and elderly group, a common cause is obstruction from gallstones or cancer. It is common for older people to have painless obstructive jaundice; bear in mind that the chances of malignancy increase with age.

Alcoholic liver disease is common and may present as chronic alcoholic cirrhosis with liver failure or as acute alcoholic hepatitis. It is worth emphasising that such patients can make a dramatic recovery when they cease drinking alcohol.

In family practice we encounter many cases of drug-induced jaundice, especially in the elderly. These drugs are outlined later in the chapter, under 'Seven masquerades checklist'.

Serious disorders not to be missed

Malignancy must always be suspected, especially in the elderly patient and those with a history of chronic active hepatitis (e.g. post hepatitis B or C infection). The former is more likely to have carcinoma of the head of the pancreas and the latter, hepatocellular carcinoma (hepatoma).

Metastatic cancer must be kept in mind, especially in those with a history of surgery, such as large bowel cancer, melanoma and stomach cancer. An enlarged, knobbly, hard liver is a feature.

Hepatic failure can be associated with severe systemic infection (e.g. septicaemia and pneumonia), and after surgery in critically ill patients. A patient

Table 58.2 Jaundice (adults): diagnostic strategy model

Probability diagnosis
Hepatitis A, B, C (mainly B, C)
Gallstones in common bile duct
Alcoholic hepatitis/cirrhosis
Serious disorders not to be missed
Malignancy:
• pancreas
• biliary tract
• hepatocellular (hepatoma)
• metastases
Severe infections:
• septicaemia
• ascending cholangitis
• fulminant hepatitis
• HIV/AIDS
Rarities:
• Wilson disease
• Reye syndrome
• acute fatty liver of pregnancy
Pitfalls (often missed)
Gallstones
Gilbert syndrome
Cardiac failure
Primary biliary cirrhosis
Autoimmune chronic active hepatitis
Primary sclerosing cholangitis
Chronic viral hepatitis
Haemochromatosis
Viral infections (e.g. CMV, EBV)
Leptospirosis
Seven masquerades checklist
Drugs (e.g. flucloxacillin)
Anaemia
Is the patient trying to tell me something?
Not usually applicable.

who has the classic Charcot triad of upper abdominal pain, fever (and chills) and jaundice should be regarded as having ascending cholangitis until proved otherwise. Wilson syndrome, although rare, must be considered in all young patients with acute hepatitis. A history of neurological symptoms, such as a tremor or a clumsy gait, and a family history is important. If Wilson disease is suspected, an ocular slit lamp examination, serum ceruloplasmin levels (low in 95% of patients) and a liver biopsy should be performed. Early diagnosis and treatment mean a better prognosis.

Reye syndrome is a rare and severe complication of influenza and some other viral diseases, especially in children when given aspirin. There is rapid development of hepatic failure and encephalopathy.

Pitfalls

Gallstones, especially in the absence of upper abdominal pain, can be overlooked, so this possibility should be kept in mind in the elderly.

Gilbert syndrome is worth considering, especially as it is the commonest form of unconjugated hyperbilirubinaemia. It affects at least 3% of the population.

Cardiac failure can present as jaundice with widespread tenderness under the right costal margin. It can be insidious in onset or manifest with gross acute failure. It can be confused with acute cholecystitis. The biochemical abnormalities seen are very variable. Usually there is a moderate rise in bilirubin and alkaline phosphatase and sometimes, in acute failure, a marked elevation of transaminase may occur, suggesting some hepatocellular necrosis.

There are many other pitfalls for a family doctor, who may encounter the conditions very rarely, if at all. Such disorders include:

- inherited conjugated hyperbilirubinaemias (Dubin–Johnson and Rotor syndromes) caused by faulty excretion by liver cells
- haemochromatosis (associated pigmentation and diabetes)
- chronic active hepatitis
- primary biliary cirrhosis
- primary sclerosing cholangitis (associated with ulcerative colitis)

General pitfalls

- Excluding jaundice by examining the sclera in artificial light
- Not realising that the sclera in elderly patients often have an icteric appearance (without jaundice)
- Omitting to take a careful history, including illicit drugs
- A liver biopsy is essential in all patients with chronic hepatitis

Seven masquerades checklist

Of this group the haemolytic anaemias and drugs have to be considered.

Drug-related jaundice

Drug-induced jaundice is common and many drugs are implicated. The patterns of drug-related liver damage include cholestasis, necrosis ('hepatitis'), granulomas, chronic active hepatitis, cirrhosis, hepatocellular tumours and veno-occlusive disease.[4,5] Some drugs, such as methyldopa, can initiate haemolysis.

The important drugs to consider are presented in TABLE 58.3. Antibiotics, especially flucloxacillin, amoxycillin + clavulanate and erythromycin, are commonly implicated.

Table 58.3 Drugs that can cause jaundice

Haemolysis
Methyldopa
Hepatocellular damage
Dose-dependent:
• paracetamol (can cause acute hepatic necrosis)
• salicylates
• tetracycline
Dose-independent:
• anaesthetics (e.g. halothane)
• antidepressants (e.g. MAOIs, duloxetine)
• anti-epileptics (e.g. phenytoin, sodium valproate, carbamazepine)
• antibiotics (a long list, e.g. penicillins, sulphonamides)
• antimalarials (e.g. Fansidar)
• antiretrovirals (e.g. efavirenz, nevirapine)
• antituberculosis (e.g. isoniazid)
• anti-inflammatories (e.g. NSAIDS, various)
• carbon tetrachloride
• cardiovascular (e.g. amiodarone, methyldopa, hydralazine, perhexiline)
• statins (e.g. simvastatin)
Cholestasis
Antithyroid drugs
Chlorpromazine
Erythromycin estolate
Penicillins, esp. flucloxacillin
Gold salts
Oral contraceptives/oestrogens
Synthetic anabolic steroids (e.g. methyltestosterone)
Hypoglycaemic drugs (e.g. chlorpropamide)
Amitriptyline
Others
Allopurinol
Cimetidine (aggravated by alcohol)
DMARDs (e.g. methotrexate, azathioprine, ipilimumab)
Immunomodulators (e.g. interferon, TNF-alpha I)
Etretinate
Nitrofurantoin
Illicit drugs e.g. MDMA/ecstasy, cocaine
Vitamin A (mega dosage)
Various complementary medicines (e.g. herbal agents)

Haemolysis

The patient may present with the symptoms of underlying anaemia and jaundice with no noticeable change in the appearance of the urine and stool. The degree of haemolysis may vary from the lemon-yellow tinge of pernicious anaemia in an elderly patient to a severe haemolytic crisis precipitated by drugs or broad beans (favism) in a patient with an inherited red cell deficiency of glucose-6-phosphate dehydrogenase (G6PD). More common causes include the hereditary haemolytic anaemias, such as congenital spherocytosis and thalassaemia major. Acquired causes include incompatible blood transfusions, malignancies (such as lymphoma), severe sepsis and some drugs.

Splenomegaly occurs in most patients with haemolytic anaemia, and decreased red cell survival can be measured.

Psychogenic considerations

This is not really applicable for an organic problem such as jaundice. Nevertheless, the cause may be related to factors in the patient's lifestyle, such as homosexuality, sexual promiscuity or intravenous drug abuse, and the patient may be reluctant to offer this information. Discreet, concerned probing will be necessary.

Red flag pointers for jaundice

- Unexplained weight loss
- Progressive jaundice including painless jaundice
- Oedema
- Cerebral dysfunction (e.g. confusion, somnolence)

The clinical approach

History

The history should include questioning about the following:

- any episodes of jaundice
- change in colour of faeces and urine
- anorexia, sore throat, weight loss, pruritus
- abdominal pain
- residence and members of household
- contact with patients with hepatitis or jaundice
- recent overseas travel
- exposure to blood or blood products
- needle-stick injuries or exposure to needles, such as acupuncture, tattooing and intravenous drugs
- dietary history—shellfish, drinking water
- sexual history—evidence of promiscuity
- drug history, including alcohol, paracetamol

- recent medical history, including surgery
- family history—family contacts who have had jaundice, haemolytic disease and other genetic liver diseases
- ethnic history—liable to haemolytic disease, contact with hepatitis B
- occupational history—exposure to hazards

Significance of various symptoms

- Pain in the right hypochondrium:
  - gallstones
  - acute hepatitis (a constant ache)
  - cholecystitis
- Anorexia, dark urine, fever:
  - viral hepatitis probable
  - alcoholic liver disease possible
  - drug-induced hepatitis possible
- Pruritus:
  - cholestasis probable
  - possible with all liver diseases
- Arthralgia, rash:
  - viral hepatitis
  - autoimmune hepatitis

Examination

The abdominal examination is very important. The liver should be palpated carefully for enlargement, consistency and tenderness under the right costal margin. Search for enlargement of the gall bladder and the spleen. The gall bladder lies in the transpyloric line. A palpable gall bladder indicates extrahepatic biliary obstruction, and splenomegaly may indicate haemolytic anaemia, portal hypertension or viral hepatitis. Test for ascites.

Skin excoriation may indicate pruritus, which is associated with cholestatic jaundice. Look for evidence of chronic liver disease, such as palmar erythema, easy bruising, spider naevi and muscle wasting, and testicular atrophy and gynaecomastia. Test for hepatic flap (asterixis) and fetor, which indicate liver failure. Search for lymphadenopathy, which may be indicative of malignancy.

The examination should include dipstick urine testing for bilirubin and urobilinogen.

A summary of the possible findings is presented in FIGURE 58.2.

Investigations

The main investigations are FBE and the standard LFTs and viral serology for the infective causes, particularly hepatitis A, B and C virus (also EBV and CMV).

A summary of the general findings for liver function tests is shown in TABLE 58.4. Consideration should be given to ordering fractionalisation of bilirubin to determine whether it is conjugated or unconjugated (important in diagnosis of Gilbert syndrome).

Diagnostic markers for hepatitis

- Hepatitis A: IgM antibody (HAV Ab)
- Hepatitis B: surface antigen (HBsAg)
- Hepatitis C: HCV antibody (HCV Ab)

Hepatobiliary imaging

Tests to identify causes such as malignancy or gallstones are now sophisticated and should be chosen with care.

- X-ray: a plain abdominal X-ray shows up to 15–20% of opaque gallstones
- Transabdominal ultrasound (US): the most useful investigation for detecting gallstones and

Table 58.4 Characteristic liver function tests for selected types of liver disease

Liver function tests (serological)	Hepatocellular (viral) hepatitis	Haemolytic jaundice	Obstruction	Gilbert syndrome	Liver metastases/ abscess	Alcoholic liver disease
Bilirubin	↑ to ↑↑↑	↑ unconjugated	↑ to ↑↑↑	↑ up to 50 unconjugated	↑ to N	↑ to N
Alkaline phosphatase	↑ <2N	N	↑↑↑ >2N	N	↑↑ to ↑↑↑	↑
Alanine transferase (ALT)	↑↑↑ >5N	N	N or ↑	N	↑	↑
Gamma glutamyl transferase	N or ↑	N	↑↑	N	↑	↑↑↑
Albumin	N or ↓	N	N	N	N to ↓	N to ↓↓
Globulin	N or ↑	N	N	N	N	N to ↑

N: is within normal limits

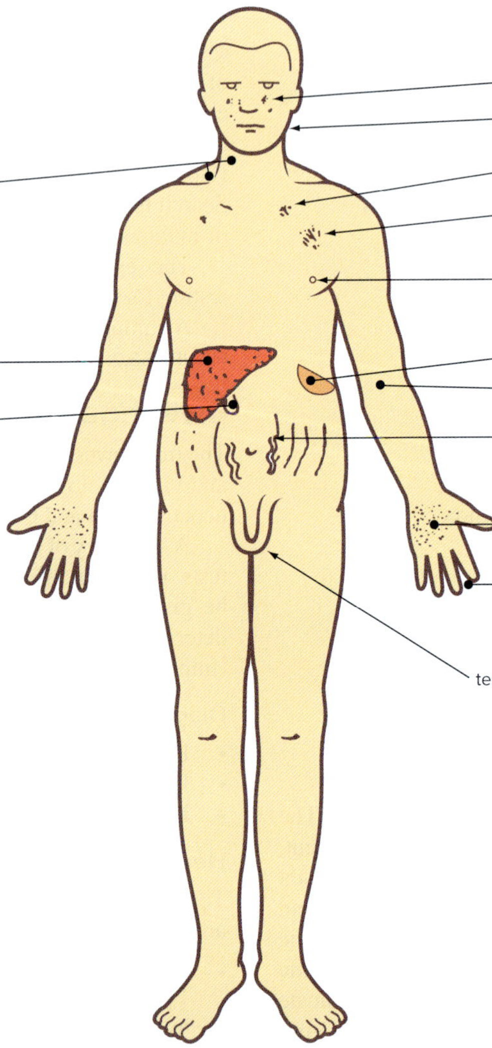

FIGURE 58.2 Possible findings on examining the jaundiced patient

dilatation of the common bile duct; also detects liver metastases and other diffuse liver diseases

- HIDA scintiscan: useful in diagnosis of acute cholecystitis
- CT scan: for diagnosis of enlargement of the head of the pancreas and other pathology; indicated if US unsatisfactory
- PTC: percutaneous transhepatic cholangiography: shows imaging of biliary tree
- ERCP: endoscopic retrograde cholangiopancreatography; PTC and ERCP (best) determine the cause of the obstruction and relieves it by sphincterotomy and removal of CBD stones
- MRCP: magnetic resonance cholangiography provides non-invasive planning for obstructive jaundice
- Liver isotopic scan: useful for liver cirrhosis, especially of the left lobe
- Fibroscan (transient elastography) to measure liver fibrosis

Specific tests

Some specific tests include:

- auto-antibodies for autoimmune chronic active hepatitis and primary biliary cirrhosis
- carcinoembryonic antigen to detect liver secondaries, especially colorectal
- serum iron studies, especially transferrin saturation—elevated in haemochromatosis
- alpha-fetoprotein—elevated in hepatocellular carcinoma; mild elevation with acute or chronic liver disease (e.g. cirrhosis)

- serum ceruloplasmin level—low in Wilson disease
- liver biopsy
- EBV/cytomegalovirus serology (consider if hepatitis serology negative)

Jaundice in children

JAUNDICE IN THE INFANT

Jaundice in the newborn is clinically apparent in 50% of term babies and more than 80% of preterm.[6] Icterus is therefore common and invariably physiologically benign. However, it is a cause for concern as there are many other causes and investigation is needed to determine whether the bilirubin is conjugated (always pathological) or unconjugated. If conjugated, consider the serious biliary atresia (stools are white); also a cyst obstructing the bile duct or neonatal hepatitis. Prompt referral is essential.

Jaundice occurring in the first 24 hours after birth is not due to immature liver function but is pathological and usually due to haemolysis consequent on blood group incompatibility. In primigravidas it is usually due to ABO incompatibility. Causes of pathological jaundice are presented in TABLE 58.5 Such causes demand referral.

Table 58.5 Pathological neonatal jaundice: diagnostic strategy model (brief)

Probability diagnosis
Physiological: day 2–5
ABO incompatibility: first 24 hours
Breast milk jaundice: late first week
Serious disorders not to be missed
ABOI: first 24 hours
Biliary atresia (conjugated)
Haemolysis: ABOI, G-6-DPD
Sepsis
Seven masquerades checklist
Drugs
Hypothyroidism
Hereditary spherocytosis, other inherited disorders
Polycythemia

Bilirubin encephalopathy

Unconjugated bilirubin can be regarded as a neurological poison. With increasing serum levels an encephalopathy (which may be transient) can develop, but if persistent can lead to the irreversible brain damage known as kernicterus. The level of bilirubin causing kernicterus is totally unpredictable, but a guideline as a cause for concern in babies with Rh disease is a serum unconjugated bilirubin of 340 μmol/L (20 mg/dL).

Guidelines for treatment for hyperbilirubinaemia (at 24–36 hours)—an example:

- >285 μmol/L—phototherapy
- >360 μmol/L—consider exchange transfusion

An example of a normogram is presented in FIGURE 58.3.

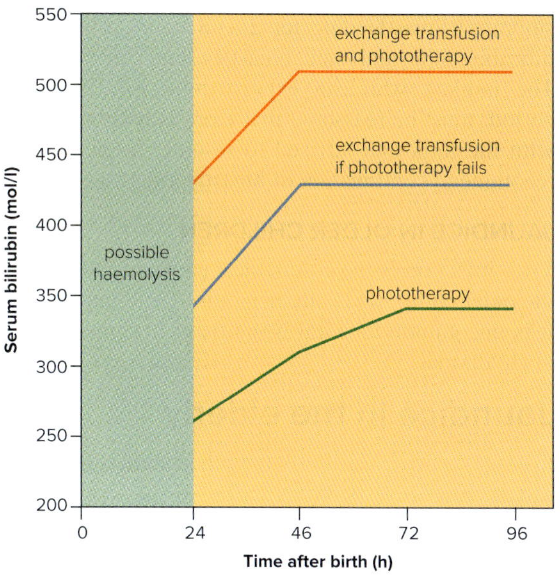

FIGURE 58.3 Typical normogram for decision making in healthy infants with jaundice

Physiological jaundice

This mild form of jaundice, which is very common in infants, is really a diagnosis of exclusion. In a term infant the serum bilirubin rises quickly after birth to reach a maximum by day 3–5, then declines rapidly over the next 2–3 days before fading more slowly for the next 1–2 weeks. Management includes phototherapy.

ABO blood group incompatibility

This is antibody-mediated haemolysis (Coomb test positive):

- Mother is O
- Child is A or B

Jaundice develops within first 24 hours.

Treatment

- Perform a direct Coomb test on infant.
- Phototherapy is required immediately.
- These children require follow-up developmental assessment including audiometry.

Breast milk jaundice

If the secondary causes of prolonged jaundice are excluded, the baby is well and breastfeeding, the likely cause of unconjugated elevated bilirubin is breast milk jaundice. It occurs in 2–4% of breastfed infants. It usually begins late in the first week and peaks at 2–3 weeks. Diagnosis is confirmed by suspending (not stopping) breastfeeding for 24–48 hours. The serum bilirubin falls and then breastfeeding can continue. The mother, who can express milk for this short period, must be reassured that there is nothing wrong with the milk and advised to resume. Some doctors recommend continuation of breastfeeding.

JAUNDICE IN OLDER CHILDREN

Viral infection is the commonest cause of jaundice in the older child, especially hepatitis A and hepatitis B. It is uncommon for viral hepatitis to become chronic in childhood.

Jaundice in the elderly

If an elderly person presents with jaundice the usual causes and investigations have to be considered. Obstructive jaundice is the commonest form of jaundice in the elderly and may be caused by gallstones blocking the common bile duct (may be painless) and carcinoma of the head of the pancreas, the biliary tract itself, the stomach or multiple secondaries for other sites. While it is not uncommon for a gallstone to produce marked obstructive jaundice and yet be painless, it is appropriate to adhere to the old adage that painless obstructive jaundice is due to neoplasm—particularly if the gall bladder is palpable (Courvoisier's law).

Alcoholic liver disease, although most frequently affecting patients between 40 and 60 years, can present for the first time over age 60 years. The commonest cause of hepatocellular jaundice in the elderly is probably alcoholic cirrhosis; hepatitis A is still relatively uncommon in old persons.

Drugs do not cause jaundice in the elderly as frequently as they once did, particularly as phenothiazines, especially chlorpromazine, are not prescribed as often as previously. However, drugs should be considered as a potential cause and a careful check of the drug history is important.

Infective causes of jaundice

A generation ago hepatitis A (infectious hepatitis or yellow jaundice) was the commonest recognised form of viral hepatitis, presenting usually with an abrupt onset of fever, anorexia, nausea and vomiting. It usually occurred in epidemics and hence was common in overcrowded institutions and camps. Now hepatitis B and C are the most commonly reported types of viral hepatitis with an onset that is more insidious and with a longer incubation period.[4,7] Symptoms include malaise, anorexia, nausea and polyarthritis. Acute hepatitis C is often subclinical.

The various forms of hepatitis are summarised in TABLE 58.6. All forms of hepatitis are common in developing countries and travellers are at risk of contracting these infections: hepatitis A and E from faeco-oral transmission; and hepatitis B, C, D and G from intravenous drugs and bodily fluids (from sexual transmission, in particular, for hepatitis B).

Evidence points to more viruses causing non-ABC hepatitis.[8] Hepatitis F virus has been claimed to be transmitted enterically while the newly designated hepatitis G virus (HGV) is transmitted parenterally. It does not appear to cause a severe illness in recipients. It can be predicted that the hepatitis alphabet will continue to expand.

In hepatitis A, liver damage is directly due to the virus, but in hepatitis B and C it is due to an immunologic reaction to the virus.

Other infections that can present with jaundice as part of a systemic disease are malaria, Epstein–Barr mononucleosis, cytomegalovirus, Q fever, toxoplasmosis, leptospirosis and, rarely, measles, varicella, yellow fever, rubella, herpes simplex, dengue fever, Lassa fever and Marburg and Ebola virus.

Hepatitis A

Hepatitis A is becoming relatively less prevalent in developed countries. It is enterically transmitted and arises from the ingestion of contaminated food, such as shellfish, or water. There is no carrier state and it does not cause chronic liver disease. Hepatitis A most often causes a subclinical or self-limited clinical illness.

Clinical features

Pre-icteric (prodromal) phase:

- anorexia, nausea ± vomiting
- malaise
- headache
- distaste for cigarettes in smokers

Table 58.6 Characteristic profiles of viral hepatitis A–E

Characteristic	Hepatitis A	Hepatitis B	Hepatitis C	Hepatitis D	Hepatitis E
Pseudonyms	Infectious hepatitis	Serum hepatitis	Parenterally transmitted non-A, non-B	Delta hepatitis	Enterically transmitted non-A, non-B
Agent (virus)	27 nm RNA	42 nm DNA	50 nm RNA	35 nm RNA	30 nm RNA
Transmission	Faecal–oral Contaminated water/food	Blood and other body fluids Mother to child	Infected blood ? Other body fluids	Blood and other body fluids	Faecal–oral Contaminated water/food
Incubation period	15–45 days	40–180 days	14–180 days	30–50 days	15–45 days
Severity of acute illness	Mild to moderate; often subclinical—no jaundice	Mild to severe; jaundice common; arthralgia and rash common	Mild to moderate; often subclinical	Moderate to severe; high mortality; usually jaundice	Mild to moderate; often subclinical
Chronic liver disease	No	Yes 10–15%	Yes 65–80%	Yes Potentially worst	No
Carrier state	No	Yes	Yes	Yes	No
Risk in travellers	Yes, applies to all A–E: East and South-East Asia, Asian subcontinent (e.g. India), South Pacific Islands (e.g. Fiji), sub-Saharan Africa, Mexico, Russia, other developing countries. A and E with poor sanitation; B, C, D also with IV drug use; B, D sexual contact.				
Antigens	HAV Ag	HBsAg, HBcAg, HBeAg	HCV Ag	HDV Ag	HEV Ag
Diagnosis—antibodies	anti-HAV	HBsAg anti-HBc anti-HBs	anti-HCV	anti-HDV	anti-HEV
Vaccine	Hepatitis A vaccine	Hepatitis B vaccine	None	Hepatitis B vaccine	None

- mild fever
- ± diarrhoea
- ± upper abdominal discomfort

Icteric phase (many patients do not develop jaundice):

- dark urine
- pale stools
- hepatomegaly
- splenomegaly (palpable in 10%)

Recovery usually in 3–6 weeks.

Fulminant hepatitis with liver coma and death may occur but is rare.

Investigations

LFTs and viral markers confirm the diagnosis. The antibodies to HAV are IgM, which indicates active infection, and IgG antibodies, which means past infection and lifelong immunity and which is common in the general population. Ultrasound is useful to exclude bile duct obstruction, especially in an older patient.

Outcome and treatment

Hepatitis A has an excellent prognosis with most patients making a complete recovery, and patients should be reassured. The mortality is less than 0.5%. Admission to hospital is not usually necessary. There is no specific treatment, so management is as follows.

- Provide appropriate reassurance and patient education.
- Rest as appropriate.
- Follow a fat-free diet.
- Avoid alcohol, smoking and hepatotoxic drugs (until recovery).
- Advise on hygiene at home to prevent spread to close contacts and family members. Recent evidence indicates that it can be spread sexually and by IV drugs.

- Wash hands carefully after using the toilet and disinfect them with antiseptic.
- Do not handle food for others with your fingers.
- Do not share cutlery and crockery during meals.
- Do not use tea-towels to dry dishes.

Prevention

Simple health measures such as good sanitation, effective garbage disposal and hand washing are probably responsible for the major decrease in the disease. Immune serum globulin (0.03–0.06 mL/kg IM) confers satisfactory passive immunity for close contacts (within 2 weeks of contact) and for travellers to endemic areas for up to 3 months. An active vaccine consisting of a two-dose primary course is the best means of prevention.

Hepatitis B

Hepatitis B has protean clinical manifestations. Transmission is by blood spread, percutaneous, sexual transmission, perinatal spread or by close prolonged family contact. Infection may be subclinical or self-limited acute hepatitis. Fulminant hepatitis is rare. Five per cent of subjects go on to become chronic carriers of the virus. Most are 'healthy carriers' but some may develop chronic active hepatitis, cirrhosis and hepatoma. The serology of hepatitis B involves antibody responses to the four main antigens of the virus (core, DNA polymerase, protein X and surface antigens). Passive and active vaccines are available, and should be used freely in groups at risk, including babies of infected mothers. High-risk groups are presented in TABLE 58.7. The clinical features are the same as those found in hepatitis A infection but may be less abrupt in onset but more severe in the long term.[7] A serum sickness-like immunological syndrome may be seen with transient rashes (e.g. urticaria or a maculopapular rash), and polyarthritis affecting small joints in up to 25% of cases in the prodromal period.

Investigations[5,9,10]

The main viral investigation for HBV is HBsAg (surface antigen), which is searched for routinely. If detected, indicating hepatitis B positive or carrier, a full viral profile is then formed.

HBsAg may disappear or persist. Its presence indicates a current or chronic infection as well as a carrier state (see FIG. 58.4). Chronic hepatitis B (carriage) is defined as the presence of HBsAg for at least 6 months.

Table 58.7 Higher-risk groups for contracting hepatitis B (vaccination advisable)[7]

Babies born to hepatitis B positive (carrier) mothers
Garbage collectors
Health care workers
Household contacts of hepatitis B carriers
Institutionalised intellectually disabled patients
Intravenous drug users
Kidney dialysis patients
Male homosexuals
Prisoners
Recipients of blood or blood products (prior to testing)
Sex industry workers
Sexual partners of hepatitis B carriers (especially acute HBV)
Travellers to endemic areas

HBeAg is a soluble protein from the pre-core and core. Antibodies develop to both HBsAg and HBeAg.

Serological patterns

Acute hepatitis B
HBsAg +ve, anti-HBcIgM +ve, anti-HBs –ve
Chronic hepatitis B
HBsAg +ve, anti-HBcIgG +ve, anti-HBs –ve
Resolved hepatitis B
HBsAg –ve, anti-HBcIgG +ve, anti-HBs +ve

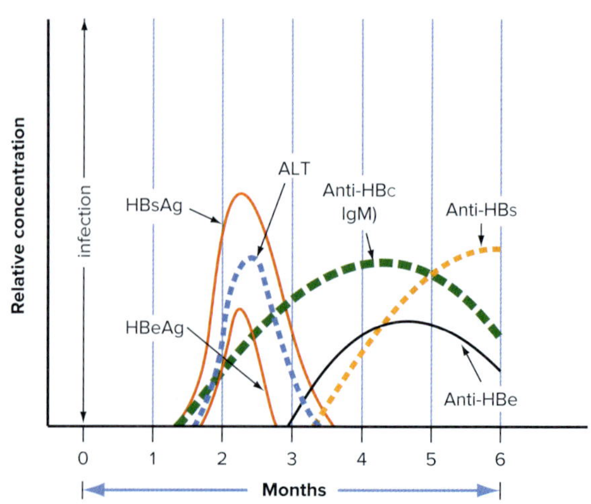

FIGURE 58.4 Time course of acute hepatitis B infection

Monitoring and outcome[9,10]

The possible course of events is shown in FIGURE 58.5. The majority of patients recover completely with the outcome depending on several factors, including the virulence of the virus and the immune state and age of the patient. Some will develop chronic hepatitis, some will develop a fulminant course, and others will become asymptomatic carriers and present a health risk to others.

Monitor progress with 6–12 monthly LFTs, HBeAg and HBV DNA.

- Negative HBsAg and HBV DNA (with anti-HBe) = resolving, with anti-HBs = full recovery.
- Positive HBsAg and HBV DNA = replicating and infective—refer.
- Monitor LFTs every 6 months. Refer if ALT elevated.

Treatment[5]

There is no specific treatment initially—being similar to hepatitis A, appropriate reassurance and patient education are necessary. Advise avoidance of alcohol. Avoid certain drugs, e.g. sedatives, NSAIDs, OCP, until recovery (normal LFTs). Advise about prevention of transmission, especially safe sex and sharing needles. Refer to a liver transplantation centre if encephalopathy or severe coagulopathy develop. Treatment of chronic hepatitis B infection (abnormal LFTs) is with the immunomodulatory and antiviral agents—pegylated interferon alpha and entecavir, tenofovir or other agents. This is expensive but it achieves permanent remission in 25% of patients, and temporary remission in a further 25%.[7] Liver transplantation has been performed, but is often followed by recurrence of hepatitis B in the grafted liver. Follow up with regular LFTs and alpha-fetoprotein screening. It is appropriate to refer any HBsAg positive patient with an abnormal ALT and/or signs of chronic liver disease to a specialist since the evaluation of chronic hepatitis B can be complex.[4]

Serology guidelines

HBsAg = acute or persistent infection
anti-HBs = past infection and immunity
HBeAg = highly infectious
HBV DNA = circulating and replicating virus
anti-HBc IgM = recent and continuing infection
anti-HBc IgG = past infection
anti-HBe = seroconversion

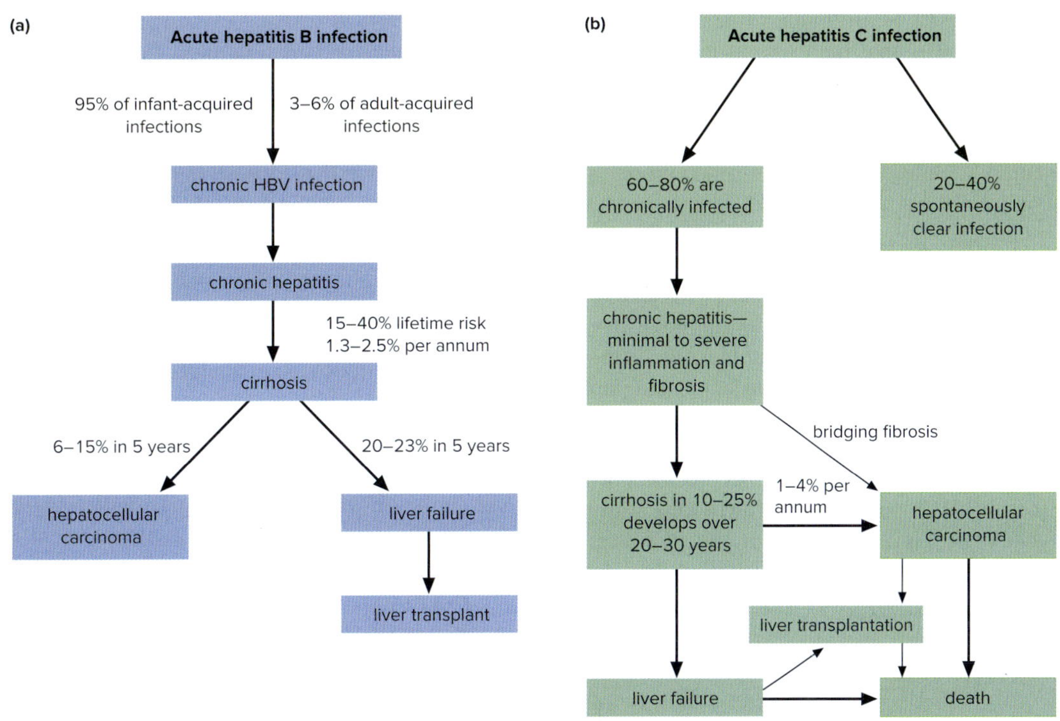

FIGURE 58.5 Natural history of **(a)** hepatitis B infection; **(b)** hepatitis C infection

Source: W Sievert, B Katz, Department of Gastroenterology, Monash Medical Centre

58

Prevention

Active immunisation through hepatitis B vaccination has been a major breakthrough in the management of this serious illness. There is a course of three injections. If there is a negative antibody response after 3 months, revaccinate with a double dose. If the response is positive, consider a test in 5 years with a view to a booster injection.

For non-immune patients at risk (e.g. after a needle-stick injury), hepatitis B immunoglobin (HBIg), which contains a high level of HBV surface antibody, is appropriate.

Prenatal screening of pregnant women and appropriate use of HBIg and HB vaccine is useful in preventing perinatal vertical transmission of HBV.

Hepatitis C[5,9,11,12]

Hepatitis C virus is responsible for most cases of viral hepatitis in Australia. It is primarily contracted from intravenous drug use or tattooing. It does not seem to be spread very readily by sexual contact although there is a small risk during heterosexual and homosexual intercourse. It is also not readily spread perinatally.

Clinical symptoms of hepatitis C are usually minimal (often asymptomatic), and the diagnosis is often made after LFTs are found to be abnormal. An important feature is that there are at least six major genotypes of HCV and treatment decisions are based on the genotype; thus, patients with acute hepatitis C should have HCV genotype testing.

Hepatitis C infection may be self-limiting, but more commonly (in about 70% of cases) causes a slow, relentless progression to chronic hepatitis, cirrhosis (20%) and also hepatoma.[7] See FIGURE 58.6. The severity of hepatic fibrosis can be assessed by liver biopsy or, preferably, by a non-invasive device called a FibroScan that assesses 'hardness or stiffness' of the liver via the technique of transient elastography. A raised ALT level that is tested three times over the next 6 months implies disease activity. HCV RNA (a PCR test) is present when the ALT becomes abnormal while the anti-HCV rises more slowly and may not be detectable for several weeks. If the PCR test is negative, the hepatitis C infection has resolved.

Diagnosis and progress

This is by serology:

- HCV Ab (anti-HCV) +ve = exposure (current or past)
- HCV-RNA +ve = chronic viraemia
  −ve = spontaneous clearance

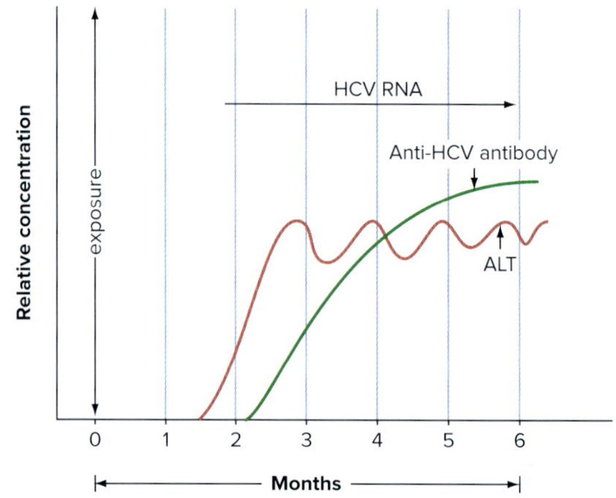

FIGURE 58.6 Time course of active hepatitis C infection

- CD_4/HCV = viral load
- ALTs on LFTs indicate disease activity (tested 3 times over next 6 months)
  ALT persistently normal = good prognosis
  ALT ↑ ↑ = requires referral for treatment
- If PCR +ve + significant viral load + ALT ↑ perform HCV genotype—determines treatment
- PCR −ve, ALT −ve = infection clear

Treatment[5,12]

The current standard treatment for chronic hepatitis C is direct-acting antivirals (DAAs) taken daily by mouth. These agents are now supplanting interferon-based therapy. The determination of genotype and viral load, as well as hepatic status, will identify those most likely to respond to therapy.

Examples of DAAs are:

- protease inhibitors, e.g. simeprevir
- nucleotide polymerase inhibitors, e.g. sofosbuvir
- non-nucleotide inhibitors, e.g. dasabuvir
- NS5A inhibitors, e.g. daclatasvir, ledipasvir

These agents are given in combination according to the genotype. Cure rates are in the order of 95%. Treatment can be managed within general practice, in collaboration with a specialist gastroenterologist.[13]

The recommended steps for pretreatment assessment are:[13,14]

1. Confirm the diagnosis of chronic HCV infection.
2. Test for hepatitis C virus genotype and viral load.
3. Document the HCV treatment history.
4. Evaluate comorbidity and liver status, especially cirrhosis (refer if present), FBE, APRI, LFTs, blood glucose, creatinine U and E, HIV, HBV.
5. Discuss contraception and pregnancy (if applicable).

6. Consider concomitant medication.
7. Assess adherence to treatment.
8. Select treatment regimen (8 or 12 weeks) and review potential drug interactions.
9. Consult with a specialist.
10. Treat and monitor.

Cure is defined as undetectable plasma HCV RNA at least 12 months after treatment.

Those at increased risk of having hepatitis B and C

- Blood transfusion recipients (prior to HBV and HCV testing)
- Intravenous drug users (past or present)
- MSM who have practised unsafe sex
- Kidney dialysis patients
- Sex industry workers
- Those with abnormal LFTs with no obvious cause
- Tattooed people/body piercing

Prevention of transmission of hepatitis B and C viruses

Advice to those who are positive for HCV:

- Do not donate blood or any body organs or tissues.
- Do not share needles.
- Advise health care workers, including your dentist.
- Do not share intimate equipment such as toothbrushes, razors, nail files and nail scissors.
- Wipe up blood spills in the home with household bleach.
- Cover up cuts or wounds with an adequate dressing.
- Dispose of bloodstained tissues, sanitary napkins and other dressings safely.
- Use safe sex practices such as condoms.
- Avoid tattooing.

Hepatitis D

Hepatitis D is a small defective virus that lacks a surface coat. This is provided by hepatitis B virus, and so hepatitis D infection occurs only in patients with concomitant hepatitis B.

It is usually spread parenterally and if chronic is usually associated with progressive disease with a poor prognosis. Treatment with interferon has a variable success rate. Antibodies to the delta virus, both anti-HDV and anti-HDV IgM (indicating a recent infection) as well as HDV Ag can be measured.[15] Referral to a specialist is recommended.

Hepatitis E

Hepatitis E is an enterically transmitted virus that occurs in outbreaks in certain countries with a poor water supply, such as some Asian subcontinent countries. Epidemiologically, HEV behaves like HAV, with well-documented water-borne epidemics in areas of poor sanitation. There is a high case fatality rate in endemic areas (10–20%) and in pregnant females.

Hepatitis F

Researchers claim to have identified HGF virus, which is spread enterically.[16] Treatment can be comfortably managed within general practice.

Hepatitis G

HGV has been identified as a transfusion-spread virus. It has subsequently been found to be prevalent among Queensland blood donors.[10,17]

Cholestatic jaundice

Cholestasis refers to the syndrome of biliary obstructive jaundice whereby there is obstruction to the flow of bile from the hepatocyte to the duodenum, thus causing bilirubin to accumulate in the blood. It is classified into two main groups:

- intrahepatic cholestasis—at the hepatocyte or intrahepatic biliary tree level
- extrahepatic cholestasis—obstruction in the large bile ducts by stones or bile sludge

The significant causes are listed in TABLE 58.8.

Table 58.8 Significant causes of cholestasis in adults

Intrahepatic
Alcoholic hepatitis/cirrhosis
Drugs
Primary biliary cirrhosis
Viral hepatitis
Extrahepatic
Cancer of bile ducts
Cancer of pancreas
Other cancer: primary or secondary spread
Cholangitis
Primary sclerosing cholangitis (? autoimmune) IgG_4-related disease
Common bile duct gallstones
Pancreatitis
Post-surgical biliary stricture or oedema

58

Symptoms

- Jaundice (greenish tinge)
- Dark urine and pale stools
- Pruritus—worse on palms and soles
- Pain varies from nil to severe

Gallstones and jaundice

Gallstones can be found in the following (see FIG. 58.7):

- gall bladder (asymptomatic up to 75%)—the majority remain here
- neck of gall bladder (biliary 'colic' or acute cholecystitis)
- cystic duct (biliary 'colic' or acute cholecystitis)
- common bile duct—may cause severe biliary 'colic', cholestatic jaundice or cholangitis

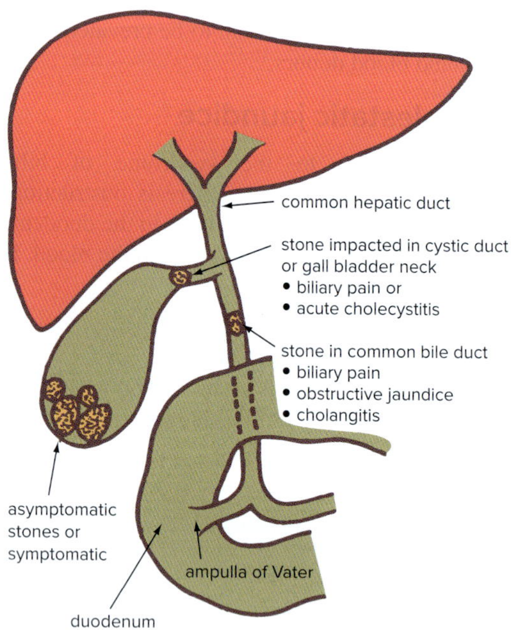

FIGURE 58.7 Clinical presentation of gallstones

Acute cholecystitis is accompanied by mild jaundice in 25% of cases, due to accompanying common duct stones.[15]

Common bile duct stones may be asymptomatic or may present with any one or all of the triad of abdominal pain, jaundice and fever. The jaundice varies, depending on the amount of obstruction. The liver is moderately enlarged if the obstruction lasts for more than a few hours.

The investigations of choice for cholestatic jaundice are ultrasound and ERCP.

Acute cholangitis

This is due to bacterial infection of the bile ducts secondary to abnormalities of the bile duct, especially gallstones in the common duct. Other causes are neoplasms and biliary strictures.

Charcot triad (present in 70%) is shown in the diagnosis box.

DxT fever (often with rigor) + upper abdominal pain + jaundice ➜ acute cholangitis

Older patients can present with circulatory collapse and Gram-negative septicaemia. Urgent referral is necessary.

Carcinoma of head of the pancreas

Pancreatic cancer is the fourth commonest cause of cancer death in the UK and US.[15]

Clinical features

- M > F
- Mainly >60 years of age
- Obstructive jaundice
- Pain (over 75%)—epigastric and back
- Enlarged gall bladder (50–75%)

Possible features

- Weight loss, malaise, diarrhoea
- Migratory thrombophlebitis
- Palpable hard, fixed mass
- Metastases (e.g. left supraclavicular gland of Virchow—Troisier sign)
- Occult blood in stool
- Glycosuria

Diagnosis

- Scanning by ultrasound or CT scan may show mass
- ERCP

DxT jaundice + constitutional symptoms (malaise, anorexia, weight loss) + epigastric pain (radiating to back) ➜ pancreatic cancer

Prognosis

Prognosis is very poor: 5-year survival is 5%.

Cirrhosis of the liver

Cirrhosis is accompanied by jaundice as a late and serious manifestation with the exception of primary biliary cirrhosis, where jaundice appears before advanced liver failure. The development of jaundice usually indicates that there is minimal hepatic reserve and is therefore found in conjunction with other signs of liver failure (see FIG. 58.8).

Causes

Common:

- alcohol excess
- chronic viral hepatitis (esp. HBV, HCV)

Others:

- autoimmune chronic active hepatitis
- primary biliary cirrhosis (autoimmune)
- haemochromatosis
- Wilson disease
- drugs (e.g. methotrexate)
- cryptogenic (no cause found)

Clinical features

- Anorexia, nausea ± vomiting
- Swelling of legs
- Abdominal distension
- Bleeding tendency
- Drowsiness, confusion or coma (if liver failure)

Signs

- Spider naevi (distribution of superior vena cava)
- Palmar erythema of hands
- Peripheral oedema and ascites
- Jaundice (obstructive or hepatocellular)
- Enlarged tender liver (small liver in long-term cirrhosis)
- Ascites
- Gynaecomastia
- ± Splenomegaly (portal hypertension)

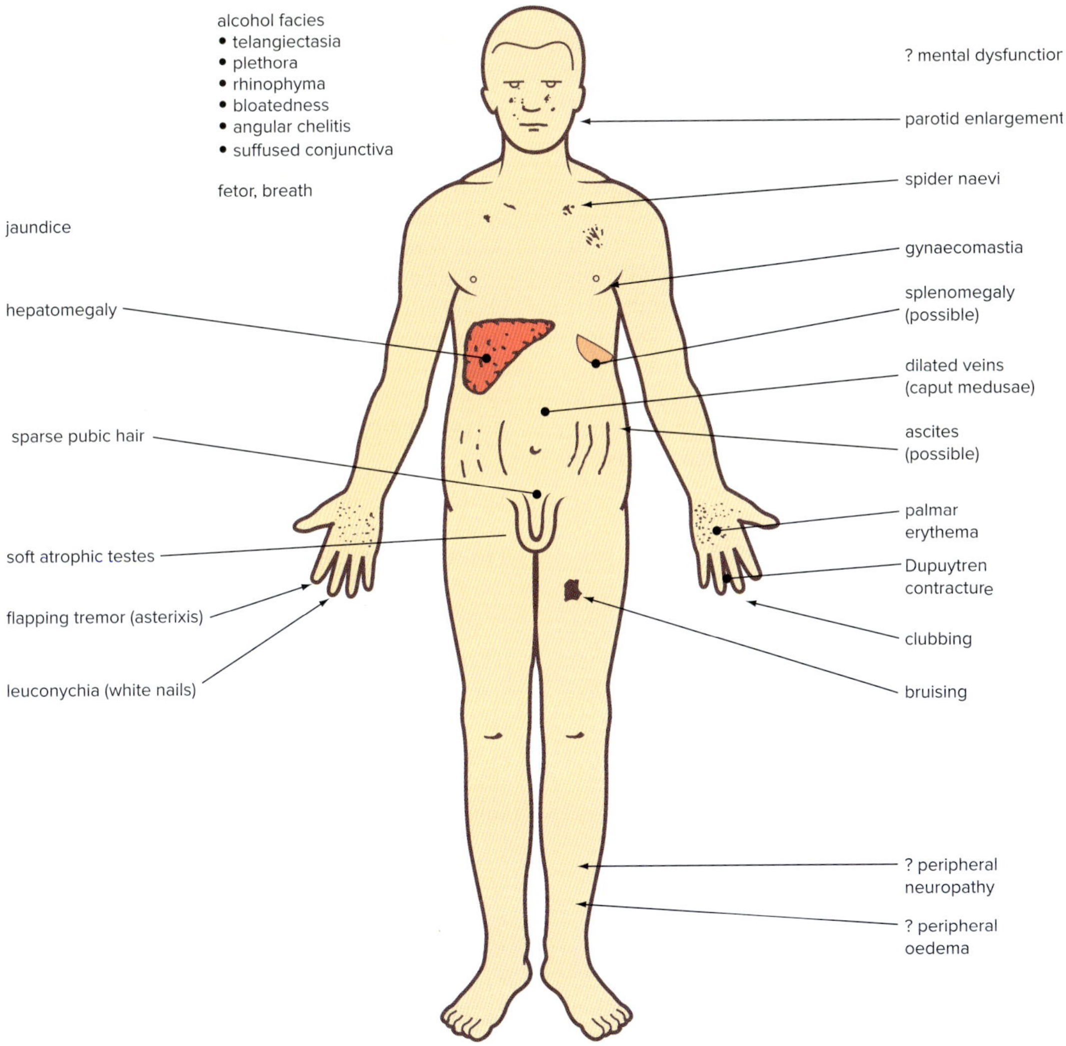

FIGURE 58.8 Possible features of chronic alcoholic liver disease

Complications

- Ascites
- Portal hypertension and GIT haemorrhage
- Portosystemic encephalopathy
- Hepatoma
- Kidney failure

Autoimmune chronic active hepatitis (ACAH)[5]

Also termed idiopathic ACAH, this usually affects young females (10–40 years) who present insidiously with progressive fatigue, anorexia and jaundice. Diagnosis is made by abnormal LFTs (which should raise suspicion), positive smooth muscle antibodies, a variety of other autoantibodies and a typical liver biopsy. If untreated, most patients die within 3–5 years. Treatment is with prednisolone orally, monitored according to serum alanine aminotransferase levels, and supplemented with azathioprine or mercaptopurine. About 80% respond, while 20% develop chronic liver disease. Specialist referral is advisable.

Primary sclerosing cholangitis[5]

This uncommon inflammatory disorder of the biliary tract presents with progressive jaundice and other features of cholestasis such as pruritus. It is often associated with ulcerative colitis. Diagnosis is based on characteristic cholangiopancreatography findings. There is no specific therapy, but refer for possible ERCP. Ursodeoxycholic acid may benefit some patients. Patients have an increased risk of colorectal cancer.

Primary biliary cirrhosis[5]

This is an uncommon cause of chronic liver disease that often presents with pruritis, malaise and an obstructive pattern of liver biochemistry. Found mainly in women. Treatment is with ursodeoxycholic acid orally.

Alcoholic liver disease

The main effects of alcohol excess on the liver are:

- acute alcoholic liver disease
- fatty liver
- alcoholic hepatitis (progresses to cirrhosis if alcohol consumption continues)
- alcoholic cirrhosis

If diagnosed, patients are advised to stop drinking alcohol for life except for fatty liver when small amounts can be drunk later.

Fatty liver

Alcohol can cause hepatic steatosis (fatty liver), which is almost universal in obese alcoholics. Non-alcoholic causes include obesity, diabetes mellitus, hypertriglyceridaemia and corticosteroids. A significant number with this very common condition (one in five Australians) will develop cirrhosis. Fatty liver is usually asymptomatic but some complain of malaise and tiredness. Serology is unhelpful. Diagnosis is by liver biopsy and perhaps CT scan. The treatment is weight loss through diet, which improves liver function and reduces fatty deposits.

Haemochromatosis

See CHAPTER 18.

Special patient groups

The returned overseas traveller

The overseas traveller presenting with jaundice may have been infected by any one of the viruses—hepatitis A, B, C, D or E. All are prevalent in developing countries, especially in south-eastern and eastern Asia, some Pacific islands and Africa.

Other causes to consider are malaria, ascending cholangitis and drug-induced hepatic damage due to, for example, the antimalarials, including mefloquine (Lariam) and Fansidar. Refer to CHAPTERS 14 and 15.

The pregnant patient

Important hepatic disorders in pregnancy leading to jaundice are intrahepatic cholestasis of pregnancy, acute fatty liver of pregnancy and severe pre-eclampsia. Delivery is advisable at 37–38 weeks.

Postoperative jaundice

There are many possible causes of postoperative jaundice either in the immediate or the long-term postoperative phase. Hypoxia associated with shock in a severely ill patient or in a patient with cardiopulmonary disease may lead to transient abnormalities in liver function. Other causes include:

- post-transfusion hepatitis
- coincident viral hepatitis
- drugs, including anaesthetics
- transfusion overload (haemolysis)
- sepsis
- unmasked chronic liver disease and biliary tract disease
- cholestasis: post major abdominal surgery

Neonates of HBeAg positive mothers

The neonates should have the following (see CHAPTER 109):

- hepatitis B immunoglobulin IM within 24 hours of birth
- hepatitis B vaccine at birth, 1 month and 6 months

This is not 100% effective because some infants can be infected in utero.

When to refer

- All patients with fulminant hepatitis
- All patients with chronic liver disease
- Painless obstructive jaundice
- Evidence of malignancy
- Symptomatic gallstones
- Patients with cirrhosis
- Acute fatty liver of pregnancy (very urgent)
- Suspected rare conditions (e.g. Wilson syndrome)

Practice tips

- All drugs should be suspected as potential hepatotoxins.
- With hepatitis A, the presence of IgM antibodies reflects recent infection, and IgG antibodies indicate past infection and lifelong immunity.
- There is no chronic carrier state of hepatitis A and E.
- All patients with jaundice should be tested for hepatitis B surface antigen (HBsAg).
- Hepatitis B infection is usually benign and short-lived, but it can be fatal if chronic hepatitis develops, which may lead later to cirrhosis and hepatocellular carcinoma.
- Up to 5% of patients with hepatitis B will become chronic carriers (especially drug addicts).
- Such carriers are identified by persistent titres of HBsAg and possibly HBeAg, the latter indicating the presence of the whole virus, and active replication and high infectivity.
- A raised gamma glutamyl transferase accompanied by a raised MCV is a good screening test for alcohol abuse.
- A systolic murmur may be heard over the liver in alcoholic hepatitis and hepatoma.
- A distaste for smoking (with jaundice) suggests acute viral hepatitis.

Patient education resources

Hand-out sheets from *Murtagh's Patient Education* 7th edition:

- Gallstones
- Hepatitis A
- Hepatitis B
- Hepatitis C

References

1. Kincaid-Smith R, Larkins R, Whelan G. *Problems in Clinical Medicine.* Sydney: McLennan & Petty, 1989: 251.
2. Coffman D, Chalstrey J, Smith-Laing G. *Gastrointestinal Disorders.* Edinburgh: Churchill Livingstone, 1986: 106.
3. Sandler G, Fry J. *Early Clinical Diagnosis.* Lancaster: MTP Press, 1986: 468–90.
4. Croagh C, Desmond D. Viral hepatitis: an A, B, C guide. Medicine Today, 2007; 8 (7): 47–56.
5. Expert group for Gastrointestinal. Viral hepatitis. In: eTG complete [Internet]. Melbourne: Therapeutic Guidelines Ltd. Available from: <www.tg.org.au>, accessed October 2017.
6. Gwee A, Rimer R, Marks M. *Paediatric Handbook* (9th edn). Melbourne: Blackwell Science, 2015: 335–6.
7. Ruff TA, Gust I. Hepatitis, viral (acute and chronic). In: *MIMS Disease Index* (2nd edn). Sydney: IMS Publishing, 1996: 226–30.
8. Bowden DS, Moaven LD, Locarnini SA. New hepatitis viruses: are there enough letters in the alphabet? Med J Aust, 1996; 164: 87–9.
9. Cossart Y. Recent advances in diagnosis and management of viral hepatitis. Common sense pathology. RCPA + Australian Doctor, 2006: 2–8.
10. McCaughan G, Levy M. Hepatitis B infection: how to treat. Australian Doctor, 16 January 2004: 28–32.
11. Singal DK, George J. Chronic hepatitis C. Australian Doctor, 15 February 2001: i–viii.
12. Mahady S, George J. Hepatitis C infection. Australian Doctor, 5 February 2010: 19–26.
13. Baker D. Curing hepatitis C in general practice. A 12-step guide. Medicine Today, 2016; 17 (10): 14–22.
14. Strasser S. Managing hepatitis C in general practice. Aust Prescr, 2017; 40: 64–9.
15. McPhee SJ, Papadakis MA et al. *Current Medical Diagnosis and Treatment* (49th edn). New York: The McGraw-Hill Companies, 2010: 636.
16. Deka N, Sharma MD, Mukerjee R. Isolation of the novel agent from human stool that is associated with sporadic human hepatitis. J Virol, 1994; 68: 7810–15.
17. Moaven LD et al. Prevalence of hepatitis G virus in Queensland blood donors. Med J Aust, 1996; 165: 369–71.

59 Nasal disorders

The face of Mrs Gamp—the nose in particular—was somewhat red and swollen, and it was difficult to enjoy her society without becoming conscious of the smell of spirits.

CHARLES DICKENS (1812–70), *MARTIN CHUZZLEWIT*

Disorders of the nose, which include the everyday problems of rhinitis, postnasal drip, epistaxis, folliculitis and disorders of smell, are very common in everyday general practice.

The main functions of the nose are:

- airflow
- filtration—of dust, organisms and other air-borne particles
- olfaction (smell)
- self-cleansing and moisturising of the mucous membrane
- humidification and warming of air in its passage to the lungs
- vocal resonance

The main symptoms of nasal disorders are discharge, blockage, sneezing, anosmia, itching, postnasal drip, bleeding and snoring (see TABLE 59.1).[1]

Nasal discharge is a common and important symptom to evaluate. The characteristics of nasal discharge are summarised in TABLE 59.2.

Table 59.1 Typical symptoms for nasal disorders[2]

Foreign body	Unilateral discharge, unilateral blockage
Acute sinusitis	Facial pain, toothache, nasal discharge, postnasal drip
Allergic rhinitis	Sneezing, rhinorrhoea, itch, eye irritation
Infective rhinitis	Blockage, purulent discharge, postnasal drip
Deviated septum	Blockage, postnasal drip
Nasal polyps	Blockage, reduced sense of smell
Nasal tumour	Blockage, unilateral discharge, epistaxis
Adenoidal hypertrophy	Bilateral blockage, snoring, halitosis
Nasal vestibulitis	Local pain, crusting, malodour

Table 59.2 Characteristics of nasal discharge

Nature of discharge	Think of
Blood	Neoplasia, trauma, bleeding disorder, rhinitis, infection, hypertension
Mucopurulent	Bacterial rhinitis, foreign body
Serosanguineous	Neoplasia, foreign body
Watery/mucoid	Viral rhinitis, allergic rhinitis, vasomotor rhinitis, CSF

A major presenting problem is nasal obstruction with the complaint of a blocked or 'stuffy' nose. Common causes are physiological (the nasal cycle), rhinosinusitis (allergic or non-allergic), polyps, adenoid hypertrophy and mechanical such as septal deformity.

Red flag pointers for nasal disorders

- Unilateral nasal 'polyp'
- Unilateral blood-stained discharge
- Toddler with offensive nasal discharge esp. unilateral
- Post-traumatic periseptal swelling
- Rhinitis medicamentosa
- Chronic sinusitis + LRTI = ? Wegener granulomatosis

Disorders of smell

The basic sense of smell is detected in the olfactory region by the olfactory nerve (cranial nerve I) while irritant sensors in the nose, mediated by the maxillary branch of the trigeminal nerve (cranial nerve V), detect some noxious odours.

The disorders can be classified as:[3]

- anosmia—no smell
- hyposmia—reduced smell
- hyperosmia—increased sensitivity to odours

- dysosmia—distortion of smell perception
  - cacosmia—normal odours seem foul or unpleasant
  - parosmia—a perverse sense of smell

Disorders of smell can be caused by conductive or sensorineural disturbances or considered as idiopathic (see TABLE 59.3). Conductive disorders present as anosmia or hyposmia, while sensorineural disorders can present with all of the above disorders.[3] Most cases of idiopathic anosmia are considered to be viral neuropathies and may last from a few days to several months. Head trauma, which can cause conductive or sensorineural disturbances, is considered to be caused either from a fracture of the skull involving the cribriform plate or, more commonly, by posterior head trauma. Some patients will never recover their sense of smell. Patients with anosmia lack flavour discrimination and often have accompanying loss of sense of taste. They are also vulnerable to an unawareness of smoke, gas, dangerous chemicals and unhealthy food.

Table 59.3 Causes of reduced sense of smell

Conductive defects
Head trauma
Nasal polyps
Septal deviation
Rhinitis and sinusitis
Rare (not to be missed)
Nasal tumour
Wegener granulomatosis
Central/sensorineural defects
Ageing
Chemicals (e.g. benzene, chlorine, formaldehyde, cement dust)
Cigarette and other smoking/inhalation
Drugs
Endocrine disorders (e.g. diabetes, hypothyroidism)
Frontal lobe tumour
Parkinson disease
Head trauma
Kallmann syndrome (anosmia + hypogonadism)
Nutritional deficiencies
Viral infections

The clinical approach

- History: head injury or surgery, recent URTI, drugs, occupation including chemical exposure
- Physical examination, including inspection via a Thudicum nasal speculum
- Sniff test—qualitative and quantitative odours (e.g. coffee, cloves, lemon, peppermint, water placebo). Ammonia (for irritant sensation)
- Investigations (e.g. CT scan for sinus disease, nasal polyps)

Treatment[2,4]

- Explanation and reassurance
- Education about smoke detectors, caution about chemicals including gas, excessive perfume, food safety including milk and meat contamination
- Consider dietary supplement with daily zinc sulphate, vitamin A and thiamine
- For chronic anosmia following an URTI: prescribe a nasal decongestant such as Spray-Tish Menthol for 5–7 days

59

Rhinitis

Rhinitis is inflammation of the nose causing sneezing, nasal discharge or blockage for more than an hour during the day. Rhinitis is subdivided into various types:

- According to time span:
  - seasonal rhinitis: occurs only during a limited period, usually springtime
  - perennial rhinitis: present throughout the year
- According to pathophysiology:
  - allergic rhinitis: an IgE-mediated atopic disorder
  - vasomotor rhinitis: due to parasympathetic overactivity

Both allergic and vasomotor rhinitis have a strong association with asthma.

The classification can be summarised as:

- seasonal allergic rhinoconjunctivitis = hay fever
- perennial rhinitis
  - allergic (usually due to house dust mites)
  - non-allergic = vasomotor: eosinophilic, non-eosinophilic

Note: allergic rhinitis (hay fever) is presented in detail in CHAPTER 80.

Clinical features

Nasal symptoms:

- sneezing
- nasal obstruction and congestion
- hypersecretion—watery rhinorrhoea, postnasal drip

- reduced sense of smell
- itching nose (usually allergic)

Throat symptoms:

- dry and sore throat
- itching throat

Irritated eyes (allergic)

Abnormal nasal mucous membrane—pale, boggy, mucoid discharge. A transverse nasal crease indicates nasal allergy, especially in a child.

Allergens

- Pollens from trees (spring) and grass (in summer)
- Moulds
- House dust mites (perennial rhinitis)
- Hair, fur, feathers (from cats, dogs, horses, birds)
- Some foods (e.g. cow's milk, eggs, peanuts, peanut butter)

Diagnosis

Allergic rhinitis—nasal allergy:

- detection of allergen-specific IgE antibodies (not specific)
- RAST test or skin testing for specific allergens (can get false negatives)

Vasomotor rhinitis—a diagnosis of exclusion.

Other causes of rhinitis

- Chronic infection (viral, bacterial, fungal)
- Rhinitis of pregnancy
- Rhinitis medicamentosa—following overuse of OTC decongestant nasal drops or oxymetazoline sprays
- Drug-induced rhinitis:
  - various antihypertensives
  - aspirin
  - phenothiazines
  - oral contraceptives
  - cocaine, marijuana
- Chemical or environmental irritants (vasomotor rhinitis):
  - smoke and other noxious fumes
  - paints and sprays
  - cosmetics

Factors aggravating rhinitis (vasomotor)

- Emotional upsets
- Fatigue
- Alcohol
- Chilly damp weather
- Air-conditioning
- Sudden changes in temperature and humidity

RHINOSINUSITIS

Acute sinusitis

Acute sinusitis is acute inflammation in the mucous membranes of the paranasal sinuses. About 5% of URTIs are complicated by an acute sinusitis,[4] which is mainly viral initially while secondary bacterial infection commonly follows. Any factor that narrows the sinus openings into the nasal cavity (the ostia) will predispose to acute sinusitis.

The two prime clinical presentations are:

1. an URTI persisting for longer than 10 days
2. an URTI that is unusually severe with pyrexia and a purulent nasal discharge

Refer to CHAPTER 52 for features of acute maxillary sinusitis.

Chronic sinusitis

Chronic sinusitis is the most common complication of acute sinusitis. In chronic sinusitis, the symptoms and signs of inflammation persist for more than 8–12 weeks and are more likely to be associated with factors that impair drainage via the osteomeatal complex, including nasal polyps.

Treatment

- Amoxycillin 500 mg (o) 8-hourly for 10–14 days, possibly for longer periods of 3–6 weeks[5]
- Consider decongestant spray (e.g. xylometazoline) for maximum of 5 days and intranasal steroids
- Steam inhalations three times daily
- Nasal saline sprays

Chronic rhinosinusitis

If the above therapies are ineffective, a mechanical saline sinus irrigation procedure to remove stagnant mucus is beneficial.[6]

Refer urgently:

- for surgical drainage if there is no response to the above regimen
- those with orbital or facial cellulitis

Nasal polyps

Nasal polyps are round, soft, pale, pedunculated outgrowths arising from the nasal or sinus mucosa. They are basically prolapsed, congested, oedematous mucosa, described by some as 'bags of water' (see FIG 59.1). They occur in patients with all types of rhinitis, but especially in allergic rhinitis (see FIG. 59.2). Polyps usually arise from the middle meatus and turbinates.

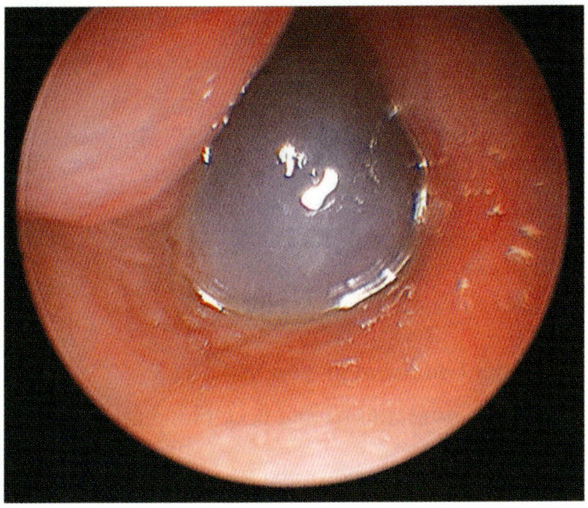

FIGURE 59.1 Nasal polyp in right nasal cavity in a patient with inflamed mucosa from allergic rhinitis

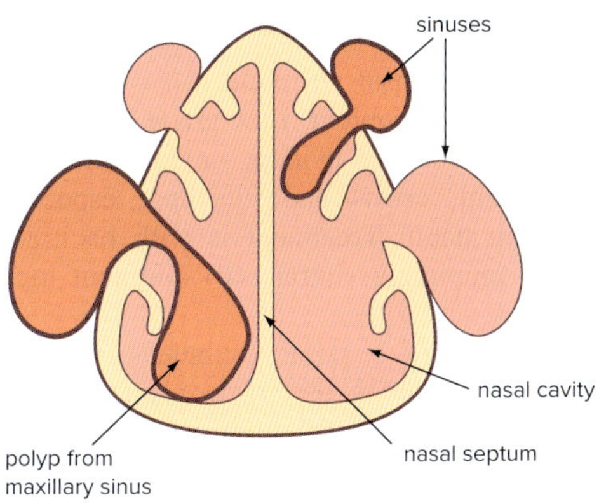

FIGURE 59.2 Cross-section of nose, demonstrating origin of nasal polyps

Symptoms include nasal obstruction, watery discharge, postnasal drip and loss of smell.

Note:

- Nasal polyps may be associated with asthma and aspirin sensitivity.
- Cystic fibrosis should be considered in any child with nasal polyps.
- A polyp that does not have the typical smooth, pale appearance may be malignant.
- A unilateral 'polyp' may be a neoplasm.
- If there is a purulent discharge, swab and give antibiotics.

Treatment

The initial treatment should be medical.[7] A medical 'polypectomy' can be achieved with oral steroids, for example, prednisolone 50 mg daily for 7 days. Supplement this with a corticosteroid spray such as betamethasone, starting simultaneously and continuing for at least 3 months.[8] Give antibiotics for any purulent nasal discharge.

Simple polyps can be readily snared and removed, but referral to a specialist surgeon is advisable for surgical intervention since the aim is to remove the polyp with the mucosa of the sinuses (often ethmoidal cells) from which it arises. This complex procedure reduces the incidence of recurrence.

Epistaxis[9]

This common emergency should, in some instances, be treated as a life-threatening problem. The common situation is intermittent anterior bleeding from Little area, seen in children and the young adult (90% of episodes), while posterior epistaxis (10%) is more common in the older hypertensive patient. It has a strong association with higher URTI (rhinitis, sinusitis), hot dry climates and trauma. Neoplasms should be kept in mind. Bleeding often occurs at night due to vascular vasodilation. Causes of epistaxis are presented in the diagnostic strategy model in TABLE 59.4). The secret of

Table 59.4 Epistaxis: diagnostic strategy model
Probability diagnosis
Idiopathic: spontaneous from Little area
URTI: common cold, influenza, sinusitis
Rhinitis
Vestibulitis
Trauma (incl. nose picking, nose injury)
Drugs (e.g. anticoagulants, aspirin)
Serious disorders not to be missed
Vascular:
• hypertension and arteriosclerosis
Infection:
• systemic febrile illness (e.g. malaria)
• HIV/AIDS
Cancer/neoplasia:
• tumours of nose/sinuses/nasopharynx
• intercranial tumours
• leukaemia
Other:
• thrombocytopenia
• coagulopathy (e.g. haemophilia, liver disease)
Pitfalls (often missed)
Exposure to toxic agents
Vitamin deficiencies: C and K
Septal granulomas and perforations
Foreign bodies (esp. in children)
Cocaine abuse
Rarities:
• hereditary haemorrhagic telangiectasia

good management is to have the right equipment, good lighting and effective local anaesthesia.

Diagnostic tips

- Recent onset of persistent bleeding in elderly points to carcinoma.
- Severe epistaxis is often caused by liver disease coagulopathy.
- Difficult-to-control posterior bleeding is a feature of the hypertensive elderly.

Ideal equipment

Head light, Thudicum nasal speculum, Tilley nasal packing forceps, suction cannula and tubing, Co-Phenylcaine forte spray ± 5% cocaine solution.

Tamponade options (for difficult bleeding)

Merocel expandable pack, Kaltostat, BIPP (bismuth iodoform paraffin paste) with ribbon gauze, Foley catheter (no. 12, 14 or 16) with a 30 mL balloon and self-sealing rubber stopper, anterior/posterior balloon, Epistat catheter with or without Kaltostat.

Treatment

Simple tamponade:

- Pinch 'soft' part of nose below the nasal septum between thumb and finger for 5 minutes
- Apply ice packs to bridge of nose

Simple cautery of Little area (see FIG. 59.3) (under local anaesthetic e.g. Co-Phenylcaine forte nasal spray ± 5% cocaine solution):

- use one of three methods: electrocautery trichloracetic acid or silver nitrate stick (preferred)

Persistent anterior bleed

Merocel (surgical sponge) nasal tampon or Kaltostat pack

'Trick of the trade' for intermittent minor anterior epistaxis:

topical antibiotic (e.g. Aureomycin ointment) bd or tds for 10 days
or (better option)
Nasalate nasal cream tds for 7–10 days
or
Rectinol ointment or Vaseline

Avoid digital trauma and nose blowing.

Severe posterior epistaxis

Use a Foley catheter or an Epistat catheter plus anterior pack.

Nasal vestibulitis

Infection of the nasal vestibule can cause a tender, irritating, crusty problem. Low-grade infections and *folliculitis*, which are evident on inspection, cause localised pain, crusts and bleeding, especially if picked from habit. Treatment is with bacitracin or preferably mupirocin (intranasal) ointment topically for 5–7 days.

Furunculosis of the nasal vestibule is usually due to *Staphylococcus aureus*. It starts as a small superficial abscess in the skin or the mucous membrane and may develop into a spreading cellulitis of the tip of the nose. The affected area becomes tender, red and swollen. It is best treated by avoiding touching it, hot

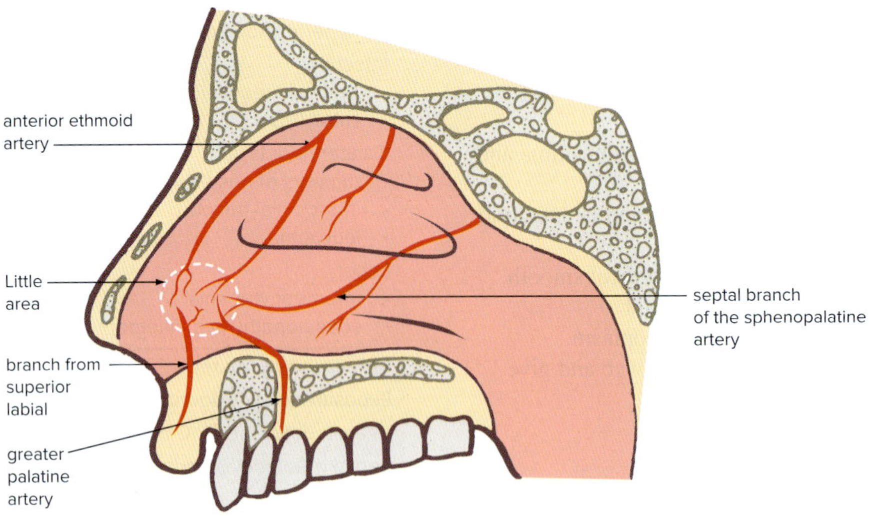

FIGURE 59.3 Little area on the nasal septum where several blood vessels anastomose. Bleeding is common here, especially in young people

soaks and systemic antibiotics such as dicloxacillin or as determined by culture from swabs of the vestibule.

Tip: Staphylococcus aureus colonises the nose of 20–30% of the population.[8] Carriers are prone to transmit nosocomial infection and have an increased risk of serious infections in the presence of serious medical disorders. Treatment includes strict hygiene and eradication with an agent such as mupirocin ointment (match-head size) 2–3 times daily for 5–7 days (max. 10 days).[6]

Fissure: Painful fissures often develop at the mucocutaneous junction. They may become crusted and chronic. Fissures can be treated by keeping the area moist with petroleum jelly (Vaseline) or saline gel, using hot compresses and the use of an antibiotic or antiseptic ointment if necessary.

Offensive smell from nose

This may be caused by vestibulitis but ensure no foreign body is present.

Treatment

- Take nasal swab for culture.

  consider mupirocin 2% nasal ointment, instilled 2–3 times a day for 10 days

  or

  Kenacomb ointment, instil 2–3 times a day

Rhinophyma

This disfiguring swelling of the nose is due to hypertrophy of the nasal sebaceous glands. There is no specific association with alcohol. It is almost exclusive to men over the age of 40 years. Rhinophyma may be associated with rosacea.

Treatment

- Good control of rosacea may reduce the risk (see CHAPTER 121).
- If surgical correction is warranted, refer to a specialist.
- Carbon dioxide laser therapy is the treatment of choice.
- Shave excision is another effective therapy.

Nasal septal deviation

This causes blockage as a solitary symptom. Mild septal deviation tends to cause alternating blockage while severe deviation causes persistent blockage on one side.

The septum can be divided into anterior and posterior segments. The anterior portion is necessary to support the cartilaginous pyramid of the nose whereas the posterior portion has no supporting role and can be removed without disturbing the support of the nose. The classic submucous resection operation is therefore suitable for posterior septal deviations. Repair of anterior septal deviations is more complex.

Nasal cosmetic surgery

Rhinoplasty is undertaken to improve the function of an obstructed nasal airway or for cosmetic reasons. In counselling for rhinoplasty it is important to undertake careful planning with realistic anticipated outcomes. The GP should provide non-judgmental support for the patient's decision on cosmetic surgery before referral to an expert in rhinoplasty. Each case has to be assessed individually and the surgery tailored to the deformity. Attention to surgery to the airway is important, otherwise the nose may become partially obstructed and stuffy after cosmetic surgery alone.

59

Septal perforation

A hole in the nasal septum is commonly caused by chronic infection, including tuberculosis, repeated trauma such as vigorous nose 'picking' or following nasal surgery. Rarely, it is encountered in syphilis and Wegener granulomatosis (see CHAPTER 32). It is a known occupational hazard, particularly among chrome workers, and is seen in drug users who sniff cocaine. In about 5–10% of cases, perforation is a result of malignant disease.[4] The condition may be asymptomatic depending on the cause, but there is often an irritating nasal crust and a whistling sound on nasal inspiration. It can be demonstrated by looking in one nares while a light is shone in the opposite one. The cartilaginous part is usually involved.

If not due to a serious cause, treat with Vaseline or saline gel and topical antibiotics for any infection. Refer if malignancy is suspected, otherwise treat symptomatically.

Nasal fractures[2,9]

Fractures of the nose can occur in isolation or combined with fractures of the maxilla or zygomatic arch. They may result in nasal bridge bruising, swelling, non-alignment and epistaxis. Always check for a compound fracture or head injury and, if present, leave alone and refer. If the patient is seen immediately (such as on a sports field) with a straightforward lateral displacement, reduction may be attempted 'on the spot' with digital manipulation before distortion from soft tissue swelling. This involves simply using the fingers to push laterally on the outside of the nose towards the injured side.[2]

Tips:

- X-rays are generally unhelpful unless excluding other facial skeletal injuries and for legal reasons.
- If a deformity is present, refer the patient within 7 days, ideally from days 3–5.
- Skin lacerations, i.e. compound fracture, usually require early repair.
- The optimal time to reduce a fractured nose is about 10 days after injury. There is a window period of 2–3 weeks before the fracture unites.
- Closed reduction under local or general anaesthetic is the preferred treatment.
- Open reduction is more suitable for bilateral fractures with significant septal deviation, bilateral fractures with major dislocations or fractures of the cartilaginous pyramid.

Refer:

- septal haematoma
- uncontrolled epistaxis
- recurrent epistaxis
- concern about cosmetic alignment
- CSF rhinorrhoea

Haematoma of nasal septum

Septal haematoma following injury to the nose can cause total nasal obstruction. It is easily diagnosed as a marked swelling on both sides of the septum when inspected through the nose (see FIG. 59.4).

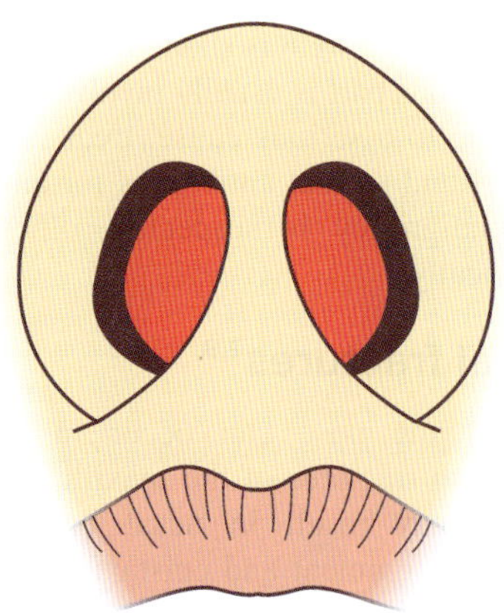

FIGURE 59.4 Inferior view of nasal cavity showing bilateral swelling of septal haematoma

It results from haemorrhage between the two sheets of mucoperiosteum covering the septum. It may be associated with a fracture of the nasal septum.

Note: This is a most serious problem as it can develop into a septal abscess. The infection can pass readily to the orbit or the cavernous sinus through thrombosing veins and may prove fatal, especially in children. Otherwise it may lead to necrosis of the nasal septal cartilage followed by collapse and nasal deformity.

Treatment

- Remove blood clot through an incision, under local anaesthetic.
- Prescribe systemic (oral) antibiotics (e.g. penicillin or erythromycin).
- Treat as a compound fracture if X-ray reveals a fracture.
- ENT specialist advice as necessary.

Stuffy, running nose in adults

For simple post-URTI rhinitis, blow the nose hard into disposable paper tissue or a handkerchief until clear, instil a nasal decongestant for 2–3 days and also have steam inhalations with Friar's Balsam or menthol preparations.

RHINORRHOEA

This can be normal or abnormal. There is a 'nasal cycle' in which there is nasal congestion and decongestion that alternates from side to side and leads to rhinorrhoea. Other causes of normal discharge include vasomotor reactions to external environmental stimuli, such as cold wind and irritants, and postnasal drip (2 L of mucus pass down the back of the nose each day). The diagnostic model for rhinorrhoea is presented in TABLE 59.5.

Senile rhinorrhoea

This is a common, distressing problem in the elderly, caused by failure of the vasomotor control of the mucosa. It may be associated with a deviated septum and dryness of the mucosa. There are few physical signs apart from the nasal drip. The treatment is to keep the nasal passages lubricated with an oil-based preparation, e.g. insufflation with an oily mixture (a sesame oil-based preparation, e.g. Nozoil, is suitable) or petroleum jelly. Topical decongestants cause serious side effects in the elderly.

CSF rhinorrhoea

Following head injury, clear dripping fluid (+ve for glucose or beta-2 transferrin, a more specific test) may indicate a fracture of the roof of the ethmoid. A

Table 59.5 Nasal drip (rhinorrhoea) diagnostic strategy model
Probability diagnosis
URTI (esp. common cold)
Rhinitis (acute infective, allergic, vasomotor)
Vasomotor stimulation (e.g. cold wind, smoke, irritants)
Sinusitis → postnasal drip
Senile rhinorrhoea
Serious disorders not to be missed
Vascular: • cluster headache
Infection: • chronic infective granulomas, e.g. TB
Cancer/tumours: • malignancy (nasal fossa, sinus, nasopharynx)
Other: • CSF rhinorrhoea (post-head injury) • Wegener granulomatosis
Pitfalls (often missed)
Nasal foreign body, e.g. in toddlers
Trauma ± blood
Adenoid hypertrophy
Illicit drugs (e.g. cocaine, opioids, esp. heroin)
Inhaled irritant gases or vapour
Rarities: • choanal atresia • barotrauma
Seven masquerades checklist
Drugs: topical OTC → rhinitis medicamentosa; narcotics
Hyperthyroidism

useful test is the 'halo' or double-ring test, where a blood-stained drop is placed on tissue paper and shows separation of blood and straw-coloured CSF. Refer for assessment, although spontaneous healing can occur.

Neoplasia

Malignant nasal disease, which is uncommon, may cause nasal discharge that may be clear at first, becoming thick and offensive. Malignancy should be suspected in the presence of blood. The growth may be in the nasal fossa, sinus or nasopharynx.

Benign tumours include papilloma, fibroma, osteoma, juvenile fibroangioma of puberty and nasal polyps. Fibroangiomas occur exclusively in males between the ages of 9 and 24. Patients present with unilateral nasal obstruction and recurrent epistaxis.

Malignant tumours include nasopharyngeal carcinoma, with the maxillary sinus being the most common site. Squamous cell carcinoma is the most common, followed by adenocarcinoma melanoma and lymphoma. Malignant or non-healing granuloma, sometimes called 'midline granuloma', is a slowly progressing ulceration of the face starting in the region of the nose.[4] It may represent a form of T cell malignant lymphoma, which responds to radiotherapy. The differential diagnosis is Wegener granulomatosis (see CHAPTER 32). Diagnosis is by CT scan and biopsy. Treatment of nasopharyngeal and sinonasal carcinoma depends on the site, size and histology, but usually involves a combination of surgery and postoperative radiotherapy.

NASAL DISORDERS IN CHILDREN

Nasal problems, especially nasal discharge (rhinorrhoea), are very common in children but the pattern of presentation is usually different from that of adults. Sinusitis is uncommon in children under the age of 10, and allergic nasal polyps are relatively rare. If a child presents with polyps, consider the possibility of cystic fibrosis or neoplasia. Rhinitis, epistaxis and nasal foreign bodies are common.

Abnormal causes

- Adenoid hypertrophy causing postnasal space obstruction
- Foreign body in nose—usually unilateral discharge
- Allergic rhinitis
- Unilateral choanal atresia
- Sinusitis (possible but rare)
- Tumour (also rare—consider fibroangioma)

Diagnosis may be enhanced by spraying with a vasoconstricting agent and getting the child to blow the nose. A tumour, foreign body or polyp may become visible.

Choanal atresia

Acute bilateral nasal obstruction may occur in newborns with congenital bilateral choanal atresia. This leads to anterior nasal discharge and to acute respiratory distress. Immediate investigation and relief are essential and a finger in the corner of the mouth can be life-saving as can passing a nasal probe down one nostril and perforating the membrane.

Sinusitis

Although rare, sinusitis can represent a serious emergency. Red flags requiring consideration include a sick child, pyrexia, rapid onset, unilateral and deteriorating airway obstruction.

Blocked nose and snoring

The above causes of nasal blockage may lead to snoring, mouth breathing, reduced sense of smell, dribbling and possibly obstructive sleep apnoea.

Nasal trauma and fractures[10]

59

Areas of concern associated with nasal fractures, which are uncommon, are possible child abuse, open fracture, septal haematoma or abscess and eye or facial changes. If a fracture is undisplaced, the treatment is pain relief, ice compresses and rest. If displaced, refer for closed reduction under general anaesthetic within 1–2 weeks (ideally at 10 days).[10] If associated epistaxis does not settle with pressure, temporary packing may be required.

Epistaxis

Epistaxis is usually intermittent anterior bleeding from Little area and may follow trauma including nose picking. Bleeding often occurs at night due to vascular vasodilatation. At first, try correction with simple measures (see earlier in chapter) such as pinching below the nasal septum for 5 minutes, supplemented by cold packs. Vaseline applied in the nose at night tends to prevent bleeding, while an antibiotic ointment twice daily for 7–10 days may help.

If problematic, refer for an ENT appointment.

Tip: Think of a bleeding disorder or a tumour, e.g. juvenile angiofibroma.

Snoring and obstructive sleep apnoea

Generally, these problems in children are almost always due to adenotonsillar hypertrophy and most cases are relieved by surgery; CPAP is rarely necessary. Sleep studies are performed to confirm clinical features and allay parental concerns. See CHAPTER 71.

The snuffling infant

Snuffling in infants is usually caused by rhinitis due to an intercurrent viral infection. The presence of yellow or green mucus should not usually be a cause for concern.

Treatment

Reassure the parents.

- Paracetamol mixture or drops for significant discomfort.
- Get the parents to perform nasal toilet with a salt solution (1 teaspoon of salt dissolved in some boiled water); using a cotton bud, gently clear out nasal secretions every 2 waking hours.
- Once the nose is clean, saline nose drops or spray (e.g. Narium nasal mist) can be instilled.
- Stronger decongestant preparations are not advised unless the obstruction is causing a significant feeding problem, when they can be used for up to 4–5 days.

Foreign bodies in the nose

The golden rule is 'a child with unilateral nasal discharge has a foreign body (FB) until proved otherwise'. Such foreign bodies usually consist of beads, pebbles, peas, pieces of rubber, plastic and paper or other small objects handled by the child. A rhinolith may develop in time on the foreign body. In adults, foreign bodies are often rhinoliths, which are sometimes calcium deposits on pieces of gauze or other material that has been used to pack the nose.

Removal of foreign bodies

Removal of FBs from the nose in children is a relatively urgent procedure because of the risks of aspiration. A disc/button battery such as a hearing aid battery in the nose is a medical emergency requiring urgent removal under anaesthetic.[10]

The nose should be examined using a nasal speculum under good illumination. The tip of the nose should be raised and pressed with the tip of a thumb. At first, spray a topical decongestant into the nose and see if the child can blow it out after waiting 10 minutes. Do not attempt to remove FBs from the nose by grasping with 'ordinary forceps'.

Methods of removal

1. Spray with decongestant, wait 10 minutes, then ask the child to blow out the FB.
2. It is best to pass an instrument behind the FB and pull or lever it forward.
   Examples of instruments are:
   - a Eustachian catheter
   - a probe to roll out the FB
   - a bent hairpin
   - a bent paperclip
3. Snaring the FB
   This is the appropriate method for soft, irregular FBs such as paper, foam rubber and cotton wool that are clearly visible. Examples of instruments are:
   - a foreign-body remover
   - crocodile forceps
   - fine nasal forceps

4 Glue on a stick
Apply SuperGlue to the plastic end of a swab stick. Apply it to the FB, wait about 1 minute and then gently extract the FB.

5 Rubber catheter suction technique
The only equipment required is a straight rubber catheter (large type) and perhaps a suction pump. This method involves cutting the end of the catheter at right angles, smearing the rim of the cut end with petroleum jelly and applying this end to the FB, then providing suction. Oral suction may be applied for a recently placed or 'clean' object, but gentle pump suction, if available, is preferred.

6 Irritation of the nose
Some practitioners sprinkle white pepper into the nose to induce sneezing.

7 The 'kiss and blow' technique
This mouth-to-mouth method is used for a cooperative child with a firm, round foreign body such as a bead impacted in the anterior nares. It is best to supervise the child's mother to perform the technique, but the practitioner or practice nurse can perform it.

Method

- Use a nasal decongestant spray.
- After 20 minutes lay the child on an examination couch with a pillow under the head.
- Obstruct the normal nostril with a finger from the side.
- Place the mouth over the child's mouth, blowing into it until a slight resistance is felt (this indicates that the glottis is closed).
- Then blow hard with a high-velocity puff to cause the FB to 'pop out'.

To encourage cooperation with the technique, the child can be asked to give mother (or other) a 'kiss'. More than one attempt may be needed, but it is usually very successful and avoids the necessity for a general anaesthetic.

Patient education resources

Hand-out sheets from *Murtagh's Patient Education* 7th edition:

- Hay fever
- Nosebleed
- Nose: stuffy, running nose
- Sinusitis

References

1 Kalish L, Da Cruz M. Nasal obstruction. Medicine Today, March 2009; 10 (3): 41–52.

2 Mendelsohn M, Ruhno J. The nose—form and function. Australian Doctor, 2 October 2004: 31.

3 Porter RS, Kaplan JL. *The Merck Manual of Diagnoses and Therapy* (19th edn). New Jersey: Merck, Sharp & Dohme Corp., 2011: 466–8.

4 Burton M (ed.). *Hall and Coleman's Diseases of the Ear, Nose and Throat* (15th edn). Edinburgh: Churchill Livingstone, 2000: 107–17.

5 Expert group for Respiratory. Rhinosinusitis. In: eTG complete [Internet]. Melbourne: Therapeutic Guidelines Ltd. Available from: <www.tg.org.au>, accessed October 2017.

6 Harvey RJ. Differentiating chronic sino-nasal complaints. Australian Doctor, 6 February 2009: 27–32.

7 Lund JL. Diagnosis and treatment of nasal polyps. BMJ, 1995; 311: 1411–4.

8 Martinez-Devesa P, Patiar S. Oral steroids for nasal polyps (Cochrane Review). Cochrane Database. Syst Rev. 2011, Issue 6. Art No. CD005232.

9 Barnes ML at al. Epistaxis: a contemporary evidence based approach. Otolaryngol Clin North Am, 2012; 45 (5):1005–17.

10 Buckley N (Chair). *Australian Medicines Handbook*. Adelaide: Australian Medicines Handbook Pty. Ltd, 2016: 429.

11 Oates K, Currow K, Hu W. *Child Health: A Practical Manual for General Practice*. Sydney: MacLennan & Petty, 2001: 328–30.

12 Hansen G. *Practice Tips*. Aust Fam Physician, 1982; 11: 867.

60 Nausea and vomiting

Nausea, retching and hypersalivation frequently precede the act of vomiting, which is a highly integrated sequence of involuntary visceral and somatic motor events.

HARRISON'S PRINCIPLES OF INTERNAL MEDICINE, 1994

Vomiting or emesis is a rather dramatic event with a diverse number of causes. It is usually preceded by nausea.

Definitions

Haematemesis Vomiting of blood. It is presented in CHAPTER 55.

Nausea The unpleasant sickly sensation that can herald the onset of vomiting or can be present without vomiting.

Regurgitation The effortless passage of gastric contents into the mouth in the absence of nausea and without diaphragmatic muscular contractions.

Retching An involuntary act with all the movements of vomiting without the expulsion of gastric contents because the cardiac orifice remains closed.

Rumination The effortless regurgitation of recently ingested food into the mouth, followed by rechewing and reswallowing or spitting out.[1]

Vomiting The forceful expulsion of gastric contents through a relaxed upper oesophageal sphincter and out of the mouth.

Key facts and checkpoints

- Nausea and vomiting have a wide range of potential causes emanating from every body system.
- The common cause of acute nausea and vomiting in most age groups is gastroenteritis.
- The most common causes of vomiting in children are infections—viral (especially) and bacterial—including otitis media and urinary infection.
- Drug ingestion is a common cause of nausea and vomiting; thus, a drug history is vital in assessment.
- Vomiting is commonly associated with migraine and may be the only symptom of a variety of migraines. Children with cyclical vomiting syndrome may have a genetic association with migraine.
- The nature of the vomitus provides a clue:
  - faecalent = intestinal obstruction
  - blood = bleeding from oesophagus, stomach or duodenum (mostly)
  - coffee-grounds = bleeding from stomach or duodenum

The clinical approach

History

A careful history is essential with an emphasis on drug intake, possible psychogenic factors, including self-induced emesis, weight loss, other GIT symptoms or symptoms suggestive of systemic disease.

Examination

If fever is present possible sources of infection (e.g. middle ear, meninges and urinary tract) should be checked.

A careful abdominal examination is appropriate in most instances and this includes urinalysis. Look particularly for scars indicating previous surgery. Look for a succussion splash—this indicates pyloric obstruction.

A neurological examination needs to be considered, including ophthalmoloscopy. Consider raised intracranial pressure.

No examination is complete without assessment of the patient's physical fitness, including the level of hydration, especially in infants and the very old. In these age groups the history may be difficult to obtain and the consequences of fluid loss are more complicated. Always be mindful of the possibility of pregnancy in the female patient. Look for acid dental erosion as a marker of bulimia.

Investigations

These should consider the underlying cause and also biochemical abnormalities resulting from fluid and electrolyte loss.

The following need to be considered:

- pregnancy test (all females of child-bearing age)
- microscopy and culture of stools
- radiology of GIT
- endoscopy
- oesophageal motility studies
- neurological investigation for suspected intracranial pressure (e.g. CT scan, MRI)
- drug toxicity studies
- biochemistry
- cortisol/short synacthen test

Red flags for vomiting

- Marked pallor
- Signs of hypovolaemia
- Peritoneal signs
- Headache, stiff neck, confusion
- Distended tympanic abdomen

Diagnostic guidelines

- Surgical GIT causes are unlikely in the absence of abdominal pain.
- Vomiting without bile-stained vomitus = pyloric obstruction.
- Vomiting of bile = obstruction below duodenal ampulla.
- Vomiting of ingested food = oesophageal obstruction.
- Vomiting without nausea and possibly projectile = ↑ intracranial pressure.

A summary of the diagnostic strategy model is presented in TABLE 60.1.

Vomiting in infancy

Common causes in infants

- feeding problems
- food intolerance
- physiological, e.g. posseting, simple reflux
- gastro-oesophageal reflux
- gastroenteritis
- viral respiratory infections

Table 60.1 Vomiting in adults: diagnostic strategy model

Probability diagnosis

Acute gastroenteritis/gastritis
Drugs and toxins/alcohol intoxication
Motion sickness
Pregnancy
Migraine/cyclical vomiting
GORD

Serious disorders not to be missed

Bowel obstruction:
- severe constipation
- malignancy (e.g. oesophagus, stomach)

Severe infection:
- botulinum poisoning
- septicaemia
- meningitis/encephalitis
- infective endocarditis
- others (e.g. acute viral hepatitis)

Malignancy
Intracranial disorders: malignancy, cerebellar haemorrhage
Acute appendicitis
Acute pancreatitis/biliary colic
Acute myocardial infarction (e.g. painless)

Pitfalls (mainly adults)

Pregnancy (early)
Organ failure: liver, kidney (uraemia), heart, respiratory
Labyrinthine disorders: Ménière syndrome, labyrinthitis
Poisoning: food, chemicals, alcohol
Gut motility disorders: achalasia
Paralytic ileus
Acute glaucoma
Substance abuse
Radiation therapy
Hypercalcaemia
Chronic idiopathic nausea and vomiting
Functional obstruction: diabetic gastroparesis, idiopathic gastroparesis

Seven masquerades checklist

Depression (possible)
Diabetes (ketoacidosis)
Drugs (various, e.g. cytotoxics, digoxin)
Anaemia
Thyroid and other endocrine disorders (Addison disease)
UTI

Is the patient trying to tell me something?

Possibly: extreme stress (e.g. panic attacks, anxiety).
Consider bulimia (self-induced vomiting) and functional (psychogenic).

Is the vomiting bile-stained?

- Green vomiting = urgent surgical referral for possible intestinal malrotation with volvulus (6 hours leeway before gangrene of bowel)[2] Other causes: meconium ileus, small bowel atresia
- Non bile-stained vomitus (curdled milk): consider pyloric stenosis, GORD, feeding problems, concealed infection (e.g. UTI, meningitis). Both pyloric stenosis and GORD cause projectile vomiting.

Important warning signs in neonates

- Excessive drooling of frothy secretions from mouth
- Bile-stained vomitus—always abnormal
- Delayed passage of meconium (beyond 24 hours)
- Inguinal hernias

Refer to surgical emergencies in children (CHAPTER 96).

Specific conditions

Oesophageal atresia

- Vomiting occurs with the first feeding.
- There is excessive drooling of frothy secretions from the mouth.
- Pass a French gauge 10 catheter through the mouth to aid diagnosis.

Congenital hypertrophic pyloric stenosis

- Usually sudden onset 3rd–6th week
- Projectile vomitus
- Failure to thrive
- Male:female = 5:1
- Gastric peristalsis during test feeding (L → R):
  - feel for pyloric tumour either during test feeding or immediately after vomiting (deep in right epigastrium)—see FIGURE 60.1; once felt, further investigation is not necessary
- Biochemistry:
  - metabolic alkalosis: sodium usually <130 mmol/L, chloride <100 mmol/L
- Special investigations (if necessary):
  - barium meal (string sign)—concern about aspiration
  - abdominal ultrasound
- Treatment:
  - correct fluid and electrolyte deficiency (hypochloraemic alkalosis) before surgery
  - appropriate fluid is $\frac{N}{2}$ (half normal) saline with 5% dextrose
  - surgical management (longitudinal pyloromyotomy)

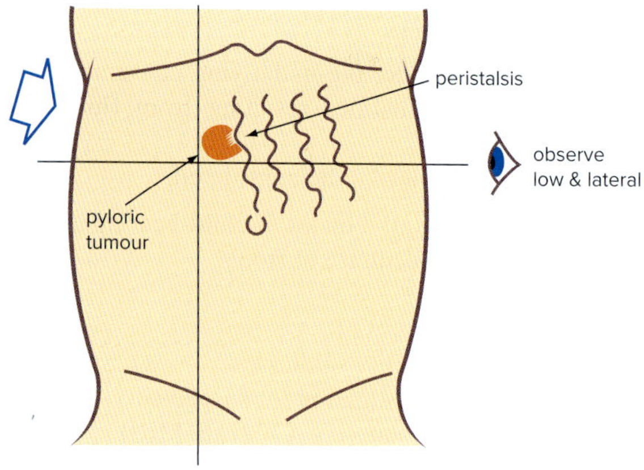

FIGURE 60.1 Signs of pyloric stenosis

Acute gastroenteritis

See CHAPTER 44.

Intussusception

See CHAPTER 34.

Vomiting in the older child

Common causes

- acute gastroenteritis
- acute viral infections
- other common infections, e.g. otitis media
- travel/motion sickness
- migraine/cyclical vomiting
- drugs and toxins, e.g. snake bite

Not to be missed

- acute appendicitis/peritonitis
- strangulated inguinal hernia
- other surgical emergencies
- raised intracranial pressure, e.g. head injury
- serious infection, e.g. pneumonia, meningitis, sepsis
- diabetes/ketoacidosis
- haemolytic uraemic syndrome
- eating disorders: binging/purging

Cyclical vomiting[7]

Features:

- severe, unexplained vomiting or nausea occurring at varying intervals in a healthy person
- lasts hours to days
- most common in children (mean age 5 years)
- ± severe abdominal pain, photophobia, headache
- regarded as a migraine variant
- usually remits in adulthood—may persist
- treated with antimigraine therapy

Gastroparesis (adults)[3]

Gastroparesis (gastropathy) or severely delayed gastric emptying is a moderately common condition, which is a cause of nausea and vomiting.

Causes include:

- diabetic gastroparesis
- postsurgical gastroparesis, e.g. vagotomy (complete or partial), fundoplication
- trauma
- idiopathic (de novo)

Less common causes include:

- connective tissue disorders (e.g. scleroderma)
- vasculitides
- myopathic disorders (e.g. muscular dystrophy)
- thyroid dysfunction
- hypokalaemia
- pancreatitis

Symptoms

- Upper abdominal discomfort/bloating
- Early satiety
- Nausea
- Postprandial vomiting (1–3 hours after meals)
- Abdominal pain

Diagnosis

- Endoscopy → significant gastric residue
- Barium swallow with follow through
- Nuclear medicine gastric emptying test (gastric retention of 60% after 2 hours is abnormal)

Special problems

- Malnutrition
- Dehydration

Management

- Advise patients to eat small, frequent meals, with careful chewing of food.
- Avoid large pieces of bread especially doughy bread (encourage toasting).
- Avoid fat, especially French fries, raw fruit and vegetables.
- Refer diabetic patients to a dietitian for advice.

Medications[4,5]

domperidone 10–20 mg (o) tds, 15–30 minutes before meals

or

metoclopramide 5–10 mg (o) tds, 30 minutes before meals

or

erythromycin (has prokinetic properties) 125 mg (o) tds, 15 minutes before meals (rapidly develops tolerance)

consider cisapride 10 mg (o) tds before meals (with caution)

Other measures

- Injection of botulinum toxin into the pylorus
- Gastric pacing with internally implanted neurostimulators[6]

Chronic idiopathic nausea and vomiting[4]

60

This term is applicable to those patients who experience chronic nausea and vomiting without an identifiable cause or precipitant.

Dietary modification with CBT is recommended. Anti-emetic or antidepressant medication can be considered.

Complications of vomiting

These include dehydration, metabolic alkalosis, hypokalaemia, aspiration, mucosal tear of gastro-oesophageal junction, rupture of the oesophagus (Boerhaave syndrome).

Symptomatic relief of vomiting

The first-line management is to ensure that any fluid and electrolyte imbalance is corrected and that any underlying cause is identified and treated. Various anti-emetics can give symptomatic relief.

Note: Avoid the use of centrally acting dopamine antagonist drugs (DADS, e.g. metoclopramide and prochlorperazine) in children because of risk of extrapyramidal side effects (EPSE), usually acute dystonic reactions. Elderly also at risk. EPSE rare with domperidone because it does not cross the blood–brain barrier. Other DADS include haloperidol and droperidol (limited use).

Serotonin 5-HT_3 antagonists

These include ondansetron, granisetron, dolasetron, palonosetron and tropisetron and are effective at preventing chemotherapy- and radiotherapy-induced emesis when initiated prior to treatment. Dexamethasone enhances the effect of 5-HT_3 agents. Ondansetron can be used in children with gastroenteritis, preferably in wafer format.

Drug-induced nausea and vomiting[4]

metoclopramide 10 mg (o) or IM 8-hourly prn
For cytotoxic drugs (e.g. cisplatin) and radiotherapy:
metoclopramide 10 mg (o) or IM 1–2 hours prior to therapy then 8-hourly (if mild)
For severe cases:
ondansetron 8 mg (o) or IV prior to therapy then two doses 6-hourly
plus
dexamethasone 8 mg IV 30 minutes prior to therapy, then two doses 6-hourly

Note: Restrict ondansetron to 8 mg daily for those with hepatic dysfunction.

A list of some drugs that can cause nausea and vomiting is presented in TABLE 60.2.

Table 60.2	Some drugs that can cause nausea and vomiting
Alcohol (including binge drinking)	
Antibiotics (various) esp. erythromycin	
Antidepressants (e.g. serotonin reuptake inhibitors)	
Antidiabetic agents (e.g. metformin, acarbose)	
Antihypertensives (e.g. CCBs, beta blockers)	
Codeine	
Colchicine	
Corticosteroids	
Cytotoxic agents and immunosuppressants	
Digoxin	
Iron preparations	
Levodopa, other antiparkinsonism drugs (e.g. bromocriptine)	
Nicotine and nicotine gum	
NSAIDs (e.g. indomethacin, COX-2 inhibitors)	
Opioids (e.g. morphine, codeine)	
Oral contraceptives	
Salicylates	
Tamoxifen	
Theophylline	

Motion sickness

Refer to CHAPTER 14.

promethazine theoclate 25 mg (o) 60 minutes prior to travel
or
dimenhydrinate 50 mg (o) 60 minutes prior to travel
or
hyoscine 300–600 mcg (o) 30 minutes prior to travel
or
hyoscine 1.5 mg dermal disc: applied to dry hairless skin behind the ear 5–6 hours before travel (effective for 72 hours)[4]

For treatment: repeat oral presentations 4–6-hourly during trip (max. 4 doses in 24 hours).

Vestibular disturbances[4]

The phenothiazine derivatives are the most effective, while the dopamine D2-receptor antagonists are relatively ineffective. Refer to CHAPTER 46.

prochlorperazine 5–10 mg (o) or 10 mg rectally, SC or IM 4 times daily prn
or
promethazine theoclate 25 mg (o) or IM 4-hourly prn (max. 100–150 mg per 24 hours)

Note: Beware of tardive dyskinesia with prolonged use.

Gastroenteritis

For severe cases in adults:
metoclopramide 10 mg (o) or IM 8-hourly prn

Pregnancy

pyridoxine hydrochloride 25 mg (o) tds
plus
doxylamine 25 mg (o) nocte
if still ineffective add
metoclopramide 10 mg (o) tds or IM (if oral intolerance)
if response still unsatisfactory
ondansetron tablet or wafer 4–8 mg (o) bd to tds

Postoperative vomiting[4]

metoclopramide 10 mg IM or IV (slowly), 8-hourly prn
or
prochlorperazine 12.5 mg IM, 8-hourly prn

Chemotherapy and radiotherapy

ondansetron 4 mg (o or SL) bd
plus
dexamethasone 4 mg (o) daily

Practice tips

- Consider the possibility of anorexia nervosa and bulimia in adolescent females with a history of vomiting immediately after meals, especially after binge eating.
- If weight loss accompanies nausea and vomiting, consider GIT malignancy and obstruction as well as the above psychogenic conditions.
- Early-morning nausea and vomiting can be caused typically by alcohol, pregnancy, kidney failure and raised intracranial pressure.
- Intracranial space-occupying lesions can cause vomiting without associated anorexia or nausea.
- Gastroparesis commonly occurs in longstanding diabetes, following surgery or may be idiopathic. Intense nausea and anorexia are features.
- Anti-emetic drug therapy should not be used in infants and children with gastroenteritis.
- Anti-emetic treatment (see TABLE 60.3) must be tailored to the specific cause of the problem.
- Cannabinoids such as tetrahydrocannabinol, long advocated for cancer-associated emesis, appear to be effective in selected patients but are associated with central nervous system side effects in most patients.[8]
- The major complications of severe vomiting include trauma of the distal oesophagus, such as a Mallory–Weiss tear, and severe fluid and electrolyte disturbances.

Table 60.3 Anti-emetic medications in common use

Anti-emetic	Receptor antagonist	Route
Promethazine	H_1; D_2	O, IM, IV
Metoclopramide	D_2 + 5-HT_3	O, IV, IM
Prochlorperazine	D_2 (central)	O, IM, PR
Domperidone	D_2 (peripheral)	O
Droperidol	D_2 (central)	IV
Haloperidol	D_2 (central)	O, IM
Ondansetron	5-HT_3	O, IV

Important side effects: dystonia, dyskinesia, drowsiness, anti-cholinergic, hyperprolactinaemia

5-HT_3 = 5 hydroxytryptamine type 3, D_2 = dopamine D_2

References

1 Duggan A, Al-Sohaily S. Nausea: how to treat. Australian Doctor, 23 March 2007: 25–32.

2 Thompson K, Tey D, Marks M. *Paediatric Handbook* (8th edn). Melbourne: Wiley-Blackwell, 2009: 537–8.

3 Hebbard G. Gastroparesis. Diabetes Management Journal, 2005; 10: 6–7.

4 Expert group for Gastrointestinal. Nausea and vomiting. In: eTG complete [Internet]. Melbourne: Therapeutic Guidelines Ltd. Available from: <www.tg.org.au>, accessed October 2017.

5 Talley NJ. Diabetes gastropathy and prokinetics. Am J Gastroenterol, 2003; 98: 264.

6 Abell T et al. Gastric electrical stimulation for medically refractory gastroparesis. Gastroenterology, 2003: 125–421.

7 Lindley KJ, Andrews PL. Pathogenesis and treatment of cyclical vomiting. J Pediatr Gastroenterol Nutr, 2005; 41 (Suppl. 1): 38–40.

8 Papadakis MA, McPhee S. *Current Medical Diagnosis and Treatment* (56th edn). New York: McGraw-Hill Education, 2017: 583.

61 Neck lumps

There are approximately 800 lymph nodes in the body; no fewer than 300 of them lie in the neck and inflammation of these is exceedingly common.

McNeil Love, Co-editor of *Bailey & Love's Short Practice of Surgery*, 1965

In the management of lumps in the neck it is important to distinguish between the various midline and lateral causes, especially cervical lymphadenopathy, which may be caused by occult malignancy, such as in the aerodigestive tract. With increasing ageing in the population the number of patients presenting with a malignant neck lump is also increasing. The neck is divided into anterior and posterior triangles by the sternomastoid muscle and the anatomical areas are helpful in identifying the origin of the primary lesion (see FIG. 61.1).

Key facts and checkpoints

- Most neck lumps are reactive lymph nodes—to concurrent infection.
- Lymph nodes are normally palpable in children between 3 and 8 years of age; soft, mobile nodes up to 1 cm in diameter are commonly felt in the anterior and posterior triangle. A node >2 cm is considered to be enlarged. Some cervical glands are very prominent, especially tonsillar nodes.
- These prominent nodes often enlarge during intercurrent viral infection.
- Causes of neck swellings are lymph nodes 85%, goitres 8%, others 7%.[1]
- Solitary nodules in the thyroid move on swallowing.
- Consider the possibility of tuberculosis, especially with exposure in endemic areas and in immunocompromised people.
- A knowledge of the areas drained by lymph nodes is important (see FIG. 61.1).
- Examination must extend beyond the neck for lymphadenopathy.
- To examine cervical nodes, slightly rotate head and palpate with palmar aspect of fingers.
- Palpate submental area with head slightly flexed.
- Biopsy of a complete lymph node is necessary to establish diagnosis for unknown or suspicious causes but do not consider it as the first step in diagnosis.[2]
- Other investigations are chest X-ray and FBE. Bone marrow biopsy or fine-needle aspiration of thyroid nodule or other masses may be considered. Fine-needle aspiration biopsy (FNAB), which is a relatively simple procedure, is the single most helpful investigation for diagnosing the cause.[3] If cytology reveals malignant squamous cells, the primary lesion may lie in the skin, lung, larynx, pharynx, ear or oesophagus.

A diagnostic approach

A summary of the diagnostic strategy model is presented in TABLE 61.1.

The key components of the history, examination and investigations follow.

History

This depends on the age of the patient but should include in all ages a history of upper respiratory infection, lower respiratory infection, possible Epstein–Barr, HIV, cytomegalovirus and tuberculosis infection. Consider red flags such as weight loss, dysphagia, history of cancer and increasing size of the lump. Note any response to antibiotics given for a throat or upper airways infection.

Examination

- Careful palpation of lymph node areas and matching the site of any lymphadenopathy with a 'map' of areas drained by the nodes
- Examine the lump according to the classic rules of look, feel, move, measure, auscultate and transilluminate
- Palpate the midline anterior area for thyroid lumps and the submental area for submandibular swellings
- Note the consistency of the lump: soft, firm, rubbery or hard

Table 61.1	Neck lumps: diagnostic strategy model

Probability diagnosis

Lymphadenitis (reaction to local infection)

- acute: viral or bacterial
- chronic: MAIS (atypical tuberculosis), viral (e.g. EBM, rubella)

Prominent normal lymph nodes

Goitre

Sebaceous cyst

Dermoid cyst

Lipoma

Sternomastoid tumour (neonates)

Serious disorders not to be missed

Vascular:

- carotid body tumour or aneurysm

Infection:

- 'collar stud' abscess (atypical TB)
- tuberculosis of cervical nodes (scrofula)
- HIV/AIDS of nodes
- actinomycosis

Cancer/tumour

- lymphoma (e.g. Hodgkin)
- leukaemia
- thyroid nodule (adenoma, cancer, colloid cyst)
- metastatic nodes
- salivary gland tumours

Pitfalls (often missed)

Parotitis

Thyroglossal cyst

Lymphatic malformation (children)

Cervical rib

Rarities:

- sarcoidosis
- cystic hygroma
- branchial cyst (child)
- torticollis

Investigations

- FBE
- ESR/CRP
- CXR
- TFTs (of thyroid swelling)
- Fine needle aspiration biopsy of thyroid nodules
- Lymph node biopsy

Thyroid and primary tumours: imaging techniques (if necessary to assist diagnosis) include:

- ultrasound
- axial CT scan (esp. in fat necks)
- MRI scan (distinguishes a malignant swelling from scar tissue or oedema)
- tomogram of larynx (malignancy)
- barium swallow (pharyngeal pouch)
- sialogram
- carotid angiogram

Red flag pointers for neck lumps

- >40 years, esp. >70 years
- Nodes >2.5 cm
- Nodes >3–4 cm ? malignancy
- Tender mass
- Purple discolouration (collar-stud abscess)
- Single, gradually enlarging node
- Fixed to skin without punctum
- Associated dysphagia
- Hard midline thyroid lump
- Patient at risk of malignancy and HIV
- Exposure to tuberculosis

61

The 20:40 and 80:20 rules[3,4]

- The age of the patient is a helpful guide, as causes of neck lumps can be roughly categorised by the '20:40 rule':
  - 0–20 years: congenital, inflammatory, lymphoma, tuberculosis
  - 20–40 years: inflammatory, salivary, thyroid, papillary thyroid cancer, lymphoma
  - >40 years: lymphoma, metastases, i.e. neck lumps are malignant until proven otherwise
- Most neck lumps (80%) are benign in children while the reverse applies to adults.
- Imaging techniques that may assist diagnosis include axial CT scan (especially in fat necks), MRI scan (distinguishes a malignant swelling from scar tissue or oedema), tomogram of larynx (laryngocele or malignancy), barium swallow (pharyngeal pouch), sialogram and carotid angiogram.[5]

A basic suggested approach for the patient presenting with a neck lump is summarised in FIGURE 61.2.

CERVICAL LYMPHADENOPATHY

- There are many causes, varying from local infections to lymphoproliferative disorders.
- Most malignant nodes in the supraclavicular area have their primary tumour below the clavicle.
- Eighty-five per cent of malignant nodes in the anterior triangle have their primary tumour in the head and neck.[2]

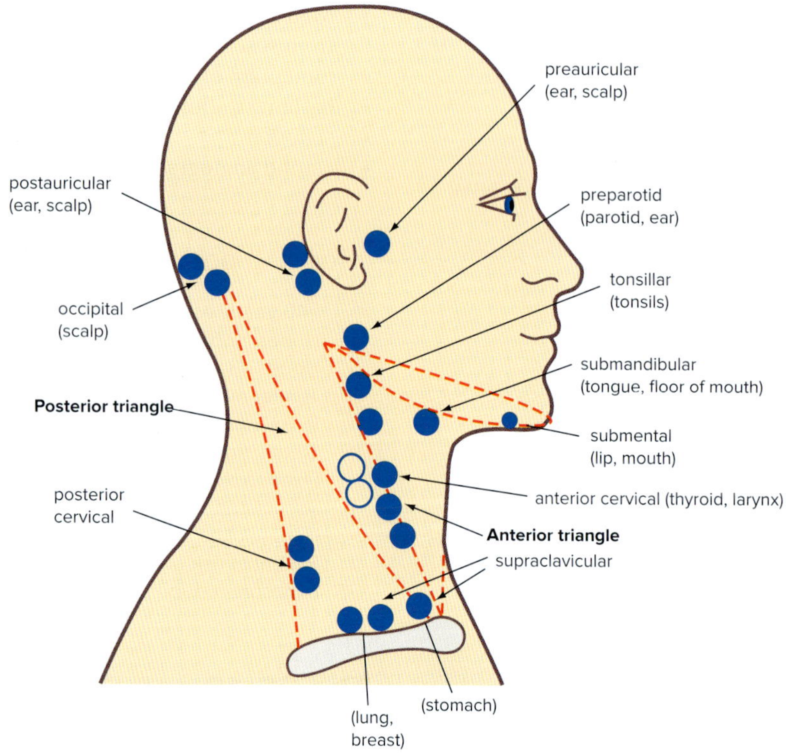

FIGURE 61.1 Lymph glands (site of the nodes) of the neck including common sources of adenopathy (excluding lymphomas)

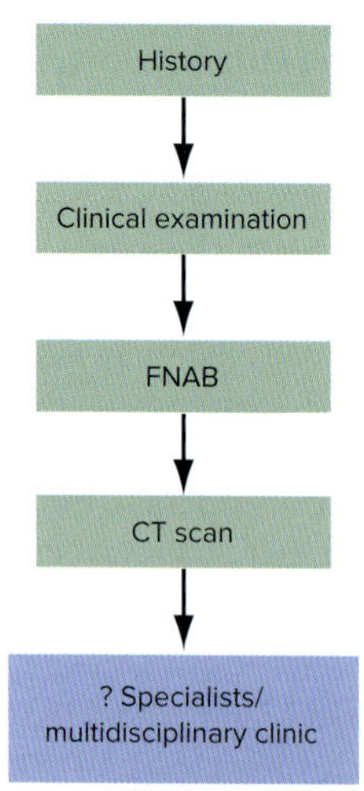

FIGURE 61.2 A basic approach for patients presenting with a neck lump[4]

- Always search for:
  - other nodes at distant sites
  - possible primary source of infections or neoplasia
  - hepatosplenomegaly
- Hodgkin lymphoma usually presents with rubbery, painless nodes in the neck.
- Most swellings are lateral.

Consistency of enlarged nodes

Rules of thumb are:[5,6]

- hard: secondary carcinoma
- rubbery: lymphoma
- soft: sarcoidosis or infection
- tender and multiple: infection

Causes of cervical lymph node enlargement (lateral cervical swelling)

Acute cervical lymphadenitis

- Acute viral lymphadenitis
- Acute bacterial lymphadenitis—coccal infection

Chronic lymph node infection

- MAIS lymphadenitis (atypical tuberculosis)
- Tuberculosis
- Viral infection, e.g. EBM (see FIG. 61.3), rubella, cytomegalovirus, HIV

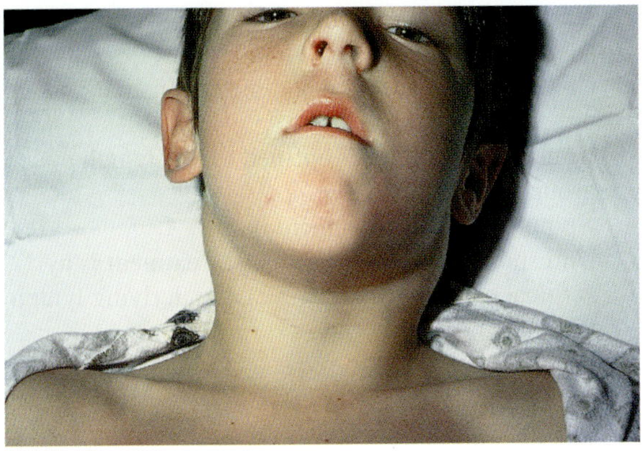

FIGURE 61.3 Cervical lymphadenopathy associated with Epstein–Barr mononucleosis

- *Toxoplasma gondii* infection
- Cat-scratch disease—*Bartonella henselae* infection

Neoplastic lymphadenopathy

- Lymphomas, esp. Hodgkin lymphoma
- Leukaemia

Metastatic

- Check mouth, pharynx, sinuses, larynx, scalp, oesophagus, stomach, breast, lungs, thyroid and skin. A working rule is upper neck—from skin to upper aerodigestive tract; lower neck—from below clavicles (e.g. lung, stomach, breast, colon).
- Examples:
  - occipital or pre-auricular—check scalp
  - submental—check mouth, tongue, teeth
  - submandibular—check floor of mouth
  - left supraclavicular (under sternomastoid)—consider stomach (Troisier sign)
  - deep anterior cervical—consider larynx, thyroid, oesophagus, lungs

NECK LUMPS NOT DUE TO LYMPH NODE SWELLING[7]

Types and causes

Widespread

- Sebaceous cysts
- Lipomas

Midline

- Thyroid nodule (moves upon swallowing)
- Thyroglossal cysts (moves upwards on tongue protrusion)
- Dermoid cyst (beneath chin)

Anterior triangle

- Branchial cyst (in upper part):
  - usually adulthood (20–25 years)
- Carotid body tumour:
  - opposite thyroid cartilage
  - smooth and pulsatile
  - can be moved laterally but not vertically
  - usually 40–60 years
  - requires excision (with care)
- Carotid aneurysm
- Lateral thyroid tumours

Posterior triangle

- Developmental remnants:
  - cystic hygroma
  - branchial sinuses and cysts
- Pancoast tumour (from apex lung)
- Cervical rib

Submandibular swellings

- Submandibular salivary gland
- Cervicofacial actinomycosis (lumpy jaw syndrome):
  - chronic granulomatosis infection due to Gram-positive *Actinomyces israelii*
  - forms a multilocular abscess (pus has 'sulphur granules')
  - infection follows dental extraction or poor dental hygiene, esp. severe caries
  - treat with high-dose penicillin G, 4 months

Sternomastoid tumour

Refer CHAPTER 91.

Pharyngeal pouch

- A soft, squelchy, indefinite mass
- Base of left neck
- History of difficulty in swallowing

Thyroid nodule

The most likely cause of a solitary thyroid nodule is the dominant nodule in a multinodular goitre.

Other causes include a true solitary nodule—adenoma, follicular carcinoma or solitary carcinoma—and a colloid cyst. Malignancy must be excluded.

Investigations

- Ultrasound
- FNAB (may resolve a cystic lesion)
- TFTs

61

Neck lumps in children

Eighty per cent of neck lumps are benign while 20% are malignant. Benign lumps usually occur in the anterior triangle, while malignant lumps are more likely in the posterior triangle. The common midline lump in children is the thyroglossal cyst.[3] Consider sternomastoid tumour (fibrosis) in infants (see CHAPTER 92).

Lymphadenopathy

- Most enlarged lymph nodes are either 'normal' or local infections (mainly viral), especially if <2 cm diameter, and not hard or fixed.
- Inflammatory nodes may be caused by infection in the tonsils, the teeth or other oral or nasopharyngeal cavities.
- They are of concern if supraclavicular node enlargement and fever <1 week.
- Suspicious nodes are >2.5 cm, with firmer consistency than normal and less mobility (investigate especially with biopsy).
- Consider bacterial infection with abscess formation in infants and children with large (2–4 cm) tender masses.

MAIS lymphadenitis[4,8]

- Child usually 2–3 years of age
- Caused by *Mycobacterium avium-intracellulare-scrofulaceum* (MAIS) infection
- Produces chronic cervical lymphadenitis and collar stud abscesses
- A relatively common infection of cervical nodes, yet often unrecognised
- Painless swelling due to development of a cold abscess in healthy child
- Nodes enlarge over 4–6 weeks prior to erupting into a 'cold' abscess and the overlying skin has a purplish discolouration, which is an indication for surgical treatment
- Common sites are submandibular, tonsillar and pre-auricular nodes
- Invariably unilateral, confined to one lymph node group
- No pulmonary involvement
- Unresponsive to antimicrobials: treatment is by surgical excision of abscess and underlying lymph nodes

Acute bacterial lymphadenitis

- Usually coccal infections—*Staphylococcus, Streptococcus*
- Can progress to abscess formation (fluctuant): requires drainage

When to refer

- A persisting lump, depending on its location and size
- A lymph node or group of nodes that are abnormally enlarged and fail to respond to antibiotics

References

1 Fry J, Berry H. *Surgical Problems in Clinical Practice.* London: Edward Arnold, 1987: 38.
2 Coman WB. Neck lumps in adults. In: *MIMS Disease Index* (2nd edn). Sydney: IMS Publishing, 1996: 340–1.
3 Cole IE, Turner J. Neck lumps: clues to the diagnosis and management. Modern Medicine Australia, 1997; April: 37–55.
4 Grace PA, Borley NR. *Surgery at a Glance* (3rd edn). Oxford: Blackwell, 2006: 10–11.
5 Hughes C, O'Brien C. Neck lumps: how to treat. Australian Doctor, 5 August 2005: 31–8.
6 Larkins R, Smallwood R. *Clinical Skills.* Melbourne: Melbourne University Press, 1993: 133–4.
7 Hobbs C, Bova R. Neck lumps: a guide to assessment and management. Medicine Today, 2010; 11 (4); 26–34.
8 Gwee A, Rimer R, Marks M. *Paediatric Handbook* (9th edn). Melbourne: Wiley-Blackwell, 2015; 291.

Neck pain

We have all heard of the courtiers who mimicked the wry neck of Alexander the Great.

WILLIAM HEBERDEN (1710–1801)

Neck pain is a very common symptom in both sexes at all ages and although most pain is experienced in the posterior aspect of the neck, anterior neck pain can occur from causes that overlap between front and back. The main cause of neck pain is a disorder of the cervical spine, which usually manifests as neck pain but can refer pain to the head, shoulders and chest. Such pain usually originates from the facet (apophyseal) joints but can arise from other musculoskeletal structures, such as the intervertebral discs and the muscles or ligaments (see FIG. 62.1). The other major symptom is limited movement or stiffness.

General causes of neck pain are presented in TABLE 62.1.

Key facts and checkpoints

- According to an Australian study, about 18% of people wake with some degree of neck pain and 4% experience neck pain or stiffness for all of the day.[1]
- The commonest cause of neck pain is idiopathic dysfunction of the facet joints, also called 'non-specific', without a history of injury, with a prevalence peak at 45 years.
- Disorders of the intervertebral discs are common, especially in the lower cervical spine, and may cause unilateral pain, paraesthesia or anaesthesia in the arm.
- In a UK study, radiological cervical disc degeneration was present in 40% of males and 28% of females between 55 and 64 years.[2]
- Strains, sprains and fractures of the facet joints, especially after a 'whiplash' injury, are difficult to detect and are often overlooked as a cause of persistent neck pain.
- Cervical spondylosis is a disorder of ageing: radiological signs occur in 50% of people over the age of 50 and in 75% over the age of 65 years.[3]

continued

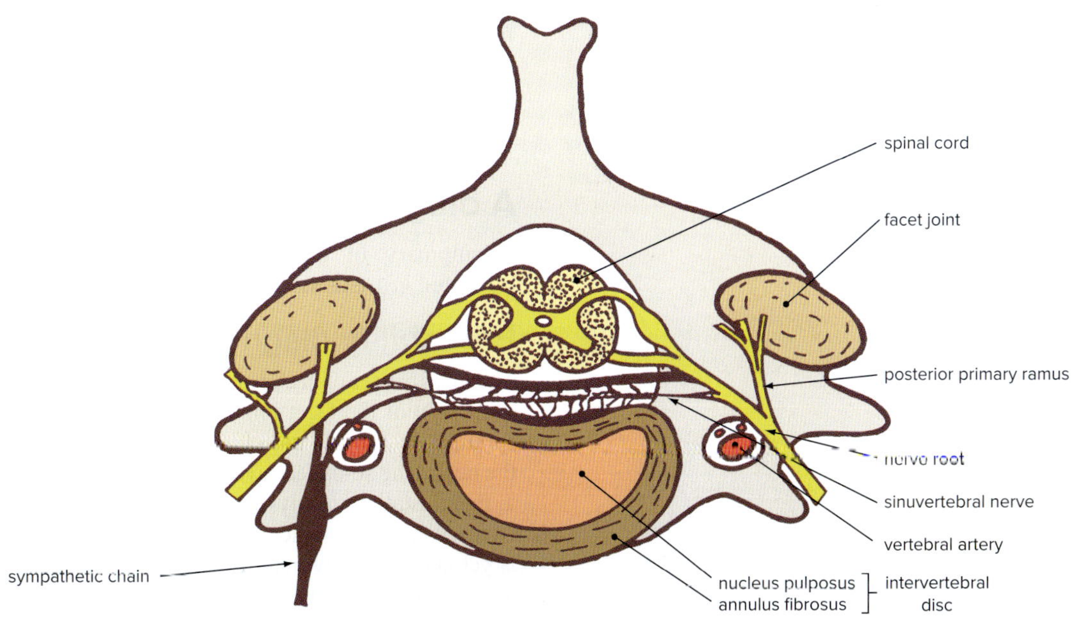

FIGURE 62.1 Transverse section illustrating the functional unit and nervous network of the cervical spine

continued

- In cervical spondylosis, osteophytic projections may produce nerve root and spinal cord compression, resulting in radiculopathy and myelopathy respectively.
- Radiculopathy can be caused by a soft disc protrusion (usually unilateral), a hard, calcified lump and osteophytes (may be bilateral).
- Cervical disorders are aggravated by vibration (e.g. riding in a motor vehicle).
- Always determine the C2, C6 and C7 levels by finding the relevant spinous processes (easily palpable landmarks) prior to palpation.
- Palpation of the neck is the cornerstone of cervical management. Palpate gently—the more one presses the less one feels.
- Most episodes of neck pain, including acute torticollis, are transient, lasting from about 2–10 days.
- In one study, 70% of people with neck pain who sought medical attention had recovered or were recovering within 1 month.[2]
- Effective management of neck pain is based on the theoretical principle that stiff dysfunctional joints are painful and restoration of normal movement may be associated with resolution of pain.
- The optimal treatment for dysfunctional joints (without organic disease or radiculopathy) is active and passive mobilisation, especially exercising.

Table 62.1 Causes of neck pain (a pathological classification)

Musculoskeletal/structural
Joint dysfunction:
- apophyseal
- intervertebral disc

Muscular/ligamentous strains or sprains
Trauma:
- 'whiplash'
- fracture
- other disorders

Inflammation
Osteoarthritis*
Rheumatoid arthritis
Spondyloarthropathies (e.g. ankylosing spondylitis, psoriasis, reactive arthritis)
Polymyalgia rheumatica
Thyroiditis

Infective
Spinal:
- osteomyelitis
- tuberculosis
- herpes zoster

Extraspinal:
- epidural abscess
- cervical adenitis
- poliomyelitis
- tetanus

Extracervical:
- meningitis
- febrile states (e.g. meningism, malaria)

Degenerative
Spondylosis*

Metabolic
Paget disease

Neoplasia
Benign
Malignant

Fibromyalgia syndrome

Psychogenic

Referred visceral
Heart:
- IHD
- pericarditis

Oesophagus
Lung cancer
Acute pancreatitis

Referred cranial
Haemorrhage (e.g. subarachnoid)
Tumour
Abscess

**Osteoarthritis, or spondylosis, is inflammatory and degenerative.*

A diagnostic approach

A summary of the diagnostic strategy model is presented in TABLE 62.2.

Probability diagnosis

The main causes of neck pain are vertebral dysfunction, especially of the facet joints, and traumatic strains or sprains affecting the musculoligamentous structures of the neck. The so-called myofascial syndrome is mainly a manifestation of dysfunction of the facet joints. Acute wry neck (torticollis), which is quite common, is yet another likely manifestation of apophyseal joint dysfunction. Spondylosis, known also as degenerative osteoarthrosis and osteoarthritis, is also a common cause, especially in the elderly patient.

Table 62.2 Neck pain: diagnostic strategy model

Probability diagnosis
Vertebral dysfunction (non-specific neck pain)
Traumatic 'strain' or 'sprain'
Cervical spondylosis

Serious disorders not to be missed
Cardiovascular:
- angina
- subarachnoid haemorrhage
- arterial dissection/leaking aortic aneurysm

Neoplasia:
- primary metastasis
- Pancoast tumour

Severe infections:
- osteomyelitis
- meningitis

Vertebral fractures or dislocation

Pitfalls (often missed)
Disc prolapse
Myelopathy
Cervical lymphadenitis
Fibromyalgia syndrome
Outlet compression syndrome (e.g. cervical rib)
Polymyalgia rheumatica
Ankylosing spondylitis
Rheumatoid arthritis
Oesophageal foreign bodies and tumours
Paget disease

Seven masquerades checklist
Depression
Thyroid disorder (thyroiditis)
Spinal dysfunction

Is the patient trying to tell me something?
Highly probable. Stress and adverse occupational factors relevant.

Intervertebral disc disruption is also a relatively common phenomenon in the cervical spine, especially at the lower levels C5–6 and C6–7.[4]

Serious disorders not to be missed

Conditions causing neck pain and stiffness may be a sign of meningitis or of cerebral haemorrhage, particularly subarachnoid haemorrhage, or of a cerebral tumour or retropharyngeal abscess.

Angina and myocardial infarction should be considered in anterior neck pain. Other visceral disorders can refer pain to the neck.

Arterial dissection of the internal carotid artery or vertebral artery should be kept in mind in patients presenting with acute neck pain, especially without musculoskeletal symptoms or signs.

Tumours are relatively rare in the cervical spine but metastases do occur and should be kept in mind, especially with persistent neck pain present day and night.

Metastasis to the spine occurs in 5–10% of patients with systemic cancer, making it the second most common neurological complication of cancer. The cervical spine accounts for some 15% of spinal metastases.[3]

The commonest primary tumours are the breast, prostate or lung. Other primaries include the kidney, thyroid and melanoma.

Red flag pointers for neck pain

- History of major trauma; vertebral fracture
- Age >50 years
- Constant pain (day and night)
- Fever >38°C
- Anterior neck (throat) pain
- Pain at multiple sites
- History of cancer
- Unexplained weight loss
- Neurological deficit
- Spinal cord pathology
- Radicular pain in arm
- Rheumatoid arthritis and ankylosing spondylitis
- Down syndrome

62

Pitfalls

There are many pitfalls in the clinical assessment of causes of neck pain, many of them related to inflammation.

Rheumatoid arthritis is the prime severe inflammatory arthropathy that involves the neck but the neck can be affected by the seronegative spondyloarthropathies, particularly ankylosing spondylitis, psoriasis and the inflammatory bowel disorders.

While polymyalgia rheumatica affects mainly the shoulder girdle, pain in the lower neck, which is part of the symptom complex, is often overlooked. Diffuse neck pain in myofascial soft tissue with tender trigger areas is part of the uncommon but refractory fibromyalgia syndrome.

General pitfalls

- Failing to appreciate how often the benign problem of facet joint dysfunction occurs in the neck, causing pain and limited movement. This involves failure to appreciate the value of physical therapy, especially exercise programs, in alleviating the problem.

- Failing to adhere to the idiom: one disc—one nerve root. Involvement of more than one nerve root in the upper limb may mean a neoplastic disorder such as metastatic disease, lymphoma in the thoracic outlet and similar serious diseases.
- Missing the insidious onset of myelopathy, especially the spasticity component, caused by rheumatoid arthritis, osteophytic overgrowth or, rarely, a soft disc prolapse.

Seven masquerades checklist

Cervical spinal dysfunction is the obvious outstanding cause. Thyroiditis may cause neck pain, as in the extremely rare cases of acute specific infection in the thyroid (e.g. syphilis, pyogenic infections), which cause severe pain; non-specific thyroiditis (de Quervain thyroiditis) produces painful swelling with dysphagia. The association between depression and neck pain is well documented.

Psychogenic considerations

The neck is one of the commonest areas for psychological fixation following injury. This may involve perpetuation or exaggeration of pain because of factors such as anxiety and depression, conversion reaction and secondary gain.

The psychological sequelae that can follow a whiplash injury and chronic neck problems such as spondylosis serve as a reminder that the state of the patient's cervical spine can profoundly affect his or her life and that we should always be aware of the whole person. A feeling of depression is a very common sequel to such an injury and these patients demand our dutiful care and understanding.

The clinical approach

History

It is important to analyse the pain into its various components, especially the nature of its onset, its site and radiation, and associated features. The diurnal pattern of the pain will provide a lead to the diagnosis (refer to FIG. 38.3: the patterns are similar to low back pain).

Key questions

- Can you point to exactly where in your neck you get the pain?
- Do you wake up with pain in the morning?
- Does the pain come on when you have to look up for a while?
- Do you have trouble reversing your car?
- Can you recall an injury to your head or neck such as hitting your head on an overhead bar?
- Does your neck grate or get stiff?
- Do you get headaches or feel dizzy?
- Is the pain present day and night?
- Do you get pain or pins and needles or numbness in your arms?
- Does the pain come on with activity?
- Does the pain wake you at night?
- Do you feel pain on both sides of your neck and over your shoulders?
- Do your hands or arms feel weak or clumsy?

Examination

It is appropriate to follow the traditional rule for examination of any joint or complex of joints: *look, feel, move, measure, test function, look elsewhere* and X-*ray*. Careful examination of the cervical spine is essential for the correct diagnosis and for specific treatment at the painful level.

Three objectives of the examination are to:

- reproduce the patient's symptoms
- identify the level of lesion or lesions
- determine the cause (if possible)

A neurological examination is essential if radicular pain is present, or weakness or other upper limb symptoms, including any pain or paraesthesia that extends below the elbow.

Inspection

The patient should be examined sitting on a couch, rather than on a chair. The body should be fully supported with the hands resting on the thighs. The following should be noted:

- willingness to move the head and neck
- level of the shoulders
- any lateral flexion
- contour of the neck from the side

In the patient with torticollis the head is held laterally flexed with, perhaps, slight rotation to one side—usually away from the painful side. Patients suffering from whiplash injury and severe spondylosis tend to hold the neck stiff and the head forward, and tend to turn the trunk rather than rotate the neck.

Palpation

For this vital component of the examination it is essential to know the surface anatomy of the neck so that the affected level can be determined.

Method

The patient lies prone on the examination couch with the forehead resting on the hands (palms up). The neck should be flexed forward and the shoulders relaxed.

1. Central digital palpation
   Systematically palpate the first spinous processes of the cervical vertebrae.
   - C2 (axis) is the first spinous process palpable beneath the occiput.
   - C7 is the largest 'fixed' and most prominent process—situated at the base of the neck.
   - C6 is also prominent but usually 'disappears' under the palpating finger with extension of the neck.
   - The spinous processes of C3, C4 and C5 are difficult to palpate because of cervical lordosis but their level can be estimated (see FIG. 62.2).

   Standing at the patient's head, place opposed pulps of the thumbs on the spinous processes (starting at C2) and then move down the middle line to C7. Press firmly over each and with arms straight oscillate with moderate firmness three or four times to assess pain, stiffness or muscle spasm.
2. Lateral digital palpation
   The facet joints lie in sequence (called the articular pillar) about 2 to 3 cm from the midline. Press with opposed thumbs against this pillar in a systematic manner on either side of the midline (top to base) to determine any painful area. Palpation should be extended to include the anterior neck, searching for evidence of lymphadenitis, muscle spasm, thyroid disorder and other problems.

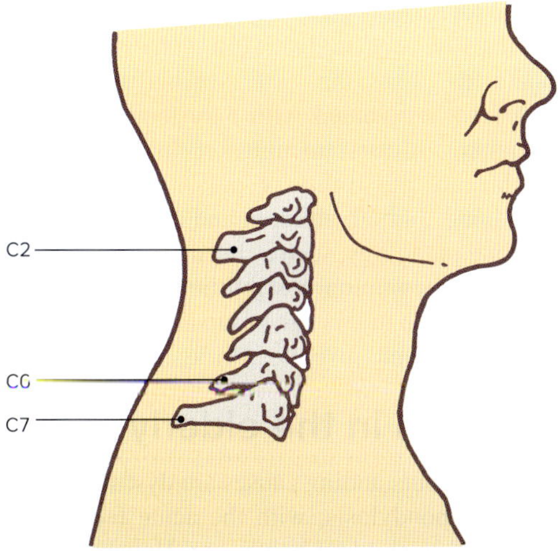

FIGURE 62.2 Relative sizes of spinous processes of the cervical spine

Movement

Active movements are observed with the patient sitting on the couch. The movements are as follows with normal range indicated:

- flexion—45°
- extension—50°
- lateral flexion (R and L)—45°
- rotation (R and L)—75°

Lhermitte sign is an electric shock-like pain throughout the body (especially in the legs) upon flexion of the neck. It indicates cervical pathology.

If there is a full range of pain-free movement, apply overpressure slowly at the end range and note any pain.

The range of movements can be plotted on a special grid called a direction of movement (DOM) diagram (see FIG. 62.3). This provides a ready reference for serial assessments.

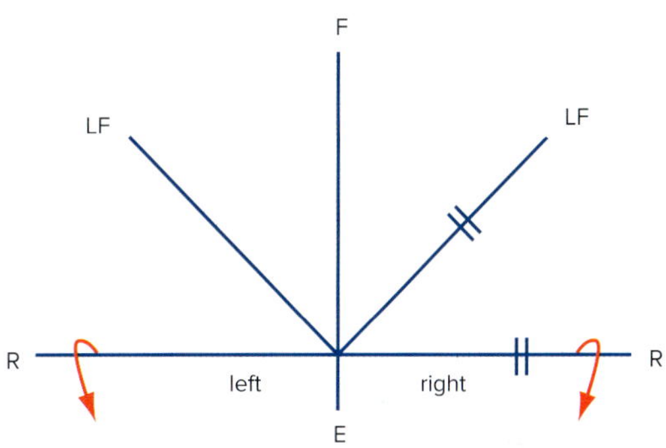

FIGURE 62.3 Direction of movement diagram to record movements of the neck. This record shows restricted and painful movements (indicated by II) in right lateral flexion and right rotation; the other movements are free

Neurological examination

A neurological examination for nerve root lesions (C5 to T1) is indicated if the clinical assessment identifies the presence of neurological symptoms and signs such as pain, paraesthesia or anaesthesia in the arm. Nerve root pressure is indicated by:

- pain and paraesthesia along the distribution of the dermatome
- localised sensory loss
- reduced muscular power (weakness or fatigue or both)
- hyporeflexia (reduced amplitude or fatigue or both)

It is necessary to know the sensory distribution for each nerve root and the motor changes. This is summarised in TABLE 62.3. The dermatomes are illustrated in FIGURE 62.4.

62

Table 62.3 Cervical nerve root syndromes

Nerve root	Sensory change	Muscle power	Power loss	Reflex
C5	Outer arm	Deltoid	Abduction arm	Biceps jerk (C5, 6)
C6	Outer forearm/thumb/ index finger	Biceps	Elbow flexion Extension wrist	Biceps + brachioradialis (C5, 6)
C7	Hand/middle and ring fingers	Triceps	Elbow extension	Triceps (C7–8)
C8	Inner forearm/little finger, e.g. pad of finger	Long flexors finger, long extensors thumb	Grip	Fingers (C8)
T1	Inner arm	Interossei	Finger spread	

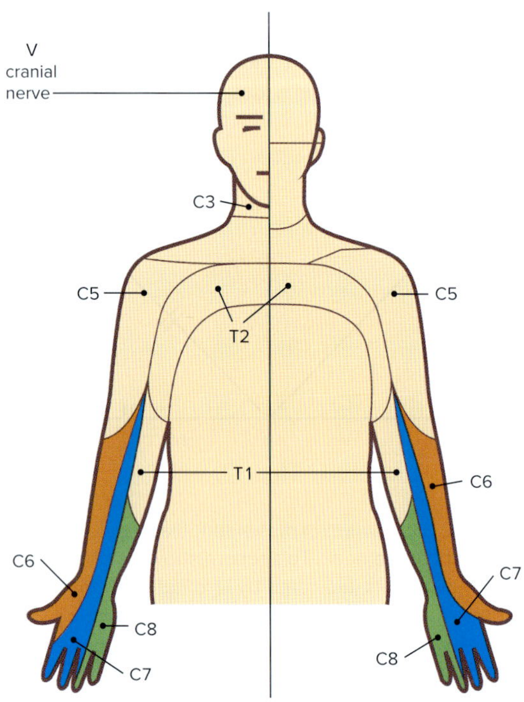

FIGURE 62.4 Dermatomes of the upper limb, head and neck

Investigations

The investigations are directed to diagnosing the painful condition and determining if suspected or true organic disease is present in the spine. It is inappropriate to perform sophisticated investigations such as CT scans on most patients. Scanning should be reserved where surgery is contemplated and serious disease is suspected but not confirmed by plain X-ray.

Investigations to consider include:

- haemoglobin, film and WCC
- ESR/CRP
- rheumatoid arthritis factor
- HLA-B_{27} antigen
- radiology:
  - plain X-ray (not indicated in absence of red flags and major trauma)
  - CT scan (good for bone definition)
  - CT scan and myelogram (if cervical disc surgery contemplated)
  - radionucleide bone scan (for suspected metastatic disease)
  - MRI: the investigation of choice for cervical radiculopathy, myelopathy, suspected spinal infection and tumour

These should be selected conservatively. CT imaging has high radiation levels.

Neck pain in children

In children and adolescents, neck pain, often with stiffness, may be a manifestation of infection or inflammation of cervical lymph nodes, usually secondary to an infected throat—for example, tonsillitis or pharyngitis. However, it is vital to consider the possibility of meningitis. Sometimes a high fever associated with a systemic infection or pneumonia can cause meningism. In the presence of fever the rare possibility of poliomyelitis should be kept in mind. In both children and adults the presence of cerebral pathology, such as haemorrhage, abscess or tumour are uncommon possibilities.[5] Acute torticollis is quite common in this age group and the neck may be involved in chronic juvenile arthritis.

Neck pain in the elderly

In adults the outstanding causes are dysfunction of the joints and spondylosis, with the acute febrile causes encountered in children being rare. However, cerebral and meningeal disorders may cause pain and stiffness in the neck.[5]

Rheumatoid arthritis is the prime severe inflammatory arthropathy that involves the neck, but the neck can be affected by the spondyloarthropathies (e.g. ankylosing spondylitis). The painful, acute wry neck can affect all ages and is considered to be caused mainly by acute disorders of the apophyseal joints rather than disc prolapse. However, disc lesions do occur and can cause referred pain or radicular pain. In the elderly, radicular pain can also be caused by impingement of the nerve root in the intervertebral foramen that has become narrowed from the degenerative changes of longstanding spondylosis.

Problems with a higher probability with increasing age include:

- cervical spondylosis with radiculopathy or myelopathy
- atlantoaxial subluxation complicating rheumatoid arthritis
- polymyalgia rheumatica
- metastatic cancer
- Pancoast tumour of the lung
- angina and myocardial infarction
- pharyngeal and retropharyngeal infection and tumour

Clinical problems of cervical spinal origin

Pain originating from disorders of the cervical spine is usually, although not always, experienced in the neck. The patient may experience headache, or pain around the ear, face, arm, shoulder, upper anterior or posterior chest.[5]

Possible symptoms include:

- neck pain
- neck stiffness
- headache
- migraine-like headache
- facial pain
- arm pain (referred or radicular)
- myelopathy (sensory and motor changes in arms and legs)
- ipsilateral sensory changes of scalp
- ear pain (peri-auricular)
- scapular pain
- anterior chest pain
- torticollis
- dizziness/vertigo
- visual dysfunction

FIGURE 24.1 in CHAPTER 24 indicates typical directions of referred pain from the cervical spine. Pain in the arm (brachialgia) is common and tends to cover the shoulder and upper arm as indicated.

CERVICAL DYSFUNCTION

Dysfunction of the 35 intervertebral joints that comprise the cervical spine complex is responsible for most cases of neck pain. The problem can occur at all ages and appears to be caused by disorder (including malalignment) of the many facet joints, which are pain-sensitive. Dysfunction of these joints, which may also be secondary to intervertebral disc disruption, initiates a reflex response of adjacent muscle spasm and myofascial tenderness.

Acute neck pain

Acute neck pain (ANP) is most commonly idiopathic or due to a whiplash accident. Serious causes are rare.[6] Dysfunction can follow obvious trauma such as a blow to the head or a sharp jerk to the neck, but can be caused by repeated trivial trauma or activity such as painting a ceiling or gentle wrestling. People often wake up with severe neck pain and blame it on a 'chill' from a draught on the neck during the night. This is incorrect because it is usually caused by an unusual twist on the flexed neck for a long period during sleep.

Clinical features[7]

- Typical age range 12–50 years
- Dull ache (may be sharp) in neck
- May radiate to occiput, ear, face and temporal area (upper cervical)
- May radiate to shoulder region, especially suprascapular area (lower cervical)
- Rarely refers pain below the level of the shoulder
- Pain aggravated by activity, improved with rest
- Various degrees of stiffness
- Neck tends to lock with specific movements, usually rotation
- Localised unilateral tenderness over affected joints
- Variable restriction of movement but may be normal
- X-rays usually normal: plain X-rays are not indicated for the investigation of ANP in the absence of 'red flags' and a history of trauma[6]

Management

The aim of treatment is to reduce pain, maintain function and minimise the risk of chronicity.

- Provide appropriate reassurance, information and support.

62

- Give advice to the patient about rules of living, including the following:
  Do:
  - Stay active and resume normal activities.
  - Keep your neck upright in a vertical position for reading, typing and so on.
  - Keep a good posture—keep the chin tucked in.
  - Sleep on a low, firm pillow or a special conforming pillow.
  - Sleep with your painful side on the pillow.
  - Use heat and massage: massage your neck firmly three times a day using an analgesic ointment.

  Don't:
  - Look up in a strained position for long periods.
  - Twist your head often towards the painful side (e.g. when reversing a car).
  - Lift or tug with your neck bent forwards.
  - Work, read or study with your neck bent for long periods.
  - Become too dependent on 'collars'.
  - Sleep on too many pillows.
- Monitor the patient's progress without overtreatment.
- Analgesia:[7]
  - first line: paracetamol 1 g (o) qid or 1.33 g (o) 8-hourly
  - consider tricyclic antidepressant for night pain or resistant pain
- Prescribe an exercise program as early as possible; start with gentle exercises and maintain them at home. Suitable exercises are shown in FIGURE 62.5.
- Refer to an appropriate therapist for cervical mobilisation for persisting pain. Mobilisation combined with exercises can be an effective treatment. Occasionally, manipulation may help with a stubborn 'locked' neck but should be left to an expert. If manipulation, which carries the rare but real risk of vertebral artery dissection and stroke, is to be performed, informed consent and an experienced therapist are required.[8]

Approximately 40% of patients recover fully from acute idiopathic ANP, about 30% continue to have mild symptoms, while 30% continue to have moderate or severe symptoms.[6]

> **Evidence of benefit (in summary)[6]**
>
> - Staying active: resuming normal activities
> - Exercises
> - Combined cervical passive mobilisation/exercises
> - Pulsed electromagnetic therapy (up to 12 weeks)

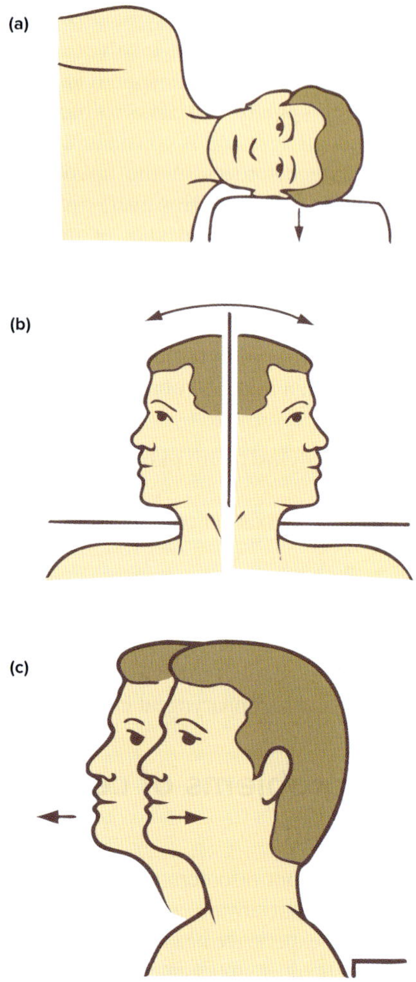

FIGURE 62.5 Examples of exercises for the neck: **(a)** resisted side bending, **(b)** rotation, **(c)** chin retraction

Chronic non-specific pain (lasting more than 3 months)[7]

Continue normal activities and exercises.

Additional treatment modalities to consider include:

- a course of antidepressants
- TENS, especially when drugs are not tolerated
- hydrotherapy
- acupuncture (may provide short-term relief)
- corticosteroid facet injections (ideally under image intensification)
- facet joint denervation with percutaneous radiofrequency (if nerve block provides relief)
- multidisciplinary rehabilitation program

Cervical spondylosis[7]

Cervical spondylosis following disc degeneration and apophyseal joint degeneration is far more common than lumbar spondylosis and mainly involves the C5–6 and C6–7 segments. The consequence is narrowing of the intervertebral foramen with the nerve roots of C6 and C7 being at risk of compression.

Cervical spondylosis is generally a chronic problem but it may be asymptomatic. In some patients the pain may lessen with age, while stiffness increases.

Clinical features

- Dull, aching suboccipital neck pain (see FIG. 62.6)
- Stiffness
- Worse in morning on arising and lifting head
- Improves with gentle activity and warmth (e.g. warm showers)
- Deteriorates with heavy activity (e.g. working under car, painting ceiling)

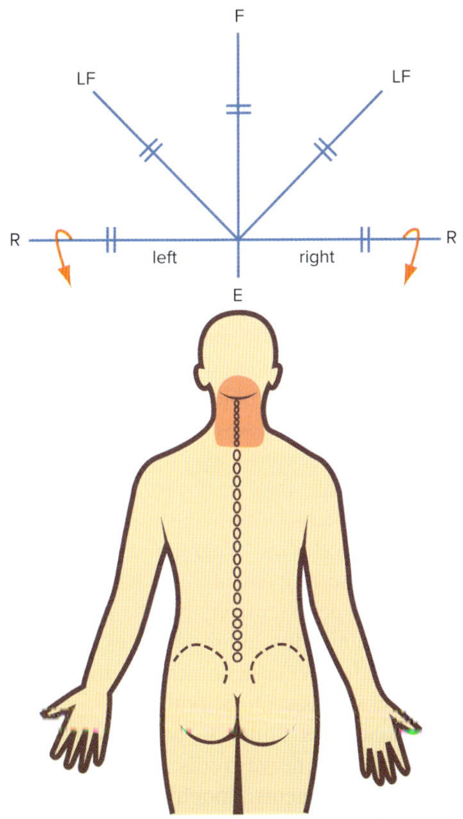

FIGURE 62.6 Cervical spondylosis: typical pain distribution with direction of movement diagram indicating painful and restricted movements

- Usually unilateral pain—may be bilateral
- Pain may be referred to head, arms and scapulae
- May wake patient at night with paraesthesia in arms
- C6 nerve root most commonly involved
- Acute attacks on chronic background
- Aggravated by flexion (reading) and extension
- Associated vertigo or unsteadiness
- Restricted tender movements, especially rotation/lateral flexion
- Joints tender to palpation
- X-ray changes invariable

Treatment

- Provide appropriate reassurance, information and support.
- Refer for physiotherapy, including warm hydrotherapy.
- Use regular mild analgesics (e.g. paracetamol).
- Use NSAIDs: a trial for 2 weeks and then review.
- Prescribe gentle mobilising exercises as early as possible.
- Give passive mobilising techniques.
- Outline general rules to live by, including advice regarding sleeping and pillows, and day-to-day activities.

Complications

- Radiculopathy (unilateral or bilateral)
- Myelopathy—pressure on spinal cord
- Spinal canal stenosis

Acute torticollis

Torticollis (acute wry neck) means a lateral deformity of the neck. This is usually a transient self-limiting acutely painful disorder with associated muscle spasm of variable intensity.

Clinical features

- Age of patient between 12 and 30 years
- Patient usually awakes with the problem
- Pain usually confined to neck but may radiate
- Deformity of lateral flexion and slight flexion/rotation
- Deformity usually away from the painful side
- Loss of extension
- Mid-cervical spine (C2–3, C3–4, C4–5)
- Any segment between C2 and C7 can cause torticollis
- Usually no neurological symptoms or signs

The exact cause of this condition is uncertain, but both an acute disc lesion and apophyseal joint lesion are implicated, with the latter the more likely cause. Acute torticollis is usually a transient and self-limiting condition that can recover within 48 hours. Sometimes it can last for about a week. Encourage heat massage and early mobility. Avoid cervical collars. Management by mobilisation and muscle energy therapy is very effective.

Muscle energy therapy

This amazingly effective therapy relies on the basic physiological principle that the contracting and stretching of muscles leads to automatic relaxation of agonist and antagonist muscles.[9,10] Lateral flexion or rotation or a combination of movements can be used, but treatment in rotation is preferred. The direction of contraction can be away from the painful side (preferred) or towards the painful side, whichever is most comfortable for the patient.

62

Method

1. Explain the method to the patient, with reassurance that it is not painful.
2. Rotate the patient's head passively and gently towards the painful side to the limit of pain (the motion barrier).
3. Place your hand against the head on the side opposite the painful one. The other (free) hand can be used to steady the painful level—usually C3–4.
4. Request the patient to push the head (in rotation) as firmly as possible against the resistance of your hand. The patient should therefore be producing a strong isometric contraction of the neck in rotation away from the painful side (see FIG. 62.7A). Your counterforce (towards the painful side) should be firm and moderate (never forceful) and should not 'break' through the patient's resistance.
5. After 5–10 seconds (average 7 seconds) ask the patient to relax; then passively stretch the neck gently towards the patient's painful side (see FIG. 62.7B).
6. The patient will now be able to turn the head a little further towards the painful side.
7. This sequence is repeated at the new improved motion barrier. Repeat three to five times until the full range of movement returns.
8. Ask the patient to return the following day for treatment, although the neck may be almost normal.

The patient can be taught self-treatment at home using this method.

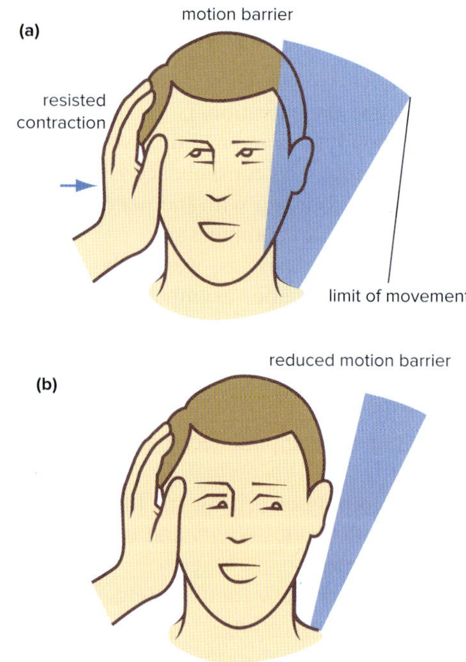

FIGURE 62.7 Muscle energy therapy for acute torticollis: **(a)** isometric contraction phase for problem on the left side, **(b)** relaxation phase towards the affected (left) side

Acceleration hyperextension (whiplash) injury

Patients with the whiplash syndrome, preferably referred to as an acceleration hyperextension injury, typically present with varying degrees of pain-related loss of mobility of the cervical spine, headache and emotional disturbance in the form of anxiety and depression. The problem can vary from mild temporary disability to a severe and protracted course.

The injury occurs as a consequence of hyperextension of the neck followed by recoil hyperflexion, typically following a rear-end collision between motor vehicles. There is a reversal of the sequence of these movements in a head-on collision. In addition to hyperextension, there is prolongation or anterior stretching plus longitudinal extension of the neck.[8] It can also occur with other vehicle accidents and in contact sports such as football.

Whiplash causes injury to soft tissue structures, including muscle, nerve roots, the cervical sympathetic chain, ligaments, apophyseal joints and their synovial capsules and intervertebral discs. Damage to the apophyseal joints appears to be severe, with possible microfractures (not detectable on plain X-ray) and long-term dysfunction.

Pain and stiffness of the neck are the most common symptoms. The pain is usually experienced in the neck and upper shoulders but may radiate to the suboccipital region, the interscapular region and down the arms. The stiffness felt initially in the anterior neck muscles shifts to the posterior neck.

Headache is a common and disabling symptom that may persist for many months. It is typically occipital but can be referred to the temporal region and the eyes.

Nerve root pain can be caused by a traction injury of the cervical nerve roots or by inflammatory changes or direct pressure subsequent to herniation of a disc.

Paraesthesia of the ulnar border of the hand, nausea and dizziness are all relatively common symptoms.

Delayed symptoms are common. A patient may feel no pain until 24 (sometimes up to 96) hours later; most experience symptoms within 6 hours. Complications of whiplash are summarised in TABLE 62.4.

Table 62.4 Complications of whiplash
Referred pain (headache, arm pain)
Visual problems
Vertigo
Dysphagia
Depression
Compensation neurosis
Disc rupture increasing to nerve root pain
Osteoarthritis becomes symptomatic

The Canadian guidelines (1995) for whiplash are:

- Grade I—neck pain, stiffness or tenderness
- Grade II—neck symptoms + musculoskeletal signs (e.g. decreased range of motion, point tenderness)
- Grade III—neck symptoms + neurological signs
- Grade IV—neck symptoms + fracture or dislocation

Management principles

The objective of treatment is to obtain a full range of free movement of the neck without pain by attending to both the physical and the psychological components of the problem. Other objectives include an early return to work and discouragement of unnecessary and excessive reliance on cervical collars and legal action.

Treatment

- Establish an appropriate empathy and instil patient confidence with a positive, professional approach. Discourage multiple therapists.
- Provide appropriate reassurance and patient education.
- Encourage normalisation of activities as soon as possible.
- Compare the problem with a sprained ankle, which is a similar injury.
- Inform that an emotional reaction of anger, frustration and temporary depression is common (lasts about 2 weeks). Offer psychotherapy, e.g. CBT for evidence of post-traumatic stress.
- X-ray is required for 'red flags'.
- Prescribe rest only for grades II and III (max. 4 days).
- Use a cervical collar (limit to 2 days) for grades II and III. Provide collar and refer for grade IV.
- Use analgesics (e.g. paracetamol)—avoid narcotics.
- Use a trial of NSAIDs for 14 days (poor evidence).
- Use tranquillisers, mild—up to 2 weeks.
- Refer for physiotherapy.
- Provide neck exercises (as early as possible).
- Use heat and massage—'spray and stretch'—or ice.
- Give passive mobilisation (not manipulation).[9]

Recovery can take any time from 1–2 weeks up to about 3 months. A valuable reference is *Update Quebec Task Force Guidelines for the Management of Whiplash—Associated Disorder* at <www.nhmrc.gov.au/guidelines/>.

Cervical disc disruption

Disruption of a cervical disc can result in several different syndromes.

1 Referred pain over a widespread area due to pressure on adjacent dura mater.
Note: A disc disruption is capable of referring pain over such a diffuse area (see FIG. 62.8) that the patient is sometimes diagnosed as functional (e.g. hysterical).
2 Nerve root or radicular pain (radiculopathy). The pain follows the dermatomal distribution of the nerve root in the arm.
3 Spinal cord compression (myelopathy).

Radiculopathy

Apart from protrusion from an intervertebral disc, nerve root pressure or irritation causing arm pain can be caused by osteophytes associated with cervical spondylosis. Uncommon causes include various tumours involving the vertebral segment, the meninges and nerves or their sheaths. The pain follows

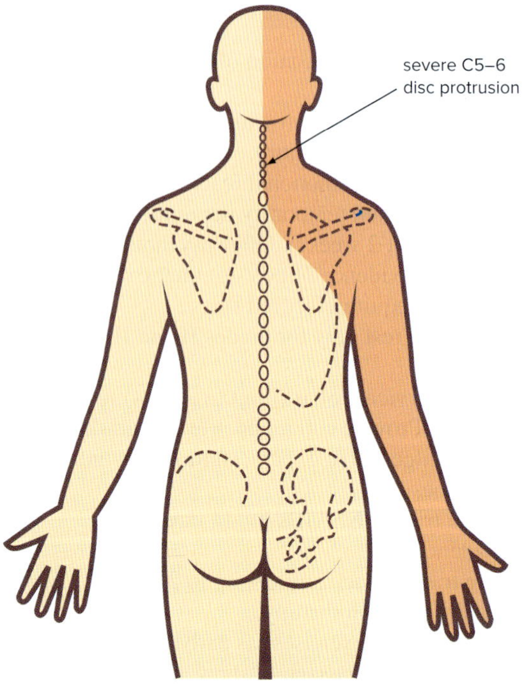

FIGURE 62.8 Zone of possible referred pain distribution caused by a cervical disc lesion on the right side

neurological patterns down the arm, being easier to localise with lower cervical roots, especially C6, C7 and C8.

1 The cervical roots exit above their respective vertebral bodies. For example, the C6 root exits between C5 and C6 so that a prolapse of C5–6 intervertebral disc or spondylosis of the C5–6 junction affects primarily the C6 root (see FIG. 62.4).
2 One disc—one nerve root is the rule.
3 Spondylosis and tumours tend to cause bilateral pain (i.e. more than one nerve root).

Clinical features

- A sharp aching pain in the neck, radiating down one or both arms
- Onset of pain may be abrupt, often precipitated by a sudden neck movement on awakening
- Paraesthesia in the forearm and hand (in particular)—in 90% with proven disc prolapse[9]
- Stiffness of neck with limitation of movement
- Nocturnal pain, waking patient during night
- Pain localised to upper trapezius and possible muscle spasm

Investigations

- Plain X-ray (AP, lateral extension and flexion, oblique views to visualise foramina); not required before 6–8 weeks unless red flags present; not useful for diagnosis or for surgery
- Plain CT scan
- CT scan and myelogram—excellent visualisation of structures but invasive
- MRI—excellent but expensive, sometimes difficult to distinguish soft disc from osteophytes
- Electromyography—may help delineate lesions requiring surgery

Treatment

Many patients respond to conservative treatment, especially from a disc prolapse. It is basically a self-limiting disorder—about 10% remain severely disabled:[10]

- bed rest
- soft cervical collar
- analgesics (according to severity—see CHAPTER 38)
- consider a course of corticosteroids for severe neck radicular pain, e.g. prednisone 30 mg (o) daily for 5–10 days then taper off to 3 weeks (limited evidence)[8]
- tranquillisers, especially at night
- traction (with care)
- careful mobilisation (manipulation is contraindicated)

CERVICAL SPONDYLITIC MYELOPATHY

Sometimes the presence of large or multiple osteophytes or in the presence of a narrowed spinal canal symptoms of spinal cord involvement may develop.[11,12] The common cause is a hard mass of material projecting from the posterior aspect of the vertebral body to indent the spinal cord and possibly the nerve roots at the exit foramina. This resultant spinal cord compression may result in several different clinical presentations, notably myelopathy in particular, but also central cord and anterior cord syndrome. A full neurological assessment is necessary.

Clinical features

- Older patients, typically men >50 years
- Insidious onset—symptoms over 1–2 years
- Numbness and tingling in fingers
- Leg stiffness
- Gait disturbance
- Numb, clumsy hands, especially with a high cervical lesion

- Signs of UMN: spastic weakness, increased tone and hyper-reflexia (arms > legs) ± clonus
- Neurological deficit, which predicts the level with reasonable accuracy
- Bowel and bladder function usually spared

Note: LMN signs occur at the level of the lesion, and UMN signs and sensory changes occur below this level.

Causes

- Cervical spondylosis
- Atlantoaxial subluxation: rheumatoid arthritis, Down syndrome
- Primary spinal cord tumours (e.g. meningiomas)
- Metastasis to cervical spine → epidural spinal cord compression

Investigations

- MRI scan
- CT scan with myelogram (most accurate)

Central cord syndrome[12]

This rather bizarre condition occurs classically in a patient with a degenerative cervical spine following a hyperextension injury that causes osteophytes to compress the cord anteriorly and posteriorly simultaneously.

The maximum damage occurs in the central part of the cord, leading to sensory and motor changes in the upper limbs with relative sparing of the lower limbs due to the arrangements of the long tracts in the cord.

Fortunately, the prognosis is good, with most patients achieving a good neurological recovery.

Anterior cord syndrome

Anterior cord syndrome occurs with hyperflexion injuries that produce 'teardrop' fractures of the vertebral bodies or extrusion of disc material. The syndrome can also be produced by comminuted vertebral body fractures.

It is characterised by complete motor loss and the loss of pain and temperature discrimination below the level of the injury, but deep touch, position, two-point discrimination and vibration sensation remain intact.

Because it is probably associated with obstruction of the anterior spinal artery, early surgical intervention to relieve pressure on the front of the cord may enhance recovery. Otherwise the prognosis for recovery is poor.

Down syndrome

One of the more sinister problems with trisomy 21 syndrome is hypoplasia of the odontoid process, leading to C1–2 subluxation and dislocation. If unrecognised in the early stages, sudden death can occur in these children. If suspected, flexion–extension lateral views of the cervical spine will highlight the developing instability and the need for early specialist opinion.

Rheumatoid arthritis[7,15]

Involvement of the cervical spine is usually a late manifestation of rheumatoid arthritis (RA). It is important to be aware of the potentially lethal problem of C1–2 instability due to erosion of the major odontoid ligaments in the rheumatoid patient. These patients are especially vulnerable to disasters when under general anaesthesia and when involved in motor vehicle accidents. Early cervical fusion can prevent tragedies, especially with inappropriate procedures such as cervical manipulation. It is imperative to perform imaging of the cervical spine of all patients with severe RA before major surgery to search for C1–2 instability. Lateral plain X-rays in flexion and extension may reveal increased distance in the atlanto–dens interval. This can be assessed further with MRI or CT scanning in a specialist clinic.

62

Treatment of spondylitic myelopathy

Conservative (may help up to 50%):[2]

- soft cervical collar
- physiotherapy for muscle weakness
- analgesics and/or NSAIDs

Surgery is indicated when the myelopathy interferes with daily activities. One procedure is the Cloward method, which is anterior decompression with discectomy and fusion. The aim of surgery is to halt deterioration.

When to refer

- Persisting radicular pain in an arm despite conservative treatment
- Evidence of involvement of more than one nerve root lesion in the arm
- Severe symptoms with motor weakness
- Evidence of myelopathy, such as weakness, numbness or clumsiness of the upper limbs

- Evidence, clinical or radiological, of cervical instability in post-accident victims, or people with Down syndrome or rheumatoid arthritis

Practice tips

- 'One disc—one nerve root' is a working rule for the cervical spine.
- The patient should sit on the couch with the thighs fully supported for inspection and movements of the neck.
- Be alert for patients with RA and Down syndrome who have cervical instability. Physical treatments such as cervical manipulation may easily cause quadriplegia.
- All acutely painful conditions of the cervical spine following trauma should be investigated with a careful neurological examination of the limbs, sphincter tone and reflexes. Plain film radiology is mandatory.
- In conscious patients, flexion and extension lateral cervical spinal plain films are useful for diagnosing instability of spinal segments with or without associated spinal fractures.
- The so-called whiplash syndrome is a diagnosis of exclusion of spinal fractures or severe ligamentous disruption causing instability, and even then, for medicolegal and psychological reasons, would best be termed a 'soft tissue injury of the cervical spine'.
- Most 'soft tissue cervical spine injuries' heal within 3 months with conservative treatment. If severe pain persists, follow-up investigations may be required.
- Dysfunction of the cervical spine is an underestimated cause of headache.
- Always consider dysfunction of the cervical spine as a possible cause of shoulder pain.
- Strains and fractures of the apophyseal joints, especially after a whiplash injury, are difficult to detect, and are often overlooked causes of neck and referred pain.

Patient education resources

Hand-out sheets from *Murtagh's Patient Education* 7th edition:

- Exercises for your neck
- Neck: painful neck
- Whiplash
- Wry neck (torticollis)

References

1. Gordon SJ, Trott P, Grimmer KA. Waking cervical pain and stiffness, headache, scapula or arm pain: gender and age effects. Australian Journal of Physiotherapy, 2002; 48 (1): 9–15.
2. Cohen ML. Neck pain. Modern Medicine Australia, 1989; November: 44–53.
3. Payne R. Neck pain in the elderly: a management review. Modern Medicine Australia, 1988; July: 56–67.
4. Bogduk N. Neck pain. Aust Fam Physician, 1984; 13: 26–9.
5. Hart FD. *Practical Problems in Rheumatology.* London: Dunitz, 1985: 10–14.
6. Australian Acute Musculoskeletal Pain Guidelines Group, National Health and Medical Research Council. *Evidence-Based Management of Acute Musculoskeletal Pain: A Guide for Clinicians.* Canberra: Australian Government, 2003: 36–43.
7. Global Burden of Disease Study 2013 Collaborators. Global, regional, and national incidence, prevalence, and years lived with disability for 301 acute and chronic diseases and injuries in 188 countries, 1990–2013: a systematic analysis for the Global Burden of Disease Study 2013. The Lancet, 2015; 22: 743–800.
8. Moulds R (Chair). *Therapeutic Guidelines: Rheumatology* (Version 2). Melbourne: Therapeutic Guidelines Ltd, 2010.
9. Vincent K et al. Systematic review of manual therapies for nonspecific neck pain. Joint Bone Spine, 2013; 80 (5): 508–15.
10. Beran RG et al. Serious complications with neck manipulation and informed consent. Med J Aust, 2000; 173: 213–14.
11. Kenna C, Murtagh J. *Back Pain and Spinal Manipulation* (2nd edn). Oxford: Butterworth-Heinemann, 1997: 83–99.
12. Bogduk N. *Medical Management of Acute Cervical Radicular Pain: An Evidence Based Approach.* Newcastle: Newcastle Bone and Joint Institute, 1999: 5–59.
13. Porter RS, Kaplan JL. *The Merck Manual* (19th edn). Whitehorse Station: Merck, Sharpe & Dohme Corp., 2011: 1808–9.
14. Young D, Murtagh J. Pitfalls in orthopaedics. Aust Fam Physician, 1989; 18: 645–6.
15. Zhang T, Pope J. Cervical spine involvement in rheumatoid arthritis over time: results from a meta-analysis. Arthritis Res Ther, 2015; 17: 148.

Shoulder pain

63

Search for clues—difficulty reaching into the hip pocket to remove a wallet may indicate loss of function due to total rupture of the supraspinatus tendon, while a complete rotator-cuff tear may lead the patient to lift the affected limb to the clothes line and leave it suspended there by the hand while hanging out the laundry.

MICHAEL HAYES 1996

The painful shoulder is a relatively common and sometimes complex problem encountered in general practice. The diagnostic approach involves determining whether the disorder causing the pain arises from within the shoulder structures or from other sources such as the cervical spine (see FIG. 63.1), the acromioclavicular (AC) joint or diseased viscera, especially the heart, lungs and sub-diaphragmatic structures.

Key facts and checkpoints

- Virtually all shoulder structures are innervated by the fifth cervical vertebra (C5) nerve root. Pain present in the distribution of the C5 nerve can arise from the:
  - cervical spine
  - upper roots of brachial plexus
  - acromioclavicular joint
  - glenohumeral joint
  - rotator cuff tendons, especially supraspinatus
  - biceps tendon
  - soft tissue (e.g. polymyalgia rheumatica)
  - viscera, especially those innervated by the phrenic nerve (C3, C4, C5)
- The visceral diseases causing a painful shoulder include cardiac disorders, such as angina and pericarditis; lung diseases, especially Pancoast tumour; mediastinal disorders; and diaphragmatic irritation, as from intra-abdominal bleeding or a subphrenic abscess.
- A careful history should generally indicate whether the neck or the shoulder is responsible for the patient's pain.
- By the age of 50, about 25% of people have some wear and tear of the rotator cuff, making it more injury-prone.[1]
- Disorders of the rotator cuff are common, especially supraspinatus tendonopathy. The most effective tests to diagnose these problems are the resisted movement tests.[1]
- Injections of local anaesthetic and long-acting corticosteroid produce excellent results for inflammatory disorders around the shoulder joint, especially for supraspinatus tendonopathy.
- The diagnosis is usually made on the history and examination. Blood tests are usually not necessary and imaging has a limited place and value.[2]

Note: The term tendonopathy or tendonosis is preferred to tendonitis since it has been shown that overuse tendon conditions generally have a non-inflammatory pathology.

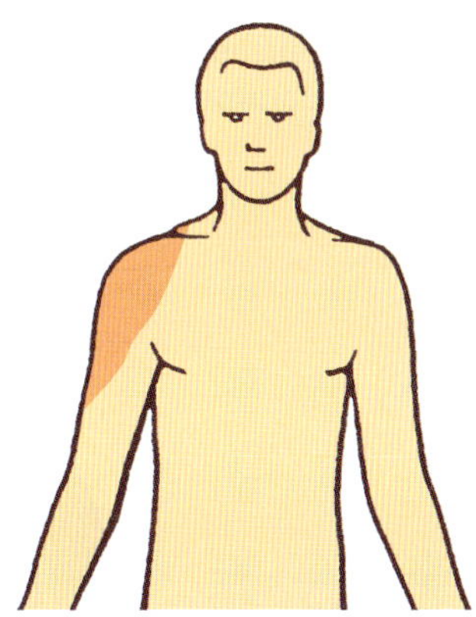

FIGURE 63.1 Typical pain zone arising from disorders of the shoulder joint and the lower cervical spine (C5 level)

Functional anatomy of the shoulder

A working knowledge of the anatomical features of the shoulder is essential for understanding the various disorders causing pain or dysfunction of the shoulder. Apart from the AC joint there are two most significant functional joints—the glenohumeral (the primary joint) and the subacromial complex (the secondary joint) (see FIG. 63.2). The glenohumeral joint is a ball and socket joint enveloped by a loose capsule. It is prone to injury from traumatic forces and develops osteoarthritis more often than appreciated. Two other relevant functional joints are the scapulothoracic and sternoclavicular joints.

The clinically important perihumeral space lies above the glenohumeral joint (GHJ) between the head of the humerus and an arch formed by the bony acromion, the thick coracoacromial ligament and the coracoid process. This relatively tight compartment houses the subacromial bursa and the rotator cuff, particularly the vulnerable supraspinatus tendon.[3] Excessive friction and pinching in this space render these structures prone to injury.

There is a critical zone of relative ischaemia that appears to affect the rotator cuff about 1 cm medial to the attachment of the supraspinatus tendon,[4] and this area is compromised during adduction and abduction of the arm due to pressure on the rotator cuff tendons from the head of the humerus. The so-called 'impingement interval' is the space between the undersurface of the acromion and the superior aspect of the humeral head. This space is normally narrow (6–14 mm), especially when the arm is abducted.

63

Such factors are largely responsible for the many rotator cuff syndromes, including subacromial bursitis and lesions of the supraspinatus tendon and also bicipital tendonopathy.

A diagnostic approach

A summary of the diagnostic strategy model is presented in TABLE 63.1.

Probability diagnosis

The commonest causes of pain in the shoulder zone (see FIG. 63.1) are cervical disorders and periarthritis (i.e. soft tissue lesions involving the tendons around the glenohumeral joint). The outstanding common disorders of the shoulder joint are the rotator cuff disorders and adhesive capsulitis. Of these, supraspinatus tendon disorders are the commonest. It is obvious that the supraspinatus tendon is subjected to considerable friction and wear and tear. For acute shoulder pain presentation consider rotator cuff disorders (including calcific tendonitis and an acute tear) and adhesive capsulitis.

Serious disorders not to be missed

As usual it is important to exclude any malignancy or septic infection, be it septic arthritis or osteomyelitis. Lung cancer (Pancoast syndrome), myeloma and bony metastases should be kept in mind. For pain in the region of the left shoulder the possibility of myocardial ischaemia has to be considered. Referred pain to the right shoulder from myocardial ischaemia is rare, occurring about once for every 20 episodes of left shoulder referral.

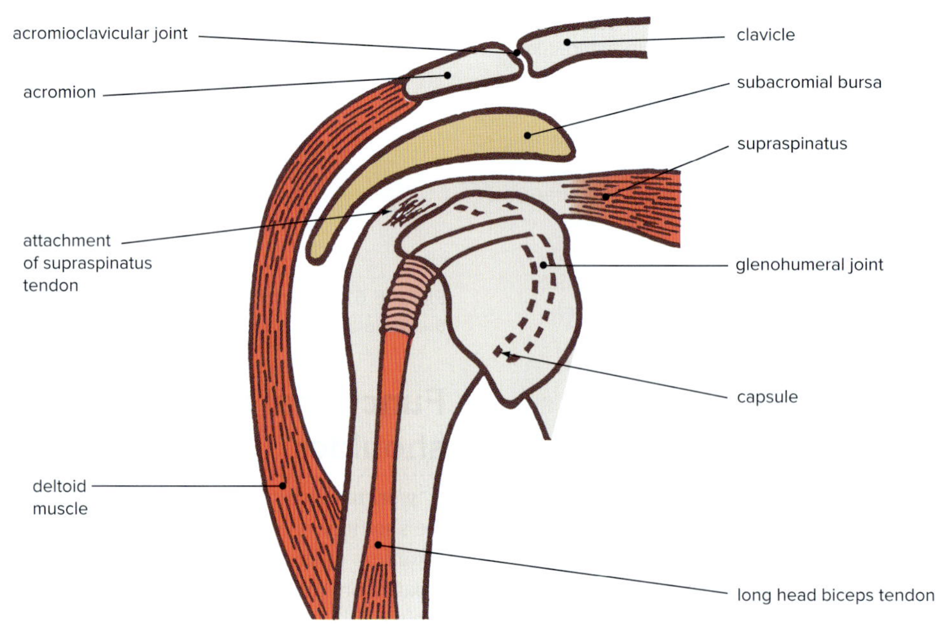

FIGURE 63.2 The basic anatomical structures of the shoulder joint

Table 63.1	Shoulder pain: diagnostic strategy model
Probability diagnosis Cervical spine dysfunction (referred pain) Rotator cuff tendonopathy ± a tear Adhesive capsulitis AC joint disorders Glenoid labral tears	
Serious disorders not to be missed Cardiovascular: • angina • myocardial infarction Neoplasia: • Pancoast tumour • primary or secondary in humerus Severe infections: • septic arthritis (especially children) • osteomyelitis Axillary vein thrombosis Rheumatoid arthritis Intra-abdominal pathology e.g. bleeding	
Pitfalls (often missed) Polymyalgia rheumatica Cervical dysfunction Gout/pseudogout (uncommon) Osteoarthritis of acromioclavicular joint Bicipital tendon lesions Winged scapula—muscular fatigue pain	
Seven masquerades checklist Depression Diabetes Drugs Thyroid disorder (rarely) Spinal dysfunction	
Is the patient trying to tell me something? Shoulder is prone to (uncommonly) psychological fixation for secondary gains, depression and conversion reaction.	

Referred pain from the diaphragm and intra-abdominal disorders (e.g. biliary, perforated ulcer, splenic rupture) should be kept in mind.

With an acute onset of painful capsulitis the possibility of rheumatoid arthritis (or even gout) is worth considering.

Pitfalls

The shoulder is notorious for diagnostic traps, especially for referred pain from visceral structures, but polymyalgia rheumatica is the real pitfall. A good rule is to consider it foremost in any older person (over 60) presenting with bilateral shoulder girdle pain that is worse in the morning.

Specific pitfalls include:

- misdiagnosing posterior dislocation of the shoulder joint
- misdiagnosing recurrent subluxation of the shoulder joint
- overlooking an avascular humeral head (post fracture)
- misdiagnosing rotator cuff tear or degeneration

Seven masquerades checklist

Of the seven primary masquerades, spinal dysfunction and depression are those most likely to be associated with shoulder pain. The degree to which cervical spondylosis is associated with shoulder pain is not always appreciated.

It is important to realise that patients' perception of pain in the 'shoulder' may be amazing. For example, pain in the lower border of the scapula may be referred to as shoulder pain.

Diabetics have a higher incidence of adhesive capsulitis. Drugs are relevant as corticosteroids can cause avascular necrosis of the humeral head and anabolic steroids (weight-lifters) can cause osteolysis of the AC joint.

A summary of common shoulder conditions is presented in TABLE 63.2.

The clinical approach

History

In analysing the pain pattern it is appropriate to keep the various causes of shoulder pain in mind (see TABLE 63.3). Many of these conditions, such as rheumatoid arthritis, osteoarthritis and gout, are relatively uncommon.

A careful history should generally indicate whether the neck or the shoulder (or both) is responsible for the patient's pain. Enquire about features of movement:

- stiffness and restriction
- excessive movement/instability
- weakness
- rough versus smooth

Red flag pointers for shoulder pain[6]

- Fever (septic arthritis, osteomyelitis)
- Skin redness or swelling
- History of trauma (dislocation, fracture, rotary cuff tear)
- History of inflammatory arthritis
- Past history cancer
- Motor or sensory loss in arm

Table 63.2 Common shoulder conditions (after Murrell)[5]

Problem	Structure affected	Typical age group	Symptoms	Diagnostic pointers
Instability	Labrum/capsule	15–35	Dislocations	History of dislocation, apprehension sign
Stiffness	Capsule	40–60	Pain, night pain, loss of movement	Loss of external rotation
Impingement	Rotator cuff (fatigue)	30–60	Night pain, pain with overhead activities	Impingement signs
Rotator cuff tear	Rotator cuff esp. supraspinatus	50 +	As above	Impingement signs, weakness external rotation, weakness supraspinatus
Capsulitis	GHJ capsule	50–60	Constant severe pain, stiffness	Loss of all movements
AC joint pain	AC joint cartilage	25–45	Localised AC joint pain	Paxinos sign
Arthritis	GHJ cartilage	70 +	Pain, loss of movement	Crepitus

Table 63.3 Causes of shoulder pain (excluding trauma, fractures and dislocations)

Cervical:
- dysfunction
- spondylosis

Cervical radiculopathy

Polymyalgia rheumatica (bilateral)

Acromioclavicular joint:
- dysfunction
- osteoarthritis

Shoulder complex

Extracapsular:
- subacromial bursitis
- rotator cuff disorders:
    - — supraspinatus tendonopathy
    - — infraspinatus tendonopathy
    - — subscapularis tendonopathy
- bicipital tendonopathy

Intracapsular (glenohumeral joint):
- adhesive capsulitis:
    - — idiopathic
    - — blunt trauma
    - — diabetes
    - — others
- rheumatoid inflammation:
    - — rheumatoid arthritis
    - — ankylosing spondylitis
    - — psoriatic arthropathy
- osteoarthritis
- avascular necrosis
- septic arthritis

Winged scapula—muscular fatigue pain

Malignant disease:
- primary or secondary in humerus
- Pancoast (referred from lung)

Referred pain

Cardiac:
- ischaemic heart disease
- pericarditis

Gall bladder

Lung
- mediastinum, including oesophagus
- diaphragmatic irritation

Herpes zoster

Key questions

- Did you have any injury, even very minor, before your pain started?
- Does the pain keep you awake at night?
- Do you have pain or stiffness in your neck?
- Do you have pain or restriction when clipping or handling your bra or touching your shoulder blades? (indicates painful internal rotation and a problem of capsular restriction or a disorder of the acromioclavicular joint)
- Do you have trouble combing or attending to your hair? (indicates problematic external rotation—infraspinatus—and also a disorder of the capsule, e.g. adhesive capsulitis)
- Is the pain worse when you wake in the morning? (indicates inflammation)

- Do you have aching in both your shoulders or around your hips?
- Do you get pain associated with sporting activity, including weight training, or with housework, dressing or other activities?
- Do you think you can throw a ball underhand for 10–20 m and/or overhead for 20–25 m with your affected arm?
- Can you lift a full 2 L container (e.g. milk) to the level of your shoulder without bending your elbow (or to the top of your head)?
- Can you carry a 20–30 kg weight (e.g. full suitcase) by your side?
- Do NSAIDs give relief?

Examination

The diagnosis is based on systematic examination of the cervical spine followed by examination of the shoulder joint. For details of examination of the cervical spine, refer to CHAPTER 62.

Examination of the shoulder[3,6]

For the examination of the shoulder it is important to understand the functional anatomy of all important tendons. Follow rule: look, feel, move.

The tendon disorders are diagnosed by pain on resisted movement (see TABLE 63.4). A knowledge of the anatomical attachments of the rotator cuff tendons to the head of the humerus (see FIG. 63.3) provides an understanding of the shoulder movements powered by these muscles.

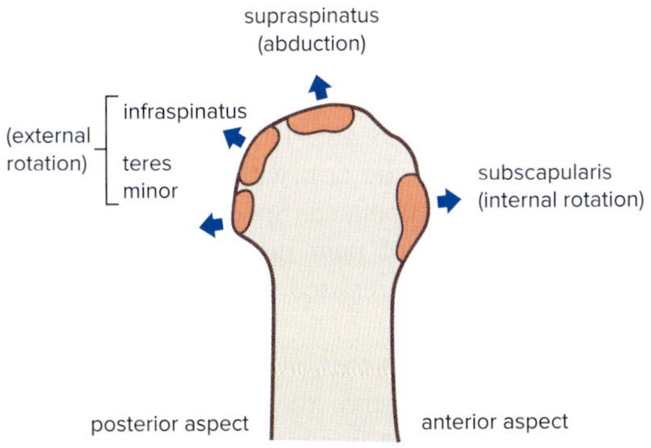

FIGURE 63.3 The attachments of the rotator cuff tendons to the head of the humerus

Source: Reproduced with permission from C Kenna and J Murtagh. *Back Pain and Spinal Manipulation.* Sydney: Butterworths, 1989

Table 63.4 Tendon disorders: determining resisted movements

Painful resisted movement at shoulder	Affected tendon
1 Abduction	Supraspinatus
2 Internal rotation	Subscapularis
3 External rotation	Infraspinatus Teres minor* Biceps*
4 Adduction	Pectoralis major Latissimus dorsi*

**Lesser role*

With tendon disorders (rotator cuff tendons or biceps) there is usually painful restriction of movement in one direction, but with capsulitis and subacromial bursitis there is usually restriction in most directions.

Inspection

Observe the shape and contour of the shoulder joints and compare both sides. Note the posture and the position of the neck and scapula. The position of the scapula provides considerable clinical information. Note any deformity, swelling or muscle wasting.

Palpation

Stand behind the patient and palpate significant structures such as the AC joint, the subacromial space, the supraspinatus tendon and the long head of biceps. The subacromial bursa is one area where it is possible to localise tenderness with inflammation. Feel also over the supraspinatus and infraspinatus muscles for muscle spasm and trigger points. The axilla should be palpated for lymphadenopathy.

Movements

The movements of the shoulder joint are complex and involve the scapulothoracic joint as well as the glenohumeral joint, with each joint accounting for about half the total range. Significant signs of a painful capsular pattern can be gained by determining the movements of flexion, abduction, external rotation and internal rotation.

For each movement, note:

- the range of movement
- any pain reproduction
- any trick movement by the patient
- scapulothoracic rotation

Movements should be tested bilaterally and simultaneously wherever possible.

Look for impingement, which is the sign of fleeting interruption of free movement by 'catching' of a tendon upon bone.

1 Active movements

- Flexion (anterior elevation) 180°
- Extension (posterior elevation) 50°

With the palm facing medially the patient moves the arm upwards through 180° to a vertical position above the head and then backwards through this plane.

- Abduction—180°
- Adduction—50° (from neutral position)

Abduction, which is initiated by the deltoid (first 15%), is possible only if the arm is fully externally rotated. It is a key combined glenohumeral and scapulothoracic movement, which should reach 180°, and these components should be differentiated if the movement is limited. This is done by fixing the scapula with one hand, holding the scapula at its inferior angle and noting the degree of movement of each component (initial glenohumeral range 85–100°). Look for the presence of a painful arc, which occurs usually between 60° and 120° of abduction (see FIG. 63.4).

The commonest cause is supraspinatus tendonopathy. Other causes include infraspinatus tendonopathy and subacromial bursitis (milder degree).

- Internal rotation—90°
- External rotation—90°

These movements are tested with the arm by the side and the elbow flexed to 90° with the palm facing medially. The hand is carried outwards to test external rotation and inwards towards the abdomen for internal rotation.

2 Resisted movements[3]

Resisted movements (isometric contractions of a muscle) are important ways of testing capsulitis and for pinpointing tenderness of muscle insertions around the shoulder joint, and no examination of the shoulder is complete without them (see TABLE 63.4).

Abduction (supraspinatus test). With the arm abducted to no more than 15° the patient pushes the elbow away from the side while the examiner's hands resist and prevent the movement, holding for 5 seconds. Compare both sides and note any reproduction of the patient's pain.

A better and more specific test for supraspinatus impingement is testing resisted elevation in the 'emptying the can' position (90° of abduction, 30° horizontal flexion and full internal rotation).

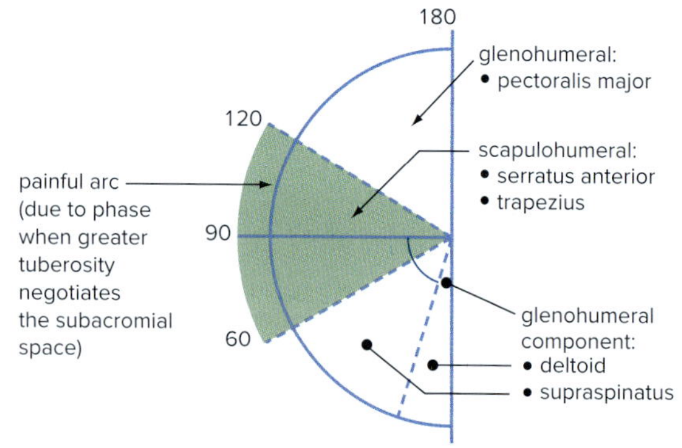

FIGURE 63.4 The painful arc syndrome

Internal rotation (subscapularis test). The examiner stands behind the patient and grasps the palmar surface of the patient's wrists (with the arm by the side and elbow at 90°). The patient attempts to move the forearm internally (medially) against resistance.

External rotation (infraspinatus test). With the examiner and patient adopting a similar position to that for internal rotation, the examiner grasps the dorsal surface of the forearm near the wrist and asks the patient to press outwards, using the forearm as a lever to produce external rotation. This test is also positive for a C5 nerve root lesion.

3 Special tests

Supraspinatus/infraspinatus rapid differentiation test. A quick test that helps to differentiate between a lesion of either of these tendons causing a painful arc syndrome is the 'thumbs up/thumbs down' abduction test. To test the supraspinatus, perform abduction with thumbs pointing upwards, and then with the thumbs pointing downwards to test the infraspinatus.

Long head of biceps test. The best test is opposed forward elevation of the arm with the elbow at right angles and forearm supinated (Speed's test). A positive test is reproduction of pain in the bicipital groove. Another useful test is resisted supination at the wrist (Yergason test).

The brachial plexus tension test. This test, devised by Elvey,[8] tests the nerve roots and sheaths of the brachial plexus without implicating the cervical spine and the glenohumeral joint. The upper cervical roots of the plexus are sometimes injured in accidents, so this test is an effective differentiation test.

Impingement test for supraspinatus lesions. See later in this chapter.

Investigations

Appropriate investigations for shoulder pain include:

- ESR (especially for polymyalgia rheumatica)/CRP
- rheumatoid factor and anti-CCP
- serum uric acid (acute pain)
- ECG (if IHD suspected)
- radiology:
  - X-ray of a specific part of the shoulder—AC joint, axillary view of glenohumeral joint (best view to show osteoarthritis)
  - X-ray of cervical spine and chest (if relevant)
  - radionuclide bone scan—to assess bone tumours
  - shoot-through axillary views (posterior dislocation)
  - high-resolution ultrasound—modern techniques make this an appropriate test to assess shoulder pain due to rotator cuff lesions, especially tears and capsulitis, especially if surgery is contemplated. However this test as sometimes reported can be misleading.
  - arthrogram of shoulder (beware of false negatives)
  - CT scan (limited use)
  - MRI—a useful imaging method but not routinely required except for the unstable joint
  - arthroscopy

Shoulder tip pain

Pain at the shoulder tip may be caused by local musculoskeletal trauma or inflammation or can be referred from blood or other irritants in the peritoneal cavity. Referred causes where the pain is unchanged by shoulder movement include:

- peptic ulceration
- diaphragmatic irritation (e.g. pneumonia)
- ruptured viscus (e.g. perforated ulcer)
- intraperitoneal bleeding (e.g. ruptured spleen)
- pneumothorax/pneumonia
- post laparoscopy (intraperitoneal gas)
- myocardial infarction/pericarditis
- ectopic pregnancy
- gall bladder disease

Shoulder pain in children

Shoulder pain in children is not a common presenting problem but the following require consideration:

- septic arthritis/osteomyelitis
- swimmer's shoulder (supraspinatus dysfunction)

Swimmer's shoulder

Although it occurs in adults, shoulder pain is the most common complaint in swimmers in the teenage years (over 12 years of age). American studies of college and national competition swimmers showed 40–60% had suffered significant pain.[9]

The problem, which is considered to be associated with abnormal scapular positioning and cervicothoracic dysfunction, occurs in the supraspinatus tendon where an avascular zone is compressed by the greater tuberosity when the arm is abducted and relieved when adducted. Swimmers' shoulders are forced through thousands of revolutions each day, so the susceptible area tends to impinge on the coracoacromial arch, leading to the impingement syndrome, which can progress with continued stress and age.[10]

Symptoms

- Stage 1: pain only after activity
- Stage 2: pain at beginning only, then after activity
- Stage 3: pain during and after activity, affects performance

Management

- Early recognition is important.
- Discuss training program with coach.
- Consider alteration of technique.
- Application of ICE after each swim.
- Use NSAIDs.
- Avoid corticosteroid injections.
- Refer for physiotherapy for scapular stabilisation and cervicothoracic mobilisation.

Shoulder pain in adults

As a rule most of the shoulder problems increase with age. Special features in the elderly are:

- polymyalgia rheumatica (increased incidence with age)
- supraspinatus tears and persistent 'tendonitis'
- other rotator cuff disorders
- stiff shoulder due to adhesive capsulitis
- osteoarthritis of AC and glenohumeral joints
- cervical dysfunction with referred pain
- the avascular humeral head

Since the rotator cuff is prone to degeneration with age, there is a high incidence of rotator cuff tears in the elderly that are mostly asymptomatic.

The avascular humeral head

The humeral head may become avascular after major proximal humeral fractures. With experience, it is usually possible to predict the fractures at special risk. Early humeral head replacement with a prosthesis can lead to excellent pain relief and to a return of good function. Once the head has collapsed, there is secondary capsular contracture. Prosthetic replacement of the head is then rarely associated with an adequate return of joint movement. Thus, early referral of comminuted proximal humeral fractures for an expert opinion in all age groups is good practice. Early replacement can improve the functional outcome.[11]

Rotator cuff tendonopathy[6]

Rotator cuff tendonopathy, also referred to as 'the subacromial impingement syndrome', is the commonest cause of shoulder pain. It can be associated with inflammation (tendonitis), a tear in a tendon (degeneration), calcification, amyloidosis or impingement under the acromion. It may involve one tendon, usually the supraspinatus, or more of the rotator cuff tendons. It is most frequently encountered in young people engaged in sport involving overhead activities and people over 50 years, in whom rotator cuff tears occur most often. The diagnosis can usually be made on the history and physical examination. A comparison between rotator cuff disease and capsulitis is presented in TABLE 63.5.

63

Table 63.5 Is it rotator cuff disease or capsulitis?[11,12]

	Rotator cuff disease	Adhesive capsulitis
Pain	Often severe Night pain Inability to sleep on affected side	Often very severe Night pain Inability to sleep on affected side
Onset	Gradual or sudden Rapid onset suggests calcific tendinitis	Usually gradual
Movement	Painful arc Aggravated by certain movements	Marked by stiffness in all directions

Supraspinatus tendonopathy

Supraspinatus tendonopathy can vary in intensity from mild to extremely severe. The severe cases usually involve calcification (calcific periarthritis) of the tendon, which has a very rapid onset, and spread to the subacromial bursa (subacromial bursitis).

The impingement tests[5]

These are effective tests for supraspinatus lesions as they force impingement of the rotator cuff and bursa under the acromion. One of these tests is the 'emptying the can' resistance test. The arm is placed in the 'emptying the can' position (90° of abduction, 30° of horizontal flexion and full internal rotation). Elevation of the arm is resisted against the therapist's downward push. This also tests the strength of supraspinatus. Impingement can also be tested in external rotation when the arm is abducted to 90° and externally rotated. Other tests include those of Neer and Hawkin.[6]

Treatment[12]

Systematic reviews to date have a lack of sufficient information to provide conclusive evidence-based recommendations for treatment.[13] For analgesia, paracetamol taken orally is first line and if inadequate, NSAIDs alone or in combination.[12] Corticosteroid injections and physiotherapy could improve range of movement. Experienced therapists believe that peritendon and subacromial corticosteroid injections are efficacious in selected patients.

- Rest during the acute painful phase
- Analgesics and NSAIDs (up to 4 weeks)
- Peritendon or subacromial injection (if no tears on ultrasound)
- Physiotherapy—an active program including scapular stabilising exercises and rotator cuff strengthening
- Surgery—consider after 3–6 months, usually subacromial decompression, sometimes excision of calcium

Injection technique

The ideal injection is a specific injection onto the tendon rather than general infiltration into the subacromial space. As a rule the therapeutic result is quite dramatic after one or two days of initial discomfort (often severe). The tendon can be readily palpated as a tender cord anterolaterally as it emerges from beneath the acromion to attach to the greater tuberosity of the humerus. This identification is assisted by depressing the shoulder via a downward pull on the arm and then externally and internally rotating the humerus. This manoeuvre allows the examiner to locate the tendon readily.

Method

- Identify and mark the tendon.
- Place the patient's arm behind the back, with the back of the hand touching the far waistline. This locates the arm in the desired internal rotation and forces the humeral head anteriorly.

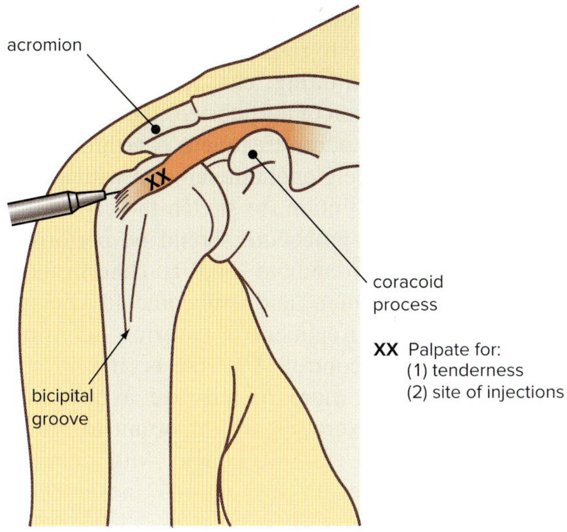

FIGURE 63.5 Injection placement for supraspinatus tendonopathy

- Insert a 23-gauge 32-mm needle under the acromion along the line of the tendon, and inject around the tendon just under the acromion (see FIG. 63.5). If the gritty resistance of the tendon is encountered, slightly withdraw the needle to ensure that it lies in the tendon sheath.
- The recommended injection is 1 mL of a soluble or long-acting corticosteroid with 5 mL of 1% lignocaine.

Persistent supraspinatus tendonopathy

There are three factors to consider with this problem:

1 A very tight subacromial space. Refer for subacromial decompression by division of the thickened coracoacromial ligament. Even in younger patients this procedure (with or without acromioplasty) may be indicated for those with pain persisting beyond 12 months.

2 Rotator cuff tear or degeneration. In middle-aged and elderly patients, persisting tendonitis is usually due to rotator cuff tear and degeneration, an underdiagnosed condition. Excellent clinical and functional results can be achieved if surgery is performed when the tear is small.

3 Calcification of the tendon. This problem usually settles but occasionally surgical intervention is necessary.

Typical pain profile—supraspinatus tendonopathy (subacromial impingement)

Site:	the shoulder and outer border of arm; maximal over deltoid insertion
Radiation:	to elbow
Quality:	throbbing pain, can be severe
Frequency:	constant, day and night
Duration:	constant
Onset:	gradual or sudden, such as straining the shoulder (e.g. dog on leash, working under car, fall onto outstretched arm)
Offset:	nil
Aggravation:	specific movements, putting on shirt, toilet activity, lying on shoulder (unable to sleep)
Relief:	analgesics only
Associated features:	trigger point over supraspinatus origin
Examination (typical features):	– painful resisted abduction – painful arc – positive impingement test – positive 'emptying the can' sign
Diagnosis:	high-resolution ultrasound

63

Other rotator cuff lesions

The patient may present with dominant signs of subscapularis or infraspinatus lesions, or a combination of two or three tendinous lesions, including the supraspinatus. This problem could be confused with milder adhesive capsulitis, hence the value of investigations such as ultrasound.

Management

A subacromial space injection of 1 mL of corticosteroid and 2–3 mL of 1% local anaesthetic, using the posterior approach, generally achieves a good result for multiple affected rotator cuff tendons with or without subacromial bursitis (aim for only one injection). Relative rest is advisable.

Method

With the patient sitting upright the large posterior gap between the medial acromial ridge and the humeral head is identified by palpation from behind. The needle (23 gauge, 32 or 38 mm long) is inserted into this gap just inferior to the acromion. The solution should flow into this space without resistance.

Rotator cuff tears

Asymptomatic rotator cuff tears are common, being present in 4% of people <40 years old and in more than

50% of those over 60 years, but a significant number will become symptomatic over time.[12] Explain to the patient that 'the rotator cuff is worn not torn', rather like the frayed heel of a sock that may have a split in it. The defect can be palpable.

Diagnostic tip: 98% specificity for all three signs:[15]

- supraspinatus weakness
- weakness in external rotation
- impingement (in external or internal rotation or both)

If two of these three tests are positive in a patient over 60 there is a 98% chance of a rotator cuff tear. Refer for surgical repair.

Subacromial bursitis

Subacromial (subdeltoid) bursitis is the more severe association of rotator cuff pathology and may require hospital admission for pain control. It is the only inflammatory disorder around the shoulder joint where localised tenderness is a reliable sign.

Management

63

- Strong analgesics (e.g. paracetamol and codeine)
- Large local injection of 5–8 mL of local anaesthetic into and around the bursa just beneath the acromion, followed immediately by 1 mL of corticosteroid (long-acting) into the focus of the lesion

Adhesive capsulitis[12]

Adhesive capsulitis or capsulosis is an acute inflammation affecting the glenohumeral joint, which becomes fibrotic and contracted. It can arise spontaneously or post injury and may be partial or global, which is the classic cause of the 'frozen shoulder'. Differential diagnoses include monoarticular rheumatoid arthritis, a crystal arthropathy such as gout, and septic arthritis. It is worse in diabetics. It is common and estimated to affect 2–5% of the general population and 10–20% of diabetes.[14] 12% develop bilaterally.

It generally occurs in three stages:[14]

1. 'freezing, frozen and thawing'—an inflammatory painful phase of 2–9 months
2. a fibrotic contracted (frozen) phase of 4–12 months
3. partial or complete resolution of 5–26 months

Treatment

For analgesia choose between paracetamol, paracetamol with NSAIDs, and NSAIDs alone (weigh the risk). For severe pain oral corticosteroids rapidly alleviate pain, improve function and may provide sustained benefit. A typical dose is prednisolone 30 mg (o) daily for 3 weeks, then taper dose over next 2 weeks and cease.[16]

This problem, which can persist for at least 18–24 months (average time to restore motion is 30 months) and is usually self-limiting, can be treated with an intra-articular injection of corticosteroid but it is often unsuccessful. The modern treatment is arthrographic hydrodilatation of the glenohumeral joint with a large quantity of sterile solution (to stretch the capsule) ± corticosteroid. This procedure should be performed slowly to produce an audible 'pop' as fluid distends into the subacromial and subcoracoid bursae. Another important treatment is severing adhesions under arthroscopic control. The rule is: if very stiff use arthroscopy; if more mobile use a distension procedure. Active exercises are important to restore function. Fifty per cent of people with adhesive capsulitis do not regain full normal movement if untreated.

Current evidence from systemic reviews indicates that both hydrodistension and intra-articular injections are likely to be beneficial.[12,17]

Exercise in the acute phase can exacerbate pain but a gentle program is useful when it settles. If stiffness persists, manipulation under anaesthesia and/or arthroscopic debridement of adhesions may be helpful.[18]

Typical pain profile—adhesive capsulitis

Usually affects people in their 40s, 50s and 60s.

Site:	around the shoulder and outer border of arm
Radiation:	to elbow
Quality:	deep throbbing pain
Frequency:	constant, day and night (severe cases)
Duration:	constant
Onset:	spontaneous, usually gradual, wakes the patient from sleep
Offset:	nil
Aggravation:	activity, dressing, combing hair, heat
Relief:	analgesics only (partial relief)
Associated features:	stiffness of arm, may be frozen
Examination (typical features):	– 'frozen' shoulder (some cases) – various active and passive movements painful and restricted, especially extension and at extremes of movement – resisted movements pain-free (patient compensates with scapulo-humeral movements)
Diagnosis:	high-resolution ultrasound (plain X-ray normal)

Bicipital tendonopathy

Bicipital tendonopathy is a lesion such as fraying or tearing of the long head of the biceps, which causes pain in front of the shoulder. Important signs include pain on resisted flexion of the elbow joint and on resisted supination with the elbow flexed to 90° (Speed test) and forearm pronated (Yergason test). A painful arc may be present when the intrascapular part is affected. Hence it is often confused with one of the rotator cuff lesions. Sometimes it is possible to elicit local tenderness by palpation along the course of the tendon in the bicipital groove. This is best done when the arm is externally rotated. Most active shoulder movements, especially external rotation, bring on the pain.

Bicipital tendonopathy usually follows chronic repetitive strains in young to middle-aged adults (e.g. home decorating, weight training, tennis, swimming freestyle, cricket bowling and baseball pitching). Two complications are complete rupture and subluxation of the tendon out of its groove.

One treatment to consider is a corticosteroid and local anaesthetic injection at the site of maximal tenderness in the bicipital groove (see FIG. 63.6). As a rule it is best to refer a significant lesion.

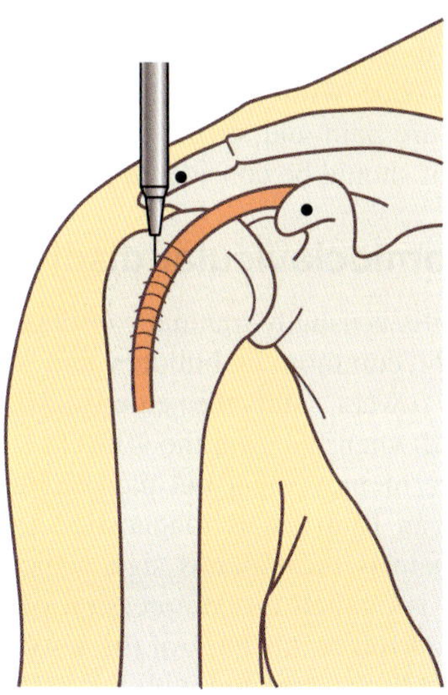

FIGURE 63.6 Injection placement for bicipital tendonopathy

Rupture of the biceps tendon

Rupture of the long head of biceps usually occurs in the older person. It may be spontaneous or occur after lifting or falling on the outstretched hand. The patient usually feels a tearing or snapping sensation in the shoulder. The shoulder may be painful and difficult to move. The upper arm looks bruised and a lump due to rolled-up belly of biceps is obvious on flexion of the elbow. Active treatment is not usually indicated but surgical intervention is appropriate for young, active people, especially those in power sports.

Polymyalgia rheumatica

It is very important not to misdiagnose polymyalgia rheumatica in the older person (over 50 years) presenting with bilateral pain and stiffness in the shoulder girdle. It may or may not be associated with hip girdle pain. Polymyalgia rheumatica sometimes follows an influenza-like illness. The patients seem to complain bitterly about their pain and seem flat and miserable. In the presence of a normal physical examination they are sometimes misdiagnosed as 'rheumatics' or 'fibrositis'.

Typical pain profile—polymyalgia rheumatica

Site:	shoulders and upper arms (see FIG. 63.7)
Radiation:	towards lower neck
Quality:	a deep, intense ache
Frequency:	daily
Duration:	constant but easier in afternoon and evening
Onset:	wakes with pain at greatest intensity
Offset:	nil
Aggravating factors:	staying in bed, inactivity
Relieving factors:	activity (slight relief)
Associated features:	severe morning stiffness 'in muscles'; malaise; ± weight loss, depression
Diagnosis:	greatly elevated ESR (can be normal)
Treatment:	corticosteroids give dramatic relief but long-term management can be problematic; regular review and support is essential (refer CHAPTER 32)

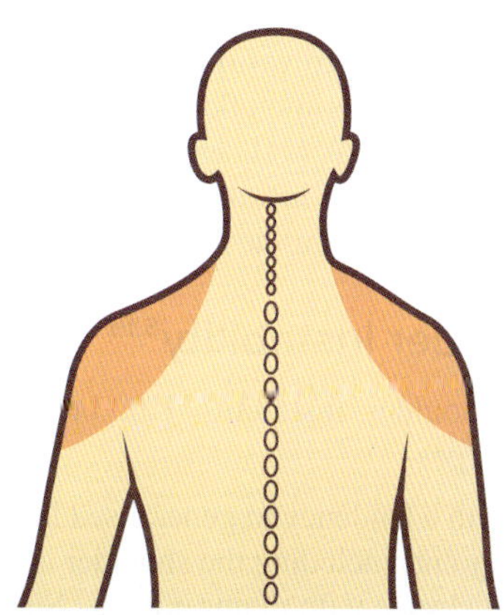

FIGURE 63.7 Polymyalgia rheumatica: typical area of pain around the shoulder girdle

63

Posterior dislocation of the shoulder

This is a rare form of shoulder instability, which is often misdiagnosed. On first inspection there may not be an obvious abnormality of the shoulder contour. Consider this condition if there is a history of electric shock or a tonic–clonic convulsion. The major clinical sign is painful restriction of external rotation, which is usually completely blocked. Routine shoulder X-rays following trauma should always include the 'axillary shoot-through' view and then the diagnosis becomes obvious. Early diagnosis and management can prevent a poor outcome and perhaps litigation.[15,19]

Recurrent subluxation

Recurrent anterior or inferior subluxations, or both, are probably more common than recurrent dislocations, yet frequently are not diagnosed. Patients who complain of attacks of sudden weakness and even a 'dead arm feeling' lasting for a few minutes with overhead activities of the arm should be investigated for this condition.

63

The disorder is usually apparent on careful stress testing of the shoulder. Air-contrast CT arthrography is considered the best investigation. Surgery is usually curative while conservative treatment often fails for younger patients.

Glenoid labrum injuries[4,7]

The glenoid labrum is the ring of fibrous tissue attached to the rim of the glenoid and provides volume to the cavity and stability to the glenohumeral joint. Injuries to the labrum are divided into superior labrum anterior to posterior (SLAP) or non-SLAP lesions and further into stable and unstable lesions.

Tests to assess these injuries are the O'Brien, Crank and Speed tests (refer to various YouTube videos).

Non-SLAP lesions include degenerative, flap and vertical labral tears as well as unstable lesions such as the classic Bankart lesion, where the labrum and capsule is detached from the rim (see CHAPTER 133).

Shoulder instability[5,16]

Recurrent shoulder instability can be divided into three main types.

1 Those with a tendency to generalised laxity of multiple joints including the shoulder and which tend to dislocate with minor injuries. Surgery is less effective and treatment is based on improving muscular stability with physiotherapy rehabilitation.
2 Those following trauma, which includes avulsion of the anterior labrum (Bankart lesion). Physiotherapy tends to be less effective and the patients often require surgical repair.
3 Those with chronic rotator cuff tendonopathy/impingement who develop subtle instability. Refer first to a sports physician or physiotherapist for assessment and management, preferably conservative initially.

The 'apprehension' test is useful to confirm the diagnosis of traumatic anterior instability. In this test the patient lies supine while the arm is externally rotated with the elbow flexed to 90°. The test is more reliable when the patient expresses apprehension that the shoulder will 'come out', rather than pain.

Osteoarthritis of the glenohumeral joint

This is usually secondary to local trauma, long-standing rotator cuff lesions and multiple surgical interventions. Shoulder movements are stiff and usually restricted in all directions. Plain X-rays show typical osteoarthritic changes. Treatment includes basic analgesics and short courses of NSAIDs plus exercises to improve mobility. Patients usually manage to cope with osteoarthritis of the shoulder, but for severe pain and stiffness arthroplasty or joint replacement should be considered.

Acromioclavicular disorders

Osteoarthritis is usually traumatic or degenerative and is relatively common in builders and sportspeople, especially rowers, and the elderly. Night pain is experienced when lying on the affected side. There is a full range of movement but pain on full elevation. The Bell–van Riet test is diagnostic. A key test for AC joint pain is the Paxinos sign, which is positive when pain is elicited on compression of the joint by placing one hand on the back of the acromion and one on the clavicle. It is treated with rest and support and analgesics. Intra-articular injections of corticosteroids can be used for resistant or severe cases. If these measures are ineffectual, pain may be relieved by excision of the lateral end of the clavicle.

When to refer

- Persisting night pain with shoulder joint stiffness
- Persisting supraspinatus tendonopathy; consider possibility of rotator cuff tear or degeneration, especially in the elderly

- Persisting restriction of movement, such as restricted cross-body flexion (indicates capsular constriction)
- Persisting supraspinatus tendonopathy or other rotator cuff problem, because decompression of the subacromial space with division of the coracoacromial ligament ± acromioplasty gives excellent results
- Confirmed or suspected posterior dislocation of the shoulder—the most commonly missed major joint dislocation
- Confirmed or suspected recurrent subluxation or avascular humeral head
- Children with shoulder joint instability
- Swimmer's shoulder refractory to changes in technique and training schedule
- Severe osteoarthritis of the glenohumeral joint (which usually follows major trauma) for consideration of prosthetic replacement
- Severe osteoarthritis of the AC or glenohumeral joint

Patient education resources

Hand-out sheets from *Murtagh's Patient Education* 7th edition:

- Exercises for your shoulder
- Polymyalgia rheumatica
- Shoulder: frozen shoulder
- Shoulder: tendonitis

Practice tips

- Consider dysfunction of the cervical spine, especially C4–5 and C5–6 levels, as a cause of shoulder pain.
- Tendonitis and bursitis are very refractory to treatment and tend to last for several months. One well-placed injection of local anaesthetic and corticosteroid may give rapid and lasting relief.
- Test for supraspinatus disorders (including swimmer's shoulder) with the impingement tests, including the 'emptying the can' test.
- Modern ultrasound is the investigation of choice for painful disorders of the rotator cuff, especially to investigate tears in tendons.
- An elderly person presenting with bilateral shoulder girdle pain has polymyalgia rheumatica until proved otherwise. Relief from corticosteroids is dramatic. Although bilateral, it may start as unilateral discomfort.
- Dysfunction of the cervical spine can coexist with dysfunction of the shoulder joints.
- Correlation between clinical symptoms and the degree of tendon injury or failure is not reliable.[18]

References

1 Sloane PD, Slatt LM, Baker RM. *Essentials of Family Medicine.* Baltimore: Williams & Wilkins, 1988: 242.
2 Buchbinder R. Acute shoulder pain: an evidence based management approach. Course Proceedings: Monash Update Course for GPs, November 2013.
3 Kenna C, Murtagh J. *Back Pain and Spinal Manipulation* (2nd edn). Oxford: Butterworth-Heinemann, 1997: 109–33.
4 Rathburn JB, Macnab I. The microvascular pattern of the rotator cuff. J Bone Joint Surg Br, 1970; 52B: 540.
5 Murrell G. Shoulder dysfunction: how to treat. Australian Doctor, 17 December 2004: 23–30.
6 Shanahan EM, Buchbinder R. The painful shoulder. Medicine Today, 2009; 11 (9): 73–9.
7 Elvey R. The investigation of arm pain. In: Grieve GP, *Modern Manual Therapy of the Vertebral Column.* London: Churchill Livingstone, 1986: 530–5.
8 Dominguez RH. Shoulder pain in swimmers. The Physician and Sports Medicine, 1980; 8: 36.
9 McLean ID. Swimmers' injuries. Aust Fam Physician, 1984; 13: 499–500.
10 Young D, Murtagh J. Pitfalls in orthopaedics. Aust Fam Physician, 1989; 18: 645–8.
11 Hermans J et al. Does this patient with shoulder pain have rotator cuff disease?: The Rational Clinical Examination systematic review. JAMA, 2013; 310 (8): 837–47.
12 Expert group for Rheumatology. Limb conditions. In: eTG complete [Internet]. Melbourne: Therapeutic Guidelines Ltd. Available from: <www.tg.org.au>, accessed October 2017.
13 Barton S (ed.). *Clinical Evidence.* London: BMJ Publishing Group, 2001; 850–63.
14 Robinson CM et al. Frozen shoulder. J Bone Joint Surg Br, 2012; 94 (1): 1–9.
15 Murrell GAC, Walton JR. Diagnosis of rotator cuff tears. The Lancet, 2001; 357: 769–70.
16 Buchbinder R, Hoving JL, Green S et al. Short course prednisolone for adhesive capsulitis (frozen shoulder or stiff painful shoulder): a randomised, double blind, placebo controlled trial. Ann Rheum Dis, 2004; 63 (11): 1460–9.
17 Buchbinder R, Green S, Forbes A et al. Arthrographic joint distension with saline and steroid improves function and reduces pain in patients with painful stiff shoulder: results of a randomised, double blind, placebo controlled trial. Ann Rheum Dis, 2004; 63 (3): 302–9.
18 Page MJ et al. Manual therapy and exercise for adhesive capsulitis (frozen shoulder). Cochrane Database. Syst Rev. 2014, Issue 8. Art No. CD011275.
19 Sher JS et al. Abnormal findings on magnetic resonance images of asymptomatic shoulders. J Bone Joint Surg Am, 1995; 77: 10–15.

64 Pain in the arm and hand

A pain in the hand is worth a look at the neck. By heck don't forget the neck!

ORTHOPAEDIC SURGEON TO STUDENTS, 1965

Pain in the arm and hand is a common problem in general practice, tending to affect the middle aged and elderly in particular.

Overview of causes of a painful arm and hand

Like pain in the shoulder, pain originating from the cervical spine and shoulder disorders can extend down the arm. While pain from disorders of the shoulder joint (because of its C5 innervation) does not usually extend below the elbow, radiculopathies originating in the cervical spine can transmit to distal parts of the arm (see FIG. 64.4, later in this chapter).

Important causes are illustrated in FIGURE 64.1. Myocardial ischaemia must be considered, especially for pain experienced down the inner left arm.

Soft tissue disorders of the elbow are extremely common, especially tennis elbow. Two types of tennis elbow are identifiable: 'backhand' tennis elbow, or lateral epicondylitis, and 'forehand' tennis elbow, or medial epicondylitis, which is known also as golfer's or pitcher's elbow.

Other significant elbow disorders include inflammatory disorders of the elbow joint, such as rheumatoid arthritis, osteoarthritis and olecranon bursitis, which may follow recurrent trauma, gout, rheumatoid arthritis or infection.

Another important group of disorders are the various regional pain syndromes around the wrists, including the common de Quervain tenosynovitis (affecting the tendons of extensor pollicis brevis and abductor pollicis longus) and to a lesser extent the extensor tendons to the fingers. Pain from these overuse syndromes can be referred in a retrograde manner into the forearm.

A fascinating and poorly understood syndrome is that related to dysfunction of the upper four vertebral segments of the thoracic spine, which can cause referred pain in the arm that does not correspond to the dermatomes. This syndrome is often confused with the more common regional pain disorders such as tenosynovitis and tennis elbow.

The various causes of the painful arm can be considered with the diagnostic strategy model (see TABLE 64.1).

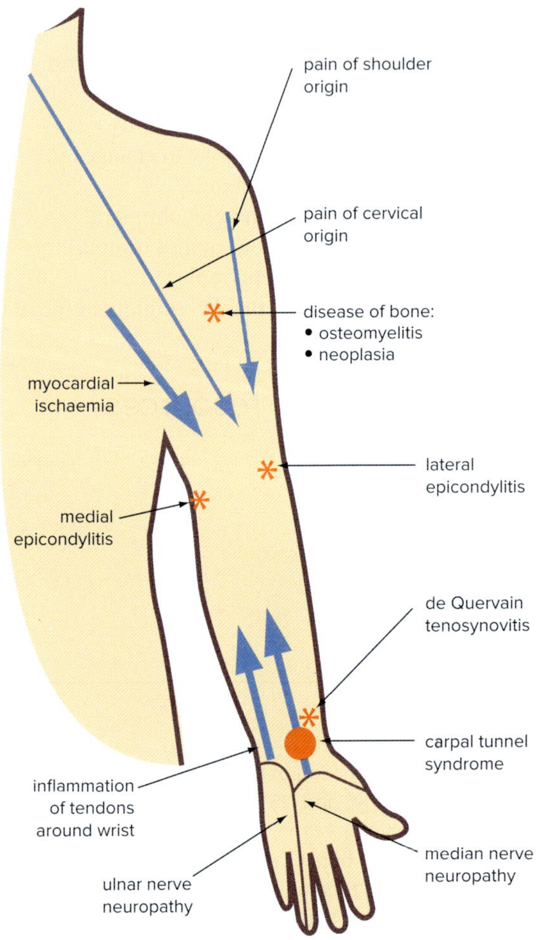

FIGURE 64.1 Important causes of arm pain (excluding trauma and arthritis)

A diagnostic approach

Probability diagnosis

The commonest causes of arm pain are referred pain and radiculopathies caused by disorders of the cervical spine, the tennis elbows (lateral and, to a lesser extent, medial epicondylitis), carpal tunnel syndrome (CTS)

Table 64.1 Pain in the arm and hand: diagnostic strategy model

Probability diagnosis
Dysfunction of the cervical spine (lower)
Disorders of the shoulder
Medial or lateral epicondylitis
Overuse tendonitis of the wrist
Carpal tunnel syndrome
Osteoarthritis of the thumb and DIP joints
Serious disorders not to be missed
Cardiovascular:
• angina (referred)
• myocardial infarction
• axillary vein thrombosis
Neoplasia:
• Pancoast tumour
• bone tumours (rare)
Severe infections:
• septic arthritis (shoulder/elbow)
• osteomyelitis
• infections of tendon sheath and fascial spaces of hand
• sporotrichosis (gardener's arm)
Pitfalls (often missed)
Entrapment neuropathies (e.g. median nerve, ulnar nerve)
Pulled elbow (children)
Foreign body (e.g. elbow)
Rarities:
• polymyalgia rheumatica (for arm pain)
• reflex sympathetic dystrophy
• thoracic outlet syndrome
• arm claudication (left arm)
• Kienböck disorder
Seven masquerades checklist
Depression
Diabetes
Spinal dysfunction
Is the patient trying to tell me something?
Possibly, especially with the so-called RSI work-related syndromes.

and regional pain syndromes caused by inflammation of the tendons around the wrist and thumb.

Disorders of the shoulder, particularly supraspinatus tendonitis, should be considered if the pain is present in the C5 dermatome distribution. Pain in the hand is commonly caused by osteoarthritis of the carpometacarpal joint of the thumb and the distal interphalangeal (DIP) joints, and also by CTS.

Serious disorders not to be missed

Like any other presenting problem, it is vital not to overlook malignant disease or severe infection. In the case of the arm, possible malignant disease includes tumours in bones, lymphoma involving axillary glands and Pancoast tumour, which may cause severe arm pain before any signs are evident.

Neoplastic tumours of the hand are uncommon and usually benign. Benign tumours include giant cell tumour of the tendon sheath, pigmented villonodular synovitis, neurilemmoma and neurofibroma. Malignant tumours are exceptionally rare but can include synovioma and rhabdomyosarcoma.

In addition, myocardial ischaemia, especially infarction in the case of pain of sudden onset, should be considered for left arm pain.

Sepsis can involve joints, the olecranon bursa and the deeper compartments of the hand, the latter leading to serious sequelae if not rapidly diagnosed and treated.

Subclavian or axillary vein thrombosis, known as 'effort thrombosis', causes swelling in the arm with pain high in the axilla. It is seen in people working constantly above their head, such as painters and basketballers. It is an emergency requiring antithrombotic therapy.

Pitfalls

Such conditions may include entrapment syndromes for peripheral nerves. If in doubt the patient should be referred for electromyography. Variations of peripheral nerve entrapments include the pronator syndrome (compression of the median nerve by the pronator teres or a fibrous band near the origin of the deep flexor muscles) and ulnar nerve entrapment at the elbow in the cubital fossa and, rarely, in the Guyon canal in the wrist.

Lesions of the nerve roots comprising the brachial plexus can also cause arm pain, especially in the C5 and C6 distribution. These can be detected by the brachial plexus tension tests.

Rarer causes of arm pain

These include polymyalgia rheumatica, although the pain typically involves the shoulder girdle, regional pain syndrome (Sudeck atrophy) and the thoracic outlet syndromes.

The thoracic outlet syndromes include problems arising from compression or intermittent obstruction of the neurovascular bundle supplying the upper extremity, for example, cervical rib syndrome, costoclavicular syndrome, scalenus anterior and medius syndrome, 'effort thrombosis' of axillary and subclavian veins and the subclavian steal syndrome.

The commonest cause of the thoracic outlet syndrome is sagging musculature related to ageing, obesity, and heavy breasts and arms, aptly described by Swift and Nichols as 'the droopy shoulder syndrome'.[1]

64

Cervical ribs are relatively common and may or may not contribute to the thoracic outlet syndrome. Often the cause is a functional change in the thoracic outlet due to the 'droopy shoulder syndrome' with no significant anatomical fault.[2]

Arm claudication is also rare. It can occur with arterial obstruction due to occlusion of the proximal left subclavian artery or the innominate artery. Exercise of the arm may be associated with central nervous system symptoms as well as claudication.

Seven masquerades checklist

Of the seven primary masquerades, spinal dysfunction and depression are those most likely to be associated with arm pain. Nerve root pain arising from entrapment in intervertebral foramina of the cervical spine or from a disc prolapse frequently leads to pain and/or paraesthesia in the arm.

Although diabetic neuropathy primarily manifests in the lower limbs it may be associated with neuropathies in the hands, including erythromelalgia (redness and burning related to heat). Hypothyroidism may cause a CTS.

Psychogenic considerations

64

The hand can be regarded as a highly emotive 'organ' that is frequently used to give outward expression to inner feelings. These can range from grossly disturbed psychiatric behaviour, manifested as a hysterical conversion disorder by a non-functioning hand, to occupational neuroses such as repetition strain injury (RSI) and malingering.[3] Experienced occupational physicians and surgeons[3] find the hand and arm a source of functional disability most often as a result of industrial injury. Of great concern are the various so-called RSI disorders, which in some people may be a means of work avoidance or a 'ticket' for compensation or both.

The clinical approach

History

The painful arm represents a real diagnostic challenge, so the history is very relevant.

It is common for arm pain to cause sleep disturbances and three causes are cervical disorders, CTS and the thoracic outlet syndrome. The working rule is:

- thoracic outlet syndrome—patients cannot fall asleep
- CTS—patients wake in the middle of the night
- cervical spondylosis—wakes the patient with pain and stiffness that persists well into the day[4]

The history should include an analysis of the pain and a history of trauma, particularly unaccustomed activity. In children evidence should be obtained about the nature of any injury, especially pulling the child up by the arms or a fall on an outstretched hand, which can cause potentially serious fractures around the elbow.

Examination

As part of the physical examination of the painful arm it may be necessary to examine a variety of joints, including the cervical spine (CHAPTER 62), shoulder (CHAPTER 63), elbow, wrist and the various joints of the hand. The arms should be inspected as a whole and it is very important to have both arms free of clothing and compare both sides.

Elbow joint

Inspection (from anterior, lateral and posterior aspects). Hold elbow in an anatomical position to measure the carrying angle of forearm—elbow fully extended, forearm supinated (palm facing forwards) normal 5–15° (greater in females). Note any swellings:

- olecranon bursitis (bursa over olecranon)
- nodules:
  - RA (subcutaneous border ulna)
  - gout
  - SLE (rare) and rheumatic fever (very rare)
  - granulomas (e.g. sarcoidosis)

Examine it from the back to assess the triangle made by the olecranon and epicondyle.

Palpation. Perform with patient supine and elbow held in approximately 70° flexion. Palpate bony landmarks and soft tissue. Note especially any tenderness over lateral epicondyle (tennis elbow) and medial epicondyle (golfer's elbow).

Movement (test active and passive). Hinge joint:

- extension—flexion (0° to 150°):
  - the arc for daily living is 30–130°
  - limitation of extension is an early sign of synovitis
- pronation—supination (rotation):
  - occurs at radiohumeral joint
  - test in two positions: 90° flexion (held to side of body) + at full extension
  - supination 85° plus
  - pronation 75° plus

Resisted movements

- Painful resisted flexion at wrist = medial epicondylitis
- Painful resisted extension at wrist = lateral epicondylitis

Wrist joint

Follow the usual rules: look, feel, move, test function, measure, look elsewhere and X-ray. Note swellings or deformities, including the 'anatomical snuff box' and distal end of radius. Feel for heat, tenderness and swelling, especially over the radial aspect of the wrist.

Movements. With elbow fixed at 90° and held into the waist:

1 compare dorsiflexion and palmar flexion on both sides (normal range extension 70–80° flexion 80–90°)
2 compare ulnar deviation (normal to 45°) and radial deviation (20°)
3 compare pronation and supination (normal to 90° for both)

Neurological examination

Test sensation, motor power and reflexes where indicated.

Summary of tests for motor power:

- C5—test resisted movement deltoid
- C6—test resisted movement biceps
- C7—test resisted movement triceps
- C8—test resisted EPL and FDL
- T1—test resisted interossei

Sensory patterns are presented in FIGURE 62.4 (CHAPTER 62).

Investigations

Pain in the arm and hand can be difficult to diagnose but the rule to follow is: 'If in doubt, X-ray and compare both sides'. This applies particularly to elbow injuries in children. The presence of a foreign body in the hand or arm also requires consideration.

Investigations to consider include:

- blood film and WCC
- ESR
- ECG
- imaging
  - plain X-rays e.g. cervical spinal
  - ultrasound
  - arthrograms (shoulder, elbow, wrist)
  - CT or MRI scanning
  - technetium bone scan
- nerve conduction studies
- electromyography

Note: Modern sophisticated ultrasound examination is becoming a vital diagnostic modality for soft tissue disorders such as tendonopathy.

Arm pain in children

The main concerns with children are the effects of trauma, especially around the elbow. Considerable awareness of potential problems and skilful management are required with children's elbow fractures. Foreign bodies in the arm also have to be considered.

Pulled elbow

This typically occurs in children under 8 years of age, usually at 2–5 years, when an adult applies sudden traction to the child's extended and pronated arm (see FIG. 64.2a): the head of the radius can be pulled distally through the annular radioulnar ligament (see FIG. 64.2b).[5]

Symptoms and signs

- The crying child refuses to use the arm.
- The arm is limp by the side or supported in the child's lap.
- The elbow is flexed slightly (any flexion will be strenuously resisted).
- The forearm is pronated or held in mid-position.
- The arm is tender around the elbow (without bruising or deformity).

Note: An X-ray is not usually necessary.

Treatment

Method

1 Gain the child's confidence.
2 The child stands facing the doctor with the parent holding the non-affected arm.
3 Place one hand around the child's elbow to give support, pressing the thumb over the head of the radius.
4 With the other hand, firmly and smoothly flex the elbow and suddenly and firmly twist the forearm into full supination (see FIG. 64.2c). A faint click (which will be painful) will be heard. After a few minutes the child will settle and resume full pain-free movement. Warn parents that recurrences are possible up to 6 years.

Alternative method

An easier method for the child is to very gently alternate pronation and supination through a small arc as you flex the elbow.

Note: Spontaneous resolution can occur eventually. Place the arm in a sling if necessary. If you cannot get the child's cooperation, send them home in a 'high' sling.

Fractures and avulsion injuries around the elbow joint, which are a major problem in children, are discussed in more detail in CHAPTER 133.[6]

64

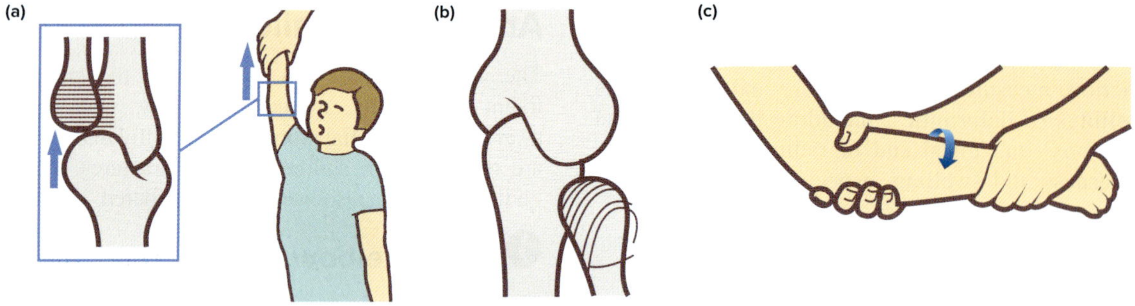

FIGURE 64.2 Pulled elbow: **(a)** mechanism of injury, **(b)** annular ligament displaced over head of radius, **(c)** reduction by supination

Arm pain in the elderly

Elderly patients are more likely to be affected by problems such as referred pain, radiculopathy or myelopathy from cervical spondylosis, tumours, polymyalgia rheumatica, entrapment neuropathies such as CTS and ulnar nerve entrapment. The latter can be related to trauma, such as Colles fractures. In addition the elderly are more prone to suffer from the thoracic outlet syndrome as previously described under 'Pitfalls'. Osteoarthritis of the hand and tenosynovitis, such as trigger thumb or finger, are more common with advancing age.

TENNIS ELBOW

Tennis elbow is caused by overuse or overload of the muscles of the forearm, especially in the middle aged. Two types of epicondylar tendonopathies are identifiable: 'backhand' tennis elbow, or lateral epicondylitis, and 'forehand' tennis elbow, or medial epicondylitis, which is also known as golfer's or pitcher's elbow. 'Backhand' tennis elbow, which will be termed lateral tennis elbow, is the common classic variety. It is an overload injury caused by excessive strain on the extensor muscles of the forearm resulting from wrist extension. Both conditions are generally self-limiting, but symptoms can persist for up to 2 years, or even much longer.

Lateral tennis elbow (lateral epicondylitis)

The patient who presents with this common and refractory problem is usually middle aged and only about one in 20 plays tennis. A typical clinical profile is presented in TABLE 64.2.

Signs

On examination the elbow looks normal, and flexion and extension are painless.

Table 64.2 Lateral tennis elbow: typical clinical profile

Age	40–60 years
Occupation	Carpenter, bricklayer, cleaner, gardener, dentist, violinist
Sport	Tennis, squash
Symptoms	Pain at outer elbow, referred down back of forearm Rest pain and night pain (severe cases) Pain in the elbow during gripping hand movements (e.g. turning on taps, turning door handles, picking up objects with grasping action, carrying buckets, pouring tea, shaking hands)
Signs	No visible swelling Localised tenderness over lateral epicondyle, anteriorly Pain on passive stretching wrist Pain on resisted extension wrist and third finger Normal elbow movement
Course	6 to 24 months
Management	Basic: • rest from offending activity • RICE* and oral NSAIDs if acute • exercises—stretching and strengthening Additional (if refractory): • corticosteroid/LA injection (max. two) • manipulation • surgery

* *RICE:* rest, ice, compression, elevation

There are three important positive physical signs:

1. localised tenderness to palpation over the anterior aspect of the lateral epicondyle
2. pain on passive stretching at the wrist with the elbow held in extension and the forearm prone (see FIG. 64.3)

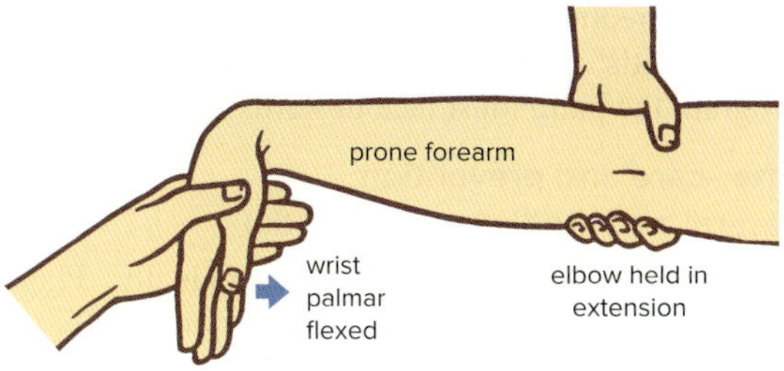

FIGURE 64.3 Lateral tennis elbow test: reproducing pain on passive stretching at the wrist

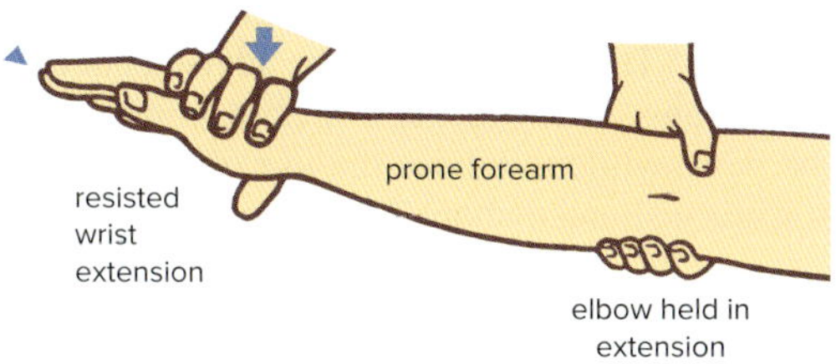

FIGURE 64.4 Lateral tennis elbow test: reproducing pain on resisted extension of the wrist

3 pain on resisted extension of the wrist with the elbow held in extension and the forearm prone (see FIG. 64.4)

Management

Although there are myriad treatments, the cornerstones of therapy are rest from the offending activity and exercises to strengthen the extensors of the wrist. The application of ice may help relieve discomfort of acute pain. Three systematic reviews have found little evidence for efficacy of any one specific intervention but short-term use of NSAIDs and progressive strengthening and stretching exercises were better than placebo.[7] A trial of oral NSAIDs or topical NSAID applied four times a day may be worthwhile.[8]

Exercises

Stretching and strengthening exercises for the forearm muscles represent the best management for tennis elbow. Three options are presented.

1 *The wringing exercise.* Chronic tennis elbow can be cured by a simple wringing exercise using a small hand towel.[9]
Method
- Roll up the hand towel.
- With the arm extended, grasp the towel with the affected side placed in neutral.
- Then exert maximum wring pressure: first flexing the wrist for 10 seconds, then extending the wrist for 10 seconds.

This is an isometric 'hold' contraction.
This exercise should be performed only twice a day, initially for 10 seconds in each direction. After each week increase the time by 5 seconds in each twisting direction until 60 seconds is reached (week 11). This level is maintained indefinitely.
Note: Despite severe initial pain, the patient must persist, using as much force as possible. Review at 6 weeks to check progress and method.

2 *Weights exercise.* The muscles are strengthened by the use of hand-held weights or dumbbells. A suitable starting weight is 0.5 kg, building up gradually (increasing by 0.5 kg) to 5 kg, depending on the patient.
Method
- To perform this exercise the patient sits in a chair beside a table.
- The arm is rested on the table so that the wrist extends over the edge.
- The weight is grasped with the palm facing downwards (see FIG. 64.5).
- The weight is slowly raised and lowered by flexing and extending the wrist.
- The flexion/extension wrist movement is repeated 10 times, with a rest for 1 minute, and the program is repeated twice.

3 *The pronating exercise.*[10] A suitable stretching exercise is to rhythmically rotate the hand and wrist inwards with the elbow extended and the forearm pronated (see FIG. 64.6). Another proven exercise program is that outlined by Nirschl[11] and this can be provided by referral to a physiotherapist familiar with the program.

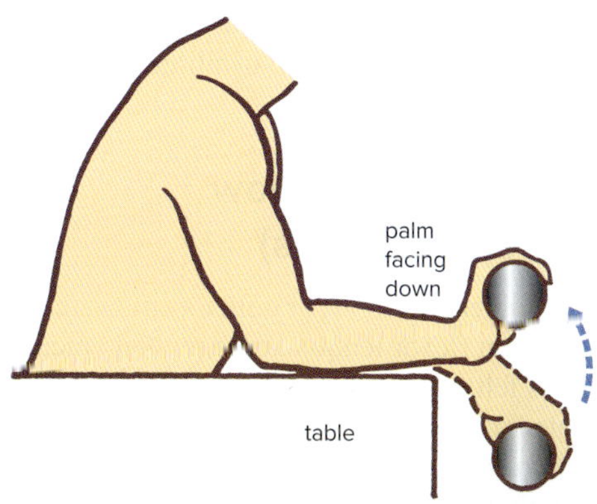

FIGURE 64.5 Lateral tennis elbow: the dumbbell exercise with the palm facing down

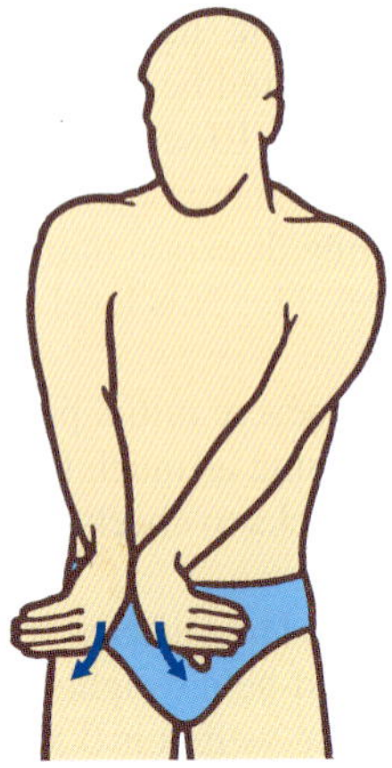

FIGURE 64.6 Tennis elbow stretching exercise: the hand and wrist are rhythmically rotated inwards until the painful point is reduced

Injection therapy

The injection of 1 mL of a long-acting corticosteroid and 1 mL of local anaesthetic should be reserved for those severe cases when pain restricts simple daily activities, and not used initially for those patients with only intermittent pain.

A Netherlands study showed that corticosteroid injections are the best short-term treatment for tennis elbow. Over the longer term, physiotherapy offers better results than injection but is on a par with a wait and see approach.[12]

Surgery

Severe and refractory cases can be referred for surgery but this is rarely indicated and there is no evidence to date on its efficacy. The usual procedure is the stripping of the common extensor origin combined with debridement of any granulation tissue.[3] Other treatments include glyceryl trinitrate patches and autologous blood injections.

Medial tennis elbow (medial epicondylitis)

In 'forehand' tennis elbow, or golfer's elbow, the lesion is the common flexor tendon at the medial epicondyle. The pain is felt on the inner side of the elbow and does not radiate far. The main signs are localised tenderness to palpation and pain on resisted flexion of the wrist.

In tennis players it is caused by stroking the ball with a bent forearm action or using a lot of top spin, rather than stroking the ball with the arm extended.

The treatment is similar to that for lateral epicondylitis except that in a dumbbell exercise program the palm must face upwards.

After-care and prevention (lateral and medial epicondylitis)

Tennis/sport should be resumed gradually. Players recovering from tennis elbow should start quietly with a warm-up period and obtain advice on style, including smooth stroke play. During a game they should avoid elbow bending and 'wristy' shots. A change to a good-quality racket (wooden or graphite frame) with a medium-sized head and suitable grip size may be appropriate.[11] The patient should be advised not to use a tightly strung, heavy racket or heavy tennis balls. It may be worthwhile to advise the use of a non-stretch band or brace situated about 7.5 cm below the elbow.

Olecranon bursitis

Olecranon bursitis presents as a swelling localised to the bursa (which has a synovial membrane) over the olecranon process. The condition may be caused by trauma, arthritic conditions (rheumatoid arthritis and gout) or infection.

Traumatic bursitis may be caused by a direct injury to the elbow or by chronic friction and pressure as occurs in miners (beat elbow), truck drivers or carpet layers. Acute olecranon bursitis with redness and warmth can occur in rheumatoid arthritis, gout, pseudogout, haemorrhage and infection (sepsis). Septic bursitis must be considered where the problem is acute or subacute in onset, and hence aspiration of the bursa contents with appropriate laboratory examination is necessary (smear, Gram stain, culture and crystal examination). Treatment depends on the cause.

Simple aspiration/injection technique

Chronic recurrent traumatic olecranon bursitis with a synovial effusion may require surgery but most cases can resolve with partial aspiration of the fluid and then injection of corticosteroid through the same needle. Sepsis must be ruled out.

Overuse syndromes of forearm muscles[8]

Pain is often experienced in the belly of a muscle, such as the flexors and extensors, following unaccustomed use of the wrists and elbows. There is pain on contraction and stretching of the muscles and tenderness on palpation. This problem can be limiting for a significant period. Early treatment includes relative rest, ice packs, analgesics (paracetamol) and gradual return to activity. Referral for physiotherapy to supervise rehabilitation is important.

Carpal tunnel syndrome

Patients with CTS complain of 'pins and needles' affecting the pulps of the thumb, and index, middle and half of the ring finger (see FIG. 64.7). They usually notice these symptoms after, rather than during, rapid use of the hands. They may also complain of pain, which may even radiate proximally as far as the shoulder, from the volar aspect of the wrist. Causes or associations of CTS are presented in TABLE 64.3.

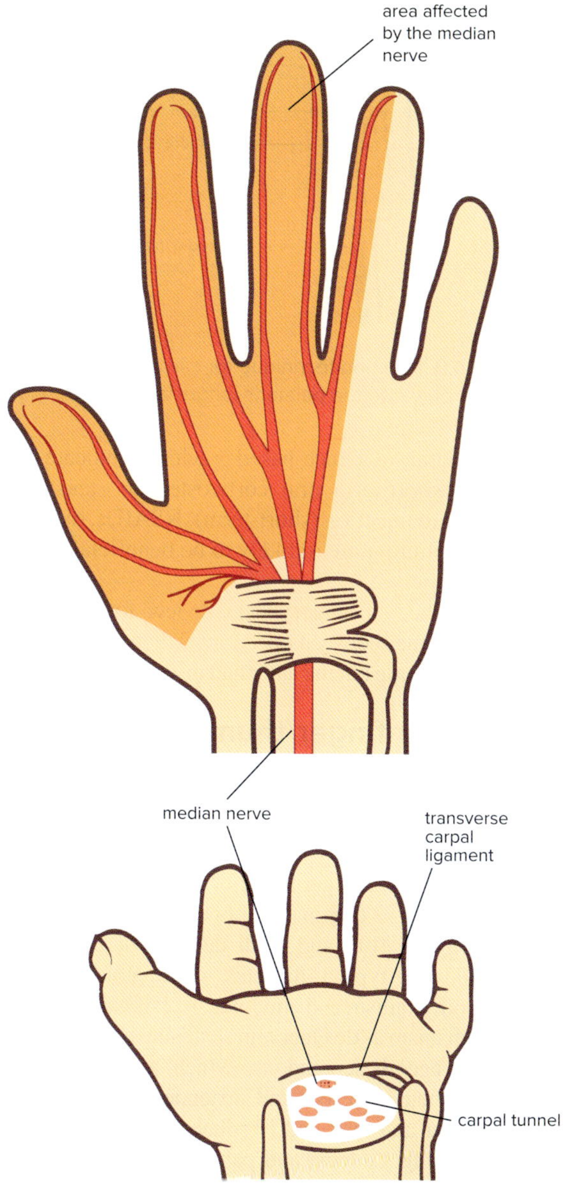

FIGURE 64.7 Carpal tunnel syndrome (median nerve compression syndrome

Table 64.3 Carpal tunnel syndrome: causes or associations
Idiopathic
Acromegaly
Amyloidosis
Consider cervical nerve root pressure
Diabetes mellitus
Fibrosis
Granulomatous disorders (TB, etc.)
Hypothyroidism
Multiple myeloma
Occupational: repetitive work with flexed wrists
Paget disease
Pregnancy
Premenstrual oedema
Rheumatoid arthritis
Tophaceous gout
Trauma

The pathognomonic symptom

Patients complain of awakening from their sleep at night with 'pins and needles' affecting the fingers. They get out of bed, shake their hands, the 'pins and needles' subside and they return to sleep. In severe cases, the patient may awaken two or three times a night and go through the same routine.

Work-related CTS

CTS is seen in many work situations requiring rapid finger and wrist motion under load, such as meat workers and process workers. A type of flexor tenosynovitis develops and thus nerve compression in the tight tunnel. It is advisable to arrange confirmatory investigations by nerve conduction studies and electromyography for this work-induced overuse disorder. This testing is also indicated where the diagnosis is uncertain or if the condition persists and numbness or weakness develops.

Diagnosis (simple clinical tests)

In the physical examination a couple of simple tests can assist with confirming the diagnosis. These are the Tinel test and Phalen test. However, they are 'soft' signs with a relatively low sensitivity and specificity.[14]

Tinel test

- Hold the wrist in a neutral or flexed position and tap over the median nerve at the flexor surface of the wrist. This should be over the retinaculum just lateral to the palmaris longus tendon (if present) and the tendons of flexor digitorum superficialis (see FIG. 64.8).

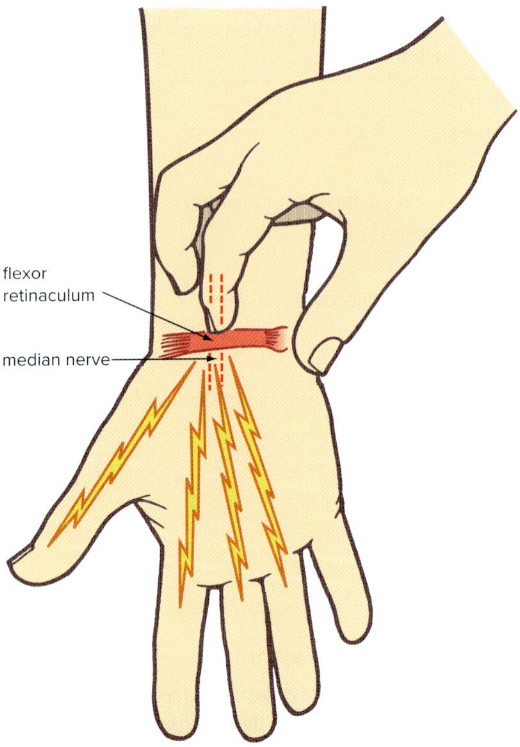

FIGURE 64.8 Carpal tunnel syndrome: Tinel sign

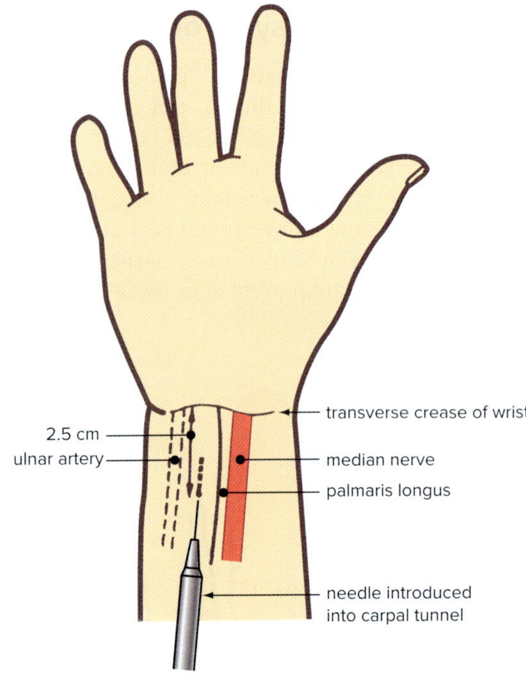

FIGURE 64.9 Injection technique for carpal tunnel syndrome: between the palmaris longus and ulnar artery

64

- A positive Tinel sign produces a tingling sensation (usually without pain) in the distribution of the median nerve.

Phalen test

- The patient approximates the dorsum of both hands, one to the other, with wrists maximally flexed and fingers pointing downwards.
- This position is held for 60 seconds.
- A positive test reproduces tingling and numbness along the distribution of the median nerve.

Two point discrimination

The test that has the highest specificity of all basic clinical tests is two point discrimination, but it has low sensitivity for CTS.[14]

Treatment

The treatment is determined by the severity. For mild cases simple rest and splinting (particularly at night) is sufficient. Carpal tunnel injection with 1 mL of corticosteroid is frequently of diagnostic as well as therapeutic value (see FIG. 64.9). Ultrasound therapy has been used with some success. Surgical release (flexor retinaculotomy) is necessary for patients with sensory or motor deficits and those with recalcitrant CTS.

Systematic evidence-based reviews indicate the benefit of short-term oral corticosteroids[7] and local corticosteroid injection (short-term). NSAIDs, diuretics and wrist splinting are unlikely to be beneficial. Avoid use of diuretics.

In reference to surgery, one review found similar clinical outcomes between open carpal tunnel release and endoscopic release but the latter had more complications.[7]

Trigger finger/thumb (flexor tenosynovitis)

In the fingers the common work-induced condition is stenosing flexor tenosynovitis, also known as trigger thumb and finger. Trigger finger or thumb has a reported lifetime risk of 2.6% in the population and is more common in the fifth and sixth decades of life.[15] It is associated with type 1 diabetes, rheumatoid arthritis, gout, hypothyroidism and amyloidosis. It is caused by the same mechanism as de Quervain stenosing tenosynovitis. In middle age these tendons, which are rapidly and constantly being flexed and extended, can undergo attrition wear and tear, and fibrillate and fragment; this causes swelling, oedema and painful inflammation and the formation of a nodule on the tendon that triggers back and forth across the thick, sharp edge of the 'pulley' (of the fibrosseous tunnel in the finger) (see FIG. 64.10).

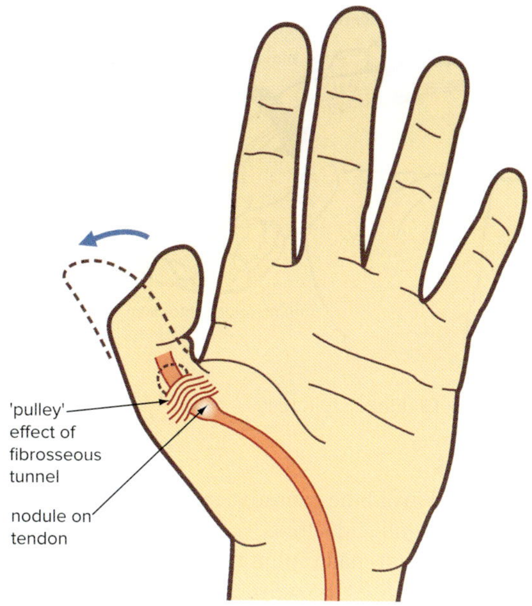

FIGURE 64.10 Trigger thumb

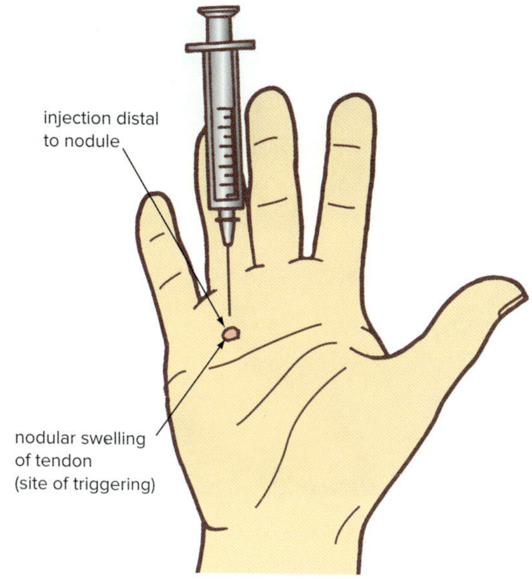

FIGURE 64.11 Injection site for trigger finger

These patients may present with a finger locked in the palm of the hand; the finger can only be extended passively (manually) with the other hand. It is easily diagnosed by triggering. If the pulp of the finger is placed over the 'pulley' crepitus can be felt and tenderness elicited. The thumb and fourth (ring) finger are commonly affected, at the level of the metacarpal head.

Treatment

Oral NSAIDs (with care) may provide pain relief.[15] Although surgery is simple and effective, treatment by injection is often very successful. The injection is made under the tendon sheath adjacent to but not into the tendon or its nodular swelling (A1 pulley). The approach can be proximal, distal or lateral to the nodule. Controlled trials report a success rate of up to 70%.[15]

Method

- The patient sits facing the doctor with the palm of the affected hand facing upwards.
- Draw 1 mL of long-acting corticosteroid solution into a syringe and attach a 25 gauge needle for the injection.
- Insert the needle at an angle distal to the nodule and direct it proximally within the tendon sheath (see FIG. 64.11). This requires tension on the skin with free fingers.
- By palpating the tendon sheath, you can (usually) feel when the fluid has entered the tendon sheath.
- Inject 0.5–1 mL of the solution, withdraw the needle and ask the patient to exercise the fingers for 1 minute.

Postinjection

Improvement usually occurs after 48 hours and may be permanent. The injection can be repeated after 3 weeks if the triggering is not completely relieved. If triggering recurs, surgery is indicated. This involves division of the thickened tendon sheath only.

64

Dupuytren contracture

Also referred to as 'Viking disease', this contracture, which causes discomfort and dysfunction rather than pain, is fibrous hyperplasia of the palmar fascia leading to nodular formation and contracture over the fourth and fifth fingers in particular (see FIG. 64.12). It occurs in about 10% of males over 65 years. The cause is unknown, but there is an AD genetic predisposition. It is associated with smoking, alcoholism, liver cirrhosis, COPD, diabetes, epilepsy and heavy manual labour. If the palmar nodule is growing rapidly, injection of corticosteroids or collagenase (e.g. Xiaflex) into the cord or nodule may be beneficial, but collagenase carries a risk of tendon rupture. Surgical intervention is indicated for a significant flexion deformity.

De Quervain tenosynovitis (washerwoman's sprain)

At the wrist, a not uncommon, work-induced condition is de Quervain stenosing tenosynovitis of the first dorsal extensor compartment tendons (extensor pollicis brevis and abductor pollicis longus), which pass along

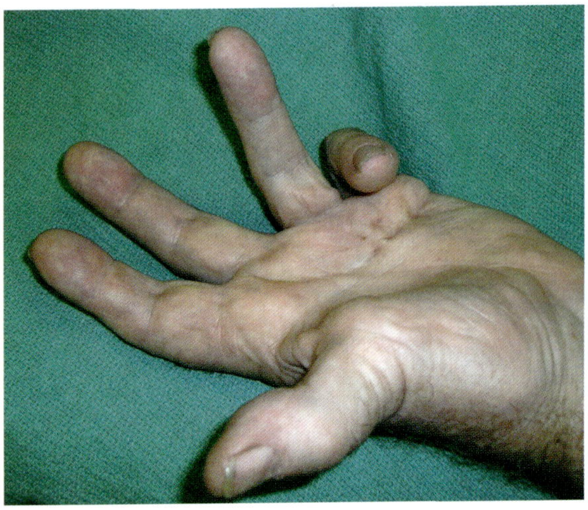

FIGURE 64.12 Dupuytren contracture showing flexion contractures of the fourth and fifth digits and a palmar cord

the radial border of the wrist to the base of the thumb. It is usually seen when the patient is required to engage in rapid, repetitious movements of the thumb and the wrist, especially for the first time, and thus is common in assembly line workers, such as staple gun operators.

64

Clinical features

- Typical age 40–50 years
- Pain at and proximal to wrist on radial border
- Pain during pinch grasping
- Pain on thumb and wrist movement
- Dull ache or severe pain (acute flare-up)
- Can be disabling with inability to use hand (e.g. writing)

Triad of diagnostic signs

- Tenderness with possible crepitations on palpation over and just proximal to radial styloid
- Firm tender localised swelling in area of radial styloid (may be mistaken for exostosis)
- Positive Finkelstein sign (the pathognomonic test)

Finkelstein test

- The patient folds the thumb into the palm with the fingers of the involved hand folded over the thumb, thus making a fist.
- Move (adduct) the wrist in an ulnar direction (towards the little finger) to stretch the involved tendons as you stabilise the forearm with the other hand (see FIG. 64.13).
- A positive test is indicated by reproduction of or increased pain.

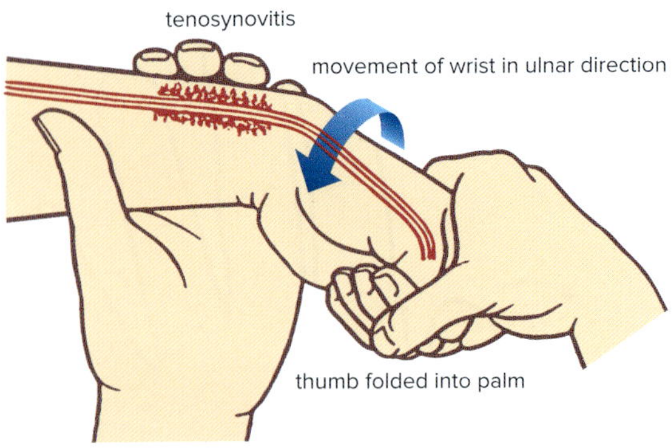

FIGURE 64.13 Finkelstein test

Treatment

- Rest and avoid the causative stresses and strains on the thumb abductors.
- Use a custom-made splint that involves the thumb and immobilises the wrist.
- Consider trial of oral or topical NSAIDs four times a day for 14–21 days.
- Local long-acting corticosteroid injection can relieve and may even cure the problem but care should be taken to inject the suspension within the tendon sheath rather than into the tendon.
- Surgical release is required for chronic cases.

Method of tendon sheath injection

- Identify and mark the most tender site of the tendon and the line of the tendon. Identify and avoid the radial artery.
- Thoroughly cleanse the skin with an antiseptic such as povidone-iodine 10% solution.
- Insert the tip of the needle (23 gauge) about 1 cm distal to the point of maximal tenderness (see FIG. 64.14).

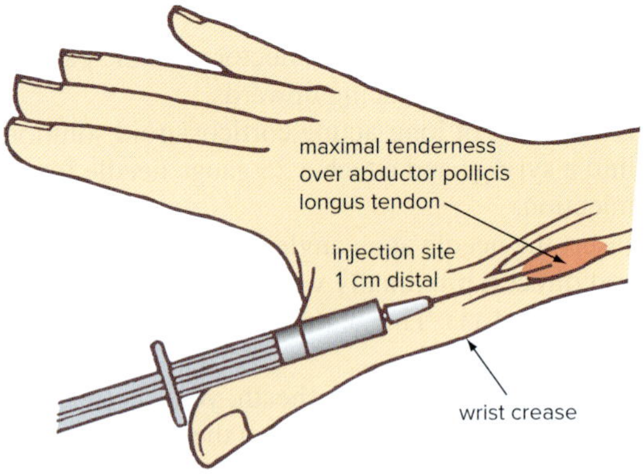

FIGURE 64.14 Tendon sheath injection

- Advance the needle almost parallel to the skin along the line of the tendon.
- Inject about 0.5 mL of the corticosteroid suspension within the tendon sheath. If the needle is in the sheath very little resistance to the plunger should be felt, and the injection causes the tendon sheath to billow out.

Tendonopathy

After excluding CTS, trigger thumb/finger, de Quervain tenosynovitis, rheumatoid and related disease, tendonitis is uncommon in the hand.[16] Tendonitis may occur in other extensor compartments of the wrist and hand with unusual repetitive stressful actions, such as power drills jamming, and in conveyor quality control where an object is picked up with the forearm prone, supinating to examine it and pronating to replace it.

Treatment is rest from the provoking activity, splintage and tendon sheath injection with long-acting corticosteroid in a manner similar to that described for de Quervain tenosynovitis.

Intersection syndrome[17]

Intersection syndrome is caused by a bursitis that develops at the site where the extensor pollicis brevis and abductor pollicis longus tendons cross over the extensor carpi radialis tendons (see FIG. 64.15). The bursitis is due to friction at the crossing point or due to tenosynovitis of the extensor tendons. On palpation tenderness is found dorsally on the radial side with swelling and crepitus. Treatment is based on relative rest, a trial of NSAIDs and an injection of local anaesthetic and corticosteroid into the bursa.

Post-traumatic chronic wrist pain[10]

Patients often present with persistent wrist pain following trauma, such as a fracture, sprain to the wrist or even a seemingly mild strain, such as falling down with the wrist flexed into the hand. An undiagnosed fracture, ischaemic necrosis or unstable ligamentous injury including a triangular fibrocartilage tear should be investigated by radiology or referral where appropriate. Look for a scapholunate ligament tear (which causes wrist instability) with tenderness 2 cm distal to the tubercle on the radial side of the lunate. For persistent tenderness an injection of corticosteroid and local anaesthetic into the tender site is advisable.[8] Imaging including MRI can be helpful but if in doubt about the diagnosis refer to a hand and wrist surgeon.

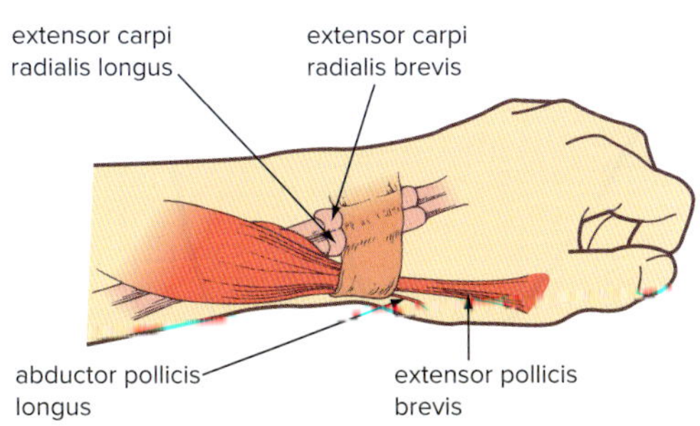

FIGURE 64.15 Intersection syndrome: pain is present over the intersection of tendons

Ulnar collateral ligaments injury ('gamekeeper's thumb')[17]

A special injury is gamekeeper's thumb (also known as skier's thumb) in which there is ligamentous disruption of the metacarpophalangeal joint with or without an avulsion fracture at the base of the proximal phalanx at the point of ligamentous attachment (Bennett fracture). This injury is caused by the thumb being forced into abduction and hyperextension by the ski pole as the skier pitches into the snow. Pinch grip is often affected.

Diagnosis is made by X-ray with stress views of the thumb. Incomplete tears are immobilised in a scaphoid type of plaster for 3 weeks, while complete tears (Stener lesions) and avulsion fractures should be referred for surgical repair.

64

Mallet finger

A mallet finger is a common sports injury caused by the ball (football, cricket ball or baseball) unexpectedly hitting the fingertip and forcing the finger to flex. Such a forced hyperflexion injury to the distal phalanx can rupture or avulse the extensor insertion into its dorsal base. The characteristic swan-neck deformity (see FIG. 64.16) is due to retraction of the lateral bands and hyperextension of the proximal interphalangeal joint.

The 45° guideline

Without treatment, the eventual disability will be minimal if the extensor lag at the distal joint is less than 45°; a greater lag will result in functional difficulty and cosmetic deformity.

Treatment

Maintain hyperextension of the distal interphalangeal joint for 6 weeks, leaving the proximal interphalangeal joint free to flex. This can be managed with non-stretched adhesive tape (see FIG. 64.17).

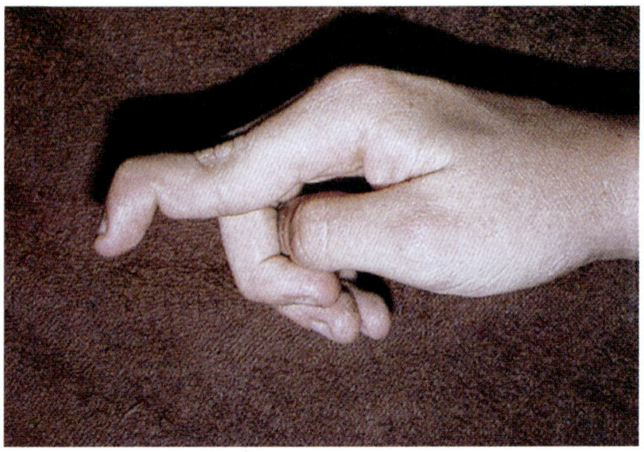

FIGURE 64.16 Mallet finger with swan-neck deformity following rupture of the extensor tendon to the distal phalanx

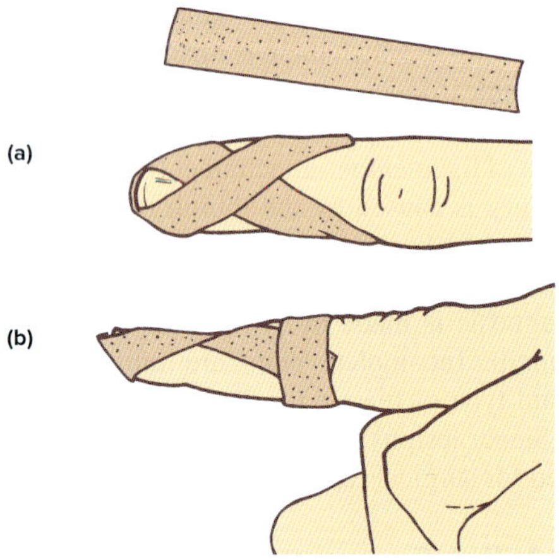

FIGURE 64.17 Mallet finger: position of finger after application of tapes

Ischaemic necrosis

Ischaemic necrosis, particularly of the scaphoid, can occur following failure to recognise a fracture. Tenderness in the 'anatomical snuff box' following trauma should be treated as a scaphoid until repeated X-rays prove negative. In children, chronic pain in the region of the lunate suggests avascular necrosis—Kienböck disease, presenting with dorsal wrist pain (see later in this chapter).

Ganglia[15]

About 60–70% of these common soft tissue tumours occur on the dorsal aspect of the wrist. The vast majority arise from the dorsal scapholunate ligament. Pain can result from compression on an adjacent nerve or joint space. If the diagnosis is uncertain, an ultrasound scan (or even an MRI) may pinpoint the tumour. See CHAPTER 124 for treatment.

Neurovascular disorders of the hand

Painful vascular disorders, which are more likely to occur in women in cold weather, include Raynaud phenomenon, erythromelalgia, chilblains and acute blue finger syndrome. Acrocyanosis is not a painful condition.

Raynaud phenomenon

The basic feature of Raynaud phenomenon, which is a vasospastic disorder, is sequential discolouration of the digits from pallor to cyanosis to rubor upon exposure to cold and other factors (a useful mnemonic is WBR, namely white → blue → red) (see FIG. 64.18). The rubor is a reactive hyperaemia when fingers become red and tender. Associated symptoms are pain, tingling and numbness. It is possible to get loss of tissue pulp at the ends of the fingers and subsequent necrotic ulcers. The benign form is the commonest, but may indicate an evolving connective tissue disorder. It is highly significant if it extends to the MCP joints (see CHAPTER 32).

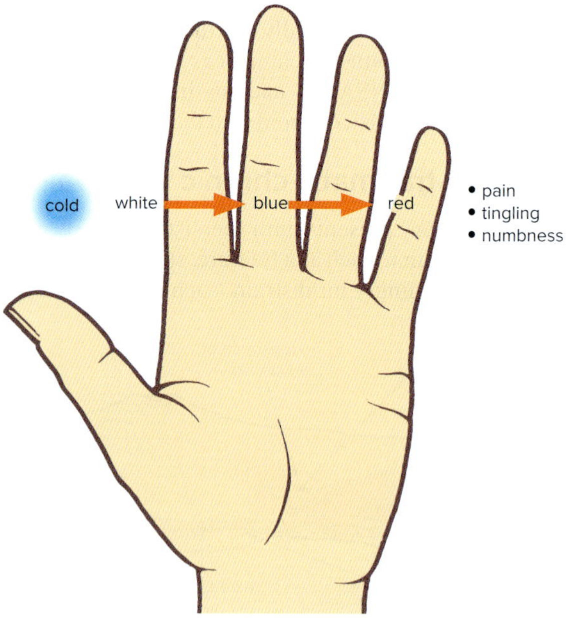

FIGURE 64.18 Raynaud phenomenon: symptoms and colour changes of fingers with cold

Causes

Primary

- Raynaud syndrome (idiopathic)

Secondary

- Occupational trauma (vibrating machinery)
- Connective tissue disorders (e.g. rheumatoid arthritis, SLE, systemic sclerosis, CREST, polyarteritis nodosa)
- Arterial disease (e.g. Buerger disease)
- Haematological disorders (e.g. polycythaemia, cold agglutinin disease, leukaemia)
- Drugs (e.g. beta blockers, sympathomimetic drugs with receptor activity, ergotamine, nasal decongestants)

Aggravating factors

- Smoking
- Cold, wet weather
- Stress or emotional upset

Differential diagnoses

- Chilblains—itchy, patchy discolouration without pallor
- Diffusely cold mottled hands—recover quickly on warming

Investigations

Exclude underlying causes with appropriate tests.

Treatment[15]

- In an attack, it is best to warm the extremities gradually.
- Total body protection from cold—wear layered clothing to prevent heat loss.
- Use an electric blanket at night, as required.
- Use mittens, fleece-lined gloves and thick woollen socks.
- Gloves or mittens should be worn when handling cold surfaces and objects, such as frozen food.
- Avoid smoking.
- Consider sympathectomy.

Vasodilators (during cold weather)[15]

topical glyceryl trinitrate 2% ointment—applied to the base of the affected fingers 2–4 times daily or applied over the radial artery or dorsum of the hand

or

amlodipine 5–20 mg (o) once daily

or

nifedipine SR 30–60 mg (o) once daily

or

diltiazem SR 180–240 mg (o) once daily

Erythromelalgia (erythermalgia)

This condition is characterised by erythema (redness), a burning sensation and swelling of the hands (and feet) after exposure to heat and exercise. It may be primary or secondary to a disease such as diabetes, haematological disorders[13] (e.g. polycythaemia rubra vera) and connective tissue disease. Treatment of primary erythromelalgia includes trials of aspirin, phenoxybenzamine (Dibenyline), methysergide or sympathectomy.

Acute blue finger syndrome in women

This unusual syndrome involves the sudden onset of pain and cyanosis of the ventral aspect of the digit initially, and then the entire digit. It lasts 2–3 days and the attacks recur one or more times per year. No abnormalities are found on physical or on laboratory examination.

The cause is probably spontaneous rupture of a vein at the base of the finger.

Chilblains (perniosis)

64

Precautions

- Think Raynaud phenomenon
- Protect from trauma and secondary infection
- Do not rub or massage injured tissues
- Do not apply heat or ice

Treatment

Physical treatment

- Elevate affected part
- Warm gradually to room temperature

Drug treatment

- Apply glyceryl trinitrate vasodilator spray or ointment or patch (use plastic gloves and wash hands for ointment)

Other treatment

- Drink rum at night
- Nifedipine SR 30 mg daily

Regional pain syndrome

The hand can be affected by complex regional pain syndrome, previously called reflex sympathetic dystrophy (RSD, also in this case Sudeck atrophy).

The patient presents with severe pain, swelling and disability of the hand. It may occur spontaneously or, more usually, it follows trauma that may even be trivial. It can occur after a Colles fracture, especially with prolonged immobilisation.

Clinical features

- Throbbing, burning pain, worse at night
- Paraesthesia
- Initial: red, swollen hand; warm, dry skin
- Later: cold, cyanosed and mottled, moist skin; shiny and stiff fingers
- Wasting of small muscles
- X-rays—patchy decalcification of bone (diagnostic)

The problem eventually settles but may take years. Patients need considerable support, encouragement, basic pain relief, mobility in preference to rest and perhaps referral to a pain clinic.

Kienböck disorder

Kienböck disease is avascular necrosis of the carpal lunate bone (see FIG. 64.19), which may fragment and collapse, eventually leading to osteoarthritis of the wrist.

64

It presents usually in young adults over the age of 15 as insidious, progressive wrist pain and stiffness that limits grip strength and hand function. Males are affected more often than females and the right hand more than the left, indicating the relationship to trauma.

Arthritic conditions of the wrist and hand

Arthritis of the hand is an inappropriate diagnosis and specificity is required to highlight the various joints that are the targets of the specific arthritides, which include osteoarthritis, rheumatoid arthritis, spondyloarthropathies, gout, haemochromatosis and connective tissue disorders. Typical target areas in the hand are shown in FIGURE 64.19.

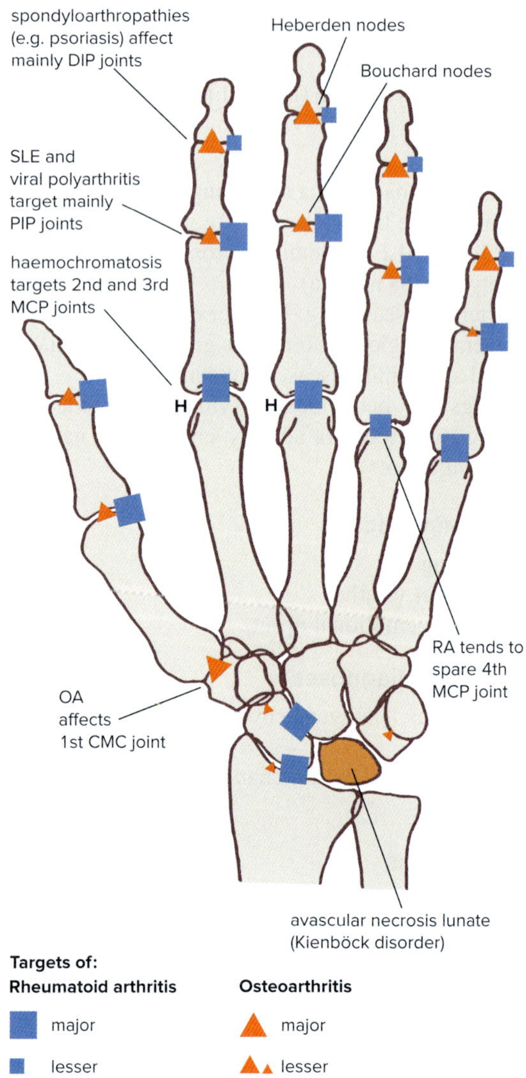

FIGURE 64.19 Typical sites of arthritic conditions and osteochondritis in the hand

Osteoarthritis

Osteoarthritis commonly involves the interphalangeal joints of the fingers (especially the DIP joints)[18] and the carpometacarpal (CMC) joint of the thumb. Degenerative changes produce bony swellings around the margins of the joints—Heberden nodes of the DIP joints and less commonly Bouchard nodes of the PIP joints. A patchy distribution occurs in metacarpophalangeal, intercarpal and wrist joints, usually related to trauma.

Osteoarthritis of the thumb

This is very common, especially in women. Pain is felt at the base of the thumb, and tenderness on palpation of the CMC joint is typical. Functional limitation is progressive, with weakness of the pinch grip and limited thumb excursion. Surgical correction may be required.

Rheumatoid arthritis

In rheumatoid arthritis, the DIP joints are often spared (only about 30% involved), but the metacarpophalangeal and proximal interphalangeal joints and wrist joints are generally affected symmetrically and bilaterally. Rheumatoid arthritis tends to affect the metacarpophalangeal joints of the fourth finger less commonly.

Gout

Gout may affect normal joints of the hand but is encountered more frequently in osteoarthritic hand joints (especially DIP joints) in elderly people taking diuretics. This clinical feature is known as nodular gout.

Seronegative arthropathies

A similar appearance to rheumatoid arthritis occurs, except that with psoriatic arthritis the terminal joints are often affected by swelling, giving the appearance of 'sausage digits'. (Refer CHAPTERS 35 and 38.)

Infections of the hand

Although not encountered as frequently as in the past, serious suppurative infections of the deep fascial spaces of the hand and tendon sheath can still occur, especially with penetrating injuries and web space infection.

Infections of the hand include:

- infected wounds with superficial cellulitis or lymphangitis (*Streptococcus pyogenes*)
- subcutaneous tissues—nail bed (paronychia), pulp (whitlow, e.g. herpes simplex)
- erysipeloid—this is a specific infection in one finger of fishers or meat handlers, caused by *Erysipelothrix insidiosa.* There is a purplish erythema that gradually extends over days. It is rapidly cured by penicillin
- tendon sheath infection (suppurative tenosynovitis)—this is a dangerous and painful infection that can cause synovial adhesions with severe residual finger stiffness. The affected finger is hot and swollen and looks like a sausage
- 'aquarium' or 'swimming pool' granuloma—non-painful infection of the tendon sheath due to *Mycobacterium marinum* following a minor cut of the finger; doxycyclin or clarithromycin is usually effective but refer to infectious disease physician
- deep palmar fascial space infection—infection from an infected tendon sheath or web space may spread to one of the two deep palmar spaces: the medial (midpalmar) space or lateral (thenar) space
- sporotrichosis (gardener's arm)—a chronic fungal infection from contaminated spikes of wood or rose thorns presenting as hard non-tender nodules in the skin of the hand and extending along the lymphatics of the arm. The diagnosis is confirmed by biopsy. Treat with itraconazole

Management of serious infection

- Early appropriate antibiotic treatment for infection and early surgical referral where necessary
- Antibiotics (adult doses)

Streptococcus pyogenes (mild to moderate cellulitis, lymphangitis)
procaine penicillin 1.5 g IM daily, 3–7 days
or
phenoxymethylpenicillin 500 mg (o) 6-hourly for 10 days
If severe, to cover both *S. pyogenes* and *Staphylococcus aureus* infection (suspected or proved)
flucloxacillin/dicloxacillin 2 g IV 6-hourly until improved, then oral for 10 days.

'Cracked' hands and fingers

- Wear protective work gloves: cotton-lined PVC gloves.
- Use soap substitutes (e.g. Cetaphil lotion, Dove).

apply 2–5% salicylic acid and 10% liq picis carb in white soft paraffin ointment.
or
corticosteroid ointment: class II–III

When to refer

- Disabling osteoarthritis of carpometacarpal joint for possible surgical repair
- Myelopathy (motor weakness) and persistent radiculopathy (nerve root pain and sensory changes) in the arm
- Unresolving nerve entrapment problems such as median and ulnar nerves
- Elbow injuries in children with proven or possible supracondylar fracture or avulsion epicondylar fractures
- Evidence or suspicion of suppurative infection of the tendon sheaths or deep palmar fascial spaces
- Septic arthritis and osteomyelitis
- Regional pain syndrome
- Other conditions not responding to conservative measures

Practice tips

- With elbow injuries in children, X-ray both elbows and compare one side with the other; this helps to determine whether there is displacement of fragments or a disturbance in the normal anatomy of the elbow.
- Tendonopathy and other entheseal problems of the arm are common and tend to take 1–2 years to resolve spontaneously, yet they resolve rapidly with rest, an exercise program or corticosteroid injections. Surgical relief is effective for refractory cases.
- The so-called thoracic outlet syndrome is probably most often caused by the 'droopy shoulder syndrome' rather than by a cervical rib.
- Consider corticosteroid injections for CTS and stenosing tenosynovitis (de Quervain and trigger finger or thumb). They are very effective and often curative.
- The site of arthritis in the hand provides a reasonable guide as to the cause.
- Always keep regional pain syndrome in mind for persistent burning pain in the hand following injury—trivial or severe.

Patient education resources

Hand-out sheets from *Murtagh's Patient Education* 7th edition:

- Carpal tunnel syndrome
- Olecranon bursitis
- Tennis elbow
- Trigger finger

References

1. Swift TR, Nichols FT. The droopy shoulder syndrome. Neurology, 1984; 34: 212–15.
2. Bertelsen S. Neurovascular compression syndromes of the neck and shoulder. Acta Chir Scand, 1969; 135: 137–48.
3. Ireland D. The hand (part two). Aust Fam Physician, 1986; 15: 1502–13.
4. Dan NG. Entrapment syndromes. Med J Aust, 1976; 1: 28–31.
5. Corrigan B, Maitland GP. *Practical Orthopaedic Medicine.* Sydney: Butterworths, 1986: 75–7.
6. Young D, Murtagh J. Pitfalls in orthopaedics. Aust Fam Physician, 1989; 18: 645–53.
7. Barton S (ed.). *Clinical Evidence.* London: BMJ Publishing Group, 2001: 717–27.
8. Expert group for Rheumatology. Upper limbs. In: eTG complete [Internet]. Melbourne: Therapeutic Guidelines Ltd. Available from: <www.tg.org.au>, accessed October 2017.
9. White ADN. Practice tip: a simple cure for chronic tennis elbow. Aust Fam Physician, 1987; 16: 953.
10. Oakes B, Fuller P, Kenihan M et al. *Sports Injuries.* Melbourne: Pitman, 1985: 51–5.
11. Ahmad Z et al. Lateral epicondylitis: a review of pathology and management. Bone Joint J, 2013; 95-B (9):1158–64.
12. Smidt N et al. Corticosteroid injections, physiotherapy or a wait and see policy for lateral epicondylitis: a randomised controlled trial. Lancet, 2002; 359: 657–62.
13. Sheon R, Moskowitz R, Goldberg V. *Soft Tissue Rheumatic Pain.* Philadelphia: Lea & Febiger, 1987: 134–40.
14. Buch-Jaeger N, Foucher G. Carpal tunnel syndrome. Hand Surgery, 1994; 19B: 72–4.
15. Expert group for Antibiotics. Soft tissue infections. In: eTG complete [Internet]. Melbourne: Therapeutic Guidelines Ltd. Available from: <www.tg.org.au>, accessed October 2017.
16. Ireland D. The hand (part one). Aust Fam Physician, 1986; 15: 1162–71.
17. Brukner P, Khan K. *Brukner & Khan's Clinical Sports Medicine* (4th edn). Sydney: McGraw-Hill, 2012: 429.
18. Myers S, Della Torre P. Hand and wrist disorders (part 2): how to treat. Australian Doctor, 11 March 2011: 32–4.

Hip, buttock and groin pain 65

Which of your hips has the most profound sciatica?

WILLIAM SHAKESPEARE (1564–1616), *MEASURE FOR MEASURE*

Pain in the hip, buttock, groin and upper thigh tends to be interrelated. Patients often present complaining of pain in the 'hip' but point to the buttock or lower back as the site of their pain. Most pain in the buttock has a lumbosacral origin. Pain originating from disorders of the lumbosacral spine (commonly) and the knee (uncommonly) can be referred to the hip region, while pain from the hip joint (L3 innervation) may be referred commonly to the thigh and the knee. Disorders of the abdomen, retroperitoneal region and pelvis may cause hip and groin pain, sometimes mediated by irritation of the psoas muscle.

Key facts and checkpoints

- Hip troubles have a significant age relationship (see FIG. 65.1).
- Children can suffer from a variety of serious disorders of the hip—such as developmental dysplasia of the hip (DDH), Perthes disease, tuberculosis, septic arthritis, slipped capital femoral epiphysis (SCFE) and inflammatory arthritis—all of which demand early recognition and management.
- SCFE typically presents in the obese adolescent (10–15 years) with knee pain and a slight limp.
- Every newborn infant should be tested for DDH, which can usually be treated successfully when diagnosed early.
- Limp has an inseparable relationship with painful hip and buttock conditions, especially those of the hip.
- The spine is the most likely cause of pain in the buttock in adults.
- Disorders of the hip joint commonly refer pain to the knee and thigh.
- If a woman, especially one with many children, presents with bilateral buttock or hip pain, consider dysfunction of the sacroiliac joints (SIJs) as the cause.
- If a middle-aged or elderly woman presents with hip pain, always consider the underdiagnosed conditions of trochanteric bursitis or gluteus medius tendonitis (greater trochanteric pain syndrome).

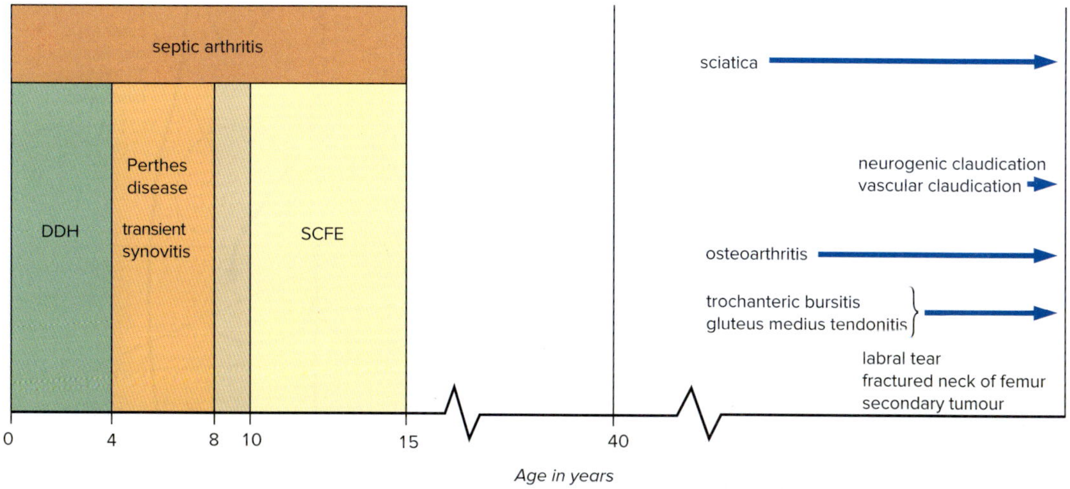

FIGURE 65.1 Typical ages of presentation of hip disorders

Table 65.1 Hip and buttock pain: diagnostic strategy model

Probability diagnosis

Traumatic muscular strains
Referred pain from spine
Osteoarthritis of hip
Greater trochanteric pain syndrome

Serious disorders not to be missed

Cardiovascular:

- buttock claudication

Neoplasia:

- metastatic cancer
- osteoid osteoma

Septic infections:

- septic arthritis
- osteomyelitis
- tuberculosis
- pelvic and abdominal infections: pelvic abscess, pelvic inflammatory disease, prostatitis
- synovial chondromatosis

Childhood disorders:

- DDH
- Perthes disease
- slipped femoral epiphysis
- transient synovitis (irritable hip)
- juvenile chronic arthritis

Pitfalls (often missed)

Polymyalgia rheumatica
Fractures:

- stress fractures femoral neck
- subcapital fractures
- sacrum
- pubic rami

Tear of hamstring
Avascular necrosis femoral head
Femoro-acetabular impingement
Torn acetabular labrum
Sacroiliac joint disorders
Inguinal or femoral hernia
Bursitis or tendonitis:

- greater trochanteric pain syndrome
- ischial bursitis
- iliopsoas bursitis

Osteitis pubis
Neurogenic claudication
Chilblains
Rarities:

- haemarthrosis (e.g. haemophilia)
- Paget disease
- nerve entrapments: sciatica 'hip pocket nerve', obturator, lateral cutaneous nerve thigh

Seven masquerades checklist

Depression
Spinal dysfunction

Is the patient trying to tell me something?

Non-organic pain may be present. Patient with arthritis may be fearful of being crippled.

65

A diagnostic approach

A summary of the diagnostic strategy model is presented in TABLE 65.1.

Probability diagnosis

The commonest cause of hip and buttock pain presenting in general practice is referred pain from the lumbosacral spine and the sacroiliac joints.[1] The pain is invariably referred to the outer buttock and posterior hip area (see FIG. 65.2). The origin of the pain can be the facet joints of the lumbar spine, intervertebral disc disruption or, less commonly, the SIJs. Much of this pain is inappropriately referred to as 'lumbago', 'fibrositis' and 'rheumatism'.

Trauma and overuse injuries from sporting activities are also common causes of muscular and ligamentous strains[2] around the buttock, hip and groin.

The hip joint is a common target of osteoarthritis. This usually presents after 50 years of age but can present earlier if the hip has been affected by another condition.

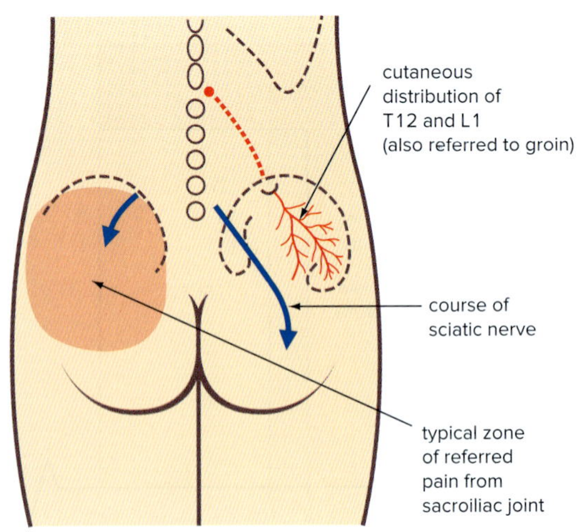

FIGURE 65.2 Referral patterns of pain from the lumbosacral spine and the sacroiliac joints

Serious disorders not to be missed

The major triad of serious disorders—cardiovascular, neoplasia and severe infections—are applicable to this area albeit limited in extent.

Aortoiliac occlusion

Ischaemic muscle pain, including buttock claudication secondary to aortoiliac arterial occlusion, is sometimes confused with musculoskeletal pain. An audible bruit over the vessels following exercise is one clue to diagnosis.

Neoplasia

Primary tumours including myeloma, lymphoma and sarcoma, can arise rarely in the upper femur and pelvis (especially the ileum). However, these areas are relatively common targets for metastases, especially from the prostate, breast and lung.

Infection

Some very important, at times 'occult', infections can develop in and around the hip joint.

Osteomyelitis is prone to develop in the metaphysis of the upper end of the femur and must be considered in the child with intense pain, a severe limp and fever. Tuberculosis may also present in children (usually under 10 years) with a presentation similar to Perthes disease.

Transient synovitis or 'irritable hip' is the most common cause of hip pain and limp in childhood.

Inflammation of the side wall of the pelvis as in a deep pelvic abscess (e.g. from appendicitis), pelvic inflammatory disease (PID) including pyosalpinx, or an ischiorectal abscess, can cause deep hip and groin pain and a limp. This pain may be related to irritation of the obturator nerve.

Retroperitoneal haematoma can cause referred pain and femoral nerve palsy.

Childhood disorders that must not be missed include:

- DDH and acetabular dysplasia
- Perthes disease
- SCFE
- stress fractures of the femoral neck

Inflammatory disorders of the hip joint that should be kept in mind include:

- rheumatoid arthritis
- juvenile chronic arthritis (JCA)
- rheumatic fever (a flitting polyarthritis)
- spondyloarthropathy

'Red flag' pointers to potentially serious hip conditions

- Swelling, redness, very limited joint motion
- Pain, fever, systemic features (in absence of trauma)
- Neurological changes (e.g. loss of power)
- Rapid joint swelling after trauma
- Constant localised pain unaffected by movement

Pitfalls

There are many pitfalls associated with hip and buttock pain and these include the various childhood problems. Fractures can be a pitfall, especially subcapital fractures.

SIJ disorders are often missed, whether it be the inflammation of sacroiliitis or mechanical dysfunction of the joint.

Inflammatory conditions around the hip girdle are common and so are often misdiagnosed. These include the common gluteus medius tendonitis and trochanteric bursitis (greater trochanteric pain syndrome).

Polymyalgia rheumatica commonly causes shoulder girdle pain in the elderly but pain around the hip girdle can accompany this important problem.

Chilblains around the upper thighs occur in cold climates and are often known as 'jodhpur' chilblains because they tend to occur during horse riding in very cold weather.

Nerve entrapment syndromes require consideration. Meralgia paraesthetica is a nerve entrapment causing pain and paraesthesia over the lateral aspect of the hip (see FIG. 66.3, CHAPTER 66).

An interesting modern phenomenon is the so-called 'hip pocket nerve' syndrome. If a man presents with 'sciatica', especially confined to the buttock and upper posterior thigh (without local back pain), consider the possibility of pressure on the sciatic nerve from a wallet in the hip pocket. This problem is occasionally encountered in people sitting for long periods in cars (e.g. taxi drivers). It appears to be related to the increased presence of plastic credit cards in wallets (see FIG. 65.3).

Paget disease can involve the upper end of the femur and the pelvis. Increased pain may indicate a fracture or malignant change causing osteosarcoma.

General pitfalls

- Failure to test the hips of neonates carefully and follow up developmental dysplasia of the hip.
- Misdiagnosis of arthritis and other disorders of the hip joint because of referred pain.

65

- Overlooking an SCFE or a stress fracture of the femoral neck in teenage boys, especially athletes. If an X-ray shows that the epiphysis is fusing or has fused, arrange a technetium bone scan.

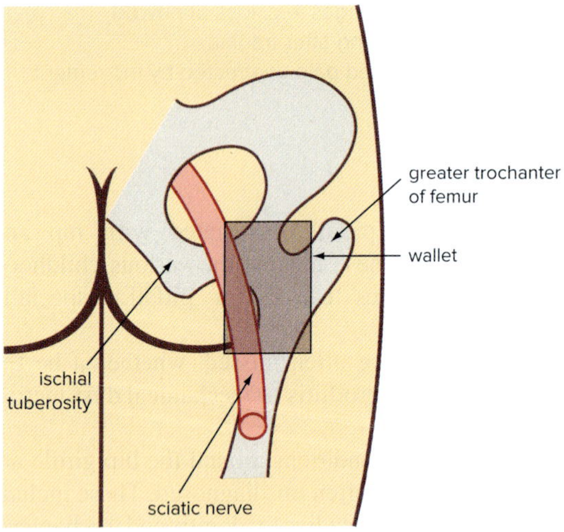

FIGURE 65.3 'Hip pocket nerve' syndrome: location and relations of sciatic nerve in the buttock

Seven masquerades checklist

The one outstanding masquerade is spinal dysfunction, which is the most likely cause of pain in the buttock. Many dermatomes meet at the buttock and theoretically pain in the buttock can result from any lesion situated in a tissue derived from L1, L2, L3, S2, S3 and S4.[1] Symptoms from L3 can spread from the outer buttock to the front of the thigh and down the leg, over the medial aspect of the knee to the calf. Such a distribution is common to an L3 nerve root lesion and arthritis of the hip.

65

Furthermore, dysfunction of the facet joints and sacroiliac joints can refer pain to the buttock. The relatively common L1 lesion due to dysfunction at the T12–L1 spinal level can lead to referred pain over the outer upper quadrant of the buttock and also to the groin (see FIG. 65.2).

Psychogenic considerations

Cyriax[1] claims that the hip shares with the back and the shoulder 'an enhanced liability to fixation' for psychological reasons. This problem is often related to work compensation factors and overpowering stresses at home. A common finding in psychoneurotic patients complaining of buttock and thigh pain is 90° limitation of flexion at the hip joint. The importance of testing passive movements of the hip joint is obvious, for often such limitation of flexion is combined with a full range of rotation. In arthritis of the hip joint internal rotation is invariably affected first.

Such patients often walk into the office with a marked limp and leaning on a thick stick. It requires great skill to evaluate and manage them tactfully and successfully.

On the other hand, patients with genuine osteoarthritis fear being crippled and ending in a wheelchair. They require considerable education and reassurance.

The clinical approach

History

Pain associated with hip joint pathology is usually described as a deep aching pain, aggravated by movement and felt in the groin and anteromedial aspect of the upper thigh, sometimes exclusively around the knee (see FIG. 66.1 in CHAPTER 66). A limp is a frequent association.

An obstetric history in a woman may be relevant for sacroiliac pain.

Key questions

- Can you tell me how the pain started?
- Could you describe the pain?
- Point to where the pain is exactly.
- Does the pain come on after walking for a while and stop as soon as you rest?
- Is there any stiffness, especially first thing in the morning?
- Do you have any difficulty climbing stairs?
- Do you get any backache?
- Do your movements feel free?
- Do you have a limp?
- Do you have a similar ache around the shoulders?
- Have you had an injury such as a fall?
- Have you lost any weight recently?
- Do you have night pain?
- Do you have trouble with shoes and socks?
- How far can you walk?
- Is it painful to lie on the affected side at night?
- Did you have a hip problem as a child?
- Does the pain respond to any treatments?

Examination

Follow the traditional methods of examination of any joint: LOOK, FEEL, MOVE, MEASURE, TEST FUNCTION, LOOK ELSEWHERE and X-RAY. The patient should strip down to the underpants to allow maximum exposure.

Inspection

Ask the patient to point exactly to the area of greatest discomfort. Careful observation of the patient, especially walking, provides useful diagnostic information. Note any antalgic (painful) gait—if walking with a limp, the leg adducted and foot somewhat externally rotated, osteoarthritis of the hip joint is the likely diagnosis.

If called to a patient who has suffered an injury such as a fall or vehicle accident, note the position of the leg. If shortened and externally rotated (see FIG. 65.4a), a fractured neck of femur is the provisional diagnosis; if internally rotated, suspect a posterior dislocation of the hip (see FIG. 65.4b). With anterior dislocation of the hip, the hip is externally rotated.

Get the patient to lie supine on the couch with the anterior superior iliac spines (ASISs) of the pelvis placed squarely and note the shape and position of the limbs. Look for muscle wasting.

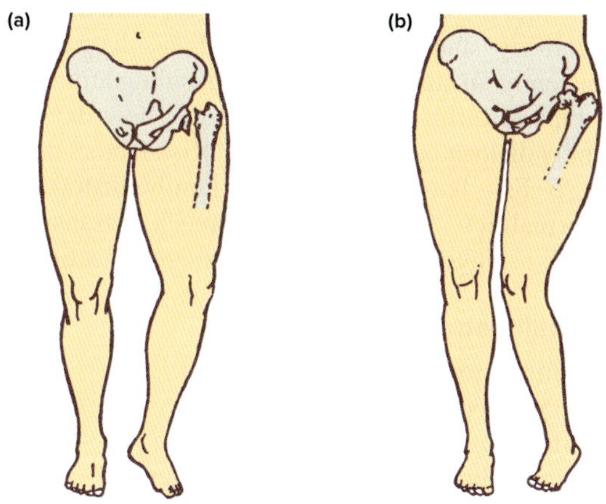

FIGURE 65.4 **(a)** General configuration of the legs for a fractured neck of femur, **(b)** general configuration for a posterior dislocated hip

Palpation

Feel one to two finger breadths below the midpoint of the inguinal ligament for joint tenderness. Check for trochanteric bursitis, gluteus medius tendonitis and other soft tissue problems over the most lateral bony aspect of the upper thigh.

Movements

- Passive movements with *patient supine* (normal range is indicated):
  - flexion with patient's knees flexed (compare both sides): 0–125°
  - external rotation (knee and hip extended in adults): 0–45°
  - internal rotation (knee and hip extended in adults): 0–45°
  - abduction (stand on same side—steady pelvis): 0–45°
  - adduction (should see the patella of the opposite leg): 0–30°

In children it is most important to measure rotation and abduction/adduction with the knee and hip flexed to detect early Perthes disease or SCFE.

- *Patient prone:*
  - extension (one hand held over SIJ): 0–20°

Note: Osteoarthritis of the hip typically affects internal rotation (IR), extension and abduction first.

Measurements

- True leg length (ASIS to medial malleolus)
- Apparent leg length (umbilicus to medial malleolus)

Note:

- Unequal true leg length = hip disease on shorter side
- Unequal apparent leg length = tilting of pelvis

Feel the height of the greater trochanter relative to the ASIS to determine if shortening is in the hip or below.

Test function including gait and special tests

Gait:

- Antalgic gait—shortened stance phase of affected leg, as patient doesn't want to stand on it, indicates pain with weight-bearing
- Coxalgic gait—upper torso shifts towards painful side due to pain in the hip
- Trendelenburg gait (the gluteus medius lurch)—similar to coxalgic but pelvis tilts
- Trendelenburg test—tests hip abductors (gluteus medius): the non-weight-bearing hemipelvis drops if abnormal
- Thomas test—tests for fixed flexion deformity
- Squeeze test for osteitis pubis
- Femoroacetabular impingement[2,3] (FAI)—get the patient to hold the hip in 90° of flexion and maximal internal rotation. Then bring the leg into adduction (FADIR test). Reproduction of pain is a positive test and indicates intra-articular hip pathology such as labral tears and a cam or Ganz (bone outgrowth) lesion. The FABERE test

(see later in chapter) also tests for this pathology. FAI causes anterior groin and trochanteric regional pain.

Look elsewhere

Examine the lumbosacral spine, SIJs, groin and knee. Consider hernias and possibility of PID. Feel pulses and test for femoral bruits.

Investigations

These can be selected from:

- serological tests: RA factor, FBE, ESR, C-reactive protein
- radiological:
  - plain AP X-ray of pelvis showing both hip joints
  - lateral X-ray ('frog' lateral best in children)
  - X-ray of lumbosacral spine and SIJs
  - CT scan: hip joint, pelvis, lumbosacral spine
  - MRI scan: stress fracture, early avascular necrosis, early osteomyelitis, labral tears of hip joint, metastases, soft tissue tumours
  - isotope bone scan; useful for whole body bony metastases
- needle aspiration of joint: if septic arthritis suspected

Role of ultrasound

Ultrasound diagnosis is now sensitive in children in detecting fluid in the hip joint, and can diagnose septic arthritis and also localise the site of an osteomyelitic abscess around a swollen joint. It can accurately assess the neonatal hip joint and confirm the position of the femoral head in children <6 months. Ultrasound is used less since increased availability of MRI.

65

Hip pain in children

Hip disorders have an important place in childhood and may present with a limp when the child is walking. These important disorders include:

- DDH
- congenital subluxation of hip and acetabular dysplasia
- transient synovitis
- Perthes disease
- septic arthritis/osteomyelitis
- SCFE
- pathological fractures through bone cyst

The important features of hip pain in children are summarised in TABLE 65.2.

Developmental dysplasia of the hip

In DDH, previously known as congenital dislocation of the hip, the underdeveloped femoral head dislocates posteriorly and superiorly. DDH is described as transiently unstable or as a mild subluxation (1 in 80 hips at birth, which stabilises in a few days) and frankly dislocated (1 in 800 hips).[4] Risk factors include the '5 Fs': female, first born, family history, foot abnormalities, 'funny' delivery (breech or transverse), as well as oligohydramnios and caesarean section.

Clinical features

- Females:males = 6:1
- Asymmetry in 40%
- Bilateral in one-third
- Tight adductors and short leg evident

Table 65.2 Comparison of important causes of hip pain in children

	DDH	Transient synovitis	Perthes	SCFE	Septic arthritis
Age (years)	0–4	4–8	4–8	10–15	Any
Limp	+	+	+	+	Won't walk
Pain	–	+	+	+	+ + +
Limited movement	Abduction	All, especially abduction and IR	Abduction and IR	All, especially IR	All
Plain X-ray	No diagnostic value in neonatal period (use ultrasound). US up to 6 months then plain X-ray	Normal	Subchondral fracture Dense head Pebble stone epiphysis	AP may be normal Frog lateral view shows slip	Normal Use ultrasound

- Diagnosed early by Ortolani and Barlow tests (abnormal thud or clunk on abduction); test usually negative after 2 months
- Ultrasound excellent (especially up to 6 months) and more sensitive than clinical examination
- X-ray difficult to interpret up to 3 months, then helpful

Note:

1 When diagnosed and treated from birth it is possible to produce a normal joint after a few months in an abduction splint.
2 Every baby should be examined for DDH during the first day of life then regularly and before discharge from hospital and at the 6-week check.[4] The Ortolani and Barlow tests remain important means of detecting an unstable or dislocated hip, but ultrasound is becoming more important and is recommended for high-risk babies (e.g. breech, family history of DDH).

Screening examination

Carry out the examination on a large firm bench with the baby stripped. Relaxation is essential; give the baby a bottle if necessary. Be gentle and have warm hands.

With the legs extended any asymmetry of the legs, especially any shortening, or skin creases is noted.

Ortolani test (IN test: gentle clunk into acetabulum)

- Hold the leg in the hand with knee flexed—thumb over groin (lesser trochanter) and middle finger over greater trochanter (see FIG. 65.5). Steady the pelvis with the other hand.
- Flex hips to about 90°, gently abduct to 45° (note any clunk or jerk as hip reduces).

Barlow test (OUT test: gentle clunk out of acetabulum)

- As one hand stabilises the pelvis, grasp the knee of the relevant leg, then flex the hip to 90°, abduct 10–20°.
- With gentle but firm backward pressure, rock the femur backwards and forwards on the pelvis by pressing forward with the middle finger and backwards with the thumb. Note any jerk or clunk as hip 'goes out' of the acetabulum. If the femoral head displaces, there is dislocation.

Plain X-ray has little or no place in the diagnosis of DDH in the neonatal period.[5] Ultrasound imaging is recommended. Early referral for treatment is essential. If not detected early the femoral head stays out of the acetabulum and after the age of 1 year the child may present with delay in walking or a limp. The diagnosis is then detected by X-ray.

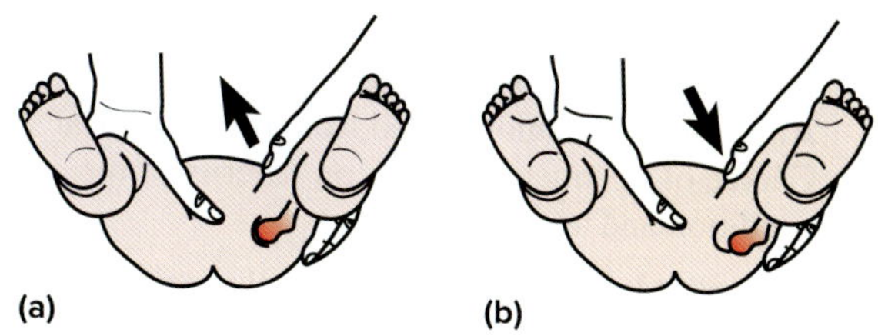

FIGURE 65.5 Screening for developmental dysplasia of the hip (left side): **(a)** Ortolani sign; **(b)** Barlow sign

Treatment (guidelines)

- DDH must be referred to a specialist[4]
- 0–6 months—Pavlik harness or abduction splint
- 3–18 months—reduction (closed or open) and cast (pelvic spica)
- >18 months—open reduction and possible osteotomy
  Slings are not recommended

Note: Despite early treatment some cases progress to acetabular dysplasia (underdevelopment of the 'roof' of the hip joint) and to premature osteoarthritis. Thus a follow-up X-ray of the pelvis during teenage years should be considered for anyone with a history of DDH.

Perthes disease

Perthes disease results in the femoral head becoming partly or totally avascular (i.e. avascular necrosis).

Clinical features

- Males:females = 4:1
- Usual age 4–8 years; range 2–12 years (rarely 2–18 years)
- Sometimes bilateral
- Presents as a limp and aching (hip or groin pain)
- May be knee pain
- 'Irritable' hip early
- Limited movement in abduction and IR

X-ray. Joint space appears increased and femoral head too lateral: typical changes of sclerosis, deformity and collapse of the femoral capital epiphysis may be delayed.

Management

- Refer urgently (provide crutches)
- Aim is to keep femoral head from becoming flat
- Choice of treatment depends on severity of the condition and age of the patient

If untreated, the femoral head usually becomes flat over some months, leading to eventual osteoarthritis. Some untreated cases of Perthes disease heal and have a normal X-ray.

Transient synovitis

This common condition is also known as 'irritable hip' or observation hip and is the consequence of a self-limiting synovial inflammation.

Clinical features

- Child aged 3–8 years (usually 6 years)
- Sudden onset of hip pain and a limp
- Child can usually walk but with pain (some may not)
- May be history of trauma or recent URTI or viral illness
- Painful limitation of movements, especially abduction and rotation
- Blood tests and X-rays normal (may be soft tissue swelling); ESR may be mildly elevated
- Ultrasound shows fluid in the joint

Differential diagnosis. This includes septic arthritis, JCA, Perthes disease.

Outcome. It settles to normal within 7 days, without sequelae.

Treatment. Refer early. Treatment is bed rest or the use of crutches and analgesics. Follow-up X-ray is needed in 4 to 6 months to exclude Perthes disease. Aspiration under general anaesthetic may be needed to exclude septic arthritis.

65

Slipped capital femoral epiphysis

One problem of the displaced capital epiphysis of the femoral head (SCFE) is when some patients develop avascular necrosis despite expert treatment. Diagnosis of the condition before major slipping is important. This necessitates early consultation with the teenager experiencing hip or knee discomfort and then accurate interpretation of X-rays.

Clinical features

- Adolescent 10–15 years, often obese
- Most common in the oversized and undersexed (e.g. the heavy prepubertal boy)
- Bilateral in 20%
- Limp and irritability of hip on movement
- Anterior hip (groin) pain
- Knee pain
- Hip rotating into external rotation on flexion and often lies in external rotation (ER)
- Most movements restricted, especially IR

Any adolescent with a limp or knee pain should have X-rays (AP and frog view) of both hips (see FIG. 65.6). Otherwise, this important condition will be overlooked. SCFE is graded I to IV. The femoral head is located posterior-inferior.

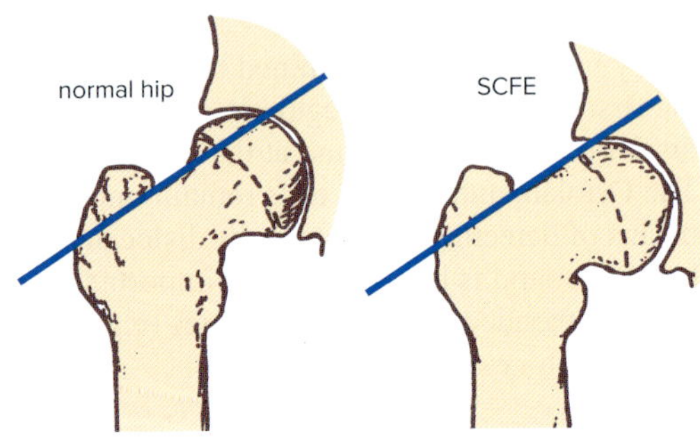

FIGURE 65.6 Appearance of a slipped capital femoral epiphysis; note that, in the normal state, a line drawn along the superior surface of the femoral neck passes through the femoral head, but passes above it with SCFE

Management

- Cease weight-bearing and refer urgently to an orthopaedic surgeon. Also refer if the clinical signs indicate SCFE but the X-rays look normal.
- If acute slip, gentle reduction via traction is better than manipulation in preventing later avascular necrosis.
- Once reduced, pinning is performed.

Septic arthritis

Septic arthritis of the hip should be suspected in all children with acutely painful or irritable hip problems. These patients may not be obviously sick on presentation, particularly in infants <2 years. A negative needle aspiration does not exclude septic arthritis. If sepsis is suspected it is better to proceed to an arthrotomy if clinically indicated.

The irritable hip syndrome should be diagnosed only after negative investigations, including plain films and ultrasound, full blood examination, ESR and bone scan. Needle aspiration has to be considered but irritable hip is often diagnosed without it, by observing in hospital in traction. If a deterioration or elevated temperature develops, needle aspiration with or without arthrotomy is indicated.

Avulsion bony injuries

Forceful contraction of muscles originating around the pelvis can lead to avulsion at their origin in those with skeletal immaturity. This causes acute pain and muscular dysfunction:

- anterior superior iliac spine (sartorius)
- anterior inferior iliac spine (long head rectus femoris)
- ischial tuberosity (hamstrings)
- lesser trochanter (psoas)

Management includes X-ray and referral. As a rule, surgical reattachment is not required.

The little athlete

The most common problem in the little athlete is pain or discomfort in the region of the iliac crest or anterior or superior iliac spines, usually associated with traction apophysitis or with acute avulsion fractures.[7] There is localised tenderness with pain on stretching and athletes should rest until they can compete without discomfort.

If there are persistent signs, pain in the knee, hip irritability or restricted range of motion, X-rays should be ordered to exclude serious problems such as SCFE or Perthes disease.

Hip and buttock pain in the elderly

The following conditions are highly significant in the elderly:

- osteoarthritis of the hip
- aortoiliac arterial occlusion → vascular claudication
- spinal dysfunction with nerve root or referred pain
- degenerative spondylosis of lumbosacral spine → neurogenic claudication
- polymyalgia rheumatica
- trochanteric bursitis
- fractured neck of femur
- secondary tumours

Subcapital fractures

The impacted subcapital fractured femoral neck can often permit weight-bearing by an elderly patient. No obvious deformity of the leg is present. Radiographs are therefore essential for the investigation of all painful hips in the elderly. Patients often give a story of two falls—the first[5] very painful, the second with the hip just 'giving way' as the femoral head fell off.

The displaced subcapital fracture has at least a 40% incidence of avascular necrosis and usually requires prosthetic replacement in patients over 70 years. MRI scan is the investigation of choice if the X-rays are normal. Intertrochanteric fractures are also common (see CHAPTER 133).

Avascular necrosis

The age of onset is usually 20–50 (average 38 years). Consider this with hip pain and deep groin pain especially with IR in those at risk: corticosteroid use, SLE, sickle cell disease, past hip fracture or dislocation, pregnancy, alcoholic liver disease. Investigate with imaging (as above) and refer.

Osteoarthritis of the hip

Osteoarthritis of the hip is the most common form of hip disorder. It can be caused by primary osteoarthritis, which is related to an intrinsic disorder of articular cartilage, or to secondary osteoarthritis. Predisposing factors to the latter include previous trauma, DDH, septic arthritis, acetabular dysplasia, SCFE and past inflammatory arthritis.

Clinical features

- Equal sex incidence
- Usually after 50 years, increases with age
- May be bilateral: starts in one, other follows
- Insidious onset
- At first, pain worse with activity, relieved by rest, and then nocturnal pain and pain after resting
- Stiffness, especially after rising
- Characteristic deformity
- Stiffness, deformity and limp may dominate (pain mild)
- Pain usually in groin—may be referred to medial aspect of thigh, buttock or knee

Examination

- Antalgic gait
- Usually gluteal and quadriceps wasting
- First hip movements lost are IR and extension
- Fixed flexion deformity
- Hip held in flexion and ER (at first)
- Eventually all movements affected
- Order of movement loss is IR, extension, abduction, adduction, flexion, ER

Treatment

- Careful explanation: patients fear osteoarthritis of hip

- Weight loss if overweight
- Relative rest
- Use crutches for acute pain
- Analgesics and NSAIDs (judicious use)
- Aids and supports (e.g. walking stick)
- Physiotherapy
- Physical therapy, including isometric exercises
- Hydrotherapy—very useful

Surgery

This is an excellent option for those with severe pain or disability unresponsive to conservative measures. Total hip replacement is the treatment of choice in older patients but a femoral osteotomy may be considered in younger patients in selected cases. In selected patients in their 30s and 40s with severe disease, total hip replacement is being performed successfully. A type of total hip replacement called hip resurfacing is becoming more popular in certain situations in patients under 60 years of age; >90% achieve a good result. Most replacements last 15–20 years.

Groin pain

All conditions involving the hip joint, especially osteoarthritis, can present with groin pain. Consider an unrecognised fracture in neck of femur, psoas abscess, Paget disease, osteitis pubis and hernias. Also consider hip labral or chondral lesions. Hip labral injuries present with inguinal pain or upper anterior thigh pain, and require investigation and referral.

65

Acute groin pain

Acute groin problems include muscular and musculotendinous strains, as well as common overuse sporting injuries such as tendonopathy and tendoperiostitis. These need to be differentiated from referred pain from the lumbosacral spine, hip and pelvis problems such as hip labral injuries. More common acute groin injuries include injuries to the following muscles and their tendons: adductor longus (e.g. musculotendinous strains causing inner thigh pain), rectus femoris, sartorius and iliopsoas. The relatively common adductor muscle or tendon injury results in upper thigh pain, local tenderness and resisted hip adduction. Ultrasound or MRI confirms the diagnosis. Treatment is based on physiotherapy, exercises and possibly a corticosteroid injection

Chronic groin pain

There are many causes of chronic groin pain, the commonest being bone and joint abnormalities. Important causes involve muscle and musculotendinous lesions, including adductor longus tendoperiostitis, osteitis pubis (pubic symphysis), iliopsoas bursitis, stress fractures (e.g. femoral neck and pubic rami), 'occult' inguinal or femoral hernias and referred pain from musculoskeletal disorders of the lumbosacral spine and hip.

Investigations include X-ray of the pelvis, tomography of the pubic symphysis (to detect osteitis pubis and pubic instability), bone scan to detect stress fractures or osteitis pubis, herniography and imaging such as CT scan, MRI or ultrasound.

Hip labral tears and FAI[9,10]

Acetabular labral tears are becoming better recognised in motor accident victims, dancers and athletes, especially with the use of MRI and hip arthroscopy. Patients may complain of sharp impingement pain in the hip and/or groin and of painful clicking, catching or locking. The impingement test should be performed (see earlier in chapter). X-rays will exclude bony hip pathology while MRI is the radiological investigation of choice. According to Paoloni, examination after hip joint anaesthetic injection is the gold standard for diagnosing hip pathology.[11] Refer for possible surgical treatment through hip arthroscopy. However, there are no proven effective treatments for FAI and hip labral tears, so any interventions should be approached cautiously.[3]

Sacroiliac pain

Pain arising from SIJ disorders is normally experienced as a dull ache in the buttock but can be referred to the groin or posterior aspect of the thigh. It may mimic pain from the lumbosacral spine or the hip joint. The pain may be unilateral or bilateral. It is worse in loading situations, e.g. walking, running, getting in and out of cars.

There are no accompanying neurological symptoms such as paraesthesia or numbness but it is common for more severe cases to cause a heavy aching feeling in the upper thigh.

Causes of SIJ disorders

- Inflammatory (the spondyloarthropathies)
- Infections (e.g. TB, *Staphylococcus aureus*—rare)
- Osteitis condensans ilii
- Degenerative changes
- Mechanical disorders
- Post-traumatic, after sacroiliac disruption or fracture
- Childbirth—in postnatal period

Examination

The SIJs are difficult to palpate and examine but there are several tests that provoke them.

Direct pressure. With the patient lying prone a rhythmic springing force is applied directly to the upper and lower sacrum respectively.

Winged compression test. With the patient lying supine and with arms crossed, 'separate' the iliac crests with a downwards and outwards pressure. This compresses the SIJs.

Lateral compression test. With hands placed on the iliac crests, thumbs on the ASISs and heels of hand on the rim of the pelvis, compress the pelvis. This distracts the SIJs.

Patrick or FABERE test. This method can provoke the hip as well as the SIJ. The patient lies supine on the table and the foot of the involved side and extremity is placed on the opposite knee (the hip joint is now flexed, externally rotated and abducted). The knee and opposite ASIS are pressed downwards simultaneously (see FIG. 65.7). If low back or buttock pain is reproduced the cause is likely to be a disorder of the SIJ.

Unequal sacral 'rise' test. Squat behind the standing patient and place hands on top of the iliac crests and thumbs on the posterior superior iliac spines (PSIS). Ask the patient to bend slowly forwards and touch the floor. If one side moves higher relative to the other a problem may exist in the SIJs (e.g. a hypomobile lesion in the painful side if that side's PSIS moves higher).

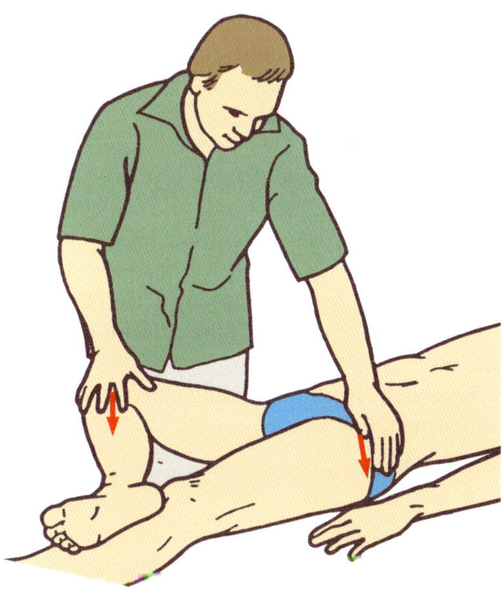

FIGURE 65.7 The Patrick (FABERE) test for right-sided hip or sacroiliac joint lesion, illustrating directions of pressure from the examiner

Mechanical disorders of the SIJ

These problems are more common than appreciated and can be caused by hypomobile or hypermobile problems.

Hypomobile SIJ disorders are usually encountered in young people after some traumatic event, especially women following childbirth (notably multiple or difficult childbirth), or after a heavy fall onto the buttocks, as well as in those with structural problems (e.g. shortened leg). Pain tends to follow rotational stresses of the SIJ (e.g. tennis, dancing). Excellent results are obtained by passive mobilisation or manipulation, such as the non-specific rotation technique with the patient lying supine.[12]

Hypermobile SIJ disorders are sometimes seen in athletes with instability of the symphysis pubis, in women after childbirth and in those with a history of severe trauma to the pelvis (e.g. MVAs, horse riders with foot caught in the stirrups after a fall). The patient presents typically with severe aching pain in the lower back, buttocks or upper thigh. Such problems are difficult to treat and manual therapy usually exacerbates the symptoms. Treatment consists of relative rest, analgesics and a sacroiliac supportive belt.

Greater trochanteric pain syndrome[13]

Pain around the lateral aspect of the hip is a common disorder, and is usually seen as lateral hip pain radiating down the lateral aspect of the thigh in older people engaged in walking exercises, tennis and similar activities. It is analogous in a way to the shoulder girdle, where supraspinatus tendonitis and subacromial bursitis are common wear-and-tear injuries.

The cause is tendonopathy of the gluteus medius tendon (considered to be the main pathology), where it inserts into the lateral surface of the greater trochanter of the femur and/or gluteus minimus tendon with or without inflammation of the trochanteric bursa. Weakness of these abductor muscles has been demonstrated. The degenerative tendon may tear, rupture or become detached. The pain of this condition tends to occur at night, especially after activity such as long walks and gardening. X-rays are usually normal but ultrasound may demonstrate the pathology.

Clinical features

- Older person especially female >45–50 years
- Pain on outside hip referred to as far as foot
- Pain on lying on hip at night
- Pain climbing stairs, getting in and out of car
- Limp
- Localised tenderness on outer border of thigh

Treatment[12]

A trial of NSAIDs (weigh the risks) is worthwhile and physiotherapy involving hip-strengthening exercises is first-line treatment. Injection therapy, including under ultrasound, is also very effective and facilitates exercises.

Method of injection without ultrasound

- Determine the points of maximal tenderness over the trochanteric region and mark them. (For tendonopathy, this point is immediately over or above the superior aspect of the greater trochanter—see FIG. 65.8).
- Inject aliquots of a mixture of 1 mL of long-acting corticosteroid with 4–5 mL of local anaesthetic into the tender area, which usually occupies an area similar to that of a standard marble.

The injection may be very effective for a variable time. Follow-up management includes sleeping with a small pillow under the involved buttock, sleeping on a sheepskin rug, and stretching the gluteal muscles with knee–chest exercises, which are the key to relief.[12] Advise the patient to walk with the feet turned out—'the Charlie Chaplin gait'. One or two repeat injections over 6 or 12 months may be required. Surgical intervention such as iliotibial band release ± bursectomy may be necessary. Local application of ice and massage therapy may provide relief. Massaging the site with fingers, a soft drink bottle or a tennis ball (while lying on the side) may also be effective.

65

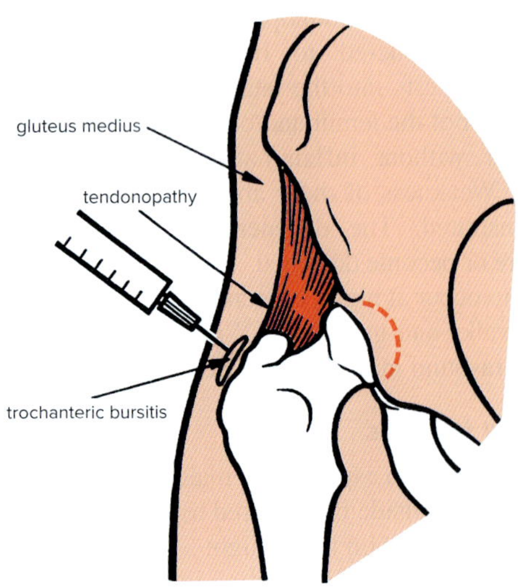

FIGURE 65.8 Injection technique for gluteus medius tendonopathy (into area of maximal tenderness)

Fascia lata syndrome

Pain in the lateral thigh can be caused by inflammation of the fascia lata. It is often due to overuse or weak musculature around the hip. Treatment is relative rest and physiotherapy.

Ischial bursitis

Tailor's bottom or 'weaver's bottom', which is occasionally seen, is a bursa overlying the ischial tuberosity. Irritation of the sciatic nerve may coexist and the patient may appear to have sciatica.

Clinical features

- Severe pain when sitting, especially on a hard chair
- Tenderness at or just above the ischial tuberosity

Treatment

- Infiltration into the tender spot of a mixture of 4 mL of 1% lignocaine and 1 mL of LA corticosteroid (avoid the sciatic nerve)
- Foam rubber cushion with two holes cut out for the ischial prominences

Snapping or clicking hip (coxa saltans)

Some patients complain of a clunking, clicking or snapping hip, either palpable and/or audible. This represents an annoying problem that may cause pain in the groin or thigh. It is more common in females with a wide pelvis.

Causes

- A taut iliotibial band (tendon or tensor fascia femoris) slipping backwards and forwards over the prominence of the greater trochanter
  or
- The iliopsoas tendon snapping across the iliopectineal eminence at the anterior brim of the pelvis
- The gluteus maximus sliding across the greater trochanter
- Joint laxity

Treatment

The basics of treatment are:

- explanation and reassurance
- exercises to stretch the iliotibial band[13]

Occasionally surgery is necessary to lengthen the iliotibial band.

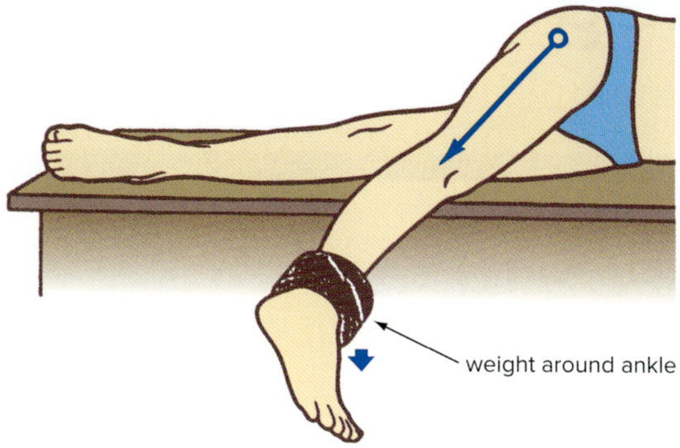

FIGURE 65.9 One treatment for the clicking hip

Exercises

- The patient lies on the 'normal' side and flexes the affected hip, with the leg straight and a weight around the ankle (see FIG. 65.9), to a degree that produces a stretching sensation along the lateral aspect of the thigh.
- This iliotibial stretch should be performed for 1–2 minutes, twice daily.

When to refer

- Clinical evidence or suspicion of severe childhood disorders: DDH, Perthes disease, septic arthritis, SCFE or osteomyelitis
- Undiagnosed pain, especially night pain
- Any fractures or suspicion of fractures such as impacted subcapital fracture or stress fracture of the femoral neck
- Patients with true claudication in buttock, whether it is vascular from aortoiliac occlusion or neurogenic from spinal canal stenosis
- Patients with disabling osteoarthritis of the hip not responding to conservative measures; excellent results are obtained from surgery to the hip
- Any mass or lump

Practice tips

- Training on a plastic DDH model should be essential for all neonatal practitioners in order to master the manoeuvres for examining the neonatal hip.
- True hip pain is usually felt in the groin, thigh and medial aspect of the knee.
- The name of the FABERE test is an acronym for **F**lexion, **Ab**duction, **E**xternal **R**otation and **E**xtension of the hip.
- Night pain adds up to inflammation, bursitis or tumour.
- The hip joint can be the target of infections such as *Staphylococcus aureus*, tuberculosis or inflammatory disorders such as rheumatoid and the spondyloarthropathies, but these are rare numerically compared with osteoarthritis.
- Psoas-related pain is an important differential diagnosis of anterior hip pain.

Patient education resources

Hand-out sheets from *Murtagh's Patient Education* 7th edition:

- Bursitis and tendonitis of outer hip
- Hip: osteoarthritis

References

1 Cyriax J. *Textbook of Orthopaedic Medicine,* Vol. 1 (6th edn). London: Balliere Tindall, 1976: 568–94.
2 Wood T (Coordinator). Sports Medicine. Check Program 453. Melbourne: RACGP, 2009: 11–13.
3 Expert group for Rheumatology. Lower limb. In: eTG complete [Internet]. Melbourne: Therapeutic Guidelines Ltd. Available from: <www.tg.org.au>, accessed October 2017.
4 Anonymous. *The Eastern Seal Guide to Children's Orthopaedics.* Toronto: Eastern Seal Society, 1982.
5 Robinson MJ. *Practical Paediatrics* (5th edn). Melbourne: Churchill Livingstone, 2003: 239–40.
6 Larkins PA. The little athlete. Aust Fam Physician, 1991; 20: 973–8.
7 Young D, Murtagh J. Pitfalls in orthopaedics. Aust Fam Physician, 1989; 18: 654–5.
8 Wood TQ, Young DA. Labral tears: understanding the significance of rim lesions. Medicine Today, 2008; 9: 71–5.
9 Wall PD et al. Surgery for treating hip impingement (femoroacetabular impingement). Cochrane Database. Syst Rev. 2014, Issue 8. Art No. CD010796.
10 Paoloni J. Hip and groin injuries in sport. Medical Observer, 9 March 2007: 27.
11 Walsh MJ, Solomon MJ. Trochanteric bursitis: misnomer and misdiagnosis. Medicine Today, 2006; 7 (12): 62–3.
12 Mellor R et al. Exercise and load modification versus corticosteroid injection versus 'wait and see' for persistent gluteus medius/minimus tendinopathy (the LEAP trial): a protocol for a randomised clinical trial. BMC Musculoskelet Disord, 2016; 17: 196.
13 Sheon RP, Moskowitz RW, Goldberg VM. *Soft Tissue Rheumatic Pain* (2nd edn). Philadelphia: Lea & Febiger, 1987: 211–12.

Resources

<http://www.ddheducation.com>

Healthy Hips Australia. <www.healthyhipsaustralia.org.au/>.

66 Pain in the leg

Thou cold sciatica
Cripple our senators, that their limbs may halt
As lamely as their manners.

WILLIAM SHAKESPEARE (1564–1616), *TIMON OF ATHENS*

Pain in the leg has many causes, varying from a simple cramp to an arterial occlusion. Overuse of the legs in the athlete can lead to a multiplicity of painful leg syndromes, ranging from simple sprains of soft tissue to compartment syndromes. A major cause of leg pain lies in the source of the nervous network to the lower limb, namely the lumbar and sacral nerve roots of the spine. It is important to recognise radicular pain, especially from L5 and S1 nerve roots, and also the patterns of referred pain, such as from apophyseal (facet) joints and sacroiliac joints (SIJs).

Key facts and checkpoints

- Always consider the lumbosacral spine, the SIJs and hip joints as important causes of leg pain.
- Hip joint disorders may refer pain around the knee only (without hip pain).
- Nerve root lesions may cause pain in the lower leg and foot only (without back pain).
- Nerve entrapment is suggested by a radiating burning pain, prominent at night and worse at rest.
- Older people may present with claudication in the leg from spinal canal stenosis or arterial obstruction or both.
- Think of the hip pocket wallet as a cause of sciatica from the buttocks down.
- Acute arterial occlusion to the lower limb requires relief within 4 hours (absolute limit of 6 hours).
- The commonest site of acute occlusion is the common femoral artery.
- Varicose veins can cause aching pain in the leg.

A diagnostic approach

A summary of the diagnostic strategy model is presented in TABLE 66.1.

Table 66.1 Pain in the leg: diagnostic strategy model

Probability diagnosis
Muscle cramps
Nerve root 'sciatica'
Osteoarthritis (hip, knee)
Exercise-related pain (e.g. Achilles tendonitis), muscular injury (e.g. hamstring)

Serious disorders not to be missed
Vascular:
- peripheral vascular disease
- arterial occlusion (embolism)
- thrombosis popliteal aneurysm
- deep venous thrombosis
- iliofemoral thrombophlebitis

Neoplasia:
- primary (e.g. myeloma)
- metastases (e.g. breast to femur)

Infection:
- osteomyelitis
- septic arthritis
- erysipelas
- lymphangitis
- gas gangrene

Pitfalls (often missed)
Osteoarthritis hip
Osgood–Schlatter disorder
Spinal canal stenosis → neurogenic claudication
Herpes zoster (early)
Greater trochanteric pain syndrome
Nerve entrapment, e.g. meralgia paraesthetica
'Hip pocket nerve': from wallet pressure
Iatrogenic: injection into nerve
Sacroiliac disorders
Sympathetic dystrophy (causalgia)
Peripheral neuropathy
Rarities:
- osteoid osteoma
- polymyalgia rheumatica (isolated)
- Paget disease
- popliteal artery entrapment
- tabes dorsalis
- ruptured Baker cyst

Seven masquerades checklist
Depression
Diabetes
Drugs (indirect)
Anaemia (indirect)
Spinal dysfunction
Is the patient trying to tell me something?
Quite possible. Common with work-related injuries.

Probability diagnosis

Many of the causes, such as foot problems, ankle injuries and muscle tears (e.g. hamstrings and quadriceps), are obvious and common. There is a wide range of disorders related to overuse syndromes in athletes.

A very common cause of acute severe leg pain is cramp in the calf musculature, the significance of which escapes some patients as judged by middle-of-the-night calls.

One of the commonest causes is nerve root pain, invariably single, especially affecting the L5 and S1 nerve roots. Tests of their function and of the lumbosacral spine for evidence of disc disruption or other spinal dysfunction will be necessary. Should multiple nerve roots be involved, other causes, such as compression from a tumour, should be considered. Remember that a spontaneous retroperitoneal haemorrhage in a patient on anticoagulant therapy can cause nerve root pain and present as intense acute leg pain. The nerve root sensory distribution is presented in FIGURE 66.1.

Other important causes of referred thigh pain include ischiogluteal bursitis (weaver's bottom) and gluteus medius tendonitis or trochanteric bursitis.

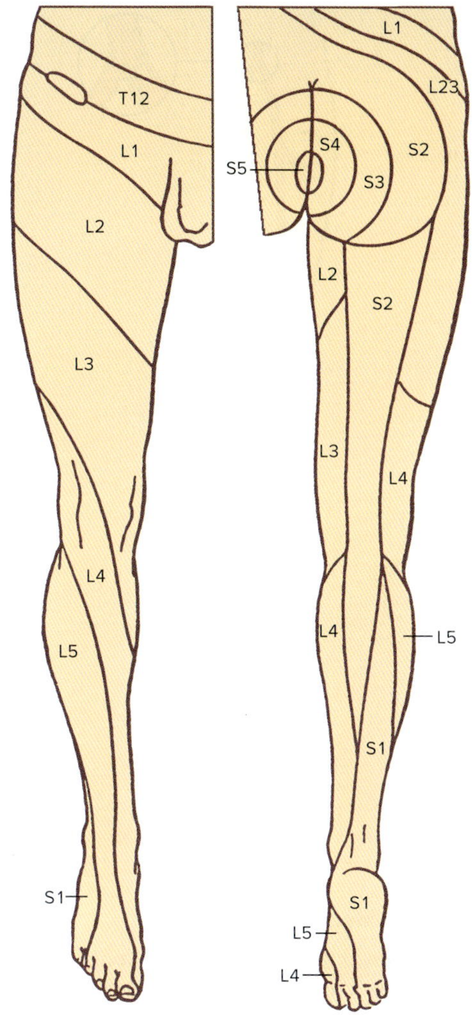

FIGURE 66.1 Dermatomes of the lower limb, representing approximate cutaneous distribution of the nerve roots

Serious disorders not to be missed

Neoplasia

Malignant disease, although uncommon, should be considered, especially if the patient has a history of one of the primary tumours, such as breast, lung or kidney. Such tumours can metastasise to the femur. Consider also osteogenic sarcoma and multiple myeloma, which are usually seen in the upper half of the femur. The possibility of an osteoid osteoma should be considered with pain in a bone relieved by aspirin.

Infections

Severe infections are not so common, but septic arthritis and osteomyelitis warrant consideration. Superficial infections such as erysipelas and lymphangitis occur occasionally.

Vascular problems

Acute severe ischaemia can be due to thrombosis or embolism of the arteries of the lower limb. Such occlusions cause severe pain in the limb and associated signs of severe ischaemia, especially of the lower leg and foot.

Chronic ischaemia due to arterial occlusion can manifest as intermittent claudication or rest pain in the foot due to small vessel disease.[1]

Various pain syndromes are presented in FIGURE 66.2. It is important to differentiate vascular claudication from neurogenic claudication (see TABLE 66.2).

66

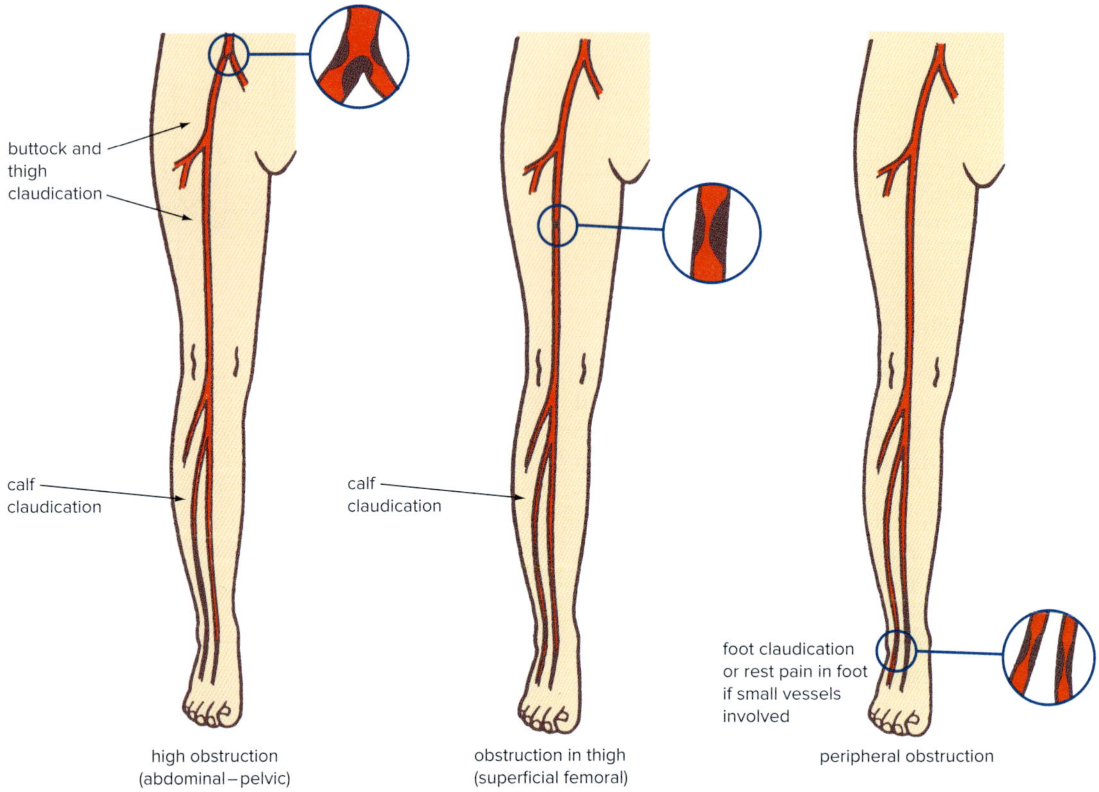

FIGURE 66.2 Arterial occlusion and related symptoms according to the level of obstruction

Venous disorders

The role of uncomplicated varicose veins as a cause of leg pain is controversial. Nevertheless, varicose veins can certainly cause a dull aching 'heaviness' and cramping, and can lead to painful ulceration.

Superficial thrombophlebitis is usually obvious, but it is vital not to overlook deep venous thrombosis. These more serious conditions of the veins can cause pain in the thigh or calf.

Pitfalls

There are many traps and pitfalls in the painful leg. Herpes zoster at the pre-eruption phase is an old trap and more so when the patient develops only a few vesicles in obscure parts of the limbs.

In future we can expect to encounter more cases of spinal canal stenosis (secondary to the degenerative changes) in the elderly. The early diagnosis can be difficult, and buttock pain on walking has to be distinguished from vascular claudication due to a high arterial obstruction.

The many disorders of the SIJ and hip region can be traps, especially the poorly diagnosed yet common gluteus medius tendonitis. Another more recent phenomenon is the 'hip pocket nerve syndrome', where a heavy wallet crammed with credit cards can cause pressure on the sciatic nerve.

One of the biggest traps, however, is when hip disorders, particularly osteoarthritis, present as leg pain, especially on the medial aspect of the knee.

Nerve entrapments (see FIG. 66.3) are an interesting cause of leg pain, although not as common as in the upper limb. Some entrapments to consider include:

- lateral cutaneous nerve of thigh, known as meralgia paraesthetica
- common peroneal nerve
- posterior tibial nerve at ankle (the 'tarsal tunnel' syndrome)
- obturator nerve, in obturator canal
- femoral nerve (in inguinal region or pelvis)

Then there are the rare causes. One overlooked problem is complex regional pain syndrome I (sympathetic dystrophy), which may follow even minor trauma to the limb. This 'causalgia' syndrome

Table 66.2 Comparison of the clinical features of neurogenic and vascular claudication

	Neurogenic claudication	Vascular claudication
Cause	Spinal canal stenosis	Aortoiliac arterial occlusive disease
Age	Over 50 Long history of backache	Over 50
Pain site and radiation	Proximal location, Initially lumbar, buttocks and legs Radiates distally	Distal location Buttocks, thighs and calves (especially) Radiates proximally
Type of pain	Weakness, burning, numbing or tingling (not cramping)	Cramping, aching, squeezing
Onset	Walking (uphill and downhill) Distance walked varies Prolonged standing	Walking a set distance each time, especially uphill
Relief	Lying down Flexing spine (e.g. squat position) May take 20–30 minutes	Standing still—fast relief Slow walking decreases severity
Associations	Bowel and bladder symptoms	Impotence Rarely, paraesthesia or weakness
Physical examination		
Peripheral pulses Lumbar extension	Present Aggravates	Present (usually) Reduced or absent in some, especially after exercise No change
Neurological	Saddle distribution Ankle jerk may be reduced after exercise	*Note:* abdominal bruits after exercise
Diagnosis confirmation	Radiological studies EMG	Duplex ultrasound Ankle brachial index Arteriography

manifests as burning or aching pain with vasomotor instability in the limbs. The essential feature is the disparity between the intensity of the pain and the severity of the inciting injury.

General pitfalls

- Overlooking beta blockers and anaemia as a precipitating factor for vascular claudication
- Overlooking hip disorders as a cause of knee pain
- Mistaking occlusive arterial disease for sciatica
- Confusing nerve root syndromes with entrapment syndromes

Seven masquerades checklist

The outstanding cause of leg pain in this group is spinal dysfunction. Apart from nerve root pressure due to a disc disruption or meralgia paraesthetica, pain can be referred from the apophyseal (facet) joints. Such pain can be referred as far as the mid-calf (see FIG. 66.4).

The other checklist conditions—depression, diabetes, drugs and anaemia—can be associated with pain in the leg. Depression can reinforce any painful complex.

Diabetes can cause discomfort through a peripheral neuropathy that can initially cause localised pain before anaesthesia predominates. Drugs such as beta blockers, and anaemia, can precipitate or aggravate intermittent claudication in a patient with a compromised circulation.

Psychogenic considerations

Pain in the lower leg can be a frequent complaint (maybe a magnified one) of the patient with non-organic pain, such as the malingerer, the conversion reaction patient (hysteria) and the depressed. Sometimes regional pain syndrome (reflex or post-traumatic) is incorrectly diagnosed as functional.

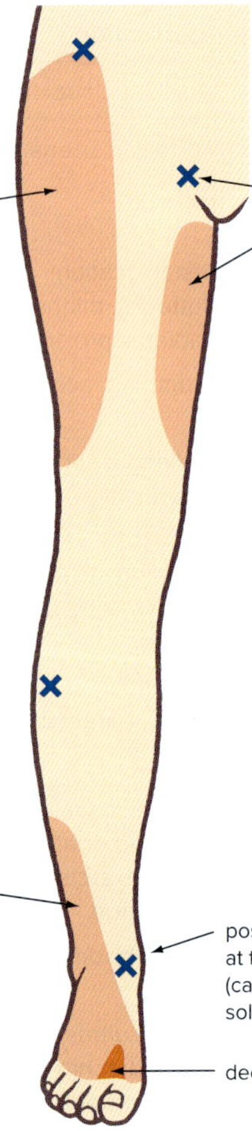

FIGURE 66.3 Distribution of pain in the leg from entrapment of specific nerves; the sites of entrapments are indicated by an X

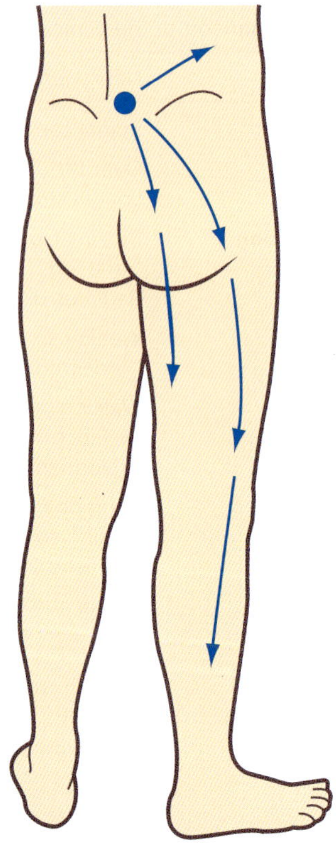

FIGURE 66.4 Possible referred pain patterns from dysfunction of an apophyseal joint, illustrating pain radiation patterns from stimulation by injection of the right L4–5 apophyseal joint

Source: Reproduced with permission from C Kenna and J Murtagh. *Back Pain and Spinal Manipulation.* Sydney: Butterworths, 1989

The clinical approach

Careful attention to basic detail in the history and examination can point the way of the clinical diagnosis.

History

In the history it is important to consider several distinctive aspects, outlined by the following questions.

- Is the pain of acute or chronic onset?
- If acute, did it follow trauma or activity?
  - If not, consider a vascular cause: vein or artery; occlusion or rupture.
- Is the pain 'mechanical' (related to movement)?
  - If it is unaltered by movement of the leg or a change in posture, it must arise from a soft tissue lesion, not from bone or joints.
- Is the pain postural?
  - Analyse the postural elements that make it better or worse.
  - If worse on sitting, consider a spinal cause (discogenic) or ischial bursitis.
  - If worse on standing, consider a spinal cause (instability) or a local problem related to weight-bearing (varicose veins).
  - If worse lying down, consider vascular origin, such as small vessel peripheral vascular disease. If worse lying on one side, consider greater trochanteric pain syndrome.
  - Pain unaffected by posture is activity-related.
- Is the pain related to walking?
  - *No:* Determine the offending activity (e.g. joint movement with arthritis).
  - *Yes:* If immediate onset, consider local cause at site of pain (e.g. stress fracture). If delayed onset, consider vascular claudication or neurogenic claudication.

- Is the site of pain the same as the site of trauma?
  - If not, the pain in the leg is referred. Important considerations include lesions in the spine, abdomen or hip and entrapment neuropathy.
- Is the pain arising from the bone?
  - If so, the patient will point to the specific site and indicate a 'deep' bone pain (consider tumour, fracture or, rarely, infection) compared with the more superficial muscular or fascial pain.
- Is the pain arising from the joint?
  - If so, the clinical examination will determine whether it arises from the joint or juxtaposed tissue.

Examination

The first step is to watch the patient walk and assess the nature of any limp.

Note the posture of the back and examine the lumbar spine. Have both legs well exposed for the inspection.

Inspect the patient's stance and note any asymmetry and other abnormalities, such as swellings, bruising, discolouration, or ulcers and rashes. Note the size and symmetry of the legs and the venous pattern. Look for evidence of ischaemic changes, especially of the foot.

Palpate for local causes of pain and if no cause is evident examine the spine, blood vessels (arteries and veins) and bone. Areas to palpate specifically are the ischial tuberosity, trochanteric area, hamstrings and tendon insertions. Palpate the superficial lymph nodes. Note the temperature of the feet and legs. Perform a vascular examination, including the peripheral pulses and the state of the veins if appropriate.

If evidence of peripheral vascular disease (PVD), remember to auscultate the abdomen and adductor hiatus, and the iliac, femoral and popliteal vessels.

A neurological examination may be appropriate, particularly to test nerve root lesions or entrapment neuropathies.

Examination of the joints, especially the hip and SIJs, is very important.

Investigations

A checklist of investigations that may be necessary to make the diagnosis is as follows:

- FBE and ESR
- radiology:
  - leg X-rays, especially knee, hip
  - plain X-ray of lumbosacral spine
  - CT scan of lumbosacral spine
  - ultrasound or MRI of greater trochanteric area
  - MRI scan of lumbosacral spine
  - bone scan
- electromyography
- vascular:
  - arteriography
  - duplex ultrasound scan
  - ankle brachial index
  - venous pool radionuclide scan
  - contrast venography
  - air plethysmograph (varicose veins)
  - D-dimer test

Leg pain in children

Aches and pains in the legs are a common complaint in children. The most common cause is soreness and muscular strains due to trauma or unaccustomed exercise. One cause of bilateral leg pain in children is leukaemia. Consider osteomyelitis (refer CHAPTER 69).

It is important to consider child abuse, especially if bruising is noted on the back of the legs.

'Growing pains'

So-called 'growing pains', or idiopathic leg pain, is thought to be responsible for up to 20% of leg pain in children.[2] Such a diagnosis is vague and often made when a specific cause is excluded. It is usually not due to 'growth' but related to excessive exercise or trauma from sport and recreation, and probably emotional factors.

The pains are typically intermittent and symmetrical and deep in the legs, usually in the anterior thighs or calves. Although they may occur at any time of the day or night, typically they occur at night, usually when the child has settled in bed. The pains usually last for 30–60 minutes and tend to respond to attention such as massage with an analgesic balm or simple analgesics (refer to CHAPTER 91).

Serious problems

It is important to exclude fractures (hence the value of X-rays if in doubt), malignancy (such as osteogenic sarcoma, Ewing tumour or infiltration from leukaemia or lymphoma), osteoid osteoma, osteomyelitis, scurvy and beriberi (rare disorders in developed countries) and congenital disorders such as sickle-cell anaemia, Gaucher disease and Ehlers–Danlos syndrome.

Leg pain in the elderly

The older the patient, the more likely it is that arterial disease with intermittent claudication and neurogenic claudication due to spinal canal stenosis will develop.

Other important problems of the elderly include degenerative joint disease, such as osteoarthritis of the hips and knees, muscle cramps, herpes zoster, Paget disease, polymyalgia rheumatica (affecting the upper thighs) and sciatica.

Spinal causes of leg pain

Problems originating from the spine are an important, yet at times complex, cause of pain in the leg.

Important causes are:

- nerve root (radicular) pain from direct pressure
- referred pain from:
  - disc pressure on tissues in front of the spinal cord
  - apophyseal joints
  - SIJs
- spinal canal stenosis causing claudication

Various pain patterns are presented in FIGURES 66.3 and 66.4.

Nerve root pain

Nerve root pain from a prolapsed disc is a common cause of leg pain. A knowledge of the dermatomes of the lower limb (see FIG. 66.1) provides a pointer to the involved nerve root, which is usually L5 or S1 or both. The L5 root is invariably caused by an L4–5 disc prolapse and the S1 root by an L5–S1 disc prolapse. The nerve root syndromes are summarised in TABLE 66.3.

A summary of the physical examination findings for the most commonly involved nerve roots is presented in TABLE 66.3.

Sciatica

See CHAPTER 38. Sciatica is defined as pain in the distribution of the sciatic nerve or its branches (L4, L5, S1, S2, S3) caused by nerve pressure or irritation. Most problems are due to entrapment neuropathy of a nerve root, in either the spinal canal (as outlined above) or the intervertebral foramen.

It should be noted that back pain may be absent and peripheral symptoms only will be present.

Treatment

Acute sciatica

A protracted course can be anticipated, in the order of 12 weeks (see CHAPTER 38). The patient should be reassured that spontaneous recovery can be expected. A trial of conservative treatment would be recommended thus:

- back care education
- relative bed rest if very painful only (2 days is optimal)—a firm base is ideal
- return to activities of daily living ASAP
- analgesics (avoid narcotic analgesics if possible)
- NSAIDs (2 weeks is recommended)
- basic exercise program, including swimming
- traction can help, even intermittent manual

Referral to a therapist of your choice (e.g. physiotherapist) may be advisable. Conventional spinal manipulation is usually contraindicated for radicular sciatica. If the patient is not responding or the circumstances demand more active treatment, an epidural anaesthetic injection is appropriate. Surgical consultation is indicated for a severe or progressive neurological deficit.

Chronic sciatica

If a trial of NSAIDs, rest and physiotherapy has not brought significant relief, an epidural anaesthetic (lumbar or caudal) using half-strength local anaesthetic (e.g. 0.25% bupivacaine HCl) and a depot corticosteroid (e.g. triamcinolone) is advisable. The lumbar route under image intensification is preferred.

Lumbar spinal canal stenosis (LSS)[3]

LSS is narrowing of the spinal canal resulting in pressure on the sciatic nerve roots and possibly the spinal canal and cord. It typically occurs in people aged over 50 years with a history of spinal degenerative changes, including osteoarthritis (see FIG. 38.9), but LSS may be congenital.

The symptoms are as outlined for neurogenic claudication in TABLE 66.2. Pain, which is usually bilateral, is in the proximal-leg buttocks, thighs and legs, radiating distally. Some 50% remain clinically stable, 25% deteriorate and about 25% improve with time. Conservative treatment includes relative rest, specific exercises, analgesics and agents for neuropathic pain. There is no evidence of the value of epidural corticosteroid injections or oral corticosteroids. Surgical consultation is indicated for severe or progressive neurological deficit or progressive pain,. The risk of surgical complications increases with age.

Referred pain

Referred pain in the leg can arise from disorders of the SIJs or from spondylogenic disorders. It is typically dull, heavy and diffuse. The patient uses the hand to describe its distribution compared with the use of fingers to point to radicular pain.

Spondylogenic pain

Non-radicular or spondylogenic pain originates from any of the components of the vertebrae (spondyles), including joints, the intervertebral discs, ligaments

Table 66.3 Comparison of neurological findings of the neurological levels L3, L4, L5 and S1

Nerve root	Pain distribution (see FIG. 67.1)	Sensory loss	Motor function	Reflex
L3	Front of thigh, inner aspect of thigh, knee and leg	Anterior aspect of thigh 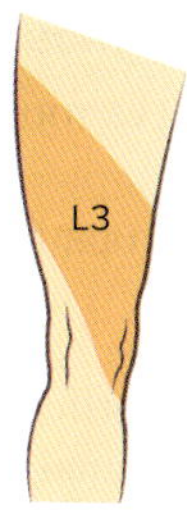	Extension of knee 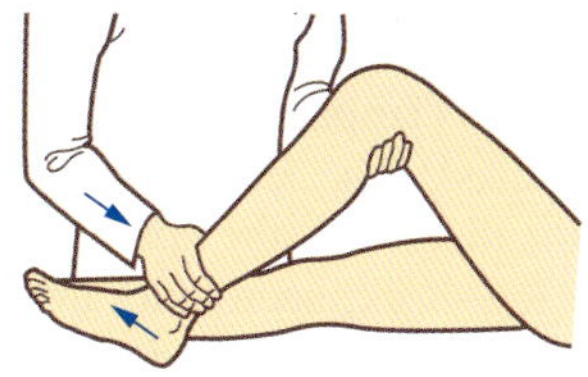	Knee jerk 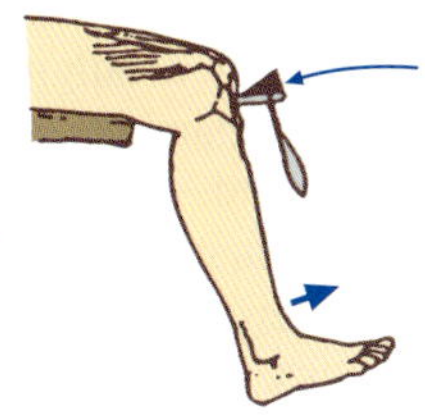
L4	Anterior thigh to front of knee	Lower outer aspect of thigh and knee, inner great toe 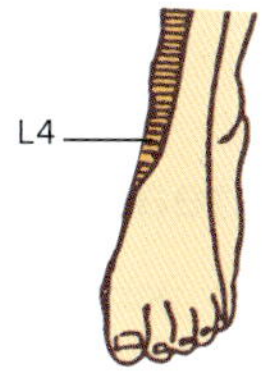	Flexion, adduction of knee, inversion of foot 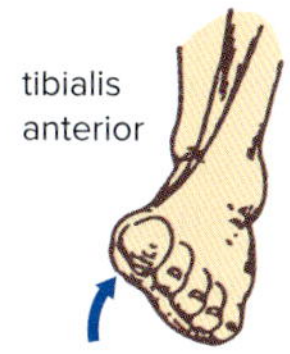	Knee jerk 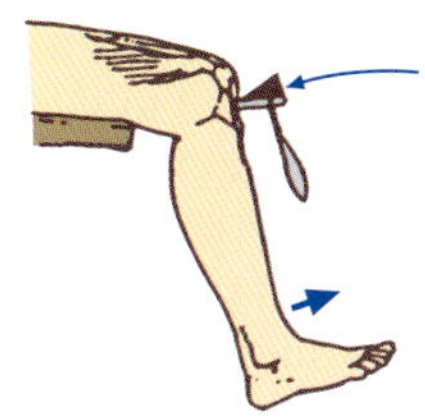
L5	Lateral aspect of leg, dorsum of foot and great toe	Dorsum of foot, great toe, 2nd, 3rd and 4th toes, anterolateral aspect of lower leg 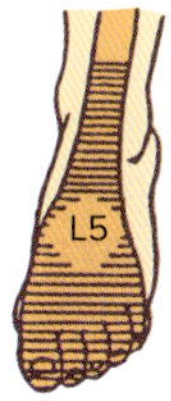	Dorsiflexion of great toe and ankle 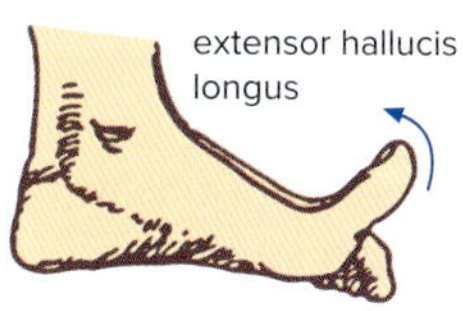	Tibialis posterior (clinically impractical) 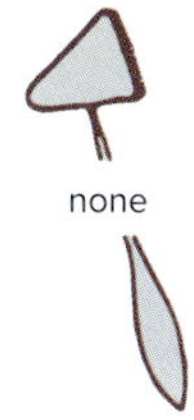
S1	Buttock to back of thigh and leg, central calf, lateral aspect of ankle and sole of foot	Lateral aspect of ankle, foot (4th and 5th toes) 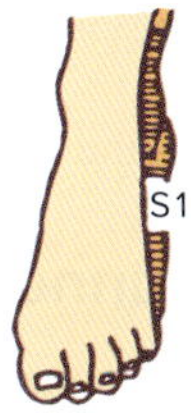	Plantar flexion of ankle and toes, eversion of foot 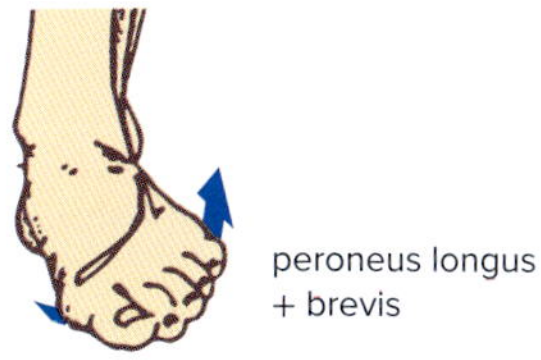	Ankle jerk 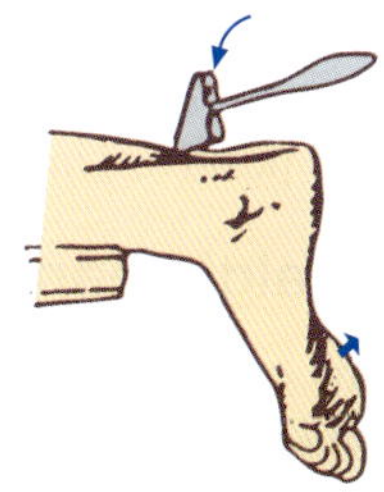

Source: Reproduced in part with permission from S Hoppenfeld. *Physical Examination of the Spine and Extremities*. Norwalk, CT: Appleton & Lange

and muscle attachments. An important example is distal referred pain from disorders of the apophyseal joints, where the pain can be referred to any part of the limb as far as the calf and ankle but most commonly to the gluteal region and proximal thigh (see FIG. 66.4).

Another source of referred pain is that caused by compression of a bulging disc against the posterior longitudinal ligament and dura. The pain is typically dull, deep and poorly localised. The dura has no specific dermatomal localisation, so the pain is usually experienced in the low back, sacroiliac area and buttocks. Less commonly, it can be referred to the coccyx, groin and both legs down to the calves. It is not referred to the ankle or the foot.

Sacroiliac dysfunction

This typically causes a dull ache in the buttock, but it can be referred to the iliac fossa, groin or posterior aspects of the thighs (see CHAPTER 65). It rarely radiates to or below the knee. It may be caused by inflammation (sacroiliitis) or mechanical dysfunction. The latter must be considered in a postpartum woman presenting with severe aching pain present in both buttocks and thighs.

Nerve entrapment syndromes

Entrapment neuropathy can result from direct axonal compression or can be secondary to vascular problems, but the main common factor is a nerve passing through a narrow rigid compartment where movement or stretching of that nerve occurs under pressure.

Clinical features

66

- Pain at rest (often worse at night)
- Variable effect with activity
- Sharp, burning pain
- Radiating and retrograde pain
- Clearly demarcated distribution of pain
- Paraesthesia may be present
- Tenderness over nerve
- May be positive Tinel sign

Meralgia paraesthetica

This is the commonest lower limb entrapment and is due to the lateral femoral cutaneous nerve of the thigh being trapped under the lateral end of the inguinal ligament, 1 cm medial to the ASIS.[4]

The nerve is a sensory nerve from L2 and L3. It occurs mostly in middle-aged people, due mainly to thickening of the fibrous tunnel beneath the inguinal ligament, and is associated with obesity, pregnancy, ascites or local trauma such as belts, trusses and corsets. Its entrapment causes a burning pain with associated numbness and tingling (see FIG. 66.3).

The distribution of pain is confined to a localised area of the lateral thigh and does not cross the midline of the thigh.

Differential diagnosis

- L2 or L3 nerve root pain (L2 causes buttock pain also)
- Femoral neuropathy (extends medial to midline)

Treatment

- Injection of corticosteroid medial to the ASIS, under the inguinal ligament
- Surgical release (neurolysis) if refractory
- Treat the cause (e.g. weight reduction, constricting belt, corset)

Note: Meralgia paraesthetica often resolves spontaneously.

Peroneal nerve entrapment

The common peroneal (lateral popliteal) nerve can be entrapped where it winds around the neck of the fibula or as it divides and passes through the origin of the peroneus longus muscle 2.5 cm below the neck of the fibula. It is usually injured, however, by trauma or pressure at the neck of the fibula.

Symptoms and signs

- Pain in the lateral shin area and dorsum of the foot
- Sensory symptoms in the same area
- Weakness of eversion and dorsiflexion of the foot (described by patients as 'a weak ankle')

Differential diagnosis

- L5 nerve root (similar symptoms)

Treatment

- Shoe wedging or other orthotics to maintain eversion
- Neurolysis is the most effective treatment

Tarsal tunnel syndrome

This is an entrapment neuropathy of the posterior tibial nerve in the tarsal tunnel beneath the flexor retinaculum on the medial side of the ankle. The condition is due to dislocation or fracture around the ankle or tenosynovitis of tendons in the tunnel from injury, or rheumatoid arthritis and other inflammations.

Symptoms and signs

- A burning or tingling pain in the toes and sole of the foot, occasionally the heel
- Retrograde radiation to the calf, perhaps as high as the buttock
- Numbness is a late symptom
- Discomfort often in bed at night and worse after standing
- Removal of shoe may give relief
- Sensory nerve loss variable, may be no loss
- Tinel test (finger or reflex hammer tap over nerve below and behind medial malleolus) may be positive
- Tourniquet applied above ankle may reproduce symptoms

The diagnosis is confirmed by electrodiagnosis.

Treatment

- Relief of abnormal foot posture with orthotics
- Corticosteroid injection into tunnel
- Decompression surgery if other measures fail

Vascular causes of leg pain

Occlusive arterial disease

Risk factors for peripheral vascular disease (for development and deterioration):

- smoking
- diabetes mellitus
- hypertension
- hypercholesterolaemia
- family history
- atrial fibrillation (embolism)

Aggravating factors:

- beta-blocking drugs
- anaemia

Acute lower limb ischaemia

Sudden occlusion is a dramatic event that requires immediate diagnosis and management to save the limb.

Causes

- Embolism—peripheral arteries
- Thrombosis: major artery, popliteal aneurysm
- Traumatic contusion (e.g. postarterial puncture)

The symptoms and signs of acute embolism and thrombosis are similar, although thrombosis of an area of atherosclerosis is often preceded by symptoms of chronic disease (e.g. claudication). The commonest site of acute occlusion is the common femoral artery (see FIG. 66.5).

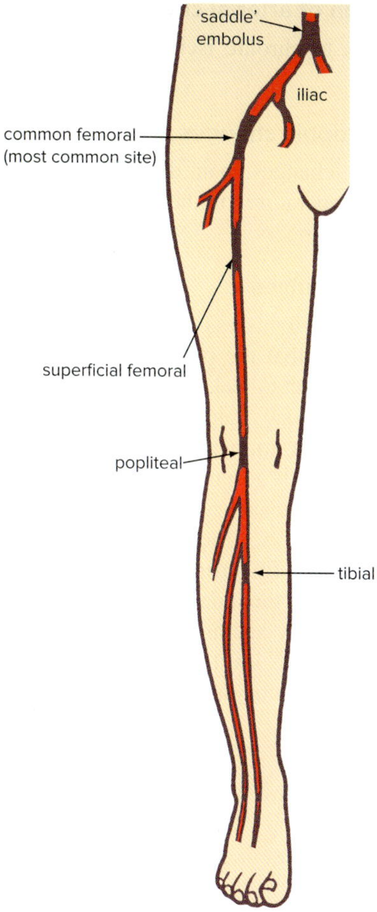

FIGURE 66.5 Common sites of acute arterial occlusion

Signs and symptoms—the 6 Ps

- Pain
- Pallor
- Paraesthesia or numbness
- Pulselessness
- Paralysis
- 'Perishing' cold

The pain is usually sudden and severe and any improvement may be misleading. Sensory changes initially affect light touch, not pinprick. Paralysis (paresis or weakness) and muscle compartment pain or tenderness are most important and ominous signs.

Other signs include mottling of the legs, collapsed superficial veins, and no capillary return. If the foot becomes dusky purple and fails to blanch on pressure, irreversible necrosis has occurred.

Note: Look for evidence of atrial fibrillation.

66

Examination of arterial circulation

This applies to chronic ischaemia and also to acute ischaemia.

Skin and trophic changes

Note colour changes, hair distribution and wasting. Note the temperature of the legs and feet with the backs of your fingers.

Palpation of pulses

It is important to assess four pulses carefully (see FIG. 66.6). Note that the popliteal and posterior tibial pulses are difficult to feel, especially in obese subjects.

Femoral artery. Palpate deeply just below the inguinal ligament, midway between the ASIS and the symphysis pubis. If absent or diminished, palpate over abdomen for aortic aneurysm.

Popliteal artery. Flex the leg to relax the hamstrings. Place fingertips of both hands to meet in the midline. Press them deeply into the popliteal fossa to compress artery against the upper end of the tibia (i.e. just below the level of the knee crease). Check for a popliteal aneurysm (very prominent popliteal pulsation).

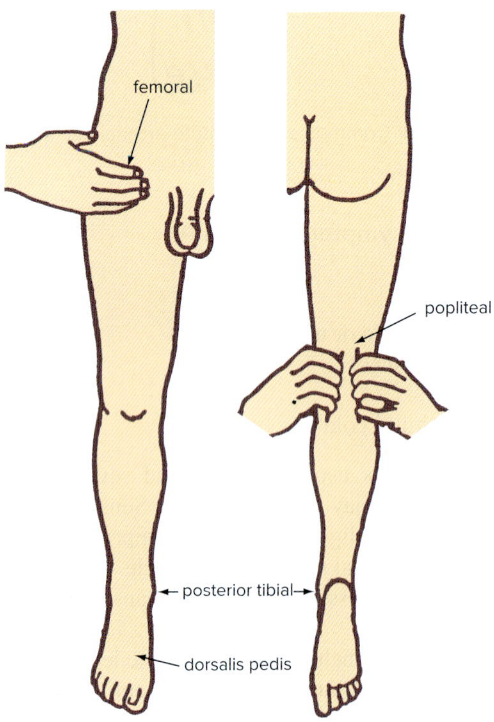

FIGURE 66.6 Sites of palpation of peripheral pulses in the leg

66

Posterior tibial artery. Palpate, with curved fingers, just behind and below the tip of the medial malleolus of the ankle.

Dorsalis pedis artery. Feel at the proximal end of the first metatarsal space just lateral to the extensor tendon of the big toe.

Oedema

Look for evidence of oedema: pitting oedema is tested by pressing firmly with your thumb for at least 5 seconds over the dorsum of each foot, behind each medial malleolus and over the shins.

Postural colour changes (Buerger test)

Raise both legs to about 60° for about 1 minute, when maximal pallor of the feet will develop. Then get the patient to sit up on the couch and hang both legs down.[4]

Note: Comparing both feet, check the time required for return of pinkness to the skin (normally less than 10 seconds) and filling of the veins of the feet and ankles (normally about 15 seconds). Look for any unusual rubor (dusky redness) that takes a minute or more in the dependent foot. A positive Buerger test is pallor on elevation and rubor on dependency and indicates severe, chronic ischaemia.

Auscultation for bruits after exercise

Listen over abdomen and femoral area for bruits.

Note: Neurological examination (motor, sensory, reflexes) is normal unless there is associated diabetic peripheral neuropathy.

Treatment

Golden rules: Occlusion is usually reversible if treated within 4 hours (i.e. limb salvage). It is often irreversible if treated after 6 hours (i.e. limb amputation).

- Intravenous heparin (immediately) 5000 U
- Emergency embolectomy (ideally within 4 hours):
  - under general or local anaesthesia
  - through an arteriotomy site in the common femoral artery
  - embolus extracted with Fogarty balloon or catheter

  or
- Stenting of vessels (a good modern option)—discuss this with an interventional cardiovascular physician or interventional radiologist (less invasive and less expensive)
- Angioplasty
- Arterial bypass if acute thrombosis in chronically diseased artery
- In selected cases, thrombolysis with streptokinase or urokinase appropriate

- Amputation (early) if irreversible ischaemic changes
- Lifetime anticoagulation with warfarin will be required

Note: An acutely ischaemic limb is rarely life-threatening in the short term. Thus, even in the extremely aged, demented or infirm, a simple embolectomy is not only worthwhile but also is usually the most expedient treatment option.

Chronic lower limb ischaemia

Chronic ischaemia caused by gradual arterial occlusion can manifest as intermittent claudication, rest pain in the foot or overt tissue loss—ulceration, gangrene (see FIG. 66.7).

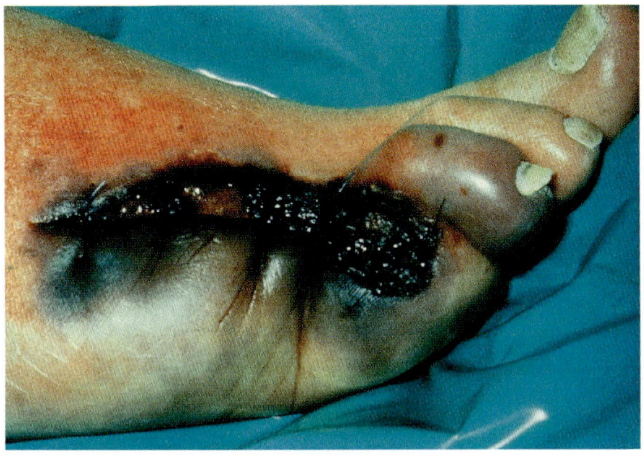

FIGURE 66.7 Gangrene of the lateral aspect of the foot following attempted amputation of an ischaemic toe. A below-knee amputation was eventually required

Intermittent claudication is a pain or tightness in the muscle on exercise (Latin *claudicare*, to limp), relieved by rest. Rest pain is a constant severe burning-type pain or discomfort in the forefoot at rest, typically occurring at night when the blood flow slows down.

The main features are compared in TABLE 66.4.

Intermittent claudication

The level of obstruction determines which muscle belly is affected (see FIGS 66.2 and 66.6).

Proximal obstruction (e.g. aortoiliac)

- Pain in the buttock, thigh and calf, especially when walking up hills and stairs
- Persistent fatigue over whole lower limb
- Impotence is possible (Leriche syndrome)

Obstruction in the thigh

- Superficial femoral (the commonest) causes pain in the calf (e.g. 200–500 m), depending on collateral circulation

Table 66.4 Comparison between intermittent claudication and ischaemic rest pain

	Intermittent claudication	Ischaemic rest pain
Quality of pain	Tightness/ cramping	Constant ache
Timing of pain (typical)	Daytime; walking, other exercise	Night-time; rest
Tissue affected	Muscle	Skin
Site	Calf > thigh > buttock	Forefoot, toes, heels
Aggravation	Walking, exercise	Recumbent, walking
Relief	Rest	Hanging foot out of bed; dependency
Associations	Beta blockers Anaemia	Night cramps Swelling of feet

- profunda femoris → claudication at about 100 m
- multiple segment involvement → claudication at 40–50 m

Causes

- Atherosclerosis (mainly men over 50, smokers)
- Embolisation (with recovery)
- Buerger disease: affects small arteries, causes rest pain and cyanosis (claudication uncommon)
- Popliteal entrapment syndrome (<40 years of age)

Note: The presence of rest pain implies an immediate threat to limb viability.

Investigations

- FBE: exclude polycythaemia and thrombocytosis
- Colour Doppler ultrasound: measure resting ankle systolic BP; determine ankle/brachial index; normal value 0.9–1.1
- Angiography: the gold standard, reserved for proposed intervention
- Digital subtraction angiography (developing)

Management of occlusive vascular disease

Prevention (for those at risk)

- Smoking is *the* risk factor and must be stopped.
- Other risk factors, especially hyperlipidaemia, must be attended to and weight reduction to ideal weight is important.
- Exercise is excellent, especially walking.

66

Diagnostic plan

- Check if patient is taking beta blockers.
- General tests: blood examination, random blood sugar, urine examination, ECG.
- Measure blood flow by duplex ultrasound examination or ankle brachial index.
- Arteriography should be performed *only* if surgery is contemplated.

Treatment

- General measures (if applicable): control obesity, diabetes, hypertension, hyperlipidaemia, cardiac failure.
- Achieve ideal weight.
- There must be absolutely no smoking.
- Exercise: daily graduated exercise to the level of pain. About 50% will improve with walking; so advise as much walking as possible.
- Try to keep legs warm and dry.
- Maintain optimal foot care (podiatry).
- Drug therapy: aspirin 150 mg daily.

Note:

- Vasodilators and sympathectomy are of little value.
- About one-third progress, while the rest regress or don't change.[5]

When to refer to a vascular surgeon

- 'Unstable' claudication of recent onset; deteriorating
- Severe claudication—unable to maintain lifestyle
- Rest pain
- 'Tissue loss' in feet (e.g. heel crack, ulcers on or between toes, dry gangrenous patches, infection)

66

Surgery. Reconstructive vascular surgery is indicated for progressive obstruction, intolerable claudication and obstruction above the inguinal ligament:

- endarterectomy—for localised iliac stenosis
- bypass graft (iliac or femoral artery to popliteal or anterior or posterior tibial arteries)

Percutaneous transluminal dilation. This angioplasty is performed with a special intra-arterial balloon catheter for localised limited occlusions. An alternative to the balloon is laser angioplasty.

Venous disorders

Varicose veins

Varicose veins are dilated, tortuous and elongated superficial veins in the lower extremity.

The veins are dilated because of incompetence of the valves in the superficial veins or in the communicating or perforating veins between the deep and superficial systems (see FIG. 66.8). The cause is a congenital weakness in the valve and the supporting vein wall, but there are several predisposing factors (TABLE 66.5), the most important being family history, female sex (5:1), pregnancy and multiparity. Previous DVT can also damage valves, especially calf perforators, and cause varicose veins.

Dilated superficial veins, which can mimic varicose veins, may be caused by extrinsic compression of the veins by a pelvic or intra-abdominal tumour (e.g. ovarian cancer, retroperitoneal fibrosis). Uncommonly, but importantly, superficial veins dilate as they become

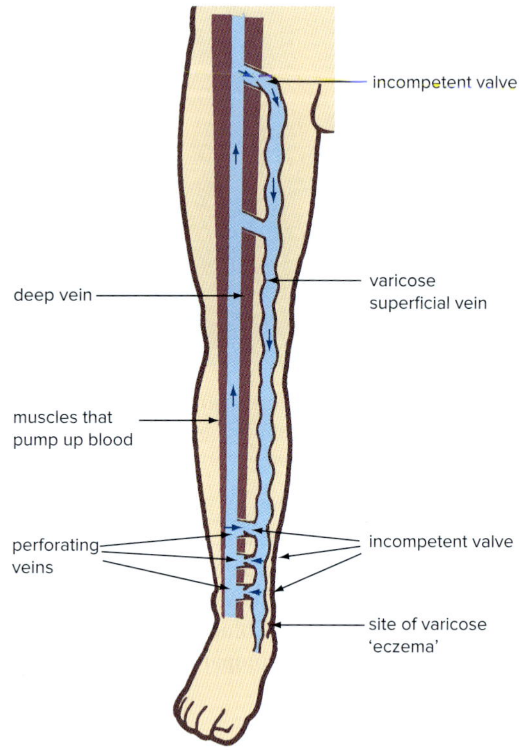

FIGURE 66.8 The common sites of varicose veins

Table 66.5 Risk factors for varicose veins
Female sex
Family history
Pregnancy
Multiparity
Age
Occupation
Diet (low fibre)

collaterals following previous DVT, especially if the iliofemoral segment is involved.

Symptoms

Varicose veins may be symptomless, the main complaint being their unsightly appearance. Symptoms include swelling, fatigue, heaviness in the limb, an aching discomfort and itching.

Varicose veins and pain

They may be painless even if large and tortuous. Pain is a feature where there are incompetent perforating veins running from the posterior tibial vein to the surface through the soleus muscle.

Severe cases lead to lower leg venous hypertension syndrome,[6] characterised by pain that is worse after standing, cramps in the leg at night, irritation and pigmentation of the skin, swelling of the ankles and loss of skin features such as hair.

A careful history will usually determine if the aching is truly due to varicose veins and not to transient or cyclical oedema, which is a common condition in women.[7]

The complications of varicose veins are summarised in TABLE 66.6.

Table 66.6 Complications of varicose veins
Superficial thrombophlebitis
Skin 'eczema' (10%)
Skin ulceration (20%)
Bleeding
Calcification
Marjolin ulcer (squamous cell carcinoma)

Examination

The following tests will help determine the site or sites of the incompetent valves.

Venous groin cough impulse. This helps determine long saphenous vein incompetence. Place the fingers over the line of the vein immediately below the fossa ovalis (4 cm below and 4 cm lateral to the pubic tubercle).[8] Ask the patient to cough—an impulse or thrill will be felt expanding and travelling down the long saphenous vein. A marked dilated long saphenous vein in the fossa ovalis (saphena varix) will confirm incompetence. It disappears when the patient lies down.

Trendelenburg test. In this test for long saphenous vein competence, the patient lies down and the leg is elevated to 45° to empty the veins (see FIG. 66.9a). Apply a tourniquet with sufficient pressure to prevent reflux over the upper thigh just below the fossa ovalis. (Alternatively, this opening can be occluded by firm finger pressure, as originally described by Trendelenburg.)

The patient then stands. The long saphenous system will remain collapsed if there are no incompetent veins below the level of the fossa ovalis. When the pressure is released, the vein will fill rapidly if the valve at the saphenofemoral junction is incompetent (see FIG. 66.9B). This is a positive Trendelenburg test.

Note: A doubly positive Trendelenburg test is when the veins fill rapidly before the pressure is released and then with a 'rush' when released. This indicates coexisting incompetent perforators and long saphenous vein.

Short saphenous vein incompetence test. A similar test to the Trendelenburg test is performed with the pressure (tourniquet or finger) being applied over the short saphenous vein just below the popliteal fossa (see FIG. 66.10).

Incompetent perforating vein test. Accurate clinical tests to identify incompetence in the three common sites of perforating veins on the medial aspect of the leg, posterior to the medial border of the tibia, are difficult to perform. The general appearance of the leg and palpation of the sites give some indication of incompetence here.

Note: Venous duplex ultrasound studies will accurately localise sites of incompetence and determine the state of the functionally important deep venous system.

Prevention

- Maintain ideal weight.
- Eat a high-fibre diet.
- Rest and wear supportive stockings if at risk (pregnancy, a standing occupation).

Treatment

- Keep off legs as much as possible.
- Sit with legs on a footstool.
- Use supportive stockings or tights (apply in morning before getting out of bed and standing up).
- Avoid scratching itching skin over veins.

Compression sclerotherapy

- Use a small volume of sclerosant (e.g. sodium tetradecyl sulphate—Fibro-vein 3%).
- It is ideal for smaller, isolated veins, particularly below the knee joint.

Surgical ligation and stripping

- This is the best treatment when a clear association exists between symptoms and obvious varicose veins (i.e. long saphenous vein incompetence).

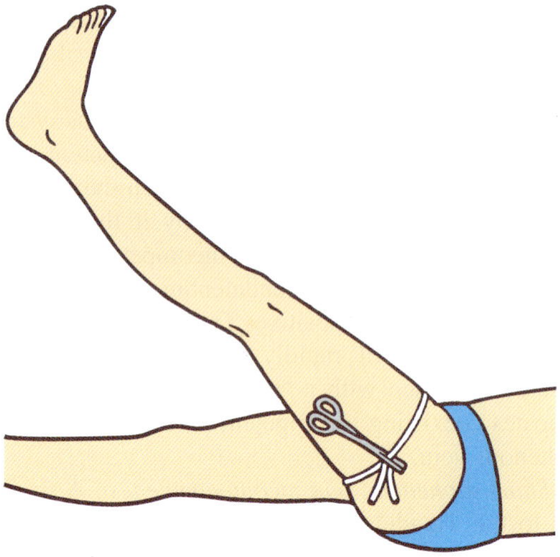

FIGURE 66.9A Trendelenburg test: the leg is elevated to 45° to empty the veins and a tourniquet applied

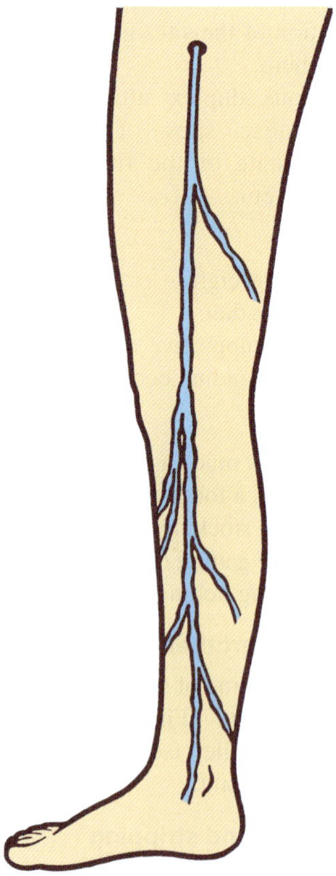

FIGURE 66.9B Trendelenburg test: test for competence of long saphenous venous system (medial aspect of knee)

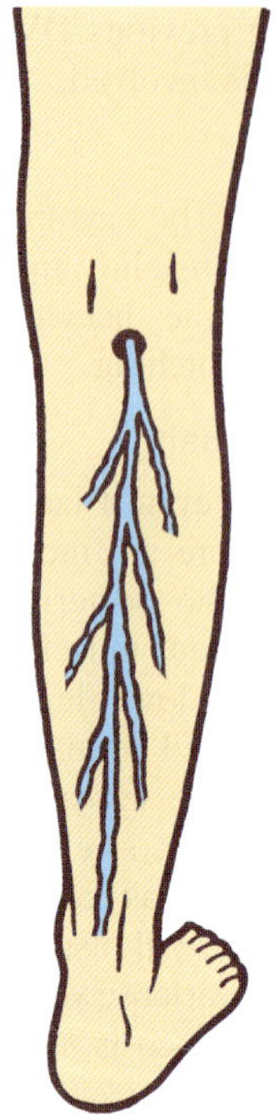

FIGURE 66.10 Testing for competence of the short saphenous vein

- Remove obvious varicosities and ligate perforators.

Note: Surgery for varicose veins may not relieve heavy, aching legs.

Superficial thrombophlebitis

Clinical features

- Usually occurs in superficial varicose veins
- Presents as a tender, reddened subcutaneous cord in leg
- Usually localised oedema
- No generalised swelling of the limb or ankle
- Requires symptomatic treatment only (see below) unless there is extension above the level of the knee, when there is a risk of pulmonary embolism
- Venous duplex scan is diagnostic and also determines:
  - extent of superficial thrombosis
  - if coexisting, unsuspected DVT is present

Treatment

The objective is to prevent propagation of the thrombus by uniform pressure over the vein.

- Cover whole tender cord with a thin foam pad.
- Apply a firm elastic bandage (preferable to crepe) from foot to thigh (well above cord).

- Leave pad and bandage on for 7–10 days.
- Bed rest with leg elevated if severe, otherwise keep active.
- If complication of IV infusion: prescribe a NSAID (e.g. diclofenac 75 mg bd or diclofenac 1% gel topically tds).[9]
- If spontaneous: LMWH (e.g. dalteparin 5000 units SC daily for 4 weeks).[9]
- The traditional glycerin and ichthyol dressings are still useful.
- Consider association between thrombophlebitis and deep-seated carcinoma.
- If the problem is above the knee, ligation of the vein at the saphenofemoral junction is indicated.

Deep venous thrombosis

Refer to CHAPTER 131.

Iliofemoral thrombophlebitis (phlegmasia dolens)[10]

This rare but life-threatening condition is when an extensive clot obstructs the iliofemoral veins (following an acute DVT) so completely that subcutaneous oedema and blanching occurs. This initially causes a painful 'milky white leg', previously termed phlegmasia alba dolens (used to be seen in late pregnancy or early puerperium). It may deteriorate and become cyanotic—phlegmasia cerulea dolens—representing incipient venous infarction. Massive iliofemoral occlusion is an emergency as such patients may develop 'shock', gangrene and pulmonary embolus. Limb amputation will usually follow.

Other painful conditions

Cellulitis and erysipelas

The causative organisms are *Streptococcus pyogenes* (commonest) and *Staphylococcus aureus*. Others include *Haemophilus influenzae, Aeromonas* and fungal infection (especially in the immunocompromised). Predisposing factors include cuts, abrasions, ulcers, insect bites, foreign matter, IV drug use and skin disorders such as eczema and tinea pedis of toe webs. Look for evidence of diabetes.

- Rest in bed.
- Elevate limb (in and out of bed).
- Use aspirin or paracetamol for pain and fever.
- Wound cleansing and dressing with non-sticking saline dressings.

Streptococcus pyogenes[11]

- If *S. pyogenes* confirmed:

  phenoxymethylpenicillin 500 mg (o) 6-hourly for 5–10 days or procaine penicillin 1.5 g IM daily for 5 days
- If organism doubtful:

  flu/dicloxacillin 500 mg (o) 6-hourly for 7–10 days
- If penicillin hypersensitive/allergic:

  cephalexin 500 mg (o) 6-hourly
  or (if severe)
  cefazolin 2 g IV 6-hourly

Staphylococcus aureus[11]

- Severe, may be life-threatening:

  flucloxacillin/dicloxacillin 2 g IV 6-hourly for 7–10 days
- Less severe:

  flucloxacillin/dicloxacillin 500 mg (o) 6-hourly for 5–10 days
  or
  cephalexin 500 mg (o) 6-hourly

Furuncle (boil) of groin

A painful furuncle caused by *S. aureus* in the hairy area of the groin is common. The aim is to treat conservatively.

- Localised:
  - local antiseptics
  - hot compresses
  - drain when 'ripe'
- Deep/extensive:
  - dicloxacillin 500 mg (o) 6-hourly for 5–7 days
  - drain when 'ripe', not before

66

Pain in the calf

Calf pain is usually not serious except if swelling is present. Some of the uncommon causes have serious implications and necessitate careful assessment.

Common causes: cramp, muscle stiffness, muscle injury e.g. gastrocnemius tear, claudication (PVD).

Not to be missed: deep venous thrombosis, cellulitis, thrombophlebitis, popliteal artery entrapment.

Other: ruptured Baker cyst, referred pain (back, knees), Achilles tendon rupture.

Torn 'monkey muscle'

The so-called torn 'monkey muscle' or 'tennis leg' is a rupture of the medial head of the gastrocnemius muscle in the lower calf. Symptoms include a sudden sharp pain in the calf with an inability to comfortably put the heel to the ground and a need to walk on tiptoe. There is localised tenderness and hardness, possible local bruising and painful dorsiflexion of the ankle. Treatment includes RICE treatment for 48 hours, ice packs every 2 waking hours, a firm elastic bandage (toes to below the knee), crutches if severe, a raised heel, active mobilisation after 48 hours' rest and physiotherapist-supervised stretching massage and exercises.

Nocturnal muscle cramps

Note: Treat cause (if known)—tetanus, drugs, sodium depletion, hypothyroidism, hypocalcaemia, pregnancy.

Physical measures

- Muscle stretching and relaxation exercises: calf stretching for 3 minutes before retiring,[11] then rest in chair with the feet out horizontal to the floor with cushion under tendoachilles for 10 minutes.
- Massage and apply heat to affected muscles.
- Try to keep bedclothes off feet and lower part of legs—a doubled-up pillow at the foot of the bed can be used.

Medication for idiopathic cramps

- Tonic water before retiring may help.
- Drug treatment:
  Consider:
  biperiden 2–4 mg nocte
  magnesium complex tablets (e.g. Crampeze)

Quinine sulphate is effective, but with a 1–3% incidence of haematological abnormalities, especially thrombocytopenia, it is no longer recommended in Australia. It is very toxic to children. More severe idiopathic cramps may respond to magnesium.[12]

66

Roller injuries to legs

A patient who has been injured by a wheel passing over a limb, especially a leg, can present a difficult problem. A freely spinning wheel is not so dangerous, but serious injuries occur when a non-spinning (braked) wheel passes over a limb and these are compounded by the wheel then reversing over it. This leads to a 'degloving' injury due to shearing stress. The limb may look satisfactory initially, but skin necrosis may follow.

- Admit to hospital for observation.
- Fasciotomy with open drainage may be an option for compartment syndrome.
- Surgical decompression with removal of necrotic fat is often essential.
- Rehydrate the patient and monitor renal function.

When to refer

- The sudden onset of pain, pallor, pulselessness, paralysis, paraesthesia and coldness in the leg
- Worsening intermittent claudication
- Rest pain in foot
- Presence of popliteal aneurysm
- Superficial thrombophlebitis above knee
- Evidence of DVT
- Suspicion of gas gangrene in leg
- Worsening hip pain
- Evidence of disease in bone (e.g. neoplasia, infection, Paget disease)
- Severe sciatica with neurological deficit (e.g. floppy foot, absent reflexes)

Practice tips

- Always X-ray the legs (including hips) of a patient complaining of unusual deep leg pain, especially a child.
- Pain that does not fluctuate in intensity with movement, activity or posture has an inflammatory or neoplastic cause.
- Hip disorders such as osteoarthritis and slipped femoral epiphysis can present as pain in the knee (usually medial aspect).
- Consider retroperitoneal haemorrhage as a cause of acute severe nerve root pain, especially in people on anticoagulant therapy.
- Avoidance of amputation with acute lower limb ischaemia depends on early recognition (surgery within 4 hours—too late if over 6 hours).

Patient education resources

Hand-out sheets from *Murtagh's Patient Education* 7th edition:

- Calf muscle injury
- Cramp
- Deep vein thrombosis
- Sciatica

References

1 House AK. The painful limb: is it intermittent claudication? Modern Medicine Australia, 1990; November: 16–26.
2 Tunnessen WW. *Signs and Symptoms in Paediatrics* (2nd edn). Philadelphia: Lippincott, 1988: 483.
3 Zaina F, Tomkins-Lane C et al. Surgical versus non-surgical treatment for lumbar spinal stenosis. Cochrane Database. Sys. Rev. 2016, Issue 1. Art No. CD010264.
4 Bates B. *A Guide to Physical Examination and History Taking* (5th edn). New York: Lippincott, 1991: 450.
5 Fry J, Berry H. *Surgical Problems in Clinical Practice.* London: Edward Arnold, 1987: 125–34.

6 Ryan P. *A Very Short Textbook of Surgery* (2nd edn). Canberra: Dennis & Ryan, 1990: 61.
7 Hunt P, Marshall V. *Clinical Problems in General Surgery.* Sydney: Butterworths, 1991: 172.
8 Davis A, Bolin T, Ham J. *Symptom Analysis and Physical Diagnosis* (2nd edn). Sydney: Pergamon, 1990: 179.
9 Expert group for Cardiovascular. Acute limb ischaemia. In: eTG complete [Internet]. Melbourne: Therapeutic Guidelines Ltd. Available from: <www.tg.org.au>, accessed October 2017.
10 Colucciello SA. Evaluation and management of deep venous thrombosis. Primary Care Rep, 1996; 2 (12): 105.
11 Expert group for Antibiotic. Skin and soft tissue infections: bacterial. In: eTG complete [Internet]. Melbourne: Therapeutic Guidelines Ltd. Available from: <www.tg.org,au>, accessed October 2017.
12 Moulds R (Chair). *Therapeutic Guidelines: Neurology* (Version 4). Melbourne: Therapeutic Guidelines Ltd, 2011: 145.

67 The painful knee

The human knee is a joint and not a source of entertainment.

Percy Hammond, 1912, review of a play

The knee, which is a gliding hinge joint, is the largest synovial joint in the body. Its small area of contact of the bone ends at any one time makes it dependent on ligaments for its stability. Although this allows a much increased range of movement it does increase the susceptibility to injury, particularly from sporting activities. Finding the cause of a knee problem is one of the really difficult and challenging features of practice. It is useful to remember that peripheral pain receptors respond to a variety of stimuli. These include inflammation due either to inflammatory disorders or chemical irritation such as crystal synovitis, traction pain (e.g. trapped meniscus stretching the capsule), tension on the synovium capsule (e.g. effusion or haemarthrosis), and impact loading of the subchondral bone.

Key facts and checkpoints

- Disorders of the knee account for about one presentation per 50 patients per year.[1]
- The commoner presenting symptoms in order of frequency are pain, stiffness, swelling, clicking and locking.[1]
- The age of presentation of a painful knee has varied significance as many conditions are age-related.
- Excessive strains across the knee, such as a valgus-producing force, are more likely to cause ligament injuries, while twisting injuries tend to cause meniscal tears.
- A ruptured anterior cruciate ligament (ACL) is a commonly missed injury of the knee.[2] It should be suspected with a history of either a valgus strain or a sudden pivoting of the knee, often associated with a cracking or popping sensation. It is often associated with the rapid onset of haemarthrosis or inability to walk or weight-bear.
- A rapid onset of painful knee swelling (minutes to 1–4 hours) after injury indicates blood in the joint—*haemarthrosis*.
- Swelling over 1–2 days after injury indicates synovial fluid—*traumatic synovitis*.
- Any collateral ligament repair should be undertaken early, but, if associated with ACL injuries, early surgery may result in knee stiffness. Thus, surgery is often delayed. With isolated ACL ruptures, early reconstruction is appropriate in the high-performance athlete; otherwise, delayed reconstruction is appropriate if there is clinical instability.[3]
- Acute spontaneous inflammation of the knee may be part of a systemic condition such as rheumatoid arthritis, rheumatic fever, gout, pseudogout (chondrocalcinosis), a spondyloarthropathy (psoriasis, ankylosing spondylitis, reactive arthritis, bowel inflammation), Lyme disease and sarcoidosis.
- Consider Osgood–Schlatter disorder (OSD) in the prepubertal child (especially a boy aged 10–14) presenting with knee pain.
- Disorders of the lumbosacral spine (especially L3 to S1 nerve root problems) and of the hip joint (L3 innervation) refer pain to the region of the knee joint.
- If infection or haemorrhage is suspected, the joint should be aspirated.
- The condition known as anterior knee pain is the commonest type of knee pain and accounts for at least 11% of sports-related musculoskeletal problems. The prime cause of this is patellofemoral dysfunction pain. It is a benign condition with a good prognosis. Consider Hoffa syndrome.

The knee and referred pain—key knowledge

Pain from the knee joint

Disorders of the knee joint give rise to pain felt accurately at the knee, often at some particular part of the joint, and invariably in the anterior aspect, very seldom in the posterior part of the knee. An impacted loose body complicating osteoarthritis and a radial tear of the lateral meniscus[4] are the exceptional disorders liable to refer pain proximally and distally in the limb, but the problems obviously originate from the knee.

Pain referred to the knee

Referred pain to the knee or the surrounding region is a time-honoured trap in medicine. The two classic problems are disorders of the hip joint and lumbosacral spine.

- The hip joint is mainly innervated by L3, hence pain is referred from the groin down the front and medial aspects of the thigh to the knee (see FIG. 67.1). Sometimes the pain can be experienced on the anteromedial aspect of the knee only. It is not uncommon for children with a slipped upper femoral epiphysis to present with a limp and knee pain.
- Knee pain can be referred from the lumbosacral spine. Patients with disc lesions may notice that sitting, coughing or straining hurts the knee, whereas walking does not.

L3 nerve root pressure from an L2–3 disc prolapse (uncommon) and L4 nerve root pain will cause anteromedial knee pain; L5 reference from an L4–5 disc prolapse can cause anterolateral knee pain, while S1 reference from an L5–S1 prolapse can cause pain at the back of the knee (see FIG. 67.1).

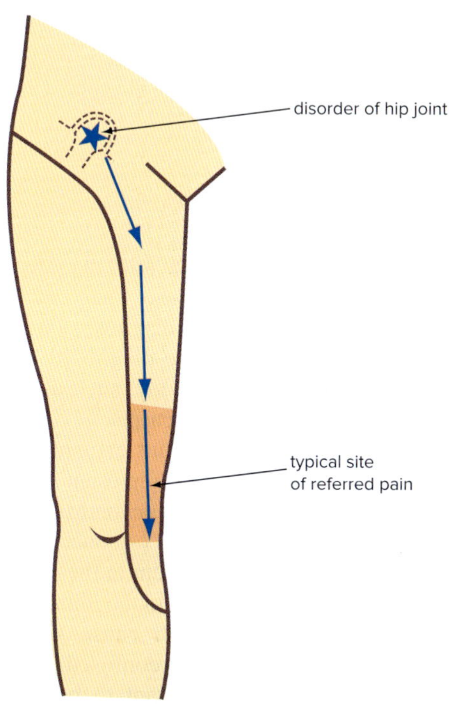

FIGURE 67.1 Possible area of referred pain from disorders of the hip joint

A diagnostic approach

A summary of the diagnostic strategy model is presented in TABLE 67.1.

Table 67.1 The painful knee: diagnostic strategy model

Probability diagnosis
Ligament strains and sprains ± traumatic synovitis
Osteoarthritis
Patellofemoral syndrome
Prepatellar bursitis
Serious disorders not to be missed
Acute cruciate ligament tear
Vascular disorders:
• deep venous thrombosis
• superficial thrombophlebitis
Neoplasia:
• primary in bone
• metastases
Severe infections:
• septic arthritis
• tuberculosis
Rheumatoid arthritis
Juvenile chronic arthritis
Rheumatic fever
Pitfalls (often missed)
Referred pain: back or hip
Foreign bodies
Intra-articular loose bodies
Osteochondritis dissecans
Osteonecrosis
Synovial chondromatosis
Osgood–Schlatter disorder
Meniscal tears including degenerative tears
Fractures around knee
Pseudogout (chondrocalcinosis)
Gout → patellar bursitis
Ruptured popliteal cyst
Hoffa fat pad syndrome
Rarities:
• sarcoidosis
• Paget disease
• spondyloarthropathy
Seven masquerades checklist
Depression
Diabetes
Drugs (indirect)
Spinal dysfunction
Is the patient trying to tell me something?
Psychogenic factors relevant, especially with possible injury compensation.

Probability diagnosis

A UK study[1] highlighted the fact that the commonest causes of knee pain are simple ligamentous strains and bruises due to overstress of the knee or other minor trauma. Traumatic synovitis may accompany some of these injuries. Some of these so-called strains may include a variety of recently described syndromes, such as the synovial plica syndrome, patellar tendonopathy and infrapatellar compressive fat-pad inflammation (see FIG. 67.2).

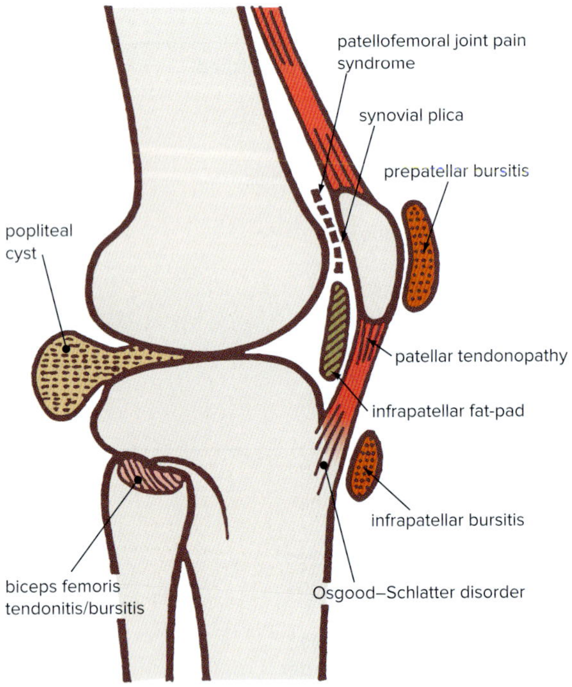

FIGURE 67.2 Lateral view of knee showing typical sites of various causes of knee pain

Low-grade trauma of repeated overuse, such as frequent kneeling, may cause prepatellar bursitis known variously as 'housemaid's knee' or 'carpet layer's knee'. Infrapatellar bursitis is referred to as 'clergyman's knee'.

Osteoarthritis of the knee, especially in the elderly, is a very common problem. It may arise spontaneously or be secondary to previous trauma with associated internal derangement and instability.

The most common overuse problem of the knee is the patellofemoral joint pain syndrome (often previously referred to as chondromalacia patellae).

Serious disorders not to be missed

Neoplasia in the bones around the knee is relatively uncommon but still needs consideration. The commonest neoplasias are secondaries from the breast, lung, kidney, thyroid and prostate. Uncommon examples include osteoid osteoma, osteosarcoma and Ewing tumour (more likely in younger people). Septic arthritis and infected bursitis are prone to occur in the knee joint, especially following contaminated lacerations and abrasions. Septic arthritis from blood-borne infection can be of the primary type in children, where the infection is either staphylococcal or due to *Haemophilus influenzae*, or gonococcal arthritis in adults. Rheumatic fever should be kept in mind with a fleeting polyarthritis that involves the knees and then affects other joints.

Inflammatory disorders such as spondyloarthropathies, sarcoidosis, chondrocalcinosis (a crystal arthropathy due to calcium pyrophosphate dihydrate in the elderly), gout and juvenile chronic arthritis have to be considered in the differential diagnosis.

Red flag pointers for knee pain

- Acute swelling with or without trauma
- Acute or acute on chronic erythema
- Systemic features (e.g. fever) in absence of trauma
- Unexplained chronic, persistent pain

Pitfalls

There are myriad pitfalls in knee joint disorders, often arising from ignorance, because there are myriad problems that are difficult to diagnose. Fortunately, many of these problems can be diagnosed by X-ray. A particular trap is a foreign body, such as a broken needle acquired by kneeling on carpet.

The presence of a spontaneous effusion demands careful attention because it could represent a rheumatic disorder or conditions such as osteochondritis dissecans (more common in the young) or osteonecrosis of the femoral condyle (a necrotic problem in the elderly) and perhaps a subsequent loose body in the joint.

A ruptured Baker cyst will cause severe pain behind the knee and can be confused with deep venous thrombosis. It is important to bear in mind complications of varicose veins, which can cause pain or discomfort around the knee joint.

General pitfalls

- Overlooking referred pain from the hip or low back as a cause of knee pain
- Failing to realise that meniscal tears can develop due to degeneration of the menisci with only minimal trauma
- Failing to X-ray the knee joint and order special views to detect specific problems, such as a fractured patella or osteochondritis dissecans

Ottawa knee rules for X-ray of an injured knee

- Patient aged 55 years or more
- Isolated tenderness of the patella
- Tenderness at the head of the fibula
- Inability to flex to 90°
- Immediate inability to weight-bear and in the emergency room (four steps: unable to transfer weight twice onto each lower limb regardless of limping).

Furthermore, a knee X-ray may be indicated following blunt trauma or a fall-type injury if the patient is:

- <12 years or >50 years
- unable to take four weight-bearing steps in front of the clinician[5]

Seven masquerades checklist

Of these, spinal dysfunction is the prime association. Diabetes may cause pain through a complicating neuropathy and drugs such as diuretics may cause gout in the elderly.

Psychogenic considerations

Patients, young and old, may complain of knee pain, imaginary or exaggerated, to gain attention, especially if compensation for an injury is involved. This requires discreet clinical acumen to help patients work through the problem.

The clinical approach

History

The history is the key to diagnosis. If any injury is involved careful description of the nature of the injury is necessary. This includes past history. A special problem relates to the elderly who can sustain knee injuries after a 'drop attack', but attention can easily be diverted away from the knee with preoccupation with the cerebral pattern.

It is relevant to define whether the pain is acute or chronic, dull or sharp, and continuous or recurring. Determine its severity and position and keep in mind age-related causes.

Key questions

Related to an injury

- Can you explain in detail how the injury happened?
- Did you land awkwardly after a leap in the air?
- Did you get a direct blow? From what direction?
- Did your leg twist during the injury?
- Did you feel a 'pop' or hear a 'snap'?
- Did your knee feel wobbly or unsteady?
- Did the knee feel as if the bones separated momentarily?
- How soon after the injury did the pain develop?
- How soon after the injury did you notice swelling?
- Have you had previous injury or surgery to the knee?
- Were you able to walk after the injury or did you have to be carried off the ground or court?
- Does this involve work care compensation?

No history of injury

- Does the pain come on after walking, jogging or other activity?
- How much kneeling do you do? Scrubbing floors, cleaning carpets?
- Could there be needles or pins in the carpet?
- Does your knee lock or catch?
- Does swelling develop in the knee?
- Does it 'grate' when it moves?
- Does the pain come on at rest and is there morning stiffness?
- Do you feel pain when you walk on steps or stairs?

67

Significance of symptoms

Swelling after injury

The sudden onset of painful swelling (usually within 60 minutes) is typical of haemarthrosis (see FIGS 67.3 and 67.4). Bleeding occurs from vascular structures such as torn ligaments, torn synovium or fractured bones, while injuries localised to avascular structures such as menisci do not usually bleed. About 75% of cases are due to ACL tears.[6] If a minor injury causes acute haemarthrosis suspect a bleeding diathesis or anticoagulant usage. The causes of haemarthrosis are listed in TABLE 67.2.

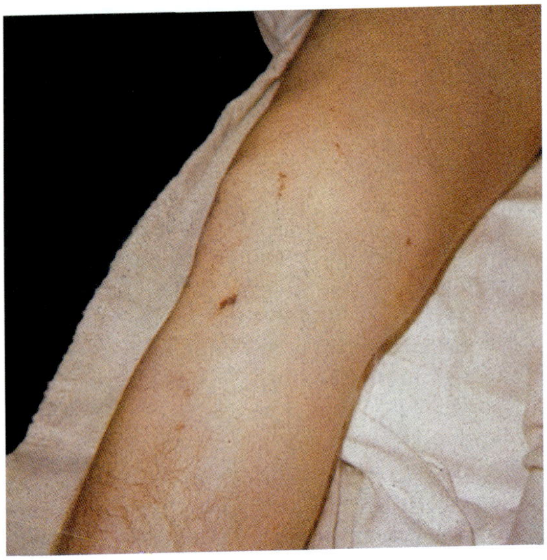

FIGURE 67.3 Haemarthrosis in a sportsman presenting with an acutely painful swollen knee

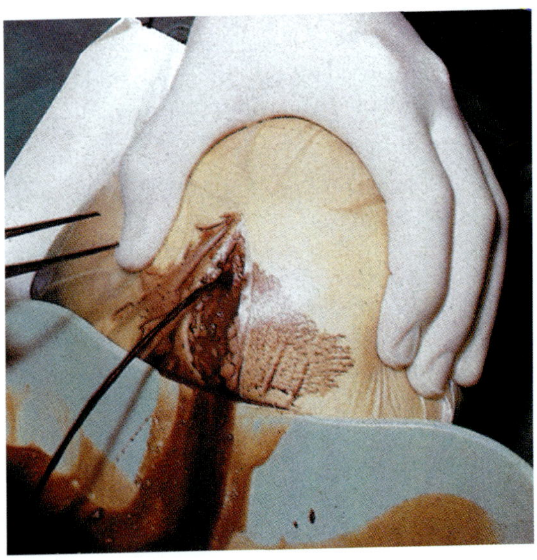

FIGURE 67.4 Haemarthrosis: Surgical release of intra-articular blood under pressure in the knee shown in FIGURE 67.3

Table 67.2	Causes of haemarthrosis
Torn cruciate ligaments, esp. ACL	
Capsular tears with collateral ligament tears	
Peripheral meniscal tears	
Dislocation or subluxation of patella	
Osteochondral fractures	
Bleeding disorders (e.g. haemophilia), anticoagulants	

Swelling of an intermediate rate of onset, stiffness and pain in the order of hours (e.g. 6–24 hours) is typical of an effusion of synovial fluid. Causes include meniscal tears and milder ligamentous injuries. Swelling gradually developing over days and confined to the anterior knee is typical of bursitis such as 'housemaid's knee'.

Recurrent or chronic swelling

This indicates intra-articular pathology and includes:

- patellofemoral pain syndrome
- osteochondritis dissecans
- degenerative joint disease including degenerative meniscus tears
- arthritides

Locking

Locking usually means a sudden inability to extend the knee fully (occurs at 10–45°, average 30°) but ability to flex fully.[7]

Causes

True locking:

- torn meniscus (bucket handle)
- loose body (e.g. bony fragment from osteochondritis dissecans)
- torn ACL (remnant)
- flap of articular cartilage
- avulsed anterior tibial spine
- dislocated patella
- synovial osteochondromatosis

Pseudo-locking:

- patellofemoral disorders
- first or second degree medial ligament tear
- strain of ACL
- gross effusion
- pain and spasm of hamstrings

Catching

'Catching' of the knee implies that the patient feels that something is 'getting in the way of joint movement' but not locking. Causes include any of the conditions that cause locking, but a subluxing patella and loose bodies in particular must be considered.

Causes of loose bodies

- Osteochondritis dissecans (usually lateral side of medial femoral condyle)
- Retropatellar fragment (e.g. from dislocation of patella)
- Dislodged osteophyte

- Osteochondral fracture—post injury
- Synovial chondromatosis

Clicking

Clicking may be due to an abnormality such as patellofemoral maltracking or subluxation, a loose intra-articular body or a torn meniscus, but can occur in normal joints when people climb stairs or squat.

Anterior knee pain[8]

Common causes include:

- fat pad disorder (inflammation)
- patellofemoral syndrome
- osteoarthritis of the knee
- patellar tendonopathy
- osteonecrosis

Lateral knee pain

Consider:

- osteoarthritis of lateral compartment of knee
- lesions of the lateral meniscus
- patellofemoral syndrome

Medial knee pain

Consider:

- osteoarthritis of medial compartment of knee
- lesions of the medial meniscus
- patellofemoral syndrome

Examination

The provisional diagnosis may be evident from a combination of the history and simple inspection of the joint but the process of testing palpation, movements (active and passive) and specific structures of the knee joint helps to pinpoint the disorder.

Inspection

Inspect the knee with the patient walking, standing erect and lying supine. Get the patient to squat to help localise the precise point of pain. Get the patient to sit on the couch with legs hanging over the side and note any abnormality of the patella. Note any deformities, swelling or muscle wasting.

The common knee deformities are genu valgum 'knock knees' (see FIG. 67.5a), genu recurvatum 'back knee' (see FIG. 67.5b) and genu varum 'bowed legs' (see FIG. 67.5c).

A useful way of remembering the terminology is to recall that the 'l' in valgus stands for 'l' in lateral.[8] In the normal knee the tibia has a slight valgus angulation in reference to the femur, the angulation being more pronounced in women.

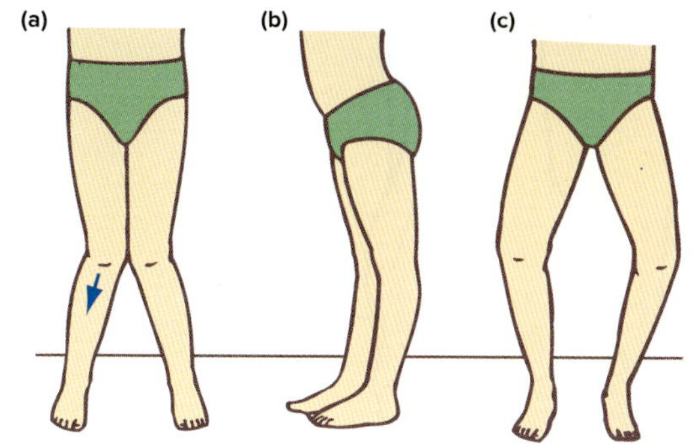

FIGURE 67.5 Knee deformities: **(a)** genu valgum ('knock knees'): tibia deviates laterally from knee, **(b)** genu recurvatum ('back knee'), **(c)** genu varum ('bowed legs')

Palpation

Palpate the knee generally, concentrating on the patella, patella tendon, joint lines, tibial tubercle, bursae and popliteal fossa.

Palpate for presence of any fluid, warmth, swelling, synovial thickening, crepitus, clicking and tenderness. Feel for a popliteal (Baker) cyst in the popliteal fossa. Draw the fingers upwards over the suprapatellar pouch: synovial thickening, a hallmark of chronic arthritis, is most marked just above the patella—it feels warm, boggy, rubbery and has no fluid thrill.

Flex the knees to 45° and check for a pseudocyst, especially of the lateral meniscus (see FIG. 67.6).

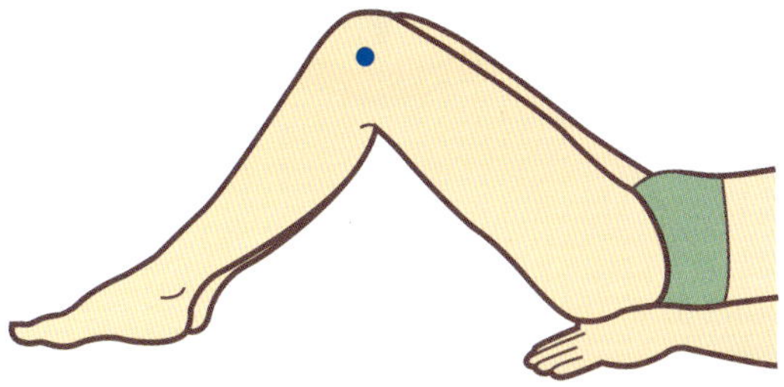

FIGURE 67.6 Pseudocyst of the lateral meniscus: flex the knees to 45° to force lump (if present) to appear

Fluid effusion

The bulge sign: compress the medial side of the joint and evacuate any fluid. The test is positive when the lateral side of the joint is then stroked and the fluid is displaced across the joint, creating a visible bulge or filling of the medial depression (see FIG. 67.7).

The test will be negative if the effusion is gross and tense, in which case the *patellar tap test* (see FIG. 67.8) is used by sharply tapping the lower pole of the patella against the femur with the index finger. A positive tap

67

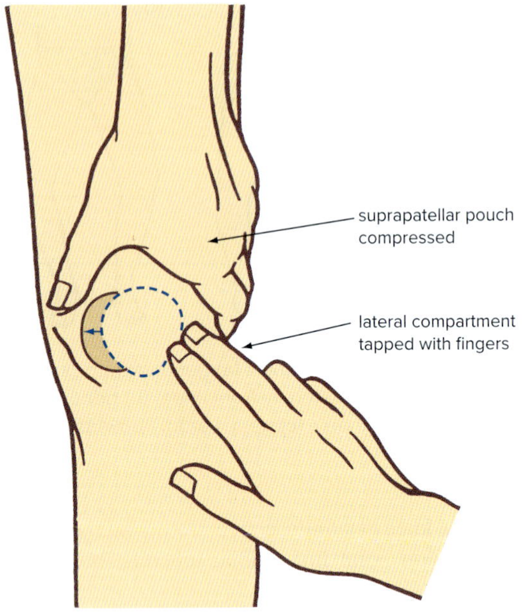

FIGURE 67.7 The bulge sign with a knee effusion: fluid bulges into the medial compartment

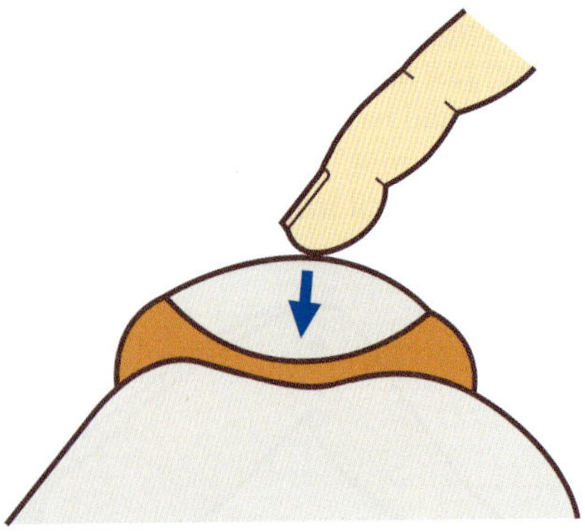

FIGURE 67.8 The patellar tap test

67

is when the patella can be felt to tap against the femur and then float free.

Movements

Extension: normal is 0–5°. The loss of extension is best measured by lifting the heel off the couch with the knee held down. In the normal knee the heel will lift 2.5–4 cm off the couch, that is, into hyperextension.

Flexion (supine or prone): normal to 135°. The normal knee flexes heel to the buttock but in locking due to medial meniscus tears there may be a gap of 5 or more centimetres between the heel and buttock.

Rotation: normal 5–10°. Test at 90° with patient sitting over the edge of the couch; rotate the feet with the hand steadying the knee.

Note: Normally, no abduction, adduction or rotation of the tibia on the femur is possible with the leg fully extended.

Ligament stability tests

Collateral ligaments. Adduction (varus) and abduction (valgus) stresses of the tibia on the femur are applied in full extension and then at 30° flexion with the leg over the side of the couch. With ligament strains there is localised pain when stressed. With a complete (third degree) tear the joint will open out. This end-point feel should be carefully noted: firmness indicates stability, 'mushiness' indicates damage (see FIG. 67.9).

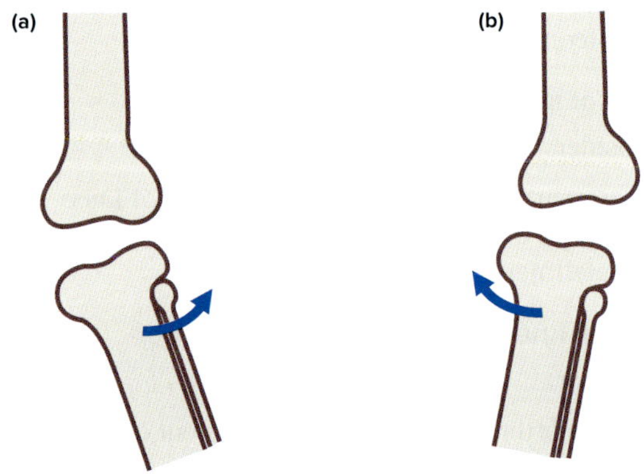

FIGURE 67.9 Medial and lateral ligament instability: **(a)** medial instability of knee joint; **(b)** lateral instability of knee joint

Cruciate ligaments. Stability of the ACL can be tested with the anterior drawer test. This is done with the patient supine and the knee flexed to 90°. The tibia is pulled forwards off the femur and in the presence of a cruciate ligament injury there will be increased gliding of the tibia on the femur. An aberrant positive sign can occur in the presence of posterior cruciate ligament (PCL) insufficiency, in which case the knee is actually brought back to its normal site from a dropped-back position. This gives the appearance of a positive anterior drawer sign. In that situation, a Lachman test will be negative. In the presence of medial ligament injury, the increased external rotation of the tibia against the femur may add to the positive drawer sign.

Specific provocation tests

The simplest menisci function tests are those outlined in TABLE 67.4, later in this chapter.

- *McMurray test.* The patient lies on the couch and the flexed knee is rotated (internally and externally) in varying degrees of abduction as it is straightened into extension. A hand over the affected knee feels for 'clunking' or tenderness.

- *Thessaly test.* The patient stands on the affected leg, flat-footed, with the knee flexed to 20°, with outstretched arms supported by the examiner's hands. The patient pivots with firm twists of the body and knee three times medially and laterally on the knee. A positive test is when the patient experiences joint line discomfort, or locking or catching. This is the most sensitive and specific clinical test for meniscal injury.[7]
- *Apley grind/distraction test.* The patient lies prone and the knee is flexed to 90° and then rotated under a compression force. Reproduction of painful symptoms may indicate meniscal tear. Then repeat the rotation under distraction—tests ligament damage.
- *Patella apprehension test.* At 15–20° flexion, attempt to push the patella laterally and note the patient's reaction.
- *Patellar tendonopathy.* Palpate patellar tendon (refer to FIG. 67.19, later in this chapter).
- *Patellofemoral pain test.* Refer to FIGURE 67.18, later in this chapter.

Examine the lumbosacral spine and the hip joint of the affected side.

Measurements

Quadriceps. For suspected quadriceps wasting, measure the circumference of the thighs at equal points above the tibial tuberosity. It is helpful to assess quadriceps function by feeling the tone.

Static Q angle (see FIG. 67.10).

If the Q angle is >15° in men and >19° in women there is a predisposition to patellofemoral pain and instability.[9]

Investigations

Investigation for the diagnosis of knee pain can be selected from:

- blood tests:
  - RA factor tests; ANA; HLA–B_{27}
  - ESR
  - blood culture (suspected septic arthritis)
- radiology[9]:
  - plain X-ray
  - special views: intercondylar (osteochondritis dissecans, loose bodies); tangential (or skyline view for suspected patella pathology); oblique (to define condyles and patella); weight-bearing views looking for degenerative arthritis

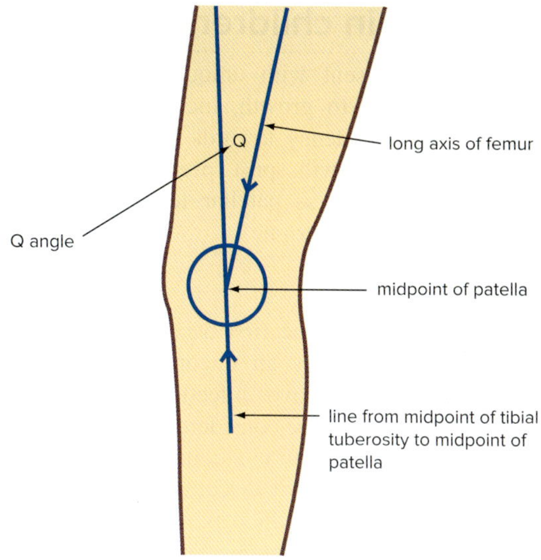

FIGURE 67.10 The Q angle of the knee gives a measure of patellar alignment

  - bone scan: for suspected tumour, stress fracture, osteonecrosis, osteochondritis dissecans
  - MRI: excellent for diagnosing cartilage and menisci disorders and ligament damage; the investigation of choice for internal 'derangement'
  - arthrography (generally superseded by arthroscopy) or MRI
  - ultrasound: good for assessment of patellar tendon, soft tissue mass, fluid collection, Baker cyst and bursae
- CT: useful for complex fractures of tibial plateau and patellofemoral joint special dysfunction
- special:
  - examination under anaesthesia
  - arthroscopy
  - knee aspiration: culture or crystal examination

Fractures that may be missed on plain films[10]

- Patellar fracture
- Tibial plateau fracture
- Tibial spine fracture
- Epiphyseal injuries in children
- Osteochondral fracture:
  - patella
  - femoral condyle
- Stress fracture upper tibia
- Avulsion fracture (e.g. Segond fracture of upper lateral tibia, with ACL tear)

Knee pain in children

Children may present with unique conditions that are usually related to growth, including epiphyseal problems. Their tendency towards muscle tightness, especially in the growth spurt, predisposes them to overuse injuries such as patellar tendonopathy and patellofemoral pain syndrome.

First decade

A painful knee during the first decade of life (0–10 years) in non-athletes is an uncommon presenting symptom, but suppurative infection and juvenile chronic arthritis have to be considered.

Genu valgum or varum is a common presentation but usually not a source of discomfort for the child. However, genu valgum, which is often seen around 4–6 years, may predispose to abnormal biomechanical stresses, which contribute to overuse-type injuries if the child is involved in sport.

Second decade

Pain in the knee presents most frequently in this decade and is most often due to the patellofemoral syndrome,[11] which is related to the retropatellar and peripatellar regions and usually anterior to the knee. It occurs in the late teenage years of both sexes.

An important problem is subluxation of the patella, typically found in teenage girls. It is caused by maltracking of the patellofemoral mechanism without complete dislocation of the patella (see FIG. 67.11).

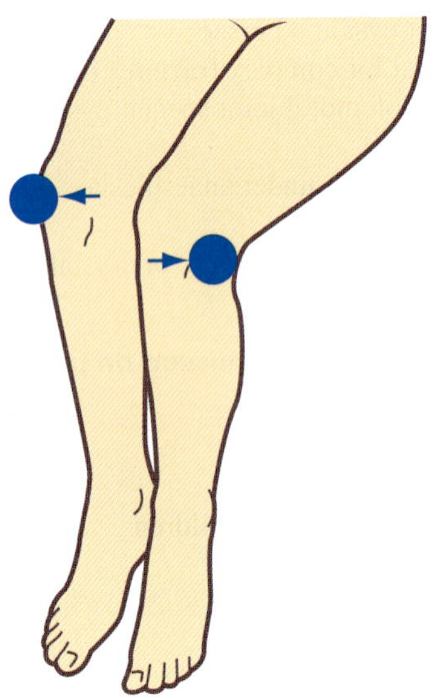

FIGURE 67.11 Lateral subluxation of the patella

On examination, the patella is usually in a high and lateral position. Surgery may be required if symptoms persist.

OSD is common in pre-pubertal adolescent boys but can occur in those aged 10–16 years.

Other conditions found typically in this age group include:

- slipped upper femoral epiphysis—usually in middle teenage years after a growth spurt
- anserinus ('goose foot') bursitis
- osteochondritis dissecans

Age-related causes of the painful knee are presented in TABLE 67.3.[11]

Table 67.3 Age-related causes of painful knee

First decade (0–10 years)
Infection
Juvenile chronic arthritis
Second decade (10–20 years)
Patellofemoral syndrome
Subluxation/dislocation of patella
Slipped femoral epiphysis (referred)
'Hamstrung' knee
Osteochondritis dissecans
Osgood–Schlatter disorder
Anserinus tendonopathy
Third decade (20–30 years)
Bursitis
Mechanical disorders
Fourth and fifth decades (30–50 years)
Cleavage tear of medial meniscus
Radial tear of lateral meniscus
Sixth decade and older (50 years and over)
Osteoarthritis
Osteonecrosis
Paget disease (femur, tibia or patella)
Anserinus bursitis
Chondrocalcinosis and gout
Osteoarthritis of hip (referred pain)

The little athlete

Children competing in sporting activities, especially running and jumping, are prone to overuse injuries such as the patellofemoral pain syndrome, traumatic synovitis of the knee joint and OSD. Haemarthrosis can occur with injuries, sometimes due to a synovial tear without major joint disruption. If knee pain persists, especially in the presence of an effusion, X-rays should be performed to exclude osteochondritis of the femoral condyle.[12]

The Ottawa knee rules

A knee X-ray series is only required for children with any of the findings in the Ottawa knee rules (see earlier in this chapter).

Osgood–Schlatter disorder

Osgood–Schlatter disorder (OSD) is a traction apophysitis resulting from repetitive traction stresses at the insertion of the patellar tendon into the tibial tubercle, which is vulnerable to repeated traction in early adolescence.

Clinical features

- Commonest in ages 10–14 years
- Boys:girls = 3:1
- Bilateral in about one-third of cases
- Common in sports involving running, kicking and jumping
- Localised pain in region of tibial tubercle during and after activity
- Aggravated by kneeling down and going up and downstairs
- Development of lump in area
- Localised swelling and tenderness at affected tubercle
- Pain reproduced by attempts to straighten flexed knee against resistance

X-ray to confirm diagnosis (widening of the apophysis and possible fragmentation of bone) and exclude tumour or fracture (see FIG. 67.12).

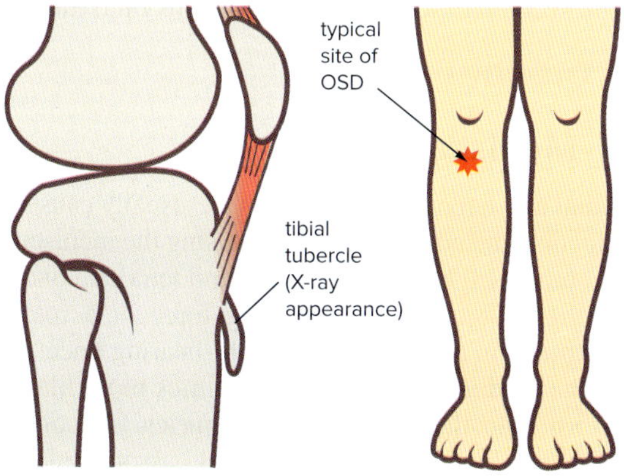

FIGURE 67.12 Features of Osgood–Schlatter disorder

Management

Treatment is conservative as it is a self-limiting condition (6–18 months: average 12 months).

- If acute, use ice packs and analgesics.
- The main approach is to abstain from or modify active sports.
- Localised treatments such as electrotherapy are unnecessary.
- Corticosteroid injections should be avoided.[13]
- Plaster cast immobilisation should also be avoided.
- Surgery may be used (rarely) if an irritating ossicle persists[13] after ossification.
- Gentle quadriceps stretching.
- Graded return to full activity.

Prevention

- Promote awareness and early recognition of OSD.
- Program of stretching exercises for quadriceps mechanism in children in sport.

Osteochondritis dissecans: juvenile form[7]

This commonly occurs in adolescent boys aged 5–16 years whereby a segment of articular cartilage of the femoral condyle (85%) undergoes necrosis and may eventually separate to form an intra-articular loose body (see FIG. 67.13).

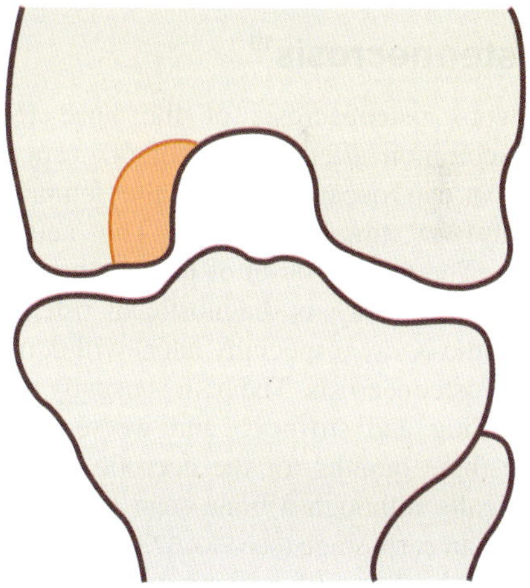

FIGURE 67.13 Osteochondritis dissecans: on X-ray, sclerosis of the lateral aspect of the medial condyle

It usually presents as pain and effusion and locking.

If the fragment has separated, surgery to reattach it can be contemplated.

Knee pain in the elderly

Rheumatic disorders are very common and responsible for considerable pain or discomfort, disability and loss of independence in the elderly.

67

Osteoarthritis is the most common cause and excellent results are now being obtained using total knee replacement in those severely affected.

The elderly are particularly prone to crystal-associated joint diseases, including monosodium urate (gout), CPPD (pseudogout) and hydroxyapatite (acute calcific periarthritis).

Chondrocalcinosis of knee (pseudogout)

The main target of CPPD is the knee, where it causes chondrocalcinosis. Unlike gout, chondrocalcinosis of the knee is typically a disorder of the elderly with about 50% of the population having evidence of involvement of the knee by the ninth decade.[14] Most cases remain asymptomatic but patients (usually aged 60 or older) can present with an acutely hot, red, swollen joint resembling septic arthritis.

Investigations include aspiration of the knee to search for CPPD crystals, and X-ray. If positive, consider an associated metabolic disorder such as haemochromatosis, hyperparathyroidism or diabetes mellitus. The treatment is similar to acute gout although colchicine is less effective. Acute episodes respond well to NSAIDs or intra-articular corticosteroid injection.

Osteonecrosis[15]

Spontaneous osteonecrosis of the knee (SPONK) is more common after the age of 60, especially in females; it can occur in either the femoral (more commonly) or tibial condyles. The aetiology is unknown. The sudden onset of pain in the knee, with a normal joint X-ray, is diagnostic of osteonecrosis. However, the X-ray (especially later) will demonstrate an area of osteonecrosis. The pain is usually persistent, with swelling and stiffness, and worse at night. It can take three months for the necrotic area to show radiologically although a bone scan or MRI may be positive at an early stage (see FIG. 67.14). The condition may resolve in time with reduction of weight-bearing. Surgery in the form of subchondral drilling may be required for persistent pain in the early stages.

67

Osteochondritis dissecans: adult form

The adult form occurs more often in males and may be the result of cysts of osteoarthritis fracturing into the joint. Up to 30% are bilateral. Symptoms depend on whether the osteochondral fragment becomes separated. A loose fragment may produce locking or collapse of the knee.

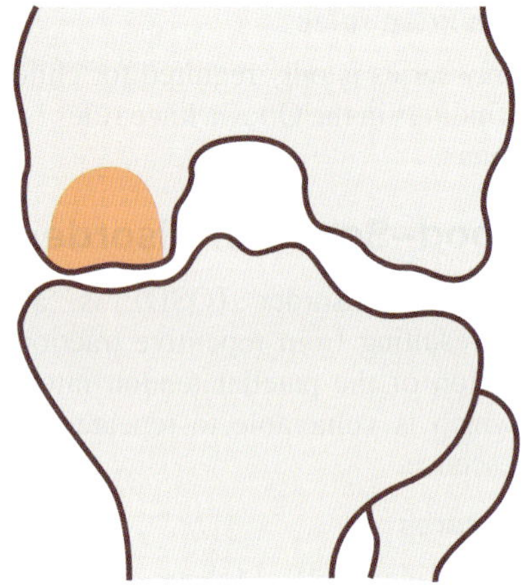

FIGURE 67.14 Osteonecrosis: necrosis in the medial femoral condyle can take three months to show radiologically

Loose bodies

The large knee joint is a 'haven' for intra-articular loose bodies, which may be formed from bone, cartilage or osteochondral fragments following injury ('chip' fragment), osteochondritis dissecans, osteoarthritis, synovial chondromatosis or other conditions. They may be asymptomatic but usually cause clicking or locking with swelling. Diagnosis is by X-ray and surgical removal is necessary for recurrent problems.

The knee 'mouse'

This common complaint is usually a result of a pedunculated fibrous lump in the prepatellar bursa, often secondary to trauma, such as falls onto the knee.

Acute injuries

Meniscal tears

Medial and lateral meniscal tears are usually caused by abduction and adduction forces causing the meniscus to be compressed between the tibial and femoral condyles and then subjected to a twisting force or a rotatory movement on a semi-flexed weight-bearing knee.

The medial meniscus is three times more likely to be torn than the lateral. These injuries are common in contact sports and are often associated with ligamentous injuries. Suspect these injuries when there is a history of injury with a twisting movement with the foot firmly fixed on the ground.

However, pain in the knee can present in the patient aged 30–50 years (and beyond 50) as the menisci degenerate, with resultant cleavage tears from the posterior horn of the medial meniscus and 'parrot-beak' tears of the mid-section of the lateral meniscus. These problems cause pain because these particular deformities create tension on the joint capsule and stretch the nerve ends. Refer to the provocation tests—Thessaly, McMurray and Apley grind tests. X-rays are not specifically useful, but an MRI scan should confirm diagnosis.

Clinical features

- General symptoms:[9]
  - joint-line pain (49%)
  - locking (17%)
  - swelling (14%)
  - loss of movement: restricted flexion, loss of last 5–10° extension
- Parrot-beak tear of lateral meniscus:
  - pain in the lateral joint line
  - pain radiating up and down the thigh
  - pain worse with activity
  - a palpable and visible lump when the knee is examined at 45°

Arthroscopic partial meniscectomy offers relief. The peripheral meniscus is vascular and can be repaired within 6–12 weeks of injury.[16]

- Cleavage tear of medial meniscus:
  - pain in medial joint line
  - pain aggravated by slight twisting of the joint
  - pain provoked by patient lying on the side and pulling the knees together
  - pain worse with activity

Arthroscopic meniscectomy is appropriate treatment, but some do settle with a trial of physiotherapy.

A diagnostic memoire

TABLE 67.4 is a useful aid in the diagnosis of these injuries. There is a similarity in the clinical signs between the opposite menisci, but the localisation of pain in the medial or lateral joint lines helps to differentiate between the medial and lateral menisci.

Note: The diagnosis of a meniscal injury is made if three or more of the five examination findings ('signs' in TABLE 67.4) are present.

Ligament injuries

Tears of varying degrees may occur in the:

- anterior cruciate ligament
- posterior cruciate ligament
- medial collateral ligament
- lateral collateral ligament

Anterior cruciate ligament rupture

This is a very serious and disabling injury that may result in chronic instability. Chronic instability can result in degenerative joint changes if not dealt with adequately. Early diagnosis is essential, but there is a high misdiagnosis rate. Sites of ACL rupture are shown in FIGURE 67.15.

Table 67.4 Typical symptoms and signs of meniscal injuries

	Medial meniscus tear	Lateral meniscus tear
Mechanism		
Twisting force on a weight-loaded flexed knee	Abduction (valgus) force Internal rotation of femur on tibia	Adduction (varus) force External rotation of femur on tibia
Symptoms		
1 Knee pain during and after activity	Medial side of knee	Lateral side of knee
2 Locking	Yes	Yes
3 Effusion	+ or –	+ or –
Signs		
1 Localised tenderness over joint line (with bucket-handle tear)	Medial joint line	Lateral joint line (may be cyst)
2 Pain on hyperextension of knee	Medial joint line	Lateral joint line
3 Pain on hyperflexion of knee joint	Medial joint line	Lateral joint line
4 Pain on rotation of lower leg (knee at 90°)	On external rotation	On internal rotation
5 Weakened or atrophied quadriceps	May be present	May be present

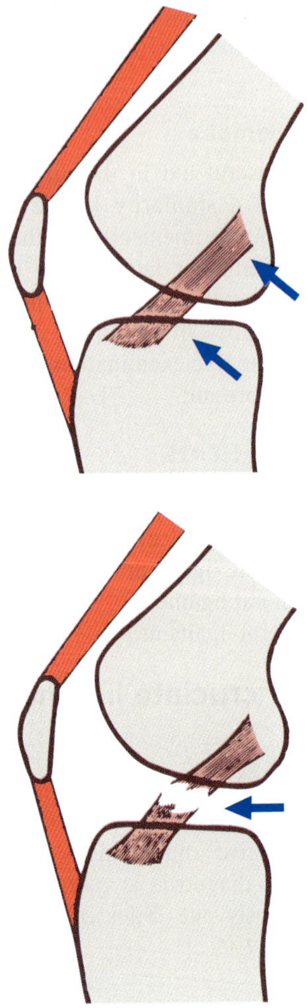

FIGURE 67.15 Sites of rupture of the anterior cruciate ligament

Mechanisms

- Sudden change in direction with leg in momentum
- Internal tibial rotation on a flexed knee (commonest) (e.g. during pivoting)
- Marked valgus force (e.g. a rugby tackle)
- May be associated with collateral ligament tears and meniscus injuries. The so-called 'unhappy triad' is a ruptured ACL, medial meniscus tear and medial collateral ligament tear.

Clinical features

- Onset of severe pain after a sporting injury, such as landing from a jump, or a forced valgus rotational strain of the knee when another player falls across the abducted leg
- Immediate effusion of blood, usually within 30 minutes
- Common sports: contact sports—rugby, football and soccer, basketball, volleyball, skiing
- Differential diagnosis is a subluxed or dislocated patella
- Subsequent history of pain and 'giving way' of the knee

Examination

- Gross effusion
- Diffuse joint-line tenderness
- Joint may be locked due to effusion, anterior cruciate tag or associated meniscal (usually medial) tear
- Ligament tests:
  - anterior drawer: negative or positive
  - pivot shift test: positive (only if instability)
  - Lachman test: lacking an end point

Note: It may be necessary to examine the knee under anaesthesia, with or without arthroscopy, to assess the extent of injury.

The Lachman test

This test is emphasised because it is a sensitive and reliable test for the integrity of the ACL. It is an anterior draw test with the knee at 15–20° of flexion. At 90° of flexion, the draw may be negative but the anterior cruciate torn.

Method—Lachman test

1. The examiner should be positioned on the same side of the examination couch as the knee to be tested.
2. The knee is held at 15–20° of flexion by placing a hand under the distal thigh and lifting the knee into 15–20° of flexion.
3. The patient is asked to relax, allowing the knee to 'fall back' into the steadying hand and roll slightly into external rotation.
4. The anterior draw is performed with the second hand grasping the proximal tibia from the medial side (see FIG. 67.16) while the thigh is held steady by the other hand. The examiner's knee can be used to steady the thigh.
5. The feel of the end point of the draw is carefully noted. Normally there is an obvious jar felt as the anterior cruciate tightens. In an anterior cruciate deficient knee there is excess movement and no firm end point. The amount of draw is compared with the opposite knee. Movement greater than 5 mm is usually considered abnormal.

67

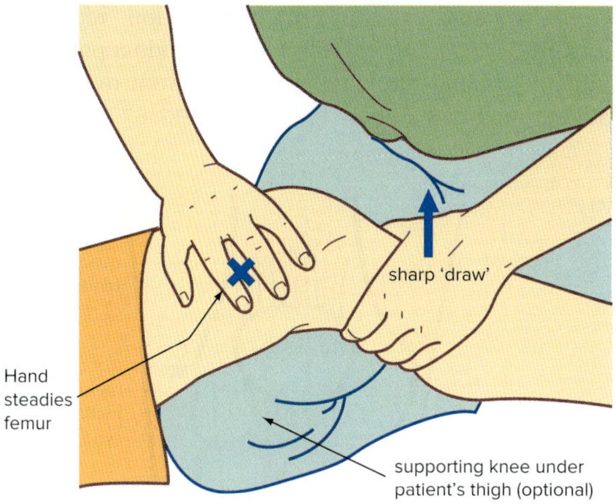

FIGURE 67.16 The Lachman test

Functional instability due to anterior cruciate deficiency is best elicited with the pivot shift test. This is more difficult to perform than the Lachman test.

Pivot shift test

This is an important test for anterolateral rotatory instability. It is positive when anterior cruciate injuries are sufficient to produce a functional instability.

Method—Pivot shift test

1. The tibia is held in internal rotation by grasping the ankle firmly, with the knee in full extension.
2. A valgus force is applied to the knee with the hand placed on the lateral aspect of the knee just below it (this maximises subluxation in the presence of an ACL tear).
3. The knee is then flexed from 0–90°, listening for a 'clunk' of reduction. The test is positive when there is a sudden change of rhythm during flexion that corresponds to relocation of the subluxed knee. This usually occurs between 30° and 45° of flexion.
4. From this flexed position, the knee is extended, seeking a click into subluxation. This is called a positive jerk test.

Management[17]

Management depends on the finding by the surgeon. Surgical repair is reserved for complete ligament tears. This usually involves reconstruction of the ligament using patellar or preferably hamstring tendons. Early reconstruction is appropriate in younger patients who participate in high levels of sporting activity for whom it can be predicted that functional instability will be a problem. In less active people, a conservative approach is appropriate. The ACL may be trimmed. Cruciate reconstruction can then be undertaken if the knee becomes clinically unstable. The presence of an ACL injury with a significant medial ligament injury will necessitate reconstructive surgery, but this is probably best delayed for some weeks as the subsequent incidence of knee stiffness is high.

Posterior cruciate ligament rupture

Mechanisms

- Direct blow to the anterior tibia in flexed knee
- Severe hyperextension injury
- Ligament fatigue plus extra stress on knee

Clinical features

- Posterior (popliteal) pain, radiating to calf
- Usually no or minimal swelling
- Minimal disability apart from limitation of running or jumping
- Pain running downhill
- Recurvatum
- Posterior sag or draw

Management

- Usually managed conservatively with immobilisation and protection for 6 weeks
- Graduated weight-bearing and exercises

Medial collateral ligament rupture

Mechanisms

- Direct valgus force to knee—lateral side knee (e.g. rugby tackle from side)
- External tibial rotation (e.g. two soccer players kicking ball simultaneously)

Clinical features

These depend on the degree of tear (1st, 2nd or 3rd degree):

- pain on medial knee
- aggravated by twisting or valgus stress
- localised swelling over medial aspect
- pseudo-locking—hamstring strain
- ± effusion
- no end point on valgus stress testing (3rd degree) (see FIG. 67.9a)

67

Note: Check lateral meniscus if MCL tear. Pellegrini–Stieda syndrome—calcification in haematoma at upper (femoral) origin of MCL—may follow.

Management

If an isolated event, this common injury responds to conservative treatment with early limited motion bracing to prevent opening of the medial joint line. Six weeks of limited motion brace at 20–70° followed by knee rehabilitation usually returns the athlete to full sporting activity within 12 weeks.

Note: The same principles of diagnosis and management apply to the less common rupture of the lateral collateral ligament, which is caused by a direct varus force to the medial side of the knee. However, lateral ligament injuries tend to involve the cruciate ligament and reconstruction of both ligaments is usually necessary.[16]

Complex regional pain syndrome I

A localised complex regional pain syndrome I (also known as reflex sympathetic dystrophy) can follow a direct fall onto the knee. (See CHAPTER 12.)

Symptoms

- Hypersensitivity
- Full extension, loss of flexion
- Possible increased sweating
- Tenderness of the joint

Overuse syndromes

The knee is very prone to overuse disorders. The pain develops gradually without swelling, is aggravated by activity and relieved with rest. It can usually be traced back to a change in the sportsperson's training schedule, footwear or technique, or to related factors. It may also be related to biomechanical abnormalities ranging from hip disorders to feet disorders.

Overuse injuries include:

- patellofemoral pain syndrome ('jogger's knee', 'runner's knee')
- patellar tendonopathy ('jumper's knee')
- anserinus tendonopathy/bursitis
- semimembranous tendonopathy/bursitis
- biceps femoris tendonopathy
- quadriceps tendonopathy/rupture
- popliteus tendonopathy
- iliotibial band friction syndrome ('runner's knee')
- the hamstrung knee
- synovial plica syndrome
- infrapatellar fat-pad inflammation

It is amazing how often palpation identifies localised areas of inflammation (tendonopathy or bursitis) around the knee, especially from overuse in athletes and in the obese elderly (see FIG. 67.17).

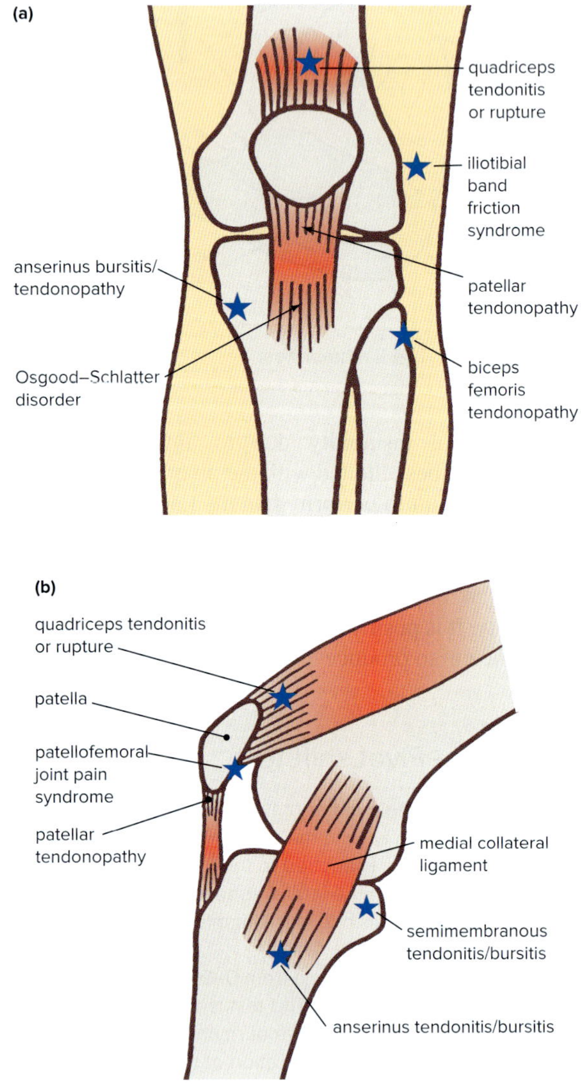

FIGURE 67.17 Typical painful areas around the knee in overuse syndromes: **(a)** anterior aspect, **(b)** medial aspect

Patellofemoral pain syndrome

This syndrome, also known as chondromalacia patellae or anterior knee pain syndrome and referred to as 'jogger's knee', 'runner's knee' or 'cyclist's knee', is the most common overuse injury of the knee. There is usually no specific history of trauma. It may be related to biomechanical abnormalities and abnormal position and tracking of the patella (e.g. patella alta). It usually presents in females aged 13–15 years with faulty knee mechanisms or in people aged 50–70 years with osteoarthritis of the patellofemoral joint.[18]

Clinical features

- Pain behind or adjacent to the patella or deep in the knee
- Pain aggravated during activities that require flexion of the knee under loading:
  - climbing stairs
  - walking down slopes or stairs
  - squatting
  - prolonged sitting
- The 'movie theatre' sign: using aisle seat to stretch knee
- Crepitus around patella may be present

Signs (chondromalacia patellae)

Patellofemoral crepitation during knee flexion and extension is often palpable, and pain may be reproduced by compression of the patella onto the femur as it is pushed from side to side with the knee straight or flexed (Perkins test).

Method for special sign—patella grind test

See FIGURE 67.18.

- Have the patient supine with the knee extended.
- Grasp the superior pole of the patella and displace it inferiorly.
- Maintain this position and apply patellofemoral compression.
- Ask the patient to contract the quadriceps (it is a good idea to get the patient to practise quadriceps contraction before applying the test).

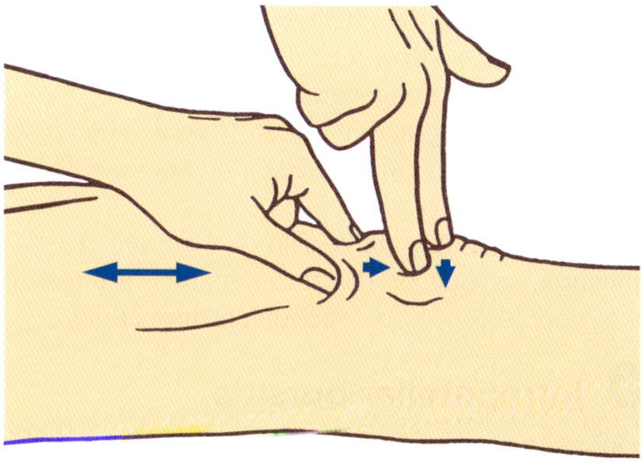

FIGURE 67.18 Special sign of the patellofemoral pain syndrome

- A positive sign is reproduction of the pain under the patella and hesitancy in contracting the muscle.

Treatment

- Give reassurance and supportive therapy.
- Reduce any aggravating activity.
- Refer to a physiotherapist.
- Correct any underlying biomechanical abnormalities such as pes planus (flat feet) by use of orthotics and correct footwear.
- Employ quadriceps (especially) and hamstring exercises.
- Consider course (trial) of NSAIDs.

Patellar tendonopathy ('jumper's knee')

'Jumper's knee', or patellar tendonopathy (see FIG. 67.2, earlier in this chapter), is a common disorder of athletes involved in repetitive jumping sports, such as high jumping, basketball, netball, volleyball and soccer. It probably starts as an inflammatory response around a small tear.

Clinical features

- Gradual onset of anterior pain
- Pain localised to below knee (in patellar tendon)
- Pain eased by rest, returns with activity
- Pain with jumping

The diagnosis is often missed because of the difficulty of localising signs. The condition is best diagnosed by eliciting localised tenderness at the inferior pole of the patella with the patella tilted. There may be localised swelling.

Method

- Lay the patient supine in a relaxed manner with the head on a pillow, arms by the side and quadriceps relaxed (a must).
- The knee should be fully extended.
- Tilt the patella by exerting pressure over its superior pole. This lifts the inferior pole.
- Now palpate the surface under the inferior pole. This allows palpation of the deeper fibres of the patellar tendon (see FIG. 67.19).
- Compare with the normal side.
- Very sharp pain is usually produced in the patient with patellar tendonopathy.

Management

Early conservative treatment, including rest from the offending stresses, is effective. Referral to a physiotherapist for exercise-based rehabilitation is

67

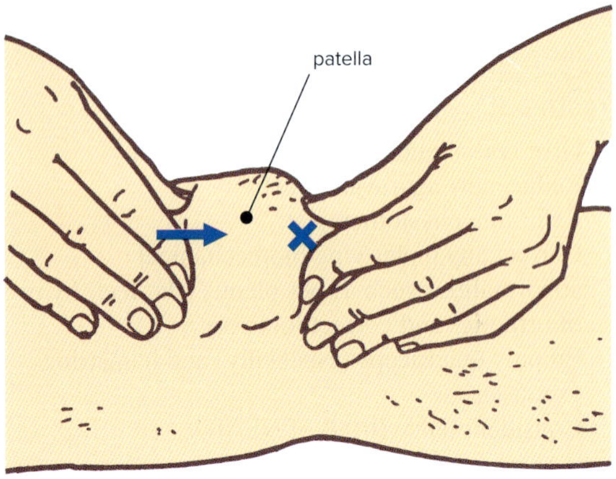

FIGURE 67.19 Patellar tendonopathy: method of palpation

appropriate. This includes adequate warm-up and warm-down. Training modification includes calf, hamstring and quadriceps muscle stretching. Modified footwear and a patellar tendon strap may be helpful in some cases. The use of NSAIDs and corticosteroid injections is disappointing. Chronic cases may require surgery.

Anserinus tendonopathy/bursitis

Localised tenderness is found over the medial tibial condyle where the tendons of the sartorius, gracilis and semitendinosus insert into the bone. It is distal to the joint line. It is a common cause of knee pain in the middle-aged or elderly, especially the overweight woman. Pain is aggravated by resisted knee flexion.

Semimembranous tendonopathy/bursitis

This inflamed area is sited either at the tendon insertion or in the bursa between the tendon and the medial head of the gastrocnemius. It is an uncommon problem. The bursa occurs on the medial side of the popliteal fossa between the medial head of the gastrocnemius and the semimembranous tendon. It often communicates with the knee joint and, if so, treat knee joint pathology. If not, one can give an injection of depot triamcinolone or betamethasone.

Biceps femoris tendonopathy/bursitis

The tendon and/or the bursa that lies between the tendon insertion and the fibular collateral ligament at the head of the fibula may become inflamed due to overuse. It is usually encountered in sprinters.

Popliteus tendonopathy

Tenosynovitis of the popliteus tendon may cause localised pain in the posterior or the posterolateral aspect of the knee. Tenderness to palpation is elicited with the knee flexed to 90°.

Iliotibial band syndrome

Inflammation develops over the lateral aspect of the knee where the iliotibial band passes over the lateral femoral condyle. An inflamed bursa can occur deep to the band. The problem, which is caused by friction of the iliotibial band on the bone, is common in long-distance runners, especially when running up and down hills, and in cyclists. It presents with well-localised lateral knee pain of gradual onset. Palpation reveals tenderness over the lateral condyle 1–2 cm above the joint line.

Treatment of tendonopathy and bursitis (small area)

Generally (apart from patellar tendonopathy), the treatment is an injection of local anaesthetic and long-acting corticosteroids into and deep to the localised area of tenderness. In addition, it is important to restrict the offending activity and refer for physiotherapy for stretching exercises. Attention to biomechanical factors and footwear is important.

If conservative methods fail for iliotibial tract tendonopathy, surgical excision of the affected fibres may cure the problem.

Prepatellar bursitis

Repetitive low-grade direct trauma, such as frequent kneeling, can cause inflammation with swelling of the bursa, which lies between the anterior surface of the patella and the skin. 'Housemaid's knee', or 'carpet layer's knee', can be difficult to treat if rest from the trauma does not allow it to subside. If persistent, drain the fluid with a 23 gauge needle and then introduce 0.5–1 mL of long-acting corticosteroid. The presence of a bursa 'mouse' and persistent bursitis usually mean that surgical intervention is required.

Acute bursitis may also be caused by acute infection, or one of the inflammatory arthropathies (e.g. gout, seronegative spondyloarthropathies).

Infrapatellar bursitis

'Clergyman's knee' is produced by the same mechanisms as prepatellar bursitis and can be involved with inflammatory disorders or infection. Treatment is also the same.

The hamstrung knee

Cross describes this condition in young active sportspeople (second decade)[9] as one that causes bilateral knee pain and possibly a limp. It is caused by a failure to warm up properly and stretch the hamstring muscles, which become tender and tight during the growth spurt. A 6-week program of straight leg raising and hamstring stretching will alleviate the pain completely.

Synovial plica syndrome

This syndrome results from a synovial fold (an embryological remnant) being caught between the patella and the femur during walking or running. It causes an acute 'catching' knee pain of the medial patellofemoral joint (see FIG. 67.2, earlier in this chapter) and sometimes a small effusion. It generally settles without treatment.

Infrapatellar fat-pad inflammation

Hoffa fat pad syndrome follows acute compression of the fat-pad, which extends across the lower patella deep to the patellar tendon and into the knee joint (see FIG. 67.2, earlier in this chapter), during a jump or other similar trauma, producing local pain and tenderness similar to the sensation of kneeling on a drawing pin.[18]

The pain usually settles without therapy over a period of days or weeks. There is localised tenderness and it can be confused with patellar tendonopathy.

Arthritic conditions

Osteoarthritis

Osteoarthritis is a very common problem of the knee joint. Symptoms usually appear in middle life or later. It is more common in women, obese people, and in those with knee deformities (e.g. genu varum) or previous trauma, especially meniscal tears. The degenerative changes may involve either the lateral or the medial tibiofemoral compartment, the patellofemoral joint or any combination of these sites.

Clinical features

- Slowly increasing joint pain and stiffness
- Aggravated by activities such as twisting, bending, prolonged walking, standing or squatting
- Descending stairs is usually more painful than ascending stairs (suggestive of patellofemoral osteoarthritis)
- Pain may occur after rest, especially prolonged flexion
- Minimal effusion and variable crepitus
- Restricted flexion but usually full extension
- Often quadriceps wasting and tender over medial joint line
- Diagnosis confirmed by X-ray (weight-bearing view)

Management options

- Relative rest
- Weight loss
- Analgesics and/or judicious use of NSAIDs
- Glucosamine: a Cochrane review showed that it is both safe and modestly effective (see CHAPTER 35)
- Walking aids and other supports
- Physiotherapy (e.g. hydrotherapy, quadriceps exercises, mobilisation and stretching techniques)
- Viscosupplementation: intra-articular injection of hylans
- Intra-articular injections of corticosteroids are generally not recommended, but a single injection for severe pain can be very effective
- Surgery is indicated for severe pain and stiffness and includes arthroscopic debridement and wash out, osteotomy, arthrodesis and total joint replacement (see FIG. 67.20) or hemiarthroplasty, especially for the medial compartment with focal arthritis and varus deformity

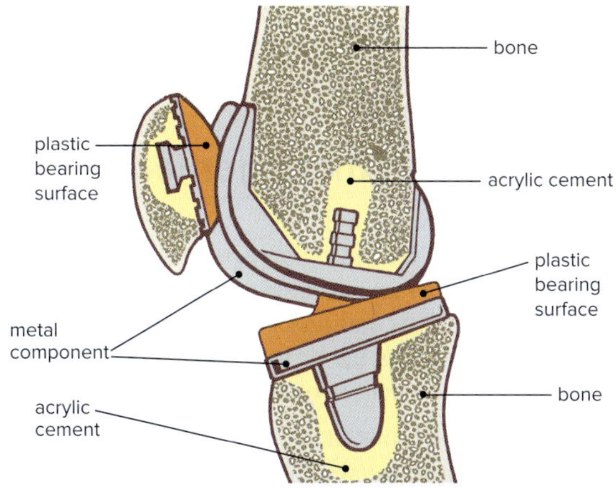

FIGURE 67.20 Total joint replacement of knee

Rheumatoid arthritis

The knee is frequently affected by rheumatoid arthritis (RA), although it rarely presents as monoarticular knee pain. RA shows the typical features of inflammation—pain and stiffness that is worse after resting. Morning stiffness is a feature.

Note: The spondyloarthropathies have a similar clinical pattern to RA.

Synovectomy is a useful option with persistent boggy thickening of synovial membrane but without destruction of the articular cartilage.[2]

Baker cyst

A popliteal cyst (Baker cyst) is a herniation of a chronic knee effusion between the heads of the gastrocnemius muscle and is usually associated with osteoarthritis (most common), rheumatoid arthritis or internal derangement of the knee. It presents as a mass behind the knee and may or may not be tender or painful.

It tends to fluctuate in size.

A Baker cyst indicates intra-articular pathology and indicates a full assessment of the knee joint.

Rupture may result in pain and swelling in the calf, mimicking DVT.

Treat underlying knee inflammation (synovitis).

Surgical removal of the cyst is advisable for persistent problems.

Septic arthritis

This tends to be more common in the knee than in other joints. Septic (pyogenic) arthritis should be suspected when the patient complains of intense joint pain, malaise and fever. In the presence of acute pyogenic infection, the joint is held rigidly. The differential diagnosis includes gout and pseudogout (chondrocalcinosis).

Principles of management

Most painful knee conditions are not serious and, providing a firm diagnosis is made and internal knee disruption or other serious illness discounted, a simple management plan as outlined leads to steady relief. For more serious injuries the primary goal is to minimise the adverse consequences of forced inactivity.

- First aid: RICE (avoid heat in first 48 hours).
- Lose weight if overweight.
- Adequate support for ligament sprains—supportive elastic tubular (Tubigrip) bandage or a firm elastic bandage over Velband.
- Simple analgesics—paracetamol (acetaminophen).
- Judicious use of NSAIDs and corticosteroid injections.
- Physiotherapy to achieve strength and stability.
- Attend to biomechanical abnormalities, inappropriate footwear and athletic techniques.
- Orthotics and braces to suit the individual patient.
- Specialised exercise techniques (e.g. the McConnell technique).[2]
- Quadriceps exercises: these simple exercises are amazingly effective.

Quadriceps exercises (examples)

- Instruct the patient to tighten the muscles in front of the thighs (as though about to lift the leg at the hip and bend the foot back but keeping the leg straight). The patient should hold the hand over the lower quadriceps to ensure it is felt to tighten. This tightening and relaxing exercise should be performed at least 6 times every 2 hours or so until it becomes a habit. It can be done sitting, standing or lying (see FIG. 67.21).
- Sitting on a chair the patient places a weight of 2–5 kg around the ankle (e.g. a plastic bag with sand or coins in a sock) and lifts the leg to the horizontal and then gently lowers it (avoid in patellofemoral problems).

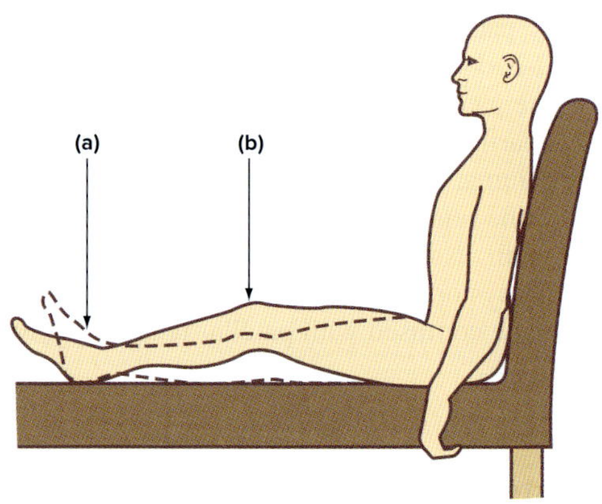

FIGURE 67.21 A quadriceps exercise: with outstretched legs the quadriceps muscle is slowly and deliberately tightened by straightening the knee to position **(a)** from the relaxed position **(b)**

When to refer

- Early referral is required for knees 'at risk' following acute injuries where one or more of the following are present:
  - – locked knee
  - – haemarthrosis
  - – instability
- Clinical evidence of a torn cruciate ligament, third degree tear of the collateral ligaments or torn meniscus
- Undiagnosed acute or chronic knee pain
- Recurrent subluxation or dislocation of the patella

67

- Suspected septic arthritis
- Presence of troublesome intra-articular loose body
- Evidence of severe osteoarthritis

Practice tips

- The absence of an effusion does not rule out the presence of severe knee injury.
- Examine the hip and lumbosacral spine if examination of the knee is normal but knee pain is the complaint.
- Always think of an osteoid osteoma in a young boy with severe bone pain in a leg (especially at night) that responds well to aspirin or paracetamol or other NSAID.
- Tears of the meniscus can occur, especially in middle age, without a history of significant preceding trauma.
- If a patient presents with a history of an audible 'pop' or 'crack' in the knee with an immediate effusion (in association with trauma), he or she has an ACL tear until proved otherwise.
- Haemarthrosis following an injury should be regarded as an anterior cruciate tear until proved otherwise.
- The 'movie theatre' sign, whereby the patient seeks an aisle seat to stretch the knee, is usually due to patellofemoral pain syndrome.
- The 'bed' sign, when pain is experienced when the knees touch while in bed, is suggestive of a medial meniscal cleavage tear.
- A positive squat test (medial pain on full squatting) indicates a tear of the posterior horn of the medial meniscus.
- Joint aspiration should not be performed on the young athlete with an acute knee injury.
- If an older female patient presents with the sudden onset of severe knee pain, think of osteonecrosis.
- Reserve intra-articular corticosteroid injections for inflammatory conditions such as rheumatoid arthritis or a crystal arthropathy: regular injections for osteoarthritis are to be avoided. Do not give the injections when the inflammation is acute and diffuse or in the early stages of injury.
- Many inflammatory conditions around the knee joint, such as bursitis or tendonopathy, respond to a local injection of local anaesthetic and corticosteroid, but avoid giving injections into the tendon, especially the patellar tendon.
- Keep in mind the technique of autologous cartilage transplantation: in this technique, cartilage cells (chondrocytes) are taken from the patient, multiplied in a laboratory and eventually implanted into the damaged area. It can be used for damage in any major joint, especially the knee, being ideal for osteochondritis dissecans.

Patient education resources

Hand-out sheets from *Murtagh's Patient Education* 7th edition:

- Baker's cyst
- Exercises for your knee
- Knee: anterior knee pain
- Osgood–Schlatter disorder

References

1 Knox JDE. Knee problems. In: *Practice*. London: Kluwer-Harrap Handbooks, 1982; 3.66: 1–5.

2 Selecki Y, Helman T. Knee pain: how to treat. Australian Doctor, 22 April 1993: i–viii.

3 McLean I. Assessment of the acute knee injury. Aust Fam Physician, 1984; 13: 575–80.

4 Cyriax J. *Textbook of Orthopaedic Medicine*, Vol. 1 (6th edn). London: Bailliere Tindall, 1976: 594.

5 Expert group for Rheumatology. In: eTG complete [Internet]. Melbourne: Therapeutic Guidelines Ltd. Available from: <www.tg.org.au>, accessed October 2017.

6 Noyes FR. Arthroscopy in acute traumatic haemarthrosis of the knee. J Bone Joint Surg, 1980: 624–87.

7 Shiraev T, Anderson SE, Hope N. Meniscal tear—presentation, diagnosis and management. Aust Fam Physician, 2012; 41 (4): 182–7.

8 Brukner P, Khan K. *Clinical Sports Medicine* (3rd edn). Sydney: McGraw-Hill, 2007: 506–37.

9 Cross MJ, Crichton KJ. *Clinical Examination of the Injured Knee*. London: Harper & Row, 1987: 21–46.

10 Lau L (ed.). *Imaging Guidelines* (4th edn). Melbourne: RAZNC Radiologists, 2001: 200–1.

11 Jackson JL, O'Malley PG et al. Evaluation of acute knee pain in primary care. Ann Intern Med, 2003; 139 (7): 575–88.

12 Larkins P. The little athlete. Aust Fam Physician, 1991; 20: 973–8.

13 Rostrom PKM, Calver RF. Subcutaneous atrophy following methyl prednisolone injection in Osgood–Schlatter epiphysitis. J Bone Joint Surg, 1979; 61A: 627–8.

14 Wilkins E et al. Osteoarthritis and articular chondrocalcinosis in the elderly. Ann Rheum Dis, 1983; 42 (3): 280–4.

15 Rush J. Spontaneous osteonecrosis of the knee. Current Orthopaedics, 1999; 13: 309–14.

16 Edwards E, Miller R. Management of acute knee injuries. Medical Observer, 17 March 2000: 67–9.

17 Frobell RB et al. Treatment for acute anterior cruciate ligament tear: five year outcome of randomised trial. BMJ, 2013; 346: f232.

18 Fricker P. Anterior knee pain. Aust Fam Physician, 1988; 17: 1055–6.

68 Pain in the foot and ankle

The victim goes to bed and sleeps in good health. About two o'clock in the morning he is awakened by a severe pain in the great toe; more rarely in the heel, ankle, or instep . . . The part affected cannot bear the weight of the bed clothes nor the jar of a person walking in the room. The night is spent in torture.

THOMAS SYDENHAM (1624–89) ON GOUT

Pain in the foot (podalgia) and ankle problems are common occurrences in general practice. Various characteristics of the pain can give an indication of its cause, such as the description of gout by Thomas Sydenham. There are many traumatic causes of podalgia and ankle dysfunction, especially fractures and torn ligaments, but this chapter will focus mainly on everyday problems that develop spontaneously or through overuse. Forefoot pain is common especially in the elderly. The forefoot comprises the toes to the middle of the metatarsals and all of the supporting structures. Metatarsalgia is a term used to describe pain in the distal aspect of one or more of the metatarsal bones during weight-bearing.[1]

Key facts and checkpoints

- Foot deformities such as flat feet (pes planus) are often painless.
- Foot strain is probably the commonest cause of podalgia.[2]
- A common deformity of the toes is hallux valgus, with or without bunion formation.
- Osteoarthritis is a common sequel to hallux valgus.
- Osteoarthritis affecting the ankle is relatively uncommon.
- All of the distal joints of the foot may be involved in arthritic disorders.
- Many foot and ankle problems are caused by unsuitable footwear and lack of foot care.
- Ankle sprains are the most common injury in sport, representing about 25% of injuries.
- Severe sprains of the lateral ligaments of the ankle due to an inversion force may be associated with various fractures.
- Bunions and hammer toes are generally best treated by surgery.

A diagnostic approach

A summary of the diagnostic strategy model is presented in TABLE 68.1.

Probability diagnosis

Common causes include osteoarthritis, especially of the first metatarsophalangeal (MTP) joint, acute or chronic foot strain, plantar fasciitis, plantar skin conditions such as warts, corns and calluses and various toenail problems.

Serious disorders not to be missed

The very important serious disorders to consider include:

- vascular disease—affecting small vessels
- diabetic neuropathy
- osteoid osteoma
- rheumatoid arthritis
- complex regional pain syndrome I

Vascular causes

The main problem is ischaemic pain that occurs only in the foot. The commonest cause is atheroma. Vascular causes include:

- acute arterial obstruction
- chilblains
- atherosclerosis, especially small vessel disease
- functional vasospasm (Raynaud)—rare

Symptoms:

- claudication (rare in isolation)
- sensory disturbances, especially numbness at rest or on walking
- rest pain—at night, interfering with sleep, precipitated by elevation, relieved by dependency

For treatment refer to CHAPTER 67.

Complex regional pain syndrome I

Also known as reflex sympathetic dystrophy or Sudeck atrophy, regional pain syndrome is characterised by severe pain, swelling and disability of the feet. It is a neurovascular disorder resulting in hyperaemia and osteoporosis that may be a sequela of trauma (often

Table 68.1	The painful foot and ankle: diagnostic strategy model
Probability diagnosis	
Acute or chronic foot strain	
Sprained ankle	
Osteoarthritis (esp. great toe)	
Plantar fasciitis	
Achilles tendonopathy	
Tibialis posterior tendonopathy	
Wart, corn or callus	
Ingrowing toenail/paronychia	
Serious disorders not to be missed	
Vascular insufficiency:	
• small vessel disease	
Neoplasia:	
• osteoid osteoma	
• osteosarcoma	
• synovial sarcoma	
Severe infections (rare):	
• septic arthritis	
• actinomycosis	
• osteomyelitis	
Rheumatoid arthritis	
Peripheral neuropathy	
Complex regional pain syndromes	
Ruptured Achilles tendon	
Ruptured tibialis posterior tendon	
Pitfalls (often missed)	
Foreign body (esp. children)	
Gout	
Morton neuroma	
Tarsal tunnel syndrome	
Deep peroneal nerve entrapment	
Chilblains	
Stress fracture (e.g. navicular)	
Erythema nodosum	
Rarities:	
• spondyloarthropathies	
• osteochondritis: navicular (Köhler), metatarsal head (Freiberg), calcaneum (Sever)	
• glomus tumour (under nail)	
• Paget disease	
Seven masquerades checklist	
Depression (?)	
Diabetes	
Drugs	
Spinal dysfunction	
Is the patient trying to tell me something?	
A non-organic cause warrants consideration with any painful condition.	

trivial) and prolonged immobilisation. Complex regional pain syndrome I usually lasts 2 years and recovery to normality usually follows.

The clinical features include sudden onset in middle-aged patients, pain worse at night, stiff joints and skin warm and red. X-rays that show patchy decalcification of bone are diagnostic. Treatment includes reassurance, analgesics, mobility in preference to rest, and physiotherapy.

Osteoid osteoma

Osteoid osteomas are rare but important little 'brain teasers' of benign tumours that typically occur in older children and adolescents. Males are affected twice as often as females. Any bone (except those of the skull) can be affected but the tibia and femur are the main sites. Nocturnal pain is a prominent symptom with pain relief by aspirin being a feature.

Diagnosis is dependent on clinical suspicion and then X-ray, which shows a small sclerotic lesion with a radiolucent centre. Treatment is by surgical excision.

Pitfalls

There are many traps in the diagnosis and management of problems presenting with a painful foot. Common problems require consideration—these include gouty arthritis, chilblains, a stress fracture and a foreign body in the foot, especially in children. Nerve entrapment, as outlined in CHAPTER 66, is uncommon but Morton neuroma is reasonably common.

Less common disorders include complex regional pain syndrome, which is often misdiagnosed, the spondyloarthropathies (psoriasis, reactive arthritis, ankylosing spondylitis and the inflammatory bowel disorders) and osteochondritis of the calcaneus, navicular bone and metatarsal head. If there is an exquisitely tender small purple–red spot beneath a toenail, a glomus tumour (a benign hamartoma) is the diagnosis. It is worth noting that most of these conditions are diagnosed by X-rays.

General pitfalls

- Failing to order X-rays of the foot.
- Failing to order X-rays of the ankle following injury.
- Failing to appreciate the potential for painful problems caused by diabetes—neuropathy and small vessel disease.
- Neglecting the fact that most of the arthritides can manifest in joints in the foot, especially the forefoot.
- Regarding the sprained ankle in adults and children as an innocuous injury: associated

injuries include chondral fractures to the dome of the talus, impaction fractures around the medial recess of the ankle, avulsion fractures of the lateral malleolus and base of fifth metatarsal.
- Misdiagnosing a stress fracture of the navicular which, like the scaphoid fracture, causes delayed union and non-union. Cast immobilisation for 8 weeks initially may prevent the need for surgery.
- Misdiagnosing a complete rupture of the Achilles tendon because the patient can plantar flex the foot.
- Overlooking tibialis posterior tendonopathy as a cause of ankle pain.

Seven masquerades checklist

The checklist has four conditions that should be considered, especially diabetes and spinal dysfunction. Diabetes may be responsible for a simple type of atherosclerotic pattern, possibly complicated by infection and ulceration. The neuropathy of diabetes can cause a burning pain with paraesthesia. It has a 'sock'-type pattern as opposed to the dermatome pattern of nerve root pressure arising from the lumbosacral spine. The common S1 pain is experienced on the outer border of the foot, into the fifth toe and on the outer sole and heel of the foot.

Drugs and anaemia could indirectly cause pain through vascular insufficiency. The drugs that could cause vasospasm include beta blockers and ergotamine. An alcoholic neuropathy also has to be considered.

Red flag pointers for foot pain

- Pain in forefoot disturbing sleep
- Fever and systemic illness with bone pain
- Localised tenderness away from heel in child
- 'Burning' feet

68

Psychogenic considerations

Any painful condition can be closely associated with psychogenic disorders, including depression.

The clinical approach

History

This is very important, as always, since various characteristics of the pain can give an indication of its cause. Questions should address the quality of the pain, its distribution, mode of onset, periodicity, relation to weight-bearing, and associated features such as swelling or colour change. It is relevant to enquire about pain in other joints such as the hand and spine, including the sacroiliac joints, which might indicate that the foot pain is part of a polyarthritis. A history of diarrhoea, psoriasis, urethritis or iritis may suggest that one of the spondyloarthropathies has to be excluded.

Key questions

The practitioner should address the following questions:

- Does the pain arise from a local condition or is it part of a generalised disease?
- Is there a history of psoriasis, chronic diarrhoea or colitis, urethritis or iritis?
- Is pain also present in other joints, thus indicating the foot pain is part of a polyarthritis, such as rheumatoid arthritis?
- Is the problem related to unsuitable footwear?
- Does the nature of the pain point to the cause?
  - throbbing pain → inflammation
  - burning pain → nerve entrapment, diabetic neuropathy or regional pain syndrome
  - severe episodic pain → gout
  - pain worse at night → ischaemia (small vessel disease), regional pain syndrome, cramps or osteoid osteoma
  - pain worse at night, relieved by aspirin → osteoid osteoma
  - pain worse on standing after sitting and getting out of bed → plantar fasciitis

For ankle injuries it is important to ask about the nature of the injury:

- Did the foot twist in (invert) or twist out (evert)?
- Was the foot pointing down or up at the time of injury?
- Point with one finger to where it hurts (the finger-pointing sign).
- What happened immediately after the injury?
- Were you able to walk straight away?
- What happened when you cooled off?

If there has been a fall onto the foot from a height, consider the possibility of a fracture of the calcaneus or talus or disruption of the syndesmosis between the tibia and fibula. Also check the lumbar spine.

Examination

Inspection

Inspect the feet with the patient standing, sitting, walking (in shoes and barefooted) and lying down (note plantar surfaces). Inspect the footwear (normally, a shoe wears first on the outer posterior margin of the heel).

Note:

- any gait abnormalities, including limping and abnormal toe in or toe out
- deformities, such as hammer toes, bunions—medial (hallux valgus) and lateral (Tailor bunion)—and claw toes
- swellings, including callosities
- muscle wasting
- skin changes and signs of ischaemia

Palpation

Systematic palpation is very useful as most structures in the foot are accessible to palpation.

Movements (active and passive)

The joints to test are:

- ankle (talar) joint
- hindfoot (subtalar) joint
- midfoot (midtarsal) joint

Movements

- Plantar flexion (normal—50°) and dorsiflexion (20°) of foot (see FIG. 68.1)
- Inversion and eversion of hindfoot (mainly subtalar joint)—hold heel and abduct and adduct (see FIG. 68.2)
- Inversion and eversion of forefoot (midtarsal joint)—hold heel in one hand to fix hindfoot, hold forefoot in the other and abduct and adduct (rotation movement) (see FIG. 68.3)
- Test other joints individually (e.g. MTP, midtarsal)

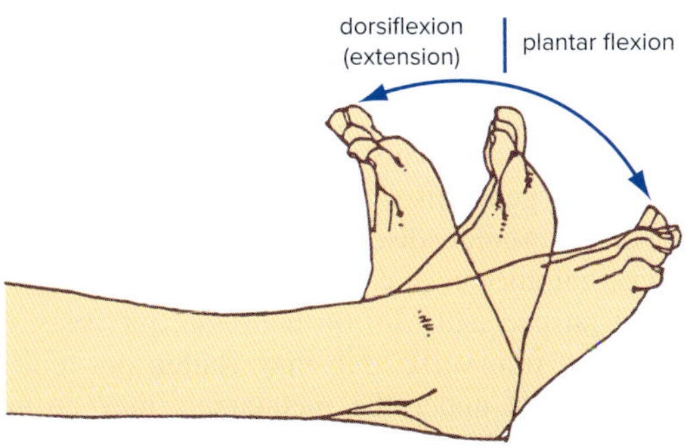

FIGURE 68.1 Dorsiflexion and plantar flexion of the ankle joint

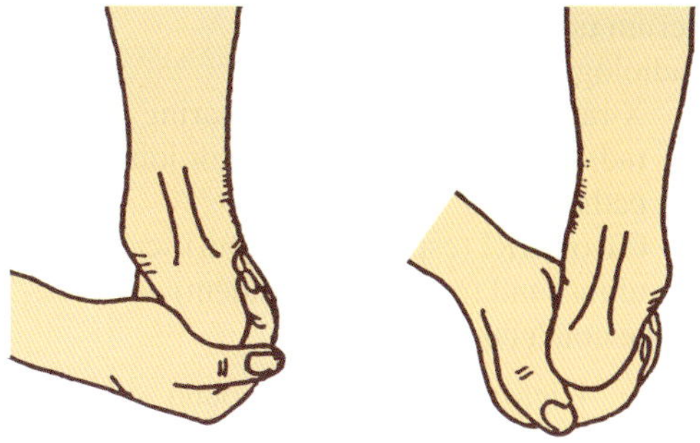

FIGURE 68.2 Testing inversion and eversion of the hindfoot

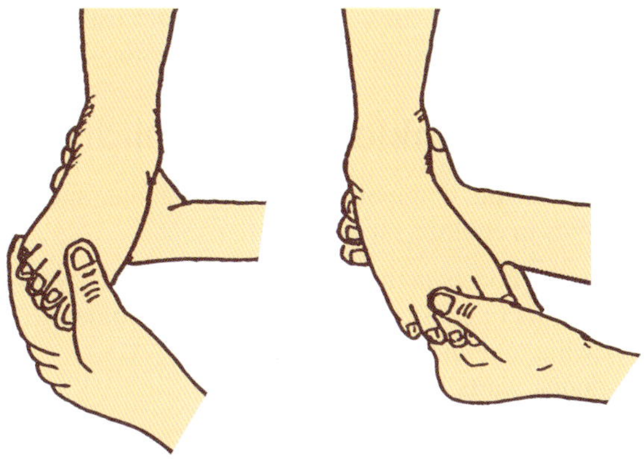

FIGURE 68.3 Testing eversion and inversion of the forefoot

Special tests

- Achilles tendon, including calf squeeze (Thompson or Simmond test)
- Compress MTP joints from above and below
- Compress metatarsals mediolaterally between thumb and forefinger
- Press upwards from sole of foot just proximal to third and fourth MTP joints—Morton test
- Check circulation—test dorsalis pedis and posterior tibial pulses
- Neurological examination, including tests for L4, L5 and S1 nerve root function

Investigations

The choice of investigations depends on the clinical features elicited by the history and examination. Select from the following list:

- for systemic diseases:
  - blood glucose
  - RA tests
  - ESR/C-reactive protein
  - HLA-B_{27}

- serum uric acid
- radiology:
  - X-ray ± stress and weight-bearing views
  - radionuclide scans (for bone or joint pathology)
  - CT or MRI (especially helpful) scans
  - ultrasound (operator dependent)
- nerve conduction studies

Note: High-resolution ultrasound is used to diagnose disorders of the Achilles and posterior tibialis tendons and to locate foreign bodies such as splinters of wood and glass.

Radionuclide scanning may detect avascular necrosis in bones, stress fractures, osteoid osteomas, inflammatory osteoarthritis and similar lesions.[3]

Foot and ankle pain in children

Apart from the common problem of trauma, special problems in children include:

- foreign bodies in the foot
- tumours (e.g. osteoid osteoma, osteosarcoma, Ewing tumour)
- plantar warts
- osteomyelitis/septic arthritis
- ingrowing toenails
- osteochondritis/aseptic necrosis
- osteochondritis dissecans of talus (in adolescents)
- pitted keratolysis and juvenile plantar dermatosis (adolescents)
- stress fractures

Think of osteoid osteoma in children with night pain.

Osteochondritis/aseptic necrosis

Three important bones to keep in mind are:

- the calcaneum—Sever disease
- the navicular—Köhler disease
- the head of the second metatarsal—Freiberg disease

Sever disease is traction osteochondritis, while the other disorders are a 'crushing' osteochondritis with avascular necrosis.

Sever disease of the heel

This is calcaneal apophysitis, which presents in a child (usually a boy) aged 7–15 years (average of 10 years) with a painful tender heel at the insertion of the tendoachilles. It is diagnosed by X-ray. The only treatment is to ensure that the child avoids wearing flat-heeled shoes and wears a slightly raised heel. Strenuous sporting activities should be restricted for 12 weeks and then reviewed.

Köhler disease of the navicular

This disorder causes a painful limp (usually mild) with some swelling and tenderness around the navicular in a child (usually a boy) aged 3–6 years, although it is seen sometimes in older children. Complete recovery occurs with temporary rest. Sometimes supportive strapping is helpful.

Freiberg disease

This problem affects the head of the second metatarsal (rarely the third), which feels tender and swollen on palpation. It is more common in girls aged 12–16 years and can present in young adults as pain aggravated by standing on the forefoot. Plain X-ray shows the characteristic collapse of the metatarsal head. The treatment is restriction of activity, protective footwear and protective padding.

Sprained ankle in a child

Children rarely sprain ligaments so it is important to assess apparent strains carefully, including an X-ray.

The little athlete

The 'little athlete' can suffer a variety of injuries from accidents and overuse. Diffuse heel pain, which is common, is most often related to Sever apophysitis of the calcaneum. Occasionally, a juvenile-type plantar fasciitis may occur. Little athletes can develop tendonitis around the ankle, either on the lateral side (peroneals) or medially (tibialis posterior). Occasionally, a stress fracture of the metatarsals or other bones can occur.[4] Special attention must be paid to any developmental structural abnormalities and to footwear.

Foot and ankle problems in the elderly

Foot problems are more prevalent in old age. Some are due to a generalised disease, such as diabetes or peripheral vascular disease, while others, such as bunions, hammer toes, calluses and corns, atrophy of the heel fat-pad and Morton neuroma, increase with ageing. The transverse arch may flatten out and the protective pads under the metatarsals may atrophy, resulting in painful callosities.

Unfortunately, many elderly people regard foot problems as a normal process but these problems actually require considerable care and attention, especially in the presence of peripheral vascular disease, diabetes or rheumatoid arthritis. Deformed toenails (onychogryphosis) are also common albeit not a painful condition.

Flat foot occurring in middle age is usually due to stretching or rupture of the tibialis posterior tendon.[5]

Sprained ankle

There are two main ankle ligaments that are subject to heavy inversion or eversion stresses, namely the lateral ligaments and the medial ligaments respectively. Most of the ankle 'sprains' or tears involve the lateral ligaments (up to 90%) while the stronger, tauter medial (deltoid) ligament is less prone to injury. It is important not to misdiagnose a complete rupture of the lateral ligaments.

Most sprains occur when the ankle is plantar flexed and inverted, such as when landing awkwardly after jumping or stepping on uneven ground. It is a very common sporting injury.

Clinical features (sprained lateral ligaments)

- Ankle 'gives way'
- Difficulty in weight-bearing
- Discomfort varies from mild to severe
- Bruising (may take 12–24 hours) indicates more severe injury
- May have functional instability: ankle gives way on uneven ground

Physical examination

Perform as soon as possible:

- note swelling and bruising
- palpate over bony landmarks and three lateral ligaments
- test general joint laxity and range of motion
- a common finding is a rounded swelling in front of the lateral malleolus (the 'signe de la coquille d'oeuf')
- test stability in AP plane (anterior draw sign)

Is there an underlying fracture?

For a severe injury the possibility of a fracture—usually of the lateral malleolus or base of fifth metatarsal—must be considered. If the patient is able to walk without much discomfort straight after the injury a fracture is unlikely. However, as a rule, ankle injuries should be X-rayed according to the Ottawa rules.

HEEL PAIN

Important causes of heel pain in adults (see FIG. 68.4)[6] include:

- Achilles tendon disorders:
  - tendonopathy/peritendonitis
  - bursitis: postcalcaneal, retrocalcaneal
  - tendon tearing: partial, complete
- bruised heel
- tender heel pad:
  - usually atrophy

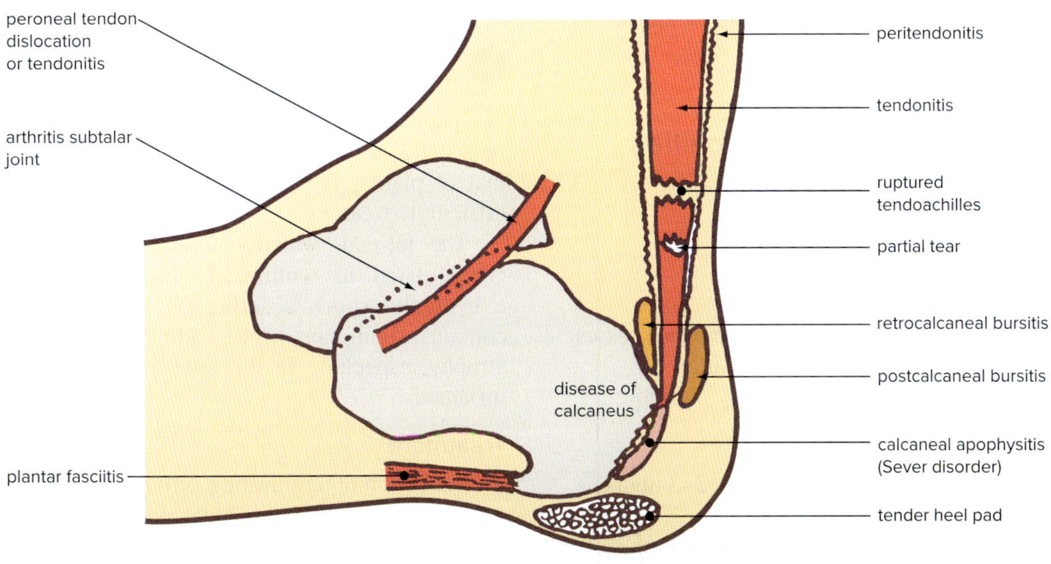

FIGURE 68.4 Important causes of the painful heel

68

- also inflammation
- neuropathies (e.g. diabetic, alcoholic)
- tenosynovitis (FHL, FDL)
- 'pump bumps'
- plantar fasciitis
- periostitis
- calcaneal apophysitis
- peroneal tendon dislocation
- nerve entrapments
  - tarsal tunnel
  - medial calcaneal nerve
  - nerve to abductor digiti minimi

Ultrasound examination is useful to differentiate the causes of Achilles tendon disorders.

Achilles tendonopathy[6]

The pathology is a combination of degenerative and inflammatory changes due to overuse and may occur either in the tendon itself or in the surrounding paratendon. It presents with tendon pain during and after weight-bearing activities with a tender local swelling of the tendon. The latter is called peritendonitis rather than tenosynovitis because there is no synovial sheath.

Management

- Relative rest
- Course of NSAIDs for acute pain
- Heel padding
- Consider heel 'raisers'
- Consider continuous topical glyceryl trinitrate as patches
- Physiotherapy for stretching and an eccentric exercise program[6]
- Physiotherapy

Complete rupture of Achilles tendon[6]

Clinical features

- Sudden onset of intense pain
- Patient usually falls over
- Feels more comfortable when acute phase passes
- Development of swelling and bruising
- Some difficulty walking, especially on tiptoe

Diagnosis

- Palpation of gap (best to test in first 2–3 hours as haematoma can fill gap)
- Positive Thompson test: compression of the calf muscles reveals an absent plantar reflex on the affected side

Treatment

- Early surgical repair (within 3 weeks)

Partial rupture

Similar history and clinical findings. Localised tenderness and very tender defect about the size of the tip of the finger.

Refer for evaluation—if gap, early surgical exploration and repair. Conservative treatment if no gap, including heel raise and crutches early.

Achilles tendon bursitis

Bursitis can occur at two sites:

- posterior and superficial—between skin and tendon
- deep (retrocalcaneal)—between calcaneus and tendon (see FIG. 68.4)

The former occurs mainly in young women from shoe friction and is readily palpated. Tenderness from the deep bursitis is elicited by squeezing in front of the tendon with the thumb and index finger: a swelling may be seen bulging on either side of the tendon.

Treatment

- Avoid shoe pressure (e.g. wear sandals)
- 1–2 cm heel raise inside the shoe
- Apply local heat and ultrasound
- NSAIDs
- Inject corticosteroid into bursa with a 25 gauge needle

Fat-pad disorders

A tender heel pad or cushion causes a dull throbbing pain under the heel. It is localised more proximal to that of plantar fasciitis. Once established, it is very difficult to treat.

The fat-pad, which consists of globules of fat encapsulated in multiple U-shaped septa, acts as a hydraulic shock absorber on heel strike. It also contains significant nerve endings.[7] It can undergo atrophy, especially in the elderly, and also become inflamed.

Treatment

- Reduction of aggravating activity
- Weight loss (if applicable)
- Simple analgesics
- Orthotic (cushioning heel cup) ± foam insert
- Good footwear

Problems are treated with an orthotic or an insert and good footwear. Corticosteroids should be avoided as they can accelerate the atrophy.[8]

Plantar fasciitis

This common condition (also known as 'policeman's heel') is characterised by pain on the plantar aspect of the heel, especially on the medial side; it usually occurs about 5 cm from the posterior end of the heel, although it can be experienced over a wide area beneath the heel. The pain radiates into the sole.

Clinical features

- Pain:
  - under the heel
  - first steps out of bed
  - relieved after walking
  - increasing towards the end of the day
  - worse after sitting
- May be bilateral—usually worse on one side
- Typically over 40 years
- Both sexes
- Sometimes history of injury or overuse
- No constant relationship to footwear

Signs[8]

- Tenderness:
  - localised to medial tuberosity
  - may be more posterior
  - may be lateral
  - may be widespread
  - not altered by tensing fascia (but this action may cause pain)
- Heel pad may bulge or appear atrophic
- Crepitus may be felt
- No abnormality of gait, heel strike or foot alignment
- Patient often obese

Treatment

Plantar fasciitis not associated with one of the spondyloarthritides tends to heal spontaneously in 12–24 months. It has a variable response to treatment with NSAIDs, injections, ultrasound and insoles. Rest from long walks and from running is important. Systematic reviews to date indicate that taping is effective for short-term relief. Plantar fascia-stretching exercises, when combined with prefabricated insoles and a short course of NSAIDs, are effective for short-term and long-term pain relief.[9] Another systematic review supports a conservative approach based on maximising comfort during the 3-month period of considerable discomfort.[10]

Protection

Symptomatic relief is obtained by protecting the heel with an orthotic pad to include the heel and arch of the foot (e.g. Rose insole). Otherwise, a pad made from sponge or sorbo rubber that raises the heel about 1 cm is suitable. A hole corresponding to the tender area should be cut out of the pad to avoid direct contact with the sole. The aim is to get all of the foot to take the stress.

Injection technique

Disabling plantar fasciitis can be treated by injecting local anaesthetic and long-acting corticosteroid into the site of maximal tenderness in the heel. An alternative is to inject the corticosteroid into the anaesthetised heel—this is usually for temporary relief.

'Cracked' heels

- Soak feet for 30 minutes in warm water containing an oil such as Alpha Keri or Derma Oil.
- Pat dry, then apply a cream such as Nutraplus (10% urea) or Eulactol heel balm. Use hydrocortisone 0.5% cream for resistant cases.
- For severe cases, use sorbolene cream with 20% glycerol and 30% urea (test skin sensitivity first).

Arthritic conditions

Arthritis of the foot or ankle is a rather meaningless diagnosis and specificity is required. Typical sites of arthritic targets are shown in FIGURE 68.5.

Osteoarthritis

Osteoarthritis may occur in any of the joints of the foot, but it commonly involves the first MTP joint, leading to hallux rigidus. It can affect the subtalar joint, but the ankle joint proper is usually not affected by osteoarthritis.

Hallux rigidus

Osteoarthritis of the first MTP joint can lead to gradual loss of motion of the toe and considerable discomfort. Roomy protective footwear and relative rest is the basis of treatment, coupled with daily self-mobilisation (stretching toe into plantar flexion morning and night). Other measures include manipulation under general anaesthesia or surgery (arthrodesis or arthroplasty) for severe cases.

Rheumatoid arthritis

Rheumatoid arthritis is typically a symmetrical polyarthritis presenting with pain in the MTP joints. It may also affect the ankle, midtarsal and tarsometatarsal joints. The interphalangeal joints are seldom affected primarily. It causes pain and stiffness under the balls of the feet, especially first thing in the morning.

68

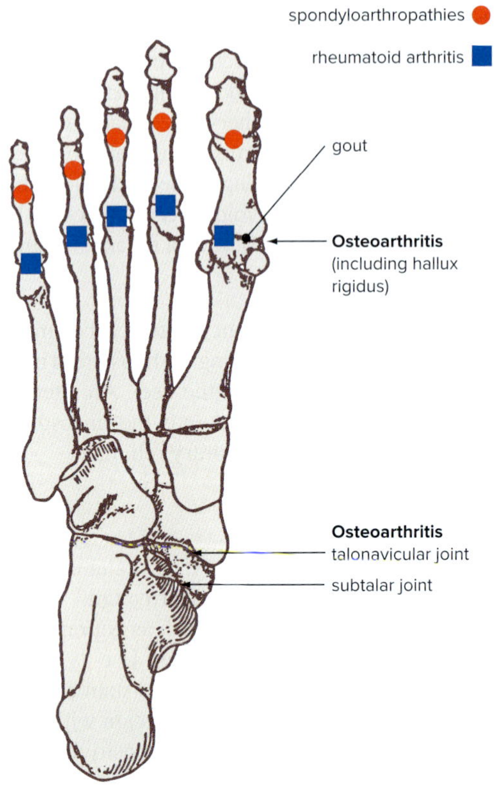

FIGURE 68.5 Typical sites of arthritic causes of podalgia on skeleton of right foot (plantar aspect)

Gout

Gout typically affects the first MTP and should be considered with the sudden onset of pain, especially in the presence of redness, swelling and tenderness. It can affect any synovial joint and occasionally may be polyarticular. Gout is often dismissed by the patient as a 'sprain'. A history of alcohol consumption or diuretic treatment is relevant.

Spondyloarthritides

This group of arthritic disorders (reactive arthritis, ankylosing spondylitis, psoriatic arthritis and arthritides associated with chronic bowel disorders) may involve peripheral joints. Other foot involvement includes plantar fasciitis, Achilles tendonitis and sausage-shaped toes due to tenosynovitis, and arthritis of the proximal interphalangeal joints.

'Burning' feet

It is not uncommon for people, especially the elderly, to present with the complaint of 'burning' feet. A careful history is needed to elicit exactly what they mean by 'burning'—is it real pain, a cold sensation or paraesthesia?

A checklist of causes is as follow:

- vascular: ischaemic rest pain from small vessel disease, chilblains or other cold reaction, functional vasospasm (Raynaud phenomenon)
- diabetic neuropathy
- tarsal tunnel syndrome
- complex regional pain syndrome I or II
- Morton neuroma (localised pain between toes)
- psychogenic, especially anxiety

It is worth considering tarsal tunnel syndrome if there is anterior burning pain in the forefoot with associated aching in the calf. It is usually present in menopausal women and worse at night. It is caused by entrapment of the posterior tibial nerve near the medial malleolus, and may be associated with rheumatoid arthritis. Treat with physiotherapy, a medial arch support and a corticosteroid injection before contemplating surgery.

Foot strain

Foot strain is probably the commonest cause of podalgia. A foot may be strained by abnormal stress, or by normal stress for which it is not prepared. In foot strain, the supporting ligaments become stretched, irritated and inflamed. It is commonly encountered in athletes who are relatively unfit or have a disorder such as flat feet, or in obese adults.

Symptoms and signs

- Aching pain in foot and calf during or after prolonged walking or standing
- Initial deep tenderness felt on medial border of plantar fascia (see FIG. 68.6)
- Worse with new shoes, especially a change to high heels

Acute foot strain

Acute ligamentous strain, such as occurs to the occasional athlete or to the person taking long unaccustomed walks. It is usually self-limiting and recovers rapidly with rest.

Chronic foot strain

Foot strain will become chronic with repeated excessive stress or with repeated normal stress on a mechanical abnormality. A common consequence is an everted foot, leading to flattening of the longitudinal arch on weight-bearing. It is important to establish whether the symptoms commenced after the patient began wearing a different type of footwear.

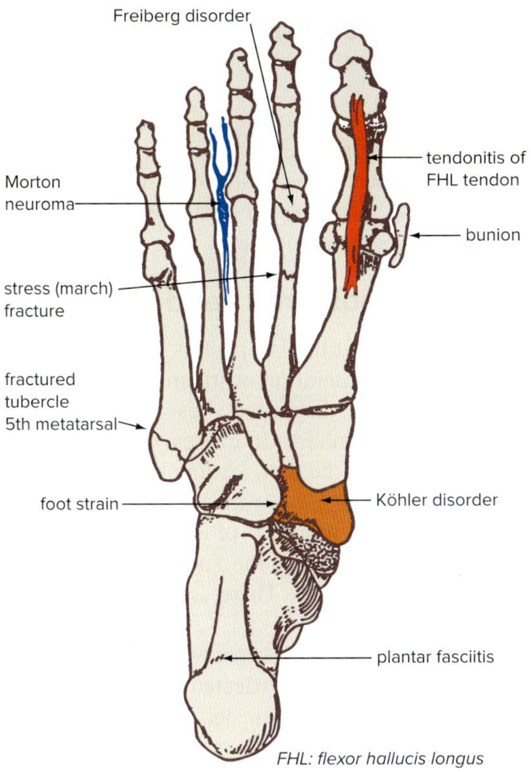

FIGURE 68.6 Typical sites of important causes of podalgia (other than arthritis)—right foot

Treatment

The treatment is basically the same as that of the adult flat foot. Acute strain is treated with rest and by reducing walking to a minimum. Try the application of cold initially and then heat. The management of chronic strain is based on an exercise program and orthotics, including arch supports, to correct any deformity.

Aching feet

- Avoid wearing high heels.
- Wear insoles to support the foot arch.
- Perform foot exercises.
- Soak the feet in a basin of warm water containing therapeutic salts (Epsom salts is suitable).
- Massage feet with baby oil followed by a special ribbed wooden foot massager.

Flat feet (pes planus)

Flat feet are normal in young children. No treatment is required in flat feet in which the arch is restored by standing on tiptoe (see CHAPTER 92). If painful, treat with exercises and insoles. Refer if concerned. Hind foot fusion can be performed for severe pain.

Claw foot (pes cavus)

High foot arch is usually of congenital origin. It may be secondary to polio or various neurological conditions. The foot is inflexible and the toes may be 'hammer' or clawed. Treatment includes special orthotics with good shock-absorbing properties, appropriate footwear, foot exercises and padding under the metatarsal heads. Operative treatment involves soft tissue release or arthrodesis to strengthen toes.

Disorders of the ankle tendons

Inflammation of a tendon sheath surrounding the ankle may result from repetitive overuse, trauma such as a sprained ankle or unaccustomed stress, including sporting injuries.

Tenosynovitis commonly involves the tibialis posterior tendon over the medial compartment or the peroneal tendons over the lateral compartment. It may also affect the tibialis anterior and extensor digitorum longus tendons. Friction at the point where the tendons become angulated at the ankle causes the inflammation. The patient presents with pain, swelling and restricted movement. On examination there is swelling and tenderness where the tendon bulges out from behind and below the malleolus.

If necessary, the diagnosis can be confirmed by ultrasound or MRI imaging.

Complications include tenovaginitis, weakness, ganglion formation, subluxation or dislocation and rupture.

Treatment of tendonitis includes partial immobilisation (rarely in a cast) or an orthotic device to support the arch of the foot.

A carefully directed injection of corticosteroid into the tendon sheath can be very effective.

Peroneal tendonitis

This occurs along the course of the tendon from behind the lateral malleolus to the outer side of the foot and is common in athletes and ballet dancers. Pain is reproduced on palpation, on stretching the tendons by passive inversion of the foot or by resisting eversion of the foot.

Peroneal tendon dislocation

This is most commonly a dislocated leg tendon as a result of forceful dorsiflexion. An audible painless snapping sensation may be experienced. Surgical repair is necessary.

Tibialis posterior tendonopathy

This is a common problem, especially in middle-aged females, in ballet dancers and in those with pes planus with a valgus deformity. The tendon (see FIG. 68.7), which is an invertor of the foot, is attached to the navicular tuberosity.[11]

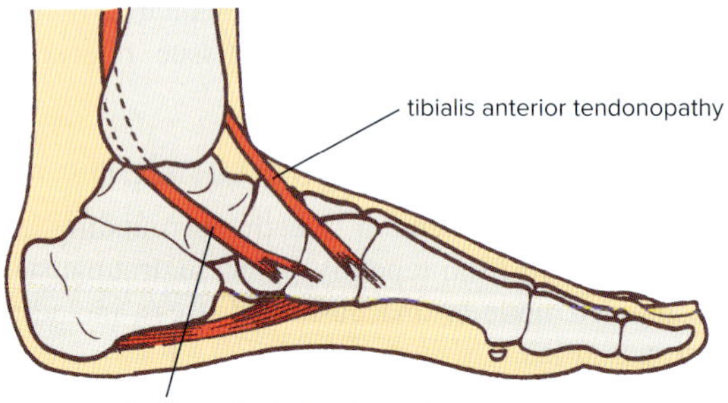

FIGURE 68.7 Medial aspect of the foot illustrating tendon disorders: tendonopathy of tibialis anterior and tibialis posterior

Clinical features[6,11]

- Pain and a feeling of weakness in the medial ankle and foot
- Pain aggravated by standing and walking
- Standing on toes is painful and difficult
- Pain on palpation anterior and inferior to the medial malleolus
- Pain on stretching into eversion
- Painful resisted active inversion
- May cause tarsal tunnel syndrome

Diagnosis

Ultrasound examination—but MRI is the gold standard for delineating tendon tears and inflammation.[12]

Treatment

68

This is basically conservative with a good outcome in 12–24 months.

- Orthotic correction (bilateral) with semi-rigid orthosis to support faulty arch
- Exercises under physiotherapist guidance
- Remedial massage

Consider ultrasonic guided injection of corticosteroids into tendon sheath (but best avoided) and a surgical opinion for failed conservative management.

Tibialis posterior tendon dislocation

This can occur with forceful ankle dorsiflexion and inversion. The patient usually experiences pain and cannot weight-bear. The dislocated tendon may be seen overlying the medial malleolus. Immediate surgical repair is recommended.

Tibialis posterior tendon rupture

Rupture of the tibialis posterior tendon after inflammation, degeneration or trauma[13] is a relatively common and misdiagnosed disorder, especially in middle-aged females. It causes collapse of the longitudinal arch of the foot, leading to a flat foot.[5]

It is uncommon for patients to feel obvious discomfort at the moment of rupture. They may subsequently present with the sudden appearance of an 'abnormal' flat foot. There is gross eversion of the foot.

A simple test is the 'too many toes' test whereby more toes are seen on the affected side when the feet are viewed from about 3 m behind the patient (see FIG. 68.8).[5]

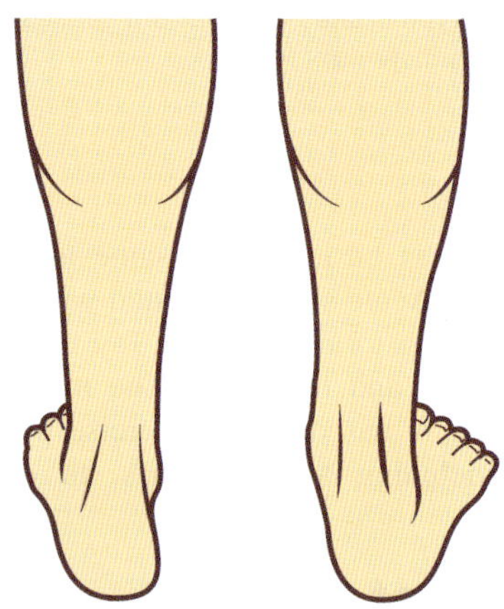

FIGURE 68.8 Tibialis posterior tendon rupture (right foot): the 'too many toes' posterior view

The single heel raise test is also diagnostic. The most useful investigation is an ultrasound examination. Minor cases can be treated conservatively with orthotics, but severe problems respond well to surgical correction.

Sesamoiditis[1]

The two sesamoids that lie beneath the head of the first metatarsal may develop painful conditions such as chondromalacia, osteoarthritis and stress fractures. A special 'sesamoid' X-ray assists diagnosis. A painful callus can develop over here in the elderly. Well-designed insoles are usually effective, as is surgical excision for persistent problems.

Metatarsalgia[1]

Metatarsalgia is a symptom rather than a disease and refers to pain and tenderness over the plantar heads of the metatarsals (the forefoot). Causes include foot deformities (especially with depression of the transverse arch), leading to painful strain, arthritis of the MTP joints, trauma, Morton neuroma, Freiberg disorder and entrapment neuropathy. However it can occur in normal feet after prolonged standing.

Depression of the transverse arch results in abnormal pressure on the second, third and fourth metatarsal heads with possible callus formation. Repetitive foot strain, pes cavus and high heels may cause a maldistribution of weight to the forefoot.

Treatment involves treating any known cause, advising proper footwear and perhaps a metatarsal bar. Flat-heeled shoes with ample width seldom cause problems in the metatarsal region.

Stress fractures[14]

Clinical features

- The aches or pains may be slow in onset or sudden
- Common in dancers, especially classical ballet, and in unfit people taking up exercise
- Examination is often unhelpful: swelling uncommon[12]
- Routine X-rays often unhelpful
- A bone scan is the only way to confirm the suspected diagnosis
- Basis of treatment is absolute rest for 6 or more weeks with strong supportive footwear
- A walking plaster is not recommended

Avulsion fracture of base of fifth metatarsal

Known also as a Jones fracture, it is usually a traumatic fracture but can be a stress fracture and associated with severe ankle sprains.

March fracture of metatarsal

Stress or fatigue fracture of the forefoot usually involves the neck of the second metatarsal (sometimes the third). Swelling typically occurs along the bone shaft. X-ray changes are often delayed. Treat conservatively with support from a firm elastic bandage; avoid painful activities. Resolution may take many months.

Tarsals, especially navicular

Stress fracture of the navicular, which is a disorder of athletes involved with running sports, presents as poorly localised midfoot pain during weight-bearing. Examination and plain X-ray are usually normal. It is a recently recognised serious disorder due to the advent of nuclear bone scans and CT scans. A protracted course of treatment can be expected.

Calcaneum

Stress fractures of the os calcis usually have an insidious onset. Osteoporosis is a predisposing factor, as is an increased training program.[14]

Morton neuroma[12]

Morton interdigital neuroma is probably misdiagnosed more often than any other painful condition of the forefoot. It is not a true neuroma but a fibrous enlargement of an interdigital nerve, and its aetiology is still uncertain. It is related to overuse and inappropriate footwear. The diagnosis is made on clinical grounds. An ultrasound examination may detect a neuroma.

Clinical features

- Usually presents in adults <50 years
- Four times more common in women
- Bilateral in 15% of cases
- Commonest between third and fourth metatarsal heads (see FIG. 68.9), and second and third (otherwise uncommon)

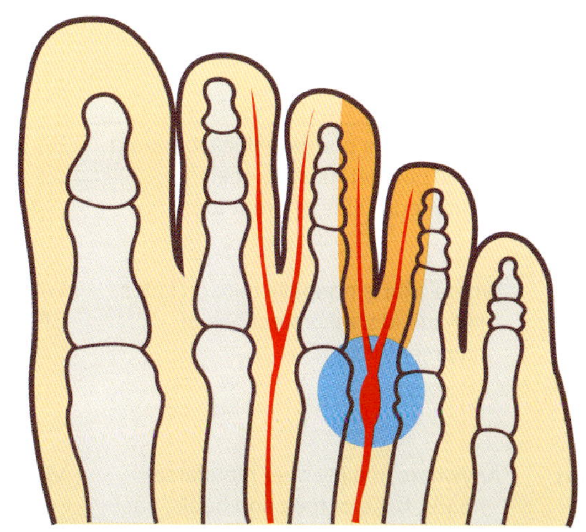

FIGURE 68.9 Morton neuroma: typical site and pain and paraesthesia distribution

68

- Severe burning pain (sometimes sharp and shooting) between third and fourth or second and third toes
- Worse on weight-bearing on hard surfaces (standing and walking)
- Aggravated by wearing tight shoes
- Relieved by taking off shoe and squeezing the forefoot
- Localised tenderness between metatarsal heads

Treatment

Early problems are treated conservatively by wearing loose shoes with a low heel and using a sponge rubber metatarsal pad. An orthosis with a dome under the affected interspace helps to spread the metatarsals and thus takes pressure off the nerve. Any biochemical abnormalities of the foot should be corrected. Most eventually require surgical excision, preferably with a dorsal approach. A corticosteroid injection can be considered.

'Turf toe'

This is a sprain of the first metatarsophalangeal joint caused by a forced hyperextension (occasionally hyperflexion) injury to the joint. It is common in football players and athletes, e.g. jamming or stubbing the great toe. There is pain, swelling and limitation of movement. Plain X-rays are unhelpful, but isotopic scans and MRI may help to diagnose the injury.

Treatment is conservative with RICE, NSAIDs and relative rest. Surgical intervention may be required.

Hallux valgus

Hallux valgus with associated bunion formation and splaying of the forefoot is common. It may be a consequence of poor-fitting footwear.

A bunionette, also caused by pressure, may form over the fifth metatarsal.

Pain, if present, may be due to shoe pressure on an inflamed bunion, a hammer toe, metatarsalgia or secondary arthritis of the first MTP joint.

Hallux valgus with bunions should be treated by correcting footwear prior to any surgical correction. Systematic evidence-based reviews found that preventive orthoses and night splints were unlikely to be beneficial but absorbable pin fixation was likely to be beneficial.[6]

Hammer toes[1]

Mainly involve the second toe with extended MTP joint, hyperflexed PIP joint and extended DIP joint. Painful corns will appear over the prominent joint. They respond well to surgery if problematic and are not helped by good footwear.

Claw toes

Often follows polio. The feature is extended MTP joint, flexion PIP and DIP. Refer for surgical opinion.

Calluses, corns and warts

The diagnosis of localised, tender lumps on the sole of the foot can be difficult. The differential diagnosis of callus, corn and wart is aided by an understanding of their morphology and the effect of paring these lumps (see TABLE 68.2).

Table 68.2 Comparison of the main causes of a lump on the sole of the foot

	Typical site	Nature	Effect of paring
Callus	Where skin is normally thick: beneath heads of metatarsals, heels, inframedial side of great toe	Hard, thickened skin	Normal skin 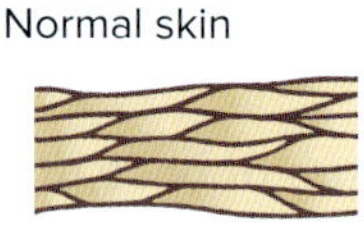
Corn	Where skin is normally thin: on soles, fifth toe, dorsal projections of hammer toes	White, conical mass of keratin, flattened by pressure	Exposes white, avascular corn with concave surface 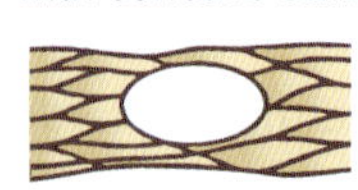
Wart	Anywhere, mainly over metatarsal heads, base of toes and heels; has bleeding points	Viral infections, with abrupt change from skin at edge	Exposes bleeding points 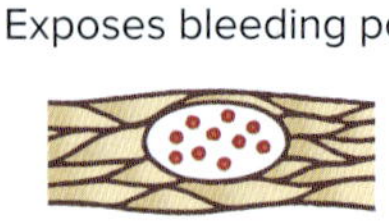

Calluses

A callus (see FIG. 68.10) is simply a localised area of hyperkeratosis related to some form of pressure and friction. It is very common under the metatarsal heads, especially the second.

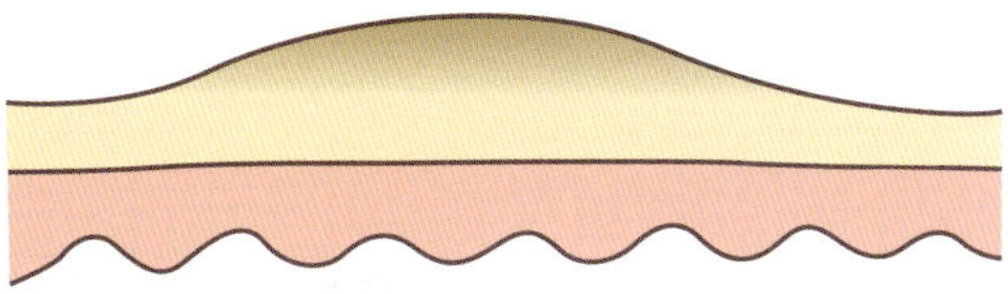

FIGURE 68.10 Callus

Treatment

No treatment is required if asymptomatic. Remove the cause. Proper footwear is essential—wide enough shoes and cushioned pads over ball of foot. Proper paring gives relief, also filing with callus files. If severe, apply daily applications of 10% salicylic acid in soft paraffin with regular paring.

Corns

A corn (see FIG. 68.11) is a small, localised, conical thickening. It is a horny plug of keratin in the epidermis. A corn develops in response to chronic irritation, usually over a bony prominence of the foot, e.g. outer distal fifth toe. It is associated with poorly fitting footwear, excessive activity or faulty intrinsic foot mechanics. It may resemble a plantar wart but gives a different appearance on paring.

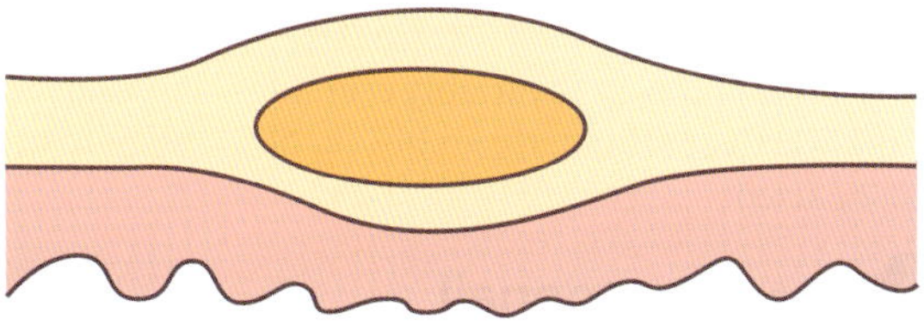

FIGURE 68.11 Corn

Treatment

Remove cause of friction and use wide shoes to allow the foot to expand to its full width. Soften corn with a few daily applications of 15% salicylic acid in collodion or commercial 'corn removers' with salicylic acid and then pare. For soft corns between the toes (usually last toe-web) keep the toe-webs separated with lamb's wool or a cigarette filter tip at all times and dust with a foot powder.

Plantar warts

A plantar wart (see FIGS. 68.12 and 68.13 and CHAPTER 124) is more invasive, and paring reveals multiple small, pinpoint bleeding spots.

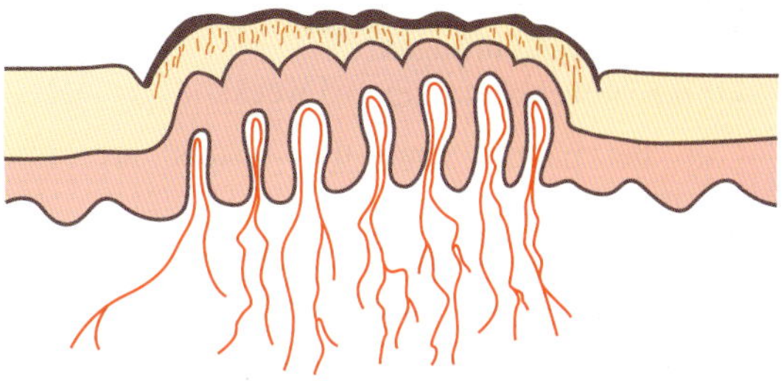

FIGURE 68.12 Plantar wart

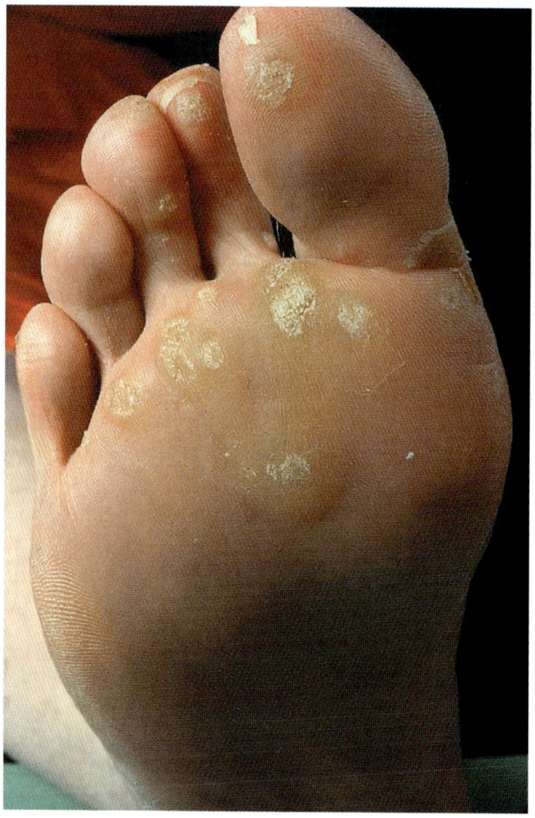

FIGURE 68.13 Plantar warts on the sole of the foot and toes showing a mosaic pattern

Methods of removal[15]

There are many treatments for this common and at times frustrating problem. A good rule is to avoid scalpel excision, diathermy and electrocautery because of the problem of scarring. One of the problems with the removal of plantar warts is the 'iceberg' configuration—not all the wart may be removed.

- Salicylic acid 17%, lactic acid 17% in collodion:
  – apply daily, dry and cover
- Liquid nitrogen:
  – pare wart (a 21 gauge blade is recommended)
  – apply liquid nitrogen
  – repeat weekly for up to 3 weeks

Can be painful and the results are often disappointing.

- Topical chemotherapy:
  – soak feet in warm water, then pare wart (particularly in children)
  – apply Upton's paste or salicylic acid (up to 27%) gel or cream to wart each night and cover
  – review if necessary

(Upton's paste comprises trichloracetic acid 1 part, salicylic acid 6 parts, glycerin 2 parts.)

- Topical chemotherapy and liquid nitrogen:
  – pare wart
  – apply paste of 70% salicylic acid in raw linseed oil
  – occlude for 1 week
  – pare on review, then apply liquid nitrogen and review
- Curettage under local anaesthetic:
  – pare the wart vigorously to reveal its extent
  – thoroughly curette the entire wart with a dermal curette
  – hold the foot dependent over kidney dish until bleeding stops (this always stops spontaneously and avoids a bleed later on the way home)
  – apply 50% trichloracetic acid to the base

Occlusion method

Occlusion with topical chemotherapy: a method of using salicylic acid alone or in a paste under a special occlusive dressing is described.

68

Equipment

- 2.5 cm (width) elastic adhesive tape
- 30% salicylic acid in Lassar's paste of plasticine consistency

Method

1 Cut two lengths of adhesive tape, one about 5 cm and the other shorter.
2 Fold the shorter length in half, sticky side out (see FIG. 68.14A).

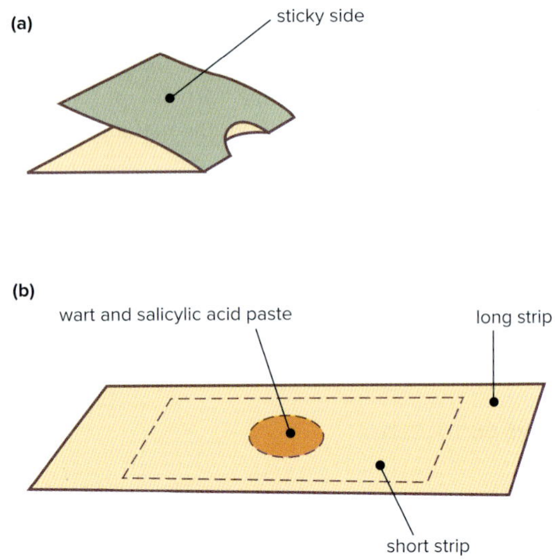

FIGURE 68.14 Treatment of plantar wart: **(a)** 'window' to fit the wart is cut out of shoulder of elastic adhesive tape, **(b)** larger strip covers the wart and shoulder strip

3 Cut a half-circle at the folded edge to accommodate the wart.
4 Press this tape down so that the hole is over the wart.
5 Roll a small ball of the paste in the palm of the hand and then press it into the wart.
6 Cover the tape, paste and wart with the longer strip of tape (see FIGS. 68.14B).

This paste should be reapplied twice weekly for 2–3 weeks. The reapplication is achieved by peeling back the longer strip to expose the wart, adding a fresh ball of paste to the wart and then recovering with the upper tape.

The plantar wart invariably crumbles, and vanishes. If the wart is particularly stubborn, 50% salicylic acid can be used.

Ingrown toenail (onychocryptosis)

Ingrown toenail is a very common condition, especially in adolescent boys. Although not so common in adults, it may follow injury or deformity of the nail bed. It is typically located along the lateral edges of the great toenail and represents an imbalance between the soft tissues of the nail fold and the growing nail edge. The basic cause is a redundant skin fold. It is exacerbated by faulty nail trimming, constricting shoes and poor hygiene. A skin breach is followed by infection, then oedema and granulation tissue of the nail fold.[5]

Initial management on presentation[14]

First-line management should be conservative. Gently lift the nail edge and pack moistened cotton wool soaked in 70% alcohol beneath the nail. Remove any nail spicules. Pack daily until healed. If bacterial infection, treat with a topical antiseptic, e.g. povidone–iodine 10% ointment under occlusion. Oral antibiotics will be required for infection such as cellulitis or suppuration.

Treat any granulation tissue with curettage or electrocautery (under local anaesthetic) and/or a silver nitrate cautery stick.

Prevention

All patients should be instructed on correct foot and nail care. Foot hygiene includes foot baths, avoiding nylon socks and frequent changes of cotton or wool socks. Cotton wool pledgets can be placed beneath the nail edge to assist separation.

It is important to fashion the toenails so that the corners project beyond the skin (see FIG. 68.15). The end of the nail (not the corners) should be cut squarely so that the nail can grow out from the nail fold. Then each day, after a shower or bath, use the pads of both thumbs to pull the nail folds as indicated.

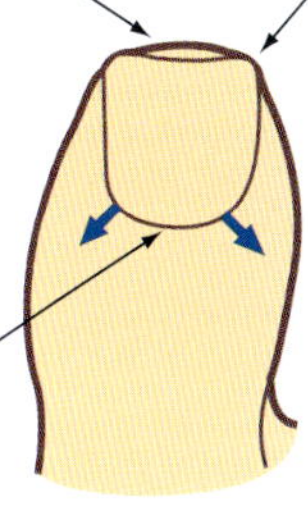

FIGURE 68.15 Method of fashioning toenails

Treatment—the spiral tape method[15]

This simple technique involves the application of strong adhesive tape such as Elastoplast or Leukosilk 12.5 mm to retract the skin off the ingrowing nail. At first, use the thumb pads, despite the discomfort, to retract the skin. The tape is then passed around the plantar surface to anchor the tape in loops around the proximal aspect of the toe (see FIG. 68.16). The application of Friar's Balsam to the distal 'anchor' gives a better grip. This process is repeated 2–4 times weekly until the problem settles.

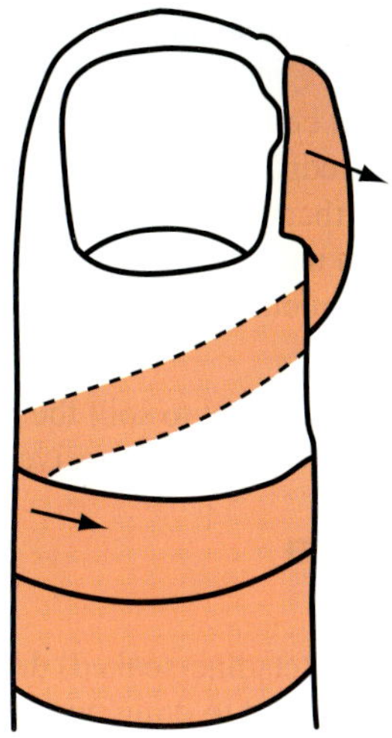

FIGURE 68.16 The spiral tape method for the ingrowing toenail

Treatment—surgical[15]

1 *Excision of ellipse of skin.* This 'army method' transposes the skin fold away from the nail. The skin heals, the nail grows normally and the toe retains its normal anatomy.
2 *Electrocautery.* This is similar in principle to the preceding method but is simple, quick and very effective with minimal after-pain, especially for severe ingrowing with much granulation tissue. Under digital block the electrocautery needle removes a large wedge of skin and granulation tissue so that the ingrown nail stands free of skin (see FIG. 68.17).
3 *Skin wedge excision.* Another similar method under digital block is to dissect away all the skin fold adjacent to the nail, starting from the nail base, extending proximally for about 4 mm and then sweeping around the side of the nail to under its tip, using a 3–4 mm margin all the way.

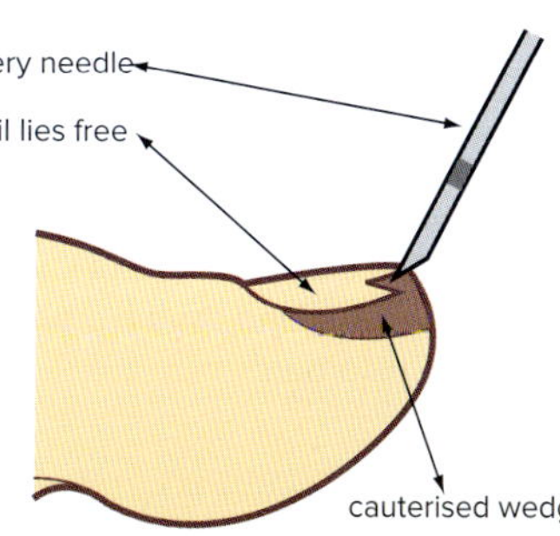

FIGURE 68.17 Treatment of ingrown toenail: electrocautery of wedge of tissue

4 *Wedge of nail excision and phenolisation.* This method uses 80% phenol (concentrated solution) to treat the nail bed following excision with scissors of a wedge for about one quarter of the length (rather than a standard wedge resection) of the ingrown nail. A cotton wool stick soaked in phenol is introduced deep into the space of the nail bed.

Warning: Take care not to spill the phenol onto the surrounding skin as it is very corrosive.

Paronychia

Initial treatment:

- antiseptic (e.g. Betadine-soaked) dressing
- elevation of nail fold to drain pus
- application of petroleum gauze dressing
- antibiotics if extensive or cellulitis developing

Sometimes the nail requires avulsion to establish free drainage of a periungual abscess. Refer to CHAPTER 127.

Practice tips

- Good-quality X-rays are mandatory in all severely sprained ankle injuries.
- If in doubt about the diagnosis of a painful foot, X-ray.
- Children rarely sprain ligaments. All joint injuries causing pain and swelling in children need to be X-rayed.
- Think of the rare problem of a dislocating peroneal tendon if a sharp click and stab of pain is experienced just behind and below the lateral malleolus.
- Paraesthesia of part or whole of the foot may be caused by peripheral neuropathy, tarsal tunnel syndrome, mononeuritis (e.g. diabetes mellitus), rheumatoid arthritis or a nerve root lesion from the lumbosacral spine.
- Avoid giving injections of corticosteroids into the Achilles tendon.
- Avoid invasive procedures such as surgical excision, diathermy or electrocautery for plantar warts. Be aware of the limitations of liquid nitrogen.
- High-resolution ultrasound can help diagnose Achilles tendon disorders.
- Keep in mind the possibility of pain around the sesamoid bones of the first metatarsal.
- Beware of acral lentiginous melanoma on the sole of the foot, especially if amelanotic (see CHAPTER 125).

Patient education resources

Hand-out sheets from *Murtagh's Patient Education* 7th edition:

- Bunions
- Calluses, corns and warts on feet
- Flat feet
- Ingrowing toenails
- Plantar fasciitis

References

1 Lam P. Forefoot pain: how to treat. Australian Doctor, 22 February 2008: 21–32.
2 Cailliet R. *Foot and Ankle Pain.* Philadelphia: FA Davis, 1983: 105–15.
3 de Jager JP. Problems with the shoulder, knee, ankle and foot. Med J Aust, 1996; 165: 570–1.
4 Larkins PA. The little athlete. Aust Fam Physician, 1991; 20: 973–8.
5 Quirk R. Flat foot in middle age: diagnosis and treatment. Modern Medicine Australia, 1995; 38 (11): 44–7.
6 Expert group for Rheumatology. Lower limb disorders. In: eTG complete [Internet]. Melbourne: Therapeutic Guidelines Ltd. Available from: <www.tg.org.au>, accessed November 2017.
7 Jahss MH et al. Investigations into the fat-pads of the sole of the foot: anatomy and histology. Foot and Ankle, 1992; 13: 233–42.
8 Brown CH. A review of subcalcaneal heel pain and plantar fasciitis. Aust Fam Physician, 1996; 25: 875–85.
9 Barton S (ed.). *Clinical Evidence.* London: BMJ Publishing Group, 2001: 742–3, 823–31.
10 Lam P. Acquired adult flatfoot deformity: how to treat. Australian Doctor, 1 May 2009: 25–32.
11 Paoloni J. Chronic foot and ankle conditions. Update. Medical Observer, 17 October 2008: 29–32.
12 Masterton E et al. The planovalgus rheumatoid foot—is tibialis tendon rupture a factor? Br J Rheumatol, 1995; 34: 645–6.
13 Quirk R. Stress fractures of the foot. Aust Fam Physician, 1987; 16: 1101–2.
14 Expert group for Dermatology. Nail disorders. In: eTG complete [Internet]. Melbourne: Therapeutic Guidelines Ltd. Available from: <www.tg.org.au>, accessed November 2017.
15 Murtagh J. *Practice Tips* (7th edn). Sydney: McGraw-Hill Education, 2017: 97–9.

Walking difficulty and leg swelling

69

Would ye not think his cunning to be great that could restore this cripple to his legs again?

William Shakespeare (1564–1616), *King Henry VI*, Part II, Act 2, Scene 1

The clinical evaluation of the patient presenting with difficulty walking can be very complex, especially for abnormal gaits caused by neurological conditions. Not all gaits fall into a single category; gait disturbances may be multifactorial, especially in the elderly.

Non-neurological conditions are the most common cause of walking difficulties. They include various arthritic conditions of the lower limbs, usually presenting as a limp, other mechanical factors, such as swelling of the legs, disorders of circulation such as intermittent claudication, and general debility (e.g. malignancy, anaemia and endocrine disorders such as hyperparathyroidism).

It is important for the general practitioner not to overlook hypokalaemia and drugs or the myopathies as a cause of walking difficulty. The drugs that require special consideration include alcohol, corticosteroids, chloroquine, colchicine, clofibrate, bretylium, HMG-CoA reductase inhibitors (the statins), gemfibrozil, penicillamine, diuretics, beta blockers and general anaesthetic agents.

Abnormal gaits

It is convenient to classify abnormal gaits as painless or painful (antalgic). With antalgic gaits the rhythm is disturbed; with painless abnormal gaits the contour is affected. One type of skeletal mechanical abnormality is described as arthrogenic (due particularly to hip disorders) and a second type as osteogenic (due to a shortened limb).

Neurogenic gaits and myogenic gaits are considered together below, under the heading 'Neurological disorders of gait'.

Psychogenic or 'hysterical' gait may have to be considered if the gait is bizarre or seems greatly exaggerated. On the other hand, loss of confidence, especially in the elderly, is an important cause of gait disturbance. However, many abnormal gaits that are caused by neurological disease may also appear bizarre, and caution is advised. Doubtful cases should be referred for an expert opinion.

Examination of gait and posture[1]

Disorders of gait and posture go hand in hand because of a common physiological process.

The source of the abnormality is indicated.

1. Ask the patient to stand.
   Note any difficulty in reaching a standing position. Difficulty = proximal muscle weakness.
2. Ask the patient to stand with eyes closed (Romberg test).
   If positive (sways or falls) = loss of proprioception (e.g. peripheral neuropathy).
3. Ask the patient to walk (ensure sufficient testing length).

Gait initiation:	hesitancy = basal ganglia or frontal cortex
Stride length:	very short = basal ganglia or frontal cortex irregular = cerebellar
Narrow or broad base:	narrow = UMN, muscle weakness, basal ganglia broad = cerebellum, proprioception, vestibular
Stiff or 'sloppy':	stiff = UMN, basal ganglia sloppy = LMN, muscle weakness
Heel strike:	loss of normal strike = UMN, LMN, myopathy
High stepping:	positive = LMN (distal), proprioception, muscle weakness
Arm swing:	decreased = basal ganglia, UMN (frontal lobes)
Pelvis control:	Trendelenburg gait = proximal muscle weakness

4. Ask the patient to walk using provocation tests.

'Tightrope' walk:	tests proprioception
Stand on tiptoes and back on the heels:	tests distal muscle weakness

Note: Peripheral neuropathy is a common cause of LMN lesion.

Neurological disorders of gait

Cerebellar (ataxic) gait

The patient has difficulty standing, has a broad-based stance and an unsteady gait, with swaying from side to side. It has been described as the 'dirty diaper' gait. The patient may stagger or bump into walls and may be accused of being drunk. When asked to walk in a straight line the patient tends to veer towards the side of the lesion. Ask the patient to walk 'heel to toe' in a straight line and perform a heel–knee–shin test to demonstrate cerebellar ataxia. Significant causes are multiple sclerosis, alcoholic cerebellar degeneration and space-occupying lesions. Cannot climb stairs.

Basal ganglia gait (Parkinson type)

Identifying this disorder in its early stages can be difficult as the first sign may be a limp with one leg being described as weak or stiff or slow.[2] However, the typical gait is a shuffling of the feet with small steps in a forward flexed posture, rather like a person walking with a belt around the ankles. This leads to a hurrying (festinant) gait as though there is an impending feeling of falling forward. There is hesitation in starting.

Spastic gait

Spastic gait may be regarded as the typical bilateral or paraplegic gait, or as a hemiplegic gait. With the former the gait affects both legs—they are stiff or weak, leading to slow, jerking walking, dragging of the feet and scraping of the toes. This scuffing can be heard as the front of the shoe drags along the ground. Every step can be a struggle and the patient may appear as though walking through glue on the floor.

A scissor-type gait will develop with bilateral hip adduction. Spasticity is caused by a UMN lesion, including multiple sclerosis and spinal cord compression. The typical UMN posture is of a flexed upper limb and an extended lower limb.

With hemiplegia the patient drags the affected leg stiffly with the hips adducted, the knee extended and the foot plantar flexed, leading to scraping of the toes. Mounting stairs can be very difficult, especially if clonus is induced with dorsiflexion of the foot.

Foot drop gait

The patient cannot dorsiflex the foot, leading to a high-stepping gait with extra flexion of the hip and knee to lift the foot off the ground. The foot then slaps down on the ground.

Vestibular gait

If unilateral the patient tends to veer off to the side of the lesion.

Apraxia

With apraxia of gait (due to a prefrontal lobe lesion) there is a failure of control of the legs. The patient may stand up and try to walk but looks with bewilderment at the legs (the 'glued to the floor' effect) and moves them in an inappropriate manner with a broad-based, small-stepping unsteady gait. Turning is difficult. Apraxia is caused by bilateral cortical involvement, such as normal pressure hydrocephalus, multi-infarct states and tumours of the corpus callosum.[2]

Neurogenic claudication

With intermittent claudication of the cauda equina, due to spinal canal stenosis, the patient develops pain in the leg after walking a certain distance. However, weakness and numbness are usually more prominent than pain.

Drop attacks

In a drop attack the patient suddenly falls to the ground, without other symptoms, and gets up almost immediately. There is no loss of consciousness. Drop attacks can be caused by disorders such as epilepsy, Parkinson disease and vertebrobasilar insufficiency. However, in most cases, particularly middle-aged and elderly women, there is no obvious cause. (See CHAPTER 54.)

Waddling (myopathic) gait

A waddling gait is usually caused by muscular dysfunction affecting the pelvic girdle muscles and trunk. There is a wide-based gait with a marked 'rocking and rolling' body swing from side to side and related compensatory movements of the pelvis, that is, a bilateral Trendelenburg gait. Cannot climb stairs.

Proximal muscle weakness

The patient may complain when getting out of a low chair or going up or downstairs. The weakness can be demonstrated by asking the patient to squat down and, after a second, rise from the squatting position.[2] Waddling of gait reflects extreme cases. Causes include myopathies, motor neurone disease and Guillain–Barré syndrome.

Distal muscle weakness

This causes a high-stepping gait as the foot is floppy and tends to flap, with walking similar to foot drop gait. Causes include peripheral neuropathy, myotonic dystrophy and peroneal muscular atrophy.

Limp

Limp is a symptom commonly associated with painful disorders of the lower limb, especially of the hip and knee joints. A limp implies an asymmetrical gait pattern caused by one of four general factors:

1. unequal leg length
2. antalgic (painful) gait (e.g. hip disorder)
3. restricted joint movement (e.g. ankylosed knee)
4. neuromuscular weakness (e.g. poliomyelitis)

Limp has an inseparable relationship with painful hip and buttock conditions, especially those of the hip. Painful hip and pelvic conditions that cause limp are presented in CHAPTER 65.

Limp in adults

In adults the cause of limp is usually more obvious than in children and is commonly due to degenerative osteoarthritis of the hip or knee, to spinal disorders, especially sciatica caused by a disc prolapse, or to overuse disorders of the knee, ankle or foot. Other causes to consider are trauma to the back and legs, vestibular ataxia, Parkinson disease and intermittent claudication.

Limp in children

The child who limps presents an interesting diagnostic dilemma. The limp must be considered to be due to a definite organic cause, although conversion reactions can be a factor.[3] It is appropriate to focus initially on the hip. The diagnostic strategy is presented in TABLE 69.1.

Limp can be considered as acute, subacute or chronic. An acute limp may be due to injury, infection (osteomyelitis, septic arthritis), spinal injuries, a fracture or an irritable hip (transient synovitis). Subacute causes include juvenile rheumatoid arthritis and tumour or leukaemia. Chronic causes include cerebral palsy, DDH, Perthes disease and chronic SCFE.

Key facts and checkpoints

- Trauma, sepsis and DDH are perhaps the most common reasons for an infant to limp and refuse to walk. However, a painless waddling gait suggests DDH or Perthes disease, which usually begins with a painless limp.
- Multiple fractures and epiphyseal separations in toddlers are highly suggestive of child battering; a skeletal survey should be ordered if this is suspected.
- Perthes disease can present from ages 4–12 years but is usually found from 4–8 years with a peak age of 5–7 years.
- Infections of and around the hip joints are most common in infancy. Classically, the hip is held immobile in about 30° of flexion with slight abduction and external rotation. The commonest organism is *Staphylococcus aureus*, followed by *Haemophilus influenzae*.
- Tuberculosis may also occur in children (usually under 10 years) with a presentation similar to Perthes disorder.
- SCFE typically presents in the obese adolescent (10–15 years) with knee pain and a slight limp.
- Growing pains are a controversial issue but do appear to exist as an aching myalgia usually manifest in the leg muscles (anterior thigh, calf, posterior knee). The pain is bilateral, non-articular and usually unrelated to activity.

A diagnostic approach

History

The age of the patient gives a diagnostic pointer. A careful history, especially of trauma, may lead to the diagnosis. A history of injury is usually but not always available. The relationship of the limp to exercise and footwear is significant. The location of any associated pain is relevant: low back pathology can refer to the buttocks and hip pathology can cause knee pain.

Examination

The hip and knee joints should be carefully examined if the source of limp has no specific localisation. Get the child to walk and run on the toes and heels (if appropriate). Note the gait and check whether it is antalgic (painful), hemiplegic (the arm is held out in a balancing action) or Trendelenburg (classic for DDH). Look for evidence of muscular dystrophy. Never forget to examine the soles of the feet and between the toes.

Investigations

The following have to be considered:

- FBE and ESR
- blood culture
- needle aspiration of joint
- radiological: plain X-ray, ultrasound, bone scan, CT or MRI scan

Table 69.1 Limp in children: diagnostic strategy model (modified)

Probability diagnosis	
Post trauma/intense exercise causing strain syndromes	
Ill-fitting shoes	
Hip disorders, esp. transient synovitis	
Heel disorders (12–14 years)	
Serious disorders not to be missed	
Toddlers	DDH Child abuse Septic arthritis Foreign body (e.g. needle in foot)
4–8 years	Perthes disorder Transient synovitis
Adolescents	SCFE Avulsion injuries (e.g. ischial tuberosity) Osteochondritis dissecans of knee Duchenne muscular dystrophy
All groups	Septic infections: • septic arthritis • osteomyelitis • tuberculosis Tumour (e.g. osteosarcoma) Juvenile chronic arthritis Spinal disorders: • discitis • fracture
Pitfalls (often missed)	
Foreign body (e.g. in foot)	
Osteochondritis (aseptic necrosis): • femoral head—Perthes disease • knee—Osgood–Schlatter disease • calcaneum—Sever disease • navicular—Köhler disease	
Myalgia = growing pains[9]	
Overuse syndrome (esp. adolescent): • patellar tendonopathy (jumper's knee)	
Stress fractures (e.g. tibia, femoral neck, navicular)	

Management

Management is based on the cause. Surgical drainage supplemented with antibiotics is essential for septic arthritis. If the child initially has a limp and cannot walk, admit to hospital for:

- skin traction
- FBE and ESR
- ultrasound of hip
- blood culture

69

Specific conditions

Osteomyelitis

Acute haematogenous osteomyelitis is mainly a disease of childhood, occurring in the proximal ends of long bones, particularly the femur and tibia. It should be suspected in a child with an acute febrile illness, unwillingness to move the limb and 'fingertip' tenderness near one of the large points (the metaphysis). Main organisms—*S. aureus*, *S. pneumonia*, *Kingella kingae*, *Propionibacterium acnes*. Sources of infection—boils, abscesses, septic toes, surgical procedures. Consider impaired immunity and diabetes.

Blood should be collected for FBE, ESR and culture (positive in 60%). A plain X-ray and nuclear scan are valuable but may not provide immediate confirmation of the diagnosis (may be normal for the first 10 days). The child should be admitted to hospital, an IV line should be inserted and IV antibiotics commenced to cover the organisms involved—empirical therapy:

> di(flu)cloxacillin:[4] 50 mg/kg up to 2 g IV 6-hourly; adjust according to the site of infection, patient's age and particularly to culture and sensitivity results[4]

Septic arthritis

Septic arthritis should be suspected in a child with pyrexia and an acute arthritis with limited motion. Manage as for osteomyelitis as causative organisms are similar.

Bone tumour

Chronic limp is a common presentation of malignant bone tumours. Radiological investigation is mandatory.

Irritable hip syndrome (transient synovitis)

Typical age is 3–8 years and the child presents with an acute limp with restricted hip motion. Plain X-ray is normal. Orthopaedic assessment is recommended.

Perthes disease, SCFE and DDH

Refer to CHAPTER 65.

Paget disease

Paget disease of bone (osteitis deformans) is a chronic focal disorder of the adult skeleton in which new soft bone replaces localised areas of normal bone. The cause is unknown but a viral aetiology is suspected. There is a great increase in bone turnover with osteoclastic resorption followed by increased but disorganised osteoblastic activity. The disorder is quite common:

- 1 in 200 of the population at 40 years
- 1 in 10 of population at 90 years

Paget disease is usually asymptomatic but some patients may present with deep aching pain in the lower back and lower limbs. They may also present with a disturbance of gait due to unequal leg length, osteoarthritis of associated joints such as the knee or hip, or a change in the distribution of mechanical forces in the lower extremities (see FIG. 69.1).

Clinical features[5]

- Male:female ratio = 2:1.
- 95% asymptomatic (discovered by X-ray or raised serum alkaline phosphatase [ALP] level).
- Symptoms may include joint pain and stiffness (e.g. hips, knees), bone pain (usually spine), deformity, headache and deafness.
- Bone pain is typically deep and aching; it occurs at rest, particularly at night.
- Signs may include deformity, enlarged skull ('hats don't fit any more'), bowing of tibia, waddling gait, hyperdynamic circulation (see FIG. 69.2).
- Bones most commonly affected, in decreasing order, are the pelvis, femur, skull, tibia, vertebrae, clavicle and humerus.
- Sensory disability—taste, smell, vision, hearing, loss or reduction of feeling in areas of the face if cranial nerves involved.

Diagnosis

- Raised serum ALP level (often very high >1000 U/L). A result >125 U/L suggests active disease.[6]

  Note: calcium and phosphate normal.
- Plain X-ray: dense expanded bone—best seen in skull and pelvis.

  Note: Can mimic prostatic secondaries, so every male Pagetic patient should have a DRE and serum PSA test.
- Bone isotopic scans: useful in locating specific areas.
- Watch for the uncommon complication of osteogenic sarcoma.

  Note: screen siblings and children every 5 years after the age of 40.[6]

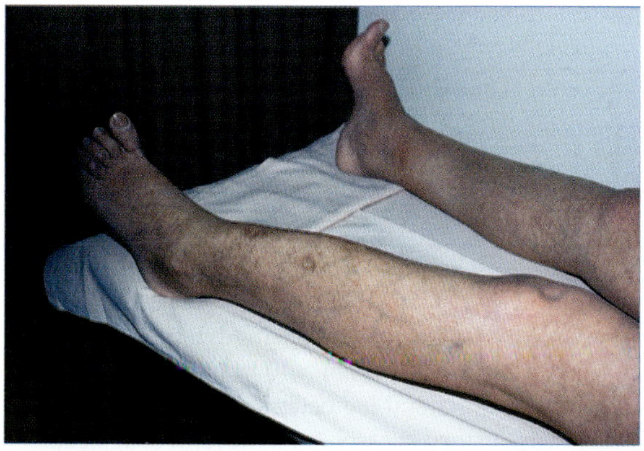

FIGURE 69.1 Paget disease of the left leg showing deformity of the tibia with a 'sabre' tibia due to its enlargement of length and bulk

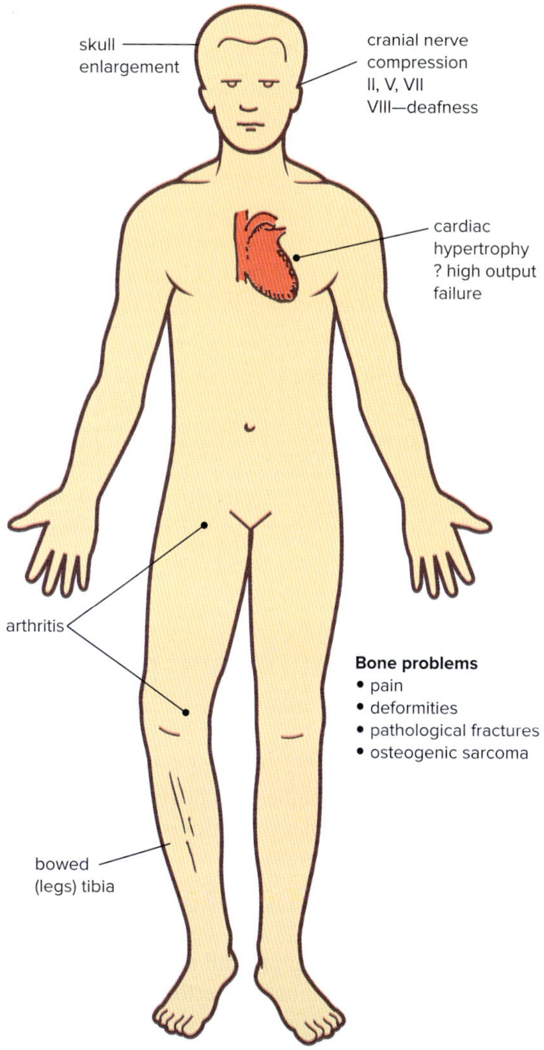

FIGURE 69.2 Paget disease: possible clinical features

Treatment[5,6]

The major goals are relief of pain, normal biochemical indices of bone turnover and prevention of long-term complications (e.g. deafness, deformities). Treatment is required for symptomatic features such as bone pain and neurological complications, and for selected asymptomatic patients such as those with active disease and <50 years.

Localised disease and most patients with asymptomatic disease require no treatment.

Three groups of drugs are currently available:

- the calcitonins
- the bisphosphonates—e.g. etidronate, pamidronate disodium (APD), alendronate, risedronate
- various antineoplastic agents (e.g. mithramycin)

Bisphosphonates have become the preferred drugs for first-line therapy, with intravenous preparations shown to be superior, including:[6]

- alendronate 40 mg (o) daily for 6 months (oesophagitis can be problematic)
- pamidronate disodium 30–60 mg IV infused over 2–4 hours (usually the preferred option)
- risedronate 30 mg (o) daily for 2 months
- tiludronate 400 mg (o) daily for 3 months
- zoledronic acid 5 mg IV over at least 15 minutes, once yearly (certain biomedical parameters must be met e.g. eGFR >35)

All oral agents should be taken on an empty stomach.

Repeated doses may rarely be required in severe cases as judged by symptoms and disease activity (e.g. monitoring with serum ALP usually 6 months post-therapy and then 2-yearly; X-rays also help monitor response).

Leg swelling

Diagnostic features and pitfalls

- Not all swollen legs require investigation and treatment.
- The significance of leg swelling varies according to the age group, whether it is bilateral or unilateral, and whether the onset is sudden or gradual (see TABLE 69.2).

69

- If the onset of oedema is acute (often <72 hours) suspect DVT.[7]
- DVT must be considered in all unilateral cases and ultrasound examination performed if appropriate.
- If a DVT is present, consider occult malignancy (e.g. pancreatic cancer).
- Consider pelvic cancer causing lymphatic obstruction in a woman >40 years presenting with painless unilateral leg oedema.
- A drug history is essential as several drugs can cause oedema.
- Pitting oedema is a feature of venous thrombosis or insufficiency, not lymphatic obstruction.

Table 69.2 Leg and ankle swelling: diagnostic strategy model

Probability diagnosis
Physiological:
• dependency/gravitational
• prolonged sitting, standing, walking
• hot weather
• pregnancy
• mechanical (e.g. constricting clothing)
Chronic venous insufficiency (varicose veins)
Congestive cardiac failure
Drugs (e.g. calcium antagonists, NSAIDs, steroids, glitazones, beta blockers)
Local trauma
Obesity
Serious disorders not to be missed
Vascular:
• deep venous thrombosis (DVT)
• inferior vena cava thrombosis
• thrombophlebitis
Infection:
• cellulitis
• tropical infections (e.g. filariasis, hookworm)
Cancer:
• obstruction from pelvic cancer
• localised malignancy
Other:
• kidney disease (e.g. nephrotic syndrome)
• liver disease (e.g. cirrhosis)
• skin allergy (e.g. angioneurotic oedema)
Pitfalls (often missed)
Idiopathic (periodic or cyclic) oedema
Protein-losing enteropathy (e.g. Crohn)
Lipoedema (fat and fluids) of legs
Lipidema (fat) of legs
Factitious oedema
Rarities:
• malnutrition
• lymphoedema: primary or secondary
Seven masquerades checklist
Diabetes
Drugs (multiple)
Thyroid/endocrine (hypothyroidism, Cushing syndrome)
Anaemia

Investigations

Select from these first-line tests:

- urinalysis (? albumin)
- FBE and ESR
- serum electrolytes, urea and creatinine
- blood sugar
- serum albumin/LFTs
- TSH level
- ultrasound (DVT screen)
- other radiographs (e.g. CT scan, venogram)

Calf swelling of sudden onset

Causes to consider:

- acute arterial occlusion
- ruptured Baker cyst
- ruptured medial head of gastrocnemius
- DVT (usually gradual)
- cellulitis/erysipelas
- compartment syndrome

Pain accompanies most of these conditions but the absence of pain does not exclude DVT or thrombophlebitis. Refer to CHAPTER 66.

Lipoedema

Lipoedema or lipedema is the development of bilateral leg swelling that does not involve the feet (in lymphoedema the swelling develops in the most distal part of the foot). Lipoedema is fat and fluid.

Clinical features

- Exclusive to obese women
- Spares the feet
- Bilateral and symmetrical distribution of fat
- The legs are often painful and bruise easily
- The Stemmer sign (the ability to pick up a fold of skin at the base of the large toe) is usually negative[8]

Patient education resources

Hand-out sheets from *Murtagh's Patient Education* 7th edition:

- Deep venous thrombosis
- Paget's disease of bone
- Parkinson disease

References

1. Horne M. Gait and postural disorders. Monash University Neurology Notes, 1996: 1–4.
2. Kincaid-Smith P, Larkins R, Whelan G. *Problems in Clinical Medicine.* Sydney: MacLennan & Petty, 1990: 190–4.
3. Gwee A, Rimer R, Marks M (eds). *Paediatric Handbook* (9th edn). Melbourne: Blackwell Science, 2015: 227–8.
4. Expert group for Antibiotic. Bone and joint infection. In: eTG complete [Internet]. Melbourne: Therapeutic Guidelines Ltd. Available from: <www.tg.org.au>, accessed October 2017.
5. Ralson D, Langston AL, Reid IR. Pathogenesis and management of Paget disease of bone. Lancet, 2008; 372 (9633): 155–63.
6. Expert group for Endocrinology. Paget disease of bone. In: eTG complete [Internet]. Melbourne: Therapeutic Guidelines Ltd. Available from: <www.tg.org.au>, accessed October 2017.
7. Diu P, Juergens C. Clinical approach to the patient with peripheral oedema. Medicine Today, October 2009; 10 (10): 37–42.
8. Piller N, Birrell S. Lymphoedema: how to treat. Australian Doctor, 6 June 2003: I–VIII.

Resource

A physician's guide to the management of Paget disease of bone. Brooklyn NY: The Paget Foundation. <pagetfdn@aol.com>

70 Palpitations

The most important requirement of the art of healing is that no mistakes or neglect occur. There should be no doubt or confusion as to the application of the meaning of complexion and pulse. These are the maxims of the art of healing.

HUANG TI (THE YELLOW EMPEROR) (2697–2597 BCE)

Palpitations are an unpleasant awareness of the beating of the heart. By definition it does not always imply 'racing' of the heart but any sensation in the chest, such as 'pounding', 'flopping', 'skipping', 'jumping', 'thumping' or 'fluttering' of the heart. The problem requires careful attention and reassurance (if appropriate) because heartbeat is regarded as synonymous with life. To the practitioner it may simply represent anxiety or it could be a prelude to a cardiac arrest. In many circumstances prompt referral to a cardiologist is imperative.

Key facts and checkpoints

- The symptom of palpitations is suggestive of cardiac arrhythmia but may have a non-cardiac cause.
- Palpitations not related to emotion, fever or exercise suggest an arrhythmia.
- Perhaps the commonest arrhythmia causing a patient to visit the family doctor is the symptomatic premature ventricular beat/complex (ventricular ectopic). Atrial fibrillation is very common.
- The commonest cause of an apparent pause on the ECG is a blocked premature atrial beat/ complex (atrial ectopic).
- A 12-lead electrocardiographic diagnosis is mandatory. If the cause is not documented, an ambulatory electrographic monitor (e.g. Holter) may be used.
- Consider myocardial ischaemia as a cause of the arrhythmia.
- Consider drugs as a cause, including prescribed drugs and non-prescribed drugs such as alcohol, caffeine and cigarettes.
- Common triggers of paroxysmal supraventricular tachycardia (PSVT) include anxiety and cigarette smoking.
- The commonest mechanism of any arrhythmia is re-entry.
- Get patients to tap out the rate and rhythm of their abnormal beat.

A diagnostic approach

A summary of the diagnostic strategy model is presented in TABLE 70.1, which includes significant causes of palpitations.

Probability diagnosis

If the palpitations are not caused by anxiety or fever, the common causes are sinus tachycardia and premature complexes/ectopics (atrial or ventricular). Sinus tachycardia, which by definition is a rate of 100–160/min, may be precipitated by emotion, stress, fever or exercise.

PSVT and atrial fibrillation are also quite common arrhythmias. Some cardiologists claim that the commonest arrhythmia causing a patient to visit the family doctor is the symptomatic ventricular ectopic beat.[1]

Sinus tachycardia can be differentiated clinically from PSVT in that it starts and stops more gradually than PSVT (abrupt) and has a lower rate of 100–150 compared with 160–220.

Important causes of tachyarrhythmias are:

- ischaemic heart disease, especially acute coronary syndromes
- hypertension
- heart failure
- mitral disease
- thyrotoxicosis
- atrial septal deficit

Serious disorders not to be missed

It is vital not to overlook acute coronary syndromes as a cause of the arrhythmia manifesting as palpitations. About 25% of infarcts are either silent or unrecognised. Sinister life-threatening arrhythmias are:

- ventricular tachycardia
- atypical ventricular tachycardia (torsade de pointes)

Table 70.1 Palpitations: diagnostic strategy model

Probability diagnosis
Anxiety
Premature beats (ectopics)
Sinus tachycardia
Drugs (e.g. stimulants)
Supraventricular tachycardia
Serious disorders not to be missed
Myocardial infarction/angina
Arrhythmias:
• atrial fibrillation/flutter
• ventricular tachycardia
• bradycardia
• sick sinus syndrome
• torsade de pointes
Long QT syndrome
Wolff–Parkinson–White (WPW) syndrome
Electrolyte disturbances:
• hypokalaemia
• hypomagnesaemia
• hypoglycaemia (type 1 diabetes)
Pitfalls (often missed)
Fever/infection
Pregnancy
Menopause (sudden vasodilatation)
Drugs (e.g. caffeine, cocaine)
Mitral valve disease
Aortic incompetence
Hypoxia/hypercapnia
Rarities:
• tick bites (T1–5)
• phaeochromocytoma
Seven masquerades checklist
Depression
Diabetes (indirect)
Drugs
Anaemia
Thyroid disorder (hyperthyroidism)
Spinal dysfunction
UTI (possible)
Is the patient trying to tell me something?
Quite likely. Consider cardiac neurosis, anxiety.

- sick sinus syndrome (SSS)
- complete heart block

  It is also important not to miss:

- hypokalaemia
- hypomagnesaemia

Pitfalls

There are many pitfalls in the diagnosis and management of arrhythmias, especially in the elderly, where symptoms of infection may be masked. Palpitations associated with the menopause can be overlooked. Valvular lesions, usually associated with rheumatic heart disease, such as mitral stenosis, and aortic incompetence may cause palpitations. The rare tumour, phaeochromocytoma, presents with palpitations and the interesting characteristic of postural tachycardia (a change of more than 20 beats/ min). The toxin from tick bites in dermatomes T1–5 can cause palpitations.

General pitfalls

- Misdiagnosing PSVT as an anxiety state
- Overlooking a cardiac arrhythmia as a cause of syncope or dizziness
- Overlooking atrial fibrillation (AF) in the presence of a slow heartbeat
- Overlooking mitral valve prolapse in a patient, especially a middle-aged woman presenting with unusual chest pains and palpitations (auscultate in standing position to accentuate click(s) ± murmurs)

Red flags for palpitations

- lightheadedness
- chest pain
- new onset of irregular heart rhythm
- heart rate >120 or <45/minute at rest
- significant underlying heart disease
- family history of sudden death

Seven masquerades checklist

Surprisingly, all the masquerades have to be considered, either as direct or indirect causes: depression, especially with anxiety and in the postpartum period; diabetes, perhaps as an arrhythmia associated with a silent myocardial infarction or with hypoglycaemia; drugs as a very common cause (see TABLE 70.2); anaemia, causing a haemodynamic effect; hyperthyroidism; spinal dysfunction of the upper thoracic vertebrae T1–5; and urinary tract infection, especially in the elderly.

PSVT has been described as resulting from injury or dysfunction of the upper thoracic spine (especially T4 and T5) in the absence of organic heart disease.[2] The author has personally encountered several cases of PSVT alleviated by normalising function of the spine.

Psychogenic considerations

Emotional factors can precipitate a tachycardia, which in turn can exaggerate the problem in an anxious person.

Table 70.2 Some drugs that cause palpitations
Alcohol
Alendronate
Aminophylline/theophylline
Amphetamines
Antipsychotics (e.g. CPZ, haloperidol, olanzapine)
Antiarrhythmic drugs
Antidepressants:
• tricyclics
• MAO inhibitors
Appetite suppressants
Atropine, hyoscine, hyoscyamine
Caffeine, including energy drinks
Cocaine
Class 1a and 1c drugs
Digitalis
Diuretics → K ↓, Mg ↓
Glyceryl trinitrate
Nicotine in cigarettes
Sympathomimetics:
• in decongestants (e.g. pseudoephedrine, ephedrine)
• β-agonists (e.g. salbutamol, terbutaline)
Thyroxine

Some people have a cardiac neurosis, often related to identification with a relative or friend. A family history of cardiac disease can engender this particular anxiety. Evidence of anxiety and depression should be sought in patients presenting with palpitations without clinical evidence of cardiovascular disease.

The clinical approach

Careful attention to basic detail in the history and examination can point the way clearly to the clinical diagnosis.

History

Ask the patient to describe the onset and offset of the palpitations, the duration of each episode and any associated features. Then ask the patient to tap out on the desk the rhythm and rate of the heartbeat experienced during the 'attack'. If the patient is unable to do this, tap out the cadence of the various arrhythmias to find a matching beat.

An irregular tapping 'all over the place' suggests atrial fibrillation, while an isolated thump or jump followed by a definite pause on a background of a regular pattern indicates premature beats (ectopics/extrasystoles) usually of ventricular origin. The thump is not the abnormal beat but the huge stroke volume of the beat following the compensatory pause.

Key questions

- Do the palpitations start suddenly? How long do they last?
- What do you think brings them on?
- Are they related to stress or worry or excitement?
- What symptoms do you notice during an attack?
- Do you have pain in the chest or breathlessness during the attack?
- Do you feel dizzy or faint during the attack?
- What medications do you take?
- How much coffee, tea, Coke do you drink?
- Have you been using nasal decongestants?
- Did you eat Chinese food before the attack?
- Do you smoke cigarettes, and how many?
- Do you take any of the social drugs, such as cocaine or marijuana?
- Have you ever had rheumatic fever?
- Have you lost weight recently or do you sweat a lot?

Chest pain may indicate myocardial ischaemia or aortic stenosis; breathlessness indicates anxiety with hyperventilation, mitral stenosis or cardiac failure; dizziness or syncope suggests severe arrhythmias such as SSS and complete heart block, aortic stenosis and associated cerebrovascular disease.

Examination

The ideal time to examine the patient is while the palpitations are being experienced. Often this is not possible and the physical examination is normal. Measurement of the heart rate may provide a clue to the problem.

As a working guide, a rate estimated to be about 150 beats/minute suggests PSVT, atrial flutter/fibrillation or ventricular tachycardia (see FIG. 70.1). A rate less than 150 beats per minute is more likely to be sinus tachycardia, which may be associated with exercise, fever, drugs or thyrotoxicosis.[3]

Assess whether the pulse is regular or irregular. If irregular, the possible causes are ectopic beats, atrial fibrillation and atrial flutter with varying degrees of block.

The nature of the pulse, especially the pulse pressure and rhythm, should be carefully evaluated (see FIG. 70.2). Look for evidence of fever and infection and features of an anxiety state or depressive illness.

Have the patient hyperventilate for 3 minutes to determine whether the arrhythmia is induced. Evidence of underlying disease such as anaemia, thyroid disorder, alcohol abuse or cardiac disease including the JVP and pulmonary congestion should be sought.

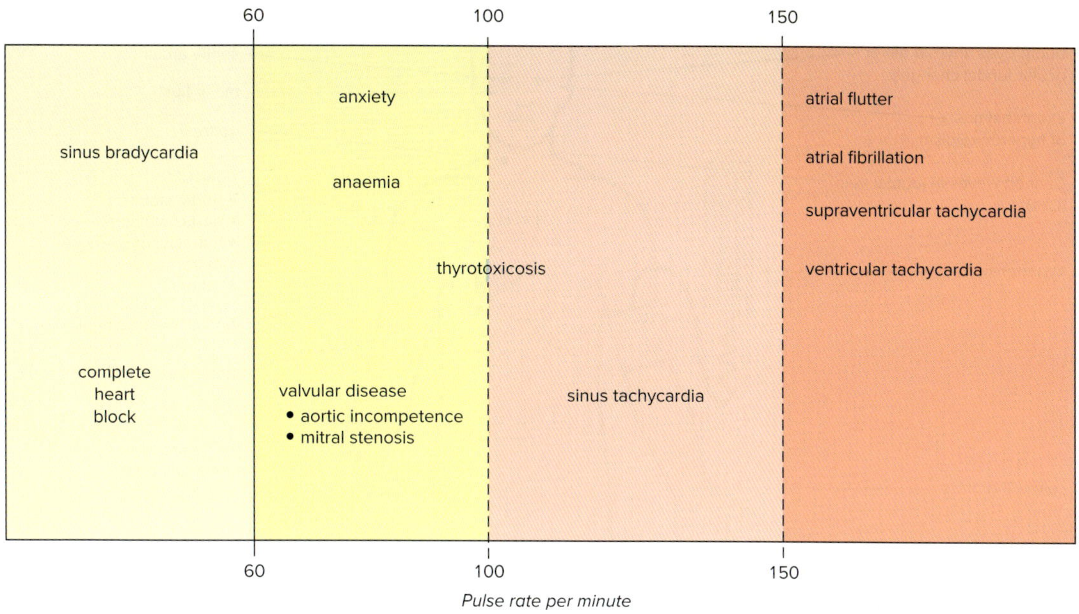

FIGURE 70.1 Heart rate guide to causes of various arrhythmias

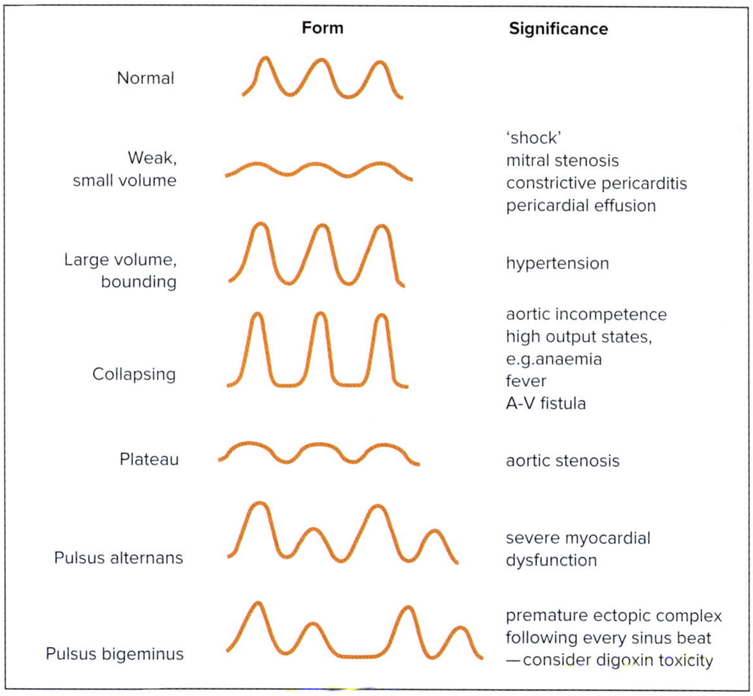

FIGURE 70.2 Various pulse forms

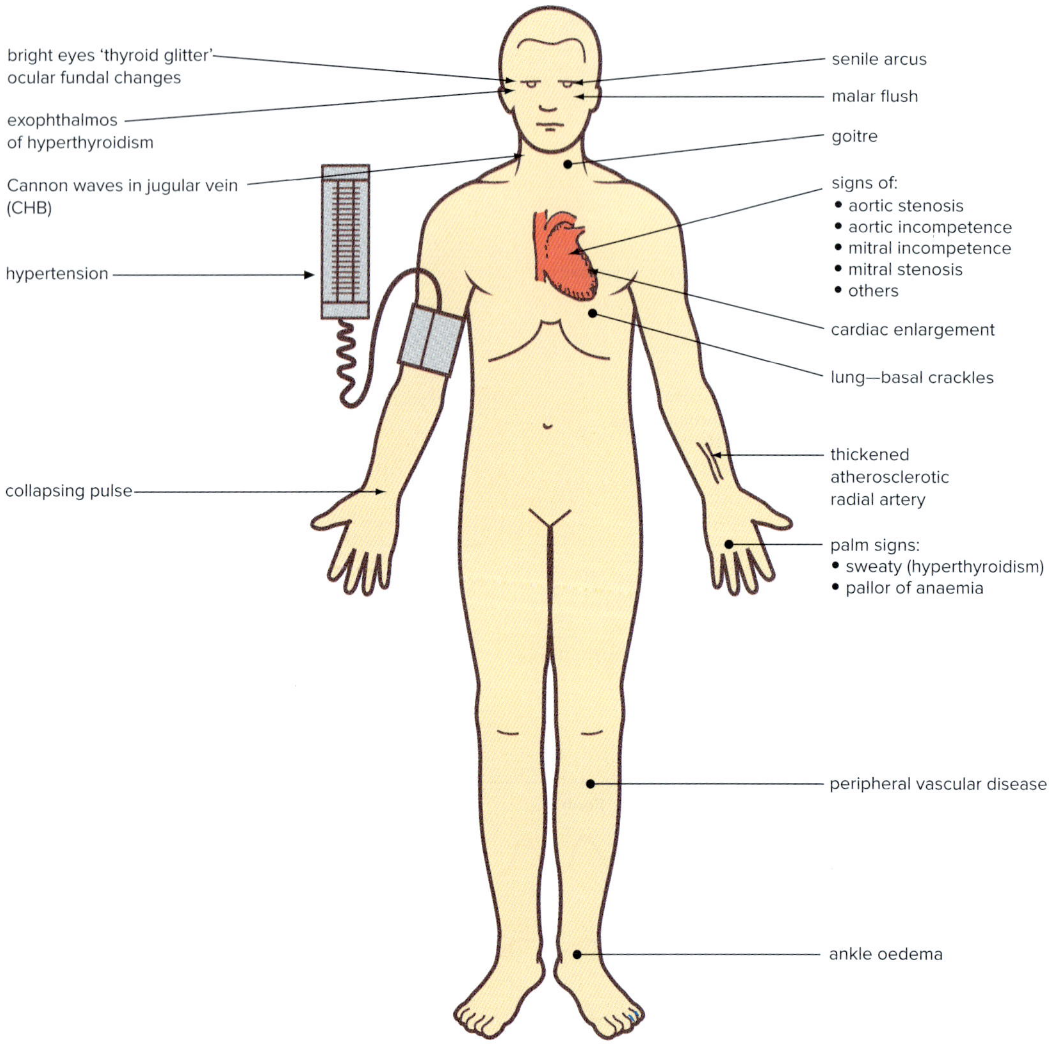

FIGURE 70.3 Signs to consider in a patient with palpitations

Also look for evidence of a mitral valve prolapse (mid-systolic click; late systolic murmur). Possible signs in the patient presenting with palpitations are shown in FIGURE 70.3.[4]

Investigations

The number and complexity of investigations should be selected according to the problem and test availability. A checklist would include:

- blood tests (for underlying disease):
  - haemoglobin and film
  - thyroid function tests
  - serum electrolytes and magnesium
  - serum digoxin ? digitalis toxicity
  - virus antibodies ? myocarditis
- chest X-ray
- cardiac (ischaemia and function):
  - ECG (12 lead)
  - ambulatory 24-hour ECG monitoring
  - echocardiography (to look for valvular heart disease and assess left ventricular function)
  - electrophysiology studies
  - exercise stress test (? underlying CAD)
  - event monitor (can record up to 2 weeks)
  - implantable monitor (may last 1 year)

Palpitations in children

Children may complain of palpitations which may be associated with exercise, fever or anxiety. Various arrhythmias can occur with three requiring special consideration—PSVT, heart block and ventricular arrhythmias.[5]

PSVT is characterised by beats at 200–300 per minute, the fastest rates occurring in infants. The cause is often not found but some children have ECG abnormalities compatible with the Wolff–Parkinson–White (WPW) syndrome. The recommended first-line treatment of PSVT is vagal stimulation via the application of ice packs to the upper face (forehead, eyes and nose) of the affected infant. Intravenous adenosine will usually terminate the episode.

A particular concern is these children who have the familial long QT syndrome. They are prone to develop ventricular tachyarrhythmias, which may lead to sudden death. Consider it in children developing syncope on exertion.

Palpitations in the elderly

The older the patient, the more likely is the onset of palpitations due to cardiac disease such as myocardial infarction/ischaemia, hypertension, arrhythmias and drugs, especially digoxin. Occasional atrial and ventricular arrhythmias, especially premature complexes (ectopics), occur in 40% of old people[6] and treatment is rarely required. Atrial fibrillation occurs in 5–10% of patients over 65 years of age, 30% of whom have no clinical evidence of cardiovascular disease. A rapid ventricular rate with symptoms is the only indication for digoxin in the elderly but beware of SSS, especially if dizziness or syncope accompanies the fibrillation.

In the elderly, thyrotoxicosis may present as sinus tachycardia or atrial fibrillation with only minimal signs—the so-called 'masked thyrotoxicosis'—so it is easy to overlook it. The only clue may be bright eyes ('thyroid glitter') due to conjunctival oedema (see CHAPTER 23).

Arrhythmias

Facts and figures

- See FIGURE 70.4 for tracings of important arrhythmias.
- Cardiac arrhythmias account for about 25% of management decisions in cardiology (see TABLE 70.3)
- Commonest are premature (ectopic) ventricular beats and atrial fibrillation.
- PSVT is next most common—6 per 1000 of population.
- The commonest mechanism of paroxysmal tachycardias is re-entry (see FIG. 70.5).

Table 70.3 Types of arrhythmias

Non-pathological sinus rhythms

Sinus arrhythmia
Sinus bradycardia
Sinus tachycardia

Pathological bradyarrhythmias

Sinus node disease (sick sinus syndrome)
Atrioventricular (AV) block:
- first-degree AV block
- second-degree AV block
- third-degree (complete) AV block

Pathological tachyarrhythmias

1 Atrial:
  - atrial premature (ectopic) complexes
  - PSVT
  - atrial flutter
  - atrial fibrillation (AF)

2 Ventricular:
  - ventricular premature (ectopic) complexes
  - ventricular tachycardia: non-sustained/sustained
  - ventricular fibrillation
  - accelerated idioventricular rhythm
  - torsade de pointes (twisting of points)

- Electrophysiological studies are the gold standard investigation for tachycardias but are rarely needed for diagnosing most arrhythmias.
- Almost all antiarrhythmic drugs have a proarrhythmic potential (i.e. they may worsen existing arrhythmias or provoke new arrhythmias in some patients) (see TABLE 70.4). Always consider the no-treatment option.
- Sinus tachycardia is usually physiological. If no obvious cause, but the symptoms are troublesome, treat with a beta blocker or verapamil.[10]
- Avoid digoxin in cases with an accessory pathway.
- If 'quinidine syncope' occurs, consider torsade de pointes as the cause.
- Any patient commencing antiarrhythmic therapy should have a 12-lead ECG 1–2 weeks later to check the QT interval. If prolonged, treatment should usually be ceased.
- The two main indications for permanent pacemaking are SSS (only if symptomatic) and complete heart block.

Management strategies

- Treat the underlying cause.
- Give appropriate reassurance.
- Provide clear patient education.
- Explain about the problems of fatigue, stress and emotion.

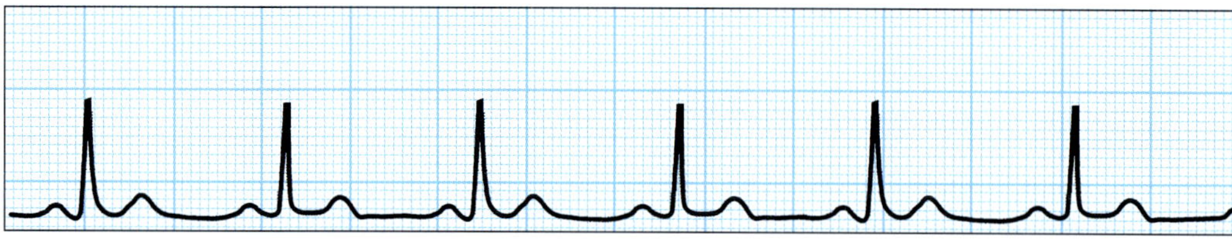

normal sinus rhythm

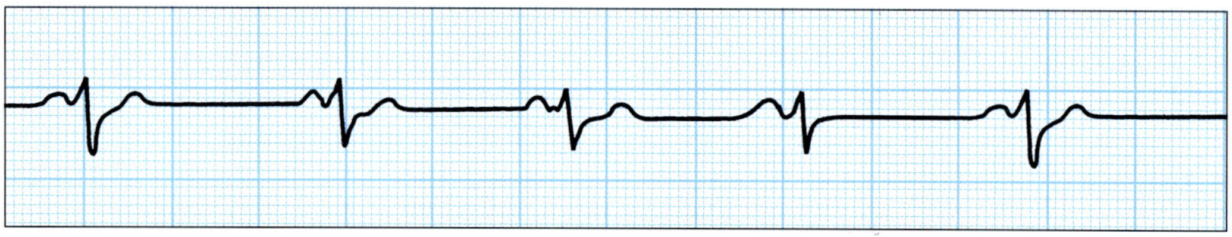

sinus bradycardia and sinus arrhythmia—rate approx. 55 per minute

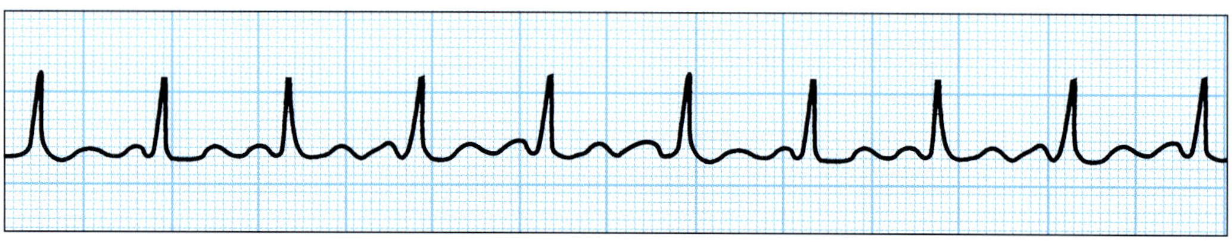

sinus tachycardia—rate approx. 100 per minute

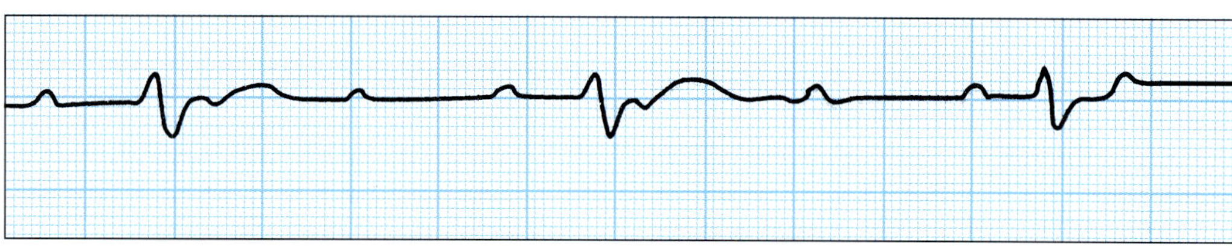

complete heart block

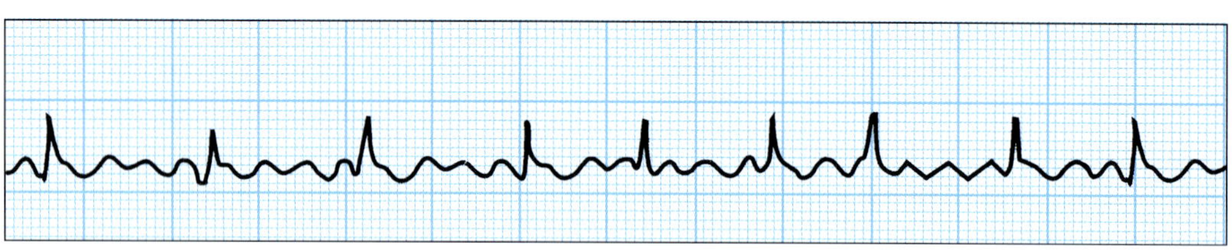

atrial flutter

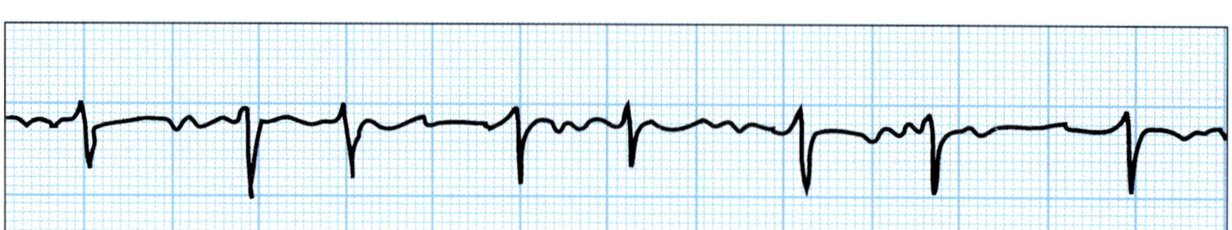

atrial fibrillation

FIGURE 70.4 Tracings of important arrhythmias

continued

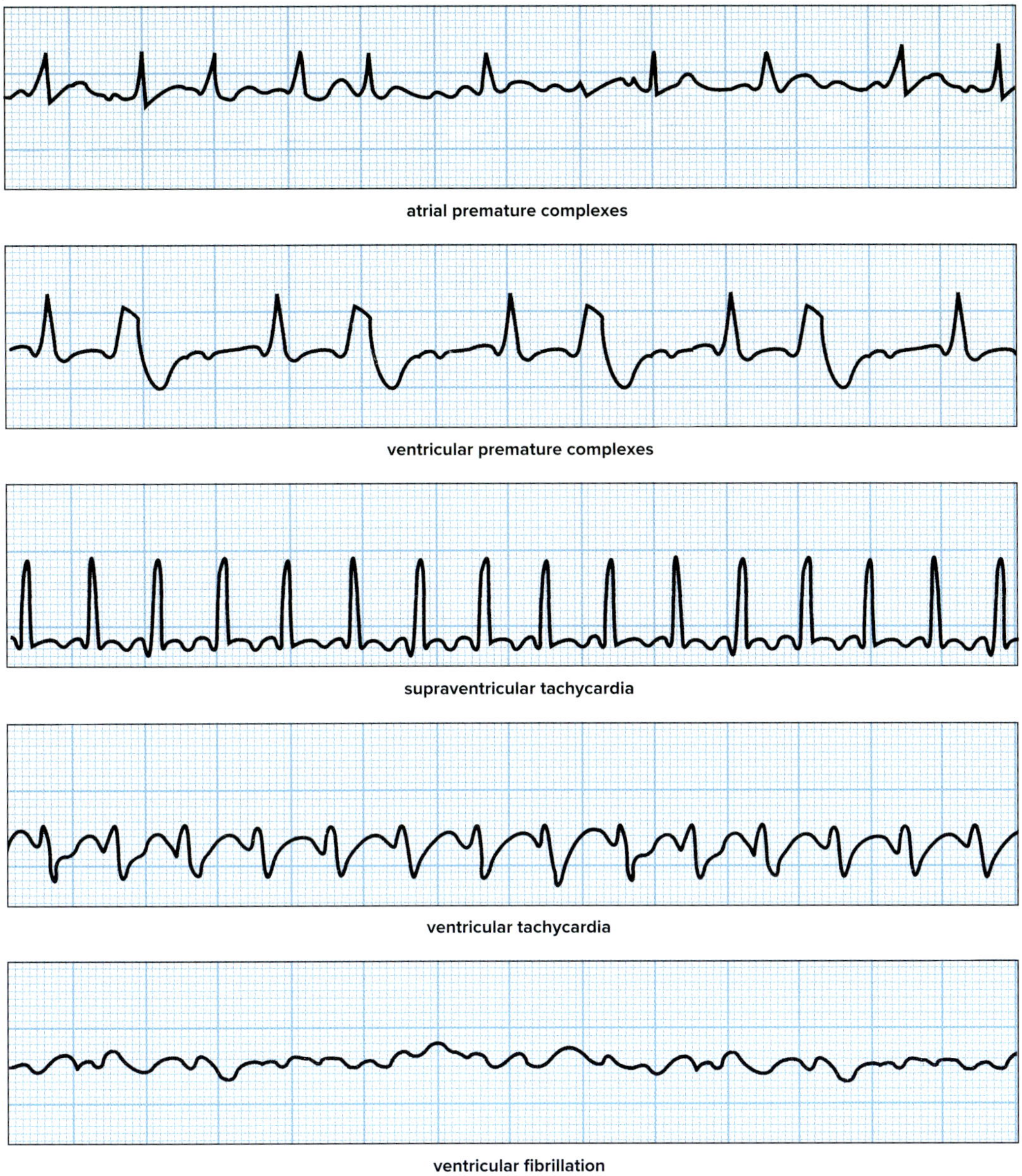

FIGURE 70.4 Tracings of important arrhythmias *continued*

- Advise moderation in consumption of tea, coffee, caffeine-containing soft drinks and alcohol.
- Advise about cessation of smoking and other drugs.

Sinus bradycardia

Look for causation (e.g. hypothyroidism and drugs). Correct the cause. Treatment is required only if symptomatic, which is uncommon at rates >40–45 beats/min. Use IV atropine if acute treatment is required. However, mild or transient bradyarrhythmias may be asymptomatic or even physiological, such as in a healthy athlete. Palpitations are not a feature but they can cause dizziness, fatigue or syncope (e.g. Stokes–Adams attack—transient bradycardia due to complete heart block).

Stokes–Adams attack

- Sudden onset without warning
- Patient falls to ground
- Collapse with loss of consciousness

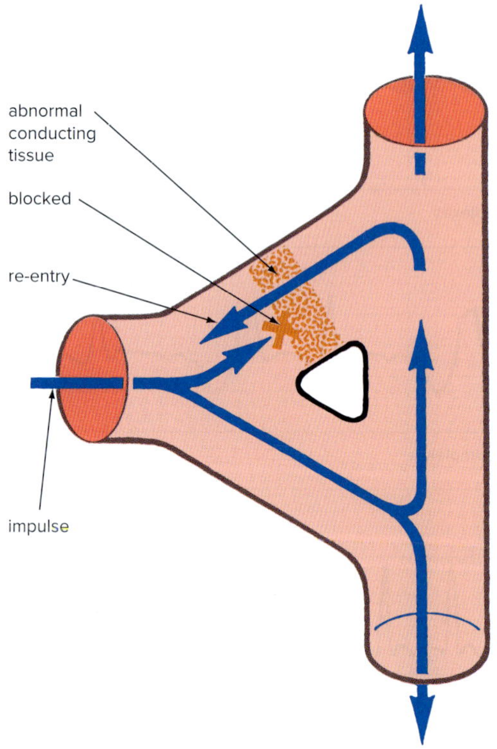

FIGURE 70.5 Diagrammatic mechanism of re-entry tachycardia

- Pallor and still as if dead with slow or absent pulse
- Recovery—in seconds back to normal
- Patient flushes as pulse increases
- Refer for management as attacks may be recurrent

PREMATURE (ECTOPIC) COMPLEXES

Premature (ectopic) atrial complexes

- These are usually asymptomatic.
- Management is based on reassurance.
- Check lifestyle factors such as excess alcohol, caffeine, stress and smoking; avoid precipitating factors.
- Treatment is rarely required and should be avoided if possible.
- At present there is no ideal anti-ectopic agent.
- They may be a forerunner of other arrhythmias (e.g. PSVT, atrial fibrillation).
- For intolerable symptoms give:[6]

  atenolol or metoprolol 25–100 mg (o) daily
  or
  verapamil SR 160–480 mg (o) daily

Table 70.4 Electrophysiological classification of common antiarrhythmic drugs (after Vaughan Williams)

Class	Drug	Usual dosage	Common side effects
I	Membrane depressant drugs (sodium-channel blockers)		
Ia	Disopyramide Procainamide Quinidine	100–200 mg qid 1 g qid IV use 2–3 SR tabs (0.25 g) bd	Blurred vision, dry mouth, urinary problems in males (avoid in men >50) Anorexia, nausea, urticaria Diarrhoea, headache, tinnitus
Ib	Lignocaine Mexiletine	IV use 200 mg tid	Nausea, dizziness, tremor Nausea, vomiting, tremor, dizziness
Ic	Flecainide	100 mg bd	Nausea, dizziness, rash
II	Beta blockers	Various	Fatigue, insomnia, nightmares, hypotension, bronchospasm Avoid in asthmatics
III	Potassium channel blockers Amiodarone Sotalol	 SVT: 200 mg daily VT: 400 mg daily 80–160 mg bd	 Rash, pulmonary fibrosis, thyroid, hepatic and CNS effects As for beta blockers
IV	Calcium channel blockers Verapamil Diltiazem	 (SR) 160–480 mg daily (CR) 180–360 mg daily	 Constipation, dizziness, hypotension Hypotension, headache

Note: Sotalol is a (beta blocker and thus is a class II and III agent. All drugs are taken orally unless IV indicated. Adenosine and digoxin are not classified.

Premature (ectopic) ventricular complexes

- These are also usually asymptomatic (90%).
- They occur in 20% of people with 'normal' hearts.
- Symptoms are usually noticed at rest in bed at night.
- Check lifestyle factors as for atrial premature beats.
- Drugs that can cause both types of premature beats include digoxin and sympathomimetics.
- Look for evidence of ischaemic heart disease, mitral valve prolapse (especially women), thyrotoxicosis and left ventricular failure.
- Ventricular premature complexes may be a forerunner of other arrhythmias (e.g. ventricular tachycardia).
- If symptomatic but otherwise well with a normal chest X-ray and ECG, reassure the patient.
- Drug therapy: never commence drug therapy without performing an echocardiograph. This will help to guide the choice of agent. Class 1 agents can make the arrhythmia worse or even life-threatening if there is reduced ventricular function. If this is the case, the patient should be referred to a cardiologist.
- For troublesome symptoms, the beta blockers atenolol or metoprolol can be used e.g. atenolol 25–100 mg (o) daily.

Supraventricular tachycardia[7,8]

- SVT can be paroxysmal or sustained.
- Rate is 160–220/min.
- There are at least eight different types of SVT with differing risks and responses to treatment.
- PSVT commonly presents with a sudden onset in otherwise healthy young people.
- Passing copious urine after an attack is characteristic of PSVT.
- Look for predisposing factors such as an accessory pathway and thyrotoxicosis.
- Approximately 60% are due to atrioventricular (AV) node re-entry and 35% due to accessory pathway tachycardia (e.g. WPW).[8]
- Look for evidence of accessory pathways after reversion because accessory pathways can lead to sudden death (avoid digoxin in WPW).
- Consider SSS in a patient with SVT and dizziness.

Wolff–Parkinson–White syndrome

The structural basis for the arrhythmia of SVT in WPW syndrome is an accessory pathway that bypasses the AV node. A typical ECG shows a short PR interval and slurred upstroke of the QRS complex (delta wave). Patients are prone to sudden attacks of SVT. Up to 30% of patients will develop atrial fibrillation or flutter. Even one episode of PSVT requires consideration for radiofrequency ablation.[9]

Management of PSVT

1 Vagal stimulation can be attempted. Carotid sinus massage was the treatment of choice, but it has fallen out of favour because of the potential for stroke. A popular method is to blow hard into the end of an empty 20 mL plastic syringe to move the plunger. Other methods of vagal stimulation include:
   - Valsalva manoeuvre (easiest for patient)
   - self-induced vomiting
   - ocular pressure (avoid)
   - cold (ice) water to face or swallowing ice
   - immersion of the face in water

2 If vagal stimulation fails

   give adenosine IV (try 6 mg first over 5–10 seconds, then 12 mg in 2 minutes if unsuccessful, then 18 mg in 2 minutes if necessary and well tolerated). Second-line treatment is verapamil IV 1 mg/min up to 10–15 mg (provided patient is not taking a beta blocker).[8]

   Precautions
   - Adenosine causes less hypotension than verapamil but may cause bronchospasm in asthmatics
   - Use only if narrow QRS and BP >80 mm Hg
   - Carefully monitor blood pressure
   - AVOID verapamil if taking beta blockers

   and

   persistent tachycardia with QRS complexes >0.14 s (suggests ventricular tachycardia)

3 In the rare event of failure of medical treatment, consider DC cardioversion or overdrive pacing.

Prevention and maintenance

To prevent recurrences (frequent episodes) use at first atenolol or metoprolol, flecainide (only if no structural heart damage) or sotalol (second line). If these agents fail, consider amiodarone. Do an echocardiograph first to exclude structural heart disease. Radiofrequency catheter ablation, which is usually curative, is indicated for frequent attacks not responding to medical therapy.

Carotid sinus massage[1]

Carotid sinus massage causes vagal stimulation and its effect on SVT is all or nothing. It has no effect on ventricular tachycardia. It slows the sinus rate and breaks the SVT by blocking AV nodal conduction.

In general, right carotid pressure tends to slow the sinus rate and left carotid pressure tends to impair AV nodal conduction. Never massage both sides simultaneously. As a rule, avoid this method and use one of the simpler alternatives.

Precautions

Avoid in the elderly (risk of embolism or bradycardia).

Ventricular tachycardia

Management requires special supervision.[9,10] It may be non-sustained, where drug treatment such as beta blockers and amiodarone may be used for symptomatic cases, or sustained, which may result in cardiac arrest. An implantable cardioverter defibrillator or radiofrequency catheter ablation may be used.

Torsades de pointes

This uncommon condition is potentially lethal as it may occasionally be prolonged or jump into ventricular fibrillation with sudden death. It is associated with disorders that prolong the QT interval. Treatment involves cessation of drugs that may prolong the QT interval, correcting electrolyte imbalance (especially potassium), cardiac pacing and IV magnesium sulphate.[10]

Atrial fibrillation

Facts and figures

- A common problem (9% incidence in the over-70 age group).
- It usually presents with an irregular ventricular rate of about 160–180 beats/minute in untreated patients with a normal AV node.
- Apart from acute AF (new onset <48 hrs), it tends to fall into one of the 'three Ps' patterns:
  - paroxysmal AF: abrupt onset, spontaneous return to normal rhythm (lasts <48 hrs)
  - persistent AF: abrupt onset, lasts >7 days
  - permanent (chronic) AF: cannot be converted to normal rhythm

All types appear to have a similar risk for thromboembolism.

- Remember to look for the underlying cause: myocardial ischaemia (15% of cases), mitral valve disease, thyrotoxicosis, hypertension, pericarditis, cardiomyopathy including chronic alcohol dependence, alcohol binge.
- No cause is found in 12%—isolated[9,10] atrial fibrillation.
- All patients should have thyroid function tests and an echocardiograph to help find a cause.
- With sustained atrial fibrillation there is a 5% chance per annum of embolic episodes. There is a fivefold risk of CVA overall.
- The risk of CVA is greater in those with previous CVA, valvular heart disease, prosthetic mitral valve and cardiac failure.
- For reversion anticoagulate with warfarin for 4 weeks beforehand and maintain for 4 weeks afterwards.
- Digoxin controls the ventricular rate but does not terminate or prevent attacks.
- Sotalol, flecainide and amiodarone are used for conversion of atrial fibrillation and maintenance of sinus rhythm. Flecainide should never be prescribed in patients with reduced LV function.
- Evidence basis: RCTs showed that digoxin was beneficial for lowering the ventricular rate in the short term but no better than placebo in restoring rhythm. Beta blockers and calcium-channel antagonists benefited rate control but verapamil was much less effective than amiodarone at restoring cardiac rhythm.[11]

Atrial flutter

The ECG of atrial flutter has a regular saw-tooth baseline ventricular rate of 150 with narrow QRS complexes. This is a 2:1 AV block. It is often misdiagnosed as SVT. Rarely, conduction occurs 1:1, giving a ventricular rate of 300/min.

Treatment for atrial fibrillation/flutter[8,9]

To address rate and rhythm control and prevent stroke it is best to refer or consult a specialist. The treatment needs to control the arrhythmia either as the rate or the rhythm and also from the viewpoint of prophylaxis against thromboembolic complications. Paroxysmal or persistent atrial fibrillation confers a risk of thromboembolism similar to permanent atrial fibrillation.[8] The AFFIRM study[12] confirmed that there was no statistically significant difference between the rate and rhythm of control groups. However, patients fare marginally better (in terms of mortality) with just rate control rather than trying to get them back into sinus rhythm if they are asymptomatic in atrial fibrillation.

Rate control

Aim for a rate <110/minute at rest.[8]

Rapid, urgent control of ventricular rate:

verapamil 1 mg/min IV up to maximum 15 mg then orally
or
metoprolol 5 mg (1 mg/min) IV to max 20 mg (provided no evidence of heart failure and well-monitored BP)

Routine control and maintenance[8]

verapamil SR 160–480 mg (o) daily
or
diltiazem CR 180–360 mg (o) daily
or
atenolol or metoprolol 25–100 mg (o) bd

Digoxin still has a place in the elderly, especially with cardiac failure:

digoxin 0.0625–0.25 mg (o) daily according to age, plasma creatinine and digoxin level

Rhythm control

This should be considered if the patient is symptomatic and the arrhythmia is of recent onset—less than 6 months.

Medical cardioversion

amiodarone or flecainide

If the rate cannot be well controlled despite maximal medical therapy, consider AV node ablation and a permanent pacemaker. Atrial fibrillation with a rapid ventricular response over a long period gradually causes left ventricular dysfunction.

Synchronised electrical DC cardioversion

This can be given for first-line treatment or for failed medical conversion.

The use of oral anticoagulation in atrial fibrillation[8]

(Refer to CHAPTER 131.)

The decision to use an oral anticoagulant or an antiplatelet agent (e.g. aspirin), especially in the younger patient, is difficult and should be made in consultation with a cardiologist. If aspirin is indicated, use:

aspirin 100–300 mg (o) daily

If oral anticoagulation is indicated, use:

warfarin—start with a low dose (e.g. 2–4 mg) and maintain a relatively low INR of 2–3 with regular checks.
or
a direct-acting oral anticoagulant (DOAC) e.g. dabigatran

Advances in treatment of arrhythmias

Apart from special rate-responsive pacemakers for bradycardia, there are several new modalities of treatment for complex arrhythmias, including means of blocking the re-entry phenomenon.

Surgery

Guided by electrophysiological monitoring, surgeons can dissect a small section of the AV ring to ensure that all aberrant connections between the atria and the underlying ventricular muscle are severed.

Catheter electrode ablation

Specific abnormal foci in the conducting pathways can be ablated using direct current electrical surgery or radiofrequency ‘burns’ via a catheter electrode. Radiofrequency ablation, which will probably supplant surgery as a form of treatment, is indicated for recurrent episodes of supraventricular tachycardia, accessory pathways and nodal re-entry tachycardia with success rates of up to 95%. Catheter ablation for atrial fibrillation is more complex and still evolving. Success rates at best are 60–80%.

Automatic implantable cardioverter defibrillator (AICD)

This expensive implant is the most effective therapy yet devised for the prevention of sudden cardiac death in patients with documented sustained ventricular tachycardia or fibrillation. Operative mortality should be less than 10%, after which survival at 1 year is over 90%. These new defibrillators incorporate an antitachycardia pacemaker. Patients can either be paced out of arrhythmia or, if they develop ventricular fibrillation, they can be defibrillated using higher energy.

TABLE 70.5 presents a summary of the treatment of arrhythmias.

Table 70.5 Summary of treatment of arrhythmias[7,8]

Arrhythmia	First line	Second line	Third line
Sinus tachycardia	Treat cause Reduce caffeine intake	Metoprolol or atenolol *or* Verapamil (rarely indicated)	
Bradycardia			
Sick sinus syndrome	Permanent pacing if symptomatic		
AV block			
First degree	No treatment		
Second degree:			
• Mobitz I	No treatment		
• Mobitz II	Consider pacing	Pacing if problematic	
Third degree:			
• acute (e.g. MI)	Temporary pacing	Adrenaline IV	Atropine
• chronic	Permanent pacing		Isoprenaline
Atrial tachyarrhythmias			
PSVT	Valsalva manoeuvre	Adenosine IV *or* Verapamil IV	DC cardioversion Class III drug? Ablation
Atrial fibrillation / Atrial flutter } Rate control	Rate control with beta blocker *or* verapamil (with care)	Add digoxin (if necessary)	AV node ablation + permanent pacemaker
Atrial fibrillation / Atrial flutter } Rhythm control	Rhythm control with cardioversion, electrical or drugs	Cardioversion → *or* Maintenance of sinus rhythm → Sotalol, flecainide, amiodarone + anticoagulation	Electrical or chemical
Atrial premature complexes	Treat cause Check lifestyle	Metoprolol or atenolol *or* verapamil	
Ventricular tachyarrhythmias			
Ventricular premature beats	Treat cause Check lifestyle	Beta blocker (especially mitral valve prolapse)	Class I or III drugs (rarely needed)
Ventricular tachycardia: • non-sustained • sustained	Beta blocker or amiodarone or sotalol if stable—if not: DC shock	Lignocaine IV	DC cardioversion
Ventricular fibrillation	DC cardioversion	IV adrenaline if fine VF then DC cardioversion	Amiodarone (maintenance) Class III (if recurrent)
Torsades de pointes	Correct cause, e.g. potassium Cease drugs if ↑ QT	Cardiac pacing, IV magnesium sulphate	IV isoprenaline

When to refer[13]

Patients should be referred to a cardiologist[12] when:

- a sustained supraventricular tachycardia is suspected
- a sustained ventricular tachycardia is suspected
- an ECG shows sustained delta waves of WPW syndrome, even if asymptomatic
- syncope or dizziness suggests a cardiovascular cause
- a paroxysmal arrhythmia may be the cause of unexplained cardiovascular symptoms
- anticoagulation has to be considered

Practice tips

- Atrial fibrillation and dizziness (even syncope) are suggestive of SSS (bradycardia–tachycardia syndrome), which is made worse by digoxin.
- Consider thyrotoxicosis as a cause of atrial fibrillation or sinus tachycardia, even if clinical manifestations are not apparent.
- Check for a history of palpitations in a patient complaining of dizziness or syncope (and vice versa). Consider an arrhythmia, especially in the elderly.
- PSVT is rarely caused by organic heart disease in young patients.
- Arrhythmia of sudden onset suggests PSVT, atrial flutter/fibrillation or ventricular tachycardia.
- A normal ECG in sinus rhythm does not exclude an accessory pathway.
- Consider conduction disorders such as the WPW syndrome in PSVT. Avoid digoxin in WPW syndrome.
- Common triggers of premature beats and PSVT are smoking, anxiety and caffeine (especially 8 or more cups a day).

Patient education resources

Hand-out sheets from *Murtagh's Patient Education* 7th edition:

- Atrial fibrillation

References

1. Boxall J. Annual update course for general practitioners. Course abstracts. Melbourne: Monash University, 2002: 16.
2. Lewit K. *Manipulative Therapy in Rehabilitation of the Motor System.* London: Butterworths, 1985: 338–9.
3. Davis A, Bolin T, Ham J. *Symptom Analysis and Physical Diagnosis* (2nd edn). Sydney: Pergamon, 1985.
4. Sandler G, Fry J. *Early Clinical Diagnosis.* Lancaster: MTP Press, 1986: 327–59.
5. Robinson MJ, Roberton DM. *Practical Paediatrics* (5th edn). Melbourne: Churchill Livingstone, 2003: 501–2.
6. Merriman A. *Handbook of International Geriatric Medicine.* Singapore: PG Publishing, 1989: 99–100.
7. O'Connor S, Baker T. *Practical Cardiology.* Sydney: MacLennan & Petty, 1999.
8. Expert group for Cardiovascular. Tachyarrhythmias. In: eTG complete [Internet]. Melbourne: Therapeutic Guidelines Ltd. Available from: <www.tg.org.au>, accessed October 2017.
9. Pedersen CT et al. EHRA/HRS/APHRS expert consensus on ventricular arrhythmias. Europace, 2014; 16 (9): 1257–83.
10. Buckley N (Chair). *Australian Medicines Handbook.* Adelaide: Australian Medicines Handbook Pty Ltd, 2016: 292–3.
11. Corcoran S, Lightfoot D. Palpitations: how to treat. Australian Doctor, 13 March 2009: 33–40.
12. Barton S (ed.). *Clinical Evidence.* London: BMJ Publishing Group, 2001: 1–6.
13. Wyse DG et al. The Atrial Fibrillation Follow-up Investigation of Rhythm Management (AFFIRM) investigators. NEJM, 2002; 347 (23): 1825–33.
14. Ross DL. Cardiac arrhythmias. In: *MIMS Disease Index* (2nd edn). Sydney: IMS Publishing, 1996: 93–6.

71 Sleep disorders

Sleep . . . is the first great natural resource to be exhausted by modern man. The erosion of the nerves, not to be halted by any reclamation project, public or private.

IRWIN SHAW, 'THE CLIMATE OF INSOMNIA', *THE NEW YORKER,* 1949

Sleep is one of the five great innate drives in humans. Disorder of this basic function is one of the most common health-related problems presenting to the GP. It may represent the clue to some very important disorders, such as depression, anxiety, adverse drug reactions, drug abuse and obstructive sleep apnoea (OSA). About half of the population report having some sleep-related problem in a year, with 25% of the Australian population reporting trouble getting enough sleep.[1] Normal sleep requirement varies considerably.

Sleep is divided into rapid eye movement (REM—also called dream sleep), as shown by EEG studies, and non-rapid REM sleep (NREM), which is subdivided into stages 1, 2, 3 and 4. Most stage 4 sleep (deepest) occurs in the first hours. REM sleep is accompanied by dreaming and physiological arousals; some dreaming occurs in NREM.

Disorders of the sleep-wake cycle, which are invariably caused by a disruption of the body's endogenous time clock, can result in insomnia or hypersomnolence (excessive sleepiness) or a combination of both. This is a feature of people experiencing the jet lag of international travel and shift workers.

Key facts and checkpoints

- Normal sleep: in a fit young person the ideal is 7.5–8 hours; latency <30 minutes; wakefulness within sleep usually <5% of time.
- Humans can stay awake without a problem for 16–18 hours. Sleepiness is wake-state instability.
- The evaluation of sleep disorders involving the sleep-wake cycle is enhanced by the patient keeping a sleep chart.
- It is important to take a drug history from patients complaining of insomnia or hypersomnolence.
- Drugs that can disturb sleep include alcohol, nicotine, antihistamines, selective serotonin reuptake inhibitors (SSRIs), caffeine, hypnotics, venlafaxine, selected β-blockers, β_2-agonists, theophylline, corticosteroids, sympathomimetic agents.
- Sleep disorders in children, including snoring, should be taken seriously and investigated. They have many consequences, such as learning difficulties, hyperactivity, behavioural disorders, failure to thrive and short stature.
- Be wary of young people and others presenting with insomnia with some urgency, especially requesting temazepam capsules—they may be dependent on benzodiazepines.
- People with OSA usually present with the TATT syndrome—'tired all the time'. These patients are often unaware of waking or becoming aroused during the night.
- A patient who snores, has witnessed apnoeas and sleepiness is likely to have OSA.
- The majority of cases of excessive somnolence are caused by OSA and narcolepsy.[2]
- Non-pharmacological therapies, which include basic education and practice of sleep hygiene and behavioural therapy, should be used in management wherever possible.
- Referral to the new generation specialist sleep disorder centres provides enhanced objective evaluation, diagnosis and treatment of the more complex disorders.
- It is illegal for a driver with a commercial driver's licence to continue to drive while suffering from untreated OSA.

Sleep-related disorders

Disorders of sleep are a common and significant contribution to community illness and death. For example, it is known that untreated moderate to severe OSA has an 11–13% 5-year mortality and a 37% 8-year mortality, mainly from cardiovascular and motor vehicle accident related deaths.[3,4] A classification of sleep disorders is presented in TABLE 71.1.[5]

Table 71.1 Classification of sleep and wake disorders (DSM-5)[5]

Insomnia disorder
Hypersomnolence disorder
Narcolepsy
Breathing-related sleep disorders
• obstructive sleep apnoea/hypopnoea
• central sleep apnoea
• central alveolar hypoventilation syndrome
Circadian rhythm sleep disorders
Non-REM* sleep arousal disorder
Nightmare disorder
REM* sleep behaviour disorder
Restless legs syndrome
Substance- or medication-induced sleep disorder

* REM = rapid eye movement

Many conditions may disturb breathing during the night (see FIG. 71.1). Nocturnal dyspnoea may result from cardiac causes (mitral stenosis, ischaemic cardiomyopathy, cardiac arrhythmias, fluid overload or retention), which usually present with orthopnoea, pulmonary crepitations and peripheral oedema. Asthma is another common cause of nocturnal dyspnoea, cough (with or without wheeze) occurring classically between 2 am and 5 am. Gastro-oesophageal reflux with or without aspiration may disturb respiration at night, but it usually presents with daytime or postural reflux. All these conditions can usually be differentiated from sleep apnoea clinically or with further investigation.

The sleep apnoea syndromes are a common group of disorders that result in periodic hypoventilation during sleep. They occur in about 2% of the general population in all age groups, and in about 10% of middle-aged men.

Insomnia

Insomnia is defined as the inability to initiate or maintain sleep. Insomniac patients may complain of difficulty getting to sleep or staying asleep, of

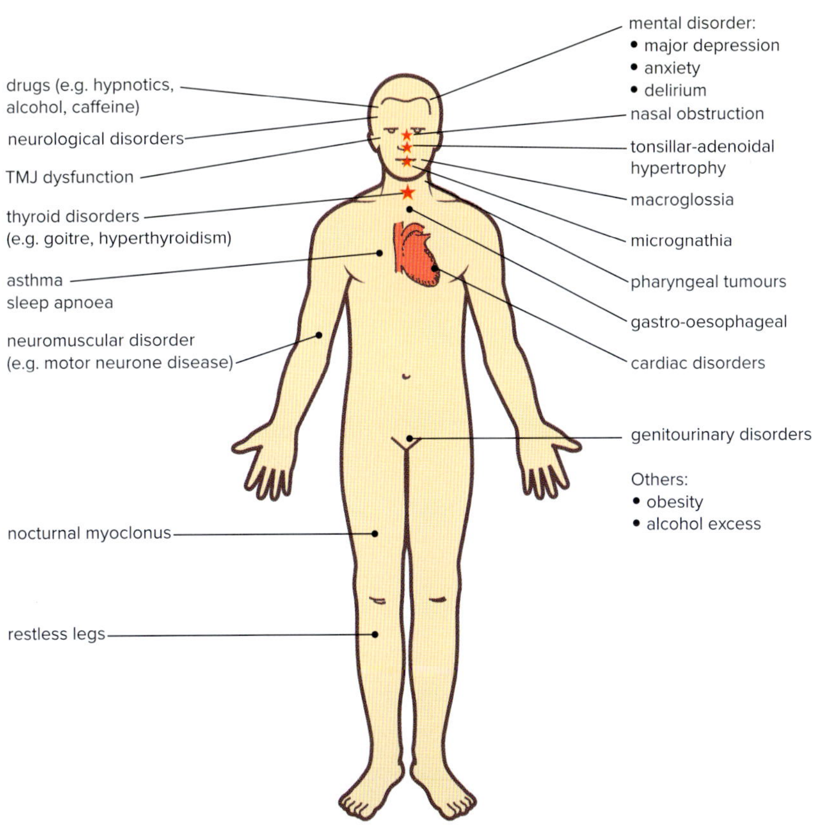

FIGURE 71.1 Significant causes of sleep disturbance

frequent intermittent nocturnal arousals, early morning awakening or combinations of these.

A careful history is required because some patients have unrealistic expectations about the required amount of sleep they need or have misperceptions of how long they have slept.

When taking the history, explore lifestyle factors, especially psychological reasons, painful conditions, drug use and abuse, appetite, energy, sexual issues and physical factors. Check thyroid status, especially hyperthyroidism.

Basic principles for managing insomnia[5,6]

- Address anxiety about sleep.
- Address maladaptive behaviours around sleep.
- Address fear of further sleep disruption.
- Consider predisposing dispositions.
- Consider comorbidities.
- Assess pharmacological options, but consider hypnotics only as a short-term measure.
- Refer to a specialist if there are ongoing symptoms despite the above considerations.

Table 71.2 Common causes of insomnia

Common causes of insomnia
Drugs (prescribed, illicit, stimulants, addictive, alcohol)
Anxiety, stress (esp. PTSD)
Depression
Inappropriate sleep hygiene or lifestyle
Delirium and dementia
Biorhythm disruption, e.g. shift work, travel
Restless legs syndrome
Pain, e.g. carpal tunnel syndrome
Sleep apnoea
Parasomnias—nightmares, sleepwalking
Physical disorders (e.g. CCF, arthritis, asthma)
Bed-wetting
Reflux disease
Thyroid disorders (e.g. thyrotoxicosis)
Menopausal symptoms
Snoring partner
Lower urinary tract symptoms with nocturia

Management[6]

1 Contract with the patient: discuss and agree to the therapeutic objective with the patient (e.g. to reinstate sleep without medication).
2 Sleep–wake history: take a sleep–wake history (preferably with a sleep diary) and evaluate daytime functioning.
3 Exclude and treat any underlying problem (see TABLE 71.2).
4 Explanation and reassurance, including patient education handout.
5 Sleep hygiene advice:
   - Try to recognise what helps patient to settle best (e.g. warm bath, listening to music).
   - Establish a routine before going to bed.
   - Regular daytime exercise.
   - Regular time of arising.
   - Avoid daytime naps.
   - Avoid strenuous exercise close to bedtime.
   - Avoid alcohol and drinks containing caffeine in the evening, especially close to retiring.
   - Avoid a heavy evening meal within 3 hours of bedtime.
   - Avoid smoking, especially in the evening.
   - Remove pets from the bedroom.
   - Use a suitable mattress and pillow for comfort and support.
   - Ensure a dark, quiet room for sleeping.
   - Avoid lights, including poorly screened windows and highly illuminated clocks in the room.

   Sleep-promoting adjuvants:
   - Try a drink of warm milk before retiring.
   - Organise a comfortable, quiet sleep setting with the right temperature.
   - Try a warm bath before bed.
6 Non-pharmacological treatment: various techniques should be adopted according to patient personality and preference, the clinician's expertise and the available resources. These include relaxation therapy, meditation and stress management, which are all highly recommended. Other measures include cognitive behaviour therapy (first-line treatment), structured problem-solving and electromyographic feedback. Hypnosis is also worth considering.
7 Pharmacological treatment:[6] it is advisable to avoid hypnotic agents as first-line treatment. If any form of continuous agent is necessary, it is best to limit it to 2 weeks.

   Options:
   temazepam 10 mg tablets (o) nocte
   or
   zopiclone 3.75 mg (o) nocte
   or
   zolpidem 5 mg (o) or CR 6.25 mg nocte
   or
   melatonin prolonged release 2 mg (o) 1–2 hrs before bedtime (best >55 years). Long-term safety and efficacy not clearly evaluated.

Note:

- The cyclopyrrolone derivative zopiclone and the imidazopyridine derivative, zolpidem, are non-benzodiazepine hypnotics with a similar action to the benzodiazepines represented by temazepam. However, warnings have been issued about adverse neurological and psychiatric reactions.[4]
- Tricyclic antidepressants with sedative effects (e.g. amitriptyline) are often used as hypnotics but should generally be avoided in the absence of depressive disorders, especially in older people.

Sleep apnoea[7]

The term 'sleep apnoea' is used to describe cyclical brief interruptions of ventilation, each cycle lasting 15–90 seconds and resulting in hypoxaemia, hypercapnia and respiratory acidosis, terminating in an arousal from sleep (often not recognised by the patient). The interruption is then followed by the resumption of normal ventilation, a return to sleep, and further interruption of ventilation.

Sleep apnoea is broadly classified into obstructive and central types.

Obstructive sleep apnoea (OSA) refers to the presence of apnoeas and hypopnoeas during sleep together with daytime dysfunction, predominantly excessive daytime sleepiness. The effects include snoring (see FIG. 71.2).

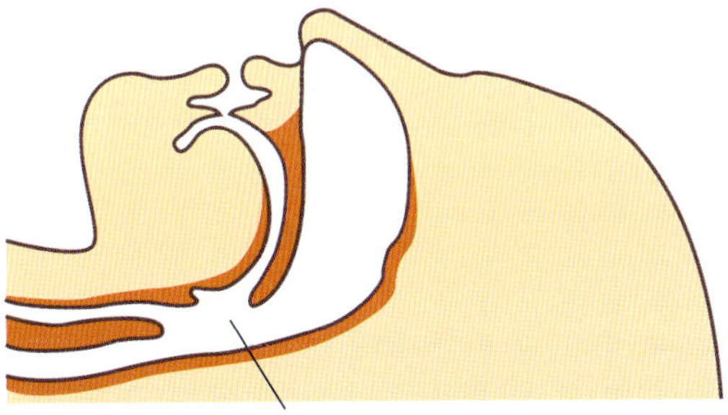

FIGURE 71.2 Normal airway when sleeping

Predisposing causes include:

- diminished airway size (e.g. macroglossia obesity, tonsillar-adenoidal hypertrophy)
- upper airway muscle hypotonia (e.g. alcohol hypnotics, neurological disorders; see FIG. 71.3)
- nasal obstruction

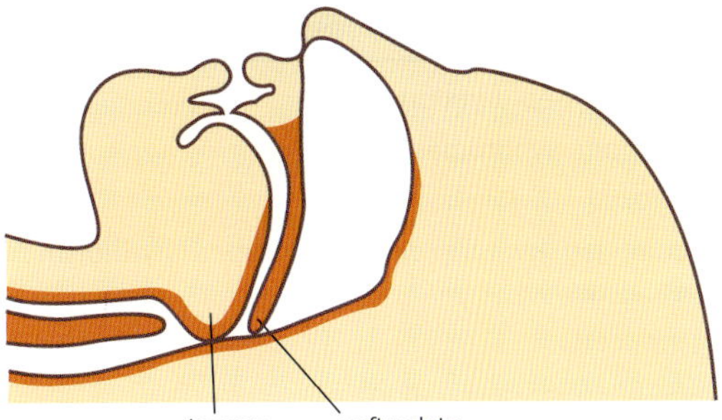

FIGURE 71.3 Sleep apnoea: obstructed airway when sleeping

Central sleep apnoea (CSA), which occurs when there is either brief or prolonged loss of breathing during sleep, is less common (accounts for <10% of sleep-disordered breathing). It is due mainly to neurological conditions such as brain stem disorders leading to reduced ventilatory drive, and neuromuscular disorders such as motor neurone disease. Cardiorespiratory disease is also a risk factor. It requires specialist referral. Treatment of CSA is based on optimal therapy for these underlying conditions and attending to lifestyle modification as outlined below.

Clinical effects of sleep apnoea syndromes[5,7]

Important clinical presentations include:

- excessive daytime sleepiness and tiredness
- nocturnal problems (e.g. loud snoring, thrashing, 'seizures', choking, pain reactions)
- morning headache
- subtle neuropsychiatric disturbance—learning difficulties, loss of concentration, personality change, depression
- sexual dysfunction
- occupational and driving problems

Causes of excessive daytime sleepiness are presented in TABLE 71.3. In OSA, sleepiness results from repeated arousals during sleep and the effects of hypoxaemia and hypercapnia on the brain. Physical examination may reveal few or no signs.

Management of sleep apnoea[7]

Referral to a comprehensive sleep disorder centre especially for sleep polysomnography (the gold standard diagnostic test) is advisable if this disorder is diagnosed or suspected. Consider also the Berlin questionnaire[8] or the Epworth sleepiness scale.[9]

Table 71.3 Causes of excessive somnolence

Inadequate sleep duration
Sleep apnoea syndromes
Narcolepsy
Endocrine (e.g. hypothyroidism, hyperparathyroidism, hypercalcaemia)
Drug induced
Purposeful sleep deprivation
Nocturnal myoclonus
Bereavement
Idiopathic

The general principles are as follows:

1 Lifestyle modification
- Weight loss (e.g. loss of 10–15%, e.g. 7–10 kg can significantly reduce severity).
- Achieve physical fitness with regular exercise.
- Good sleep hygiene and adequate sleep hours (increase time in bed).
- Reduce or cease sedatives/hypnotics.
- Avoid alcohol for up to 3 hours before going to sleep and drugs in general.
- Cease cigarette smoking (increases nasal resistance).
- Medical management of nasal obstruction (e.g. short-course nasal decongestants) or 6-week trial intranasal topical corticosteroids.
- Obtain positional therapy, avoid supine sleep—sleeping on side is best. Consider neck support.

2 Continuous positive airway pressure (CPAP)
- CPAP is currently the most effective treatment for OSA (consider it for CSA)—the gold standard treatment.
- Delivered by nasal (or facial) mask.
- Provides an air splint to the upper airway and prevents pharyngeal collapse.
- Sleepiness and neurocognitive function improved.
- Not tolerated by all patients.

3 Surgery
In children, OSA is usually due to tonsillar and/or adenoid hypertrophy and is relieved by surgery (see FIG. 71.4). In adults, depending on the cause, the options are:
- correction of the specific upper airway anatomical problem—up to 2% of problems
- correction of nasal obstruction (improves snoring and OSA)

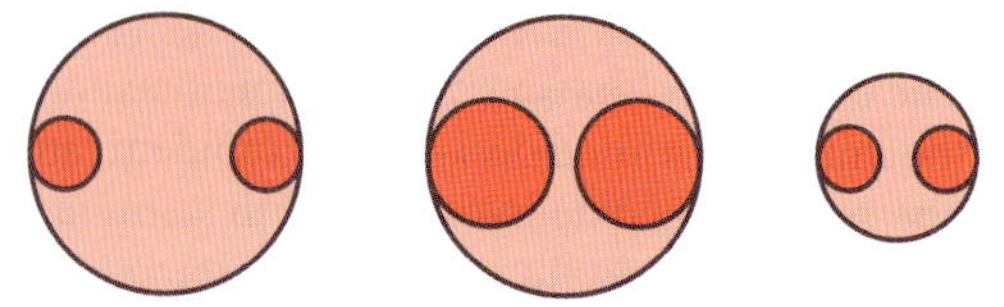

FIGURE 71.4 Influence of tonsils and adenoids on airways

- palatal surgery: uvulopalatopharyngoplasty for carefully selected patients—conventional or laser assisted
- nasal polypectomy
- tonsillectomy
- base of tongue surgery
- radiofrequency treatment to soft palate and base of tongue ('somnoplasty')

4 Oral appliances
- The mandibular advancement splint—a custom-made dental device that supports the mandible and tongue during sleep to increase pharyngeal dimensions. An effective alternative to CPAP.

5 Medication
There are no reliable drug treatment options for OSA. Consider:
- amitriptyline 25–100 mg (o) nocte, in severe cases during REM sleep and intolerance of CPAP
- trial of corticosteroid sprays in children with mild OSA

Obesity hypoventilation syndrome (OHS)—Pickwickian syndrome

OHS may occur alone or secondary to OSA. The main features of the OHS patient are:

- marked/morbid obesity
- cyanosis or plethora
- excessive daytime sleepiness
- right heart failure

There is impaired breathing leading to hypercapnia (↑ $PaCO_2$) and hypoxia. Diagnosis is by sleep studies. Treatment is weight loss plus CPAP. It is a complex problem with a risk of premature death.

Narcolepsy

Narcolepsy is a specific, permanent neurological disorder that is characterised by brief spells of irresistible sleep during daytime hours in inappropriate circumstances, even during activity and usually at times when the average person simply feels sleepy. It is uncommon with an incidence of two to five per 100 000.

Features

Usual onset between adolescence and 30 years of age—in teens and 20s (but has been reported in children as young as 2 years).

Tetrad of symptoms

- Daytime hypersomnolence: sudden brief sleep attacks (15–20 minutes).
- Cataplexy: a sudden decrease or loss of muscle tone in the lower limbs that may cause the person to slump to the floor, unable to move. These attacks are usually triggered by sudden surprise or emotional upset.
- Sleep paralysis: a frightening feeling of inability to move while drowsy (between sleep and waking).
- Hypnagogic (terrifying) hallucinations on falling asleep or waking up (hypnopompic hallucination).

  Several attacks per day are possible.

Diagnosis

The diagnosis is clinical through the taking of an appropriate history. If doubtful, include:

- EEG monitoring
- sleep laboratory studies (sleep latency test—rapid eye movement is a hallmark)

Treatment[6]

Treatment is mainly symptomatic and initiated by a consultant. Central nervous system psychostimulants are of proven effectiveness in increasing alertness:

dexamphetamine 5–10 mg (o), half an hour before breakfast and lunchtime; up to 40 mg daily may be required in slowly increasing doses

or

methylphenidate (Ritalin) 10–20 mg (o) half an hour before breakfast and lunchtime; up to 60 mg daily may be required

Drug holidays from these drugs may be necessary.

- Tricyclic antidepressants are used to treat cataplexy, sleep paralysis and hypnagogic hallucinations (e.g. clomipramine 20–100 mg (o) daily).
- Modafinil is used successfully in some countries.

  Reflect on driving licence issues as appropriate.

Idiopathic hypersomnia[10]

This type of excessive daytime sleepiness (EDS) can present similarly to narcolepsy without cataplexy. The condition, which accounts for 5–10% of patients in sleep clinics with EDS, is diagnosed despite adequate sleep and exclusion of other causes. They usually have non-refreshing deep nocturnal sleep but, unlike narcolepsy, naps are not refreshing. The onset is usually insidious before 30 years and persists for life. Treatment is usually based on psychostimulant therapy to improve EDS.

Snoring

Definition

Snoring is a sonorous sound with breathing during sleep, caused by vibrations in the upper airways from the nose to the back of the throat. It is caused by partially obstructed breathing during sleep (see FIG. 71.5).

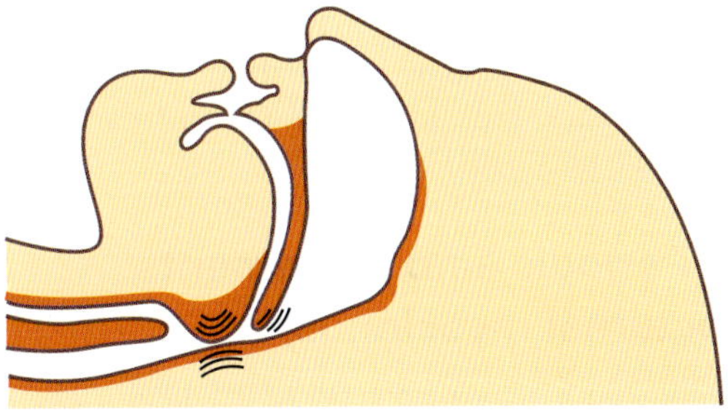

FIGURE 71.5 Snoring: vibrations of tongue and soft palate

Features

- Sometimes indicates OSA, especially in perimenopausal women[7]
- Three times more common in obese persons
- Generally harmless, but if very severe, unusual or associated with periods of no breathing (>10 s) assessment is advisable

Aggravating factors[9,11]

- Obesity
- Old age
- Sleeping on the back
- Sleep deprivation
- Excess alcohol
- Neck problems, especially a 'thick', inflexible neck
- Various drugs, especially sedatives and sleeping pills

- Hay fever and other causes of nasal congestion
- Problems in the upper airways, such as nasal polyps, enlarged tonsils or a foreign body (e.g. a piece of plastic or metal)
- Endocrine abnormalities (e.g. acromegaly, hypothyroidism)

Management

If an examination rules out a physical problem causing obstruction in the back of the nose and OSA, then the following simple advice can be given to patients.

- Obtain and keep to ideal weight.
- Avoid drugs (including sedatives and sleeping tablets), alcohol in excess and smoking.
- Treat nasal congestion (including hay fever) but avoid the overuse of nasal decongestants.
- For neck problems, keep the neck extended at night by wearing a soft collar.
- Consider a trial of an intranasal device such as the Breathing Wonder, which is a hollow intranasal plastic insert. Pharmacists can advise about the range of such devices.
- Try to sleep on your side. If you tend to roll on to your back at night, a maverick method is to consider sewing ping pong balls or tennis balls on the back of the nightwear. Others wear a bra (with tennis balls) back to front.

Periodic limb movements (nocturnal myoclonus)

Periodic limb movements (PLMs) and restless legs syndrome are important causes of insomnia and excessive daytime sleepiness. They may coexist in the same patient. Periodic limb movements, which are also referred to as nocturnal myoclonus or 'leg jerks', tend to occur usually in the anterior tibialis muscles of the leg but can occur in the upper limbs. The prevalence increases with age. Most people with PLMs are completely asymptomatic. The diagnosis is often made during sleep studies.[12] If troublesome, referral to a sleep clinic or neurologist may be appropriate.[12]

Medication

Medication that may help includes:

levodopa plus carbidopa (e.g. Sinemet 100/25, tablets before bedtime)
or
clonazepam 1 mg (o) nocte increasing to 3 mg (o) nocte
or
sodium valproate 100 mg (o) nocte

Sleep paralysis

This is the temporary inability to move or speak when falling asleep or upon awakening, with intact consciousness. It is REM atonia. It can occur in the general population (8%) and about 30% of those with narcolepsy. It can be terrifying but is not dangerous.

Treatment is educational and preventive with optimal sleep hygiene.

Restless legs syndrome (RLS)

RLS, also known as periodic limb disorder or Ekbom syndrome, is a rather common movement disorder of the nervous system where the legs feel as though they want to exercise or move when the body is trying to rest. Sensations that may be experienced include 'twitching', 'prickling' and 'creeping'.[11, 13] The major complaint of sufferers is of disruption both to sleep and of relaxing activities, such as watching television or reading a book. Prolonged car or airplane travel can be difficult.

RLS is frequently an undiagnosed disorder because people often don't complain about it to their doctor. A Canadian study reported that 15% of people sampled reported 'leg restlessness' at bedtime.

The diagnosis is made from the history—there are no special diagnostic tests.

Its prevalence increases with age so it mainly affects elderly people. Women are more prone to get RLS and it is aggravated by pregnancy. The exact cause of primary RLS is not clear. It is not related to exercise and does not appear to follow strenuous exercise.

Symptoms

There is an urge to move legs upon resting, particularly after retiring to bed. This urge is a response to unpleasant sensations in the legs, especially in the calves. The sensations are commonly and variously described as crawling, creeping, prickly, tingling, itching, contractions, burning, pulling or tugging, electric shock-like. However, sometimes patients are unable to describe the sensation or refer to it as simply a compulsion to move the legs.

In some patients the arms are affected in a similar way. The symptoms seem to be aggravated by warmth or heat. Many patients with RLS also experience nocturnal myoclonus.

Secondary (medical) causes include:

- anaemia (common)
- iron deficiency (common)
- uraemia
- hypothyroidism

- pregnancy (usually ceases within weeks of delivery)
- drugs (e.g. antihistamines, anti-emetics, selective antidepressants, lithium, selective major tranquillisers and antihypertensives)

Management

Iron studies should be performed and, if low, treat with iron and vitamin C tablets. Advise patients that although RLS can come and go for years, it usually responds well to treatment.

Self-help advice

- Perform activities that can reduce symptoms, for example, a modest amount of walking before bedtime, massage or prescribed exercises (see FIG. 71.6).
  Note: getting out of bed and going for a walk or run does not seem to help RLS.

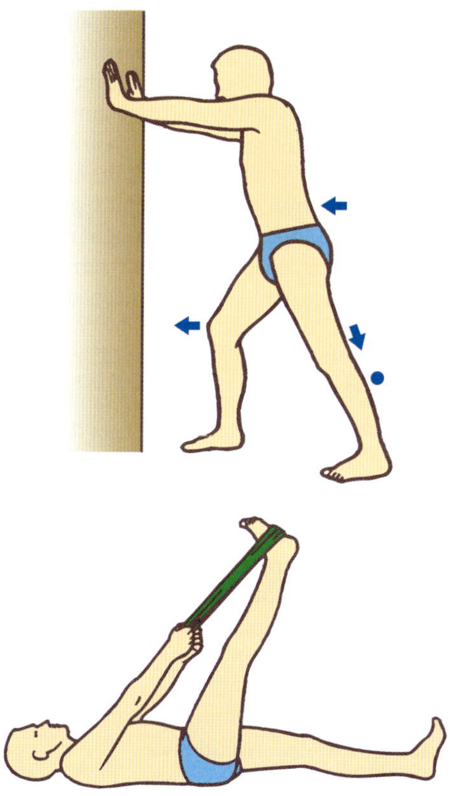

FIGURE 71.6 Stretching exercises for restless legs

- Good sleep hygiene, namely regular sleeping hours, gradual relaxation at bedtime, avoidance of non-sleep activities in bed (e.g. reading, eating).
- Diet: follow a very healthy diet. Avoid caffeine drinks, smoking and alcohol.
- Try keeping the legs cooler than the body for sleeping.
- Exercises: a popular treatment is gentle stretching of the legs, particularly of the hamstring and calf muscles, for at least 5 minutes before retiring. This can be done by using a wide crepe bandage, scarf or other length of material around the foot to stretch and then relax the legs.

Pharmacological treatment[6]

The following may be effective if simple measures fail: (taken before bedtime)

clonazepam 0.5–1 mg (o) 1 hour before retiring
or
levodopa (+ benserazide or carbidopa) 100–200 mg (o) (especially if limb movements at sleep onset are infrequent)

For more severe symptoms consider low-dose dopamine agonists:

pramipexole 0.125 mg (o) daily, increasing as tolerated to 0.75 mg
or
ropinirole 0.5 mg (o) → 4 mg daily

Cabergoline, gabapentin, codeine, baclofen and propranolol may be helpful. Carbamazepine, quinine, antipsychotics (avoid), antihistamines (avoid) and antidepressants are generally unhelpful.

Bruxism (teeth grinding)

Bruxism is the habit of grinding, clenching or tapping teeth, which may occur while awake (especially in children) or more commonly while asleep. The usual symptom is annoying, teeth-grinding noises during sleep that disturb family members. It may result in headaches and TMJ dysfunction in the person during the day. The cause may be a habit or a response to subconsciously correct a faulty bite by making contact between the upper and lower teeth when the jaws are closed. It is aggravated by stress and is more common in heavy alcohol drinkers and SSRI users.

Management

- Educate the patient to recognise, understand and try to overcome the habit.
- Practise keeping the jaws (and teeth) apart.
- Slowly munch an apple before retiring.
- Practise relaxation techniques, including meditation, before retiring.
- Consider other stress-management techniques (e.g. counselling, relaxation exercises, yoga and tai chi).

- Place a hot towel against the sides of the face before retiring to achieve relaxation.
- If this fails and bruxism is socially unacceptable, a plastic night-guard mouthpiece can be fashioned by a dentist to wear at night.

PARASOMNIAS

Parasomnias are defined as dysfunctional episodes associated with sleep, sleep stages or partial arousal. They are more common in children. Diagnosis is clinical.

Nightmares (dream anxiety)

These dream-related anxiety episodes usually occur later in the REM sleep period and are accompanied by unconscious body movements, which usually cause the person to awaken.

Associations include traumatic stress disorders, fever, drug withdrawal (e.g. alcohol, barbiturates, drugs such as zolpidem, SSRIs, beta blockers, benzodiazepines, mirtazepine). Violent behaviour can occur during these dreams due to a REM behaviour disorder and this requires a sleep study and specialist evaluation.

Psychological evaluation with cognitive behaviour therapy (CBT) is appropriate. Medications that may help include phenytoin, clonazepam or diazepam.

REM sleep behaviour disorder

A feature is complex and elaborate motor activity associated with dreams. The behaviour may be violent with profane verbalisation. It is more common in older males and among those with CNS degeneration disorders (e.g. dementia, Parkinson disease). Diagnosis is by sleep studies and treatment is low-dose clonazepam.

Somnambulism (sleepwalking)[2]

This is a complex motor activity in which the person performs some repetitive activity in bed or walks around freely while still asleep. There is amnesia for the event. No treatment is usually required but, if it is repetitive and potentially dangerous, then the sleeping environment should be rendered safe. Psychological assistance is required for recurring episodes. Benzodiazepines such as clonazepam 0.5–2 mg (o) nocte may be useful, but withdrawal usually leads to rebound problems.

Sleep-related leg cramps

Prevention is by stretching the affected muscles for several minutes before sleep. Consider magnesium. Refer to CHAPTER 68.

Sleep terrors

These are part of the same non-REM sleep cycle disorder as somnambulism. Characteristics of night terrors are sharp screams, violent thrashing movements and autonomic overactivity, including sweating and tachycardia. The sufferers, usually preadolescent, may or may not wake and usually cannot recall the event. They also require psychological evaluation and therapy. Similar medication as used for nightmares may help (e.g. a 6-week trial of phenytoin, diazepam or clonazepam).

Sleep disorders in children

Sleep disorders in children are very common in late infancy, toddlerhood and early preschool age groups. By 3 months 70% begin to sleep through the night. The majority do not sleep throughout the night until 6 months of age. Over 50% of toddlers and preschool children resist going to bed.[12] At least 30% of infants and toddlers wake at least once during the night every night. Toddlers begin to have dreams coinciding with language development in the second year of life.[14]

The child who wakes during the night needs reassurance, protection and the parent's presence, but it must be given discreetly. Although psychosocial stresses can trigger sleep problems, serious psychological problems in children with sleep disorders are uncommon.[15]

Management[14]

Aim to see both parents together and get them to agree on the approach, including sharing the workload. Advice to parents:

- Resist taking the child into bed during the night unless they are happy to encourage this.
- Avoid giving attention to the child in the middle of the night—it encourages attention seeking.
- Avoid extra feeding or other pacifiers during the night.
- Return the child to bed promptly and spend only a brief time to give reassurance.
- A rigid series of rituals performed before bedtime helps the child to develop a routine. Settling to sleep may be assisted by soft music, a soft toy and a gentle night light.
- Take the child into the bedroom while still awake.
- Encourage the parents to keep a sleep diary.

Sedative medication has a minimal place in the management of sleep disturbances,[6] and is not recommended for children <2 years although the judicious use of a sedative/hypnotic for a short term may break the sleepless cycle. Such drugs include promethazine 0.5 mg/kg (max. 10 mg) and trimeprazine (Vallergan) 1–2 mg/kg per dose (not for infants under 6 months).[14]

Parasomnias (sleep terrors, sleep walking and sleep talking)[2]

These are not true sleep disorders or night-time arousals. They occur in deep non-REM sleep. With sleep terrors, which usually develop within 2 hours of sleep and last 1–2 minutes, the child is usually inconsolable and has no memory of the event. These events cluster in age ranges:

- sleep terrors 4–8 years
- sleep walking 8–12 years
- sleep talking 6–10 years
- nightmares 3–6 years

They are self-limiting over a period of months. Usually, no active treatment is needed but for persistent, severe problems a 6-week trial of phenytoin, diazepam or imipramine is worthwhile.

Sleep problems in the elderly

The elderly constitute the bulk of long-term users of hypnotics and benzodiazepines. Two key issues to consider are sleep in the elderly and confusion in the elderly. Problems associated with long-term benzodiazepine use are dependence, confusion, memory impairment and falls.

A study of elderly patients with insomnia showed that:[16]

- 25% had insomnia either coexisting with or related to other sleep disorders, such as sleep apnoea or periodic limb movement disorder
- 10% had insomnia related to medical or psychiatric conditions
- 13% had insomnia associated with an inability to stop taking sedative-hypnotic agents

Principles of management in the elderly

- Exclude underlying causes of sleep disturbance.
- Educate patients and carers about the changing needs with ageing and the rational use of medicines.
- Avoid hypnotics if possible.
- Avoid hypnotics combined with alcohol.
- Beware of risks of long-term use and drug accumulation.
- Consider non-drug measures where possible (e.g. CBT).
- Avoid the 'why bother' factor when carers and patients are comfortable with hypnotics.
- In nursing homes, practise 'bothering' and use team effort to encourage less prescribing.

Medication[6]

If medication is necessary, prescribe a short-acting benzodiazepine for as limited a time as possible. An alternative non-benzodiazepine hypnotic (e.g. zopiclone or zolpidem) taken just before retiring may be useful in the elderly (beware of adverse effects). Consider melatonin prolonged release medication. Tricyclic antidepressants with a sedative action are frequently used, especially if there is coexistent depression, but side effects limit their use. However, commonsense prescribing needs to be used and the best option may be to continue the long-term prescribing of hypnotics in those with chronic medical problems or long-term dependents on a low effective dose.

Patient education resources

Hand-out sheets from *Murtagh's Patient Education* 6th edition:

- Sleep problems: insomnia
- Restless legs syndrome
- Sleep problems in children

References

1 Wilson CW, Lack L. Sleeping habits of people living in the Adelaide metropolitan area—a telephone survey. Australian Psychologist, 1983; 18: 368–76.

2 Tiller JWG, Rees VW. Sleep disorders. In: *MIMS Disease Index* (2nd edn). Sydney: IMS Publishing, 1996: 475–8.

3 Partinen M, Guilleminault C. Daytime sleepiness and vascular morbidity: a seven year follow-up in obstructive sleep apnoea patients. Chest, 1990; 97: 27–32.

4 Prescribing benzodiazepines—ongoing dilemma for the GP. NPS News, 2002; 24: 1–2.

5 Cunnington D, Junge M. Chronic insomnia: diagnosis and non-pharmacological management. BMJ, 2016; 355: 5819.

6 Expert group for Psychotropic. Insomnia, parainsomnia. In: eTG complete [Internet]. Melbourne: Therapeutic Guidelines Ltd. Available from: <www.tg.org.au>, accessed October 2017.

7 Expert group for Respiratory. Sleep disordered breathing. In: eTG complete [Internet]. Melbourne: Therapeutic Guidelines Ltd. Available from: <www.tg.org.au>, accessed October 2017.

8 Netzer NC et al. Using the Berlin questionnaire to identify patients at risk for the sleep apnea syndrome. Ann Intern Med, 1999;131 (7): 485–91.

9 Johns MW. A new method for measuring daytime sleepiness: the Epworth sleepiness scale. Sleep, 1991;14 (6): 540–5.
10 Desai A, Kwan B. Excessive sleepiness of non-sleep-apnoea origin: how to treat. Australian Doctor, 15 May 2009: 25–32.
11 Killick R, Grunstein R. Obstructive sleep apnoea. Medical Observer, 21 November 2008: 27–9.
12 Laks L. Sleep disorders. Check Program 346. Melbourne: RACGP, 2000: 3–10.
13 Thyragarajan D. Restless legs syndrome. Australian Prescriber, 2008; 31: 90–3.
14 Gwee K, Rimer R, Marks M. *Paediatric Handbook* (9th edn). Oxford: Wiley-Blackwell, 2015: 370-5.
15 Ramchandani P, Wiggs L et al. A systemic review of treatments for settling problems and night waking in young children. BMJ, 2000; 320: 209–13.
16 Morin CM et al. Behavioral and pharmacological therapies for late-life insomnia: a randomised controlled trial. JAMA, 1999; 281 (11): 991–9.

Sore mouth and tongue 72

The key to managing diseases of the oral mucosa is to evaluate lifestyle factors carefully, including causes of immune suppression.

Dr Jonathan Tversky 2002

Evaluating the sore mouth and tongue is basically an understanding of disorders of the oral mucosa. Disorders of the oral mucosa are a common problem in general practice, with recurrent aphthous ulceration being the most common oral mucosal disease in humans.

There are three types of stratified squamous epithelium in the oral mucosa:[1]

1 masticatory—surface layer, cornified (orthokeratinised), attached to underlying periosteum (e.g. hard palate and gingivae)
2 lining—(e.g. lip and buccal mucosa, alveolar mucosa, floor of mouth, soft palate and tongue —lateral and undersurface)
3 specialised—with taste buds and papillae, e.g. on dorsum of tongue

Key facts and checkpoints

- Dental trauma or neglect is an important cause of many oral mucosal disorders, such as ulceration, bleeding gums and hyperplasia.
- Non-healing oral ulcers warrant biopsy to exclude squamous cell carcinoma (SCC).
- If oral mucosal cancer is suspected, palpate the lesions to check for induration or a firm, discrete edge and check regional nodes.
- Erythroplasia or leucoplakia persisting for 3 weeks after injury, e.g. sharp tooth or denture, should have an incisional biopsy.
- Any oral ulcer or soft-tissue lesion that persists 3 weeks after the apparent cause has been removed should be biopsied.
- Consider Epstein–Barr virus (EBV) infection with unusual faucial ulceration and petechial haemorrhages of the soft palate.
- Aphthous ulcers are usually 3–5 mm in diameter—minor ones have an erythematous margin.
- Intraoral bony exostoses, other than palatal and mandibular tori, are often variations from normal or less commonly part of a syndrome, e.g. Gardner syndrome. No treatment is usually required.[2]
- Shared care of more complex lesions of the mouth and tongue with an oral or dental surgeon is best practice.

Red flag pointers for oral conditions

- Dehydration in children with herpetic gingivostomatitis
- Petechiae on soft palate with gingivostomatitis or pharyngotonsillitis
- Oral ulcers and skin disorders
- Oral ulcers (especially solitary) or soft tissue lesions persisting for >3 weeks
- Oral ulcers and bowel dysfunction
- Oral candidiasis (may indicate diabetes or other immunosuppression)
- Glossodynia may indicate psychological disorder (e.g. depression)

Oral ulceration

The histology of oral ulceration is usually non-specific, with fibrin slough covering granulation tissue, and the aetiology is varied. The ulceration is a breach in the epithelial compartment with inflammatory cell infiltrate in the submucosa. The most common form is recurrent aphthous ulceration. Always inquire about a history of skin problems, medication, bowel function and psychological stress.

A list of causes is presented in the diagnostic strategy model (see TABLE 72.1). Depending on the clinical picture, investigations may include FBE, swabs, autoantibody screen, syphilis serology, blood sugar, vitamin B12 and folate levels, and biopsy.

Table 72.1 Mouth ulcers: diagnostic strategy model
Probability diagnosis
Recurrent aphthous ulceration
Trauma, e.g. sharp broken tooth
Acute herpes simplex infection
Candidiasis
Serious disorders not to be missed
Cancer: SCC, leukaemia
Agranulocytosis
Severe herpetic gingivostomatitis
HIV
Syphilitic—chancre or gumma
Tuberculosis
Pitfalls (often missed)
Aspirin burn
Inflammatory bowel disease (e.g. Crohn)
Herpes zoster virus
Glandular fever (EBV)
Lichen planus
Coxsackie virus:
• herpangina
• hand, foot and mouth disease
Immunosuppression therapy
Lupus erythematosus
Coeliac disease
Rarities:
• Behçet syndrome
• pemphigoid and pemphigus vulgaris
• erythema multiforme
• radiation mucositis
Seven masquerades checklist
Diabetes (*Candida*)
Drugs
Anaemia (iron-deficiency)
Is the patient trying to tell me something?
Unlikely.

Recurrent aphthous ulceration

Aphthous ulcers are round/oval ulcers usually 3–5 mm in diameter with an erythematous margin and sloughing base.

Aphthous ulcers occur in all ages on un(para)-keratinised mucosa such as the buccal and labial mucosa and the floor of the mouth (not on orthokeratinised mucosa) (see FIG. 72.1). The frequency of aphthous ulcers in the population varies from 5% to 25% (average 20%). The cause is unknown, although human herpes virus 6 has been implicated, as have nutritional and autoimmune factors.[3] People with recurrent aphthous ulcers have a genetic predisposition.

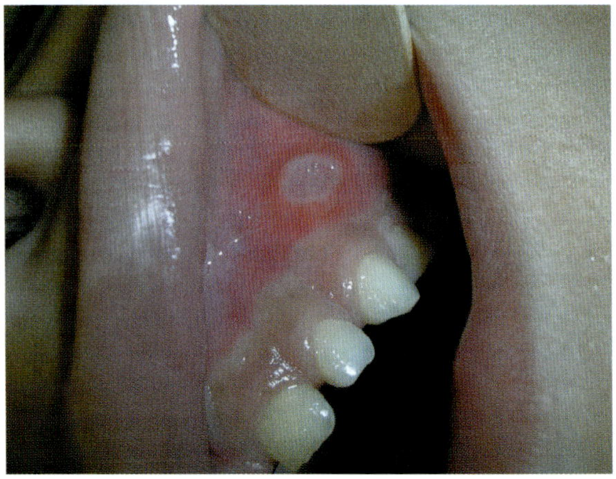

FIGURE 72.1 Apthous ulcer located on unkeratinised (movable) mucosa in a 5-year-old girl

Source: Usatine 41.4.

Precipitating factors

- Trauma (e.g. cheek and tongue biting, toothbrush, dental pressure)
- Drug reaction (e.g. new medication)
- Stress
- Allergy
- Systemic factors (e.g. iron, folate, vitamin B12 deficiency, hormonal)

Note: Exclude blood dyscrasias, Crohn disease, Behçet syndrome, coeliac disease, drug therapy (e.g. phenytoin, cytotoxics, corticosteroids, immunosuppressants).

Rules

- Minor ulcer <5 mm in diameter: lasts 5–10 days and heals without scarring
- Major ulcer >8 mm: can persist for up to 6 weeks[3]
- Major ulcers usually occur on lips, soft palate and fauces and sometimes on the tongue
- Minor ulcers are usually found on the buccal and labial mucosa and the floor of the mouth
- Non-healing ulcers: consider SCC (biopsy required)
- Recurrent ulcers: consider Behçet syndrome. Check serum iron and folate

DxT recurrent oral and genital ulcers + uveitis + arthritis → Behçet syndrome

Treatment

There are multiple methods but none are specific.

Symptomatic relief

topical lignocaine (e.g. 2% jelly or 5% ointment) with cotton bud: after 2 minutes apply lignocaine gel or paint (e.g. SM-33 adult paint formula or SM-33 gel children) every 3 hours

or

eutectic EMLA cream 5%—apply on a cotton bud or gauze for 5 minutes

Healing: options[4]

- Triamcinolone 0.1% (Kenalog in Orabase) paste, apply three times daily after meals and nocte (preferred method but be careful of herpes simplex ulcers).
- Other topical steroids (e.g. betamethasone 0.05% ointment, hydrocortisone 1%).
- Hydrocortisone lozenges (if available)—dissolve in contact with ulcer, qid.
- 10% chloramphenicol in propylene glycol—apply with cotton bud for 1 minute (after drying the ulcer) 6 hourly for 3–4 days.
- Beclomethasone dipropionate 50 mcg spray onto ulcer tds.
- Sucralfate 1 g in 20–30 mL of warm water—use this as a mouthwash.
- Diclofenac 3% in hyaluronan 2.5%.

All of the above treatments have been shown to be effective in controlled trials.

Major ulceration

Consider:

injection of steroids into the base of the ulcer

and/or

oral prednisolone 25 mg daily, 5–7 days[4]

Referral: Patients with a non-healing ulcer within 3 weeks of presentation.

Complementary measures

1. *Teabag method.* Consider applying a wet, squeezed-out, black teabag directly to the ulcer regularly (the tannic acid promotes healing). Must be used when ulcer is worse.
2. *Melaleuca (tea-tree) oil.* 1% tea-tree oil used as a mouth rinse for 1 minute has been shown to prevent secondary infection.[5]
3. *Acupuncture.* This is advocated by its protagonists. It has been proven to improve salivary flow.

Traumatic ulceration

- This is commonly caused by sporting injuries, biting of the cheek and lip, and hot food.
- Factitious causes include scratching of an 'itchy' mouth or over-brushing of the teeth.
- Other relevant causes include dentures, sharp tooth surface, orthodontic bands and sharp objects, such as pencils and hard food.
- Aspirin 'burns' are caused by people leaving salicylate-based tablets to dissolve against oral mucosa.
- Iatrogenic causes include surgical procedures, such as intubation and endoscopy, and dental treatment, such as retractors and removing dry cotton rolls.

Management[1]

- Explanation, including removal of the cause.
- Warm salt-water mouthwashes, and/or local anaesthetic mouthwashes:
  benzocaine compound (Cepacaine), swirl in mouth 10–15 mL for 10–15 seconds and expel, every 3 hours prn
  or
  benzydamine hydrochloride (Difflam), swirl in mouth 15 mL for 30 seconds and expel

  These ulcers can take up to 10 days to resolve.

Lichenoid drug reaction

Several drugs can induce a lichenoid drug reaction of the oral mucosa, that is, cause shallow mucosal erosions similar to lichen planus. The drugs include gold, the NSAIDs, carbimazole, selected antihypertensives and cytotoxics.

Herpes infection

- It is important to beware of herpes simplex virus lesions.
- Primary herpetic gingivostomatitis is usually obvious but herpes infection has an extraordinary ability to present in many ways. It can spread from the hands to the mouth.
- Application of a topical corticosteroid, such as Kenalog in Orabase, can aggravate and spread the herpetic lesion.
- Treatment: aciclovir or similar antiviral if seen early, e.g. 48 hours from onset; fluids + + + ; analgesic mouth rinses, e.g. Difflam; consider admission for IV aciclovir and hydration.
- Lesions of herpes zoster virus affecting the maxillary division of the trigeminal nerve, for example, can involve the buccal mucosa in a unilateral pattern.

Red patches

A reduction in the surface epithelial layer causes erythematous patches. Causes include trauma (e.g. cheek biting), infection (e.g. *Candida albicans*), geographic tongue, haematologic disorders, the dermatoses and neoplasia.

Neoplasia that can look red includes squamous cell carcinoma, Kaposi sarcoma and erythroplakia. Erythroplakia is similar in significance to leucoplakia except for the erythematous feature. It is an important condition to recognise since about 90% of cases are either dysplastic or cancer.[6]

White patches

White patches occur where the epithelial compartment thickens. Causes include inflammation due to trauma or infection, especially *Candida*, dermatoses and neoplasia.

An interesting condition is hyperkeratotic burns on the dependent floor of the mouth, which appear white. Causes include tea-tree oil mouthwash and the sucking of aspirin.

Leucoplakia is any white lesion that cannot be removed by rubbing the mucosal surface (unlike oral candidiasis). About 5% of cases represent either dysplasia or early SCC.[6] Any persistent white patch should be biopsied (see FIG 72.2).

Specific conditions causing red and/or white patches follow.

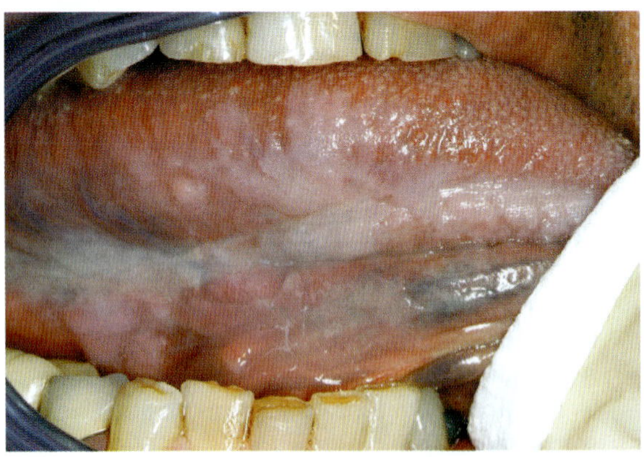

FIGURE 72.2 Leucoplakia showing white patch below tongue

Oral candidiasis (thrush)

This is usually tender and looks like white or yellowish curd-like patches overlying erythematous mucosa. Unlike lichen planus or leucoplakia, they are usually readily rubbed off and hence only the underlying red patch may be seen.

Patients may also complain of a bad metallic taste or halitosis and dysphagia. They often complain of sensitivity to toothpaste or acidic substances in general.

Consider predisposing factors:

- immunodeficiency and cytotoxic therapy
- medication, especially broad-spectrum antibiotics and corticosteroids, including inhalers
- debility and anaemia (iron, folic acid, vitamin B6 deficiency)
- diabetes mellitus and HIV infection

The carriage rate of *Candida albicans* in the oral cavity is 60–75%. The diagnosis is made clinically but a wet preparation using potassium hydroxide will reveal spores and perhaps mycelia.

Treatment

Attend to underlying cause. Consider dental hygiene multivitamin preparations. Antifungal agents should not be used until the fungal infection is confirmed.[5]

Topical therapy

nystatin suspension, rinse and swallow qid: place 1 mL under the tongue then swallow

or

miconazole oral gel (as directed by manufacturer)

or

amphotericin 10 mg or nystatin 100 000 U lozenges dissolved slowly in oral cavity, 6-hourly, for 7–14 days. Avoid with a severe dry mouth.

Oral therapy

Use if unresponsive to topical therapy and the immunocompromised:[5]

fluconazole 50 mg (o) daily for 7–14 days

Denture therapy[1]

Dentures need to be decontaminated, especially if acrylic. Use:

- chlorhexidine denture scrub (care with bleaching), or
- dilute Milton's denture scrub (e.g. ¼ teaspoon White King in a cup of water)

Keep dentures in a dry place at night when not being worn.

If oral thrush, brush the dentures each night with a thin coat of nystatin cream or oral miconazole.

Angular cheilitis

Feature is redness, soreness and maceration of the corners of the mouth. Usually associated with oral candidiasis. Consider poor-fitting dentures, diet—vitamin B deficiency, iron deficiency and atopic or seborrhoeic dermatitis. Treat with topical nystatin or miconazole. 'Golden' crusting indicates *S. aureus.*

Bleeding or painful gums

Erythematous bleeding gums are a common worldwide problem, which is almost always a localised inflammation associated with poor dental hygiene.[7] Systemic problems usually as part of a bleeding diathesis need to be considered.

The causes are summarised in the diagnostic strategy model (see TABLE 72.2).

Acute necrotising ulcerative gingivitis (Vincent infection or trench mouth) caused by anaerobic organisms is rarely seen but is more common in undernourished or ill young adults under stress.

Table 72.2	Bleeding/painful gums: diagnostic strategy model (modified)
Probability diagnosis	
Gingivitis/periodontal (gum) disease	
Trauma: poor-fitting or partial dentures	
Factitious: excessive brushing	
Drugs: warfarin overdose	
Serious disorders not to be missed	
Oral cancer/benign neoplasms (e.g. epulis)	
Blood dyscrasias (e.g. AML)	
Acute herpetic gingivostomatitis	
Pitfalls (often missed) but uncommon	
Acute ulcerative gingivitis (Vincent infection, trench mouth)	
Autoimmune disease (e.g. lichen planus, SLE)	
Hereditary haemorrhagic telangiectasia	
Malabsorption	
Scurvy	

Gingivitis

Caused by plaque (bacterial biofilm) with calculus (tartar secondary to poor oral hygiene).

Features

- Red, swollen gingivae adjacent to teeth (see FIG. 72.3)
- Bleeds with gentle probing
- Halitosis
- Usually no pain

Treatment[4,7]

- Dental care—remove plaque and clean
- Cease smoking

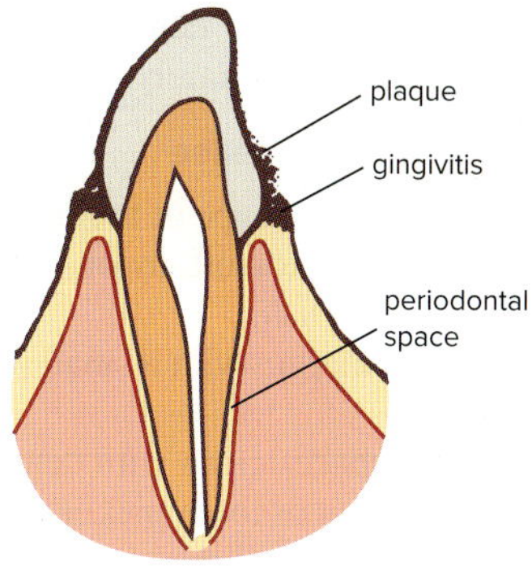

FIGURE 72.3 Gingivitis, showing plaque and gingivitis

- Mouthwash: chlorhexidine 0.2 or 0.12% aqueous solution 10 ml for 1 minute 8–12 hourly for 10 days or until pain abates (beware of superficial discolouration of teeth with prolonged use)

Acute ulcerative gingivitis

This is a very painful form of gingivitis. Treatment is as for gingivitis but add antibiotics, e.g. metronidozole 400 mg (o) 12 hourly or tinidazole 2 g (o) single dose and drain pus from abscess.[4]

Periodontitis

This is inflammation of the periodontal space. It is a sequel to gingivitis and shows periodontal ligament breakdown with recession or periodontal pocketing and alveolar bone loss. There is possible loosening of teeth and periodontal abscess formation (see FIG. 72.4). An underlying medical condition must be suspected.

Risk factors are smoking and diabetes.

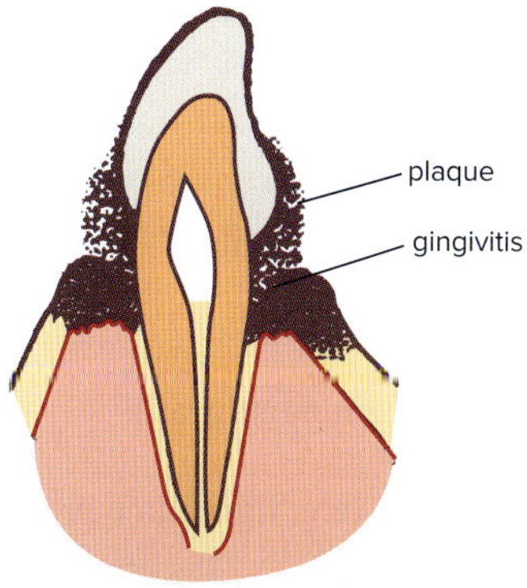

FIGURE 72.4 Periodontitis with more widespread gingival inflammation that invades the supporting alveolar bone

Treatment is meticulous dental treatment and mouthwashes. Antibiotics are rarely required.[4]

Prevention of gingival disease

- Use a fluoride, abrasive type of toothpaste.
- Brush with a medium-to-soft, nylon-tufted, small-headed toothbrush.
- Direct at gingival margin with a small horizontal motion.
- Keep interdental spaces clean with dental flossing in a vertical direction or tooth picking.
- Regular dental review—eliminate plaque.

Oral dermatoses

The dermatoses include lichen planus, pemphigus vulgaris (uncommon), mucous membrane pemphigoid (uncommon) and lupus erythematosus. The clinical appearance of these conditions in the mouth is quite different to the skin condition because of the environment, especially due to the presence of saliva.

Diagnosis

Histopathological examination (after appropriate biopsy) with immunofluorescence is recommended, especially because of the similarity of the lesions of lupus erythematosus and lichen planus, which are both considered to be potentially premalignant in the mouth.[8]

Clinical features

Lichen planus:

- affects 2% of the population, usually over 45 years
- can vary from asymptomatic to severely painful
- usually white lace-like patterns on mucosa, cheeks and tongue
- may form superficial erosions

Lupus erythematosus:

- oral lesions may be first sign of SLE
- usually on lateral aspects of the hard palate
- can resemble lichen planus

Treatment

Consider specialist referral.

Oral hygiene and pain control:

chlorhexidine mouthwash
or
tetracycline/nystatin mouthwash
or
topical analgesics (e.g. lignocaine preparation)

Corticosteroids:

- topical (e.g. Kenalog in Orabase; betamethasone dipropionate 0.05%)
- intralesional (e.g. triamcinolone 10 mg/mL, especially for lichen planus)
- systemic—may be necessary in severe cases

The painful tongue[9]

Pain in the tongue is a reasonably common symptom in general practice. The cause is usually obvious upon examination, but there are some obscure causes. As for many other oral mucosal problems, shared care with a dental or oral medical specialist is important. The causes of a sore or painful tongue are similar to that of the sore throat or mouth. Xerostomia is common in the elderly.

Investigations may include an FBE, serum vitamin B12, folate and ferritin levels, a swab or a biopsy of a suspicious lesion.

A diagnostic strategy with lists of causes is presented in TABLE 72.3.

Table 72.3 Sore tongue: diagnostic strategy model
Probability diagnosis
Geographic tongue Atrophic glossitis Trauma (bites, teeth, hot food/drink) Aphthous ulceration Herpes simplex virus (children) Fissured tongue
Disorders not to be missed
Cancer Agranulocytosis (? drug induced) HIV
Pitfalls (often missed)
Anaemia: iron, vitamins B6 and B12, folate deficiency Citric acid-containing foods Glossopharyngeal neuralgia Lichen planus Fissured tongue (rarely causes soreness) Median rhomboid glossitis Behçet syndrome Crohn disease Coeliac disease
Seven masquerades checklist
Depression Diabetes (*Candida*) Drugs (mouthwashes, aspirin) Anaemia (various)
Is the patient trying to tell me something?
Possible with glossodynia.

Tongue tips

- Look for evidence of trauma, especially from a sharp tooth.
- A miserable child with a painful mouth and tongue is likely to have acute primary herpetic gingivostomatitis or hand, foot and mouth disease.
- When taking the history, take note of self-medications, especially sucking aspirin, a history of skin lesions (e.g. lichen planus) and consider underlying diabetes or immunosuppression.
- A long history of soreness with spicy or other foods indicates benign migratory glossitis (geographic tongue) or median rhomboid glossitis (see FIG. 72.5).
- Any non-healing or chronic ulcer requires urgent referral.
- Macroglossia (large tongue): consider acromegaly, myxoedema, amyloidosis, lymphangioma.
- Strawberry tongue: consider scarlet fever, Kawasaki disease.
- Glossodynia (painful tongue): characteristically presents as a burning pain on the tip of the tongue.[9] It can be a real 'heartsink' presentation. Consider depressive illness as an underlying cause.

Erythema migrans (geographic tongue)

Also known as benign migratory glossitis, this benign condition shows changing patterns of desquamatous areas and erythema on the dorsum and edges of the tongue. With the smooth red patches and raised whitish grey edges, the pattern resembles a relief map with mountain ridges. The border changes shape within weeks. It is irregular and slightly reddened.

It is considered to be a hypersensitivity reaction but the offending allergen has not been identified. Stress, tobacco, alcohol, marijuana and spicy foods can aggravate the condition in some individuals.

Management

- The condition is self-limiting and there is no specific therapy.
- Explanation and reassurance is important.
- No treatment is recommended if asymptomatic.
- If tender, benzocaine compound (Cepacaine) gargle 10 mL tds.
- If persistent and troublesome, low-dose inhaled glucocorticoid (e.g. beclomethasone 50 mcg tds—don't rinse after use).

Black or hairy tongue

This is due to overgrowth of papillae or reduced wear of papillae, e.g. debility and lack of fibrous foods.

- Appearance: dark, elongated filiform papillae giving brownish appearance to dorsum (posterior) of tongue.
- Symptoms: bad tastes and malodorous oral cavity.

Causes

- Unknown
- Poor oral hygiene/debility
- Iatrogenic (e.g. antibiotics, major tranquillisers, corticosteroids)

Treatment

Brush or scrape tongue to remove stained papillae. Use a topical keratolytic agent such as salicylate, with pineapple being the most practical (95% cases are helped).

Method

- Cut a thin slice of pineapple into eight segments. Slowly suck a segment on the back of the tongue

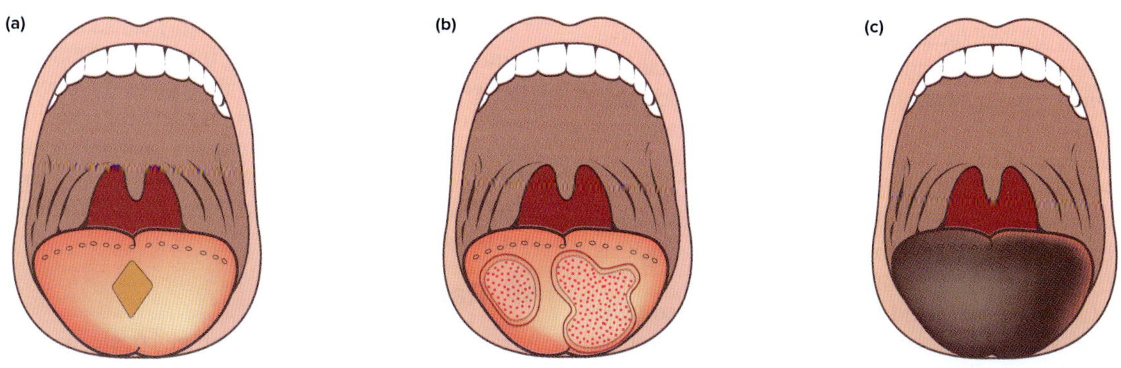

FIGURE 72.5 Disorders of the tongue: **(a)** median rhomboid glossitis, **(b)** geographic tongue, **(c)** black tongue

for 40 seconds and then slowly chew it. Repeat until all segments are completed. Do this bd for 7–10 days.[1] Repeat if recurs.

Note: The salicylate in pineapple can aggravate irritable bowel syndrome.

Consider sodium bicarbonate mouthwash.

Oral dysaesthesia ('burning mouth' syndrome)

The classic chronic burning sensation of the oral cavity appears to have a neuropathic and/or psychological basis.[1] Symptoms include:

- altered sensitivity—burning pain or 'raw' sensation, mainly of the tongue and mucosa of lips
- altered taste—sweet, salty, bitter or metallic
- altered saliva (subjective)—quality and quantity
- altered tooth sensation (e.g. 'phantom tooth pain')
- dry mouth (xerostomia)

Consider the underlying cause:

- medications
- haematinic deficiency—iron, folate, vitamin B12
- autoimmune disorder (e.g. Sjögren syndrome)
- endocrine disorder (e.g. diabetes)
- psychological disorder

Management

- Detailed history with exclusion of organic causes
- Provision of education and understanding

Consider clonazepam 0.5–1 mg bd.

Oral cancer

Cancer of the lip and oral cavity accounts for 2–3% of all newly diagnosed cancers in Australia.[10]

SCC is the most common malignancy of the oral cavity, accounting for 90% of cases. It has a 5-year survival rate of 65% without lymph node involvement and 50% with local node metastases.[11] Cancer of the lip is usually treated successfully by excisional biopsy but intraoral cancer has significant morbidity and mortality.[10]

Other malignancies include mucoepidermoid carcinoma, lymphoma, Kaposi sarcoma and malignant melanoma, which is usually found on the palate.

Predisposing or associated factors for SCC include tobacco and marijuana abuse, alcohol abuse, excessive sunlight and immune suppressive disorders such as HIV, lymphoma and various medications.

SCC is usually found as a chronic indurated ulcer on the ventral and lateral surfaces of the tongue followed by the floor of the mouth and buccal mucosa. It may present as a white patch or, more commonly, as a speckled white and red nodular patch or a red velvety patch.

The red patches of erythroplakia (in particular) and the white patches of leucoplakia may be premalignant or early invasive cancer and necessitate further investigation, particularly incisional biopsy.

Treatment for oral cancer is surgery ± radiotherapy and chemotherapy.

Benign intraoral swellings and tumours

Epulis

An epulis is a benign, localised gingival swelling. It is a very ancient term with no pathological significance, meaning a 'tumour situated on the gum'. There are two distinct types—a fibrous epulis and giant cell epulis. An epulis emerges between two teeth from the periodontal membrane where there is usually dental decay or a site of irritation, such as a partial denture. It appears to be more common during pregnancy where the epulis has a more vascular appearance.

Treatment is usually by excision, with histological examination, curettage of the origin and extracting associated teeth. The 'pregnancy' epulis should be left for several weeks after childbirth before treatment.

Typical locations of intraoral tumours are shown in FIGURE 72.6.

Pyogenic granuloma

These may occur on the gums or oral mucosa of the lips and look like pyogenic granulomas of the skin, which also are associated with minor trauma. It is best treated by excision.

Retention cysts (mucous cysts)

The oral mucosa contains numerous mucous cysts and accessory mucous and serous salivary glands.

Small retention cysts are probably caused by minor trauma to the duct. They may rupture spontaneously. They commonly occur on the mucosa of the lower lip. Treatment is by incision and enucleation under local anaesthesia. Larger ones require marsupialisation. Others occur on the tonsils where they usually appear as sessile yellow swellings. A special type of retention cyst is the ranula.

Ranula

A ranula is a large transparent mucocele occurring in the floor of the mouth. A blue colour and small tortuous veins stretched across the surface is typical.

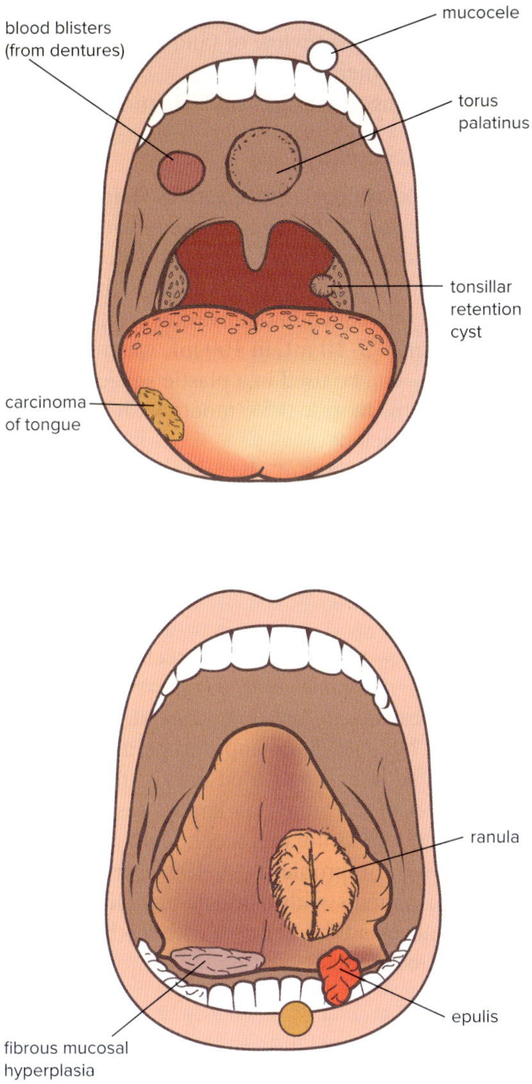

FIGURE 72.6 Typical location of swellings in the oral cavity

It is usually unilateral and simple but may extend into the tissues of the floor of the mouth and neck (plunging ranula). Patients may give a history of a cyst that bursts and then returns.

Treatment is usually by marsupialisation.

Fibrous (fibroepithelial) hyperplasia

Hyperplasia of the oral mucosa, a very common condition, is usually seen on the floor of the mouth and is due to chronic irritation from ill-fitting dentures. Removal of the offending irritation is necessary. The hyperplasia may resolve, but if it doesn't, surgical removal of the residual mass is necessary.

Haemangioma

These appear as a dark blue/purple sessile or modular swelling anywhere in and around the mouth, especially on the vermilion border of the lips, floor of the mouth and tongue. They blanch on pressure. No treatment is needed except for pressing cosmetic reasons. Copious bleeding can occur with attempted removal.

Other soft tissue swellings

Swelling that may be encountered includes squamous papillomas (like viral warts), fibroepithelial polyps (inner side cheek), mixed salivary tumours, vascular haematomas and giant cell granulomas.

The most common benign intraoral salivary neoplasm is the pleomorphic adenoma usually presenting as an asymptomatic swelling of the hard palate or cheeks.[2] Excision is recommended.

Bony exostoses

Bony outgrowths of the maxilla and mandible are reasonably common and the hard intraoral lump may cause concern. The most common is known as torus palatinus (see FIG 72.7), which is situated in the centre of the hard palate. A similar exostosis is torus mandibularis, which occurs inside the mandible, opposite the premolar teeth and is usually bilateral. These lesions are hamartomas and do not require removal except if there is impending dental obstruction.

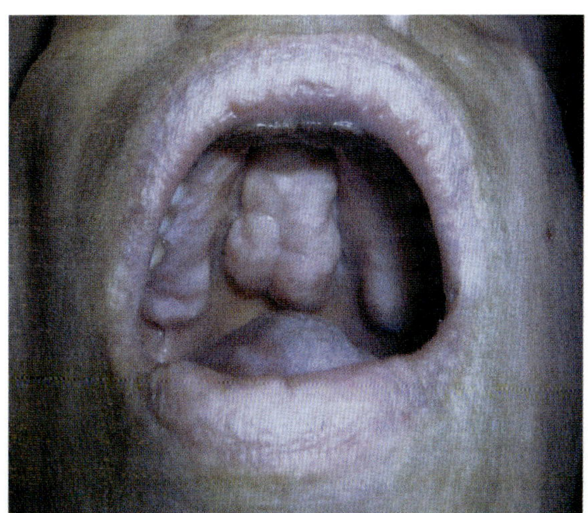

FIGURE 72.7 Torus palatinus in a woman aged 66 years. An incidental finding: it was asymptomatic

72

Xerostomia (dry mouth)

This is a symptom rather than a disease entity. It occurs in about 10% of the population and approximately 70% of patients have a systemic cause.[12]

The most common cause is a side effect of drug therapy and it is relative rather than absolute. Some patients who have a dry mouth on clinical examination do not complain of it while others who do complain of it may be found to have a normal salivary flow rate (a feature of depressive illness).

Other obvious causes are dehydration, mouth breathing and psychogenic.

Primary xerostomia

Causes

- Salivary gland atrophy due to ageing
- Salivary gland infections
- Autoimmune salivary gland disease (e.g. Sjögren syndrome)

> **DxT** dry eyes + dry mouth + arthritis ➜ Sjögren syndrome

Secondary xerostomia

Causes

- Mouth breathing
- Drugs: antidepressants (especially tricyclic agents), diuretics, anticholinergics, tranquillisers, antihistamines, anti-emetics, antihypertensives (some), antimigraine (some), antiparkinson, lithium and opioids
- Depression and anxiety (e.g. public speaking)
- Thirst/hunger
- Dehydration (e.g. diabetes, diarrhoea, kidney failure)
- Anaemias: iron, folate, vitamin B12 deficiency

Consequences[12]

Xerostomia interferes with speech, mastication and swallowing and causes difficulty in managing oral hygiene, especially dentures.

Symptoms include a burning sensation, a decrease in taste or a bad taste and fetid breath.

There is an increase in dental decay and perhaps a tendency to *Candida albicans* infection.

Treatment

This involves education, especially the need for meticulous oral hygiene, including topical fluoride preparations to the teeth and regular dental checks.

The cause must be diagnosed and treated if possible, especially a review of (and replacement of if necessary) drug therapy.

Avoid decongestants and antihistamines.

Strategies to consider

- Suck ice or lozenges, sip sugarless fluids frequently and chew sugarless gum (avoid mouthwashes containing sugars and alcohol).
- Use a saliva substitute (e.g. Aquae, Saliva Orthana) or frequent mouthwashes (e.g. lemon and glycerin, 5–10 mL in 100 mL water as required—can be used in a plastic squeeze bottle).
- Use sodium fluoride 0.5% mouthwash for 5 minutes each day.
- Topical applications of glycerin or paraffin oil to the lips.

Halitosis[4]

Causes

The diagnostic strategy model for chronic halitosis (bad breath) is presented in CHAPTER 17. The commonest causes are orodental disorders secondary to poor oral hygiene and inappropriate diet. Bacterial putrefaction of dental and food debris, together with inflammation of the gums, is largely responsible for the oral malodour. Smoking, alcohol and a dry mouth will aggravate the problem. (A 1999 survey showed that 87% of patients with halitosis had an oral cause, 8% an ear, nose and throat cause with 5% having other or unidentified causes.)

Management

- First exclude dental disease, malignancy (esp. nasopharyngeal cancer), pulmonary TB, hairy tongue, nasal and sinus infection.
- Refer for a dental check. Treat gingivitis.
- Consider drugs such as isosorbide dinitrate and various antidepressants as a cause.
- Cease smoking if this is a factor.
- Avoid or limit onions, garlic, peppers, curries, spicy salami and similar meats.
- Avoid or limit strong cheeses.
- Avoid smoking and excessive nips of alcohol.
- Brush teeth regularly during the day—immediately after meals.
- Gently brush the dorsum of the tongue with special, available soft brushes.
- Rinse mouth out with water after meals.
- Avoid fasting for long periods during the day.
- Drink copious amounts of water during the day.
- Chew sugarless gum to help moisten the mouth.

- Gargle with mouthwash regularly (e.g. Listerine; Cepacol Mint mouthwash; 0.2% aqueous chlorhexidine).
- Use dental floss regularly to clean the teeth.

Tip: use an oil/water wash (e.g. equal volumes of cetylpyridinium chloride (Cepacol) and olive oil), gargle a well-shaken mixture and spit out, qid.

Practice tips

- Recurrent herpes simplex ulceration is not common in the oral mucosa and if suspected should be confirmed by laboratory investigation. The treatment is different from aphthous ulceration so clinical distinction is important. Herpes simplex virus is aggravated by topical steroids.
- For unusual mouth ulceration, consider acute leukaemia, cancer, blood dyscrasias, Crohn disease and drug therapy such as anti-epileptics and antihypertensives.

Patient education resources

Hand-out sheets from *Murtagh's Patient Education* 7th edition:

- Aphthous ulcers
- Halitosis
- Hand, foot and mouth disease
- Tongue soreness

References

1 Tversky J. Oral mucosal disease. In: *Skin and Cancer Foundation Dermatology Conference Proceedings.* Melbourne, 2002.

2 Angel CM et al. Non-neoplastic oral swellings. Aust Fam Physician, 1992; 21: 188–9.

3 Vickers R. Oral ulcers. Medical Observer, 12 May 2000: 78–9.

4 Papadakis MA, McPhee SJ. *Current Medical Diagnoses and Treatment* (56th edn). New York: McGraw-Hill Education, 2017; 226–7.

5 Expert group for Oral and dental. Oral mucosal disease. In: eTG complete [Internet]. Melbourne: Therapeutic Guidelines Ltd. Available from: <www.tg.org.au>, accessed October 2017.

6 Rogers AH, Gully NJ. *Melaleuca* (tea tree oil) for mouth ulcers. J Dent Res, 1998; 78: 949.

7 Bastiaan RJ. Periodontal disease. In: *MIMS Disease Index* (2nd edn). Sydney: IMS Publishing, 1996: 403–4.

8 Reade PC, Rich AM. Oral dermatoses. In: *MIMS Disease Index* (2nd edn). Sydney: IMS Publishing, 1996: 362–4.

9 Hopcroft K, Forte V. *Symptom Sorter* (4th edn). Oxford: Ratcliffe Publishing, 2011; 356–8.

10 Rich AM, Reade PC. Oral cancer. In: *MIMS Disease Index* (2nd edn). Sydney: IMS Publishing, 1996: 360–1.

11 Kaplan JL, Porter R. *The Merck Manual of Diagnosis and Therapy* (19th edn). Whitehouse Station: Merck Research Laboratories, 2011; 492.

12 Abetz LM, Savage NW. Burning mouth syndrome and psychological disorders. Aust Dent J, 2009; 54 (2): 84–93.

73 Sore throat

I believe there are hundreds of young adults who have erroneously suffered tonsillectomy because of the tonsillitis of undiagnosed glandular fever.

SCEPTICAL GP (ANONYMOUS)

A sore or painful throat is one of the commonest symptoms encountered in general practice. The most usual cause is viral pharyngitis, which is self-limiting and usually only requires symptomatic treatment.

Definitions

Pharyngitis Inflammation of pharynx ± tonsils.
Quinsy A peritonsillar abscess.
Tonsillitis Inflammation of tonsils only.

Key facts and checkpoints

- In the National Morbidity Survey (UK),[1] nine episodes per annum of acute pharyngitis or acute tonsillitis were diagnosed for every 100 patients.
- Sore throats account for about 5% of consultations in general practice per annum.[2]
- In one UK general practice, it was the third most common new presenting symptom—5.4% of presenting problems.
- Although throat infections are common from infancy, children under 4 years of age rarely complain of a sore throat.
- Complaints of a sore throat are prevalent in children between 4 and 8 years and in teenagers.
- Sore throats continue to be common up to the age of 45 and then decline significantly.
- The common causes are viral pharyngitis (approximately 60–65%) and tonsillitis due to *Streptococcus pyogenes* (approximately 20%).
- The sore throat may be the presentation of serious and hidden systemic diseases, such as blood dyscrasias, HIV infection and diabetes (due to candidiasis).
- A very important cause is tonsillitis caused by Epstein–Barr mononucleosis (EBM). Treating this cause with penicillin can produce adverse effects.
- As a general rule, antibiotics should not be prescribed to treat a sore throat, excluding evidence of group A beta-haemolytic *Streptococcus* (GABHS) infection.[3]

Presentation

Sore throat may be present as part of a complex of the common upper respiratory infections, such as the common cold and influenza. However, sore throat often presents as a single symptom. The pain is usually continuous and aggravated by swallowing. In those under 4 years of age the presentation of acute pharyngitis or tonsillitis may be confusing as the presenting complaints may be vomiting, abdominal pain and fever rather than sore throat and swallowing difficulty.

It is appropriate to consider sore throat as acute or chronic. Most presentations come as acute problems, the causes of which are listed in TABLE 73.1.

A diagnostic approach

A summary of the diagnostic strategy model is presented in TABLE 73.2.

Probability diagnosis

The majority of sore throats, mainly pharyngitis, will be caused by a virus. A viral infection is supported by the presence of coryza prodromata, hoarseness, cough, conjuctivitis and nasal stuffiness.

Serious disorders not to be missed

It is vital to be aware of *Haemophilus influenzae* infection in children, especially between 2 and 4 years, when the deadly problem of epiglottitis can develop suddenly. These patients present with a short febrile illness, respiratory difficulty (cough is not a feature) and are unable to swallow.

Apart from acute epiglottitis it is important not to overlook cancer of the oropharynx or tongue, or the blood dyscrasias, including acute leukaemia (see CHAPTER 26). The severe infections not to be missed include streptococcal pharyngitis with its complications, including quinsy, diphtheria and HIV infection (including AIDS).

Table 73.1 Causes of acute sore throat

Bacteria
Beta-haemolytic streptococci (GABHS)
Diphtheria (rare)
Gonococcal pharyngitis
Haemophilus influenzae
Moraxella catarrhalis
Quinsy
Staphylococcus aureus (rare)
Syphilis (rare)
Acute ulcerative gingivitis (Vincent angina infection)
Viral
Moderate–severe soreness
Epstein–Barr mononucleosis
Herpangina (Coxsackie A or B)
Herpes simplex pharyngitis
Mild–moderate soreness
Adenovirus
Cytomegalovirus
Coronavirus
Enterovirus
Influenza virus
Picornavirus
Rhinovirus
Human immunodeficiency virus
Varicella (chicken pox)
Other infections
Candida albicans, esp. in infants
Mycoplasma pneumoniae
Chlamydia pneumoniae
Blood dyscrasias
Agranulocytosis
Leukaemia
Irritants
Tobacco smoke
Antiseptic lozenges (oral use)

A foreign body may stick in the supraglottic area and may not be seen on oral examination.

Pitfalls

There are many pitfalls, the classic being to diagnose the exudative tonsillitis of EBM as streptococcal tonsillitis and prescribe one of the penicillins, which may precipitate a severe rash. Primary HIV infection can present with a sore throat along with other symptoms. Adenovirus pharyngitis can also mimic streptococcal pharyngitis, especially in young adults.

Traumatic episodes are important but are often not considered, especially in children. They include:

- a foreign body—may cause a sudden onset of throat pain, then drooling and dysphagia

Table 73.2 Sore throat: diagnostic strategy model

Probability diagnosis
Viral pharyngitis
Streptococcal (GABHS) tonsillitis
Chronic sinusitis with postnasal drip
Oropharyngeal candidiasis
Epstein–Barr mononucleosis
Serious disorders not to be missed
Cardiovascular:
• angina
• myocardial infarction
Neoplasia:
• cancer of oropharynx, tongue
Blood dyscrasias (e.g. agranulocytosis, acute leukaemia)
Severe infections:
• acute epiglottitis (children and adults)
• peritonsillar abscess (quinsy)
• pharyngeal abscess
• diphtheria (very rare)
• HIV/AIDS
• Vincent angina
Pitfalls (often missed)
Trauma—foreign body (e.g. fish bone)
Epstein–Barr mononucleosis
Candida:
• common in infants
• steroid inhalers
STIs:
• gonococcal pharyngitis
• herpes simplex (type II)
• syphilis
Irritants (e.g. cigarette smoke, chemicals)
Reflux oesophagitis → pharyngolaryngitis
Tonsilloliths
Cricopharyngeal spasm
Kawasaki disease
Angioedema (Quinckie oedema)
Chronic mouth breathing
Aphthous ulceration
Thyroiditis
Glossopharyngeal neuralgia
Rarities:
• scleroderma
• Behçet disease
• sarcoidosis
• malignant granuloma
• tuberculosis
Seven masquerades checklist
Depression
Diabetes (*Candida*)
Drugs
Anaemia (possible)
Thyroid disorder (thyroiditis)
Spinal dysfunction (cervical)
Is the patient trying to tell me something?
Unlikely, but the association with depression is significant.

- vocal abuse—excessive singing or shouting can cause a sore throat and hoarseness
- burns—hot food and drink, acids or alkalis

Red flag pointers for sore throat

- Persistent high fever
- Failed antibiotic treatment
- Medication-induced agranulocytosis
- Mouth drooling: consider epiglottitis (don't examine the throat)
- Sharp pain on swallowing (? foreign body)
- Marked swelling of quinsy
- Candidiasis: consider diabetes or immunosuppression

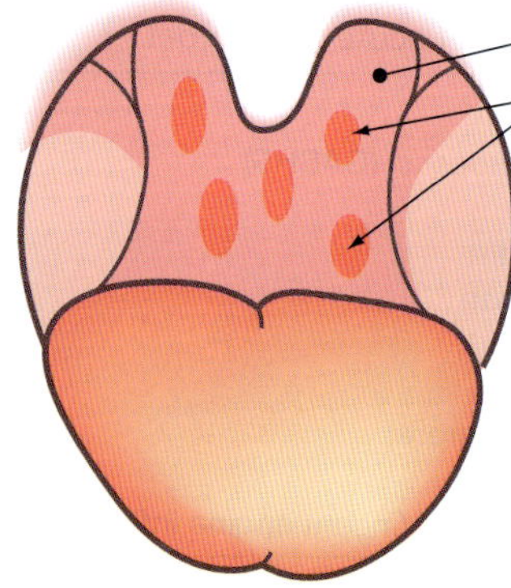

FIGURE 73.1 Viral pharyngitis: the signs may be minimal but mild redness of pharynx and prominent lymphoid patches on the oropharynx are typical

Various irritants, especially cigarette smoke in the household and smoke inhalation from fires, can cause pharyngeal irritation with sore throat, especially in children.

The mouth and pharynx may become dry and sore from mouth breathing, which is often associated with nasal obstruction (e.g. adenoid hypertrophy, allergic rhinitis).

Tonsilloliths are concretions of debris entrapped within deep tonsillar crypts. They are a common cause of halitosis, vague sore throat and possibly recurrent bouts of tonsillitis.

Seven masquerades checklist

Depression may be associated with a sore throat. Diabetes and aplastic anaemia and drugs are indirectly associated through candidiasis, neutropenia and agranulocytosis respectively. NSAIDs can cause a sore throat. The possibility of thyroiditis presenting as a sore throat should be kept in mind.

Making a diagnosis

The issues of making a reliable diagnosis and prescribing antibiotics are rather contentious and at times difficult. It is difficult to distinguish clinically between bacterial and viral causes. The main issue is to determine whether the sore throat has a treatable cause by interpretation of the clinical and epidemiological data.

The appearance of the pharynx and tonsils is not always discriminating. A generalised red throat may be caused by a streptococcal or a viral infection, as may tonsils that are swollen with follicular exudates. On probability, most sore throats are caused by a virus and generally do not show marked inflammatory changes or purulent-looking exudates (see FIG. 73.1). Such throats should be treated symptomatically.

The clinical approach

History

It is necessary to determine whether the patient has a sore throat, a deep pain in the throat or neck pain. Instruct the patient to point to exactly where the pain is experienced. Enquire about relevant associated symptoms such as metallic taste in mouth, fever, upper respiratory infection, other pain such as ear pain, nasal stuffiness or discharge and cough.

Note whether the patient is an asthmatic and uses a corticosteroid inhaler, or is a smoker, or exposed to environmental irritants. Check the immunisation history, enquiring especially about diphtheria.

The history should give a clue to the remote possibility that the painful throat is a manifestation of angina.

Examination

An inspection should note the general appearance of the patient, looking for 'toxicity', the anaemic pallor of leukaemia, the nasal stuffiness of infectious mononucleosis, the characteristic halitosis of a streptococcal throat.

Palpate the neck for soreness and lymphadenopathy, inspect the ears and check the sinus areas.

Then inspect the oral cavity and pharynx. Look for ulcers, abnormal masses and exudates. Note whether the uvula and soft palate, tonsils, fauces or pharynx are swollen, red or covered in exudate. The typical appearances of various conditions causing a sore throat are shown in FIGURES 73.1 to 73.7, and important causes to exclude in FIGURE 73.8.

Guidelines

- Small patches of exudate on the palate or other structure indicate *Candida albicans* (oral thrush) FIG. 73.2).
- A large whitish-yellow membrane virtually covering both tonsils indicates EBM (see FIG. 73.3).
- A generalised red, swollen appearance with exudate indicates GABHS infection (see FIG. 73.4 and 73.5).

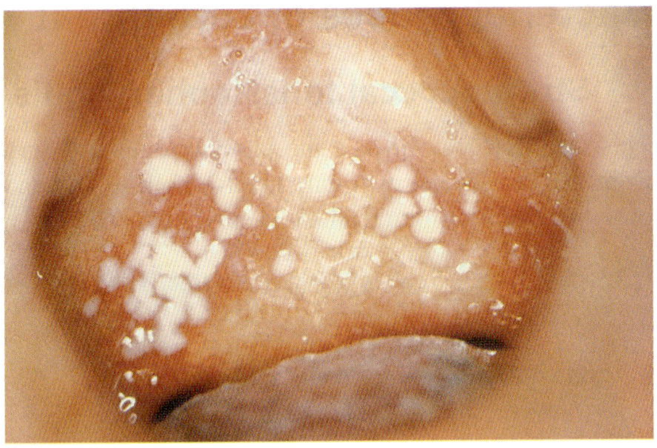

FIGURE 73.2 Oral thrush due to *Candida albicans* in a diabetic patient. Small patches of yellow–white exudate are seen on the palate, dorsum of the tongue, pharynx and mucosa

Photo courtesy Hugh Newton-John

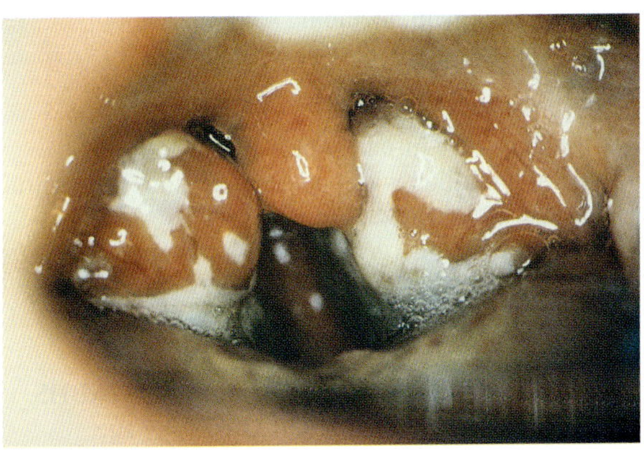

FIGURE 73.3 Tonsillitis of Epstein–Barr mononucleosis showing swollen red tonsils, with a whitish-yellow membranous exudate, swollen uvula and petechiae on the soft palate

Photo courtesy Hugh Newton-John

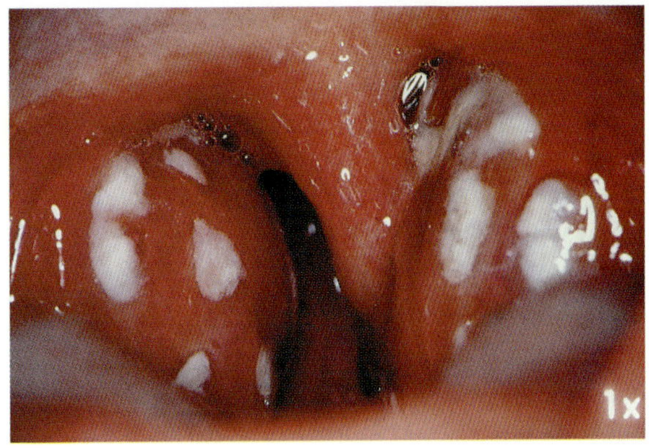

FIGURE 73.4 Acute follicular tonsillitis due to *Streptococcus pyogenes:* the tonsils are red and swollen with pockets of pus

Photo courtesy Hugh Newton-John

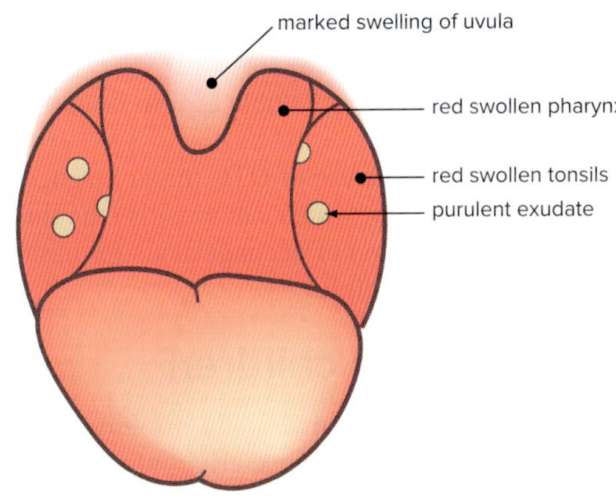

FIGURE 73.5 Streptococcal tonsillopharyngitis: severe inflammation involves both tonsils and pharynx with marked redness, swelling and exudate. Consider herpes simplex and mononucleosis as alternative diagnoses

Investigations

Investigations can be selected from:

- throat swab
- haemoglobin, blood film and white cell count
- mononucleosis test
- random blood sugar (? diabetes)
- biopsy of suspicious lesions

To swab or not to swab

Throat swabs are about 90% effective in isolating GABHS from the infected throat. Authorities are divided about management. Some recommend that throat cultures be performed for all sore throats and antibiotics given only when GABHS is found. Others regard throat cultures as being unnecessary and recommend therapy based on clinical judgments. Swabs are seldom helpful because the isolation of GABHS often represents asymptomatic carriage.[4] Still others recommend throat cultures for selected patients only.[5]

73

Generally, throat cultures are not necessary except to verify the presence of *S. pyogenes*, especially in closed institutions such as boarding schools, or if diphtheria is suspected in the non-immunised. One study has found that toothbrushes harbour GABHS and should not be shared.[6] A positive culture and a fourfold rise in the ASO titre are necessary for a precise diagnosis.

Epstein–Barr mononucleosis screening

It is important initially if tonsillar exudate is present to consider the possibility of EBM. If suspected, an IgM antibody test should be ordered, rather than the older tests, such as a Paul–Bunnell test.

Supportive symptomatic treatment

Supportive measures include:

- adequate soothing fluids, including icy poles
- analgesia: adults—2 soluble aspirin; children—paracetamol elixir (not alcohol base) or ibuprofen
- rest with adequate fluid intake
- soothing gargles (e.g. soluble aspirin used for analgesia)
- advice against overuse of OTC throat lozenges and topical sprays, which can sensitise the throat; limited use (3 days) of decongestants for nasal decongestion is helpful

Sore throat in children

An acute sore throat in a child usually means a viral or, less commonly, bacterial infection of the tonsillopharynx. A bacterial cause is more common in children aged 3–13 years than in children <3 years. Other causes to consider are:

- gingivostomatitis, especially primary herpes simplex
- epiglottitis
- laryngotracheobronchitis (croup)
- laryngitis
- oral candidiasis (more a bad taste than pain)
- aphthous ulcers
- foreign bodies
- postnasal drip (e.g. allergic rhinitis)
- irritation: low environmental humidity, smoke (e.g. household smoke)

Sore throat in the elderly

Sore throat in the elderly may be caused by a viral infection but otherwise needs to be treated with considerable respect. It is important to exclude pharyngeal cancer which can present with the classic triad.

> **DxT** painful swallowing + referred ear pain + hoarseness → pharyngeal cancer

Oropharyngeal lesions may occur with herpes zoster but vesicles are usually present on the face.

A metallic taste in the mouth with or without a complaint of a sore throat indicates *C. albicans* and hence diabetes must be excluded.

Bacterial causes of sore threat

Streptococcal tonsillopharyngitis

This infection may involve the pharynx only and vary from mild to severe, or it may involve both tonsils and pharynx. It is uncommon under 3 years or over 40 years.[7]

Guidelines for streptococcal throat

The four diagnostic features are:

- constitutional symptoms:
  - fever ≥38°C
  - toxicity
- tender anterior cervical lymphadenopathy
- tonsillar swelling and exudate
- absence of cough

Other symptoms include:

- difficulty in swallowing
- significant pain, including pain on talking
- foul-smelling breath

Examination

- Pharynx very inflamed and oedematous
- Tonsils swollen with pockets of yellow exudate on surfaces (see FIGS. 73.4 and 73.5)
- Very tender enlarged tonsillar lymph nodes

Treatment

Indications for antibiotic therapy:[4]

- severe tonsillitis with above features of GABHS
- existing rheumatic heart disease at any age
- scarlet fever
- peritonsillar cellulitis or abscess (quinsy)
- patients 2–25 years with presumptive GABHS from special communities (e.g. remote Indigenous) with a high incidence of acute rheumatic fever

One evidence-based review recommended that if a cold follows its natural course, no antibiotics will be helpful. If there is a sore throat with no cough, but fever >38°C, tender neck glands and white spots in the throat, antibiotics are indicated.[8] Treatment should be with penicillin or an alternative antibiotic (see TABLE 73.3).[4]

Table 73.3 Treatment for streptococcal throat (proven or suspected)[4]

Children

phenoxymethyl penicillin 50 mg/kg/day (o) in 2 divided doses for 10 days (to max. 1 g/day) *or* (if hypersensitive to penicillin) azithromycin 12 mg/kg up to 500 mg (o) daily for 5 days

Adults

phenoxymethyl penicillin 500 mg (o) 12-hourly for 10 days (can initiate treatment with one injection of procaine penicillin) *or* (if hypersensitive to penicillin) azithromycin 500 mg (o) daily for 5 days

In poorly compliant patients:
benzathine penicillin 900 mg IM as a single dose in adults

In severe cases:
procaine penicillin 1–1.5 g IM daily for 3–5 days *plus* phenoxymethyl penicillin (as above) for 10 days

Note: Although symptoms and most evidence will disappear within 1–2 days of treatment, a full course of 10 days should be given to provide an optimal chance of eradicating *S. pyogenes* from the nasopharynx and thus minimising the risk of recurrence or complications such as rheumatic fever.[4] Some studies indicate that 7 days may be sufficient.

Corticosteroids can be added in adults if very severe symptoms e.g. restricted swallowing.

Antibiotic treatment has a variable effect on the resolution of symptoms. It does not protect against glomerulonephritis but does protect against rheumatic fever.[7] Amoxycillin should be avoided in tonsillitis because of confusion caused should mononucleosis be present. Frequent fluids are advisable and paracetamol for pain.

Recurrent tonsillitis[4,7]

Recurrent sore throat is common in childhood and usually has a viral cause. Recurrent tonsillitis tends to be overdiagnosed. A throat swab taken during an acute episode can be helpful.[9] Only patients with more than five episodes of presumptive or proven bacterial tonsillitis in a year should be treated with prophylactic penicillin. The decision should be based on the severity of the episode, time lost from work or school, infectivity and response to antibiotics. Tonsillectomy in children results in only a modest reduction in the number of subsequent sore throats.[10]

Quinsy

Quinsy is a peritonsillar abscess characterised by marked swelling of the peritonsillar area with medial displacement of tonsillar tissue (see FIG. 73.6). It is usually caused by GABHS or anaerobes, occasionally *Staphylococcus aureus*. A typical picture of tonsillitis with severe unilateral throat pain and high fever is followed by increasing difficulty in swallowing and trismus.

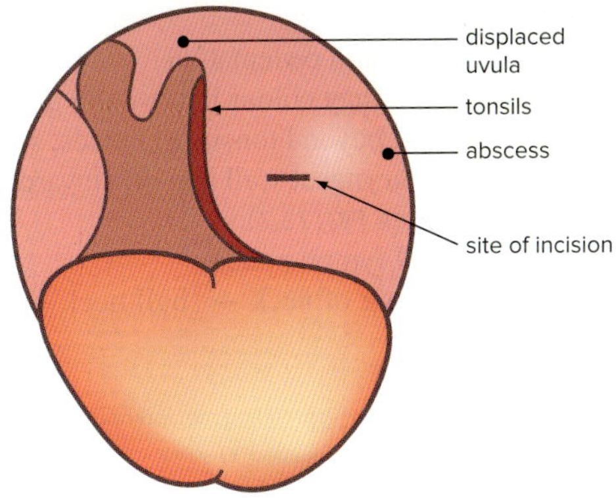

FIGURE 73.6 Peritonsillar abscess (quinsy): a tense red bulging mass is noted and the uvula is displaced from the mid-line; a site of incision for drainage is indicated

Treatment

Antibiotics (e.g. procaine penicillin IM or clindamycin) plus aspiration or drainage in hospital under local anaesthetic if it is pointing. Oral penicillin treatment is likely to fail. Subsequent tonsillectomy may, but not always, be necessary. The cover can be broadened by adding metronidazole.[4]

Acute epiglottitis

In children this is a life-threatening infection. It may be overlooked in adults where, unlike children, the airway is usually not obstructed and the patient presents with a severe sore throat, dysphagia, drooling of saliva and a tender neck. Examination of the throat may appear quite normal. However, it is a severe infection requiring hospitalisation and parenteral antibiotics (e.g. cefotaxime).

Diphtheria

Due to the bacterium *Corynebacterium diphtheriae*, the potentially fatal form of this disease almost always occurs in non-immunised people. The clinical presentation may be modified by previous immunisation or by antibiotic treatment.

Clinical features

- Insidious onset
- Mild to moderate fever
- Mild sore throat and dysphagia
- Patient looks pale and ill

- Enlarged tonsils
- Pharynx inflamed and oedematous
- Pseudomembrane (any colour but usually grey–green) can spread beyond tonsils to fauces, soft palate, lateral pharyngeal wall and downwards to involve larynx (see FIG. 73.7)
- Enlarged cervical lymph nodes
- Soft tissue swelling of neck → 'bull neck' appearance

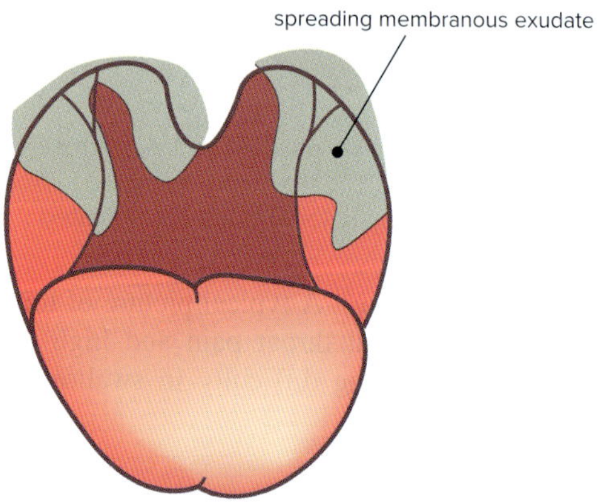

FIGURE 73.7 Diphtheria: tonsils and pharynx are red and swollen; a thick grey-green exudate forms on the tonsils as a spreading membrane

Management

- Throat swabs
- Antitoxin
- Penicillin or erythromycin 500 mg qid for 10 days
- Isolate patient

Viral causes of sore throat

Epstein–Barr mononucleosis

The angiose form of EBM is a real trap and must be considered in patients aged 15–25 years (peak incidence) with a painful throat that takes about 7 days to reach its peak. Refer to CHAPTER 28.

Clinical features

- Sore throat
- Prodromal fever, malaise, lethargy
- Anorexia, myalgia
- Nasal quality to voice
- Skin rash

Examination

- Petechiae on palate (not pathognomonic)
- Enlarged tonsils with or without white exudates (looks, but isn't, purulent)
- Peri-orbital oedema
- Lymphadenopathy, especially posterior cervical
- Splenomegaly (50%)
- Jaundice ± hepatomegaly (5–10%)

The rash

- Primary rash (5%)
- Secondary rash:

  with ampicillin, amoxycillin (90–100%)
  with penicillin (50%)

Note: This rash is not synonymous with penicillin hypersensitivity.

Diagnosis

- Blood film—atypical lymphocytes
- White cell count—absolute lymphocytosis
- Heterophil antibodies

  or

  Monospot test (Paul Bunnell)

  or

- EBV IgM test (more specific)

Treatment[4]

Symptomatic, e.g. paracetamol for pain. Parenteral corticosteroids only in most severe cases.

Herpangina

An uncommon infection caused by the Coxsackie virus. Presents as small vesicles on soft palate, uvula and anterior fauces. These ulcerate to form small ulcers. The problem is benign and rapidly self-limiting.

Herpes simplex pharyngitis

In adults primary infection is similar to severe streptococcal pharyngitis but ulcers extend beyond the tonsils.

Other viral pharyngitis

Typically, the signs are fewer than with other causes. The typical case has mild redness without exudate and prominent (sometimes pale) lymphoid patches on the posterior pharynx (see FIG. 73.1). Tonsillar lymph nodes are usually not enlarged or tender. This picture is the commonest encountered in general practice.

Candida pharyngitis

Oral candidiasis typically presents as milky-white growths on the palate, buccal and gingival mucosae, pharynx and dorsum of the tongue (see FIG. 73.2). If scraped away, a bleeding ulcerated surface remains.

A bad (metallic) taste is a feature but the patient may complain of a sore throat and tongue and dysphagia.

Causes or predisposing factors to consider:

- HIV infection
- diabetes mellitus
- broad-spectrum antibiotics
- corticosteroids, including inhalers
- dentures
- debility

Management

- Determine underlying cause.

Nystatin suspension, rinse and swallow qid
or
amphotericin 10 mg lozenge dissolved slowly in oral cavity, 6-hourly, for 7–14 days

When to refer

- Acute epiglottitis in children (a medical emergency)
- Inaccessible foreign body
- Abscess: peritonsillar or retropharyngeal
- Recurrent attacks of tonsillitis and adenoid hypertrophy for an opinion about tonsillectomy and/or adenoidectomy
- Suspicion or evidence of HIV infection or diphtheria
- Patients not responding to treatment
- Patients with more generalised disorders that are not yet diagnosed[9]

Guidelines for tonsillectomy[10]

- Repeated attacks of acute tonsillitis
- Enlarged tonsils and/or adenoids causing airway obstruction, including OSA
- Chronic tonsillitis
- More than one attack of peritonsillar abscess
- Biopsy excision for suspected new growth

Antibiotic treatment is aimed primarily at streptococcal pharyngitis and this is often based on clinical judgment.

Practice tips

- Consider severe tonsillitis with a covering membrane as EBM.
- If an adult presents with an intensely painful throat with a heavy exudate and that seems toxic, consider primary herpes simplex as well as streptococcal throat.
- Reserve swabs of the throat for verification of a streptococcal throat where it is important to do so, for suspected diphtheria and for suspicion of other serious infections such as tuberculosis.
- Be aware of possible complications, such as febrile convulsions in children and abscess formation.
- Do not misdiagnose unusual causes of a sore throat, such as cancer (see FIG. 73.8).
- The triad: hoarseness, pain on swallowing and referred ear pain = possible pharyngeal cancer.
- The two major considerations in managing the acute sore throat are:
  - Can diphtheria be excluded?
  - Should the patient be treated with an antibiotic?

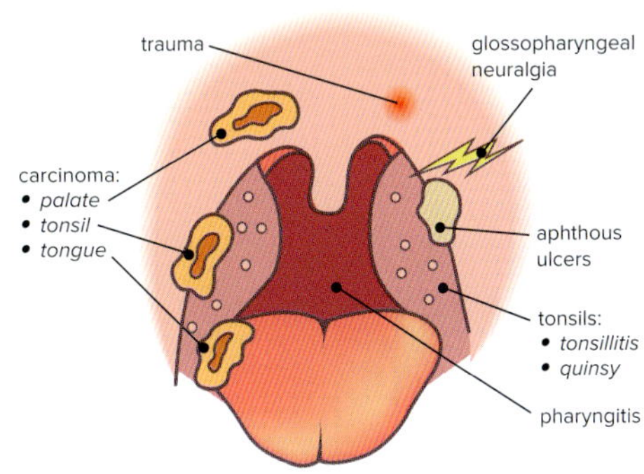

FIGURE 73.8 General causes of a sore throat: note the importance of excluding cancer

Patient education resources

Hand-out sheets from *Murtagh's Patient Education* 7th edition:

- Tonsillitis

References

1 Office of Population Censuses and Surveys. *Morbidity Statistics from General Practice Studies on Medical and Population Subjects.* No 26. London: HMSO, 1974: 33–40.
2 Cormack J, Marinker M, Morrell D. *A Handbook of Primary Medical Care.* London: Kluwer-Harrap, 1980: 3 (25): 1–7.
3 Del Mar CB, Glasziou PO, Spinks AB. *Antibiotics for Sore Throat* (Cochrane review). In: The Cochrane Library, Issue 1. Oxford: Update Software, 2002.
4 Expert group for Antibiotic. Acute pharyngitis and tonsillitis. In: eTG complete [Internet]. Melbourne: Therapeutic Guidelines Ltd. Available from: <www.tg.org.au>, accessed October 2017.
5 Yung AP, McDonald MI et al. Infectious diseases: a clinical approach. Melbourne: A Yung, 2001: 66–74.

6 Brook I, Gober AE. Persistence of group A β-hemolytic streptococci in toothbrushes and removable orthodontic appliances following treatment of pharyngotonsillitis. Arch Otolaryngol Head Neck Surg, 1998; 124: 993–5.
7 Cooper RJ, Hoffman JR et al. Principles of appropriate antibiotic use for acute pharyngitis in adults. Ann Intern Med, 2001; 134: 509–17.
8 Rosser W, Shafir MS. *Evidence-Based Family Medicine.* Hamilton: BC Decker Inc, 1998: 108–10.
9 Buckley N (Chair). *Australian Medicines Handbook.* Adelaide: Australian Medicines Handbook Pty Ltd. 2016: 430.
10 Burton MJ, Glasziou PP. Tonsillectomy or adeno-tonsillectomy versus non-surgical treatment for chronic/recurrent acute tonsillitis. Cochrane Database. Syst Rev. 2009, Issue 1. Art No. CD001802.
11 Jacobson I. Choosing the appropriate patients for tonsillectomy. Medicine Today, October 2012; 13 (10): 39–42.S

Tiredness/fatigue

74

Chronic fatigue syndrome is not tiredness: there is a difference between feeling tired and 'fatiguey'. Fatigue involves a heaviness in the limbs, a sense of inability to think or move, pain in muscles and joints, nausea etc. Please understand the difference.

CFS PATIENT TO AUTHOR, JANUARY 1995

Tiredness, which basically means 'a desire to rest', or chronic fatigue is not a diagnosis but rather a symptom of illness: it may occur as either a presenting or a supporting symptom. Tiredness is interchangeable with terms such as weariness, lethargy, loss of energy, listlessness and exhaustion. It is a common and difficult presenting symptom often known by the acronym TATT—'tired all the time'. The symptom of tiredness is likely to be 'hidden' behind the request for a tonic or a physical check-up.[1]

Tiredness can be a symptom of a great variety of serious and uncommon diseases, including malignant disease. The challenge for the family doctor is to diagnose such disorders quickly without extravagant investigation.

Key facts and checkpoints

- The commonest cause of tiredness is psychological distress, including anxiety states, depression and somatisation disorder.
- An Australian study showed that fatigue presents at a rate of 1.4 per 100 encounters.[2]
- The study by Hickie et al[3] showed that 25% of a sample of attendees visiting general practices had chronic fatigue. Of these, 70% had psychological distress. The others were more likely to have a current depressive disorder.
- In Jerrett's study,[4] no organic cause was found in 62.3% of patients presenting with lethargy; the constant factors were sleep disturbance and the presence of stress in their lives. Many of them turned out to be suffering from psychological problems or psychiatric illnesses, including depression, anxiety state or bereavement.
- An important cause of daytime tiredness is a sleep disorder such as obstructive sleep apnoea, which results in periodic hypoventilation during sleep. It occurs in 2% of the general population in all age groups and in about 10% of middle-aged men.[4] A history of snoring is a pointer to the problem. See CHAPTER 71.
- Underlying disorders that need to be considered as possible causes of chronic fatigue are endocrine and metabolic disorders, malignancy, chronic infection, autoimmune disorders, primary psychiatric disorders, neuromuscular disorders, anaemia, drugs and cardiovascular disorders.
- Prolonged or chronic tiredness is characterised clinically by disabling tiredness, typically lasting more than 2 weeks, associated with non-restorative sleep, headaches and a range of other musculoskeletal and neuropsychiatric symptoms.[3]
- Sociodemographic correlates are concurrent psychological distress, female sex, lower socioeconomic status and fewer total years of education.[3]
- Chronic fatigue syndrome (CFS) is defined as debilitating fatigue, persisting or relapsing over 6 months, associated with a significant reduction in activity levels of at least 50%, and for which no other cause can be found.

Causes of tiredness

Analysing the symptom and reaching a diagnosis demands considerable skill, since tiredness may indicate the first subtle manifestation of a serious physical disease or, more commonly, may represent a patient's inability to deal with the problems of everyday life. Chronic tiredness or fatigue is a feature of the 'high pressure' nature of many people's lifestyles.

Careful consideration must be given to the differentiation of physiological tiredness, as a result of excessive physical activity, from psychological tiredness. Furthermore, before diagnosing tiredness as psychological, pathological as well as physical causes must be excluded.

A summary of causes of chronic tiredness is presented in TABLE 74.1.

74

Table 74.1 Causes of chronic tiredness/fatigue

Psychogenic/non-organic
Psychiatric disorders: • anxiety states • depression/dysthymia • other primary disorders • bereavement • somatisation disorder Lifestyle factors: • workaholic tendencies and 'burnout' • lack of exercise/sedentary lifestyle • mental stress and emotional demands • exposure to irritants (e.g. carbon monoxide, 'lead' fumes) • inappropriate diet • obesity • sleep deprivation
Organic
Congestive cardiac failure Anaemia Malignancy HIV/AIDS Subacute to chronic infection (e.g. hepatitis, malaria, Lyme disease) Endocrine: various, especially thyroid (hyper and hypo), Addison disease and diabetes mellitus Nutritional deficiency Kidney failure Liver disorders: chronic liver failure, chronic active hepatitis Respiratory conditions (e.g. asthma, COPD) Neuromuscular (e.g. MS, myasthenia gravis, Parkinson disease) Metabolic (e.g. hypokalaemia, hypomagnesaemia Drug toxicity, addiction or side effects (see TABLE 74.3) Autoimmune disorders Sleep-related disorders Postinfectious fatigue syndrome (e.g. influenza, mononucleosis)
Unknown
Fibromyalgia Chronic fatigue syndrome Somatisation disorder Irritable bowel syndrome

A diagnostic approach

A summary of the diagnostic strategy model is presented in TABLE 74.2.

Probability diagnosis

The most probable diagnoses to consider are:

- tension, stress and anxiety
- depression

Table 74.2 Tiredness/chronic fatigue: diagnostic strategy model

Probability diagnosis
Stress and anxiety Depression Inappropriate lifestyle and psychosocial factors Viral/postviral infection Sleep-related disorders (e.g. sleep apnoea)
Serious disorders not to be missed
Vascular: • cardiac arrhythmias • cardiomyopathy • incipient CCF Infection: • hidden abscess • HIV/AIDS • hepatitis B and C • others Cancer Other: • anaemia • haemochromatosis
Pitfalls (often missed)
'Masked' depression Food intolerance Coeliac disease Chronic infection (e.g. Lyme disease) Incipient CCF Fibromyalgia Lack of fitness Drugs: alcohol, prescribed, withdrawal Menopause syndrome Pregnancy Neurological disorders: • post-head-injury • CVA • Parkinson disease Kidney failure Metabolic (e.g. hypokalaemia, hypomagnesaemia) Chemical exposure (e.g. occupational) *Rarities:* • hyperparathyroidism • Addison disease (see CHAPTER 23) • Cushing syndrome • narcolepsy • multiple sclerosis • autoimmune disorders
Seven masquerades checklist
Depression Diabetes Drugs Anaemia Thyroid disease (other endocrine) Spinal dysfunction UTI
Is the patient trying to tell me something?
Highly likely.

- inappropriate lifestyle and psychosocial factors
- viral or postviral infection
- sleep-related disorders

Research studies have reported that over 50% (and in some cases as many as 80%) of reported cases of fatigue have been of psychological causation.[3] Overwork is a common cause of fatigue and is often obvious to everyone but the patient. The modern approach to sleep-related disorders has revealed several important factors causing excessive tiredness.

Serious disorders not to be missed

Many serious disorders such as anaemia, malignant disease and subacute or chronic infections (e.g. hepatitis, bacterial endocarditis and tuberculosis) can be 'hidden' or masked in the initial stages or not readily apparent. Neuromuscular diseases such as myasthenia gravis and multiple sclerosis, connective tissue disorders and HIV infection also have to be excluded.

Pitfalls

The symptom of tiredness is fraught with pitfalls. Common ones include depression and other psychoneurotic disorders, and incipient congestive cardiac failure. Drug intake is a very common pitfall, whether it be by self-administration (including alcohol) or iatrogenic.

Tiredness is a feature of pregnancy in many women, so this association is worth keeping in mind, especially in the early stages when a change in menstrual history is not given or a young single woman will attempt to conceal the fact. It is also a presenting symptom of the menopause syndrome, which should not be misdiagnosed. Two classic causes of tiredness are haemochromatosis and coeliac disease.

Seven masquerades checklist

All these important problems are capable of being responsible for tiredness, especially depression, diabetes, drugs, anaemia and urinary infection. Thyroid disorder could certainly be responsible. Spinal pain can indirectly cause tiredness. Drugs that commonly cause tiredness are listed in TABLE 74.3.

Antihypertensives require special consideration. Drug withdrawal, especially for illicit drugs such as amphetamines, marijuana, cocaine and heroin, has to be considered.

Psychogenic considerations

Tiredness is a symptom that may represent a 'ticket of entry': a plea for help in a stressed, anxious or depressed patient. Any of the primary psychiatric disorders can present as tiredness.

Table 74.3 Drugs that can cause tiredness

Alcohol
Analgesics
Antibiotics
Anticonvulsants
Antidepressants
Anti-emetics
Antihistamines
Antihypertensives, e.g. beta blockers
Anxiolytics
Corticosteroids
Digoxin
Ergot alkaloids
Hormones (e.g. oral contraceptives)
Hypnotics
Nicotine
NSAIDs
Vitamins A and D (early toxic symptoms)

Note: Most drugs have a considerable capacity to cause tiredness.

Red flag pointers for tiredness

- Unexplained weight loss
- Sleep disturbance
- Symptoms of depression
- Drug and alcohol abuse
- Persistent fever

The clinical approach—key history

In routine history taking, it is mandatory that questions be asked about the following if the information is not volunteered by the patient:

- sleep pattern (it is not uncommon for patients to say they sleep well and yet on questioning it is found they have initial insomnia, or middle insomnia, or both, with or without early morning waking). It is most relevant to talk to any sleeping partners to obtain a history of sleep disturbance
- weight fluctuations
- energy—performance—ability to cope
- sexual activity/sexual problems
- suicidal ideas
- self-medication—OTC preparations (e.g. bromides, stimulants, analgesics, alcohol, cigarettes, other drugs); this is particularly important in the drug addiction-prone group: doctors, chemists, nurses, workers in the liquor industry, truck drivers
- fears (including phobic symptoms, hypochondriasis)

74

- precipitating factors (present in over 50% of patients with depressive illness):
  - postpartum
  - postoperative
  - associated with chronic physical illness
  - bereavement
  - pain—chronic pain conditions
  - retirement
  - medication
  - post trauma (e.g. motor vehicle accident)
  - postviral infections, especially hepatitis, mononucleosis, influenza
- work history—determine whether the patient is a workaholic; ask about bullying at work
- dietary history—determine pattern, including fad diets or skipped meals
- psychological history—stress, anxieties, phobias, depression
- menstrual history and symptoms related to the menopause syndrome
- final questions: 'Is there anything else you feel you should tell me?' 'Do you have any explanation for your tiredness?'
- self-question: 'Is this patient depressed?'

Physical examination—key features

- General inspection noting facial features, skin appearance and colour, hyperpigmentation, conjunctivae
- Vital signs
- Anthropometric measurements
- Basic respiratory and cardiovascular
- Abdominal examination with focus on masses and inguinal lymphadenopathy
- Urinalysis

Key investigations (screening) guidelines[5]

- FBE
- ESR/CRP
- Blood sugar
- Serum electrolytes, calcium, magnesium
- Kidney function tests
- Liver function tests
- Iron studies
- Gluten sensitivity screening blood tests
- Faecal occult blood
- Thyroid function tests
- CXR
- Urine—dipstick/MCU

Consider others according to clinical features e.g. chronic infection and HIV screening, autoimmune disorders, cancer markers and sleep disorder studies.

The diagnosis of CFS can be made only when the minimum investigations have been shown to be normal or to demonstrate minor abnormalities in liver function or blood film (atypical lymphocytes).

Tiredness in children

Tiredness in children is caused by a range of predictable conditions, such as physiological factors (excessive exercise, lack of sleep, poor diet), infections, allergies including asthma, drugs, depression and various illnesses in general.

Overweight children are likely to fatigue more rapidly than children of normal weight.[6] Any bacterial, viral or other infection may be associated with tiredness, with EBV being very significant in adolescents. Chronic EBV infection causing recurrent episodes of fever, pharyngitis, malaise and adenopathy can occur, especially in teenagers, who present with chronic exhaustion that is frequently mistaken for malignancy.[6]

Tiredness is a presenting feature of depression in adolescents, a serious problem that often goes unrecognised. Tonsillar–adenoidal hypertrophy may be large enough to compromise air exchange, particularly during sleep. Snoring may be a feature plus tiredness and lethargy in the waking state.

Tiredness in the elderly

Elderly people tend to tire more quickly and recover more slowly and incompletely than younger ones. Sleep in older people is generally shorter in duration and of lesser depth, and they feel less refreshed and sometimes irritable on awakening.

Fatigue may be present as a result of emotional frustration. Whenever the prospect of gratification is small, a person tends to tire quickly and to remain so until something stimulating appears. Since the prospects for gratifying experience wane with the years, easy 'fatigueability' or tiredness is common in this age group.

Bereavement

Although a bereavement reaction is common and a normal human response that occurs at all ages, it is more frequently encountered in the elderly, with the loss of a spouse or a child (young or middle-aged). Fatigue that occurs during the initial mourning period is striking and might represent a protective mechanism against intense emotional stress. With time, usually around 6 to 12 months, a compensated stage is reached, fatigue gradually abates, and the patient resumes normal activities as the conflicts of grief are gradually resolved. Freud pointed out the complexities of mourning as the bereaved person slowly adjusts to the loss of the loved one. In others, various symptoms persist as an 'abnormal grief reaction', including persistence of fatigue. Some factors that may lead to this include:

- unexpected death
- high dependence upon the dead person
- guilt feelings, especially in a love/hate relationship

Studies in general practice have shown that widows see their family doctors for psychiatric symptoms at three times the usual rate in the first 6 months after bereavement. The consultation rate for non-psychiatric symptoms also increases, by almost 50%.

Role of the family doctor

Following bereavement it is important to watch for evidence of depression, drug dependency, especially on alcohol, and suicidal tendencies. In cases of expected death, management should, if possible, start before the bereavement. Supportive care and ongoing counselling are very important.

Burnout

Definition

Burnout is a clinical syndrome with three components:

- long-term emotional exhaustion
- depersonalisation of others and
- lack of personal accomplishment[7]

It is similar to stress-related depression but mood lowering is temporary and work-specific.

Burnout is not a recognised disorder in the DSM-5 criteria, although the ICD-10 classifies it under 'problems related to life management' as a 'state of vital exhaustion'.[8]

Patients sometimes claim that they feel 'burnout'. Burnout can mean many things and include a whole constellation of psychogenic symptoms, such as exhaustion, boredom and cynicism, paranoia, detachment, heightened irritability and impatience, depression and psychosomatic complaints, such as headache and tiredness. Ellard[9] defines burnout as the syndrome that arises when a person who has a strong neurotic need to succeed in a particular task becomes confronted with the impossibility of success in that task. This seems a realistic explanation, but the important factor is to clarify the nature of the problem with care and determine whether the patient has a psychoneurotic disorder, such as hypomania, anxiety state or depression, or a personality disorder or simply unrealistic goals.

Another viewpoint is that it is caused by chronic emotional stress resulting from prolonged intensive involvement with people.[10] Burnout can be work related. Those who tend to be prone to it are musicians, authors, health professionals, teachers, athletes, engineers, emergency service workers, soldiers, reporters and high-technology professionals. Management involves appropriate counselling, which aims to help the patient to identify life stressors, set realistic personal goals and develop good support mechanisms.

74

Chronic fatigue syndrome

This complex syndrome, which causes profound and persistent tiredness, is also referred to as myalgic encephalomyelitis, chronic neuromuscular viral syndrome,[11] postviral syndrome, chronic EBV syndrome, viral fatigue state, epidemic neuromyasthenia, neurasthenia, Icelandic disease, Royal Free disease and Tapanui disease. CFS is not to be confused with the tiredness and depression that follow a viral infection such as infectious mononucleosis, hepatitis or influenza. These postviral tiredness states are certainly common but resolve within 6 months or so.

Typical features of CFS (see FIG. 74.1):[11]

- extreme exhaustion (with minimal physical effort)
- headache or a vague 'fuzzy' feeling in the head
- aching in the muscles and legs
- poor concentration and memory

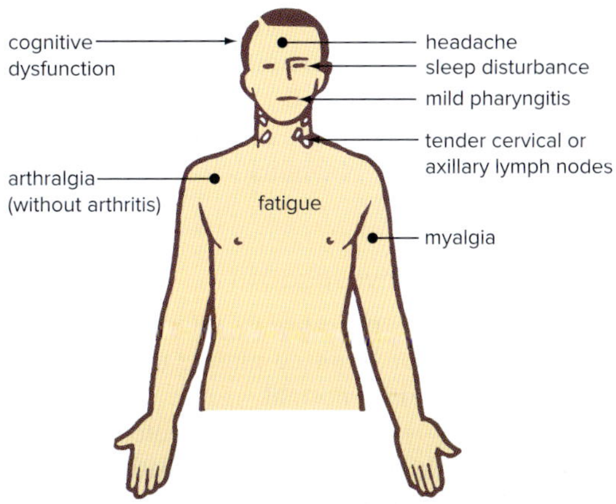

FIGURE 74.1 Chronic fatigue syndrome: characteristic symptoms

- hypersomnia or other sleep disturbance
- waking feeling tired
- emotional lability/anxiety
- depressive-type illness, mood swings
- arthralgia (without joint swelling)
- sore throat
- subjective feeling of fever (with a normal temperature)
- shortness of breath
- tender, swollen lymph nodes
- usually occurs between 20 and 40 years of age

74

Epidemiologically it has been related to Coxsackie B virus infections. The responsible organism is referred to as a slow virus infection by some authorities.[8]

In approximately two-thirds of patients the illness follows a clearly defined viral illness. However, no single virus has been consistently associated with the development of the syndrome, which is known to develop following a wide range of viral and non-viral infective illness. Immune system dysfunction with chronic overproduction of cytokines (e.g. interferon) is a possible pathogenetic mechanism.

Every family doctor probably has patients with this disorder and the syndrome has been observed in isolated endemics from time to time. Hickie et al[3] found that only 0.3% of those with prolonged fatigue had been diagnosed with CFS by their family doctor. Veterans of the Gulf War show a tenfold incidence of CFS compared with non-deployed military personnel.[10]

There is no doubt that the syndrome is real in these patients. One of the major problems confronting clinicians is that there is no diagnostic test for this illness, so it remains a clinical diagnosis backed up by normal baseline investigations.

Diagnostic criteria for CFS have been published[13] (see TABLE 74.4), which emphasise the positive clinical features of the syndrome and the chronicity of symptoms (greater than 6 months), in addition to the need for careful exclusion of alternative diagnoses by history, physical examination and laboratory investigation.

Examination and investigation

Apart from mild pharyngeal infection, cervical lymphadenopathy or localised muscle tenderness, the physical examination is normal.

Investigations should be directed towards excluding possible diagnoses for that patient, such as chronic infection, autoimmune disorders, endocrine and metabolic disorders, primary neuromuscular disorders, malignancy and primary psychiatric disorders.

Table 74.4 Criteria for the diagnosis of chronic fatigue syndrome[13]

Fatigue

Clinically evaluated, unexplained, persistent or relapsing fatigue persistent for 6 months or more, that:

- is of new or definite onset
- is not the result of ongoing exertion
- is not substantially alleviated by rest
- results in substantial reduction in previous levels of occupational, educational, social or personal activities

and

Other symptoms

Four or more of the following symptoms that are concurrent, persistent for 6 months or more and which did not predate the fatigue:

- impaired short-term memory or concentration
- sore throat
- tender cervical or axillary lymph nodes
- muscle pain
- multi-joint pain without arthritis
- headaches of a new type, pattern, or severity
- unrefreshing sleep
- post-exertional malaise lasting more than 24 hours

The last mentioned is the most difficult of the differential diagnoses and psychiatric referral will often need to be considered.

Management

Patients who have CFS are really suffering and unhappy people, similar to those with fibromyalgia (see CHAPTER 37). They require considerable understanding and support. Multidisciplinary intervention is recommended. Symptoms last approximately 2½ years.

Management strategies include:[11]

- CFS recognition—explain that the illness is real but the cause unknown and tests are likely to be normal
- explanation and reassurance that the illness is usually self-limiting with no permanent complications; and that a slow, steady improvement can be anticipated, with most CFS patients returning to normal health
- provide continued psychological support
- review for diagnostic reappraisal (examine at least every 4 months)
- avoid telling patients they are depressed
- treat symptomatically—pain relief, consider NSAIDs and antidepressants if significant depression
- refer to counselling and support groups
- provide a realistic, regular, graduated exercise program

- reduce relevant stress factors (map a realistic living program)
- psychiatric referral if appropriate
- ask the patient to keep a diary of exercise/stress and symptom severity, in particular
- avoid long-distance travel, which is poorly tolerated

Cognitive behaviour therapy appears to help some patients, as do relaxation therapy, meditation, stress management and psychotherapy, where indicated.

The emphasis should be placed on caring, rather than curing, until a scientific solution is found.

A systematic review has found that cognitive behaviour therapy administered by skilled therapists and exercise are beneficial. Although few patients are cured with CBT, the therapeutic effect is substantial.[12] There is insufficient data or evidence to support the use of antidepressants, corticosteroids, complementary therapies and dietary supplements, including vitamins B12 and C and co-enzyme Q_{10}.[5] Prolonged rest and immunotherapy was unlikely to be beneficial.[14]

Fibromyalgia

The fibromyalgia syndrome (see CHAPTER 37) bears a clinical resemblance to CFS. Musculoskeletal pain is more prominent although tiredness (fatigue) and sleep disturbance are features. According to Schwenk,[15] fibromyalgia affects 5% of the American population with a peak age of 35 years (range 20–60) and a female:male ratio of 10:1. The management is similar to CFS but the prognosis less optimistic.

Practice tips

- Always consider underlying psychological distress, especially a depressive disorder.
- Do not overlook a sleep disorder.
- Believe the patient's symptoms.
- Ask the patient what he or she believes may be the cause of the tiredness.
- Be careful of labelling a patient as having CFS.
- Restrict investigations to those that are more likely to be relevant, therapeutic and reassuring.

Patient education resources

Hand-out sheets from *Murtagh's Patient Education* 7th edition:

- Chronic fatigue syndrome

References

1. Marinker M, Watter CAH. The patient complaining of tiredness. In: Cormack J, Marinker M, Morrell D (eds). *Practice*. London: Kluwer Medical, 1982: Section 3.1.
2. Britt H, Henderson J, Charles J et al. General practice activity in Australia 2011–12. General Practice Series no. 31. Sydney: Sydney University Press, 2012.
3. Hickie IB et al. Sociodemographic and psychiatric correlates of fatigue in selected primary care settings. Med J Aust, 1996; 164: 585–8.
4. Jerrett WA. Lethargy in general practice. Practitioner, 1981; 225: 731–7.
5. National Institute for Health and Care Excellence. Chronic fatigue syndrome/myalgic encephalitis. London: NICE, 2007. Available at <www.nice.org.uk>.
6. Tennessen WW. *Signs and Symptoms in Paediatrics.* Philadelphia: Lippincott, 1988: 37–40.
7. Kirwan M, Armstrong D. Investigation of burnout in a sample of British general practitioners. Br J Gen Pract, 1995; 45: 259–60.
8. Sartorius N (Chair). *International Classification of Mental and Behavioural Disorders.* Problems related to life management. Burnout. Geneva, 2007; 273: 24v.
9. Ellard J. A note on burnout. Modern Medicine Australia, 1987; January: 32–5.
10. West CP et al. Intervention to prevent and reduce physician burnout: a systematic review and meta-analysis. Lancet, 2016; 388 (10057): 2272–81.
11. Loblay R, Stewart G (Convenors). Chronic fatigue syndrome: clinical practice guidelines 2002. RACGP/Med J Aust, 2002; 176 (Suppl.).
12. Papadakis MA, McPhee SJ. *Current Medical Diagnoses and Treatment* (56th edn). New York: McGraw-Hill Education, 2017; 37–9.
13. Fukuda K, Straus SE, Hickie I et al. The chronic fatigue syndrome: a comprehensive approach to its definition and study. International Chronic Fatigue Syndrome Study Group. Ann Intern Med, 1994; 121: 953–9.
14. Barton S. Chronic fatigue syndrome. In: *Clinical Evidence.* London: BMJ Publishing Group, 2001: 729–33.
15. Schwenk TL. Fibromyalgia and chronic fatigue syndrome: solving diagnostic and therapeutic dilemmas. Modern Medicine (US), 1992; 60: 50–60.

75 The unconscious patient

In whatever disease sleep is laborious, it is a deadly symptom; but if sleep does good, it is not deadly.

HIPPOCRATES

The state of arousal is determined by the function of the central reticular formation, which extends from the brain stem to the thalamus. Coma occurs when this centre is damaged by a metabolic abnormality or by an invasive lesion that compresses this centre. Coma is also caused by damage to the cerebral cortex.[1]

The word 'coma' is derived from the Greek *koma,* which means deep sleep. The deeply unconscious patient is not in a deep sleep. Coma is best defined as 'lack of self-awareness'.[2]

The various levels of consciousness are summarised in TABLE 75.1; the levels vary from consciousness, which means awareness of oneself and the surroundings in a state of wakefulness,[3] to coma, which is a state of unrousable unresponsiveness. Rather than using these broad terms in clinical practice it is preferable to describe the actual state of the patient in a sentence.

Key facts and checkpoints

- Always consider hypoglycaemia or opioid overdose in any unconscious patient, especially of unknown background.
- If a patient is unconscious and cyanosed, consider upper airway obstruction until proved otherwise.
- The commonest causes of unconsciousness encountered in general practice are reflex syncope, especially postural hypotension, concussion and cerebrovascular accidents (CVAs). The main causes are presented in TABLE 75.2.
- Do not allow the person who accompanies the unconscious patient to leave until all relevant details have been obtained.
- Record the degree of coma as a baseline to determine improvement or deterioration.

Urgent attention

The initial contact with the unconscious patient is invariably sudden and dramatic and demands immediate action, which should take only seconds to minutes. The primary objective is to keep the patient alive until the cause is determined and possible remedial action taken.[3]

Table 75.1 The five conscious levels

	State	Clinical features	Simplified classification
↑	1 Consciousness	Aware and wakeful	Awake
Degree of consciousness	2 Clouded consciousness	Reduced awareness and wakefulness 'Alcohol effect' Confusion Drowsiness	Confused
	3 Stupor	Unconscious Deep-sleep-like state Arousal with vigorous stimuli	Responds to shake and shout
	4 Semicomatose	Unconscious (deeper) Responds only to painful stimuli (sternal rubbing with knuckles) without arousing	Responds to pain
↓	5 Coma	Deeply unconscious Unrousable and unresponsive	Unresponsive coma

Table 75.2 Main causes of loss of consciousness

Episodic causes—blackouts

Epilepsy
Orthostatic intolerance and syncope
Drop attacks
Cardiac arrhythmias (e.g. Stokes–Adams attacks)
Vertebrobasilar insufficiency
Psychogenic disorders, including hyperventilation
Breath-holding (children)
Silent myocardial infarction
Hypoxia

Coma

(COMA provides a useful mnemonic for four major groups[1] of causes of unconsciousness)

C = CO_2 narcosis: respiratory failure

O = Overdose of drugs:
- alcohol
- opioids
- tranquillisers and antidepressants
- carbon monoxide
- analgesics
- others

M = Metabolic:
- diabetes:
  - hypoglycaemia
  - ketoacidosis
- hypothyroidism
- hypopituitarism
- hepatic failure
- Addison disease
- kidney failure (uraemia)
- others

A = Apoplexy:
- intracerebral haemorrhage
- haematoma: subdural or extradural
- head injury
- cerebral tumour
- cerebral abscess

Infratentorial (posterior fossa):
- pressure from above
- cerebellar tumour
- brain-stem infarct/haemorrhage
- Wernicke encephalopathy

Meningismus (neck stiffness):
- subarachnoid haemorrhage
- meningitis

Other:
- encephalitis
- overwhelming infection

Trauma

History

A history can be obtained from relatives, friends, witnesses, ambulance officers or others. The setting in which the patient is found is important. Evidence of discs or cards identifying an illness such as diabetes or epilepsy should be searched for. Is there a known history of hypertension, heart disease, respiratory disease or psychiatric illness?

Questions to be considered[4]

- Is the patient diabetic?
  Does the patient have insulin injections?
  Has the patient had an infection?
  Has the patient been eating properly?
- Is drug overdose possible?
  Has the patient been depressed?
  Has the patient experienced recent stress or personal 'mishaps'?
  Has the patient been on any medications?
- Is opioid usage possible in this patient?
  Are the presenting circumstances unusual?
- Is epilepsy possible?
  Was twitching in the limbs observed?
  Did the patient pass urine or faeces?
- Is head injury possible?
  Has the patient been in a recent accident?
  Has the patient complained of headache?
- Has a stroke or subarachnoid haemorrhage occurred?
  Has the patient a history of hypertension?
  Did the patient complain of a severe headache?
  Has the patient complained of weakness of the limbs?
- Has the patient bitten the tongue?

Examination

General features requiring assessment:

- breathing pattern:
  - Cheyne–Stokes respiration (periodic respiration) = cerebral dysfunction
  - ataxic respiration: shallow irregular respiration – brain stem lesion
  - Kussmaul respiration: deep rapid hyperventilation = metabolic acidosis
- breath: characteristic odours may be a feature of alcohol, diabetes, uraemia and hepatic coma
- level of consciousness: degree of coma (see TABLE 75.1); the Glasgow coma scale

(see TABLE 75.3) is frequently used as a guide to the conscious state
- skin features: look for evidence of injection sites (drug addicts, diabetics) and snake bite marks, colour (cyanosis, purpura, jaundice, rashes, hyperpigmentation) and texture
- circulation
- pulse oximetry
- temperature: consider infection such as meningitis and hyperpyrexia if raised and hypothermia (e.g. hypothyroidism) if low
- hydration: dehydration may signify conditions such as a high fever with infections, uraemia, hyperglycaemic coma

75

Examination	Action
Is the patient breathing?	If not, clear airway and ventilate.
Note chest wall movement.	Perform cardiopulmonary resuscitation if necessary.
Check pulse and pupils.	Consider naloxone.
Is there evidence of trauma?	Consider extradural haematoma.
Is the patient hypoglycaemic?	Consider glucometer estimation of blood sugar.
Evidence of diabetes (discs, etc.)	
Are vital functions present yet immediate correctable causes eliminated?	Place in coma position.

Examination of the head and neck[3,4]

The following should be considered:

- facial asymmetry
- the skull and neck: palpate for evidence of trauma and neck rigidity
- eyes, pupils and ocular fundi: look for constricted pupils in opioid overdose
- tongue
- nostrils and ears
- auscultation of the skull

Examination of the limbs

Consider:

- injection marks (drug addicts, diabetics)
- tone of the limbs by lifting and dropping (e.g. flaccid limbs with early hemiplegia)
- reaction of limbs to painful stimuli
- reflexes—tendon reflexes and plantar response

Table 75.3 Glasgow coma scale

	Score
Eye opening (E)	
Spontaneous opening	4
To verbal command	3
To pain	2
No response	1
Verbal response (V)	
Orientated and converses	5
Disoriented and converses	4
Inappropriate words	3
Incomprehensible sounds	2
No response	1
Motor response (M)	
Obeys verbal command	
Response to painful stimuli	6
Localises pain	5
Withdraws from pain stimuli	4
Abnormal flexion	3
Extensor response	2
No response	1
Coma score = E + V + M	
Minimum 3	
Maximum 15	
If 8–10: take care—monitor the airway	

General examination of the body

This should include assessment of the pulses and blood pressure.

Urine examination

Catheterisation of the bladder may be necessary to obtain urine. Check the urine for protein, sugar and ketones.

Diagnosing the hysterical 'unconscious' patient

One of the most puzzling problems in emergency medicine is how to diagnose the unconscious patient caused by a conversion reaction (hysteria). These patients really experience their symptoms (as opposed to the pretending patient) and resist most normal stimuli, including painful stimuli.

Method

- Hold the patient's eye or eyes open with your fingers and note the reaction to light.

- Now hold a mirror over the eye and watch closely for pupillary reaction. The pupil should constrict with accommodation from the patient looking at his or her own image.

Investigations

Appropriate investigations depend on the clinical assessment. The following is a checklist.

- Blood tests:
  - All patients: blood sugar; urea and electrolytes
  - Selected patients: FBE; blood gases; liver function tests; blood alcohol; serum cortisol; thyroid function tests; serum digoxin
- Pulse oximetry
- Urine tests:
  - a urine specimen is obtained by catheterisation
  - test for glucose and albumin
  - keep the specimen for drug screening
- Stomach contents: aspiration of stomach contents for analysis
- Radiology: CT or MRI scan are the investigations of choice (if available). If unavailable, X-ray of the skull may be helpful.
- Cerebrospinal fluid: lumbar puncture, necessary with neck stiffness, has risks in the comatose patient. A preliminary CT scan is necessary to search for coning of the cerebellum. If clear, the lumbar puncture should be safe and will help to diagnose subarachnoid haemorrhage and meningitis.
- Electroencephalograph
- ECG; look for ↑ QT interval, etc.

Blackouts—episodic loss of consciousness

Episodic or transient loss of consciousness is a common problem. The important causes of blackout are presented in TABLE 75.4. The history is important to determine whether the patient is describing a true blackout or episodes of dizziness, weakness or some other sensation.

The clinical features of various types of blackouts are summarised in TABLE 75.4.

Epilepsy

Epilepsy is the commonest cause of blackouts. There are various types, the most dramatic being the tonic–clonic seizure in which patients have sudden loss of consciousness without warning. See CHAPTERS 54 and 84.

The typical features (in order) of a tonic–clonic convulsion are:

- aura (sensory or psychological feelings)
- initial rigid tonic phase (up to 60 seconds)
- convulsion (clonic phase) (seconds to minutes)
- mild coma or drowsiness (15 minutes to several hours)—postictal confusion

Associated features:

- cyanosis, then heavy 'snoring' breathing
- eyes rolling 'back into head'
- ± tongue biting
- ± incontinence of urine or faeces

75

It should be noted that sphincter incontinence is not firmly diagnostic of epilepsy. In less severe episodes the patient may fall without observable twitching of the limbs.[5]

In atonic epilepsy, which occurs in those with tonic–clonic epilepsy, the patient falls to the ground and is unconscious for only a brief period.

Orthostatic intolerance and syncope

In syncope there is a transient loss of consciousness but with warning symptoms and rapid return of alertness following a brief period of unconsciousness (seconds to 3 minutes). The three main syndromes that are outlined in CHAPTER 54 are reflex syncope, postural orthostatic tachycardia syndrome and autonomic failure.

Reflex syncope

Relevant features of reflex syncope or vasovagal or common faint (see TABLE 75.4):

- occurs with standing or, less commonly, sitting
- warning feelings of dizziness, faintness or true vertigo
- nausea, hot and cold skin sensations
- fading hearing or blurred vision
- sliding to ground (rather than heavy full-length fall)
- rapid return of consciousness
- pallor and sweating and bradycardia
- often trigger factors (e.g. emotional upset, pain)

75

Table 75.4 Clinical features of blackouts

Cause	Precipitants	Subjective onset	Observation	Recovery
Reflex syncope	Posture Stress Haemorrhage Micturition	Warning of feeling 'faint', 'distant', 'clammy, sweaty'	Very pale Sweating	Gradual Feels 'terrible' Fatigue Nausea
Cardiac syncope including POTS syndrome	Various	May be palpitations	Pale	Rapid May be flushing
Autonomic syncope	Postural change orthostasis, food alcohol	Warning (feels faint)	Pale	Rapid
Respiratory syncope	Cough Weight-lifting 'Trumpet playing'	Warning (feels faint)	Pale	Rapid
Carotid sinus syncope	Carotid pressure (e.g. tight collar + turning neck) Postendarterectomy	Warning (feels faint)	Pale	Rapid
Migrainous syncope	Foods Stress Sleep deprivation	Scotomas	Pale	Nausea and vomiting Throbbing headache
Epilepsy	Stress Sleep deprivation Alcohol withdrawal Infection Menstruation Drug non-compliance	Aura with complex partial seizures (CPS)	Automatism (e.g. fidgeting, lip smacking) with CPS	Slow Confused

The patient invariably remembers the onset of fainting. Most syncope is of the benign vasomotor type and tends to occur in young people, especially when standing still (e.g. choir boys). It is the main cause of repeated fainting attacks.

The treatment is to avoid precipitating causes (e.g. prolonged standing, especially in the sun) and bend forwards with the head down or lie down with premonitory signs. 'Smelling salts' (ammonium carbonate) can be carried and used in these circumstances.

Other forms of syncope

Micturition syncope

This uncommon event may occur after micturition in older men, especially during the night when they leave a warm bed and stand to void. The cause appears to be peripheral vasodilatation associated with reduction of venous return from straining.

Cough syncope

Severe coughing can result in obstruction of venous return with subsequent blackout. This is also the mechanism of blackouts with breath-holding attacks.

Carotid sinus syncope

This problem is caused by pressure on a hypersensitive carotid sinus (e.g. in some elderly patients who lose consciousness when their neck is touched).

Effort syncope

Syncope on exertion is due to obstructive cardiac disorders, such as aortic stenosis and hypertrophic obstructive cardiomyopathy.

Choking

Sudden collapse can follow choking. Examples include the so-called 'cafe coronary' or 'barbecue coronary' when the patient, while eating meat, suddenly becomes cyanosed, is speechless and grasps the throat. This is caused by inhaling a large bolus of meat that obstructs the larynx. To avoid death, immediate relief of obstruction is necessary. An emergency treatment is the Heimlich manoeuvre, whereby the patient is grasped from behind around the abdomen and a forceful squeeze applied to try to eject the food. If this fails, the foreign body may have to be manually removed from the throat.

Drop attacks

Drop attacks are episodes of 'blackouts' in which the patient suddenly falls to the ground and then immediately gets up again. They involve sudden attacks of weakness in the legs. Although there is some doubt about whether loss of consciousness has occurred, most patients cannot remember the process of falling. Drop attacks occur typically in middle-aged women and are considered to be brain-stem disturbances producing sudden changes in tone in the lower limbs. Other causes of drop attacks include vertebrobasilar insufficiency, Parkinson disease and epilepsy.[5]

Cardiac arrhythmias

Stokes–Adams attacks (see CHAPTER 70) and cardiac syncope are manifestations of recurrent episodes of loss of consciousness, especially in the elderly, caused by cardiac arrhythmias. These arrhythmias include complete heart block, sick sinus syndrome and ventricular tachycardia. The blackout is sudden with the patient falling straight to the ground without warning and without convulsive movements. The patient goes pale at first and then flushed.

Twenty-four-hour ambulatory cardiac monitoring may be necessary to confirm the diagnosis.

Patients with aortic stenosis are prone to have exercise-induced blackouts. Consider the prolonged QT interval syndrome in all age groups when the person presents with dizziness or blackouts.

Vertebrobasilar insufficiency

Loss of consciousness can occur rarely with vertebrobasilar insufficiency (VBI) transient ischaemic attack. Typical preceding symptoms of VBI include dysphasia, dysarthria, vertigo, vomiting, hemisensory loss, ataxia and transient global amnesia.

Hypoglycaemia

Hypoglycaemia can be difficult to recognise but must be considered as it can vary from a feeling of malaise and lightheadedness to loss of consciousness, sometimes with a convulsion. There are usually preliminary symptoms of hunger, sweating, shaking or altered behaviour. Hypoglycaemic attacks are usually related to diabetes and can occur with oral hypoglycaemics as well as insulin. Causes of hypoglycaemia are presented in TABLE 75.5. Refer to CHAPTER 128.

Table 75.5 Causes of hypoglycaemia (adults)
Diabetes-related including insulin and oral hypoglycaemics
Drugs (e.g. quinine, salicylates, pentamidine)
Alcohol
Fasting
Tumours (e.g. insulinomas)
Addison disease
Hypopituitarism
Liver disease
Hypoglycaemic artefacta
Pregnancy
Post-gastrectomy
Gastric 'dumping' syndrome
Autoimmune: antibodies to insulin or insulin receptors

75

Head injuries and unconsciousness

Some non-life-threatening head injuries are sufficiently serious to cause significant loss of consciousness and retrograde amnesia. The clinical terms used to describe brain injury of concussion, contusion and laceration simply indicate minor to major degrees of a similar injury. Severe individual cases of the above can certainly result in fatal outcomes.

Concussion[6]

Concussion is a transient disturbance of neurological function induced by head injury and resulting in no persistent abnormal neurological signs. There may or may not be brief loss of consciousness. The old definition of loss of consciousness with eventual recovery applies only to more severe forms of concussion. The features of the various grades of concussion are shown in TABLE 75.6.

Take extra care in children who are more sensitive to head injury and need to be kept home for at least 3 days.

Post-concussion syndrome

Occasionally, a person who has an episode of concussion has persistence of headaches and dizziness for a number of weeks. Poor memory and concentration

Table 75.6 Classification of concussion

Grade	Clinical features
Mild (grade 1)	Stunned or dazed Sensorium clears in <60 seconds No post-traumatic amnesia ± Loss of consciousness
Moderate (grade 2)	Stunned or dazed Sensorium cloudy >60 seconds Headache Amnesia <60 minutes ± Loss of consciousness
Severe (grade 3)	Sensorium cloudy >60 seconds Irritable Persistent headache Unsteady gait ± Loss of consciousness

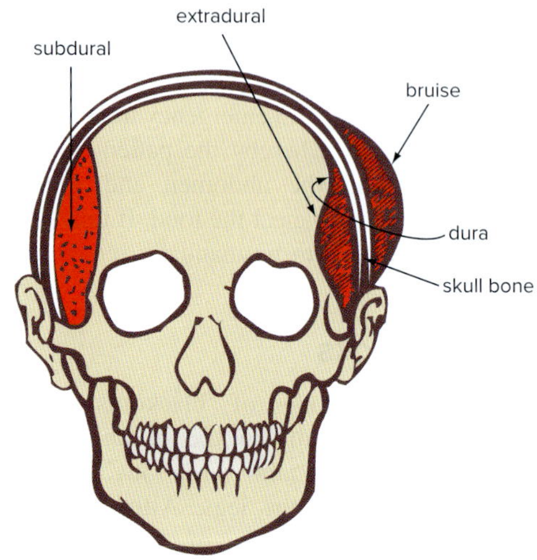

FIGURE 75.1 Illustration of sites of subdural and extradural haematomas in relation to the dura, skull and brain

and sluggish decision-making indicate impaired mental capacity. Patients with this problem should be investigated with neuropsychological testing and CT scanning or MRI of the brain.

Links to sports concussion tests[7]

- Pocket Concussion Recognition Tool
- Sports Concussion Assessment Tool 5th edn (SCAT5)

Extradural haematoma

This life-threatening head injury is caused by arterial bleeding between the skull bone and dura mater (see FIG. 75.1). Following injury there may be a short lucid interval followed by loss of consciousness. The patient is restless, confused, irritable (see FIG. 75.2), has severe headaches and develops neurological signs such as seizures, ipsilateral pupil dilatation and facial weakness. A skull X-ray and CT scan should demonstrate the haematoma. Lumbar puncture is contraindicated. Urgent decompression of the haematoma is required.

Subdural haematoma

This is due to a venous bleed between the dura and the arachnoid. It follows injury, which may be seemingly trivial, especially in the elderly, and may be acute, subacute and chronic. Consider it in a person with personality change, slowness and unsteadiness of movement, headache, irritability and fluctuating conscious level. A CT scan or MRI should reveal the haematoma and/or a midline shift. Neurological referral is urgent.

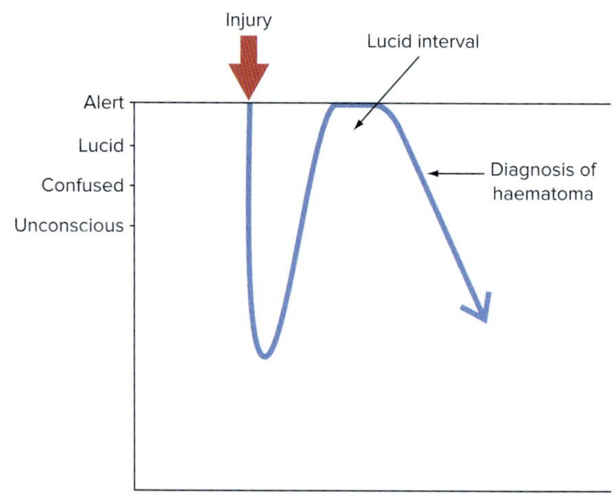

FIGURE 75.2 Classic conscious states leading to extradural haematoma after injury

Psychogenic factors

Psychogenic factors leading to blackouts represent a diagnostic dilemma, especially if occurring in patients with tonic–clonic epilepsy. If the attacks are witnessed by the practitioner then the possibility of functional origin can be determined.

Hysterical blackouts or fits are not uncommon and have to be differentiated from hyperventilation. It is unusual for hyperventilation to cause unconsciousness but it is possible to get clouding of consciousness, especially if the patient is administered oxygen.

Other features that suggest psychogenic rather than organic factors are:

- labile affect
- rapidly changing levels of consciousness
- well-articulated speech
- bizarre thought control

The patient found unconscious[7]

Most likely causes to consider

- drug overdose, including alcohol
- head injury
- postictal state (epilepsy or CVA)
- hypoglycaemia or ketoacidosis
- subarachnoid haemorrhage
- respiratory failure
- hypotension, including cardiac arrhythmias or myocardial infarction
- infection, e.g. meningitis
- psychogenic

Basic investigations

- oxygen saturation
- blood glucose
- urine or blood drug profile
- brain CT scan
- lumbar puncture (CT scan permitting)
- routine blood chemistry
- ECG

Initial management of the unconscious patient

The first principle of management of a person found unconscious is to keep the patient alive by maintaining the airway and the circulation. The basic management essentials are summarised in TABLE 75.7.

Before embarking on a secondary survey always consider giving the 'coma cocktail' (also called TONG[2]), which refers to the combination of:

T = **T**hiamine	100 mg IM or IV
O = **O**xygenation	
N = **N**aloxone	0.1–0.2 mg IV
G = **G**lucose	i.e. 50 mL, 50% dextrose

The rapid administration of these agents should be considered for any patient[3,8] with an altered level of consciousness because they may lessen or reverse metabolic insult to the brain. Some emergency physicians recommend adding flumazenil to the cocktail.

Table 75.7	Basic management essentials
Keep patient alive (maintain airway and circulation)	
Get history from witnesses	
Examine patient	
Give 'coma cocktail' (TONG)	
Take blood (for investigations)	
CT scan (if diagnosis doubtful)	

In the presence of hypoventilation, constricted pupils[10] or circumstantial evidence of opioid use, naloxone (the specific opiate antagonist) should be given intravenously. If there is no response the patient should be intubated before further naloxone is given. Use a nasogastric tube to prevent acute gastric dilatation.

Catheterise to relieve urinary distension, send a urine sample for micro and culture, pregnancy test and drug screen.

Use of flumazenil

Flumazenil is a specific benzodiazepine antagonist and may have an important use in the assessment of the unconscious patient. It can have a dramatic effect on benzodiazepine overdosage. After an initial dose of 0.2 mg IV, 0.3–0.5 mg boluses should be given every 1–2 minutes with caution until a response is observed.[9]

Opioid (heroin) overdose

A known overdose patient should be treated initially with both IV and IM naloxone:

- naloxone 0.4 mg IV (repeat in 3 minutes if necessary)
- naloxone 0.4 mg IM (to maintain cover)

Practice tips[2]

- The hypotensive patient is bleeding until proved otherwise.
- The presence of a head injury should not prevent rigorous resuscitation of the hypotensive patient.
- Always suspect cervical injury in the presence of patients who are victims of time-critical trauma.
- Tachypnoea is a sign of inadequate oxygenation and not a sign of central nerve damage.
- Always suspect opioid overdosage in the 'unknown' patient brought in with an altered conscious state.
- Consider administration of TONG—the 'coma cocktail'.

75

References

1 Talley N, O'Connor S. *Clinical Examination* (3rd edn). Sydney: MacLennan & Petty, 1996: 414.
2 Wassertheil J. Management of neurological emergencies. Melbourne: Monash University, Update for GPs: course notes, 1996: 1–10.
3 Kumar PJ, Clark ML. *Clinical Medicine* (5th edn). London: Bailliere Tindall, 2003: 1161–2.
4 Davis A, Bolin T, Ham J. *Symptom Analysis and Physical Diagnosis* (2nd edn). Sydney: Pergamon Press, 1990: 276–9.
5 Kincaid-Smith P, Larkins R, Whelan G. *Problems in Clinical Medicine*. Sydney: MacLennan & Petty, 1990: 340–7.
6 Brukner P, Khan K. *Clinical Sports Medicine* (4th edn). Sydney: McGraw-Hill, 2012: 272–87.
7 Elkington LJ, Hughes DC. Australian Medical Association position statement on concussion in sport. Med J Aust, 2017; 206 (1): 46–50.
8 Brown FT. *Emergency Medicine: Diagnosis and Management*. Oxford: Butterworth Heinemann, 2004: 43–6.
9 Webster V. Trauma. Melbourne: RACGP Check Program 293, 1996: 3–14.
10 McGirr J, McDonagh T. Management of acute poisoning. Current Therapeutics, 1995; 36 (5): 51–9.

Urinary disorders

As men draw near the common goal,
Can anything be sadder
Than he who, master of his soul,
Is servant to his bladder?

ANONYMOUS, *SPECULUM*, 1938

Disturbances of micturition are a common problem in general practice, with an annual incidence of about 20 per 1000 patients at risk.[1] Such disturbances include dysuria, frequency of micturition, difficulty or inability to initiate micturition, stress incontinence and haematuria. These symptoms are three times as common in women as in men.[1] The combination of dysuria and frequency is the most common of the symptoms with an incidence of about 14 per 1000 patients and a female:male ratio of 5:1.[1]

Among children and the elderly, the patient may complain of urinary incontinence unassociated with stress. However, with the exception of enuresis (CHAPTER 91), disturbances of micturition are uncommon in children.

Dysuria and frequency

Dysuria, or difficult and/or painful micturition, which is characterised mainly by urethral and suprapubic discomfort, indicates mucosal inflammation of the lower genitourinary tract (i.e. the urethra, bladder or prostate). The passage of urine across inflamed mucosa causes pain. Frequency can vary from being negligible to extreme. It can be 'habit frequency' or associated with anxiety, which is typically long term and worse with stress and cold weather. In these conditions urinalysis is normal. Sometimes haematuria and systemic symptoms can accompany dysuria and frequency.

A summary of the diagnostic strategy model for dysuria is presented in TABLE 76.1.

Key facts and checkpoints[1,2]

- Strangury = difficult and painful micturition with associated spasm.
- Inflammation usually results in the frequent passage of small amounts of urine and a sense of urgency.
- Urethritis usually causes pain at the onset of micturition.
- Cystitis usually causes pain at the end of micturition.
- Suprapubic discomfort is a feature of bladder infection (cystitis).
- Vesicocolonic fistulas (e.g. prostatic cancer) cause severe dysuria, pneumaturia and foul-smelling urine.
- Dysuria and frequency are most common in women aged 15–44 years.
- They are four times more common in sexually active women.
- Vaginitis is an important cause and must be considered.
- Dysuria and discomfort is a common feature of postmenopausal syndrome, due to atrophic urethritis. The urethra and lower bladder are oestrogen-dependent.
- Unexplained dysuria could be a pointer to *Chlamydia* urethritis.
- Urinary infection and other disorders can be quite asymptomatic.

Is it really a urinary tract infection?

Although UTIs account for the majority of cases of dysuria in women it must be remembered that vaginitis and postmenopausal atrophic vaginitis can cause dysuria (see FIG. 76.1). Vaginitis is the most common cause of dysuria in the adolescent age group and is a relatively common cause of dysuria in family practice, estimated at around 15%. Postmenopausal oestrogen deficiency is estimated at 5–10%.[3] In the latter it is worthwhile prescribing oestrogen, either topically or systemically. Acute bacterial cystitis accounts for about 40% of causes of dysuria.

The dysuria associated with vaginitis may be described as burning 'on the outside' with the discomfort usually felt at the beginning or end of micturition. If

76

Table 76.1 Dysuria: diagnostic strategy model
Probability diagnosis UTI esp. cystitis (female) Urethritis Urethral syndrome (female) Vaginitis
Serious disorders not to be missed Neoplasia: • bladder • prostate • urethra Severe infections: • gonorrhoea • NSU • genital herpes Reactive arthritis Calculi (e.g. bladder)
Pitfalls (often missed) Menopause syndrome Adenovirus urethritis Prostatitis Foreign bodies in lower urinary tract (LUT) Acute pelvic or retrocaecal appendicitis Acidic urine Acute fever Interstitial cystitis Urethral caruncle/diverticuli Vaginal prolapse Obstruction: • benign prostatic hyperplasia • urethral stricture • phimosis • meatal stenosis
Seven masquerades checklist Depression Diabetes Drugs UTI
Is the patient trying to tell me something? Consider psychosexual problems, anxiety and hypochondriasis.

vaginitis is suspected, a pelvic examination should be carried out to inspect the genitalia and obtain swabs.[3]

Urethral syndrome

Also known as chronic sterile inflammatory disorder and abacterial cystitis, it presents with lower urinary tract symptoms (LUTS) or symptoms of urethritis. Others refer to it as 'painful bladder syndrome' or interstitial cystitis. It affects 20–30% of adults, mainly female. Management, which is difficult, is supportive.

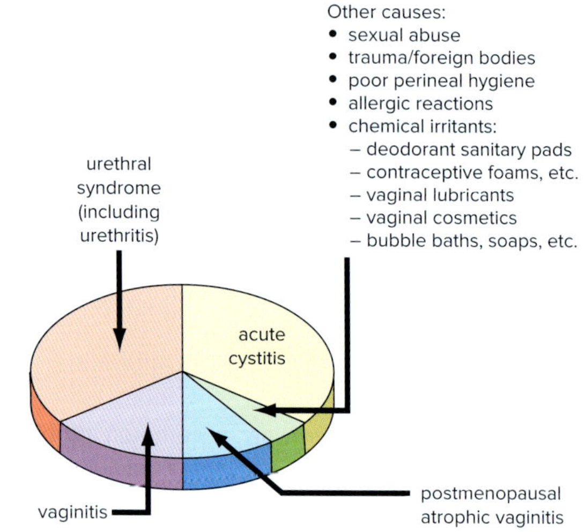

FIGURE 76.1 Relative causes of dysuria in women

The clinical approach

History

It is important to determine whether dysuria is really genitourinary in origin and not attributable to functional disorders, such as psychosexual problems. Disturbances of micturition are uncommon in the young male and if present suggest venereal infection.

Key questions

- Could you describe the discomfort?
- What colour is your urine?
- Does it have a particular odour?
- Have you noticed a discharge?
- If so, could it be sexually acquired?
- Do you find intercourse painful or uncomfortable (women)?
- Have you any fever, sweats or chills?

Examination

The general inspection and examination should include measurement of the basic parameters of pulse, temperature and blood pressure. The possibility of underlying kidney disease, especially in the presence of an obstructive component, should be kept in mind.

Abdominal palpation is important with a focus on the loins and suprapubic areas. The possibility of sexually transmitted diseases should also be considered and vaginal examination of the female and rectal and genital examination in the male may be appropriate. In the menopausal female, a dry atrophic urethral opening, a urethral caruncle or urethral prolapse may give the clue to this important and neglected cause of dysuria.

Investigations

Basic investigations include:

- dipstick testing of urine
- microscopy and culture (midstream specimen of urine, or suprapubic puncture in children), and possibly urethral swabs or first pass urine for sexually transmitted infections

Further investigations depend on initial findings and referral for detailed investigation will be necessary if the primary cause cannot be found.

The management of urinary tract infection is presented in CHAPTER 25.

Haematuria

Haematuria is the presence of blood in the urine and can vary from frank bleeding (macroscopic) to the microscopic detection of red cells. Haematuria can occur in a wide variety of disorders but a careful history and examination can often lead to the source of the bleeding and help with the selection of investigations. It is often a sign of a serious underlying disorder.

Key facts and checkpoints

- Macroscopic haematuria is the presence of blood visible to the naked eye. It is always abnormal except in menstruating women.
- Small amounts of blood (1 mL/1000 mL urine) can produce macroscopic haematuria.
- Microscopic haematuria is the presence of blood in the urine that can be detected only by microscopic or chemical methods.
- Microscopic haematuria includes the presence of red blood cells (RBC) >8000 per mL of urine (phase contrast microscopy) or >2000 per mL of urine (light microscopy) representing the occasional RBC on microscopic examination.
- Joggers and athletes engaged in very vigorous exercise can develop transient microscopic haematuria.
- Microscopic (asymptomatic haematuria) can be classified as either:
  - glomerular (from kidney parenchyma): common causes are IgA nephropathy and thin membrane disease[4]

  or
  - non-glomerular (urological): the common causes are bladder cancer, benign prostate hyperplasia and urinary calculi
- Common sources of macroscopic haematuria are the bladder, urethra, prostate and kidney.[5]
- Macroscopic haematuria occurs in 70% of people with bladder cancer and 40% with kidney cancer.[5]
- Common urological cancers that cause haematuria are the bladder (70%), kidney (17%), kidney pelvis or ureter (7%) and prostate (5%).[6]
- It is important to exclude kidney damage, so patients should have blood pressure, urinary protein and plasma creatinine levels measured as a baseline.
- All patients presenting with macroscopic haematuria or recurrent microscopic haematuria require judicious investigation, which may involve both radiological investigation of the upper urinary system and visualisation of the lower urinary system to detect or exclude pathology.
- The key radiological investigation is the intravenous urogram (pyelogram), unless there is a history of iodine allergy, severe asthma or other contraindications, when ultrasound is the next choice.

The clinical approach

History

Is it really haematuria? In many patients the underlying disorder may be suspected from a detailed enquiry about associated urinary symptoms. The presence of blood can be verified rapidly by microscopy so that red discolouration due to haemolysis or red food dye can be discounted.

The time relationship of bleeding is useful because, as a general rule, haematuria occurring in the first part of the stream suggests a urethral or prostatic lesion, while terminal haematuria suggests bleeding from the bladder. Uniform haematuria has no localising features.

The possibility of sexually acquired urethritis should be kept in mind. It is most unusual for haematuria to cause anaemia unless it is massive. Massive haematuria is a feature of radiation cystitis.

Painful haematuria is suggestive of infection, urethral caruncle, calculi or kidney infarction, while painless haematuria is commonly associated with infection, trauma, tumours or polycystic kidneys. Loin pain can occur as a manifestation of nephritis and may be a feature of bleeding in cancer of the kidney or polycystic kidney.

A drug history is relevant, especially with anticoagulants and cyclophosphamide. A diet history should also be considered.

It is worth noting that large prostatic veins, secondary to prostatic enlargement located at the bladder neck, may rupture when a man strains to urinate.

A summary of the diagnostic strategy model for haematuria is presented in TABLE 76.2.

Key questions

- Have you had an injury such as a blow to the loin, pelvis or genital area?
- Have you noticed whether the redness is at the start or end of your stream or throughout the stream?
- Have you noticed any bleeding elsewhere, such as bruising of the skin or nose bleed?
- Have you experienced any pain in the loin or abdomen?
- Have you noticed any burning or frequency of your urine?
- Have you had any problems with the flow of your urine?
- Have you been having large amounts of beetroot, red lollies or berries in your diet?
- Could your problem have been sexually acquired?
- Have you been overseas recently?
- What is your general health like?
- Have you been aware of any other symptoms?
- Do you engage in strenuous sports such as jogging?
- Have you had any kidney problems in the past?
- Are you taking blood-thinning drugs?

76

Examination

The general examination should include looking for signs of a bleeding tendency and anaemia, and recording the parameters of temperature, blood pressure and the pulse (see FIG. 76.2). The heart should be assessed to exclude atrial fibrillation or infective endocarditis with emboli to the kidney, and the chest should be examined for a possible pleural effusion associated with perinephric or kidney infections.

The abdomen should be examined for evidence of a palpable enlarged kidney or spleen. The different clinical findings for an enlarged left kidney and spleen are shown in TABLE 76.3. Kidney enlargement may be due to kidney tumour, hydronephrosis, or polycystic disease. Splenomegaly suggests the possibility of a bleeding disorder.

The suprapubic region should be examined for evidence of bladder tenderness or enlargement. In men the prostate should be examined rectally to detect benign or malignant enlargement or tenderness from prostatitis.

Table 76.2 Haematuria: diagnostic strategy model

Probability diagnosis Infection: • cystitis/urethrotrigonitis (female) • urethritis (male) • prostatitis (male) Calculi—kidney, ureteric, bladder
Serious disorders not to be missed Cardiovascular: • kidney infarction • kidney vein thrombosis • prostatic varices Neoplasia: • kidney tumour • urothelial: bladder, kidney, pelvis, ureter • prostate cancer Severe infections: • infective endocarditis • kidney tuberculosis • acute glomerulonephritis • blackwater fever IgA nephropathy Kidney papillary necrosis Other kidney disease e.g. polycystic kidneys
Pitfalls (often missed) Urethral prolapse/caruncle Pseudohaematuria (e.g. beetroot, porphyria) Haemorrhagic cystitis Benign prostatic hyperplasia Trauma: blunt or penetrating Foreign bodies Bleeding disorders Exercise Radiation cystitis Menstrual contamination *Rarities:* • hydronephrosis • Henoch–Schönlein purpura • bilharzia • schistosomiasis • polycystic kidneys • kidney cysts • endometriosis (bladder) • systemic vasculitides
Seven masquerades checklist Drugs (cytotoxics, anticoagulants) UTI
Is the patient trying to tell me something? Consider artefactual haematuria.

In women a vaginal examination should be performed to search for possible pelvic masses. The urethral meatus should be inspected to exclude a

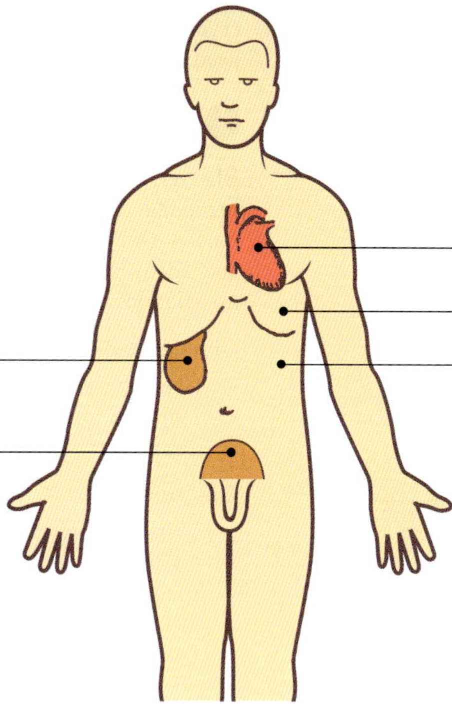

FIGURE 76.2 Features to consider in the physical examination of the patient with haematuria

Table 76.3 Differences between spleen and left kidney on abdominal examination

	Spleen	Left kidney
Palpable upper border	Impalpable	Palpable
Movement with inspiration	Inferomedial	Inferior
Notch	Yes	No
Ballotable	No	Yes
Percussion	Dull	Resonant (usually)
Friction rub	Possible	Not possible

urethral caruncle ('raspberry tumour') or urethral prolapse.

Investigations

It is important to identify the cause, especially if a possible sequel is impaired kidney function.

- Urinalysis by dipstick testing (e.g. Hemastix-affected derivatives—affected by vitamin C intake).
- Urine microscopy:
  - formed RBCs in true haematuria
  - red cell casts indicate glomerular bleeding
  - deformed (dysmorphic) red cells indicate glomerular bleeding
- Urinary culture: early culture is important because of the common association with infection and consideration of early treatment with antibiotics. If tuberculosis is suspected, three early morning urines should be cultured for tubercle bacilli.
- Urinary cytology: this test, performed on a urine sample, may be useful to detect malignancies of the bladder and lower tract but is usually negative with kidney cancer.
- Blood tests: appropriate screening tests include a full blood count, ESR and basic kidney function tests (urea and creatinine). If glomerulonephritis is suspected, antistreptolysin O titres and serum complement levels should be measured.
- Radiological techniques—available tests include:
  - intravenous urography (IVU); intravenous pyelogram (IVP)—the key investigation
  - ultrasound (less sensitive at detecting LUT abnormalities)
  - CT scanning

– kidney angiography
– retrograde pyelography
- Direct imaging techniques: these include urethroscopy, cystoscopy and ureteroscopy. In all patients, regardless of the IVU findings, cystoscopy is advisable.
- Kidney biopsy: indicated if glomerular disease is suspected, especially in the presence of dysmorphic red cells on microscopic examination.

Pseudohaematuria

Pseudohaematuria is red urine caused by pigments other than red blood cells that simply stain the culture red.

Causes include:

- anthocyanins in food (e.g. beetroot, berries)
- red-coloured confectionery
- porphyrins
- free haemoglobin (e.g. haemoglobinuria)
- myoglobin (red-black colour)
- drugs (e.g. pyridium, phenolphthalein—alkaline urine)

Exercise haematuria

Exercise or sports haematuria is the passage of a significant number of red cells in the urine during or immediately after heavy exercise. It has been recorded in a wide variety of athletes, including swimmers and rowers. Dipstick testing is usually positive in these athletes. Despite the theory that it is largely caused by the posterior wall of the bladder impacting repetitively on the base of the bladder during running, there are other possible factors and glomerular disease must be excluded in the athlete with regular haematuria, especially if dysmorphic red cells are found on microscopy.

Artefactual haematuria

Macroscopic haematuria is a common presenting ploy of people with Munchausen syndrome and pethidine addicts simulating kidney colic. If suspected, it is wise to get these people to pass urine in the presence of an appropriate witness before examining the urine.

Urethral caruncle

This is a benign granulomatous tumour about the size of a pea in the distal urethra. Almost exclusive to post-menopausal women, it is very tender and bleeds easily. The main symptom is haematuria. It may require cystoscopy and biopsy for diagnosis. Treatment includes warm salt baths and oestrogen creams. Otherwise obliteration by laser vaporisation, cryotherapy or cautery or even surgical excision is used.

Bladder cancer[7]

Bladder cancer is the seventh most common malignancy, with 90% being transitional cell carcinomas. Other forms include squamous cell carcinoma and adenocarcinoma. Smoking is the most common association.

Clinical features

- Haematuria/microhaematuria
- Irritative symptoms: frequency, urgency, nocturia
- Dysuria

Diagnosis

- Urine cytology: three specimens
- Cystoscopy and biopsy
- Imaging of upper tracts: IVU, ultrasound, but CT IVU is the gold standard
- Differential diagnosis is haemorrhagic cystitis

Management

- Cease smoking (if applicable)
- Lifestyle attention
- Drink ample purified (no chlorine) water

Treatment depends on the staging and grading.

- The common carcinoma in situ is treated with intravesical BCG immunotherapy. This 6-week course and follow-up if necessary leads to 60–75% remission
- Other intravesical agents used include various cytotoxics (e.g. mitomycin C)
- Other treatments include surgery such as tumour resection plus intravesical agents, bladder resection (partial or total) and radio–chemotherapy.

Regular patient surveillance, which may be lifelong, is essential.

Glomerulonephritis[8]

Glomerulonephritis means kidney inflammation involving the glomeruli. It can be simply classified into:

- nephritic syndrome: oedema + hypertension + haematuria
- nephrotic syndrome: oedema + hypoalbuminaemia + proteinuria
- asymptomatic kidney disease

The main causes of glomerulonephritis–nephritic syndrome are:

- IgA nephropathy (commonest)
- thin glomerular basement membrane disease (has an AD genetic link)
- post-streptococcal glomerulonephritis
- systemic vasculitis
- others

IgA nephropathy

Typically presents as haematuria in a young male adult at the time of or within 1–2 days of a mucosal infection (usually throat, influenza or URTI) and persists for several days. Other presentations are as incidentally found microscopic haematuria or as previously unsuspected chronic kidney failure.

Due to deposition of IgA antibody complexes in the glomeruli, it runs a variable course, but prognosis is usually good. There is no specific treatment to date but immune suppression may be used. Refer suspected cases immediately. Diagnosis is by biopsy.

Acute post-streptococcal glomerulonephritis

Typically seen in children (>5 years), especially in Indigenous communities following GABHS throat infection or impetigo. Presents after a gap of 7–10 days or so.

Clinical features

- Irritable, lethargic, sick child
- Haematuria: discoloured urine ('Coke' urine)
- Peri-orbital oedema (may be legs, scrotum)
- Rapid weight gain (from oedema)
- Scanty urine output (oliguria)
- Hypertension → may be complications

Usual course

- Oliguria 2 days
- Oedema and hypertension 2–4 days
- Invariably resolves
- Good long-term prognosis

Diagnosis

- GABHS antigens
- Blood urea, creatinine, $C_{3\&4}$ (complement), ASOT, anti-DNase B

Treatment

- Hospital admission
- Bed rest
- Strict fluid balance chart
- Daily weighing
- Penicillin (if GABHS +ve)
- Fluid restriction
- Low protein, high carbohydrate, low salt diet
- Antihypertensives and diuretics (as necessary)

DxT discoloured urine + peri-orbital oedema + oliguria → post-streptococcal glomerulonephritis

Follow-up: monitor BP and kidney function. Regular urinalysis (microscopic haematuria may last for years).

Proteinuria

Proteinuria is an important and common sign of kidney disease. The protein can originate from the glomeruli, the tubules or the LUT. Healthy people, however, do excrete some protein in the urine, which can vary from day to day and hour to hour; hence the value of collecting it over 24 hours. While proteinuria can be benign, it always requires further investigation. Important causes of proteinuria are presented in TABLE 76.4.

76

Key facts and checkpoints[9]

- The amount of protein in the urine is normally less than 100 mg/24 hours.
- Greater than 300 mg/24 hours is abnormal in children and adults.
- Proteinuria >1 g/24 hours indicates a serious underlying disorder.
- If accompanied by dysmorphic haematuria or red cell casts, this tends to confirm glomerular origin.
- Routine dipstick testing will detect levels greater than 300 mg/24 hours only and thus has limitations.
- In diabetics, microalbuminuria is predictive of nephropathy and an indication for early blood pressure treatment.

Predictive levels

- **Proteinuria** >150–300 mg/day
- **Microalbuminuria** 30–300 mg/day
- **Macroalbuminuria** >300 mg/day

Table 76.4 Important causes of proteinuria

Transient
Contamination from vaginal secretions
Urinary tract infection
Pre-eclampsia
These all require exclusion and follow-up.
Kidney disease
Glomerulonephritis
Nephrotic syndrome
Congenital tubular disease, e.g.
• polycystic kidney
• kidney dysplasia
Acute tubular damage
Kidney papillary necrosis, e.g.
• analgesic nephropathy
• diabetic papillary necrosis
Overflow proteinuria, e.g.
• multiple myeloma
Systemic diseases affecting the glomeruli:
• diabetes mellitus
• hypertension
• SLE
• malignancy
• drugs (e.g. penicillamine, gold salts)
• amyloid
• vasculitides
No kidney disease
Orthostatic proteinuria
Exercise
Emotional stress
Fever
Cold exposure
Postoperative
Acute medical illness (e.g. heart failure)

If proteinuria is confirmed on repeated dipstick testing it should be measured more accurately by measuring daily albumin excretion with a 24-hour urine or the albumin creatinine ratio (ACR), which is preferred as it is more accurate and avoids costly 24-hour collections. Refer to CHAPTER 31. High values require referral for investigation. The minimum investigations are microurine and assessment of kidney function (eGFR). Nephrotic range proteinuria (>3 g/24 hours) is due to one or other form of glomerulonephritis in over 90% of patients.[8] Possible contamination from vaginal secretions or from a low UTI needs to be excluded.

Orthostatic proteinuria

Orthostatic proteinuria is the presence of significant proteinuria after the patient has been standing but is absent from specimens obtained following recumbency for several hours, such as an early morning specimen.

It occurs in 5–10% of people,[6] especially during their adolescent years. In the majority it is of no significance and eventually disappears without the development of significant kidney disease. However, in a small number the proteinuria can foreshadow serious kidney disease.

Diabetic microalbuminuria

The presence of protein in the urine is a sensitive marker of diabetic nephropathy, so regular screening for microalbuminuria in diabetics is regarded as an important predictor of nephropathy and other possible complications of diabetes. Dipstick testing for microalbuminuria is now available but more accurate measurement can be performed with radioimmunoassay techniques. The use of ACE inhibitors at the microalbuminuria stage may slow the development of overt nephropathy. The gold standard is a 24-hour collection.

Consequences of proteinuria

While proteinuria is usually simply a marker of kidney disease, heavy proteinuria in excess of 3 g/24 hours may have severe clinical consequences, including oedema, intravascular volume depletion, venous thromboembolism, hyperlipidaemia and malnutrition.

Minimal change glomerulonephritis is the commonest cause of the nephrotic syndrome in childhood and accounts for about 30% of adult nephrotic syndrome.[7] It is steroid responsive.

Nephrotic syndrome[8,9]

DxT proteinuria + generalised oedema + hypoalbuminaemia ➔ nephrotic syndrome

Nephrotic syndrome occurs at any age but is more common in children and has primary and secondary causes that require elucidation.

Clinical features

- Proteinuria >3 g/day (3–4[1] on dipstick)
- Swelling of eyelids and face
- Generalised oedema, especially peripheral oedema
- Hypoalbuminaemia <30 g/L
- Hypercholesterolaemia >4.5 mmol/L
- Waxy pallor
- Normal BP
- Dyspnoea
- Frothy urine

Predisposes to sepsis (e.g. peritonitis, pyelonephritis, thromboembolism).

Causes

- 1 in 3 (approx.):
  - systemic kidney disease (e.g. diabetes, SLE, amyloid)
- 2 in 3 (approx.):
  - idiopathic nephrotic syndrome (based on kidney biopsy)
  - minimal change disease (commonest)
  - focal glomerular sclerosis
  - membranous nephropathy
  - membranoproliferative glomerulonephritis
- Others: drugs, malignancy, infection, e.g. malaria

Treatment

- Referral to renal physician or unit
- Bed rest
- Diet: low fluid, high protein, low salt
- *Medication may include*
- Diuretics
- Prednisolone
- Phenoxymethylpenicillin
- Aspirin

URINARY INCONTINENCE

Definitions

Functional incontinence Loss of urine secondary to factors extrinsic to the urinary tract.

Nocturnal enuresis (or bed-wetting) Involuntary urine loss during sleep.

Overactive bladder (detrusor instability) The commonest cause of urge incontinence; synonymous with an irritable or unstable bladder; characterised by involuntary bladder contractions, resulting in a sudden urge to urinate.

Overflow incontinence Escape of urine following poor bladder emptying.

Stress incontinence The involuntary loss of urine on coughing, sneezing, straining or lifting, or any factor that suddenly increases intra-abdominal pressure.

Urge incontinence An urgent desire to void followed by involuntary loss of urine.

Urinary incontinence The involuntary loss of urine during the day or night.

Voiding dysfunction Includes urinary difficulties, detrusor instability and overflow incontinence.

Table 76.5 Types of incontinence and their implied causes

Type of incontinence	Likely cause
Simple stress incontinence (with cough/sneeze)	Sphincter incompetence
Urge incontinence Giggle incontinence Stress and urge incontinence Enuresis Complex stress incontinence (with exercise)	Unstable bladder, with or without sphincter weakness
Quiet dribble incontinence	Sphincter incompetence and unstable bladder or overflow
Continuous leakage	Fistula, ectopic ureter, patulous urethra
Reflex incontinence	Neuropathic bladder

A summary of the types of incontinence and their causes is presented in TABLE 76.5.

The basic requirements for continence are:

- adequate central and peripheral nervous function
- an intact urinary tract
- a compliant stable bladder
- a competent urethral sphincter
- efficient bladder emptying

Female urinary incontinence

Urinary leakage affects at least 37% of women in Australia.[11] Successful treatment depends on accurate assessment of the LUT storage and emptying functions. The most common contributing factor is weakness of the pelvic floor muscles.

Assessment

The basic assessment of the incontinent patient requires a careful history and examination, exclusion of infection and keeping of a micturition or bladder chart. Use of a severity index questionnaire is very helpful. Drugs that adversely affect urinary function are presented in TABLE 76.6. Investigations, particularly urodynamic studies, may be required to dispel doubt about the diagnosis or to exclude intravesical or kidney disorders: these include cystometry, uroflowmetry, cystourethroscopy, fluoroscopy, micturating cysto-urethrogram, IVU and also residual volume (>100 mL is abnormal).

Table 76.6 Drugs that can cause or aggravate incontinence

- ACE inhibitors
- phenoxybenzamine (Dibenyline)
- prazosin
- labetalol

Bladder relaxants → overflow incontinence:

- anticholinergic agents
- tricyclic antidepressants

Bladder stimulants → urge incontinence:

- cholinergic agents
- caffeine

Sedatives → urge incontinence:

- antidepressants
- antihistamines
- antipsychotics
- hypnotics
- tranquillisers

Others → urge incontinence:

- alcohol
- loop diuretics (e.g. frusemide), other diuretics
- lithium

Causes of incontinence (a mnemonic: DIAPPEERSS)[10,11]

D = **D**elirium/dementia
I = **I**nfection of urinary tract
A = **A**trophic urethritis
P = **P**harmacological (e.g. diuretics)
P = **P**sychological (e.g. acute distress)
E = **E**ndocrine (e.g. hypercalcaemia, diabetes insipidus)
E = **E**nvironmental (e.g. unfamiliar surrounds)
R = **R**estricted mobility
S = **S**tool impaction
S = **S**phincter damage or weakness

The severity index questionnaire

- How often do you experience urine leakage?
  0 = never
  1 = less than once a month
  2 = one or several times a month
  3 = one or several times a week
  4 = every day and/or night
- How much urine do you lose each time?
  1 = drops or little
  2 = more

The total score is the score for the first question multiplied by the score for the second question.

0 = dry, 1–2 = slight, 3–4 = moderate, 6–8 = severe

Management

1 Exclude UTI and drug causes.
2 Is it stress incontinence?
   - key symptoms: involuntary loss with coughing, jumping, etc.
   - demonstrable (e.g. patient coughs when standing with full bladder—check for leakage)

   Treatment[12]
   - Weak pelvic floor—exercises
   - Obesity—weight reduction
   - Menopause—HRT/vaginal oestrogen creams
   - Chronic cough—physiotherapy
     If urodynamic studies of LUT function show genuine stress incontinence (GSI) due to urethral sphincter weakness, consider surgery (e.g. suprapubic urethral suspension—better than vaginal repair).

3 Is it urge incontinence?
   - urge symptoms prominent
   - no residual urine
   - urodynamic studies to confirm GSI

   Treatment
   - neurological signs → neurologist
   - abnormal voiding pattern → bladder retraining (e.g. void more urine less frequently)
   - surgery (e.g. Burch procedure)

4 Is it voiding dysfunction?
   - symptoms of voiding difficulty (e.g. frequency, urgency, nocturia, incomplete emptying)
   - large residual urine

   Treatment
   - Neurological signs → neurologist
   - Gynaecological cause (e.g. pelvic mass) → gynaecologist
   - If bladder atony → anticholinergic drugs
   - Intravesical treatment:
     – oxybutynin
     – botulinum toxin
     – others, e.g. capsaicin
   - May require catheterisation

Anticholinergic/antispasmodic drugs[13]

These may be worth a trial for bladder instability or voiding dysfunction:

- solifenacin 5–10 mg (o) daily
- propantheline 15 mg (o) bd or tds
- oxybutynin 2.5–5 mg (o) bd or tds
- tolterodine 2 mg (o) bd
- imipramine 10–75 mg (o) nocte
- mirabegron 25–50 mg (o) daily

The future:

- neuromodulation (e.g. sacral nerve)

Pelvic floor muscle training[13,14]

- The mainstay of treatment of most problems, especially GSI (e.g. 40 'squeezes' daily).
- 75% improved and 25% cured.
- Best in motivated young women with bladder GSI.
- At least 3 months trial with supervision (physiotherapist or continence nurse adviser).

Basic techniques:

- Advise the patient to pull up her pelvic muscles to imagine herself stopping passing urine (or controlling diarrhoea) and hold the 'squeeze' for a count of 10. Repeat many times daily. Refer to *Patient Education.*
- Bladder retraining includes getting the patient to delay micturition for 10–15 minutes whenever she wishes to void.

Bladder dysfunction (in women during night)

Women with urethral syndrome constantly wake at night with urge to micturate but produce only a small dribble of urine.

- Instruct patient to perform a pelvic tilt exercise by balancing on upper back, lifting her pelvis with knees flexed and holding position for 30 seconds
- Squeeze pelvic floor inwards (as though holding back urine or faeces)
- Repeat a few times

Uterovaginal prolapse[15]

Uterovaginal prolapse is very common, affecting 50% of parous women. The main complaint is of 'heaviness' in the vagina and a sensation of 'something coming down'. Relevant symptoms that are of considerable distress for the patient and, depending on the type of prolapse, include voiding difficulties, urinary stress incontinence, faecal incontinence, incomplete rectal emptying and recurrent cystitis. Backache is a common associated symptom, usually relieved by lying down.

Classification of prolapse

See FIGURE 76.3.

- Cystocele—bladder descends into vagina
- Urethrocele—urethra bulges into vagina
- Rectocele—rectum protrudes into vagina
- Enterocele—loop of small intestine bulges into vagina (usually posterior wall)

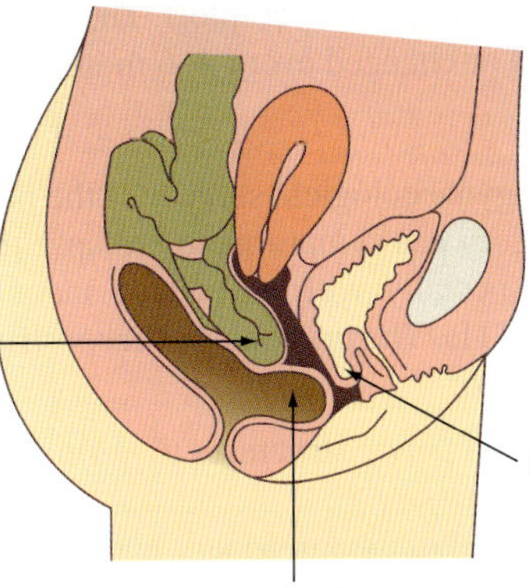

FIGURE 76.3 Uterovaginal prolapse

- Uterine—uterus and cervix descend toward vaginal introitus:
  - first degree—cervix remains in vagina
  - second degree—cervix protrudes on coughing/straining
  - third degree (procidentia)—uterus lies outside vagina

Examination

This is best performed with women in the left lateral position using a Sims speculum or posterior blade of the Graves speculum. Ask the patient to cough or bear down (several times)—observe anterior, posterior and lateral vaginal walls and descent of cervix.

Management

As a rule asymptomatic prolapse does not need invasive treatment, just basic reassurance and education, including pelvic floor exercises (see earlier in this chapter). Consider referral to a physiotherapist. Lifestyle measures include optimal nutrition, weight loss if obese, smoking cessation and exercise. Aggravating comorbidities such as constipation, menopause/atrophic vaginitis and COPD require optimal treatment. Consider topical oestrogens.

Prevention

Promote optimal obstetric management, especially postpartum exercises, lifelong pelvic floor exercises, ideal weight and sensible bladder and bowel function.

Ring pessaries

Pessaries are an option for those who are poor anaesthetic risks, too frail for surgery, don't want surgery, are young and have not completed their family or are awaiting surgery. Each patient needs to be fitted individually with the correct-sized pessary. Topical oestrogens will improve comfort. The pessary needs to be cleaned or changed every 4–6 months.

Surgery

Refer to a gynaecological surgeon if the patient who is fit for surgery has symptomatic prolapse that warrants surgery especially with associated incontinence and recurrent UTIs. The principles of reconstructive pelvic surgery are to:

- reposition pelvic structures to normal anatomical relationships
- restore and maintain urinary and/or faecal continence
- maintain coital function
- correct coexisting pelvic pathology

Options include repair procedures (vaginally, sometimes abdominally, per laparoscopy), colpo/vaginal suspension, hysteroscopy and hysterectomy (vaginal or abdominal).

Patient education resources

Hand-out sheets from *Murtagh's Patient Education* 7th edition:

- Incontinence of urine

References

1 Cormack J, Marinker M, Morrell D. *Practice. A Handbook of Primary Medical Care.* London: Kluwer-Harrap Handbooks, 1980: 3.51: 1–10.

2 Kincaid-Smith P, Larkins R, Whelan G. *Problems in Clinical Medicine.* Sydney: MacLennan & Petty, 1990: 105–8.

3 Sloane PD, Slatt PD, Baker RM. *Essentials of Family Medicine.* Baltimore: Williams & Wilkins, 1988: 169–74.

4 Mathew T. Microscopic haematuria: how to treat. Australian Doctor, 27 April 2007: 27–34.

5 Walsh D. *Symptom Control.* Boston: Blackwell Scientific Publications, 1989: 229–33.

6 George C. Haematuria and proteinuria: how to treat. Australian Doctor, 15 March 1991: I–VIII.

7 Gray S, Frydenberg M. Bladder cancer: how to treat. Australian Doctor, 21 November 2008: 29–36.

8 Faull R. Glomerulonephritis: how to treat. Australian Doctor, 8 February 2002: I–VIII.

9 Thomson N. Managing the patient with proteinuria. Current Therapeutics, 1996; 9: 7–28.

10 Jayasuriya P. Urinary incontinence: how to treat. Australian Doctor, 11 May 2001: I–VIII.

11 Whishaw DMK. Urinary incontinence in the frail female: how to treat. Australian Doctor, 25 July 2008: 29–36.

12 Qaseem A et al. Nonsurgical management of urinary incontinence in women: a clinical practice guideline from the American College of Physicians. Ann Intern Med, 2014; 161 (6): 429–40.

13 Haylen B. Advances in incontinence treatment. Australian Doctor, 10 September 1999: 66–70.

14 Mazza D. *Women's Health in General Practice* (2nd edn). Sydney: Elsevier Australia, 2011: 288–94.

15 Haylen B. Pelvic organ prolapse. Australian Doctor, 21 February 2014: 23–30.

Visual failure

All those, therefore, who have cataract see the light more or less, and by this we distinguish cataract from amaurosis and glaucoma, for persons affected with these complaints do not perceive the light at all.

PAUL OF AEGINA (615–690 CE)

The commonest cause of visual dysfunction is a simple refractive error. However, there are many causes of visual failure, including the emergency of sudden blindness, a problem that requires a sound management strategy. Apart from migraine, virtually all cases of sudden loss of vision require urgent treatment.

The 'white' eye or uninflamed eye presents a different clinical problem from the red or inflamed eye.[1] The 'white' eye is painless and usually presents with visual symptoms and it is in the 'white' eye that the majority of blinding conditions occur.

Criteria for blindness and driving

This varies from country to country. The WHO defines blindness as 'best visual acuity less than 3/60', while in Australia eligibility for the blind pension is 'bilateral corrected visual acuity less than 6/60 or significant visual field loss' (e.g. a patient can have 6/6 vision but severely restricted fields caused by chronic open-angle glaucoma). The minimum standard for driving is 6/12 (Snellen system).

Key facts and checkpoints

- The commonest cause of blindness in the world is trachoma. The other major causes of gradual blindness are cataracts, onchocerciasis and vitamin A deficiency.[2]
- In Western countries, the commonest causes are senile cataract, glaucoma, age-related macular degeneration, trauma and the retinopathy of diabetes mellitus.[2]
- The commonest causes of sudden visual loss are transient occlusion of the retinal artery (amaurosis fugax) and migraine.[3]
- 'Flashing lights' are caused by traction on the retina and may have a serious connotation: the commonest cause is vitreoretinal traction, which is a classic cause of retinal detachment.
- The presence of floaters or 'blobs' in the visual fields indicates pigment in the vitreous: causes include vitreous haemorrhage and vitreous detachment.
- Posterior vitreous detachment is the commonest cause of the acute onset of floaters, especially with advancing age.
- Retinal detachment has a tendency to occur in short-sighted (myopic) people.
- Suspect a macular abnormality where objects look smaller or straight lines are bent or distorted.

The clinical approach

History

The history should carefully define the onset, progress, duration, offset and the extent of visual loss. An accurate history is important because a longstanding visual defect may only just have been noticed by the patient, especially if it is unilateral. Two questions need to be answered:

- Is the loss unilateral or bilateral?
- Is the onset acute, or gradual and progressive?

The distinction between central and peripheral visual loss is useful. Central visual loss presents as impairment of visual acuity and implies defective retinal image formation (through refractive error or opacity in the ocular media) or macular or optic nerve dysfunction. Peripheral field loss is more subtle, especially when the onset is gradual, and implies extramacular retinal disease or a defect in the visual pathway.

It is important to differentiate the central field loss of macular degeneration from the hemianopia of a CVA.

A drug history is very important (see TABLE 77.1). Treatment for tuberculosis with ethambutol or

Table 77.1 Visual disorders associated with drugs

Disorder	Drug
Corneal opacities	Amiodarone Hydroxychloroquine Chlorpromazine Vitamin D Indomethacin Chlorpropamide
Precipitating of acute narrow angle glaucoma	Mydriatic drops Tricyclics Antihistamines
Refractive changes	Thiazides
Lens opacities	Corticosteroids Phenothiazines
Retinopathy	Hydroxychloroquine Chloroquine Thioridazine (other phenothiazines less commonly) Tamoxifen
Papilloedema (secondary to benign intracranial hypertension)	Oral contraceptives Corticosteroids Tetracyclines Nalidixic acid Vitamin A Nitrofurantoin
Optic neuropathy	Ethanol Tobacco Ethambutol Disulfiram

Source: Reprinted from *Central Nervous System: Clinical Algorithms*, published by the BMJ, with permission

treatment with quinine/chloroquine has to be considered as these drugs are oculotoxic. The family history is relevant for diabetes, migraine, Leber hereditary optic atrophy, Tay–Sachs disease and retinitis pigmentosa.

Questions directed to specific symptoms

- Presence of floaters → normal ageing (especially ≥55 years) with posterior vitreous detachment or may indicate haemorrhages or choroiditis
- Flashing lights → normal ageing with posterior vitreous detachment or indicates traction on the retina (? retinal detachment)
- Coloured haloes around lights → glaucoma, cataract
- Zigzag lines → migraine
- Vision worse at night or in dim light → retinitis pigmentosa, hysteria, syphilitic retinitis
- Headache → temporal arteritis, migraine, benign intracranial hypertension
- Central scotomata → macular disease, optic neuritis
- Pain on moving eye → retrobulbar neuritis
- Distortion, micropsia (smaller), macropsia (larger) → macular degeneration
- Visual field loss:
  - central loss—macular disorder
  - total loss—arterial occlusion
  - peripheral loss

It is worth noting that if a patient repeatedly knocks into people and objects on a particular side (including traffic accidents), a bitemporal or homonymous hemianopia should be suspected.

Diseases/disorders to exclude or consider

- Diabetes mellitus
- Giant cell (temporal) arteritis
- Hypopituitarism (pituitary adenoma)
- Cerebrovascular ischaemia/carotid artery stenosis (emboli)
- Multiple sclerosis
- Cardiac disease (e.g. arrhythmias, and SBE—emboli)
- Anaemia (if severe can cause retinal haemorrhage and exudate)
- Marfan syndrome (subluxated lenses)
- Malignancy (the commonest cause of eye malignancy is melanoma of the choroid)

Examination

The same principles of examination should apply as for the red eye. Testing should include:

- visual acuity (Snellen chart)—with pinhole testing
- pupil reactions, to test afferent (sensory) responses to light
- confrontation fields (using a red pin)
- colour vision (Ishihara chart)
- Amsler grid (or graph paper)
- fundus examination with dilated pupil (ophthalmoscope), noting:
  - the red reflex
  - appearance of the retina, macula and optic nerve
- tonometry

General examination

General examination should focus on the general features of the patient, the nervous system, endocrine system and cardiovascular system.

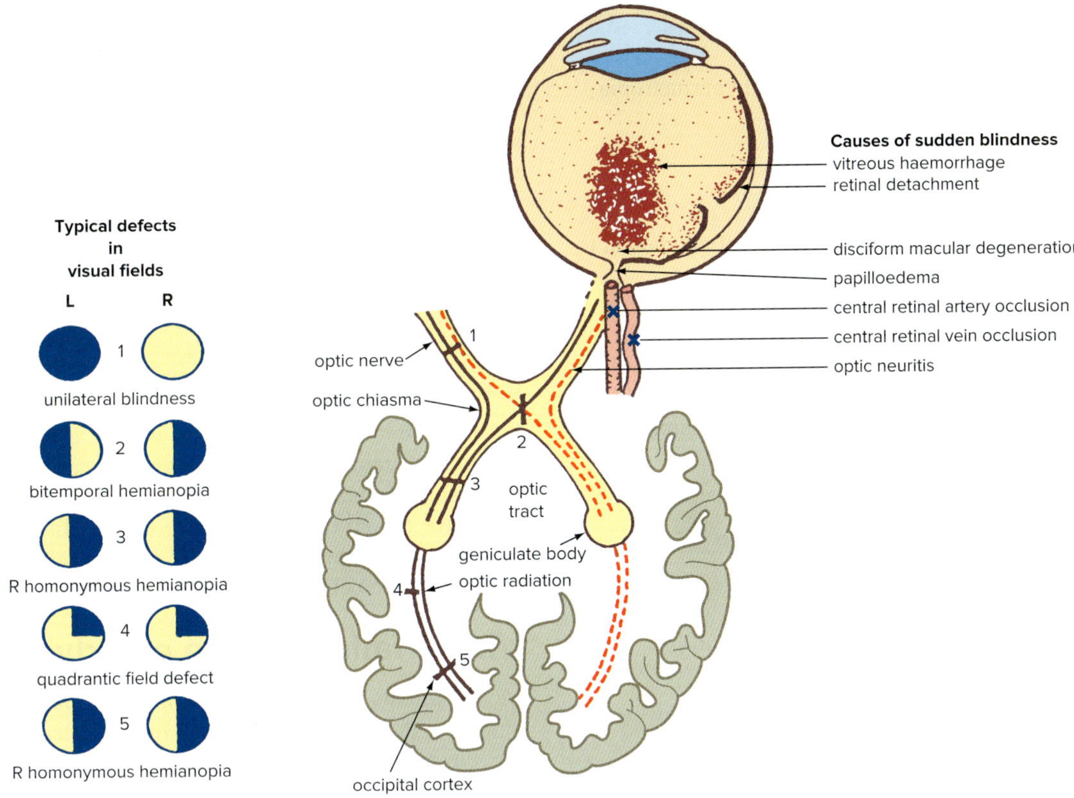

FIGURE 77.1 Diagrammatic representation of important causes of sudden painless loss of vision (right side) and typical defects in the visual fields (left side)

Perimetry

Various defects in the visual fields are depicted in FIGURE 77.1.

Investigations

Depending on the clinical examination the following tests can be selected to confirm the diagnosis:

- blood tests:
  - full blood (? anaemia, lead poisoning, leukaemia)
  - ESR (? temporal arteritis)
  - blood sugar (? diabetes mellitus)
- temporal artery biopsy (? temporal arteritis)
- CT/MRI scan (? CVA, optic nerve lesions, space-occupying lesions)
- formal perimetry and Bjerrum screen
- fluorescein angiography (? retinal vascular obstruction, diabetic retinopathy)
- visual evoked responses (? demyelinating disorders)
- carotid Doppler ultrasound
- B-scan ocular ultrasound

Visual failure in children

There are long lists of causes for visual failure or blindness in children. An approximate order of frequency of causes of blindness in children is cortical blindness, optic atrophy, choroidoretinal degeneration, cataract and retinopathy of prematurity. Almost half the causes of blindness are genetically determined, in contrast to the nutritional and infective causes that predominate in third world countries.[4] About 3% of children will fail to develop proper vision in at least one eye.

The eyes of all babies should be examined at birth and at 6 weeks.

Amblyopia

Amblyopia, referred to as 'lazy eye', is defined as a reduction in visual acuity due to abnormal visual experience in early childhood. It is the main reason for poor unilateral eyesight until middle age and is usually caused by interference with visual development during the early months and years of life.

The common causes are:

- strabismus
- large refractive defect, especially hypermetropia
- congenital cataract

Principles of management[5]

- Most cases are treatable.
- Early diagnosis and intervention is fundamental to achieving useful vision.
- No child is too young to have the visual system assessed.
- The good eye should be patched in order to utilise the affected eye.
- Remove a remedial cause such as strabismus.
- Correct any refractive error, usually by prescription of glasses.

Some important guidelines in children

Referral

Refer if any of the following are present in infants:

- nystagmus
- a wandering eye
- a lack of fixation or following of movements
- photophobia
- opacities (seen with ophthalmoscope set on +3, held 30 cm from baby's eye)
- delayed development

Strabismus

- The two serious squints are the constant and alternating ones, which require early referral. Transient squint and latent squint (occurs under stress e.g. fatigue) usually are not a problem.
- Always refer children with strabismus (squint) when first seen to exclude ocular pathology such as retinoblastoma, congenital cataract and glaucoma, which would require emergency surgery.
- Children with strabismus (even if the ocular examination is normal) need specialist management because the deviating eye will become amblyopic (a lazy eye with reduced vision, i.e. 'blind', if not functioning by 7 years of age). The younger the child, the easier it is to treat amblyopia; it may be irreversible if first detected later than school age. Surgical correction of a true squint is preferred at 1–2 years of age. (See also CHAPTER 92.)

Cataracts

Children with suspected cataracts must be referred immediately; the problem is very serious as the development of vision may be permanently impaired (amblyopia).[2] Cataracts are diagnosed by looking at the red reflex and this should be a routine part of the examination of a young child. Common conditions causing cataracts are genetic disorders and rubella but most causes are unknown. Rarer conditions, such as galactosaemia, need to be considered.

Refractive errors

Refractive errors, with the error greater in one eye, can cause amblyopia. Detection of refractive errors is an important objective of screening.

Retinoblastoma

Retinoblastoma, although rare, is the commonest intraocular tumour in childhood. It must be excluded in any child presenting with a white pupil. Such children also have the so-called 'cat's eye reflex'. In 30% of patients the condition is bilateral with an autosomal dominant gene being responsible.

Visual failure in the elderly

Most patients with visual complaints are elderly and their failing vision affects their perception of the environment and their ability to communicate effectively. Typical problems are cataracts, vascular disease, macular degeneration, chronic simple glaucoma and retinal detachment. Retinal detachment and diabetic retinopathy can occur at any age, although they are more likely with increasing age. Macular degeneration in its various forms is the commonest cause of visual deterioration in the elderly. For the elderly with cataracts the decision to operate depends on the patients' vision and their ability to cope. Most patients with a vision of 6/18 or worse in both eyes usually benefit from cataract extraction, but some can cope with this level of vision and rely on a good, well-placed (above and behind) reading light.[6]

Sudden loss of vision in the elderly is suggestive of temporal arteritis or vascular embolism, so this problem should be checked.

Floaters and flashes

When the vitreous gel shrinks as part of the normal ageing process, it tugs on the retina (rods and cones), causing flashing lights. When the gel separates from the retina, floaters (which may appear as dots, spots or cobwebs) are seen. Floaters are more commonly seen with age, but are also more common in people who are myopic or who have had eye surgery such as removal of cataracts. It is important to consider retinal detachment but if floaters remain constant there is little cause for concern. The appearance of a fresh onset of flashes or floaters is of concern.

Refractive errors

Indistinct or blurred vision is most commonly caused by errors of refraction—the commonest being myopia.

In the normal eye (emmetropia) light rays from infinity are brought to a focus on the retina by the cornea (contributing about two-thirds of the eye's refractive power) and the lens (one-third). Thus, the cornea is very important in refraction and abnormalities such as keratoconus may cause severe refractive problems.[6]

The process of accommodation is required for focusing closer objects. This process, which relies on the action of ciliary muscles and lens elasticity, is usually affected by ageing, so that from the age of 45 close work becomes gradually more difficult (presbyopia).[6]

The important clinical feature is that the use of a simple 'pinhole' in a card will usually improve blurred vision or reduced acuity where there is a refractive error only.[1]

Myopia (short/near-sightedness)

Close objects appear clearly but far objects are blurred. This is usually progressive in the teens. Highly myopic eyes may develop retinal detachment, macular degeneration or glaucoma.

Management

- Glasses with a concave lens
- Contact lenses
- Consider radial keratotomy or excimer laser surgery

Hypermetropia (long/far-sightedness)

This condition is more susceptible to closed angle glaucoma. In early childhood it may be associated with convergent strabismus (squint). The spectacle correction alone may straighten the eyes. It is mostly overcome by the accommodative power of the eye, though it may cause reading difficulty. Typically, the long-sighted person needs reading glasses at about 30 years. A convex lens is used for correction.

Presbyopia

There is a need for near correction with loss of accommodative power of the eye in the 40s.

Astigmatism

There is non-spherical (variable) curvature of the lens or cornea. This creates the need for a corrective lens that is more curved in one meridian than another because the cornea does not have even curvature. If uncorrected, this may cause headaches of ocular origin. Conical cornea is one cause of astigmatism.

Keratoconus

Keratoconus is a bulging, slowly progressive thinning and distortion of the cornea, leading to loss of visual acuity—commonly irregular astigmatism. It usually appears between the ages of 10 and 25 and seems to be genetically determined. Frequent changes of glasses is a feature and contact lenses may help. If not, corneal transplant surgery may be necessary.

Pinhole test

The pinhole reduces the size of the blur circle on the retina in the uncorrected eye. A pinhole acts as a universal correcting lens. If visual acuity is not normalised by looking through a card with a 1 mm pinhole, then the defective vision is not solely due to a refractive error. The pinhole test may actually help to improve visual acuity with some cataracts. Further investigation is mandatory.

Cataract

The term 'cataract' describes any lens opacity. The symptoms depend on the degree and the site of opacity. Cataract causes gradual visual loss with normal direct pupillary light reflex.

The prevalence of cataracts increases with age: 65% at age 50–59, and all people aged over 80 have opacities.[3] Significant causes of cataracts are presented in TABLE 77.2 and causes of progressive visual loss in TABLE 77.3.

Typical symptoms:

- reading difficulty
- difficulty in recognising faces
- problems with driving, especially at night
- difficulty with television viewing
- reduced ability to see in bright light
- may see haloes around lights

The type of visual distortion seen by patients is illustrated in FIGURE 77.2.

Examination

- Reduced visual acuity (sometimes improved with pinhole)
- Diminished red reflex on ophthalmoscopy
- A change in the appearance of the lens

Table 77.2 Causes of cataracts

Advancing age
Diabetes mellitus
Smoking cigarettes
Steroids (topical or oral)
Radiation: long exposure to UV light
TORCH organisms → congenital cataracts
Trauma
Uveitis
Dystrophia myotonica
Galactosaemia

Table 77.3 Progressive bilateral visual loss

Globe	Chronic glaucoma
	Senile cataracts
Retina	Macular degeneration
	Retinal disease: • diabetic retinopathy • retinitis pigmentosa • choroidoretinitis
Optic nerve	Optic neuropathies
	Optic nerve compression (e.g. aneurysm, glioma)
	Toxic damage to optic nerves
Optic chiasma	Chiasmal compression: pituitary adenoma, craniopharyngioma, etc.
Occipital cortex	Tumours
	Degenerative conditions

Note: Unilateral causes (e.g. cataract, refractive errors, uveitis, glaucoma, progressive optic atrophy and tumours) can affect the second eye.

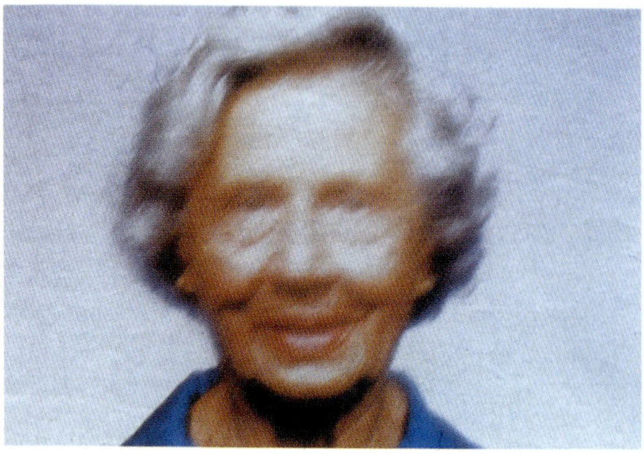

FIGURE 77.2 Blurred vision: appearance of a subject through the eyes of a person with cataracts.
Photo courtesy Allergan Pharmaceuticals

The red reflex and ophthalmoscopy

The 'red reflex' is a reflection of the fundus when the eye is viewed from a distance of about 60 cm (2 feet) with the ophthalmoscope using a zero lens. This reflex is easier to see if the pupil is dilated. Commencing with the plus 15 or 20 lens, reduce the power gradually and, at plus 12, lens opacities will be seen against the red reflex, which may be totally obscured by a very dense cataract. The setting up of the ophthalmoscope to examine intraocular structures is illustrated in FIGURE 77.3.

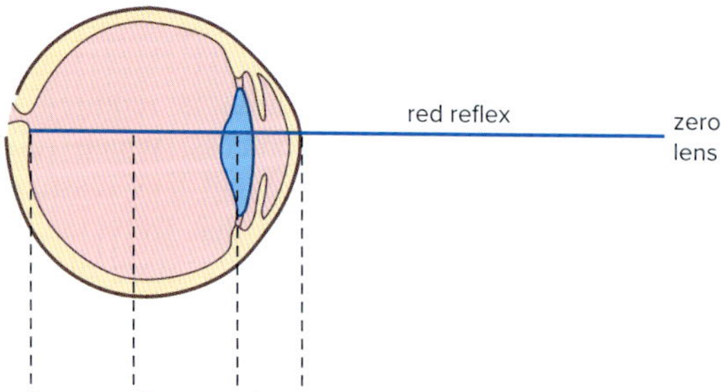

FIGURE 77.3 Settings of the ophthalmoscope used to examine intraocular structures

Management

Advise extraction of the cataract when the patient cannot cope. Contraindications for extraction include intraocular inflammation and severe diabetic retinopathy. There is no effective medical treatment for established cataracts. The removal of the cataractous lens requires optical correction to restore vision and this is usually performed with an intraocular lens implant. Full visual recovery may take 2–3 months. Complications are uncommon yet many patients may require YAG laser capsulotomy to clear any opacities that may develop behind the lens implant.

Postoperative advice to the patient

- Avoid bending for a few weeks.
- Avoid strenuous exercise.
- The following drops may be prescribed:
  - steroids (to reduce inflammation)
  - antibiotics (to avoid infection)
  - dilators (to prevent adhesions)

Prevention

Sunglasses, particularly those that wrap around and filter UV light, may offer protection against cataract formation.

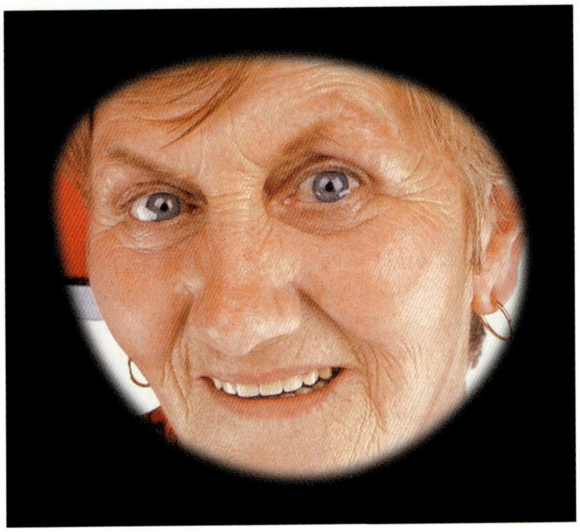

FIGURE 77.4 Typical visual field loss for chronic simple glaucoma; a similar pattern occurs with retinitis pigmentosa and hysteria

Glaucoma

Glaucoma, which is caused by raised intraocular pressure, is categorised as open-angle or closed-angle and further as primary or secondary and acute or chronic. Open-angle glaucoma, also known as chronic simple glaucoma is the commonest cause of irreversible blindness in middle age.[1] At a very late stage, it presents as difficulty in seeing because of loss of the outer fields of vision due to optic atrophy (see FIG. 77.4). Acute glaucoma, on the other hand, has a relatively rapid onset over a few days.

Clinical features (chronic glaucoma)

- Familial tendency
- No early signs or symptoms
- Central vision usually normal
- Insidious progressive restriction of visual field resulting in 'tunnel vision'

Investigations

Tonometry

- Upper limit of normal is 22 mmHg

Ophthalmoscopy

- Optic disc cupping >30% of total disc area

Screening

- Adults 40 years and over: 2–5 yearly (at least 2 yearly over 60)
- Start about 30 years, then 2 yearly if family history

Management

- Treatment can prevent visual field loss
- Medication (for life) usually selected from:[7]
  - timolol or betaxolol drops bd
    Note: These beta blockers can cause systemic complications, e.g. asthma
  - latanoprost (or other prostaglandin analogue) drops, once daily
  - pilocarpine drops qid
  - dipivefrine drops bd
  - brimonidine drops bd
  - acetazolamide (oral diuretics)
- Surgery or laser therapy for failed medication

Retinitis pigmentosa

Primary degeneration of the retina is a hereditary condition characterised by a degeneration of rods and cones associated with displacement of melanin-containing cells from the pigment epithelium into the more superficial parts of the retina.

Typical features

- Begins as night blindness in childhood
- Visual fields become concentrically narrowed (periphery to centre)
- Blind by adolescence (sometimes up to middle age)
- Irreversible course—may be delayed by vitamin A

Examination (ophthalmoscopic)

- Irregular patches of dark pigment, especially at periphery
- Optic atrophy

Trauma

Trauma to the eye may cause only a little discomfort so it is important to keep this in mind.

Intraocular foreign body

A small metal chip may penetrate the eye with minimal pain and the patient may not present with an ocular problem until the history of injury is long forgotten.

If infection does not supervene, presentation may be delayed for months or years until vision deteriorates due to metal degradation. The iris becomes rust-brown. It is important to X-ray the eye if it has been struck by a hammered fragment or if in any doubt at all about the mechanism of the injury.[1]

Chronic uveitis

Pain and redness may be minimal with this chronic inflammation. If untreated, visual loss often develops

77

from secondary glaucoma and cataract. The pupil is bound to the lens by synechiae and is distorted.

HIV infection

AIDS may have serious ocular complications, including Kaposi sarcoma of the conjunctivae, retinal haemorrhage and vasculitis.[3] Another problem is ocular cytomegalovirus infection, which presents as areas of opacification with haemorrhage and exudates.

Sudden loss of vision

It is important to remember that the problem is alarming and distressing to the patient; considerable empathy is needed and care must be taken not to diagnose seemingly inappropriate behaviour as of psychogenic origin.

A comparison of bilateral and unilateral causes of sudden loss of vision is presented in TABLE 77.4, and the diagnostic strategy model in TABLE 77.5. A simplified classification is:

77

unilateral:	retinal detachment
	retinal artery occlusion
	retinal vein thrombosis
	temporal arteritis
	optic neuritis
	migraine
bilateral:	bilateral optic nerve lesion
	hysteria

A flow chart for the diagnosis of painless loss of vision is presented in FIGURE 77.5.

Amaurosis fugax

Amaurosis fugax is transient loss of vision (partial or complete) in one eye due to transient occlusion of a retinal artery. It is painless and lasts less than 60 minutes. It is usually caused by an embolus from an atheromatous carotid artery in the neck. The most common emboli are cholesterol emboli, which usually arise from an ulcerated plaque.[7] Other causes include emboli from the heart, temporal arteritis and benign intracranial hypertension. Other symptoms or signs of cerebral ischaemia, such as transient hemiparesis, may accompany the symptom. The source of the problem should be investigated. The risk of stroke after an episode of amaurosis fugax appears to be about 2% per year.[7]

Transient ocular ischaemia

Unilateral loss of vision provoked by activities such as walking, bending or looking upwards is suggestive of ocular ischaemia.[7] It occurs in the presence of severe extracranial vascular disease and may be triggered by postural hypotension and stealing blood from the retinal circulation.

Retinal detachment[8]

Retinal detachment may be caused by trauma, thin retina (myopic people), previous surgery (e.g. cataract operation), choroidal tumours, vitreous degeneration or diabetic retinopathy.

Table 77.4 Causes of sudden loss of vision[7]

	Bilateral	Unilateral: Transient	Unilateral: Permanent
Vascular causes	Occipital cortex ischaemia Pituitary apoplexy Homonymous hemianopia—vascular	Amaurosis fugax Transient ocular ischaemia Retinal emboli Malignant hypertension	Central retinal artery occlusion Central retinal vein occlusion Vitreous haemorrhage Ischaemic optic neuropathy
Other causes	Bilateral optic neuritis Toxic damage to optic nerve: • methanol • ethanol • tobacco • lead Leber optic atrophy Quinine poisoning of retina Cerebral oedema Occipital lobe trauma Craniopharyngioma Hysteria	Acute angle closure glaucoma Uhthoff phenomenon Papilloedema Posterior vitreous detachment	Optic neuritis Retinal detachment Optic nerve compression Carcinomatous optic neuropathy Intraocular tumour

Table 77.5	Acute or subacute painless loss of vision: diagnostic strategy model
Probability diagnosis Amaurosis fugax Migraine Retinal detachment 'Wet' macular degeneration	
Serious disorders not to be missed Cardiovascular: • central retinal artery occlusion • central retinal vein occlusion • hypertension (complications) • CVA Neoplasia: • intracranial tumour • intraocular tumour: — primary melanoma — retinoblastoma — metastases Vitreous haemorrhage AIDS Temporal arteritis Acute glaucoma Benign intracranial hypertension	
Pitfalls (often missed) Papilloedema Optic neuritis Intraocular foreign body Posterior uveitis	
Seven masquerades checklist Diabetes (diabetic retinopathy) Drugs (quinine) Thyroid disorder (hyperthyroidism)	
Is this patient trying to tell me something? Consider 'hysterical' blindness, although it is uncommon.	

Clinical features

- Sudden onset of floaters or flashes or black spots
- Blurred vision in one eye becoming worse
- 'A curtain came down over the eye', grey cloud or black spot
- Partial or total loss of visual field (total if macula detached)

Ophthalmoscopy may show detached retinal fold as large grey shadow in vitreous cavity.

Management

- Immediate referral for sealing of retinal tears
- Small holes treated with laser or freezing probe
- Pneumatic retinopexy is an option
- True detachments usually require surgery

Vitreous haemorrhage

Haemorrhage may occur from spontaneous rupture of vessels, avulsion of vessels during retinal traction or bleeding from abnormal new vessels.[6] Associations include ocular trauma, diabetic retinopathy, tumour and retinal detachment.

Clinical features

- Sudden onset of floaters or 'blobs' in vision
- May be sudden loss of vision
- Visual acuity depends on the extent of the haemorrhage; if small, visual acuity may be normal

Ophthalmoscopy may show reduced light reflex: there may be clots of blood that move with the vitreous (a black swirling cloud).

Management

- Urgent referral to exclude retinal detachment
- Exclude underlying causes such as diabetes
- Ultrasound helps diagnosis
- May resolve spontaneously
- Bed rest encourages resolution
- Surgical vitrectomy for persistent haemorrhage

77

Central retinal artery occlusion

The cause is usually arterial obstruction by atherosclerosis, thrombi or emboli. There may be a history of TIAs. Exclude temporal arteritis (perform immediate ESR).

Clinical features

- Sudden loss of vision like a 'curtain descending' in one eye
- Vision not improved with 1 mm pinhole
- Usually no light perception

Ophthalmoscopy

- Initially normal
- May see retinal emboli
- Classic 'red cherry spot' at macula

Management

Urgent referral to an ophthalmologist but if seen early, or opthalmologist delayed, use this procedure within 30 minutes:

- massage globe digitally through closed eyelids (use rhythmic direct digital pressure)—may dislodge embolus

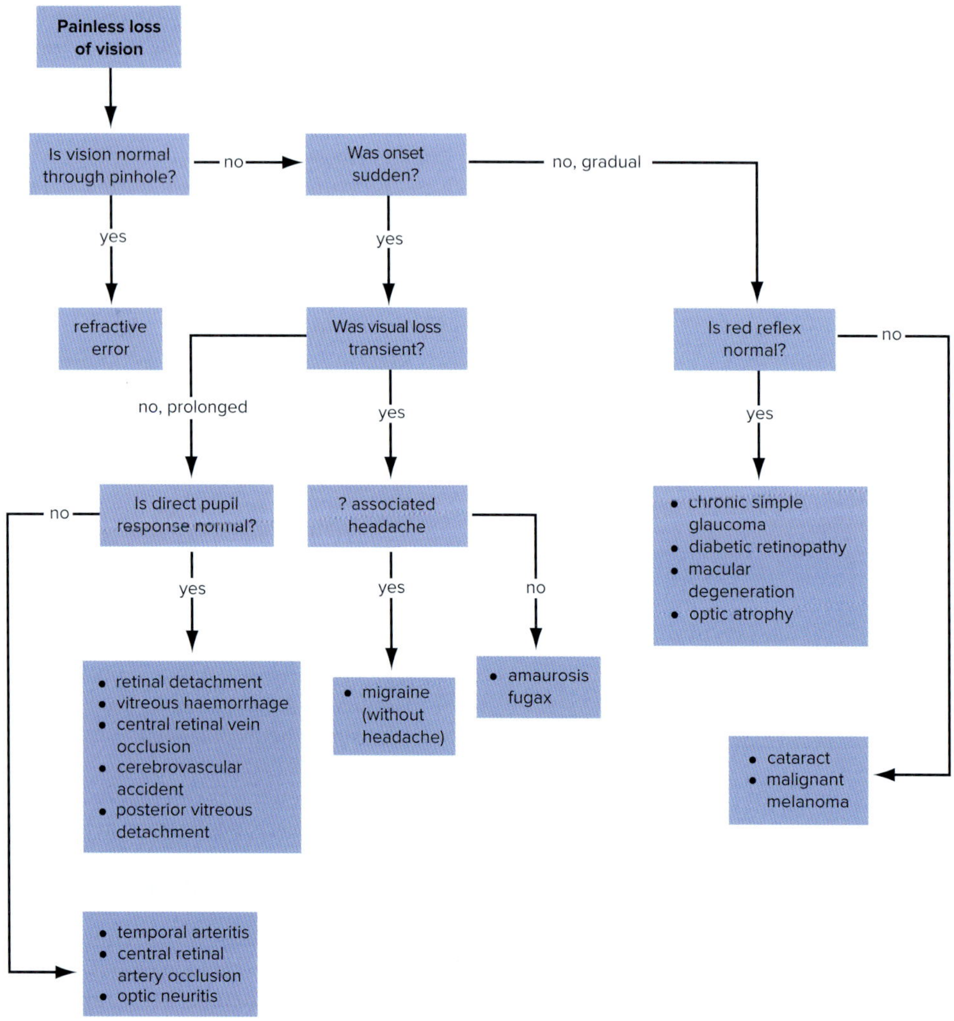

FIGURE 77.5 Diagnosis of painless loss of vision

Source: Reproduced with permission of Dr J Reich and Dr J Colvin

- rebreathe carbon dioxide (paper bag) or inhale special CO_2 mixture (carbogen)
- intravenous acetazolamide (Diamox) 500 mg
- refer urgently (less than 6 hours)—exclude temporal arteritis

Prognosis is poor. Significant recovery is unlikely unless treated immediately (within 30 minutes).

Central retinal vein thrombosis

Thrombosis is associated with several possible factors, such as hypertension, diabetes, thrombocytopenia, glaucoma and hyperlipidaemia. It usually occurs in elderly patients.

Clinical features

- Sudden loss of central vision in one eye (if macula involved): can be gradual over days
- Vision not improved with 1 mm pinhole

Ophthalmoscopy shows swollen disc and multiple retinal haemorrhages, 'stormy sunset' appearance.

Management

Refer to an ophthalmologist. No immediate treatment is effective. The cause needs to be found first and treated accordingly. Some cases respond to fibrinolysin treatment. Laser photocoagulation may be necessary in later stages if neovascularisation develops to prevent thrombotic glaucoma.

Macular degeneration

There are two age-related types: exudative or 'wet' (acute), and pigmentary or 'dry' (slow onset).

- 'Wet' MD is caused by choroidal neovascular membranes that develop under the retina of the macular area and leak fluid or bleed. It is a serious disorder.
- 'Dry' MD (9 out of 10 cases of MD) develops slowly and is always painless.
- More common with increasing age (usually over 60), when it is termed 'age-related MD', and in those with myopia (relatively common).
- May be familial.

Clinical features

- Sudden fading of central vision (see FIG 77.6)
- Distortion of vision
- Straight lines may seem wavy and objects distorted
- Use a grid pattern (Amsler chart): shows distorted lines
- Central vision eventually completely lost
- Peripheral fields normal

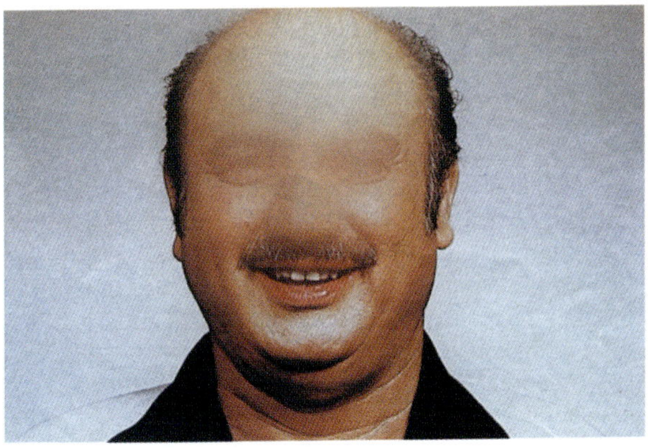

FIGURE 77.6 Appearance of a subject through the eyes of a person with age-related macular degeneration

Photo courtesy Allergan Pharmaceuticals

Ophthalmoscopy

- White exudates, haemorrhage in retina
- Macula may look normal or raised

Management

No treatment is available to stop or reverse MD. For 'wet' MD refer urgently for treatment, which is currently based on injection of antivascular endothelial growth factor drugs (e.g. ranibizumab, bevacizumab) into the vitreous humour.[9] The Age-Related Eye Disease Study provided confirmatory evidence that the chronic pigmentation type responds to free-radical treatment with the antioxidants vitamins A, C, E, and zinc using beta-carotene, 15 mg; vitamin C, 500 mg; vitamin E, 400 IU; and 80 mg zinc oxide.[10] Advise patient to cease smoking if applicable.[11]

Temporal arteritis

With temporal arteritis (giant cell arteritis) there is a risk of sudden and often bilateral occlusion of the short ciliary arteries supplying the optic nerves, with or without central retinal artery involvement.[12]

Clinical features

- Usually older person: over 65 years
- Sudden loss of central vision in one eye (central scotoma)
- Can rapidly become bilateral
- Associated temporal headache (not invariable)
- Temporal arteries tender, thickened and non-pulsatile (but often normal)
- Visual acuity severely impaired
- Afferent pupil defect on affected side
- Usually elevated ESR >40 mm

Ophthalmoscopy shows optic disc swollen at first, then atrophic. The disc may appear quite normal.

Management

- Other eye must be tested
- Immediate corticosteroids (60–100 mg prednisolone daily for at least 1 week)
- Biopsy temporal artery (if there is a localised tender area)

Retinal migraine

Migraine may present with symptoms of visual loss. Associated headache and nausea may not be present.

Clinical features

- Zigzag lines or lights
- Multicoloured flashing lights
- Unilateral or bilateral field deficit
- Resolution within a few hours

Posterior vitreous detachment

The vitreous body collapses and detaches from the retina. It may lead to retinal detachment.

Clinical features

- Sudden onset of floaters
- Visual acuity usually normal
- Flashing lights indicate traction on the retina

77

Management

- Refer to an ophthalmologist urgently.
- An associated retinal hole or detachment needs exclusion.

Optic (retrobulbar) neuritis

Causes include multiple sclerosis, neurosyphilis and toxins. A significant number of cases eventually develop multiple sclerosis.

Clinical features

- Usually a woman 20–40 years
- Loss of vision in one eye over a few days
- Retro-ocular discomfort with eye movements
- Variable visual acuity
- Usually a central field loss (central scotoma)
- Afferent pupil defect on affected side

Ophthalmoscopy

- Optic disc swollen if 'inflammation' anterior in nerve
- Optic atrophy appears later
- Disc pallor is an invariable sequel

Management

- Test visual field of other eye
- Consider MRI
- Most patients recover spontaneously but are left with diminished acuity
- Intravenous steroids hasten recovery and have a protective effect against the development of further demyelinating episodes

Corneal disorders

Patients with corneal conditions typically suffer from ocular pain or discomfort and reduced vision. The common condition of dry eye may involve the cornea while contact lens disorders, abrasions/ulcers and infections are common serious problems that threaten eye sight. Inflammation of the cornea—keratitis—is caused by factors such as ultraviolet light, e.g. 'arc eye', herpes simplex, herpes zoster ophthalmicus and the dangerous 'microbial keratitis'. Bacterial keratitis is an ophthalmological emergency that should be considered in the contact lens wearer presenting with pain and reduced vision. Topical corticosteroids should be avoided in the undiagnosed red eye.

Refer to CHAPTER 51 for corneal lesions.

Pitfalls

- Mistaking the coloured haloes of glaucoma for migraine.
- Failing to appreciate the presence of retinal detachment in the presence of minimal visual impairment.
- Omitting to consider temporal arteritis as a cause of sudden visual failure in the elderly.
- Using eyedrops to dilate the pupil (for fundal examination) in the presence of glaucoma.

When to refer

- Most problems outlined need urgent referral to an ophthalmologist.
- Acute visual disturbance of unknown cause requires urgent referral.
- Any blurred vision—sudden or gradual, painful or painless—especially if 1 mm pinhole fails to alter visual acuity.
- Refer all suspicious optic discs.

Practice tips

- Tonometry is advised routinely for all people over 40 years; those over 60 years should have tests every 2 years.
- Any family history of glaucoma requires tonometry from 40 years onwards.
- Sudden loss of vision in the elderly suggests temporal arteritis (check the ESR and temporal arteries). It requires immediate institution of high-dose steroids to prevent blindness in the other eye. A time-scale guide showing the rate of visual loss is presented in TABLE 77.6.
- Temporal arteritis is an important cause of retinal artery occlusion.
- Suspect field defect due to chiasmal compression if people are misjudging when driving.
- Pupillary reactions are normal in cortical blindness.
- Central retinal artery occlusion may be overcome by early rapid lowering of intraocular pressure.
- Retinal detachment and vitreous haemorrhage may require early surgical repair.
- Keep in mind antioxidant therapy (vitamins and minerals) for chronic macular degeneration.
- Consider multiple sclerosis foremost if there is a past history of transient visual failure, especially with eye pain.
- If the patient has been using a hammer, always X-ray if a fragment of metal has hit the eye but nothing can be seen.

Table 77.6 Time-scale guide for rate of visual loss[3,7]

Sudden: less than 1 hour
Amaurosis fugax
Central retinal artery occlusion
Hemianopias from ischaemia (emboli)
Migraine
Vitreous haemorrhage
Acute angle glaucoma
Papilloedema
Within 24 hours
Central retinal vein occlusion
Hysteria
Less than 7 days
Retinal detachment
Optic neuritis
Acute macular problems
Up to several weeks (variable)
Choroiditis
Malignant hypertension
Gradual
Compression of visual pathways
Chronic glaucoma
Cataracts
Diabetic maculopathy
Retinitis pigmentosa
Macular degeneration
Refractive errors

Patient education resources

Hand-out sheets from *Murtagh's Patient Education* 7th edition:

- Cataracts
- Floaters and flashes
- Glaucoma
- Macular degeneration

References

1. Colvin J, Reich J. Check Program 219–220. Melbourne: RACGP, 1990: 1–32.
2. Hopcroft K, Forte V. *Symptom Sorter* (4th edn). Oxford: Ratcliffe Publishing, 2010: 138.
3. Enoch B. Painless loss of vision in adults. Update, 1987; 5 June: 22–30.
4. Robinson MJ, Roberton, DM. *Practical Paediatrics* (5th edn). Melbourne: Churchill Livingstone, 2003: 756–70.
5. Cole GA. Amblyopia and strabismus. In: *MIMS Disease Index* (2nd edn). Sydney: IMS Publishing, 1996: 20–4.
6. Elkington AR, Khaw PT. *ABC of Eyes*. London: British Medical Association, 1990: 20–38.
7. Li T et al. Comparative effectiveness of first-line medications for primary open-angle glaucoma: a systematic review and network meta-analysis. Ophthalmology, 2016; 123 (1): 129–40.
8. King J. Loss of vision. Mod Med Aust, 1990; May: 52–61.
9. Hodge C, Ng D. Eye emergencies. Check Program 400. Melbourne: RACGP, 2005: 1–34.
10. Bunting R, Guymer R. Treatment of age-related macular degeneration. Aust Prescr, 2012; 35: 90–3.
11. Age-Related Eye Disease Study Research Group. A randomised, placebo-controlled, clinical trial of high dose supplementation with vitamins C and E, beta-carotene, and zinc for age-related macular degeneration and vision loss. Arch Ophthalmol, 2001; 119: 1417–36.
12. Warne R, Prinsley D. *A Manual of Geriatric Care*. Sydney: Williams & Wilkins, 1988: 191–5.

78 Weight gain

Persons who are naturally very fat are apt to die earlier than those who are slender.

HIPPOCRATES

Obesity is the most common nutrition-related disorder in the Western world; as Tunnessen puts it, 'Obesity is the most common form of malnutrition in the United States'.[1] Most overweight adults and children who are obese have exogenous obesity, which tends to imply that 'they ate too much', but the problem is more complex than relative food input. Physical activity and environmental and genetic influences must also be taken into account. However, only a small percentage (4–6%) of human obesity is thought to be due to a single gene mutation.[2] There is still a persisting tendency of affected families to blame 'glandular' problems as a cause of obesity. It is now considered that there is a strong genetic basis to obesity and that attributing it to overeating and lack of exercise is an overly simplistic viewpoint.

Key facts and figures

- Two-thirds of the Australian population are overweight or obese and only 2–4% underweight.[3]
- Abdominal obesity gives a higher cardiovascular risk at any weight.
- The onset of obesity can occur at any age.
- Secondary or pathologic causes are rare.
- Less than 1% of obese patients have an identifiable secondary cause of obesity.[2]
- Two conditions causing unexplained weight gain that can be diagnosed by the physical examination are Cushing syndrome and hypothyroidism.
- After pregnancy, obesity may result from a failure to return to prepartum energy requirements.
- Even small weight losses are effective in preventing diabetes and improving the cardiovascular risk profile.[4]

A diagnostic approach

A summary of the diagnostic strategy model is presented in TABLE 78.1.

Table 78.1 Weight gain: diagnostic strategy model

Probability diagnosis
Exogenous obesity
Alcohol excess
Drugs
Serious disorders not to be missed
Cardiovascular:
• cardiac failure
Hypothalamic disorders (hyperphagia):
• craniopharyngiomas
• optic gliomas
Liver failure
Nephrotic syndrome
Pitfalls (often missed)
Pregnancy (early)
Endocrine disorders:
• hypothyroidism
• Cushing syndrome
• insulinoma
• acromegaly
• hypogonadism
• hyperprolactinaemia
• polycystic ovarian syndrome
Idiopathic oedema syndrome
Klinefelter syndrome
Congenital disorders:
• Prader–Willi syndrome
• Laurence–Moon–Biedl syndrome
Seven masquerades checklist
Depression
Drugs
Thyroid disorder (hypothyroidism)
Is the patient trying to tell me something?
Yes: the reasons for obesity should be explored.

Probability diagnosis

The outstanding cause of weight gain in exogenous obesity is excessive calorie intake coupled with lack of exercise. This is determined largely by environmental influences. Overweight people often deny overeating but the true situation can be determined by recording actual food intake and energy expenditure, and by interviewing reliable witnesses.

Serious causes not to be missed

It is important not to misdiagnose hypothalamic disorders, which may result in hyperphagia and obesity. Injury to the hypothalamus may occur following trauma and encephalitis and with a variety of tumours, including craniopharyngiomas, optic gliomas and pituitary neoplasms. Some of these tumours may cause headaches and visual disturbances.

It is also important not to overlook major organ failure and kidney disorders as a cause of increased body weight, especially cardiac failure, liver failure and the nephrotic syndrome. The associated increase in body water needs to be distinguished from increased body fat. Consider the obesity hypoventilation syndrome (Pickwickian syndrome) in Grade III obese patients.

Pitfalls

Endocrine disorders

The endocrine disorders that cause obesity include Cushing syndrome, hypothyroidism, insulin-secreting tumours and hypogonadism. They should not represent difficult diagnostic problems.

An insulin-secreting tumour (insulinoma) is a very rare adenoma of the B cells of the islets of Langerhans. The main features are symptoms of hypoglycaemia and obesity.

Congenital disorders

The rare congenital disorders that cause obesity, such as Prader–Willi and Laurence–Moon–Biedl syndromes, should be easy to recognise in children (see CHAPTER 18 and later in this chapter).

Chromosomal abnormalities

An important abnormality to bear in mind is Klinefelter syndrome (XXY karyotype), which affects one out of every 400–500 males. The boys show excessive growth of long bones and are tall and slim. Without testosterone treatment they become obese as adults.

Some girls with Turner syndrome (XO karyotype) may be short and overweight.

Some gender pointers

Consider polycystic ovarian syndrome in women and obstructive sleep apnoea in obese men.

Seven masquerades checklist

The important masquerades include hypothyroidism and drug ingestion. Hypothyroidism is usually not associated with marked obesity. Drugs that can be an important contributing factor include tricyclic antidepressants, mirtazapine, corticosteroids, pizotifen, thioridazine, haloperidol, Depo-Provera and the contraceptive pill. Obesity (overeating) may be a feature of depression, especially in the early stages. Prescribed tricyclic antidepressants may compound the problem.

Psychogenic considerations

An underlying emotional crisis may be the reason for the overweight patient to seek medical advice. It is important to explore diplomatically any hidden agenda and help the patient to resolve any conflict.

The clinical approach

A careful history is very valuable in ascertaining food and beverage intake and perhaps giving patients insight into their calorie intake, since some deny overeating or will underestimate their food intake.[4] Enquire about gynaecological and family history, e.g. diabetes, cardiac disease.

Relevant questions

- Do you feel that you have an excessive appetite?
- Tell me in detail what you ate yesterday.
- Give me an outline of a typical daily meal.
- Tell me about snacks, soft drink and alcohol that you have.
- What exercise do you get?
- Do you have any special problems, such as getting bored, tense and upset or depressed?
- What drugs are you taking?

Examination

In the physical examination it is very important to measure body weight and height and calculate the BMI, and assess the degree and distribution of body fat and the overall nutritional status. A person's adiposity is more important than body weight.[5] Record the blood pressure and test the urine with dipsticks. Keep in mind that a standard blood pressure cuff on a large arm may give falsely elevated values. Remember the rare possibilities of Cushing syndrome, acromegaly and hypothyroidism. Search for evidence of atherosclerosis and diabetes and for signs of alcohol abuse.

An extensive working up of the CNS is not indicated in obesity without the presence of suspicious symptoms such as visual difficulties.

Investigations

It is essential to perform two measurements:

- weight and height (to calculate BMI)
- waist circumference

Important investigations

- Cholesterol/triglycerides
- Glucose (fasting)
- Liver function tests
- Electrolytes and urea

Investigations to consider

- Thyroid function tests
- Cortisol (if hypertensive)
- Testosterone (suspected sleep apnoea)
- ECG and chest X-ray (older than 40)

Anthropometric measurements[5]

Useful measuring instruments include:

- BMI: 'healthy' range is between 20 and 25
- Waist circumference: increased risk of comorbidities and is critical when considering cardiometabolic risk
  – in men >94 cm (>102—high risk)
  – in women >80 cm (>88—high risk)
  Measure waist halfway between inferior margin of last rib and crest of ilium in mid-axillary line over bare skin; use a stretch-resistant tape.
- Waist–hip circumference ratio (W/H ratio): healthy range <0.9—a better predictor of cardiovascular risk than BMI
- Single skinfold thickness (>25 mm suggests increased body fat)
- Upper arm circumference
- 4 skinfold thickness (sum of suprailiac, subscapular, triceps and biceps skinfolds)—for calculation of percentage body fat

Abdominal fatness, which is defined as a W/H ratio of >0.85 in women and >0.95 in men, is a more accurate indicator of the complications of diabetes. In practice, the combination of waist circumference and BMI is the most useful indicator of risk and relative change.[5]

Body mass index

The easiest and possibly most accurate assessment of obesity is the BMI (refer to Appendix V):

$$\text{BMI} = \frac{\text{weight (kg)}}{\text{height (m}^2)}$$

Table 78.2 Classification of obesity (based on WHO guidelines)[6]

BMI	Grading	Suggested therapy
<18.5	Underweight	Diet and counselling
18.5–25	Healthy weight	
25–30	Overweight	More exercise Diet: less alcohol
30–35	Class I: mildly obese	Combined program: • behaviour modification • diet • exercise
35–40	Class II: moderately obese	Consider medical therapy if >35
≥40	Class III: severely obese	Combined program plus medical therapy Consider gastric surgery

The RACGP recommends measuring the above two parameters every 2 years and recording them in the medical record.[9]

Garrow[6] has produced a simple classification of the BMI associated with the relative degree of risk increase and suggested therapy (see TABLE 78.2).

The BMI has limitations. It doesn't distinguish between men and women or between body types and it doesn't work for children.

Weight gain in children

Various studies have found that approximately 10% of prepubertal and 15% of adolescent age groups are obese.[1]

Obesity in children is a BMI for age >95th percentile while overweight is >85th percentile. There is a risk of obesity-associated diseases and carrying the problem into adulthood, with a greater risk of obesity, premature death and disability.

Childhood obesity is rising at an alarming rate worldwide—the figure is reportedly ten times higher than it was in 1970. The WHO reported that over 340 million children and adolescents aged 5–19 years were overweight or obese in 2016, with almost half of them living in Asia (WHO MONICA project).

Raising the issue with parents and child requires sensitivity and discretion. Parents often blame obesity in children on their 'glands', but endocrine or metabolic causes are rare and can be readily differentiated from exogenous obesity by a simple physical examination and an assessment of linear growth. Children with exogenous obesity tend to have an accelerated linear growth whereas children with secondary causes are usually short.

Congenital or inherited disorders associated with obesity

Prader–Willi syndrome

The characteristic features are bizarre eating habits (e.g. binge eating), obesity, hypotonia, hypogonadism, intellectual disability, small hands and feet and a characteristic facial appearance (narrow bifrontal diameter, 'almond-shaped' eyes and a 'tented' upper lip). Progressive obesity results from excessive intake in addition to decreased caloric requirements (see CHAPTER 18).

Laurence–Moon–Biedl syndrome

The characteristic features are obesity, intellectual disability, polydactyly and syndactyly, retinitis pigmentosa and hypogonadism.

Beckwith–Wiedemann syndrome

Characteristics include excessive growth, macrosomia, macroglossia, umbilical hernia and neonatal hypoglycaemia. Children appear obese as they are above the 95th percentile by 18 months of age. Intelligence is usually in the normal range.

Endocrine disorders

Endocrine disorders in children that can rarely cause obesity include hypothyroidism (often blamed as the cause but seldom is), Cushing syndrome, insulinomas, hypothalamic lesions, Fröhlich syndrome (adiposogenital dystrophy) and Stein–Leventhal syndrome (PCOS) in girls.

Managing obesity in children

Childhood obesity usually reflects an underlying problem in the family system. It can be a very difficult emotional problem in adolescents, who develop a poor body image. An important strategy is to meet with family members, determine whether they perceive the child's obesity as a problem and whether they are prepared to solve the problem. The family dynamics will have to be assessed and strategies outlined. This may involve referral for expert counselling. It is worth pointing out that children eat between one-third and two-thirds of their meals at school so schools should be approached to promote special programs for children who need weight reduction.

Conventional therapy by dietary modification, increasing energy expenditure by increasing activity, reducing sedentary behaviour, behaviour modification and family involvement is recommended. The best outcomes are achieved with a specialist team working with the whole family.[5] Some authorities emphasise that weight maintenance rather than weight loss is appropriate since many children will 'grow into their weight'.[7]

Cushing syndrome

Cushing syndrome is the term used to describe the chemical features of increased free circulating glucocorticoid. The most common cause is iatrogenic with the prescribing of synthetic corticosteroids. The spontaneous primary forms such as Cushing disease (pituitary dependent hyperadrenalism) are rare. As the disorder progresses the body contour tends to assume the often quoted configuration of a lemon with matchsticks (see CHAPTER 23).

Clinical features

- Change in appearance
- Central weight gain (truncal obesity)
- Hair growth and acne in females
- Muscle weakness
- Amenorrhoea/oligomenorrhoea (females)
- Thin skin/spontaneous bruising
- Polymyalgia/polydipsia (diabetes mellitus)
- Insomnia
- Depression

Signs

- Moon face
- 'Buffalo hump'
- Purple striae
- Large trunk and thin limbs: the 'lemon with matchsticks' sign

The patient should be referred for diagnostic evaluation, including plasma cortisol and overnight dexamethasone suppression tests.

Untreated Cushing syndrome has a very poor prognosis, with premature death from myocardial infarction, cardiac failure and infection; hence early diagnosis and referral is essential.

Obesity

Obesity and overweight are the most common pathological conditions in our society, creating on increasing public health problem. Worldwide in 2016, 39% of adults aged 18 years and over were overweight (39% of men and 40% of women) and 13% were obese (11% of men and 15% of women). Caused by an accumulation of adipose tissue, the problem is described as a 'global health epidemic' and also as a chronic disease (see TABLE 78.3). Each

Table 78.3 Factors predisposing to primary obesity

Genetic	Familial tendency
Sex	Women more susceptible
Activity	Lack of physical activity
Psychogenic	Emotional deprivation, depression
Socioeconomic status	Lower
Alcohol	Problem drinking
Smoking	Cessation of smoking
Prescribed drugs	Tricyclic derivatives

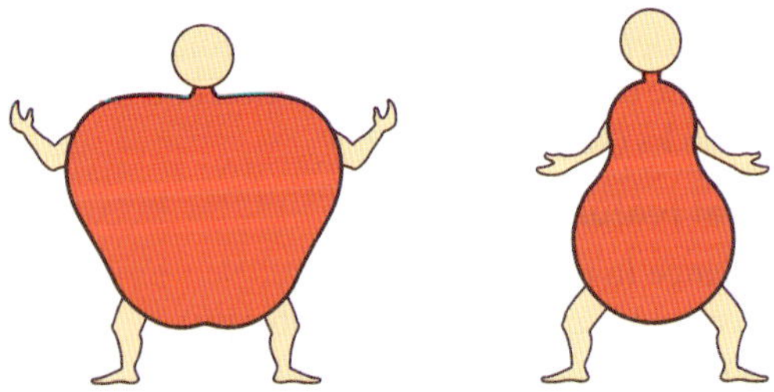

FIGURE 78.1 Comparison of two types of obesity according to distribution of body fat

year, more than a million adults die due to conditions associated with obesity. It is not the extra weight per se that causes problems, but the excess fat. Calculating the BMI gives a better estimate of adiposity, and it is convenient and preferable to use this index when assessing the overweight and obese. However, recent data suggest that the distribution of body fat is as important a risk factor as its total amount. Abdominal fat (upper body segment obesity, or 'apple' obesity) is considered a greater health hazard than fat in the thighs and buttocks (lower body segment obesity, or 'pear' obesity) (see FIG. 78.1).

Obese patients with high waist–hip ratios (>1.0 in men and >0.9 in women) have a significantly greater risk of diabetes mellitus, stroke, coronary artery disease and early death than equally obese people with lower waist–hip ratios.[2]

In regard to the BMI reference scale it is worth noting that the risks follow a J-shaped curve (see FIG. 78.2) and are only slightly increased in the overweight range but increase with obesity so that a BMI of >40 carries a threefold increase in mortality.

The consequences of obesity include:

- cardiovascular:
  - increased mortality (stroke, ischaemic heart disease, etc.)
  - hypertension*
  - varicose veins

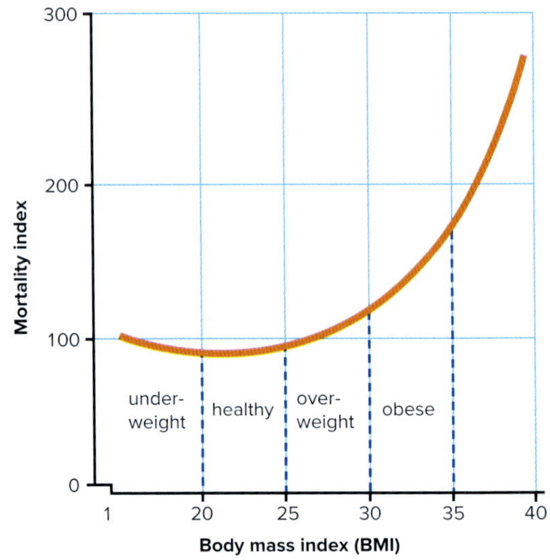

FIGURE 78.2 Body mass index (BMI) reference scale

- metabolic:
  - dyslipidaemia*
  - type 2 diabetes*
  - insulin resistance
  - hyperuricaemia/gout
  - infertility
  - PCOS
- mechanical:
  - osteoarthritis
  - obstructive sleep apnoea*
  - restrictive pulmonary disease
  - spinal dysfunction
  - low back pain
  - urinary incontinence
- other:
  - hiatus hernia/GORD
  - gall bladder disease*
  - fatty liver
  - cancer (various)
  - kidney disease (check microalbuminuria)
  - excessive daytime sleepiness
  - erectile dysfunction/subfertility
  - psychological problems/depression/anxiety

Indicates relative risk > 3

Obesity is responsible for 80% of type 2 diabetes, 35% of ischaemic heart disease and 55% of hypertension in European adults.

Management

An imperative of treatment is to address the serious comorbidities of type 2 diabetes and insulin resistance. Lifestyle changes are fundamental to outcomes.

Treatment is based on four major interventions, the choice of which depends on the degree of obesity, the associated health problems and the health risk posed. Both the WHO and the NHMRC recommend the approach to obesity and overweight being based on these lifestyle changes, but with an emphasis on realistic goals.

1 reduction in energy (calorie) intake
2 change in diet composition including reduced fat intake
3 increased physical activity
4 behavioural therapy

Pharmacological agents are not used for first-line therapy although they may have a place in management, especially at grade III level of obesity. Surgery is an option for the treatment of morbid obesity.

There is no single effective method for the treatment of obesity, which is a difficult and frustrating problem. A continuing close therapist/patient contact has a better chance of success than any single treatment regimen.

Goals

1 no further weight gain
2 loss of 5–10% initial body weight
3 improve activity

Most successful programs involve a multidisciplinary approach to weight loss, embracing the four major interventions. The first goal should be no further weight gain. Emphasis must be on maintenance of weight loss. Behaviour modification is important and the most valuable strategy is to emphasise planning and record keeping with a continuous weekly diary of menus, exercise and actual behaviour.

Social support is essential for a successful weight loss program. A better result is likely if close family members, especially the chief cook, are involved in the program, preferably striving for the same goals.[2]

A doctor–patient strategy

A close therapeutic supportive relationship with a patient can be effective using the following methods:[8]

1 *Promote realistic goals.* Lose weight at the same rate that it was gained (i.e. slowly)—for example, 5–10 kg a year. A graph can be used for this purpose with an 'exaggerated' scale on the vertical axis so that small variations appear highly significant and encouraging (see FIG. 78.3).

Promote the equation:
Energy In = Energy Out + Energy Stored

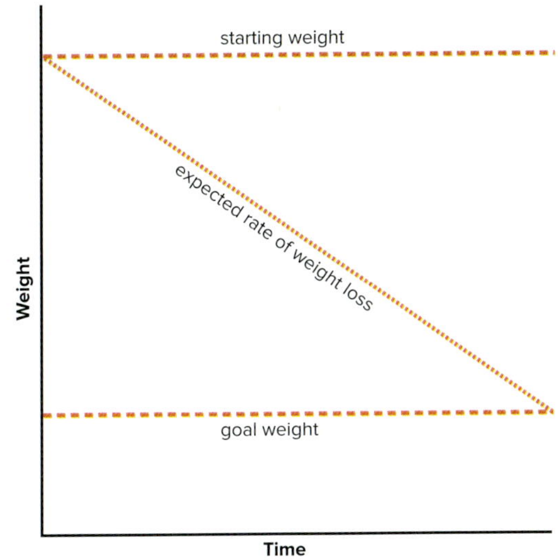

FIGURE 78.3 Weight loss chart to encourage patient
Source: After Kaczmarczyk[8]

The appropriate way to reduce the stored energy (fat) is either to reduce energy in (eat less) or increase energy out (exercise).

2 *Dietary advice.* It is important to be realistic and allow patients to eat their normal foods but advise them about quantity and frequency. Give advice on simple substitutions (e.g. fortified skim milk in place of whole milk, high-fibre wholemeal bread instead of white bread, and fruit and vegetables instead of biscuits and cakes as in-between snacks).[8] Reduce fat intake to <30% of total calorie intake.[7] A strategy that seems to work effectively is to advise patients, especially those who are overweight (and grade I obesity), to eat one-third less than they usually do and discipline themselves not to 'pick' and to avoid second helpings.

3 *Counselling* is simple and commonsense. It involves being supportive, interested and encouraging. A list of tips on coping is provided (see below 'A practical plan' for grade II and III obesity) and the patient advised to keep a food, exercise and behaviour diary.

4 *Review.* 'Review is the most vital part of the weight loss programme as it stimulates and revitalises motivation and enables assessment of progress.'[8] It should be frequent initially (e.g. fortnightly), then monthly until the goal weight has been achieved and then 3-monthly. It is important never to be judgmental or critical if progress is unsatisfactory.

78

A practical plan

The following patient education sheet to be handed to patients represents useful advice to offer the obese patient.[8] The emphasis is on a healthy lifestyle program.

Physical activity

- A brisk walk for at least 20–30 minutes each day is the most practical exercise.
- Other activities such as tennis, swimming, golf and cycling are a bonus.

Dietary advice

Provide patients with a glycaemic index guide (see CHAPTER 10).

Breakfast:

- oatmeal (soaked overnight in water); after cooking, add fresh or dried fruit; serve with fat-reduced milk or yoghurt
  or
- muesli (homemade or from a health food store)—medium serve with fat-reduced milk, perhaps add extra fruit (fresh or dried)
- slice of wholemeal toast with a thin scraping of margarine, spread with Vegemite, Marmite or sugar-free marmalade
- fresh orange juice or herbal tea or black tea/coffee

78

Morning and afternoon tea:

- piece of fruit or vegetable (e.g. carrot or celery)
- freshly squeezed juice or chilled water with fresh lemon

Midday meal:

- salad sandwich with wholemeal or multigrain bread and thin scraping of margarine (for variety use egg, salmon, chicken or cheese fillings)
- drink as for breakfast

Evening meal:

- Summer (cold)—lean meat cuts (grilled, hot or cold), poultry (skin removed) or fish; fresh garden salad; slices of fresh fruit
- Winter (hot)—lean meat cuts (grilled), poultry (skin removed) or fish; plenty of green, red and yellow vegetables and small potato; fruit for sweets

Weight-losing tips[9]

- Have sensible goals; do not 'crash' diet but have a 6–12 month plan to achieve your ideal weight.
- Go for natural foods; avoid junk foods.
- Select fish, poultry and lean meats.
- Trim excess fat from meat and skin from poultry.
- Eat more breads (wholemeal), cereals, fruit and vegetables.
- Increase intake of complex carbohydrates that contain starch and fibre.
- Plant food is good for you; have it as part of breakfast.
- Eat less sugar; avoid lollies and syrups.
- Avoid alcohol, sugary soft drinks and high-calorie fruit juices.
- Strict dieting without exercise fails.
- If you are mildly overweight, eat one-third less than you usually do.
- Do not eat biscuits, cakes, buns, etc. between meals (preferably at no time).
- Limit the intake of full-cream products, fried foods and fatty take-away meals.
- Limit the amount of butter or margarine on vegetables and bread.
- Reduce calorie intake; reduce fat intake to <30% of total calorie intake.
- What you usually eat matters most, not what you eat occasionally.
- Use high-fibre foods to munch on.
- Drink copious water—at least 2 L a day.
- A small treat once a week may add variety.
- Avoid seconds and do not eat leftovers.
- Avoid non-hungry eating.
- Eat slowly—spin out your meal.

Pharmacological agents

A variety of these adjuvant agents are available or imminent but they have limitations and need to be used with caution, if at all. Adverse effects can be problematic. Consider for those with a BMI >30 kg/m^2 and failed well-supervised lifestyle measures.

The agents are:[4,5,9,10]

- Local, acting on GIT:
  - bulking agents (e.g. methylcellulose)
  - lipase inhibitor—orlistat (Xenical) 120 mg (o) tds ac (used with a low-fat eating program)
- Centrally acting agents:
  - amphetamine derivatives (reduce hunger): phentermine 15–40 mg (o) daily (limited use and not recommended)
  - serotonin analogues (enhance satiety): fluoxetine 20–40 mg (o) daily in depressed patients but only temporary weight reduction[7]
  - other SSRIs, e.g. sertraline
  - sibutramine 10–15 mg (o) daily (monitor BP)

A summary of systemic reviews to date indicates that the effectiveness of serotonin analogues is unknown or, with sibutramine and phentermine, of some benefit, which has to be weighed against adverse effects, including the potentially fatal serotonin syndrome. The same applies to orlistat, which, together with a low-fat eating program, does produce extra weight loss over placebo.[11] Drugs should not be expected to have a continuing effect after therapy ceases.

Inappropriate drug treatment includes bulk-forming laxatives, thyroxine, diuretics, complementary and alternative medicines (which may cause adverse cardiovascular effects).[7]

Meal replacements

Food replacement agents such as Optifast have been promoted but there is insufficient evidence so far to evaluate their effectiveness and the reduced intake of key vitamins. Long-term results are disappointing.

Surgery (bariatric surgery)[5,7]

Surgery is the most effective treatment for obesity, but is associated with risks such as malabsorption[4] and nutritional deficiency.[12] In those with morbid obesity (about 2% of the population) unresponsive to behaviour modification therapy and a course of pharmacological agents for 3 months or so, gastric banding has a place. It is recommended in those with a BMI >40 or >35 with at least one severe comorbidity such as poorly controlled diabetes or severe OSA.[13,14] One example is Lap-Band, which is inserted laparoscopically and can be adjusted and eventually removed with minimal significant residual adverse defect left in the stomach. It appears to be effective for 10 years.[5,14] Sleeve gastrectomy gastric bypass such as Roux-en-Y bypass and other techniques can be considered.

Oedema

Oedema (dropsy) is an excessive accumulation of fluid in tissue spaces. It may be generalised or localised—periorbital, peripheral or an arm (lymphoedema, refer CHAPTER 69).

Generalised oedema

The site of generalised oedema is largely determined by gravity. It is due to an abnormal excess of sodium in the body, which leads to accumulation of water. The causes can be generally divided into two groups—oedema associated with a decreased plasma volume and oedema associated with an increased plasma volume (see TABLE 78.4).

Table 78.4 Causes of generalised oedema

Decreased plasma volume
Hypoalbuminaemia (e.g. nephrotic syndrome, chronic liver disease, malnutrition)
Increased plasma volume
Congestive cardiac failure
Chronic kidney failure
Drugs (e.g. corticosteroids, NSAIDs, certain antihypertensives, oestrogens, lithium, others)
Idiopathic oedema

Diagnosis

Clinical examination, including urinalysis, is usually sufficient to establish the cause of the oedema. In other cases, investigation of kidney or liver function may be required.

Treatment

- Treat the cause where known
- Salt (sodium) restriction
- Diuretics:
  - a loop diuretic (e.g. frusemide)
  - a potassium-sparing diuretic (e.g. spironolactone)

Idiopathic oedema

Idiopathic oedema, also known as cyclical or periodic oedema, is a common problem and the diagnosis is made on a characteristic history:

- exclusive to women
- may be cyclical or persistent
- usually unrelated to menstrual cycle
- excessive diurnal weight gain (worse on prolonged standing)
- abdominal bloating
- may affect hands and face as well as feet
- often made worse by diuretics
- may be associated with headache, depression, tension

Treatment of this condition is difficult. Most diuretics can aggravate the problem. Supportive stockings and a nutritious diet (with restricted sodium intake) are recommended as first-line treatment. A trial of spironolactone is often recommended.

Swelling (puffiness) of the face and eyelids

The causes are similar to those for generalised oedema. Important specific causes to consider are:

78

- kidney disease (e.g. nephrotic syndrome, acute nephritis)
- hypothyroidism
- Cushing syndrome and corticosteroid treatment
- mediastinal obstruction/superior vena cava syndrome
- angio-oedema
- skin sensitivity (e.g. drugs, cosmetics, hair dryers)
- carotico-cavernous fistula

Swelling of the legs

Refer to CHAPTER 69.

'Cellulite'

'Cellulite' refers to a characteristic form of dimpling seen in the subcutaneous tissues of hips, buttocks and thighs of females. The dimpling pattern is related to the manner of attachment of fibrous septae that contain the fat. Many patients seek advice about 'cellulite' in the buttocks and thighs in particular. Explain that the best way to overcome it is to maintain an ideal weight. If overweight, lose it slowly and exercise to improve the muscle tone in the buttocks and thighs.

When to refer

- Patients with grade II or III obesity (BMI >35) who are resistant to simple weight control measures.[5]
- Patients with associated medical problems such as angina or severe osteoarthritis who require relatively rapid weight reduction.
- Possibility of endocrine cause of obesity.
- Suspicion of congenital or inherited disorder in children.

Practice tips

- Avoid a critical or judgmental attitude to the overweight patient.
- Diplomatically seek independent information from a spouse or parent about food and beverage intake.
- Obtain a chronological history of the patient's weight from infancy onwards and attempt to correlate any significant changes with stressful life events.
- Central or visceral obesity carries a large risk factor for medical complications. People are advised to keep the waist circumference to less than 100 cm, and ideally less than 80 cm in women and 94 cm in men.
- The best approach is to focus on fitness, with dietary advice on fresh vegetables and fewer 'empty' calories (soft drinks, snack foods). It is much better to be overweight and fit than to be normal weight and unfit.[3]
- What you usually eat matters most, not what you occasionally eat.

Patient education resources

Hand-out sheets from *Murtagh's Patient Education* 7th edition:

- Obesity: how to lose weight wisely
- BMI calculator

References

1 Tunnessen WW Jr. *Signs and Symptoms in Paediatrics* (2nd edn). Philadelphia: JB Lippincott, 1988: 33–41.
2 Papdakis MA, McPhee SJ. *Current Medical Diagnosis and Treatment* (52nd edn). New York: McGraw-Hill Lange, 2013: 1259.
3 Funder J. Weighing it up. RACGP: Good Practice, 2014; 4: 13.
4 Caterson ID. Weight management. Australian Prescriber, 2006; 29: 43–7.
5 Expert group for Cardiovascular. Overweight and obesity. In: eTG complete [Internet]. Melbourne: Therapeutic Guidelines Ltd. Available from: <www.tg.org.au>, accessed October 2017.
6 WHO Technical Report Series Number 894. Geneva: WHO, 2000.
7 Buckley N (Chair). *Australian Medicines Handbook*. Adelaide: Australian Medicines Handbook Pty Ltd, 2016: 550.
8 Kaczmarczyk W. The obese patient. In: How I manage my difficult problems. Aust Fam Physician, 1991; 20: 417–21.
9 RACGP. *Guidelines for Preventive Activities in General Practice* (Red book) (9th edn). Melbourne, 2016: 69–72.
10 Padwal R, Li SK, Lau DC et al. Long term pharmacotherapy for obesity and overweight (Cochrane Review). Cochrane Database. Sept. Rev. 2008, Issue 1. Art No. CD 004094.
11 Arterburn D, Noel P. Obesity. In: Barton S, ed., *Clinical Evidence* (issue 5). London: BMJ Publishing Group, 2001: 412–19.
12 Sjostrom L et al. Bariatric surgery and long-term cardiovascular events. JAMA, 2012; 307 (1): 56–65.
13 Preda TC, Preda VA, Lord RV. What's new in weight loss management and surgery? Medicine Today, 2017; 18 (10): 54–60.
14 Dixon J, O'Brien P et al. Adjustable gastric banding and conventional therapy for type 2 diabetes: a randomised controlled trial. JAMA, 2008; 299 (3): 316–22.

Resources

NHMRC Obesity Guidelines. <www.health.gov.au/internet/main/publishing.nsf/Content/obesityguidelines-index.htm>.

RACGP Red book: the 5 As approach. <www.racgp.org.au/your-practice/guidelines/snap/2-approach-to-preventive-care-in-general-practice/21-the-5as/>.

WHO MONICA project. MONICA Monograph & Multimedia Sourcebook. Geneva: WHO, 2003.

Weight loss

79

Among young women dieters in modern society about 1 in 20 will become preoccupied with their appearance and progress to the eating disorders of anorexia nervosa and bulimia.

PROFESSOR DORIS YOUNG, 1988

In family practice complaints of loss of weight are more frequent than complaints about being too thin. Of great significance is the problem of recent loss of weight. A very analytical history is required to determine the patient's perception of weight loss. The equivalent problem in children is failure to gain weight or thrive.

Weight loss is an important symptom because it usually implies a serious underlying disorder, either organic or functional. It may or may not be associated with anorexia and thus diminished food intake.

Key facts and checkpoints

- Any loss of more than 5% of normal body weight is significant.
- The most common cause in adults of recent weight loss is stress and anxiety.[1]
- Serious organic diseases to consider are:
  - malignant disease
  - diabetes mellitus
  - chronic infections (e.g. tuberculosis)
  - thyrotoxicosis
- The most important variable to consider in evaluating weight loss is appetite. Eating and weight go hand in glove.
- Two conditions commonly associated with weight loss are anaemia and fever; they must be excluded.
- Early detection of eating disorders improves outcome.

A diagnostic approach

A summary of the diagnostic strategy model is presented in TABLE 79.1.

Probability diagnosis

Excluding planned dietary restriction, psychological factors are the most common cause, particularly recent stress and anxiety.[1] Elderly people with adverse psychological factors, neglect and possibly drug effects can present with wasting.

Serious disorders not to be missed

Many of the problems causing weight loss are very serious, especially malignant disease.

Malignant disease

Weight loss may be a manifestation of any malignancy. With cancer of the stomach, pancreas and caecum, malignant lymphomas and myeloma, weight loss may be the only symptom. Occult malignancy must be regarded as the most common cause of weight loss in the absence of major symptoms and signs. The mechanisms may be multiple, with anorexia and increased metabolism being important factors.

Chronic infections

These are now less common but tuberculosis must be considered, especially in people from less developed countries. Some cases of infective endocarditis may progress only very slowly with general debility, weight loss and fever as major features.[2]

Other infections to consider are brucellosis, and protozoal and systemic fungal infection. Infection with HIV virus must be considered, especially in high-risk groups.

Pitfalls

Drug dependency, including alcohol and narcotic drugs, must be considered, especially when the problem may result in inappropriate nutrition. Apart from malignant disease there is a whole variety of gastrointestinal disorders that require consideration—these include malabsorption states, gastric ulceration, and intestinal infestations, especially in people returning from a significant stay in tropical and under-developed countries.

Table 79.1 Weight loss: diagnostic strategy model (other than deliberate dieting or malnutrition)

Probability diagnosis

Stress and anxiety (e.g. redundancy, divorce)
Depressive illness
Non-coping elderly/dementia
Eating disorders: anorexia nervosa/bulimia

Serious disorders not to be missed

Chronic congestive heart failure
Malignant disease, including:

- stomach
- pancreas
- lung
- myeloma
- caecum
- lymphoma

Chronic infection:

- HIV infections (AIDS, AIRC)
- tuberculosis
- hidden abscess
- infective endocarditis
- brucellosis
- others, e.g. overseas acquired infection

Pitfalls (often missed)

Drug dependence esp. alcohol
Malabsorption states:

- ? intestinal parasites/infestations
- coeliac disease

Other GIT problems
Chronic kidney failure
Connective tissue disorders (e.g. SLE, RA)
Dementia
Rarities:

- malnutrition
- Addison disease
- hypopituitarism

Seven masquerades checklist

Depression
Diabetes
Drugs
Anaemia
Thyroid disorder (hyperthyroidism)
UTI

Is the patient trying to tell me something?

A possibility. Consider stress, anxiety and depression. Anorexia nervosa and bulimia are special considerations.

79

Addison disease (CHAPTER 23) can be very difficult to diagnose. Symptoms include excessive fatigue, anorexia, nausea and postural dizziness. Hyperpigmentation is a late sign.

Seven masquerades checklist

Depression and the endocrine disorders, diabetes mellitus and hyperthyroidism, are important causes.

Diabetes

The diabetic who presents with weight loss will be young and insulin-dependent. The initial presentation may be ketoacidosis. The triad of symptoms is thirst + polyuria + weight loss.

Hyperthyroidism

This is usually associated with weight loss although in some, such as an elderly male, it may not be obvious. An important clue will be weight loss in the presence of an excellent appetite and this helps to distinguish it from a psychoneurotic disturbance.

Depression

Weight loss is a common feature of depression and is usually proportional to the severity of the disease. In the early stages of depression, weight gain may be present but when the classic loss of the four basic drives (appetite, energy, sleep and sex) becomes manifest, weight loss is a feature.

Drugs

Any prescribed drugs causing anorexia can cause weight loss. Important drugs include digoxin, narcotics, cytotoxics, NSAIDs, some antihypertensives and theophylline. Be mindful of inappropriate use of thyroxine and laxatives.

Red flag pointers for weight loss

Weight loss per se is a big red flag

- Rapid weight loss with malaise
- Acid dental erosion on surfaces of upper teeth: think bulimia
- Weakness and malaise in young females: consider eating disorder and hypokalaemia
- Evidence of abuse in a child

Psychogenic considerations

Weight loss is a feature of anxiety as well as depression. Some patients with psychotic disturbances, including schizophrenia and mania, may present with weight loss.

Anorexia nervosa is quite common and is almost entirely confined to females between the ages of 12 and 20 years. The main differential diagnosis is hypopituitarism, although anorexia nervosa can cause endocrine disturbances through the hypothalamic pituitary axis.

The clinical approach

History

It is important to document the weight loss carefully and evaluate the patient's recordings. The same set of scales should be used. It is also important to determine the food intake. However, in the absence of an independent witness such as a spouse or parent, this can be difficult. Food intake may be diminished with psychogenic disorders and cancer but increased or steady with endocrine disorders, such as diabetes and hyperthyroidism, and with steatorrhoea. FIGURE 79.1 shows the possible causes of weight loss.

General questions

- Exactly how much weight have you lost and over how long?
- Have you changed your diet in any way?
- Has your appetite changed? Do you feel like eating?
- Have your clothes become looser?
- What is your general health like?
- How do you feel in yourself?
- Do you feel uptight (tense), worried or anxious?
- Do you get very irritable or tremulous?
- Do you feel depressed?
- Do you ever force yourself to vomit?
- Are you thirsty?
- Do you pass a lot of urine?
- Do you have excessive sweating?
- Do you experience a lot of night sweats?
- What are your motions like?
- Are they difficult to flush down the toilet?
- Do you have a cough or bring up sputum?
- Do you get short of breath?
- Do you have any abdominal pain?
- Are your periods normal (for females)?
- What drugs are you taking?
- How many cigarettes do you smoke?

Examination

A careful general examination is essential with special attention to:

- vital parameters, e.g. BMI, temperature, BP
- the thyroid and signs of hyperthyroidism

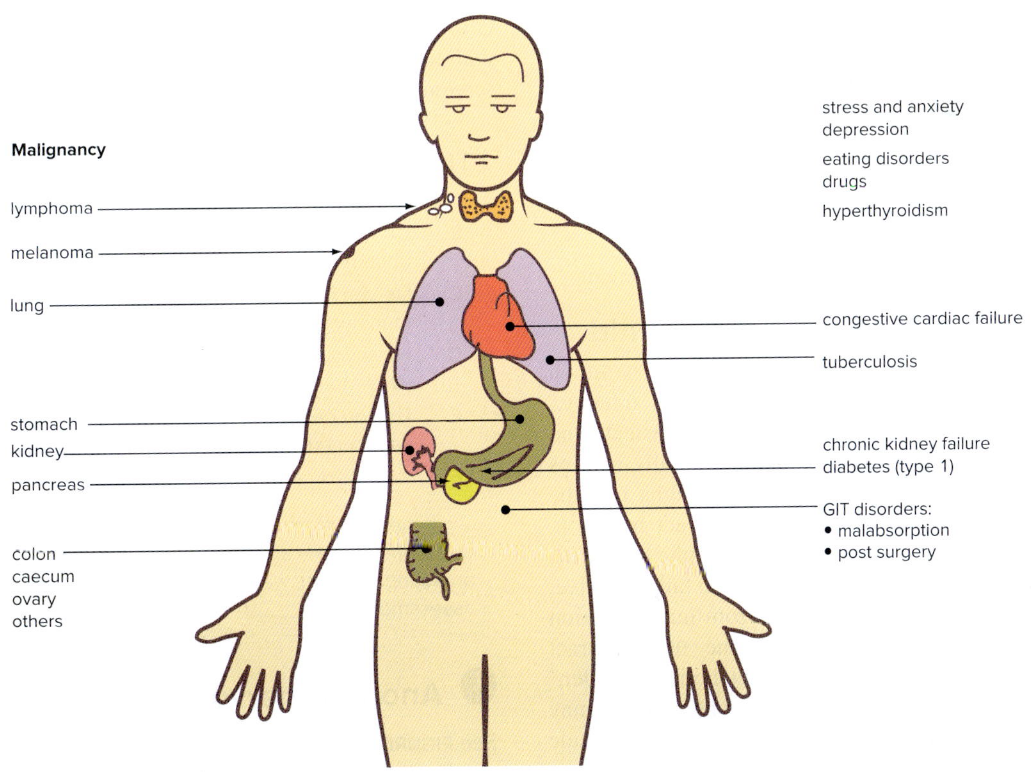

FIGURE 79.1 Weight loss: causes to consider

79

- the abdomen (check liver, any masses and tenderness)
- rectal examination (test stool for occult blood)
- reflexes
- look for acid dental erosion on surface of upper teeth (bulimia)

Investigations

Basic investigations include:

- haemoglobin, red cell indices and film
- white cell count
- ESR/CRP
- thyroid function test
- random blood sugar
- urea and electrolytes
- chest X-ray
- urine analysis
- faecal occult blood

Others to consider:

- upper GIT (endoscopy or barium meal)
- HIV serology
- ultrasound of abdomen (or CT if suspected abnormality not found)
- colonoscopy
- LFTs
- tumour markers, e.g. CA-125, CEA

79

Weight loss in children

Weight loss in children can be considered as:

1 failure to thrive (FTT): the child up to 2 years below 3rd percentile (refer to CHAPTER 91)
2 weight loss in a child after normal development

Loss of weight in the older child

Acute or chronic infections are the most common causes of weight loss in children beyond infancy.[3] In acute infections the weight loss is transient, and once the infection clears the child generally regains the lost weight. In chronic infections signs may be more difficult to detect (e.g. urinary tract infection, pulmonary infection, osteomyelitis, chronic hepatitis). In common with the younger child who fails to thrive, the older child may be suffering from malabsorption syndrome, chronic infection of the urinary tract or a rare chromosomal or metabolic disorder.[4] Tuberculosis, diabetes and malignant disease may present as weight loss and it is necessary to exclude organic disease before considering the more common emotional disorders.

Eating disorders in the adolescent

Concerns about body image and dieting are very common among young women in modern society. Among these dieters 5–10% become abnormally preoccupied with dieting and slimness and progress to the eating disorders of anorexia nervosa and bulimia. Sufferers often have extremely low self-esteem and feel ineffective. They tend to be perfectionists with obsessive–compulsive traits. A history of childhood sexual abuse may be relevant. Media images alone do not cause eating disorders but have a role—genetic vulnerability, temperament, psychological and environmental factors also mediate these illnesses: 'Genes load the gun—the environment pulls the trigger'.

The DSM-5 criteria for diagnosing these disorders, which have serious physical and psychological consequences, are presented in TABLE 79.2. The differential diagnosis of anorexia nervosa includes most of the problems listed in TABLE 79.1.

The history[5]

These patients are often secretive, tend to minimise their symptoms and may be in denial of their problem. Dr Suzy Redston and psychiatric colleagues encourage GPs to engage these patients and keep in close contact with them, referring them as necessary. The validated screening tool SCOFF is recommended.

The SCOFF screening tool

S Do you make yourself **S**ick because you feel uncomfortably full?

C Do you worry you have lost **C**ontrol over how much you eat?

O Have you recently lost more than 6.35 kg (**O**ne stone) in a 3-month period?

F Do you believe yourself to be **F**at when others say you are too thin?

F Would you say **F**ood dominates your life?

If the patient answers Yes to two or more questions, there is a high index of suspicion for an eating disorder, warranting a more detailed assessment.

Anorexia nervosa

See FIGURE 79.2.

Anorexia nervosa is a syndrome characterised by the obsessive pursuit of thinness through dieting with

Table 79.2 DSM-5 criteria for diagnosing anorexia nervosa and bulimia

Anorexia nervosa	
A	Restriction of energy intake relative to requirements leading to significantly low body weight in context of age, sex and physical health. That weight is less than minimally normal or expected
B	Intense fear of gaining weight or becoming fat, despite current underweight status
C	Disturbance of body image (body size or shape) or persistent lack of recognition of seriousness of low body weight
Types	Restricting type—no binge eating or purging binge eating/purging type
Bulimia nervosa	
A	Recurrent episodes of binge eating, that is: 1 eating in a discrete period of time an abnormal quantity of food compared with the average person 2 a sense of lack of control during the binge
B	Recurrent inappropriate compensatory behaviour to prevent weight gain (e.g. self-induced vomiting; misuse of laxatives, diuretics, enemas etc.); fasting or excessive exercise
C	A and B both occur, on average, at least twice a week for 3 months
D	Self-evaluation is unduly influenced by body shape and weight
E	Does not occur exclusively during periods of anorexia nervosa
Types	Purging, non-purging (e.g. fasting, excessive exercise)

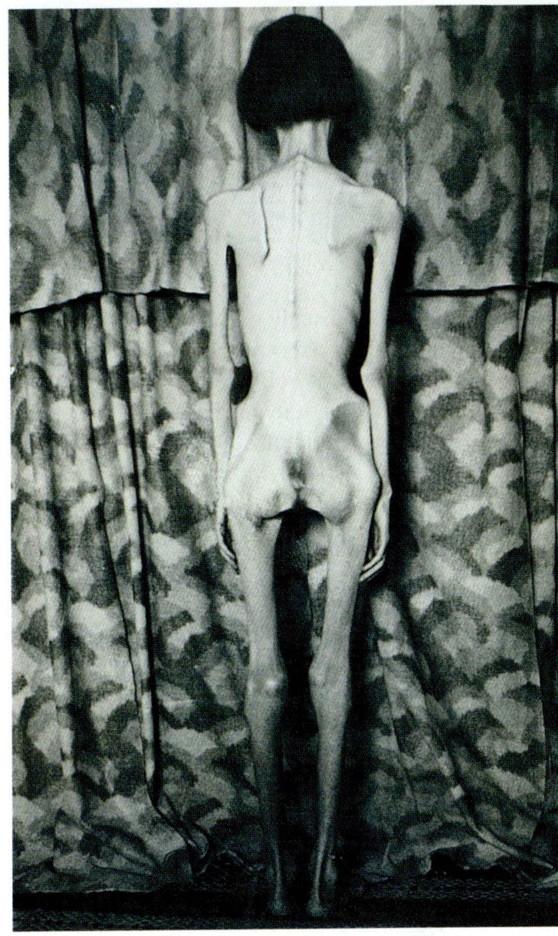

FIGURE 79.2 18-year-old adolescent with severe anorexia nervosa (BMI 7.7). This patient survived after care by her GP

Photo and history courtesy Dr MM O'Brien

extreme weight loss and disturbance of body image.[7] The main symptoms are anorexia and weight loss. The mortality rate may be as high as 18%. It has the highest mortality and suicide rate of any psychiatric disorder.[6]

Typical features

- Adolescent and young adult females
- Up to 1% incidence among schoolgirls aged 16[8]
- Bimodal age of onset: 13–14 and 17–18 years[6]
- Unknown cause
- Poor insight
- Severe emaciation
- Amenorrhoea
- Loss of body fat
- Sallow, dry and scaly skin, hair loss
- Increased lanugo body hair
- BMI <17.5
- Continuing behaviour directed at weight loss

Bulimia nervosa

Bulimia is episodic secretive binge eating followed by self-induced vomiting, fasting or the use of laxatives or diuretics. This binge–purge syndrome is also referred to as bulimarexia. It is more difficult to detect than anorexia nervosa but has a higher incidence. There are two types—the purging type and the non-purging type where fasting or excessive exercise are the compensatory behaviours. The purging type is the most life-threatening behaviour because of the danger of hypokalaemia.

Typical features[6]

- Young females (F:M ratio 10:1)
- Begins at later age, usually 17–25 years
- Associated psychoneurotic disorders
- Family history
- Fluctuations in body weight without extreme loss or gain
- Menstrual history usually normal but periods may be irregular—amenorrhoea rare
- Physical complications of frequent vomiting (e.g. dental decay, effects of hypokalaemia)
- Recurrent laxative, stimulant or enema abuse
- Preoccupation with food
- Exaggerated weight/body shape concern
- Impulse control disorders (e.g. gambling, substance abuse)
- Depressed mood with guilt after a binge

Laboratory evaluation should include electrolytes, FBE, iron studies, TFTs, kidney function tests, coeliac disease screening and LFTs, ESR.

Note: The other main eating disorder is 'binge eating disorder', which is defined as recurrent episodes of binge eating in the absence of regular use of inappropriate compensatory behaviours characteristic of bulimia nervosa. However, most of these patients are obese.

Management of eating disorders

Early detection and intervention are essential to reduce the risk of chronicity. Treatment can be conducted on an outpatient basis but if there are marked trends, such as severe weight loss, a family crisis, severe depression and a suicide risk, the patient requires hospital admission. The burden on caregivers of people with eating disorders is high. There are often problematic family interrelationships that require exploration.

Important goals are:

- establish a good and caring relationship with the patient
- resolve underlying psychological difficulties
- restore weight to a level between ideal and the patient's concept of optimal weight
- provide a balanced diet of at least 3000 calories per day (anorexia nervosa)

Structured behavioural therapy, intensive psychotherapy and family therapy may be tried but supportive care by physicians and allied health staff appears to be the most important feature of therapy.[9] Psychotherapy may be arranged by referral to a psychologist or psychiatrist. The patient may need admission to hospital, especially if dehydration and hypokalaemia (from purging) and also suicide are concerns. Rapid weight loss, vomiting, especially with poor insight, are also 'red flags' for hospital admission. Antidepressants, especially of the SSRI group, may be helpful for selected patients with a comorbid depressive illness. Fluoxetine is the preferred agent for bulimia. It is important to provide ongoing support for both patient and family.

Weight loss in the elderly

General weight loss is a relatively common physiological feature of many elderly people. However, abnormal weight loss is commonly encountered in the socially disadvantaged elderly, especially those who live alone and lack drive and interest in adequate food preparation. Other factors include relative poverty and poor dentition, including ill-fitting and painful false teeth. An important cause that should always be considered is malignant disease. Consider depression, dementia and drug interactions as potential causes of weight loss. Depression is the most common reversible cause of weight loss in elderly people, occurring in up to 30% of all medical outpatients presenting with undernutrition.[10] Weight loss of more than 5% body weight in 6 months is significant and suggests undernutrition.[10]

Congestive cardiac failure, especially secondary to ischaemic heart disease, is a common cause of weight loss. This is due to visceral congestion.

Gastrointestinal causes of weight loss

The following conditions may lead to weight loss:

- coeliac disease
- poor oral hygiene
- chronic vomiting or diarrhoea (e.g. pyloric stenosis)
- gastric ulcer
- cancer of the stomach, oesophagus, large bowel
- problem alcohol drinking
- partial or total gastrectomy
- other GIT surgery
- inflammatory bowel disease (e.g. Crohn disease, ulcerative colitis)
- steatorrhoea
- lymphoma of the gut

- parasitic infestation
- cirrhosis of the liver

The mechanisms of weight loss include anorexia, malabsorption, obstruction with vomiting and inflammation.

When to refer

- Any unexplained weight loss, especially if an endocrine cause or malignancy is suspected
- Weight loss related to a serious psychological illness
- A serious eating disorder

Practice tips

- Ask patients what they really believe is the cause of their weight loss.
- An anxiety state and hyperthyroidism can be difficult to differentiate. Consider the latter and perform thyroid function tests.
- Laboratory tests are rarely needed to establish the diagnosis of an eating disorder. Hormonal levels return to normal following weight gain.
- A high index of suspicion by the family doctor is required to diagnose eating disorders. Think of it in a mid-teen female; weight loss through dieting; wide fluctuation in weight; amenorrhoea and hyperactivity.

Patient education resources

Hand-out sheets from Murtagh's Patient Education 7th edition:

- Eating disorders

References

1 Hopcroft K, Forte V. *Symptom Sorter* (4th edn). Oxford: Radcliffe Publishing, 2010: 226–7.

2 Beck ER, Francis JL, Souhami RL. *Tutorials in Differential Diagnosis* (2nd edn). Edinburgh: Churchill Livingstone, 1988: 117–20.

3 Tunnessen WW. *Symptoms and Signs in Paediatrics* (2nd edn). Philadelphia: Lippincott, 1988: 25–8.

4 Robinson MJ, Roberton DM. *Practical Paediatrics* (5th edn). Melbourne: Churchill Livingstone, 2003: 140–4.

5 Redston S et al. 'Help us, she's fading away'. How to manage the patient with anorexia nervosa. Aust Fam Phys, 2014; 43 (8): 531–6.

6 Young D. Eating disorders. In: Jones R et al, *Oxford Textbook of Primary Medical Care*. Oxford: Oxford University Press, 2004: 972–5.

7 Smink FR et al. Epidemiology, course and outcome of eating disorders. Curr Opin Psychiatry, 2013; 26 (6): 543–8.

8 Crisp AH, Palmer RL, Kalucy RS. How common is anorexia nervosa? A prevalence study. Br J Psychiatry, 1976; 128: 549–54.

9 Papadakis MA, McPhee SJ. *Current Medical Diagnosis and Treatment*. New York: McGraw-Hill Lange, 2013: 1262.

10 Szonyi G, Pokorny CS. Investigating weight loss in the elderly. Medicine Today, 2004; 5 (9): 53–8.

Part 4

Chronic disorders: continuing management

80 Allergic disorders including hay fever

The nostril membrane is so irritable that light dust, contradiction, an absurd remark—anything—sets me sneezing and I can be heard in Taunton with a favourable wind, a distance of six miles. Turn your mind to this little curse. If consumption is too powerful for physicians, at least they should not suffer themselves to be outwitted by such little upstart disorders as the hay fever.

SYDNEY SMITH, LETTER TO DR HOLLAND, 1835

Allergic disorders affect approximately 20% of the population. The clinical spectrum of allergic disorders includes asthma, rhinitis, atopic dermatitis, drug allergy, food allergy, insect sting allergy and anaphylaxis.[1] The most common allergies are those associated with IgE-mediated (immediate or type 1) hypersensitivity, such as allergic rhinoconjunctivitis (hay fever), atopic dermatitis (eczema) and allergic asthma.[2]

Less commonly encountered but of increasing clinical importance in the community are IgE-mediated allergies to foods such as peanuts and/or other nuts and seafoods (crustaceans or molluscs), which may cause urticaria, angioedema, anaphylaxis and even death. Peanuts are one of the most common causes of food-induced anaphylaxis in adults. A clinically significant cross-reactivity between peanuts and other legumes is uncommon, but allergy to tree nuts such as almonds and walnuts may occur in up to 50% of those with peanut allergy.[1] Another special case is the oral allergy syndrome, in which people with some degree of seasonal allergy to grass pollens or birch pollen suffer oral itch and swelling when they come into contact with certain fruits. This problem may be alleviated by desensitisation to pollens.[1]

Natural rubber latex allergy is an increasingly important cause of type 1 hypersensitivity, affecting particularly medical and paramedical personnel, and patients who have had multiple operations or procedures. Diagnosis is suggested by history and confirmed by specific skin tests or the detection of serum-specific IgE. The development of urticaria on contact with latex is highly suggestive of underlying type 1 hypersensitivity. An interesting association between latex allergy and sensitivity to fruit occurs most commonly with banana, kiwifruit or avocado.[1]

Atopy

Atopy occurs in those 45% of the population who have an inherited tendency for an exaggerated IgE antibody response to common environmental antigens.[2] It is not a disease. There will be a positive response to one or more allergen skin-prick tests and usually a family history of allergic disorders. Of those who are atopic, one-half to one-third manifest an allergic disorder, most commonly allergic rhinitis, asthma, atopic dermatitis or allergic gastroenteropathy.

Common allergens causing immediate hypersensitivity

It is helpful to consider important allergen exposure during history taking. TABLE 80.1 lists sources of common allergens.

Table 80.1 Sources of common allergens[1,2]

Source	Allergens
Inhalants	Pollens, domestic animals, house dust mites, mould spores, cockroaches
Foods	Peanuts, fish, shellfish, milk, eggs, wheat
Other	Drugs, latex, insect venoms, occupational

Inhalant allergies

Allergic rhinoconjunctivitis and asthma are the main manifestations. The history provides a strong pointer to the causative allergen. If symptoms are seasonal, pollen allergy is most likely; perennial symptoms may indicate an allergy to dust mites, household pets or moulds. Certain activities that precipitate symptoms may also provide a clue—these include mowing lawns, dusting and vacuuming.

FOOD ALLERGY AND INTOLERANCE[3]

Food allergy usually manifests in infancy and childhood, with symptoms ranging from severe urticarial-type reactions to gastrointestinal symptoms such as anorexia, nausea, vomiting and spitting up of food, colic, diarrhoea and failure to thrive.

Commonly implicated foods include milk and other dairy products, eggs and peanuts. Other foods include oranges, soy beans, nuts, chocolate, fish, shellfish and wheat.

The allergic reactions are not to be confused with non-immunological food intolerances such as lactose intolerance.

A food intolerance is an adverse reaction to a specific food or food ingredient. It is regarded as a food allergy if the reaction is immune based. Food allergies can be simply classified as:

- immediate reactions—occurring within 2 hours
- delayed reactions—occur up to 24 hours after ingestion

IgE-mediated food reactions[3]

These are immediate immune-mediated responses to a foreign glycoprotein which are relatively easy to diagnose.

Clinical features

- Typically in infants and toddlers
- Usually occur within 30–60 minutes
- Due to release of mast cell mediators
- Produce flushing or blotchiness/pallor (if severe)
- Itchy oropharynx
- Itchy, runny nose and eyes
- Wheeze
- Dizziness and confusion
- Urticaria—facial or generalised (see FIG. 80.1)
- Feeling of intense fear (angor animi)
- Angioedema of face and airway
- Vomiting, diarrhoea and abdominal colic (immediate or soon after)
- ± Anaphylaxis with wheezing, etc.
- Death can occur (especially if asthma history)
- Big three foods—cow's milk, egg, peanuts
- Also: soy beans; fish, especially shellfish; wheat; tree nuts; various fruits and vegetables
- Cow's milk can cross-react with goat's milk and soy protein
- Frequently resolves by 3–5 years
- In adults the foods are mainly peanuts, tree nuts, fish and shellfish

Management

- Document diet, symptoms, past history, family history
- Refer for specialist allergy advice
- Provide patient education sheet
- Advise avoidance of suspected food
- IgE reactions investigated with skin testing
- Consider provision of an adrenaline auto-injector

Non-IgE-mediated food reactions[3]

These are less common and are usually delayed, occurring within 24–48 hours of food ingestion—but some reactions may be immediate. The real explanation is not clear. This includes cow's milk protein intolerance with both breast milk- and formula-fed infants. It affects 2% of infants under 2 years with most resolving by 2–3 years of age.

Clinical features

- Gastrointestinal symptoms (e.g. vomiting, diarrhoea, abdominal colic)
- May be malabsorption, weight loss, failure to thrive (rare)
- Aggravation of atopic dermatitis
- Severe reactions possible
- Main foods—cow's milk, soy proteins
- Uncommon after 3 years of age

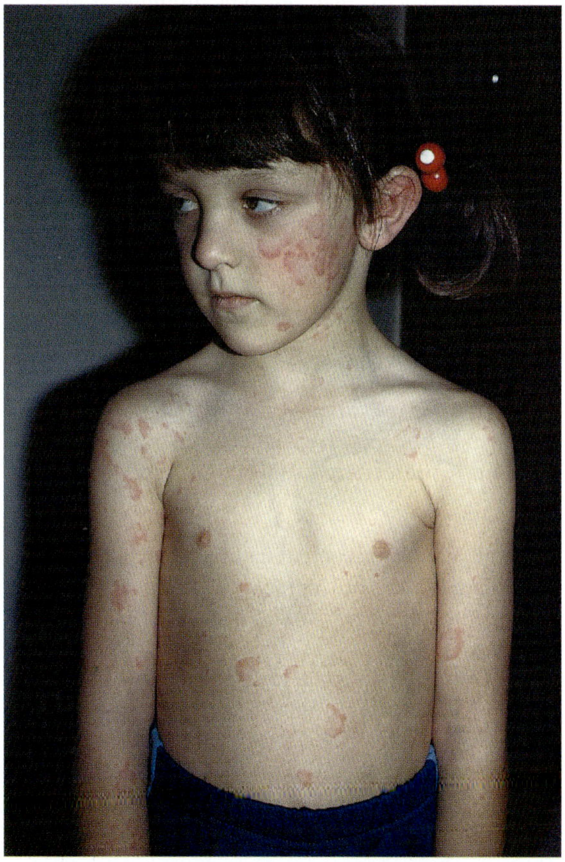

FIGURE 80.1 Acute urticaria in a child caused by a sensitivity to aspirin

80

Management

- Elimination of suspected food, then formal food challenge
- For milk protein intolerance first-line treatment is a formula containing cow's milk protein hydrolysate. Don't use soy-based formulas under 6 months since many are also soy protein intolerant.
- Skin testing usually not helpful and may be risky

Food protein-induced enterocolitis syndrome (FPIES)

This is seen in young infants usually <6 months and is usually due to cow's milk, soy or cereals. It can be seen in breastfed infants and older children. A typical reaction is delayed onset of projectile vomiting and protracted diarrhoea. The stool contains blood and eosinophils. Treatment is with substance elimination.

Food intolerances[4]

In general practice it is common to see a variety of food intolerances that are not immune (allergic) or psychologically based. The food constituents represent an important group. The intolerances can be grouped as:

- fructose intolerance from excessive ingestion of fruit juices and soft drinks
- lactase deficiency from milk
- histamine-related reactions from strawberries, tomatoes
- chemical triggers:
  - aspirin, tartrazine, sodium metabisulphite—triggering rhinitis and asthma
  - aspirin, tartrazine, benzoic acid—triggering chronic urticaria
- others—salicylates (manufactured or natural), amines, preservatives and colourings

  Note:
- foods with high-content natural salicylate include: dried fruits, pineapple, apricots, oranges, cucumbers, grapes, honey, olives, tomato sauce, wines, tea, herbs
- foods likely to contain tartrazine (food colouring) include: bottled sauces, cakes (from shops), coloured fizzy drinks, fruit cordial, custard, coloured sweets, ice-cream and lollies, jam

Symptoms

There can be a variety of symptoms:

- irritability, behavioural problems
- gastrointestinal (e.g. infant colic, diarrhoea, irritable bowel syndrome)
- respiratory—rhinitis, asthma
- headache/migraine

Management

- Document diet, reactions, past/family history
- Elimination diet and controlled food challenge
- Referral for specialist allergy advice
- Radioallergosorbent (RAST) testing is indicated where skin testing contraindicated

Peanut allergy

Peanuts are one of the most common causes of food-induced allergy including anaphylaxis in adults. The diagnosis is confirmed by demonstration of peanut-specific IgE by either skin-prick tests with peanut extract or RAST testing. Reaction to peanuts usually begins within minutes of ingestion, the first symptoms being oropharyngeal itching or burning. Flushing, urticaria, wheeze, stridor, angioedema and collapse may follow.[5] The combination of peanut allergy and asthma is dangerous, as evidenced by fatal or near-fatal reactions in young children.[6] The key to management is avoidance of peanut-containing foods. Desensitisation is currently not recommended. Those at risk should carry an anaphylaxis kit (see TABLE 80.2).

Table 80.2 Adult anaphylaxis kit[2]

Item	Instructions
Autoinjector 300 mcg adrenaline 1:1000 IM injection	Inject into outer thigh muscle at first sign of swelling of throat or tongue, or other reaction (e.g. breathlessness)
Medihaler-Epi MDI (adrenaline metered aerosol spray)	Spray 10–20 times in milder reactions only (e.g. local lip tingling or swelling)
Oral antihistamines	e.g. 10 mg loratadine tablets (× 2) Take 1 tablet after adrenaline injection
Prednisolone 25 mg tablets (× 2)	Take immediately after adrenaline

Doses for children: 15–30 kg—150 mcg; 30 kg—300 mcg

Risk-minimisation strategies for food anaphylaxis[1]

- Achieve optimal asthma control (unstable asthma is the major risk factor)
- Notify others: school, homes, restaurants
- Carry treatment: action plan and adrenaline

80

- 'Touch test' food on external lip before consumption
- Avoid skin preparations containing natural foods

Egg allergy

Previous advice was to avoid introducing potentially allergenic foods to babies. The evidence now shows that babies who are given foods such as peanuts, eggs and seafoods in the first year of life develop fewer allergies than babies where these foods are strictly avoided. The Australian Society of Clinical Immunology and Allergy (ASCIA) has detailed information about introducing foods on its website.[7]

Current vaccinations do not include egg; it is present in only minute amounts in the MMR vaccine.

Latex allergy

The clinical manifestations of type 1 hypersensitivity reactions to latex protein are wide-ranging, from urticaria to life-threatening anaphylaxis and death. It is believed that some episodes of intra-operative anaphylaxis are due to the patient—who has been sensitised to latex—reacting after mucosal contact with gloves worn by operating staff. Some institutions now provide latex-free operating suites in response to this serious problem.[8]

Latex allergy is thus a significant problem for at-risk people, including health care workers, patients with spina bifida or other spinal cord abnormalities, and those who have had multiple operations. The greatest risk is contact with 'dipped' rubber products (e.g. gloves, condoms, balloons). Some hard rubber products may not pose a risk.

Symptoms

- Contact dermatitis (type 4 hypersensitivity), urticaria, worsening atopic dermatitis, allergic rhinoconjunctivitis, asthma, allergy to multiple fruits and possibly anaphylaxis

Diagnosis

Skin-prick tests (dangerous and best left to experts) are more sensitive than blood tests at this stage but carry a risk of anaphylaxis. Measurement of serum specific IgE is safe although less sensitive. Contact allergy (type 4) is identified by patch testing.

Management

Health care workers who are allergic can never again wear latex gloves.[9]

Tests for specific IgE

Skin-prick tests

This is the preferred method as results can be read at the first consultation, provided high-quality allergen preparations are used. A positive test alone may be of no diagnostic significance if the patient is asymptomatic to the specific allergens. A negative test is very useful for excluding IgE-mediated allergy.

Detection of serum-specific IgE

A number of tests, including RAST tests[1] and ELISA tests, measure allergen-specific IgE in the serum. They are no more accurate than skin testing, are expensive and do not provide an immediate result.

Indications include: history and skin tests not matching, extensive eczema, dermographism, infants and very young children, immunotherapy work-up, antihistamine use in past 48 hours.

Management principles[1]

Allergen avoidance

If relevant from history and skin-prick testing, special attention should be paid to reducing exposure to house dust mites and mould, to pet selection and specific food avoidance. Change of occupation and environment may be necessary for some people.

Pharmacotherapy

Drugs are used to alleviate symptoms where avoidance methods have failed or are impractical. Examples include antihistamines (H_1-receptor and H_2-receptor antagonists), adrenaline (emergency use), sodium cromoglycate, corticosteroids, some anticholinergics and sympathomimetics.

80

Immunotherapy (desensitisation)

This involves repeated administration of small, increasing doses of allergen by subcutaneous injection. This is the treatment of choice for severe wasp or bee venom allergy and for resistant allergic rhinoconjunctivitis where a single causative allergen can be identified. Patients should be observed for at least 45 minutes after each injection and adequate resuscitation facilities are essential.

Management of specific allergic disorders

- Asthma—see CHAPTER 82
- Atopic dermatitis—see CHAPTER 121

- Urticaria—see CHAPTER 120
- Anaphylaxis and angioedema—see CHAPTER 128

Rhinitis

Refer to CHAPTER 59.

The classification of rhinitis can be summarised as:

- seasonal allergic rhinoconjunctivitis = hay fever
- perennial rhinitis:
  - allergic (often due to house dust mites)
  - non-allergic = vasomotor: eosinophilic, non-eosinophilic

ALLERGIC RHINITIS[9,10]

> **Definition**
>
> **Allergic rhinitis** May be seasonal or perennial. It can be classified as either intermittent (lasting for <4 days of the week or <4 weeks) or persistent (lasting >4 days of the week or >4 weeks).

The severity of symptoms is classified as either mild (normal function including sleep and only slightly troublesome symptoms) or moderate/severe (troublesome symptoms with impairment of activities).[9] Its prevalence has increased worldwide, affecting 20% of the adult population and up to 40% in children; 60% have a family history. It varies from 5–20% with a peak prevalence in children and young adults up to 20%.[11] The symptoms are caused by release of powerful chemical mediators such as histamine, serotonin, prostaglandins and leukotrienes from sensitised mast cells.[11]

80

Seasonal allergic rhinoconjunctivitis (hay fever)

This is the most common type of allergic rhinitis and is due to a specific allergic reaction of the nasal mucosa, principally to pollens. The allergens responsible for perennial allergic rhinitis include inhaled dust, dust mite, animal dander and fungal spores.

Most cases of hay fever begin in childhood with one-half of eventual cases having the problem by the age of 15 and 90% by the age of 30.[12] Approximately 20% suffer from asthma.

While patients with hay fever tend to have widespread itching (nose, throat and eyes), those with perennial rhinitis rarely have eye or throat symptoms but mainly sneezing and watery rhinorrhoea. Nasal polyps are associated with this disorder (refer to CHAPTER 59).

Management

Management consists of four main areas:

1. appropriate explanation and reassurance
2. allergen avoidance
3. pharmacological treatment
4. immunotherapy

Intranasal corticosteroids which reduce inflammation and nasal secretions are first-line treatment for moderate to severe cases.[14]

Advice to patients

- Keep healthy, eat a well-balanced diet, avoid 'junk food' and live sensibly with balanced exercise, rest and recreation. If your eyes give you problems, try not to rub them, avoid contact lenses and wear sunglasses.
- Avoid using decongestant nose drops and sprays: although they soothe at first, a worse effect occurs on the rebound.
- Avoidance therapy: avoid the allergen, if you know what it is (consider pets, feather pillows and eiderdowns).
- Sources of the house dust mite are bedding, upholstered furniture, fluffy toys and carpets. Seek advice about significantly reducing the dust in your bedroom or home, especially if you have perennial rhinitis.
- Pets, especially cats, should be kept outside.
- Avoid chemical irritants such as aspirin, smoke, cosmetics, paints and sprays.

Allergen avoidance

This is difficult during the spring pollen season, particularly where patients are living in high-pollen (e.g. country farming) areas, or spending considerable time outdoors in the course of work or sporting and recreational activities.

Treatment (pharmacological)[9]

Therapy can be chosen from:

1. antihistamines:
   - oral (not so effective for vasomotor rhinitis)
   - intranasal spray (rapid action)
   - ophthalmic drops
2. decongestants (oral or topical)
3. sodium cromoglycate
   - intranasal: powder insufflation or spray
   - ophthalmic drops for associated conjunctivitis
4. corticosteroids
   - intranasal (not so effective for non-eosinophilic vasomotor rhinitis)

- oral (very effective if other methods fail)
- ophthalmic drops for allergic conjunctivitis

Immunotherapy

Consider hyposensitisation/immunotherapy when specific allergens are known (very important) and conventional response is inadequate. Immunotherapy to grass pollen is generally very effective and should be considered in moderate to severe springtime hay fever. Immunotherapy by injection or oral administration can be labour-intensive, often taking years.

Antihistamines

Oral antihistamines are the first line of treatment for seasonal hay fever and are generally effective where symptoms are intermittent, or when used prophylactically before periods of high pollen exposure. The newer 'non-sedating' antihistamines that do not cross the blood–brain barrier are used in preference to the first-generation drugs, although some degree of sedation may occur even with these. A list of non-sedating antihistamines is presented in TABLE 80.3. It is claimed by some that the newer topical preparations, levocabastine and azelastine, as intranasal sprays, are rapidly effective for an exacerbation of symptoms. If sedation is desirable (e.g. overnight), a sedating antihistamine can be used.

Table 80.3 Less sedating antihistamines (oral regimens)

Generic name	Onset	Adult dosage
Cetirizine	Rapid	10 mg daily
Desloratadine	Very rapid	5 mg daily
Fexofenadine	Rapid	60 mg bd
Loratadine	Very rapid	10 mg daily

Oral decongestants

Oral sympathomimetics, either used alone or in combination with antihistamines (where they may help reduce drowsiness), may be of some value, particularly where nasal discharge and stuffiness are major symptoms. Side effects include nervousness and insomnia. They should be used cautiously in patients with hypertension, heart disease, hyperthyroidism, glaucoma and prostatic hypertrophy.

Examples:
pseudoephedrine HCl 60 mg (o) tds (max. 240 mg/day), or 120 mg controlled release (o) bd

Intranasal therapy[9,10]

Intranasal decongestants should be used for limited periods only (i.e. less than a week) or intermittently (3–4 doses per week) because of the potential problems with rebound congestion and rhinitis medicamentosa. They are often of particular value during the first week of treatment with intranasal corticosteroids (where the onset of action is delayed several days), improving nasal patency and allowing more complete insufflation of the corticosteroids. Adverse reactions similar to those of oral decongestants may occur.

Intranasal sodium cromoglycate acts by preventing mast cell degranulation and is effective without serious side effects. The capsule variety must be used (the spray form requires 1–2 hourly dosage to be effective); it is useful in perennial allergic rhinitis but is not as effective as intranasal corticosteroids for springtime hay fever.

Intranasal corticosteroid sprays are the most effective agents for treating seasonal allergic rhinitis. Side effects are minimal and adrenal suppression is not a problem with normal usage. Patients should be informed that these medications will not give immediate relief (often taking 10–14 days to have peak effect) and must be used continuously throughout the hay fever season for at least 6–8 weeks. Local side effects include dryness and mild epistaxis.

Intranasal antihistamines group—includes azelastine and levocabastine—are effective at relieving itching and sneezing.

TABLE 80.4 lists intranasal preparations for rhinitis.

Ophthalmic preparations

Sodium cromoglycate eyedrops are usually very effective for springtime conjunctivitis. They can be used as necessary (no dosage limit) and are most helpful when used prophylactically before periods of high pollen exposure. Decongestant eyedrops may also be helpful (care with narrow angle glaucoma), while corticosteroid eyedrops are reserved for resistant allergic conjunctivitis and should be used with care to exclude infection and glaucoma. Antihistamine eyedrops antazoline and levocabastine are yet another option.

Other treatments

Corticosteroids (oral)

These can be very effective where other treatments or methods have failed. A 6–10 day short course can be used. An example of a 6-day 'rescue course' is prednisolone 25, 25, 20, 15, 10, 5 mg daily doses.

Table 80.4 Intranasal preparations for rhinitis

	Brand name	Dosage	Comments
Sodium cromoglycate	Rynacrom powder (capsules)	Insufflate 1 capsule, qid 2%	Compliance a problem
	Rynacrom nasal spray	Spray 4–6 times daily 4%	
		Spray 2–4 times daily	
Beclomethasone dipropionate 50 mcg/spray	Beconase Hayfever	100 mcg spray each nostril bd or tds	
Budesonide 64 mcg/spray	Budamax nasal	1–2 sprays each nostril daily	
	Rhinocort nasal		
Ciclesonide 50 mcg/spray	Alvesco, Omnaris	2 sprays each nostril daily	
Fluticasone furoate 27.5 mcg/spray	Avamys	2 sprays each nostril daily, reducing to 1 spray	
Fluticasone propionate 50 mcg/spray	Beconase Allergy 24 hour aqueous	2 sprays each nostril daily reducing to 1 spray	
Mometasone furoate 50 mcg/spray	Nasonex	2 sprays per nostril daily	
Triamcinolone 55 mcg/spray	Telnase	2 sprays each nostril daily reducing to 1 spray	
Ipratropium bromide	Atrovent	1–2 sprays per nostril tds prn	Useful for vasomotor rhinitis and profuse rhinorrhoea
			Care needed with elderly
Azelastine	Azep	1 spray each nostril bd	Antihistamine
Levocabastine 0.05%	Livostin	2 sprays each nostril bd	Antihistamine, max. 8 weeks
Various sympathomimetics (e.g. phenylephrine)		2, 3 or 4 times daily (max. 7 days)	Short-term use only Care with elderly, prostatic hypertrophy

Ipratropium bromide (Atrovent)[13]

80

The nasal preparation of this topical anti-cholinergic is often very effective when rhinorrhoea is the major problem.

Leukotriene receptor antagonist

Regarded as equivalent to oral antihistamines, they have a place in the management of children with concurrent asthma and hay fever (e.g. montelukast).

Surgery

Inferior turbinate reduction aims to reduce the size of turbinates and so reduce nasal obstruction when congested.

Guidelines from elite task force[15]

1. For initial treatment of seasonal allergic rhinitis in people aged 12 or older, routinely prescribe monotherapy with an intranasal corticosteroid rather than an intranasal corticosteroid in combination with an oral antihistamine.
2. For initial treatment of seasonal allergic rhinitis in those aged 15 or more, recommend an intranasal corticosteroid over a leukotriene receptor antagonist.
3. For treatment of moderate to severe seasonal allergic rhinitis in people 12 or older, you may recommend the combination of an intranasal corticosteroid and an intranasal antihistamine initially.

TABLE 80.5 summarises recommended steps in management.

When to refer

- Where surgical intervention is required, such as with nasal obstruction from polyps, bulky nasal turbinates and deviated septum
- For immunotherapy

Table 80.5 Summary of recommended treatment steps for allergic rhinitis[9]

Patient education
Allergen avoidance (if possible)

Mild cases:

- less sedating antihistamines including levocabastine nasal spray ±
- decongestant (e.g. pseudoephedrine)

Moderate to severe (persistent):

- intranasal corticosteroids (as preventer—the most effective)
- sodium cromoglycate (Opticrom) eyedrops
- oral corticosteroids (if topicals ineffective)
- immunotherapy if applicable

Practice tips

- Avoid long-term use of topical decongestant nasal drops.
- Avoid topical antihistamine preparations.
- Prescribe sodium cromoglycate eyedrops for the hay fever patient with itchy eyes.
- Be careful of severe systemic reactions that can occur with intradermal skin testing and with immunotherapy. Resuscitation facilities should be available.

References

1. O'Hehir R. Update in allergic diseases. In: *Update Course for GPs handbook*. Melbourne: Monash University, 2016 (available on request).
2. Loblay RH. Allergies (type 1). In: *MIMS Disease Index* (2nd edn). Sydney: IMS Publishing, 1996: 12–15.
3. Thomson K, Tey D, Marks M. *Paediatric Handbook* (8th edn). Oxford: Wiley-Blackwell, 2009: 229–32.
4. Joshi P. Does my child have a food allergy? Medicine Today, Jan 2011; 12 (1): 20–25.
5. Douglas R, O'Hehir R. Peanut allergy. Med J Aust, 1997; 166: 63–4.
6. Sampson HA, Mendleson L, Rosen JP. Fatal and near fatal anaphylactic reactions to food in children and adolescents. N Engl J Med, 1992; 327: 380–4.
7. ASCIA, Information on how to introduce solid foods to babies for allergy prevention. Available from: <www.allergy.org.au/patients/allergy-prevention/ascia-how-to-introduce-solid-foods-to-babies>, accessed March 2018.
8. Katelaris CH et al. Prevalence of latex allergy in a dental school. Med J Aust, 1996; 164: 711–14.
9. Walls RS. Latex allergy: a real problem. Med J Aust, 1996; 164: 707.
10. Expert group for Respiratory guidelines. Rhinitis. In: eTG complete. Melbourne: Therapeutic Guidelines Ltd. Available from: <www.tg.org.au>, accessed September 2017.
11. Baumgart K. Allergic rhinitis: update. Medical Observer, 28 September 2012: 28–30.
12. Scoppa J. Rhinitis (allergic and vasomotor). In: *MIMS Disease Index* (2nd edn). Sydney: IMS Publishing, 1996: 450–1.
13. Fry J. *Common Diseases* (4th edn). Lancaster: MTP Press, 1985: 134–8.
14. Buckley N (Chair). *Australian Medicines Handbook*. Adelaide: Australian Medicines Handbook Pty Ltd, 2016: 391–2.
15. Wallace DV et al. Pharmacological treatment of seasonal allergic rhinitis: synopsis of guidance from the 2017 joint task force on practice parameters. Ann Internal Med, 19 December 2017; 167(12): 876–881.

Resource

Australasian Society of Clinical Immunology and Allergy <www.allergy.org.au>

81 Anxiety disorders

Anxiety is a thin stream of fear trickling through the mind. If encouraged, it cuts a channel into which all other thoughts are drained.

Arthur Somers Roche (1883–1935)

Anxiety is a normal human physiological response that helps us respond to potential threats or dangers. We cannot get by without it. With an increase in anxiety, our performance should increase accordingly (e.g. preparing for exams). When we have too much anxiety, however, a further increase in anxiety will lead to our performance dropping off, described by the Yerkes–Dodson curve (see FIG. 81.1). The optimal place to be on the curve is to the left of the peak, so we have a positive response in our performance to an increase in stress. Being at the peak or to the right will make us vulnerable to stress.

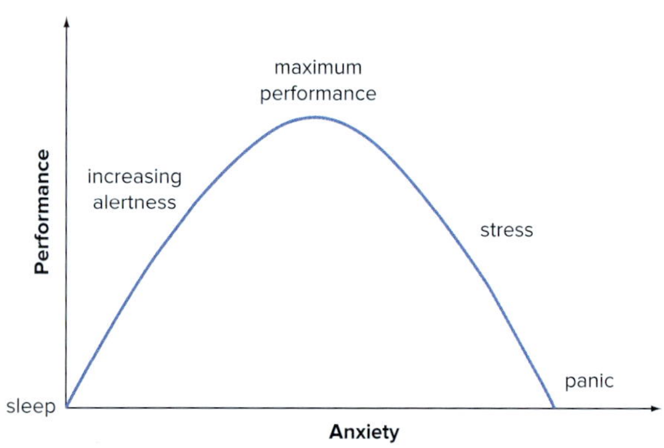

FIGURE 81.1 Yerkes–Dodson curve

Anxiety becomes a problem when the stressor overwhelms us, resulting in poor performance, or if the unwanted consequences of the anxiety response give us undesirable physiological consequences. The stressor causes limbic activation, which in turn leads to autonomic and neuro-endocrine activity (down-regulation) that causes various physiological responses, including activation of the hypothalamic–pituitary axis. Blood flows from the gut to the skeletal muscles, smooth muscle contracts in the bowels and increases nausea, muscle tension increases, pupils dilate, the heart rate increases and blood pressure rises. These changes account for various somatic symptoms commonly seen in anxiety disorders (e.g. tension headaches, palpitations, eye strain and irritable bowel-like symptoms). In high stress situations, a flight–fright–freeze response can ensue.

The physiological role of anxiety and the way in which excess anxiety can cause these physical symptoms can be explained to patients suffering from anxiety disorders—and the GP is very well placed to conduct such psycho-education. Patients suffering from somatic symptoms are often unaware of the physiological consequences of anxiety and usually find this clarification comforting. It can help motivate patients to pursue strategies to reduce them.

Prevalence and classification of anxiety

Anxiety disorders affect 14% of the population,[1] with many people fulfilling the criteria for multiple anxiety disorders and/or a common co-diagnosis of depression.[2] The criteria for defining anxiety, as for many mental health disorders, have broadened over time, so it is difficult to compare historic prevalence figures. Specific phobia is the most commonly reported anxiety-related diagnosis (1 in 5 women and 1 in 10 men), and PTSD is the most common disorder (over 6%).[1] Anxiety disorders listed in the DSM-5 are:[3]

- separation anxiety disorder
- selective mutism
- specific phobia
- social anxiety disorder (social phobia)
- panic disorder
- panic attack (specifier)
- agoraphobia
- generalised anxiety disorder

- substance/medication-induced anxiety disorder
- anxiety due to another medical condition
- other specified anxiety disorder
- unspecified anxiety disorder

Other conditions discussed in this chapter include:

- obsessive–compulsive disorder
- body dysmorphic disorder (see CHAPTER 45)
- post-traumatic stress disorder
- acute stress disorder
- adjustment disorder with anxious mood
- somatic symptom disorder

Generalised anxiety disorder

Generalised anxiety .comprises excessive anxiety and worry about various life circumstances and is not related to a specific activity, time or event such as trauma, obsessions or phobias. It affects up to 5% of the population. There is an overlap between generalised anxiety disorder (GAD) and other anxiety disorders.

General features:

- persistent unrealistic and excessive anxiety
- worry about a number of life circumstances for 6 months or longer

Diagnostic criteria for generalised anxiety disorder

Three or more of:

- restless, 'keyed up' or 'on edge'
- easily fatigued
- difficulty concentrating or 'mind going blank'
- irritability
- muscle tension
- sleep disturbance

Clinical features

Psychological

- Apprehension/fearful anticipation
- Irritability
- Exaggerated startle response
- Sleep disturbance and nightmares
- Impatience
- Panic
- Sensitivity to noise
- Difficulty concentrating or 'mind going blank'

Physical

- Motor tension:
  - muscle tension/aching
  - tension headache
  - trembling/shaky/twitching
  - restlessness
  - tiredness/fatigue
- Autonomic overactivity:
  - dry mouth
  - palpitations/tachycardia
  - sweating/cold, clammy hands
  - flushes/chills
  - difficulty swallowing or 'lump in throat'
  - diarrhoea/abdominal distress
  - frequency of micturition
  - difficulty breathing/smothering feeling
  - dizziness or lightheadedness

Symptoms and signs according to systems

- *Neurological:* dizziness, headache, trembling, twitching, shaking, paraesthesia
- *Cardiovascular:* palpitations, tachycardia, flushing, chest discomfort
- *Gastrointestinal:* nausea, indigestion, diarrhoea, abdominal distress
- *Respiratory:* hyperventilation, breathing difficulty, air hunger
- *Cognitive:* fear of dying, difficulty concentrating, 'mind going blank', hypervigilance

Diagnosis of generalised anxiety disorder

The diagnosis is based on:

- history—it is vital to listen carefully to what the patient is saying
- exclusion of organic disorders simulating anxiety by history, examination and appropriate investigation
- exclusion of other psychiatric disorders, especially depression and adjustment disorder with anxious mood

Note: Anxiety and major depression often co-exist.

Main differential diagnoses (note that this conforms to the seven masquerades list):

- depression
- alcohol or drug (including benzodiazepine) dependence/withdrawal
- hyperthyroidism
- angina and cardiac arrhythmias
- iatrogenic drugs
- caffeine intoxication

Important checkpoints

Five self-posed questions should be considered by the family doctor before treating an anxious patient:

- Is this hyperthyroidism?
- Is this depression?
- Is this normal anxiety?
- Is this mild anxiety or simple phobia?
- Is this moderate or severe anxiety?
- Is this an adjustment disorder?

Management

The management applies mainly to generalised anxiety, as specific psychotherapy is required in other types of anxiety. Much of the management can be carried out successfully by the family doctor using brief counselling and support. Cognitive behaviour therapy (CBT), in which maladaptive thinking, feelings, perceptions and related behaviours are identified, assessed, challenged and modified, can be of considerable benefit.[4] Exercise, both low or high intensity, has been shown to decrease anxiety symptoms. Hence psychological therapy and non-drug strategies are first-line therapy for most anxiety disorders.[5]

Principles of management

- Psychological interventions (e.g. 'life coaching' and CBT) are first line.
- Give careful explanation and reassurance:
  - explain the reasons for the symptoms
  - be aware that patients often 'worry about worrying' (e.g. that anxiety is dangerous, that they are going crazy or 'losing it')[6]
  - reassure the patient about the absence of organic disease (can only be based on a thorough examination and appropriate investigations)
  - direct the patient to appropriate resources to give insight and support
- Provide practical advice on ways of dealing with the problems.
- Advise on the avoidance of aggravating substances such as caffeine, nicotine and other drugs.
- Advise on general measures such as stress management techniques, relaxation programs, mindfulness and regular exercise and if possible organise these for the patient (don't leave it to the patient).

81

Table 81.1 Significant differential diagnoses of anxiety

Psychiatric disorders
Depression
Drug and alcohol dependence/withdrawal
Benzodiazepine dependence/withdrawal
Schizophrenia
Acute or chronic organic brain disorder
Early dementia
Organic disorders
Drug-related:
• amphetamines
• bronchodilators
• caffeine excess
• ephedrine/pseudoephedrine
• levodopa
• thyroxine
Cardiovascular:
• angina
• cardiac arrhythmias
• mitral valve prolapse
Endocrine:
• hyperthyroidism
• phaeochromocytoma
• carcinoid syndrome
• hypoglycaemia
• insulinoma
Neurological:
• epilepsy, especially complex partial seizures
• acute brain syndrome
Respiratory:
• asthma
• acute respiratory distress
• pulmonary embolism

- Advise on coping skills, including personal and interpersonal strategies, to manage difficult circumstances and people (in relation to that patient).
- Provide ongoing supportive psychotherapy.

TABLES 81.2 and 81.3 list a number of good sources of reliable information about anxiety.[7]

Pharmacological treatment[8,9]

The key principles of using medication for anxiety disorders are:

- Non-pharmacological management is first line for a reason. Do not rush into using medication and repeatedly reassess whether to continue prescribing.

Table 81.2 Australian websites providing information about anxiety

Provider and hosting organisation	Website
beyondblue, The National Depression Initiative	www.beyondblue.org.au/home www.youthbeyondblue.com (for young people aged 12–25 years)
Black Dog Institute, Prince of Wales Hospital, University of New South Wales	www.blackdoginstitute.org.au www.biteback.org.au (for young people aged 12–18 years)
Centre for Clinical Interventions, Government of Western Australia, Department of Health	www.cci.health.wa.gov.au
Clinical Research Unit for Anxiety and Depression (CRUfAD), St Vincent's Hospital, Sydney	www.crufad.org
e-hub, Australian National University	www.bluepages.anu.edu.au
Inspire Foundation	http://au.reachout.com (for young people aged 14–25 years)
National e-Therapy Centre, Swinburne University	www.anxietyonline.org.au

Table 81.3 Openly accessible Australian-based interactive internet programs for anxiety

Organisation and program name	Website
CRUfAD clinical programs	www.crufad.org*
e-hub Australian National University, MoodGYM	www.moodgym.anu.edu.au

*in-house clinical support is supplied, but costs apply

- Of the medications, SSRIs are regarded as first line and other antidepressants such as SNRIs, e.g. duloxetine and venlafaxine, have shown some benefit in anxiety disorders (see TABLES 81.4 and 81.6), but their benefits are not as long-lasting as psychological and behavioural approaches.[10,11]
- Assess efficacy of antidepressants after at least 12 weeks (in contrast to 6–8 weeks when treating major depression) and, if of clear benefit, treat for at least 6 months.

Table 81.4 Dosage recommendations for SSRIs in anxiety disorders[10]

Drug	Initial dose	Maximum dose
citalopram	10 mg	40 mg
escitalopram	5 mg	20 mg
fluoxetine	10 mg	80 mg
fluvoxamine	50 mg	300 mg (split dose to bd over 150 mg)
paroxetine	10 mg	60 mg
sertraline	25 mg	200 mg

Table 81.5 Initial medication options for anxiety disorders[10]

Condition	Medication options
Generalised anxiety disorder	SSRI, duloxetine (30–120 mg), venlafaxine controlled release (75–225 mg)
Panic disorder	SSRI, venlafaxine controlled release (75–225 mg)
Obsessive-compulsive disorder	SSRI
Agoraphobia (without panic)	none
Social anxiety disorder (generalised)	SSRI, venlafaxine controlled release (75–225 mg)
Social anxiety disorder (non-generalised)	propranolol 10–40 mg orally, 30–60 minutes before the social event or performance
Specific phobias	not recommended
Post-traumatic stress disorder	SSRI, mirtazapine

Note: not every SSRI has Australian TGA approval for use for each anxiety disorder; the TGA website can provide up-to-date information on this changing landscape. There is insufficient evidence to differentiate between efficacy of the individual SSRIs.

- The cessation of an SSRI commonly causes withdrawal symptoms. A common trap (for doctor and/or patient) is to interpret these symptoms as a recurrence of the underlying anxiety and as evidence that the drug continues to be required.
- Propranolol is of benefit in social anxiety disorder, particularly with anticipated stressful events (e.g. public speaking, presenting at work events).
- Benzodiazepines have a limited role in anxiety disorders. If used, they should be reserved for people who have not responded to at least

2 therapies (e.g. psychological therapy and antidepressant) and used only in the short term (stop within 6 weeks). They can also be used for specific phobias (e.g. fear of flying, agoraphobia and MRI machines).
- Consider buspirone, which has negligible potential for tolerance or dependence.

Panic attack[8]

A panic attack is defined[3] as a discrete period of intense fear or discomfort in which four (or more) of the following symptoms develop abruptly and reach a peak within 10 minutes:

- shortness of breath or smothering sensations
- dizziness, unsteady feelings, lightheadedness or faintness
- palpitations or accelerated heart rate
- trembling or shaking
- sweating
- feeling of choking
- nausea or abdominal distress
- depersonalisation or derealisation
- numbness or tingling sensations (paraesthesia)
- flushes (hot flashes) or chills
- chest pain or discomfort
- fear of dying
- fear of going crazy or of doing something uncontrolled

Organic disorders that simulate a panic attack are hyperthyroidism, phaeochromocytoma and hypoglycaemia.

Note: A single panic attack is not synonymous with panic disorder, which is characterised by recurrent panic attacks. Some 40% of young people have had at least one spontaneous panic attack. Panic disorder is when there are recurrent attacks that are followed by at least a month of worrying about future attacks and/or the consequences of them. Panic disorder can occur with or without associated agoraphobia, though >90% of people with agoraphobia develop it as a result of recurrent panic attacks.[10]

81

Management

Reassurance, explanation and support (as for generalised anxiety). This is the mainstay of treatment. A patient who is experiencing a panic attack should be taught breathing techniques to help control hyperventilation (e.g. timing breaths, breathing through nose, slow inspiration, measured medium-sized breaths). Relaxation techniques can also be employed, such as progressive muscle relaxation, and patients can teach themselves these techniques via online resources (see TABLES 81.2 and 81.3). Rebreathing into a paper bag is rarely indicated in a general practice setting[9,10] as the hyperventilation has usually settled by the time the patient presents. The above breathing techniques can be used by the patient anywhere and are more socially acceptable than breathing noisily into a paper bag when an attack is feared.

The danger in a panic attack is the danger *to the self by the self*[8] (e.g. fleeing into danger, non-intentional overdose).

Cognitive behaviour therapy (CBT)

(See CHAPTER 5.)

CBT aims to reduce anxiety by teaching patients how to identify, evaluate, control and modify their negative, fearful thoughts and behaviour. If simple psychotherapy and stress management fail then patients should be referred for CBT, usually to a psychologist (or occasionally psychiatrist), although some GPs have a particular interest in providing CBT.

Patients' fears, especially if irrational, need to be clearly explained by the therapist, examined rationally and challenged, then replaced by positive calming thoughts.

Pharmacological treatment

Pharmacological treatment is rarely of benefit in the acute attack, as the attacks occur too quickly for their effect to be of use. For ongoing treatment of panic disorder with or without agoraphobia, there is little good quality evidence comparing medication to CBT.[9]

Continual use of benzodiazepines (BDZs, e.g. alprazolam or clonazepam) has previously been utilised in panic and other anxiety disorders but is now no longer recommended.[10] Problems associated with benzodiazepine use include:

- impaired alertness, oversedation
- dependence
- increased risk of accidents
- adverse effects on mood and behaviour
- interaction with alcohol and other drugs
- potential for abuse and overdose
- risks during pregnancy and lactation
- muscle weakness
- sexual dysfunction
- diminished motivation
- lowered sense of competency
- lower self-esteem

Some principles of using BDZs in anxiety disorders[10] are:

- always check for a history of problem alcohol or drug use
- be wary of prescribing to unfamiliar patients, especially if asking for a particular drug by name (may indicate drug-seeking behaviour)
- carefully discuss the potential for addiction with the patient
- avoid using short-acting drugs as they are the most highly addictive
- prescribe only small quantities of medication at a time
- use only as short-term treatment
- ensure regular review of the patient and continuity of care

If already being used, BDZs should be tapered very slowly (this may take 6–12 months or longer). A benzodiazepine withdrawal syndrome, which can include rebound anxiety, depression, confusion, insomnia and seizures, may occur. However, the doctor's fear of being responsible for a withdrawal syndrome has also been used as leverage by those seeking drugs. If in doubt, seek specialist drug and alcohol advice.

Phobic disorders

In phobic states, the anxiety is related to specific situations or objects. Phobic disorders include agoraphobia, social anxiety disorder (otherwise known as social phobia) and specific phobias. Patients avoid these objects or situations, become anxious when they anticipate having to meet them and/or endure them with intense distress.

Common phobias are spiders, people and social situations, flying, open spaces, confined spaces, heights, cancer, thunderstorms, death and heart disease. The problem is seldom encountered in practice and there is usually no call for drug therapy.

Agoraphobia

Avoidance includes staying away from many situations where there are issues of distance from home, crowding or confinement. Typical examples are travel on public transport, crowded shops and confined places. Patients fear they may lose control, faint and suffer embarrassment.

Social anxiety disorder

Social anxiety disorder is experienced in anxiety-provoking social situations in which the person feels subject to critical public scrutiny (e.g. canteens, restaurants, staff meetings, speaking engagements). It can either be generalised (fear of numerous social situations, including both performance and interactional situations) or non-generalised (fear of one or just a few situations or performance type). The treatments for the two subtypes are quite different (see TABLE 81.5). The sufferer may be a shy, self-conscious, premorbid personality. Social phobias, including performance anxiety and symptoms, are often related to sympathetic overactivity.

Management

The basis of treatment for all phobias is psychotherapy that involves behaviour therapy (e.g. graduated exposure therapy) and cognitive therapy.

Obsessive–compulsive disorder (OCD)

Anxiety is associated with obsessive thoughts and compulsive rituals.

The obsessions are recurrent and persistent intrusive ideas, thoughts, impulses or images that are usually resisted by the patient. Compulsions are repetitive, purposeful and intentional behaviours conducted in response to an obsession to prevent a bad outcome for the person (e.g. excessive washing of the genitals).

Mild obsessional or compulsive behaviour can be regarded as normal in response to stress.

Management

Optimal management is a combination of psychotherapeutic—particularly CBT—and pharmacological treatment, namely:

- cognitive behaviour therapy for obsessions
- exposure and response prevention for compulsions

Body dysmorphic disorder

The person with this disorder has an exaggerated preoccupation with an imagined defect in appearance (see CHAPTER 45).

Patients may be helped by counselling and psychotherapy.

Acute stress disorder

This is defined as a constellation of abnormal anxiety-related symptoms lasting at least 3 days and occurring within 4 weeks of a traumatic event. The symptoms can include a sense of numbing, altered sense of reality, amnesia of the event, intrusive memories or dreams of the event, dissociative reactions, physiological reactions to triggers, avoidance of reminders, sleep disturbance, hypervigilance, anger and aggression, exaggerated startle response and agitation. It is appropriate to provide people with an acute stress reaction with debriefing and counselling (if agreeable); pharmacological intervention is rarely indicated.

Post-traumatic stress disorder (PTSD)

PTSD is defined somewhat differently, in terms of time lapses from the traumatic event. It refers to a similar constellation of symptoms that persist for 1 month after exposure:

- acute PTSD: duration of symptoms <3 months
- chronic PTSD: duration of symptoms ≥3 months
- delayed onset PTSD: onset of symptoms at least 6 months after the stressor

Typical distressing recurrent symptoms:

- intrusive features—recollections, nightmares, flashbacks
- avoidance of events that symbolise or resemble the trauma
- persistent negative alterations in cognitions and mood
- hyperarousal phenomena: exaggerated startle response, irritability, anger, difficulty with sleeping and concentrating, hypervigilance, reckless or self-destructive behaviour

Treatment

This is difficult and involves counselling, the basis of which is facilitating abreaction of the experience by individual or group therapy. The aim is to allow the patient to face up openly to his or her memories. Persistent symptoms are an indication for referral for focused psychological intervention therapy.

Pharmacological treatment

SSRIs have limited evidence of some benefit, but response is slower than for their use in depression (trial for 8–12 weeks) and, if effective, they should be used for at least 12 months.[10,11]

Hyperventilation

Hyperventilation syndrome can be a manifestation of anxiety. The main symptoms are:

- lightheadedness, faintness or dizziness
- breathlessness
- palpitations
- sweating
- dry mouth with aerophagy
- agitation
- fatigue and malaise

Other symptoms include paraesthesia of the extremities, peri-oral paraesthesia and carpopedal spasm (see FIG. 81.2).

Carpopedal spasm: biochemical explanation

CO_2 loss from hyperventilation

Equation: $H^+ + HCO^-_3 \rightleftharpoons CO_2 + H_2O$

$p\,CO_2 \downarrow \rightarrow HCO^-_3 \downarrow$ and $pH \uparrow$ (respiratory alkalosis)

H^+ depleted and replenished from plasma proteins

$H(\text{protein}) \rightleftharpoons H^+ + Pr^-$

Protein anions accumulate and take up calcium

$Ca^{++} + 2\,Pr^- \rightleftharpoons Ca(Pr)_2$

Thus ionised calcium is depleted causing hypocalcaemic tetany.

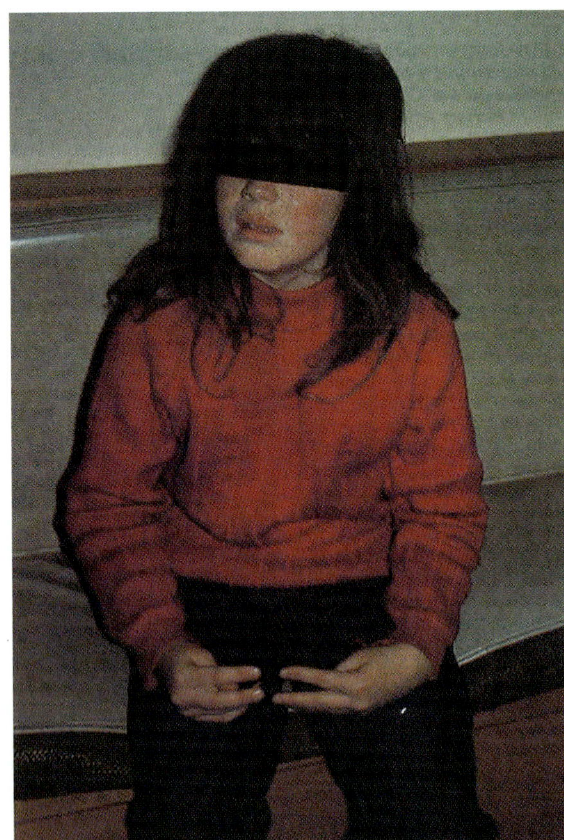

FIGURE 81.2 Carpopedal spasm (showing carpal spasm) in an anxious and agitated 10-year-old girl

Management

- Reassure.
- Encourage patients to identify the cause and then control their rate and depth of breathing.

Adjustment disorder with anxious mood

This term is reserved for patients who present with anxiety symptoms within 3 months of response to an identifiable psychosocial stressor. It is a common presentation of anxiety symptoms and should be regarded as a separate entity to a generalised anxiety disorder.

The symptoms are in excess of the normal expected reaction to the stressor but have persisted for less than 6 months following the removal of the stressor.

The basic treatment is non-pharmacological: counselling, relaxation and stress management. A short-term course of drug treatment, e.g. diazepam for 2 weeks, can be used in severe or persisting cases.

Somatic symptom disorder (DSM–5)

Somatic symptom disorder (SSD) is defined as the tendency to experience, conceptualise and communicate mental states and distress as physical symptoms or altered bodily function. It is associated with excessive illness, worry and abnormal illness behaviour. SSD is persistent with a history of numerous unsubstantiated physical complaints over several years beginning before the age of 30. Previously called somatisation disorder in the DSM-IV-TR, or hysteria in the past, SSD has 2 subtypes: those with predominantly somatic complaints and those with predominantly pain issues (previously known as pain disorder).

Symptoms include:

- gastrointestinal—nausea, vomiting, abdominal pain
- genital/sexual—dysmenorrhoea, dyspareunia, genital pain, anorgasmia
- cardiovascular—palpitations, shortness of breath, chest pain
- pseudoneurological—amnesia, loss of voice, dizziness, difficulty walking/talking/swallowing
- pain—diffuse, neck/back ache, joint/limb pain, headaches
- other—fatigue, globus, fainting

None of these symptoms has an adequate physical explanation. SSD is more common in females. There is persistent refusal to be reassured that there is no explanation for the symptoms. There is associated impaired social, occupational and family functioning.

Management involves skilful counselling, explanation for symptoms, searching for and treating comorbid conditions (e.g. depression, anxiety) and CBT. It is preferable to be managed by a single supportive doctor. It is not malingering.

Anxiety in children

Anxiety disorders can occur in childhood and, if left untreated, may persist into adolescence and adulthood. Panic attacks are not uncommon. Other disorders include GAD, social phobia, obsessive–compulsive disorder, PTSD, selective mutism and separation anxiety disorder. Non-pharmacological approaches are preferred, and may require input from an educational and developmental psychologist. Separation anxiety disorder for real, threatened or imagined separation is the most common anxiety disorder; if severe and persistent, treatment (under specialist supervision) with one of the SSRIs could be considered.

When to refer

- If the diagnosis is doubtful
- If drug and alcohol dependence or withdrawal complicate the management
- If psychosis appears to be involved
- Failure of response to basic treatment

Note: The threshold for referral varies depending on the GP's confidence and experience in dealing with anxiety, and the available referral pathways.

Practice tips

- Be careful not to confuse depression with anxiety.
- A depressive disorder can be the cause of anxiety symptoms.
- For anxiety, especially with cardiovascular symptoms (palpitations and/or flushing), always consider the possibility of hyperthyroidism and order thyroid function tests.
- Always try non-pharmacological measures to manage anxiety whenever possible.
- Be careful with the use of benzodiazepines: aim for short-term treatment only.

Tips to beat stress

- Get enough sleep and rest.
- Listen to music.
- Do things that you enjoy.

- Look at positives.
- Develop strategies to laugh.
- Go to the movies or a show weekly.
- Consider getting a pet.
- Remember that your job is what you do (not who you are).
- Have regular chats with close friends.
- Exercise for 30 minutes, 4 or 5 times a week. There is good evidence this helps.
- Learn to meditate.
- Avoid interpersonal conflicts.
- Learn to accept what you cannot change.

Patient education resources

Hand-out sheets from *Murtagh's Patient Education* 7th edition:

- Anxiety disorder
- Phobias
- Post-traumatic stress disorder
- Stress: coping with stress

References

1 Australian Bureau of Statistics. Survey of Mental Health and Wellbeing: Summary of Results, 2007. Available from: <www.abs.gov.au/ausstats/abs@.nsf/mf/4326.0>, accessed February 2018.

2 Tiller J. Depression and anxiety. MJA Open, 2012; 1 (Suppl. 4): 28–32.

3 American Psychiatric Association. *Diagnostic and Statistical Manual for Mental Disorders: DSM-5.* Available from: <www.dsm5.org/Pages/Default.aspx>, accessed February 2018.

4 Covin R et al. A meta-analysis of CBT for pathological worry among clients with GAD. J Anxiety Disord, 2008; 22(1): 108–16.

5 Deacon B, Abramowitz J. Cognitive and behavioural treatments for anxiety disorders: a review of meta-analysis findings. J Clin Psychol, 2004; 60: 429–41.

6 Kyrios M. Anxiety disorders: assessment and management in general practice. Aust Fam Physician, 2011; 40(6): 370–4.

7 Reynolds J, Griffiths K, Christensen H. Anxiety and depression: online resources and management tools. Aust Fam Physician, 2011; 40(6): 382–6.

8 Royal Australian and New Zealand College of Psychiatrists. Australian and New Zealand clinical practice guidelines for the treatment of panic disorder and agoraphobia. Aust N Z J Psychiatry, 2003; 37: 641–56.

9 Imai H et al. Psychological therapies versus pharmacological interventions for panic disorder with or without agoraphobia in adults. Cochrane Database of Systematic Reviews 2016, Issue 10.

10 Expert group for Psychotropic guidelines. Anxiety disorders. In: eTG complete. Melbourne: Therapeutic Guidelines Ltd. Available from: <www.tg.org.au>, accessed January 2018.

11 Buckley N (Chair). *Australian Medicines Handbook.* Adelaide: Australian Medicines Handbook Pty Ltd, 2016: 821.

Asthma

82

After I'd written to you yesterday I had an attack of asthma and an incessantly running nose, which forced me to tramp about, lighting cigarettes at every tobacconist etc. And worse was to come: I went to bed about midnight, feeling all right after spending a long time inhaling smoke, but 3 or 4 hours later came the real attack of the summer.

MARCEL PROUST, LETTER TO HIS MOTHER, 1901

Asthma, which is an inflammatory disorder, is defined by the presence of both of the following:[1]

- excessive variation in lung function ('variable airflow limitation', i.e. variation in expiratory airflow that is greater than that seen in healthy people)
- respiratory symptoms (e.g. wheeze, shortness of breath, cough, chest tightness) that vary over time and may be present or absent at any point in time

In young children in whom lung function testing is not feasible, including most preschool children, asthma is defined by the presence of variable respiratory symptoms.

Key facts and checkpoints

- Asthma continues to be underdiagnosed and undertreated.[2] It is increasing worldwide.
- It has an unacceptable mortality rate: 455 deaths in Australia in 2016 (1.9 per 100 000).[3]
- One child in nine (age 0–14 years) reports having asthma (usually in a mild form).[4]
- It tends to develop between the ages of 2 and 7 years, but can develop at any age.
- Most children present with a cough.
- Most children are free from it by puberty.
- About one adult in eight has or has had asthma.
- The focus of management should be on prevention; an acute asthmatic attack represents failed treatment.
- Measurement of function is vital as 'objective measurement is superior to subjective measurement'.
- Spirometry is the key investigation.
- Inhaled corticosteroids are the cornerstone of asthma treatment.
- Medicines should be prescribed at the lowest strength that works. Patients should not be left on combination or high-dose inhalers without regular review.
- Avoid concomitant medication that may exacerbate asthma (e.g. beta blockers, aspirin, NSAIDs).

Pathophysiology[1]

Chronic asthma is an inflammatory disease with the following pathological characteristics:

- infiltration of the mucosa with inflammatory cells (especially eosinophils) and cellular elements
- airway hyper-responsiveness[5]
- intermittent airway narrowing (due to bronchoconstriction, congestion or oedema of bronchial mucosa or a combination of these) (see FIG. 82.1)

Causes of asthma

No single cause for asthma has been found, but a variety of factors may trigger an attack. These include specific factors such as viruses, allergens and non-specific factors such as temperature or weather changes and exercise. A checklist of *trigger factors* includes:

A allergens—pollens, animal dander, dust mites, mould
B bronchial infection
C cold air, exercise
D drugs—aspirin, NSAIDs, beta blockers
E psychosocial problems, emotion—stress, laughter
F food—sodium metabisulphate, seafood, nuts, monosodium glutamate
G gastro-oesophageal reflux
H hormones—pregnancy, menstruation
I irritants—smoke, perfumes, smells
J job—wood dust, flour dust, isocyanates, animals

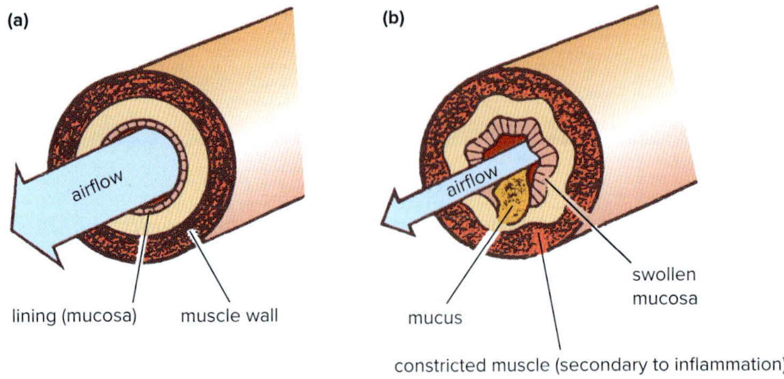

FIGURE 82.1 Airway changes in asthma: (a) normal airway, (b) airway in asthma

Additional points

- Patients with asthma must never smoke.
- Atopic patients should avoid exposure to furred or feathered domestic animals if they have problems.
- About 90% of children with atopic symptoms and asthma demonstrate positive skin-prick responses to dust mite extract. Total eradication of house dust mite from the home is difficult.

Clinical features

The classic symptoms are:

- wheezing
- coughing (chronic, esp. at night)
- tightness in the chest
- breathlessness

Asthma is likely if more than one of the above is present. Other supporting features:

- symptoms recurrent or seasonal
- worse at night or early morning
- history of allergies
- family history of asthma or allergies
- widespread audible wheeze on chest auscultation
- symptoms rapidly relieved by a short-acting beta agonist bronchodilator (SABA)

82

Note: Asthma should be suspected in children with recurrent nocturnal cough and in people with intermittent dyspnoea or chest tightness, especially after exercise.

Severe symptoms and signs are presented in the section on dangerous asthma later in this chapter.

Examination[6]

Physical signs may be present if the patient has symptoms at the time of examination.

The absence of physical signs does not exclude a diagnosis of asthma as the chest examination may be normal between attacks. During an attack, auscultation usually reveals diffuse, high-pitched wheezes throughout inspiration and most of expiration, which is usually prolonged. If wheeze is not present during normal tidal breathing it may become apparent during a forced expiration or after asking the child to exercise for 1–2 minutes. Wheeze does not necessarily indicate asthma.

Absence of wheeze in a breathless person is a serious sign.

Investigations

- Spirometry: a value of <75% for FEV_1/VC ratio indicates obstruction (a relatively accurate test and recommended for those who can perform it, i.e. most adults and children >6 years; see CHAPTER 49)
- Measurement of peak expiratory flow rate (PEFR) or spirometry before and after SABA: has a characteristic improvement >15% in FEV_1 and PEFR
- Bronchial provocation tests: airway reactivity is tested in a respiratory laboratory to inhaled histamine, methacholine or hypertonic saline (rarely required, but sometimes useful to confirm diagnosis)
- Fractional exhaled nitric oxide test
- An exercise challenge may also be helpful
- Allergy testing may be appropriate
- Chest X-ray: not routine but useful if complications suspected or symptoms not explained by asthma

Significant historical advances in asthma management

1 The realisation that asthma is an inflammatory disease—the appropriate first- or second-line treatment in moderate to severe asthma is inhaled sodium cromoglycate (especially in children) or inhaled corticosteroids (ICS)
2 The regular use of spirometry
3 The use of spacers attached to inhalers/puffers
4 Improved and more efficient inhalers
5 Combined long-acting relievers and preventers including combinations of long-acting beta agonists (LABA) and ICS—the fixed-dose inhalers

Reasons for suboptimal asthma control are presented in TABLE 82.1.

Table 82.1 Reasons for suboptimal asthma control[2,4]
Poor compliance
Inefficient use of inhaler devices—poor technique
Procrastination in introducing optimal therapy
Failure to prescribe preventive medications, particularly inhaled corticosteroids for chronic asthma
Using bronchodilators alone and repeating these drugs without proper evaluation
Reliance on inappropriate alternate therapies
Patient fears:
• concerns about corticosteroids
• overdosage
• developing tolerance
• embarrassment
• peer group condemnation
Doctor's reluctance to:
• use corticosteroids
• recommend obtaining a mini peak flow meter
• recommend obtaining a spacer
Medical factors:
• obesity
• rhinosinusitis
• GORD
• sleep apnoea
• vocal cord dysfunction
• smoking/COPD

Treating inflammatory airways disease

If inflammatory airways disease is undertreated there is the risk of fixed irreversible airways obstruction from submucosal fibrosis. One of the most common mistakes in medical practice is to fail to introduce inhaled corticosteroids for the management of patients with moderately severe asthma.

Measurement of peak expiratory flow rate

Patients with moderate to severe chronic asthma require regular measurement of PEFR, which is more useful than subjective symptoms in assessing asthma control. This allows the establishment of a baseline of the 'patient's best', monitors changes, and allows the assessment of asthma severity and response to treatment.

Spirometry including FEV_1 is the gold standard (see CHAPTER 49). Peak flow meters are not a substitute for spirometry. There is considerable variation between users and instruments. However, they have a place in helping patients self-manage their asthma by serially recording their PEFR and comparing this with the best peak flow.

Spacers[7]

Large volume spacers

Some people who have trouble using metered dose inhalers (MDIs) can have a spacer fitted onto the mouthpiece of the inhaler. One puff at a time is put in the spacer. The patient breathes in from its mouthpiece, taking 1–2 very deep breaths, or 4–6 normal breaths (especially in children). This method is useful for adults having trouble with the MDI and for younger children (older than 3 years). Spacers are very efficient, overcome poor technique and cause less irritation of the mouth and throat (see FIG. 82.2).

They allow increased airway deposition of inhalant and less oropharyngeal deposition.

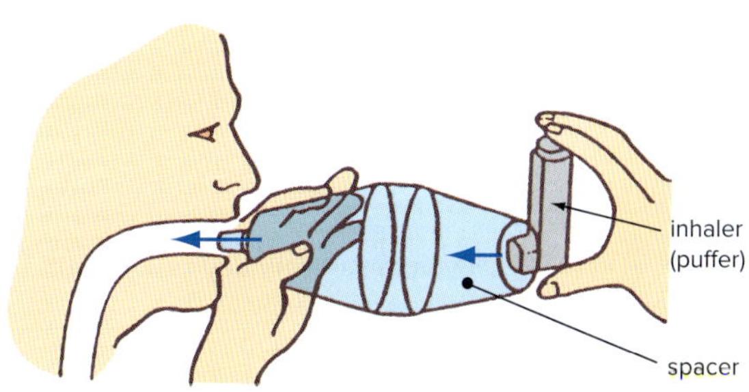

FIGURE 82.2 Using a spacer device. Rules: children—single puff, then 4–6 normal breaths; adults—single puff then 1–2 deep breaths

82

Note: It is recommended to dip plastic spacers into water with ordinary household detergent and dry in sunlight (no rinsing, no wiping) every 10 days or at least monthly.

Small volume spacers

Children under 5–6 years and/or 20 kg can use an MDI and a small volume valved spacer (AeroChamber, Breath-A-Tech) with a face mask.

Management principles

Starting treatment[1]

- Confirm the diagnosis.
- Assess recent asthma control and risk factors (see TABLE 82.2).
- Choose initial treatment appropriate to the above.
- Avoid the use of LABA on its own (i.e. without ICS), as it is associated with an increased risk of asthma death.
- Document evidence (patient's notes).
- Identify management goals in collaboration.
- Provide clear written patient information.
- Educate and review regularly.

Goals of management:

- absent or minimal daytime symptoms and no nocturnal symptoms; restore normal airway function (>80% of predicted)
- maintain best possible lung function at all times—keep asthma under control
- reduce morbidity

Table 82.2 Asthma severity classification for an untreated newly diagnosed adult asthma patient[8]

Severity/ grade	Status before treatment	Lung function FEV_1 or PEFR (% predicted)	Recommended β_2-agonist	Estimated starting daily dose range of ICS required to achieve good control
Intermittent	Episodic Symptoms <weekly Night symptoms <2 per month Mild occasional symptoms with exercise	≥ 80%	SABA prn	Regular ICS not required Add preventer if ≥3 uses of SABA/week
Mild persistent	Symptoms >weekly, not every day Night symptoms >2 per month Symptoms regularly with exercise	≥ 80%	SABA prn	<250 mcg beclomethasone <400 mcg budesonide <250 mcg fluticasone <160 mcg ciclesonide Increase dose if >2 SABA 2–3 times daily
Moderate persistent	Symptoms every day Night symptoms >weekly Several known triggers apart from exercise	60–80 %	LABA + SABA prn	250–400 mcg beclomethasone 400–800 mcg budesonide 250–500 mcg fluticasone 160–320 mcg ciclesonide
Severe persistent	Symptoms every day Wakes frequently at night with cough/ wheeze Chest tightness on waking Limitation of physical activity	<60%	LABA + SABA prn	>400 mcg beclomethasone >800 mcg budesonide >500 mcg fluticasone >320 mcg ciclesonide

- control asthma with the use of regular anti-inflammatory medication and relieving doses of β_2-agonist when necessary

  Long-term goals:

- achieve use of the least drugs, least doses and least side effects
- reduce risk of fatal attacks
- reduce risk of developing irreversible abnormal lung function

Good asthma control

- minimal symptoms day and night
- no nocturnal waking due to asthma
- no limitation of normal activity or exercise
- minimal need for reliever medication
- no exacerbation
- normal or near-normal lung function (FEV_1 and/or PEFR >80% of predicted or best)
- no side effects of medication

Questions to assess asthma control[1]

Ask about:

- limitation of daily activities
- shortness of breath
- sleep disturbance
- use of reliever medication
- perceived level of asthma control

Pharmacological agents to treat asthma

Simple classification

- Reliever = bronchodilator
- Preventer = anti-inflammatory
- Symptom controller = long-acting β_2-agonist (LABA)

It is useful to teach patients the concept of the 'preventer' and the 'reliever' for their asthma treatment. The pharmacological treatment of asthma is summarised in TABLE 82.3.

'Preventer' drugs: anti-inflammatory agents

These medications are directed towards the underlying abnormalities—bronchial hyper-reactivity and associated airway inflammation. Treatment with a 'preventer' is recommended if asthma episodes are >3/week or those who use SABA >3 times a week.

Corticosteroids

Inhaled (ICS)

Types:

- beclomethasone
- budesonide
- ciclesonide (single daily dose)
- fluticasone

  Dose range:

- 400–1600 mcg (adults); aim to keep below 500 mcg children and 1000 mcg (adults)

  Availability:

- MDI
- Turbuhaler
- Autohaler
- Accuhaler

  Frequency:

- once or twice daily (helps compliance)

  Side effects:

- oropharyngeal candidiasis, dysphonia (hoarse voice)—less risk with once daily ciclesonide
- bronchial irritation: cough
- adrenal suppression (doses of 2000 mcg/daily; sometimes as low as 800 mcg)

Note: Rinse mouth with water and spit out after using inhaled steroids.

ICSs have a flat dose–response curve so it may not be necessary to prescribe above ICS doses considered high—beclomethasone or budesonide 1000 mcg/day or fluticasone 500 mcg/day. For newly diagnosed patients with mild-to-moderate asthma 'start low and step up prn' (e.g. 250–400 mcg/day).[6] Step down the dose when safe to do so.

Note: Most adults and older adolescents with asthma should be on long-term inhaled corticosteroid therapy.[1]

Oral

Prednisolone is used mainly for exacerbations. It is given with the usual inhaled corticosteroids and bronchodilators.

Dose:

- up to 1 mg/kg/day (usual max. 50 mg) for 3 days to 2 weeks

Table 82.3 Pharmacological treatment of asthma[5]

	Generic types	Examples	Vehicle of administration: Nebulising solution	Oral	Aerosol (metered dose inhalation)	Dry powder (inhalation)	Injection
Bronchodilators							
1 β_2-adrenoceptor agonists	Salbutamol	Ventolin	✓	✓	✓	✓	✓
	Salmeterol	Serevent			✓	✓	
	Terbutaline	Bricanyl	✓	✓		✓	✓
	Eformoterol	Foradile, Oxis				✓	
	Indacaterol	Onbrez					
	Adrenaline						✓
2 Anticholinergics	Ipratropium bromide	Atrovent	✓		✓		
3 Methylxanthines	Theophylline	Nuelin		✓			
	Aminophylline						✓
Mast cell stabilisers							
	Sodium cromoglycate	Intal	✓		✓ ✓	✓	
	Nedocromil sodium	Tilade			✓		
Corticosteroids—for inhalation							
	Beclomethasone	QVAR			✓	✓	
	Budesonide	Pulmicort	✓		✓	✓	
	Ciclesonide	Alvesco			✓		
	Fluticasone	Flixotide	✓		✓	✓	
Combination reliever (LABA) + preventer (ICS)—fixed combination MDI							
Salmeterol + fluticasone (Seretide)					✓	✓	
Eformoterol + fluticasone (Flutiform)					✓		
Eformoterol + budesonide (Symbicort)					✓	✓	
Vilanterol + fluticasone (Breo ellipta)						✓	
Leucotriene antagonists							

Side effects:

- these are minimal if drug is used for short periods
- long-term use has significant side effects: osteoporosis, glucose intolerance, adrenal suppression, thinning of skin and easy bruising

Note: Short-term oral corticosteroids can be ceased abruptly.

Cromolyns

These are sodium cromoglycate (SCG) and nedocromil sodium. SCG is available as dry capsules for inhalation, metered dose aerosols and a nebuliser solution. They are often inhaled via a spacer in children. Adverse effects are uncommon; local irritation may be caused by the dry powder. Systemic effects do not occur.

Nedocromil is used for frequent episodic asthma in children over 2 years of age for the prevention of exercise-induced asthma and the treatment of mild-to-moderate asthma in some adults. The initial dose is 2 inhalations qid. Adverse effects are uncommon.

Leucotriene antagonists

These drugs, which include montelukast and zafirlukast, are very useful for seasonal asthma and aspirin-sensitive asthma and reduce the need for inhaled steroids or offer an alternative for those who cannot tolerate ICSs or have trouble using an inhaler. Favourable evidence is based on a small number of trials only, mostly in children but some adults benefit.[9] Montelukast is taken as a 5 or 10 mg chewable tablet once daily.

Indications for preventive therapy[10]

Guidelines for introducing preventive asthma therapy in adults and children include any of the following:

- requirement of β_2-agonist >2 days per week or >1 canister every 3 months (excluding pre-exercise)
- symptoms (non-exercise) >2 times per week between attacks
- any symptoms during the night or on waking
- spirometry showing reversible airflow obstruction during asymptomatic phases
- asthma significantly interfering with physical activity despite appropriate pre-treatment
- asthma attacks ≥twice per month
- infrequent asthma attacks but severe or life-threatening

'Reliever' drugs or bronchodilators

The three groups of bronchodilators are:

- the β_2-adrenoceptor agonists (β_2-agonists)—short acting (SABA) and long acting (LABA)
- methylxanthines—theophylline derivatives
- anticholinergics

β_2-agonists

These drugs stimulate the β_2 adrenoreceptors and thus relax bronchial smooth muscle. Inhalation is the preferred route of delivery; the vehicles of administration include metered dose inhalation, a dry powder, and nebulisation where the solution is converted to a mist of small droplets by a flow of oxygen or air through the solution.

Oral administration of β_2-agonists is not required. The inhaled drugs produce measurable bronchodilation in 1–2 minutes and peak effects by 10–20 minutes. The traditional agents such as salbutamol and terbutaline are short-acting preparations. The new longer-acting agents (LABA) include salmeterol, eformoterol and vilanterol.

These are to be used in combination with an ICS, not as monotherapy.[11]

Theophylline derivatives

These oral drugs may have complementary value to the inhaled agents but tend to be limited by side effects and efficacy.

Anti-IgE monoclonal antibodies

These newer agents (e.g. omalizumab) bind IgE without activating mast cells. They are directed for use in patients >12 years of age with moderate to severe allergic eosinophilic asthma who have been treated by ICS and who have raised serum IgE levels. They are given by SC injection.

Antibiotic use for chronic asthma[12]

Antibiotics are not recommended apart from clinical evidence of super-respiratory infection. However, a recent Australian study concluded that 'adults with persistent symptomatic asthma experience fewer exacerbations and improved quality of life when treated with oral azithromycin (500 mg tds) for several weeks'. Its clinical use remains uncertain.

Starting treatment

Current treatment supports the initial treatment (summarised in TABLE 82.2) of a SABA with low to moderate doses of ICS with estimated equivalent doses shown in the table.

Initiate therapy sufficient to achieve best lung function promptly.

Wean inhaled corticosteroids to the minimum dose needed to maintain adequate asthma control.

Prophylactic agents

This term is reserved for those medications that are taken prior to known trigger factors, particularly for exercise-induced asthma.

Exercise-induced asthma (options)

- β_2-agonist inhaler (puffer): two puffs 5 minutes immediately before exercise last 1–2 hours. LABA such as salmeterol and eformoterol are more effective if used with ICS.

- SCG or nedocromil, two puffs
- Combination β_2-agonist + SCG (5–10 minutes beforehand)
- Montelukast 10 mg (less in children ≥2 years) oral daily or 1–2 hours beforehand
- Paediatricians often recommend a non-drug warm-up program as an alternative to medication.

Ongoing management

The three-step asthma control plan[13,14]

The National Asthma Council of Australia has developed the following follow-up plan, summarised in FIGURE 82.3.

Step 1: Assess asthma symptom control and identify the patient's risk factors.

- Assess asthma symptom control over the previous 4 weeks.
- Assess the patient's risk factors.
- Exclude factors contributing to poor control before intensifying preventer treatment:
  - check adherence
  - check inhaler technique
  - check inhaler device is appropriate
  - consider that symptoms may be due to alternative or comorbid diagnoses

Step 2: Treat and adjust to achieve good control.

- All patients should have a reliever inhaler for as-needed use.
- Most patients can achieve well-controlled asthma with low-dose ICS.
- Trial low-dose ICS before ICS/LABA fixed combination therapy[15]
- Reserve ICS/LABA as a later option. This combination is too readily used in Australia.
- Where appropriate, step down treatment.
- Schedule follow-up visit.

See TABLE 82.3.

Step 3: Review response and monitor to maintain control.

- Review diagnosis and treatment regularly.
- Monitor to maintain control.

A general management plan for chronic asthma is summarised in FIGURE 82.4.

> **Practice tips**
>
> - For breakthrough asthma or persistent poorly controlled asthma with poor compliance switch to combined medication (e.g. Seretide MDI Accuhaler, or Symbicort).

Correct use of the asthma MDI (puffer)

Did you know that:

- faulty inhaler technique occurs in at least one-third of users?
- in faulty technique, up to 90% of the medication sticks to the mouth and does not reach the lungs?

82

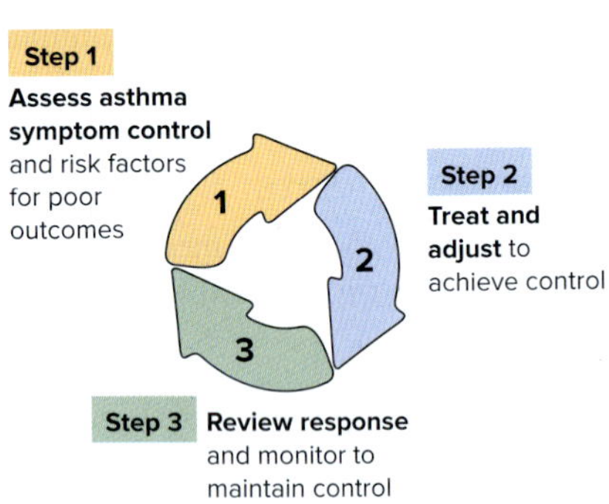

FIGURE 82.3 Asthma: ongoing management steps

Source: Reprinted with permission from NPS Medicine Wise

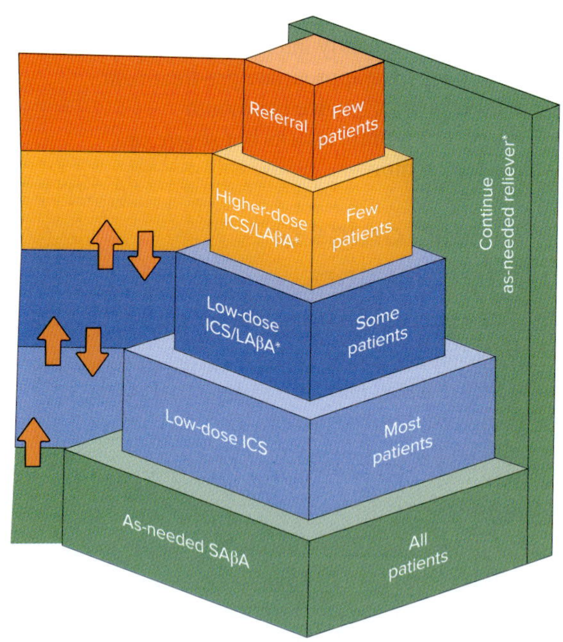

FIGURE 82.4 Stepped approach to adjusting asthma medication in adults[14]

Source: Reprinted with permission from NPS Medicine Wise

- it is the inhalation effort—not the pressure from the aerosol—that gets the medication to the lungs?
- it is important to instruct patients properly and check their technique regularly?

The two main techniques

The open-mouth technique and the closed-mouth technique are the main methods, and both are effective but the closed-mouth technique is preferred. Both techniques are suitable for most adults. Most children from the age of 7 can learn to use puffers quite well.

The closed-mouth technique

See FIGURE 82.5.

Instructions for patients:

1. Remove the cap. Shake the puffer vigorously for 1–2 seconds. Hold it upright (canister on top).
2. Place the mouthpiece between your teeth (do not bite it) and close your lips around it.
3. Breathe out slowly and gently to a comfortable level.
4. Tilt your head back slightly with your chin up.
5. Just as you then start to breathe in (slowly) through your mouth, press the puffer firmly, once. Breathe in as far as you can over 3–5 seconds. (Do not breathe in through your nose.)
6. Remove the puffer from your mouth and hold your breath for about 10 seconds; then breathe out gently.
7. Breathe normally and then repeat the inhalation if you need to.

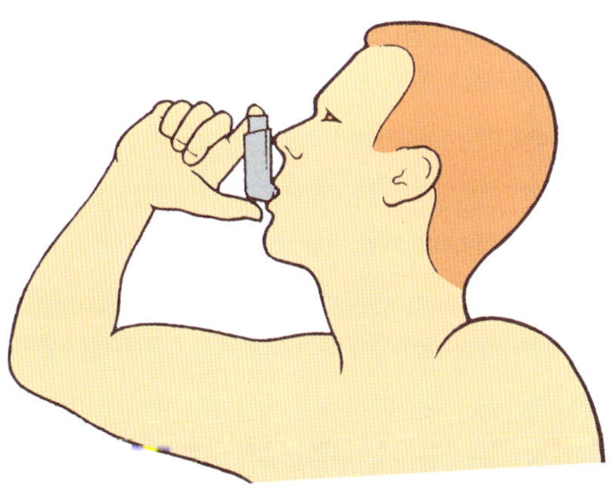

FIGURE 82.5 Using the metered dose inhaler: the closed-mouth technique

Extra points

- The usual dose of standard MDI is one or two puffs (adult) every 3–4 hours for an attack (four puffs in children).
- If you do not get adequate relief from your normal dose, contact your doctor.
- It is quite safe to increase the dose, such as to 4–6 puffs.
- If you are using your inhaler very often, it usually means your other asthma medication is not being used properly. Discuss this with your doctor.

Autohaler

The Autohaler is a breath-activated MDI which can improve lung deposition in patients with poor inhaler technique.

The Turbuhaler

The Turbuhaler is a dry powder delivery system that is widely used as an alternative to the MDI. It is a breath-activated device.

Other dry powder devices are the Accuhaler and Diskhaler.

Spacers versus nebulisers

Both MDIs via a spacer and dry powder inhalers are at least as effective as a nebuliser for treating acute exacerbations in both adults and children.[16] They are considerably cheaper and more readily available than an electrically powered device.

Summary of devices

- Breath-activated MDIs: Autohaler
- Breath-activated dry powder inhalers: Accuhaler, Aerolizer, Diskhaler, Rotahaler, Spinhaler, Turbuhaler
- Large-volume spacer: Nebuhaler, Volumatic
- Small-volume spacer: Aerochamber, Breath-A-Tech

82

Dangerous asthma

Failure to recognise the development of a severe attack has cost the lives of many asthmatics. A severe attack can start suddenly (even in mild asthmatics) and catch people by surprise.

High-risk patients

People who have experienced one or more of the following are more likely to have severe attacks:

- previous severe asthma attack

- previous hospital admission, especially admission to intensive care
- hospital attendance in the past 12 months
- long-term oral steroid treatment
- carelessness with taking medication
- night-time attacks, especially with severe chest tightness
- recent emotional problems
- frequent SABA use

Early warning signs of a severe asthma attack:

- symptoms persisting or getting worse despite adequate medication
- increased coughing and chest tightness
- poor response to two inhalations
- benefit from inhalations not lasting 2 hours
- increasing medication requirements
- sleep being disturbed by coughing, wheezing or breathlessness
- chest tightness on waking in the morning
- low PEFR readings

Thunderstorm asthma[17]

One theory is that this occurs when the high winds preceding a storm whip up massive quantities of rye grass pollens which absorb moisture and rupture, releasing allergens. People most vulnerable to an asthma attack are those with a history of allergy and poorly controlled asthma in particular. When an attack is imminent, at-risk people should stay inside with windows and doors closed, take preventer medication, follow action plans and ensure reliever drugs are readily available. Treatment is with a salbutamol spray followed by corticosteroids.

Seasonal allergic rhinitis patients not on constant intranasal corticosteroids (INCS) should start taking them 6 weeks before the pollen season and continue until pollen levels abate. For those with asthma include a combination of an INCS and intranasal antihistamine if symptoms are severe or not controlled by INCS alone.[1]

Dangerous signs

- Marked breathlessness, especially at rest
- Sleep being greatly disturbed by asthma
- Asthma getting worse quickly rather than slowly, despite medication
- Feeling frightened
- Difficulty in speaking; unable to say more than a few words
- Pulsus paradoxus
- Exhaustion and sleep deprivation
- Drowsiness or confusion
- Chest becoming 'silent' with a quiet wheeze, yet breathing still laboured
- Cyanosis
- Chest retraction
- Respiratory rate greater than 25 (adults) or 50 (children)
- Pulse rate >120 beats/min
- Peak flow <100 L/min or <40% predicted FEV_1
- Oximetry on presentation (SaO_2) <90%

Asthma action plans

Examples of action plans for patients are presented below. Having a written asthma action plan as part of self-management reduces asthma-related mortality and morbidity.[18]

Action plan

If you are distressed with severe asthma:

- call an ambulance and say 'severe asthma attack' (best option)

  or
- call your doctor

  or
- if you are having trouble finding medical help, get someone to drive you to the nearest hospital

Follow the '4 × 4 × 4' plan with your reliever medication, but keep using it continuously if you are distressed.

The following is an example of an asthma action plan that the patient keeps on a card for easy reference. Remember to have extra prednisolone and salbutamol in a household where you may be staying.

Asthma first aid action plan

Name ____________________

Contacts:

Dr ____________ Tel ____________

Ambulance tel (000)

1 Sit upright and stay calm.
2 Take 4 separate puffs of a reliever puffer (one puff at a time) via a spacer device. Just use the puffer on its own if you don't have a spacer. Take 4 breaths from the spacer after each puff
3 Wait 4 minutes. If there is no improvement, take another 4 puffs. (The 4 × 4 × 4 rule)
4 If little or no improvement CALL AN AMBULANCE IMMEDIATELY (dial 000 and/or 112 from mobile phone) and state that you are having an asthma

attack. Keep taking 4 puffs every 4 minutes until the ambulance arrives.

See your doctor immediately after a serious asthma attack.

The acute severe asthma attack

Summary (adult dosage):[6,8]

- continuous nebulised salbutamol (or terbutaline) with oxygen flow rate 6–8 L/min if nebuliser available (or 12 puffs of β_2-agonist inhaler, with spacer, using one loading puff at a time followed by 4–5 normal tidal breaths)

Ipratropium bromide may be mixed with β_2-agonist for concurrent nebulisation.

- parenteral β_2-agonist (e.g. salbutamol 500 mcg IM, SC)
- corticosteroids, e.g. prednisolone 50 mg (o) statim then daily until resolved

or

- hydrocortisone 250 mg IV or IM, 6 hourly
- oxygen 8 L/min by face mask to maintain SpO_2 >92–95% or at least 95% in children
- monitor PEFR

Further deterioration:

- magnesium sulphate 25–100 mg/kg (max. 2 gm) IV over 20 min
- adrenaline 0.5 mg 1:1000 SC, IM or 1:10,000 IV

Guidelines for spacer use in severe asthma[8]

- Frequency—every 20 minutes (first hour)
- One puff actuation at a time
- 4–5 normal breaths each time
- 25 kg or <6 years:
  - 6 puffs—salbutamol
  - 2 puffs—ipratropium
- 25–35 kg:
  - 8 puffs salbutamol
  - 3 puffs ipratropium
- >35 kg:
  - 12 puffs—salbutamol
  - 4 puffs—ipratropium
- For moderate asthma use salbutamol only

The management of severe asthma is presented in CHAPTERS 96 and 128.

Asthma in children

The prevalence of asthma is increasing in childhood and the management (especially in infants) is always a concern for the family doctor. The aim of treatment is to enable children to enjoy a normal life, comparable with that of non-asthmatic children, with the least amount of medication and at minimal risk of adverse events. Maintenance should be determined by symptom control and lung function, especially using clinical criteria since PEFR is unreliable. A diagnosis of asthma should not be made if cough is the only or predominant symptom and no signs of airflow limitation.

Key checkpoints

- Seek specialist advice for children under 6 months of age.
- Bronchodilators, inhaled or oral, are ineffective under 12 months.
- The delivery method is a problem in children and TABLE 82.4 gives an indication of what systems can be used at various levels.
- In the very young (e.g. 1–2 years old), a spacer with a face mask such as Aerochamber or Breath-A-Tech can deliver the aerosol medication.
- The PEFR should be measured in all asthmatic children older than 6 years. Children under 6 years generally cannot cope with the meters and those with mild asthma don't usually need PEFR measurement.
- The Turbuhaler is usually not practical under 7–8 years.

Prophylaxis in children

The non-steroidal medications, montelukast (oral) and SCG and/or nedocromil sodium by inhalation, are the prophylactic drugs of choice in childhood chronic asthma of mild-to-moderate severity.

If there is no clinical response to these agents in 4 weeks, consider use of inhaled corticosteroids, but the risks versus benefits must always be considered. Any dose equal to or greater than 400 mcg in children can have side effects, including growth suppression and adrenal suppression. Aim for a maintenance of 100–400 mcg, which keeps the child symptom-free. Once this stage is reached, consider stopping treatment or changing to the non-steroidal options.

Leucotriene antagonists taken orally for children aged 6 years and above is another option.

Delivery systems for children are presented in TABLE 82.4. Guidelines for the management of asthma in children are summarised in TABLE 82.5.

Table 82.4 Delivery systems for asthma in children

Vehicle of administration	Age in years: Under 2	2–4	5–7	8 and over
MDI (puffer) alone			*	✓
MDI + small volume spacer** + face mask	✓	✓		
MDI + large volume spacer**		✓	✓	✓
Nebuliser/air compressor/face mask	✓	✓	✓	✓
Dry powder inhalers (e.g. Turbuhaler, Rotahaler)			*	✓
Breath-activated device			*	✓

*Possible in some individual children
**Small volume spacer—2 tidal breaths; large volume—3

Table 82.5 Stepwise interval management plan for children[8,16]

Grade of asthma	Therapeutic agents
Mild—infrequent episodic: • attacks not severe • >6–8 weeks apart	SABA prn
Moderate—frequent episodic: • attacks <6 weeks apart • average every 4–6 weeks • attacks more troublesome	SABA prn *and* (trial of) • montelukast especially 2–5 yo: 4 mg (o) nocte 6–14 yo: 5 mg (o) nocte *or* • cromolyn stepped-up regular preventer • ICS—minimum effective dose, e.g. beclomethasone 100–200 mcg/day budesonide 200–400 mcg/day
Severe—persistent asthma: • symptoms most days • nocturnal asthma >1 per week • multiple ED visits	Referral SABA prn *and* • ICS (as above) • consider combination LABA + ICS (>6 yo) Add: • ipratropium bromide (nebuliser) • oral prednisolone (when required)

Practice tips

- Reassure the patient that 6–10 inhaled doses of a β_2-agonist is safe and appropriate for a severe attack of asthma.
- It is important to achieve a balance between undertreatment and overtreatment.
- Beware of patients, especially children, manipulating their peak flow meter results.
- Get patients to rinse out their mouth with water and spit it out after inhaling corticosteroids.
- Patients who are sensitive to aspirin/salicylates need to be reminded that salicylates are present in common cold cure preparations and agents such as Alka-Seltzer.[2]
- Aspirin-sensitive asthma usually manifests late in life with associated rhinitis. It cross-sensitises with NSAIDs.
- Possible side effects of inhaled drugs can be reduced by always using a spacer with the inhaler, using the medication qid rather than bd, rinsing the mouth, gargling and spitting out after use, and using corticosteroid sparing medications.

When to refer

- If you are doubtful about the diagnosis
- For problematic children
- For advice on management when asthmatic control has failed or is difficult to achieve

Patient education resources

Hand-out sheets from *Murtagh's Patient Education* 7th edition:

- Asthma
- Asthma: correct use of your aerosol inhaler
- Asthma: dangerous asthma

References

1 National Asthma Council of Australia. *Australian Asthma Handbook* (Version 10). Melbourne, 2014: updated 2017. <www.asthmahandbook.org.au>

2 Seale JP. Asthma. In: *MIMS Disease Index*. Sydney: IMS Publishing, 1991–92: 59–65.

3 Australian Bureau of Statistics. ABS mortality rate 2016. Available from: <https://assets.nationalasthma.org.au/resources/ABS-Mortality-Report-2016.xlsx>, accessed March 2018.

4 Australian Bureau of Statistics. Prevalence of asthma, by age and sex, 2014–15. Available from: <www.aihw.gov.au/reports/asthma-other-chronic-respiratory-conditions/asthma/dat>a, accessed March 2018.

5 Global strategy for asthma management and preventing: global initiative for asthma (GINA). Updated 2009. <www.ginasthma.com>

6 Rees J, Price J. *ABC of Asthma* (2nd edn). London: BMJ Publishing Group, 1989: 1–34.

7 National Asthma Council Australia. Australian Asthma Handbook. Use and care of spacers. Available from: <www.asthmahandbook.org.au/management/devices/spacers>, accessed February 2018.

8 Expert group for Respiratory guidelines. Asthma. In: eTG complete. Melbourne: Therapeutic Guidelines Ltd. Available from: <www.tg.org.au>, accessed February 2018.

9 Ducharme F, Hicks GC. Anti-leukotriene agents compared to inhaled corticosteroids in the management of recurrent and/or chronic asthma. In: The Cochrane Library, Issue 1, 2002. Oxford: Update Software.

10 Improve asthma control with six-step management plan. NPS News, 23; 2002: 1–6.

11 Worsnop C. Combination inhalers for asthma. Australian Prescriber, 2005; 28: 26–8.

12 Gibson PG et al. Efficacy of azithromycin on asthma exacerbations and quality of life in adults with persistent uncontrolled asthma (AMAZES): a randomised, double blind, placebo-controlled trial. Lancet, 12 Aug 2017, 390(10095): 659–68.

13 Global strategy for asthma management and prevention. Bethesda MD: Global Initiative for Asthma, 2012.

14 Asthma: steps to control. NPS Medicine Wise, April 2014: 1–6.

15 Ni Chroinin M et al. Addition of long acting beta-2 agonists to inhaled steroids. Cochrane Database Syst Rev. 2009: October: CD005307.

16 Cates CJ et al. Holding chambers versus nebulisers for beta-agonist treatment of acute asthma. In: The Cochrane Library, Issue 2, 2002. Oxford: Update Software.

17 Lindstrom SJ, Silver J et al. Thunderstorm outbreak of November 2016: a natural disaster requiring planning. MJA, 18 September 2017; 207(6): 235–7.

18 Gibson PE et al. Barriers to improved asthma outcomes. Cochrane Database Syst Rev. 2003: July: CD001117.

19 Buckley N (chair). *Australian Medicines Handbook*. Adelaide: Australian Medicines Handbook Pty Ltd, 2016: 845–8.

83 Chronic obstructive pulmonary disease

Tobacco drieth the brain, dimmeth the sight, vitiateth the smell, hurteth the stomach, destroyeth the concoction, disturbeth the humors and spirits, corrupteth the breath, induceth a trembling of the limbs, exsiccateth the windpipe, lungs and liver, annoyeth the milt, scorcheth the heart, and causeth the blood to be adusted.

TOBIAS VENNER (1577–1660), *VIA RECTA AD VITAM LONGAM*

Chronic obstructive pulmonary disease (COPD) is described by the Global Initiative for Chronic Obstructive Lung Disease (GOLD) as a 'common, preventable and treatable disease characterised by non-fully reversible persistent airflow limitation that is usually progressive and associated with an enhanced chronic inflammatory response in the airways and the lung to noxious particles or gases. It is basically a structural disease. Exacerbations and comorbidities contribute to the overall severity in individual patients'.[1]

COPD typically affects middle-aged and older people with the usual age of onset in the fifth and sixth decades. It is the fourth leading cause of death and the third leading burden of disease in Australia, affecting 12.4% of Australians between 45 and 70 years. Early diagnosis and treatment is important to outcome and the provisional diagnosis should be based on the clinical features of breathlessness and cough in a smoker or ex-smoker.

Cigarette smoking is undoubtedly the major cause of both chronic bronchitis and emphysema, although only 10–15% of smokers develop the diseases.[2] Chronic bronchitis is defined as >3 episodes per year for 2 years while emphysema is destruction of alveoli. The clinical differences between asthma and bronchitis are summarised in CHAPTER 49. Patients experiencing overlap of asthma and COPD should be identified and treated differently to patients with either condition alone.

Lifelong passive smoking exposure increases COPD risk by 2.2 to 4.0 times.

FIGURE 83.1 illustrates the influence of smoking on lung function.

Factors in causation

- Cigarette smoking (usually 20/day for 20 years or more)[4]
- Natural fuel—wood, twigs, crop residue
- Air pollution (outdoor and indoor)
- Airway infection/chronic bronchitis
- Occupation: related to cadmium, silica, dusts
- Familial factors: genetic predisposition
- $Alpha_1$-antitrypsin deficiency (emphysema)
- Bronchial hyper-responsiveness

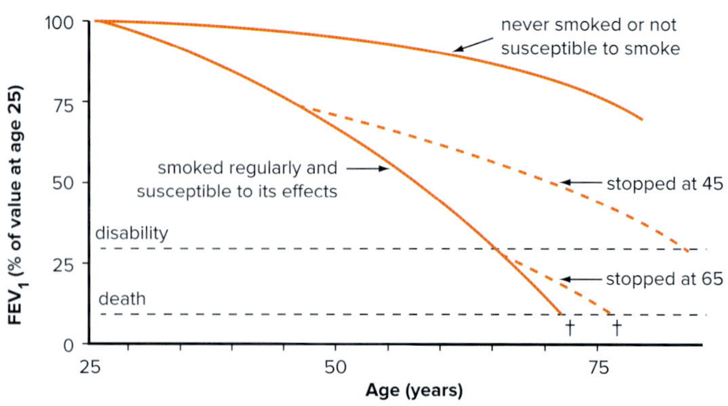

FIGURE 83.1 Decline of FEV_1 with age

Source: Adapted from Fletcher and Peto[3]

Diagnosis and management of COPD

The COPDX Plan guidelines[5] developed by the Australian Lung Foundation and the Thoracic Society of Australia and New Zealand provide an appropriate framework for diagnosis and management. The key recommendations are: Confirm diagnosis, Optimise function, Prevent deterioration, Develop a self-management plan and manage eXacerbations.

C—Confirm diagnosis and assess severity

Symptoms

- Breathlessness
- Cough
- Sputum production

} main symptoms

- Chest tightness
- Wheezing
- Airway irritability
- Fatigue
- Anorexia
- Weight loss

} with advanced disease

Consider the diagnosis of COPD in all smokers and ex-smokers older than 35 years. The diagnosis of COPD rests on the demonstration of airflow obstruction.

The sensitivity of the physical examination for detecting mild to moderate COPD is poor.

Signs

The signs vary according to the nature of the disease and the presence of infection. Signs may be completely absent in the early stages of COPD: chronic bronchitis may present only with wheezing, while dyspnoea is a feature of associated airflow obstruction.

Signs may include:

- tachypnoea
- reduced chest expansion
- hyperinflated lungs
- hyper-resonant percussion
- diminished breath sounds ± wheeze
- 'pink puffer'—always breathless
- 'blue bloater'—oedematous and central cyanosis
- signs of respiratory failure
- signs of cor pulmonale

The diagnosis is usually clinical with a history of increasing dyspnoea and sputum production in a lifetime smoker with no features of asthma. It is imprudent to make a diagnosis of chronic bronchitis and emphysema in the absence of cigarette smoking unless there is a family history suggestive of alpha$_1$-antitrypsin deficiency.[6]

At diagnosis, up to 50% of lung function may have been lost.

Investigations

Pulmonary function tests

Spirometry remains the gold standard for diagnosing, assessing and monitoring COPD. Post-bronchodilator forced expiratory ratio (FER) <0.7 is required for diagnosis.

> **Definition**
>
> COPD Post-bronchodilator FEV_1/FVC of <0.70 (<70%) and FEV_1 <80% predicted.

The Australian stages of severity based on FEV_1% predicted are mild (60–80%), moderate (40–50%) and severe (<40%), while the GOLD[1] staging is 1. mild (≥80%), 2. moderate (50–80%), 3. severe (30–50%), 4. very severe (<30%).

Chest X-ray

This can be normal (even with advanced disease) but characteristic changes occur late in disease. May exclude lung cancer >1 cm.

Blood gases

- May be normal
- $PaCO_2$ ↑; PaO_2 ↓ (advanced disease)

Gas transfer factor

- A reduced diffusing capacity of the lungs for carbon monoxide (DLCO) is a feature of COPD. DLCO is not reduced in asthma.

ECG

- This may show evidence of cor pulmonale

Sputum culture

- If resistant organism suspected

FBE

- To identify anaemia and polycythaemia
- Haemoglobin and PCV may be raised in COPD

O—Optimise function

The principal goals of therapy are to stop smoking, to optimise function through relief of symptoms with

Table 83.1 SMOKES, a consultation checklist for chronic obstructive pulmonary disease[7]

S	= **S**moking cessation
M	= **M**edication—inhaled bronchodilator, vaccines (influenza, pneumococcus), corticosteroids (if indicated)
O	= **O**xygen—is it needed?
K	= **K**omorbidity—cardiac dysfunction, sleep apnoea, osteoporosis, depression, asthma, GORD
E	= **E**xercise and rehabilitation
S	= **S**urgery—bullectomy, lung volume reduction surgery, single-lung transplantation

medication and pulmonary rehabilitation, and to prevent or treat aggravating factors and complications.

TABLE 83.1 is a useful consultation checklist mnemonic.[7]

Long-term treatment

Advice to patient

- If you smoke, you must stop (persuading the patient to stop smoking is the key to management). The only treatment proven to slow the progression of COPD is smoking cessation.[3] Consider smoking cessation medications.
- Avoid places with polluted air and other irritants, such as smoke, paint fumes and fine dust.
- Go for walks in clean, fresh air.
- A warm, dry climate is preferable to a cold, damp place (if prone to infections).
- Get adequate rest.
- Avoid contact with people who have colds or flu.
- Optimal diet—reduce weight if necessary.

Physiotherapy

Refer to a physiotherapist for chest physiotherapy, breathing exercises and an aerobic physical exercise program.

Drug therapy[6]

83

In the long-term treatment of COPD, bronchodilators are recommended for the relief of wheezing and shortness of breath. Bronchodilation is important to allow 'lung emptying' and reduce gas trapping. These include: short-acting β_2-agonists (SABAs, e.g. salbutamol, terbutaline) and short-acting anticholinergic drugs (ipratropium bromide); long-acting β_2-agonists (LABAs, e.g. eformoterol, salmeterol, indacaterol, vilanterone); long-acting anticholinergic drugs with muscarinic antagonist action (LAMAs, e.g. tiotropium, glycopyrronium, umeclidinium) which block parasympathetic bronchial constriction; and corticosteroids.

The preferred route of administration of bronchodilator is by inhalation, which requires correct device technique.

Inhaled drugs can be administered by MDIs, dry-powder devices or nebulisers. The evidence suggests that an MDI and spacer are as effective as a nebuliser—they are also simpler and cheaper—but the appropriate method depends on patient needs and preference.

The usefulness of a bronchodilator for an individual can only be assessed by a therapeutic trial, accepting either objective improvement in lung function or improvement in symptom control as endpoints.

Short-acting bronchodilator therapy

Most studies suggest that short-acting β_2-agonists and ipratropium bromide are equally efficacious in patients with COPD. If patients do not respond adequately to one of these bronchodilators then it is appropriate to consider a trial of a combination of the two classes of bronchodilator with objective monitoring of response.

Use the following by inhalation:[6]

> salbutamol 100–200 mcg, up to 4 times daily
> *or*
> terbutaline 500 mcg, up to 4 times daily
> *or (with and without)*
> ipratropium bromide 40–80 mcg, up to 4 times daily

For patients unable to use an MDI or a spacer, a nebuliser should be used, with the following doses:

> salbutamol or terbutaline 2.5 to 5 mg
> *and/or*
> ipratropium bromide 250 to 500 mcg by nebuliser, up to 4 times a day

Long-acting bronchodilator therapy

Long-acting β_2-agonists can be used in patients who remain symptomatic despite treatment with combinations of short-acting bronchodilators and those with frequent exacerbations. Used regularly they can be effective and may be more convenient than using short-acting bronchodilators.[8] Long-acting anticholinergic therapy[2] with tiotropium bromide (taken by inhalation) has been proven to reduce the frequency of exacerbations with COPD compared with short-acting anticholinergic drugs. The choice of drug can be determined by the patient's response to a trial of the drug, the drug's adverse effects and cost including PBS listing.

Table 83.2 Long-acting bronchodilators[7]

LABAs*	
eformoterol	12 mcg twice daily
salmeterol	50 mcg twice daily
indacaterol	150–300 mcg daily
olodaterol	5 mcg daily
LAMAs**	
aclidinium	322 mcg twice daily
tiotropium	18 mcg daily
glycopyrronium	50 mcg daily
umeclidinium	62.5 mcg daily

Source: Based on Table 9.24[6]

*LABA = long-acting β_2-agonist

**LAMA = long-acting muscarinic antagonist

For treatment with long-acting bronchodilator by inhalation, see TABLE 83.2.

Corticosteroids[6]

Only 10% of patients with stable COPD benefit in the short term from inhaled corticosteroids (ICS). There are no distinguishing clinical features to predict in advance which patients may respond. The aim of treatment is to reduce exacerbation rates and slow the decline of the disease. The effect of ICS on mortality is uncertain, and there is some evidence that ICS use may increase rates of pneumonia. Note that asthma can possibly coexist with COPD. Benefits are not seen in patients who continue to smoke.

If corticosteroids are to be used, usual practice is ICS/LABA combination inhalers (fluticasone/salmeterol, fluticasone/vilanterol or budesonide/eformoterol), which are available on the PBS for use in symptomatic patients with moderate to severe COPD (FEV_1<50% predicted).[9]

In this group, tiotropium combined with an ICS/LABA combination inhaler (triple therapy) is more beneficial than the individual treatments alone.[9] Combining LAMA and LABA provides a modest additive effect.[10]

Inhaled corticosteroids

Guidelines for prescription include:

- documented but limited evidence of responsiveness to inhaled corticosteroids, including functional status
- those with an FEV_1 ≤50% predicted
- two or more exacerbations requiring oral steroids in 12 months

There is no role for ICS monotherapy in the treatment of COPD. Oral corticosteroids are not recommended for maintenance therapy in COPD, although they may be needed in patients with severe COPD where corticosteroids cannot be withdrawn following an acute exacerbation. A stepwise approach to management is outlined in FIGURE 83.2.

P—Prevent deterioration[5]

Reducing risk factors for COPD is a priority, and smoking is the most important and prime target if this continues to be a problem. Stopping is the only measure that slows the progression of COPD. Reinforce patient education programs, and avoid exposure to passive smoke as far as possible.

Annual influenza vaccination

Influenza vaccination reduces the risk of exacerbations, hospitalisation and death. It should be given in early autumn to all patients with COPD.

Pneumococcal vaccination

Vaccination (23vPPV) to prevent invasive bacteraemic pneumococcal pneumonia is recommended, with a booster at 5 years.[11]

Long-term oxygen therapy

Long-term oxygen therapy (LTOT) reduces mortality in COPD. Long-term continuous therapy given for at least 15 hours a day (as close as possible to 24 hours a day)

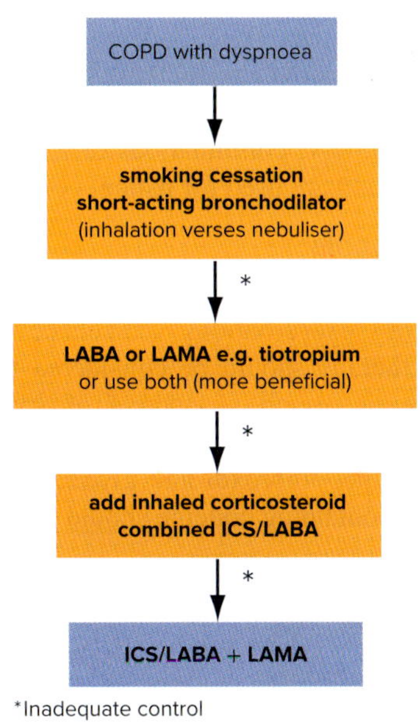

FIGURE 83.2 Stepwise approach to management of COPD.

83

prolongs life in hypoxaemic patients—those who have PaO_2 consistently <55 mm Hg (7.3 KPa; SpO_2 88%) when breathing air. At assessment for ongoing therapy, the patient's condition must be stable and the patient must have stopped smoking at least 1 month previously. Flow should be set at the lowest rate needed to maintain a resting PaO_2 of 60 mm Hg. A flow rate of 0.5–2.0 L/min is usually sufficient. Best used for at least 18 hours a day.[6] There is no clear-cut evidence about the effectiveness of intermittent ambulatory domiciliary oxygen therapy, but patients with hypoxaemia during sleep may require nocturnal oxygen therapy.

Check current smoking status

Smoking cessation clearly reduces the rate of decline of lung function. GPs and pharmacists can help smokers quit. Brief counselling is effective and every smoker should be offered at least this intervention at every visit.

Refer to strategies in CHAPTER 21, including effectiveness of treatment for nicotine dependence.

Antibiotics

Current evidence does not support long-term antibiotic use to prevent exacerbations, but they should be used in exacerbations with an increase in cough, dyspnoea, sputum volume or purulence.

Corticosteroids

No medication has yet been shown to prevent the long-term decline in lung function. Inhaled corticosteroids (ICS) are indicated for patients with a documented response or those who have moderate to severe COPD with frequent exacerbations. ICS use has been observed to be associated with increased rates of pneumonia.

Note: fixed-dose combinations of LABA and ICS (see CHAPTER 82) are used for patient convenience.[6]

Mucolytic agents

Mucolytic agents may reduce the frequency and duration of exacerbations (evidence level I). Mucolytic therapy should be considered for patients with a chronic cough productive of sputum. Oral mucolytics include potassium iodide, bromhexine, N-acetylcysteine, ambroxol and glyceryl guaiacolate. Compounds containing codeine should be avoided.

Antitussive agents

Regular use of antitussives in stable COPD is contraindicated.

Regular review

Regular review with objective measures of function is recommended in anticipation of reducing complications, frequency and severity of exacerbations and admissions to hospital. Regular schedules for follow-up visits are appropriate. Medication review should involve consideration of deprescribing as well as prescribing.

Lung surgery[12]

The options are bullectomy, lung volume reduction surgery and transplantation. Patients should be referred for consideration for bullectomy if they have a single large bulla on CT scan associated with breathlessness and an FEV_1 <50% predicted. Other lung surgery should be considered in patients with severe COPD who remain breathless with marked restriction of their activities of daily living, despite maximal therapy. Emphysema mainly involving the upper lobes with $PaCO_2$ <55 mm Hg and FEV >20% predicted are some factors required for lung volume reduction surgery.

D—Develop support network and self-management plan[5]

COPD imposes a considerable handicap on patients and carers, with heavy psychosocial issues including fears about the outcome of the disease.

Respiratory physician referral

Early referral to a respiratory physician is appropriate in order to clarify the diagnosis, consider other therapies, consider long-term home oxygen and facilitate organisation of pulmonary rehabilitation.

Pulmonary rehabilitation

One highly effective strategy is pulmonary rehabilitation, which aims to increase patient and carer knowledge and understanding, reduce carer strain and develop positive attitudes toward self-management and exercise. Integrated programs include education, exercise, behaviour modification and support, which are more effective than any separate component.

The support team and multidisciplinary care plans

As the patient's primary health care provider, the GP is uniquely placed to identify smokers and help them quit, facilitate early diagnosis and coordinate the support team. The support team can enhance the quality of life and reduce morbidity for the COPD patient. The support team can include a nurse/respiratory educator, physiotherapist, occupational therapist, social worker, clinical psychologist, speech pathologist, pharmacist and dietitian.

Government and community support services such as Home Care, home maintenance, exercise programs, Meals on Wheels and support groups can be galvanised to provide support.

Self-management plans

Patients should be encouraged to take appropriate responsibility for their own management. The primary care team, supported by Extended Primary Care item numbers, should develop systems to identify those with more severe COPD who might benefit from more focused education and training in self-management skills.

Psychological issues

The issues facing the COPD patient include fear, stress, sleep disturbance, anxiety, panic and depression. Proactive management, including optimal care of these problems as they arise, will facilitate coping. Management also focuses on symptom control and maximising the quality of life. These patients have to face palliative care at the end stage and ethical issues have to be handled sensitively.

Referral to in-patient care

The management plan should include the identification of clinical markers indicating more intensive hospital treatment.

Indications for hospitalisation include:[5]

- rapid rate of onset of acute exacerbation with increased dyspnoea, cough or sputum
- inability to cope at home
- inability to walk between rooms when previously mobile
- severe breathlessness leading to inability to eat or sleep
- inadequate response to ambulatory treatment
- altered mental status suggestive of hypercapnia
- significant comorbidity (e.g. cardiac disease)
- new arrhythmia
- cyanosis

X—manage eXacerbations[5]

Diagnosis of an exacerbation is symptomatically the acute onset over minutes to hours of:

- increasing dyspnoea including use of accessory muscles at rest
- increased sputum
- more purulent sputum

Fever may be present, but fever and chest pain are uncommon symptoms. One-third have no identifiable cause, but infections and heavy pollutants can cause the exacerbation. Consider investigating with pulse oximetry, chest X-ray and sputum culture.

Patients should be treated with a bronchodilator, preferably with a large-volume spacer. If nebulisers are used they should be driven by compressed air (to avoid the problem of potentially adverse oxygenation). Systemic glucocorticoids reduce the severity and shorten recovery.

Ventilatory support may be used if hypercapnia develops or worsens despite optimal drug therapy. Non-invasive ventilatory support may avoid the need for intubation.

Treatment in summary[6,14]

Bronchodilators

Initial therapy by SABA inhalation:

salbutamol 100 mcg MDI, up to 8 to 10 inhalations, repeat as required

or

terbutaline 500 mcg DPI, 1 to 2 inhalations, repeat as required

or

ipratropium bromide 20 mcg MDI, up to 4–6 inhalations, repeat as required

If control is inadequate, combine salbutamol or terbutaline with ipratropium bromide.

If a nebuliser is used (which is usually the case upon hospitalisation), use salbutamol 2.5–5 mg, terbutaline 2.5–5 mg or ipratropium bromide 250–500 mcg, as required.

Oxygen therapy[6]

Controlled oxygen delivery—28% via Venturi mask or 2 L/min via nasal prongs should be commenced if the patient is hypoxaemic (oxygen saturation >92% with pulse oximetry). Maintain the arterial oxyhaemoglobin saturation at 90%. It is important to obtain a direct measurement of arterial blood gases to confirm the degree of hypoxaemia and if hypercapnia or acidosis is present.

Note that patients with severe COPD are prone to hypercapnia if they breathe high oxygen concentrations. Supplemental oxygen should be kept to a minimum. If hypercapnia develops assisted ventilation may be required.

Corticosteroids

Corticosteroids should be used routinely for severe exacerbations. Use:

prednisolone or prednisone 30–50 mg (o), daily

If oral medication cannot be tolerated, use:

hydrocortisone 100 mg IV 6 hourly (or equivalent dose of alternative corticosteroid)

Conversion from IV to oral corticosteroid should occur as soon as practicable.

The duration of oral corticosteroid therapy for exacerbations of COPD is not well established; however, courses of 7 to 14 days are commonly used.

A tapering dose schedule is not required for short courses.

Antibiotics[6]

The use of antibiotics for exacerbations is not routinely indicated as many episodes are due to viral infections. Some patients have repeated exacerbations due to bacterial infection (usually *Haemophilus influenzae, S. pneumoniae* or *Moraxella catarrhalis*) where antibiotics have been proven to be beneficial, reducing the risk of mortality by 77%.[13]

The indication for antibiotic treatment is:

- increased cough and dyspnoea, *together with*
- increased sputum volume and/or purulence

When indicated, use:

amoxycillin 500 mg (o), 8 hourly for 5 days

or

doxycycline 200 mg (o) as 1 dose on day 1, then 100 mg (o) daily for a further 5 days

or

azithromycin 500 mg (o) daily for 5 days

A stepwise approach is summarised in FIGURE 83.3.

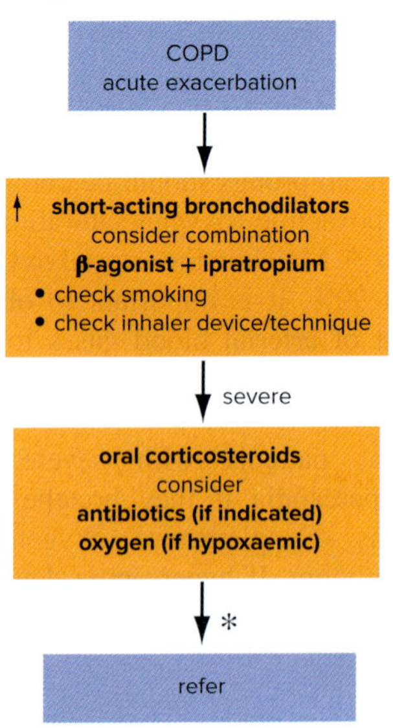

*Inadequate control

FIGURE 83.3 Management plan for acute exacerbation of COPD

Evidence update[15,16]

Evidence indicates that regular treatment with long-acting β_2-agonists is more effective than treatment with short-acting agents (evidence level I) and is associated with improved quality of life (evidence level II), although they are more costly and do not significantly improve lung function. Current recommended guidelines based on the severity of disease are summarised in TABLE 83.3.

Table 83.3 COPD therapy according to severity of disease[9,15]

Stage of COPD		Treatment
0	At risk	Avoidance of risk factors, esp. smoking
		Influenza and pneumococcal vaccination. ? *Haemophilus influenzae* vaccination
1	Mild	**Add** short-acting bronchodilator
2	Moderate	**Add** long-acting bronchodilators LAMA + LABA
		Consider LABA/ICS and referral
		Add pulmonary rehabilitation
3	Severe	**Add** inhaled corticosteroids LABA/ICS + LAMA
4	Very severe	**Add** long-term oxygen (if chronic respiratory failure)
		Consider theophylline (o) or roflumilast
		Consider surgical referral

Practice tips

- The key triad of treatment is: inhaled bronchodilators, smoking cessation and exercise.
- The two priorities are improving lung function and reducing exacerbations. LAMA is a cornerstone of COPD treatment.
- COPD patients should be referred early for rehabilitation. Contact your respiratory physician or hospital for help.
- Pulmonary rehabilitation programs benefit most patients with pulmonary disease.
- Rehabilitation teams are interdisciplinary, usually comprising a rehabilitation physician, physiotherapist, occupational therapist, social worker and dietitian.
- Patients with COPD commonly present in the fifth decade with productive cough or an acute chest illness.[4]

- Diagnosis can only be established by objective measurement using spirometry with FEV_1 being the preferred parameter.
- Non-invasive positive pressure ventilation (NPPV) reduces mortality and hospital stay in patients with acute failure; it is also an effective weaning strategy for patients who require intubation.[13]
- The only treatment proven to slow the progression of COPD is smoking cessation.
- It is very difficult at times to distinguish COPD from the persistent airflow limitation of chronic asthma in older patients (see TABLE 49.3).
- COPD is reportedly 'massively' underdiagnosed—screening with good quality spirometry is important.

Patient education resources

Hand-out sheets from *Murtagh's Patient Education* 7th edition:

- Chronic obstructive pulmonary disease
- Bronchitis: chronic bronchitis

References

1 Global Initiative for Chronic Obstructive Lung Disease (GOLD). Global strategy for the diagnosis, management and prevention of Chronic Obstructive Lung Disease (updated 2018). Global Initiative for Chronic Obstructive Lung Disease Inc, 2014. Available from: <www.goldcopd.org>, accessed January 2018.

2 McPhee SJ, Papadakis MA. *Current Medical Diagnosis and Treatment* (56th edn). New York: McGraw-Hill Lange, 2017: 257.

3 Fletcher C, Peto R. The natural history of chronic airflow obstruction. BMJ, 1977: 1645–48.

4 National Prescribing Service. COPD. NPS News, 2008; 58: 1–4.

5 McKenzie DK, Firth PA, Burdon JG et al. *The COPDX Plan: Australian and New Zealand Guidelines for the Management of Chronic Obstructive Pulmonary Disease 2003.* Med J Aust (Suppl 17 March), 2003: 178.

6 Expert group for Respiratory guidelines. COPD. In: eTG complete. Melbourne: Therapeutic Guidelines Ltd. Available from: <www.tg.org.au>, accessed September 2017.

7 Gibson PG. Management of chronic obstructive pulmonary disease. Australian Prescriber, 2001; 24(6): 152.

8 Dahl R, Greefhorst LA, Nowak D et al. Inhaled formoterol dry powder versus ipratropium bromide in COPD. Am J Respir Crit Care Med, 2001; 164: 778–84.

9 Yang I, Jenkins C. COPD management: an integrated approach. Medicine Today, Sept 2013: 3–7.

10 MacDonald M. Handbook notes. Annual Update Comms for GPs. Melbourne: Monash University, 2015 (available on request).

11 Australian Technical Advisory Group on Immunisation (ATAGI). *The Australian immunisation handbook* (10th edn). Canberra: Australian Government Department of Health, 2017: 4.13 Pneumococcal disease.

12 Snell GI, Solin P, Chin W. Lung volume reduction surgery for emphysema. Med J Aust, 1997; 167: 529–32.

13 Ram FSF, Rodriguez-Roisin R, Granados-Navarrete A et al. Antibiotics for exacerbations of chronic obstructive pulmonary disease. Cochrane Database of Systematic Reviews 2006, Issue 2. Art. No.: CD004403.

14 Buckley N (Chair). *Australian Medicines Handbook.* Adelaide: Australian Medicines Handbook Pty Ltd, 2016: 848–50.

15 Abramson MJ, Crockett AJ, Frith PAet al. COPDX Plan (version 2,37): Australian and New Zealand guidelines for the management of chronic obstructive pulmonary disease. Milton: Lung Foundation Australia, April 2014.

16 NHLBI/WHO Workshop Report. *Global Initiative for Chronic Obstructive Lung Disease (GOLD): Global Strategy for the Diagnosis, Management and Prevention of Chronic Obstructive Pulmonary Disease.* Bethesda, MD: National Institute of Health—National Heart, Lung and Blood Institute, 2005. <www.goldcopd.org>

84 Epilepsy

The fit makes the patient fall down senseless; and without his will or consciousness presently every muscle is put in action; as if all the powers of the body were exerted to free itself from some great violence. In these strong and universal convulsions, the urine, excrements and seed, are sometimes forced away, and the mouth is covered with foam, which will be bloody, when the tongue is bit, as it often is in the agony.

William Heberden (1710–1801)

Epilepsy is defined as a 'tendency to recurrence of seizures'. It is a symptom, not a disease. A person should not be labelled as having epilepsy until at least two attacks have occurred.[1] Epilepsy is common and affects about one person in 50. Both sexes are about equally involved, and some forms run in some families. Famous people who have had epilepsy include Julius Caesar, Thomas Edison and George Frideric Handel.

The most important factors in the management of epilepsy are the accurate diagnosis of the type of seizures; identification of the cause and appropriate investigation; the use of first-line drugs as the sole therapy of some weeks; and adjustment of the dose, according to clinical experience and plasma levels, to give maximum benefit.

To be accurate in diagnosing seizures the diagnosis must be based on:[2]

- the patient's memory of the seizure
- the patient's history (e.g. family history, toxin exposure, accidents, febrile convulsions, eclampsia)
- the observation of a witness to the seizure
- a general and neurological examination
- an EEG, although this has considerable limitations
- a CT scan or preferably MRI (especially if the EEG is focal and a tumour is suspected)

Long-term ambulatory EEG recording now provides more information and, coupled with video monitoring, provides a permanent record of the seizure which can be reviewed at will. The CT or MRI scan is necessary to exclude a focal cause (such as a cyst, tumour, malformation or abscess) which might be treatable by surgery. The MRI scan can indicate developmental migration disorders.

The scan may identify mesotemporal sclerosis (an abnormality in the hippocampus due to birth hypoxia), thereby making some 'idiopathic' seizures into secondary seizures from a known cause.

Epilepsy usually starts in early childhood.

Optimal management includes adequate psychosocial support with education, counselling, advocacy and appropriate referral. Advice about appropriate lifestyle using the NEAT approach (see CHAPTER 7) is important.

An underlying organic lesion becomes more common in epilepsy presenting for the first time in patients over the age of 25 years, and thus more detailed investigation is required.[1]

Secondary causes of seizures include:

- trauma—head injuries
- postcerebral surgery
- metabolic (e.g. calcium and sodium electrolyte disturbances, hypoglycaemia, uraemia, hepatic failure)
- drugs and other toxins (e.g. alcohol, amphetamines including withdrawal)
- intracerebral infections (e.g. meningitis, cysticercosis-specific refugees)
- autoimmune encephalitis (CHAPTER 29)
- vascular—cerebrovascular, arteritis, hypertension
- eclampsia
- MELAS syndrome (CHAPTER 18)
- hypoxia
- degenerative diseases
- sleep deprivation
- prescribed drugs, including antidepressants (e.g. SSRIs, TCAs, venlafaxine, mirtazapine), antibiotics (e.g. norfloxacin, ganciclovir, isoniazid), amantadine, antipsychotics, chloroquine, interferons, pizotifen, promethazine, theophylline

Types of epileptic seizures/ syndromes

Epileptic seizures are classified in general terms as generalised and partial (see TABLE 84.1). Some others are unclassifiable. Partial seizures are about twice as common as generalised seizures and are usually due

Table 84.1 Classification of epileptic seizures[2]

1 Generalised seizures

Motor—convulsive:
- tonic–clonic (previously called grand mal)
- clonic
- myoclonic
- secondary generalised

Motor—non-convulsive:
- tonic (drop attacks)
- atonic (drop attacks)

Non-motor (absence):
- typical absence—childhood (petit mal) and juvenile
- atypical absence
- eyelid myoclonia

2 Focal (partial) seizures

Simple partial (consciousness retained):
- with motor signs (Jacksonian)
- with somatosensory symptoms
- with psychic symptoms

Complex partial (consciousness impaired)

to acquired pathology.[2] Epilepsy syndromes including those first encountered in children are presented in CHAPTER 54.

Generalised seizures

Generalised seizures arise in both cerebral hemispheres simultaneously from the outset. The seizure may be primary with generalised onset (no focus), or secondary, which starts focally and spreads to become secondary and may be due to acquired cerebral pathology.

The main features are:

- abrupt impairment or loss of consciousness
- possible bilateral symmetrical motor events

Types

- Tonic–clonic (formerly called grand mal) seizure: this is the classic convulsive seizure with muscle jerking (see CHAPTER 54)
- Tonic seizure: stiffness only, often with a 'drop' (hallmark of Lennox–Gastaut syndrome)
- Clonic seizure: jerks only
- Atonic seizure: loss of tone, and 'drops'
- Absence seizure (formerly called petit mal): involves loss of consciousness with no or only very minor bilateral muscle jerking, mainly of the face[2]
- Myoclonic seizure: bilateral discrete muscle jerks, which may be very severe, and loss of consciousness

Partial seizures

In partial seizures the epileptic discharge begins in a localised focus of the brain and then spreads out from this focus. The clinical pattern depends on the part of the brain affected:

- simple partial seizures: consciousness is retained (see CHAPTER 54)
- complex partial seizures: consciousness is clouded so that the patient does not recall the complete seizure (see CHAPTER 54)

Both these types of partial seizure can evolve into a bilateral tonic–clonic seizure; this is termed a secondary generalised seizure and is usually due to diffuse brain pathology.[1]

Investigations

Standard minimum investigations are:

- serum calcium, magnesium and electrolytes
- fasting glucose
- EEG (usually with sleep deprivation)
- syphilis serology

Other tests may include:

- chest X-ray
- ECG (? ↑ QT interval)
- video EEG (limited mainly to frequent seizures or to diagnostic dilemmas)
- MRI
- CT scanning (if MRI unavailable)
- other cerebral imaging (e.g. SPECT and PET)

A patient presenting with the first seizure after the age of 25 years will require more detailed investigation.

The single unprovoked seizure: to treat or not[3]

Starting drugs after a single afebrile seizure can be a difficult decision. It basically depends on the EEG findings and also on whether the impact of further seizures outweighs the risk of treatment. If not treated, the risk of recurrence over a 3-year period is 40% with a risk of approximately 25% if treated.[4] The lowest recurrence rates are associated with a normal EEG. Drug therapy should be offered to the patient following two or more seizures within 6–12 months except when there is a clear avoidable precipitant.

Approaches to management

- Shared care between GP and consultant is optimal management.
- An accurate diagnosis of the seizure type is essential.

- An underlying brain disease has to be investigated and treated.
- Treatment is based on drugs and lifestyle management. Alcohol abstinence is preferable.
- Aim for monotherapy.
- A decision has to be made about whether drug therapy is appropriate. Pharmacotherapy should be offered if the patient has had two or more seizures within 6–12 months.[4,5] Treatment is usually commenced after the second seizure. Most seizures require long-term anti-epileptic (anticonvulsant) drug therapy aimed at suppressing the underlying seizure activity in the hope that it may subside, so that 'cure' ultimately occurs and treatment may be ceased. A summary of anti-epileptic drugs is presented in TABLE 84.2.
- The choice of drug depends on the seizure type, the age and sex of the patient, and efficacy in relation to toxicity.
- Treatment should be initiated with one drug and pushed until it controls the events or causes side effects, irrespective of the medication blood level. The disorder can usually be controlled by one drug, provided adequate serum or plasma concentrations are reached.[5] Seventy to eighty per cent of people will have no seizures after treatment with a first-line drug (see TABLE 84.3).
- If a maximum tolerated dosage of this single drug fails to control the seizures, replace it with an alternative agent with a different action. Add the

Table 84.2 Anti-epileptic drugs

The following anti-epileptic drugs are used

Benzodiazepines:
- clobazam
- clonazepam
- diazepam
- midazolam
- nitrazepam

Carbamazepine

Tetracosactrin

Phenobarbitone and related drugs:
- methylphenobarbitone
- primidone

Phenytoin

Sodium valproate (valproate)—avoid in reproductive phase. If necessary, ensure adequate contraception.

Succinimides:
- ethosuximide

Newer drugs (mainly as 'added on' therapy)

Gabapentin

Lacosamide

Lamotrigine

Levetiracetam

Oxcarbazepine

Perampanel

Pregabalin

Sulthiame

Tiagabine

Topiramate

Vigabatrin

Zonisamide

Cannabinoids (evidence is emerging, e.g. Dravet syndrome)

Table 84.3 Recommended selection of anti-epileptics in epilepsy[4,5]

Type of seizure	First-line therapy	Second-line therapy (select from)
Tonic–clonic	Valproate	Carbamazepine Phenytoin Oxcarbazepine Lamotrigine Levetiracetam Topiramate Phenobarbitone
Absence (petit mal)	Ethosuximide Valproate (especially if associated with other seizure type)	Clobazam Clonazepam Lamotrigine
Myoclonic	Valproate	Clobazam Clonazepam Levetiracetam Phenobarbitone
Simple partial (Jacksonian) and complex partial	Carbamazepine	Phenytoin Valproate Topiramate Gabapentin Lamotrigine Tiagabine Phenobarbitone
Infantile spasms	Tetracosactrin Prednisolone	Clonazepam Valproate Nitrazepam Vigabatrin

second drug and obtain a therapeutic effect before removing the first drug.

- An example of an initial drug regimen in a young man with idiopathic generalised tonic–clonic seizures is: valproate 500 mg (o) daily for 2 weeks, then bd, up to 3 g or more per day. *If not controlled, second-line (add on):* lamotrigine 12.5 mg (o) once daily for 2 weeks, increasing up to 100 mg.
- Pay special attention to the adverse psychological and social effects of epilepsy. Emotional and social support is important and advice about epilepsy support groups is appropriate.

A flow chart for the initial management of epilepsy is presented in FIGURE 84.1.

Drug therapy

The following are important specific considerations:

- The basic aim is to prevent seizure recurrence preferably with monotherapy and to minimise adverse effects.
- It is best to select the most effective recommended drug for a specific seizure type (see TABLE 84.3).
- Carbamazepine is the initial choice for focal (partial) seizures, while valproate is the first choice for generalised seizures.[6]
- Young women usually prefer carbamazepine to phenytoin because of the adverse effects of gingival hypertrophy and hirsutism of phenytoin.
- Each drug has specific adverse effects while all drugs tend to be sedating, especially phenobarbitone and its derivatives.
- Twice daily dosage is usually practical.
- Phenytoin (Dilantin) is no longer a first-line agent because of saturable metabolism and the range of unwanted side effects.[6]
- Phenytoin or carbamazepine will bring about control in at least 80% of patients with tonic–clonic seizures.[1] Do not use these drugs together as they have a similar action.

Cessation of drug therapy

It is important to review the need for anti-epileptics every 12 months. The only way to find out if drug therapy is still needed is to withdraw it. It may be ceased if the patient has been free of seizures for at least 2–3 years, particularly if epileptiform activity has disappeared from the EEG (best under specialist supervision). Up to 60% of children have a mild, self-limiting condition and can settle after medication is withdrawn. It is usual to wean children off drugs after 2–3 years (seizure free) and advise about buccal midazolam in the event of a seizure.

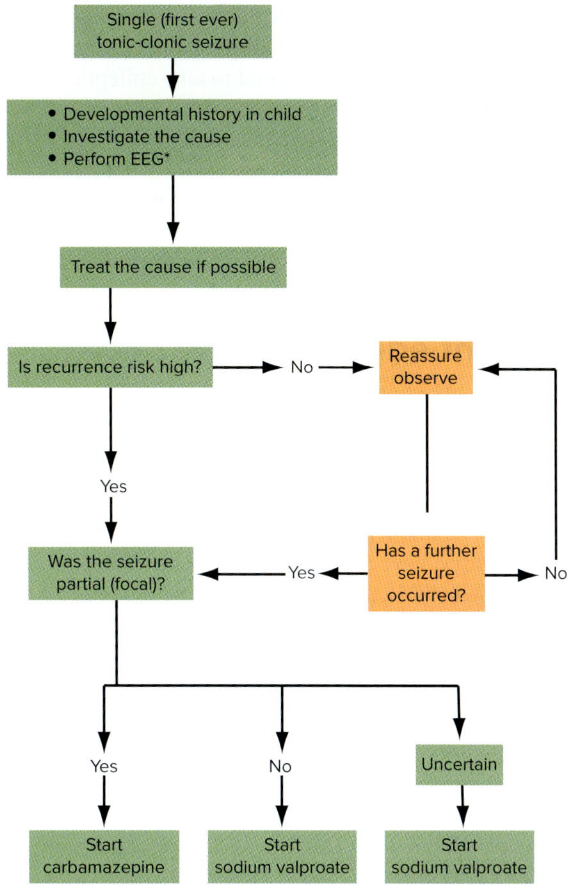

*EEG—electroencephalography

FIGURE 84.1 Initial management of epilepsy

Source: Adapted with permission from Neurology Expert Group. Initial management of epilepsy (Figure 7.1) [revised June 2011]. In: eTG complete. Melbourne: Therapeutic Guidelines Ltd, March 2015.

Adverse drug reactions

Patients should be warned about significant side effects:

- nausea, dizziness, ataxia, visual disturbance or excessive tiredness/fatigue indicate excessive dosage of carbamazepine or phenytoin
- most drugs can cause a rash
- gingival hyperplasia is a classic effect of phenytoin
- hirsutism can occur with phenytoin while hair loss can occur with sodium valproate
- sodium valproate has rare but potentially serious toxic effects
  - liver toxicity
  - dysmorphogenic effects (specifically spina bifida) on fetus during pregnancy. Therefore

it is a risk in women of child-bearing age, especially if inadvertent pregnancy occurs due to pill failure related to anti-epileptic interaction. If valproate is considered necessary, strongly consider long-acting reversible contraceptives.

- LFTs should be performed every 2 months for 6 months after starting sodium valproate;[1] liver toxicity is much more common in the under-2-years age group

Patient education

The following points are worth emphasising.

- Most patients can achieve complete control of seizures, but medication compliance is essential.
- Most people lead a normal life—they can expect to marry, have a normal sexual life and have normal children.
- Patients need good dental care, especially if taking phenytoin.
- A seizure in itself will not usually cause death or brain damage unless prolonged or in a risk situation such as swimming.

Table 84.4 Commonly used anti-epileptics: usual oral dose

	Usual starting adult dose
Carbamazepine	100 bd, increasing gradually to control (max. 2 g/day) Usual range: 400 mg–1.2 g daily
Clonazepam	0.25 mg bd increasing to control
Ethosuximide (used only in absence seizures)	20–30 mg/kg/day in 2 divided doses Usual starting dose: 250 mg bd
Gabapentin	300 mg bd or tds, increasing to 3.6 g daily (max.)
Lamotrigine	25 mg/day increasing to 100–200 mg/day
Levetiracetam	250 mg bd for 7 days increasing to 500 mg bd (max 3 g/day)
Phenobarbitone	60–240 mg daily at bed time Usual dose: 60–120 mg
Phenytoin	5 mg/kg/day in 2 divided doses Average adult: 300 mg
Sodium valproate	500 mg daily for 7 days then bd, increasing to achieve control (up to 2–3 g/day)

- Patients cannot swallow their tongue during a seizure.
- Take special care with open fires.
- Encourage patients to cease intake of alcohol. Intoxication is very harmful.
- Adequate sleep is important. Deprivation is harmful.
- Avoid fatigue.
- Advise showering in preference to bathing.

Driving

One has to be very careful about driving. Most people with epilepsy can drive but each case has to be considered individually. Applicants for a learner's licence need to be seizure-free for 2 years (varies between states/territories), with an annual medical review for 5 years following receipt of the licence. Restrictions range from 1 month to 2 years, depending on the circumstances of the seizures. For a new patient the usual rule is suspension of driving until 3–6 months seizure free.[7]

Employment

People with epilepsy can hold down most jobs, but if liable to seizures they should not work close to heavy machinery, in dangerous surroundings, at heights (such as climbing ladders) or near deep water. Careers are not available in some services, such as the police, military, aviation (pilot, traffic controller) or public transport (e.g. bus driver).

Sport and leisure activities

Most activities are fine, but people with epilepsy should avoid dangerous sports such as scuba diving, hang-gliding, parachuting, rock climbing, car racing and swimming alone, especially surfing.

TABLE 84.5 outlines contraindications for sporting activities. These apply to patients who suffer from very frequent seizures, especially the complex partial seizures with prolonged postictal states.[5]

Avoid trigger factors

- Fatigue
- Lack of sleep
- Physical exhaustion
- Stress
- Excess alcohol
- Prolonged flashing lights if photosensitive (e.g. video games—this applies to those with a proven response to a proper EEG with photic stimulation)

Table 84.5 Sporting activities: contraindications[8]

Absolute contraindications
Flying and parachuting
Motor racing
Mountain and rock-climbing
High diving
Scuba diving
Underwater swimming, especially competitive
Hang-gliding
Abseiling
Relative contraindications
Aiming sports such as archery and pistol shooting
Contact sports such as boxing, rugby, football, including soccer, where heading the ball is involved
Competitive cycling for children with absence epilepsy
Bathing and swimming
Gymnastics, especially activities such as trampolining and climbing on bars
Ice skating and skiing
Javelin throwing

Epilepsy in children

Refer to CHAPTER 54.

Single (first) episode tonic–clonic seizure in school-aged child

1 Take a comprehensive history: family history, past history, developmental history, any loss of skills, recent head injury, headache, drowsiness, dizziness, recent school performance
2 Investigations:
- biochemistry (glucose, electrolytes incl. Ca^{++}, Mg^{++})
- ECG (? QT interval)
- EEG (specialist input)
- Imaging—brain CT or MRI

3 Management:
- Reassure may be one-off event
- Usually no medication
- If recurs, start sodium valproate (see FIG. 84.1)

Photosensitive epilepsy in children

Some children suffer from photosensitive epilepsy related to exposure to computer and video games and 3D television. There is some evidence that such children may not have seizures if they keep one eye covered. If television provokes seizures, strategies such as watching it with ambient lighting and using the remote control rather than approaching the set will minimise the problem.

Epilepsy in the elderly

The elderly require the same diagnostic approach as any other age group. However, they are sensitive to side effects of drugs and may require a lower dose than younger patients. Remember that antidepressant or major tranquiliser drugs can precipitate a generalised seizure.

Menstrual period and epilepsy

Should seizures occur only during the menstrual period, then the addition of clobazam 1–2 days before the period and 1–2 days into the menses may be all that is required.[6]

Pregnancy and epilepsy[5,9]

Pregnancy is associated with a 30% increase in seizures. Although the outcome is successful for more than 90% of women with epilepsy, there is a slightly increased risk of prematurity, low birthweight, mortality, defects and intervention. About 45% of women have an increased number of seizures, due mainly to a fall in anti-epileptic drug levels.

All anti-epileptic drugs are potentially teratogenic, with different drugs being related to different defects: phenytoin has been related to cleft lip and palate and congenital heart disease, while sodium valproate (in particular) and carbamazepine have been associated with spina bifida. Sodium valproate should be avoided unless other drugs are unlikely to prevent seizures. All anti-epileptic drugs are expressed in breast milk but in such reduced concentrations as not to preclude breastfeeding, although it is preferable for mothers taking lamotrigine and levetiracetam to abstain from breastfeeding.[10]

Neurosurgical treatment

Surgical techniques are based on resection such as for temporal lobe epilepsy for a highly select group of patients and also on disconnection techniques. The latter includes corpus callosotomy, multiple subpial transection, hemispherectomy and vagal nerve stimulation. The treatments are limited to a select group with poorly controlled seizures who require detailed evaluation in a specialist centre.

Pitfalls in management of epilepsy[4]

Misdiagnosis

The main pitfall associated with seizure disorders and epilepsy is misdiagnosis. It should be realised that not all seizures are generalised tonic–clonic in type. The most common misdiagnosed seizure disorders are complex partial seizures (an underdiagnosed disorder) or the tonic or atonic seizures.

The diagnosis of epilepsy is made on the history rather than the EEG so a very detailed description of the events from eyewitnesses is important.

The features of complex partial seizure (described in CHAPTER 54) have many variations, the commonest being a slight disturbance of perception or consciousness. The complex partial seizure may evolve to a generalised tonic–clonic seizure. A simple partial seizure may also do this.

In tonic–clonic seizures the patient may become momentarily rigid or fall to the ground and perhaps have one or two jerks only.

Misdiagnosing behavioural disorders

It is important to differentiate between a fit and a behavioural disorder, but it can be difficult. About 20% of apparently intractable 'seizures' are considered to be non-epileptic (pseudoseizures, i.e. emotionally based).[10] These often resemble tonic–clonic seizures but usually there are bizarre limb movements. Ancillary testing, especially with video EEG recording, can help overcome these diagnostic problems but the differentiation may be difficult as the most common situation for pseudoseizures is in the person who has real fits.

Overtreatment

Polypharmacy

Polypharmacy may be counterproductive for the patient and the seizure disorder. This is especially applicable to drugs with a high incidence of side effects. If a patient is taking several medications, management of the case needs questioning and perhaps reconsidering with a consultant's help.

Seizure control may be improved by reducing polypharmacy. When initiating treatment it is best to select one drug and increase its dose until its maximum recommended level, the onset of side effects or appropriate control. If control is not obtained, the drug should be replaced with an alternative agent but a crossover period is essential. Monotherapy is preferred but combination therapy is often acceptable.

84

Prolonged treatment

The question should be asked at some stage 'Does this patient really need medication?' Some patients are kept on anti-epileptics for too long without any attempt being made to wean them off medication or to transfer them onto anti-epileptics less prone to side effects. Patients should not be left on inappropriate drugs especially if side effects and drug interactions are a problem.

Drug interactions

Drug interactions with anti-epileptics should always be kept in mind. The most serious of all is the interaction with the oral contraceptive pill because pregnancy can occur. Erythromycin and carbamazepine interact.

Management of status epilepticus[3,4]

Definition

Status epilepticus is the situation in which a patient suffers from two or more generalised seizures without regaining consciousness between seizures, or suffers from continuous partial seizures;[4] refer to CHAPTER 128.

Focal status

- A high index of suspicion is needed to diagnose
- Oral medication usually adequate
- Avoid overtreatment

Generalised status

Absence attacks (petit mal)

- Hospitalisation
- IV diazepam

Note: These can cause long-term damage.

Tonic–clonic (dangerous!)

Give a benzodiazepine followed by an anti-epileptic agent. Ensure adequate oxygenation: attend to airway (e.g. Guedel tube); give oxygen plus:

midazolam 5–10 mg (child: 0.15–0.2 mg/kg up to 10 mg) IM or IV, over 2–5 minutes

or

midazolam 5–10 mg (child: 0.2–0.3 mg/kg up to 10 mg) buccally or intranasally. One drop = 0.3 mg. Repeat once 15 minutes later if seizure continues

or

diazepam 10–20 mg (child: 0.1–0.25 mg/kg up to 20 mg) IV, over 2–5 minutes (max. 5 mg/min). Repeat once 15 minutes later if seizure continues (beware of respiratory depression)

or
clonazepam 1 mg (child 0.25–0.5 mg) IV over 2–5 minutes. Repeat once 15 minutes later if necessary
followed immediately (for all of above) by an anti-epileptic:
phenytoin 15–20 mg/kg IV in a glucose-free solution over 30 minutes (child 25 mg/min) careful monitoring of ECG and BP
or
sodium valproate 10 mg/kg (child: 15–30 mg/kg up to 800 mg by slow IV injection

Note: Midazolam is suitable for all types of seizures and can be given IM, buccally or intranasally.

Diazepam can be given rectally. In an adult, 10 mg is diluted in 5 mL of isotonic saline and introduced via the nozzle of the syringe into the rectum. The dose in children is 0.5 mg/kg.

Intranasal midazolam (0.2–0.3 mg/kg/dose) up to maximum of 10 mg may be given in children.

DOs and DON'Ts for the onlookers of a seizure

- Don't move the person to another location (unless necessary for safety).
- Don't force anything into the person's mouth.
- Don't try to stop the fit.
- Do roll the person on to his or her side with the head turned to one side and chin up.
- Do call for medical help if the seizure lasts longer than 10 minutes or starts again.
- Do remove false teeth and help clear the airway once the fit is over.

Recurrent prolonged or repetitive status epilepticus

Patients having recurrent prolonged convulsive seizures or serial seizures can be given the following medication options (following appropriate training of carers):

midazolam 10 mg buccally
or
diazepam 10–20 mg rectally (may be available from hospital pharmacies)

When to refer[2]

Specialist referral is advisable under the following circumstances:

- uncertainty of diagnosis
- at onset of seizure disorder to help obtain a precise diagnosis
- when seizures are not controlled by apparently suitable therapy. ? wrong drug ? suboptimal dose ? progressive underlying disorder
- when the patient is unwell, irrespective of laboratory investigation
- when a woman is considering pregnancy (preferable) or has become pregnant: to obtain therapeutic guidance during a difficult phase of management
- for assessment of the prospects for withdrawing treatment after some years of absolute seizure control

Practice tips

- The EEG has considerable limitations in diagnosis. It is diagnostic in less than 50%,[1] although more diagnostic if conducted under sleep deprivation. An accurate eyewitness account of the seizure is the most reliable diagnostic aid.
- During evaluation look for evidence of neurofibromatosis.
- Beware of interactions between anti-epileptics and the oral contraceptive pill.
- Interactions between erythromycin and carbamazepine can cause toxicity.
- Always aim to achieve monotherapy.
- An important toxic reaction can occur with combined phenytoin and carbamazepine.
- Patients should not drive while medication is being adjusted, particularly if weaning is being attempted. Patients must not drive if they do not meet national guidelines on seizure-free periods.[7]
- The development of sophisticated surgical techniques means that surgery can be used in selected patients with poor control. Evaluation for surgery is a very specialised area.

Patient education resources

Hand-out sheets from *Murtagh's Patient Education* 7th edition:

- Epilepsy

References

1 Scott AK. Management of epilepsy. In: *Central Nervous System.* London: BMJ Publishing Group, 1989: 1–2.
2 Beran R. Management of epilepsy. Update 2008. Part 1. Medical Observer, 11 July: 31–3.
3 Berg AT, Shinnar S. The risk of seizure recurrence following a first unprovoked seizure: a quantitative review. Neurology 1991; 41(7): 965–72.
4 Expert group for Neurology guidelines. Epilepsy and seizures. In: eTG complete. Melbourne: Therapeutic Guidelines Ltd. Available from: <www.tg.org.au>, accessed September 2017.

5 Buckley N (Chair). *Australian Medicines Handbook*. Adelaide: Australian Medicines Handbook Pty Ltd, 2016: 718–2.
6 Beran R. Management of epilepsy. Update 2008. Part 2. Medical Observer, 18 July: 27–9.
7 Austroads. Assessing Fitness to Drive for commercial and private vehicle drivers 2016 (as amended up to August 2017), Part 6.2 Seizures and epilepsy. Available from: <www.austroads.com.au/drivers-vehicles/assessing-fitness-to-drive>, accessed April 2018,
8 Cordova F. Epilepsy and sport. Aust Fam Physician, 1993; 22: 558–62.
9 Kilpatrick C. Epilepsy poses special problems. Australian Doctor Weekly, 1993; 19 February: 48.
10 Ahmed R, Apen K, Endean C. Epilepsy in pregnancy. Aust Fam Physician, 2014; 43(3): 112–6.
11 Theodore HR. Neurotrek: a PC based system for automated recording of epileptic seizures and similar events. Patient Management, 1992; 16: 15–16.

Cardiovascular disease 85

Of all the ailments which may blow out life's little candle, heart disease is the chief.

WILLIAM BOYD (1885–1979), *PATHOLOGY FOR THE SURGEON*

Cardiovascular disease includes mainly:

- coronary heart disease—myocardial ischaemia (CHAPTER 40)
- cerebrovascular disease—strokes and transient ischaemia (CHAPTER 130)
- peripheral vascular disease (CHAPTER 66)

The number one cause of death in the world is coronary heart disease (CHD),[1] whether from sudden fatal acute coronary events, particularly myocardial infarction (CHAPTER 40) or blocked arteries causing angina and eventually cardiac failure (CHAPTER 88). CHD is responsible for about 3 in 10 deaths in Australia.[2] However, there has been a pleasing reduction in deaths from coronary heart disease and stroke in recent years because of improved preventive measures. Continuing emphasis on behavioural modification of risk factors and healthy habits is essential to continue this trend.

Risk factors for CVD

Modifiable:

- Hypertension (CHAPTER 86)
- Dyslipidaemia (CHAPTER 87)
- Smoking (CHAPTER 21)
- Diabetes (CHAPTER 20) with microalbuminuria
- Obesity (CHAPTER 78)
- Sedentary lifestyle
- Alcohol excess (CHAPTER 21)
- Poor nutrition (CHAPTER 10)
- Mental stress[3] (CHAPTER 81)

Non-modifiable

- Family history
- Increasing age
- Male gender
- Social history, inc. cultural/ethnic identity

Related conditions:

- Chronic kidney disease (CHAPTER 31) with microalbuminuria

Assessment of absolute cardiovascular risk

The risk of having a cardiovascular event over the next 5 years (or sometimes 10) is an important assessment which should be estimated before deciding on preventative medication as it greatly influences the pros and cons of screening investigations and treatment. The following target groups should be reassessed every 2 years:

- all adults ≥45 years without known history of CVD
- Aboriginal and Torres Strait Islander people ≥35 years

People for whom a high CVD risk can be assumed (e.g. diabetes, established CVD, hypertension) do not need an absolute CVD risk assessment using the Framingham Risk Equation.[4]

Specific screening recommendations[4]

- Blood pressure should be measured in all adults from age 18 years at least every 2 years.
- Adults should have their fasting blood lipids assessed starting at age 45 years, every 5 years (Aboriginal and Torres Strait Islander people from 35 years).
- Adults should be screened for diabetes (fasting plasma glucose or HbA1c) every 3 years from age 40 years (Aboriginal and Torres Strait Islander people from 18 years).
- Adults at high risk should be screened for kidney disease every 1–2 years (ACR ratio and eGFR).

Estimation of cardiovascular risk guidelines based on the key parameters—hypertension, diabetes, smoking, total cholesterol:HDL ratio, age and sex—are presented in FIGURES 85.1 and 85.2. Note that BMI, ethnicity and sedentary lifestyle do not form part of the estimates below (or in many other cardiovascular risk tools) even though in practice they may independently influence risk.

85

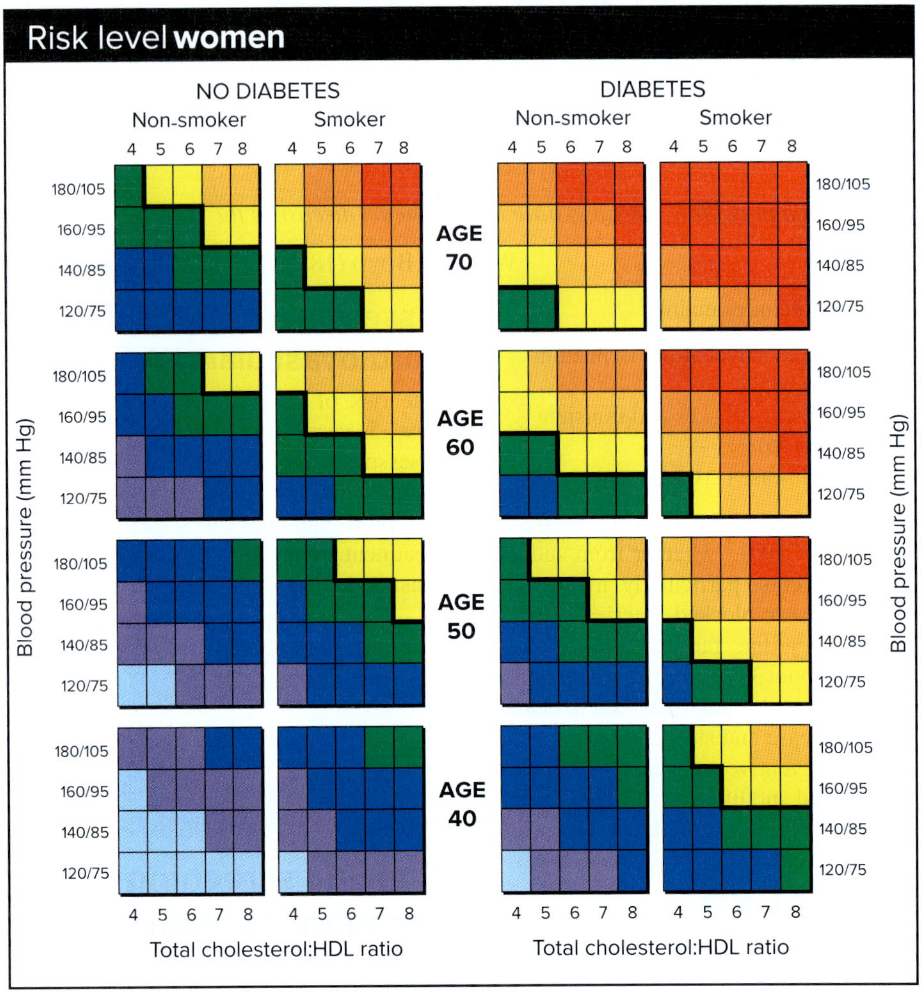

Risk level (for women and men)

5-year cardiovascular disease (CVD) risk (non-fatal and fatal)

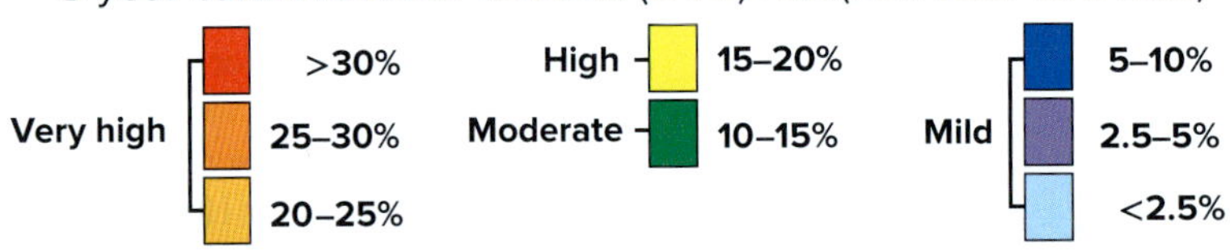

How to use the charts

Σ Identify the chart relating to the person's sex, diabetic status, smoking history and age.

Σ Within the chart choose the cell nearest to the person's age, blood pressure (BP) and TC:HDL ratio. When the systolic and diastolic values fall in different risk levels, the higher category applies.

Σ For Example, the lower left cell contains all non-smokers without diabetes who are less than 45 years and have a TC:HDL ratio of less than 4.5 and a BP of less than 130/80 mm Hg. People who fall exactly on a threshold between cells are placed in the cell indicating higher risk.

Certain groups may have CVD risk underestimated using these charts, see TABLE 86.8 in CHAPTER 86 for recommended adjustments.

FIGURE 85.1 Estimation of cardiovascular risk—women

Source: New Zealand Guidelines Group. *New Zealand Cardiovascular Guidelines Handbook: Developed for primary care practitioners.* Wellington: June 2005 <www.nzgg.org.nz>. Courtesy of the New Zealand Ministry of Health

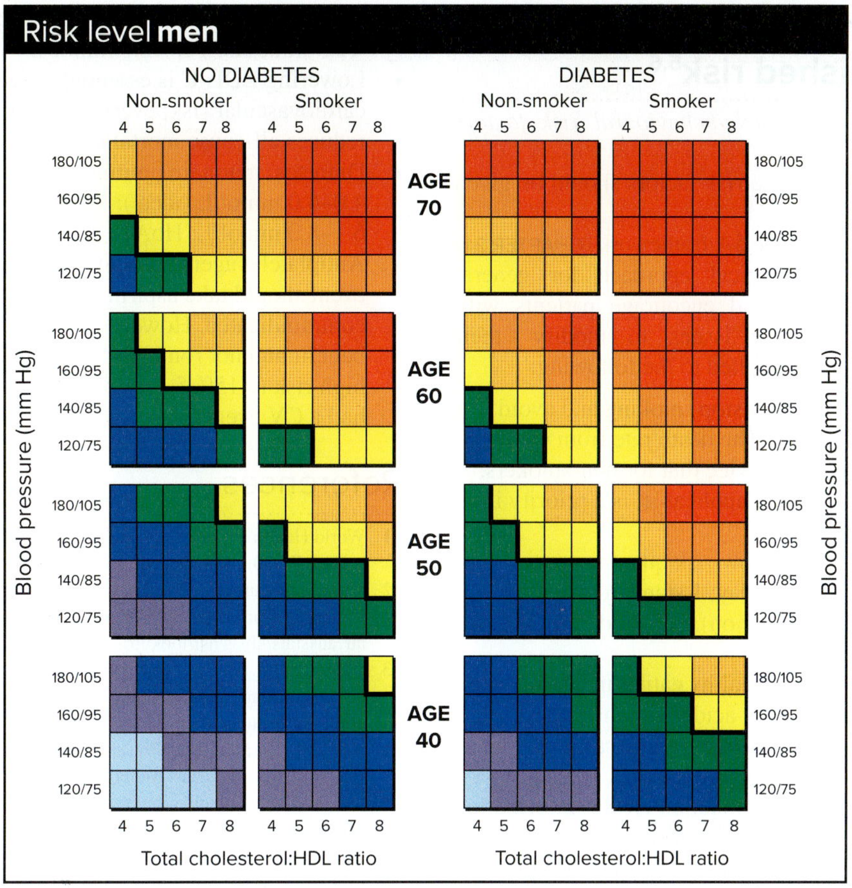

Risk level: 5-year CVD risk (fatal and non-fatal)	**Benefits: NNT for 5 years to prevent one event** (CVD events prevented per 100 people treated for 5 years)		
	1 intervention (25% risk reduction)	**2 interventions (45% risk reduction)**	**3 interventions (55% risk reduction)**
30%	13 (7.5 per 100)	7 (14 per 100)	6 (16 per 100)
20%	20 (5 per 100)	11 (9 per 100)	9 (11 per 100)
15%	27 (4 per 100)	15 (7 per 100)	12 (8 per 100)
10%	40 (2.5 per 100)	22 (4.5 per 100)	18 (5.5 per 100)
5%	80 (1.25 per 100)	44 (2.25 per 100)	36 (3 per 100)

Based on the conservative estimate that each intervention: aspirin, blood pressure treatment (lowering systolic blood pressure by 10 mm Hg) or lipid modification (lowering LDL-C by 20%) reduces CV risk by about 25% over 5 years.

Note: Cardiovasular events are defined as myocardial infarction, new angina, ischaemic stroke, transient ischaemic attack (TIA), peripheral vascular disease, congestive heart failure and cardiovascular-related death.

NNT = Number needed to treat

FIGURE 85.2 Estimation of cardiovascular risk—men

Source: New Zealand Guidelines Group. *New Zealand Cardiovascular Guidelines Handbook: Developed for primary care practitioners.* Wellington: June 2005 <www.nzgg.org.nz>. Courtesy of the New Zealand Ministry of Health

85

Secondary prevention of CHD for established risk[5,6]

1 Management of lifestyle/behavioural risk factors with goals

All patients who have risk factors should be given lifestyle advice.

Intervention using the 5A framework (CHAPTER 21) is an appropriate practical approach for general practitioners to assist and encourage patients with behavioural risk factor issues to modify[7] their behaviour, and can be applied to the following:

- smoking—completely stop smoking and avoid second-hand smoke. The death rate from CHD for smokers is about twice that for non-smokers. Smoking cessation, if applicable, is a priority in risk factor reduction.
- alcohol—consume a low-risk quantity (max. 2 standard drinks per day; 1 standard drink for women with hypertension). See guidelines in CHAPTER 21.
- nutrition—maintain healthy eating including limiting saturated fatty acid and trans fat and salt intake to ≤4 g/day.[7] Aim for a low carbohydrate, healthy fat Mediterranean-type diet. Arrange access to the Heart Foundation Health Information Services and/or refer to a dietitian.
- physical activity—if possible, at least 30 minutes of moderate-intensity physical activity on most days of the week (min. 150 minutes/week). If feasible arrange an appointment with an accredited exercise physiologist as well as a local activity program.
- healthy weight—waist measurement (men <94 cm, women <80 cm; BMI range 18.5–25). The benefits of weight reduction include improved insulin resistance, decreased LDL-C and triglycerides, and increased HDL-C.
- stress management—encourage promotion of recreation, relaxation techniques, meditation and social support. Treat anxiety disorders and depression with counselling if appropriate.

Additionally, patients at high risk (>15% 5-year CV risk or previous CV event) should have specific parameters treated.

2 Management of biomedical risk factors with targets

- Blood pressure: <130/80 mmHg
  Lipids: total C <4 mmol/L; LDL-C <2 mmol/L; HDL-C ≥1.0 mmol/L; non-HDL-C <2.5 mmol/L; TG <2.0 mmol/L[5]
- Lowering LDL-C is essential to reduce cardiovascular risk; every decrease of 1 mmol/L reduces all-cause mortality by 10%[8]
- Diabetes: maintain optimal blood sugar level 4.0–6.0 mmol/L (ideal); compare NHMRC 6.1–8.0 mmol/L; HbA1c ≤7%
- Antiplatelet agent: patients with a previous CV event should take aspirin 75–150 mg/day unless contraindicated. However, aspirin is of limited benefit and not routinely recommended in those at high risk (>15% 5-year or diabetes) who have not had a CV event.[9]

References

1 World Health Organization: fact sheet 310, July 2013. <www.WHO.int/mediacentre/factsheets/fs310>

2 Australian Bureau of Statistics. Leading causes of death 2012. Canberra: Commonwealth of Australia, 2014. <www.abs.gov.au?ausstats/abs@nsf/lookup>

3 Weissman M, Markowitz J et al. Panic disorder and cardiovascular/cerebrovascular problems: results from a community survey. Am J Psych, 1990; 147(11): 1504–5.

4 RACGP. *Guidelines for Preventive Activities in General Practice* (9th edn). East Melbourne: RACGP, 2016.

5 National Heart Foundation of Australia and Cardiac Society of Australia and New Zealand. Reducing risk in heart disease, 2012. <www.heartfoundation.org.au>

6 Franklin BA, Cushman M. Recent advances in preventive cardiology and lifestyle medicine: a themed series. Circulation, 2011; 123(20): 893–905.

7 Expert group for Cardiovascular guidelines. Behavioural risk factor modification. In: eTG complete. Melbourne: Therapeutic Guidelines Ltd. Available from: <www.tg.org.au>, accessed October 2017.

8 Baigent C et al. Cholesterol Treatment Trialists (CTT) Collaboration. Lancet, 2010; 376(9753): 1670–81.

9 National Vascular Disease Prevention Alliance. Guidelines for the management of absolute cardiovascular disease risk, 2012. Available from: <www.heartfoundation.org.au/images/uploads/publications/Absolute-CVD-Risk-Full-Guidelines.pdf>, accessed April 2018.

Resource

National Vascular Disease Prevention Alliance, Guidelines for the management of absolute cardiovascular disease risk. <www.heartfoundation.org.au/images/uploads/publications/Absolute-CVD-Risk-Full-Guidelines.pdf>, accessed April 2018.

Hypertension

86

The greatest danger to a man is that someone will discover hypertension and some fool will try to reduce it.

JOHN HAY 1931

Hypertension is a serious community disorder and the most common condition requiring long-term drug therapy in Australia. It is a silent killer because most people with hypertension are asymptomatic and unaware of their problem. Epidemiological studies have demonstrated the association between hypertension and stroke, coronary heart disease, kidney disease, heart failure and atrial fibrillation. Treatment may be lifelong, hence the need for careful work-up.

- Target organs that can be damaged by hypertension include the heart (failure, LVH, ischaemic disease), kidney (kidney insufficiency), retina (retinopathy), blood vessels (peripheral vascular disease, aortic dissection) and brain (cerebrovascular disease).
- Deaths in hypertensive patients have been shown to be due to stroke 45%, heart failure 35%, kidney failure 3% and others 17%.[1]
- Almost half of the Australian cardiovascular disease burden is due to hypertension.[2]
- Factors increasing the chances of dying in hypertensive patients are: male, onset at a young age, family history, increased diastolic pressure.[2]

Definitions and classification

- The various categories of BP are arbitrarily defined according to BP values for both diastolic and systolic readings (see TABLE 86.1).[4,5]

For adults aged 18 years and older, hypertension is repeated measurements of:

- diastolic pressure >90 mmHg, and/or
- systolic pressure >140 mmHg

- Isolated systolic hypertension is that of ≥140 mmHg in the presence of a diastolic pressure <90 mmHg.

Table 86.1 Definition and classification of blood pressure adults aged 18 years and older measured as sitting blood pressure (mmHg)[4,5]

Category	Systolic	Diastolic
Optimal	<120	<80
Normal	120–129	80–84
High normal	130–139	85–89
Grade 1 hypertension (mild)	140–159	90–99
Grade 2 hypertension (moderate)	160–179	100–109
Grade 3 hypertension (severe)	≥180	≥110
Isolated systolic hypertension	≥140	<90

When a patient's systolic and diastolic BPs fall into different categories, the higher category should apply.

- Hypertension is either essential or secondary (see TABLE 86.2).
- Essential hypertension is the presence of sustained hypertension in the absence of underlying, potentially correctable kidney, adrenal or other factors.

Table 86.2 Causes of hypertension

Essential (90–95%)
Secondary (approx. 5–10%)
Kidney <3%
- glomerulonephritis
- reflux nephropathy
- kidney artery stenosis (see later in this chapter)
- other renovascular disease

Endocrine: 0.3–1%
- primary aldosteronism (Conn syndrome) (see CHAPTER 23)
- Cushing syndrome (see CHAPTER 23)
- phaeochromocytoma (see CHAPTER 23)
- oral contraceptives
- other endocrine factors

Coarctation of the aorta
Immune disorder (e.g. polyarteritis nodosa)
Drugs (e.g. NSAIDs, corticosteroids)
Pregnancy

- Malignant hypertension is that with a diastolic pressure >120 mmHg and exudative vasculopathy in the retinal and kidney circulations.
- Refractory hypertension is a BP >140/90 mmHg despite maximum dosage of two drugs for 3–4 months.

Risk stratification and calculation of cardiovascular risk[4,5]

Treatment of hypertension is generally indefinite (or until old age and frailty render the risks of treatment greater than the benefits). It is important to establish the risk status and the prognosis prior to commencing therapy, especially if hypertension is an isolated factor. The World Health Organization–International Society of Hypertension (WHO–ISH) recommendation is that decisions about management of patients with hypertension should not be based on BP alone but also on the presence or absence of other risk factors, including age, diabetes and smoking. This is because the benefits of treatment are less in those with low cardiovascular risk. CV risk should be stratified according to the BP level and the presence of:

- absolute cardiovascular risk factors
- associated clinical conditions
- target organ damage (see TABLE 86.3)

A practical approach to stratifying total cardiovascular risk is proposed in TABLE 86.4. The terms 'low', 'moderate' (medium), 'high' and 'very high' added risk are calibrated to indicate an absolute 5-year risk of cardiovascular disease of <10%, 10–15%, 15–20% and >20% respectively (based on Framingham criteria).[6] For example, 'low risk' indicates consideration of treatment and monitoring; 'high risk' indicates treating immediately.

Risk estimation can be determined by referring to various cardiovascular risk tables on the website (and in CHAPTER 85). A commonly used tool in Australasia is the modified New Zealand Cardiovascular Risk Charts (www.nzgg.org.nz or www.heartfoundation.com.au). See CHAPTERS 20 and 85.

It is important to collaborate with patients in decision making, and thus discussing cardiovascular

Table 86.3 Factors influencing prognosis in hypertension[4]

Risk factors for cardiovascular disease used for stratification	Associated clinical condition (ACC)	Target organ damage (TOD)
Levels of systolic and diastolic BP Male >55 years Female >65 years Smoking Diabetes mellitus Dyslipidaemia (total cholesterol >6.5 mmol/L, >250 mg/dL or LDL-cholesterol >4.0 mmol/L, >155 mg/dL or HDL-cholesterol M <1.0, F <1.2 mmol/L Family history of premature cardiovascular disease (at age <55 years M, <65 years F) Abdominal obesity (abdominal circumference M ≥102 cm, F ≥88 cm) C-reactive protein ≥1 mg/dL	Cerebrovascular disease: • ischaemic stroke • cerebral haemorrhage • transient ischaemic attack Heart disease: • myocardial infarction • angina • coronary revascularisation • congestive heart failure Kidney disease: • diabetic nephropathy • kidney impairment • proteinuria (>300 mg/24 h) Peripheral vascular disease Advanced retinopathy: • haemorrhages or exudates • papilloedema	Left ventricular hypertrophy Microalbuminuria and/or proteinuria and/or eGFR <60 ml/minute Ultrasound or angiographic evidence of atherosclerotic disease Hypertensive retinopathy (grade II or more)
Other factors affecting prognosis Excessive alcohol intake Specific complementary medicines, e.g. containing tyramine Sedentary lifestyle High-risk socioeconomic group High-risk ethnic group		

Table 86.4 Stratification of cardiovascular risk to quantify prognosis[5]

Other risk factors and disease history	Normal BP	High normal BP	Mild hypertension	Moderate hypertension	Severe hypertension
No other risk factors	Low risk	Low risk	Average risk	Moderate risk	High risk
1 or 2 risk factors but not diabetes	Low risk	Low risk	Moderate risk	Moderate risk	Very high risk
3 or more risk factors or target organ damage or diabetes mellitus	Moderate risk	High risk	High risk	High risk	Very high risk
Associated clinical conditions	High risk	Very high risk	Very high risk	Very high risk	Very high risk

risk assessment and blood pressure (BP) level should be the starting point when discussing the risks and benefits of treatment.

Secondary hypertension

Secondary hypertension may be suggested in patients below 40 years by the history (see TABLE 86.5), physical examination, severity of hypertension or the initial laboratory findings. It is also more likely where BP is responding poorly to drug therapy, and in patients with accelerated or malignant hypertension.[5]

The most common causes of secondary hypertension are various kidney diseases, such as renovascular disease, chronic glomerulonephritis, and chronic pyelonephritis (often associated with reflux nephropathy).[1] There will often be no physical findings to suggest the existence of such kidney diseases, but an indication will generally be obtained by the presence of one or more abnormalities when the urine is examined. Clinical pointers include proteinuria, an abnormal urine sediment, general atheroma, smokers and abdominal bruit. Consider sleep apnoea, and take a comprehensive medication history, including illicit drugs and alternative remedies.

Table 86.5 Clinical features suggesting secondary hypertension[3]

Clinical features	Likely cause
Abdominal systolic bruit	Renal artery stenosis
Proteinuria, haematuria, casts	Glomerulonephritis
Bilateral kidney masses with or without haematuria	Polycystic disease
History of claudication and delayed femoral pulse	Coarctation of the aorta
Progressive nocturia, weakness	Primary aldosteronism (check serum potassium)
Obesity, snoring, daytime sleepiness	Sleep apnoea
Recreational drugs, complementary or prescribed therapies	Stimulants, diet pills, OCP, energy drinks
Paroxysmal hypertension with headache, pallor, sweating, palpitations	Phaeochromocytoma

Physical findings that may suggest secondary hypertension include epigastric bruits (indicating possible kidney artery stenosis) and abdominal aortic aneurysm. Less common findings include abdominal flank masses (polycystic kidneys), delayed or absent femoral pulses (coarctation of the aorta), truncal obesity with pigmented striae (Cushing syndrome), and tachycardia, sweating and pallor (phaeochromocytoma). Endocrine causes are presented in CHAPTER 23.

Further investigation will be required to confirm or reveal secondary hypertension.

Renal artery stenosis

Atherosclerotic kidney artery stenosis accounts for the majority of cases, while fibromuscular dysplasia remains an important cause. Doppler ultrasound is a highly sensitive and specific investigation.

Detection of hypertension[1]

Hypertension can only be detected when BP is measured. Therefore frequent opportunities should be taken to measure BP: every 6–12 weeks in high-risk patients; every 6–12 months in moderate-risk patients.[7]

Diagnosis should not be made on the basis of a single visit. Initial raised BP readings should be confirmed on at least two other visits within the space of 3 months; average levels of 90 mmHg diastolic or more, or 140 mmHg systolic or more, are needed before hypertension can be diagnosed. This will avoid the possibility of an incorrect diagnosis, committing an asymptomatic, normotensive individual to unjustified, lifelong treatment.

Measurement guidelines[4,5]

BP varies continuously and can be affected by many outside factors. Care should therefore be taken to ensure that readings accurately represent the patient's usual pressure.

BP measurement recommendations[6]

- All people aged 18 years and over
- Frequency—every 2 years

Office BP measurement guidelines[5]

- Allow the patient to sit quietly for several minutes.
- Use a validated (calibrated) device.
- Take at least two measurements spaced by 60 seconds.
- Use a standard bladder (12–13 × 35 cm), but a larger one for big arms.
- Have the cuff at the heart level (see FIG. 86.1).
- Deflate the cuff slowly (2 mmHg/s).
- Measure BP also in standing position in elderly patients and diabetic patients.

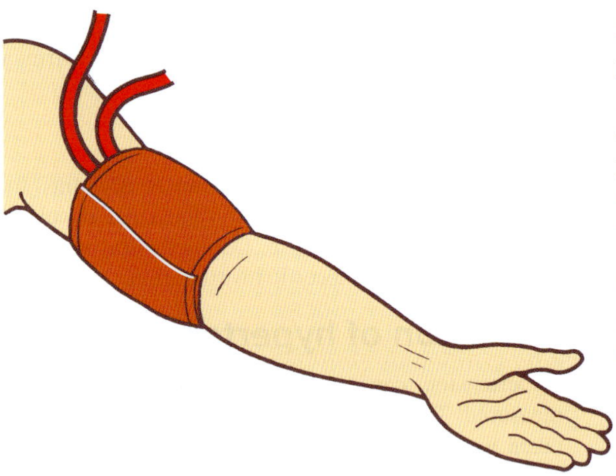

FIGURE 86.1 Correct placement of the cuff

Recording

On each occasion when the BP is taken, two or more readings should be averaged. Wait at least 30 seconds before repeating the procedure. If the first two readings differ by more than 6 mmHg systolic or 4 mmHg diastolic, more readings should be taken.

Both systolic and diastolic levels should be recorded. For the diastolic reading the disappearance of sound (Phase 5)—that is, the pressure when the last sound is heard and after which all sound disappears—should be used.[8] This is more accurate than the muffling of sounds (phase 4) (see FIG. 86.2), which should only be used if the sound continues to zero.

Heart rate and pulse

At the same time the BP is measured, the heart rate and rhythm should be measured and recorded. A high heart rate may indicate undue stress that is causing the associated elevated BP reading. An irregular heart rhythm may cause difficulty in obtaining an accurate BP reading.

BP modifying factors

Apprehension	Patient should be rested for at least 5 minutes and made as relaxed as possible.
Caffeine	Patients should not take caffeine for 4–6 hours before measurement.
Smoking	Patients should avoid smoking for 2 hours before measurement.
Eating	Patients should not have eaten for 30 minutes.

Strategies for high initial readings

If the initial reading is high (DBP >90 mmHg, SBP >140 mmHg) repeat the measures after 10 minutes of quiet rest. The 'white coat' influence in the medical practitioner's office may cause higher readings so measurement in other settings such as the home or the workplace should be managed whenever possible.

Confirmation and follow-up[1]

Repeated BP readings will determine whether initial high levels are confirmed and need attention, or whether they return to normal and need only periodic checking. Particular attention should be paid to younger patients to ensure that they are regularly followed up.

Initial diastolic BP readings of 115 mmHg or more, particularly for patients with target organ damage, may need immediate drug therapy.

Once an elevated level has been detected, the timing of subsequent readings should be based on the initial pressure level, as shown in TABLE 86.6.

If mild hypertension is found, observation with repeated measurement over 3–6 months should be followed before beginning therapy. This is because levels often return to normal.

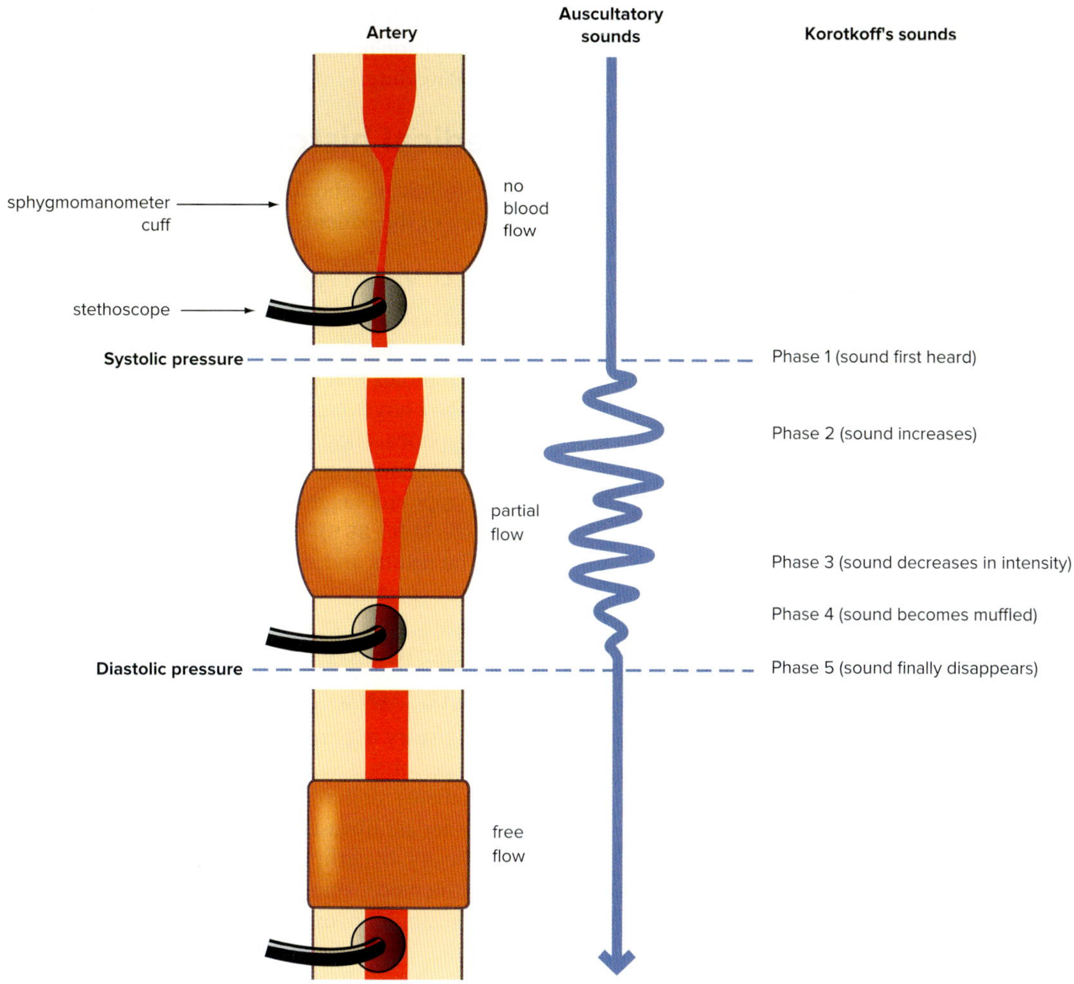

FIGURE 86.2 Illustration of blood pressure measurement in relation to arterial blood flow, cuff pressure and auscultation

Ambulatory 24-hour monitoring

This is required for the diagnosis and follow-up of patients with fluctuating levels, borderline hypertension or refractory hypertension (especially where the 'white coat' effect may be significant). Studies have shown that this method provides a more precise estimate of BP variability than casual recordings.

Guidelines for ambulatory BP measurement:

- unusual variability of office BP
- marked discrepancy between office and home BP
- resistance to drug treatment
- suspected sleep apnoea
- when two BP readings >140/90

'White coat' hypertension

This group may comprise up to 25% of patients presenting with hypertension. These people have a type of conditioned response to the clinic or office setting, yet their home BP and ambulatory BP profiles are normal. They appear to be at low risk of cardiovascular disease but may progress to sustained hypertension. Ambulatory 24-hour monitoring can be useful.

Masked hypertension

This is where office measurements are normal but ambulatory BP is elevated. Prognosis is relatively poor. Suspect it if evidence of end organ damage but normal office BP.

Table 86.6 Follow-up criteria for initial blood pressure measurement for adults 18 years and older[9]

Systolic (mmHg)	Diastolic (mmHg)	Action/recommended follow-up*
<120	<80	Recheck in 2 years
120–139	80–89	Recheck in 1 year—lifestyle advice
140–159	90–99	*Confirm within 2 months—lifestyle advice
160–179	100–109	*Evaluate (or refer) within 1 month—lifestyle advice
≥180	≥110	*Further evaluate and refer within 1 week (or immediately depending on clinical situation)
		If BP has been confirmed at ≥180 mm Hg systolic and/or ≥110 diastolic mmHg (after multiple readings and excluding 'white coat' hypertension), commence drug treatment

If systolic and diastolic categories are different, follow recommendations for shorter follow-up (e.g. for BP 160/86 mmHg evaluate or refer within 1 month).

**Note:* Earlier initiation of drug therapy may be indicated for some patients.

Isolated systolic hypertension

Isolated systolic hypertension is most frequently seen in elderly people. It is not benign.

> **Definition**
>
> SBP ≥140 mmHg with a DBP <90 mmHg

If a trial of non-pharmacological therapy fails, then drugs are used to cautiously reduce the systolic BP to between 140 and 160 mmHg.

Evaluation

As well as defining the BP problem, the clinical evaluation for suspected hypertension should also determine:

- whether the patient has potentially reversible secondary hypertension
- whether target organ damage is present
- whether there are other potentially modifiable cardiovascular risk factors present, and
- what comorbid factors exist

These factors markedly influence the weighing up of benefit versus risk when deciding whether to commence (or increase) antihypertensive medication. That decision needs to take into account more than just the BP reading.

Medical history

The following should be included in the medical history of the patient.

History of hypertension

- Method and date of initial diagnosis
- Known duration and levels of elevated BP
- Symptoms that may indicate the effects of high BP on target organ damage, such as headache, dyspnoea, chest pain, claudication, ankle oedema and haematuria
- Symptoms suggesting secondary hypertension (see TABLE 86.5)
- The results and side effects of all previous antihypertensive treatment

Presence of other diseases and risk factors

- A history of cardiovascular, cerebrovascular or peripheral vascular disease, kidney disease, diabetes mellitus or recent weight gain
- Other cardiovascular risk factors, including obesity, hyperlipidaemia, carbohydrate intolerance, smoking, salt intake, alcohol consumption, exercise levels and analgesic intake
- Other relevant conditions, such as asthma or psychiatric illness (particularly depressive illness)

Family history

Particular attention should be paid to the family history of hypertension, cardiovascular or cerebrovascular disease, hyperlipidaemia, obesity, diabetes mellitus, kidney disease, alcohol abuse and premature sudden death.

Medication history

A history of all medications, including over-the-counter products, should be obtained because some can raise BP or interfere with antihypertensive therapy. Prohypertensive substances include:

- alcohol
- oral and depot contraceptives
- hormone replacement therapy
- steroids/corticosteroids
- NSAIDs/COX–2 inhibitors
- sympathomimetics, nasal decongestants and other cold remedies, pseudoephedrine

86

- appetite suppressants
- stimulants, e.g. amphetamines
- irreversible monoamine oxidase inhibitors
- analgesics
- ergotamine
- cyclosporin
- tacrolimus
- natural liquorice
- bupropion/clozapine
- SNRIs, e.g. venlafaxine (dose-related)

Alcohol intake[1]

Alcohol has a direct pressor effect that is dose-related. An assessment of the average daily number of standard drinks is important—more than two standard drinks (20 g alcohol) a day is significant.

Examination

The approach to the physical examination is to detect possible target organ damage and possible causes of secondary hypertension. The main features to consider are illustrated in FIGURE 86.3.

The four grades of hypertensive retinopathy are illustrated in FIGURE 86.4.

Leg pulses and pressure

To assess the remote possibility of coarctation of the aorta in the hypertensive patient, perform at least one observation comparing:

1. the volume and timing of the radial and femoral pulses
2. the BP in the arm and leg
3. comparison of BP in the two arms

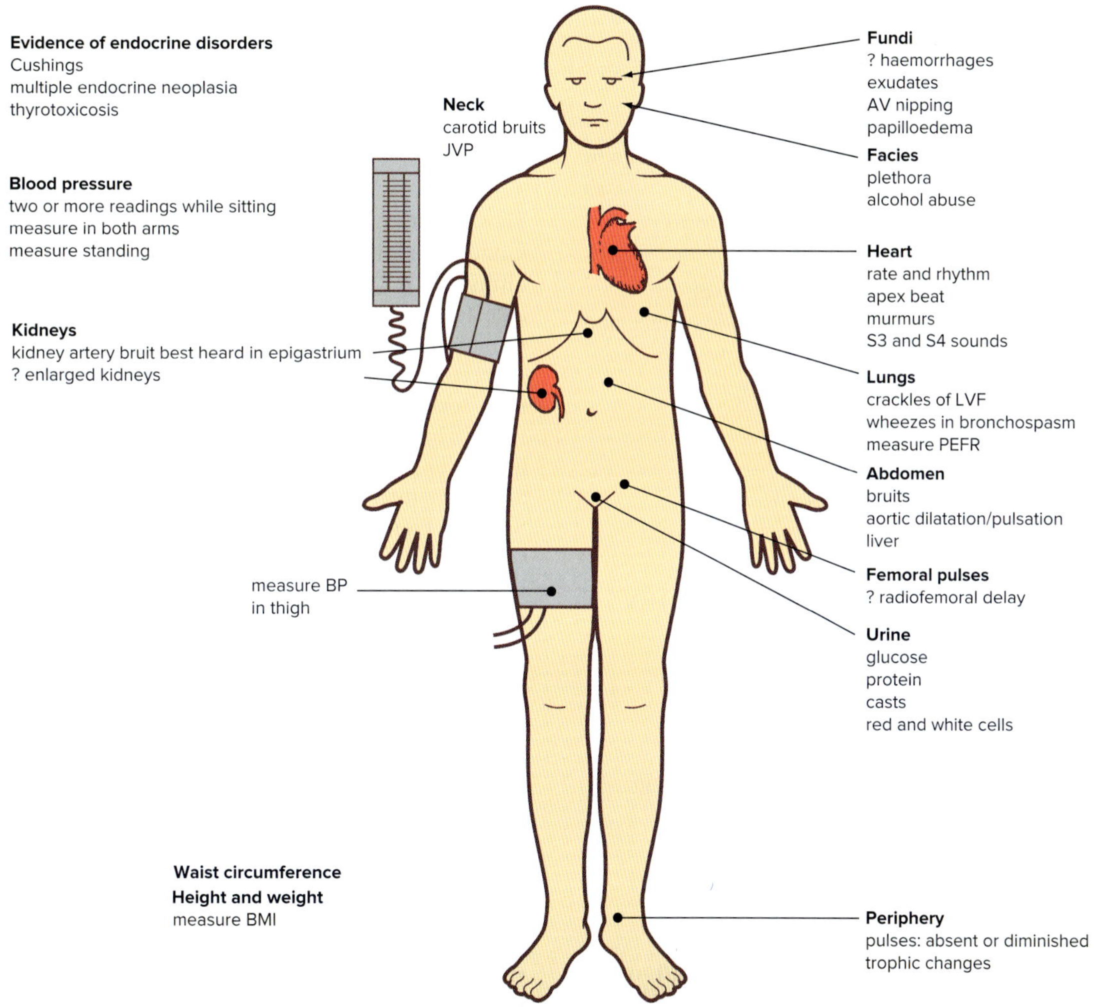

FIGURE 86.3 Examination of patient with hypertension: what to look for

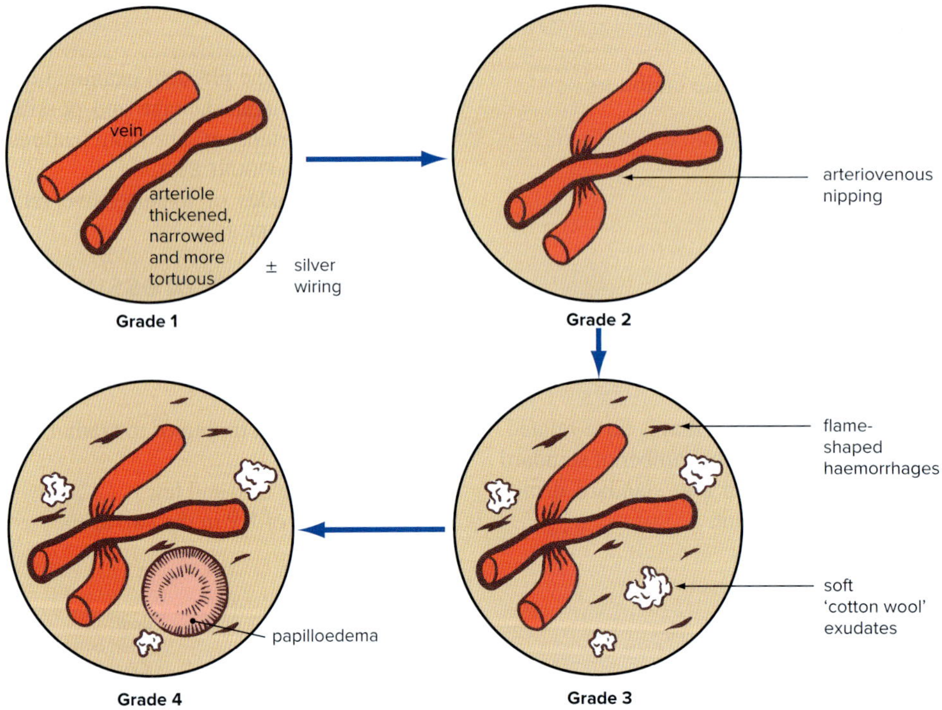

FIGURE 86.4 The four grades of hypertensive retinopathy

Blood pressure measurement in the leg

- Place the patient prone.
- Use a wide, long cuff at mid-thigh level.
- Position the bladder over the posterior surface and fix it firmly.
- Auscultate over the popliteal artery.

Investigations[3,5,7]

Recommended tests

- Chest X-ray
- Plasma glucose (preferably fasting)
- Serum total and high-density lipoprotein (HDL) cholesterol, fasting serum triglycerides
- Serum creatinine/eGFR/ACR
- Serum uric acid
- Serum potassium and sodium
- Haemoglobin and haematocrit
- Urinalysis (dipstick test and urinary sediment)
- Electrocardiogram

Other tests to consider

- Echocardiogram
- Carotid (and femoral) ultrasound
- HbA1c (when fasting glucose ≥6.1 mmol/L or 110 mg/dL)
- Fundoscopy (in severe hypertension)

These other investigations, including echocardiography, kidney imaging studies (especially kidney doppler ultrasound), 24-hour urinary catecholamines, aldosterone and plasma renin, are not routine and should be performed if specifically indicated (e.g. suspected primary hyperaldosteronism). A chest X-ray may serve as a baseline against which to measure future changes. However, if a chest X-ray shows the heart is enlarged, it is more likely to represent chamber dilatation than increased ventricular wall thickness.[1] Specific kidney studies now favoured include isotope scans, duplex ultrasound studies of kidney arteries and kidney arteriography.

Treatment

A correct diagnosis is the basis of management. Assuming that the uncommon secondary causes are identified and treated, treatment will focus on essential hypertension.

Benefits of treatment

Trials have shown that lowering BP reduces:

- cardiovascular and total mortality
- stroke
- coronary events

Benefits have been proven:

- in patients with systolic/diastolic hypertension
- in elderly patients with isolated systolic hypertension

Principles of management[3]

- The overall goal is to improve the long-term survival and quality of life.
- Promote an effective physician–patient working relationship.
- Aim to reduce the levels to 140/90 mmHg or less (ideal).
- Undertake a thorough assessment of all cardiovascular risk factors.
- Instruct all patients in the use of non-drug treatment strategies and their potential benefits. The benefits of exercise and healthy diet go far beyond what will be measurable by merely observing their effect on hypertension.
- In patients with mild-to-moderate hypertension and no target organ damage, consider ambulatory or home BP monitoring before deciding to start medication.
- Drug therapy should be given to those with:
  - sustained high initial readings (e.g. DBP 100 mmHg)
  - target organ damage
  - failed non-drug measures
- Make a careful selection of an antihypertensive drug and an appraisal of the side effects against the benefits of treatment.
- Avoid drug-related problems such as postural hypotension.
- Avoid excessive lowering of BP—aim for steady and graduated control.
- Aim to counter the problem of patient non-compliance.
- Be aware of factors that may contribute to drug resistance.

Patient education

Patient education should include appropriate reassurances, clear information and easy-to-follow instructions. It is important to establish patients' understanding of the concept of hypertension and its consequences by quizzing them about their knowledge and feelings.

Correction of patients' misconceptions[1]

Patients are likely to have several misconceptions about hypertension that may adversely affect their treatment. For example, they might believe that:

- hypertension can be cured
- they do not need to continue treatment once BP is controlled
- they do not have a problem because they do not have symptoms
- they need to take additional pills, or stop treatment in response to symptoms they believe are caused by high or low BP levels
- they need not take prescribed pills if they attend to lifestyle factors such as exercise and diet
- they can gauge their BP by how they feel

Tips for optimal compliance

- Establish a good, caring rapport.
- Give advice about pill-taking times.
- Set therapeutic goals.
- Establish a recall system.
- Provide patient education material.

On review:

- Ask if any pills were missed by accident.
- Attempt to reduce waiting time to a minimum (e.g. direct a patient to a spare room on arrival).
- Review all cardiovascular risk factors.
- Enquire about any side effects.

Non-pharmacological (lifestyle) management measures

If the average diastolic BP at the initial visit is 90–100 mmHg, and there is no evidence of end organ damage, non-pharmacological therapy is indicated for a 3-month period without use of antihypertensive drugs. Remember to remove, revise or substitute drugs that may be causing hypertension (e.g. NSAIDs, corticosteroids, oral contraceptives, hormone replacement therapy).

Behaviour intervention measures

- *Weight reduction*
  There is considerable evidence that weight loss and gain are linked to a corresponding fall and rise in BP. Hovell has estimated that for every 1 kg of weight lost, BP dropped by 2.5 mmHg systolic and 1.5 mmHg diastolic.[10] The BMI should be calculated for all patients and where appropriate a weight loss program organised to target waist measurement to <94 in males and <80 in females or reduce the BMI to around 25.
- *Reduction of excessive alcohol intake*[1]
  The direct pressor effect of alcohol is reversible. Drinking more than 20 g of alcohol a day raises BP and makes treatment of established

hypertension more difficult. People with hypertension should limit their alcohol intake to one or two standard drinks (10–20 g) per day. Reduction or withdrawal of regular alcohol intake reduces BP by 5–10 mmHg.

- *Reduction of sodium intake to ≤4 g/day*
  Some individuals seem to be more sensitive to salt restriction. Advise patients to put away the salt shaker and use only a little salt with their food. Reduction of sodium intake to less than 100 mmol sodium per day is advised. Special care should be taken with processed and take-away foods.
- *Increased exercise and regular physical activity*
  Regular aerobic or isotonic exercise helps to reduce BP.[9] Hypertensive patients beginning an exercise program should do so gradually. Walking is an appropriate exercise, ideally 150–300 minutes each week.
- *Reduction of particular stress*
  If avoiding stress or overwork is difficult, recommend relaxation and/or meditation therapy.
- *Other dietary factors for a healthy eating plan*
  There is evidence that lacto–vegetarian diets and diets high in vegetables, fruits and whole grains can reduce BP.[3] A diet high in calcium, and low in fat and caffeine, may also be beneficial. Avoid or minimise liquorice.
- *Smoking*
  Smoking causes acute rises in BP but does not appear to cause sustained hypertension. However, the elimination of smoking is important as it is a strong risk factor for cardiovascular disease and continuing to smoke may negate any cardiovascular benefits of antihypertensive therapy.[1]
- *Management of sleep apnoea*
  A 2014 systematic review found that CPAP reduces BP in those with obstructive sleep apnoea and hypertension, although only by a small amount (2–3 mmHg).[11]

Pharmacological therapy

The benefits of drug therapy appear to outweigh any known risks to individuals with a persistently raised diastolic pressure >95 mmHg. Although the ideal antihypertensive drug has yet to be discovered, there are many effective drugs available from all the major classes of antihypertensive drugs.[12] Deciding which one to use first involves an assessment of the patient's general health, the medication's known side effects, the simplicity of its administration and its cost. A useful plan is outlined in FIGURE 86.5.

Various disorders such as diabetes, asthma, COPD, Raynaud phenomenon, heart failure, and elevated serum urate and/or lipid levels may restrict the use of some classes of drugs.

When to treat

- Failed genuine non-pharmacological trial
- For those with >10% 5-year CV risk, treat if SBP >140 mmHg or DBP >90 mmHg
- For those with <10% 5-year CV risk, treat if SBP >160 mmHg or DBP >100 mmHg (see TABLE 86.7)

Guidelines[13]

- Start with a single drug at low dose.
- A period of 4–6 weeks is needed for the effect to become fully apparent.
- If ineffective, consider increasing the drug to its maximum recommended dose, or add an agent from another compatible class, or substitute with a drug from another class.
- Use only one drug from any one class at the same time.
- A summary of first-line therapy options and the uses of the various pharmacological agents is shown in TABLE 86.8.
- Measure the BP at the same time each day.
- Consider asking patients to self-measure.
- Patients commonly require two or more agents to reach BP targets.

Starting regimens

In patients with uncomplicated hypertension, ACE inhibitors or ARBs, calcium channel blockers and thiazides are all suitable first-line antihypertensive drugs, either as monotherapy or in some combinations unless contraindicated.

Table 86.7 BP treatment targets for adults (mm Hg)[3,13]

People with proteinuria >1 g/day (with or without diabetes)	<125/75
People with associated condition(s) or end-organ damage: • coronary heart disease • diabetes • chronic kidney disease • proteinuria (>300 mg/day) • stroke/TIA	<130/80
People with none of the above	<140/90 or lower if tolerated

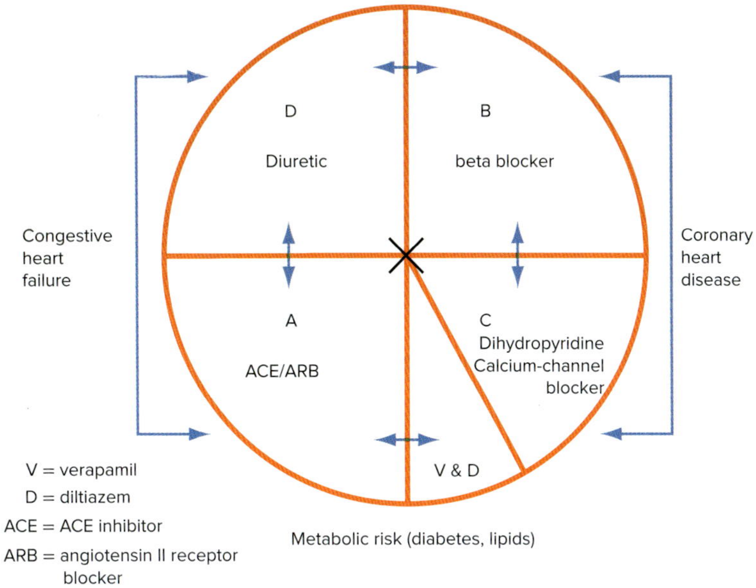

FIGURE 86.5 Common combinations of the therapeutic drug classes used for first-line therapy of hypertension

- Adjacent drug classes are useful combinations in that effects on BP are additive but adverse effects are no more likely than with either drug used alone.
- Non-dihydropyridine CCBs: verapamil (V) and diltiazem (D) generally should not be used with β_2-antagonists (beta blockers).
- Drug groups that are diametrically located on the diagram may be used together, but may not have fully additive effects.
- Drugs on the left side should be combined in patients with hypertension and heart failure, and those on the right side are useful in patients with hypertension and coexisting coronary disease.
- Drug groups in the lower half lack metabolic effects and may be preferred combinations in the presence of diabetes or lipid abnormalities as well as hypertension.
- Do not combine ACE with ARB (increased side effects for little benefit).
- β_2-antagonists are not routine first-line treatment unless they will also be useful for a coexisting condition.
- Prazosin and other α-antagonists are also sometimes used as monotherapy and may be combined with any of the above drug groups.
- Small doses of centrally acting anti-adrenergic drugs (e.g. methyldopa, clonidine) can probably also be used with any of the other agents although data on their use in combination are scarce with the newer drug groups.

Source: Adapted from Management of hypertension: a consensus statement, Med J Aust, 1994, 160: Supplement 21 March.

The traditional method has been to use stepwise therapy until ideal control has been reached, commencing with:

Starting medication

1. ACE inhibitor or ARB especially if ≥55 years
   or
   calcium channel blocker (CCB)
   or
   low-dose thiazide diuretic
   (if aged ≥65 years)
2. If target not reached after 3 months: combination
   ACEI or ARB + CCB (best evidence)[14]
   or
   ACEI or ARB + thiazide
   or
   ACEI or ARB + beta blocker
3. If target not reached:
   ACEI/ARB + CCB + thiazide
4. If still not reached use spironolactone or seek specialist advice

Table 86.8 First-line pharmacological options for the management of hypertension[3,13,16] (standard doses)

Drug class				
Thiazide diuretic	Beta blocker	Calcium channel blocker	ACE inhibitor	ARB (sartans)
Typical examples and starting dose (oral therapy)				
Chlorthalidone 12.5–25 mg daily Hydrochlorothiazide 12.5 mg daily Indapamide(SR) 1.5 mg daily Indapamide 1.25–2.5 mg daily	Atenolol 25–50 mg daily Metoprolol 50 mg daily Pindolol 5 mg daily Propranolol 40 mg daily	*Dihydropyridine CCBs* Amlodipine 2.5 mg daily Felodipine SR 2.5 mg daily Lercanidipine 10 mg daily Nifedipine CR 20 mg daily *Non-dihydropyridine* Diltiazem CD 180 mg daily Verapamil SR 120–180 mg daily	Captopril 6.25 mg bd Enalapril 5 mg daily Lisinopril 5 mg daily Perindopril 2.5 mg daily Ramipril 2.5 mg daily Fosinopril 10 mg daily Quinapril 5 mg daily Trandolapril 1 mg daily	Candesartan 8 mg daily Eprosartan 600 mg daily Irbesartan 150 mg daily Losartan 50 mg daily Olmesartan 10 mg daily Telmisartan 40 mg daily Valsartan 80 mg daily
Recommended in				
Heart failure (mild) Older patients	Pregnancy Glaucoma Stable angina Postmyocardial infarction Migraine	Asthma Stable angina PVD Raynaud phenomenon	Left ventricular heart failure PVD Diabetes Raynaud Post AMI	Left ventricular heart failure Diabetes PVD ACEI-induced cough Post AMI
Contraindications				
Type 2 diabetes Hyperuricaemia/gout Kidney failure	Asthma/COPD History of wheeze Heart failure Heart block (2nd and 3rd degree) PVD Brittle type I diabetes	Heart block 2nd and 3rd degree Heart failure (verapamil, diltiazem) Tachyarrhythmias	Bilateral kidney artery stenosis Pregnancy Hyperkalaemia Angioedema	Pregnancy Severe kidney failure Hyperkalaemia
Precautions				
Hypokalaemia Thiazides + ACE inhibitors Kidney failure	Avoid abrupt cessation with angina Caution using with verapamil, NSAIDs and in smokers	Caution using with beta blockers, digoxin and in CCF	Chronic kidney disease Caution using with K-sparing diuretics and NSAIDs	Electrolyte imbalance Renal impairment Hepatic impairment
Important side effects				
Rashes Sexual dysfunction Weakness Blood dyscrasias Muscular cramps Hypokalaemia Hyponatraemia Hyperuricaemia Hyperglycaemia Lipid metabolism effect	Fatigue Insomnia Vivid dreams Bronchospasm Cold extremities Sexual dysfunction Lipid metabolism effect	Headache Flushing Ankle oedema Palpitations Dizziness Nausea Constipation (verapamil) Nocturia, urinary frequency Gum hyperplasia	Cough Weakness Rash Dysgeusia (taste) Hyperkalaemia First dose hypotension Angioedema	Headache Dizziness Orthostatic hypotension Fatigue Weakness Hyperkalaemia Allergies Angle closure glaucoma

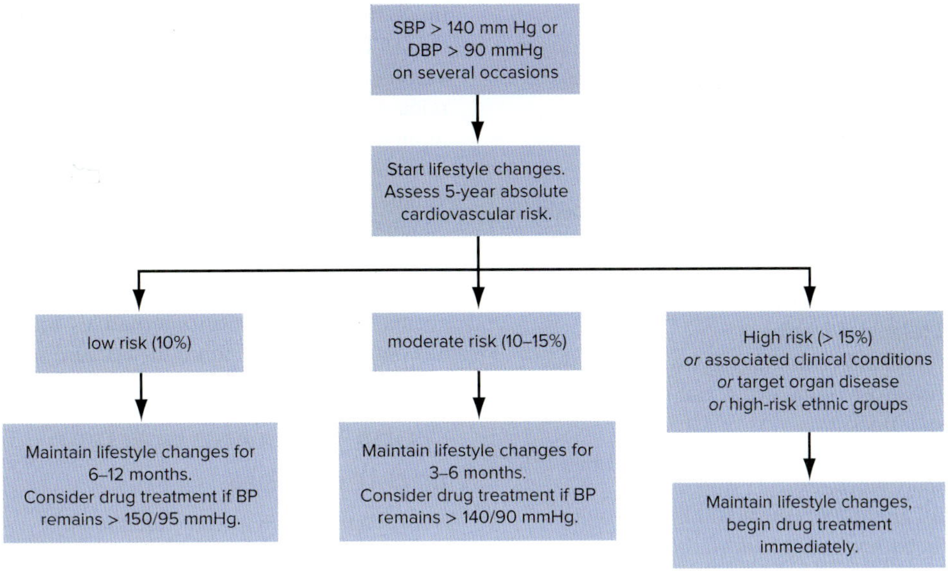

FIGURE 86.6 Decision tree for managing hypertension[2]

As recommended by the National Heart Foundation (updated December 2010)

The following are useful combinations:[9,15]

Initial agent	Additional drugs
Thiazide diuretic	ACEI/ARB *or* CCB *or* beta blocker
Beta blocker	Diuretic *or* dihydropyridine calcium channel blocker
ACE inhibitor or ARB	Diuretic *or* beta blocker *or* calcium channel blocker

Relatively ineffective combinations[9]

- Diuretic and calcium channel blocker
- Beta blockers and ACE inhibitors

Undesirable combinations[9,13]

- More than one drug from a particular pharmacological group:
  - beta blockers and verapamil (heart block, heart failure)
  - potassium-sparing diuretics and ACE inhibitors or ARB (hyperkalaemia)
  - ACEI and ARB

Diuretics[9,16]

- Thiazides are good first-line therapy for hypertension.
- Hypokalaemia can be corrected with potassium-sparing diuretics or by changing to another first-line drug.
- Loop diuretics are less potent as antihypertensive agents but are indicated where there is concomitant cardiac or kidney failure and in resistant hypertension.
- Thiazides are less effective where there is kidney impairment.
- Thiazides may precipitate acute gout.
- NSAIDs may antagonise the antihypertensive and natriuretic effectiveness of diuretics.
- A diet high in potassium and magnesium should accompany diuretic therapy (e.g. lentils, nuts, high fibre).
- Avoid use if significant dyslipidaemia.
- Indapamide has different properties to the thiazide and loop diuretics and has less effect on serum lipids.

Beta blockers

- NSAIDs may interfere with the hypotensive effect of beta blockers.
- If BP is not reduced by one beta blocker it is unlikely to be reduced by changing to another.
- Verapamil plus a beta blocker may unmask conduction abnormalities causing heart block.

- In patients with ischaemic heart disease, or susceptibility to it, treatment must not be stopped suddenly—this can precipitate angina at rest.

Calcium channel blockers

- These drugs reduce BP by vasodilatation.
- The properties of individual drugs vary, especially their effects on cardiac function.
- The dihydropyridine compounds (nifedipine and felodipine) tend to produce more vasodilatation and thus related side effects.
- Unlike verapamil or diltiazem (which slow the heart), dihydropyridine drugs can be used safely with a beta blocker.
- Verapamil is contraindicated in second and third degree heart block.
- Verapamil and diltiazem should be used with caution in patients with heart failure.
- These drugs are efficacious with ACE inhibitors, beta blockers, prazosin and methyldopa.

ACE inhibitors

Angiotensin-converting enzyme (ACE) is responsible for converting angiotensin I to angiotensin II (a potent vasoconstrictor and stimulator of aldosterone secretion) and for the breakdown of bradykinin (a vasodilator). ACE inhibitors are effective in the elderly; improve survival and performance status in cardiac failure; are protective of kidney function in diabetes; and are cardioprotective after myocardial infarction.

Disturbance in taste is usually transitory and may resolve with continued treatment. Cough, which occurs in about 15% of patients, may disappear with time or a reduction in dose but it often persists and requires a change in drug in some patients. Angioedema, a potentially life-threatening condition, may occur in 0.1–0.2% of subjects. Like cough, it is a class effect and will mitigate against use of any ACE inhibitor in patients with such an adverse effect. The Heart Outcomes Prevention Evaluation (HOPE)[17] trial demonstrated that the ACE inhibitor ramipril reduces the number of cardiovascular deaths, non-fatal myocardial infarctions, non-fatal strokes and instances of new onset heart failure in a high-risk population. The data also indicated that all diabetic patients with microalbuminuria or pre-existing vascular disease will benefit from ACE I treatment, even if normotensive.[15,17]

Angiotensin II receptor antagonists (sartans)

These agents competitively block the binding of angiotensin II to type I angiotensin receptors and block the effects of angiotensin more selectively than the ACE inhibitors. This reduces angiotensin-induced vasoconstriction, sodium reabsorption and aldosterone release. The action of the ACEIs and ARBs on the renin–angiotensin–aldosterone pathway system is illustrated in FIGURE 86.7. They have a similar adverse kidney and other effects to the ACE inhibitors but cough does not appear to be a significant adverse effect. This group is used for mild-to-moderate hypertension alone or with other antihypertensive agents. They are useful alternatives for patients who discontinue an ACE inhibitor because of cough. They may be used in combination with thiazide diuretics.

Alpha blockers: prazosin and terazosin

Not recommended as first-line therapy.

A specific problem of alpha blockers is the 'first-dose phenomenon'; this involves acute syncope about 90 minutes after the first dose, hence treatment is best initiated at bedtime. Prazosin potentiates beta blockers and works best if used with them. It is a useful second-line therapy in patients who are unsuitable for diuretic or beta blocker therapy (e.g. those with diabetes, asthma or hyperlipidaemia).

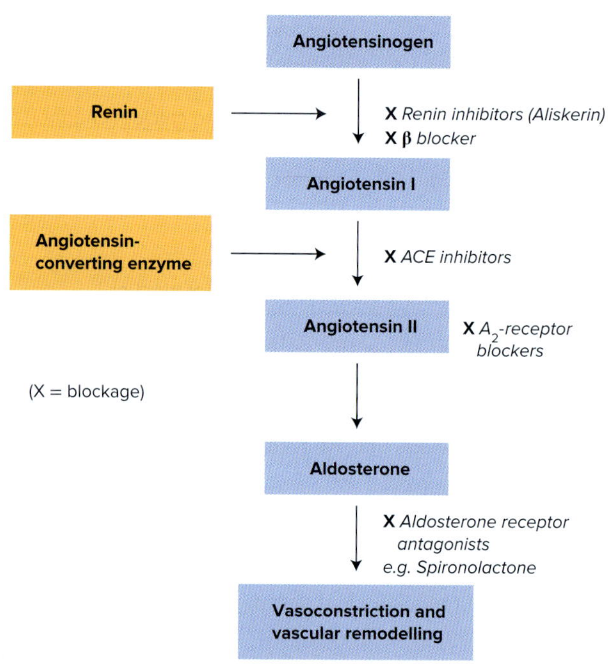

FIGURE 86.7 Drugs targeting the renin–angiotensin–aldosterone system

Vascular smooth muscle relaxants

Other than calcium channel blockers these include hydralazine, minoxidil and diazoxide, which are not used for first-line therapy but for refractory hypertensive states and hypertensive emergencies.

Sympathetic nervous system inhibitors

A newer class of antihypertensive agents has been developed to reduce peripheral sympathetic activity by inhibiting the sympathetic nervous system. Methyldopa and clonidine may be used during pregnancy.

Hypertensive emergencies[13]

A hypertensive emergency occurs when high BP causes the presenting cardiovascular problem. Typical presentations of hypertensive emergencies (which are rare) include hypertensive encephalopathy, acute stroke, heart failure, dissecting aortic aneurysm and eclampsia. Symptomatically patients may present with headache and confusion.

In all such cases referral to an emergency department is essential and the patient should be hospitalised immediately for monitoring and treatment. Treatment must be individualised, mindful of the nature of the underlying problem and associated disorders.

The BP lowering must be gradual because a sudden fall can precipitate a stroke. Aim to reduce the BP by no more than 25% within the first 2 hours then towards 160/100 mmHg within 2 to 6 hours.[13]

Treatment is with a dihydropyridine CCB and/or an ACE inhibitor. Otherwise, sodium nitroprusside IV in an intensive care setting is the optimal treatment.

Magnesium sulphate reduces the risk of eclampsia and maternal death in women with pre-eclampsia (see CHAPTER 108).

Refractory hypertension

Refractory hypertension exists where control has not been achieved despite reasonable treatment for 3–4 months. A review of a possible secondary causes is appropriate. Consider non-compliance, sleep apnoea, hypertensive effects of other drugs, undisclosed use of alcohol and recreational drugs, and also spurious factors (e.g. instrument factors such as small cuff, 'white coat' hypertension).

When adequate control is not possible and the cause is not obvious, the patient should be referred to a specialist. Measurement outside the clinic may help in the assessment of such people, as may 24-hour ambulatory monitoring.

Hypertension in children and adolescents

BP is less frequently measured in children for a number of reasons, including the lower chances of finding any abnormality, the unavailability of an appropriately sized cuff or difficulty in measuring BP in the infant or toddler.

The children of parents with hypertension should be closely watched. Those at risk of secondary hypertension (e.g. kidney or cardiovascular disease, urological abnormalities and diabetes mellitus) should have routine measurements. Children with visual changes, recurrent headache or abdominal pain, seizures, and those on drugs such as corticosteroids or oral contraceptives, should have their BP checked regularly.

Although secondary causes of hypertension are proportionally more common in children than in adults, young people are still more prone to developing essential rather than secondary hypertension. Kidney parenchymal disease and kidney artery stenosis are the major secondary causes.

The upper limits of normal BP for children in different age groups are:[1]

Age (in years)	Arterial pressure (mmHg)
5 or less	110/75
6–9	120/80
10–13	125/85
14–18	135/90

The proper cuff size is very important to avoid inaccurate readings and a larger rather than a smaller cuff is recommended. The width of the bladder should cover 75% of the upper arm. In infants and toddlers, use of an electronic unit may be necessary. Although cessation of sound (phase 5) is the better reflection of true diastolic pressure, there is often no disappearance of sound in children and so estimation of the point of muffling (phase 4) is recorded instead.

Diagnostic evaluation and drug treatment for children are similar to those for adults. Strongly consider specialist referral. When a child is obese, reduction in weight may adequately lower BP. ACE inhibitors or calcium channel blocking agents are preferable in the young hypertensive, with diuretics a second agent. ACE inhibitors should be avoided in postpubertal girls.

Hypertension in the elderly

BP shows a gradual increasing linear relationship with age.

86

Guidelines for treatment

- Isolated systolic hypertension is worth treating.[18]
- Older patients may respond to non-pharmacological treatment.
- Reducing dietary sodium is more beneficial than with younger patients.
- If drug treatment is necessary, commence with half the normal recommended adult dosage—'start low and go slow'.
- Patients over 75 years and in good health should be treated the same as younger patients. Studies indicate that benefits are still significant. However, weigh this against the fact that harms (e.g. falls risk) may be greater.
- A gradual reduction in BP is recommended.
- Drug reactions are a limiting factor.
- Drug interactions are also a problem: these include NSAIDs, antiparkinson drugs and phenothiazines.

Specific treatment

- *First-line choice:* indapamide (preferred) or thiazide diuretic (low dose);[1] check electrolytes in 2–4 weeks: if hypokalaemia develops add a K-sparing diuretic rather than K supplements. Diuretics may aggravate bladder difficulties (e.g. incontinence).
- *Second-line choice:* ACE (or ARB) inhibitors (especially with heart failure)

Other effective drugs (especially for isolated systolic hypertension):

- beta blockers (low dose) where diuretic cannot be prescribed or if angina
- calcium channel blockers

Both these groups are generally well tolerated but constipation may be a problem with verapamil.

Kidney function and electrolytes should be monitored when ACE inhibitors are started.

Special management problems

These conditions are summarised in TABLE 86.9.

Step-down treatment of mild hypertension[9]

This is an important concept that recognises that drug treatment need not necessarily be lifelong. If BP has been well controlled for several months to years it is often worth reducing the dosage or the number of drugs.

Table 86.9 Choice of drugs in patients with coexisting conditions[1]

	Diuretic	ACE inhibitors ARBs	Calcium channel blockers	Beta blockers
Asthma/COPD	✓	✓	✓	✗ Caution
Bowel disease/constipation	✗	✓	✗	✗
Bradycardia/heart block	✓	✓	Care	✗
Cardiac failure	✓*	✓*	Care	✗
Depression	✓	✓	✓ Care	✗
Diabetes	✗	✓*	✓	✗ Care
Dyslipidaemia	✗	✓	✓	✗
Hyperuricaemia/gout	✗	✓*	✓*	✗
Impotence	✗	✓	✓	✗
Ischaemic heart disease	✓	✓	✓*	✓*
Peripheral vascular disease	✓	✓	✓*	✗
Pregnancy	✗	✗	✓	✓ Not in late term
Raynaud phenomenon	✓	✓	✓*	✗
Kidney artery stenosis	✓	✗	✓* Care	✓* Care
Kidney failure	✓	Care	✓	✓
Tachycardia (resting)	✗	✗	Care	✓*

*Drugs of choice
Calcium channel blockers need to be selected with care—some are suitable, others not.

The general 'deprescribing' rule of thumb is that a drug (or its specific dosage) should only be continued if the expected benefits justify its continuation.

A 'drug holiday' (cessation of treatment) can be hazardous, however, because satisfactory control may be temporary and hypertension will re-emerge. Careful monitoring under such circumstances is mandatory.

When to refer

- Refractory hypertension—adequate control not possible and cause not obvious
- Suspected 'white coat' hypertension—for ambulatory BP monitoring
- Severe hypertension—diastolic BP >115 mmHg
- Hypertensive emergency
- Evidence of ongoing target organ impairment and BP inadequately controlled
- Significant kidney impairment eGFR <30 mL/min
- A treatable cause of secondary hypertension is found

Practice tips

- Hypertension should not be diagnosed on a single reading.
- At least two follow-up measurements with average systolic pressure >140 mmHg or diastolic pressures >90 mmHg are required for the diagnosis.
- Beware of using beta blockers in a patient with a history of wheezing.
- Add only one agent at a time and wait about 4 weeks between dosage adjustments.
- Excessive intake of alcohol can cause hypertension and make treatment difficult.
- If hypertension fails to respond to therapy, an underlying kidney or adrenal lesion may have been missed.
- The low-pitched bruits of kidney artery stenosis are best heard by placing the diaphragm of the stethoscope firmly in the epigastric area.
- Older patients may respond better to diuretics, calcium channel blockers and ACE inhibitors.
- Younger patients may respond better to beta blockers or ACE inhibitors.

Patient education resources

Hand-out sheets from *Murtagh's Patient Education* 7th edition:

- Hypertension

References

1. Sandler G. High blood pressure. In: *Common Medical Problems.* London: Adis Press, 1984: 61–106.
2. Nichols M et al. Australian heart disease statistics 2015. Melbourne: National Heart Foundation, 2016.
3. National Heart Foundation of Australia. Guideline for the diagnosis and management of hypertension in adults 2016. Melbourne: National Heart Foundation of Australia, 2016. Available from: <www.heartfoundation.org.au/for-professionals/clinical-information/hypertension>, accessed April 2018.
4. Practice guidelines for primary care physicians: 2003 ESH/ESC Hypertension Guidelines. J Hypertens, 2003; 21(10): 1779–86.
5. Guidelines Subcommittee 1999. WHO–ISH guidelines for the management of hypertension. J Hypertens, 1999; 17: 151–83.
6. National Vascular Disease Prevention Alliance. Guidelines for the management of absolute cardiovascular disease risk 2012. National Stroke Foundation, 2012: 6–7. Available from: <www.heartfoundation.org.au/images/uploads/publications/Absolute-CVD-Risk-Full-Guidelines.pdf>, accessed April 2018.
7. Royal Australian College of General Practitioners. *Guidelines for Preventive Activities in General Practice* (9th edn). Melbourne: RACGP, 2016: 87–9.
8. Bates B. *A Guide to Physical Examination and History Taking* (5th edn). Philadelphia: Lippincott, 1991: 284.
9. National Heart Foundation of Australia. *Guide to Management of Hypertension.* Canberra: National Heart Foundation of Australia, 2008 (updated 2014).
10. Hovell MF. The experimental evidence for weight loss treatment of essential hypertension: a critical review. Am J Public Health, 1982; April 72(4): 359–68.
11. Fava C et al. Effect of CPAP on blood pressure in patients with OSA/hypopnea. Chest, 2014; 145(4): 762.
12. Jennings G, Sudhir K. Initial therapy of primary hypertension. Med J Aust, 1990; 152: 198–202.
13. Expert group for Cardiovascular guidelines. Hypertension. In: eTG complete. Melbourne: Therapeutic Guidelines Ltd, 2015. Available from: <www.tg.org.au>, accessed September 2017.
14. Law MR, Morris JK, Wald NJ. Use of blood pressure lowering drugs in prevention of cardiovascular disease: meta analysis of 147 randomised trials in the context of expectations from prospective epidemiological studies. BMJ, 2009 May 19; 338: b1665.
15. Kjeldsen SE, Jamerson KA, Bakris GL et al. **A**voiding **C**ardiovascular events through **COM**bination therapy in **P**atients **LI**ving with **S**ystolic **H**ypertension investigators. Predictors of blood pressure response to intensified and fixed combination treatment of hypertension: the ACCOMPLISH study. Blood Press, 2008; 17: 7–17.
16. Buckley N (Chair). *Australian Medicines Handbook.* Adelaide: Australian Medicines Handbook Pty Ltd, 2017: 241–3.
17. Yusef S et al. Effects of an angiotensin-converting inhibitor, ramipril, on cardiovascular events in high risk patients. The Heart Outcomes Prevention Evaluation Investigations. N Engl J Med, 2000; 342: 145.
18. SHEP Cooperative Research Group. Prevention of stroke by antihypertensive drug treatment in older persons with isolated systolic hypertension. JAMA, 1991; 265: 3255–64.
19. Wright JT et al. Systolic Blood Pressure Intervention Trial (SPRINT). Hypertension 68(2): 318–23.

87 Dyslipidaemia

The landmark Scandinavian Simvastatin Survival Study (4S) published in 1994, may well be remembered as the study that finally put to rest many of the apprehensions and misconceptions regarding lipid-lowering therapy.

DUFFY AND MEREDITH 1996[1]

Dyslipidaemia is the presence of an abnormal lipid/lipoprotein profile in the serum and can be classified as:

- predominant hypertriglyceridaemia
- predominant hypercholesterolaemia
- mixed pattern with elevation of both cholesterol and triglyceride (TG)

Modern epidemiological studies have established the facts that elevated plasma cholesterol causes pathological changes in the arterial wall leading to CAD, and that lipid-lowering therapy results in reduction of coronary and cerebrovascular events with improved survival.

A Cochrane systematic review[2] of 18 large RCTs found high quality evidence that statins reduce all-cause mortality and major vascular events. The number needed to treat (NNT) with statins varies markedly depending on the risk category the person falls into (see TABLE 87.1).

The main focus of treatment will be on primary dyslipidaemia but secondary causes (see TABLE 87.2) also need to be addressed. LDL-C is the lipid with the highest correlation with CHD and its level remains the primary target of lipid modifying therapy. The statins are the first-line therapy for a raised level. Like total cholesterol measurement, LDL-C should not be used in isolation.

Table 87.1 Number needed to treat (NNT) with a statin for 1 year to prevent 1 death[2]

Risk level	NNT
<5% five-year CV risk	835
5–10% five-year CV risk	335
Previous cardiovascular event—high risk[3]	165

Established facts[4,5,6]

- Major risk factors for CAD include:
  - increased LDL cholesterol + reduced HDL cholesterol
  - ratio LDL-C:HDL-C >4

Table 87.2 Common causes of secondary dyslipidaemia

Hypothyroidism
Nephrotic syndrome
Type 2 diabetes
Cholestasis
Anorexia nervosa
Obesity
Kidney impairment
Smoking
Alcohol excess
Oestrogen therapy
Obstructive liver disease

- Risk increases with increasing cholesterol levels
- TG level >10 mmol/L increases risk of pancreatitis
- Management should be correlated with risk factors
- 10% reduction of total cholesterol gives 20% reduction in CAD after 3 years
- LDL-C reduction with statin therapy reduces heart attacks, stroke, the need for revascularisation and death
- Screening is recommended 5 yearly from age 45 years (Aboriginal and Torres Strait Islander people from 35 years)

Investigations[5]

The following fasting tests are recommended in patients every 5 years, starting at age 45 years:

- serum cholesterol level, HDL-C, LDL-C and triglyceride (TG)

Confirm an initial high result with a second test at 6–8 weeks. Those at moderate risk (5-year CV risk >10%) should have a screening test every two years. Commence testing at 35 years of age if Aboriginal or Torres Strait Islander.

All patients should receive advice and support regarding lifestyle risk management. Patients requiring pharmacological treatment are summarised in TABLE 87.3.

Table 87.3 Patients requiring treatment (PBS guidelines)[4]

Risk category	Initiate drug therapy if lipid level (mmol/L) is
Patients with existing symptomatic coronary heart disease, peripheral vascular disease and cerebrovascular disease. Patients with diabetes plus one of microalbuminuria; age >60; Aboriginal or Torres Strait Islander Family history of coronary heart disease (one first-degree relative <45 years of age, or two <55 years)	Any level
Aboriginal and Torres Strait Islander patients with hypertension Family history of coronary heart disease (one first-degree relative <60 years of age, or one second-degree relative <50 years)	Cholesterol >6.5 mmol/L *or* Cholesterol >5.5 mmol/L *and* HDL <1 mmol/L
Patients with HDL <1 mmol/L	Cholesterol >6.5 mmol/L
Patients not eligible under the above: • men 35–75 years • postmenopausal women up to 75 years	Cholesterol >7.5 mmol/L *or* Triglyceride >4 mmol/L
Patients not otherwise included in the above	Cholesterol >9 mmol/L *or* Triglyceride >8 mmol/L

Recommended treatment goals[7]

- Total cholesterol <4.0 mmol/L
- LDL-C <2.0 mmol/L*
- HDL-C ≥1.0 mmol/L
- non-HDL-C <2.5 mmol/L
- TG <2 mmol/L

NVDPA guidelines[7] note there appears to be no major difference between dose titration regimens or use of a fixed dose in studies of longer duration. The majority of benefit from statins results at the lower doses, with less added benefit as doses are increased towards maximum. Therefore treatment should aim towards these targets rather than consider them definitive.

Non-pharmacological measures[6]

- Dietary measures:
  - keep to ideal weight (as for cardiovascular disease, see CHAPTER 85)
  - reduce saturated and trans fat intake, especially dairy products and meat
  - avoid fast foods and deep-fried foods
  - replace saturated fats with mono or polyunsaturated fats
  - use approved cooking methods (e.g. steaming, grilling)
  - trim fat off meat, remove skin from chicken
  - avoid biscuits and cakes between meals
  - high-fibre diet, especially fruit and vegetables (to increase soluble fibre)
  - introduce plant sterol-enriched milk, margarine or cheeses
  - alcohol intake 0–2 standard drinks/day
  - drink more water
- Encourage physical activity: regular exercise program
- Cease smoking
- Cooperation of family is essential
- Exclude secondary causes (e.g. kidney disease, type 2 diabetes, hypothyroidism, obesity, alcohol excess—especially ↑ TG), specific diuretics

Checkpoints

- Diet therapy effective (TG ↓, LDL-C ↓) within 6–8 weeks
- Continue at least 6 months before considering drug therapy in all but the highest-risk category

Pharmacological measures

The choice of the lipid-lowering agent depends on the pattern of the lipid disorder.[5,6] See TABLE 87.4. Use the following agents in addition to diet.

Treatment should commence with a statin. If LDL-C levels are not reduced to target levels or a maximally tolerated dose on a statin, add one of ezetimibe,[5,8] bile acid binding resin or nicotinic acid.

87

Table 87.4 Lipid-lowering drugs

Drug	Dose (average)	Usage	Adverse effects	Safety monitoring
The statins	**Dose range from starting**			
Atorvastatin Pravastatin Simvastatin Fluvastatin Rosuvastatin	10–80 mg 20–80 mg 10–80 mg 20–80 mg 5–40 mg	↑ cholesterol (total or LDL-C)	Muscle pains, raised liver enzymes	Liver enzymes: creatine kinase and ALT
Bile acid binding resins				
Cholestyramine Colestipol	4–8 g daily–bd 5–10 g daily–bd	↑ cholesterol	GIT dysfunction, drug interactions	
Fibrates				
Gemfibrozil Fenofibrate	600 mg bd 145 mg daily	↑ triglycerides mixed hyperlipidaemia	GIT dysfunction, myositis; Gemfibrozil relatively contraindicated with statins	Liver enzymes coagulation
Other agents				
Ezetimibe	10 mg daily	↑ cholesterol	Arthralgia, myalgia, myositis, liver dysfunction	Liver enzymes
Nicotinic acid	250 mg bd to 1000 mg bd–tds	↑ cholesterol and triglycerides	Flushing (common), raised glucose, urate and liver enzymes	Glucose urate Liver enzymes Increase dose slowly
Fish oils n-3 fatty acids	2 g daily	↑ triglycerides	Minimal	Bleeding time

These agents can be used as monotherapy if statins cannot be tolerated.

Hypercholesterolaemia especially ↑ LDL-C

Choose from the following.[6,9]

First-line agent

1 HMG-CoA reductase inhibitors (statins—see TABLE 87.4): supported by evidence but be cautious in patients with muscle or hepatobiliary disease. Typical reduction is 30–50%.[9]
- adverse effects: GIT side effects, myalgia, abnormal liver function (uncommon)
- monitor: measure LFTs (ALT and CPK) and CK as baseline
- repeat LFTs after 4–8 weeks. It is no longer recommended to continue to monitor these unless patient becomes symptomatic.[5]

Additional drug therapy (options):

2 Ezetimibe 10 mg daily (especially if statin-intolerant). Reduces LDL by about 18%.[9]

3 Combination: ezetimibe + statin (consider if cholesterol above target)[8]

4 Bile acid binding resins (typically reduce LDL by 15–24%):
- e.g. cholestyramine 4 g daily in fruit juice increasing to maximum tolerated dose (often poorly tolerated)
- adverse effects: GIT side effects (e.g. constipation, offensive wind)

5 Fibrates: consider if above drugs not tolerated (e.g. fenofibrate 145 mg (o) daily—special care with renal impairment)
6 Nicotinic acid
   - nicotinic acid 250 mg (o) bd with food daily, increase gradually to max. 1000 mg tds if necessary (effective lipid reduction)
   - adverse effects: flushing (common), gastric irritation, gout
   - minimise side effects with gradual introduction; take with food
7 Evolocumab: a new monoclonal antibody agent for familial hypercholestoerolaemia and muscle-related statin intolerance[10]

Resistant LDL-C elevation

1 Combination statin + ezetimibe
2 Combined statin and resin
   cholestyramine 4–8 g (o) mane
   plus
   a statin

Moderate to severe (isolated or predominant) TG elevation[6]

Fibrate:

gemfibrozil 600 mg (o) bd
or
fenofibrate 145 mg (o) daily

Note: Slow response; monitor LFTs; predisposes to gallstones and myopathy
and/or

n-3 fish oil concentrate 6 g (o) daily in divided doses to max. 15 g/day
add
nicotinic acid if insufficient response

Note: Reduction in alcohol intake is important.

Massive hypertriglyceridaemia (TG) 10 mmol/L:

- fibrate plus fish oil plus (if necessary) nicotinic acid

Mixed hyperlipidaemia (↑ TG + ↑ LDL-C)

- If TG <4: a statin
- If TG >4: a fibrate

Consider combination therapy, e.g.:

- fish oil + statin
- fibrate + resin

Note: Statin + gemfibrozil increases risk of myopathy and should ideally be avoided.

Familial hypercholesterolaemia[11]

This is a dominant inherited condition causing accelerated cardiovascular disease by 20–40 years. Diagnosis requires exclusion of secondary causes, e.g. nephrotic syndrome. Refer to Dutch lipid diagnostic criteria.[11]

Special considerations

The decision to commence drug therapy should be based on at least two separate measurements at an accredited laboratory.

Be careful with beta blockers and diuretics affecting lipid levels.

Length of treatment

Possibly lifelong, although the need to consider deprescribing may become the priority with age over 75 years and increasing frailty or reduced life expectancy.

Follow-up investigations

- Serum lipids (overly frequent testing is widespread—for those on therapy, don't monitor levels more often than 6–12 monthly without good reason)
- LFTs (ALT and CPK)
- Possibly CK
- Biochemical monitoring

Special groups

Children

In general there is little justification for using lipid-regulating drugs in children, especially as the drugs have been shown to reduce heart disease within 2–5 years in adults.[6] Initial dietary advice and avoidance of smoking is recommended. Bile acid binding resins are safe to use.

The elderly

The role of lipid therapy remains unclear. Generally, elderly patients with established CHD should receive standard lipid management unless their general medical status is poor or the potential harms start to outweigh potential benefits.

Pregnancy[6]

As a general rule the increase in cholesterol level associated with pregnancy subsides after delivery.

Systemically absorbed lipid-lowering agents may be unsafe during pregnancy and should be avoided.

Complementary therapy

Claims have been made for the cholesterol-lowering properties of policosanol (derived from sugar cane), fish oils, plant sterols, vitamin E, garlic and lecithin. The evidence from RCTs to date indicates a modest benefit from policosanol, fish oils (consuming a fish-based meal at least twice a week is recommended) and plant sterols but there is insufficient evidence to recommend vitamin E, garlic and lecithin.[12]

Patient education resources

Hand-out sheets from *Murtagh's Patient Education* 7th edition:

- Cardiovascular (including coronary) risk factors
- Cholesterol: how to lower cholesterol

References

1 Duffy SJ, Meredith IJ. Treating mildly elevated lipids. Current Therapeutics, 1996; 37(4): 49–58.

2 Taylor F et al. Statins for the primary prevention of cardiovascular disease. Cochrane Database of Syst Rev. 2013; (1).

3 Cheung B et al. Meta-analysis of large randomized controlled trials to evaluate the impact of statins on cardiovascular outcomes. Br J Clin Pharmacol, May 2004; 57(5): 640–51.

4 The Pharmaceutical Benefits Scheme. General statement for lipid-lowering drugs prescribed as pharmaceutical benefits. Available from: <www.pbs.gov.au/info/healthpro/explanatory-notes/gs-lipid-lowering-drugs>, accessed March 2018.

5 The Royal Australian College of General Practitioners. *Guidelines for preventive activities in general practice.* (9th edn). East Melbourne: RACGP, 2016.

6 Expert group for Cardiovascular guidelines. Dyslipidaemia. In: eTG complete. Melbourne: Therapeutic Guidelines Ltd. Available from: <www.tg.org.au>, accessed January 2018.

7 National Vascular Disease Prevention Alliance. Guidelines for the management of absolute cardiovascular disease risk, 2012. Available from: <www.heartfoundation.org.au/images/uploads/publications/Absolute-CVD-Risk-Full-Guidelines.pdf>, accessed April 2018.

8 Baigent C, Landray MJ et al. The effects of lowering LDL cholesterol with simvastatin plus ezetimibe in patients with chronic kidney disease: a random placebo-controlled trial. Lancet 2001; 377(9784): 2182–92.

9 Buckley N (Chair). *Australian Medicines Handbook.* Adelaide: Australian Medicines Handbook Pty Ltd, 2016: 302–4.

10 Sabatine MS, Guigliano RP. Evolocumab and clinical outcome in patients with cardiovascular disease. N Eng J Med, 2017; 376: 1713–22.

11 Watts GF, Sullivan DR et al. Familial hypercholesterolaemia: a model of care for Australasia. Atherosclerosis Supplement, October 2011; 12(2): 221–63.

12 Managing dyslipidaemia. NPS News, 2002; 20: 5–6.

Chronic heart failure

In the year 1775 my opinion was asked concerning a family recipe for the cure of the dropsy. I was told that it had long been kept a secret by an old woman in Shropshire who had sometimes made cures after the more regular practitioners had failed—this medicine was composed of twenty or more different herbs and the active herb could be no other than the Foxglove.

WILLIAM WITHERING (1741–99), *ON THE USE OF FOXGLOVE (DIGITALIS) IN THE TREATMENT OF HEART DISEASE*

Heart failure occurs when the heart is unable to maintain sufficient cardiac output to meet the demands of the body for blood supply during rest and activity.

Chronic heart failure (CHF) remains a very serious problem with a poor prognosis. It has a 50% mortality within 3 years of the first hospital admission.[1] Australian and overseas data indicate that 1.5% of the adult population have heart failure. The prevalence of CHF has been shown to increase from approximately 1% in those aged 50–59 years to over 5% in those 65 and older, to over 50% in those 85 years and older.[2] Australian research suggests that under-treatment with the all-important ACE inhibitors continues to be a problem. ACE inhibitors (or ARBs) and beta blockers are the gold standard for treating systolic heart failure, with aldosterone antagonists providing added benefit if symptoms persist.[3] The clinical diagnosis is based on a careful history and examination. A major goal of management of CHF is the identification and reversal where possible of underlying causes and/or precipitating factors. CHF is characterised by two pathophysiological factors: fluid retention and reduction in cardiac output.

Diagnosis

The clinical diagnosis is based on a careful history and examination. The classic symptom of CHF is dyspnoea on exertion but symptoms may be reported relatively late, particularly with a sedentary lifestyle. Dyspnoea can progress as follows: exertional dyspnoea → dyspnoea at rest → orthopnoea → paroxysmal nocturnal dyspnoea.

Symptoms in summary

Fluid accumulation:

- Dyspnoea and orthopnoea (as above)
- Dry irritating cough (especially at night)
- Lethargy/fatigue
- Weight change: gain (mainly) or loss
- Ankle oedema
- Abdominal discomfort: hepatic congestion

Poor cardiac output:

- Dizzy spells/syncope
- Weakness
- Fatigue

Note: The irritating cough due to left ventricular failure can be mistaken for asthma, bronchitis or ACE-inhibitor-induced cough. Poor cardiac output causes fatigue and weakness.

Examination

The physical examination is very important for the initial diagnosis and evaluation of progress. The signs are as follows.

Signs

There may be no abnormal signs initially. It is helpful clinically to differentiate between the signs of right and left heart failure:

Left heart failure

- Tachycardia
- Low volume pulse (pulse pressure <25 mm Hg)
- Tachypnoea
- Laterally displaced apex beat
- Bilateral basal crackles
- Gallop rhythm (3rd heart sound)
- Pleural effusion
- Poor peripheral perfusion—cool, pale extremities

Right heart failure

- Elevated jugular venous pressure
- Right ventricular heave
- Peripheral/ankle oedema
- Hepatomegaly
- Ascites

Auscultation is important to identify adventitious sounds, a third heart sound and possible underlying valvular disease.

Systolic versus diastolic heart failure

The classic heart failure is systolic failure due to an inadequate pumping action of the heart. The ventricle is dilated and contracting poorly (left ventricular ejection fraction <40%).[4]

Diastolic heart failure is due to impairment of left ventricular filling with preserved systolic function. A substantial proportion of heart failure presentations are due to diastolic heart failure (impaired ventricular relaxation).[2] It should be suspected in the elderly with hypertension and a normal heart size on chest X-ray who present with dyspnoea or pulmonary oedema.[3] It is particularly common in elderly females.

Note: Patients can have simultaneous systolic and diastolic failure.

88

The oedema of heart failure

Peripheral oedema appears initially on the lower legs as 'pitting'. To assess the presence of pitting, which is usually graded on a four-point scale, press firmly yet gently with the thumb for 5–10 seconds over the dorsum of the feet, behind each medial malleolus and over the shins. With increasing severity of failure the oedema extends proximally to involve the abdomen. In the recumbent position it may be apparent over the sacrum.[5]

Determining severity of heart failure

The severity of heart failure can be considered from three different perspectives: the severity of the symptoms, the degree of impairment of cardiac function and the severity of the congestive state. The severity of the symptoms or the degree of functional disability is usually described according to the New York Heart Association criteria (see TABLE 88.1).[6] The left ventricular ejection fraction provides an indication of cardiac function.

Causes of heart failure

Causes of CHF can be classified under systolic heart failure (impaired ventricular contraction) and diastolic heart failure (impaired ventricular relaxation and filling despite normal contractions). Diagnosis is based on echocardiography.

Systolic heart failure

Ischaemic heart disease, including previous myocardial infarction, is the most common cause, accounting for approximately two-thirds. There is often a history of at least one myocardial infarction.[2] Essential hypertension is the other common cause.

Other causes:

- valvular heart disease, mainly aortic and mitral incompetence
- high output states (e.g. anaemia, hyperthyroidism, Paget disease)
- non-ischaemic idiopathic dilated cardiomyopathy
- viral cardiomyopathy
- alcoholic cardiomyopathy
- other cardiomyopathies—diabetic, familial
- persistent arrhythmias, especially atrial fibrillation
- other systemic illness (e.g. sarcoidosis, SLE, scleroderma, myxoedema)
- chemotherapy
- peripartum

Diastolic heart failure

- Obesity, hypertension and diabetes significant risk factors
- Familial: more common in women and the elderly

Table 88.1 New York Heart Association (NYHA) functional classification of CHF symptoms[2,6]

Class	Disability	Approximate 1-year mortalities
I (asymptomatic)	No limitation: cardiac disease present, but ordinary physical activity causes no symptoms such as fatigue, dyspnoea or palpitation, or rapid forceful breathing	5%
II (mild)	Slight limitation: ordinary activity (moderate exertion) causes symptoms but patients comfortable at rest	10%
III (moderate)	Marked limitation: symptoms with less than ordinary physical activity (mild exertion) although patients still comfortable at rest	20%
IV (severe)	Unable to carry out any physical activity without symptoms; may have symptoms at rest	50%

- Common causes include ischaemic heart disease, systemic hypertension, aortic stenosis, atrial fibrillation (inadequate filling), hypertrophic cardiomyopathy, pericardial disease
- Significant morbidity and difficult to diagnose

Investigations

The following should be considered:

- Echocardiography[2]—the transthoracic echocardiogram is the investigation of choice to measure ventricular function. It can differentiate between systolic dysfunction and those with normal systolic function but abnormal diastolic filling. It gives information about left and right ventricular systolic and diastolic function, left and right ventricular size, volumes, thickness, structure and function. It also provides information about cardiac valves, congenital heart defects and pericardial disease.
- Electrocardiogram—a key investigation to look for evidence of ischaemia, conduction abnormalities, arrhythmias and LV hypertrophy
- Chest X-ray to look for:
  - cardiomegaly and interstitial oedema
  - upper lobe blood diversion
  - fluid in fissures
  - oedema in perihilar area with prominent vascular markings
  - small basal pleural effusions
  - Kerley B lines = raised pulmonary venous pressure
  - frank pulmonary oedema

  Note: a normal CXR does not exclude CHF.
- Spirometry/respiratory function testing—to detect associated airways dysfunction
- B-type natriuretic peptide—a hormone secreted from the ventricular myocardium is an indicator of severity of CHF and prognosis

Peripheral markers

- FBE and ESR: anaemia can occur with CHF; severe anaemia may cause CHF
- Serum electrolytes: usually normal in CHF, important to monitor management
- Kidney function tests: for monitoring drug therapy
- Liver function tests: congestive hepatomegaly gives abnormal LFTs
- Urinalysis
- Thyroid function tests, especially if atrial fibrillation
- Viral studies: for suspected viral myocarditis

Specialised cardiac investigation (specialist directive)

- Coronary angiography—for suspected and known ischaemia. CT angiography and cardiovascular MRI preferred
- Haemodynamic testing
- Endomyocardial biopsy
- Nuclear cardiology

Treatment of heart failure

88

The treatment of heart failure includes determination and treatment of the cause, removal of any precipitating factors, appropriate patient education, general non-pharmaceutical measures and drug treatment. Studies have shown the benefit of an integrated, multidisciplinary approach to management.

Prevention of heart failure

The emphasis on prevention is very important since the onset of heart failure is generally associated with a poor prognosis. Approximately 50% of patients with heart failure die within 5 years of diagnosis.[7]

The scope for prevention includes the following measures:[8]

- dietary advice (e.g. achievement of ideal weight, optimal nutrition)
- emphasising the dangers of smoking and excessive alcohol
- control of hypertension
- control of other risk factors (e.g. hypercholesterolaemia)
- early detection and control of diabetes mellitus
- early intervention during myocardial infarction to preserve myocardial function (e.g. thrombolytic therapy)
- secondary prevention after the occurrence of myocardial infarction (e.g. beta blockers, ACE inhibitors and aspirin)
- appropriate timing of surgery or angioplasty for ischaemic or valvular heart disease

Treatment of causes and precipitating factors

Any underlying cause should be identified and treated, if possible. Precipitating factors that should be treated include:

- arrhythmias (e.g. atrial fibrillation)
- electrolyte imbalance, especially hypokalaemia
- anaemia

- myocardial ischaemia, especially myocardial infarction
- dietary factors (e.g. malnutrition, excessive salt or alcohol intake)
- adverse drug reactions (e.g. fluid retention with NSAIDs and COX-2 agents) (see TABLE 88.2)[9]
- infection (e.g. bronchopneumonia, endocarditis)
- hyper- and hypothyroidism
- lack of compliance with therapy
- fluid overload

Note: Be mindful of complementary medications.

88

General non-pharmacological management

- Education and support
- Smoking: encourage no smoking
- Refer for a rehabilitation program with interdisciplinary care
- Encourage physical activity especially when symptoms absent or mild
- Rest while symptoms are severe
- Weight reduction, if patient obese
- Advice on food supplementation—dietitian
- Salt restriction: advise no-added-salt diet (<2 g or 60–100 mmol/day)
- Water restriction: water intake should be limited to 1.5–2 L/day or less in patients with advanced heart failure, especially when the serum sodium level falls below 130 mmol/L[7]
- Limit caffeine to 1–2 cups coffee/tea a day
- Limit alcohol to 1 standard drink a day
- Fluid aspiration—if pleural or pericardial effusion present

Table 88.2 Drugs that can aggravate CHF

NSAIDs including COX-2 inhibitors
Corticosteroids
Tricyclic antidepressants
Calcium channel blockers (verapamil and diltiazem)
Selected anti-arrhythmics (e.g. quinidine)
Macrolide antibiotic
Macrogol
Type 1 antihistamines
Clozapine
H_2-receptor antagonists
Thiazolidinediones (glitazones)
TNF-alpha inhibitors (e.g. etanercept, infliximab)
Ethanol or illicit drug (e.g. cocaine) use

- Daily weighing—check significant weight gain or loss

Other general measures[1]

- Optimise cardiovascular risk factors (e.g. BP, lipids, HbA_{1C})
- Monitor emotional factors including depression
- Regular review
- Vaccination: annual influenza, 5-yearly pneumococcus
- 2-yearly echocardiography (or more) as indicated
- Pleurocentesis or pericardiocentesis (if applicable)
- Treat co-existing obstructive sleep apnoea

Drug therapy of heart failure due to left ventricular systolic dysfunction

Any identified underlying factor should be treated.

Evidence from RCTs shows the beneficial results from ACE inhibitors[2,9] (or angiotensin II blockers), digoxin (improves outcome in people already receiving diuretics and ACE inhibitors), beta blockers and spironolactone (in severe heart failure).

Atrial fibrillation should be treated with digoxin. Vasodilators are widely used for heart failure and angiotensin converting enzyme inhibitors (ACEI) are currently the most favoured vasodilator.

Note: Monitor and maintain normal potassium level in all patients.

ACE inhibitors improve prognosis in all grades of heart failure and should be employed as the initial therapy in all patients, except where contraindicated (e.g. kidney artery stenosis, angioedema).

Diuretics have an important place in patients with fluid overload. As a rule they should be added to an ACEI to achieve euvolaemia. Diuretics should be used in moderation and excessive doses of a single drug avoided. In patients with systolic LV dysfunction they should not be used as monotherapy.[8] Close monitoring of weight, kidney function and electrolytes is required. Loop diuretics such as frusemide, bumetanide or ethacrynic acid are commonly used, especially for heart failure of moderate severity.[8] Thiazide and related diuretics produce a gradual diuresis and are recommended for mild heart failure. Examples include hydrochlorothiazide, bendrofluazide, chlorthalidone or indapamide.

Initial therapy of heart failure[7,10]

1 ACE inhibitor (start low, aim high)

Dosage of ACE inhibitor: commence with ¼ to ½ lowest recommended therapeutic dose and then adjust it for the individual patient by gradually increasing it to the maintenance or maximum dose (see TABLE 88.3). Once-daily agents are preferred. Use an ARB if cough is problematic.

ACE inhibitors

- ACE inhibitors are regarded as the agents of first choice because they correct neuroendocrine abnormalities and reduce cardiac load by their vasodilator action.
- Every effort should be made to up-titrate to the highest tolerated dose.
- Consider giving the first dose at bedtime if there is a risk of orthostatic hypotension.
- If the ACEI is not tolerated (e.g. due to cough) consider an angiotensin II receptor blocker (ARB) as they have proven benefit in CHF.[11]
- In practice the usual initial treatment of heart failure is an ACE inhibitor plus diuretic. This combination optimises response and improves diuretic safety.
- Consider stopping any diuretic for 24 hours before starting treatment with an ACEI.
- Potassium-sparing diuretics or supplements should not be given with ACEI (or should at least be used with caution) because of the danger of hyperkalaemia.
- Kidney function and potassium levels should be monitored in all patients.

2 Add a diuretic (if congestion):

loop diuretic (preferred)
frusemide 20–40 mg (o) once or twice daily
or
ethacrynic acid 50 mg (o) daily

Table 88.3 Some ACE inhibitors in common usage[6]

ACE inhibitor	Initial daily oral dose	Usual maintenance dose
Captopril	6.25 mg	25 mg tds
Enalapril	2.5 mg	10 mg bd
Fosinopril	5 mg	20 mg daily
Lisinopril	2.5 mg	5–20 mg daily
Perindopril	2 mg*	4 mg* daily
Quinapril	2.5 mg	20 mg daily
Ramipril	1.25 mg	5 mg daily
Trandolapril	0.5 mg	2–4 mg daily

*2 mg perindopril erbumine = 2.5 mg perindopril arginine

or
(thiazide-type diuretic)
hydrochlorothiazide 25–50 mg (o) daily (or other thiazide)
or
indapamide 1.5–2.5 mg (o) daily

3 Add an aldosterone antagonist diuretic (if fluid overload not controlled):

spironolactone 12.5–50 mg (o) daily
or
eplerenone 25–50 mg (o) daily

Some authorities are concerned about the over-reliance on diuretics and also about compliance as well as side effects. Once the diuretic effect has been achieved, diuretics may be withdrawn and fluid restriction advised. The ACEI is then used alone or with a beta blocker.

88

Beta blockers

Selective beta blockers have been shown to prolong survival of patients with mild to moderate CHF taking ACE inhibitors who are stabilised. Start with extremely low doses (see TABLE 88.4). Commence when patient stable and euvolaemic.

Digoxin

Digoxin was the mainstay of treatment of heart failure for decades prior to the use of ACE inhibitors. It was an effective agent but limited. The two indications for its current use are in patients with atrial fibrillation to control rapid ventricular rate and in patients with sinus rhythm not adequately controlled by the other agents above it in FIGURE 88.1. Most patients are started on a low dose digoxin:

62.5–250 mcg (o) daily

New agents[7]

Ivabradine is a direct sinus node inhibitor which can be added to a beta blocker in patients with continuing

Table 88.4 Beta blockers approved to treat heart failure

Beta blocker	Initial daily dose	Target dose
Bisoprolol	1.25 mg (o) daily	10 mg (o) daily
Carvedilol	3.125 mg (o) bd	25 mg (o) daily
Metoprolol extended release	23.75 mg (o) daily	190 mg (o) daily
Nebivolol	1.25 mg (o)	10 mg (o) daily

symptoms of moderate to severe failure, or where beta blockers are contraindicated or not tolerated. Other new agents to consider for optimal treatment include sacubitril/valsartan (Entresto)—an angiotension/neprilysin inhibitor.

Heart failure (unresponsive to first-line therapy)—stepwise strategy[2,7]

ACE inhibitor
plus
frusemide 40–80 mg (o) bd
plus
spironolactone 12.5 (starting)—25 mg (o) daily (monitor potassium and RFTs), if still congestion
plus
a selective beta blocker (if patient euvolaemic)
plus
digoxin (if not already taking it):[7] loading dose:

- 0.5–0.75 mg (o) statim (depending on kidney function)
- then 0.5 mg (o) 4 hours later
- then 0.5 mg the following day
- then individualise maintenance

Severe heart failure[7,10]

Seek specialist advice.

Hospital with bed rest.
ACE inhibitor to maximum tolerated dose
plus
frusemide to max. 500 mg/day
plus
spironolactone (low dose) 25 mg/day
If poorly controlled, consider adding:

- thiazide diuretic
- spironolactone—doses up to 100–200 mg daily
- a beta blocker
- digoxin
- heparin (if confined to bed)

Vasodilators

If still uncontrolled consider vasodilators other than ACEIs or ARBs:

isosorbide dinitrate 20–40 mg (o) 6 hourly
plus
hydralazine 50–100 mg (o) 6 hourly

A glyceryl nitrate patch can be used for the relief of symptoms, especially nocturnal dyspnoea.

Consider cardiac transplantation for appropriate patients with end-stage heart failure (e.g. patients under 50 with no other major disease). Other surgical options include heart valvular surgery, coronary artery bypass surgery and surgical ventricular restoration (surgical reduction of an enlarged left ventricle).

A flow chart for the basic management of heart failure is presented in FIGURE 88.1.

Diastolic heart failure[2,8]

Management is based on treating the cause such as hypertension, ischaemia and diabetes. The basic treatment is with inotropic agents such as calcium channel blockers (verapamil or diltiazem) and beta blockers. If possible avoid diuretics (except for congestion), digoxin, nitrates/vasodilators and nifedipine. Excessive diuresis from overzealous diuretic therapy can cause severe consequences for cardiac output. ACE inhibitors can be used with caution.

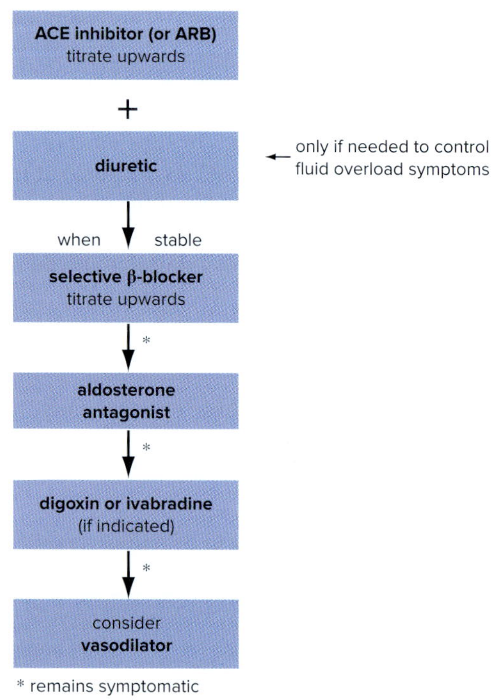

FIGURE 88.1 A stepwise pharmacological management approach to systolic heart failure[10,12]

Pitfalls in management

- The most common treatment error—excessive use of diuretics[3]
- Giving an excessive loading dose of ACE inhibitor
- Failure to correct remedial causes or precipitating factors
- Failure to measure left ventricular function
- Failure to monitor electrolytes and kidney function

Acute severe heart failure

For the treatment of acute pulmonary oedema refer to CHAPTER 128.

ACE inhibitors, beta blockers and spironolactone have been shown to improve survival in CHF.[9]

Device-based heart failure treatments[1]

The use of mechanical devices to treat patients with severe failure is gaining momentum. Devices include:

- implantable cardiac defibrillators
- biventricular pacemakers
- left ventricular assist devices (definitive VentrAssist)

The evidence for the efficacy of these devices is good, but limitations include cost and infection. Biventricular pacing or cardiac resynchronisation therapy resynchronises cardiac contraction in patients with systolic CHF and left branch bundle block. VentrAssist is based on a continuous flow rotary blood pump that is surgically implanted in the abdominal wall and attached to the apex of the ventricle.

When to refer

- Age <65 years
- Uncertainty of diagnosis, especially diastolic heart failure
- Complex management issues (especially with beta blockers, digoxin)
- Familial screening (where appropriate)
- Acute decompensation
- Refractory symptoms
- Device implantation or cardiac transplantation

Practice tips

- Echocardiography is the gold standard for diagnosing CHF.
- Early diagnosis and then optimal therapy is the key to prevent or slow progression.
- Use a multidisciplinary team approach for the patient with CHF and refer early and readily for specialist advice.
- ACE inhibitors, if tolerated, are recommended for all patients with heart failure, whether symptoms are mild, moderate or severe.[1]
- The primary reason for prescribing an ACE inhibitor is to reduce the risk of death or hospitalisation.
- Diuretics are very effective in the presence of fluid overload, but should be used in combination with an ACE inhibitor—not as monotherapy.
- Drug treatment should include an ACE inhibitor and selective beta blocker wherever possible.[1]
- Beware of hyperkaelaemia with the combination of an ACEI or ARB with an aldosterone antagonist.
- Device-based heart failure therapy is an expanding field and includes three major groups of devices: biventricular pacemakers (cardiac resynchronisation therapy), implantable cardiac defibrillators and left ventricular assist devices.[1]

88

Patient education resources

Hand-out sheets from *Murtagh's Patient Education* 7th edition:
- Heart failure

References

1 Piterman L, Zimmet H, Krum H et al. Chronic heart failure: optimising care in general practice. Aust Fam Physician, 2005; 34(7): 547–53.

2 National Heart Foundation of Australia and the Cardiac Society of Australia and New Zealand. Diagnosis and management of chronic heart failure, 2011. <www.heartfoundation.org.au>

3 Krum H, Tonkin AM, Currie R et al. Chronic heart failure in Australian general practice: the Cardiac Awareness Survey and Evaluation (CASE) Study. Med J Aust, 2001; 174: 439–44.

4 Lemanna A, Atherton JJ. Prevention and management of heart failure. Medicine Today, June 2010; 11(6): 56–68.

5 Davis A, Bolin T, Ham J. *Symptom Analysis and Physical Diagnosis* (2nd edn). Sydney: Pergamon Press, 1990: 173.

6 Piterman L, Zimet H, Krum H. Chronic heart failure. Check Program 410. Melbourne: RACGP, 2006: 5.

7 Expert group for Cardiovascular guidelines. Heart failure. In: eTG complete. Melbourne: Therapeutic Guideline Ltd, 2015. Available from: <www.tg.org.au>, accessed September 2017.

8 Kumar P, Clark M. *Clinical Medicines* (9th edn). London: Elsevier Saunders, 2009: 129.

9 Sindone A. Investigation and management of chronic heart failure. Medicine Today, 2008; 9(1): 27–37.

10 Buckley N (Chair). *Australian Medicines Handbook*. Adelaide: Australian Medicines Handbook Pty Ltd, 2016: 228–9.

11 Granger CB, McMurray JJV, Yusuf S et al. Effects of candesartan in patients with chronic heart failure and reduced left-ventricular systolic function intolerant to angiotensin-converting-enzyme inhibitors: the CHARM-alternative trial. Lancet, 2003; 362: 772–6.

12 The National Collaborating Centre for Chronic Conditions. NICE Guideline No. 5. *Chronic Heart Failure. National Clinical Guideline for Diagnosis and Management in Primary and Secondary Care,* 2011. Further information: <www.heartfoundation.com.au/downloads>.

89 Osteoporosis

Like bones which, broke in sunder, and well set, knit the more strongly . . . but old bones are brittle.

JOHN WEBSTER (1580–1625)

Osteoporosis, which literally means porous bone, is reduced bone mass per unit volume (see FIG. 89.1), thus predisposing the person with it to an increased risk of fracture. It also refers to the increased bone fragility that accompanies ageing and many illnesses. Following menopause, women begin to lose calcium from their bone at a much faster rate than men, presumably in response to low levels of oestrogen. By the age of 65 the rate of fractures in women has increased to 3–5 times that of men.[1] However, a third of all hip fractures in the community occur in men.

In recent decades osteoporosis was largely prevented by correction of oestrogen deficiency through the use of hormone replacement therapy but the balance has changed since the controversial association of HRT with breast cancer was reported.

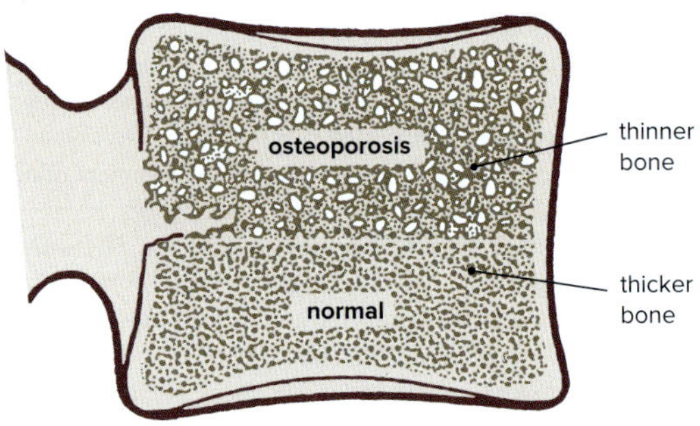

FIGURE 89.1 Osteoporosis is reduced bone mass per unit volume

Key facts and checkpoints

- Osteoporosis is silent, common, measurable, treatable and potentially lethal.[2]
- Osteoporosis is commonest in postmenopausal women.
- Up to 50% of women will develop fragility fractures in their lifetime and 30% of all women reaching 90 years of age will suffer a hip fracture.[1,3]
- Osteoporosis leads to reduced bone strength and susceptibility to fracture, even with minor trauma.
- Osteoporosis usually causes pain when complicated by fracture.
- First presentation is usually a fracture (Colles, femoral neck and vertebra) or height shrinkage.
- Vertebral collapse is the hallmark of osteoporosis.
- For osteoporosis in a vertebra including a pathological fracture, multiple myeloma needs exclusion.
- The first step in prevention is regular exercise, an adequate dietary intake of calcium (1500 mg per day) and maintenance of adequate serum vitamin D levels.

Classification[4]

Primary

Type 1: Postmenopausal (vertebral or distal forearm fractures between the ages of 51 and 75). Due to increased osteoclast activity. It is six times more common in women than men.

Type 2: Involutional or senile osteoporosis (fracture of proximal femur and other bones). It affects patients over 60 years and is twice as common in women as in men.

Idiopathic osteoporosis: Occurs in children and young adults of both sexes with normal gonadal function.

Secondary

Secondary to various endocrine disorders, malabsorption and malignancies. Various causes and risk factors are presented in TABLE 89.1.

Investigations

- Plain radiography is of limited value. Osteoporosis is not detectable until 40–50% of bone is lost.
- 25-hydroxy vitamin D (most useful test): normal range 75–250 nmol/L.

Table 89.1 Osteoporosis: risk factors and/or causes[3]

Constitutional and non-modifiable
Female sex
Ageing: M >60, F >50 (including sarcopenia)
Thin build; low BMI <20; short stature
Race: Asian, Caucasian
Family history (e.g. maternal hip fracture <75 yrs)
Premenopausal oestrogen deficiency (e.g. amenorrhoea)
Late menarche
Early menopause <45 years (natural or surgical)
Modifiable lifestyle factors
Cigarette smoking
High alcohol intake >2 standard drinks per day
Low calcium intake
Lack of vitamin D
Physical inactivity
Medical causes
Eating disorders (e.g. anorexia nervosa)
Malabsorption syndrome (e.g. coeliac disease)
Endocrine disorders:
• Cushing syndrome
• diabetes mellitus
• hyperparathyroidism
• thyrotoxicosis
• amenorrhoea in elite athletes
• hypogonadism/sex hormone deficiency
• acromegaly
Connective tissue disorders (e.g. RA)
Chronic organ failure (kidney, liver, heart, lungs)
Drugs causing bone loss:
• corticosteroids >3 months ≥7.5 mg/day
• anti-epileptic drugs, especially hepatic enzyme inducers
• thiazolidinediones for diabetes
• long-term heparin
• excessive thyroid hormone replacement
• prostate cancer hormone therapy
• breast cancer hormone therapy
Prolonged immobilisation

- Plasma calcium, phosphate and alkaline phosphatase, parathyroid hormone (usually normal).
- Thyroid stimulating hormone.
- Parathyroid hormone.
- Consider tests for multiple myeloma in an osteoporotic area.
- Densitometry can predict an increased risk of osteoporosis and fracture, the best current modality being dual energy X-ray absorptiometry (DEXA scan) in a facility with high-standard quality control.[3] The spine and femoral neck are targeted: the femoral neck is the most useful index.

DEXA, T scores and Z scores[5]

DEXA is the current gold standard for the diagnosis of osteoporosis. It assesses both whole-body and regional bone mass (lumbar spine and proximal femur). Bone mass is measured as bone mineral density (BMD) in g/cm^2 and the lower the BMD, the higher the risk of fracture. There are actually different normal ranges of BMD for each bone and for each type of DEXA measuring machine.

The BMD 'T score' is the number of standard deviations (SD) away from the mean BMD of a 30-year-old adult (see TABLE 89.2). Osteopenia (low bone density) is 1–2.5 SDs below the young adult standard mean. Osteoporosis is >2.5 SD below this mean. This is a strong indicator of bone fragility. Consider treatment if T score is <−2.5.

The BMD 'Z score' is the number of SDs away from the age- and sex-matched mean BMD. The Z score is used to express bone density in patients <50 years, premenopausal women, younger men and children. If low (<−2) it indicates prompt investigation for underlying causes of a bone deficit.

BMD is subsidised under the MBS[6] for:

- people over the age of 70 years (2- or 5-yearly screening, depending on first T score)
- diagnosis of osteoporosis following a low-impact fracture

Table 89.2 Interpretation of T scores (WHO criteria)

T score	Interpretation
≥−1.0	Normal
−1 to −2.5	Osteopenia
≤−2.5	Osteoporosis
<−2.5 with fracture	Severe osteoporosis

89

- screening for people with specific medical conditions or treatments likely to cause osteoporosis (annual)
- subsequent monitoring of low BMI

The decision whether to measure BMD in non-subsidised situations, and whether to treat a low BMD, may also be guided by an assessment of absolute fracture risk. The FRAX tool is commonly used, although somewhat controversially was developed by manufacturers of osteoporosis medication.[7]

Treatment

The management of osteoporosis starts with restoring mobility and instituting measures to prevent falls. Underlying diseases that may be responsible for increased bone fragility should be identified and treated where possible. Carefully consider deprescribing medications adding to the risk of osteoporosis and falls.

89

The goal of drug treatment is to prevent osteoporosis or reduce further loss. Eliminate risk factors where possible and focus on optimal lifestyle measures as a baseline for management. No treatment has been shown to replace lost bone effectively. Anabolic agents such as nandrolone decanoate may reduce further loss but the side effects are problematic. The list of recent recommendations from the American College of Physicians is noteworthy.

Recommendations of American College of Physicians[5]

- Treat women who have known osteoporosis with alendroate, risedronate, zoledronic acid or denosumab to reduce the risk for hip and vertebral fractures
- Treatment should last 5 years (oral) or 3 years (annual IV), then usually cease unless recent fracture
- Menopausal hormone therapy should not be prescribed to treat osteoporosis in women
- BMD monitoring during the 5-year treatment period is not advised as evidence suggests that women see fracture reduction benefits regardless of BMD changes
- Offer bisphosphonate therapy to men with clinically recognised osteoporosis
- For osteopenic women ≥65 at high fracture risk, decisions to treat should take into account patient preference, fracture-risk profile, benefits, harms and price of medications
- Denosumab can cause hypocalcaemia which could lead to heart failure

Medications of value in decreasing further loss[3]

The following medications may be valuable in preventing further bone loss, possibly reversing the osteoporosis process and preventing further fractures.

- HRT (long-term use is not recommended but weigh potential benefits versus harms with female patients)[8]

  or
- bisphosphonates (decrease bone absorption)[3]—can be used alone or combined with other agents (take care with potential adverse effects of oesophagitis and osteonecrosis of jaw):
  - alendronate 70 mg (o) once weekly on an empty stomach (take care with potential side effect of oesophagitis)

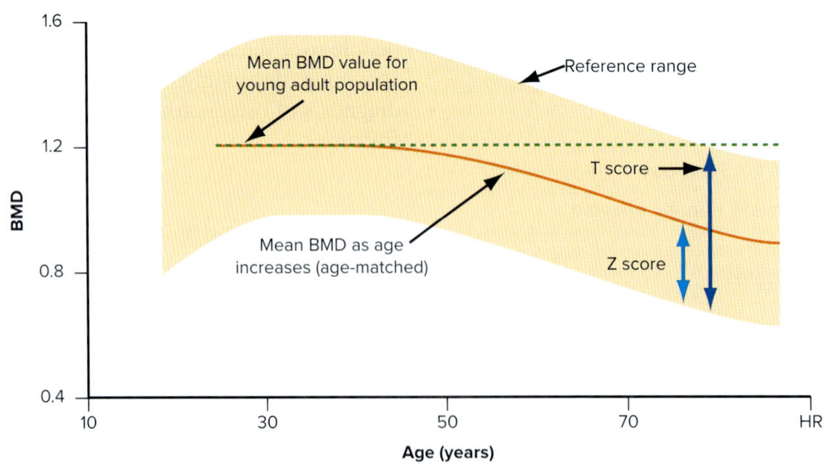

FIGURE 89.2 Illustration of T scores and Z scores

  - risedronate 150 mg (o) once monthly or 35 mg (o) once weekly or in combination therapy with calcium carbonate ± vitamin D
  - zoledronic acid, single annual IV injection
- raloxifene (a selective oestrogen-receptor modulator) (SERM) 60 mg (o) daily
- teriparatide (a synthetic form of human parathyroid hormone) increases bone formation—give 20 mcg SC once daily
- denosumab (a monoclonal antibody) 60 mg SC, once every 6 months, once calcium intake and vitamin D levels are optimal—a potential risk factor for osteonecrosis of the jaw especially in patients with bone cancer

The choice depends on the clinical status, such as the age of the patient and the extent of disease, the patient's tolerance of drugs and further clinical trials of these drugs.

Recommendations for prevention[3,7,8,9]

- lifestyle factors: stop smoking, limit caffeine and alcohol (2 SDs/day)
- maintain adequate nutrition: aim for ideal body weight with recommended waist measurements (preferable) or BMI 18–25
- adequate dietary intake of calcium:
  - at least 1000 mg/day in women <50 years and men <70 years; 1300 mg in women >50 years and men >70 years
  - dairy food is the main source of dietary calcium and people should meet their requirements with a good diet; supplementation in non-institutionalised people is not required
  - oral calcium supplements may be necessary where a person's diet does not meet their daily calcium requirements, particularly in postmenopausal women
- calcium citrate is better absorbed than carbonate[3]—recommend: calcium citrate 2.38 g (= 500 mg elemental calcium) daily
  or
  calcium carbonate 1.5 g (= 600 mg elemental calcium) daily with food
- calcium-rich foods include low-fat calcium-enriched milk (500 mL contains 1000 mg), other low-fat dairy products (e.g. yoghurt or cheese), fish (including tinned fish such as salmon with the bone), citrus fruits, sesame and sunflower seeds, almonds, brazil nuts and hazel nuts
- vitamin D deficiency and sunlight[9,10]: there is evidence we need significant exposure to sunlight of the face, bare arms and hands to produce natural vitamin D (e.g. for those at risk—in summer 6–7 minutes mid-morning or mid-afternoon; in winter 7–40 minutes at noon with as much bare skin as possible). Refer to regional recommendations.[11] Measure serum 25-hydroxy vitamin D and ideally maintain it at >50 nmol/L. Mild deficiency is 30–49 nmol/L, moderate 12.5–29, severe <12.5. If supplementation is required use cholecalciferol 25–50 mcg (1000–2000 IU) (o) daily.[3]
- exercise: moderate exercise against gravity—walking (brisk walking for 30 minutes 4 times a week) or jogging may make a small contribution to retarding bone loss, but also help reduce falls. Highly osteogenic exercise includes basketball, tennis, dancing and gymnastics.
- attention to falls prevention, including avoiding falls (refer to CHAPTER 8)[12]
- 'hip protectors' for osteoporotic patients at increased falls risk have some weak evidence, but adherence can be poor

89

Natural remedies

An Australian review investigating the effect of natural remedies on BMD commented that there is good evidence that exercise increases BMD in postmenopausal women with osteoporosis, little good-quality empirical evidence to support the use of natural progesterone cream and insufficient evidence to support the use of boron, cod liver oil or chelated calcium supplements (as opposed to calcium carbonate).[13]

There is no evidence that complex mineral preparations have added benefit and often they contain less elemental calcium than simple preparations.[3]

Monitoring osteoporosis treatment[3]

Recommendations are to measure BMD at the lumbar spine and hip:

- 2 years after therapy begins
- 1–2 years after therapy changes significantly or where high risk of bone loss (long-term glucocorticoids or post-transplant)

Osteoporosis in children

The main problem in children is secondary osteoporosis, which is usually related to chronic inflammatory disorders which require treatment with corticosteroids and/or cause reduced mobility. Other medical causes are malignancy, malabsorption syndromes, poor nutrition, anorexia nervosa and hypogonadism. Use DEXA to assess and monitor BMD and Z scores. Refer for treatment, which may be based on bisphosphonates.

Osteoporosis in men

Refer to CHAPTER 110.

When to refer

- Refer postmenopausal women and older men to a specialist according to individual needs
- Osteoporosis appears to be secondary to an underlying illness
- Advice is required about the management of a patient with pathological osteoporotic fractures or loss of height

Patient education resources

Hand-out sheets from *Murtagh's Patient Education* 7th edition:

- Osteoporosis

References

1 Seeman E, Young N. Osteoporosis. In: *MIMS Disease Index* (2nd edn). Sydney, IMS Publishing, 1996: 368–71.
2 Phillips P. Osteoporosis. Check Program 366. Melbourne: RACGP, 2002: 5–31.
3 Expert group for Endocrinology guidelines. Osteoporosis. In: eTG complete. Melbourne: Therapeutic Guidelines Ltd, 2016. Available from: <www.tg.org.au>, accessed September 2017.
4 Porter RS, Kaplan JL. *The Merck Manual* (19th edn). Whitehorse Station: Merck Research Laboratories, 2011: 356.
5 Gupta A, March L. Treating osteoporosis. Aust Prescr, 2016: 40–6.
6 Department of Health. Bone densitometry. Available at <http://www.health.gov.au/internet/main/publishing.nsf/content/diagnosticimaging-bd.htm> accessed March 2018
7 Cassels A. WHO exposes deceptive promotion of industry-supported FRAX osteoporosis screening tool. Health News Review 2016, available at <https://www.healthnewsreview.org/2016/12/frax-osteoporosis-screening-tool/>
8 Ensrud KE, Grandall CJ. Osteoporosis. Ann Intern Med, 1 Aug 2017; 167(3): 17–32.
9 Newson CA, McGrath JJ, Ebeling PR et al. Vitamin D and health in adults in Australia and New Zealand: a position statement. Med J Aust, 2012; 196(11): 656–7.
10 Diamond TH, Eisman JA et al. Working Group of the Australian and New Zealand Bone and Mineral Society, Endocrine Society of Australia and Osteoporosis Australia. Vitamin D and adult bone health in Australia and New Zealand: a position statement. Med J Aust, 2005; 182: 281–4.
11 Ebeling PR, Daly RM et al. An evidence informed strategy to prevent osteoporosis in Australia. Med J Aust, 2013; 198(2): 90–1.
12 Gillespie LD, Robertson MC et al. Interventions for preventing falls in older people living in the community. Cochrane Database Syst Rev. 2012; (9): CD007146.
13 Del Mar CB et al. Natural remedies for osteoporosis in postmenopausal women. Med J Aust, 2002; 176: 182–3.

Resources

NICE Fragility fracture risk (2012). <https://www.nice.org.uk/guidance/CG146>, accessed April 2018.

Part
5

Child and adolescent health

90 An approach to the child

In every child who is born, under no matter the circumstances, and of no matter what parents, the potentiality of the human race is born again; and in him, too, once more, and of each of us, our terrific responsibility towards human life; towards the utmost idea of goodness.

James Agee (1909–55)

Seeing a child as a patient means you are dealing with at least one extra person in the room. Communication and rapport building need to be undertaken with both the child and those who have brought the child (usually the parents). By engaging the child, you will usually win over the parent. Parents are often apprehensive about bringing their child to the doctor, concerned to the child might misbehave or do or say something to embarrass them. By displaying a natural interest in and ease with the child, a tolerance of child behaviour (or misbehaviour) and being generally 'child friendly', the consultation is more likely to be successful.

Engaging children can be done from the moment they are called from the waiting room. All of the usual rapport-building skills we use for adults (see Chapter 4) can be utilised with children. Respect, genuine interest in them, active listening and use of body language all matter with children, perhaps even more so than for adults as children naturally have less developed communication skills.

There is also a different style of communication required and this is age dependent. Infants will be dominated by emerging object permanence skills (e.g. playing peek-a-boo), attachment (they will constantly refer to their parent), separation and stranger anxiety. Toddler and preschooler communication is dominated by play, particularly 'pretend' or 'imaginative' play. Pretending to be a scary bear, to see animals in their ears when you examine them or to believe they are a different age from what they actually are will fire their imagination and make them curious in and more comfortable with you.

Primary school-aged children are old enough to have conversations about their pets, favourite toys, TV shows or movies (merchandised clothing they are wearing or accessories they are holding can give clues to these), their friends, teachers or school. Other rapport-building strategies include:

- greeting children as well as parents
- asking their name (even though you already know it) and/or what they like to be called
- asking their age (even though you already know it)
- asking about their pets
- if present, engaging the siblings too (e.g. asking a small child whether he or she is helping Mummy with the new baby)
- talking at their level, not down to them (e.g. child sitting on parent's knee, or the doctor squatting down or sitting on the floor)
- having a vague idea of current children's films, TV shows and their characters (e.g. Disney movies, Thomas the Tank Engine, The Wiggles)
- having toys in the room, both displayed for them to play with and for you to bring out as a surprise
- having special stickers or stamps (e.g. for the backs of hands)
- blowing bubbles (particularly to distract post-vaccination)[1]
- showing them and letting them hold examination equipment before you use it
- treating them as individuals to be engaged, not clinical puzzles to be solved (this is especially important for children with special needs, who may have greater communication challenges and may also be more used to being treated as a medical condition)

All of this effort will help set the scene for easier history taking and physical examination.

Parent–child interaction

It is advisable to observe carefully the parent–child interaction at all times, including in the waiting room (sometimes you will hear a dysfunctional parent–child interaction before you see it!). The parent's manner in talking to and handling the child will provide useful clues about any possible problems in terms of the parent's ability to nurture the child adequately, and how well they are coping, especially in the postnatal period.[2]

An approach to the parent

Parenting has recently become a lot more complicated. Controversies have arisen and flourished, such as those over vaccination and supposed adverse reactions or parenting styles (e.g. 'attachment parenting'). Much of this is driven by information on the internet, with mothers in particular increasingly spending time on 'mummy blogs' and parenting websites.

Cultural backgrounds also often strongly influence attitudes to aspects of parenting such as how to communicate with children, diet, discipline and punishment, and the role of the mother or father.

Being a parent is laden with intense emotion, and this intensity can lead to very concrete beliefs about different parenting issues (e.g. that MMR vaccination causes autism, that hitting a child improves behaviour). Being aware of these possibilities and not 'putting your foot in it' by making assumptions about parenting attitudes can help avoid communication breakdowns with the parents of your paediatric patients.

History

Obtaining information in the following sequence is recommended:

- *presenting problem* or problems (focus on this first):
  - allow the parents to elaborate without interruption
  - be a listener
  - never judge a parental concern as trivial (especially with a new parent)
- *past history:*
  - medical and surgical history
  - pregnancy, birth and neonatal history
  - vaccination history, medications and allergies
- *family history* (e.g. inherited disorders)
- *growth* (percentiles) and feeding/diet
- *development:*
  - gross motor
  - fine motor
  - speech and communication
  - social skills
- *family and social function* (relationships, behaviour, sleep)

Physical examination

As mentioned above, the approach to the child and parent from the waiting room will help determine the ease or difficulty of examining a child. A good aphorism is 'Win the child, win the mother (parent)'.

Observation

As always, observation is critical. Not only looking at the parent–child interaction, but closely observing the appearance and behaviour of a child can give a multitude of clues as to how unwell the child is. What is the child's general appearance? How active and alert is the child? How interactive is he or she with you and the parents? Is he or she breathing comfortably? Does the child look distressed? This information should be recorded in the medical record as the first line of examination (i.e. above the 'obs').

Growth and development should always be assessed when seeing a child (see below) and the growth parameters are part of the general measurable observations. Temperature should be recorded, but the presence of fever, the degree of fever and the response to antipyretics are poor predictors of serious disease.[3] Also, the thermometers parents and GPs use are often unreliable—tympanic and per axilla thermometers miss a lot of raised temperatures found on PR measurement.[4] A raised temperature tells you something is going on, and not much else. Caveats to this are children in the first 3 months of life, or those in special circumstances (such as those who are immunocompromised) or the worrying presentation of fever combined with drowsiness and pallor (see CHAPTER 96).

90

Increasingly, oxygen saturation measurement is being incorporated into the general observations of children in general practice, especially in children with a significant respiratory infection.

Observations of the child, parents and their interactions are also important in picking up clues concerning psychosocial issues, such as family dysfunction (e.g. marital issues, drug and alcohol abuse in parents, mental health issues in parents), attachment issues, neglect or child abuse (see CHAPTER 95).

Achieving cooperation of small children

Children, especially if they are sick and irritable, can be very difficult to examine and may be most uncooperative, particularly if distressed by past experiences. However, they can be readily distracted, a characteristic that the family doctor can use effectively to achieve some degree of cooperation.

It is generally better to examine younger children on their parent's lap. An older child can be made to feel 'grown up' and important by being examined on the couch (a good strategy if unsure is to ask them what they would prefer first).

Distraction and humour

A variety of techniques can be used to distract the small child or make a game of the physical examination. Individual doctors will often develop their own repertoire of jokes, pretend play and sleight of hand to get the job done without distressing child and parent. Apart from the distress, it is easier to get a good look at an eardrum or to hear a heart murmur when a child is not crying or fighting your invasion of their personal space.

Techniques include:

- tickling games
- peek-a-boo
- using pretend animal noises
- looking for/hearing animals, fairies, monsters, trains (or whatever the child is most interested in at the time) in the child's ears, mouth, chest or abdomen
- getting the older child to block the non-examined ear with a finger to stop the light going through his or her head
- toys (including those that make a noise) being held by your non-examining hand, the parent, a nurse or medical student
- bubbles (and games popping bubbles)
- animal images on stethoscope heads
- images drawn on the unused end of spatulas[5]
- a musical or moving toy above an examination couch
- distracting conversation while examining an abdomen ('how old are you *really?*')
- distracting images (such as a home page of their favourite TV or film character) on your computer screen

Despite your best efforts, sometimes it just doesn't work, especially with a sick child. In these circumstances, you should give clear instructions in advance to the parent (who will often be flustered) on how to best restrain the distressed child. Talk slowly, simply and, if necessary, loudly (if the child is crying), so the parent can understand. Don't ask the child for permission in these circumstances; the answer will be no! The doctor's tone of voice and body language should display to both parent and child that he or she is calm, in charge and not bothered by crying, screaming or lashing out by the child. Getting angry at the child can make the situation worse.

Growth and development

Checking a child's growth and development is a core role of the GP, as we will generally see an infant in our practice quite frequently. By definition, the neonatal period is 28 days post-birth, while infancy is 1–12 months of age. The immunisation visits, routine baby and child checks in the Personal Health Record (PHR, see below) and other visits for viral URTIs and other presentations provide perfect opportunities for GPs to assess appropriate growth and development over time.

This longitudinal monitoring is more reliable at picking up issues than screening programs, which are a mere snapshot. That is why growth parameters (weight, height/length and head circumference, known as anthropometric data) and a quick developmental check at each visit should be done.

In terms of growth, if there are concerns—either of crossing growth percentiles, or worse, of decreasing growth parameters—then obviously further exploration and possible investigation is warranted (see the section on failure to thrive in CHAPTER 91).

Development is normally thought of in 4 domains: gross motor, fine motor, speech/communication and social development. Even if not doing a formal screening check from the PHR or other sources, a few screening questions from each domain will help pick up developmental concerns (see TABLE 90.1). Gross motor and fine motor are grouped together, as are speech/communication and social development for simplicity, and useful screening questions at each visit on the Australian Immunisation Program are suggested). A useful standardised screening tool to use for further evaluation in a GP setting, if there are concerns regarding development, is the Denver-II Developmental Screening Test,[6] and any significant concerns regarding development should have specialist review.

Gross motor development

The neurological control of the infant's body travels from the top down (caudo-equinal) and the inside out (see FIG. 90.1). It is analogous to a flag unfolding. If you are in an art class drawing an adult, you will draw the hips at the halfway point, the nipple line a quarter of the way down and the knees three-quarters of the way down. If you divide the first 12 months of a child's life into quarters, you will quite conveniently find the gross motor development roughly progressing down at these points (see FIG. 90.1). That is, at 3 months a baby should have control of his or her chest, at 6 months the hips (sitting usually happens at 7–8 months; see FIG. 90.2), at 9 months the knees (e.g. crawling, bum-shuffling or commando crawling), and at 1 year the feet (standing holding on, not necessarily walking).[7,8]

Table 90.1 Developmental milestones to check at vaccination visits

Age	Gross motor/fine motor milestones	Social/speech/communication milestones
6 weeks	• Eyes mostly moving together • Some head control—not flopping everywhere • Symmetrical movements of limbs	• Cooing (vowels) emerging • Starting to smile (probably) • Some brief eye contact
4 months	• Hands to midline and then to mouth • Has hand regard • Lifts knees • Tracks objects through 180 degrees • Lifts head up 90 degrees when lying prone • Grasps objects handed to him or her	• Cooing well established • Social smiling (smiling in response to a smile) and laughs • Eye contact more prolonged at times • Babble (consonants) emerging (possibly)
6 months	• Propped up sitting (independent sitting 7–8 months) • Hands down in front of him or her, hands to feet • Keeping head level with body when pulled to a sitting position • Rolling-up on extended arm when placed in prone and creeping when placed in prone • Possibly bangs objects on a surface	• Babbling well established • Quietens and attends when spoken to (listening) • 'Vocal play'—experimenting with new sounds (e.g. blowing raspberries) • Enjoys interactive games • Smiles when sees parent • Laughs/squeals with delight
12 months	• Takes weight on feet when feet plonked on ground in standing position (parachutes them) or standing holding onto furniture • Transitions by moving in and out of positions • Cruising (probably) and crawling • Points and follows a point (possibly) • Grasps with index and thumb • Claps hands • Waves goodbye	• Lots of conversational babble • A couple of words ('Mum', 'Dad', other) probably • Possible separation and/or stranger anxiety • Looks for objects out of direct line of vision (dropped toy) • Co-looking at pictures in books or objects (shared attention) • Possible pointing or following a point ('look at the . . .') • Waves bye-bye
18 months	• Walks well and probably holding hand upstairs • Climbs on and off everything • Attempts a jump • Isolated 'tip to tip' pincer • Bilateral play—hands doing different things • Eyes point, focus and track a moving object • Posting objects into containers	• Follows 1-step commands (when he or she wants to) • Does pretend play—tea sets, dolls, kitchen toys • Interested in everything, especially people • Pointing and following a point well established • Good understanding of what is said, maybe developing lots of words (or soon) • Points to body parts • Uses at least 2 words by 16.5 months
3.5–4 years	• Moves towards learning to ride a bike • Catches a ball onto chest • Catches a larger ball with the hands • Throws a ball overarm • Hops • Washes and dries hands • Does puzzles independently	• Clear and intelligible speech • Able to have a long reciprocal (back and forth) conversation with parents and siblings/peers • Plays with siblings/peers • Unwanted behaviours not standing out among peers (e.g. childcare, preschool)

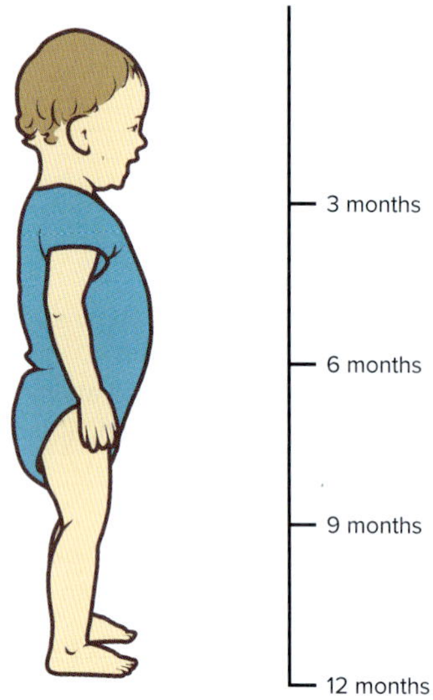

FIGURE 90.1 With gross motor development, at 3 months you are at the chest, at 6 months the hips, at 9 months the knees and at 12 months you have control of the feet

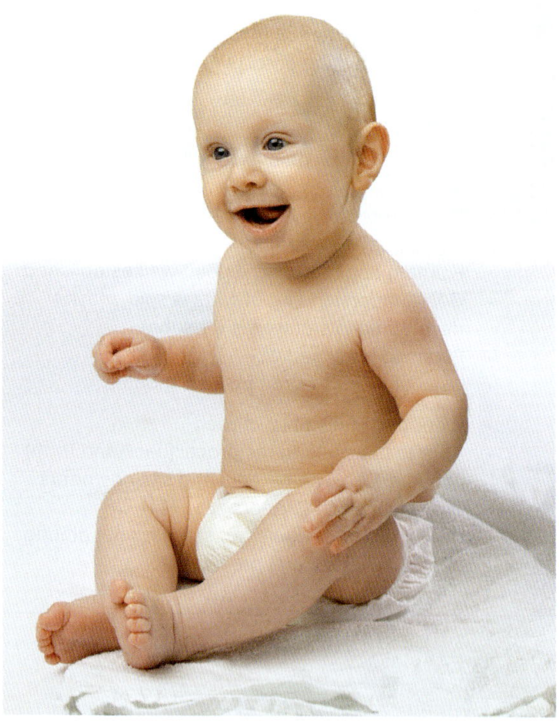

FIGURE 90.2 Normally a child will sit without support at 7–8 months

Beyond 12 months, children will expand this neurological connection into increasingly complex activities (see TABLE 90.2).

Table 90.2 Gross motor skills we want to see emerge (12 months to 6 years)

- **2 years**—walking up stairs holding onto an adult hand, and possibly attempting alternating feet with each stair
- **2½ years**—observing a child being able to jump
- **3 years**—starting to try and to use a tricycle
- **5–6 years**—weaning the trainer wheels off the bike
- **6 years**—skipping

Note: any loss of gross motor (or any other developmental) skill is a red flag.

Fine motor development

Fine motor development mimics that of gross motor, with a steady progression down the body over the first year of life then an 'unfolding' pattern of control of movement with extension and opening out of joints (particularly hands and fingers) followed by an increasing complexity of movements. An easy way to remember the principles of fine motor development is to think of the first 9 months in terms of whole-hand activity, and the second 9 months (9–18 months of age) as individual digit activity[7,8] (see TABLE 90.3).

Speech and communication development

Newborns squawk, squeak and cry. At around 1–2 months, cooing (vowels that use the vocal cords) will start to appear, much to the parents' delight. Between 3 and 6 months, babble (using consonants—that is, involving the tongue and lips to change sounds) will appear. The babble then becomes something the baby starts to play with, and then banters back-and-forth with the parent and others. This 'conversational babble' becomes more sophisticated over the second half of the first year. Into this conversational babble, the first words appear, usually at the end of the first year.

In the second year, there is frequently a rapid expansion in vocabulary around the middle of the year, with girls often having this expansion earlier than boys. Receptive language usually precedes expression, so at the 18-month check, even if a child is not saying many words, his or her increasing understanding of speech should be evident.

Between 18 months and 3 years, the combination of words and small sentences and increasingly

Table 90.3	Fine motor skills we like to see emerge over the first 18 months
Whole-hand activities (0–9 months)	
• **3–6 months**—includes grasping objects passed to the child, looking at objects he or she is holding ('object regard') and banging objects onto a surface, such as a tray in a high chair. • **6–9 months**—banging objects together. By 9 months, babies should be doing hand-to-hand transfers and purposefully releasing objects.	
Individual finger activities (9–18 months)	
• **Pinching** (pulp-to-pulp), **pincing** (tip-to-tip with curled fingers) and **pointing**, all of which can emerge progressively. • **Pointing** is an important milestone, and is often there by 12 months and should be there by 18 months. Prior to children developing their own point, they will reach out towards things, straightening out their fingers as they reach. This action will be followed by the index finger being straightened in isolation while the other fingers are curled. We start in the first year of life by 'following a point'; that is, looking at an object when someone says 'look at the . . .' As well as following a point, children will often point at themselves by 12 months. A young child points for several different reasons. Sometimes it is to share something interesting with another person, sometimes it is to get something they want and sometimes it is to find out what something is called.	

reciprocal (back-and-forth) conversation expand markedly. Articulation also improves over this time, with around 25% of articulation intelligible at 18 months, 50–75% intelligible at 2 years and 75–100% at 3 years. Other articulation issues such as lisps and stutters can also be important.

Social development

As a species, human beings are very socially immature at the time of birth. We are completely dependent on our carer, and remain so for a long time. Soon, though, through attachment, a baby will learn social skills from his or her parents by having a *shared understanding*. This is where the baby's and (usually) the mother's thoughts connect—a 'meeting of minds'.[2]

At around 6 months of age, separation anxiety[9] will usually appear. Separation anxiety is a normal developmental phenomenon as the infant becomes more aware of object permanence (something existing when it is out of sight). Parents, particularly mothers, may worry that they are doing something wrong by causing distress through separation (e.g. leaving the baby in the cot to self-settle), though this is something that we want the child to learn to handle. A stepladder approach (gently increasing the exposure to separation as the child increases the skill to cope) will help. Separation anxiety often peaks around 14–18 months and then decreases through the preschool years.

Stranger anxiety,[10] usually appearing around 7–9 months and reducing after 14 months of age, is similar in many ways to separation anxiety. It too is best managed through a gradual exposure, especially when the child is feeling comfortable.

Tantrums,[11] which are common between 18 months and 3 years (or older), occur because the child lacks the skills to deal with an emotionally challenging event. If a child is not developing some coping skills through this period, his or her social development should be assessed.

In the second year of life, two emerging skill sets dominate social development: speech and play, particularly pretend play.[2,7,8] Play is far more important than children simply acting out their wishes. It's the training ground for life, it's how children learn to interact with others and the world. Deficits in the social use of speech and pretend play should alert the GP to consider autism (see Red flags for autism box, and CHAPTER 94).

GUIDELINES FOR FEEDING INFANTS

The benefits of breastfeeding

For the infant, the benefits include a potential lower risk of:

- gastrointestinal and respiratory infections
- asthma
- otitis media
- urinary tract infections
- necrotising enterocolitis
- insulin-dependent diabetes
- inflammatory bowel disease
- lymphoma
- atopy

The benefits for the mother include:

- a potential lower risk of postpartum bleeding
- delayed resumption of ovulation
- improved bone mineralisation postpartum
- potential lower risk of ovarian and postmenopausal breast cancer

Breastfeeding also improves bonding, is less costly and is beneficial to the environment. Most

(96%) Australian women initiate breastfeeding, but almost a third will have introduced formula or stopped breastfeeding by 3 months, and few will achieve the goal of exclusive breastfeeding to 6 months (EBF6). This goal is recommended in the WHO and NHMRC guidelines and endorsed by the RACGP, but other guidelines suggest exclusive breastfeeding to 4–6 months (EBF4-6), with the introduction of solids at this age. It is also recommended that the woman continues to breastfeed while introducing appropriate solid food until 12 months of age and beyond, and for as long as the mother and infant desire. Exclusively breastfed infants do not require additional fluids up to 6 months of age.

Formulas

If formula is used, a cow's milk-based type should be used up until 12 months (note: all infant formulas available in Australia are iron-fortified). Specialty formulas are indicated only for confirmed pathology. If a woman cannot or chooses not to breastfeed, it is important that she does not feel that she is being judged, as postpartum women are vulnerable to suggestions of lactation failure, which is a risk factor for postnatal depression.

Cow's milk itself should not be given as the main drink to infants under 12 months, though small amounts may be used in the preparation of solid foods. The only other fluid besides breast milk and formulas suitable to be given to infants is boiled and cooled tap water (i.e. no bottled water, juice, cordial or other beverages).

Starting solid foods

Taking into account allergic considerations and best research evidence, the Murdoch Children's Research Institute recommends:

- solid foods should be introduced at around 6 months
- these should include cooked egg, peanut butter, dairy and wheat products
- this advice applies to all babies, including those at risk of allergy, as research shows that early exposure may reduce the risk of eczema and food allergies
- women are advised against hypoallergenic hydrolysed formula to prevent allergy

Solids should be introduced one at a time. They should be offered after a feed or between feeds of milk.

Examples of solid foods for beginners are:

- baby rice cereal mixed with the usual milk or cooled boiled water
- fruits such as banana, cooked apple or pear
- pureed meat and poultry dishes

The texture should be pureed (no lumps) at first. Introduce a new food only after 3–4 days, early in the day. Start with 1–2 teaspoons of solids and build up to three meals a day at your baby's own pace. Lumpy foods can be introduced at 6–9 months, as by this time babies learn to chew.

By 9–10 months, more solids should be eaten each mealtime and the milk gradually decreased. Foods with poor nutritional value and high saturated fats, added sugars (which will increase risk of dental caries) and added salt should be avoided. Honey should be avoided because of the risk of botulism. Hard, small, round (e.g. whole nuts) and/or sticky foods are not recommended because of choking and aspiration risk. Low-fat milks should not be used in the first 2 years of life, and soy and other milks (e.g. goat's milk, sheep's milk, coconut milk, almond milk) are inappropriate alternatives to breast or formula or pasteurised whole cow's milk.

From 12 months onwards, cow's milk can be introduced and more solid foods, especially meats, vegetables and fruits. From 12 months, milk and other drinks should be offered in a cup rather than a feeding bottle (i.e. no need for tipping cups or transitional bottles) and toddler milks and supplements are not required for healthy children.

Toilet training

As a rule, children will learn to use the toilet when they are ready.

The ages by which most children are fully trained are:

- daytime—between 2½ and 4 years
- night-time—by 8 years of age

Once they start training it can take weeks to months to achieve dryness or the ability to open their bowels on the toilet.

General rules for parents

- Be relaxed about toilet training.
- Avoid rushing toilet training.
- Do not force your child to go to the toilet.
- Nagging does not work; a positive-reinforcement approach is far better. This can include reward systems such as reward charts and stickers.
- Punishing will not work.

Indications that a child is ready to start toilet training

- Interest in others going to the toilet
- Has a dry nappy for 1–2 hours or more

- Tells you when they have wet or soiled their nappy or are about to go
- Doesn't like wearing a nappy, especially when it is wet or soiled
- Has the motor skills to pull training pants up and down and get on and off the toilet (may need a step) or potty

Best times to sit children on the toilet

- First thing in the morning
- After meals
- When you sense their need to go
- Before going out
- Upon returning home

Key points for parents

- Consider using a potty or toilet with a seat ring and a step.
- Explain the process in simple terms (there are good resources available, such as books suitable for children of this age).
- Sit both boys and girls on the toilet to pass urine.
- Do not force them if they refuse to use it.
- Help the child relax on the toilet (e.g. using distraction, or having favourite toys).
- Stop using nappies (except when sleeping).
- Don't make a fuss if there are any accidents.
- If the training upsets them, wait for a month and try again.

Child safety

Parents will often be bombarded with child safety messages, many of them valid but many of them not. An excellent resource to point them towards is <www.kidsafe.com.au>, which gives reliable advice on child safety issues.

Table 90.4 Accidents don't have to happen: key points

- Have cupboards in which medicines and household chemicals are stored made child-resistant. Pesticides and petroleum products should be locked away in the shed. Don't store them in ordinary food and drink containers.
- Fires and radiators should be adequately guarded.
- Cords on electrical food and drink heaters need to be shortened or hooked up out of toddlers' reach. Do not use tablecloths. Put hot food and drinks into the centre of the table.
- Fit dummy plugs in unused power points.
- Restrain children in cars according to child-restraint guidelines.
- Infants are safest if they remain in a rear-facing restraint as long as they still fit into it.
- Supervise your toddler at all times in or near water. The swimming pool needs to be adequately fenced in (on all four sides and with a secure gate)—and never leave a child alone in the bath.
- Keep matches and lighters locked away and out of reach. Put scissors, knives, needles and pins well out of reach, too.
- Have the play yard safely fenced in, away from the street.
- Parents: walk right round your car before reversing down the drive, or place your child in the car first.

Personal health record

Many children have a personal health record (PHR), which is given to the child's parents or carers as a means of improving health care delivery, including the enhancement of preventive care. The PHR is a small, loose-leaf booklet with a sturdy plastic cover that can be easily carried around by the parent. The contents can vary from one state to another (as does the colour of the cover) and from edition to edition but generally it contains:

- records of birth details and newborn examination
- percentile charts for weight gain
- visual check
- hearing check
- developmental check
- immunisation schedules and recordings
- progress notes
- advice on accident prevention (see TABLE 90.4)
- other health educational material

The PHR provides a very practical method of promoting communication between various health professionals involved in the child's care and also between the family and their doctor. It promotes the concept of self-care by encouraging a sense of responsibility in parents for the child's health and is also a medium for enhancing preventive care, especially with regard to immunisation, growth and development.

Immunisation schedule

Refer to CHAPTER 9 and <www.immunise.health.gov.au> for updates.

Diagnostic triads for children

The following is a selection of childhood disorders. The arrow represents a pointer to a possible diagnosis and is of course not conclusive.

90

Acute–subacute onset

DxT Arthralgia (lower limbs) + rash (buttocks, legs) ± abdominal pain ➜ Henoch–Schönlein purpura
DxT Pallor + drowsiness + fever ➜ meningitis
DxT Pallor + abdominal pain (severe and intermittent) + inactivity ➜ intussusception
DxT (<12 months): drowsiness + cough + wheezing ➜ bronchiolitis
DxT (<3 months, usually male): weakness + weight loss + vomiting (severe, intermittent) ➜ pyloric stenosis
DxT (Neonate): vomiting (after first feeds) + drooling + abdominal distension ➜ oesophageal or duodenal atresia
DxT Malaise + pallor + bone pain ➜ acute lymphatic leukaemia
DxT Malaise + pallor + oral problems (gingival hypertrophy, bleeding, ulceration) ➜ acute myeloid leukaemia
DxT Abdominal pain + pallor + a/n/v ➜ acute appendicitis
DxT Abdominal pain + malar flush + fever ± URTI ➜ mesenteric adenitis
DxT Drowsiness + tachypnoea + chest wall recession ➜ pneumonia
DxT Drowsiness + fever + purpuric rash ➜ meningococcal infection
DxT URTI + brassy cough + inspiratory stridor ➜ croup
DxT Coughing + wheezing + chest wall recession ➜ asthma or aspirated foreign body
DxT Fever + conjunctivitis + skin changes (cracked red lips, maculopapular rash, erythema of palms/soles, desquamation of fingertips) ➜ Kawasaki syndrome

Congenital syndromes

DxT Large ears + long narrow face + large genitals ➜ fragile X syndrome
DxT Small extremities (hands, feet, genitals) + narrow forehead + eating disorder ➜ Prader–Willi syndrome
DxT 'Elfin' face + low-set ears + cardiac murmur ➜ Williams syndrome
DxT (Female): short + webbed neck + pigmented naevi ± cardiac disorder ➜ Turner syndrome
DxT Short + webbed neck + facial disproportion (broad forehead, ptosis, low-set ears, etc.) ± cardiac disorder ➜ Noonan syndrome

Chronic

DxT Malaise + abdominal pain (vague) + abnormal behaviour ➜ lead poisoning
DxT (<2 years): lethargy + irritability + pallor ➜ iron deficiency anaemia
DxT Fever + malaise (extreme) + a/n/v ± anaemia ➜ neuroblastoma
DxT Headache + a/n/v + ataxia ➜ medulloblastoma
DxT Speech communication skills + poor socialisation + repetitive/obsessive behaviour/restriction of interests ➜ autism spectrum disorder

Older children

DxT (Male): snorting, blinking, etc. + oral noises (e.g. grunts, hisses) ± loud expletives ➜ Tourette syndrome
DxT Mid to low back pain/discomfort + inability to touch toes + kyphosis ➜ Scheuermann disorder
DxT Knee pain (after activity) + tender knee 'lump' + pain on kneeling ➜ Osgood–Schlatter disorder
DxT (Adolescent): limp + knee pain + hip pain ➜ slipped capital femoral epiphysis

Patient education resources

Hand-out sheets from *Murtagh's Patient Education* 7th edition:

- Feeding your baby
- Normal development in children
- Toilet training your child

References

1 Harrison D et al. Pain management strategies used during early childhood immunisation in Victoria. J Paediatr Child Health, 2013; 41 (4): 313–18.
2 Berk LE. *Awakening Children's Minds.* New York: Oxford University Press, 2001.
3 Royal Children's Hospital. *Clinical Practice Guidelines: Fever,* October 2011 <www.rch.org.au/clinicalguide/guideline_index/Febrile_Child/> (accessed 15/6/2014).
4 Canadian Paediatric Society. Temperature measurement in paediatrics. Paediatr Child Health, 2000; 5 (5): 273–6.
5 Malcher G. Spatula sketches for children. Aust Fam Physician, 1990; 19: 1441.
6 Glascoe F et al. Accuracy of the Denver-II in developmental screening. Pediatrics, 1992; 89 (6): 1221–5.

7 The Developmental Medicine Center, Children's Hospital Boston. Development screening tool kit for primary care providers <www.developmentalscreening.org/> (accessed 23/6/2014).
8 Raising Children Network. Your guide to child development, 27 June 2014 <www.raisingchildren.net.au/articles/grow_and_learn_together_child_development_guide.html> (accessed 3/7/2014).
9 Women and Children's Health Network. Parenting and child health: separation anxiety, 3 October 2013 <www.cyh.com/HealthTopics/HealthTopicDetails.aspx?p=114&np=141&id=1848> (accessed 23/6/2014).
10 Raising Children Network. Stranger anxiety, 24 August 2011 <www.raisingchildren.net.au/articles/fear_of_strangers.html> (accessed 23/6/2014).
11 Women and Children's Health Network. Parenting and child health: tantrums, 30 January 2014 <www.cyh.com/HealthTopics/HealthTopicDetails.aspx?p=114&np=141&id=1775> (accessed 23/6/2014).
12 Wray J, Knott H, Silove N. Language disorders and autism. Med J Aust, 2005; 182 (7): 354–60.
13 Royal Australian College of General Practitioners. Position statement on breastfeeding, 2007 <www.racgp.org.au/download/documents/Policies/Clinical/breastfeeding_position_statement.pdf> (accessed 29/6/2014).
14 National Health and Medical Research Council. Eat for health: infant feeding guidelines: information for health workers, summary, 2013. <www.nhmrc.gov.au/_files_nhmrc/publications/attachments/n56b_infant_feeding_guideline_summary.pdf> (accessed 29/6/2014).
15 Australian Society of Clinical Immunology and Allergy. Infant feeding advice, 2010. <www.allergy.org.au/images/stories/aer/infobulletins/2010pdf/ASCIA_Infant_Feeding_Advice_2010.pdf> (accessed 29/6/2014).
16 Raising Children Network. Toilet training, 25 October 2010. <www.raisingchildren.net.au/articles/toilet_training.html> (accessed 29/6/2014).
17 NHS choices. Potty problems and toilet training tips, 4 February 2013. <www.nhs.uk/Conditions/pregnancy-and-baby/pages/potty-training-tips.aspx#close> (accessed 29/6/2014).
18 National Guidelines for Safe Restraint of Children Travelling in Motor Vehicles. Neuroscience Research Australia, 2 July 2013 <www.neura.edu.au/crs-guidelines> (accessed 29/6/2014).

Resources

The Australasian Society for Clinical Immunology and Allergy (ASCIA) Guidelines

91 Specific problems of children

Children are not simply micro-adults, but have their own specific problems.

BELA SCHICK (1877–1967)

The family doctor usually treats children for common minor complaints such as non-serious viral respiratory infections and minor skin problems, offering parental advice and reassurance. Many of these everyday problems are discussed in this chapter, while immunisations (CHAPTER 9) and more complicated problems such as anaemia, diarrhoea and chronic cough are covered elsewhere (see PART 3, Problem solving in general practice).

Crying and fussing in infants

Crying and fussing is a very common concern in the infant in the first few months. The term 'colic' (which is still widely used) needs to be used with caution, as it infers something is wrong with the gut of the infant, when most of the time this is not the case.[1]

The normal pattern is for crying to start increasing around two weeks of age, to peak around two months, and then settle down around three to four months of age, perhaps five. On average, a baby cries or fusses for 3 hours a day. The amount of crying varies from baby to baby, but all babies cry—and not just human babies; in the early months babies of other mammal species cry as well. This is a survival instinct, to get the full attention of the carer and to establish attachment. It can also cause a great deal of distress for a mother or other carer, so active listening, careful assessment to exclude other causes and advice and reassurance are important.

Management

- History—crying pattern and duration, assessment of the child's temperament and parents' coping abilities.
- Perform careful physical examination, including growth parameters, feeding and settling pattern, and development.
- Reassure parents that extra attention will not affect the baby but overstimulation should be avoided.
- Give parental reassurance and education (including advice on soothing techniques and coping strategies).

Practice tip—the period of purple crying[1]

A useful term developed by specialists in this area is 'the period of PURPLE crying' <www.purplecrying.org>. The letters of the word 'purple' stand for characteristics of this period of crying, namely:

P = **P**eak—your baby may cry more each week, the most at 2 months, then less at 3–5 months
U = **U**nexpected—crying can come and go and you won't know why
R = **R**esists soothing—your baby may not stop crying no matter what you try
P = **P**ain-like face—babies may look like they are in pain, even when they're not
L = **L**ong-lasting—crying can last as much as 5 hours a day, or more
E = **E**vening cluster—your baby may cry more in the late afternoon or evening

Causes (to exclude)

- Cow's milk intolerance
- Lactose intolerance
- Gastro-oesophageal reflux
- Pain from UTIs and other infections, bowel obstruction/hernias, other causes

Soothing techniques

- Gentle stroking and cuddling
- Providing close contact or skin-to-skin contact
- Talking to them, singing to them, smiling at them and rocking them
- Repetitive rocking movements help calm an overstimulated baby's brain

Coping strategies[1]

- Increase carry, comfort, walk and talk responses—the baby may still continue to cry, but there is a reasonable chance the parents may be able to soothe him or her.
- It's okay to walk away—it's important for parents to calm themselves before trying to calm their baby.

- Never shake or hurt a baby—advise that shaking a baby is a critically dangerous thing to do.

It is also useful to advise a parent to try and learn their baby's signals and body language, which are unique for every infant. Some typical body language patterns include:

- tired—stiff, jerky movements, being quiet or still, blank faced, rubbing eyes, moodiness, droopy eyelids or slow blinking and crying
- hungry—open mouth, eager expression and crying
- ready for action—wide open eyes, alert expression and kicking legs
- upset—jerky movements, turning away and crying

Teething

Baby teeth (milk or deciduous teeth)

- Babies usually cut their teeth from age 6 months until 2–3 years.
- The first teeth to appear (which seldom cause discomfort) are usually the lower incisors (during the first year).
- The first and second molars (ages 1–3) tend to cause problems.
- Usually the first set (20 teeth) is complete soon after the second birthday (see FIG. 91.1).

Symptoms

- The gum is slightly swollen and red
- This may cause little or no discomfort but may be quite tender
- The child may be more clingy and fretful, and dribbling more than usual
- Chews and mouths (though mouthing fingers, hands and other objects is a normal infant behaviour, especially from 4 months onwards)
- Irritability and crying (on and off for no more than a few days)

Treatment

Parents are often misinformed about the importance and consequences of teething pain. Reassure parents that teething rarely results in anything more than minor distress, that it does not cause fever, rashes or diarrhoea, and that it will usually settle quickly.

Soothing methods

- Gentle massaging of the gum with the parent's forefinger wrapped in a soft cloth or gauze pad is comforting.
  or
- Allow the baby to chew on a clean, cold, lightly moistened facewasher (a piece of apple can be placed inside the facewasher).
  or
- Give the baby a teething ring (kept cold in the refrigerator) or a teething biscuit.

Medication

Medicine is usually not necessary for teething. Paracetamol should be used only for significant discomfort. Teething gels are salicylate-based and are not recommended.

91

Pitted dark teeth and bruised teeth

Some children who are breastfed for long periods (e.g. 3 years) may develop unsightly pitting of the front surface of their teeth. This will not go away but parents should be reassured that the adult teeth will be normal when they appear.

Bruised teeth can result from minor trauma, with the tooth appearing a grey-brown colour. While a cosmetic issue for some parents, these too are not a concern and the adult tooth will appear and develop normally.

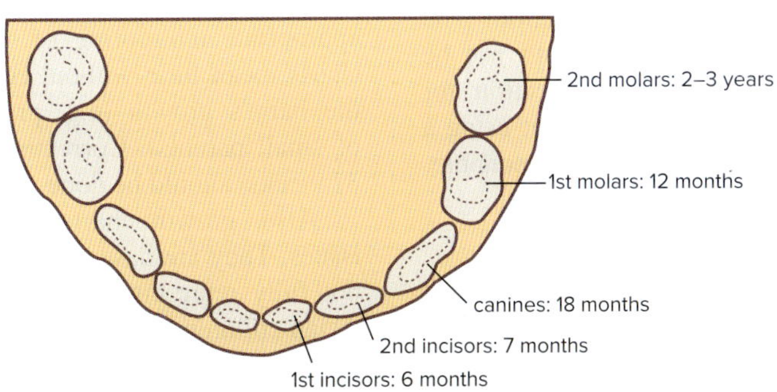

FIGURE 91.1 The lower set of primary teeth with average times of eruption

Thumb sucking

Thumb sucking involves placing the thumb or finger on the roof of the mouth behind the teeth (hard palate) and sucking with the mouth closed. Sucking is a normal and soothing behaviour for the infant, but it can become an entrenched habit. It occurs in children up to the age of 12 years but is most common under the age of 4 years. It usually settles by the early primary school years, and will sometimes stop if the child becomes self-conscious because other children notice. It can cause problems with the child's bite, especially as the adult teeth appear, at about age 7. One effect is that the pressure on the front teeth may cause protrusion of the front teeth (i.e. buck teeth); another is a narrowing of the bite with a gap between the top and bottom incisors, referred to as an open anterior bite. This can also happen with pacifiers. The best approach is for parents to notice when the child is doing it less, and to comment on how grown up the child is becoming, rather than scolding or overly drawing attention to the behaviour.

91

Advice to parents

- No special diet or medication is necessary. Unpleasant-tasting topical applications to the pacifier or thumb are counter-productive.
- For a child over 6 years, carefully observe trigger factors and find ways of avoiding them. Provide distractions.
- Help the child explore other solutions to sooth themselves.
- Give praise and rewards for efforts to stop.

Snuffling infants

Snuffling frequently occurs in normal babies in the few weeks after birth and is not a problem unless it affects feeding. Infants and small children have particularly small noses, which block easily.

Snuffling in older infants is usually caused by rhinitis due to an intercurrent viral infection. The presence of yellow or green mucus should not be a cause for concern and is not an indication for antibiotics. Give reassurance, and advise that using a saline nasal solution to clear congestion is reasonable.

Blocked nasolacrimal duct

About 20% of infants develop watery eyes, but most resolve by 12 months. Excessive eye watering in infants is the key sign that there is inherited narrowing of the nasolacrimal ducts (see FIG. 91.2). It usually becomes obvious in infants between 3 and 12 weeks

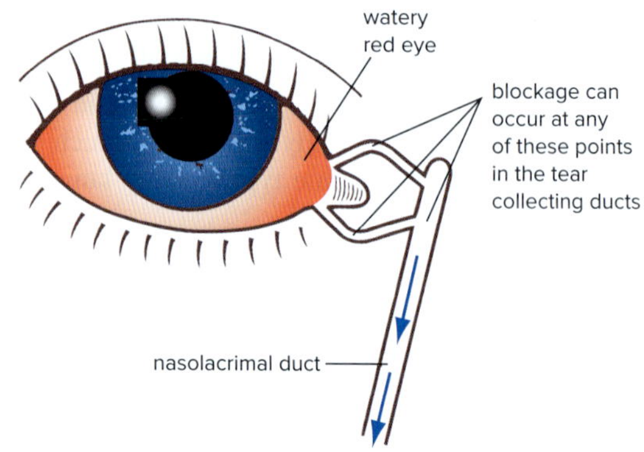

FIGURE 91.2 Blocked nasolactimal duct

and affects one or both eyes. Mucus and mucopus may appear in the tears. The discharge is worse on waking. In some infants, watering and discharge soon after birth indicate that the ducts have failed to open. Infection may intervene (refer to CHAPTER 51) and conjunctivitis can be problematic.

Outcome

In most cases the problem improves spontaneously. Self-correction usually occurs from 6 months of age onwards or even earlier. It remains a matter of controversy whether massage helps or not.

Minor infection can be treated with warm cotton-wool soaks. For more severe blockage, recurrent conjunctivitis or when eye watering has not settled by 12 months, referral to an ophthalmologist for consideration of whether probing is warranted.

Failure to thrive (FTT)[2,3]

It is essential to monitor growth of children, particularly infants (see CHAPTER 90). The sequential plotting of the weight, length and head circumference (anthropometric criteria) on growth charts (see Appendices I–IV) in the personal health record (PHR) and/or the doctor's medical file on the child enables appropriate monitoring of this growth. The growth charts mean little without considering the context of the baby's growth (e.g. premature babies, children of small parents). Correcting for prematurity (under 37 weeks) should be done until the age of 24 months.

Also, growth charts themselves have reliability issues. They are based on Caucasian children and are not fully representative for some other groups (e.g. Asian children tend to be smaller). Growth charts can also vary depending on whether they use data based on populations of exclusively breastfed infants or include formula-fed infants (who tend to grow faster).

Classically, failure to thrive (FTT) has been defined as children whose weight <3rd percentile on ≥2 occasions, or whose weight crosses two centile lines over time. These criteria, however, are met by 5% of infants at some stage, many of whom do not have concerning growth progression; they will also fail to pick up all children who may not be growing adequately. It is therefore important to consider the contextual issues of measurement mentioned above, as well as taking into account the overall clinical picture of the growth over time (e.g. how quickly is the percentile change happening) and the general health and development of the child. While FTT is a useful term to help identify and describe infants and children that may have growth issues, it is not a diagnosis in itself.

Average weight gain/week:

0–3 months	180 g/week
3–6 months	120 g/week
6–9 months	80 g/week
9–12 months	70 g/week

Weight gain slows further after 12 months of age.

Causes

Traditionally, FTT was divided into organic and non-organic causes. It is becoming increasingly recognised that in many cases the cause is multifactorial, including biological, psychosocial and environmental contributors. A practical way of considering potential causes is looking at caloric intake, absorption and expenditure. In many cases (>80%) no cause is found.

Table 91.1	Failure to thrive: causes to consider[2]
Inadequate caloric intake/retention (most common)	• Inadequate amount of food provided • Breastfeeding issues • Physical reasons baby can't feed well (e.g. cleft palate) • Persistent vomiting • Chronic disease causing anorexia
Inadequate absorption	• Coeliac disease • Chronic liver disease • Pancreatic insufficiency (e.g. CF) • Chronic diarrhoea (e.g. protein-losing enteropathy)
Excessive caloric utilisation	• UTIs • Chronic respiratory disease (e.g. severe asthma, bronchiectasis) • Congenital heart disease • Diabetes mellitus • Hyperthyroidism
Other medical causes	• Genetic disorders • Inborn errors of metabolism
Psychosocial factors	• Parental depression • Coercive feeding (feeding becomes a battle) • Distractions at meal times • Poverty (the single biggest risk factor in both developed and developing countries) • Behavioural disorders • Poor social support • Neglect and abuse (risk of child abuse is 4x higher in children with FTT)

History

- Antenatal/birth/postnatal history—including growth parameters
- Feeding history (most important aspect)
  - Infants—BF/attachment, formula feeding, timing, volumes (e.g. weigh infant before and after, mother expressing and measuring breast milk), vomiting?, solids introduction (see CHAPTER 90)
  - Toddlers—types and amounts of foods/liquids (see CHAPTER 90), especially iron-containing foods, food intake inside and outside home, mealtime battles, distractions, food refusal, milk volume, parental food attitudes
- Medical history
- Developmental history (e.g. regression, specific known syndromes)
- Family history (e.g. mid-parental height, parents' or siblings' childhood weight gain)
- Social history (e.g. finance, supports)

Examination

- Growth charts (refer to FIG. 91.3)
- General appearance (does the child look sick/irritable/lethargic? dehydration? loss of subcutaneous fat? pallor? inappropriate bruising or affect)
- Observation of infant feeding and child–parent interaction (a home visit, or assessment by a lactation consultant/early childhood nurse may be useful here)
- Dysmorphic features
- Developmental assessment
- Jaundice/bruising/scratches
- Skin, hair and nails
- ENT

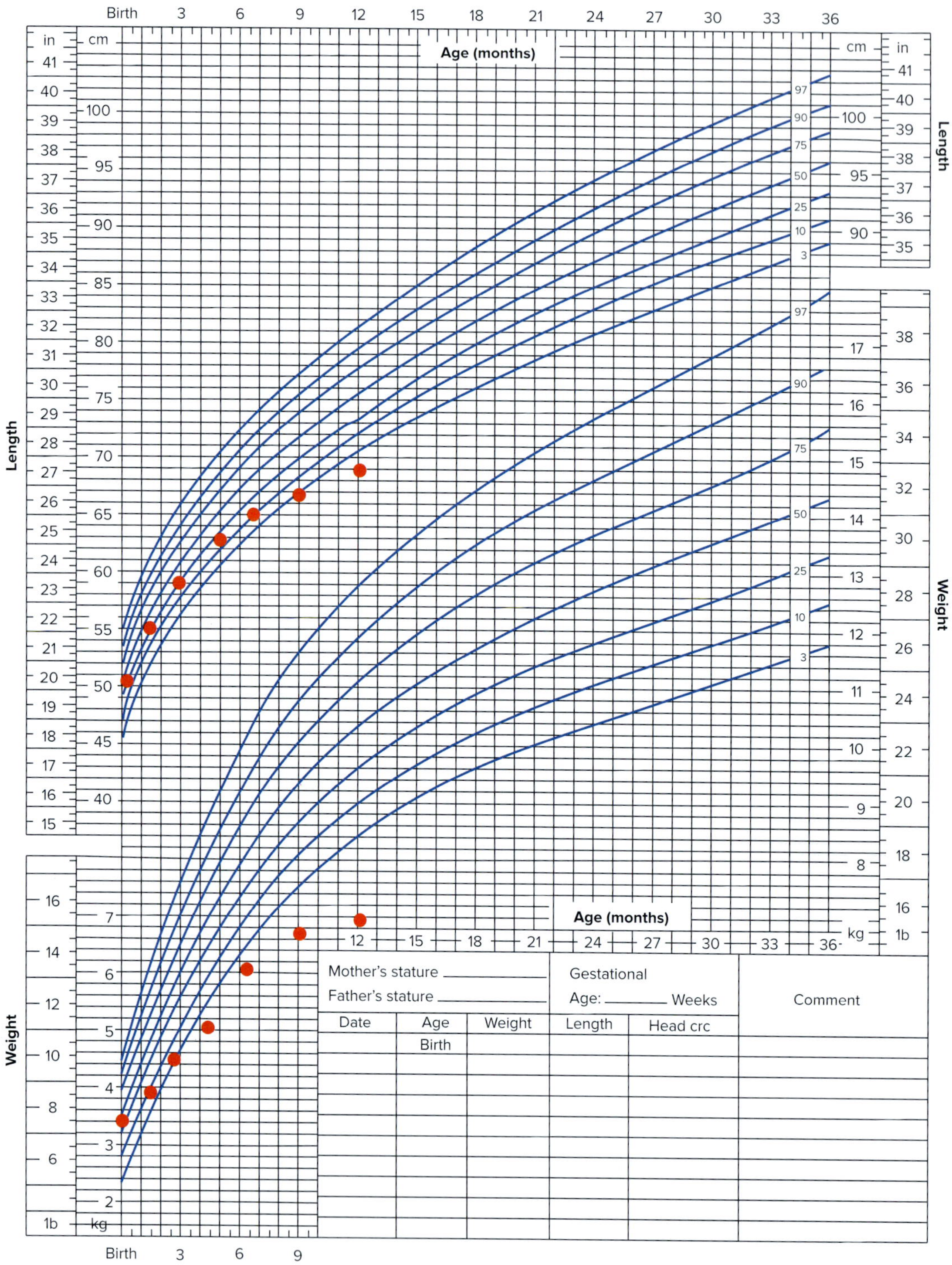

FIGURE 91.3 Example of growth chart with FTT from inadequate calorie intake (the red dots indicate FTT). Note how the weight drop is more marked than the length drop.

- Cardiac/respiratory
- Abdomen (e.g. distention, organomegaly)
- Endocrine (e.g. goitre, urinalysis, finger prick glucose)
- Lymphadenopathy

Investigations

In a healthy infant with no concerns found on history and examination, no investigations are required, and reassuring the family and further monitoring is appropriate. If concerns are found, targeted investigation for these should be done. Simple first-line investigations may include:

- FBC, CRP
- iron studies
- UEC/LFTs
- urine MC&S
- coeliac screen
- stool fat globules/fatty acid crystals

Other issues to consider

Frequent weighing of children may exacerbate parental anxiety. Babies under 3 months of age should not be weighed more than weekly, and not more than fortnightly after that. A paediatric review may be required in more significant FTT situations, and occasionally admission to hospital to further assess feeding, psychosocial aspects and other medical causes. In difficult cases, a team-based approach potentially using paediatricians, lactation consultants, dietitians, early childhood nurses, speech pathologists or psychologists as well as the family doctor can be utilised.

Short stature[4,5,6]

Short stature is considered to be below the 3rd percentile. In general, it is important to differentiate between normal physiological variants of growth and pathological causes.

Causes

1 Familial short stature—this follows the family trend of a genetically small family.
2 Constitutional delay in maturation—a common and normal variant in which the growth spurt is later than average. Bone age is delayed.
3 Pathological causes—of the many causes, some are rare but serious conditions, such as coeliac disease, Crohn disease and chronic kidney failure. These may present with slow growth as the only abnormal sign.

> **Rough rule for expected adult height based on parental height**
>
> - Boys—mean of parents' heights + 5 cm
> - Girls—mean of parents' heights – 5 cm

Recombinant human growth hormone treatment for those children with idiopathic short stature (ISS, a diagnosis of exclusion) increases height in some children, with the range of benefit usually between 3 cm and 7 cm. It is expensive, and while considered safe in the short term, long-term safety is lacking. Specialist advice is recommended.

Tall stature

Tall stature is considered to be above the 97th percentile. It is not a common presenting childhood problem in general practice. The estimated mature height is:

- females: 182.9 cm
- males: 193.1 cm

Causes

- familial (predicted final height should roughly match mid-parental height)
- precocious puberty
- growth hormone excess (pituitary gigantism)
- hyperthyroidism
- syndromic: Marfan, Klinefelter, homocystinuria

Management

As tall stature is generally socially acceptable, reassurance, counselling and education may alleviate the family's concerns. If treatment is considered appropriate, high-dose oestrogen is used in very tall girls (accelerates epiphyseal maturation and reduces final height) while high-dose testosterone is used for boys. The management should be undertaken by endocrinologists. The ideal time to commence hormone therapy is just after the appearance of the first pubertal changes.

Overweight and obese children

Approximately a quarter of Australian children are overweight or obese.[7] A recent national nutrition survey showed that children eat too much saturated fat and sugar and regularly exceed the recommended maximum times spent watching screens.[8] Obesity in childhood increases the risk of adult obesity. Nutritional obesity is associated with growth acceleration and advancement of bone age, while endocrine obesity has the opposite effect. Refer to CHAPTER 78.

Delayed puberty[9]

This is the absence of pubertal development (testicular enlargement in boys or breast development in girls) in:

- girls >13 years
- boys >14 years

Significant causes include:

- constitutional delay of growth and puberty (CDGP) is usually familial and the commonest cause. It is associated with delayed growth and bone age
- chronic illness (e.g. severe asthma, cystic fibrosis, kidney failure)
- poor nutrition and exercise
- anorexia nervosa

Other less common causes include chromosomal abnormalities (e.g. Turner syndrome) and gonadal hormone deficiency (e.g. Kallmann syndrome, post-chemotherapy). Consider referral to a paediatric endocrinologist for investigation and management, which can include testosterone for boys and oestrogen for girls.

Precocious puberty[10]

Puberty is trending earlier than in previous generations, known as the 'secular trend', and is presumed to be due to improved nutrition and absence of chronic disease. True precocious puberty is considered to be:

- girls <8 years
- boys <9 years

Growth spurts will be earlier and bone growth will be advanced, though final adult height may be reduced from what would otherwise be expected due to premature fusion of the long bones (height issues may determine the need for treatment). True precocious puberty is 20 times more common in girls than boys. It is usually idiopathic, though pituitary adenomas are a rare cause and more common as a cause in boys (boys always require brain imaging). Treatments are often not required, but may include gonadotrophin releasing hormone (GnRH) analogues and cyproterone.

Premature thelarche[10]

This is breast development in girls under 8 years old without other pubertal signs. It usually occurs in girls under 3 years and spontaneous regression can be expected. It may present at birth. Observation with reassurance for this benign condition is appropriate.

Premature adrenarche[10]

This is the isolated appearance of pubic hair in boys or girls aged 6–9 years old. There are no other features of virilisation or oestrogenisation, and the hair remains until other signs of puberty appear at the normal time. It is usually a normal variant (no specific treatment necessary) but may rarely signify atypical congenital adrenal hyperplasia. Referral is indicated if any concerns.

Pubertal gynaecomastia[10]

This is a normal variant of male puberty, with a prevalence of about 40–50% and is usually a transient phenomenon, subsiding in 2–3 years.

There is a palpable and/or visible disc of breast tissue, which in boys may feel quite firm and needs to be distinguished from adipose tissue in overweight boys. There is no hormonal or medical treatment and surgical removal is rarely necessary. Advice regarding clothes (e.g. loose T-shirts for social activities or swimming) or explanatory letters to school can be helpful.

Asymmetrical breast development[10]

This may occur in both sexes—in males being a variant of pubertal gynaecomastia and in females part of a normal development process—and reassurance that the breast sizes will usually normalise in time is all that is required. If the discrepancy persists and is causing psychological problems, further strategies, such as prostheses or reconstructive surgery, may be advised by specialists.

Infant breast hyperplasia

A breast 'bud' is common in most term babies and may enlarge with breastfeeding (see FIG. 91.4). Milk may discharge from some ('witches' milk) but reassurance is all that is required (see CHAPTER 101).

Growing pains[11,12]

Growing pains (benign nocturnal limb pains) are real and common (around 1 in 5 children).

Features

- Typical age 3–12 years
- Positive family history
- Usually bilateral and non-articular

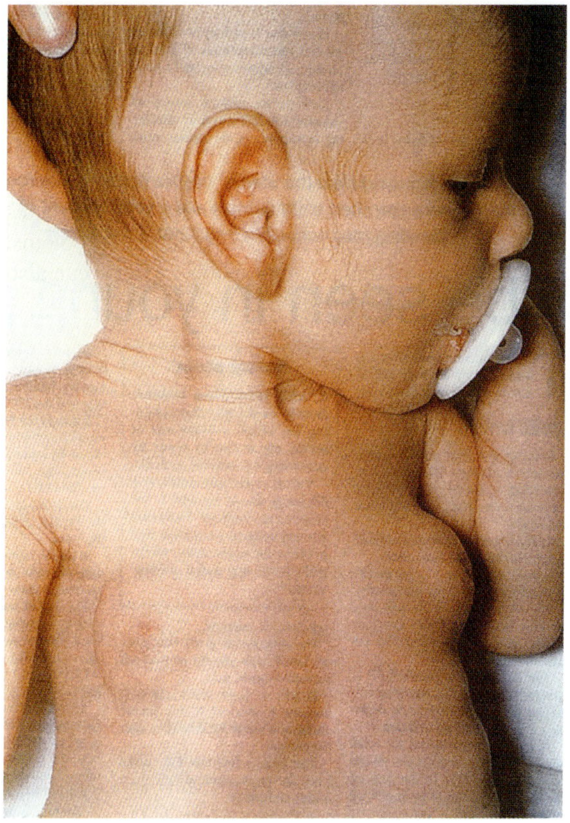

FIGURE 91.4 Breast hyperplasia in a 15-week-old child

- Poorly localised in leg—typical sites include shins, calves, thighs, popliteal fossa (see FIG. 91.5)
- Episodic, with pain-free intervals from weeks to months
- Last minutes to hours, regardless of treatments, and usually gone by the morning
- Usually occur late in the day or during the night
- Normal examination
- No associated symptoms
- No pain or disability next morning (runs okay)
- Very active days or being moody may lead to a 'bad' night

Management

- Problem resolves spontaneously in time
- Reassurance
- Consider analgesic and heat packs (usually unsuccessful)
- Massage is a reasonable option—appears to help
- Check ESR if in doubt

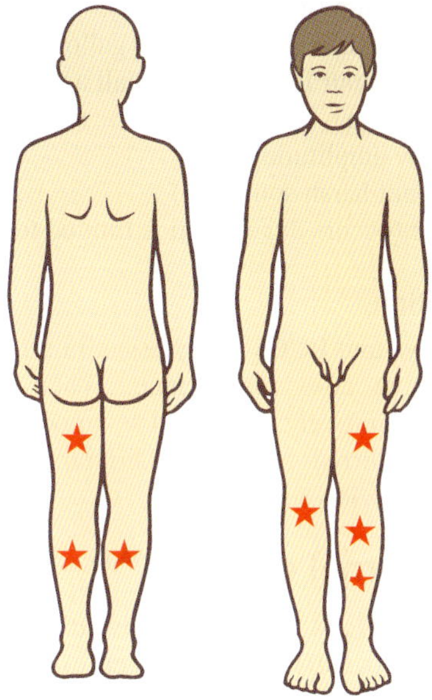

FIGURE 91.5 Growing pains: typical sites of pain

Childhood cardiac murmurs

Many children and infants will be found to have systolic murmurs on routine examination, especially in the presence of a fever, anxiety or fear. The majority, which will be innocent or physiological, are found in asymptomatic children and due to normal turbulence of flow within the heart and great vessels.

Innocent murmurs[13]

An innocent murmur can be diagnosed in children over 12 months of age if the following 4 criteria are met:

- there are no other abnormal physical findings
- the child is asymptomatic (e.g. no dyspnoea, palpitations, fatigue, nausea/vomiting, ongoing cough)
- no history of risk factors for structural heart disease (e.g. family history, maternal gestational DM/alcohol abuse, previous Kawasaki disease/ rheumatic fever, genetic disorders, prematurity)
- auscultatory features typical of an innocent murmur (see 7 Ss below)

In murmurs heard in infants under 12 months of age, the risk of asymptomatic structural heart disease is higher, and further assessment is warranted.

The 7 Ss of innocent murmurs:

1 **S**ensitive (changes with child's position or with respiration)

2 **S**hort duration (not holosystolic)
3 **S**ingle (no associated clicks or gallops)
4 **S**mall (murmur limited to a small area and non-radiating)
5 **S**oft (low amplitude)
6 **S**weet (not harsh sounding)
7 **S**ystolic (occurs during and is limited to systole)

Investigation

Chest X-rays and ECGs rarely assist in the diagnosis, and can give false reassurance. When a murmur cannot be definitively diagnosed as innocent, the child should be referred for echocardiography, paediatric cardiologist review or both.

Nocturnal enuresis[14,15]

Nocturnal enuresis (NE), or bedwetting, is urinary incontinence occurring during sleep in a child with a developmental age of 5 or older. An absence of other urinary symptoms (e.g. frequency, urgency, straining or daytime wetting) is referred to as monosymptomatic NE, but if present then the term non-monosymptomatic NE is used. Primary enuresis (80% of cases) occurs in a child who has never had urinary continence for 6 months, and secondary enuresis (20%) occurs after 6 months or more of day and night dryness, and is more commonly associated with organic or psychological causes.

What is normal?

Prevalence:

- 15–20% of 5 year olds
- 5% of 10 year olds
- 1–2% of 15 year olds

The spontaneous resolution of NE is 15% per year. Boys are affected 3 times as much as girls, and there is a strong familial tendency (75% have an affected first degree relative, with maternal enuresis a greater risk factor than paternal enuresis). Twenty per cent of children with NE will also have daytime symptoms.

Aetiology

The causes of NE are not fully understood, but are thought to be multifactorial, including:

- disturbance in arousal—children with NE often do not wake adequately in response to a full bladder
- overactive bladder—which leads to a reduced bladder capacity. Children in this situation will often have daytime symptoms or other urinary symptoms (e.g. urgency, frequency)
- nocturnal polyuria—this is caused by reduced nocturnal vasopressin (which normally reduces nocturnal urine production)

Other common contributing factors include constipation (more than a third of patients) and obstructive sleep apnoea. Both of these should be carefully enquired about in the history. UTIs, diabetes and psychopathology (e.g. behavioural problems, ADHD, stress or trauma, depression, anxiety) can also contribute to and/or are associated with NE.

Assessment

As well as assessing for the above contributing factors, a detailed history of the urinary symptoms and pattern should be taken. This is greatly assisted by getting the parents (and child if old enough) to complete a 48-hour time and volume chart of fluids and urine (including urine symptoms).

Physical examination should include ENT examination (looking for large tonsils or nasal obstruction causing OSA), abdominal examination (large bladder, faecal loading) and a focused neurological examination.

Urinalysis and culture can help detect infection. Blood tests, imaging and urodynamics are not usually required for uncomplicated primary NE. If there are daytime symptoms, significant other urinary symptoms, history or diagnosis of UTIs, structural abnormalities of the urinary system or genitals, secondary enuresis or refractory problems, then further investigations and/or specialist review is warranted.

Advice for parents/child: 'they/you will very likely grow out of it'

Both the parents and child should be reassured that primary NE is common, unlikely to be a medical concern, not the child's fault and will nearly always resolve by itself with time. If the issue is not bothering the child then treatment is not needed. If conducted, treatment should be delayed until the child is able and willing to comply, which is generally around age 7 years.

Tips to help the family deal with the situation

- Do not scold or punish the child.
- Praise the child if achieving dryness.
- Use a night light to help the child who wakes.
- Use absorbent 'pyjama pants' or mattress protectors (absorbent underlays), which can help reduce distress for parents and child, and will not contribute to the enuresis.
- Make sure the child has a shower or bath before going to kindergarten or school (to avoid teasing).

Treatment

The treatment of primary monosymptomatic NE requires educated and motivated child and parents. Guilt, shame and punishment need to be avoided. The child should be involved in the treatment (even though the child didn't cause the problem, he or she has a role in treating it).

Urotherapy

Urotherapy, or improving urination habits, includes increasing daytime fluid intake (to increase bladder capacity and awareness of bladder fullness). Six to eight reasonable-sized drinks spaced throughout the day (not just after school) are recommended (50 ml/kg/day). Regular voiding every 2–3 hours will help the child become more cognitively aware of the bladder sensations.

Promptly and aggressively treating constipation will help bladder capacity and control.

Alarm therapy

Alarms can be obtained through enuresis clinics, pharmacies and community health clinics. They can be body-worn, or bed alarms, and work on operant conditioning. The buzzer goes off and wakes the child when urine is passed.

Alarms take effort and commitment. It takes around 3 weeks for the child to recognise the sensation of a full bladder, and around 12 weeks to achieve dryness (success is measured as 14 consecutive dry nights). If dryness is achieved it is either through the child waking to urinate (a third of children) or sleeping through dry (two-thirds).

The success rate is around two-thirds of children, and half of these remain dry. 'Overlearning' (giving additional fluids at bedtime to those who achieve dryness) can improve the child's response to a full bladder signal and reduce the risk of relapse, especially in those who are sleeping through dry. If bedwetting restarts after stopping treatment, alarm training can be retried.

Medications

Desmopressin acetate: while this vasopressin analogue is very effective, it has a high relapse rate. It comes in tablets, melts and nasal spray, with the tablets and melts preferable as they have a lower risk of hyponatraemia. Fluids need to be restricted from 1 hour before taking to 8 hours after the dose. It is very useful for children in school camps or having sleepovers.

Other treatment options include using anticholinergics, tricyclic antidepressants, combinations of alarms and medications, or combinations of medications. These options should be undertaken by a specialist or through an enuresis clinic.

Constipation in children[16,17,18]

Constipation is quite common in children, although no cause has been discovered in 90–95% of cases. Constipation usually appears between 2 and 4 years of age, and up to a third of primary school-aged children will report constipation over a 12-month period. In toddlers, the gender distribution is equal, but by age 5, boys are more likely to get constipation than girls, with the frequency of faecal incontinence three times higher in boys. The most common factor is diet. Organic causes of chronic constipation are rare.

Refer to CHAPTER 41 for detailed information.

COMMON SKIN PROBLEMS[19,20,21]

91

Many of the common problems (e.g. acne, psoriasis, atopic dermatitis, seborrhoeic dermatitis) are covered in more detail in CHAPTER 121. The following are specifically (or usually) disorders of the neonatal period and early infancy.

Toxic erythema of newborn

This benign condition occurs in around half of babies, usually 1–2 days after birth (but may appear up to 2 weeks later) with 2–3 mm erythematous macules and papules developing into pustules, with a surrounding blotchy area of erythema, described as a 'flea-bitten' appearance. The rash starts on the face and spreads to the torso and proximal limbs, and spares the palms and soles. The rash usually fades over a week, but may recur for a few weeks. No treatment is required.

Salmon patch (naevus flammeus nuchae)

These are flat patches of pink or red skin with poorly defined borders. They occur in 40% of all newborns, and are seen at the nape of the neck ('stork bite') or between the eyebrows/on the eyelids ('angel's kiss') (see FIG. 91.6). They are more prominent when the child is crying. They fade over 6–12 months but neck patches may persist into adult life. No treatment is required.

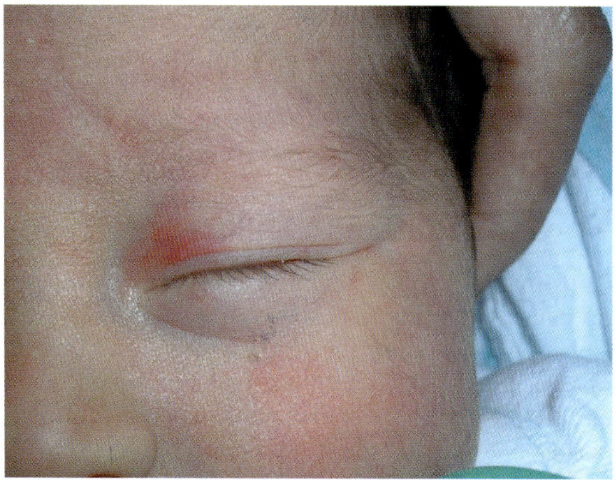

FIGURE 91.6 Salmon patch on the upper eyelid: called an 'angel's kiss'

Infantile haemangioma

Infantile haemangiomas can be superficial ('strawberry haemangioma', flat or lumpy, resembling strawberry jam splashed on the skin, see FIG. 91.7) or deep

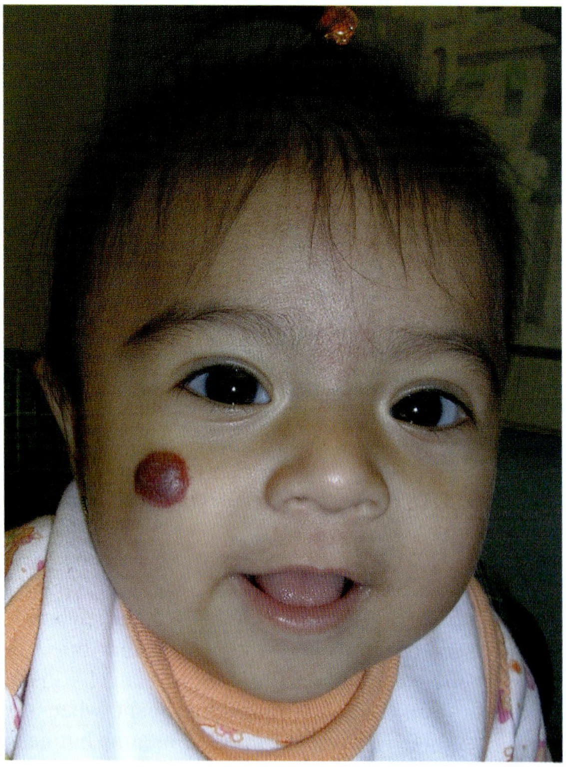

FIGURE 91.7 Strawberry haemangioma on the face of a child

('cavernous haemangioma', a bluish swelling). They usually appear after birth, and occur in 10% of infants.

Some 80% occur on the head and neck and 80% of their growth occurs in the first 3 months (most stop by 5 months, though some continue until 18 months). They usually involute and disappear (50% by 5 years, 70% by 7, 90% by 10), though regression of bulky ones tends to be incomplete, and they often leave an atrophic 'dented' scar. Large, deep or multiple haemangiomas can be associated with malformations of organs, and referral of these, those causing cosmetic issues (such as being prominent on the face), those that impair vision/hearing/breathing or feeding, or that are in other important locations (e.g. perineum or sacrum) is recommended. Active non-treatment is the rule, but beta blockers have proven effectiveness. Propanolol is useful, especially if used early in the growth phase, and is now usually preferred over oral steroids. Preparations include oral propanolol (with caution) and topical timolol drops or gel.[22]

Capillary vascular malformation ('port wine stain')

These dark red to purple lesions (a type of naevus flammeus) are present from birth and affect 3 in 1000 neonates. They are usually flat at birth, though they can become lumpy. There is an association with vascular syndromes, including Sturge–Weber syndrome, where a port wine stain on the skin supplied by the ophthalmic division of the trigeminal nerve is accompanied by glaucoma and seizures, and patients are at increased risk of developmental delay and hemiplegia. Port wine stains will often respond well to pulse dye laser (the treatment of choice). Cosmetic camouflage is useful.

Lymphatic malformation (lymphangioma)

These are present at birth but can subsequently grow. They can vary from large fluid-filled spaces (cystic hygromas) down to clusters of small firm blisters resembling frogspawn. They can be skin-coloured, red or purple (if associated vascular involvement) or brown or black. Surgical excision may be required.

Dermal melanocytosis ('Mongolian spot')

This condition presents as blue-grey discolouration of the skin over the lower back and sacrum in babies of east Asian and other dark-skinned ethnic backgrounds. These are of no clinical significance but may be mistaken for bruising or non-accidental injury. They usually disappear by 4 years of age.

Sebaceous hyperplasia

Hyperplastic sebaceous glands appear as tiny yellow–white papules on the nose or forehead. They disappear in several weeks.

Milia

Blocked sebaceous glands, leading to pearly-white lumps under the skin, especially on the face, are present in 50% of neonates. The firm, white papules are about 1–2 mm in diameter and differ from the yellowish papules of sebaceous hyperplasia. These also disappear after several weeks, and usually no treatment is required (see FIG. 91.8).

Miliaria ('sweat rash')

This is related to overheating and occurs in skin folds such as around the neck and armpits, but also on the face. It appears as two types:

- 'crystallina'—beads of sweat trapped under the epidermis with surrounding erythema
- 'rubia'—itchy red papules

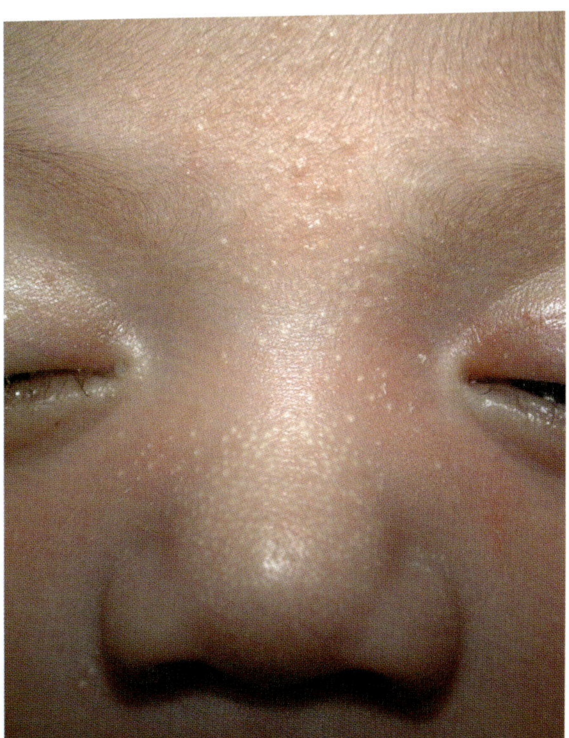

FIGURE 91.8 Milia on the face of a 2-week-old infant

It is a benign condition that disappears after a few weeks.

If problematic:

- keep skin dry and cool (e.g. fan, air-conditioner)
- dress in loose-fitting cotton clothing
- avoid frequent bathing and overuse of soap
- mild topical steroids (e.g. hydrocortisone) can help if inflamed

Suckling 'blisters'

These are a hyperplastic response to suckling, and are common on the upper lip. Reassure that these will settle.

Umbilical discharge

When the umbilical stump first separates, some granulation and mild exudate can be present until healing occurs. If the umbilicus is discharging pus and there is surrounding erythema in the neonate, infection should be considered, and a bacterial swab taken and appropriate antibiotics given. Be watchful for urine or faecal discharge.

91

Bleeding umbilical cord

Small amounts of bleeding may occur as the cord is separating and requires no treatment unless it is more profuse (if so, consider infection or a bleeding disorder).

Umbilical granuloma

These common fleshy pink-red growths can cause a persisting seropurulent discharge after the separation of the umbilical stump. The granuloma is often seen only by carefully examining the base of an 'innie' umbilicus. Drying out of the granulomatous tissue and healing can be achieved by the parent airing regularly, applying salt twice a day at home for a week or two (followed by irrigation), or the GP using a silver nitrate stick or copper sulphate crystals every few days until healing occurs. Protect the surrounding skin with Vaseline. Large pedunculated and persistant granulomas may be helped by applying a double ligature to the neck of the granuloma.

Pityriasis alba

- These are round or oval pale skin patches usually on the face of children and adolescents, and are more visible in tanned or dark-skinned patients.
- They can occur on the neck and upper limbs, occasionally on the trunk.

- Full repigmentation occurs after a couple of years
- They may start out pale pink then fade to white, and can leave slight depigmentation.

Treatment

- Reassurance
- Simple emollients
- Restrict use of soap and washing
- Mild steroids if scaly and itchy (rarely necessary)

Atopic dermatitis (eczema)

See FIGURE 91.9.

This common condition may appear typically in infants on the cheeks of the face, the folds of the neck and scalp and extensor surface of the limbs. For further information on its manifestation in children and management refer to CHAPTER 121.

Seborrhoeic dermatitis

See FIGURE 91.10.

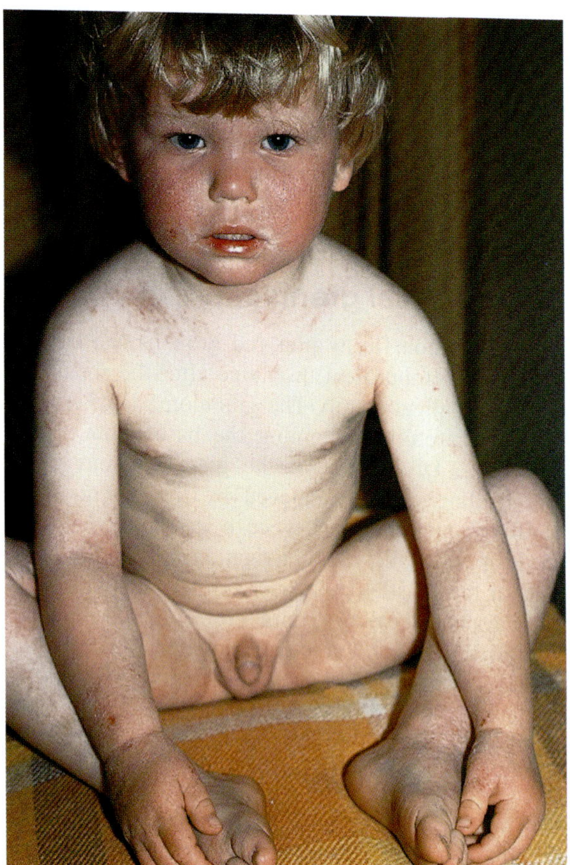

FIGURE 91.9 Atopic dermatitis (eczema) in a 3-year-old child with widespread distribution and severe pruritus

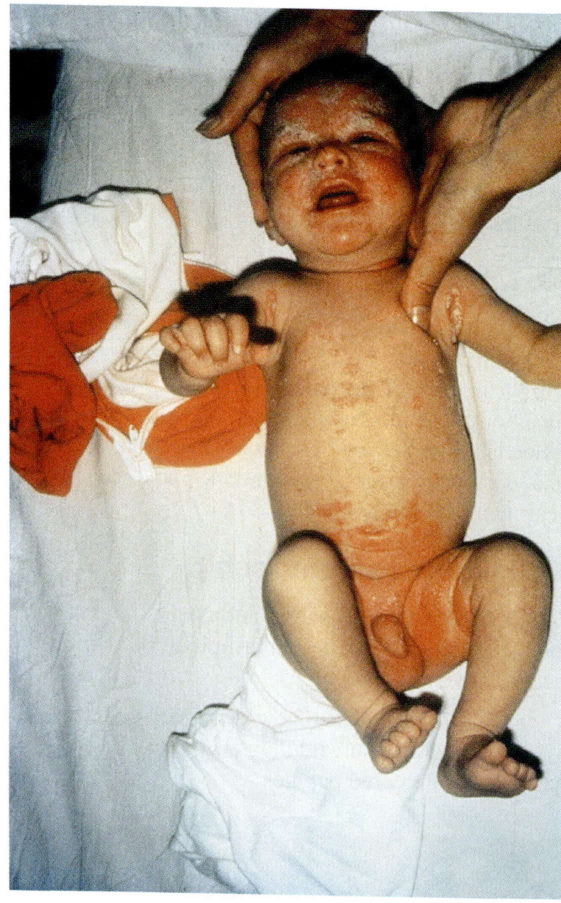

FIGURE 91.10 Seborrhoeic dermatitis in a 10-week-old child, showing a red, scaly rash affecting the scalp, forehead, face, axillae and nappy area. Both cradle cap and nappy rash are present.

This is quite different from adult seborrhoeic dermatitis and appears in the first 2 to 3 months.

Refer to CHAPTER 121.

Nappy rash

Nappy rash occurs under the nappy in response to wetness. The most common cause is contact dermatitis from urine and faeces, which will inevitably cause a rash if left on the skin for long enough. This will lead to the dull red rash being most prominent where the nappy contacts the skin, and sparing the folds. Sometimes ammonia is formed, resulting in a chemical burn (hence the alternative term ammoniacal dermatitis).

Nappy rash in the folds is more commonly found in infants with cradle cap and seborrhoeic dermatitis. Thrush can also coexist, with the rash appearing more bright red, and often having satellite lesions or pustules around the main rash. Bacterial superinfection (impetigo, see later in this chapter) can occur, with crusting, pustules and irregular blisters. Swabs should be taken for this if suspected. Other conditions such as psoriasis and atopic dermatitis also need to be considered, especially for resistant or recurrent nappy rash.

Advice to parents

- Keep the area dry. Air dry when possible (e.g. lying on towel without a nappy).
- Do not use powder, which can irritate the skin.
- Change wet or soiled napkins promptly—disposable ones with their absorbent hydrocellulose gel are very effective.
- If using cloth nappies, nappy liners can help keep the skin dry. Do not use plastic pants around them.
- Give evening fluids early to reduce night-time wetting, and change the nappy before parents go to bed.
- Wash gently with warm water and pat dry (do not rub).
- Avoid excessive bathing and soap.
- Use moisturisers to keep skin lubricated (e.g. zinc oxide and castor oil cream). Silicone barrier creams can also help.

Treatment

- Hydrocortisone and/or antifungal cream while rash is present.
- Antifungal can be continued for a few more days if thrush suspected.
- Do not use strong steroid creams on baby's bottom.

Cradle cap

Cradle cap is infantile seborrhoeic dermatitis confined to the scalp. The seborrhoeic dermatitis may also involve other areas (see CHAPTER 121). Cradle cap is very common, usually occurring in the first 6 weeks of life and settling over the next few weeks to months, but it sometimes takes much longer.

Greasy yellow scales are formed in response to sebum combining with old skin cells as they try to dry and fall off. The yeast *Malassezia furfur* may be involved. It is not usually itchy or distressing to the child.

Treatment

- Reassurance and watchful waiting (if not too bad, given the natural history is to improve with time)
- Use vegetable oil overnight to soften scales and then gently brush off (not olive oil; this encourages *Malassezia*)
- Baby shampoos and then gentle brushing off of scales
- 2% ketoconazole shampoo (Nizoral) twice weekly
- Apply hydrocortisone cream to red and inflamed areas

Molluscum contagiosum in children[23]

Molluscum is usually diagnosed by its distinct pink pearly appearance and central punctum (see CHAPTER 124). It is very common in children (up to 10% of the paediatric population have it at any given time), and is usually spread by direct contact, sharing towels and bath toys, or through water (e.g. sharing baths or swimming).

The rash lasts weeks to months, or occasionally a couple of years. Molluscum rarely leaves tiny pit-like scars. It can have a reactive dermatitis surrounding the lesions (especially in children prone to atopic dermatitis) and hydrocortisone cream can be used to help this.

Advice to parents

- Give the child a shower instead of a bath (the bath can spread the virus to other parts of the body).
- Don't share baths.
- Wash and dry bath toys after use.
- After showers/baths/swimming, dry areas with molluscum last and don't share/re-use towels.
- Wash hands after touching molluscum.
- Don't exclude children from school or playing together.
- If swimming, reasonable precautions include covering the lesions with waterproof tape and having personal kick-boards.

Treatment

The most common approach in children is to leave the rash alone and wait for it to clear. Treatments designed to irritate the lesion can make the rash clear more quickly (see CHAPTER 124) but can be distressing to the child and so are not normally done.

Warts in children[24]

Warts affect about 10% of children. Even without treatment, 50% of them will go in 6 months, and 90% in 2 years. It is therefore best to avoid painful treatments unless the parent and child are motivated (e.g. for cosmetic reasons, or uncomfortable plantar warts). A reasonable option that can help the wart disappear faster is to cover with occlusive tape (e.g. duct tape) 24 hours a day.

Refer to CHAPTER 68 (plantar warts) or CHAPTER 124 (general warts) for more active treatment options.

Hair problems in children

Refer to CHAPTER 126.

Lead poisoning[25]

- Young children are susceptible to lead poisoning. They are more likely than adults to be exposed to lead because of their exploratory and mouthing behaviour and because they absorb more of any ingested dose. The most common source seen in general practice is home renovation, involving paint removal in houses built before the 1980s.
- All Australians should have a blood lead level below 10 mcg/dL (though there is no known safe level of lead).
- Some communities are more susceptible to lead exposure due to industrial or mining activity, and some occupations and hobbies can also increase risk to household members. These include home and furniture restoration, soldering, burning of plastics and paints and cigarette smoking. Other potential sources include imported toys containing lead or coated with lead-based paints, some 'traditional' medicines and improperly fired ceramic cookware (e.g. imported tagines).
- Levels of lead have increased in the biosphere 1000-fold in the past 300 years, especially during the second half of the twentieth century, but the elimination of lead in petrol has helped reduce the exposure risk.
- Levels above 10 mcg/dL are associated with adverse neurocognitive effects including decreased IQ levels and behavioural issues, and it is uncertain whether levels below this also cause problems.
- When symptoms appear, they are usually non-specific and may include lethargy, intermittent abdominal pain, irritability, headache, abnormal behaviour and, in acute high-level exposure (rare), encephalopathy.
- High blood lead levels should be considered in the presence of unexplained iron-deficiency anaemia.
- Advise parents or parents-to-be to reduce exposure to lead by testing paint (particularly old or peeling paint) in houses (testing kits are readily available in paint shops), painting over old paint, being careful with old furniture and imported toys, and avoiding exposure to smoking or other sources.

Patient education resources

Hand-out sheets from *Murtagh's Patient Education* 7th edition:

- Bed-wetting (enuresis)
- Crying and unsettled baby
- Dyslexia and other SLDs
- Faecal incontinence in children (encopresis)
- Growing pains
- Infant colic
- Nappy rash
- Seborrhoea in infants
- Snuffling infant
- Tear duct blockage
- Teething
- Thumb sucking

References

1 The National Center on Shaken Baby Syndrome. The period of purple crying <www.purplecrying.org> (accessed 5/7/2014).

2 The Royal Children's Hospital, Melbourne. *Failure to thrive—initial management,* May 2014 <www.rch.org.au/clinicalguide/guideline_index/Failure_to_thrive_initial_management/> (accessed 5/7/2014).

3 Cole S, Lanham J. Failure to thrive: an update. Am Fam Physician, 2011; 83 (7): 829–34.

4 Cohen L. Idiopathic short stature: a review. JAMA 2014; 311 (17): 1787–96.

5 Allen D. Short stature in childhood—challenges and choices. N Engl J Med, 2013; 368 (13): 1220–8.

6 Nwoso B, Lee M. Evaluation of short and tall stature in children. Am Fam Physician, 2008; 78 (5): 597–604.

7 Australian Institute of Health and Welfare. Overweight and obesity, 2013 <www.aihw.gov.au/overweight-and-obesity/> (accessed 1/6/2014).

8 Department of Health, Canberra. 2007 Australian National Children's Nutrition and Physical Activity Survey—Key Findings <www.health.gov.au/internet/main/publishing.nsf/Content/phd-nutrition-childrens-survey-keyfindings> (accessed 1/6/2014).

9 Australian Paediatric Endocrine Group. Hormones and me: delayed puberty, 2011 <www.apeg.org.au/Portals/0/Resources/Hormones_and_Me_6_Delayed_Puberty.pdf> (accessed 6/7/2014).

10 Australian Paediatric Endocrine Group. Hormones and me: puberty and its problems, 2011 <www.apeg.org.au/Portals/0/resources/hormones&me5_puberty&its_problems.pdf> (accessed 6/7/2014).

11 Uziel Y, Hashkes P. Growing pains in children. Pediatr Rheumatol, 2007; 5: 5.

12 Raising Children Network. Growing pains, June 2011 <www.raisingchildren.net.au/articles/growing_pains.html> (accessed 12/7/2014).

13 Frank J, Jacobe K. The evaluation and management of heart murmurs in children. Am Fam Physician, 2011; 84 (7): 793–800.

14 Hahn D, Caldwell P. Nocturnal enuresis. Medical Observer, August 2013 <www.medicalobserver.com.au/news/nocturnal-enuresis> (accessed 12/7/2014).

15 Ramakrishnan K. Evaluation and treatment of enuresis. Am Fam Physician, 2008; 78 (4): 489–96.

16 The Royal Children's Hospital Melbourne. *Clinical Practice Guidelines: constipation,* December 2013 <www.rch.org.au/clinicalguide/guideline_index/Constipation_Guideline/#fu> (accessed 12/7/2014).

17 Biggs W, Dery W. Evaluation and treatment of constipation in infants and children. Am Fam Physician, 2006; 73 (3): 469–77.

18 The Royal Children's Hospital Melbourne. *Constipation management.* <www.rch.org.au/uploadedFiles/Main/Content/clinicalguide/guideline_index/CONSTIPATION%20HOME%20MANAGEMENT%20-%20poomeds%20revised.pdf> (accessed 12/7/2014).

19 DermNet NZ: the dermatology resource. <www.dermnetnz.org/> (accessed 12/7/2014).

20 O'Conner N, O'Gloughlin M, Ham P. Newborn skin, part 1: common rashes. Am Fam Physician, 2008; 77 (1): 47–52.

21 O'Conner N, O'Gloughlin M. Newborn skin, part 2: birthmarks. Am Fam Physician, 2008; 77 (1): 56–60.

22 Parker SL, Hildebrand GD. Review of topical beta blockers as treatment for infantile hemangiomas. Surv Ophthalmol, 2016; 61 (1): 51–8.

23 Center for Disease Control. Recommendations: patients with molluscum contagiosum and swimming pool safety, March 2013 <www.cdc.gov/ncidod/dvrd/molluscum/swimming/swimming_recommendations.htm> (accessed 12/7/2014).

24 The Royal Children's Hospital Melbourne. *Fact sheet: warts,* November 2010 <www.rch.org.au/kidsinfo/fact_sheets/Warts/> (accessed 12/7/2014).

25 National Health and Medical Research Council. Information paper—blood lead level for Australians, July 2014 <www.nhmrc.gov.au/guidelines/publications/eh55> (accessed 12/7/2014).

92 Surgical problems in children

A surgeon should have three diverse properties in his person. That is to saie, a harte as the harte of a lyon. His eyes like the eyes of a hawke, and the handes of a woman.

JOHN HALLE (1529–68)

An imperative task for the GP is not only to diagnose surgical conditions in infancy and children as early as possible, but to be aware of the degree of urgency and the optimal times for intervention. In many instances the emphasis should be placed on a non-surgical solution using natural resolution with time and simple 'tricks of the trade'.

HEAD DEFORMITY

The neonate's head may become distorted because of the position in utero or after the passage through the birth canal. The head shape can recover to a normal shape within about 8 weeks following birth. If the abnormal shape persists consider deformational plagiocephaly or craniostenosis.

Plagiocephaly (flat head sydrome)

This is asymmetry of the skull with a normal head circumference. The shape can be likened to a tilted parallelogram (see FIG. 92.1); it is the most common cause of an abnormal head shape. On the side with the flat frontal area, the ear and the parietal eminence sit more posteriorly. It affects 1 in 5 infants and is either congenital or acquired and often results from the infant sleeping in one position, usually on their back. There is usually no impairment of cerebral development or intellect. If the sutures are ridged or the sleeping position causation is ruled out, a skull X-ray should be performed. Management involves initially changing the side to which the child usually faces for sleeping, then regularly changing sides and encouraging time in the prone position while awake. If not responsive, a cranial remodelling helmet can be tried—best from 4 to 8 months.[1]

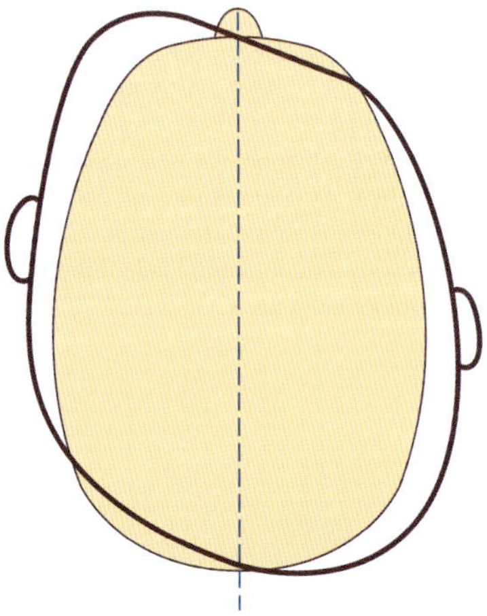

FIGURE 92.1 Plagiocephaly, congenital or acquired. The long axis is deflected from the saggital plane. In this case the right ear is more posterior.

Craniostenosis

This is premature fusion of one or more sutures of the cranial vault and base, which act as lines of growth. The abnormality of head shape depends on the sutures involved. The diagnosis is confirmed by radiography. Prompt referral to a paediatric craniofacial surgeon is necessary as planning for possible complex surgery, best at 5 to 10 months, is required.

Hydrocephalus

This condition, which is due to an imbalance between the production and absorption of CSF, usually caused by obstruction to circulation, requires early referral for diversion of ventricular fluid. Prognosis is generally good with early intervention and regular supervision.

Macrocephaly and microcephaly

Macrocephaly and microcephaly are defined as a head circumference greater than the 97th percentile and less than the 3rd percentile respectively. Infants whose head circumference measurements cross these percentile lines require expert assessment and investigation. It is appropriate to undertake regular head circumference measurements in the early childhood years.

EARS, NOSE, FACE AND ORAL CAVITY

Prominent bat/shell ears

The ears are almost adult size and firmness by 5 to 6 years of age but the ear cartilage is not strong enough to cope with surgery under 3 years. For this reason, and because it is best to correct the problem when the child is in a position to support a decision to operate, the optimal time for surgical correction is after 5 to 6 years. It may be possible to correct an ear deformity by moulding the ear with tape or splinting within the first 6 months of life.[1]

Facial deformity

It is best to refer any facial deformity as soon as it is detected.

External angular dermoid

This dermoid cyst, which has a readily identifiable constant position, lies in the outer aspect of the eyebrow. It is noticed in infancy as it progressively enlarges. Excision is advisable, but check with ultrasound examination because of the possibility of an intracranial extension.

Cleft lip and cleft palate

Congenital clefts of the lip and palate occur in approximately 1:600 of all births. It is very important that the simplest and least obvious form should be recognised in time for adequate repair. This is the submucus cleft, frequently not recognised in infancy because the palate appears to be intact.[2] The submucus cleft can be diagnosed on close inspection as the uvula is bifid and there is a deep groove in the midline of the palate covered only by mucous membrane. The ideal age for repair of the cleft lip is under 3 months of age. Secondary surgery can then be performed at various ages. The repair of the palate, which requires preliminary diagnostic ultrasound, is best performed before the child begins to speak. The optimal time is 6 to 12 months of age.

Nasal disorders

Rhinoplasty is best deferred to late adolescence. If performed early there is a higher incidence of secondary surgery.

Choanal atresia may be unilateral, leading to delayed diagnosis, or bilateral, where there is no instinctive reaction to breathe through the mouth, leading to asphyxia. Since the obstruction is usually by a very thin membrane one side can be perforated with a urethral sound as an emergency procedure.

Septoplasty can be considered if the problem is symptomatic.

Tongue tie (ankyloglossia)

Early signs:

- tongue may appear heart-shaped
- infants unable to protrude the tongue over the lower lip
- breastfeeding problems

The ideal time to release the 'tie' is in infancy, under 4 months.[3] As the frenulum is thin and avascular, simple frenulotomy by snipping with sterile scissors (with care) is advisable (see FIG. 92.2). Otherwise surgery should be left until after 2 years of age. The conditions may not be noticed until later in life. A useful guideline is a strong family history of speech problems corrected by tongue tie surgery.

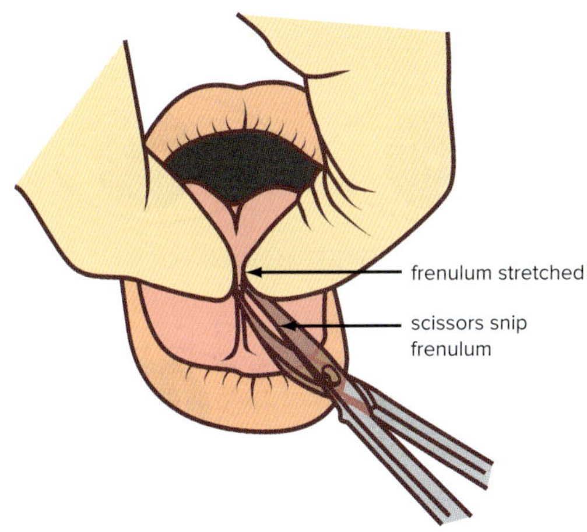

FIGURE 92.2 Tongue tie release in infant

Pre-auricular sinus

This common condition can get recurrently infected with pus discharge from a small opening immediately anterior to the ear at the level of the meatus in front of the upper crus of the helix. It also causes cosmetic problems. It is not a branchial sinus. It can be associated with kidney abnormalities. Refer when diagnosed for surgical excision, although it can be left alone if it is causing no problems.

Branchial sinus/cyst/fistula

This is a rare condition and is located inferior to the external auditory meatus or anterior to the

92

sternomastoid muscle. The opening may discharge mucopus. A skin tag or cartilage remnant may be present. Refer when diagnosed for excision.

Strabismus (squint)

A squint is rarely obvious in the first weeks of life, but tends to show up when the baby learns to use the eyes, from about 2 weeks to 3 or 4 months of age. However, it may appear late, even as an adult. Vision, which is present at birth, continues to develop until 7–8 years of age.

Main types of squint

See FIGURE 92.3.

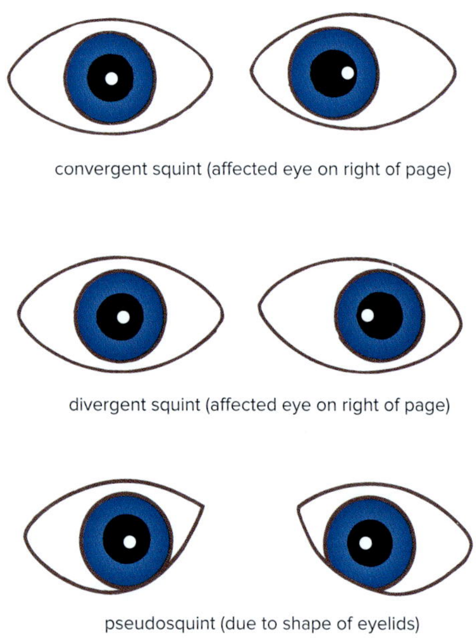

FIGURE 92.3 Types of squint

- *Constant or true squint* is one that is permanent—always present.
- *Latent squint* is one that only appears under stressful conditions such as fatigue.
- *Transient squint* is one that is noticeable for short periods and then the eye appears normal.
- *Alternating squint* is one that changes between the eyes so the child can use either eye to fix vision.
- *Pseudosquint* is not a true squint but only appears to be one because of the shape of the eyelids, i.e. broad epicanthic folds.

A useful way to differentiate a true squint from a pseudosquint is to observe the position of the light in the eyes (corneal reflections) when a torch is shone into them from about 40 cm away. This light reflex will be in exactly the same position in both eyes in the pseudosquint but in different spots with the true squint.

- If one eye is 'lazy' (that is, not being used), it is standard practice to wear a patch (maybe on glasses) over the good eye for long periods in order to use the inactive eye and have both eyes eventually capable of vision.
- The two serious squints are the constant and alternating ones, which require early referral. Transient squint and latent squint usually are not a problem.
- Always refer children with strabismus (squint) when first seen to exclude ocular pathology such as retinoblastoma, congenital cataract and glaucoma, which would require emergency surgery.
- Children with strabismus (even if the ocular examination is normal) need specialist management because the deviating eye will become amblyopic (a lazy eye with reduced vision, i.e. 'blind', if not functioning by 7 years of age). The younger the child, the easier it is to treat amblyopia; it may be irreversible if first detected later than school age. Surgical correction of a true squint is preferred at 1–2 years of age.

Blocked nasolacrimal duct

Refer CHAPTER 91.

NECK LUMPS

Sternomastoid tumour/fibrosis

Features in infants:

- hard painless lump (2–3 cm long) within sternomastoid muscle
- tight and shortened sternomastoid muscle
- usually not observed at birth
- appears at 20–30 days of age
- associated torticollis—head turned away from but tilted towards the tumour
- restricted head rotation to side of tumour

Most tumours resolve spontaneously within 1 year. The mother or baby's carer should be reassured and the child referred to a physiotherapist early. The mother or carer should frequently gently massage the lump, rotate the head to the side of the lesion and then side-flex (stretch) away from that side. Repeat several times twice daily. Encourage the baby to look towards the affected side. If surgery for a persistent fibrotic shortened muscle is required it is best before 12 months.

Older children can present with torticollis and a tight, short fibrous sternomastoid muscle. It is associated with rotation of the head to the affected side, hemihypoplasia of the face and a wasted ipsilateral trapezius muscle. It requires surgical repair.

Thyroglossal cyst

This is the most common childhood midline neck swelling. It moves with swallowing and tongue protrusion. It is prone to infection, including abscess formation. The cyst and its tract are best excised before it becomes infected.

Lymphatic malformation/ lymphangioma/cystic hygroma

These usually present as soft cystic tumours of the neck, face or oral cavity. They resemble clusters of vesicles and are often poorly localised. Some have visible red dots due to haemangiomatous inclusions. If located in the floor of the mouth or peripharyngeal area they endanger the airway and can precipitate an emergency requiring surgery. Surgery is advisable in the early years.

Cervical lymphadenopathy

Refer to CHAPTER 61.

BIRTHMARKS AND SKIN TUMOURS

Infantile haemangioma (strawberry naevus)

See CHAPTER 91. These start soon after birth as a red pinpoint lesion and grow rapidly for the first 6 months, then involute and become pale. Full resolution may take several years. Reassure parents and demonstrate how to stop any bleeding by applying pressure. Possible treatment options include oral or intralesional steroids, vascular laser, interferon and surgery. Surgical intervention is usually not necessary. Exceptions are locations in critical areas such as periorbital, nose, lips and face. Refer lesions on the eyelid early since visual obstruction can lead to amblyopia. Stridor accompanying a haemangioma on the face is suggestive of laryngeal haemorrhage, so refer urgently.

Capillary vascular malformation (port wine stain)

These are present from birth and surgical intervention is inadvisable. They may be treated by pulsed dye laser, which is best initiated as early as possible as the response is best in the first 2 years[4] (see CHAPTER 91).

Venous malformations

These are aggregations of abnormal subcutaneous veins that may infiltrate deeper tissues. In the past these lesions were treated surgically, but now the emphasis is on specialised sclerosant agents injected under fluoroscopic guidance and specialised laser techniques. Referral to Vascular Malformation Clinics in larger centres is worthy of enquiry.

Lymphatic malformation

These appear sometimes as skin lesions because of the red discolouration on the surface of the tumour. Management is as described above.

Congenital naevi

These have to be treated on an individual basis. If giant naevi they can be dermabraded at ideally less than 6 weeks.

Benign juvenile melanoma (Spitz naevus)

These pigmented lesions, which typically appear on the face, are usually surgically excised because of their rapid growth and family concerns.

CHEST AND BREAST DISORDERS

Breast asymmetry

If necessary surgery should be performed in late adolescence after breast development is complete. It can take the form of a unilateral implant, different-sized bilateral implants or unilateral breast reduction.

Macromastia

Reduction surgery should also be delayed until breast growth is complete, at late adolescence.

Gynaecomastia

This is not to be confused with pseudogynaecomastia due to fat in obese preadolescents. However, gynaecomastia in thin boys does occur and requires referral for assessment if it cannot be attributed to drugs such as oestrogen. If it develops in the pubertal stage, gynaecomastia may resolve spontaneously within 1 or 2 years. If necessary, simple mastectomy can be performed, if no cause can be found.

Subareolar hyperplasia in boys

This presents as a firm discoid subareolar lesion similar to premature breast hyperplasia of girls. It typically occurs at about 12–14 years. There is no indication for surgical treatment. Give an explanation with reassurance that the problem will dissipate.

Chest wall skeletal deformity

Surgical correction is best performed in adolescence.

Poland syndrome

This syndrome is an absent sternal head of pectoralis major with associated chest wall deformity plus a hypoplastic or absent breast and nipple–areolar complex. Surgical correction can be undertaken from 10 to 20 years.

CONGENITAL HEART DISORDERS

GPs have an important role in the diagnosis of congenital heart disorders as many of the affected infants develop cyanosis, murmurs or congestive heart failure. Early diagnosis and intervention helps prevent serious problems such as bacterial endocarditis and paradoxical emboli.

Ventricular septal defect (VSD)

VSD is the commonest congenital heart lesion (1:500 births).

The defect connects the two ventricles with a L → R shunt (see FIG. 92.4).

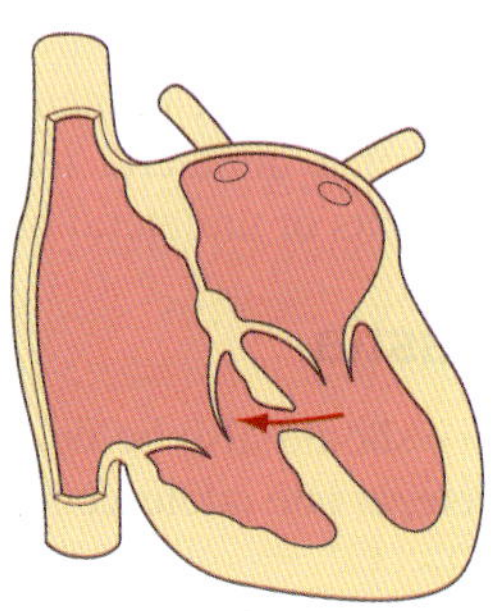

FIGURE 92.4 Ventricular septal defect: defect in muscle wall

Symptoms and signs depend on size of hole. All have a palpable thrill at the left sternal edge and a pansystolic murmur down right sternal edge.

Small VSD ('maladie de Roger'): harsh murmur, usually asymptomatic and closes spontaneously.

Larger VSD: symptoms appear in infancy.

- Breathlessness on feeding and crying (i.e. early CHF)
- Recurrent chest infections
- Failure to thrive
- Heart failure from about 3 months with large defects

Refer early, especially if failure—early surgery performed by 6 months but can be performed at any age from the newborn period. A patch can close the defect through open-heart surgery. Some may be closed by sealing with an occlusive device through a percutaneous cardiac catheter. A cardiologist will make the appropriate decision. As a general rule about 50% of all VSDs will close spontaneously. The membraneous type, unlike the muscular type, is less likely to close spontaneously.

Atrial septal defect (ASD)

In ASD the defect connects the two atria with two distinct types—ostium secundum with holes higher in the septum (most common) and ostium primum with holes lower in the septum (more serious) (see FIG. 92.5). Signs are a mid-systolic murmur in the pulmonary area, a split 2nd sound and a loud P2. An echocardiogram is diagnostic.

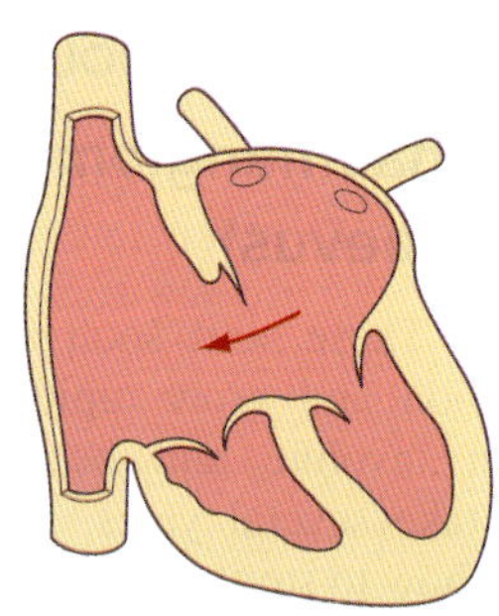

FIGURE 92.5 Atrial septal defect: primum defect

Symptoms are uncommon in infancy and childhood with ostium secundum but heart failure with pulmonary hypertension develops early with ostium primum.

Refer these patients early. Prophylactic antibiotics are needed for patients with ostium primum. Follow other cases with regular echocardiograms and growth/development monitoring. Closure is advisable where there is evidence of a troublesome shunt. Options are repair by direct surgical suture or an insertion of a patch or a device closure using a self-expanding 'double umbrella device' manipulated into the defect via cardiac catheterisation.

All patients require prophylactic antibiotics before procedures.

Patent ductus arteriosus

The ductus fails to close after birth. A loud, continuous machinery murmur is heard. Symptoms relate to shunt size. The child presents with a murmur with possible respiratory infections, failure to thrive and heart failure. Refer for possible surgical closure by ligation. Alternatives include device closure with placement of an occlusive device or by embolisation coils.

Coarctation of the aorta

This usually presents in infancy with heart failure. Refer for early surgery to remove the narrowed portion of the aorta.

HERNIAS AND GENITAL DISORDERS

Inguinal hernias

These usually present in the first 3 to 4 months with an incidence of 1 in 50 males and 1 in 500 females (see FIG. 92.6).

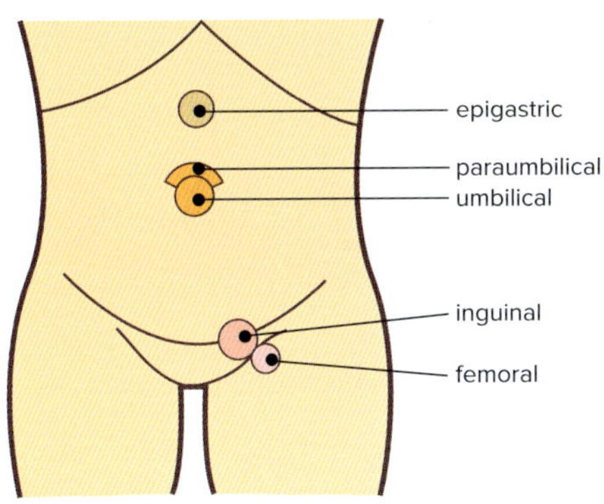

FIGURE 92.6 Sites of common hernias

Inguinal and femoral hernias should be referred urgently as early surgery is advisable to avoid the high risk of bowel incarceration or strangulation and ovarian entrapment and ischaemia in females. It is useful to follow the '6–2' rule (see CHAPTER 112).

Hydroceles

Scrotal hydroceles are painless cystic swellings around the testis. The opening of the processus vaginalis is narrow and often closes spontaneously. Two types can be identified—slack, often bilateral, which disappear within 12 months, and tense, often unilateral, which often persist after the first year. Ninety per cent resolve by 18 months of age; for those that persist, referral is recommended with a view to surgical intervention if present for longer than 2 years.

Undescended testes

Testes can still descend up to 3 months after birth. Refer by 6 months with a view to correction between 9 and 12 months but definitely before 2 years (see CHAPTER 112).

Hypospadias

Refer to disorders of the penis (see CHAPTER 113). Look for other abnormalities. Refer as soon as possible if the child is not producing a good urinary stream. Non-urgent cases should be evaluated by 6 months with a view to surgery at around 12 months; these patients should not be circumcised.

The foreskin and circumcision

For more detail refer to penile problems (see CHAPTER 113). If not circumcised in the neonatal period it is best performed under general anaesthetic after 6 months of age following consultation, counselling and with the consent of both parents.

92

Phimosis

Real phimosis is uncommon and almost all cases of tight foreskin with narrowing of the preputial orifice resolve naturally. Treatment with corticosteroid creams should be considered (see CHAPTER 113). Probably the only indication for circumcision is persistent difficulty in passing urine.

Paraphimosis

Management of this painful condition is outlined in CHAPTER 113.

Umbilical hernia

Surgery is not usually required for umbilical herniae as most close naturally by 4 years of age (95% resolve spontaneously by 2–3 years). Refer for possible repair if still present at 4 years of age. A good guideline is that if the hernial orifice is greater than 1 cm at 12 months then surgical intervention is a possibility. It is usual to operate at 4–5 years.

Umbilical granuloma

Refer CHAPTER 91.

Para-umbilical hernia

This is due to a defect in the linea alba adjacent to the umbilicus proper. Most lie just above the umbilicus. The defect is felt like an elliptical slit with firm edges. Spontaneous closure rarely occurs and they are more likely to incarcerate. Refer for operation at any age preferably after 6–12 months.

Epigastric hernia

An epigastric hernia (not to be confused with divarification of the rectus muscles) lies between the umbilicus and the xiphisternum. It is unlikely to close naturally, is likely to incarcerate and causes pain by strangulation of herniated fat. Indications for repair are pain (reproducible on palpation of the hernia) and cosmetic.

Anal fissure

Anal fissures are often seen in infants and toddlers with uncomfortable defecation and minimal bright bleeding. The anal mucosa is split in the midline either anterior or posterior. It is caused by the passage of hard stool. The fissure usually heals within a few days.

Fused labia (labial agglutination)

Labial fusion is caused by adhesions considered to be acquired from perineal inflammation (see CHAPTER 107). They are certainly not present at birth. Most authorities recommend no treatment if the child can void readily and allow natural healing to occur.

Penile problems

Refer CHAPTER 113.

CHILDHOOD LEG AND FOOT DEFORMITIES

Developmental dysplasia of hip

- Detected by clinical examination (Ortolani and Barlow tests) and ultrasound examination (see CHAPTER 65).
- Infants are usually treated successfully by abduction splinting (e.g. Pavlik harness).
- Open reduction may be required, especially in older babies and toddlers.

Bow legs (genu varum)

- Most are physiological (which are symmetrical) and improve with age.
- Consider rickets in children at risk.
- Toddlers are usually bow-legged until 3 years of age.
- Resolve spontaneously by 3 years except in severe cases.
- Monitor intercondylar separation (ICS): distance between medial femoral condyles.
- Refer when ICS >6 cm at 4 years, not improving or asymmetric (see FIG. 92.7).

Knock knees (genu valgum)

- Most are physiological and children are usually knock-kneed from 2–8 years (maximal 3–4 years).
- Running is awkward, but improves with time.
- Reassure parents about spontaneous improvement.
- Monitor intermalleolar separation (IMS): distance between medial malleoli.
- Refer if IMS >8 cm (see FIG. 92.7).

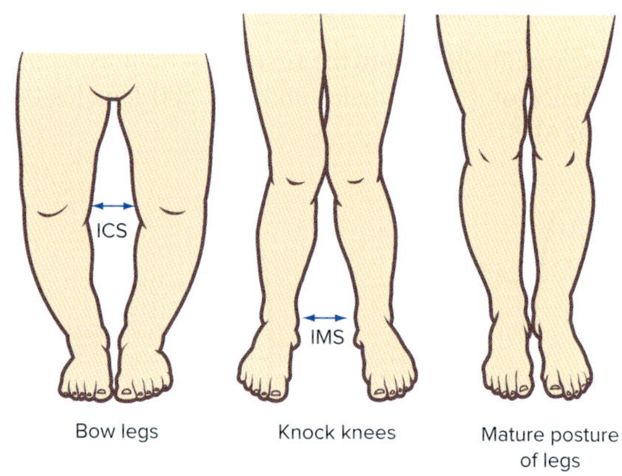

FIGURE 92.7 Postural variance of lower limbs

In-toeing (pigeon toes)

In-toeing does not cause pain or affect mobility.

Causes of in-toeing (see FIG. 92.8) are metatarsus varus, internal tibial torsion and medial femoral torsion. Children with femoral torsion tend to sit in a characteristic 'W' sitting position (see FIG. 92.9). These features are compared in TABLE 92.1.[5]

Out-toeing

Infants

- Have restricted internal rotation of hip due to an external rotation contracture
- Exhibit a 'Charlie Chaplin' posture between 3 and 12 months—up to 2 years

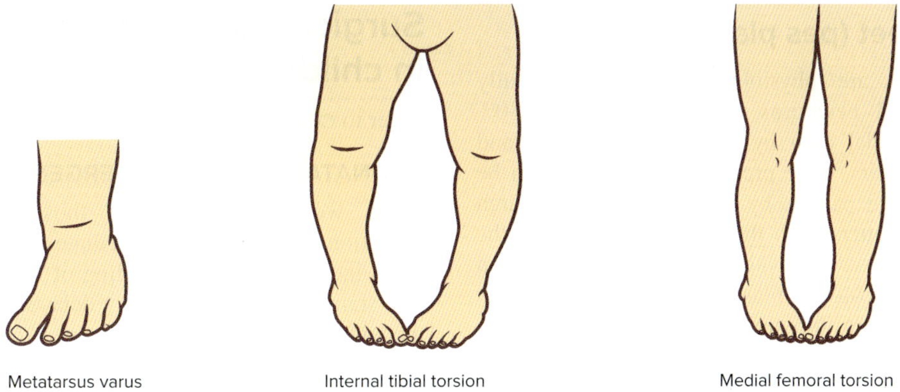

FIGURE 92.8 Causes of in-toeing

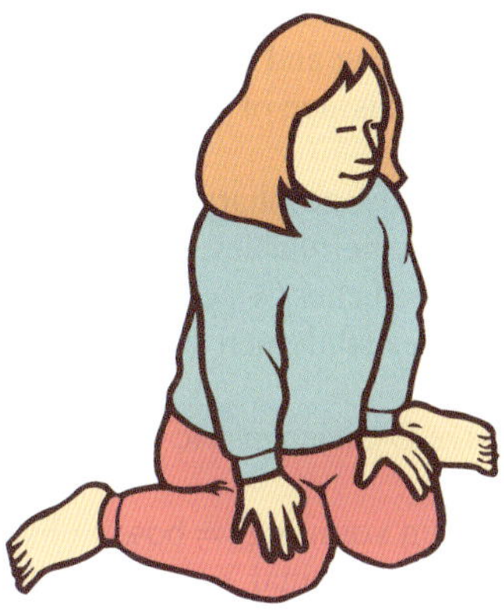

FIGURE 92.9 The classic 'W' position of femoral torsion (inset hips)

- Child weight-bears and walks normally
- No treatment required as spontaneous resolution occurs

Surgery may be necessary in older children.

Club foot (congenital talipes equinovarus)

Most abnormal-looking feet in infants are not a true club foot deformity; the majority have postural problems referred to as 'postural talipes' such as talipes calcaneovalgus, metatarsus varus and postural talipes equinovarus. Such conditions are usually quite mobile and mild, and all resolve spontaneously without treatment. True club foot deformity is usually stiff and severe, and requires orthopaedic correction.[5]

92

Inset hips (medial femoral torsion)

In children with inset hips, the femur tends to rotate inwards especially when the child is about 5–6 years old and is normal up to 12 years. The children tend to sit in a 'W' position (see FIG. 92.9). Fortunately, most children outgrow this condition before the age of 12.

Table 92.1 In-toeing in childhood

	Metatarsus varus	Internal tibial torsion	Medial femoral torsion
Synonyms	Metatarsus adductus		Inset hips
Age at presentation	Birth	Toddler	Child
Site of problem	Foot	Tibia	Femur
Examination	Sole of foot bean-shaped	Thigh–foot angle is inwards	Arc of hip rotation favours internal rotation
Management	Observe or cast	Observe and measure	Observe, rarely surgery
Resolution (usually by)	3 years	3–4 years	8–9 years
When to refer if not resolved	3 months after presentation	6 months after presentation	8 years after presentation

Source: Reprinted from D Efron. *Paediatric Handbook*. Melbourne: Blackwell Science, 1996 with permission

Flat feet (pes plano valgus)

The majority are physiological and are usually hereditary. All newborns have flat feet but 80% develop a medial arch by their sixth birthday and most by 11 years.[5] The presence of the arch can be demonstrated to parents by the tiptoe test. The arch can be seen better when the feet are hanging in the air and even better still when the child is standing on tiptoes (see FIG. 92.10). Flat feet are present in about 10% of teenagers. No treatment is required unless painful and stiff. Good roomy footwear is important. Studies in California have shown no benefit from wearing orthoses or other forms of arch supports. Arches develop naturally.

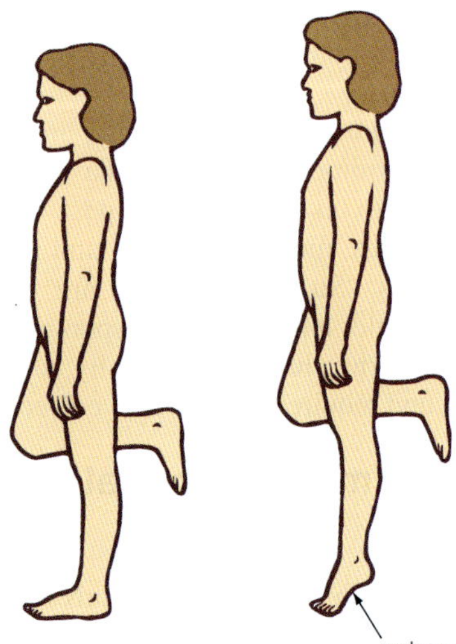

FIGURE 92.10 The tiptoe test for flat feet

92

Curly toes

Usually the third toe curls inward under the second toe so that the second toe lies above the level of the first and third toes. The toes can usually be straightened if necessary, so ignore the problem until 2 years. Refer if necessary to have a severe deformity corrected by flexor tenotomy.

A summary of optimal signs for surgical intervention in children's surgical disorders is presented in TABLE 92.2.

Appendicitis in children

Refer to CHAPTER 34.

Surgical causes of vomiting in children

Refer to CHAPTER 60.

NEONATAL SURGICAL EMERGENCIES

It is worthwhile knowing those non-traumatic conditions that demand immediate attention. Danger signs include excessive drooling of frothy secretions, bile-stained vomiting and delayed passage of meconium.

Neonatal gut obstruction—consider meconium ileus, volvulus, small bowel atresia.

Neonatal emergencies[6,7]

- Oesophageal atresia: rattling respiratory distress + excessive drooling and secretions + choking with feeding (passage of 10F catheter stops about 10 cm)
  Action: nil orally, oropharyngeal suction, IV fluids
- Diaphragmatic hernia: severe respiratory distress + barrel-shaped chest + scaphoid abdomen (X-rays of chest/abdomen show loops of bowel in chest)
  Action: Give O_2, nasogastric tube (avoid bag and mask)
- Bilious (green vomiting) = bowel obstruction or malrotation (abdominal X-ray)
  Action: nasogastric drainage and refer (do not feed)
- Neonatal intestinal obstruction including volvulus, Hirschsprung disorder, atresia and meconium ileus: bilious vomiting (green bile) + distension + delayed stools
  Action: nasogastric tube, IV fluids, refer
- Imperforate anus and rectum
  Action: refer for surgery on day of birth, anoplasty for low lesions; complex surgery for high lesions
- Bile duct atresia: neonatal jaundice (conjugated bilirubin) (usually 4–6 weeks) → white stools
  Action: refer early for precise diagnosis and surgical correction
- Congenital lobar emphysema: respiratory distress + cyanosis + signs of emphysema
  Action: refer early for urgent assessment and surgery to remove diseased lung
- Congenital cystic disease of the lungs: respiratory distress soon after birth
  Action: as above
- Congenital heart disease (severe forms)
  Action: refer early for medical treatment and assessment

Table 92.2 Optimal times for surgery/intervention in children's surgical disorders

Disorder	Surgery/intervention
Squint (fixed or alternating)	12–24 months: absolutely before 7 years
Tongue tie	3–4 months or 2–6 years
Ear deformity	After 6 years
Cleft lip	Less than 3 months
Cleft palate	6–12 months
Inguinoscrotal lumps:	Best assessed before 6 months
• undescended testes	Surgery best at 6–12 months Don't leave >12 months
• inguinal hernia	ASAP, especially infants and irreducible hernias Reducible hernias: the '6–2' rule Birth–6 weeks: surgery within 2 days 6 weeks–6 months: surgery within 2 weeks Over 6 months: surgery within 2 months
• femoral hernia	ASAP
• torsion of testicle	Surgery within 4 hours (absolutely 6 hours)
• hydrocele	Leave to 12 months, then review (often resolve; if not, repair by 2 years)
• varicocele	Leave and review
Other hernias:	
• umbilical hernia	Leave to age 4 Surgery after 4 if persistent (tend to strangulate) Never tape down
• para-umbilical hernia	Any age—best after 6 months
• epigastric hernia	Any age—best after 6 months
Leg and foot development problems:	
• developmental dysplasia hip	Most treated successfully by abductor splinting (e.g. Pavlik harness)
• bow legs (genu varum)	Normal up to 3 years Usually improve with age: refer if ICS > 6 cm
• knock knees	Normal 3–8 years, then refer if IMS > 8 cm
• flat feet	No treatment unless stiff and painful
• internal tibial torsion	Refer 6 months after presentation if unresolved
• medial femoral torsion	Leave to 8 years, then refer if unresolved
• metatarsus varus	Refer 3 months after presentation if unresolved

- Exomphalos (intestinal contents in a sac)
  Action: nasogastric tube, IV dextrose drip, temperature control, refer
- Gastroschisis (exposed bowel contents through anterior wall defect)
  Action: as for exomphalos; cover with plastic wrap
- Pierre–Robin syndrome: micrognathia + cleft palate + respiratory obstruction from tongue
  Action: early referral
- Tension pneumothorax
  Action: intercostal needle/catheter with aspiration
- Myelomeningocele and meningocele
  Action: early neurosurgical referral

Note the importance of plain X-rays as urgent first-line investigations and early surgical referral.

92

Other important childhood emergencies

- Pyloric stenosis: projectile vomiting weeks 2–6, epigastric 'tumour' (CHAPTER 60)
- Torsion of testis: severe groin/low abdominal pain + vomiting
- Intussusception: pallor + abdominal pain (severe and intermittent) + inactivity
- Acute appendicitis: abdominal pain + a/n/v + guarding
- Peritonitis
- Intestinal obstruction: colicky pain + vomiting + distension
- Irreducible inguinal hernia
- Paraphimosis
- Cerebral abscess
- Meckel diverticulum—diverticulitis or haemorrhage
- Various neoplasias

References

1 MacGill KA. Paediatric plastic surgery. Australian Doctor, 9 September 2005: 32.
2 Hutson JM, Woodward A, Beasley SW. *Jones Clinical Paediatric Surgery*. Oxford: Blackwell Publishing, 2003: 18–72.
3 Lalakea ML, Messner AH. Ankyloglossia: does it matter? Pediatr Clin North Am, 2003; 50: 381–97.
4 Expert group for Dermatology. In eTG complete [Internet]. Melbourne: Therapeutic Guidelines Ltd. Available from: <www.tg.org.au> (accessed November 2017).
5 Kerr G, Barnett P. Orthopaedic conditions. In: Smart J (ed), *Paediatric Handbook* (6th edn). Melbourne: Blackwell Science, 2000; 454–9.
6 Jones PG. *Clinical Paediatric Surgery*. Sydney: Ure Smith, 1970: 16–19.
7 Gwee A, Rimer R, Marks M. *Paediatric Handbook* (9th edn). Oxford: Wiley-Blackwell, 2015: 220–5.

Common childhood infectious diseases (including skin eruptions)

93

The physical signs of measles are nearly the same as those of smallpox, but nausea and inflammation is more severe. The rash of measles usually appears at once, but the rash of smallpox spot after spot . . .

AVICENNA (980–1037)

Chickenpox (varicella)

Epidemiology

Chickenpox has become much less common since the introduction of the varicella vaccine in 2000 and its inclusion on the National Immunisation Program in 2005, because of both individual and herd immunity.[1] Prior to this, nearly all children acquired it (<80% of the Australian population were seropositive by their teens). Chickenpox has a complication of only 1%, and is often thought of as not being a serious disease—which mostly it isn't—but because it was so common prior to the vaccine's introduction it resulted in 1500 hospital admissions and 7–8 deaths a year.[1]

Chickenpox is a highly contagious infection caused by the varicella zoster virus, a DNA virus within the herpes virus family. Primary infection causes chickenpox (varicella), with the virus establishing latency in the dorsal root ganglia. Reactivation leads to herpes zoster (shingles), which is relatively uncommon in children and can be more difficult to diagnose as it often presents with only a few lesions.

Note: shingles *can* happen in childhood.

See CHAPTER 122.

Clinical features

The clinical features of varicella are shown in TABLE 93.1 and the complications in TABLE 93.2. Children are not normally very sick but tend to be lethargic and have a mild fever. Adults have an influenza-like illness. The typical distribution is shown in FIGURES 93.1 and 93.2.

Congenital varicella syndrome can occur from varicella in pregnancy, and may result in skin scarring, limb defects, ocular anomalies and neurological malformations, with the risk highest in the second trimester. Intrauterine exposure also increases the risk of shingles in infancy. Severe neonatal varicella infection can result from perinatal varicella in the mother (especially if contracted from 5 days before the birth to 2 days after).

Table 93.1 Clinical features of varicella

Onset
Children: no prodrome
Adults: prodrome (myalgia, fever, headaches) for 2–3 days
Rash
Centripetal distribution, including oral mucosa (see FIG. 93.1)
Lesions can become infected
'Cropping' phenomenon: vesicles, papules, crusting lesions present together
Pruritic
Degrees of severity
Number of vesicles can vary from fewer than 10 to thousands (usually 200–500)[1]
Mild cases can be missed
More severe in adults and the immunocompromised
Viral pneumonia rare in children, uncommon in adults
Death rare except in the immunocompromised and neonates with congenital varicella

Treatment

Treatment is symptomatic and usually no specific therapy is required. Antiviral therapy is used in patients with complications or those at high risk (e.g. immunocompromised people). Many people, especially parents, worry about scarring but the lesions invariably heal, leaving normal skin, unless they become infected.

Advice to parents

- The patient should rest until feeling well.
- Give paracetamol for the fever (avoid aspirin in children due to the possibility of Reye syndrome).

Table 93.2 Complications of varicella
Common
Bacterial infection of cutaneous lesions (usually staphylococcal or streptococcal); can take form of cellulitis or bullous impetigo
Can leave pitted scars
Uncommon
Viral pneumonia
Eczema herpeticum
Thrombocytopenia
Birth defects with neonatal infection
Acute cerebellitis (ataxia, normal mental state)
Rare
Meningoencephalitis
Purpura fulminans

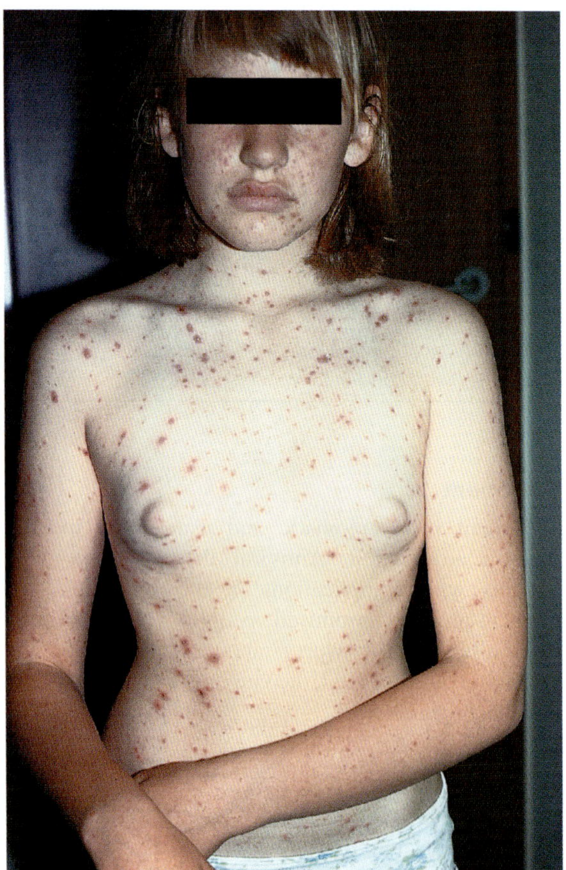

FIGURE 93.1 Varicella (chickenpox) in a 12-year-old girl showing a maculopapular vesicular rash with a centripetal distribution

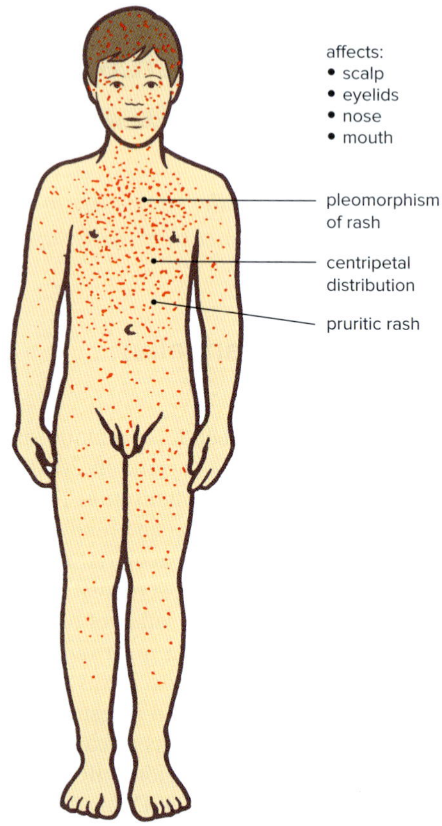

FIGURE 93.2 Chickenpox: typical distribution

- Daub calamine or a similar soothing lotion to relieve itching, although the itch is usually not severe.
- Avoid scratching; clean and keep the fingernails short. Provide cotton mittens if necessary.
- Daily bathing is advisable, with the addition of mild antiseptic or sodium bicarbonate if pruritic (add half a cup to the bath water). Pat dry with a clean, soft towel; do not rub.

Medication

Antihistamines can be prescribed for itching. Aciclovir or similar agents can be life-saving in the immunocompromised host. Antibiotics (e.g. flucloxacillin/dicloxacillin) are reserved for bacterial skin infection. Use hydrogel for sore wounds.

Exclusion from school[2]

Exclusion is recommended until the blisters have dried, usually at least 5 days in unimmunised children but possibly shorter in those immunised. Except for immunocompromised children, contacts should not be excluded from school.

Exclusion and incubation times for chickenpox (and other basic childhood infectious diseases) are given in TABLE 93.3.

Prevention

Prevention in contacts who are immunocompromised or at high risk (e.g. neonates) and in contact with varicella, is possible with zoster immune globulin (ZIG). An attenuated live virus vaccine is available and suitable for healthy children from the age of 12 months up to and including 13 years. It is given routinely at 18 months with the immunisation schedule. Vaccination of household contacts and post-exposure vaccination will reduce risk and also result in less serious disease if it does occur.

Reye syndrome and aspirin

There is concern over children with febrile illness ingesting aspirin because of the suspected causal relationship between aspirin and Reye syndrome, particularly in those with varicella, influenza and other viral diseases. The syndrome includes nausea and vomiting with the rapid development of encephalopathy, hepatic failure, seizures and coma.

Measles

Measles (rubeola) is a highly contagious disease caused by an RNA paramyxovirus. It presents as an acute febrile exanthematous illness with characteristic lesions on the buccal mucosa called Koplik spots (tiny white spots like grains of salt, opposite the molars).

The disease is endemic throughout the world and complications are usually respiratory in nature. If an acute exanthematous illness is not accompanied by a dry cough and red eyes, it is unlikely to be measles. Laboratory diagnosis is by serology, with IgM rising 3–5 days after the onset of the rash.

Table 93.3 Basic childhood infectious diseases: incubation periods, minimum exclusion periods from school, preschool and child care centres (times in days)[1,2]

	Incubation period (days)	Patient exclusion (least time from onset of rash or symptoms) (days)	Contact exclusion (days)
Measles	10–14	4	14 in non-immunised
Glandular fever	? 30–50	Nil	Nil
Mumps	12–25	9	Nil
Pertussis	7–20	5 (after starting antibiotics) or 21 from onset of cough	Non-immunised household contacts—until have had 5 days of antibiotics or 21 days after exposure finishes
Parvovirus B19 (erythema infectiosum)	4–20	Nil	Nil
Roseola infantum	7–17	Nil	Nil
Rubella	14–21	4	Nil
Scarlet fever	1–7	24 hours (after starting antibiotics and feeling well)	Nil
Impetigo	1–3 for strep, 4–10 for staph	Until treatment commenced (cover sores)	Nil
Meningococcus	1–10 (commonly 3–4)	Until antibiotic therapy complete	Check with consultant
Varicella and zoster	10–21	Until blisters have dried	Only those immune deficient
Hepatitis			
A	15–50	7 or recovery	Nil
B	45–180	Nil	Nil
C	14–180	Nil	Nil
Infective diarrhoea	Varies	24 hours after cessation of diarrhoea	Nil

Epidemiology

Measles is transmitted by patient-to-patient contact through oropharyngeal and nasopharyngeal droplets expelled during coughing and sneezing.

The incubation period is 10–14 days and the patient is infectious until about 4 days after the onset of the rash, but especially just before the appearance of the rash. Morbidity and mortality are high in countries with substandard living conditions and poor nutrition.

Immunity appears to be lifelong after infection. Measles, like smallpox, could be eradicated with public health measures. While vaccination programs have been very successful worldwide, there has been a recent resurgence of measles in developed countries due to falling vaccination rates in some areas.

Clinical features

The clinical presentation can be considered in three stages.

1 *Prodromal stage.* This usually lasts 3–4 days. It is marked by fever, malaise, anorexia, diarrhoea and 'the three Cs': cough, coryza and conjunctivitis (see FIG. 93.3). Sometimes a non-specific rash appears a day before the Koplik spots.
2 *Exanthema (rash) stage.* Identified by a typically blotchy, bright red maculopapular eruption; this stage lasts 4–5 days. The rash begins behind the ears; on the first day it spreads to the face (see FIG. 93.4), the next day to the trunk and later to the limbs. It may become confluent and blanches under pressure. The patient's fever usually subsides within 5 days of the onset of the rash.
3 *Convalescent stage.* The rash fades, leaving a temporary brownish 'staining'. The patient's cough may persist for days, but usually good health and appetite return quickly, with recovery in about 7–10 days.

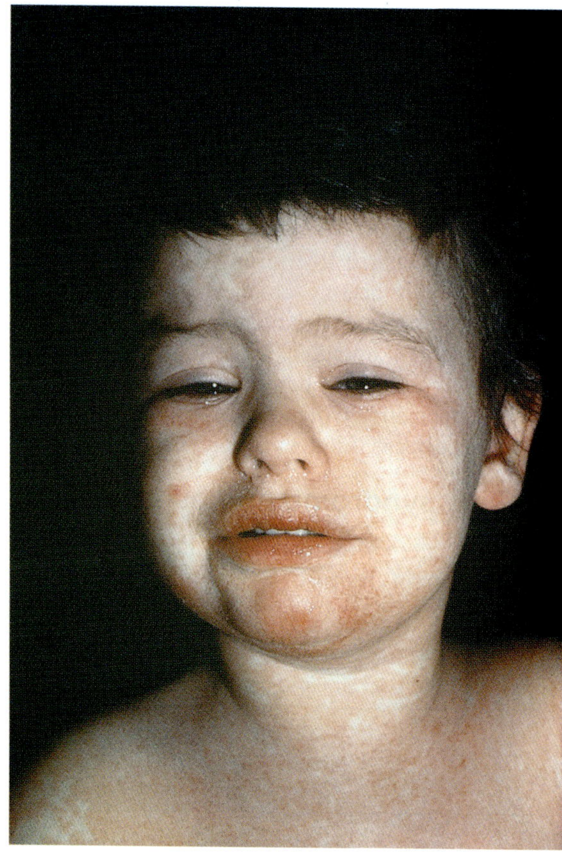

FIGURE 93.3 Measles showing the typical blotchy, bright red maculopapular rash on the face of a miserable child with the three Cs (cough, coryza and conjunctivitis)

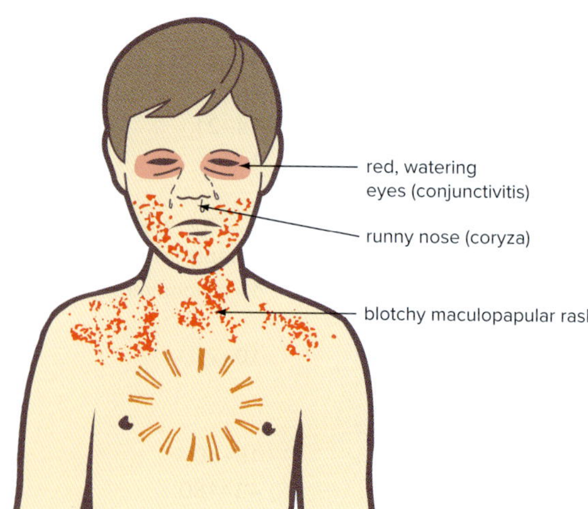

FIGURE 93.4 Measles typical symptoms. Note the 3Cs: cough, coryza, conjunctivitis.

Complications

Measles is often a serious disease, and complications are common.[1] These include otitis media (9%), pneumonia (6%) and diarrhoea (8%). Children under 5 and adults and patients with chronic disease are more prone to complications. For every 1000 children who get measles, 1 to 2 will die,[3] with the majority of deaths occurring from pneumonia. Infection during pregnancy can lead to miscarriage or premature delivery, but is not associated with congenital malformation.

Central nervous system

Encephalitis has an incidence of 1 in 1000, and has a mortality of 10–15% and also a high rate of permanent brain damage. Subacute sclerosing panencephalitis (SSPE) is a late complication, occurring on average 7 years after infection in 0.5–1/100 000 cases, and is manifested by universally fatal progressive brain damage.

Treatment

There is no specific treatment although some symptoms can be relieved (e.g. a linctus for the cough, paracetamol for fever). The patient should rest quietly, avoid bright lights and stay in bed until the fever subsides. Oral vitamin A has been reported to reduce complications.

Prevention

Vaccination should be given to any child over 12 months, or any teenager or adult born since 1966 who does not have a documented record of 2 MMR-containing vaccines (or serological evidence of protection for measles, mumps and rubella).[1] Live attenuated measles virus vaccinations combined with mumps and rubella (MMR) are recommended at the age of 12 months and then MMRV (with varicella) at 18 months. Consider normal immunoglobulin for infants under 12 months and the immunocompromised when MMR is contraindicated, given as soon as possible after exposure.

Rubella

Rubella (German measles) is a viral exanthema caused by a togavirus. It is a minor illness in children and adults, but devastating when transmitted in utero. Congenital rubella syndrome (CRS) occurs in up to 90% of infants born to mothers contracting rubella in the first trimester. Multiple features of CRS are usually evident, which include intellectual disabilities, cataracts, deafness, cardiac abnormalities, intrauterine growth disorders (IUGR) and inflammatory lesions of the brain, liver, lungs and bone marrow. It is completely preventable. The risk declines rapidly after the first trimester.

All women of child-bearing age should have 2 documented doses of rubella-containing vaccines and if not their immune status should be assessed serologically. If not immune, they should be vaccinated and retested 6–8 weeks later and revaccinated if they have negative or low levels. No antibody response to 2 doses may represent a false negative result. Rubella-containing vaccinations are contraindicated in pregnant woman and pregnancy should be avoided for 28 days after vaccination.[1] Once the baby arrives, postpartum vaccination of those mothers not fully immune should be done immediately (breastfeeding is not a contraindication).

Epidemiology

CRS is rare in Australia due to vaccination. Only 2.5% of women of child-bearing age are seronegative, though the risk is higher in women born overseas. Intra-uterine infection occurs via the placenta.

Approximately one-third of infections are asymptomatic (subclinical). Infection usually confers lifelong immunity. Incubation period is 14–21 days.

Clinical features

The clinical features of rubella are presented in TABLE 93.4 and FIGURE 93.5 and the complications in TABLE 93.5.

Table 93.4 Clinical features of rubella

There is no prodrome.
A generalised, maculopapular rash, sometimes pruritic, may be the only evidence of infection.
Other symptoms are usually mild and short-lived.
There is often a reddened pharynx but sore throats are unusual. An exudate may be seen as well as palatal exanthem.
Fever is usually absent or low-grade.
Other features: headache, myalgia, conjunctivitis and polyarthritis (small joints).
Lymphadenopathy may be noted; usually postauricular, suboccipital and postcervical.
The patient is infectious for a week before and at least 4 days after the onset of the rash.
The rash
A discrete pale pink maculopapular rash (not confluent as in measles).
Starts on the face and neck—spreads to the trunk and extremities.
Variable severity: may be absent in subclinical infection.
Exaggerated on skin exposed to sun.
Brief duration—usually fades on the third day.
No staining or desquamation.

Treatment

Treatment is symptomatic, especially as rubella is a mild disease. Patients should rest quietly until they feel well and take paracetamol for fever and aching joints. Prevention is by vaccination, recommended at 12 and 18 months.

School exclusion

The child is usually excluded until fully recovered or for at least 4 days from the onset of the rash.

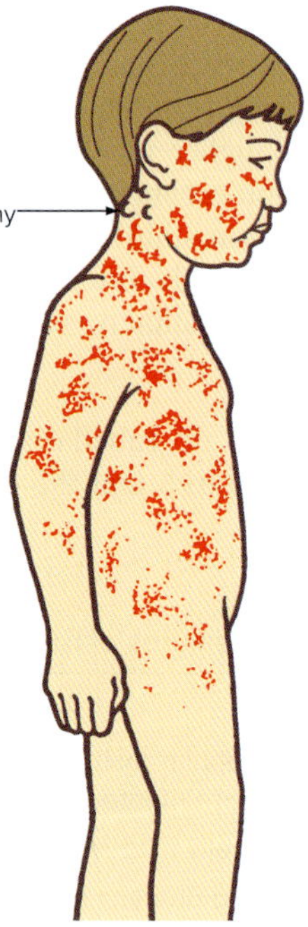

FIGURE 93.5 Rubella: typical symptoms

Table 93.5 Complications of rubella
Encephalitis (rare)
Polyarthritis, especially in adult women (this complication abates spontaneously)
Thrombocytopenia (rare)
Congenital rubella syndrome

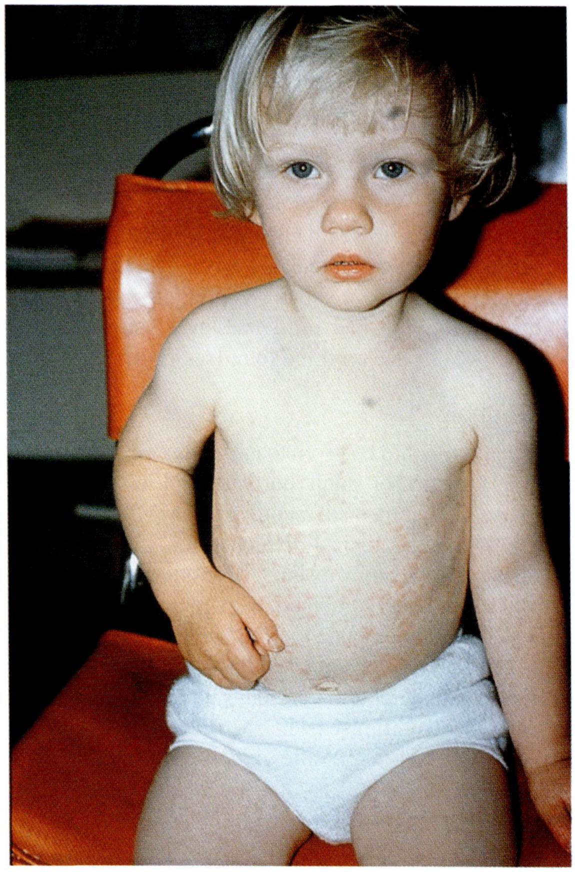

FIGURE 93.6 Viral exanthema (fourth syndrome). This mild rubella-like maculopapular rash, which may be caused by a number of viruses, is usually non-pruritic

93

Viral exanthema (fourth syndrome)

This mild childhood infection may be caused by a number of viruses, especially the enteroviruses, and produces a rubella-like rash that may be misdiagnosed as rubella. The rash, which is usually non-pruritic and mainly confined to the trunk, does not desquamate and often fades within 48 hours (see FIG. 93.6). The child may appear quite well or can have mild constitutional symptoms, including diarrhoea.

Parvovirus B19 (erythema infectiosum, fifth disease)

Parvovirus, also known as 'slapped cheek' syndrome, is a childhood exanthem caused by parvovirus strain B19. It occurs typically in young school-aged children. The incubation period is 4–20 days. Non-specific prodromal symptoms (fever, runny nose, headache, nausea) are followed 2–5 days later by the rash. The bright macular rash erupts on the face first (see FIG. 93.7) then, after a day or so, a maculopapular rash appears on the limbs.[1] The rash lasts for only a few days but may recur for several weeks. By the time the rash appears the individual usually is no longer infective.

Clinical features

- Mild fever (30%) and malaise
- Runny nose, headache, nausea
- Possible lymphadenopathy (especially cervical)

The rash (see FIG. 93.8):

- bright red flushed cheeks with circumoral pallor for 2–3 days
- maculopapular rash on limbs (especially) and trunk (sparse)
- reticular appearance on fading
- may be pruritic

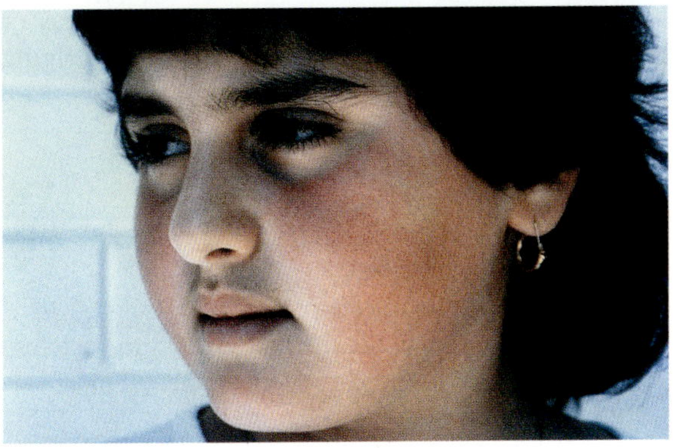

FIGURE 93.7 Parvovirus, showing the typical slapped cheek appearance

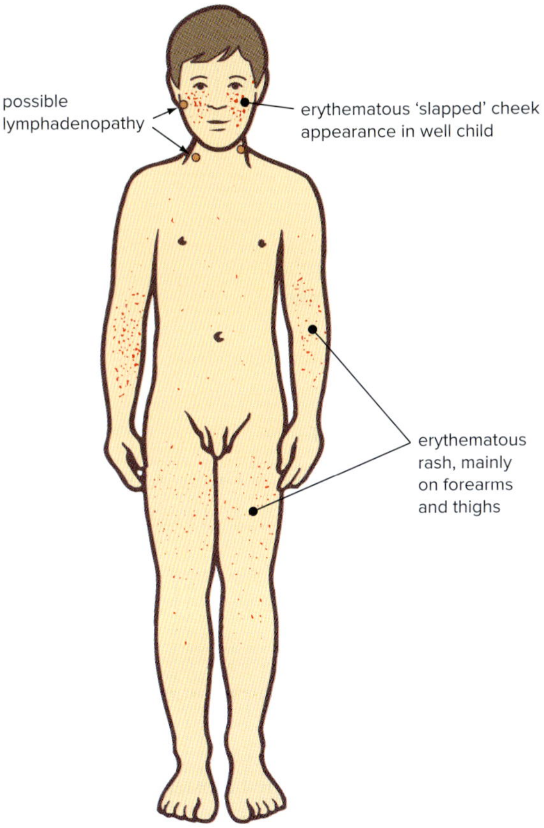

FIGURE 93.8 Parvovirus: typical distribution of rash

Typically, the cheeks become reddened again for the next few weeks on exposure to sunlight or wind or after a hot bath. Adults can be infected and the side effects, especially arthritis, can be quite severe.

Parvovirus in pregnancy[4]

Erythema infectiosum is a mild illness but, if the parvovirus infection occurs during pregnancy, fetal complications including miscarriage can occur. It is advisable to avoid close contact with pregnant women (see CHAPTER 108). Some 50% of young adult females are susceptible to parvovirus infection. About 50% of susceptible household contacts will become infected, and around 20% of classroom contacts.

Pregnant women should be tested for parvovirus IgM and IgG if:

- in the same room as the infected person for >15 minutes
- face-to-face contact
- household contact

The results are interpreted as:

- IgG alone detected—immune
- IgM detected—false positive or early infection. Repeat in 2 weeks to see if rising IgG levels
- IgM and IgG not present—susceptible. If susceptible and becomes unwell, repeat test

If infection occurs in the first half of pregnancy, the fetus may become anaemic (the virus replicates in erythroid progenitor cells) and hydrops fetalis and miscarriage can occur. Women in this situation should be reassured that <5% of women will miscarry, though ultrasound monitoring is recommended. Parvovirus in pregnancy is not associated with fetal anomalies. If exposure or infection is suspected in the second half of pregnancy, investigation is still warranted as there may be errors in the gestational age and the risk to other pregnant women in health settings needs to be managed.

Treatment

Treatment is symptomatic.

- Ample fluid intake
- Paracetamol for fever
- If itchy, daub a soothing anti-itch lotion such as Pinetarsol or calamine lotion
- Wear a broad-brimmed hat when outside

Adults may need stronger analgesics or NSAIDs for arthralgia (more common in adult women).

Roseola (roseola infantum, exanthema subitum or sixth disease)

Roseola is a viral infection (human herpes virus 6) of infancy, affecting children at the age of 6 months and 2 years; 95% of children have had it by this time, and it is rare after this. Constitutional symptoms are generally mild.

Clinical features

- *Sudden* high fever (up to 40°C)
- Runny nose
- Temperature falls after 3 days (or so) *then*
- Red macular or maculopapular rash appears

The rash:

- largely confined to the trunk and limbs (see FIG. 93.9)
- usually spares face
- appears as fever subsides
- blanches on pressing
- disappears within 2 days
- no desquamation
- mild cervical lymphadenopathy

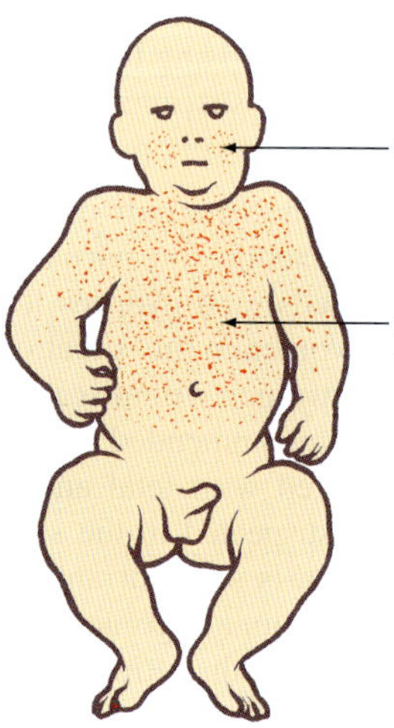

FIGURE 93.9 Roseola: typical distribution of rash

The infection runs a benign course, although a febrile convulsion can occur. The child will no longer be infectious by the time the symptoms appear. Treatment is symptomatic. Encourage high fluid intake.

Hand, foot and mouth (HFM) disease

This is a mild vesicular eruption caused by enteroviruses, the most common being Coxsackie A-16, with EV-71 being less common. HFM disease affects both children and adults but typically children under the age of 10. Sometimes referred to as 'crèche disease', it often occurs among groups of children in child care centres. Transmission is through respiratory secretions, touch contact with the blistered areas or faeco-oral transmission (hand washing after changing nappies is important to reduce transmission).

Clinical features

- Incubation period 3–5 days
- Initial fever, headache and malaise
- Sore mouth and throat
- The rash appears after 1 or 2 days
- Starts as a red macule, then progresses to vesicles
- Vesicles lead to shallow ulcers on buccal mucosa, gums and tongue
- Greyish vesicle with surrounding erythema
- On hands, palms and soles (usually lateral borders)
- May appear on limbs especially buttocks and genitals
- Lesions resolve in 3–5 days
- Healing without scarring
- Virus excreted in faeces and saliva for several weeks
- Children are infectious until the blisters have disappeared
- Diagnosis is clinical, investigations usually unnecessary

Management

- Reassurance and explanation
- Symptomatic treatment
- Careful hygiene
- Exclusion until blisters have dried up

Scarlet fever

Scarlet fever results when a Group A *Streptococcus pyogenes* organism produces erythrogenic toxin. The prodromal symptoms prior to the acute exanthem comprise malaise, sore throat, fever (may be rigors) and vomiting. A throat swab should be taken.

Features of the rash

- Appears 12–24 hours after the start of the fever
- First appears on neck
- Rapidly generalised
- Punctate and red, a 'boiled lobster' or sunburnt appearance
- Blanches on pressure
- Prominent on neck, in axillae, cubital fossa (Pastia lines), groin, skinfolds (see FIG. 93.10)
- Absent or sparse on face, palms and soles
- Circumoral pallor
- Feels like fine sandpaper
- Lasts about 5 days
- Fine desquamation

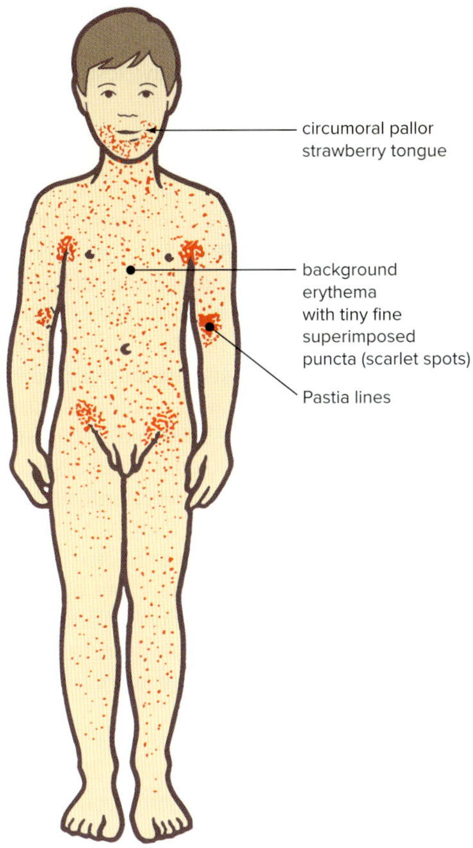

FIGURE 93.10 Scarlet fever: typical presentation of rash

Treatment

Phenoxymethylpenicillin (dose according to age) for 10 days with rapid resolution of symptoms, although resistance is increasingly common. Children can return to school 24 hours after taking antibiotics and feeling well.

Kawasaki disease[5,6]

This is an uncommon but important systemic vasculitis that typically affects the coronary arteries, usually in children under 5 years of age and likely caused by an infection, though the presumed agent remains unknown. It is characterised by an acute onset of fever >39°C of 5 days or more and accompanied by 4 out of 5 of the following features:

- polymorphous rash
- bilateral (non-purulent) conjunctival infection
- mucous membrane changes, e.g. reddened or dry cracked lips, strawberry tongue, diffuse redness of oral or pharyngeal mucosa
- peripheral changes, e.g. erythema of the palms or soles, oedema of the hands or feet (and in convalescence desquamation)
- an 'unusual' nappy rash
- cervical lymphadenopathy (>15 mm diameter, usually unilateral, single, non-purulent and painful)

Diagnosis is basically a clinical one. Other diseases with similar signs should be excluded (e.g. staph or strep infections, measles, viral exanthems, drug reactions or JRA).

Kawasaki disease can be elusive as there are variations with atypical or incomplete manifestations. Think of it in a miserable child with a high fever ≥5 days and arrange for paediatric review if suspicious. Blood results will also help contribute to the diagnosis and management decisions (e.g. ESR and CRP usually raised, thrombocytosis often raised in second week, neutrophilia, normochromic normocytic anaemia, hypoalbuminuria, abnormal LFTs).

The disease is often benign and self-limiting but it is important to make an early diagnosis because early treatment may prevent complications (which also occur in the atypical cases). The major complication is vasculitis, which causes coronary aneurysms and ectasia in 15–25% of untreated cases, and which can lead to ischaemic heart disease and sudden death either at the time or years later. The aneurysms usually develop between the second week and the second month of the illness. Early treatment with immunoglobulin, oral aspirin and possibly IV methylprednisolone has been shown to be effective in reducing the prevalence of coronary artery abnormalities. Echocardiography is used to detect the aneurysms and determine prognosis.

93

Mumps[1]

Mumps is an acute infectious disease caused by a paramyxovirus with an affinity for the salivary glands and meninges. It is usually transmitted by respiratory secretions or saliva. A third of infections are asymptomatic, and most of the others have non-specific symptoms, such as fever, headache, malaise, myalgia and anorexia. The classic parotitis occurs in only two-thirds of clinical cases and is usually bilateral. The submandibular and sublingual glands are less commonly involved. About 6% of patients will have presternal oedema resembling cellulitis of the neck.

Mumps can result in spontaneous abortion if contracted in the first trimester of pregnancy. Maternal infection is not associated with an increased risk of congenital malformations.

Prior to vaccination, cases peaked in the 5–9-year age group; however, since 2000 it is now most commonly seen in adolescents and young adults. Recent outbreaks have occurred in the developed world in areas of declining vaccination rates.

Clinical diagnosis

Enlargement of the cervical lymph glands can be mistaken for parotitis but the correct diagnosis is indicated by the anatomy of this area. Lymph nodes are posteroinferior to the ear lobe; the parotid gland is anterior and, when enlarged, obscures the angle of the mandible.

Bacterial (suppurative) parotitis is associated with toxaemia and results in a high leucocyte count. The skin over the parotid gland is tense and shiny and the Stensen duct might discharge pus.

Rare disorders such as Sjögren syndrome can be misdiagnosed as mumps.

Complications

The complications are summarised in TABLE 93.6.

Orchitis, usually unilateral, occurs in 15–30% of postpubertal males, developing 3–4 days after parotitis. Subsequent sterility is rare, even if both testes are affected.

Aseptic meningitis is common but benign. Many patients suffer transient abdominal pain and vomiting.

Table 93.6 Complications of mumps

Common
Orchitis
Meningeal symptoms (10%)
Abdominal pain (transient)
Rare
Oophoritis
Encephalitis
Arthritis (one or several joints)
Deafness (usually transient)
Pancreatitis

Management

Treatment is symptomatic. Paracetamol may be prescribed for fever, meningitis and orchitis. The patient with orchitis should use supportive underwear. Children should be excluded until 9 days after the onset of the parotitis.

Epstein–Barr mononucleosis

Although glandular fever is more common in adolescents and young adults, it can occur in young children but is often asymptomatic or atypical. The differential diagnosis includes cytomegalovirus infection and acute lymphatic leukaemia. Diagnosis is confirmed by specific antibody tests. Refer to CHAPTER 28.

Pertussis[1,7]

Pertussis (whooping cough) is a respiratory infection (a bronchitis) caused by *Bordetella pertussis* and occurs worldwide. Other organisms (*Bordetella parapertussis, Mycoplasma pneumoniae, Chlamydia pneumoniae*) can cause a pertussis-like syndrome. Despite vaccination, pertussis remains prevalent in Australia, and is the least well-controlled vaccine-preventable disease. Between 2000 and 2010 multiple epidemics caused over 139 000 confirmed cases.

The greatest risk of severe infection and complications is to infants with their soft and easily damaged airways, especially before the first 2 vaccine doses are administered. Adolescents and adults with waning immunity (both from vaccination and previous infection) are often the source of infection, in particular the parents (>50% of identified primary cases).

Clinical features

Pertussis is highly infectious, with *B. pertussis* spreading to >90% of household contacts. The incubation period is 7 to 20 days. The classical paroxysmal cough followed by an inspiratory whoop is less common in older children and adults, or children who have partial immunity from vaccination. A prolonged cough may be the only presenting feature, and in local epidemics every cough needs to be approached with the suspicion of pertussis.

B. pertussis accounts for 7% of cough illnesses in adults, and given that each year 25% of adults have a cough ≥5 days duration, many cases go undiagnosed. The primary goal of preventing complications and deaths is centred on protecting children, particularly infants (see Prevention below). The fatality rate in unvaccinated infants less than 6 months is 8 per 1000 cases. The most common cause of death is pertussis pneumonia, sometimes complicated by seizures and hypoxic encephalopathy. Apnoea and cyanosis from coughing spasms are also common in the very young.

Even in adults the cough can be very distressing and prolonged. Pertussis is also referred to as the '100 day cough'. This can lead to issues with sleep disturbance, work performance (especially when dealing with machinery or driving) and rarely rib fractures.

Classic whooping cough is characterised by cough and coryza for 1 week (catarrhal phase) followed by paroxysms of a more pronounced cough (paroxysmal phase). Fever is uncommon, there are often no other clinical signs, and children are well between coughing paroxysms. Vomiting may follow a coughing spasm (a 'cough-vomit').

Diagnosis

As well has having a high index of suspicion with coughing patients (both immunised and non-immunised), particularly in outbreaks, any suspicion should lead to PCR testing of nasopharyngeal aspirate/swab.

Complications

- Neurological: asphyxia, hypoxia, seizures, cerebral haemorrhages
- Pulmonary: atelectasis, pneumonia, pneumothorax, bronchiectasis

Treatment[7,8]

Treatment during the catarrhal phase or early in the paroxysmal stage may ameliorate symptoms. Treatment early in the disease will help reduce infectiousness; however, once the cough has been present for 3 weeks there is little risk of infectiousness. Options include:

- azithromycin
  - <6 months: 10 mg/kg daily for 5 days
  - >6 months: 10 mg/kg on day 1 (up to 500 mg) then 5 mg/kg (up to 250 mg) for a further 4 days
- clarithromycin
  - >1 month: 7.5 mg/kg (up to 500 mg) bd for 7 days
- erythromycin
  - >1 month: 10 mg/kg (up to 250 mg, or 400 mg if ethyl succinate) qid for 7 days

Cough mixtures are ineffective. Good ventilation is important: avoid dust and smoke, and also emotional excitement and overfeeding during the paroxysmal phase.

All infants under 6 months and older children with complications (e.g. apnoea, cyanosis, pneumonia, encephalopathy) require admission to hospital.

Treatment of contacts[8]

High-risk contacts of a pertussis case (those with close/household contact and who may be vulnerable to complications, or transmit to others who are vulnerable) should be treated with the same medications, dosage and duration as above. There is little evidence that prophylactic antibiotic treatment of contacts reduces secondary transmission outside of household settings (i.e. not in child-care centres, preschools, schools or workplaces). State public health officers should be contacted to determine which contacts require prophylaxis.

Prevention[8]

Active immunisation with pertussis vaccine is given at 2, 4 and 6 months, then at 4 years as per the NIP schedule. Other strategies to reduce the incidence of pertussis and its complications, particularly in infants, include:

- a 'cocoon' strategy of vaccinating any adults who are or will be in close contact with an infant. Fathers and other adult contacts can be vaccinated before the birth
- mothers should be vaccinated in pre-pregnancy planning or straight after delivery. Alternatively, if more than 5 years has elapsed since their last previous dose, a pertussis vaccine should be given in their third trimester (which will boost maternal antibodies that are transmitted in utero to the about-to-be-newborn)
- a single booster dose of pertussis-containing vaccine is recommended in health care workers and other adults in regular contact with young children (booster required after 10 years)

Herpes simplex[9]

93

Herpes simplex virus (HSV) infection is common and widespread. Primary HSV infection is usually a disease of childhood readily transmitted through direct contact, with the majority of the population being infected in early childhood. Many cases are asymptomatic or non-specific. The specific gingivostomatitis occurs in 25–30% of cases and can be severe and acute.

Clinical features

Typical clinical features of the primary infection:

- children 1–3 years
- fever and refusal to feed
- ulcers on gums, tongue and palate
- prone to dehydration
- may be lesions on face and conjunctivae
- resolution over 7–14 days

Pushing fluids and monitoring for dehydration is important. Topical lignocaine preparations can help. Paracetamol is often not useful, though if the child is very distressed, combined ibuprofen and paracetamol compounds can be considered. Topical antivirals usually do not contribute and are not recommended.

Serious complications (seek specialist advice):

- encephalitis can develop in otherwise healthy children (see CHAPTER 30)
- eczema herpeticum—children with eczema can get widespread severe herpetic lesions
- disseminated HSV infection in neonates (avoid contact until recovered)
- HSV can be a serious issue in the immunocompromised patient

Impetigo[10]

Impetigo (school sores) is a contagious superficial bacterial skin infection caused by *Streptococcus pyogenes* or *Staphylococcus aureus* or a combination of these two virulent organisms.

There are two common forms:

1. vesiculopustular with honey-coloured crusts (either strep or staph)
2. bullous type, usually *S. aureus*

Treatment

If mild with small lesions and a limited area:

- soak a clean cloth in a mixture of ½ cup white vinegar and 1 L of tepid water. Apply the compress to moist areas for 10 minutes several times a day then wipe off crusts (alternatively just use soap and water)
- antiseptic (povidone iodine, chlorhexadine) or mupirocin (Bactroban), a small amount tds for 10 days. Topical antibiotics other than mupirocin 2% (Bactroban) are not recommended
- general measures while still oozing or crusted:
  - cover the sores
  - avoid close contact with others (especially touch and bathing contact)
  - regular hand washing
  - use separate towels and cloths
  - change and launder clothes and linen daily

If extensive and causing systemic symptoms:

flucloxacillin/dicloxacillin 12.5 mg/kg up to 500 mg) 6 hourly for 10 days
or
cephalexin 25 mg/kg up to 1 g 12 hourly for 10 days

Boils (furunculosis) and carbuncles can use the same treatment as impetigo.

The child should be excluded from child-care settings until antibiotic treatment has commenced. Any sores on exposed skin should be covered with a watertight dressing.[2]

93

Head lice[11]

Head lice is an infestation caused by the louse *Pediculus humanus capitis* (see FIG. 93.11). The head louse is about 1–3 mm in length, white to grey, wingless and has a flat elongated body. They spread through close contact, and do not jump or fly. The female louse lays eggs (or 'nits'), which are glued to the hairs a few millimeters from the scalp. The nit moves away from the scalp as the hair grows. They hatch at around 8 days, mature into adults in about 10 days and live for about a month.

Head lice spread from person to person by direct contact, such as sitting and working very close to one another. They can also spread by the sharing of combs, brushes and headwear, especially within the family. Children are the ones usually affected, but people of all ages and from all walks of life can be infested. It is more common in overcrowded living conditions but is not a reflection of poor hygiene. Resistance to the usual agents is becoming a problem.

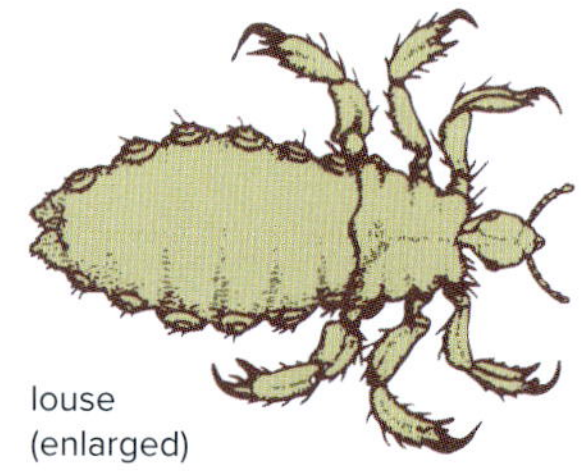

FIGURE 93.11 Louse (enlarged)

Clinical features

Infestations can vary from a few dozen to hundreds of lice and eggs.

- Asymptomatic or itching of scalp
- White spots of nits can be mistaken for dandruff
- Unlike dandruff, the nits cannot be brushed off
- Diagnosis by finding lice (or nits)
- Occasionally the eyelashes can be affected (use physical removal methods outlined below)
- 'Wet combing' (see below) improves detection rate

Treatment

Treatment can be based on physical methods, chemical methods or both (the most effective).

Physical methods

Wet combing:

- Inspection—look for both lice and nits behind and above the ears and at the back of the scalp.
- Treat all members of family at the same time.

- Have ready a metal nit comb (available at pharmacies), a good light, some paper towels or tissues and lots of cheap hair conditioner. Sitting a child in front of the TV will help them keep still (it takes around 30 minutes).
- Wet the hair with a handful or two of conditioner.
- Work through the hair in sections, removing resistant nits by combing down the hair towards the shaft.
- Wipe the conditioner onto tissues or paper towels, where the lice and nits will be visible.

Repeat the combing routine for at least 2 more consecutive nights. Repeat weekly until no lice are found on 3 consecutive nights (nits may persist but do not necessarily mean active infection—they may be empty or dead eggs). Other physical measures include:

- machine wash bed-linen, clothes, towels in hot water
- items that can't be washed such as soft toys/helmets should be placed in an airtight plastic bag for two weeks
- vacuum pillows
- spray hairbrushes and combs with fly spray

Chemical treatments

Insecticides used to treat head lice include:

- malathion
- permethrin
- phenothrin

These applications can be irritating to the scalp, so use caution in children prone to atopic dermatitis; following the manufacturer's instructions carefully is important. A second application 7 days after the first may be required.

Many other methods are used and recommended for head lice, both commercially available or 'home remedies', which may or may not be useful. These include suffocating agents (e.g. mayonnaise, olive oil, petroleum jelly), natural oils and cutting the hair short (especially in boys e.g. a No. 1 cut).

Treatment failure and/or reinfestation is common. The former can be from inappropriately applied treatments, resistance to chemical treatments or misdiagnosis of old nits as active infection. Cotrimoxazole can be trialled for resistant head lice. Community or school-wide education programs can also keep infestation rates down.

Patient education resources

Hand-out sheets from *Murtagh's Patient Education* 7th edition:

- Chickenpox (varicella)
- Hand, foot and mouth disease
- Lice: head lice
- Herpes simplex (cold sores)
- Impetigo
- Measles
- Mumps
- Roseola
- Rubella
- Slapped cheek disease
- Whooping cough (pertussis)

References

1 National Health and Medical Research Council. *The Australian Immunisation Handbook* (10th edn, updated January 2014).

2 National Health and Medical Research Council. *Staying Healthy in Child Care—Preventing Infectious Diseases in Child Care* (4th edn), December 2005.

3 The Center for Disease Control. Measles (home page), July 2014 <www.cdc.gov/measles/> (accessed 27/7/2014).

4 The Center for Disease Control. Pregnancy and fifth disease, February 2012 <www.cdc.gov/parvovirusB19/pregnancy.html> (accessed 27/7/2014).

5 The Royal Children's Hospital Melbourne. *Clinical Practice Guidelines: Kawasaki Disease,* December 2012 <www.rch.org.au/clinicalguide/guideline_index/Kawasaki_Disease_Guideline/> (accessed 28/7/2014).

6 American Academy of Pediatrics. Diagnosis, treatment, and long-term management of Kawasaki disease: a statement for health professionals. Pediatrics, 2004; 114 (6): 1708–33.

7 The Royal Children's Hospital Melbourne. *Clinical Practice Guidelines: Whooping Cough (Pertussis),* May 2014 <www.rch.org.au/clinicalguide/guideline_index/Whooping_Cough_Pertussis/> (accessed 28/7/2014).

8 Expert group for Antibiotic. ENT: pertussis. In: eTG complete [Internet]. Melbourne: Therapeutic Guidelines Limited. Available from: <www.tg.org.au> (accessed November 2017).

9 The Royal Children's Hospital Melbourne. *Clinical Practice Guidelines: HSV Gingivostomatitis,* November 2013 <www.rch.org.au/clinicalguide/guideline_index/HSV_Gingivostomatitis/> (accessed 29/7/2014).

10 Expert group for Antibiotic. Skin and soft tissue infections: impetigo. In: eTG complete [Internet]. Melbourne: Therapeutic Guidelines Limited. Available from: <www.tg.org.au> (accessed November 2017).

11 DermNet NZ: the dermatology resource <www.dermnetnz.org/> (accessed 30/7/2014).

94 Behavioural and developmental issues and disorders in children

Although the world is full of suffering, it is full also of the overcoming of it.

HELEN KELLER, 1903

Many behavioural issues in children arise because of (and in the context of) factors such as the child's temperament, parental schema and child–parent attachment. These factors determine, in the beginning, how the parent–child relationship will evolve, and also strongly affect the psychological development of the child.

Temperament

Temperament refers to the personality characteristics you are born with—what is innate rather than learned. An awareness of the fact that children are born with characteristics over which parents have no control can be liberating, especially for parents of children with challenging temperaments.

The best-known description of temperament is based on the work of Thomas and Chess from the 1970s[1] (TABLE 94.1). They found that about two-thirds of children can be classified into one of three categories: easy, difficult and slow to warm up. Of these, about 15% were considered easy, 70% slow to warm up and 15% difficult. A child with a difficult temperament will be emotionally labile and have difficulty coping with new experiences. A child with a slow-to-settle temperament will have some difficulty coping with new experiences, but will eventually manage after repeated exposures. A child with an easy temperament will cope easily with new experiences and will have a calm nature.

Easy doesn't mean good, and difficult doesn't mean bad. These children may just require more patience and a thoughtful and paced approach to parenting. Further, the characteristics that can make a child 'difficult' can be the flipside of other characteristics that lead them to achieve success (if appropriately nurtured and guided). A stubborn child may have good persistence, and a distractible child may be artistic and expressive.

Of course, most children will have a few 'difficult' characteristics, but some will have more than others. Raising parents' awareness of this, getting them to think about the innate characteristics of their child (which may or may not be similar to their siblings or one or both of the biological parents) and to adjust their parenting style accordingly will help them deal more effectively with the challenges of raising their child.

Table 94.1 Easy and difficult temperament characteristics

Easy temperament characteristic	Difficult temperament characteristic
Generally happy	Generally serious
Goes with the flow	Inflexible
Laid-back	In-your-face
Patient	Impulsive
Flexible	Stubborn
Friendly	Shy
Calm body movements	Restless
Persistent	Gives up easily
Calm nature	Hot-tempered
Expressive	Reserved
'Even' mood	Up and down mood
Thick-skinned	Over-sensitive
Good concentration	Distractible
Regular body clock	Chaotic body clock
Tolerates sensations well	'Sensory defensiveness' (light, sounds, tastes, textures)

Parental schema

Schema is the view you have of the world based on your own experiences; it is the 'soup in your head'. Parental schema is how parents view how they should parent, and is often based on how they were brought up themselves. Parental schemas may not match, and this can cause relationship issues. Parental attitudes to issues such as communication, emotion sharing and discipline can fundamentally affect the behaviour and psychological health of a child. Parental schema can also commonly be influenced by cultural factors.

Child–parent attachment

An infant first has to learn how to connect with other minds. A child does this in their first relationship, usually with their mother. This is attachment.

It's important to note that attachment is an ongoing phenomenon, even into adulthood. Children attach not only to their mother, but to other people from whom they can 'gather strength'. Children's attachment to their two parents may differ and can also change over time.

A secure attachment is achieved if a parent responds to a child's cries *promptly*, *consistently* and *appropriately*. The three main ways in which attachment can go wrong are:

- Carer not responding—this can result in a lack of emotional depth in the child.
- Carer responding inconsistently—this can lead to uncertainty and anxiety in the child.
- Carer responding inappropriately—such as with aggression or anger. This is obviously very damaging, and happens in situations of emotional abuse, particularly with mental health or drug and alcohol issues in the carer. It creates a terrible and *unsolvable paradox* for children, where the person on whom they are completely reliant to teach them how to relate to the world is also a threat.

Observing how carers, particularly mothers, respond and interact to their child can give the family doctor insight into this relationship. Gently advising and encouraging appropriate responses to the child's needs can be beneficial, particularly in a mother with poor parenting capabilities and/or difficult circumstances (e.g. very young mothers, socially isolated, postnatal depression, drug using or alcoholic parents, violence in the household). In high-risk situations, further referral to support services or even protective agencies may be required (see CHAPTER 95).

Child behaviour and discipline[2,3]

Issues around child behaviour and how to deal with unwanted behaviours commonly arise and are often a source of conflict and angst. It is normal for children, especially toddlers, to have resistant and oppositional behaviour. The word 'discipline' comes from the Latin *disciplina*, which means 'to teach'. The purpose of disciplining a child is to guide and teach, so they know what is allowed and what is not allowed, what 'works' in the world and what will not.

Parents can teach children in a variety of ways. The most effective forms of discipline are actually praise and encouragement—of wanted behaviours. However, when children are doing something that they should not—an unwanted behaviour—they need to learn that this is the case. The challenge for parents is to get this message across to them clearly and effectively.

A simple equation sums up the best way to deliver this message:

> unwanted behaviour = unwanted (by your child) outcome

Educating parents to recognise that the thing a child desires most in the world is the attention (this is a survival instinct) and approval of their parents will help them understand how to reinforce desired behaviours, and extinguish unwanted behaviours. That is, pay attention to when the child is behaving, and even praise particularly wanted behaviours, and ignore unwanted behaviours.

Consequences[3]

Consequences work only with children >3 years of age, and should be used solely in response to a small fraction of a child's behaviour, regardless of the child's temperament. If consequences are overused, their effectiveness diminishes and family relationships can be damaged.

There are three types of consequences that work (in decreasing order of usefulness):

- *Natural consequences:* where there is a natural flow from the misdemeanour to the consequence. For example, if a child refuses to have dinner, he or she goes to bed hungry. Natural consequences have a momentum of their own and, assuming they do not result in harm, can provide many valuable lessons.
- *Related consequences:* where there is some link between the unwanted behaviour and the result. This is also sometimes called a 'logical consequence'. For example, if a child makes a mess, he or she must clean it up. Or, if two children are fighting over a toy, the toy gets taken away for a while.

  Related and natural consequences allow a child to link the unwanted behaviour with the consequence.
- *Losing a privilege:* This can be a very powerful technique as it focuses the child's attention but is more punitive than natural and related consequences. Also, there is no logical link between behaviour and consequence. Parents should only withdraw a privilege with care as it

can cause resentment, and the child should be warned beforehand that he or she is going to lose a particular privilege for a particular unwanted behaviour.

Time-outs[4] are another response to unwanted behaviours. Time-outs are useful from 2–3 years of age, and can take the heat out of a situation, for both the parent and child. Time-outs should be consistent, enforced promptly and calmly, even with empathy, and short—a good rule of thumb is a minute per year of age.

Responses that don't work when disciplining children include: screaming, constantly explaining, repeatedly warning, threatening, pleading, arguing, bribing and giving in, as well as smacking.[5] Most parents who are struggling with behaviour and discipline issues respond with relief when provided with a set of alternative responses for disciplining children, though care needs to be used when raising these issues, as they can be highly emotional and confronting topics for parents.

Maltreatment

GPs should consider maltreatment of the child if there is behaviour change inconsistent with age or development and which is not explained by a problem such as autism or by a stressful situation such as parental separation.

Tantrums[6]

94 Tantrums are when we lose control of our feelings and behaviour. Everyone, including adults, is capable of tantrums. Tantrums are what we use to deal with an emotionally confronting situation when we have no other option—the emotional response of last resort. They are more common in toddlers (particularly between 18 months and 3 years of age) because they have not learned any or many other emotional responses to challenging situations, such as ignoring, negotiating, reconsidering or reframing a situation. There is a lot of misinformation about tantrums, frequently over-emphasising control rather than guidance. They may be a pointer to autism.

Diverting a child from predictable tantrum triggers, 'scaffolding' (giving necessary support) to handle the event (e.g. a 5-minute warning), distraction or active listening in the build-up to a tantrum can be useful strategies to employ.

Once a child is mid-tantrum, any attempts at negotiation will be ineffective. Afterwards, an unemotional and calm response from the parent will tell the child that tantrums don't work (though, of course, this can be difficult for a stressed parent). Skill-building toddlers in how to handle emotionally challenging situations (i.e. expanding their repertoire beyond tantrums) is best done either before or after ('What else could you have done?'). Rousing at a child is counter-productive; they are still learning to control their emotions, and this will just increase the risk of them becoming demoralised and losing self-esteem.

Breath-holding attacks[7]

Breath-holding is common (around 5% of children do so at some stage), and occurs between 6 months and 6 years (peak at age 2). While frightening to watch, such attacks are harmless, and no treatment or action is required. There are two types:

- blue spells (more common)—these happen in response to being upset or angry. The child cries loudly then holds his or her breath at the end of expiration
- pale spells—these happen in response to pain or a fright

They can last from 10–60 seconds, and can cause the child to faint or, rarely, fit. They cause no harm, and parents should be reassured. Approaches to discipline should not change because of them. There is no need to blow air or splash water in the child's face, and the child should be treated as if the breath-holding has not occurred (i.e. no discussion or punishment).

Head banging and rocking[8]

Head banging and rocking, which usually occur before the child goes to sleep, are common. Head banging occurs in up to 30% of normal infants and toddlers, and rocking is even more prevalent. They are more frequent in children with developmental disability and autism, where these behaviours may be more pervasive through the day.

Features

- Usually starts after 8–9 months, and is rare after 2 years of age
- Usually prior to going to sleep
- Child usually not distressed and rarely self-injurious

Management

There is no need to try to stop the behaviour, and attempting to do so is often not successful.

- Reassure parents that it's a self-limiting behaviour and usually settles by 2 years.

- Avoid reinforcing behaviour by excessive attention or punishment.
- Ignore the behaviour.
- Place the bed or cot in the middle of the room away from a wall (reduces disruption from noise).
- Monitor the condition of the cot, to ensure screws and hinges are not being loosened.

Sibling rivalry

Sibling rivalry is very common and can cause a lot of disruption in the family. A toddler may pinch, prod and even attempt to smother a new baby, so providing the toddler with attention from the mother and encouraging the child to see that it is his or her baby too can ease the jealousy. In school-age children the following tips are useful:[9]

- Be fair.
- Avoid making comparisons between your children.
- Encourage the children to work out their own differences.
- Avoid taking sides in sibling conflicts. Set guidelines on how children can disagree and resolve conflicts.
- Discourage telling tales on each other.
- When it is necessary to punish or reprimand, do it with the child alone in a quiet, private place.
- Use regular family meetings to establish family rules and negotiating conflicts.

Stuttering/stammering

Stuttering (also known as stammering)[10] usually begins at age 2–4 years, as children start to use more words and longer sentences. It can start suddenly or develop slowly. Up to 12% of children will stutter by the age of 4.

Stutters can be repetitions (of a sound, word or phrase), prolongations of a sound (e.g. 'aaaand'), a block (where no sounds comes out) or combinations of these. There is no known cause, though it can run in families. Stutters are not associated with other disabilities, though they may cause psychological distress for the child. They are not caused by anxiety or stress, but can be more prominent when the child is excited.

A child developing a stutter should see a speech pathologist as soon as possible, as early treatment is more successful. The most common program used in Australia to treat stuttering is the Lidcombe Program, which is often successful and can even sometimes stop the stutter.

Habit cough

This is a common problem usually affecting school-age children and occurs in the absence of underlying disease. It occurs only when the child is awake—not during sleep.

There are two common types of habit cough:

1 A honking-type cough (heard from the waiting room) in teenage girls. There is no dyspnoea or sputum production.
2 A throat-clearing cough commonly seen in boys aged 7–10. This is related to a transient tic disorder.

Habit cough is a diagnosis of exclusion and there should be a careful assessment to exclude other causes such as respiratory disorders or pertussis. Underlying triggers include inter-family problems and bullying or other perceived stress or anxiety. Management includes explanation, reassurance and CBT.

Referral for resistant cases is appropriate.

Other functional respiratory problems:

- hyperventilation
- sighing dyspnoea
- vocal cord dysfunction (see CHAPTER 57)

Sleep disorders in children

See CHAPTER 71.

Bullying[11,12]

There are varying figures on how common bullying is, but most suggest more than a quarter of children are significantly bullied at some stage. It is more common in the early school years, but can happen at any age. Bullying differs from conflict, in that there is an imbalance of power between the perpetrator and the victim. It is a deliberate behaviour repeatedly done and intended to harm the victim. It is a power play, constructed on contempt, not anger, and this is what can make it so damaging.

Types of bullying include physical harm, verbal assaults, hidden bullying (e.g. exclusion or spreading rumours) and cyberbullying (now the most common form of bullying). The latter is particularly insidious as it is difficult to detect and follows the victim home and even into their bedroom via social media or phones. Bullying can lead to physical, psychological and social consequences, and in extreme cases depression and even suicide. Despite this, less than half of bullying is reported (with boys reporting less than girls) due to fear of retaliation or not being believed.

Bullies themselves tend to be assertive, impulsive and aggressive, with little empathy for their victims or remorse for their actions. They often come from dysfunctional backgrounds, and their bullying tendency may have been learned from being modelled by parents or peers.

If bullying is raised, the child should be believed, and a history carefully, gently and non-judgmentally extracted. Parents should be encouraged to stay calm, involve other adults in the environment (e.g. teachers at school) and to formally address the issue after educating themselves on the best approach. There are many good resources available for this, such as the National Centre Against Bullying at <www.ncab.org.au>. A vigilant approach to this common and serious problem by GPs and parents should be employed, especially in those particularly vulnerable to bullying, such as children who are shy, lacking in confidence, children with disabilities or who physically or socially stand out in some way (e.g. children with speech disorders). Indicative signs to watch out for include:

- school phobia: sham sickness and other excuses
- being tense, tearful and miserable after school
- reluctance to talk about happenings at school
- poor appetite
- functional symptoms (e.g. habit cough)
- repeated abdominal pains/headache
- unexplained bruises, injuries, torn clothing, damaged books
- lack of a close friend; not bringing peers home
- crying during sleep
- restless sleep with bad dreams
- appearing unhappy or depressed
- unexpected irritability and moods; temper outbursts

Referral to a psychologist should be considered in severe cases, in those that fail to be resolved, or if there are other psychological or family issues. If child abuse is suspected, appropriate action should be taken (see CHAPTER 95).

BEHAVIOURAL AND DEVELOPMENTAL DISORDERS

Developmental disability and delay

The family doctor is in an ideal position to recognise and initiate evaluation of the child with a developmental disability, whether it is a physical disability or delay, an intellectual disability or a learning disability. All children with a suspected developmental delay should be promptly evaluated by a paediatrician or a multidisciplinary developmental assessment team, and the family doctor should remain a key player in the long-term management both of the child and the family.

Many developmental problems will be obvious but others are subtle. Several disabilities may evade a diagnosis. Transient developmental delay may be associated with factors such as prematurity, family stress, physical illness and learning opportunities, while persistent delay can be caused by intellectual disability, cerebral palsy, autism and hearing and visual impairment.

Many rare dysmorphic syndromes are becoming more recognised and defined with the rapid advances in genetics, and referral to genetic disorder units will help in getting an appropriate evaluation.

Evaluation

An appropriate history includes a careful look at developmental milestones, social and behavioural issues, and family history (see CHAPTER 9). A new diagnosis of developmental delay of any sort can have a massive impact on family members, especially parents, and the family doctor should keep a watchful eye on how they are coping and reacting to the diagnostic process.

The physical examination includes growth parameters, assessment of all developmental domains, looking for dysmorphic features, testing of hearing and vision, examining for neurocutaneous stigmata (e.g. café-au-lait spots, neurofibromas, hypopigmented macules) and careful systems examination, including cardiac and neurological examination. Eyes, ears, mouths (including teeth), hands and feet, and genitals should all be examined.

Investigations are usually coordinated via specialist services, but often include bloods (including karyotyping and genetic tests), urinary metabolic screening, and imaging such as cerebral MRI (which may require a general anaesthetic).

Intellectual disability

Intellectual disability (ID) is a neurodevelopmental disorder characterised by deficits in intellectual and adaptive functioning that present before 18 years of age.[13] The term replaces and improves upon the older term 'mental retardation'. The term 'global developmental delay' (GDD) is usually used to describe children <5 years of age who fail to meet expected developmental milestones in several areas of development. Not all children with GDD will meet criteria for ID as they grow older.

Presentations include learning difficulties, language delay and behavioural problems.

The two most common causes are trisomy 21 (see CHAPTER 18) and fragile X syndrome.

Fragile X syndrome, Prader–Willi syndrome and Williams syndrome are presented in CHAPTER 18.

Cerebral palsy[14]

Cerebral palsy (CP) is a physical disability that affects movement and posture, and is the most common physical disability in childhood (2 in 1000 live births). Its cause is usually unknown, but CP is associated with numerous antenatal and perinatal factors, including antenatal infections (e.g. rubella, CMV), birth defects, preterm birth, IUGR, multiple pregnancy, perinatal hypoxia and postnatal head trauma or cerebral infection. It is more common with low birth weight or low socioeconomic status. It can vary from minimal to profound disability.

Definition

There are 5 key elements:

1 It is an umbrella term for a group of disorders.
2 It is permanent, but not unchanging.
3 It involves a disorder of movement and/or posture and of motor function.
4 It is due to a non-progressive interference, lesion or abnormality.
5 The interference, lesion or abnormality originates in the immature brain.

Associated impairments

- 3 in 4 are in pain
- 1 in 2 has an intellectual disability
- 1 in 3 cannot walk
- 1 in 3 requires a hip replacement
- 1 in 4 cannot talk
- 1 in 4 has epilepsy
- 1 in 4 has a behavioural disorder
- 1 in 4 has bladder control problems
- 1 in 5 has a sleep disorder
- 2 in 5 dribble
- 1 in 10 is blind
- 1 in 15 is tube fed
- 1 in 25 is deaf

Classification

Many different classification systems are used for CP. These include those based on:

- *severity*—mild (no restriction of activities and mobile without aids), moderate (some assistance/ aids required), severe (wheelchair and marked restriction of activities)
- *topographic location:*
  - paresis (weakened) vs plegia (paralysis)
  - terms include: mono- (one limb), di- (two, usually legs), hemi- (arm and leg), para- (lower body), quadri- (4 limbs) and penta- (4 limbs and also head and neck/breathing issues)
- *motor function*—spastic (pyramidal) versus non-spastic (extra-pyramidal)
- *muscle tone*—hypertonic or hypotonic

Other terms used include 'ataxic', 'dyskinetic' and 'athetoid'.

Diagnosis

Severely affected children are often picked up soon after birth, but mildly affected cases may not be diagnosed for years. A family doctor who has any suspicion of a disorder in movement or posture should refer the child for specialist assessment, which may include a paediatrician, a paediatric physiotherapist or a multidisciplinary team assessment.

Depending on the clinical presentation, multiple investigations may be undertaken, including visual and hearing tests, pathology tests (e.g. karyotyping, genetic testing, urine metabolic screening) or imaging such as a cerebral MRI.

Management

Management of motor and posture issues is largely the domain of therapists and specialist clinics such as a cerebral palsy clinic in a major hospital. Multiple team members may be involved, and the family doctor may be required to take a team management and coordination role. Other responsibilities that may be met by the family doctor include:

- facilitating access to funding streams and services
- diet and growth monitoring
- monitoring and treating bladder issues, including UTIs
- managing constipation issues
- dealing with pressure sores
- addressing sleep issues
- helping with behaviour issues
- looking at pain management
- addressing family issues, such as parents coping or sibling dynamics
- dealing with normal paediatric issues in general practice (e.g. immunisations, treating commonplace infections and injuries). These may present special challenges, depending on the level and type of CP

Autism spectrum disorder

In May 2013, the DSM-5[13] made significant changes to autism terminology and classification that reflected recent research. Autism spectrum disorder (ASD) superseded autistic disorder, pervasive developmental disorder not otherwise specified (PDD-NOS) and Asperger disorder, though the latter term is also still widely used by clinicians and the public. This resulted in a change in the way autism was diagnosed, with three domains (social deficits, communication deficits and repetitive behaviour) reducing to two (social–communication deficits and repetitive behaviour). Another change is a 'severity' criterion that is designed to better capture the 'spectrum' nature of the disorder: level 3 (very substantial support), level 2 (substantial support) and level 1 (some support).

ASDs are common, with the latest Australian data putting the incidence at 1 in 160 children.[15] While autism diagnoses are much more common in recent decades compared to previously (it was first described as a disorder only in 1944), whether there has been a true increase in incidence is unknown, as increasing awareness and widened diagnostic criteria make comparison with previous prevalence data unreliable.

Identification

When an autism spectrum disorder (ASD) is suspected, a GP is likely to face one of three different scenarios:

A A family member presents with his or her own concerns about their child's development.

B A family member reports that a third party, such as a child-care worker or teacher, has expressed concerns about their child's development.

94

C The GP himself/herself identifies concerns with a child's social and language development through routine developmental screening or general observation.

Scenario A should always be taken seriously, as the concerns of parents are commonly justified. Many parents present to their GP during the second to third year of their child's life when it becomes apparent that the child's development has stalled compared with his or her peers. While social deficits of ASD (such as delayed or absent joint attention—see below) often present earlier, they frequently go unrecognised by parents and it is usually speech delay that prompts a visit to the doctor.

Other parents may request a hearing assessment, thinking their child is deaf because he or she doesn't respond to their name. In about 25–30% of cases there may be actual regression, with the child beginning to say words but stopping, commonly between the ages of 15 and 24 months. Parents may also report loss of eye contact and gestures such as waving or pointing.

When to suspect ASD

A typically developing child should smile in response to a familiar caregiver's smile or 'baby talk' by 2–4 months. At 8 months, an infant will follow a parent's gaze, that is, look in the same direction as the parent is looking. Children should be able to follow their parent's point by 10–12 months and start pointing themselves by 12–14 months. They then begin to point to share ('look at this') by 16 months. As they point, children will look back and forth between the object and their parent—it's the shared social experience, not the tangible object, the child seeks. These joint attention behaviours are often absent or reduced in a child with ASD.

Social deficits

Younger children with ASD often appear to have little desire to connect with others. They may have problems imitating actions (such as clapping). As they get older, individuals may have difficulty understanding the perspective of others, commonly called theory-of-mind, which in turn leads to difficulties with empathy and sharing. Affected children will often have few or no friends; higher-functioning children may desire friendship but approach peers in an inappropriate way. Inappropriate social behaviours (e.g. commenting loudly on someone's physical appearance) can lead to problems at school. Frequently, individuals become overwhelmed by social or sensory stimulation, such as loud sounds.

Communication deficits

Communication deficits in ASD include deficits in both non-verbal and verbal communication, and expressive and receptive language. Some individuals remain mute throughout life. Although present, language may not be functional—children may be able to rote learn shapes and numbers, but not follow one-step commands. Stereotyped and repetitive language, including echolalia ('parroting' of learned phrases or scripts) is common. Other signs include unusual vocal qualities, such as tone or speed, and pronoun reversal (e.g. saying 'you' instead of 'I').

Affected individuals frequently have a very concrete and literal understanding of language, such as not understanding idioms, lies or jokes, and miss social cues such as body language and tone of voice. Even relatively mildly affected children (and adults) may have difficulty initiating and sustaining two-way conversations.

Children with ASD tend not to play imaginatively (e.g. pushing the car along and saying 'brrm') and instead will engage in unusual repetitive play, such as lining up toys, or spinning the wheels of a car. They frequently show little interest in social play (e.g. peek-a-boo or pattycake) and their play is often object-focused (e.g. computer games) rather than people-focused.

The following red flags[16] are absolute indications for referral for an autism-specific assessment:

Red flags for autism

- Lack of babbling, gesturing or pointing by 12 months
- No sharing of interest in objects or activities with another person
- No single words by 16 months, or no two-word (non-echoed) phrases by 24 months
- Any loss of language or social skills at any age

A GP-friendly screening tool for ASD is the Checklist for Autism in Toddlers (CHAT)—abbreviated version (see TABLE 94.2).[17] This can be administered at approximately 18 months of age and takes only a couple of minutes.

If a child fails all three items, referral is indicated, as the chances of *autism* are high. If a child fails only 1 or 2 items, still refer as the chances of *developmental delay* are high.

Further assessment

If there are concerns that a child may have ASD, it is essential that the child is promptly referred to a general or developmental paediatrician, or to a developmental assessment unit, for an autism-specific diagnostic assessment. Taking a 'wait and see' approach, or saying 'come back in 6 months and we'll reassess', is not acceptable. Getting hearing checked or assessments from speech therapists, occupational therapists (OTs) or psychologists may also be done in this work-up phase.

Management

Intensive early intervention for ASD, which is what guidelines[18] recommend as gold standard and does improve long-term outcomes, involves intensive and often expensive behavioural/developmental therapies,

Table 94.2 Checklist for Autism in Toddlers (CHAT)—abbreviated version

Section A: Ask the parent	Section B: GP's observation
1 Does your child ever pretend, for example, to make a cup of tea using a toy cup and teapot, or pretend to do other things?	Get the child's attention, then give the child a miniature toy cup and teapot and say, 'Can you make a cup of tea?' Does the child pretend to pour out tea, drink it, etc.? (If you can elicit an example of pretending in some other game, score a YES for this item.)
2 Does your child ever use his/her index finger to point, to ask for something?	Get the child's attention, then point across the room at an interesting object and say 'Oh look! There's a (name of toy)!' Watch the child's face. Does the child look across to see what you are pointing at? (To record a YES for this item, ensure the child has not simply looked at your hand, but has actually looked at the object at which you are pointing.)
	Say to the child, 'Where's the light?', or 'Show me the light'. Does the child point with his or her index finger at the light? (If the child does not understand 'light', repeat this with 'Where's the teddy?' or other unreachable object.) (To record a YES for this item, the child must have looked up at your face around the time of pointing.

and the earlier it commences the better. However, this type of therapy may be beyond the organisational and financial capability of the family, so care should be taken in what is recommended. Parents should be directed to reliable information sources[17,18] on these options, which they may find daunting. There is also a lot of misinformation on autism, particularly regarding complementary and alternative therapies, for which there is no evidence of efficacy.[18] State-based autism associations can also help with advice. If the waiting times for diagnostic assessment are long (as is often the case), families should be referred to early intervention services while they wait.

The role of the GP in management

A child being diagnosed with ASD can have a massive impact on the family. GPs should monitor how family members are coping, and provide a 'medical home' for reliable advice on management options. Children with autism also have particular vulnerability to certain medical issues, and the GP will be involved in the management of these. These include:

- minor traumas and injuries
- restricted diet (due to sensory issues or special diets used by some families)
- behavioural issues
- constipation (due to sensory issues causing voluntary faecal retention, or from medications used for co-diagnoses)
- dental issues (sensory issues making brushing difficult, or grinding)

When consulting children with autism, special tactics can be employed to help things run smoother. Alerting front desk staff so they are aware of potential behavioural issues, allowing easier access for families in stress (e.g. calling the patient from the car if behaviour in the waiting room is problematic) and reassuring parents that challenging behaviour by the child is not an issue will help. The decreased eye contact and interaction means that the GP needs to work harder to engage these children, but it can be done, and parents will appreciate any effort made. Adjusting for sensory issues, for example, letting children hold and examine equipment before it is used, can also help.

Dyspraxia

Dyspraxia (from the Greek, meaning 'disorder of practising') is a disorder of the planning, organising and carrying out of motor tasks. It can affect articulation and speech, perception and thought, though it is not associated with decreased intelligence. It can vary from difficulties with simple motor movements, such as waving goodbye or clapping, to more complex issues such as handwriting or riding a bike. It is more common in males. Another term that is used is developmental coordination disorder (DCD).

If there is an issue with motor skills being delayed (without associated social and communication delay beyond motor skills) then referral to physiotherapists, occupational therapists and speech therapists, depending on the type of motor issues involved, is advisable. A delay in fine and gross motor skills can become a barrier to socialisation (e.g. not being able to play or perform in team sports) or academic achievement (e.g. writing) and can have flow-on effects on self-esteem and mood.

Specific learning disorders

A specific learning disorder (SLD) is characterised by persistent difficulties in reading, writing, arithmetic and mathematical reasoning skills during school years.[13] The difficulties must result in abilities well below what is expected in culturally and linguistically appropriate testing. The learning issues should not be explained by other developmental, neurological, sensory (such as vision or hearing problems) or motor disorders and must significantly interfere with academic achievement, occupational performance, or activities of daily living. Dyslexia and dyscalculia are examples of SLDs.

Dyslexia

Dyslexia (from the Greek, meaning 'disorder of words') is an SLD of reading and spelling, while still having otherwise normal learning abilities. The condition was originally called 'word blindness'. Also referred to as developmental reading disorder, it is not a problem of comprehension, but of the speed and accuracy of decoding (converting letters and words to sounds) and spelling (converting sounds to their correct written symbols). It can run in families. Individuals with dyslexia can have different or compensatory learning styles, but may also be helped with input from an occupational therapist or speech therapist and a dyslexia clinic.

Attention deficit hyperactivity disorder

Attention deficit hyperactivity disorder (ADHD) is a disorder affecting attention, hyperactivity and impulse control.[19] It can also affect children's learning, social skills and family functioning. It is very common, affecting 3–5% of Australian children. It is much more common in boys. There are 3 types: predominantly hyperactive/impulsive; predominantly inattentive; and mixed, with the latter being the most common. To meet DSM-5 criteria, symptoms must be present before the age of 12, and often persist into adulthood.

Criteria[13]

Hyperactive/impulsive—6 out of 9 of the following:

- often fidgets with hands or feet or squirms in a seat
- often leaves seat in classroom or in other situations in which remaining seated is expected

- often runs about or climbs excessively during inappropriate situations (in adolescents or adults, may be limited to subjective feelings of restlessness)
- often has difficulty playing or engaging in leisure activities quietly
- is often on the go
- often talks excessively
- often blurts out answers before questions have been completed
- often has difficulty awaiting turn
- often interrupts or intrudes on others (e.g. butts into conversations or games)

Inattentive—6 out of 9 of the following:

- often fails to pay close attention to detail or makes careless mistakes in schoolwork, work or other activities
- often has difficulty sustaining attention in tasks or play activities
- often does not seem to listen when spoken to directly
- often does not follow through on instructions and fails to finish schoolwork, chores or duties in the workplace (not due to oppositional behaviour or failure to understand instructions)
- often has difficulty organising tasks and activities
- often avoids, dislikes or is reluctant to engage in tasks that require sustained mental effort (such as schoolwork or homework)
- often loses things necessary for tasks or activities
- is often easily distracted by extraneous stimuli
- is often forgetful in daily activities

Mixed—meets both hyperactive/impulsive and inattentive criteria.

Diagnosis

While most young children have short attention spans and are impulsive, children who meet the above criteria will stand out, and the symptoms should be displayed in more than one environment (e.g. home and school). The issue is usually raised by the parents to the GP, and a query may have been raised by an early childhood worker or teacher. Symptoms often become apparent when the child starts school, or as academic expectations start to rise around age 7–8 years. The diagnosis should be made only by appropriately experienced psychologists, paediatricians or child psychiatrists, and will require information gathered from parents, teachers or other important adults in the child's life.[19]

Treatment

Children with ADHD often find their condition distressing and demoralising, and need support and understanding from family and teachers. Behavioural strategies (see TABLE 94.3) should be offered to all children, even those who do not strictly meet the diagnostic criteria but have these types of behaviours. Individual or family counselling should be considered.

Medication[20,21]

Stimulants are the single most effective treatment for ADHD, and became the standard treatment in the 1980s. Controversy remains in the media, and the public are often wary, with concerns about addiction and other safety issues often raised by parents, but these fears are unfounded. While there are potential side effects, these are mostly not serious. Stimulants are often useful, and 1–2% of Australian children are put on them at some stage. Parents (and children) will frequently report a positive experience, reflecting that their previous concerns were unfounded. Eight out of ten children will find a significant improvement in their concentration, impulse control and overactivity.

Medications (4 years and older: as a rule, avoid stimulants under 4 years):

- methylphenidate (Ritalin, short acting, effect duration 3–4 hours); therapy should be started with this immediate-acting preparation
- slow-release methylphenidate (Ritalin LA 6–8 hours, Concerta 10 hours)
- dexamphetamine
- atomoxetine (Strattera)

Issues related to medication

- Can normally be prescribed only by paediatricians, child psychiatrists or neurologists
- Mechanism of action—increases noradrenalin and/or dopamine at the synapse
- Common side effects:
  - decreased appetite
  - poor weight gain
- Uncommon side effects:
  - headache/dizziness
  - stomach aches
  - insomnia
  - irritable, withdrawn or highly emotional
- Slight growth stunting (rarely a problem clinically)
- Slight increase in heart rate/blood pressure (not an issue unless underlying cardiac issues)

Fish oil

- Sometimes suggested for ADHD, but research is unclear about existence of and/or extent of benefit
- Contains high amounts of omega-3 fatty acids
- May help improve symptoms in some children

Table 94.3 Behavioural strategies for ADHD[20]

Verbal instructions	Keep brief and clear
	State name or tap on shoulder before giving instructions
	Keep eye contact
Written work	Use highlighters
	Use *asterisks*, UPPER CASE, or **bold** layout techniques
Other learning strategies	Use one-on-one teaching where possible
	Use class 'buddies' to help
	Use activities with 'hands-on' involvement
	Most important learning is done when concentrating best (usually morning)
	Use checklists
	Sit front and centre in class, not near friends
	Homework done in clutter-free environment (no distractions, no unnecessary screens nearby or available)
	Organised bag, organised diary, organised desk, organised locker
	Regular scheduled homework time
Reduce overactivity/fatigue	Regular rest breaks
	Physically active breaks (e.g. delivering notes, taking lunch orders)
Keeping structure	Fixed routine
	Activities predictable (home and school)
	Display schedules and rules (home and school, in multiple places)
	Tell about changes to activities/schedules/rules in advance
	Use countdowns (e.g. 5-minute warnings)
	Keep choices to a minimum
Self-esteem	Set up for success (i.e. achievable goals)
	Acknowledge achievements (by written and verbal means) and regularly review achievements
	Acknowledge effort
	Ensure participation in classroom and positive feedback for effort
	Address any specific learning difficulties promptly
Social skills	Expose to small groups rather than large
	Reward appropriate social behaviour (e.g. sharing)
	Teach problem-solving skills when provoked
	Encourage 'supervised socialisation' (e.g. sport, Scouts/Girl Guides)
	Regularly discuss consequences of his or her actions
	Use visual prompts to think before acting (e.g. STOP, THINK, DO)
Communication between home and school	Have formal communication portal (e.g. diary, online parent forum) and use regularly
	Communicate positive and negative behaviours

Oppositional defiant disorder

Oppositional defiant disorder (ODD) is defined as an ongoing pattern of anger-guided disobedience and hostile and defiant behaviour towards authority figures that goes beyond the bounds of normal childhood behavior.[13] In the DSM-5, symptoms are grouped into three types: angry/irritable mood, argumentative/defiant behaviour and vindictiveness, reflecting the disorder having emotional and behavioural symptomatology. While such behaviours are common in early childhood, ODD should be considered when they are consistently displayed, and are impacting the family and the child's social and educational functioning.

ODD is common (with an incidence estimated at 5–10%)[22] and often undiagnosed, and has a large incidence of co-diagnosis with ADHD, with many of the symptoms crossing over between the two conditions. The onset is usually gradual, becoming evident before the age of 8. Children with ODD have a higher incidence of child abuse, school dropout and long-term mental health problems. ODD is caused by a combination of difficult temperament traits (see earlier in this chapter) and environmental factors, such as poor attachment, parenting styles or family conflict/mental health issues in parents.

Management[21]

For parents:

- improve positive parenting skills
- enhance skills in problem-solving, conflict resolution and communication

For the child:

- develop communication, problem-solving and anger management skills

For the family:

- counselling and support regarding relationships and home environment

In the classroom:

- teacher or school counsellor to provide social skills/conflict resolution skills training

There is strong evidence that psychological strategies and interventions reduce the impact of ODD on the child and family, and the earlier the better. They can also prevent progression to more serious disorders[13] such as:

- *Disruptive mood dysregulation disorder (DMDD)*—characterised by severe and recurrent temper outbursts greatly out of proportion in intensity or duration to the situation >3/week for >12 months
- *Conduct disorder*—where there is behaviour that violates the rights of others or societal norms, such as aggression directed towards people, animals or property, often with a callous manner and lack of empathy

Tic disorders[23]

Tics are sudden, rapid, recurrent involuntary vocalisations or movements usually appearing in bouts that wax and wane in intensity, frequency and type of tic. They include behaviours such as grunting, blinking, shrugging shoulders, humming, yelling out a word or phrase or clearing the throat. Tic disorders are classified into:[13]

- *Tourette syndrome*—motor *and* vocal tics for >1 year
- *persistent motor* or *vocal tic disorder*—motor *or* vocal tics for >1 year
- *provisional tic disorder*—motor and/or vocal tics for <1 year

Characteristics of tic disorders:

- average age of onset 5–6 years
- average of 5 years from onset to diagnosis
- associated with psychosocial distress and poor functioning
- strong genetic component (first-degree relatives have 10–100-fold increased risk of tics)
- associated with ADHD and OCD
- can be simple (one muscle group) or complex
- examples of complex tics (which are different from compulsions in OCD in that they are not cognitive, preplanned or anxiety reducing) include:
  - copropraxia (making obscene gestures)
  - echopraxia (copying others)
  - wounding oneself
  - echolalia (repeating others)
  - palilalia (repeating oneself)
  - coprolalia (uttering obscenities)
- unknown aetiology
- 80% decrease in adolescence and adulthood to no longer be an impairment
- 20% do not decrease, and may increase
- there is no treatment, other than psychosocial support and treating comorbidities

Patient education resources

Hand-out sheets from *Murtagh's Patient Education* 6th edition:

- Attention deficit hyperactivity disorder
- Autism

- Autism: Asperger's syndrome
- Bullying of children
- Stuttering
- Tantrums

References

1 Thomas A, Chess S. *Temperament and Development.* New York: Bruner/Mazel, 1977.

2 American Academy of Pediatrics Committee on Psychosocial Aspects of Child and Family Health. Guidance for effective discipline. Pediatrics, 1998; 101: 723–28 (reaffirmed Pediatrics, 2012; 130: e467).

3 Raising Children's Network. Consequences, June 2011 <www.raisingchildren.net.au/articles/consequences.html> (accessed 3/8/2014).

4 Raising Children's Network. Time out, June 2010 <www.raisingchildren.net.au/articles/time_out.html> (accessed 3/8/2014).

5 The Royal Australian College of Physicians. Paediatric & Child Health Division. Position statement: physical punishment of children, July 2013 <www.racp.edu.au/page/paed-policy> (accessed 3/8/2014).

6 Women and Children's Health Network. Parenting and child health: tantrums <http://www.cyh.com/HealthTopics/HealthTopicDetails.aspx?p=114&np=141&id=1775> (accessed 20/11/2017).

7 The Royal Children's Hospital Melbourne. *Kids health info: breath holding.* <www.rch.org.au/kidsinfo/fact_sheets/Breath_holding/> (accessed 18/11/2017).

8 Women and Children's Health Network. Parenting and child health: head banging and rocking, November 2013 <http://www.cyh.com/HealthTopics/HealthTopicDetails.aspx?p=114&np=141&id=2958> (accessed 20/11/2017).

9 American Academy of Pediatrics. Healthy children: dealing with sibling rivalry, November 2013 <www.healthychildren.org/English/family-life/family-dynamics/Pages/Dealing-with-Sibling-Rivalry.aspx> (accessed 9/8/2014).

10 Raising Children's Network. Stuttering, November 2013 <www.raisingchildren.net.au/articles/stuttering_an_overview.html> (accessed 9/8/2014).

11 The National Centre Against Bullying, Alannah & Madeline Foundation <www.ncab.org.au/> (accessed 2/12/2017).

12 Briggs, F. *Smart Parenting for Safer Kids.* Melbourne: JoJo Publishing, 2011.

13 American Psychiatric Association. *Diagnostic and Statistical Manual of Mental Disorders* (5th edn), 2013.

14 Australian Cerebral Palsy Register Group, report 2013.

15 Wray J, Williams K. The prevalence of autism in Australia. Report commissioned by the Australian Advisory Board on Autism Spectrum Disorders, 2007.

16 Wray J et al. Language disorders and autism. MJA, 2005; 182 (7): 354–60.

17 Raising Children's Network. Children with autism, September 2016 <www.raisingchildren.net.au> (accessed 19/11/2017).

18 Prior M et al. The Australian Society for Autism Research. A review of the research to identify the most effective models of practice in early Intervention for children with autism spectrum disorders. Report commissioned by the Australian Government Department of Families, Housing, Community Services and Indigenous Affairs (FaHCSIA), 2011.

19 The Royal Children's Hospital Melbourne. *Kids health info: ADHD—an overview,* September 2012. <www.rch.org.au/kidsinfo/fact_sheets/ADHD_an_overview/> (accessed 13/8/2014).

20 The Royal Children's Hospital Melbourne. *Kids health info: ADHD—ways to help children with ADHD,* September 2012. <www.rch.org.au/kidsinfo/fact_sheets/ADHD_ways_to_help_children_with_ADHD/> (accessed 17/11/2017).

21 Expert group for Psychotropic. Disorders usually first diagnosed in childhood and adolescence. In: eTG complete [Internet]. Melbourne Therapeutic Guidelines Limited. Available from: <www.tg.org.au> (accessed December 2017).

22 Fraser A, Wray J. Oppositional defiant disorder. Aust Fam Physician, 2008; 37 (4): 402–5.

23 ESSTS guideline group. European clinical guidelines for Tourette syndrome and other tic disorders. Eur Child Adolesc Psychiatry, 2011; 20: 155–71.

Child abuse

It is customary, but I think it is a mistake, to speak of happy childhood. Children, however, are often overanxious and acutely sensitive. Man ought to be man and master of his fate; but children are at the mercy of those around them.

SIR JOHN LUBBOCK, BARON AVEBURY (1834–1913)

Public and medical awareness of child abuse has markedly increased in recent decades, and the possibility of child abuse and neglect has to be kept in mind by the family doctor. It may surface in families from all walks of life and where a good trustful relationship exists between parents or children and doctor.

While reporting rates continue to increase (at 34 per 1000 Australian children in 2012[1]), the true incidence of child abuse is much greater and also difficult to assess.

The various types of abuse[1] (and their estimated incidence[2]) are shown in FIGURE 95.1.

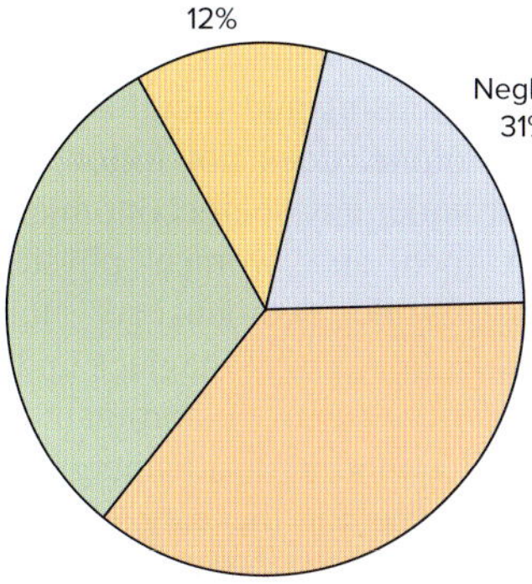

FIGURE 95.1 Percentage breakdown of primary substantiated harm types in Australia in 2011–12[4]

Source: Based on Australian Institute of Health and Welfare material.

Facts on child abuse[1,4,5]

- The younger the child the greater the risk.
- The more disabled the more vulnerable.
- Indigenous children are 8 times more likely to be the subject of substantiated abuse than non-Aboriginal children.
- The number of children who are deemed at risk and placed in out-of-home care (OOHC) has increased in recent years, with the rate in 2012 at 7.7 per 1000 Australian children nationally. Roughly half of these are in foster care, and half in relative/kinship care, with a small (5%) proportion in residential (paid workers) care.

Definitions[6]

Child abuse and neglect are collectively referred to as child maltreatment. This refers to any non-accidental behaviour by parents or other adults or adolescents that is outside the norms of conduct and entails a substantial risk of causing physical or emotional harm to a child or young person. Such behaviours may be intentional or unintentional, and can be through omission (i.e. neglect) or commission (i.e. abuse).

Deciding whether behaviour constitutes maltreatment can depend on:

- cultural issues (e.g. corporal punishment)
- developmental age of the child
- the severity, frequency and duration of the behaviour
- the behaviour itself, or the result of the behaviour (a definition issue)

Physical abuse (non-accidental injury)

Physical abuse is defined as the non-accidental use of physical force against a child that results in harm to the child. It include behaviours such as hitting, shoving, slapping, shaking, throwing, punching, kicking, biting, burning, strangling and poisoning. Munchausen syndrome by proxy (see below) is considered physical abuse.

Neglect

Neglect is defined as the failure by a parent/caregiver to provide a child (when they are in a position to do so) with the conditions that are culturally accepted as being essential for the child's physical and emotional development and well-being.

Emotional maltreatment

This is where a parent or caregiver conducts inappropriate verbal or symbolic acts towards a child, and/or there is a pattern or failure over time to provide a child with adequate non-physical nurture and emotional availability. This can take the form of rejecting, isolating, terrorising, ignoring or corrupting, and can damage the child's self-esteem and social functioning.

Sexual abuse

Sexually abusive behaviour refers to any sexual activity between an adult and a child below the age of consent; non-consensual sexual activity between minors (e.g. a 14-year-old and a 10-year-old); or any sexual activity between a child under 18 years of age and a person in a position of power or authority (e.g. parent, teacher).[2] It is sometimes difficult to determine whether a behaviour constitutes sexual abuse, depending on variables such as age, development and cultural norms.

Behaviours can include fondling of genitals, masturbation, oral sex, vaginal or anal penetration by a penis, finger or any other object, fondling of breasts, voyeurism, exhibitionism or exposure to pornography. In contrast to other forms of maltreatment, the labelling of an act as sexual abuse also depends on the relationship between perpetrator and victim (e.g. age difference, being related).

Other types of child maltreatment

- Munchausen syndrome by proxy—this is the term used when a parent or guardian creates an illness in a child so that the perpetrator can develop or maintain a relationship with medical staff or transfer his or her responsibilities. A 'devoted parent' may continually present a child for medical treatment yet deny the origin of the problem—namely, the parent. Often the mother is the abuser. The abuse may be of physical or medical neglect. The masquerade may be simple or very sophisticated. Children may be indirectly abused by the lengthy or invasive investigations. Be cautious where there has been unexplained illness or death of a sibling.
- Incest—defined as intercourse between biological family members.
- Fetal abuse behaviour, such as smoking, drinking or illicit drug use, during pregnancy that endangers a fetus.
- Bullying, or peer abuse (see CHAPTER 94)
- Sibling abuse
- Witnessing community violence
- Institutional abuse
- Organised exploitation (e.g. child sex rings, child prostitution)
- State-sanctioned abuse (e.g. female genital mutilation in parts of Africa, the Stolen Generations in Australia)

Female genital mutilation

This comprises all procedures involving partial or total removal of the female external genitalia or other injuries to the female genital organs, whether for cultural or other non-therapeutic reasons (WHO definition).

It is also referred to as female circumcision.

Abuse: who and why?

The real cause seems to be a combination of several interrelated factors: personal, familial, social/cultural and societal stress. Abused children exist at all levels of society, although the majority of abused children who come to the attention of authorities are from families where there is high mobility, lack of education, loneliness, poverty, unemployment, inadequate housing and social isolation. Sexual abuse, occurring alone, does not follow these patterns and can occur under any socioeconomic circumstance.

Both men and women physically abuse their children. While women are the parents most responsible in cases of neglect and emotional abuse (probably because of a dominant role in childcare, social and economic disadvantage and being the only one responsible for the care of children in a single parent arrangement), men are more likely to abuse their own or other's children sexually.

The child can be abused at any age (even adolescents can be victims of abuse and neglect). It is important to keep this in mind—*it does happen.*

Underdiagnosing and under-reporting

Although the medical profession remains the foremost focus of child abuse reporting (they are the most likely to encounter injured children and are the most qualified to diagnose abuse), they still contribute only a small percentage of the total reporting to central registries.[7] This could be because there is underdiagnosis of the problem but it could also be because of under-reporting.

Reasons given[7] as to why GPs don't report more cases of child abuse include:

- concern about drain on time and finances
- breaching doctor–patient confidentiality
- lack of undergraduate education on the topic
- risk of alienation and stigmatisation to the family
- the feeling by some GPs that they can work on the problem with the family without outside intervention
- a breakdown of the doctor–patient relationship
- uncertainty about *what* to do
- personal and legal risks (e.g. fear of court, libel suits, irate parents), especially if they 'get it wrong'
- reluctance until absolutely certain of diagnosis

It will always be difficult to take the first step but it is important and it can help, no matter how small that first step is.

Interviewing parents or guardians

A skilled, sensitive, diplomatic interview is fundamental to management. Guidelines include:

- a relaxed, non-judgmental approach
- sensitivity to all people involved
- appropriate questions—open-ended, not leading
- using verbatim quotes from the child where possible and waiting silently for a reaction
- recording notes carefully

Physical abuse[8,9]

Physical abuse should be suspected, especially in a child aged under 2 years, if certain physical or behavioural indicators in either the child or the parents are present. Inflammation, bruising, abrasions and lacerations are the most common presentations of the physically abused child, with equal incidence in boys and girls. As well as the consequences of the physical injuries, victims of physical abuse are more likely to develop a variety of behavioural and functional problems including conduct disorders, physically aggressive behaviour (e.g. become bullies), poor academic performance and decreased cognitive functioning. Children suffering traumatic brain injuries from physical abuse (e.g. hitting head or shaking) are at risk of disabilities including ADHD, seizures, spasticity, blindness, paralysis and developmental delay.

Parents and carers can tend to misinterpret normal child behaviours (e.g. crying and tantrums) and respond to them inappropriately. A vigilant GP can actually help prevent abuse by providing 'anticipatory guidance' to parents on normal child behaviour, educating them on appropriate responses to behaviours, and offering themselves as a resource to which they can turn if the child's behaviour becomes unmanageable or overwhelming.

Risk factors:

- maternal smoking
- >2 siblings
- low infant birth weight
- unmarried mother
- poverty
- significant life stressors in parents
- caregiver role conflicts
- living in house with unrelated adult (50 times more likely to die from inflicted injuries)

Physical abuse indicators

Accidental injuries such as bruises or fractures are common in children, but tend to follow certain patterns. A GP should be aware of cases where the injury or injuries suggest a non-accidental cause is possible, when the history doesn't match up with the injury or developmental age of the child, or when the behaviour of the parent and/or child is suggestive of non-accidental injury.

Bruises

Bruises are commonly found on the front of the body over bony prominences (e.g. forehead in toddlers, knees and shins in older children). Suspicious bruises include:

- finger-shaped bruises (e.g. thumb grip marks)
- multiple bruises/welts of different ages (the colour of a bruise doesn't reliably indicate when it occurred)
- bruises in premobile children
- bruises away from bony prominences—face, scalp, neck, buttocks (see FIG. 95.2), genitalia, earlobes, behind the ears
- abdominal bruising (consider damage to internal organs, including organ rupture)
- multiple bruises of uniform shape
- multiple bruises in clusters

Scalds and burns

Beware of:

- a scald of uniform depth, sparing flexures, uniform burn line demarcation, bilateral and no splash marks (suggests forced immersion)

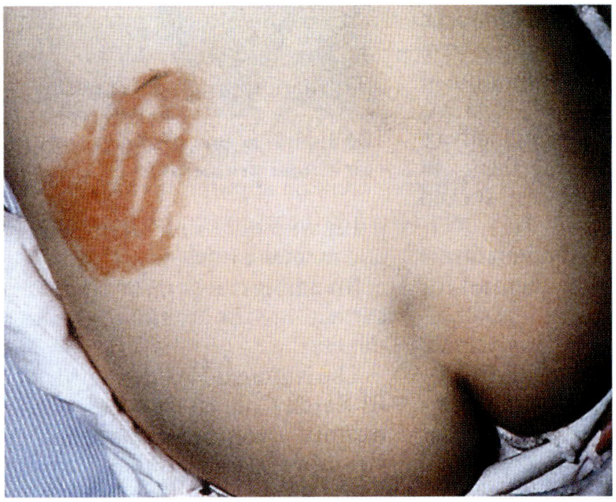

FIGURE 95.2 Physical abuse: imprint of a boot on the buttock of a child

- unusual position (e.g. back of hand, genitals)
- cigarette butt-type burns

Fractures

Look out for:

- metaphyseal fractures of the proximal humerus and proximal or distal tibia are highly suggestive
- other fractures commonly non-accidental: rib (especially posterior), clavicle, vertebral body, sternum, scapula
- multiple, especially bilateral
- complex or multiple skull fractures

Shaking and brain injury

Shaking a baby is a critically dangerous thing to do, a danger often underestimated by perpetrators. The relatively large head size and weak neck muscles can easily lead to serious injury. Suspicion of traumatic brain injury should be raised when there is:

95

- unexplained encephalopathy
- unexplained vomiting, irritability and apnoeas
- altered states of consciousness
- neurological symptoms and signs
- torn frenulum or retinal damage

History

- Unexplained injury
- Different explanations offered
- Vague or changing history
- Injury unlikely to have occurred in manner stated
- Unreasonable delays between injury and presentation
- Presentation inconsistent with child's developmental capabilities
- Evidence of neglect (clues include failure to thrive, dental caries, severe nappy rash, poor wound care)

  Remember Munchausen syndrome by proxy.

Behavioural indicators

- Wariness of adult contacts
- Inappropriate clothing (e.g. long sleeves on a hot day)
- Apprehension when other children cry or shout
- Behavioural extremes
- Fear of parents
- Afraid to go home
- Child reports injury by parents or gives inappropriate explanation of injury
- Excessive compliance
- Extreme wariness
- Attaches too readily to strangers

Management

If suspected or disclosed, a thorough assessment, with detailed documentation (including measurement and photography of bruises/other injuries) of findings should be undertaken. A detailed history and thorough examination of all areas of the body is required. In a general practice setting, getting help with this difficult situation would often be useful. Discussing (immediately) with colleagues or child protection authorities is advisable, with the safety of the child (and other cohabiting children) being ensured at all stages. Verbatim comments should be written down and, if possible, information gathered from other sources or witnesses.

The family doctor should diplomatically confront the parents and/or carers and always act in the best interests of the child. Offer to help the family. An approach would be to say, 'I am very concerned about your child's injuries as they don't add up—these injuries are not usually caused by what I'm told has been the cause. I will therefore seek assistance—it is my legal obligation. My duty is to help you and, especially, your child.'

Acquiring essential help

- Psychosocial assessment of child and family: involves social worker and multidisciplinary assessment
- Admission to hospital: for moderate and severe injuries
- Investigations done in conjunction with specialists

- Case conference (where appropriate)
- Mandatory reporting: notify child protection authorities

Emotional abuse

Physical indicators

- There are few physical indicators, but emotional abuse can cause delay in physical, emotional and mental development.

Behavioural indicators

- Extremely low self-esteem.
- Compliant, passive, withdrawn, tearful and/or apathetic behaviour.
- Aggressive or demanding behaviour.
- Anxiety.
- Serious difficulties with peers and/or adult relations.
- Delayed or distorted speech.
- Regressive behaviour (e.g. soiling).

Neglect

Poor parenting or neglect occurs in at least 5% of children under 5 years.[10]

Physical indicators

- Consistent hunger.
- Failure to thrive, or malnutrition.
- Poor hygiene.
- Inappropriate clothing.
- Consistent lack of supervision.
- Unattended physical problems or medical needs.
- Abandonment.
- Dangerous health or dietary practices.

Behavioural indicators

- Stealing food.
- Extending stays at school.
- Consistent fatigue, listlessness or falling asleep in class.
- Alcohol or drug abuse.
- Child states there is no caregiver.
- Aggressive or inappropriate behaviour.
- Isolation from peer group.

Sexual abuse[3,5]

- Only 6% of child sexual abuse is by strangers. Most are known by parents and child; that is, familiar people in familiar environments, especially within the family.
- A child may disclose up to 12 times before they are believed (listen for hints).
- Most (but not all) of the adults who sexually abuse are men.
- Boys are assaulted less commonly than girls, but are less likely to disclose if they are assaulted.
- Adolescents are perpetrators in at least 20% of cases.
- Child sexual abuse is usually about power rather than sexual gratification.

Sexual abuse presents in three main ways:

- Allegations by the child or an adult
- Injuries to the genitalia or anus
- Suspicious presentations, especially:
  - genital infection (see FIG. 95.3)
  - recurrent urinary infection
  - unexplained behavioural changes/ psychological disorders

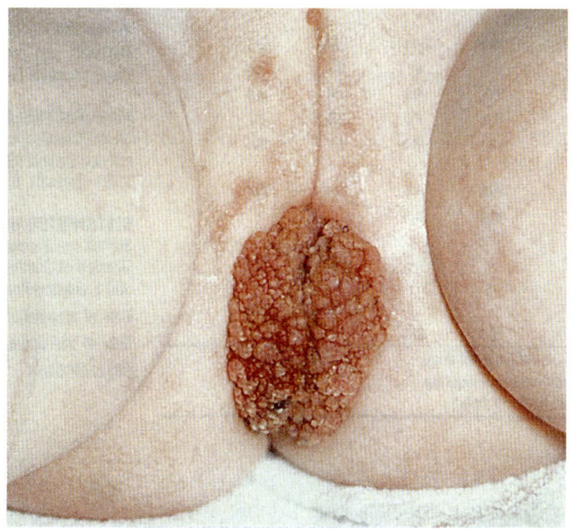

FIGURE 95.3 Genital human papillomavirus infection—a sign of sexual abuse in a child

Clinical indicators that may suggest child sexual abuse are presented in TABLE 95.1.

Clinical approach

Ideally, the child should be assessed by experienced medical officers at the regional sexual assault service, so the temptation for the inexperienced GP to have a quick look should be resisted. For the practitioner having to assess the problem, a complete medical and social history, including a behavioural history, should be obtained prior to examination.

Table 95.1	Clinical indicators that may suggest child sexual abuse

Child disclosing abuse (rarely invented, and the majority of presentations)

Parent or adult disclosing abuse allegation

Vaginal discharge

Sexually transmitted infections (acquired in 5% of sexually abused children)

Urinary tract infection

Unexplained genital trauma

Unexplained perianal trauma

Overt sexual play

Pregnancy in an adolescent

Deterioration in school work

Family disruption

Indiscriminate attachment

Abnormal sexualised behaviour (many abused children do not do this)

Poor self-esteem

Psychological disorders:

- behaviour disturbances
- regression in behaviour
- sleep disturbances
- abnormal fears/reactions to specific places or persons
- psychosomatic symptoms
- anxiety
- lack of trust
- overcompliance
- aggressive behaviour

Depression:

- self-destructive behaviour
- substance abuse
- suicidal tendencies

Non-specific physical problems:

- abdominal pain
- enuresis (especially secondary)
- encopresis

95

Examination (abnormal findings uncommon)

Genital trauma

Perforated hymen/lax vagina (may be normal variant)

Perianal trauma

Vaginal discharge

Look for semen and STIs

The child's history must be obtained carefully, honestly, patiently and objectively, without leading the child. The history is more important than the physical findings as there are no abnormal physical findings in many confessed cases.

Examination

A parent or legal guardian must give informed consent before the child is physically examined. It is recommended that the physical examination of any child suspected of being sexually abused is performed by a paediatrician or forensic physician experienced in the area of sexual abuse.

> **Point of caution:**
>
> Perianal erythema due to streptococcal infection (GABHS) (see FIG 95.4) or threadworms and non-specific vulvovaginitis (see CHAPTER 107) can be misinterpreted as sexual abuse.

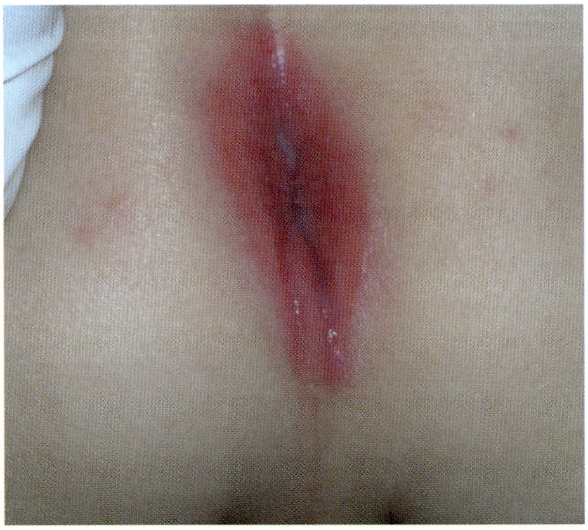

FIGURE 95.4 Perianal dermatitis with erythema caused by group A beta-haemolytic streptococcal infection

The crisis situation

It is important to realise that the child will be in *crisis*. Children are trapped into the secrecy of sexual abuse, often by a trusted adult, through powerful threats of the consequences of disclosure. They are given the great responsibility of keeping the secret and holding the family together or disclosing the secret and disrupting the family. A crisis occurs when these threats become reality.

Management

It is important to act responsibly in the best interests of the child. When we encounter real or suspected child abuse, immediate action is necessary. The child needs an advocate to act on its behalf and our intervention actions may have to override our relationship with the family.

Some golden rules are:

- Never attempt to solve the problem alone.
- Do not attempt confrontation and counselling in isolation (unless under exceptional circumstances).
- Seek advice from experts (only a telephone call away).
- Avoid telling the alleged perpetrator what the child has said.
- Refer to a child sexual assault centre or Protective Services Unit where an experienced team can take the serious responsibility for the problem.

Supporting the child

- Acknowledge the child's fear and perhaps guilt.
- Assure the child it is not his or her fault.
- Tell the child you will help.
- Obtain the child's trust.
- Tell the child it has happened to other children and you have helped them.

Prevention of child abuse

Prevention of abuse, particularly self-perpetuating abuse, can be helped by creating awareness through media attention, programs in schools and the community in general, and increased knowledge and surveillance by all professionals involved with children. Clear guidelines on reporting and the accessibility of child abuse clinics are important for the strategies to be effective. Teaching children how to protect themselves offers the greatest potential for prevention.[5]

Counselling the secondary victims

Non-offending parents, who are the secondary victims of the abused child, will require help and guidance from their family doctor on how to manage the crisis at home.[3] Parents should be advised to reassure the child of support and safety and to maintain usual routines. The child should be allowed to set the pace, without overattention and pressure from the parents. Siblings should be informed that something has happened but that the child is safe. Ensure that the child will inform if the perpetrator attempts further abuse. Parents need substantial support, including alleviation of any guilt.

An unhappy consequence of the crisis is the problem of broken relationships, which may involve the separation of the child from the family. At least one hitherto unsuspecting parent will be devastated if a parent is responsible for the abuse. The sexually abused child needs to be living with a protective parent or carer, with the abusive parent living separately.

Support for doctors

The attending doctor also requires support, and sharing the problem with colleagues, mentors and family is recommended. Some helpful guidelines are as follows.

- Carefully record all examination findings (take copious notes).
- Always keep to the facts and be objective.
- Do not become emotionally involved.
- Work with (not for) the authorities.
- Avoid making inappropriate judgments to the authorities (e.g. do not state 'incest was committed', but rather say 'there is evidence (or no evidence) to support penetration of . . .').
- If called to court, be well prepared; rehearse presentation; be authoritative and keep calm without allowing yourself to be upset by personal affronts.

The main difficulty in diagnosing child abuse is denial that it could be possible.

Adult survivors of child abuse[10]

All forms of child abuse can result in PTSD (from a single incident) or complex trauma (cumulative). Because of the high rate of child abuse, much of it unreported and hidden away for many years, adult survivors of child abuse are likely to be presenting to GPs on a frequent basis, often unknowingly.

The effect is more likely to be noticed in adulthood. We may encounter the sequelae of the issue, for the first time, in women in their early 30s and men in their late 60s.[11]

Childhood trauma, especially in the first few years during formative brain development, can lead to lifelong problems with dealing with stress. Unresolved trauma restricts the capacity to respond flexibly to life challenges. Patients may present with diverse and puzzling symptoms, including medically unexplained symptoms. Substance abuse, mood disorders and other psychological impairments may result.

A GP should be aware of this possibility, and screen for trauma from child abuse in patients presenting with such issues. Take particular care with physical examination, particularly in sensitive areas or involving internal examination, and realise that many patients on whom we are doing Pap tests or rectal examinations may be survivors of child abuse. Procedures can also cause pain, and may re-traumatise such a patient. Practising in a 'trauma informed' manner involves paying attention to the way we perform a service or procedure, as well as what it comprises, and being sensitive to the context of what may have come before. Trauma from previous child abuse can often be helped by appropriately targeted counselling and psychological therapies.

Basic rules

- Suspect child abuse.
- Recognise child abuse.
- Consult the child protection authorities.

Mandatory reporting

In most states of Australia and in many areas throughout the world it is mandatory to notify the relevant statutory authorities about suspected child abuse. All family doctors should become familiar with the appropriate local legislation.

Practice tips and guidelines

- A child's statement alleging abuse should be accepted as true until proved otherwise.
- Children rarely lie about sexual abuse.
- False allegations, however, are a sign of family disharmony and an indication that the child may need help.
- Do not insist that the child has 'got it wrong', even if you find the actions by the alleged perpetrator unbelievable.
- Do not procrastinate—move swiftly to solve the problem.
- The genitalia are normal in the majority of sexually abused children.
- Be supportive to the child by listening, believing, being kind and caring.

When to refer

Unless there are exceptional circumstances, referral to an appropriate child abuse centre, where an expert team is available, is recommended. If doubtful, relatively urgent referral to a paediatrician is an alternative. There is also the National Child Abuse Helpline: phone, 1800 99 10 99, email helpline@childwise.org.au.

References

1 Australian Institute of Family Studies. Child abuse and neglect statistics, May 2013 <www.aifs.gov.au/cfca/pubs/factsheets/a142086/> (accessed 18/8/2014).
2 Australian Institute of Family Studies. The prevalence of child abuse, March 2013 <www.aifs.gov.au/cfca/pubs/factsheets/a144254/index.html> (accessed 18/8/201).
3 Kellogg N. The evaluation of sexual abuse in children. Pediatrics, 2005; 116: 506–12.
4 Australian Institute of Health and Welfare. Child Protection Australia 2011–2012, March 2013 <www.aihw.gov.au/publication-detail/?id=60129542755> (accessed 18/8/2014).
5 Briggs F. *Smart Parenting for Safer Kids*. Melbourne: JoJo Publishing, 2011.
6 Australian Institute of Family Studies. Child abuse and neglect statistics, May 2013 <www.aifs.gov.au/cfca/pubs/factsheets/a142091/> (accessed 18/8/2014).
7 Bird S. Child abuse: mandatory reporting requirements. Aust Fam Physician, 2011; 40 (11): 921–6.
8 Kellogg N. Evaluation of suspected child physical abuse. Pediatrics, 2007; 119: 1232–41.
9 Smith A. Nonaccidental injury in childhood. Aust Fam Physician, 2011; 40 (11): 858–61.
10 Adults surviving child abuse (ASCA). ASCA factsheet for general practitioners: understanding complex trauma, 2014 <www.asca.org.au/video/primary-care-practitioners.aspx> (accessed 25/8/2014).
11 Paulton R, Moffitt TE, Silva PA. The Dunedin Multidisciplinary Health and Development Study: overview of the first 40 years, with an eye to the future. Soc Psychiatry Psychiatr Epidemiol, 2015; 50 (5): 679–93.

Resources

The Royal Children's Hospital Melbourne, *Clinical Practice Guidelines: Child Abuse*, <https://www.rch.org.au/clinicalguide/guideline_index/Child_abuse/> (accessed 14/5/2018).

Emergencies in children

We can say with some assurance that, although children may be the victims of fate, they will not be the victims of our neglect.

John F Kennedy (1917–63)

Important serious emergencies in children include:

- trauma, especially head injuries and intra-abdominal injuries
- painful conditions
- swallowed foreign bodies (FB)
- respiratory problems:
  - bronchial asthma
  - epiglottitis
  - croup
  - inhaled FB
  - acute bronchiolitis
- severe gastroenteritis
- septicaemia (e.g. meningococcal septicaemia)
- myocarditis
- immersion
- poisoning
- bites and stings
- seizures
- febrile convulsions
- sudden infant death syndrome (SIDS) and apparent life-threatening episode (ALTE)
- child abuse:
  - emotional
  - physical
  - sexual
  - neglect
  - potential
- psychogenic disturbances
- anxiety/hyperventilation
- suicide/parasuicide

Survey by age group

The author's study analysed emergencies into three groups:[1] preschool (0–5 years), primary school (6–12), adolescence (13–17).

The commonest emergency calls in the 0–5 years group were poisoning, accidents and violence, dyspnoea, fever/rigors, convulsions, abdominal pain, earache, vomiting.

In the 6–12 years age group: accidents and violence, dyspnoea, abdominal pain, vomiting, acute allergy, bites and stings, earache.

In the 13–17 years age group: accidents and violence, abdominal pain, psychogenic disorders, acute allergy, bites and stings, epistaxis.

The signs and symptoms of a serious illness

Babies who are febrile, drowsy and pale are at very high risk and require hospital admission.

The busy GP will see many sick children in a day's work, especially in the winter months with the epidemic of URTIs. It is vital to be able to recognise the very sick child who requires special attention, including admission to hospital. It is unlikely that the commonplace robust, lustily crying, hot, red-faced child is seriously ill but the pale, quiet, whimpering child spells danger. These rules are particularly helpful in the assessment of babies under six months of age.[2,3] The presence of a fever in itself is not necessarily an indication of serious illness but rather that the baby has an infection.[2]

The features of a very sick infant include:

- inactive, lying quietly, uninterested
- increased respiratory rate
- increased work of breathing
- noisy breathing:
  - chest wall or sternal retraction
  - wheezes, grunting, stridor
- tachycardia
- sunken eyes
- cold, pale skin
- cold extremities
- drowsiness
- poor perfusion (reduced capillary refill time)

A Melbourne study[4] of the sensitivity of clinical signs in detecting serious illness in infants identified five key signs or markers:

Marker	Risk to baby
Drowsiness	58%
Pallor	49%
Chest wall retraction	41%
Temperature >38.9°C or <36.4°C	42%
Lump >2 cm	42%

If sepsis suspected, investigate with:

- blood culture
- FBE/ESR/CRP
- lumbar puncture
- urine culture
- chest X-ray

Serious infectious illnesses to consider include:

- *Haemophilus influenza* type B (Hib) infection:
  - acute epiglottitis
  - meningitis

  (now uncommon since Hib immunisation)
- acute bacterial meningitis
- septicaemia:
  - meningococcaemia
  - toxic shock syndrome
  - other bacterial sepsis
- acute viral encephalitis
- acute myocarditis
- asthma/bronchitis/bronchiolitis
- pneumonia
- intussusception/bowel obstruction/appendicitis
- severe gastroenteritis

Strategic approach[5]

It is useful to have a systematic mnemonic for appraisal of the sick child. One general pattern (ABCDEFG) for the primary survey is:

- **A**irway
- **B**reathing
- **C**irculation
- **D**isability (neurological assessment)
- **E**xposure
- **F**luids: in and out
- **G**lucose

Another is the ABCD assessment (see below). Blood glucose should not be overlooked:

- normal random range
  - children 3.5–5.5 mmol/L
  - neonates 2.9–7 mmol/L
- hyperglycaemia >12 mmol/L
- hypoglycaemia <2.5 mmol/L

Two main groups of signs are good indicators of serious illness.[2]

Group 1: common features with reasonable risk and indicator of toxicity

Here a useful mnemonic is ABCD:

A = poor **A**rousal, **A**lertness and **A**ctivity
B = **B**reathing difficulty
C = poor **C**irculation (persistent pallor, cold legs to knees)
D = **D**ecreased fluid intake and/or urine output

Note: The more signs present, the greater the risk.

Children with any of these signs must be seen early, investigated and treated as a priority.

Group 2: uncommon features with high risk requiring urgent referral

- Respiratory: apnoea, central cyanosis, respiratory grunt
- GIT: persistent bile-stained vomiting, mass >2 cm other than hydrocele or umbilical hernia, significant faecal blood
- CNS: convulsions
- Skin: petechial rash

Airway and breathing[5]

Assessment of the airway and breathing is an important barometer of life-threatening illness and impending cardiac arrest due to hypoxia. The effort and efficacy of breathing must be assessed in the sick infant and child.

Important signs to observe with indicators

- Inspiratory noises with obstruction
  - bubbly noises—partial obstruction with fluid
  - snoring—decreased level of consciousness
  - stridor—partial obstruction to larynx or trachea
- Apnoea—no respiratory effort for >20 seconds
- Bradypnoea—respiratory rate < normal for age
- Tachypnoea—rate > normal for age (indicates need to ↑ O_2 and ↓ CO_2)
- Chest recession—on inspiration
- Tracheal tug—downward pull on inspiration
- Accessory muscle use
- Nasal flaring
- Gasping—severe hypoxia; impending arrest
- Grunting—expiration against obstructed glottis
- Oxygen saturation—efficacy of breathing; use oximetry only as an adjunct to clinical assessment
- Cyanosis

Secondary signs of worsening obstruction

- Increased respiratory rate or effort
- Decreased oxygen saturation
- Increasing tachycardia
- Deterioration of colour
- Development of agitation or decreased level of consciousness

Pulse oximetry and oxygen saturation

The pulse oximeter measures arterial saturation of arterial blood (SpO_2). In healthy young people, the SpO_2 should be 97–99%. The ideal value is 97–100%. The median value in neonates is 97%, in young children 98% and in adults 98%. A level less than 95% and particularly 92% is a serious concern. The aim of treatment, including for asthma, is to keep it above 94%.

Indications for investigations are presented in TABLE 96.1.

Table 96.1 Indications for investigations in the sick child[2]

Urine microscopy, culture and sensitivity	All with fever
Full blood examination	All <4 weeks Risk factors present Doctor uncertain
Blood microscopy, culture and sensitivity	All <3 months Risk factors present Doctor uncertain
Faecal microscopy, culture and sensitivity	All with diarrhoea
Chest X-ray	All with significant respiratory track symptoms and signs
C-reactive protein	Those on antibiotics Doctor uncertain
CSF examination (lumbar puncture contraindicated in the unresponsive febrile patient)	Suspected meningitis (infant drowsy, pale and febrile) Convulsion in febrile child and: • source of fever unknown • receding drowsiness and pallor • infant <6 months, child >5 years • prolonged convulsion (>10 minutes) • postictal phase longer than usual (>30 minutes)

Collapse in children

Collapse in children is a very dramatic emergency and often represents a life-threatening event. It is important to remember that the child's brain requires two vital factors: oxygen and glucose.

There is only a 2-minute reserve once cerebral blood flow stops. Bacterial meningitis should be considered as a cause.

Important causes of collapse are presented in TABLE 96.2. Keep in mind child abuse as a cause of collapse.

Table 96.2 Collapse in children: causes to consider

Anaphylaxis	Penicillin injection Stings
Asphyxia	Near drowning Strangulation
Airways obstruction	Asthma Epiglottitis Croup Inhaled foreign body
CNS disorders	Convulsions Meningitis Encephalitis Head injury
Severe infection	Gastroenteritis → dehydration Septicaemia Myocarditis
Hypovolaemia	Dehydration (e.g. heat) Blood loss (e.g. ruptured spleen)
Cardiac failure	Arrhythmias Cardiomyopathy
Metabolic	Acidosis (e.g. diabetic coma) Hypoglycaemia Hyponatraemia
Poisoning	Drug ingestion Envenomation
SIDS	Near miss
Functional	Breath-holding attacks Conversion reaction Vasovagal

Note: Consider child abuse.

Initial basic management[6]

1. Lay child on side.
2. Suck out mouth and nasopharynx.

3 Rescue breaths.
4 Intubate or ventilate (if necessary).
5 Give oxygen 8–10 L/min by mask.
6 Pass a nasogastric tube:
 0–3 years 12 FG
 4–10 years 14 FG
7 Attend to circulation: IV access
 ? give blood, Haemaccel or N saline.
8 Take blood for appropriate investigations.
9 Consider 'blind' administration of IV glucose.
10 A pulse oximeter is ideal.

Cardiopulmonary resuscitation[6]

Sudden primary cardiac arrest is rare in children. It is mostly due to hypoxia. Asystole or severe bradycardia is the usual rhythm at the time of arrest.

The following basic life support plan should be followed:

- Check breathing and pulse.
- Inspect oropharynx and clear any debris using suction if necessary.
- Basic life support outside the hospital setting is 30:2 compression ventilation ratio, including two initial rescue breaths. The ratio of 30:2 is recommended for all ages regardless of the number of revivers present <www.resus.org.au/policy/guidelines/index.asp>.
- Tilt head backwards, lift chin and thrust jaw forwards (the sniffing position).
- Ventilate lungs at about 20 inflations/min with bag-valve-mask or mouth to mask or mouth to mouth. An Air-viva using 8–10 L/min of oxygen is ideal if available.
- Intubate via mouth and secure, if necessary (must pre-oxygenate).
- If intubation not possible, use a needle cricothyroidotomy as an emergency.
- Start external cardiac compression immediately if pulseless or <60 beats/min (see TABLE 128.2 in CHAPTER 128). Use two fingers or thumbs for infants <1 year and heel of one hand for children 1–8 years.
- If >8 years use a two-handed technique. Avoid pressure over ribs and abdominal viscera. The compression ratio for children is 100 per minute (one per 0.6 seconds).

96

Guidelines

Differences in children's airways for intubation:

- epiglottis longer and stiffer, more horizontal
- larynx more anterior → difficult to intubate 'blind'
- cricoid ring is narrowest position → cuffed tube not required
- shorter trachea → increased risk intubating right main bronchus
- narrow airway → increased airway resistance

Rule for endotracheal tube (ETT) size (internal diameter in mm)

- ETT (mm) = (age in years ÷ 4) + 4
  or
  the size of the child's little finger or nares
- ETT length (cm) oral = (age in years ÷ 2) + 12 from lower lip; nasal—add 3 cm

For endotracheal size refer to TABLE 96.3 and for a basic schedule for CPR refer to TABLE 128.2.

Table 96.3 Childhood intubation: endotracheal tube size and insertion distance[6]

Age	Internal diameter (mm)	Length to lip (cm)
Newborn	3.0	8.5
1–6 months	3.5	10
6–12 months	4.0	11
2 years	4.5	12
4	5.0	14
6	5.5	15
8	6.0	16
10	6.5	17
12	7.0	18
14	7.5	19
Adult	8.0	20

Drugs that can be administered through the ETT can be considered under the mnemonic NASALS:

N = **N**aloxone
A = **A**tropine
S = **S**albutamol
A = **A**drenaline
L = **L**ignocaine
S = **S**urfactant

Paediatric advanced life support

- Compression ventilation ratio of 30:2 for infants and children should be used in an advanced life support situation (i.e. in a hospital setting).

- Give a single shock instead of stacked shocks (single shock strategy) for ventricular fibrillation/pulseless ventricular tachycardia.
- Where the arrest is witnessed by a health care professional and a manual defibrillator is available, then up to three shocks may be given (stacked shock strategy) at the first defibrillation attempt.
- Monophasic or biphasic defibrillation: first shock—2 J/kg, subsequent shocks—4 J/kg.

Poisoning

Poisoning in children is a special problem in toddlers (accidental) and in adolescents (deliberate). Children aged 1–6 years are most prone to accidental poisoning, with a peak at 2 years. The most common cause of death in comatose patients is respiratory failure.

The common dangerous poisons in the past were kerosene and aspirin. Excluding household chemicals, camphor/moth balls, pesticides, insecticides, organophosphates and opioids, the most dangerous drugs or substances, even in small doses, are:

- antidepressants, especially tricyclics
- antihistamines
- antihypertensives
- antipsychotics
- anxiolytics (e.g. benzodiazepines/barbiturates)
- beta blockers
- calcium channel blockers
- chloral hydrate
- clonidine
- disc (button) batteries
- digoxin
- dishwashing powder
- iron tablets
- Lomotil (diphenoxylate)
- opiates/'designer' drugs
- paracetamol/acetaminophen (the most common in Australia)
- paraquat
- potassium tablets
- quinine/quinidine/chloroquine
- salicylates (e.g. aspirin)
- selective serotonin reuptake inhibitors
- tricyclic antidepressants

Be mindful of the serotonin syndrome (see CHAPTER 19).

In a UK study[7] the main cause of deaths from poisoning were (in order) tricyclics, salicylates, opioids including Lomotil, barbiturates, digoxin, orphenadrine, quinine, potassium and iron. Another study highlighted, in addition, carbon monoxide and corrosive substances.

Principles of treatment[8,9]

The vast majority of paediatric exposures are benign, and do not require hospital referral for observation or assessment. The management of childhood poisoning has undergone a transformation, with the cornerstone being conservative–supportive and symptomatic care.[8]

Early discussion with a poisons information centre is appropriate and will often help direct management. Key initial steps are to identify the poison and rapid triage of the child.

In an emergency, call for an ambulance and consult your local emergency department or poisons information centre. The process is:

- Identify the poison
- Rapid triage
- Support vital functions—ABCD:
  Airway—relieve any obstruction
  Breathing—ventilate with oxygen
  Circulation—treat hypotension/arrhythmias
  Detect and treat seizures and/or hypoglycaemia (consider dextrose)
- Administer antidote early if indicated (see TABLE 96.4)

Note: Emesis, gastric lavage and charcoal are not routinely recommended and are best given on the advice of a poisons information centre.[7]

- Treat any complications:
  - respiratory failure: hypoventilation, apnoea
  - pulmonary aspiration of gastric contents
  - arrhythmias
  - hypotension
  - seizures
  - delayed effects (e.g. paracetamol—hepatotoxicity; tricyclics—arrhythmia)

Investigations

- Drug levels (e.g. paracetamol, aspirin, iron)
- Blood gas analysis
- X-ray:
  - chest
  - abdomen (e.g. radio-opaque iron tablets)
  - skull
- ECG

Psychosocial care

The reasons for the poisoning need to be carefully evaluated and proper support and advice given.

Table 96.4 Important antidotes for poisons[10]

Poison	Antidote
Amphetamines (cause hypertension)	Glyceryl trinitrate IV Sodium nitroprusside
Benzodiazepines	Flumazenil
Beta blockers	Glucagon Isoprenaline
Calcium blocker	Calcium chloride IV *or* Calcium gluconate IV
Carbon monoxide	Oxygen 100% Hyperbaric oxygen
Cyanide	Hydroxocobalamin Dicobalt edetate Sodium nitrite IV Sodium thiosulphate IV
Digoxin	Digoxin-specific antibodies Magnesium sulphate
Heavy metals (e.g. Pb, As, Hg, Fe)	Chelating agents, e.g. dimercaprol
Heparin	Protamine IV
Iron	Desferrioxamine
Isoniazid	Pyridoxine
Methanol, ethylene glycol	Ethanol (ethyl alcohol) Fomepizole
Narcotics/opioids	Naloxone (Narcan)
Organophosphates	Atropine Pralidoxime (2-PAM)
Paracetamol (acetaminophen)	Acetylcysteine (IV) (effective within 12 hours) consider up to 36 hours
Phenothiazines	Benztropine
Potassium	Calcium gluconate Kayexalate Sodium bicarbonate (if acidosis) Salbutamol aerosol
Tricyclic antidepressants	Sodium bicarbonate IV
Warfarin	Fresh frozen plasma Vitamin K

96

Swallowed foreign objects

A golden rule

The natural passage of most objects entering the stomach can be expected. Once the pylorus is traversed the FB usually continues.

This includes:

- coins
- buttons
- sharp objects
- open safety pins
- glass (e.g. ends of thermometers)
- drawing pins

Special cases are:

- very large coins: watch carefully
- hair clips (usually cannot pass duodenum if under 7 years)

Management

- Manage conservatively.
- X-ray all children (mouth to anus, especially chest and abdomen) on presentation (the oesophagus is a concern).
- Investigate unusual gagging, coughing and retching with X-rays of the head, neck, thorax and abdomen (check nasopharynx and respiratory tract).
- Watch for passage of the FB in stool (usually 3 days). Defecate into a container.
- If not passed, order X-ray in 1 week.
- If a blunt FB has been stationary for 1 month without symptoms, remove at laparotomy.

Button and disc battery ingestion

If not in stomach these (especially lithium batteries) create an emergency if in the oesophagus because electrical current generated destroys mucous membranes and perforates within 6 hours (must be removed endoscopically ASAP). This also applies to the ear canal and nares.

Fever[11]

Fever, which is commonly defined as a temperature >38°C, is a significant symptom in a child, especially in neonates (see CHAPTER 53). If an infant aged less than 3 months presents with a fever but no focus of infection, consider bacteraemia. One recommendation is that all febrile neonates should have a full septic work-up and be admitted for parenteral antibiotics.

Not to be missed

- Meningitis/encephalitis
- Sepsis
- Pneumonia
- Osteomyelitis/septic arthritis
- Pertussis
- Urinary infection (especially if no focus)

Febrile convulsions

Diagnosis based on presence of fever, short duration and no clinical evidence of CNS pathology.

Clinical features

- The commonest cause is an URTI (e.g. the common cold or similar viral syndrome).
- About 5 per 100 incidence in children.
- Rare under 6 months and over 5 years.
- Commonest age range 9–20 months.
- Recurrent in up to 50% of cases.
- Consider meningitis and lumbar puncture after first convulsion if under 2 years or cause of fever not obvious.
- Epilepsy develops in about 2–3% of such children.

Management of the convulsion (if prolonged >15 minutes), also for status epilepticus

- Undress the child to singlet and underpants or light clothing but take care to prevent the child getting cold.
- Maintain the airway and prevent injury.
- Place patient chest down with head turned to one side.
- Oxygen 8 L/min by mask.
- Give midazolam or diazepam.
- Give midazolam by one of four routes:

  IV 0.15 mg/kg, IM 0.2 mg/kg, buccal 2–5 mg/dose or (preferable) intranasal 0.3 mg/kg undiluted (use 1 mL of drops from vial) Buccal and nasal routes slower response—IM may be most practical.

- Give diazepam by one of two routes:

  IV 0.2 mg/kg, undiluted or diluted (10 mg in 20 mL N saline)
  or
  rectally 0.5 mg/kg (dilute with saline or in pre-prepared syringe) up to 10 mg or with suppository or rectal gel.

Note: Although the IV route is preferred, the rectal route is ideal in a home or office situation; for example consider a 2-year-old child (weight 12 kg) with a persistent febrile convulsion. The dose of diazepam injectable is 0.5 mg/kg, so 6 mg (1.2 mL) of diazepam is diluted with isotonic saline (up to 10 mL of solution) and the nozzle of the syringe pressed gently but firmly into the anus and injected slowly. *Observe carefully for respiratory depression.*

rectal paracetamol 15 mg/kg statim

The anti-epileptics can be repeated in 5 minutes if fitting continues.

Check blood glucose: if <3.5 give a bolus dose of IV dextrose.

If still fitting, admit to an appropriate unit and rapidly induce 'coma' with thiopentone or propofol (preferred) followed by intubation.

Explain risk of later epilepsy is small: <3%.

Meningitis or encephalitis

Diagnosing meningitis and encephalitis requires a high level of clinical awareness and watchfulness for the infective problem that appears more serious than normal. Follow the appropriate guidelines: ABCDEFG (see earlier in this chapter). Refer also to CHAPTER 30.

Bacterial meningitis[12]

Bacterial meningitis is basically also a childhood infection. Neonates and children aged 6–12 months are at the greatest risk. For clinical features see CHAPTER 30. Meningococcal disease can take the form of either meningitis or septicaemia (meningococcaemia) or both. Most cases begin as septicaemia, usually via the nasopharynx.

Treatment for suspected meningitis (summary)[9]

First—oxygen and IV access (interosseous if difficult):

- take blood for culture (within 30 minutes of assessment)
- for child give bolus of 10–20 mL/kg of N saline
- admit to hospital for lumbar puncture when patient is resuscitated and stable and without signs of raised ICP
- dexamethasone 0.15 mg/kg up to 10 mg IV
- ceftriaxone 100 mg/kg up to 4 g, IV statim then daily for 3–5 days
  or
  cefotaxime 50 mg/kg up to 2 g, IV statim then 6 hourly for 3–5 days

  Neonates to 3 months:
- ampicillin/amoxycillin (or benzylpenicillin) + cefotaxime

Meningococcaemia[12,13]

Note: Treatment is urgent once sepsis suspected (e.g. petechial or purpuric rash on trunk and limbs). It should be given before reaching hospital according to the following plans (see CHAPTER 30).

- Antibiotics:
  ceftriaxone 100 mg/kg IV or IM (max. 4 g) or cefotaxime statim then daily for 5 days

or
benzylpenicillin 60 mg/kg IV (max. 1.8 g), 4-hourly for 3–5 days. Give IM if IV access not possible

- Admit to hospital
- Continue antibiotics for 7–10 days

Treat contacts who:

- live in the household and <24 months
- have kissed patient in the previous 10 days
- have attended the same day-care centre

For prophylaxis—rifampicin dose:
adult — 600 mg bd for 3 days
child <1 month—5 mg/kg
child >1 month—10 mg/kg
give bd for 2 days
or (if unsuitable)
ceftriaxone 1 g (child: 25 mg/kg up to 1 g) IM daily for 2 days
ciprofloxacin 500 mg (o) as single dose (child 125 mg)
give meningococcus type C vaccine

A simple plan for children (prehospital): benzylpenicillin[13]

- infants <1 year: 300 mg IV or IM
- 1–9 years: 600 mg
- ≥ 10 years: 1200 mg

Other septicaemic shock

- take blood for culture
- if unknown pathogen, give flucloxacillin IV plus cefotaxime IV

Practice point

In a very sick child with fever give IV antibiotics while awaiting culture.

Acute epiglottitis

96

Acute epiglottitis due to *H. influenzae* is a life-threatening emergency in a child. A toxic febrile illness, with sudden onset of expiratory stridor, should alert one to this potentially fatal condition. A high index of suspicion of epiglottitis is always warranted in such presentations. This is uncommon since Hib immunisation.

Differential diagnosis

The main alternative diagnosis is viral laryngotracheobronchitis (croup). There are, however, significant clinical differences.

Epiglottitis is characterised by fever, a soft voice, lack of a harsh cough, a preference to sit quietly (rather than lie down) and especially by a soft stridor with a sonorous expiratory component.

Croup is distinguished by a harsh inspiratory stridor, a hoarse voice and brassy cough.

Other differential diagnoses include tonsillitis, infectious mononucleosis and bacterial tracheitis.

Diagnostic tip

Children with epiglottitis usually sit still with their mouth open, drooling saliva, and their eyes follow you around the room because limited head movement protects the compromised airway.

DO NOT EXAMINE THE THROAT IN THE OFFICE

A swollen, cherry-red epiglottis recognised on examination of the nasopharynx confirms the diagnosis. However, the initial diagnosis should be made on the clinical history and appearance of the child.

Management

Admit the child to hospital for the following:

- Intubation: in theatre suck away profuse secretions and perform nasotracheal intubation
- Antibiotics:[13]
  cefotaxime 25 mg/kg up to 1 g IV for 5 days 8 hourly
  or
  ceftriaxone 50 mg/kg to max. 1 g/day IV daily for 5 days

Croup[14]

Croup refers to a symptom complex with a harsh, brassy cough, usually with an inspiratory stridor and with or without respiratory difficulty.

Clinical features of viral laryngotracheitis:

- caused by parainfluenzal and other viruses e.g. RSV
- most common type of childhood croup
- usually 6 months to 6 years—peak incidence 1–2 years
- prodrome of URTI or coryza for 2 days
- fever variable—rarely above 39°C
- loud barking cough—increased if upset
- usually self-limiting

Treatment[14,15,16]

The grading system for croup is outlined in TABLE 96.5.

Table 96.5 Grading system for croup	
Croup score	
Grade 1: mild	Stridor at rest without retractions and no distress
Grade 2: moderate	Stridor at rest with sternal and chest wall retractions
Grade 3: severe	Marked respiratory distress indicated by irritability, pallor, cyanosis, tachycardia and exhaustion (i.e. impending airway obstruction)

Grade 1 croup

Mild croup (barking cough, no stridor or stridor at rest without chest retraction, hoarse voice):

- manage at home if no signs of Grade 2 or 3 croup, keep child relaxed
- consider oral steroids (e.g. dexamethasone 0.15–0.3 mg/kg/dose or prednisolone 1 mg/kg/dose) if stridor and chest wall retraction develop

A randomised controlled trial showed no additional benefit from mist (supersaturated air) therapy when coupled with oral corticosteroids (level II evidence).[16,17]

Grade 2 croup

Moderate croup (inspiratory stridor when upset or at rest with chest wall retractions):

- admit to hospital (e.g. emergency department)
- cool humidified air
- oral steroids
  dexamethasone 0.6 mg/kg
  or
  prednisolone (tablets or oral solution)1 mg/kg (2–3 doses)
  and/or (for children 2 or more years)
  budesonide 100 mcg × 20 puffs or 2 mg nebulised
- nebulised adrenaline—if poor response to steroids
- observe for at least 4 hours

Grade 3 croup

Severe croup (inspiratory stridor at rest, use of accessory muscles, patient restless and agitated). Adrenaline is first-line therapy:

- nurse in intensive care
- oxygen
- nebulised adrenaline 1:1000 solution
  0.5 mL/kg/dose (to max. 5 mL)
  (beware of possible rebound effect after 2–3 hours—must be observed)

Note: Can use 4 ampoules of 1:1000 solution in a nebuliser run with oxygen 8 L/min. Repeat the dose if no response at 10–15 minutes, do not dilute solution.

- dexamethasone 0.2 mg/kg IV
  or
  0.6 mg/kg IM
  followed by oral steroids
- have facilities for artificial airway
- may need endotracheal intubation (if going into respiratory failure) for 48 hours. Use a tube 0.5–1 mm smaller than normal for age.

There is no place for cough medicines or antibiotics. Steaming methods are discouraged.

Wheezing in an infant < 12 months

Probability diagnosis: bronchiolitis

Not to be missed:

- foreign body
- anaphylaxis
- heart failure
- pneumonia
- apnoea
- smokers in the household (consider)
- immune deficiency

Clinical signs to cause concern:

- grunting
- apnoea (ex premature)
- low oxygen saturation
- reduced feeds and wet napkins

Bronchiolitis[18]

- An acute viral illness usually due to RSV
- The commonest acute LRTI in infants
- Usual age 2 weeks to 9 months (up to 12 months)
- Prodromal symptoms for 48 hours (e.g. coryza, irritating cough, then 3–5 days of more severe symptoms)
- Wheezy breathing—often distressed
- Signs of hypoxia (restlessness, agitation, drowsiness)
- Tachypnoea
- Hyperinflated chest: barrel-shaped, usually subcostal recession

Note: All that wheezes is not necessarily asthma.

Auscultation

- Widespread fine inspiratory crackles (not with asthma)
- Frequent expiratory wheezes

X-ray. Hyperinflation of lungs with depression of diaphragm—but chest X-ray should not be used for diagnosis or routinely performed.[19]

Virus identified by PCR on nasopharyngeal aspirate. Rapid RSV viral test available. Blood glucose should be assessed in all sick patients.

Management

Admission to hospital is usual, especially with increasing respiratory distress reflected by difficulty in feeding (particularly less than half normal over 24 hours). Dehydration is a serious problem, especially with exhausted infants.

- Minimal handling/good nursing care
- Careful observation: colour, pulse, respiration, oxygen saturation (pulse oximetry)
- Oxygen (preferably warmed and humidified) for signs of hypoxia: by nasal prongs or even simple facemask to maintain P_aO_2 above 90% (preferably ≥ 95%), O_2 not required if P_aO_2 >95% in room air
- Fluids IV preferably or by nasogastric tube if unable to feed orally
- Antibiotics not indicated unless secondary bacterial infection. There is no evidence to support the routine use of nebulised adrenaline, bronchodilators or corticosteroids.[14]

Note: Increased tendency to asthma later.

Very severe asthma[20]

See CHAPTER 82.

Observe closely according to the ABCD rule. Very severe asthma in children should be referred to an intensive care unit; stepwise action includes:

- inhaled salbutamol (4–8 puffs) from spacer, or
- continuous nebulised 0.5% salbutamol via mask[4]
- oxygen flow 6 L/min through the nebuliser (best option)
- IV infusion of

  salbutamol 5 mcg/kg/min
  hydrocortisone 4 mg/kg IV statim then 6 hourly

96

Common mistakes

- Using assisted mechanical ventilation inappropriately (main indications are physical exhaustion and cardiopulmonary arrest—it can be dangerous in asthma)
- Not giving high flow oxygen
- Giving excessive fluid
- Giving submaximal bronchodilator therapy

Acute heart failure

Clinical features (infants)

- Increasing fatigue, dyspnoea, poor feeding
- Failure to thrive
- Tachycardia, cardiomegaly, gallop rhythm
- Fine basal crackles
- Hepatomegaly
- Usually no peripheral oedema or wheezing

Causes include:

- congenital (e.g. VSD)
- cardiomyopathy
- tachyarrhythmias
- postprocedural myocardial dysfunction

Management

- Admit to hospital
- Pulse oximetry, ECG, CXR and echocardiography
- Diuretic (frusemide and spironolactone)
- ACE inhibitors—consider digoxin
- Oxygen to maintain P_aO_2 at 85–95%
- CPAP

Breath-holding attacks

This is a dramatic emergency. There are two types: one is related to a tantrum (description follows) and the other is a simple faint.

Clinical features

- Age group—usually 6 months to 6 years (peak 2–3 years)
- Precipitating event (minor emotional or physical)
- Children emit a long loud cry, then hold their breath
- They become pale and then blue
- If severe, may result in unconsciousness or even a brief tonic–clonic fit
- Lasts 10–60 seconds

Management

- Reassure the parents that attacks are self-limiting, not harmful and not associated with epilepsy or intellectual disability.
- Advise parents to maintain discipline and to resist spoiling the child.
- Try to avoid incidents known to frustrate the child or to precipitate a tantrum.

Note: Important childhood emergency drugs with dosages are presented in TABLE 96.6.

Table 96.6 Important childhood emergency drugs[21]

Drug	Route	Dose	Notes
Adrenaline 1:10 000 Adrenaline 1:1000	IV IM	0.1 mL/kg/dose 0.01 mL/kg/dose	Anaphylaxis, asystole (repeat every 5 minutes until response)
Adrenaline 1:1000	Nebuliser	0.5 mL/kg/dose (max. 5 mL)	LTB* (patient must be admitted)
Aminophylline	IV slowly	5 mg/kg loading	Moderate to severe asthma
Atropine	IV	0.02 mg/kg	Bradycardia producing shock
Calcium gluconate 10%	IV	0.5 mL/kg (max. 20 ml)	Hyperkalaemia, hypocalcaemia
Dextrose 50%	IV	1 mL/kg	Hypoglycaemia
Diazepam	IV PR	0.2 mg/kg	Seizures
Fentanyl citrate	IV	1.2 mcg/kg (intranasal effective)	Pain control
Glucagon	IV or IM	0.1 mg/kg (max. 1 mg)	Hypoglycaemia
Hydrocortisone	IV	4 mg/kg	Anaphylaxis, asthma
Midazolam	IV or IM, intranasal	0.15–0.2 mg/kg/dose	Seizures
Morphine	IV or IM	0.1–0.2 mg/kg	Sedation, pain relief
Naloxone	IV or IM	0.01 mg/kg (max. 2 mg)	Opioid overdose
Paracetamol	O	15–20 mg/kg loading	Fever
Paraldehyde	PR	0.3 mL/kg (dilute 1:2 in peanut oil)	Seizures
Salbutamol	Nebuliser	0.3 mL/kg	Asthma
	Spacer	<6 yrs 6 puffs >6 yrs 12 puffs	
	IV	5 mcg/kg	
Sodium bicarbonate 8.4%	IV	2 mL/kg	Titrate against blood gases
Soluble insulin	IV infusion	0.1 U/kg/h	Only if glucose >14 mmol/L

*LTB = laryngotracheal bronchitis (croup)

Note: Volume resuscitation: IV fluid bolus 20 mL/kg statim of crystalloid (e.g. N saline)

Source: After Pitt[21]

Aspirated foreign body

Parents or guardians may not be able to give a history of inhalation. One in eight episodes is not witnessed.

Symptoms

- Choking or coughing episodes while eating nuts or similar food or while sucking a small object (e.g. plastic toy)
- Persistent coughing and wheezing ('all that wheezes is not asthma')
- Sudden onset of first wheezing episode in a toddler with no past history of allergy, especially after a choking bout

Signs

- Reduced or absent breath sounds over whole or part of a lung
- Wheeze

Investigations

Chest X-ray (full inspiration and full expiration) to exclude an area of collapse or obstructive hyperinflation.

Note: Normal X-rays do not absolutely exclude an FB.

Management

First aid:

- most cough out the FB, so encourage coughing
- a finger sweep helps, as do back slaps, lateral chest compression and the Heimlich manoeuvre if >8 years (take care with viscera). A good rule is the rule of 5s—5 breaths, 5 back blows, 5 chest thrusts, 5 abdominal thrusts (older child).

If complete obstruction—attempt removal of the FB with forceps. If unsuccessful, perform a tracheostomy or cricothyroidotomy.

Note: Once an FB has passed through the larynx it is very rare for there to be an immediate threat to life, so referral is usually quite safe.

Note: Do not instrument the airways if the child is coping.

Bronchoscopy

Bronchoscopy is necessary in almost every child where there is a strong suggestion of an inhaled FB. It is difficult and requires an expert with appropriate facilities.

> **Prevention**
>
> - No child <15 months should have popcorn, hard lollies, raw carrots and apples
> - Children <4 years—no peanuts
> - Children <3 years—no toys with small parts

Anaphylaxis[5]

The management of airway obstruction and hypotension can be summarised as:

- oxygen 6–8 L/min by mask
- adrenaline 0.01 mL/kg of 1:1000 IM; 0.05–0.1 ml if <1 year
  (repeat adrenaline every 5 minutes as necessary)
  if no improvement set up a continuous infusion (1 mg adrenaline in 1000 mL N saline)
  avoid SC use
- autoinjector e.g. Epipen
  <10 kg: not recommended
  10–20 kg: 150 mcg
  >20 kg: 300 mcg
- nebulised salbutamol for bronchospasm
- admit to hospital (observe at least 4 hours)
- colloid or crystalloid solution IV: give repeated boluses 10–20 mL/kg
- only if necessary: corticosteroid 4 mg/kg IV

96

If persistent upper airways obstruction—try nebulised 1% adrenaline (max. 4 mL); intubation may be necessary. Admit to hospital and observe for at least 12 hours.

Status epilepticus/prolonged seizure[22]

Ensure adequate oxygenation: attend to airway (e.g. Guedel tube): give oxygen. Check blood glucose.

Antiepileptic options include:[5]

midazolam 0.1–0.2 mg/kg IV or 0.2 mg/kg IM *or* 0.3 mg/kg intranasal
diazepam 0.2 mg/kg IV or 0.5 mg/kg per rectum
clonazepam 0.25 mg (<1 year), 0.5 mg (1–5 years), 1 mg (>5 years)
phenytoin 15 mg/kg slowly over 20–30 minutes
thiopentone: titrate the dose (usually 2–5 mg/kg)

If refractory (up to 60 minutes), use full anaesthetic with intubation.

Consider hyponatraemia as the cause of convulsions with meningitis. Perform an ECG (look for prolonged QT interval). Consider IV ceftriaxone if meningitis suspected.

Drowning

The differences between salt-water and freshwater drowning are usually not clinically significant. If global hypoxic cerebral ischaemia and pulmonary aspiration, treat as follows:[6]

- adequate oxygenation and ventilation
- decompress stomach with nasogastric tube
- support circulation with IV infusion of colloid or IV saline solution and dopamine (dobutamine) 5–20 mcg/kg per minute
- mannitol 0.25–0.5 g/kg IV if cerebral oedema
- correct electrolyte disturbances (e.g. hypokalaemia)
- give prophylactic penicillin

Intraosseous infusion[3]

In an emergency situation where intravenous access in a collapsed person (especially children) is difficult, parenteral fluid can be infused into the bone marrow (an intravascular space). Intraosseous infusion is preferred to an intravenous cutdown in children under 5 years. It is useful to practise the technique on a chicken bone.

Site of infusion

- Adults and children over 5: distal end of tibia
- Children under 5: proximal end of tibia
- The distal femur: 2–3 cm above condyles in midline is an alternative

Avoid growth plates, midshaft and the sternum.

Method for proximal tibia

Note: Strict asepsis is essential (skin preparation and sterile gloves).

- Inject local anaesthetic (if necessary).
- Choose 16 gauge intraosseous needle (Dieckmann modification, e.g. Cook critical

needle 15.5 gauge) or a 16–18 gauge lumbar puncture needle (less expensive).
- Hold it at right angles to the anteromedial surface of the proximal tibia about 2 cm below the tibial tuberosity (see FIG. 96.1). Point the needle slightly downwards, away from the joint space (<90° to long axis).
- Carefully twist the needle to penetrate the bone cortex; it enters bone marrow with a sensation of giving way.
- Remove the trocar, aspirate a small amount of marrow to ensure its position.
- Hold the needle in place with a small plaster of Paris splint.
- Fluid, including blood, can be infused with a normal IV infusion—rapidly or slowly.
- The infusion rate can be markedly increased by using a pressure bag at 300 mmHg pressure.

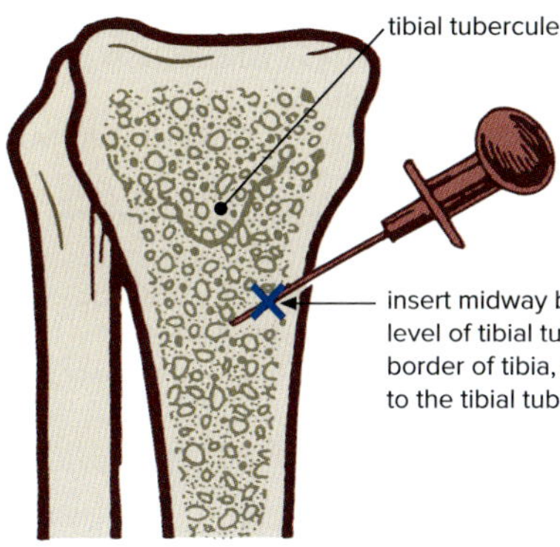

FIGURE 96.1 Intraosseous infusion

SERIOUS GASTROENTEROLOGICAL CONDITIONS

GIT conditions that cause vomiting require careful evaluation because of potentially fatal outcomes.

Gastroenteritis[23]

This condition should not be treated lightly. Assessment of general signs such as arousal, presence of pallor, degree of weight loss, fluids in and fluids out is important (see CHAPTER 44). If concerned or in doubt, arrange hospitalisation. The social situation needs to be taken into account.

Intussusception

It is important to recognise this condition as about 50% of infants with intussusception are not diagnosed on initial presentation.[2] Characteristic features include sudden-onset pallor that persists, episodic crying and vomiting. Rectal bleeding and an abdominal mass (see CHAPTER 34) are present in only 40% of cases.

Pyloric stenosis

Pyloric stenosis, which appears from 2 weeks to 3 months of age, should be suspected with projectile vomiting, acute weight loss and alkalosis. It must not be confused with projectile vomiting from overfeeding. If in doubt, expert ultrasound examination of the pylorus will assist diagnosis (refer to CHAPTER 60).

Red flag pointers for GIT conditions

- Bile-stained vomitus: indicates urgent referral to consider possible intestinal malrotation and mid-gut volvulus
- Failure to pass meconium beyond 24 hours: may represent congenital intestinal atresia and stenosis, meconium ileus or Hirschsprung disorder

Sudden infant death syndrome (SIDS)

- SIDS is the major cause of death between 1 and 12 months of age (peak incidence 4 months).
- The incidence is around 1 per 500 live births but improving.
- The causes are unknown, but risk factors have been identified. Overwhelming infection is a possibility.
- No investigations have identified susceptible infants.
- Although SIDS can recur in a family, the risk is small.
- There is an association with low socioeconomic status.

Risk factors

- Prone sleeping position
- Smothered airways (debatable)
- Artificial feeding (possible)
- Passive smoking (before or after birth)
- Hyperthermia or excess warmth
- Extreme prematurity <32 weeks
- Parental narcotic/cocaine abuse
- Intercurrent viral infections

Preventive advice

After baby is born:

- Place baby to sleep on its back (preferable) with no pillow (unless special reason for placing it on its stomach, e.g. gastro-oesophageal reflux).
- Ensure the head is uncovered.
- Encourage breastfeeding.
- Ensure the baby is not exposed to cigarette smoking (before and after birth).
- Ensure the baby does not get overheated (sweating around the head and neck indicates the baby is too hot).
- Ensure bed coverings are no more than adults require.
- Advise nothing else in cot (e.g. soft toys).

Reactions of bereaved parents

- May be hostility to GP, especially if recent examination
- May 'hear' the baby cry
- Distressing dreams
- Guilt/self-blame, especially mother
- Psychiatric morbidity
- Other stages of bereavement: denial, anger, bargaining, depression, acceptance

Management of SIDS

- Allow the parents to see or hold baby.
- Give explanations, including reasons for coroner's involvement.
- Provide bereavement counselling.
- Early contact with counsellors and continuing support.
- Contact the SIDS support group.
- Revisit the home.
- Provide hypnotics (limited).
- Offer advice on lactation suppression (see CHAPTER 109).
- Remember: siblings can also experience grief reactions.
- The police and coroner must be notified—the law requires an autopsy.

Apparent life-threatening episode

ALTE, or 'near-miss SIDS', is defined as a 'frightening' encounter of apnoea, colour change or choking. At least 10% will have another episode. Management includes admission to hospital for investigation and monitoring.

Guidelines for home apnoea monitoring

- ALTE
- Subsequent siblings of SIDS victims
- Twin of SIDS victim
- Extremely premature infants

Obstructive sleep apnoea syndrome

A childhood disorder of breathing during sleep characterised by noisy, disturbed breathing and periods of apnoea. Leads to daytime sleepiness, disturbed behaviour and cognitive dysfunction. Requires referral.

References

1 Murtagh J. The anatomy of a rural practice. Aust Fam Physician, 1981; 10: 564–7.

2 Hewson P, Oberklaid F. Recognition of serious illness in infants. Modern Medicine Australia, 1994; 37 (7): 89–96.

3 Tibballs J. Endotracheal and intraosseous drug administration for paediatric CPR. Aust Fam Physician, 1992; 21: 1477–80.

4 Hewson P et al. Recognition of serious illness in babies. J Paediatr Child Health, 2000; 36: 221–5.

5 NSW Ministry of Health: NSW health policy statements for children and infants. Recognition of a sick baby or child in the emergency department, June 2011 <www.health.NSW.gov.au/policies/> (accessed September 2014).

6 Gwee A, Rimer R, Marks M. *Paediatric Handbook* (9th edn). Oxford: Wiley-Blackwell, 2015: 1–8.

7 Fraser NC. Accidental poisoning deaths in British children 1958–77. BMJ, 1980; 280: 1595.

8 Expert group for Toxicology and Wilderness. Paediatric poisoning. In eTG complete [Internet]. Melbourne: Therapeutic Guidelines Ltd. Available from: <www.tg.org.au> (accessed November 2017).

9 Yuen A. Accidental poisoning in children. Patient Management, 1991; November: 39–45.

10 Fulde G. *Emergency Medicine*. Sydney: Elsevier, 2007: 601–5.

11 NSW Ministry of Health: NSW health policy statements for children and infants. Fever—acute management, October 2010 <www.health.NSW.gov.au/policies/> (accessed 25/11/2017).

12 NSW Ministry of Health: NSW health policy statements for children and infants. Bacterial meningitis—acute management, July 2014 <www.health.NSW.gov.au/policies/> (accessed 25/11/2017).

13 Spicer J (Chair). *Therapeutic Guidelines: Antibiotics* (Version 13). Therapeutic Guidelines Ltd, Melbourne: 2006: 55–247.

14 NSW Ministry of Health: NSW health policy statements for children and infants. Croup—acute management, August 2010 <www.health.NSW.gov.au/policies/> (accessed 25/11/2017).

15 Fitzgerald DA, Kilhan HK. Croup: assessment and evidence-based management. Med J Aust, 2003; 179: 372–7.

16 Mazza D, Wilkinson F et al. Evidence based guidelines for the management of croup. Aust Fam Physician, Special issue, 2008; 37 (6): 14–19.

17 Neto GM, Kentab O et al. A randomised controlled trial of mist in the acute treatment of moderate croup. Acad Emerg Med, 2002; 9: 873–9.

18 NSW Ministry of Health: NSW health policy statements for children and infants. Bronchiolitis—acute management,

October 2012 <www.health.NSW.gov.au/policies/> (accessed 25/11/2017; reviewed 19/1/2017).

19 Turner T, Wilkinson F et al. Evidence based guidelines for the management of bronchiolitis. Aust Fam Physician, Special issue, 2008; 37 (6): 6–13.

20 NSW Ministry of Health: NSW health policy statements for children and infants. Asthma—acute management, October 2012 <www.health.NSW.gov.au/policies/> (accessed 25/11/2017).

21 Pitt R. Common paediatric emergencies. Aust Fam Physician, 1989; 18: 1228–34.

22 NSW Ministry of Health: NSW health policy statements for children and infants. Seizures—acute management, October 2009 <www.health.NSW.gov.au/policies/> (accessed December 2014).

23 NSW Ministry of Health: NSW health policy statements for children and infants. Gastroenteritis—acute management, February 2010 <www.health.NSW.gov.au/policies/> (accessed September 2014).

Resources

ViCTOR: Victorian Children's Tool for Observation and Response <https://www.victor.org.au/>, including Back to Basics videos <https://www.victor.org.au/implementing-victor/victor-back-to-basics/> (accessed 14/5/2018).

97 Adolescent health

The feeling of apartness from others comes to most with puberty, but it is not always developed to such a degree as to make the difference between the individual and his fellows noticeable to the individual.

W Somerset Maugham (1874–1965), *Of Human Bondage*

Adolescence is the transitional period of development between relatively dependent childhood and relatively independent adulthood. The time of onset and duration varies from one person to another but it is generally considered to occur between the ages of 10 and 19 years.[1] It is a critical period of transition in the human lifespan, marked by rapid growth and physical and mental changes second only to infancy.

While biological changes drive this transition, the duration and characteristics of adolescence can vary depending on cultural and socioeconomic settings. Adolescence has also altered over the past century, occurring earlier and being influenced by societal changes such as later marriage, increased urbanisation, global communication, information technology, social networking and changing sexual attitudes and behaviours.[1,2]

Adolescent patients require special understanding and caring from their family doctor. They can present very challenging and sometimes confronting issues. A profound increase in mental health issues (particularly mood disorders)[3] in adolescents has exacerbated the frequency of challenging adolescent consultations in general practice. Another common difficulty is establishing rapport and trust with adolescents, who may be trying to break away from the adult world to establish their own sense of adult self, so it can be vitally important to address confidentiality issues. Actively raising and clarifying confidentiality parameters and doing so at the beginning of the consultation can greatly assist the interaction with an adolescent patient.

In recent times, reference is made to the young person in the context of health policies. Young people are defined as those between the ages of 12 and 24 years and youths as those between 15 and 24 years.[2] Some 18% of the population are young people, and they tend to have a low rate of GP visits; if they do visit, it is usually for physical reasons, despite the fact that the largest health burden for adolescents is actually mental health issues.

Adolescent development periods[4]

Early adolescence (10–14 years): *'Am I normal?'*

This stage is dominated by adjustment to physical and psychosexual changes and by the beginnings of psychological independence from parents. Girls generally advance through this stage more rapidly than boys.

Middle adolescence (14–17 years): *'Who am I?'*

Middle adolescence is a time when boys have caught up physically and psychologically with girls, so that peer group sexual attractions and relationships are common preoccupations at this stage. It is a phase of peer group alliances, clothes, music, jargon and food and drink. The average age for first sexual intercourse for both sexes is 16 years. It is a stage where intellectual knowledge and cognitive processes become quite sophisticated. Experimentation and risk-taking behaviour is a feature, and confidentiality issues are often important.

Late adolescence (17–19 years): *'Where am I going?'*

This is the stage of reaching maturity and leads to more self-confidence with relationships and successful rapport with parents. Thought is more abstract and reality-based. Relationships may become more intimate, moral value systems are more established, and vocational and educational goals become more central.

Major areas of health problems

- Psychological health problems with high rates of first onset in adolescence include depression, self-harm, anxiety disorders, behavioural disorders (e.g. ADHD, conduct disorders) and eating disorders. More than 80% of mental illness starts under the age of 25

- Other areas of concern: substance abuse, schizophrenia and drug-related psychosis
- Eating disorders, including obesity, fast food, bulimia nervosa and anorexia nervosa (refer to CHAPTERS 78 and 79)
- Injuries, including sporting injuries, motor vehicle accidents and interpersonal violence
- Risk-taking behaviour, including drug abuse
- Sexual adjustment, including unsafe sexual practices and teenage pregnancy
- Chronic illness and disability, including survivors of inherited disorders
- Asthma, which is a leading cause of hospital admissions for both sexes in the 10–14 years age group
- Overexposure to sunlight
- Acne, which can be very distressing for adolescents. Severe acne can increase the risk of suicide[5]

Myths about the adolescent patient

The following are myths that some practitioners feel apply to the adolescent:

- different from adults in needs
- 'superficial' thinkers
- represent a 'quick' consultation
- shun personal questions
- resent invasion of space

It is important to treat adolescents as normal human beings.

Age and informed consent

As a rule, parents and physicians should not exclude children and adolescents from decision making without persuasive reasons. Across Australia, common law states that 18 years of age is the age of consent. It also states that consent *may* be given under 18 years, but that the nature of the medical intervention and the ability of the young person to fully understand need to be taken into consideration. A concept that can be applied to this is the Gillick test, which prescribes that the parental right to determine their child's treatment terminates once an adolescent under the age of 16 is capable of fully understanding the medical treatment proposed. Two questions that GPs may be confronted with are:

- When can a young person under 18 years of age consent to medical treatment?
- When can parents or guardians consent to medical treatment for young people under 18 years of age?

When considering these questions, a competency assessment of the adolescent should be undertaken that includes considering:

- age
- level of independence
- level of schooling
- maturity
- ability to express own wishes

In NSW and South Australia, additional laws allow for those aged 14 years (NSW) and 16 years (SA) and over to consent to their own treatment. GPs in these states should familiarise themselves with these laws in situations where consent is problematic.

What do adolescents value and what are they concerned about?

A large ongoing survey by Mission Australia[6] on 15–19-year-olds shows that these adolescents most value:

- friendships
- family relationships
- school and study satisfaction
- physical and mental health

The top issues of personal concern include:

- coping with stress (increasing from 19% to 38% from 2009 to 2013)
- school or study problems (37%)
- body image (31%)

Some 20% were also extremely or very concerned about family conflict.

The internet is the number one source of information for young people, 20% of whom spend >20 hours a week on social network sites.

Access to general practice

There can be many barriers to adolescents accessing general practice. This is especially so for those marginalised by factors such as homelessness or risk of homelessness, involvement in the juvenile justice system, disability, same-sex attraction, or being from an Indigenous, non-English-speaking or refugee background. Barriers include:[7]

- knowledge of services
- concerns about confidentiality
- availability of services, particularly in regional, rural and remote areas

- cost
- poor previous experiences
- location of services
- complicated systems and referral processes

Because of these significant barriers, improving adolescents' access to health services in general, and specifically to general practice, is essential. While youth-specific services such as the national headspace initiative <www.headspace.org.au> have gained momentum in recent years, general practice remains the cornerstone of primary health care for young people.[6] The characteristics of a youth-friendly practice have been defined[7] as having:

- accessibility to young people (e.g. visual appearance, online services, registering for Medicare)
- youth participation in the practice (e.g. involving adolescents in policy development, employing adolescent/young person staff)
- collaboration and partnerships (e.g. with housing or mental health services)
- professional development in youth service provision
- evaluation by the practice of services provided to young people
- evidence-based approaches to the health of adolescents
- sustainability of these approaches

Teenagers want to be asked about sexual health, mental health and substance use, even if they present to their GP for other reasons, according to Tasmanian research. They also want non-judgmental doctors who 'avoid medical jargon, listen, assure them about confidentiality and respect their views and choices'.[8]

A video for GPs and young people about being and implementing a youth-friendly practice is available through NSW Kids and Families <www.kidsfamilies.health.nsw.gov.au/current-work/youth-health-and-wellbeing/>. It includes issues such as adolescents accessing Medicare and the all-important issue of confidentiality.

The clinical approach

Confidentiality

97

Confidentiality is a major issue when seeing adolescent patients, especially those who are new to the practice or who have had negative experiences with authority previously (e.g. involvement in community services or the juvenile justice system) or in cases where other members of a family (particularly the parents) are also your patients. The whole concept of adolescents struggling to establish an identity separate from their carers is tied up in the burgeoning relationship with the GP, and the rules of medical confidentiality, well known to most adults, are often a mystery to young people.

Some tips on reassuring adolescents on confidentiality issues[7,9] include:

- having a practice confidentiality policy visible for all patients to see (e.g. online, in waiting room, in practice information leaflets/orientation pack)
- talking about or defining what medical confidentiality means (and the boundaries or exceptions to this—see TABLE 97.1) up front, i.e. before the first consult starts, especially if you suspect the patient may be worried about such issues
- reinforcing these principles when sensitive issues arise through the evolving GP–patient relationship (e.g. contraceptive or other sexual health issues, mental health issues)

Table 97.1 Three main exceptions to confidentiality[4]

1	If the young person discloses suicidal intent or is threatening significant self-harming behaviour
2	If someone else is threatening or harming them (e.g. physical, sexual or emotional abuse)
3	If the young person is at risk of physically harming someone else (e.g. assault, abuse)

Note: Other exceptions exist (e.g. notification of infectious diseases) but these can be explained if and when necessary. The above are recommended exceptions to explain up front.

Cost

One of the major barriers to adolescents accessing primary care is cost. They are often unaware of how Medicare operates and how to access a card. Adolescents can acquire their own Medicare card from the age of 15. Having application forms available in the surgery (you need photo identification) can help. Young people should be made aware that they do not need to have the card on them to see the doctor. Medicare doesn't reveal to anyone (including parents) who has used the card, provided they are over the age of 14.

Who is in the room and who talks?

An adolescent may present alone or accompanied by others, including, often, a parent. The parent may take a dominating role, doing the talking for the adolescent. Teasing out the two roles (that of the adolescent and that of the parent) as two separate entities can be a challenge, and needs to be done sensitively. The objective of the GP should be to establish rapport and a patient–doctor relationship with the adolescent him or herself, while not threatening the role of the parent.

Most parents will be aware of and sensitive to this, and may even encourage the adolescent to talk for themselves or offer to leave the consulting room. An offer like this should be taken up, with a view to bringing the parent back into the room after a private conversation with the adolescent. It should be made clear exactly what the adolescent will and will not allow to be revealed to the parent (once he or she returns) during the private conversation.

Asking a parent to leave (if no offer is made) may surprise an anxious or overbearing parent, and should be negotiated carefully. Normalising this early in the consultation, as your usual approach, can help.[4] 'Normally when seeing a young patient like your son/daughter, I like to see them by themselves at some stage in the consultation and then get the parent back in afterwards. Is that okay by you?'

If a parent does not want to leave the room, or continues to talk for or over the top of the adolescent, a more forthright approach may be warranted, though this is unusual. It will be difficult to foster a patient–doctor relationship with the adolescent in such circumstances.

Communication and rapport with adolescents

> The single most crucial role of a GP caring for an adolescent, regardless of their presenting complaint, is to foster and develop a relationship of trust.[10]

Tips for fostering engagement with adolescents[3] include:

- Treat the young person as responsible and capable of contributing to decision making.
- Take a curious, non-intrusive and respectful stance.
- Be open and honest as much as possible.
- Clarify what the young person wants from you.
- Establish agreed goals or explain clearly why you cannot help.
- Be honestly interested in what the young person has to say.
- Be yourself, don't fake it.
- Use metaphor and humour (where appropriate) to build rapport.
- Use language that is clear and easily understood and avoid jargon; overuse of slang is probably worse than not using it at all.
- Warn the young person if you are going to ask questions about topics that may be difficult (e.g. sexual matters).
- Avoid getting into a controlling, authoritarian position.
- Remember that engagement may wax and wane.

HEEADSSS[4]

HEEADSSS is a guide (not a script or tick list) that can be useful for a GP when conducting a psychosocial assessment of an adolescent. It is a framework designed to progress from the (usually) less sensitive to more sensitive areas of potential concern in an adolescent. It does not have to be covered all in one consultation, and the areas that are covered may be tailored to the individual patient and his or her circumstances. A shortcut on clinical software may prompt the GP to use HEEADSSS. It has recently been expanded to reflect the major causes of adolescent morbidity and mortality.

H = **H**ome
E = **E**ducation and **E**mployment
E = **E**ating and **E**xercise
A = **A**ctivities and peer relationships
D = **D**rug use, cigarettes and alcohol
S = **S**exuality
S = **S**uicide and depression (including mood and possible psychiatric symptoms)
S = **S**afety

Physical examination

Adolescents are often very sensitive about their bodies and physical appearance, especially when going through puberty. When physically examining adolescents:

- carefully explain what you are going to do before you do it
- obtain consent for examining adolescents
- consider offering a chaperone for examining breasts or genitals, especially a male doctor and female adolescent patient
- gender and cultural differences and norms should be considered prior to physical examination

Note: The new cervical screening test is not required until the age of 25.

Risk behaviours

Risk behaviours are common in adolescents and should be actively but sensitively screened for.

The HEEADSSS model can be employed to do this screening. If there are risk behaviours:

- Assess how high the risk is (e.g. multiple risk behaviours? is it escalating? aware of the risk and potential consequences?).
- What are possible protective factors (e.g. support from family, school, positive peer relationships or culture)?
- Focus on strengths and abilities the adolescent may have.
- Build motivation and reinforce capacity to change.
- Actively promote behaviour change by using guided decision making.
- Provide appropriate information and education on the risk behaviour and potential consequences.
- If high-risk behaviours are identified, referral to appropriate services (e.g. drug and alcohol, psychologists) while the GP maintains a case management role.

Developing a management plan[4]

Informing an adolescent of your assessment and actively involving him or her in the development of your management plan will help improve trust and compliance. It is also useful to:

- identify risk behaviours—provide relevant information and education
- set realistic treatment goals appropriate to your adolescent patient
- where appropriate, discuss how much he or she wants parents to be informed and involved
- guide parents in how to best support their adolescent child and best respond to risk-taking behaviours

MENTAL HEALTH IN ADOLESCENTS[4]

- Up to 25% of adolescents suffer from a mental health and/or substance abuse problem.
- Mental health in adolescents is worsening.
- Many chronic mental health issues have their onset in adolescence.
- Anxiety and depression are the leading mental health problems in adolescents (17% of the male disease burden and 32% of the female).
- Behavioural disorders are also common (8% of 12–17-year-olds have ADHD, and 3% have conduct disorders) as are eating disorders.
- There is a marked increase in risk factors and risk-taking behaviours for mental health in adolescence (e.g. substance abuse, peer conflicts).
- Mental health issues in adolescents can present differently from in adults, with mood swings, poor school performance or attendance, irritability, anger, substance abuse, somatic complaints, risk-taking behaviours or conflict with peers or family being more common.
- Adolescents are generally ill informed about mental health (<25% seek help).

Depression in adolescents[3,4]

(See CHAPTER 19 for a discussion on depression.)

- Up to 24% of adolescents will have suffered an episode of major depression by the age of 18.
- Depression can be more masked by the patient and harder to detect in adolescents, so requires more active screening.
- Psychosocial development may be compromised by depression in adolescence.
- Effective engagement and developing a trusting therapeutic alliance are critical in managing depressed adolescents.
- Using the HEEADSSS tool can help in assessment.
- Comorbidity with other mental health issues (anxiety disorders, behavioural disorders, eating disorders, substance abuse) is common.
- It helps to encourage protective factors such as positive peer relationships, support from schools or families, regular sleep patterns and pleasurable activity scheduling.
- Counselling and psychological treatments are first line in the treatment of adolescents with depression.
- Using mental health Medicare item numbers may help improve access to services.

Use of antidepressants in adolescents

In major depression in adolescents, treatment with fluoxetine can be considered. There appears to be an age-related mechanism linking SSRI treatment with an increased risk of suicidal thinking, with adolescents being at greatest increased risk. Because of this, if pharmacological therapy is warranted, it should be prescribed by a practitioner who is very familiar with the range of adverse effects and able to monitor the young person appropriately. Close monitoring for suicidality is especially important in the first 4 weeks. If there are concerns regarding severe symptoms or risk of suicide, referral to a psychiatrist who treats adolescents is recommended.

Suicidality in adolescents[4]

- Hospital rates for suicide attempts are 3 times higher in females, but suicide deaths are 3 times higher in males (males use more lethal means).

- More than half of all adolescents who try to kill themselves will have visited a GP within the previous month (i.e. GPs can play a very important preventive role, see TABLE 97.2).

Table 97.2	Warning signs of potential suicide in adolescents[11]
Change in behaviour (e.g. risk taking, isolation, giving away possessions, losing interest in activities)	
Change in mood (e.g. hopelessness)	
Change in thinking (e.g. guilt, bizarre thoughts)	
Preoccupation with death	
Talk of suicide	
Perceived intolerable loss or stress	
Apparent resolution (e.g. sudden calmness/happiness after other warning signs)	

Risk factors

- Previous suicide attempt/self-harm
- History of previous attempts in family/friends
- Concrete suicide plan
- Underlying mental disorders—e.g. depression, anxiety, substance abuse
- Comorbid conditions—e.g. eating disorder, conduct disorder
- Recent stressful life events (e.g. relationship breakdown, humiliation, school problem, conflict with peers)
- Ongoing family problems
- Victim of bullying
- Lesbian, gay, bisexual, transexual (LGBT) orientation
- Cultural conflicts or concerns

Management

- Fully explore the adolescent's thoughts, plans and actions. Assess his or her level of risk.
- Do not agree to secrecy.
- Confidentiality is over-ridden if there is serious or imminent danger of suicide. Gently explain this to the adolescent while trying to maintain and protect a therapeutic alliance.
- Contact and mobilise family and social supports.
- Get help from peers or other health providers where possible. Mental health services such as crisis teams may need to be involved.
- If possible, remove or limit access to means of self-harm (e.g. medications).
- Consider (in conjunction with other therapeutic approaches) a 'no-suicide contract'. Usually verbal, this is an agreement for the adolescent to commit to you that he or she will not act on any suicidal thoughts until you next see them. This should be done for only a short (<1 week) period.

Anxiety disorders in adolescents

In a similar fashion to depression, anxiety disorders in adolescents are common, hard to detect and heavily reliant on the GP having a trusting relationship with the adolescent; they also have psychological therapies as the first-line treatment. See CHAPTER 81 for further discussion on anxiety disorders.

Eating disorders

Anorexia nervosa and bulimia nervosa arise usually in the early to mid-teens (see CHAPTER 79). There are many sub-syndromal variations that threaten to develop into a serious state but these can settle, especially with early identification and counselling.

Practice tips in handling adolescents

- Confidentiality is of great importance to adolescents.
- Barriers to adolescents accessing general practice should be removed wherever possible.
- Seeing adolescents by themselves at some stage in the consultation is desirable.
- Developing a relationship of trust is critical when dealing with adolescents in general practice.
- HEEADSSS is a useful tool for conducting a psychosocial assessment.
- Mental health problems in adolescents are common, often hard to detect, and are heavily reliant on the GP having a trusting relationship with the adolescent.
- Adolescents need support and understanding.

Adolescent violence in the home

Adolescent violence towards parents is defined as 'any act of a child that creates fear in, and is intended to hurt parents'. It usually refers to behaviours by adolescents between 12 and 18 years of age.

Victoria Police has reported a 40% plus increase over the past six years in family violence incident reports where the perpetrator was under the age of 18 (Victoria Police 2012). This is repeated in other states. (*Violence toward parents,* Parent Easy Guide 17, Department for Health and Ageing, South Australia)

Types of adolescent violence include physical, psychological/emotional, financial and sexual behaviours.

Help guidelines include:

- Emergency lifeline 13 11 14
- Parent line 13 22 89
- Kids helpline 1800 551 800
- Relationships Australia 1300 364 277.

References

1 World Health Organization. Adolescent health, 2014 <www.who.int/maternal_child_adolescent/topics/adolescence/dev/en/> (accessed 3/9/2014).

2 Australian Institute of Health and Welfare. Young Australians: their health and wellbeing, 2011 <www.aihw.gov.au/publication-detail/?id=10737419261> (accessed 3/9/2014).

3 McDermott B, Baigent M, Chanen A et al. Clinical practice guidelines: depression in adolescents and young adults. Melbourne: beyondblue: the national depression initiative, 2011: 143.

4 NSW Centre for the Advancement of Adolescent Health, the Children's Hospital at Westmead. Adolescent Health, GP resource kit (2nd edn), 2008 <www.schn.health.nsw.gov.au/files/attachments/complete_gp_resource_kit_0.pdf> (accessed 3/9/2014).

5 Sundstrom et al. Association of suicide attempts with acne and treatment with isotretinoin: retrospective Swedish cohort study. BMJ, 2010; 341: c5812.

6 Mission Australia. Annual Youth Survey 2013 <www.missionaustralia.com.au/what-we-do-to-help-new/young-people/understanding-young-people/annual-youth-survey> (accessed 3/9/2014).

7 Cummings M, Kang M. Youth health services: improving access to primary care. Aust Fam Physician, 2012; 41 (5): 339–41.

8 Turner L, Spencer L, Strugnell J et al. Young people have their say: what makes a youth-friendly general practice? Aust Fam Physician, 2017; 46 (1): 70–4.

9 New South Wales Kids + Families. Youth health and wellbeing <www.kidsfamilies.health.nsw.gov.au/publications/nsw-youth-health-policy-2011-2016/> (accessed 3/9/2014).

10 Bennett DL, Kang M. Communicating with adolescents in general practice. In: *The Missing Link—Adolescent Mental Health in General Practice.* Sydney: Alpha Biomedical Communications, 2001.

11 Martin G. Management of depression and suicide in general practice. In: *The Missing Link—Adolescent Mental Health in General Practice.* Sydney: Alpha Biomedical Communications, 2001.

Part 6

Women's health

98 Cervical cancer screening

We are forecasting that over the next 30–40 years, rates of cervical cancer will drop from around the current 1000 cases a year in Australia to just a few . . . we are well positioned to be the first country to effectively end this deadly cancer.

Professor Suzanne Garland, 2018

Cervical cancer

Cervical cancer is the fourth most common cause of cancer death in women worldwide, especially in developing countries.[1] It is the most common cancer in women in Eastern and Middle Africa, and the 14th most common in Australian women.[1,2] Australia has the second lowest incidence of cervical cancer in the world as a result of the success of the National Cervical Screening Program introduced in 1991, which has halved its incidence.[3]

The most common cervical cancer is squamous cell carcinoma (SCC), accounting for 80% of cases. Adenocarcinoma is less common and more difficult to diagnose because it starts higher in the cervix. Cervical cancer almost exclusively occurs in women who have been sexually active, due to exposure to human papillomavirus (HPV). Other risk factors include smoking, use of combined oral contraception >5 years, immunosuppression and exposure to diethylstilboestrol in utero.[4]

Since the introduction of the human papillomavirus (HPV) vaccine in Australia in 2007, the incidence of low- and high-grade abnormalities has significantly reduced in vaccinated populations. Studies have revealed reductions as high as 45% for low-grade abnormalities and 85% for high-grade abnormalities.[5] Recent modelling suggests that, with the tools available, elimination of cervical cancer in local populations is achievable within our lifetime.[6]

Cervical cancer and human papillomavirus[7]

It is now well established that the primary cause of cervical cancer is human papillomavirus. There are approximately 200 different types of HPV, 40–50 of which specifically infect the anogenital area. These types are mainly spread by skin contact during sexual activity.

Of the genital HPV types, 15 are classified as 'high risk', as they are associated with anogenital cancer (including squamous and adenocarcinoma of the cervix). HPV 16 and 18 are responsible for around 70% of invasive cervical cancers and 50% of high-grade lesions.

Prior to immunisation, infection with HPV was common and mostly transient, with 80% of women being infected with at least one genital type of HPV in their lifetime without ever knowing it. Cervical cancer is a rare outcome of HPV infection. Most cervical HPV infections are cleared or suppressed by cell-mediated immunity within 1–2 years of exposure. Persistent infection of the cervix with a high-risk HPV is known to cause high-grade cervical changes that, if left untreated, can progress to cervical cancer. More than 99.7% of cervical cancers test positive for HPV DNA.[8]

Basic pathology

The focus of attention is the transformation zone (see FIG. 98.1), where columnar cells lining the endocervical

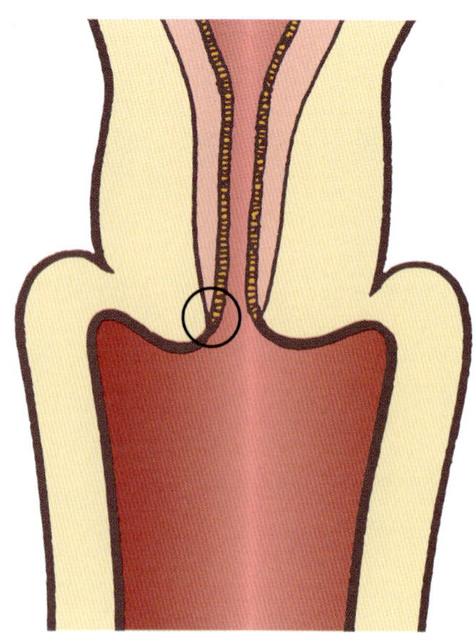

FIGURE 98.1 The transformation zone: it is vital that cells are taken from this zone in cervical screening tests

canal undergo metaplasia to squamous cells in the region of the squamocolumnar junction. It is important clinically to realise that this transformation zone can extend with progressive metaplasia of columnar epithelium and so the squamocolumnar junction may recede into the endocervical canal. This is a feature in postmenopausal women (see FIG. 98.2). As squamous cell carcinoma almost always arises in the transformation zone, it is vital that cells from this area are sampled.

HPV and the natural history of cervical neoplasia[9]

Low-grade squamous intraepithelial lesions (LSILs) represent an acute HPV infection of the transformation zone. LSILs are seen with both low- and high-risk HPV types. Most women will clear the virus over about 10 months with no lasting effect. Persistent infection with an oncogenic HPV type causes precancerous changes (high-grade squamous–intraepithelial lesion or HSIL).

HSILs may return to normal, persist or eventually progress to invasive cervical cancer. The average duration between HSILs and cancer is between 10 and 15 years. However, women with histologically confirmed moderate to severe dysplasia require a colposcopic assessment. FIGURE 98.3 and TABLE 98.1 illustrate the disease spectrum of cervical neoplasia.

Clinical presentation

Many patients with cervical cancer are asymptomatic and when early symptoms do arise they are often dismissed as of little consequence.

Symptoms, if present, may be:

- irregular vaginal bleeding, especially postcoital or intermenstrual bleeding
- postmenopausal bleeding
- vaginal discharge
- symptoms of advanced disease (e.g. back pain, fatigue, vaginal fistula)

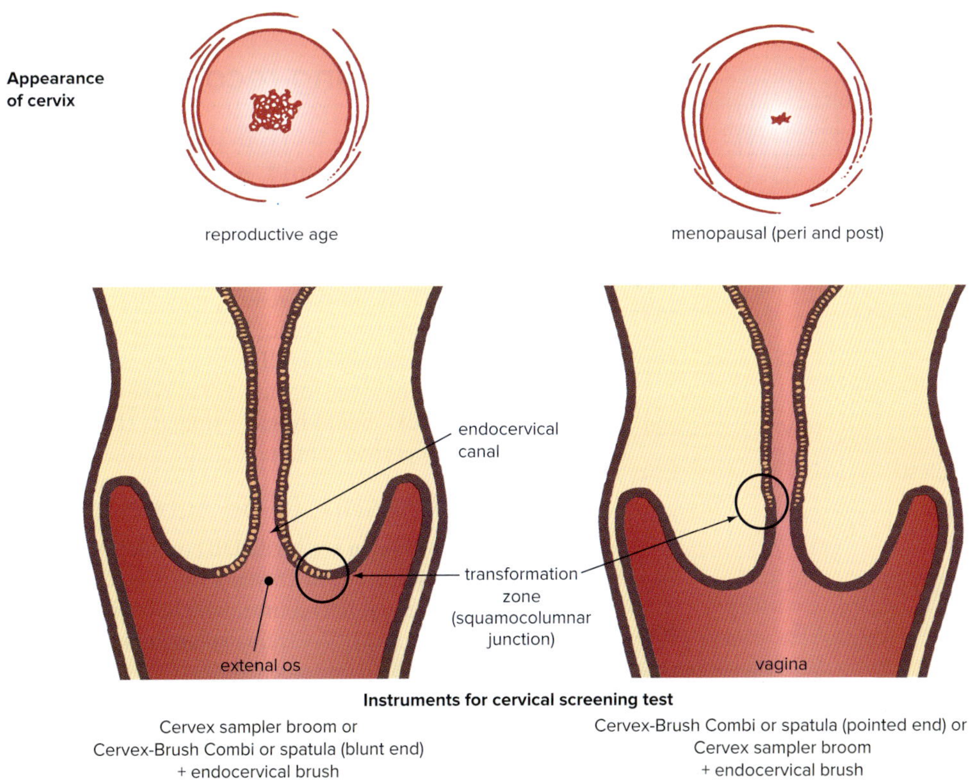

FIGURE 98.2 Changing position of the transformation zone with age, and a selection of sampling instruments according to its position

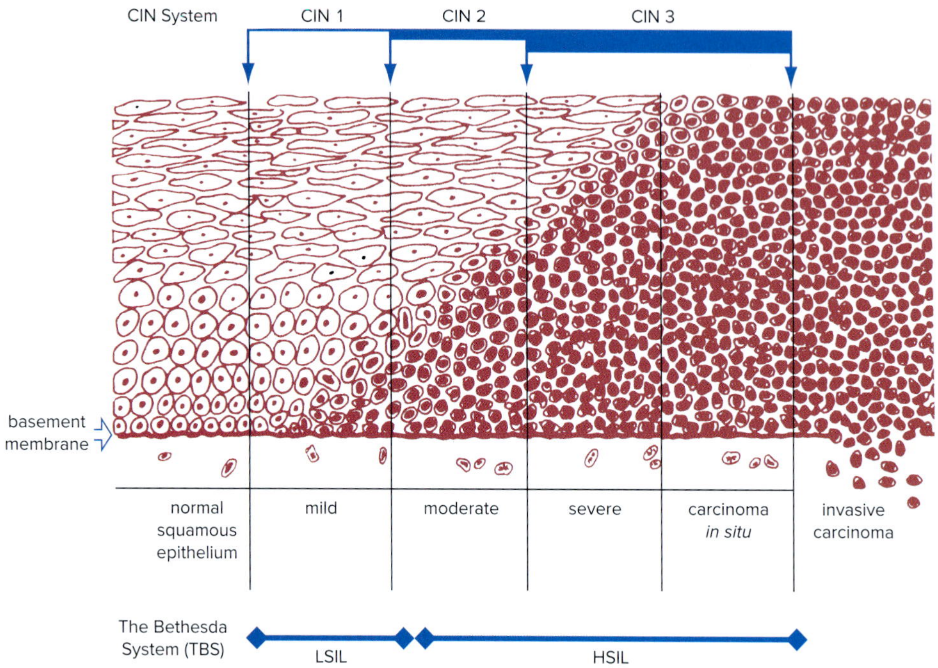

FIGURE 98.3 Illustration of the various grades of squamous intraepithelial lesions and CIN (comparison of nomenclature)

Table 98.1 Squamous cell abnormalities and the different nomenclatures[8]

	Description	CIN grade	Australian modified Bethesda system
1	Normal	Normal	Within normal limits
2	Atypia: reactive or neoplastic	Atypia	ASCUS
3	HPV	HPV	LSIL
4	Mild dysplasia	CIN 1	LSIL
5	Moderate dysplasia	CIN 2	HSIL
6	Severe dysplasia	CIN 3	HSIL
7	Carcinoma in situ	CIS	HSIL
8	Invasive carcinoma	Invasive carcinoma	Invasive carcinoma

ASCUS = **A**typical **s**quamous **c**ells of **u**ndetermined **s**ignificance
CIN = **C**ervical **i**ntraepithelial **n**eoplasia
CIS = **C**arcinoma **i**n **s**itu
HSIL = **H**igh-grade **s**quamous **i**ntraepithelial **l**esion
LSIL = **L**ow-grade **s**quamous **i**ntraepithelial **l**esion

Screening recommendations

Cervical screening test[10]

In December 2017, the National Cervical Screening Program changed from the two-yearly Papanicolaou smear (or Pap test) to a five-yearly cervical screening test. The cervical screening test uses a primary HPV test with partial genotyping. This test will separately identify oncogenic HPV types 16 and 18, and 12 other oncogenic HPV types (not 16/18). All women who have oncogenic HPV types detected will have 'reflex' liquid-based cytology (LBC) performed on the cervical sample, to guide further management.

Who should be screened?[4]

- Women are invited to commence cervical screening at 25 years (or two years after first sexual intercourse, whichever is later).
- Both HPV-vaccinated and non-vaccinated women should be screened.
- An exit test can be performed at age 70–74 years.
- Women aged 75 years or older may request screening.
- Screening applies only to asymptomatic women. Women with postcoital or persistent intermenstrual bleeding require a co-test (both HPV test and diagnostic LBC), and referral for an

appropriate investigation to exclude malignancy should be considered.[10]

- For women who experienced first sexual activity at a young age (<14 years) and who had not received the HPV vaccine before sexual debut, a single HPV test between 20 and 24 years of age could be considered on an individual basis.[10]

Screening in particular groups[10]

Hysterectomy. Cervical screening is still required if the cervix was not completely removed. Vaginal vault co-tests (HPV and LBC) may be indicated if there is a history of gynaecological dysplasia or malignancy.

Pregnancy. Cervical screening can be safely performed at any time during pregnancy, provided that the correct sampling equipment is used. An endocervical brush or Cervex-Brush Combi should not be inserted into the cervical canal because of the risk of associated bleeding, which may distress the patient.

Postmenopausal women. Postmenopausal women may benefit from a short course of topical vaginal oestrogen before their cervical screening test. This may improve the quality of the test and comfort of the examination. Treatment should be stopped approximately 3 days before the test to ensure it does not interfere with the test interpretation.

Immune-deficient women. Woman with HIV or who are solid organ transplant recipients should be screened every 3 years with HPV testing.

Exposure to diethylstilboestrol (DES) in utero. An annual co-test (HPV and LBC) and colposcopic examination of both the cervix and vagina should be offered indefinitely.

Women with abnormal vaginal bleeding. A co-test is indicated and should not be delayed due to the presence of blood. Women with postcoital bleeding or persistent and/or unexplained intermenstrual bleeding require referral for colposcopy regardless of the result. However, premenopausal women who have a single episode of postcoital bleeding, a clinically normal cervix and negative co-test do not need to be referred for colposcopy. Postmenopausal women with any vaginal bleeding should be referred for a specialist gynaecological assessment to exclude genital tract malignancy.

Underscreened populations[8]

Special attention should be focused on screening the following women:

- Aboriginal and Torres Strait Islander women (mortality of cervical cancer five times that of other women in Australia)
- Women from culturally and linguistically diverse backgrounds
- Women in rural and remote areas
- Women with disabilities
- Women who have experienced sexual trauma and/or domestic violence
- Those who identify as lesbian, gay, bisexual, transgender, queer or questioning and intersex (LGBTQI)

The Cervical Screening Test consultation

The Cervical Screening Test consultation provides an excellent opportunity to perform a general women's health check. For women of reproductive age, it is important to take a focused menstrual history, specifically enquiring about intermenstrual or postcoital bleeding. Consider discussing contraception use and the need for STI screening, especially for women aged under 30 years. Opportunistic discussions regarding family planning, breast awareness and breast screening are often appropriate.

Enquire about previous cervical screening results and whether the woman has found cervical screening difficult. Some women may be highly anxious, and identifying this early allows the clinician to address fears sensitively and discuss strategies that may help them feel more comfortable. Women with atrophic vaginitis often benefit from topical oestrogen in the immediate weeks prior to cervical screening.

Clinician-collected samples

The optimal cervical screening test contains:

- sufficient mature and metaplastic squamous cells to indicate adequate sampling from the whole of the transformation zone
- sufficient endocervical cells to indicate that the upper limit of the transformation zone was sampled; and to provide a sample for screening of adenocarcinoma and its precursors

Optimal timing of specimens

- Avoid performing a cervical screening test during menstruation.
- Avoid in the presence of obvious vaginal infection.
- Avoid within 48 hours of use of vaginal creams or pessaries or douching.

Communicating with the pathologist

Good communication with the pathologist is essential. It is important to provide basic details and the clinical history on the pathology form sent to the laboratory. It is especially important to include whether the patient is symptomatic, as this changes the testing procedure. Include the patient's age, current hormonal state, such as pregnancy, the postpartum period or if they are postmenopausal, the presence of an IUD, previous abnormal results and clinical findings.

The method

1 *Explanation and history*
Take time to explain the reason for the cervical screening test, especially if it is the first. Anatomical models are useful in describing the procedure.
Explain that it usually does not take long, that it may be uncomfortable but should not be painful. Slow, deep breathing often helps relax the pelvic floor, allowing for easier speculum insertion.
Take a brief history as previously outlined, enquire about previous cervical screening results (if any), as well as direct questions about any intermenstrual or postcoital bleeding. Verbal consent should be obtained.[5]
Encourage the woman to empty her bladder if she desires and ensure privacy before asking her to undress below the waist. A gown or cover sheet should be provided.
Check if the woman would like a chaperone to be present during the examination.

2 *Equipment*[6]
Wash hands and prepare the following equipment:
- adequate light source
- appropriate-sized speculum (small for women having a first test, wider for women with poor vaginal tone)
- water-based lubricant if using a plastic speculum
- non-sterile gloves for both hands
- vial of liquid medium
- swabs for STI screening if required
- cervical screening implements; choose from:
  - cervical sampler broom
  - endocervical brush
  - Cervex-Brush Combi
  - spatula

  (refer to FIGURE 98.2 for recommended choice)

  Special notes:
- pregnancy—avoid use of the endocervical brush and the Cervex-Brush Combi
- eversion—take care to sample the squamocolumnar junction

3 *Positioning*
The supine position is usually best (see FIG. 98.4). The left lateral position can be used if smears are difficult to obtain (e.g. older women with lax anterior vaginal walls, older women with poor hip mobility). The Sims exaggerated left lateral position (see FIG. 98.5) provides better exposure

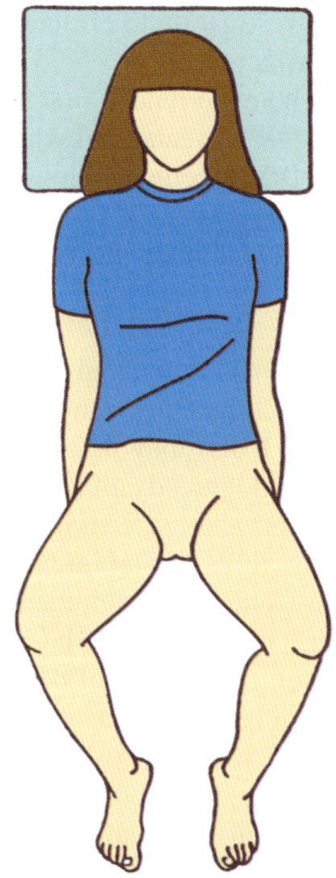

FIGURE 98.4 The supine or dorsal position is the best position for the speculum examination and subsequent bimanual palpation (patient should be appropriately clothed and/or draped)

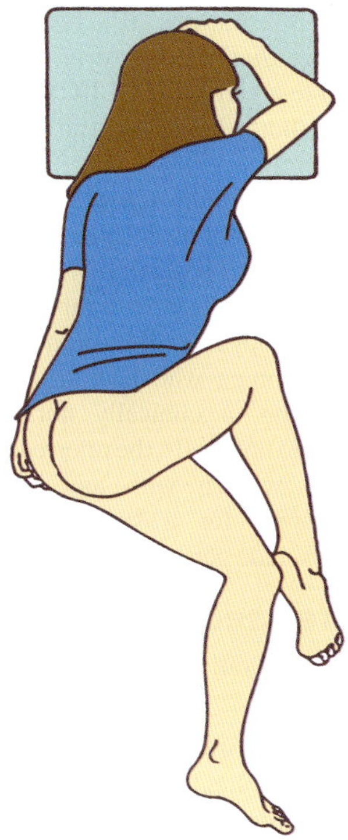

FIGURE 98.5 The Sims exaggerated left lateral position

of the vulva but requires more manipulation of the patient. Better visualisation of the cervix is obtained if the patient elevates her buttocks with her fists, a small pillow or towel.

4 *Inspection of external genitalia*
Observe any skin conditions or lesions, any intra-oital bleeding or vaginal discharge.

5 *Inserting the speculum*
A metal speculum should be warmed with lukewarm water. A small amount of water-based lubricant is appropriate for a plastic speculum. Gently spread the labia with a gloved hand and introduce the speculum with the blades remaining horizontal and closed. Gently advance the speculum into the vagina guided by the posterior wall. Open the blades of the speculum slightly to guide the visual location of the cervix. Remember that the cervix is situated in the upper sixth of the anterior vaginal wall (not in the apex of the vagina).

6 *Visualising the cervix*
When the cervix is visualised, lock the blades to keep the speculum in position. Good lighting and exposure of the cervix is essential. Note any significant features or abnormalities of the cervix. A cervical ectropion is normal in most premenopausal women.

7 *Taking the sample*
There are a variety of sampling instruments to choose from.
Cervical sampler broom: can be used alone if the transformation zone is visible. Insert the central part of the brush into the os and rotate for 3–5 turns (FIG. 98.6A).
Spatula: take care to keep contact with the ecto-cervix and rotate once or twice. Use

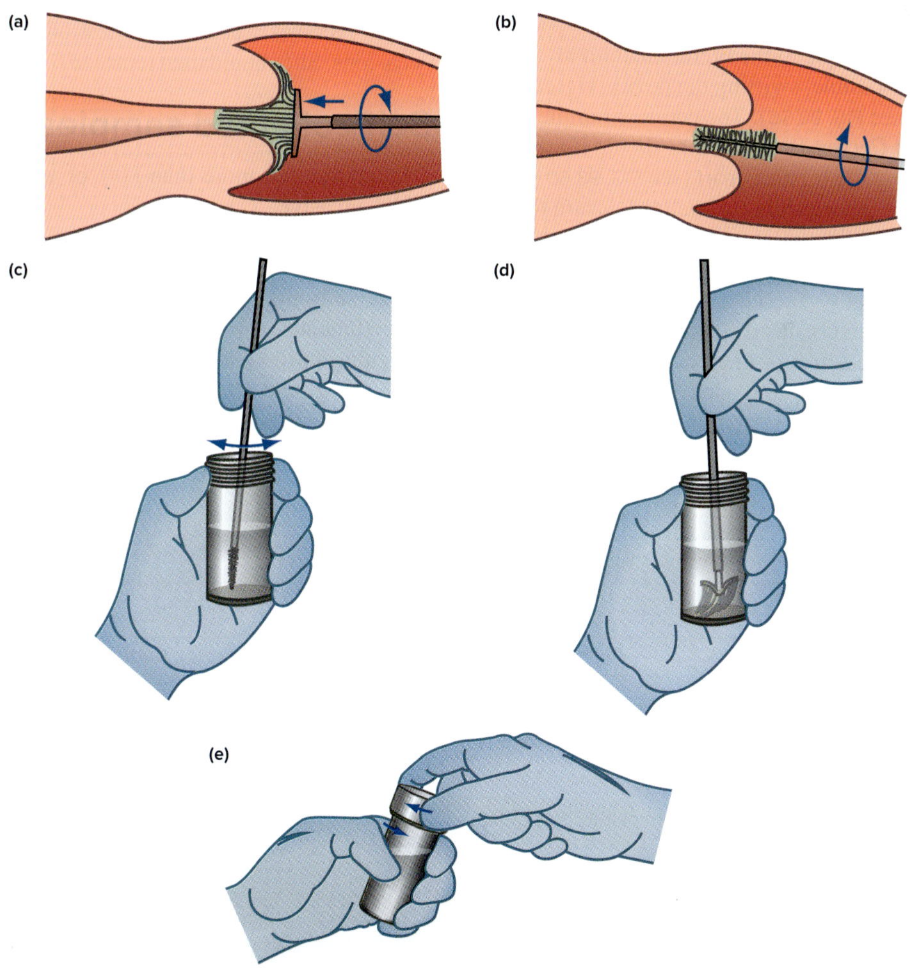

FIGURE 98.6 Method of taking and transferring an endocervical sample[11]

with the endocervical brush to maximise endocervical sampling.
Endocervical brush should be advanced until only the lower bristles are still visible, then rotated for a quarter of a rotation (see FIG. 98.6B). The endocervical brush should be avoided in pregnant women as it tends to cause bleeding.
Cervex-Brush Combi combines features of the cervical broom and endocervical brush. Insert the central part of the brush into the os and rotate for two turns. It is not advised in pregnancy.
It is common practice to use either the cervical sample broom or spatula first, followed by the endocervical brush. Use of the Cervex-Brush Combi alone is an alternative.
After removing the speculum, perform a bimanual pelvic examination if appropriate. A bimanual examination may assist in locating the cervix if it could not be visualised at the initial speculum examination.[5]

8 *Transferring the sample*
Transfer the sample to the liquid medium as quickly as possible, swirling the device vigorously 10 times (see FIG. 98.6C). The cervical sample broom and Cervex-Brush Combi should hit the base, forcing the bristles apart (see FIG. 98.6D). Remove the device from the vial and ensure the cap is secured tightly (see FIG. 98.6E).
Follow-up
Discuss mutually suitable arrangements to ensure that the woman obtains the result of the test, whether it is positive or negative. Inform her when her next test is likely to be due (special cards are available) and have a system in place to send a reminder note.
The explanation of the results and follow-up required, especially if there is an abnormality present, should be crystal-clear to the patient. Common medicolegal claims made against GPs include poor communication regarding cervical screening tests and failure to arrange adequate specialist referral for women with abnormal results or a clinically suspicious cervical lesion.

Management of results

Follow the guidelines in TABLE 98.2 and FIGURE 98.7 for management of results.

Post-treatment assessment of HSIL[10]

A woman treated for HSIL should complete a test of cure surveillance to confirm her treatment has been successful. Test of cure surveillance is a co-test (HPV and liquid-based cytology test) performed 12 months after treatment, and annually thereafter, until the patient receives a negative co-test on two consecutive occasions. She should then return to 5-yearly screening.

Self-collected samples[10,12]

Data shows that more than 80% of women diagnosed with invasive cervical cancer have never been screened or were more than 6 months overdue for a screening test at the time of diagnosis. Providing HPV self-collection kits to never-screened and underscreened women has been shown to improve screening participation in international studies. HPV tests using self-collected samples are considered to have moderate-to-high sensitivity and comparably high specificity for detecting CIN2+.

Table 98.2 Guidelines for positive cervical screening tests[10]

Cervical screening test result	Investigation and management
HPV not detected	Repeat in 5 years
Unsatisfactory HPV test	Repeat test in 6–12 weeks
HPV not 16/18 detected	
Negative cytology	Repeat HPV test in 12 months
Possible low-grade intra-epithelial lesion (pLISIL) and definite LSIL	Repeat HPV test in 12 months
High-grade epithelial lesion (HSIL)	Refer for colposcopy
Unsatisfactory cytology result	Repeat test in 6–12 weeks
HPV 16/18 detected	
All cytology results	Refer for colposcopy

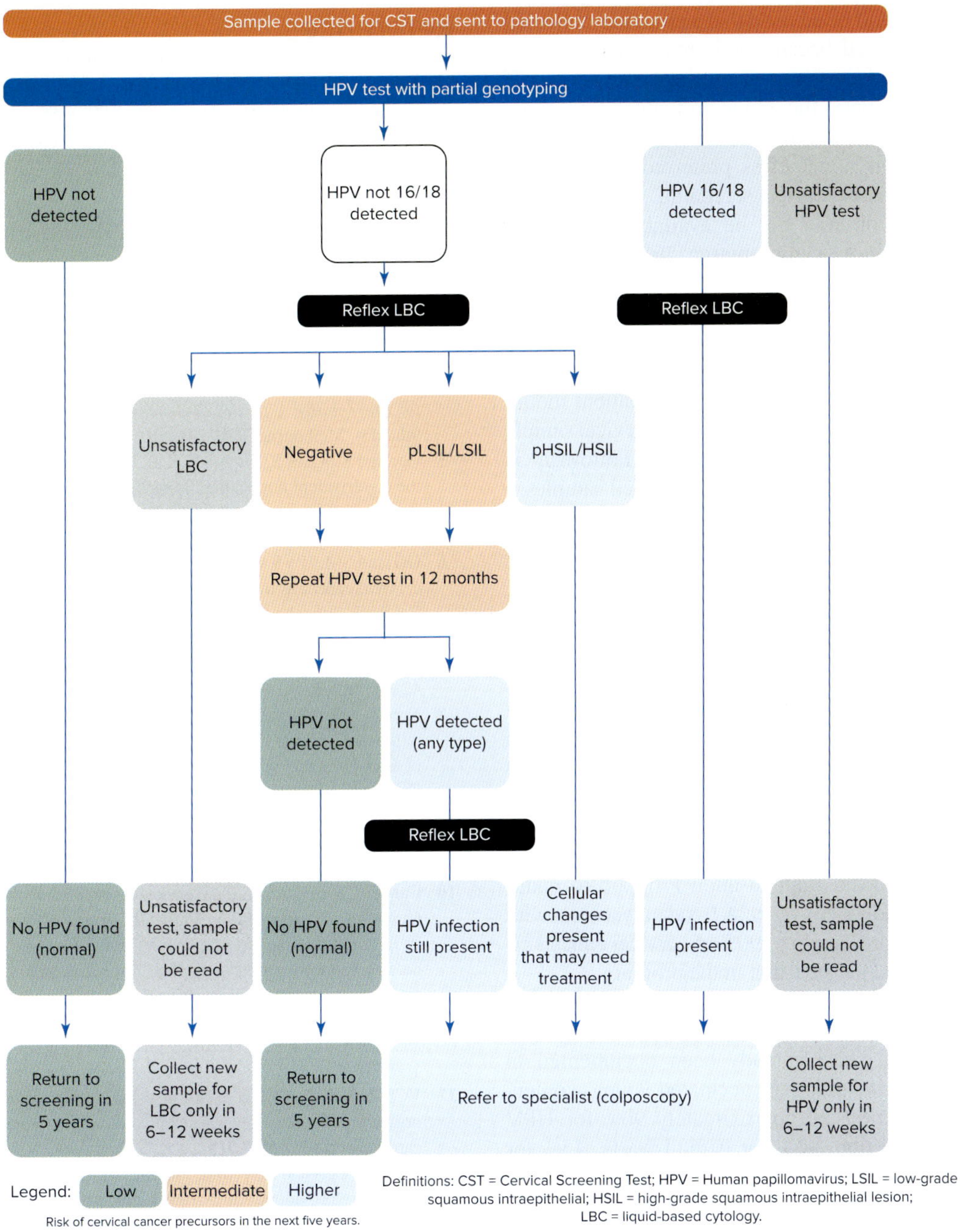

FIGURE 98.7 Cervical screening pathway for clinician-collected sample[12]

Source: Diagram adapted from Cervical Screening Guidelines 2016.

Under the renewed National Cervical Screening Program, HPV testing on self-collected samples will be available to some women aged 30–74 years under the supervision of a health care professional who also offers cervical screening. The following groups of women will be eligible:

- women who have never participated in cervical screening and are aged 30 or over
- women who are overdue for cervical screening by 2 years or longer and are aged 30 years or over

98

Women should be advised that a clinician-collected sample is preferred because it is more effective and reflex LBC can be performed on the same sample. If the woman declines the clinician-collected sample, she will be able to submit a self-collected sample. Self-collection is nonetheless preferred compared to non-participation in cervical screening.

Self-collection will not be available to women who are pregnant, symptomatic, have undergone hysterectomy with a history of HSIL and women exposed to DES in utero.

If HPV (not 16/18) is detected on a self-collected sample, a clinician-collected liquid-based cytology is advised. If HPV 16 or 18 is detected, the patient should be referred directly for colposcopy and a cervical sample for LBC will be collected at that visit. Follow-up is otherwise the same as for clinician-collected samples.

At the time of writing, self-collection is not yet available as laboratories require validation of HPV analysers on self-collected swabs.

HPV vaccination[10]

In 2007, Australia led the world with its national publicly funded HPV vaccination program, using a three-dose schedule of the quadrivalent HPV vaccine that protects against HPV types 16 and 18 (high risk for cervical cancer) and types 6 and 11 (which cause genital warts). Vaccination ideally occurs before first sexual activity. Currently, the HPV vaccine (Gardasil®) is administered through the National Immunisation Program to males and females aged 12–13 years. A 9-valent vaccine, with the capacity to prevent up to 90% of cervical cancers, is being considered for inclusion in the program.

Since 2007, reductions in the prevalence of HPV types 16 and 18, anogenital warts and histologically confirmed HSIL have already been documented in young women, including unvaccinated young women. Maximal reductions of approximately 90% for HPV 6/11/16/18 infection, 90% for genital warts, 45% for low-grade cytological cervical abnormalities and 85% for high-grade cervical abnormalities have been reported.[5] Women who have been immunised still require cervical screening because the vaccine does not prevent all HPV types that cause cervical cancer.

References

1 Ferlay J, Soerjomataram I, Ervik M et al. GLOBOCAN 2012 v1.0, Cancer incidence and mortality worldwide: IARC CancerBase No. 11 (online). Lyon, France: International Agency for Research on Cancer, 2013 <http://globocan.iarc.fr> (accessed 5/10/2014).

2 Australian Government, Cancer Australia. Cervical cancer statistics. Cervical cancer in Australia. Updated 30 January 2018. <https://cervical-cancer.canceraustralia.gov.au/statistics> (accessed 15/5/2018).

3 Australian Institute of Health and Welfare. Cervical screening in Australia 2010–2011. Cancer series 76. Cat. no. CAN 72. Canberra: AIHW; 2013.

4 Royal Australian College of General Practitioners. *Guidelines for Preventative Activities in General Practice* (the Red Book; 9th edn). Melbourne: RACGP, 2016.

5 Garland S, Kjaer S, Munoz N et al. Impact and effectiveness of the quadrivalent human papillomavirus vaccine: a systematic review of 10 years of real-world experience. Clinical Infectious Diseases, 2016; 63 (4): 519–27.

6 Garland SM. IPVS statement moving towards elimination of cervical cancer as a public health problem. Papillomavirus Research, June 2017; 5: 87–8.

7 Heley S. HPV testing in the National Cervical Screening Program: when is it recommended? Aust Fam Physician, 2013; 42 (7): 463–6.

8 National Health and Medical Research Council. Screening to prevent cervical cancer. Guidelines for the management of asymptomatic women with screen detected abnormalities. Canberra: NHMRC, 2005.

9 Bateson D, Bower H, Stewart M. Cervical screening in the HPV era: don't ditch the Pap test! Medicine Today, 2011; 12 (10): 42–52.

10 Cancer Council Australia, Cervical Cancer Screening Guidelines Working Party. National Cervical Screening Program: guidelines for the management of screen-detected abnormalities, screening in specific populations and investigation of abnormal vaginal bleeding. Sydney: Cancer Council Australia, 2016. <https://wiki.cancer.org.au/australia/Guidelines:Cervical_cancer/Screening> (accessed 15/5/2018).

11 VCS Pathology. Cervix sampling card. <www.vcspathology.org.au/practitioners/renewal-documents/cervix-sampling-card> (accessed 15/5/2018).

12 National Cervical Screening Program. A guide for healthcare providers. <http://www.cancerscreening.gov.au/internet/screening/publishing.nsf/Content/C2058A7D155867ACCA2581C400082790/$File/CAN174-Understanding-the-National-Cervical-Screening-Program-Management-Pathway.pdf> (accessed 15/5/2018).

Family planning 99

The Membranous Envelope (condom) is prepared from the bladder of a fish caught in the Rhine. Its extreme thinness does not in the least interfere with the pleasure of the act . . . [its use] is of the greatest utility because, while it is a sure preventive of conception, it also prevents either party from contracting disease.

EDWARD BLISS FOOTE, *MEDICAL COMMON SENSE*, 1864

The classic family planning consultation is the presentation of a young woman for contraceptive advice. It is a very critical visit and provides an excellent opportunity to develop a good rapport with the patient and provide education on important health concerns, such as sexual health, fertility, pregnancy prevention, STI prevention, immunisation and cervical screening.

In counselling and treating patients, especially teenagers, confidentiality is of paramount importance. Keep in mind the Gillick test of competency for females aged under 16 (see CHAPTER 97). Contraceptive methods can be confusing, so careful education using charts and other aids is recommended to enhance the therapeutic relationship and ensure the patient understands the best options available to them.

Fertility control

The choice of contraceptive methodology will be determined not only by individual needs, personal preference and resources but also by its effectiveness, safety and incidence of side effects.

In developed countries of the Western world, the most widely used methods in order of preference are the male condom, combined oral contraceptive pill, intra-uterine device (IUD), female sterilisation and withdrawal.[1]

The past decade has seen a wider availability of long-acting reversible contraception (LARC). LARC methods are defined as non-permanent contraception administered less frequently than once a month. They include implants, IUDs and injectables. LARC methods are the most effective reversible contraceptives, with failure rates for typical use virtually the same as for perfect use. For this reason, LARC plays an important public health role in reducing unintended pregnancies.[2] Approximately half the pregnancies in the US are unintended and occur because of non-use of contraception, failure of a specific method or discontinuation of contraception.[3] While many women are satisfied with oral contraceptives or barrier methods, it is important to check their awareness of LARC proactively.[4]

A comparison of the failure rates of the various contraceptive methods is presented in TABLE 99.1.

It should be noted that condoms are the only contraception that protect against STIs. For women at risk of acquiring STIs, dual protection should be recommended. This involves use of condoms in addition to an effective form of contraception, offering both STI and pregnancy protection.[6]

> **Practice tip**
>
> Long-acting reversible contraception (LARC) methods include implants, IUDs and injectables. LARC methods are the most effective reversible contraceptives and have the potential to reduce unintended pregnancy rates.

Safe prescribing[4]

Most women of reproductive age can safely use all contraceptive methods. However, there are some conditions, risk factors and concurrent medications that make a particular method unsuitable. Medical Eligibility Criteria (MEC) tables for contraceptive use are an internationally recognised system to guide clinicians in the safe provision of contraceptive methods. Conditions affecting eligibility are classified under one of four categories: MEC 1—no restrictions; MEC 2—the benefits generally outweigh the risks; MEC 3—the risks generally outweigh the benefits; MEC 4—an absolute contraindication. A full listing of the UK MEC is available at <http://ukmec.pagelizard.com/2016>;

Table 99.1 Effectiveness of contraceptive methods

Contraceptive method	Failure rate (%) during first year of use: Typical use	Perfect use (consistent and correct)
No method	85	85
Fertility awareness-based methods	24	0.4–5
Withdrawal	22	4
Barrier		
• Female:		
— diaphragm with spermicide	12	6
— condom	21	5
• Male:		
— condom	18	2
Intrauterine contraceptive device		
• copper	0.8	0.6
• levonorgestrel	0.2	0.2
Vaginal ring	9	0.3
Combined oral contraceptive pill	9	0.3
Injection (medroxyprogesterone acetate)	6	0.2
Implant (etonogestrel)	0.05	0.05
Sterilisation		
• female	0.5	0.5
• male	0.15	0.1

Source: Adapted from Trussell J. Contraceptive efficacy. In: Hatcher RA, Trussell J, Nelson AL et al., *Contraceptive Technology* (20th edn). New York: Ardent Media, 2011[5]

Note: Failure rate is the percentage of women who have an unintended pregnancy during the first year of use of the contraceptive method. United States data

see also the WHO MEC at <www.who.int/reproductivehealth/publications/family_planning/MEC-5/en/>.

Hormonal contraception

Methods of hormonal contraception include:[7,8]

- Progestogen-only contraceptives:
  - etonogestrel implant (Implanon NXT)
  - levonorgestrel-releasing IUD (Mirena)
  - depot medroxyprogesterone acetate (DMPA)
  - progestogen-only pill (POP or 'mini-pill')
- Combined hormonal contraceptives:
  - combined oral contraceptive pill (COC or 'the pill')
  - vaginal ring (NuvaRing)
- Emergency contraception:
  - levonorgestrel emergency contraceptive pill (ECP)
  - ulipristal acetate

Progestogen-only contraception[7,8]

Progestogen-only methods include the progestogen-only pill, implant, IUD and injection. These methods are safe in women who are breastfeeding or have a contraindication to taking oestrogen. Progestogen-only contraception is contraindicated in women with active breast cancer within the past 5 years (MEC 4), but has relatively few other contraindications. The harms outweigh the benefits in the following conditions (MEC 3): antiphospholipid antibodies with systemic lupus erythematosus, unexplained vaginal bleeding, ischaemic heart disease or stroke, severe cirrhosis or hepatocellular carcinoma.

Use of progestogen-only contraception is not associated with an increased risk of venous thromboembolism. Women taking liver enzyme-inducing drugs are not advised to use the POP or etonogestral implant due to reduced effectiveness.

DMPA and the levonorgestrel IUD are appropriate for use with liver enzyme-inducing drugs. If emergency contraception is required, a double dose of the levonorgestrel-ECP is recommended.

Etonogestrel implant (Implanon NXT)[7]

This is a subdermal contraceptive implant; it is a 3-year system consisting of a single rod containing the progestogen etonogestrel. It inhibits ovulation and has an anti-cervical mucus effect. Irregular bleeding is the most common side effect, with one in 5 women experiencing frequent or prolonged bleeding episodes. Twenty-two per cent of women are amenorrhoeic within 12 months. Several treatments (e.g. cyclical use of a COCP; mefenamic acid; tranexamic acid) are safe to use to reduce troublesome bleeding in the short term. Approximately 20–25% of women request the implant to be removed within 12 months and it is important to provide information about expected bleeding patterns prior to insertion. It requires a minor surgical procedure to insert it and also to remove it. The pregnancy rate is the lowest of all contraceptives at <1:1000 over 3 years of use.

Intra-uterine contraceptive devices[7]

IUDs are highly effective LARCs that are increasingly used worldwide by women of all reproductive ages, including young and nulliparous women. They are made of an inert material to which may be added a bioactive substance such as copper (e.g. Multiload Cu375) or a progestogen (e.g. Mirena). All IUDs prevent pregnancy by inhibiting sperm migration and ovum transport and preventing implantation. The levonorgestrel IUD also causes endometrial suppression and cervical mucus thickening and may prevent or delay ovulation.

Efficacy:

- copper IUDs: 99.4% perfect use; 99.2% typical use
- levonorgestrel IUDs: 99.8% perfect and typical use

Absolute contraindications include active PID, undiagnosed abnormal genital tract bleeding and current or past history of breast cancer for those considering levonorgestrel IUD (MEC 4).

Recommended use time: copper IUD 5–10 years depending on brand, Mirena 5 years.

Side effects and complications of IUD use

The biggest difference between copper and hormonal IUDs is the effect on bleeding patterns and pain. Women with a copper IUD will have their usual menstrual periods, usually with an increase in menstrual loss and dysmenorrhoea. Spotting, heavier and prolonged bleeding are common in the first 3–6 months but usually decrease with time.

The levonorgestrel IUD results in a reduction of blood loss. Sixty-five per cent of women are amenorrhoeic or have light bleeding only after the first year of use. For this reason, the hormonal IUD is particularly suitable for women with heavy menstrual bleeding. Persistent light vaginal bleeding and/or spotting are common initially for the first 3–5 months.

Menstrual bleeding and pain are the most common reason for IUD discontinuation. Discontinuation rates for both IUDs are similar.

Pregnancy/ectopic pregnancy

If pregnancy occurs there is an increased risk of abortion and intra-uterine sepsis during the second trimester. Early removal of the IUD is essential. Since the IUD prevents intra-uterine rather than tubal pregnancies, the proportion of ectopic pregnancy is higher in the case of IUD failure, although the absolute risk is low compared to the risk for women using no contraception.

Pelvic inflammatory disease

There is a small increased risk of PID in the first 20 days post-insertion. Subsequent risk of PID reverts to baseline and is related to the risk of STIs.

Extrusion, perforation of uterus and translocation

Spontaneous extrusion occurs in about 5% with the highest risk within the first year. Perforation of the uterus occurs in up to 2.3 in 1000 insertions.[7] Factors that increase risk of perforation include breastfeeding, first 6 months postpartum and previous caesarean section. If translocation of the IUD outside the uterus is proved by X-ray and pelvic ultrasound, referral for removal is mandatory. The woman should attend for a follow-up visit between 3–6 weeks after insertion specifically to exclude infection, perforation or expulsion.

Injectable contraceptives

Depot medroxyprogesterone acetate

Depot medroxyprogesterone acetate (DMPA) is the only injectable intramuscular contraceptive available in Australia. It is very effective for up to 14 weeks. Although DMPA is technically a LARC, it is not immediately reversible and is less effective than implants and IUDs due to the need for repeated injections.

- Dose: 150 mg by deep IM injection in first 5 days of the menstrual cycle. The same dose is given every 12 weeks ± 2 weeks to maintain contraception.
- Effectiveness: perfect use 99.8%; typical use 94%.

Side effects include a disrupted menstrual cycle (amenorrhoea rate 50–70% by 12 months), weight gain (average 2–6%), breast tenderness, mood changes and a delay in return of fertility (mean time 8 months).[7] Long-term use is associated with accelerated bone loss, but this is not clinically significant and does not translate into fracture risk. However, for this reason it is not recommended as a first-line contraceptive for women less than 18 and more than 45 years.

Progestogen-only contraceptive pill

The POP (mini-pill) is most commonly prescribed for breastfeeding women for whom an oestrogen contraceptive would potentially suppress milk supply. It is safe from 6 weeks postpartum.

The two common formulations are:

- levonorgestrel 30 mcg/day
- norethisterone 35 mcg/day

The primary mechanism of action is cervical mucus thickening, preventing sperm penetration. In addition, POPs prevent ovulation in up to 60% of cycles.[8]

Efficacy is 99.7% in perfect use and 91% in typical use.[7] The failure rate is lower in women >40 years compared to younger women. The POP is considered to have a more vulnerable efficacy, and it is important that the woman strictly adheres to taking the pill within a daily 3-hour timeframe for maximum efficacy. The POP is effective after 3 tablets have been taken.[4]

Compliance can be a problem because of cycle irregularity. Twenty per cent of women will be amenorrhoeic on the POP, 40% will have regular bleeding and 40% will have irregular bleeding.[7]

Combined hormonal contraception (CHC)[7]

Combined hormonal contraceptives contain an oestrogen and progestogen, and their main mode of action is inhibition of hypothalamic and pituitary function leading to anovulation. They are available as a combined oral contraceptive pill (COC) and the vaginal ring. COCs and vaginal rings work in the same way and are treated similarly in terms of contraindications, complications, side effects and drug interactions.

Combined oral contraception (COC)

COCs in Australia contain ethinyloestradiol (EE), oestradiol valerate (EV), oestradiol (E2) or mestranol and one of a range of progestogens. Efficacy is 99.7% with perfect use, 91% with typical use.

Which oestrogen to use[7]

Type

EE is the most commonly used oestrogen. The active oestrogen in the newer E2 and EV pills is structurally identical to the E2 produced by the ovaries. They have a theoretical but unproven benefit in terms of venous thromboembolism (VTE) risk, and it will be some years before there is any evidence of VTE rates in women using these pill preparations. Both E2 and EV are associated with a moderately high rate of amenorrhoea during the hormone-free break.

Dose

It is recommended to use a dose of 35 mcg EE or less. There is some association between increasing EE dose and risk of venous thromboembolism (VTE). Formulations containing 50 mcg EE are no longer recommended because there is no known additional benefit from their use and they are associated with an increased risk of VTE. Women starting on a 20 mcg EE pill are likely to have fewer hormonally related side effects such as headaches or mood swings, but have a higher chance of discontinuation due to breakthrough bleeding.

Which progestogen to use[7]

The early progestogens include levonorgestrel and norethisterone. Newer progestogens have been developed over recent decades to reduce androgenic side effects and to minimise the effect EE has on lipids. Nomogestrol acetate, gestodene, desogestrel and etonogestrel are less androgenic, while cyproterone acetate, drospirenone and dienogest are anti-androgenic. Drospirenone is an analogue of spironolactone and has a mild diuretic effect. There is insufficient data to initially prescribe newer progestogens in preference to older versions.

Table 99.2 Combined oral contraceptive pill formulations available in Australia[7]

Oestrogen	Dose (mcg)	Progestogen	Dose (mcg)	Trade name
Monophasic				
Ethinyloestradiol	20	Drospirenone	3000	YAZ, YAZ Flex
Ethinyloestradiol	20	Levonorgestrel	100	Femme-Tab ED 20/100, Lenest 20, Loette, Microgynon 20, Microlevlen, Micronelle 20
Ethinyloestradiol	30	Levonorgestrel	150	Eleanor 150/30, Evelyn 150/30, Femme-Tab 30/150, Lenest 30, Levlen, Microgynon 30, Micronelle 30, Monofeme, Nordette,
Ethinyloestradiol	10, 30	Levonorgestrel	150	Seasonique*
Ethinyloestradiol	30	Dienogest	2000	Valette
Ethinyloestradiol	30	Gestodene	75	Minulet
Ethinyloestradiol	30	Desogestrel	150	Marvelon
Ethinyloestradiol	35	Cyproterone acetate	2000	Brenda-35, Carolyn-35, Chelsea-35, Diane-35, Estelle-35, Juliet-35, Laila-35, Jene-35
Ethinyloestradiol	35	Norethisterone	500	Brevinor, Norimin
Ethinyloestradiol	35	Norethisterone	1000	Brevinor-1, Norimin-1
Ethinyloestradiol	30	Drospirenone	3000	Yasmin, Petibelle
Ethinyloestradiol	50	Levonorgestrel	125	Microgynon 50
Mestranol	50	Norethisterone	1000	Norinyl-1
Oestradiol	1500	Nomegestrol acetate	2500	Zoely
Triphasic				
Ethinyloestradiol	30, 40	Levonorgestrel	50, 75, 125	Logynon, Trifeme, Triphasil, Triquilar
Ethinyloestradiol	35	Norethisterone	500, 1000	Improvil
Quadraphasic oestradiol valerate	1000–3000	Dienogest	2000, 3000	Qlaira

*Seasonique has an extended regimen, with each pack consisting of 91 tablets—made up of 84 hormonal tablets containing 30 mcg EE and 150 mcg levonorgestrel plus 7 10 mcg EE tablets

Various COC preparations available in Australia are listed in TABLE 99.2.

Starting the pill: which COC to use[7]

The past menstrual and medical history of the woman should be documented and contraindications excluded.

A suitable first choice is a monophasic pill containing 30 mcg or 35 mcg ethinyloestradiol (EE) with levonorgestrel or norethisterone (e.g. Nordette, Microgynon 30, Monofeme, Levlen ED, Brevinor).

Education and counselling are very important for the woman starting the pill. Suitable patient education should be given. Pill swatches produced by manufacturers are a useful aid. Cover starts immediately if a hormone (active) pill is commenced on day 1–5 of the menstrual cycle (except the quadriphasic pill Qlaira—refer to product information).

Note: A 'quick-start' technique, described by Westhoff, can be used to start the COC on the day of the consultation. If commenced at any time other than day 1–5 of the menstrual cycle, abstinence/condoms are required for the first 7 days after the start.[9]

Specific patient groups[4,7]

Adolescents. There is no lower age limit if the young woman has started menstruating.

99

Acne and hirsuitism. The oestrogen in any CHC may improve acne and hirsuitism via increased sex hormone binding globulin (SHBG) levels and reduction of free testosterone. COCs containing an anti-androgenic progestogen have a theoretical advantage for women who request management of androgenic symptoms. Any beneficial effect may take up to 6 months.

Women over 35 years. CHC use is safe for healthy non-smoking women until 50 years (MEC 2 for women over 40). CHC is not recommended if a woman is over 35 years and has multiple cardiovascular risk factors, including obesity, smoking, diabetes and hypertension (MEC 3/4).

Women taking liver enzyme-inducing drugs. Alternative contraception is strongly advised. The only hormonal contraceptives not affected by liver enzyme-inducing drugs are DMPA and IUDs. Current evidence suggests that most antibiotics do not interact with combined hormonal contraceptives. The only exceptions are liver enzyme-inducing rifabutin and rifampicin. Other liver enzyme-inducing drugs include many of the older anti-epileptics (e.g. phenytoin, carbamazapine), St John's wort and protease inhibitors. For women who still request the use of COC, an extended or tricycling regime of a higher dose pill (e.g. containing at least 50 mcg EE) may be effective. Further guidance on drug interactions is provided by the UK Faculty of Sexual Health & Reproductive Healthcare at <https://www.fsrh.org/standards-and-guidance/documents/ceu-clinical-guidance-drug-interactions-with-hormonal/>.

Contraindications to CHC usage are shown in TABLE 99.3.

Non-contraceptive advantages of CHCs[7]

A number of significant beneficial effects arising from the use of COCs have now been documented:

- Reduction in most menstrual cycle disorders, including dysmenorrhoea, symptoms of endometriosis and heavy menstrual bleeding
- Reduction in the incidence of functional ovarian cysts and benign ovarian tumours
- Reduced incidence of ovarian and endometrial cancer
- Can reduce acne
- Can be useful in managing symptoms of polycystic ovarian syndrome
- Can assist with perimenopausal symptoms
- Can be used to manage premenstrual syndrome (PMS) and its more severe form (PMDD) in some women
- Can reduce the risk of bowel cancer

Table 99.3 Contraindications for the use of COC[7]

Absolute (MEC 4)
First 2 weeks postpartum, 6 weeks if breastfeeding
≥35 years and smoking ≥15 cigarettes/day
History of thomboembolic disease, including known thrombophilia
Cerebrovascular disease
Ischaemic heart disease
Uncontrolled hypertension
Complicated valvular heart disease
Cardiomyopathy
Migraine with aura
Malignancy of the breast or genital tract
Severely impaired liver function
Major surgery with prolonged immobilisation
Positive antiphospholipid antibodies
Relative (MEC 3)
BMI >35 kg/m^2
Multiple risk factors for cardiovascular disease
First-degree relative who had a VTE <45 years
Undiagnosed abnormal vaginal bleeding
Past history of migraine with aura, none for 5 years
Known gene mutation associated with breast cancer
Gall bladder disease
Controlled hypertension
Long-term immobilisation

Note: Adapted from UK Medical Eligibility Criteria (UKMEC) 2016 for CHCs. Full listing available at <www.ukmec.pagelizard.com/2016>

Serious side effects of CHCs

The most serious side effects to be considered are the effects of COCs on the circulatory system and the incidence of cancer.

The following circulatory disorders have been linked with pill usage.

- Venous deep vein thrombosis, pulmonary embolism, *rarely:* mesenteric, hepatic and kidney thrombosis
- Arterial myocardial infarction, thrombotic stroke, haemorrhagic stroke, *rarely:* retinal and mesenteric thrombosis

The risk of circulatory disease has not been related to duration of use and there is no increased risk in perpetual users.

The oestrogen content of the pill is considered to be the aetiological factor and the problem is increased in women taking high oestrogen-content COCs, but now that the oestrogen content of each pill has been reduced to 35 mcg EE or less, these risks of morbidity and mortality have been reduced.

The progestogen effect on lipid metabolism is not considered significant in the aetiology of circulatory disease. Circulatory diseases have now been recognised as occurring predominantly in certain high-risk groups—the 'at-risk female', particularly the smoker over 35 years of age.

Other at-risk groups include those with thrombophilia, hyperlipidaemia, diabetes, hyperstension and a family history of cardiovascular disease or immobilisation.

Venous thromboembolism[8]

Venous thromboembolism (VTE) risk is increased 2–3 times in users of CHCs compared to non-users, with an increase of between one and three extra cases per 10 000 women in a year. The risk is highest in the first 4 months of use and gradually decreases with duration of use. Studies have shown that COCs containing cyproterone, desogestrel, drospirenone or gestodene have a higher risk of VTE than COCs containing levonorgestrel or other progestogens. However, the absolute risk of VTE in users of any CHC is very low and much lower than the risk associated with pregnancy and the postpartum period. Women who are eligible for an oestrogen-containing method of contraception can safely use any pill on the market with 35 mcg EE or less.

CHC and cancer[7]

Women who have used CHC have an overall lower risk of cancer compared to women who have not.

- Possible very small increased risk:
  - cervix (benefits of use outweigh the risk with a low- or high-grade squamous intra-epithelial lesion)
  - breast
- Protective effect:
  - endometrial
  - epithelial ovarian
  - bowel

Common side effects

The relatively minor side effects listed in TABLE 99.4 may discourage women from persisting with oral

Table 99.4 Management of common side effects of COC[4,8]

Symptom	Change
Acne	Change to a pill containing an anti-androgenic (drospirenone, dienogest or cyproterone acetate) or less androgenic (gestodene, desogestrel or etonogestrel) progestogen
Breakthrough bleeding	Exclude underlying causes (e.g. chlamydia, pregnancy, missed pills, malabsorption, diarrhoea or vomiting, concurrent medications) Increase oestrogen if taking a pill with 20 mcg EE to a maximum of 35 mcg EE Change progestogen if already taking a pill with 30 or 35 mcg EE Consider vaginal ring
Breast tenderness	Decrease oestrogen and/or progestogen dose Consider change of formulation Consider using pill containing drospirenone
Chloasma	Change to non-oestrogen-containing contraception Avoid direct sun (use blockout)
Amenorrhoea	Exclude pregnancy Absence of withdrawal bleed is not harmful and occurs in 6% of cycles with EE and 20–30% of EV or E2 pills Switch to a pill with a more predictable bleeding pattern
Lowered libido, mood changes	No evidence of a difference between COCs Trial a change of formulation
Headache	Any new headache or marked changes in headache should be evaluated Reduce oestrogen dose If occurs in pill-free week, consider a pill with a reduced number of placebo pills, an extended regimen, running packs together or giving an oestrogen supplement in the pill-free weeks (100 mcg oestrogen patch or 2 mg or 4 mg oestradiol)
Nausea/vomiting	Reduce oestrogen Take the pills at night
Weight gain	Evidence does not support an increase in weight related to COCs Drospirenone pills are associated with a small, unsustained average weight loss of 0.5 kg in the first year and may be useful for some women

contraception in the absence of appropriate explanation and reassurance. Management of these side effects is listed in the same table. It is useful in practice to have this list available as a ready reference for manipulating the COC if necessary. A common nuisance side effect is breakthrough bleeding in the first 2 months.

Important advice for the patient

- Diarrhoea and vomiting may reduce the effectiveness of the pill. If a woman vomits within 2 hours of taking an active pill, she should take an additional active pill.
- Withdrawal bleeds can be skipped for a woman's convenience, by going straight from the last active pill in the cycle to the first active pill in the next cycle. Running packs of multiphasic pills together can result in unpredictable bleeding as a result of the fluctuating dose of hormones.[10] A Cochrane Review did not demonstrate any additional safety concerns for women taking CHCs continuously without placebo breaks for up to 12 months.[11] An extended-regimen pill with 84 active pills plus 7 inactive pills is now available.

Missed pills

A missed pill is defined as one that is taken more than 24 hours late (>48 hours since last pill was taken). The advice is to take the missed pill as soon as possible, even if it means taking two pills in one day. Any previously missed pills should be discarded and the usual pill-taking schedule resumed. Condoms or abstinence should be used for 7 days (the 'Seven-day rule'). This advice does not apply to the quadriphasic pill Qlaira and the product information should be consulted. Refer to FIGURE 99.1.

If the pill is missed with <7 pills left before the next placebo break, skip placebos and continue active pills.

If <7 active pills were taken before the missed pill, consider emergency contraception if unprotected sex took place in the past 5 days. If ulipristal acetate emergency contraception is used, the woman needs to wait 5 days before restarting the pill.

Pill failure[7]

Causes of oral contraceptive failure include errors in administration, decreased absorption, missed pills and use of liver enzyme-inducing drugs. If the woman prefers to use a CHC, tricycling the COC or vaginal ring packs and having a shorter placebo break should be considered.

Vaginal ring[7]

The first available contraceptive vaginal ring is NuvaRing®, a flexible polymer ring with 15 mcg EE and 120 mcg etonogestrel being released per 24 hours. Metabolic effects and side effects are virtually the same as for the COC. It is immediately protective when inserted on days 1–5 of the menstrual cycle. It is then removed after 21 days with a break of

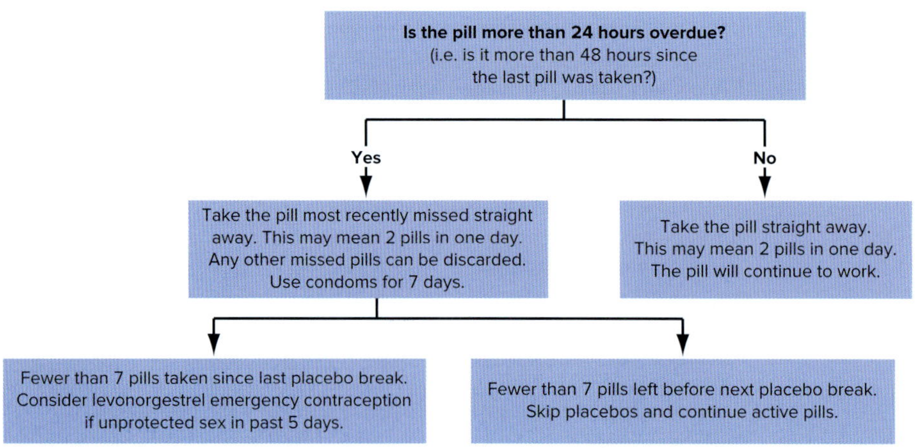

FIGURE 99.1 Missed combined oral contraceptive pill[7]

Source: Adapted from *Contraception: An Australian Clinical Practice Handbook* and reproduced with permission © 2012: Family Planning NSW, Family Planning Victoria and Family Planning Queensland

Note: These instructions do not apply to the quadriphasic pill Qlaira. See product information for advice

7 days or can be used 'back-to-back'. The cycle control is good, with a reduced incidence of irregular bleeding. This method may be useful for women who prefer the COC but are prone to missing pills, or women with inflammatory bowel disease or other malabsorption syndromes. It is recommended that the vaginal ring is not removed for intercourse.

> **Practice tip**
>
> Delaying a period:
>
> - prescribe norethisterone 5 mg bd or tds for 3 days prior to expected period
> - period resumes 2–3 days after stopping tablets

Emergency contraception[7]

- Ulipristal acetate 30 mg orally as a single dose within 5 days
- Levonorgestrel 1.5 mg as a single dose
- 25 levonorgestrel POPs (25 × 30 mcg) as an initial dose, repeating the same dose 12 hours later
- Yuzpe method: a large initial dose of COC, which is repeated 12 hours later, with each dose containing at least 100 mcg of EE and 500 mcg of levonorgestrel (example: 4 tablets of either Microgynon 30 or 5 tablets of Microgynon 20)
- Copper IUD inserted within 5 days

Uliprisital acetate is a selective progesterone receptor modulator that acts by preventing or delaying ovulation. It does this more effectively than the levonorgestrel emergency contraceptive pill (LNG-ECP), which is licensed for use only up to 72 hours after intercourse. Effectiveness for both is improved the earlier they are taken.

The Yuzpe method has an efficacy of 57–74% and is reserved only for when levonorgestrel is unavailable. The copper IUD is highly effective at 99% and can provide very reliable ongoing contraception. It may be appropriate to advise the woman seeking postcoital contraception to return for pregnancy testing in 3–4 weeks, depending on her risk. STI screening and the need for ongoing contraception need to be considered.

Barrier methods[7]

Barrier methods include male and female condoms and vaginal diaphragms. If used correctly, male condoms are very effective contraceptives with an efficacy of 98% with perfect use and 82% with typical use.

Condoms are also very effective in preventing the spread of STIs, including HIV infection. The main disadvantage is that they are mainly reliant on the cooperation of the user.

Diaphragms are inserted at any convenient time before intercourse and removed after 6 hours have elapsed since the last act of intercourse. Their presence on the Australian market in the future remains uncertain.

Fertility awareness methods

These methods require high motivation and some require regular menstrual cycles.

Basal body temperature method

Coitus should occur only after there has been a rise in basal body temperature of 0.2°C for 3 days (72 hours) above the basal body temperature measurement during the preceding 6 days, until the onset of the next menstrual period.

Calendar or rhythm method

The woman reviews and records six cycle lengths and then selects the shortest and longest cycles. She then subtracts 21 from the shortest cycle and 10 from the longest cycle to work out fertile and safe days (i.e. for a 26 to 30-day cycle: fertile days 5–20; for regular 28-day cycle: fertile days 7–18).

Billings ovulation method[7,12]

This method is based on keeping a daily record of the sensation at the vulva and the appearance of the mucus, so that ovulation can be recognised and intercourse, in the pre-ovulatory time, can be confined to when the record shows an unchanging pattern, signalling unchanging hormones and thus infertility. The fertile phase commences when there is a change in the sensation or mucus, correlating with a rise in oestrogen. This sensation at the vulva will become progressively more lubricative and will be followed by a definite change to being no longer slippery (caused by rising progesterone). The peak day of fertility is the last day of the slippery sensation, with or without the visual presence of mucus. The postovulatory infertile phase begins on the fourth day after the peak day. Regular cycles are not required for successful use of the Billings ovulation method.

Withdrawal method or coitus interruptus

Male withdrawal before ejaculation is still a widely used method of contraception and will continue to have a definite place in contraceptive practice.

Lactational amenorrhoea method (LAM)[8]

LAM is as reliable as hormonal methods of contraception if the baby is younger than 6 months, is exclusively breastfed with no long intervals between feeds (no more than 4 hours during the day or 6 hours at night) and the woman remains amenorrhoeic postpartum. Lactation is not a reliable contraceptive method once any of these criteria is not met—if the mother is still breastfeeding, a progestogen-only method is advised. Since some women may ovulate prior to the onset of menses, an additional method of contraception should be advised to reduce the risk of another pregnancy.

Ceasing contraception and menopause[13]

Women using non-hormonal contraception (i.e. barrier, copper IUD, rhythm) can be advised that contraception is no longer required once they have been amenorrhoeic for 12 months over the age of 50 years and after two years before the age of 50.

Oestrogen-containing contraception and DPMA injections are not recommended after 50 years. After this age, women should switch to an alternative progestogen-only or non-hormonal method.

Women over the age of 50 who are amenorrhoeic while using progestogen-only contraception are advised to continue the method for a further 12 months UNTIL they have two follicle stimulating hormone levels of 30 IU/L or above taken 6 weeks apart. Contraception is not required beyond the age of 55 years.

Permanent contraceptive methods

Vasectomy[14]

A vasectomy involves interruption or occlusion of the vas deferens, preventing the passage of sperm from the testes to the penis. The procedure is generally performed in an outpatient setting under local anaesthesia. It is important to confirm the absence of spermatozoa in the ejaculate 2–3 months after the operation, before ceasing other contraceptive methods. It takes about 12–15 ejaculations to clear the remaining sperm from the semen.

For the average man undergoing vasectomy reversal, pregnancy rates range between 50 and 70%. This rate decreases as the interval between vasectomy and its reversal increases.

Tubal ligation

Female sterilisation is usually performed by mini-laparotomy or laparoscopy, at which time clips are applied to each fallopian tube. This is a potentially reversible method of contraception with 50% of women achieving pregnancy after reversal. Efficacy is >99.5%.[7]

Hysteroscopic transcervical occlusive sterilisation

This procedure—Essure—involves the placement of a flexible titanium micro-insert into each fallopian tube. The insert expands and over time reactive tissue growth occludes the tubes.

This irreversible method requires alternative contraception until complete tubal occlusion is confirmed radiologically at 12 weeks.

Unintended pregnancy

Up to 51% of Australian women have experienced an unplanned pregnancy.[15] It is estimated that 1 in 4 pregnancies in Australia end in termination, and adoption is now an unusual outcome. It is important not to make assumptions about the 'wantedness' of a pregnancy.

Termination of pregnancy is lawful under certain circumstances; however, the law is different in every state and territory. The main methods used are the traditional surgical methods such as suction curettage and medical abortion. Surgical abortions can be performed from 6–7 weeks. There is an increased risk of continuing pregnancy if performed before 6 weeks. Medical abortions are usually performed before 9 weeks using mifepristone, an anti-progesterone, and then the prostaglandin analogue misoprostol 36–48 hours later. Bleeding and cramping usually occur within 4–6 hours and a check-up visit is required in two weeks.

Ideally, unintended pregnancies should be prevented through appropriate community education and contraception counselling. LARC methods are considered to play a vital role.

References

1 United Nations Publications: World Contraceptive Patterns, 2013 <www.un.org/en/development/desa/population/publications/pdf/family/worldContraceptivePatternsWallChart2013.pdf> (accessed 7/9/2014).

2 Black KI, Bateson D, Harvey C. Australian women need increased access to long-acting reversible contraception. Med J Aust, 2013; 199 (5): 317–8.

3 Gold RB et al. *Next Steps for America's Family Planning Program: Leveraging the Potential of Medicaid and Title X in an Evolving Health Care System.* New York: Guttmacher Institute, 2009.
4 Bateson D, McNamee K, Harvey C et al. Contraception: a practice-based update: how to treat. Australian Doctor, 4 May 2012: 25–32.
5 Trussell J. Contraceptive efficacy. In: Hatcher RA, Trussell J, Nelson AL et al., *Contraceptive Technology* (20th edn). New York: Ardent Media, 2011.
6 Mazza D. *Women's Health in General Practice* (2nd edn). Sydney: Elsevier, 2011: 37–85.
7 Family Planning New South Wales, Family Planning Victoria and True Relationships and Reproductive Health. *Contraception: An Australian Clinical Practice Handbook* (4th edn). Ashfield NSW, 2016.
8 Expert group for Endocrinology. In: eTG complete [Internet]. Melbourne: Therapeutic Guidelines Ltd. Available from: <www.tg.org.au> (accessed May 2018).
9 Westoff C et al. Quick start: a novel oral contraceptive initiation method. Contraception, 2002; 66: 141–8.
10 Moore P. Recent developments in contraception: how to treat. Australian Doctor, 3 April 2009: 25–32.
11 Edelman AB, Gallo MF, Nesen JT et al. Continuous or extended cycle vs. cyclic use of combined oral contraceptives for contraception. Cochrane Database Syst Rev. 2005, Issue 3. Article No. CD004695.
12 Billings E, Westmore A. *The Billings Method.* Melbourne: Anne O'Donovan, 1992: 11–49.
13 Bateson D, McNamee K, Harvey C et al. Contraception for women aged over 40. Medicine Today, 2012; 13 (8): 27–36.
14 Woolcott R. Vasectomy reversal: how to treat. Australian Doctor, 4 July 2014: 19–26.
15 What women want when faced with an unplanned pregnancy. Research by WebSurvey, commissioned by Marie Stopes International Australia, November 2006 <www.mariestopes.org.au/data-and-research/what-women-want-when-faced-with-unplanned-pregnancy/> (accessed 29/9/2014).

100 Breast pain (mastalgia)

Many women suffer breast pain so severe that it affects their lifestyles, marriages and sexual relationships, and even prevents them from hugging their children.

DR JOHN DAWSON, 1990

Breast pain, or mastalgia, is a common problem, accounting for at least 50% of breast problems presenting in general practice and 14% of referrals to an Australian breast clinic.[1] It can vary from localised breast pain due to an infection or a breast cyst to diffuse bilateral pain. If no obvious physical cause is found, the problem is all too often dismissed, without appropriate empathy and reassurance, as a normal physiological effect. However, its aetiology is not clear.

A careful, sympathetic clinical approach, however, followed by reassurance after examination, will be sufficient treatment for most patients.

Symptoms

Mastalgia usually presents as a heaviness or discomfort in the breast or as a pricking or stabbing sensation. The pain may radiate down the inner arm when the patient is carrying heavy objects or when the arm is in constant use, as in scrubbing floors.

Key facts and checkpoints

- The typical age span for mastalgia is 30–50 years.
- The peak incidence is 35–45 years.
- There are four common clinical presentations:
  1. diffuse, bilateral cyclical mastalgia
  2. diffuse, bilateral non-cyclical mastalgia
  3. unilateral diffuse non-cyclical mastalgia
  4. localised breast pain
- The specific type of mastalgia should be identified.
- The commonest type is cyclical mastalgia.
- Premenstrual mastalgia (part of type 1) is common.
- An underlying malignancy should be excluded.
- Less than 10% of breast cancers present with localised pain.
- Only about 1 in 200 women with mastalgia are found to have breast cancer.
- The problems, especially types 2 and 3, are difficult to alleviate.

A diagnostic approach

A summary of the diagnostic strategy model for mastalgia is presented in TABLE 100.1.

Probability diagnosis

In the non-pregnant patient, generalised pain, which may be cyclical or non-cyclical, is commonest. Typical patterns are illustrated in FIGURE 100.1.

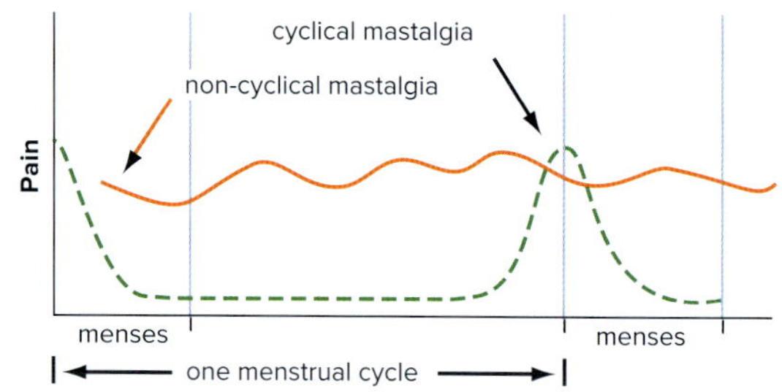

FIGURE 100.1 Pain patterns for cyclical and non-cyclical mastalgia

Cyclical mastalgia is the commonest diffuse breast pain. It occurs in the latter half of the menstrual cycle, especially in the premenstrual days, and subsides with the onset of menstruation. It obviously has a hormonal basis, which may be an abnormality in prolactin secretion. The main underlying disorder is benign mammary dysplasia, also referred to as fibroadenosis, chronic mastitis, cystic hyperplasia or fibrocystic breast disease.

Non-cyclical mastalgia, which is pain that does not vary within the menstrual cycle, is also quite common and the cause is poorly understood. It may be associated with mammary duct ectasia (see CHAPTER 101).

Serious disorders not to be missed

The three important serious disorders not to be missed with any painful chest condition—neoplasia, infection and myocardial ischaemia—are applicable for breast pain.

Table 100.1	Mastalgia: diagnostic strategy model
Probability diagnosis Pregnancy Cracked or inflamed nipple Cyclical mastalgia: • benign mammary dysplasia	
Serious disorders not to be missed Vascular: • acute coronary insufficiency • thrombophlebitis (Mondor disease) Infection: • mastitis • breast abscess Cancer: • breast (uncommon presentation) • mastitis carcinomatosa	
Pitfalls (often missed) Pregnancy Chest wall pain (e.g. costochondritis) Pectoralis muscle spasm Referred pain, esp. thoracic spine Bornholm disease (epidemic pleurodynia) Herpes zoster Mechanical: • bra problems • pendulous breasts stretching Cooper's ligaments • weight change • trauma *Rarities:* • hyperprolactinaemia • nerve entrapment • mammary duct ectasia • sclerosing adenosis • ankylosing spondylitis	
Seven masquerades checklist Depression Drugs (e.g. OCP, HRT, marijuana) Spinal dysfunction	
Is the patient trying to tell me something? Yes. Fear of malignancy. Consider psychogenic causes.	

Neoplasia

We must avoid the trap of considering that breast pain is not compatible with malignancy. Mastalgia can be a presenting symptom (although uncommon) of breast cancer. 'Mastitis carcinomatosa', which is a rare florid form of breast cancer found in young women, often during lactation, is red and hot but not invariably painful or tender.[2] Pain may also be a symptom in juvenile fibroadenoma, a soft rapidly growing tumour in adolescents, and in the fibroadenoma of adult women.

Infection

Mastitis is common among nursing mothers. It should be regarded as a serious and urgent problem because a breast abscess can develop quickly. Apart from bacterial infection, infection with *Candida albicans* may occur following the use of antibiotics. *Candida* infection usually causes severe breast or nipple pain, producing a feeling like 'hot cords', especially during and after feeding.

Myocardial ischaemia

A constricting pain under the left breast should be regarded as myocardial ischaemia until proved otherwise.

Pitfalls

These include various causes of apparent mastalgia, such as several musculoskeletal chest wall conditions and referred pain from organs such as the heart, oesophagus, lungs and gall bladder and, in particular, from the upper thoracic spine.

Musculoskeletal conditions include costochondritis, pectoralis muscle strains or spasm, and entrapment of the lateral cutaneous branch of the third intercostal nerve. Ankylosing spondylitis can affect the chest wall under the breasts. Mastalgia may be the first symptom of pregnancy. Pregnancy should be excluded before commencing drug treatment.

Seven masquerades checklist

Of these, depression, drugs and spinal dysfunction are probable causes. Drugs that can cause breast discomfort include oral contraceptives, HRT and methylxanthine derivatives such as theophylline. Drugs that cause tender gynaecomastia (more applicable to men) include digoxin, cimetidine, spironolactone and marijuana.

Dysfunction of the upper thoracic spine and even the lower cervical spine can refer pain under a breast. If suspected, these areas of the spine should be examined.

Psychogenic considerations

The symptoms may be exaggerated as a result of an underlying psychogenic disorder, but with a symptom such as breast pain most women fear malignancy and need reassurance.

The clinical approach

History

It is important to relate the pain to the menstrual cycle and determine whether the patient is pregnant or not.

Key questions

- Could you be pregnant?
- Is your period on time or overdue?
- Is the pain in both breasts or only one?
- Do you have pain before your periods (cyclical mastalgia) or all the time during your menstrual cycle?
- Do you have pain in your back or where your ribs join your chest bone?

Examination

The breasts should be systematically palpated to check for soreness or lumps. The underlying chest wall and thoracic spine should also be examined.

Investigations

The following specialised tests could be considered.

Mammography should be considered in older women. It is unreliable in young women. With few exceptions it should not be used under 40 years.

Ultrasound can be complementary to mammography as it is useful to assess a localised mass or tender area. It is inappropriate to evaluate a diffuse area. It is not so useful for the postmenopausal breast, which is fatty and looks similar to cancer on ultrasound.

FNA excision biopsy can be useful for an area of localised pain, especially in the presence of a possible mass.

Consider a chest X-ray and ECG.

Mastalgia in children

Breast pain is uncommon in children, including puberty, but it may be a presenting problem in the late teens. Pubertal boys may complain of breast lumps under the nipple (adolescent gynaecomastia) but these are rarely tender and do not require specific treatment.

Mastalgia in the elderly

Breast pain is rare after the menopause but can be associated with HRT use, where it tends to present as the diffuse bilateral type. If the problem is related to the introduction of HRT, the oestrogen dose should be reduced or an alternative preparation used.

Cyclical mastalgia

The features of cyclical mastalgia are:

- the typical age is 30–40 years (mean 35)
- discomfort and sometimes pain are present
- usually bilateral but one breast can dominate (usually upper outer quadrant)
- related to the menstrual cycle, mainly premenstrual
- usually resolves on commencement of menstruation
- breasts may be diffusely nodular or lumpy
- variable relationship to the pill

Cyclical mastalgia is rare after the menopause.

Non-cyclical mastalgia

The features of non-cyclical mastalgia are:

- the typical age is the early 40s (median age 41 years)
- bilateral and diffuse
- continuous or intermittent
- pain present throughout the cycle
- no obvious physical or pathological basis

Management for mastalgia (both types)

After excluding a diagnosis of cancer and aspirating palpable cysts, various treatments are possible and can be given according to severity.[3]

Acknowledge the condition and its discomfort.

Approach to treatment[4]

- Reassurance—explain high remission rate
- Regular review and breast self-examination
- Proper brassiere support—expert fitting
- Cease smoking (if applicable)
- Aim at ideal weight
- Adjust oral contraception or HRT (if applicable)
- Analgesia (e.g. paracetamol 0.5–1 g (o) 4–6 hourly prn)

Many products have been promoted and tried but there is no convincing evidence to support the use of vitamins B1, B6, B12 and E, diuretics, NSAIDs, narcotics, caffeine reduction and even evening primrose oil, which is a favoured product and has been helpful for many women.[5,6,7]

Evening primrose oil contains an essential fatty acid claimed to be lacking in the diet, and replacement allows for the production of prostaglandin E, which counters the effect of oestrogen and prolactin on the breast. However, according to the multi-centred

European RCT, it is no more effective than placebo,[1] but the placebo effect in these trials was strong.[6,7]

A dose of 1000 mg three times daily for 3–4 months is recommended if a trial of treatment is planned.[6] There is some evidence to support the use of a topical NSAID medication (e.g. diclofenac gel).[5]

Recent systemic reviews from RTCs assessed the effectiveness of danazol,[8] bromocriptine and tamoxifen and showed that all provided significant relief, but that all have the potential for severe adverse effects.

For very severe mastalgia it is recommended to refer to a breast specialist to consider prescribing tamoxifen or danazol.[6]

Non-cyclical mastalgia is very difficult to treat, being more refractory than cyclical mastalgia.

Local lesions

Surgical excision may be required for local lesions. If there is no discrete lesion but a tender trigger point (including costochondritis), the injection of local anaesthetic and corticosteroid may relieve the problem.

Costochondritis (Tietze syndrome)

This is a common cause of referral to a breast pain clinic. The cause is often obscure, but the costochondral junction may become strained in patients with a persistent cough. The pain can appear to be in the breast with intermittent radiation round the chest wall and is initiated or aggravated by deep breathing and coughing.

Features:

- the pain is acute, intermittent or chronic
- the breast is normal to palpation
- palpable swelling about 4 cm from sternal edge due to enlargement of costochondral cartilage
- X-rays are normal
- it is self-limiting, but may take several months to subside

Treatment. Infiltration with local anaesthetic and corticosteroid with care. Otherwise use NSAIDs or paracetamol.

Mastitis

Mastitis is basically cellulitis of the interlobular connective tissue of the breast. Mostly restricted to lactating women, it is associated with a cracked nipple or poor milk drainage, including poor infant positioning. The infecting organism is usually *Staphylococcus aureus.* Mastitis is a serious problem and requires early treatment. Breastfeeding from the affected side can continue as the infection is confined to interstitial breast tissue and doesn't usually affect the milk supply.

Clinical features

- A lump and then soreness (at first)
- A red tender area

Possibly

- Fever, tiredness, muscle aches and pains

Note: Candida infection usually causes severe breast or nipple pain—a feeling like a hot knife or hot shooting pains, especially during and after feeding. It may occur after a course of antibiotics.

Prevention (in lactation)

- Maintain free breast drainage—keep feeding
- Encourage milk expression from the infected breast manually or by breast pump
- Attend to breast engorgement and cracked nipples

Treatment

If systemic symptoms develop:

- antibiotics: resolution without progression to an abscess will usually be prevented by antibiotics[7]
  di/(flu)cloxacillin 500 mg (o) 6 hourly for at least 5, and up to 10, days
  or (if hypersensitive to penicillin),[9,10] cephalexin 500 mg (o) 6 hourly for at least 5 days
  If severe cellulitis, di/(flu)cloxacillin 2 g (IV) 6 hourly, then switch to oral therapy when symptoms are resolving
- therapeutic ultrasound (2 W/cm^2 for 6 minutes) daily for 2–3 days
- ibuprofen or paracetamol for pain
- for *Candida albicans* infection of the breast:
  fluconazole 150 mg (o) every second day for 1–2 weeks followed by a course of nystatin 1 000 000 U (o) tds[11]

Breast abscess

If tenderness and redness persist beyond 48 hours and an area of tense induration develops, then a breast abscess has formed (see FIG. 100.2).

The preferred treatment is serial aspiration drainage with a large bore needle under ultrasound guidance. Often 3 or 4 aspirations are required. Adjunct treatment is antibiotics, rest and complete emptying of the breast. Breastfeeding can continue, with provision of lactation support. Surgical drainage may be required but should be avoided if possible because fistula formation is common.

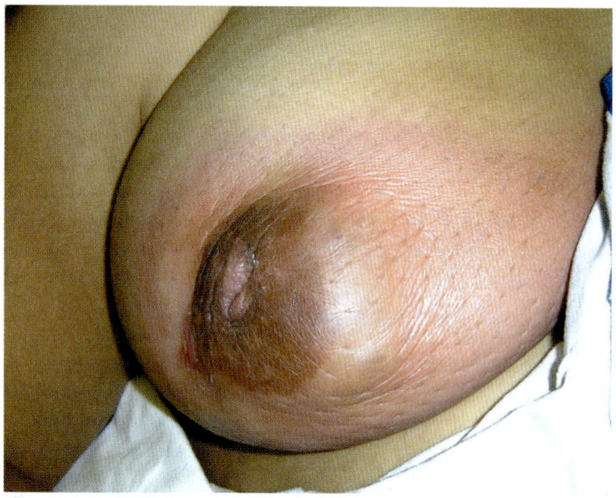

FIGURE 100.2 Localised cellulitis and breast abscess in a breastfeeding mother

Inflammatory breast cancer

Also referred to as 'mastitis carcinomatosa', this rare condition develops quickly with florid redness, swelling, dimpling and heaviness of the breast. It is not as painful as it appears and can be confused with mastitis but does not respond to antibiotics.

Refer immediately.

When to refer

- Undiagnosed localised breast pain or lump

Practice tips

- The basis of management for benign mastalgia is firm reassurance.
- Although breast cancer rarely causes mastalgia, it should be excluded.
- Think of *C. albicans* if mastitis is very severe with hot shooting pains, especially after antibiotic treatment.
- Look for underlying disorders of the chest wall if examination of the breasts is normal.
- Consider caffeine intake as a cause of benign diffuse mastalgia.
- Mastitis should be treated vigorously—it is a serious condition.
- Fibroadenomas and breast cysts are capable of causing localised pain and tenderness.

Patient education resources

Hand-out sheets from *Murtagh's Patient Education* 7th edition:

- Painful breasts

References

1 Brennan M. Mastalgia: an approach to management (update). Medical Observer, 2008: 1–3.
2 Ryan P. *A Very Short Textbook of Surgery* (2nd edn). Canberra: Dennis & Ryan, 1990: 10.
3 Barraclough B. The fibrocystic breast—clinical assessment, diagnosis and treatment. Modern Medicine Australia, 1990; 33 (4): 16–25.
4 Rosolowich V, Saettler E, Szuck B et al. Mastalgia. J Obstet Gynaecol Can, 2006; 28 (1): 49–57.
5 Mazza D. *Women's Health in General Practice* (2nd edn). Sydney: Churchill Livingstone, Elsevier, 2011: 189.
6 Cusack L, Brennan M. Breast symptoms. Check Unit 474, Melbourne: RACGP, 2011: 13–14.
7 Blommers J, de Lange-de Klerk ES, Kuik DJ et at. Evening primrose oil and fish oil for severe chronic mastalgia: a randomized, double-blind, controlled trial. Am J Obst Gynecol, 2002; 187: 1389–94.
8 Srivasta A, Mansel RE, Arvind N et al. Evidence based management of mastalgia: a meta analysis of randomised trials. Breast, 2007; 16 (5): 503–12.
9 Expert group for Antibiotic. Mastitis. In: eTG complete [Internet]. Melbourne. Therapeutic Guidelines Ltd. Available from <www.tg.org.au>, accessed April 2018.
10 Jahanfar S, Ng CJ, Teng CI. Antibiotics for mastitis in breastfeeding women. Cochrane Database Syst. Rev. 2009, Issue 1. Article No. CD005458.
11 The Royal Women's Hospital. Policy, Guideline and Procedure Manual. Infant feeding—breast and nipple thrush, 2017. <https://thewomens.r.worldssl.net/images/uploads/downloadable-records/clinical-guidelines/breast-and-nipple-thrush_160517.pdf> (accessed 25/4/2018).

Lumps in the breast 101

Neither the cause of breast cancer, one of the most feared and emotion-engendering diseases, nor the means of preventing it are absolutely known.

ANONYMOUS LECTURER ON BREAST CANCER

Breast lumps are common and their discovery by a woman provokes considerable anxiety and emotion (which is often masked during presentation) because, to many, a breast lump means cancer. Many of the lumps are actually areas of thickening of normal breast tissue. Many other lumps are due to fibrocystic disease with either fibrosis or cyst formation or a combination of the two producing a dominant (discrete) lump. However, a good working rule is to consider any lump in the breast as cancer until proved otherwise. See TABLE 101.1 for causes of breast lumps in a specific outpatient study.

The genetic predisposition to breast cancer continues to be delineated with the strong predisposition from mutations in the genes *BRCA1* and *BRCA2*. Refer to CHAPTER 18.

Key facts and checkpoints

- The commonest lumps are those associated with mammary dysplasia (32%).[1] See TABLE 101.1.
- Fibrocystic disease is also a common cause of cysts, especially in the premenopause phase.
- Over 75% of isolated breast lumps prove to be benign, but clinical identification of a malignant tumour can only definitely be made following aspiration biopsy or histological examination of the tumour.[1]
- The investigation of a new breast lump requires a very careful history and the triple test.
- Breast cancer is the most common cancer in females. The risk of developing breast cancer before age 85 in Australian women is 1 in 8.[2]
- Breast cancer is uncommon under the age of 30 but it then steadily increases to a maximum at the age of about 60 years, being the most common cancer in women over 50 years. The average age of diagnosis is 60.7 years.[3] FIGURE 101.1 highlights the changing frequencies of different discrete breast lumps with age.[4]
- About 25% of all new cancers in women are breast neoplasms.
- A 'dominant' breast lump in an older woman should be regarded as malignant.

Table 101.1 Causes of breast lumps in women: diagnostic strategy model

Probability diagnosis
Fibrocystic disease (32%)
Fibroadenoma (23%)
Cancer (22%)
Cysts (10%)
Breast abscess/periareolar inflammation
Lactation cyst (galactocele)
Serious disorders not to be missed
Vascular:
• thrombophlebitis (Mondor disease)
Infection:
• mastitis/breast abscess
• tuberculosis
Cancer:
• carcinoma
• ductal carcinoma in situ
• Paget disease of the nipple
• sarcoma
• lymphoma
• mastitis carcinomatosa
Other:
• phyllodes tumour
Pitfalls (often missed)
Duct papilloma
Lipoma
Mammary duct ectasia
Fat necrosis/fibrosis

Note: Statistics for probability diagnosis courtesy MA Henderson, PBR Kitchen, PR Hayes, University of Melbourne Department of Surgery, Breast Clinic, St Vincent's Hospital, Melbourne

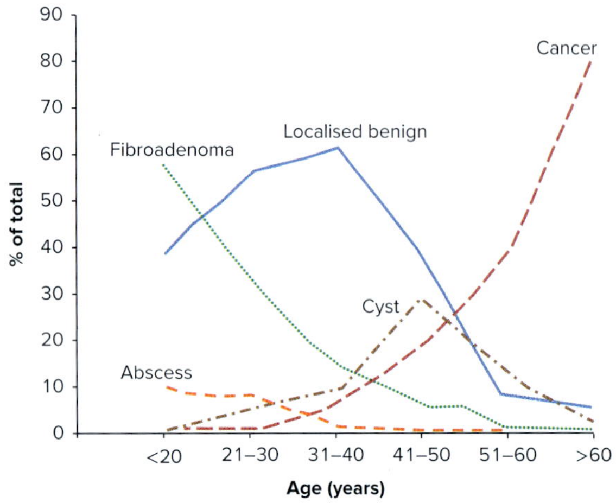

FIGURE 101.1 Changing frequencies of different discrete breast lumps with age

Source: From Dixon & Mansel.[4] Courtesy of Anthea Carter

> **The triple test**
>
> 1 History and clinical breast examination
> 2 Imaging—mammography and/or ultrasound ± MRI
> 3 Fine-needle aspiration cytology and/or core biopsy

The clinical approach

This is based on following a careful history and examination.

History

The history should include a family history of breast disease and the patient's past history, including trauma, previous breast pain, and details about pregnancies (complications of lactation such as mastitis, nipple problems and milk retention).

Key questions[1]

- Have you had any previous problems with your breasts?
- Have you noticed any breast pain or discomfort?
- Do you have any problems such as increased swelling or tenderness before your periods?
- Is the lump constant or changing?
- Have you noticed lumpiness in your breasts before?
- Has the lumpy area been red or hot?
- Have you noticed any discharge from your nipple or nipples?
- Has there been any change in your nipples?
- Does/did your mother or sisters or any close relatives have any breast problems?

Breast symptoms[5]

- Lump (76%)
- Tenderness or pain (10%)
- Nipple changes (8%)
- Nipple discharge (2%)
- Breast or nipple asymmetry or skin dimpling (4%)
- Periareolar inflammation
- Skin thickening or ridging

Important 'tell-tale' symptoms are illustrated in FIGURE 101.2.

Nipple discharge[6]

The diagnostic strategy is outlined in TABLE 101.2.

The discharge may be intermittent, from one or both nipples. It can be induced by quadrant compression.

Table 101.2 Nipple discharge: diagnostic strategy model

Probability diagnosis
Physiological
Pregnancy
Intraduct papilloma
Lactation/lactation cysts
Mammary dysplasia
Serious disorders not to be missed
Infection:
• acute mastitis/discharging breast abscess
• areolar abscess (infected gland of Montgomery)
• tuberculosis abscess
Cancer:
• intraduct carcinoma
• invasive carcinoma
• Paget disease of nipple
Other:
• hyperprolactinaemia
• hypothyroidism
Pitfalls (often missed)
Mammary duct ectasia
Drugs (e.g. chlorpromazine, metoclopramide, OCP, cimetidine, opiates, amphetamines, CCBs, SSRIs, tricyclic antidepressants, phenothiazine)
Rarities:
• mammary duct fistula
• mechanical stimulation

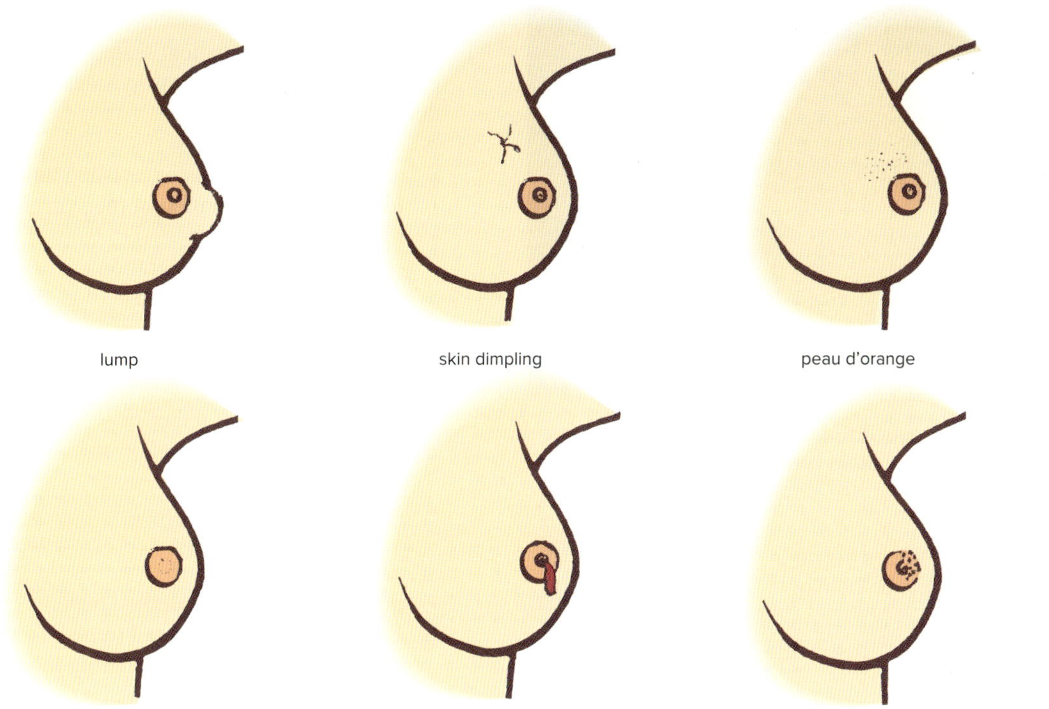

FIGURE 101.2 Important 'tell-tale' symptoms of breast cancer

A common reason is physiological, which is usually part of a normal hormonal process.

Types of discharge

- Bloodstained:
  - intraduct papilloma (commonest)
  - intraduct carcinoma
  - fibrocystic breasts
- Green–grey:
  - fibrocystic breasts
  - mammary duct ectasia
- Yellow:
  - fibrocystic breasts
  - intraduct carcinoma (serous)
  - breast abscess (pus)
- Milky white (galactorrhoea):
  - lactation cysts
  - lactation
  - hyperprolactinaemia
  - drugs (e.g. antipsychotic, cocaine)

Periareolar inflammation

This presents as pain around the areola with reddening of the skin, tenderness and swelling. Causes may be inverted nipple or mammary duct ectasia.

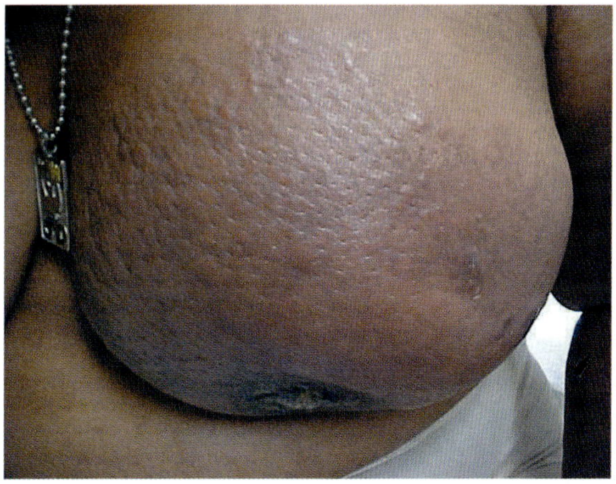

FIGURE 101.3 Woman with advanced breast cancer showing peau d'orange sign, brawny oedema and breast retraction

Paget disease of the nipple

This rare but interesting sign and condition usually occurs in middle-aged and elderly women (see FIG. 101.4). It starts as an eczematous-looking, dry scabbing red rash of the nipple and then proceeds to ulceration of the nipple and areola (see TABLE 101.3). It is always due to an underlying malignancy.

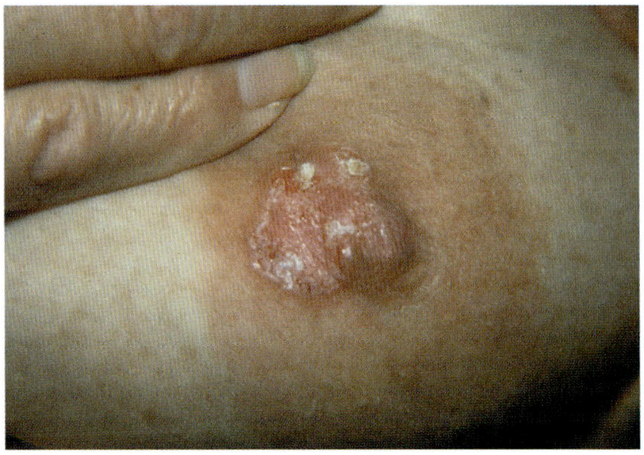

FIGURE 101.4 Paget disease of the breast: note the erythematous, eczematous, scaly appearance of the nipple

Table 101.3 Differences between Paget disease and eczema of the nipple[6]

Paget disease	Eczema
Unilateral	Bilateral
Older patients	Younger: reproductive years
Ulceration	Ulceration rare
Possible nipple discharge	No discharge
Not pruritic	Pruritic
No pustules or vesicles	Pustules and vesicles
Deformity of nipple	Normal nipple
Possible palpable lump	No lump
Mammographic changes	Normal mammogram

Examination of the breasts

Objectives

- Identify a dominant lump (one that differs from the remainder of the breast tissue).
- Identify a lump that may be malignant.
- Screen the breasts for early development of cancer.

Time of examination: ideally, 4 days after the end of the period.

Red flag pointers for breast lumps

- Hard and irregular lump
- Skin dimpling and puckering
- Skin oedema ('peau d'orange') (FIG. 101.3)
- Nipple discharge
- Nipple distortion
- Nipple eczema
- Postmenopausal women

Method[1]

1 Inspection: sitting—patient seated upright on side of couch in good light, arms by sides, facing the doctor, undressed to waist.

A *Note:*

- asymmetry of breasts or a visible lump
- localised discolouration of the skin
- nipples:
  - for retraction or ulceration
  - for variations in the level (e.g. elevation on one side)
  - or discharge (e.g. blood-stained, clear, yellow)
- skin attachment or tethering → dimpling of skin (accentuate this sign by asking patient to raise her arms above her head)
- appearance of small nodules of growth
- visible veins (if unilateral they suggest a cancer)[7]
- peau d'orange due to dermal oedema

B Raise arms above the head (renders variations in nipple level and skin tethering more obvious). Hands are pressed on the hips to contract pectoralis major to note if there is a deep attachment of the lump.

2 Examination of lymph glands in sitting position: patient with hands on hips. Examine axillary and supraclavicular glands from behind and front.

Note: The draining lymphatic nodes are in the axillae, supraclavicular fossae and internal mammary chain.

3 Palpation:

A Patient still seated: palpate breast with flat of hand and then palpate the bulk of the breast between both hands.

B In supine position:

- patient lies supine on couch with arms above head
- turn body (slight rotation) towards midline so breasts 'sit' as flat as possible on chest wall

Method

- Use the pulps of the fingers rather than the tips with the hand laid flat on the breast.
- Move the hand in slow circular movements.
- Examine up and down the breast in vertical strips beginning from the axillary tail (see FIG. 101.5).
  - Systematically cover the six areas of the breast (see FIG. 101.6):
    - the four quadrants
    - the axillary tail
    - the region deep to the nipple and areola

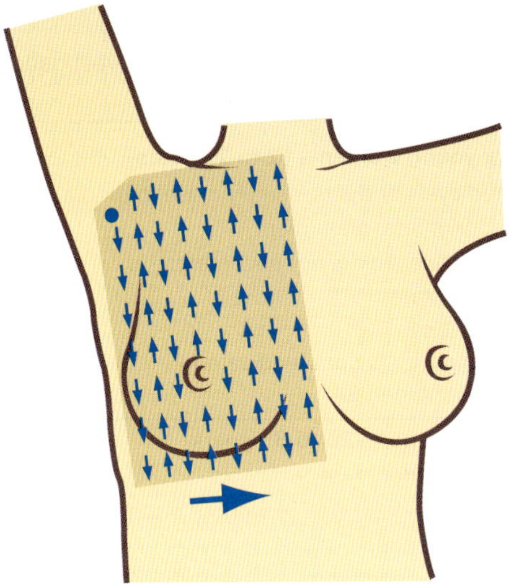

FIGURE 101.5 Systematic examination of the breast

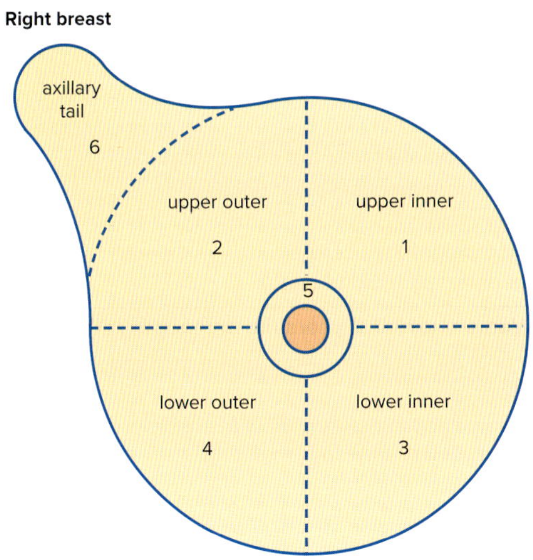

FIGURE 101.6 The six areas of the breast

4 If a suspicious lump is present, inspect liver, lungs and spine.

Note:

- Most cancers occur in the upper outer quadrant (see FIG. 101.7).[6]
- A useful diagram to record the findings is shown in FIGURE 101.8.
- Lumps that are usually benign and require no immediate action are: tiny (<4 mm) nodules in subcutaneous tissue (usually in the areolar margin); elongated ridges, usually bilateral and in the lower aspects of the breasts; and rounded soft nodules (usually <6 mm) around the areolar margin.[8]
- A hard mass is suspicious of malignancy but cancer can be soft because of fat entrapment.
- The inframammary ridge, which is usually found in the heavier breast, is often nodular and firm to hard.
- Lumpiness (if present) is usually most marked in the upper outer quadrant.

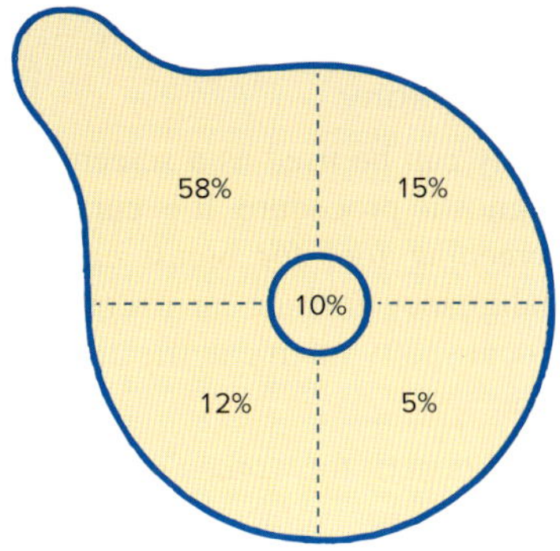

FIGURE 101.7 Relative frequencies of breast cancer at various anatomical segments

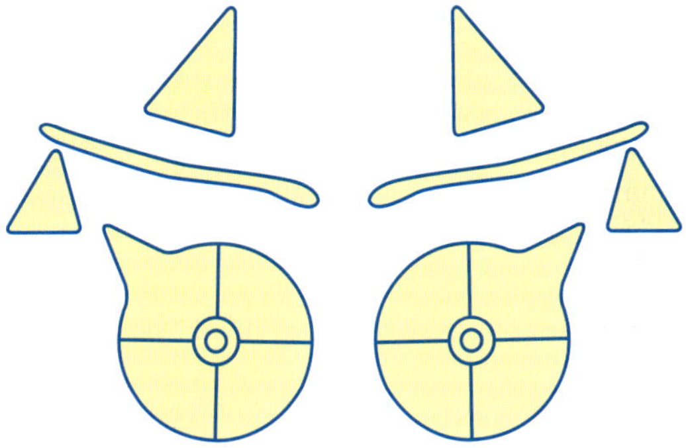

FIGURE 101.8 Diagrammatic scheme for recording the features of breast lumps and any lymphadenopathy (axilla and supraclavicular triangles)

If a solitary lump is present, assess it for:

- position (breast quadrant and proximity to nipple)
- size and shape
- consistency (firm, hard, cystic, soft)
- tenderness
- mobility and fixation
- attachment to skin or underlying muscle

Investigations

X-ray mammography

Mammography can be used as a screening procedure and as a diagnostic procedure. It is currently the most effective screening tool for breast cancer.[9] Positive signs of malignancy include an irregular infiltrating mass with focal spotty microcalcification.

Screening:

- established benefit for women over 50 years
- possible benefit for women in their 40s
- follow-up in those with breast cancer, as 6% develop in the opposite breast
- localisation of the lesion for fine-needle aspiration

Breast ultrasound

This is mainly used to elucidate an area of breast density and is the best method of defining benign breast disease, especially with cystic changes. It is generally most useful in women less than 35 years old (as compared with X-ray mammography).

Useful for:

- pregnant and lactating breast
- differentiating between fluid-filled cysts and solid mass
- palpable masses at periphery of breast tissue (not screened by mammography)
- for more accurate localisation of lump during fine-needle aspiration

Note: CT and MRI have limited use. An age-related schemata for likely diagnosis and appropriate investigations is presented in TABLE 101.4.

> **Breast imaging for palpable lumps—summary**
>
> - <35 years: bilateral ultrasound; bilateral mammography if ultrasound suspicious
> - 35–50 years: bilateral mammography + bilateral ultrasound
> - >50 years: bilateral mammography ± bilateral ultrasound

Needle aspiration and biopsy techniques

- Cyst aspiration
- Fine-needle aspiration biopsy: this is a very useful diagnostic test in solid lumps, and has an accuracy of 90–95% (better than mammography)[6]
- Large needle (core needle) biopsy
- Incision biopsy

Table 101.4 Age-related schemata for likely diagnoses and appropriate investigations (after Hirst)[8]

1 Very young women—12 to 25 years

Inflamed cysts or ducts, usually close to areola
Fibroadenomata, often giant
Hormonal thickening, not uncommon
Malignancy rare
Investigations:

- mammography contraindicated
- ultrasound helpful

2 Young women—26 to 35 years

Classic fibroadenomata
Fibrocystic disease with or without discharge
Cysts uncommon
Malignancy uncommon
Investigations:

- mammography: breasts often very dense
- ultrasound often diagnostic

3 Women—36 to 50 years (premenopausal)

Cysts
Fibrocystic disease, discharges, duct papillomas
Malignancy common
Fibroadenomata occur but cannot assume
Inflammatory processes not uncommon
Investigations:

- mammography useful
- targeted ultrasound useful

4 Women—over 50 years (postmenopausal)

Any new discrete mass—malignant until proven otherwise
Any new thickening—regard with suspicion
Inflammatory lesions—probably duct ectasia (follow to resolution)
Cysts unlikely
Investigations:

- mammography usually diagnostic (first line)
- ultrasound may be useful

5 Women—over 50 years, on hormones

Any new mass—regard with suspicion
Cysts may occur—usually asymptomatic
Hormonal change not uncommon
Investigations:

- mammography usually diagnostic but breast may become more dense
- ultrasound may be useful if above normal or unhelpful and lump suspicious

Source: After Hirst.[8] Reprinted with permission

Tumour markers

Oestrogen receptors are uncommon in normal breasts but are found in two-thirds of breast cancers, although the incidence varies with age. They are good prognostic indicators. Progesterone receptors can also be estimated.

Fine-needle aspiration of breast lump

This simple technique is very useful, especially if the lump is a cyst, and will have no adverse effects if the lump is not malignant. If it is, the needle biopsy will help with the preoperative cytological diagnosis.

Follow-up: the plan for aspiration is outlined in FIGURE 101.9.

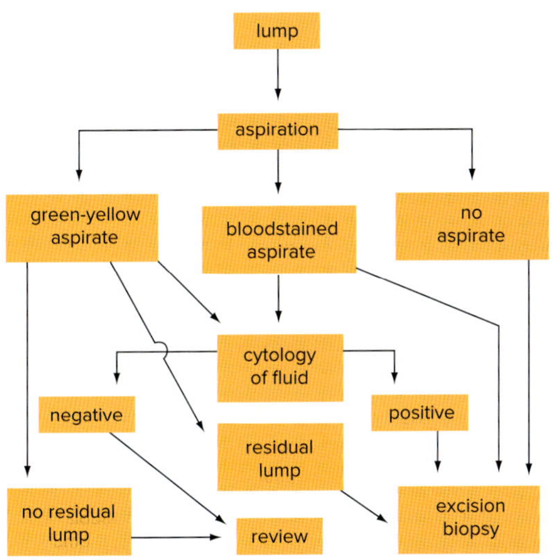

FIGURE 101.9 Scheme for management of a breast lump by fine-needle aspiration

Summary: investigation of a breast lump

If the patient presenting with a breast lump is younger than 35, perform an ultrasound;[10] if older than 35 perform a mammogram and an ultrasound. If the lump is cystic—aspirate; if solid—perform a fine-needle biopsy and then manage according to outcomes. If it is suspicious, an excisional biopsy is the preferred option.

More than 99% of breast cancers will be detected if any component of an appropriately performed triple test is positive.[11]

Indications for biopsy or excision of lump

- The cyst fluid is bloodstained.
- The lump does not disappear completely with aspiration.
- The swelling recurs within 1 month.

Breast cancer

Breast cancer is uncommon under the age of 30 but it then steadily increases to a maximum at the age of about 60 years.[6] About one-third of women who develop breast cancer are premenopausal and two-thirds postmenopausal. Ninety per cent of breast cancers are invasive ductal carcinomas, the remainder being lobular carcinoma, papillary carcinomas, medullary carcinomas and colloid or mucoid carcinomas.[1]

Risk factors include:

- increasing age (>40 years)
- living in a Western population
- pre-existing benign breast lumps
- alcohol intake >2 SDs/day
- use of menopause hormonal therapy (MHT) (combined oestrogen and progestogen) >5 years
- personal history of breast cancer
- family history in a first-degree relative (raises risk about threefold)
- known genetic mutations *BRCA1* or *BRCA2*
- nulliparity
- late menopause (after 53)
- obesity
- childless until after 30 years of age
- early menarche[9]
- ionising radiation exposure
- Ashkenazi Jewish ancestry

Familial breast cancer

Up to 5% of cases are familial, with most being autosomal dominant. Refer to CHAPTER 18.

Clinical features

- The majority of patients with breast cancer present with a lump (76%).[6]
- The lump is usually painless (10% associated with pain).
- Usually the lump is hard and irregular.
- Nipple changes, discharge, retraction or distortion.
- Rarely cancer can present with Paget disease of breast (nipple eczema) or inflammatory breast cancer (see CHAPTER 100).
- Rarely it can present with bony secondaries (e.g. back pain, dyspnoea, weight loss, headache).

Note: There are basically three presentations of the disease:

- the vast majority present with a local breast lump[1]
- ductal carcinoma in situ
- some present with metastatic disease

Of those who present with local disease, approximately 50% will develop metastatic disease.

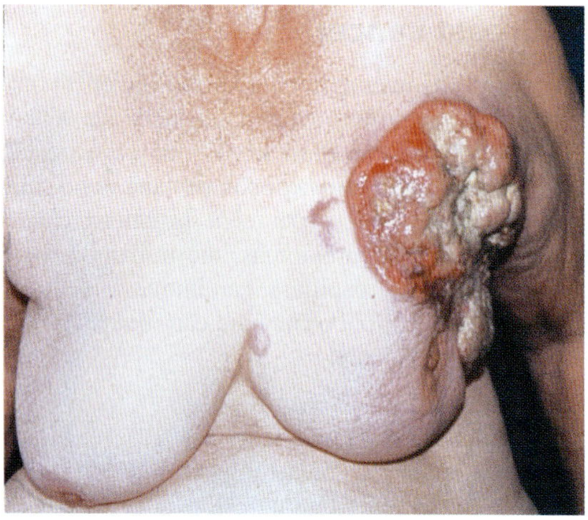

FIGURE 101.10 Advanced adenocarcinoma of breast in patient showing denial for a problem of 2 years' duration.
Photo courtesy Dr Victor Vanco

Management

Immediate referral to an expert surgeon on suspicion or proof of breast cancer is essential.

Guidelines for referral include:[11]

- any positive component of the triple test
- incomplete cyst aspiration
- spontaneous unilateral bloody or serious discharge from a single duct (especially in women aged 60 years and over)
- persistent eczematoid changes of nipple that do not respond to topical treatment
- unresolving inflammatory mastitis

The treatment has to be individualised according to the nature of the lump, age of the patient and staging. Accurate staging requires knowledge of whether the draining lymph nodes are involved with the tumour, as this is the single most powerful predictor of subsequent metastases and death. Staging for systemic disease also requires full blood examination and liver function tests (including alkaline phosphatase). A bone scan may be used as a valuable baseline. Size and histological grading of tumour plus nodal status and receptor status are the most important prognostic factors.

Optimal management of locally advanced breast cancer is a combined approach that uses chemotherapy, radiotherapy, surgery and/or endocrine therapy if applicable (level IV evidence).

Surgical options are:

- lumpectomy to negative margin
- mastectomy
- mastectomy with reconstruction

Most relapses[12] after surgery occur in the first 3 years.

Ductal carcinoma in situ

DCIS is a non-invasive abnormal proliferation of milk duct epithelial cells within the ductal–lobular system and is a precursor lesion for invasive breast cancer. Since mammography screening it is readily detected and now comprises about 20% of breast cancer. It may present clinically with a palpable mass or nipple discharge or Paget disease of the nipple with or without a mass.

Management

Management decisions are challenging, with options being total mastectomy or breast-conserving therapy with or without radiotherapy. Patients usually have an excellent outcome with low local recurrence rates and a survival of at least 98%.[13]

Adjuvant therapy for breast cancer

The consultant will choose the most appropriate surgical and adjuvant treatments (which are designed to treat and destroy micrometastatic disease) for the individual patient.

The National Breast Cancer Consensus report emphasised that 'continuing care should be coordinated through the patient's GP as the impact of treatment may last longer than therapy and support must continue'. The report made the following recommendations:[14]

- Tumour excision followed by whole breast irradiation was the most preferred local therapy for most women with stage I or II cancer.
- Total mastectomy and breast-conservation surgery had an equivalent effect on survival.
- Total mastectomy is preferred for a large tumour, multifocal disease, previous irradiation and extensive tumour on mammography.
- Recommendations for radiotherapy after mastectomy are:[15]
  - tumours >4 cm in diameter
  - axillary node involvement of >3 nodes
  - the presence of positive or close tumour margins
- Intraoperative radiotherapy following tumour excision is one of several techniques for partial breast irradiation.[16]
- Cytotoxic chemotherapy has an important place in management, especially in young, healthy women who are E receptor negative and have visceral spread.[17]

- Adjuvant hormonal therapy by the anti-oestrogen agent tamoxifen 20 mg (o) daily if E receptor +ve, which is a specific modulating agent, is widely used and is most suitable in postmenopausal women. The usual course is 5 years.

  Adjunct agents available for treatment include:[18,19]

- anti-oestrogens (E receptor blockers or SERMS): tamoxifen, toremifene
- aromatase inhibitors (for hormone receptor +ve cancer in postmenopausal women): anastrozole, letrozole, exemestane
- monoclonal antibodies: trastuzumab (Herceptin) or pertuzumab (Perjeta)
- bisphosphonates: recommended for women with bony metastases since evidence indicates reversal of bone density loss and cancer recurrence[17,18]
- progesterones (e.g. medroxyprogesterone acetate)
- the OCP (if taken) should be ceased, and pregnancy is inadvisable

  Guidelines for adjuvant treatments can be accessed at <guidelines.nbocc.org.au/guidelines/guideline_2.pdf>.

Fibrocystic breasts

Synonyms: fibroadenosis, chronic mastitis, mammary dysplasia, cystic hyperplasia, fibrocystic disease.

Clinical features

- Most common in women between 30 and 50 years
- Hormone-related (between menarche and menopause)
- Pain and tenderness and swelling
- Premenstrual discomfort or pain and increased swelling
- Fluctuation in the size of the mass
- Usually settles after the period
- Unilateral or bilateral
- Nodularity ± a discrete mass
- Ache may extend down inner aspect of upper arm
- Nipple discharge may occur (various colours, mainly green–grey)
- Most cysts are premenopausal (final 5 years before menopause)

Examination. Look for lumpiness in one or both breasts, usually upper outer quadrant.

Management

- Consider mammography if diffuse lumpiness is present in patient >40 years.
- Perform needle biopsy if a discrete lump is present and aspirate palpable cysts.
- Reassure patient that there is no cancer.
- Give advice to alleviate mastalgia (see treatment for cyclical mastalgia in CHAPTER 100).
- Use analgesics as necessary.
- Surgically remove undiagnosed mass lesions.

Breast cyst

- Common in women aged 40–50 years (perimenopausal)
- Rare under 30 years
- Associated with mammary dysplasia
- Tends to regress after the menopause
- Pain and tenderness variable, most asymptomatic
- Has a 1 in 1000 incidence of cancer
- Usually lined by duct epithelium

Examination. Look for a discrete mass, firm, relatively mobile, that is rarely fluctuant.

Diagnosis

- Mammography
- Ultrasound (investigation of choice)
- Cytology of aspirate

Management

- Drainage with a fine needle
  Surgery is rarely required.

Localised nodularity

Usually:

- in upper outer quadrant of breast
- a physiological change to breast
- managed with clinical surveillance
- investigate with imaging in older women if asymmetric or perceived change

Lactation cysts (galactoceles)

- These milk-containing cysts arise during pregnancy and present postpartum with similar signs to perimenopausal cysts.
- They vary from 1–5 cm in diameter.
- Treat by aspiration: fluid may be clear or milky.

Fibroadenoma

Clinical features

- A discrete, asymptomatic lump
- Usually in 20s (range: second to sixth decade, commonly 15–35 years)
- Firm, smooth and mobile (the 'breast mouse')
- Usually rounded
- Usually in upper outer quadrant
- May double in size every 12 months[7]

Management

Ultrasound and fine-needle aspiration or core biopsy with cytology are recommended plus mammography in older women. If needle aspiration or core biopsy is negative, the patient can be reassured and followed up until the fibroadenoma is deemed stable. A repeat ultrasound and examination within 6–12 months is ideal. Excision biopsy if large (>3–4 cm), continues to enlarge, suspicious biopsy or woman >40 years.

Phyllodes tumour[20]

These are giant fibroadenoma-like tumours that are usually benign but 25% are malignant and metastasise. They are completely excised with a rim of normal breast tissue.

Fat necrosis

Fat necrosis is usually the end result of a large bruise or trauma that may be subtle, such as protracted breastfeeding. The mass that results is often accompanied by skin or nipple retraction and thus closely resembles cancer. If untreated it usually disappears but the diagnosis can only be made on excision biopsy.

The full triple test is required.

Duct papillomas

These are benign hyperplastic lesions within large mammary ducts and are not premalignant (nor usually palpable). They present with nipple bleeding or a bloodstained discharge and must be differentiated from infiltrating carcinoma. Mammography and ductography are usually of limited value. The involved duct and affected breast segment should be excised.[20]

Mammary duct ectasia

Synonyms: plasma cell mastitis, periductal mastitis.

In this benign condition a whole breast quadrant may be indurated and tender. The larger breast ducts are dilated. The lump is usually located near the margin of the areola and is a firm or hard, tender, poorly defined swelling. There may be a toothpaste-like nipple discharge. It is a troublesome condition with a tendency to repeated episodes of periareolar inflammation with recurrent abscesses and fistula formation. Many cases settle but sometimes surgical intervention is necessary to make the diagnosis. The condition is most common in the decade around the menopause.

The problem of mammary prostheses[8]

Clinical examination is still necessary and fortunately the residual mammary tissue is usually spread over the prosthesis in a thin, easily palpable layer. The areas of clinical difficulty lie at the margin of the prosthesis, especially in the upper outer quadrant where most of the breast tissue is displaced. It should be noted that mammography may be of limited value in the presence of prostheses, especially if a fibrous capsule exists around the prosthesis. Ultrasound examination may be helpful.

Lymphoedema of arm

This is a long-term complication of surgery plus irradiation for breast cancer treatment when there is a failure of the lymphatic system to adequately drain extracellular fluid. The limb feels tight and heavy with decreased mobility. Exclude obstruction of the deep venous system by Doppler ultrasound.

Skin changes can occur from long-term lymphoedema without treatment, and cellulitis from abrasions and wounds is a concern.

Management

- Encourage movement; elevation of the arm on a pillow at night; avoid slings
- Physiotherapy: a reduction phase with non-elasticised bandages then maintenance with graduated pressure support sleeves
- Elastic sleeves worn all day but not at night
- Lymphoedema massage at home
- Skin hygiene: regular use of non-perfumed emollients, prevention of infection and injury. Avoid sunburn and insect bites
- Avoid BP measurement, venesection and IV therapy in that arm
- Consider diuretics to relieve pressure

Breast lumps in children

There are several benign conditions that can cause a breast lump in children, although the commonest presentation is a diffuse breast enlargement.

Neonatal enlargement[21]

Newborn babies of either sex can present with breast hyperplasia and secretion of breast milk (see CHAPTER 91). This is due to transplacental passage of lactogenic hormones. The swelling usually lasts 7–10 days if left alone. Any attempts to manipulate the breasts to facilitate emptying will prolong the problem.

Premature hyperplasia[21]

The usual presentation is the development of one breast in girls commonly 7–9 years of age but sometimes younger. The feature is a firm discoid lump 1–2 cm in diameter, situated deep to the nipple. The same change may follow in the other breast within 3–12 months. Reassurance and explanation is the management and biopsy must be avoided at all costs.

Counselling of patients

'Treat the whole woman, not merely her breasts.'[8] Extreme anxiety is generated by the discovery of a breast lump and it is important that women are encouraged to visit their doctor early, especially as they can learn that there is a 90% chance of their lump being benign. It is possible that denial may be a factor or there is a hidden agenda to the consultation. The decision to perform a lumpectomy or a mastectomy should take the patient's feelings into consideration—many do fear that a breast remnant may be a focus for cancer. Long-standing doctor–patient relationships are the ideal basis for coping with the difficulties.

Screening

For asymptomatic, low-risk women, screening mammography is advised every 2 years between the ages of 50 and 74 (see CHAPTER 9). In Australia, screening mammography is optional for women aged between 40 and 49. Technically, it is a better diagnostic tool in older women because of the less dense and glandular breast tissue. It has a specificity of around 90%.

The Familial Risk Assessment—Breast and Ovarian Cancer (FRA–BOC) online tool can be used to guide screening for women at increased risk. This can be accessed at <https://canceraustralia.gov.au/clinical-best-practice/gynaecological-cancers/familial-risk-assessment-fra-boc>.

A FRA–BOC risk assessment places women in one of three categories:

- Category 1—at (or slightly above) average risk. Optional 2-yearly mammograms from 40 years, routinely recommended from age 50.
- Category 2—moderately increased risk. Annual mammograms from age 40 may be recommended if the woman has a first-degree relative <50 years diagnosed with breast cancer. Otherwise, routine 2-yearly mammograms are advised.
- Category 3—potentially high risk. Referral to a family cancer clinic recommended for possible genetic testing. Increased surveillance is determined on an individual basis.

Breast self-examination is a controversial issue and has no proven benefit in reducing morbidity and mortality. The false positive rate is high, especially in those under 40 years. There is also insufficient evidence to support routine clinical breast examination, although there may be a role for it in the case of women who are not participating in regular mammographic screening. Breast awareness, which involves being familiar with the look and feel of one's breasts and presenting early if a change is detected, should be promoted to all women.

101

When to refer

- Patients with a solitary breast mass
- Following cyst aspiration:
  - blood in aspirate
  - palpable residual lump
  - recurrence of the cyst
- Patients given antineoplastic drugs, whether for adjuvant therapy or for advanced disease, require skilled supervision

Lumps that require investigation and referral are presented in TABLE 101.5.

Table 101.5 Lumps that require investigation and referral[8]

Lumps that require investigation and referral
A stony, hard lump or area, regardless of size, history or position
A new palpable 'anything' in a postmenopausal woman
A persisting painless asymmetrical thickening
An enlarging mass—cyclic or not
A 'slow-to-resolve' or recurrent inflammation
A bloodstained or serous nipple discharge
Skin dimpling, of even a minor degree, or retraction of the nipple
A new thickening or mass in the vicinity of a scar

Source: After Hirst[8]

Practice tips

- Any doubtful breast lump should be removed.
- Fibroadenomas commonly occur in women in their late teens and 20s, benign breast cysts between 35 years and the menopause, and cancer is the most common cause of a lump in women over 50 years.[6]
- Never assume a palpable mass is a fibroadenoma in any woman over 30 years of age.[8]
- Gentle palpation is required. Squeezing breast tissue between finger and thumb tends to produce 'pseudolumps'.

continued

continued

- Any eczematous rash appearing on the nipple or areola indicates underlying breast cancer.
- Mammary duct ectasia and fat necrosis can be clinically indistinguishable from breast cancer.
- Nine out of 10 women who get breast cancer do not have a strong family history.
- The oral contraceptive pill has been generally shown *not* to alter the risk of breast cancer.
- Never assume that a lump is due to trauma unless you have seen the bruising and can observe the lump decrease in size.[8]
- Never assume a lesion is a cyst—prove it with ultrasound or successful aspiration.[8]
- Never ignore skin dimpling even if no underlying mass is palpable.[8]
- Never ignore a woman's insistence that an area of her breast is different or has changed.[8]
- Mammography can detect breast cancers that are too small to feel.
- Mammography is not a diagnostic tool.
- Mammography screening recommended for low-risk women aged 50–74 years and those aged 40–49 who request it.

Patient education resources

Hand-out sheets from *Murtagh's Patient Education* 7th edition:

- Breast cancer
- Breast lumps
- Breast awareness and breast self-examination

References

1 Green M. Breast cancer. In: *MIMS Disease Index* (2nd edn). Sydney: IMS Publishing, 1996: 83–5.

2 Australian Cancer Incidence and Mortality (ACIM) books. Breast Cancer for Australia (ICD-IO C50) <www.aihw.gov.au/acim-books/> (accessed March 2014).

3 Australian Institute of Health and Welfare & Australasian Association of Cancer Registries 2012. Cancer in Australia: an overview, 2012. Cancer Series No. 74, Cat. No. CAN 70. Canberra: AIHW.

4 Dixon JM, Mansel RE. Congenital problems and aberrations of normal breast development. In: Dixon JM, ed., *ABC of Breast Diseases*. London: British Medical Journal Publishing Group, 1995.

5 Mazza D. *Women's Health in General Practice* (2nd edn). Sydney: Elsevier, 2011: 185.

6 Fox J. Breast problems. In: Smith JA et al. (eds), *Hunt and Marshall's Clinical Problems in General Surgery* (2nd edn), Sydney: Elsevier, 2010: 67–76.

7 Talley N, O'Connor S. *Clinical Examination* (7th edn). Sydney: Elsevier, 2010: 435–7.

8 Hirst C. Managing the breast lump. Solving the dilemma—reassurance versus investigation. Aust Fam Physician, 1989; 18: 121–6.

9 Barraclough B. The fibrocystic breast—clinical assessment, diagnosis and treatment. Modern Medicine Australia, 1990; April: 16–25.

10 Crea P. Benign breast diseases: a management guide for GPs. Modern Medicine Australia, 1995; 38 (8): 74–88.

11 Cancer Australia, Australian Government. *The investigation of a new breast symptom: a guide for general practitioners*, 2017. <https://canceraustralia.gov.au/publications-and-resources/cancer-australia-publications/investigation-new-breast-symptom-guide-general-practitioners> (accessed 16/5/2018).

12 National Health and Medical Research Council. *Management of Advanced Breast Cancer: Clinical Practice Guidelines.* NHMRC Clinical Practice Guidelines 2001. Canberra: NHMRC, 2001.

13 Stuart K, Boyages J, Brennan, M et al. Ductal carcinoma in situ. Aust Fam Physician, 2005; 34 (11): 949–53.

14 Coates A. Breast Cancer Consensus report. Med J Aust, 1994; 161: 510–13.

15 Wetzig NR. Breast cancer: how to treat. Australian Doctor, 19 October 2001: I–VIII.

16 Buglar L, James T et al. Breast cancer for GPs. Australian Doctor (Suppl), March 2008: 10–13.

17 Crea P, Segelov E, Yeo B. Breast cancer—part 2: how to treat. Australian Doctor, 20 Nov 2010: 23–9.

18 Buckley N (Chair). *Australian Medicines Handbook*. Adelaide: Australian Medicines Handbook Pty Ltd, 2013: 559–63.

19 Boyages J, Prassar G. Adjuvant hormonal treatment of breast cancer. Medical Observer, 3 August 2012: 27–9.

20 Burkitt H, Quick C, Gatt D. *Essential Surgery* (2nd edn). Edinburgh: Churchill Livingstone, 1996: 542.

21 Hutson JM, Beasley SW, Woodward AA. *Jones Clinical Paediatric Surgery*. Melbourne: Blackwell Scientific Publications, 1992: 266–7.

Abnormal uterine bleeding 102

The classification system for abnormal uterine bleeding uses nine basic categories, separated into structural and non structural conditions: (PALM-COEIN) ***P****olyp,* ***A****denomyosis,* ***L****eiomyoma,* ***M****alignancy–* ***C****oagulopathy,* ***O****vulatory disorders,* ***E****ndometrium,* ***I****atrogenic and* ***N****ot otherwise specified.*

FEDERATION OF GYNAECOLOGY AND OBSTETRICS, 2011

Abnormal uterine bleeding is a common problem encountered in general practice. Heavy menstrual bleeding is the commonest cause of iron-deficiency anaemia in the Western world. A classification of abnormal uterine bleeding is presented in TABLE 102.1.

Table 102.1 Classification of abnormal uterine bleeding

Abnormal rhythm
Irregularity of cycle
Intermenstrual bleeding (metrorrhagia)
Postcoital bleeding
Postmenopausal bleeding
Abnormal amount
Increased amount = menorrhagia/heavy menstrual bleeding
Decreased amount = hypomenorrhoea
Combination (rhythm and amount)
Irregular and heavy periods = metromenorrhagia
Irregular and light periods = oligomenorrhoea
Absence of periods = amenorrhoea

Key facts and checkpoints

- Up to 20% of women in the reproductive age group complain of increased menstrual loss.[1]
- At least 4% of consultations in general practice deal with abnormal uterine bleeding.
- Up to 50% of patients who present with perceived menorrhagia (or excessive blood loss) have a normal blood loss when investigated.[1]
- The possibility of pregnancy and its complications, such as ectopic pregnancy, miscarriage (threatened, complete or incomplete), hydatidiform mole or choriocarcinoma should be kept in mind.[2]
- A menstrual record is a useful way to calculate blood loss.
- The mean blood loss in a menstrual cycle is 30–40 mL.
- Blood loss is normally less than 80 mL.
- Heavy menstrual bleeding (menorrhagia)—HMB—is a menstrual loss of more than 80 mL per menstruation.
- HMB disposes women to iron-deficiency anaemia.
- Two common organic causes of HMB are fibroids and adenomyosis (presence of endometrium in the uterine myometrium).[3]
- Various drugs can alter menstrual bleeding (e.g. anticoagulants, cannabis, steroids).

Defining what is normal and what is abnormal

This feature is based on a meticulous history, an understanding of the physiology and physiopathology of the menstrual cycle and a clear understanding of what is normal. Most girls reach menarche by the age of 13 (range 10–16 years).[1] Dysfunctional bleeding is common in the first 2–3 years after menarche due to many anovulatory cycles resulting in irregular periods, heavy menses and probably dysmenorrhoea.

Once ovulation and regular menstruation are established the cycle usually follows a predictable pattern and any deviation can be considered as abnormal uterine bleeding (see TABLE 102.2). It is abnormal if the cycle is less than 21 days, the duration of loss is more than 7 days, or the volume of loss is

Table 102.2 Normal menstruation in the reproductive age group

	Mean	Range
Length of cycle	26–28 days	21–35 days
Menstrual flow	3–4 days	2–7 days
Normal blood loss	30–40 mL	20–80 mL

Source: After Fung[1]

such that menstrual pads of adequate absorbency cannot cope with the flow or clots.[4]

A normal endometrial thickness, as measured by ultrasound (best on days 4–7 of cycle), is between 6 and 12 mm in premenopausal women, <5 mm in perimenopausal women and ≤4 mm in postmenopausal women.

Relationship of bleeding to age

Dysfunctional uterine bleeding (DUB) is more common at the extremes of the reproductive era (see FIG. 102.1).[2,3] The incidence of malignant disease as a cause of bleeding increases with age, being greatest after the age of 45, while endometrial cancer is predicted to be less than 1 in 100 000 in women under the age of 35.[1]

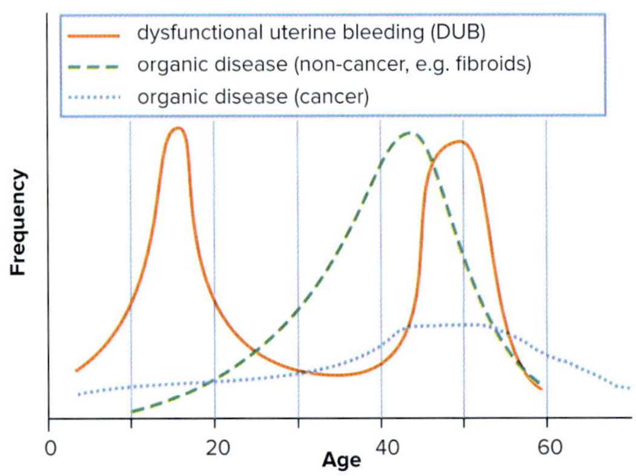

FIGURE 102.1 The relationship between age and various causes of abnormal uterine bleeding. Dysfunctional uterine bleeding is more common in the extremes of the reproductive era, while the incidence of cancer as a cause of bleeding is greatest in the perimenopausal and postmenopausal phases.

Source: After Mackay et al[2]

Heavy menstrual bleeding (HMB)

Heavy menstrual bleeding is:

- blood loss >80 mL per menstrual cycle
- bleeding that persists >7 days
- bleeding that is unacceptable to the woman

Menorrhagia[4] is essentially caused by excessive local production of prostaglandins in the endometrium and myometrium and/or excessive local fibrinolytic activity. Heavy bleeding, possibly with clots, is the major symptom of menorrhagia. Dysmenorrhoea may accompany the bleeding and, if it does, endometriosis or PID should be suspected. With care a 60–80% accuracy can be achieved in clinical assessment.[4] A summary of the diagnostic strategy model is presented in TABLE 102.3.

By far the most common single 'cause' of menorrhagia is ovulatory dysfunctional uterine bleeding (DUB). Anovulatory DUB occurs at the extremes of the reproductive period—around menarche and perimenopausally. The most common organic causes are fibromyomatas (fibroids), endometriosis,

Table 102.3 HMB: diagnostic strategy model
Probability diagnosis
Dysfunctional uterine bleeding—ovulatory
Fibroids
Complications of hormone therapy
Adenomyosis
Serious disorders not to be missed (see TABLE 101.4)
Disorders of pregnancy:
• ectopic pregnancy
• abortion or miscarriage
Neoplasia:
• cervical cancer
• endometrial cancer
• oestrogen-producing ovarian tumour (cancer)
• gestational trophoblastic disease
• leukaemia
• benign tumours (polyps, etc.)
Endometrial hyperplasia
Severe infections:
• PID
Pitfalls (often missed)
Genital tract trauma
Copper IUD
Adenomyosis/endometriosis
SLE
Rarities:
• endocrine disorders (e.g. thyroid disease)
• bleeding disorder (e.g. von Willebrand disease)
• liver disease
Seven masquerades checklist
Depression (association)
Diabetes
Drugs
Anaemia (association)
Thyroid disorder (hypothyroidism)
Is the patient trying to tell me something?
Consider exaggerated perception. Note association with anxiety and depression.

Table 102.4 Important 'not to miss' causes of irregular bleeding[5]

15–20	20–30	30–45	45–55	55 + (years)
Chlamydia/PID			Endometrial/ovarian cancer	
Pregnancy and pregnancy complications				
		Endometrial polyps		
		Endometrial hyperplasia		
Cervical cancer[5] →				

adenomyosis ('endometriosis' of the myometrium), endometrial polyps and PID.[2]

Acute heavy bleeding or 'flooding' most often occurs in pubertal girls before regular ovulation is established. Rarely, a coagulopathy may be the cause in young women with acute severe bleeding.

History

Bear in mind that abnormal uterine bleeding is a subjective complaint, and a detailed history is the key initial step in management. The patient's perception of abnormal bleeding may be misleading and education about normality might be all that is necessary. A meticulous history should include details of the number of tampons or pads used and their degree of saturation. Ask about clotting, flooding and simultaneous use of pads and tampons. A pictorial blood assessment chart can be a very useful guide.

Enquire about contraceptive use and dyspareunia and take a sexual history. A history of smoking and psychosocial factors should also be checked. For unknown reasons, cigarette smokers are five times more likely to have abnormal menstrual function.[1]

> **Practice tip**
>
> Clots, flooding and the need for simultaneous use of pads and tampons are good indicators of HMB.

Questions need to be directed to rule out:[1]

- pregnancy or pregnancy complications (e.g. ectopic pregnancy)
- trauma of the genital tract
- medical disorders (e.g. bleeding disorder)
- endocrine disorders
- cancer of the genital tract
- complications of hormonal contraception or replacement therapy

Examination[1]

A general physical examination should aim at ruling out anaemia, evidence of a bleeding disorder and any other stigmata of relevant medical or endocrine disease.

Specific examinations include:

- speculum examination: ? ulcers (cervical cancer) or polyps
- cervical screening test (if due)
- abdominal examination (an enlarged fibroid uterus may be palpable)
- bimanual pelvic examination: ? uterine or adnexal tenderness, size and regularity of uterus

It is prudent to avoid vaginal examination in selected patients, such as a young virgin girl, as the procedure is unhelpful and unnecessarily traumatic.

Investigations

Investigations, especially vaginal ultrasound scans, should be selected very carefully and only when really indicated. Abnormal pelvic examination findings, persistent symptoms, older patients and other suspicions of disease indicate further investigation to confirm symptoms of menorrhagia and exclude pelvic or systemic pathology.

Consider foremost:

- full blood count (to exclude anaemia and thrombocytopenia)
- iron studies: serum ferritin

Special investigations (only if indicated):

- first pass urine or vaginal swabs for STIs (chlamydia, gonorrhoea, mycoplasma)
- pregnancy testing (beta-hCG)
- serum biochemical screen
- coagulation profile screen
- thyroid function tests, especially TSH
- tests for SLE: antinuclear antibodies
- transvaginal ultrasound

Transvaginal ultrasound: reserved for women who fail conservative treatment or who are at increased risk of endometrial cancer (see later in this chapter). It is best performed in the first 4 to 7 days of the menstrual cycle when endometrial thickness is most easily assessed. An endometrial thickness >12 mm for premenopausal women or ≥5 mm for perimenopausal women, endometrial biopsy (with or without hysteroscopy) is indicated.

Note: Hysteroscopy and D&C remain the gold standard for abnormal uterine bleeding.[6]

102

Dysfunctional uterine bleeding

DUB, which is a diagnosis of exclusion, is defined as 'excessive bleeding, whether heavy, prolonged or frequent, of uterine origin, which is not associated with recognisable pelvic disease, complications of pregnancy or systemic disease'.[2]

Clinical features

- It is a working clinical diagnosis based on the initial detailed history, normal physical examination and normal initial investigation.
- Very common: 10–20% incidence of women at some stage. It is more common in ovulatory (regular) rather than anovulatory (irregular) cycles.
- Peak incidence of ovulatory DUB in late 30s and 40s (35–45 years).
- Anovulatory DUB has two peaks: 12–16 years and 45–55 years. The bleeding is typically irregular with spotting and variable menorrhagia.
- Up to 40% with the initial diagnosis of DUB will have other pathology (e.g. fibroids, endometrial polyps) if detailed pelvic endoscopic investigations are undertaken.

Symptoms

- Heavy bleeding: saturated pads, frequent changing, 'accidents', 'flooding', 'clots'
- Prolonged bleeding:
  - menstruation >7–8 days

  or
  - heavy bleeding >4 days
- Frequent bleeding—periods occur more than once every 21 days
- Pelvic pain and tenderness are not usually prominent features

Medical and surgical management[4,7,8]

Medical

Treatment regimens are presented in TABLES 102.5 and FIGURE 102.2. First-line treatment is with fibrinolytic inhibitors or antiprostaglandin agents, given as soon as possible and throughout the menses. The agent of first choice is usually mefenamic acid, which reduces blood loss by 20–25% as well as helping dysmenorrhoea. Second-line treatment is tranexamic acid, which reduces blood loss by about 50%. Treatment needs to start just before or with the onset of menstrual bleeding and continue for up to 5 days. These agents are simple to use, generally very safe and can be used over long periods of time.

Table 102.5 Regimens used in management of HMB[4] (includes options)

Therapy	Mean reduction[8] in blood loss 80 mL/cycle %
Levonorgestrel (IUD) Mirena 52 mg	94
Oral progestogen: • norethisterone 5mg tds on days 5–26 of cycle	83
Tranexamic acid 1 g (o) 6 hourly on days 1–4 of menstruation	47
Combined oral contraceptive pill	43
NSAIDs (oral): • ibuprofen 400 mg 3–4 times daily • naproxen 500 mg statim then 250 mg every 6–8 hours • mefenamic acid 500 mg tds	29

*Effectiveness supported by EBM[7]

If non-hormonal options are ineffective, consider the use of hormonal agents such as oral progestogens and the combined oral contraceptive pill (COCP). Danazol is another option, but it is infrequently used due to androgenic adverse effects.

The vaginal ring is an appropriate alternative to the COCP and both have the benefit of providing contraception, being short-acting and reversible. Running hormone pills or vaginal rings together in an extended regimen may also be helpful. The oestradiol valerate quadraphasic pill is particularly effective for HMB.

Oral progestins administered to women from day 5 to day 26 of their cycle result in a significant reduction in menstrual blood loss. However, this is less than is achieved with the use of the levonorgestrel intra-uterine system. Adverse side effects of oral progestins include weight gain, bloating, breast tenderness, headaches, acne and depressed mood, rendering it more suitable for short-term therapy.

Intramuscular medroxyprogesterone acetate (Depo-Provera) will induce amenorrhoea in approximately 50% of users within 1 year; however, studies for its use in HMB are limited.

If hormonal methods are ineffective, consider the use of the levonorgestral intra-uterine system (Mirena), which is regarded as the most efficacious of the medical treatments, with a mean blood loss of 94%.[7]

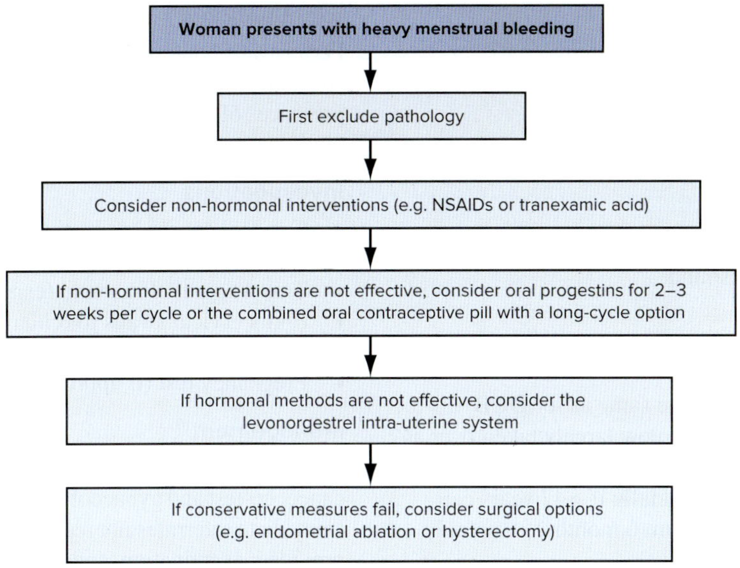

FIGURE 102.2 Treatment regimen for women experiencing heavy bleeding[8]

Source: Adapted from Baber R. What's new in the management of heavy menstrual bleeding? Medicine Today, 2011; 12 (12): 61-4.

Surgical treatment

This is indicated if menorrhagia interferes with lifestyle despite medical treatments. The surgical options are:

- endometrial ablation—to produce amenorrhoea
- hysterectomy; this requires a very carefully planned approach. It is preferred to drug therapy for women with endometrial hyperplasia with atypia

Practice tip

Emergency menorrhagia (acute flooding)[4]
First line:

- tranexamic acid 10 mg/kg IV, every 8 hours until bleeding stops
  or
- tranexamic acid 1–1.5 g (o) 6–8 hourly until bleeding stops

If above unavailable or not tolerated, other options are:

- norethisterone 5–10 mg 4 hourly (o) until bleeding stops
  or
- ethinyloestradiol 30–35 mcg combined oral contraceptive pill, 6 hourly until bleeding stops, re-evalute after 48 hours

General guidelines for surgical intervention

Women who:[4]

- no longer wish to be able to conceive
- are perimenopausal
- have poorly controlled symptoms
- have adverse effects from medical treatment

Uterine fibroids (leiomyoma)

Fibroids are benign tumours of smooth muscle of the myometrium. They are classified according to their location: subserosal, intramural, subendometrial or intra-uterine. They are oestrogen-dependent and shrink with the onset of menopause.

Clinical features

- Lifetime incidence of 60–70% in Caucasian women
- Only 1 in 800 develop malignancy
- Usually asymptomatic

Symptoms

- Often asymptomatic if small
- Menorrhagia
- Dysmenorrhoea
- Pelvic discomfort ± pain (pressure) including dyspareunia
- Bladder dysfunction
- Pain with torsion of pedunculated fibroid
- Pain with 'red degeneration'—only in pregnancy (pain, fever, local tenderness)

Other features

- Infertility (acts like IUCD if submucosal)
- Calcification

Examination

- Bulky uterus

Investigations

- Transvaginal ultrasound
- FBE ? anaemia

Management

- Medical management the same as for DUB
- Levonorgestrel IUD has now largely taken over as the preferred treatment
- GnRH analogues—especially if >42 years can shrink fibroids (maximum 6 months)—use only immediately pre-operative
- Surgical options:
  - myomectomy (remove fibroids only, esp. child-bearing years)
  - hysteroscopic resection/endometrial ablation
  - hysterectomy
- Other option: uterine embolisation

Intermenstrual bleeding (IMB) and postcoital bleeding (PCB)

It is important to note that genital tract malignancy is an uncommon cause of bleeding at any stage, but must be considered in all patients. In particular, postcoital bleeding (PCB) is regarded as a cardinal symptom of cervical cancer.

Causes[10]

- Periovulatory bleeding (normal variant)
- Defective luteal phase (causes premenstrual spotting)
- Endometriosis (causes pre- and postmenstrual spotting)
- Hormonal contraceptives and copper IUD
- Menopausal hormone therapy
- Pregnancy—early loss or ectopic
- Cervical ectropian
- STIs causing cervicitis or PID (especially if PCB)
- Polyps—cervical, endometrial
- Uterine fibroids
- Cervical cancer
- Endometrial/myometrial hyperplasia and malignancy

Examination

Perform an abdominal, bimanual pelvic examination and speculum examination. Check for cervical ectropian, presence of polyps, vaginal discharge and cervical tenderness. Note any friability of the cervix.

Investigations

- Cervical cancer 'co-test' (i.e. HPV and liquid-based cytology)
- Transvaginal ultrasound (especially for IMB)
- Endocervical swabs for chlamydia and gonorrhoea PCR
- Pregnancy test (if appropriate)

Management[10]

All women with persistent PCB require the cervical cancer co-test and gynaecologist referral for colposcopy. Immediate referral is not required after a single episode, provided examination and the co-test are normal. A second episode mandates referral.[11]

If the suspected cause of PCB is a cervical ectropian, persistent bleeding still requires referral. Various ablative treatment methods are available, but are appropriate only once pathology has been excluded.

While irregular bleeding is common with many hormonal therapies, investigation is required and referral should be considered if bleeding is excessively frequent, prolonged or new in onset.

Persistent IMB requires gynaecologist referral for hysteroscopy with endometrial biopsy.

Postmenopausal bleeding[12]

Postmenopausal bleeding suggests cervical or endometrial/myometrial cancer in up to 25% of cases.[2] Other causes include polyps, atrophic vaginitis, menopausal hormone therapy, endometrial hyperplasia and urethral caruncle. It is worth noting that tamoxifen can increase the risk of endometrial cancer. Earlier referral is an indication for women on tamoxifen who present with PMB.

Transvaginal ultrasound should be performed. Gynaecologist referral is not immediately indicated if the ultrasound reveals an endometrial thickness ≤4 mm and there are no suspicious features. However, if endometrial thickness is >4 mm or there is persistent bleeding, referral is indicated with a view to a diagnostic procedure (hysteroscopy and D&C).

Cervical cancer

This should be the diagnosis until proved otherwise for postcoital bleeding.

Clinical features

- Peak incidence in sixth decade
- 80% due to squamous cell carcinoma
- Risk factors (refer CHAPTER 98)

Symptoms

- Postcoital bleeding
- Intermenstrual bleeding
- Vaginal discharge—may be offensive

Mainly diagnosed on routine screening.

Examination

- Ulceration or mass on cervix
- Bleeds readily on contact—may be friable

Management

- Urgent gynaecological referral

Endometrial cancer

This is the diagnosis until proved otherwise in any woman presenting with postmenopausal bleeding.

Clinical features

- Peak incidence 50–70 years
- Risk factors:
  - age
  - obesity
  - nulliparity
  - late menopause
  - diabetes mellitus
  - history of chronic anovulatory bleeding
  - polycystic ovarian syndrome
  - drugs (e.g. unopposed oestrogen, tamoxifen)
  - family history—breast, ovarian, endometrial or colon cancer (Lynch syndrome)

Symptoms

Ninety per cent present with abnormal bleeding, especially postmenopausal bleeding.[3]

Note: intermenstrual bleeding or persistent bleeding in postmenopausal women should be treated with suspicion.

Examination

- Uterus usually feels normal, but may be bulky.

Investigations

- Cervical cytology (after pregnancy excluded)—detects some cases. Endometrial cancer is not excluded by normal cervical cytology
- Transvaginal ultrasound/endometrial biopsy

Management

- Urgent gynaecological referral

Amenorrhoea and oligomenorrhoea[10]

Amenorrhoea is classified as primary or secondary. Primary amenorrhoea is the failure of the menses to start by 16 years of age.[2] Secondary amenorrhoea is the absence of menses for over 6 months in a woman who has had established menstruation.

102

Primary amenorrhoea

The main approach is to differentiate primary amenorrhoea from delayed puberty, in which there are no signs of sexual maturation by age 13. Causes include:

- hypothalamic amenorrhoea:
  - excessive exercise
  - low body mass
  - severe chronic illness
  - psychological stress
- PCOS
- imperforate hymen
- congenital absence of uterus or vagina
- chromosomal anomalies (e.g. Kallman syndrome, Turner syndrome)
- pituitary tumours

Diagnostic tests include serum FSH, LH, prolactin, oestradiol and also chromosome analysis. Early referral is appropriate.

Secondary amenorrhoea

The most common causes in general practice are PCOS and hypothalamic amenorrhoea.

- hypothalamic amenorrhoea:
  - excessive exercise
  - low body mass
  - severe chronic illness
  - psychological stress
- PCOS
- pregnancy
- hyperprolactinaemia
- premature ovarian insufficiency
- medication (e.g. hormonal contraception, antipsychotics, opiates, chemotherapy)
- thyroid dysfunction
- adrenal disorders (e.g. Cushing disease, congenital adrenal hyperplasia)
- Asherman syndrome (following gynaecological surgery)

Gynaecological intervention is appropriate for women with prolonged amenorrhoea due to the increased risk of endometrial cancer.

Oligomenorrhoea

Infrequent and usually irregular periods, where the cycles are between 6 weeks and 6 months. PCOS is the most common cause.

Premature ovarian insufficiency

Apart from iatrogenic causes, this may be caused by idiopathic early menopause and autoimmune ovarian failure. Other genetic associations are Turner syndrome and Fragile X pre-mutation. It is considered a hormonal deficiency and requires hormonal therapy with either combined oral contraception or menopausal hormonal therapy.[4]

When to refer

- Women with persistent IMB and/or PCB
- Women with persistent postmenopausal bleeding
- Women with persistent increased endometrial thickness on transvaginal ultrasound
- Possibility of intra-uterine pathology
- The patient does not respond to initial therapy
- There is evidence of underlying disease (e.g. endometriosis, SLE)
- Surgery is indicated

Practice tip

- Non-menstrual bleeding suggests cancer until proved otherwise: it may be postcoital (cervical cancer); intermenstrual (common with hormonal contraception); postmenopausal (endometrial cancer).

Patient education resources

Hand-out sheets from *Murtagh's Patient Education* 7th edition:

- Fibroids
- Menorrhagia (heavy periods)
- Understanding your menstrual cycle

References

1. Fung P. Abnormal uterine bleeding. Modern Medicine Australia, 1992; May: 58–66.
2. Mackay EV, Beischer NA, Pepperell RJ et al. *Illustrated Textbook of Gynaecology* (2nd edn). Sydney: WB Saunders, 1992: 77–107.
3. O'Connor V, Kovacs G. *Obstetrics, Gynaecology and Women's Health.* Cambridge: Cambridge University Press, 2003: 466–8.
4. Expert group for Endocrinology. In: eTG complete [Internet]. Melbourne: Therapeutic Guidelines Ltd. Available from: <www.tg.org.au>, accessed May 2018.
5. Read C, May T, Stellingwerff M. Irregular vaginal bleeding: how to treat. Australian Doctor, 18 May 2007: 27–32.
6. Barton S (ed.). *Clinical Evidence.* London: BMJ Publishing Group, 2001: 1311–16.
7. Quinlivan J, Petersen RW. Menorrhagia. Medical Observer, 16 April 2004: 31–4.
8. Baber R. What's new in the management of heavy menstrual bleeding? Medicine Today, 2011; 12 (12): 61–4.
9. Farquhar C, Brown J. Oral contraceptive pill for heavy menstrual bleeding. Cochrane Database Syst Rev. 2009, Issue 4. Art No. CD00154.
10. Family Planning NSW. *Reproductive and Sexual Health: An Australian Clinical Practice Handbook* (3rd edn). Sydney: Family Planning NSW, 2016.
11. Cancer Council Australia Cervical Cancer Screening Guidelines Working Party. National Cervical Screening Program: guidelines for the management of screen-detected abnormalities, screening in specific populations and investigation of abnormal vaginal bleeding. Sydney: Cancer Council Australia, 2016. <www.wiki.cancer.org.au/australia/Guidelines:Cervical_cancer/Screening> (accessed 16/5/2018).
12. Cancer Australia. Abnormal vaginal bleeding in post-menopausal women. A diagnostic guide for general practitioners and gynaecologists. <www.canceraustralia.gov.au/sites/default/files/publications/ncgc-vaginal-bleeding-flowcharts-march-20111_504af02038614.pdf> (accessed 16/5/2018).

Lower abdominal and pelvic pain in women

103

Man endures pain as an undeserved punishment, woman accepts it as a natural heritage.

ANONYMOUS

Pain in the lower abdomen and pelvis is one of the most frequent symptoms experienced by women. The diagnostic approach requires a wide variety of consultative skills, especially when the pain is chronic. The examination of acute abdominal pain has been simplified by sensitive serum pregnancy tests, ultrasound investigation and laparoscopy. However, an accurate history and examination for all types of pain will generally pinpoint the diagnosis. The ever-present problem of PID, the leading cause of infertility in women, demands an early diagnosis and appropriate management.

Key facts and checkpoints

- A distinction has to be made between acute, chronic and recurrent pain.
- Ectopic pregnancy remains a potentially lethal condition and its diagnosis still requires a high index of suspicion.
- Sudden sharp pain in the pelvis that becomes more generalised indicates rupture of an ectopic pregnancy or an ovarian cyst.
- Recurrent sharp, self-limiting pain indicates a ruptured Graafian follicle (mittelschmerz).
- Recurrent pain related to menstruation is typical of dysmenorrhoea or endometriosis.
- A UK study[1] of chronic lower abdominal pain in women showed the causes were adhesions (36%), no diagnosis (19%), endometriosis (14%), constipation (13%), ovarian cysts (11%) and PID (7%). An Australian study found that endometriosis accounted for 30% and adhesions 20%.[2]
- The principal afferent pathways of the pelvic viscera arise from T10–12, L1 and S2–4. Thus disorders of the bladder, rectum, lower uterus, cervix and upper vagina can refer pain to the low back, buttocks and posterior thigh.[3]

A diagnostic approach

A summary of the diagnostic strategy model is presented in TABLE 103.1.

Table 103.1 Lower abdominal and pelvic pain in women: diagnostic strategy model

Probability diagnosis
Primary dysmenorrhoea
Mittelschmerz
Pelvic/abdominal adhesions
Endometriosis

Serious disorders not to be missed
Ectopic pregnancy
Neoplasia:
- ovary
- cervix and uterus
- other pelvic structures

Severe infections:
- PID
- pelvic abscess

Acute appendicitis
Internal iliac claudication

Pitfalls (often missed)
Endometriosis/adenomyosis
Torsion of ovary or pedunculated fibroid
Constipation/faecal impaction
Irritable bowel syndrome
Misplaced IUCD
Nerve entrapment
Referred pain (to pelvis):
- appendicitis
- cholecystitis
- diverticulitis
- urinary tract disorders

Transvaginal mesh complications
Ovarian vein incompetence/pelvic congestion syndrome

Seven masquerades checklist
Depression
Drugs
Spinal dysfunction (referred pain)
UTI

Is the patient trying to tell me something?
May be relevant.

Probability diagnosis

The commonest causes are primary dysmenorrhoea, the pain of a ruptured Graafian follicle (mittelschmerz), endometriosis and adhesions. In many instances of pain no diagnosis is made as no pathological cause can be found.

Serious disorders not to be missed

The potentially lethal problem of a ruptured ectopic pregnancy must not be missed, hence the axiom 'be ectopic minded'. PID can be overlooked, especially if chronic, and requires early diagnosis and aggressive treatment. Neoplasia must be considered, especially malignancy of pelvic structures, including the 'silent' ovarian cancer.

Pitfalls

Several disorders are very difficult to diagnose and these include haemorrhage into the ovary or a cyst, torsion of the ovary or pedunculated fibroid. Endometriosis may be missed so it is important to be familiar with its symptoms. Chronic constipation may be a trap.

Seven masquerades checklist

Two important conditions to consider are urinary tract infection and spinal dysfunction. Just as disorders of the pelvic organs, such as endometriosis and PID, can refer pain to the low back and buttocks, so can disorders of the lumbosacral spine cause referred pain to the lower abdomen and groin.

Psychogenic considerations

These can be extremely relevant. Problems in the patient's social, marital or sexual relationships should be evaluated, especially in the assessment of chronic pain. Patients with chronic pelvic pain may have experienced difficulties in personal development, relationships, sexual confidence, educational and financial opportunities. Such issues can have implications for medical management and need to be handled with sensitivity and tact.[4]

The clinical approach

History

The pain should be linked with the menstrual history, coitus and the possibility of an early pregnancy. For recurrent and chronic pain, it is advisable to instruct the patient to keep a diary over two menstrual cycles. The severity of the pain can be assessed as follows:[2]

- does not interfere with daily activity
- results in days off work
- results in confinement to bed

In this way the pain can be classified objectively as mild, moderate or severe.

The typical pain patterns in relation to menstruation are shown in FIGURE 103.1.

Examination

One objective is to correlate any palpable tenderness with the patient's statement of the severity of the pain. Use the traditional abdominal and pelvic examination to identify the site of tenderness and rebound tenderness,

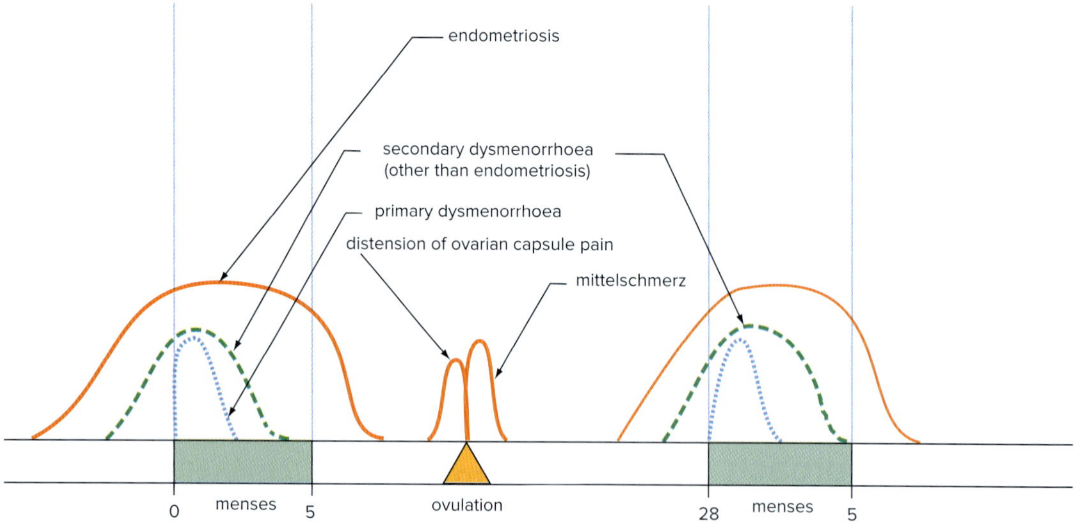

FIGURE 103.1 Typical pain patterns for menstrual cycle related gynaecological pain

and any abdominal or pelvic masses. The pelvis should be examined by speculum (preferably bivalve type) and bimanual palpation.

Proper assessment can be difficult if the patient cannot relax, if there is abdominal scarring or obesity, or if extreme tenderness is present. It is therefore important, especially in the younger and apprehensive patient, to conduct a gentle, caring vaginal examination with appropriate explanation and reassurance. Explanation of the procedure during vaginal examination, preferably using eye contact with the patient, can help her relax and be more confident in the procedure.

Investigations

Investigations may be selected from:

- haemoglobin level
- white blood cell count (limited value)
- haematocrit
- ESR/CRP
- microbiology (limited value):
  - urine for microscopy and culture ± *Chlamydia* PCR
  - endocervical and vaginal swabs
- serum β-hCG assay
- urinary hCG tests (can be negative in the presence of an ectopic pregnancy)

Diagnostic imaging:

- vaginal ultrasound—to define a gestation sac
- pelvic ultrasound—to differentiate a cystic from a solid pelvic mass. Indicated for:
  - pelvic pain
  - a palpable pelvic mass
  - a palpable lower abdominal mass
  - ascites

Laparoscopy is indicated if the history and examination are suggestive of ectopic pregnancy and ultrasound fails to confirm an intra-uterine pregnancy.

Acute pain

The causes of acute pain are summarised in TABLE 103.2. The patient is usually young (20–30 years old), sexually active and distressed by the pain, and should be considered foremost to have a bleeding ectopic pregnancy. Important differential diagnoses include acute PID, rupture or torsion of an ovarian cyst and acute appendicitis. Cases of acute ruptured ectopics are obviously easier to diagnose in the presence of circulatory collapse.

Table 103.2 Causes of acute lower abdominal and pelvic pain in women[3]

Genital
Acute salpingitis
Pelvic peritonitis
Bleeding
Rupture or torsion of ovarian cyst
Threatened or incomplete abortion
Rupture or aborting tubal ectopic pregnancy
Rupture or bleeding endometrioma
Non-genital
Acute appendicitis
Bowel obstruction
Urinary tract infection (cystitis)
Ureteric colic (calculus)
Functional
Primary dysmenorrhoea
Retrograde menstruation

Source: After Soo Keat Khoo[3]

Chronic pain

Chronic pelvic pain is constant or recurrent pain of at least 6 months' duration.

Features

- Incidence 15% in 18–50-year-olds
- Endometriosis causes 33%, adhesions 24%
- It is the reason for up to 40% of gynaecological laparoscopies
- Reason for 15% of hysterectomies

The pain can be cyclical (e.g. endometriosis, mittelschmerz) or continuous.

The common causes of chronic pain are listed in TABLE 103.3. Chronic pain is more difficult to diagnose and it is often difficult to differentiate between problems such as endometriosis, PID, an ovarian neoplasm and the irritable bowel syndrome. A comparison of the clinical features of endometriosis and PID is presented in TABLE 103.4. Furthermore it is difficult to distinguish clinically between endometriosis of the uterus (adenomyosis) and pelvic congestion syndrome. Both conditions are associated with dysmenorrhoea and a tender normal-sized uterus.

Table 103.3 Causes of chronic lower abdominal and pelvic pain in women[3]

Genital
Endometriosis/adenomyosis
Pelvic inflammatory disease (chronic; adhesions)
Ovarian neoplasm
Fibromyomata (rarely)
Non-genital
Diverticulitis
Bowel adhesions
Irritable bowel syndrome
Urinary disorders e.g. urethral syndrome
Functional
Secondary dysmenorrhoea—IUCD, polyp
Irritable bowel, chronic bowel spasm

Ectopic pregnancy

Ectopic pregnancy occurs approximately once in every 100 clinically recognised pregnancies. If ruptured it can be a rapid, fatal condition so we have to be 'ectopic minded'. It is the commonest cause of intraperitoneal haemorrhage. There is usually a history of a missed period but a normal menstrual history may be obtained in some instances.

Clinical features of a ruptured ectopic pregnancy

- Average patient in mid-20s
- First pregnancy in one-third of patients
- Patient at risk
  - previous ectopic pregnancy
  - previous PID
  - previous abdominal or pelvic surgery, especially sterilisation reversal
  - IUCD use
  - in-vitro fertilisation

Table 103.4 Comparison of clinical features of PID and pelvic endometriosis

Feature	Chronic PID	Endometriosis
History	Acute pelvic infection (e.g. ruptured appendix) IUCD usage	Dysmenorrhoea Subfertility Dyspareunia Pelvic pain
Pelvic pain	+ to ++ (mild to moderate) Premenstrual Lower abdominal location	++ to +++ (moderate to severe) Premenstrual and menstrual Acute pain if rupture of endometrioma
Backache	+ mild	++ moderate Low sacral pain with menstruation
Secondary dysmenorrhoea	Moderate to severe From onset of acute PID Decreases with menstruation	Moderate to severe Gradual onset increases in severity throughout menstruation
Menstruation	Irregular and heavy	Heavy
Dyspareunia	Moderate	Often severe
Infertility	+++	++
Urinary symptoms	—	Frequency, dysuria and haematuria if bladder wall involved
Bowel symptoms	—	Painful defecation if rectal wall involved
Vaginal symptoms	May be chronic purulent discharge or leucorrhoea	—

> **DxT** amenorrhoea (65–80%) + lower abdominal pain (95 + %) + abnormal vaginal bleeding (65–85%) → ectopic pregnancy

- Pre-rupture symptoms (many cases):
  - abnormal pregnancy
  - cramping pains in one or other iliac fossa
  - vaginal bleeding
- Rupture:
  - excruciating pain (see FIG. 103.2)
  - circulatory collapse

  Note: In 10–15% there is no abnormal bleeding.
- Pain may radiate to rectum (lavatory sign), vagina or leg
- Signs of pregnancy (e.g. enlarged breasts and uterus) usually not present

Examination

- Deep tenderness in iliac fossa
- Vaginal examination:
  - tenderness on bimanual pelvic examination (pain on cervical provocation, i.e. cervical motion tenderness)
  - palpable adenxal mass
  - soft cervix
- Bleeding (prune juice appearance)
- Temperature and pulse usually normal early

Diagnosis[5]

It is possible to diagnose ectopic pregnancy at a very early stage of pregnancy.

- Urine pregnancy test (positive in most ectopics)
- Serum β-hCG assay—may need serial quantitative tests to distinguish an ectopic from a normal intra-uterine pregnancy (IUP). If it is >2000 IU/L an IUP should be visible on vaginal ultrasound. If the uterus is empty, ectopic is more likely. If <2000 IU/L, repeat every second day to see if it is increasing normally as expected in a normal IUP.
- Transvaginal ultrasound can diagnose at 5–6 weeks (empty uterus, tubal sac, fluid in cul-de-sac)
- Laparoscopy (the definitive diagnostic procedure)

103

Ectopic pregnancy diagnosis

- beta-hCG assay
- Transvaginal ultrasound
- Laparoscopy

Management

Possible options are surgery, medical or watchful expectancy. Treatment may be conservative (based on

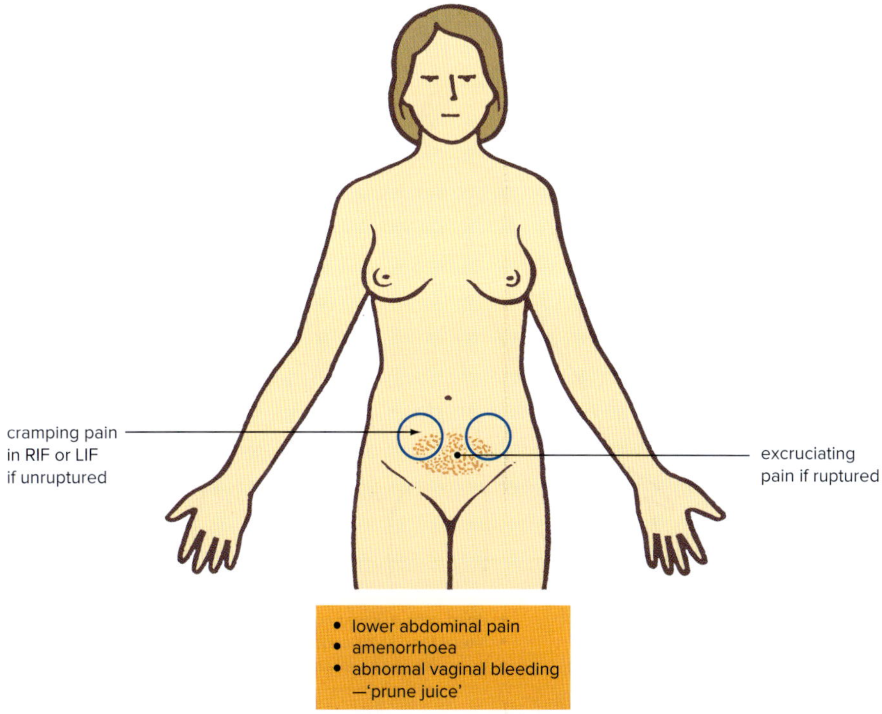

FIGURE 103.2 Clinical features of ectopic pregnancy

ultrasound and β-hCG assays); medical, by injecting intramuscular methotrexate; laparoscopic removal; or laparotomy for severe cases. Rupture with blood loss (usually about 7% of cases[6]) demands urgent surgery. Organise blood and contacts, resuscitate as necessary.

Post management

- Successful pregnancy 60–65%
- Subsequent risk of ectopic pregnancy 10–15%

Ruptured ovarian (Graafian) follicle (mittelschmerz)

When the Graafian follicle ruptures a small amount of blood mixed with follicular fluid is usually released into the pouch of Douglas. This may cause peritonism (mittelschmerz), which is different from the unilateral pain experienced just before ovulation due to distension of the ovarian capsule.

Clinical features

- Onset of pain in mid-cycle
- Deep pain in one or other iliac fossa (RIF > LIF)
- Often described as a 'horse kick pain'
- Pain tends to move centrally (see FIG. 103.3)
- Heavy feeling in pelvis
- Relieved by sitting or supporting lower abdomen
- Pain lasts from a few minutes to hours (average 5 hours)
- Patient otherwise well

Note: Sometimes it can mimic acute appendicitis.

Management

- Explanation and reassurance
- Simple analgesics: aspirin or paracetamol
- 'Hot water bottle' comfort if pain severe

OVARIAN TUMOURS

Benign ovarian tumours, particularly ovarian cysts, may be asymptomatic but will cause pain if complicated. They are common in women under 50 years of age. Ovarian cysts are best defined by vaginal ultrasound, which can identify whether haemorrhage has occurred inside or outside the cyst.

Symptoms

- Pain (usually torsion or haemorrhage)
- Pressure symptoms
- Menstrual irregularity

Ruptured ovarian cyst

The cysts tend to rupture just prior to ovulation or following coitus.

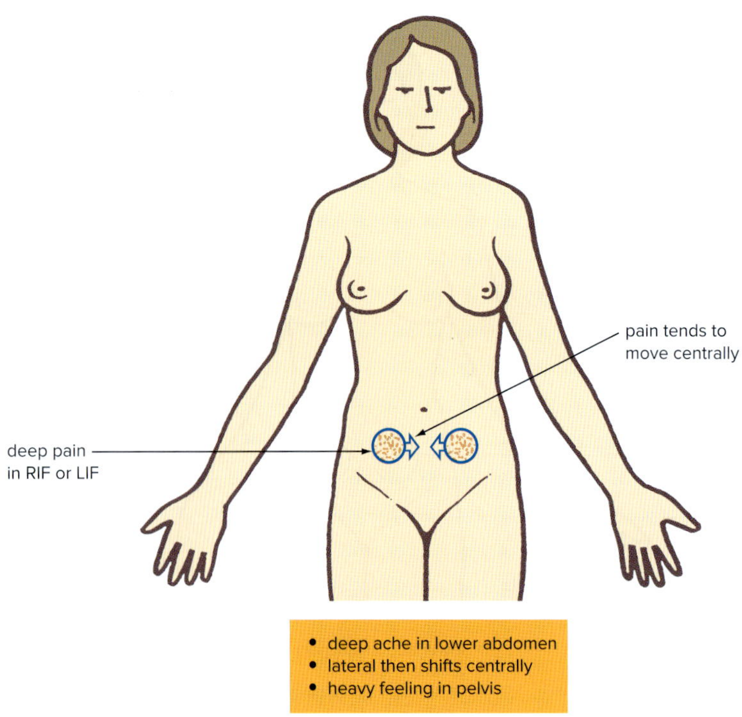

FIGURE 103.3 Typical clinical features of a ruptured Graafian follicle (mittelschmerz)

Clinical features

- Patient usually 15–25 years
- Sudden onset of pain in one or other iliac fossa
- May be nausea and vomiting
- No systemic signs
- Pain usually settles within a few hours

Signs

- Tenderness and guarding in iliac fossa
- PR: tenderness in rectovaginal pouch

Investigation

- Pelvic ultrasound (transvaginal and transabdominal views)

Management

- Appropriate explanation and reassurance
- Conservative:
  - simple cyst <4 cm
  - internal haemorrhage
  - minimal pain
- Needle vaginal drainage by ultrasonography for a simple larger cyst
- Laparoscopic surgery:
  - complex cysts
  - large cysts
  - external bleeding

Acute torsion of ovarian cyst

Torsions are mainly from dermoid cysts and, when right-sided, may be difficult to distinguish from acute pelvic appendicitis.

Clinical features

- Severe cramping lower abdominal pain (see FIG. 103.4)
- Diffuse pain
- Pain may radiate to the flank, back or thigh
- Repeated vomiting
- Exquisite pelvic tenderness
- Patient looks ill

Signs

- Smooth, rounded, mobile mass palpable in abdomen
- May be tenderness and guarding over the mass, especially if leakage

Diagnosis

- Pelvic ultrasound

Treatment

- Laparoscopy and surgical correction

103

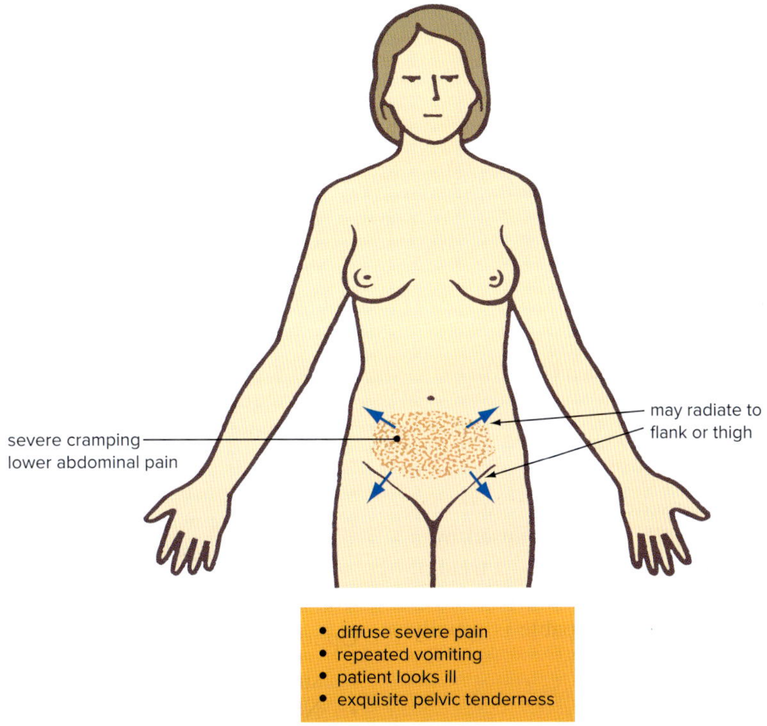

FIGURE 103.4 Typical clinical features of acute torsion of an ovarian cyst

Malignant ovarian tumours

Ovarian cancer has an incidence of 10 cases per 10 000 women per year and accounts for 5% of all cancers in women and 20% of all gynaecological cancers. It is responsible for more gynaecological cancer deaths because the tumour is often well advanced at the time of clinical presentation. Earlier discovery may sometimes be made on routine examination or because of investigation of non-specific pelvic symptoms.

Ovarian cancer tends to remain asymptomatic for a long period. No age group is spared but it becomes progressively more common after 45 years (peak incidence 60–65 years) (see CHAPTER 26).

The familial causes and relationship to breast and colorectal cancer are being delineated. Refer to CHAPTER 18.

Risk factors

- Age
- Family history
- Nulliparity
- BRCA1 and BRCA 2 gene mutations
- Ashkenazi Jewish ancestry

Protective factors

- COC pill
- Pregnancy

Clinical features

- Constitutional symptoms: fatigue, anorexia
- Ache or discomfort in lower abdomen or pelvis
- Abdominal bloating and 'fullness'
- Gastrointestinal dysfunction (e.g. epigastric discomfort, diarrhoea, constipation, wind)
- Sensation of pelvic heaviness
- Genitourinary symptoms (e.g. frequency, urgency, prolapse)
- ± Abnormal uterine bleeding
- Postmenopausal bleeding
- Dyspareunia and/or dysmenorrhoea (10–20%)
- ± Weight loss
- A bimanual examination assists diagnosis. Look for mass, ascites, pleural effusion

A pelvic mass plus ascites usually indicates ovarian cancer but occasionally may be caused by a benign ovarian fibroma (Meigs' syndrome—a triad of benign ovarian tumour + ascites + pleural effusion).

Note: Any ovary that is easily palpable is usually abnormal (normal ovary rarely >4 cm).

Diagnosis

- Pelvic ultrasound with transvaginal and transabdominal views
- Tumour markers such as CA-125, β-hCG (choriocarcinoma), human epididymis protein 4 (HE4) and alpha-fetoprotein should be measured only if the ultrasound raises suspicion of malignancy[7]

Refer urgently to gynaecologist. Treatment is usually laparoscopy ± adjuvant chemotherapy.

DYSMENORRHOEA

Dysmenorrhoea (painful periods) may commence with the onset of the menses (menarche) when it is called primary dysmenorrhoea, or later in life when the term secondary dysmenorrhoea is applied.

Primary (functional) dysmenorrhoea

This is menstrual pain associated with ovular cycles without any pathologic findings. The pain usually commences within 1–2 years after the menarche and becomes less severe with age. It affects about 50% of menstruating women and up to 95% of adolescents.

Clinical features

- Low midline abdominal pain
- Pain radiates to back or thighs (see FIG. 103.5)
- Varies from a dull dragging to a severe cramping pain
- Maximum pain at beginning of the period
- May commence up to 12 hours before the menses appear
- Usually lasts 24 hours but may persist for 2–3 days
- May be associated with nausea and vomiting, headache, syncope or flushing
- No abnormal findings on examination

Management

- Full explanation and appropriate reassurance
- Promote a healthy lifestyle:
  - regular exercise
  - avoid smoking and excessive alcohol
- Recommend relaxation techniques such as yoga
- Avoid exposure to extreme cold
- Place a hot water bottle over the painful area and curl the knees onto the chest

Medication

Options include (trying in order):

- simple analgesics (e.g. aspirin or paracetamol)
- NSAIDs
  - naproxen 500 mg (o) initially then 250 mg every 6—8 hours (max 1250 mg/day)

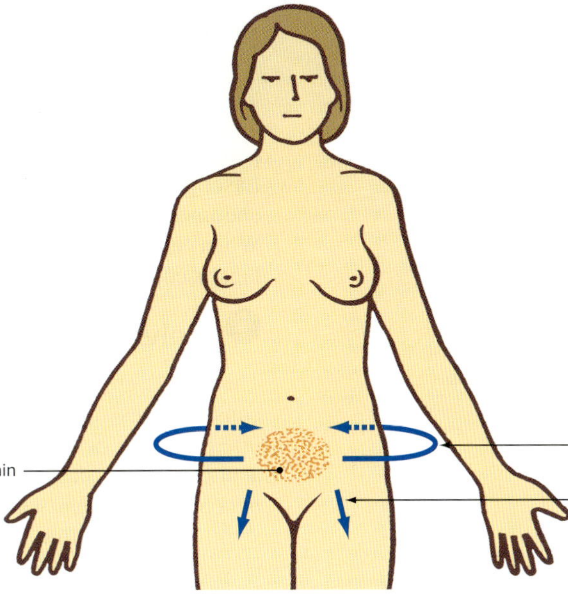

FIGURE 103.5 Typical pain of dysmenorrhoea

103

- or ibuprofen 200–400 mg (o) tds (max 1600 mg/day)
- commence at first suggestion of pain in the first 3 days of the period (if simple analgesics ineffective)

- combined oral contraceptive pill
- progestogen-medicated IUCD

If not helped by these treatments, further investigation is required.

A Cochrane review found that the most beneficial medication was the NSAIDs, and vitamin B1 and magnesium also proved effective. There is no evidence so far that vitamin B6, vitamin E or herbal remedies are effective. Spinal manipulation is unlikely to be beneficial.[8]

Secondary dysmenorrhoea

Secondary dysmenorrhoea is menstrual pain for which an organic cause can be found. It usually begins after the menarche following years of pain-free menses; the patient is usually over 30 years of age. The pain begins as a dull pelvic ache 3–4 days before the menses and becomes more severe during menstruation.

Commonest causes:

- endometriosis (a major cause)
- PID (a major cause)
- IUCD (copper)
- submucous myoma
- intra-uterine polyp
- pelvic adhesions

Investigations

Investigations include laparoscopy, ultrasound and (less commonly) assessment of the uterine cavity by dilation and curettage, hysteroscopy or hysterosalpingography.

Management involves treating the cause.

Pelvic adhesions

Pelvic adhesions may be the cause of pelvic pain, infertility, dysmenorrhoea and intestinal pain. They can be diagnosed and removed laparoscopically when the adhesions are well visualised and there are no intestinal loops firmly stuck together.

Endometriosis

Endometriosis is the condition where ectopically located endometrial tissue (usually in dependent parts of the pelvis and in the ovaries) responds to female sex hormone stimulation by proliferation, haemorrhage, adhesions and ultimately dense scar tissue changes. The average time to diagnosis is 10 years. The diagnosis is masked by taking NSAIDs and the COC.

Patients experience varying degrees of symptoms and loss of gynaecological function according to the site and severity of the endometriosis deposits. Pregnancy is beneficial but recurrence can follow.

Clinical features[9]

- 5–10% incidence
- Puberty to menopause, peak 25–35 years

- Secondary dysmenorrhoea
- Painful defecation during menses
- Urinary symptoms; dysuria, frequency
- Pain may radiate to lower back, legs or rectum
- Subfertility
- Dyspareunia
- Non-specific pelvic pain
- Menorrhagia
- Acute pain with rupture of endometrioma
- Premenstrual spotting

DxT dysmenorrhoea + menorrhagia + dyspareunia = abdominal/pelvic pain → endometriosis

Possible signs

- Fixed uterine retroversion
- Tenderness and nodularity in the pouch of Douglas/retrovaginal septum
- Uterine enlargement and tenderness

Adenomyosis: this is endometriosis of the myometrium affecting the endometrial glands and stroma. The symptoms are similar to endometriosis plus an enlarging tender uterus.

Differential diagnosis

- PID—see TABLE 103.4
- Ovarian cysts or tumours
- Uterine myomas
- Irritable bowel syndrome (a common misdiagnosis)

Diagnosis

- Usually by direct visual inspection at laparoscopy (the gold standard)
- Transvaginal ultrasound (usefulness not well established, may identify ovarian endometrioma or rectal endometriosis)
- Curettage (not routinely performed) shows small sensory C nerve fibres in the endometrium

Treatment

- Careful explanation
- NSAIDs (first line), can be supplemented by paracetamol
- Treatment can be surgical or medical

  Medical:[10] To induce amenorrhoea (only two-thirds respond to drugs):
  - COC: once daily continuously—long term
  - levonorgestrel-releasing IUCD (Mirena) 5-yearly and indefinite
  - progestogens (e.g. medroxyprogesterone acetate—Depo-Provera) or orally 10 mg bd for up to 6 months
  - GnRH analogues, e.g. goserelin, 3.6 mg SC implant every 28 days for up to 6 months, nafarelin (limited by adverse effects)

Surgical: Surgical measures depend on the patient's age, symptoms and family planning. Laser surgery, diathermy ablation and excision of endometriomata can be performed via laparoscopy. When endometriosis is associated with infertility, laparoscopic surgery is preferred to drug therapy.

Pelvic inflammatory disease

There are great medical problems in the serious consequences of PID, namely tubal obstruction, infertility and ectopic pregnancy. PID may be either acute, which causes sudden severe symptoms, or chronic, which can gradually produce milder symptoms or follow an acute episode. Acute PID is a major public health problem and is the most important complication of STIs among young women. The majority are young (less than 25 years), sexually active women who are also nulliparous. PID is usually polymicrobial, caused by sexually acquired pathogens and/or vaginal flora.[11]

Some patients may experience no symptoms but others may have symptoms that vary from mild to very severe. The clinical diagnosis can be difficult as signs and symptoms can be nonspecific and correlate poorly with the extent of the inflammation.

Clinical features

Acute PID

- Fever ≥38°C
- Moderate to severe lower abdominal pain

Chronic PID

- Ache in the lower back
- Mild lower abdominal pain

Both acute and chronic

- Dyspareunia
- Menstrual problems (e.g. painful, heavy or irregular periods)
- Intermenstrual bleeding
- Abnormal, perhaps offensive, purulent vaginal discharge
- Painful or frequent urination

The diagnostic criteria for acute PID are presented in TABLE 103.5.

Examination

- In acute PID there may be lower abdominal tenderness ± rigidity.

Table 103.5 Diagnostic criteria for acute PID[3,12]

All three of the following should be present
1 Lower abdominal tenderness (with or without rebound)
2 Cervical motion tenderness
3 Adnexal tenderness (may be unilateral) plus
One of the following should be present
1 Temperature ≥ 38°C
2 White blood cell count ≥ 10 500/mm^2
3 Purulent fluid obtained via culdocentesis
4 Inflammatory mass present on bimanual pelvic examination and/or sonography
5 ESR ≥ 15 mm/h or CRP >1.0 mg/dL
6 Isolation of *N. gonorrhoeae* and/or *C. trachomatis*
7 Histological evidence of infection (e.g. plasma cells)

- Pelvic examination: in acute PID there is unusual vaginal warmth, cervical motion tenderness and adnexal tenderness. Speculum examination usually reveals a red inflamed cervix and a purulent discharge.

Causative agents

These can be subdivided into three broad groups:

1 *Exogenous organisms:* those which are community acquired and initiated by sexual activity. They include the classic STIs, *Chlamydia trachomatis* (the most common causative organism) and *Neisseria gonorrhoeae*. This usually leads to salpingitis.

2 *Endogenous infections:* these are normal commensals of the lower genital tract, especially *Escherichia coli* and *Bacteroides fragilis*. They become pathogenic under conditions that interrupt the normal cervical barrier, such as recent genital tract manipulation or trauma (e.g. abortion, presence of an IUCD, recent pregnancy or a dilatation and curettage). The commonest portals of entry are cervical lacerations and the placental site. These organisms cause an ascending infection and can spread direct or via lymphatics to the broad ligament, causing pelvic cellulitis (see FIG. 103.6).

3 *Actinomycosis:* very rare cause of a chronic polymicrobial inflammatory mass that can mimic pelvic malignancy. Due to prolonged IUCD use. Look for *Actinomyces israelii* on culture if suspected and seek expert advice.

103

Investigations

Diagnosis is clinical. A definitive diagnosis is difficult since routine specimen collection has limitations in assessing the organisms. Definitive diagnosis is by

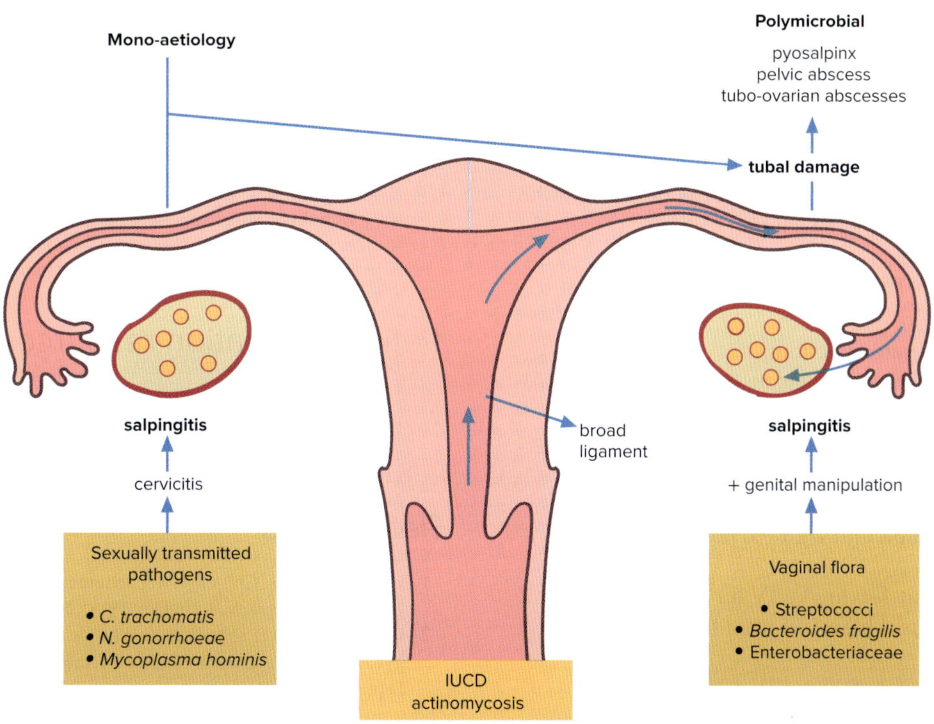

FIGURE 103.6 The pathogenesis of PID

laparoscopy but this is not practical in all cases of suspected PID.

- Endocervical swabs for NAAT (e.g. PCR) *N. gonorrhoeae, C. trachomatis* and *M. genitalium*
- Endocervical swab for culture
- Blood culture if febrile
- Pelvic ultrasound to detect alternative causes of pain

Treatment

Note: Any IUCD should be removed if there is no response to treatment in 48 to 72 hours. A new IUCD can be inserted once the infection has resolved. Current sexual partners should be treated with agents effective against *C. trachomatis* (and *N. gonorrhoeae* if likely), irrespective of test results.

Sexually acquired infection[11]

Mild to moderate infection (treated as an outpatient):
ceftriaxone 500 mg (in 2 ml 1% lignocaine) IM or 500 mg IV, as a single dose (for gonorrhoea)
plus
metronidazole 400 mg (o) 12 hourly for 14 days
plus
doxycycline 100 mg (o) 12 hourly for 14 days
Severe infection (treated in hospital):
ceftriaxone 2 g IV daily or cefotaxime 2g IV tds
plus
azithromycin 500 mg IV daily
plus
metronidazole 500 mg IV 12 hourly
until there is substantial clinical improvement, when the oral regimen above can be used for the remainder of the 14 days

Infection non-sexually acquired (related to genital manipulation)

Mild to moderate infection:
amoxycillin + clavulanate (875 mg/125 mg) (o) 12 hourly for 14 days
plus
doxycycline 100 mg (o) 12 hourly for 14 days
Severe infection (including septicaemia):
amoxy/ampicillin 2 g IV 6 hourly
plus
gentamicin 4–6 mg/kg IV for 1 dose, then 1 or 2 further doses based on renal function
plus
metronidazole 500 mg IV 12 hourly

When to refer

- All cases of 'unexplained infertility'
- All teenagers with dysmenorrhoea sufficient to interfere with normal school, work or recreational activities, and not responding to prostaglandin inhibitors
- Patients with dysmenorrhoea reaching a crescendo mid-menses
- Patients with dysmenorrhoea and unexplained bowel or bladder symptoms
- Patients with positional dyspareunia
- Patients with cyclic pain or bleeding in unusual sites

Note: Pelvic disease that can be treated by advanced laparoscopy surgery includes ectopic pregnancy, ovarian cysts, endometriosis and endometriomas, fibromyomata, pelvic adhesions and hydrosalpinx.

Practice tips

- Think of endometriosis and ovarian cysts in any woman with lower abdominal pain.
- In any woman whose normal activities are disturbed by dysmenorrhoea unrelieved by NSAIDs, endometriosis should be suspected.
- If an ectopic pregnancy is suspected and there are no facilities for resuscitation, digital vaginal examination should be deferred as it may provoke rupture.[2]
- Acute abdominal and pelvic pain in the presence of a negative β-hCG is most often due to an ovarian cyst.
- A positive β-hCG plus an empty uterus and an adnexal mass are the classic diagnostic features of ectopic pregnancy.

Patient education resources

Hand-out sheets from *Murtagh's Patient Education* 7th edition:
- Dysmenorrhoea (painful periods)
- Endometriosis
- Pelvic inflammatory disease

References

1 Foy A, Brown R. Chronic lower abdominal pain in gynaecological practice. Update, 1987; 27 March: 19–25.
2 Forbes KL. Lower abdominal and pelvic pain in the female: a gynaecological approach. Modern Medicine Australia, 1991; September: 24–31.

3 Soo Keat Khoo. Lower abdominal pain in women. Patient Management (Suppl), 1990; August: 13–23.

4 Evans, S. Management of persistent pelvic pain in girls and women. Aust Fam Physician, July 2015; 44 (7): 454–9.

5 O'Connor V, Kovacs G. *Obstetrics, Gynaecology and Women's Health.* Cambridge: Cambridge University Press, 2003: 325–7.

6 Porter R, Kaplan J. *The Merck Manual of Diagnosis and Treatment* (19th edn). Whitehouse station, 2011: 2664–5.

7 Yeoh M. Investigation and management of an ovarian mass. Aust Fam Physician, Jan/Feb 2015; (44) 1: 48–52.

8 Barton S (ed.). *Clinical Evidence.* London: BMJ Publishing Group, 2001: 1255–63.

9 Johnson NP, Hummelshoj L, The World Endometriosis Society Montpellier Consortium. Consensus on current management of endometriosis. Hum Reprod, 2013; 28 (6): 1552–68.

10 Expert group for Endocrinology guidelines. In: eTG complete [Internet}. Melbourne: Therapeutic Guidelines Ltd. Available from: <www.tg.org.au>, accessed April 2018.

11 Expert group for Antibiotic guidelines. In: eTG complete [Internet]. Melbourne: Therapeutic Guidelines Ltd. Available from: <www.tg.org.au>, accessed April 2018.

12 O'Connor V, Kovacs G. *Obstetrics, Gynaecology and Women's Health.* Cambridge: Cambridge University Press, 2003: 476–97.

104 Premenstrual syndrome

Shivering, lassitude and heaviness of the head denotes the onset of menstruation . . . mistiness of vision is relieved by menstruation.

HIPPOCRATES, 400 BCE

Premenstrual syndrome (PMS) is defined as a disorder of non-specific somatic, psychological or behavioural symptoms occurring during the late luteal phase of the menstrual cycle.[1]

The pathogenesis of PMS is still uncertain. Among the proposed causes are pyridoxine deficiency, excess prostaglandin production, hypoglycaemia and neurotransmitter (in particular, GABA) abnormalities. However, PMS is most probably related to enhanced sensitivity to progestogen with an underlying serotonin deficiency.[2]

Key facts and checkpoints

- PMS increases in incidence after 30 years, with a peak incidence in the 30–40 years age group.
- PMS also occurs in the 45–50 years age group, when it may alternate with menopausal symptoms, causing clinical confusion.[3]
- The symptoms of PMS decrease in severity just before and during menstruation.
- The symptoms cannot be explained by the presence of various psychological or psychiatric disorders.
- The severe form of PMS is classified in the *Diagnostic and Statistical Manual of Mental Disorders* (4th and 5th edns) as premenstrual dysphoric disorder (PMDD).

Incidence

Up to 90% of women may experience premenstrual symptoms, which can vary from moderately severe in 20–40% of women to disabling in 2–9%.[4] And perhaps 2–5% of women experience symptoms so debilitating as to significantly reduce their quality of life. In this case, they are considered to have premenstrual dysphoric disorder (PMDD).[1]

Symptoms

Various symptoms from among the 150 reported are summarised in FIGURE 104.1.

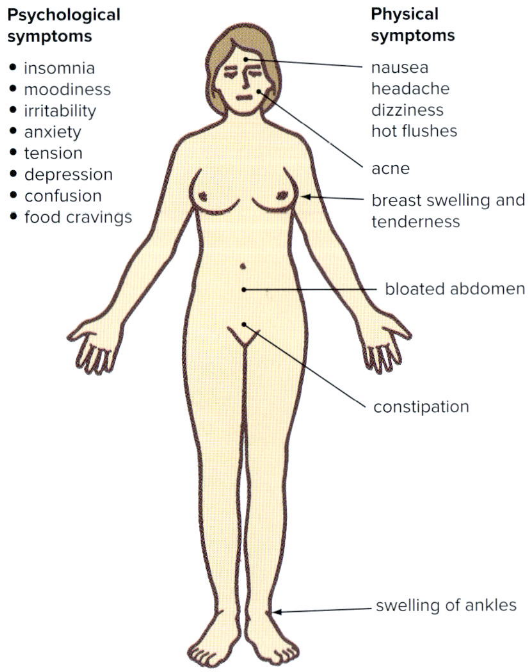

FIGURE 104.1 Symptoms of premenstrual syndrome

Symptoms usually reach a peak during the last 5 premenstrual days and remit within a few days of menstruation. Typically, they recur in subsequent cycles, although variation between cycles is common. The most common psychological symptoms are depression and irritability, while headache, bloating and breast tenderness are the most common physical symptoms.

Classification of PMS

It is convenient to classify PMS in terms of severity of symptoms.[3]

1 *Mild:* symptoms signal onset of menstruation. No medical advice sought or needed.
2 *Moderate:* symptoms annoying but insufficient to interfere with function at home or work. Medical advice sought in about one-third.

3 *Severe:* symptoms are such that functions at work or home are disrupted. Medical advice is usually sought. This disruptive form is labelled PMDD (see TABLE 104.1).

Differential diagnosis[3]

- Endometriosis
- Menopause
- Mastalgia
- Other causes of fluid retention—kidney or adrenal
- Thyroid disorder (hyper- or hypo-activity)
- Anaemia
- Polycystic ovarian syndrome
- Psychiatric disorders: depression, mania

Diagnosis

- Thorough history—including diet, exercise habits, psychosocial background, emotional influences and family history

Table 104.1 Summary of PMDD criteria*[5]

A	Symptoms must occur during the week before menses and start to improve within a few days after onset of menses.
B	One (or more) of the following symptoms must be present and marked: 1 Affective lability 2 Irritability or anger 3 Depressed mood or dysphoria 4 Anxiety, tension or feelings of being on edge
C	One or more of the following to reach a total of 5 symptoms when combined with those from criterion B above: 1 Decreased interest in usual activities 2 Concentration difficulties 3 Marked lack of energy; lethargy 4 Marked change in appetite, overeating, or food cravings 5 Hypersomnia or insomnia 6 Feeling overwhelmed or out of control 7 Other physical symptoms (e.g. breast tenderness, bloating)
D	Symptoms must interfere with work, school, productivity, usual activities or relationships
E	Symptoms must not merely be an exacerbation of another disorder such as major depression
F	Criteria for A must be confirmed by prospective daily ratings for at least two cycles
G	The symptoms are not attributable to the physiological effects of a substance or other medical condition

*Adapted from *DSM-5-TR*

- Menstrual calendar—for 3 months, showing timing of the three main symptoms[3]
- Physical examination to exclude gynaecological, endocrine or other systemic disease; and also include:
  - breast examination (if breast tenderness)
  - cervical screening test
- Investigations (to exclude other causes):
  - thyroid function tests
  - full blood count
  - electrolytes and creatinine
  - FSH and oestradiol—if perimenopause suspected
  - serum androgens—if oligomenorrhoea present

Management[2,4]

The basic aim of management is to reassure and treat the woman in such a way that she makes changes in her lifestyle to cope with the hormonal dysfunction rather than rely on medication. The management strategies include the following, with the emphasis on lifestyle factors.

104

Explanation, reassurance and insight

Cognitive-based therapy, which has been shown to have a positive effect in several RCTs,[4] is very helpful for the patient to understand the nature of her symptoms and to receive appropriate support and rapport. Advise her to be open about her problem and inform her family and close friends about her symptoms.

Keeping a diary[3]

Advise the patient to keep a daily diary of all her symptoms and when they occur over a 2–3 month period. This information should help her to plan around her symptoms: for example, avoid too many social events and demanding business appointments at the time when PMS symptoms are worst.

Dietary advice[1]

Advise the patient to eat regularly and sensibly; eat small, frequent meals and aim for ideal weight.

Increase amount of low-GI complex carbohydrates, leafy green vegetables and legumes.

Decrease or avoid: refined sugar, salt, alcohol, caffeine (tea, coffee, chocolate), tobacco, red meat and excessive fluid intake during premenstrual phase. Decrease total protein to 1 g/kg/day; decrease fats.[6]

Exercise

Recommend a program of regular exercise such as swimming, aerobics, jogging or tennis. Such exercise has been proven to decrease depression, anxiety and fluid retention premenstrually.[6]

Relaxation

Advise patients to plan activities that they find relaxing and enjoyable at the appropriate time. Consider stress reduction therapy, including meditation, yoga, relaxation techniques and appropriate counselling.

Appropriate dress

Advise sensible dressing to manage breast tenderness and a bloated abdomen, such as a firm-fitting bra and loose-fitting clothes around the abdomen.

Medication

104

Pharmaceutical agents that have been used with success in some patients and little or no relief in others include diuretics (e.g. spironolactone), vitamins and minerals (e.g. pyridoxine and evening primrose oil), simple anti-inflammatories (e.g. aspirin, mefenamic acid) and hormonal preparations such as the OCP. A combination of agents may have to be used.

It is worth noting that progestins used alone are ineffective and may even aggravate symptoms, but can be used in conjunction with oestrogen to protect the endometrium.[4]

Supplements

Women often enquire about the use of vitamins, minerals and herbal remedies for PMS. The evidence base for symptom relief so far is as follows:[1,7]

- pyridoxine/vitamin B6 up to 100 mg daily (evidence limited, beware nerve damage to hands/feet with higher doses)
- elemental calcium, 1200 mg to 1500 mg daily (two randomised controlled trials have shown significant benefit)
- elemental magnesium up to 400 mg daily (minimal evidence)
- evening primrose oil 500 mg daily (no benefit over placebo)
- *Agnus castus* (Premular®) is an extract of the berries from the chaste tree (several small randomised controlled trials have indicated some benefit over placebo)

Oral contraception[4]

It is appropriate to use a COC-containing ethinyloestradiol and drospirenone since a meta-analysis of drospirenone, which is a progestogen derivative of spironolactone, concluded that it was effective in reducing the severe symptoms of PMDD.

ethinyloestradiol 20 mgm + drospirenone 3 mg (o) once daily on days 1–24 of a 28-day cycle

Moderate to severe symptoms[4,8]

A trial of an SSRI is warranted in women with incapacitating PMDD who are unresponsive to other treatments.

fluoxetine 20 mg mane for 14 days before the anticipated onset of menstruation[4]

or

sertraline 50 mg daily for 14 days before the anticipated onset of menstruation

> **Practice tip**
>
> Moderate to severe PMDD:
>
> - fluoxetine 20 mg (o) or sertraline 50 mg (o) daily in morning for 14 days before anticipated onset of menstruation and through to the first full day of menses of each cycle

When to refer[3]

- If the recommended approach of support, education, reassurance and stress management is still not effective.
- Refer to a gynaecologist if underlying disease is suspected or proven (e.g. polycystic ovarian syndrome, endometriosis)
- Refer to an endocrinologist if an endocrine disorder such as adrenal, pituitary or thyroid is suspected or proven
- Consider referral if depression or psychosis worsens or is not cyclical

> **Practice tips**
>
> - Keeping a daily diary of symptoms is very helpful for both patient and clinician.
> - Aim for lifestyle changes and commonsense non-pharmacological management.
> - Allow at least three cycles of treatment to provide reasonable time for a particular medication to take effect.
> - High doses of pyridoxine, such as 500 mg a day, are associated with peripheral neuropathy so the dosage should be kept at or below 100 mg a day.
> - Be careful of overdiagnosing PMS and overlooking disorders such as depression, which may be exacerbated in the premenstrual phase.

Patient education resources

Hand-out sheets from *Murtagh's Patient Education* 7th edition:

- Premenstrual syndrome

References

1 Foran T. Management of premenstrual syndrome: how to treat. Australian Doctor, 28 November 2013.
2 Mazza D. *Women's Health in General Practice* (2nd edn). Sydney: Elsevier, 2011: 16–21.
3 Smith M. Premenstrual syndrome. In: *MIMS Disease Index*. Sydney: IMS Publishing, 1991–92: 439–41.
4 Expert group for Endocrinology guidelines. In: eTG complete [Internet]. Melbourne: Therapeutic Guidelines Ltd. Available from: <www.tg.org.au>, accessed April 2018.
5 Premenstrual dysphoric disorder. In: *Diagnostic and Statistical Manual of Mental Disorders* (5th edn). Arlington: American Psychiatric Association, 2013: 191–4.
6 Papadakis MA, McPhee SJ. *Current Medical Diagnosis and Treatment* (52nd edn). New York: The McGraw-Hill Companies, 2013: 749–50.
7 Wyatt K et al. Premenstrual syndrome. Clinical Evidence, 2000; 4: 1121.
8 Brown J et al. Selective serotonin reuptake inhibitors for premenstrual syndrome. Cochrane Database Syst Rev. 2009 Apr 15, Issue 2. Art No. CD006586 (PMID 193706 44).

Resource

National Association of Premenstrual Syndrome <www.pms.org.uk>

105 The menopause

Every woman should use what Mother Nature gave her before Father Time takes it away.

LAURENCE J PETER, 1977

Definitions

The WHO has defined the menopause as signifying the permanent cessation of menstruation, resulting from the loss of ovarian follicular activity.[2] In most Western women, it occurs between the ages of 45 and 55 years, with an average age of 51.5 years.[1] Premature menopause (or premature ovarian insufficiency) is menopause occurring before age 40, while early menopause occurs before 45.

The term is used in a broader sense to include the perimenopausal phase when ovarian function waxes and wanes and the periods become irregular. This may last 2–5 years and sometimes longer and involves the premenopausal and menopausal phases.

The postmenopause is the period following the menopause but cannot be defined until after 12 months of spontaneous amenorrhoea, except in women who have had an oophorectomy.

Surgical menopause is known as bilateral oophorectomy.

Summary

The climacteric can be subdivided into four phases:

Phase 1 Premenopausal: up to 5 years before the last menstrual period.

Phase 2 Perimenopausal: the presence of early menopausal symptoms with changes in menstrual cycle.

Phase 3 Menopausal: the last menstrual period.

Phase 4 Postmenopausal: the phase beginning 12 months after the last menstrual cycle.

Osteoporosis

Osteoporosis, which literally means porous bone, is reduced bone mass per unit volume. Osteoporosis is usually addressed in the context of the menopause because the drop in oestrogen levels causes accelerated loss of bone mass (10% the first 5 years after menopause). Loss of bone density can be largely prevented by correcting oestrogen deficiency.

Physiology of the menopause

FIGURE 105.1 provides an overview of how menopausal symptoms are related to ovarian follicular activity and hormonal activity.

Women are born with their total complement of ovarian primary follicles. The peak number is reached at about 20 weeks' gestation, while in their mother's womb, with an average number of 6 million. From this point, a female constantly loses gametes, reaching 1 million at birth and about 400 000 by puberty. A woman will ovulate 400–500 times in her lifetime and will begin the menopause transition when there are only a few thousand follicles remaining.

The number of follicles declines rapidly as the menopause approaches, with an insufficient number to stimulate cyclical activity. Oestrogen levels fall and this has a positive feedback on the pituitary, increasing FSH levels to 10–15 times that of the follicular phase of the cycle, while LH levels rise about threefold. The ovary secretes minimal oestrogen but continues to secrete significant amounts of androgens. Reduced oestrogen is the main cause of menopausal symptoms such as hot flushes.

Clinical features

In the early menopausal transition, the cycle length may vary by about 7 days (e.g. a 28-day cycle becomes 21). The late menopausal transition is characterised by two or more skipped menstrual cycles.[4] Variability of the heaviness of periods is common and the pattern can be erratic, with prolonged bleeding episodes or scanty menses, interspersed with regular ovarian activity. Uncommonly, women may experience regular periods until complete cessation.

Because small amounts of oestrogen are still being produced in the adrenal glands, symptoms other than cessation of periods may be mild or absent. Around 20% will have no symptoms at all, while another 20% will be severely affected, with symptoms continuing into their 60s or later.[5] Up to 80% of women experience vasomotor symptoms for an average duration of 5 years (range 1–10 years).[3]

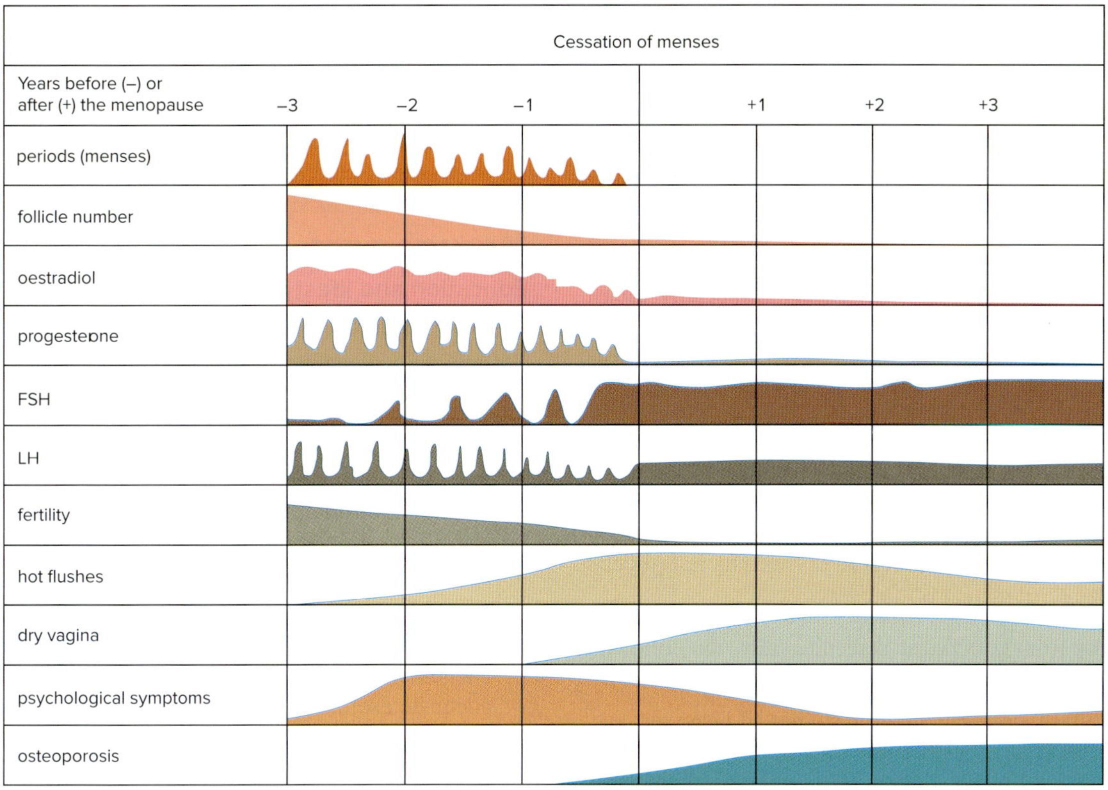

FIGURE 105.1 Schematic representation of some clinical, biological and endocrinological features of the perimenopausal and postmenopausal phases
Source: After Burger[3]

Symptoms

Vasomotor:[2]

- hot flushes (80%)
- night sweats (70%)
- palpitations (30%)
- lightheadedness/dizziness
- migraine

Psychological:

- irritability
- depression
- anxiety
- tearfulness
- loss of concentration
- poor short-term memory
- unloved feelings
- sleep disturbances
- mood changes
- loss of self-confidence
- decline in libido

Urogenital (60%):

- atrophic vaginitis
- vaginal dryness (45%); itching; burning
- dyspareunia/sexual dysfunction
- bladder dysfunction (e.g. frequency, dysuria)
- stress incontinence/prolapse

Musculoskeletal:

- non-specific muscular aches
- non-specific joint aches and pains

Skin and other tissue changes:

- dry skin
- formication (17%)
- new facial hair
- breast glandular tissue atrophy

Other:

- unusual tiredness
- headache

Clinical approach

A thorough evaluation of the patient is important, including a good history.

History

Enquire about any symptoms related to oestrogen deficiency, with an emphasis on the menstrual history and vasomotor symptoms. Take a general medical and gynaecological history, including sexual history, contraception, smoking, drug and alcohol, sleep, micturition and social history, including relationships. Enquire about mental state symptoms, such as irritability, depression, anxiety and loss of self-esteem. Ask how the symptoms are affecting quality of life, particularly sleep disturbance. A symptom score card is a helpful aid.

Consider all women at the menopause to be at risk for cardiovascular disease, cancer (especially breast, ovary and cervix), diabetes and osteoporosis.[1]

Information on family history of osteoporosis, cancer and cardiovascular disease should be sought.

Physical examination

The general examination should include measurement of blood pressure, weight, height and waist circumference. Consider breast examination, abdominal palpation, vaginal examination and cervical screening test (if due).

Investigations[1]

105

Apart from a cervical screening test, the following tests should be considered:

- full blood count and iron studies (if heavy or abnormal menstrual bleeding)
- fasting lipids including HDL and fasting glucose
- liver function tests
- thyroid stimulating hormone (TSH)
- urinalysis (if urinary symptoms)
- screening mammography (if due)
- transvaginal ultrasound (if abnormal vaginal bleeding)
- bone density study (if risk factors)

Diagnosis

Menopause is a retrospective diagnosis, which can be made after 12 months of amenorrhoea in women over 50 and after 2 years in women younger than 50. The diagnosis of perimenopause is made by taking a thorough menstrual history.

Investigating hormone levels is usually unnecessary and often unhelpful, with frequent fluctuations during perimenopause. Testing may be appropriate for younger patients (<45 years), amenorrhoeic women with a levonorgestrel IUD and women who have undergone hysterectomy. For these women, it is common practice to check for an elevated FSH (>30) and confirm with a repeat level at least 1 or 2 months later. An isolated elevated FSH is not proof of the occurrence of menopause.

Differential diagnosis of menopause syndrome

- Depression
- Anaemia
- Thyroid dysfunction
- Hyperparathyroidism
- Diabetes
- Medications (e.g. SSRIs)
- Gynaecological disorders
  - dysfunctional uterine bleeding

Management

Education and lifestyle

Patients should receive adequate understanding, support and explanation, with the emphasis being that the menopause is a natural life transition. It is also important to provide education on long-term health implications, such as cardiovascular disease risk and osteoporosis.

Always consider this as an opportunity to holistically review a woman's health and reinforce the importance of a healthy lifestyle, including:

- healthy, balanced diet
- maintain a healthy weight
- adequate relaxation
- adequate exercise (especially weight-bearing)
- adequate calcium intake (3 serves per day)
- smoking cessation
- safe alcohol intake

Menopausal hormone therapy

The principle indication of menopausal hormone therapy (MHT) is for the relief of troublesome vasomotor symptoms. The regimen is tailored to the individual patient and depends on several factors, including previous hysterectomy, menopausal phase, predominant symptoms and age. MHT has also been known as hormone replacement therapy (HRT).

The Women's Health Initiative study[6]

The arguably flawed Women's Health Initiative (WHI) trial investigated the use of long-term MHT in postmenopausal women with an intact uterus using long-term combined oral oestrogen and progesterone. The study raised concerns about the safety of MHT, with an increased risk of breast cancer (1.26-fold), coronary heart disease (1.29-fold), stroke (1.41-fold) and pulmonary embolism (2.13-fold) with prolonged use greater than 5 years.[7] The study also found a reduction in risk of bowel cancer and fracture in these women. The trial did not include people using other forms of MHT, such as patches, gels or implants.

The recently published long-term follow-up of WHI participants found no difference in the rate of all-cause mortality between women randomised to MHT or placebo. Moreover, for women aged 50–59 years who were randomised to MHT, the hazard ratio for all-cause mortality during the intervention phase of the study was 0.69.[8]

Studies show that the influence of the WHI study has resulted in women being inappropriately discouraged from the use of MHT.[9]

Benefits and risks of MHT

MHT is the most effective method for relieving distressing symptoms such as hot flushes, urogenital symptoms, sleeplessness and joint symptoms (level I and II evidence) (NHMRC criteria).[10]

Risks differ depending on the age of the woman and the route of administration. The recent National Institute for Health and Care Excellence (NICE) guideline on menopause management concluded the following:[9]

- MHT was the most appropriate treatment for menopausal symptoms.
- MHT improved bone density and reduced fracture.
- CVD risk was not increased among women using MHT and may be reduced (in normal target population).
- Venous thromboembolism (VTE) risk was increased among women using oral MHT but not among women using non-oral therapy.
- Breast cancer risk was not increased for women taking oestrogen but was increased with long-duration use in women taking combined oestrogen and progestin therapy. The effect reduced after ceasing therapy.

The International Menopause Society advises that MHT carries few risks when prescribed for symptomatic women without contraindications if initiated in women aged under 60 years or within 10 years of menopause.

> **Practice tip**
>
> In women without contraindications, MHT carries few risks if initiated before the age of 60 or within 10 years of menopause.

Contraindications to MHT[1]

Important contraindications to MHT are listed in TABLE 105.1. The main absolute contraindications are active oestrogen-dependent neoplasms, such as endometrial and breast cancer, deep venous thrombosis, acute thrombophlebitis and undiagnosed, abnormal vaginal bleeding. MHT is protective for bowel cancer but not ovarian cancer.

Table 105.1 Contraindications (absolute or relative) to MHT

History of oestrogen-dependent tumour: • endometrial cancer • breast cancer
Recurrent thromboembolism
Acute ischaemic heart disease (absolute)
History of coronary artery disease (relative)
Cerebrovascular disease
Uncontrolled hypertension
Undiagnosed vaginal bleeding
Active liver disease
Active SLE
Pregnancy
Otosclerosis
Acute intermittent porphyria

105

MHT regimens

The appropriate regimen depends on presence of a uterus and whether the woman is perimenopausal or postmenopausal. Current regimens include the following hormonal treatments:

- oestrogen
- progestogen
- selective oestrogen receptor modulator (SERM)
- tibolone

> **Golden rule**
>
> A progestogen must be used with oestrogen if the woman still has a uterus.

Oestrogen

Oestrogen comes in various preparations: oral, transdermal (patches, gels) and topical vaginal preparations (see TABLE 105.2). Topical preparations are appropriate for women with genitourinary symptoms only and will be discussed later in the chapter. Oestrogen implants are no longer available in Australia. A goal of therapy is to prescribe the lowest possible dose to relieve symptoms. Oestrogenic side effects include breast tenderness and nausea.

Table 105.2 Oestrogens used in the menopause[11]

Generic name	Daily dose range	Trade name
Oral preparations		
Conjugated equine oestrogen (CEE)	0.3–1.25 mg	Premarin
Oestradiol	0.5–2 mg	Estrofem Zumenon
Oestradiol valerate	0.5–2 mg	Progynova
Transdermal patch		
Oestradiol	25–100 mcg	Climara, Estraderm, Estradot
Transdermal gel		
Oestradiol hemihydrate	0.5–1.5 mg	Sandrena

Table 105.3 Progestogens used in the menopause[10,11]

Generic name	Daily dose range	Trade name
Oral preparations		
Medroxyprogesterone acetate	2.5–20 mg	Provera, Rolvera
Norethisterone	1.25–5 mg	Primolut N
Micronised progesterone	100–200 mg	Prometrium
Intrauterine device		
Levonorgestrel (LNG) IUD	20 mcg	Mirena

105

Progestogen

Progestogen is given to women with a uterus and may be given continuously or cyclically (see TABLE 105.3). If a progestogen is not used in addition to oestrogen, many women will develop endometrial hyperplasia and there is a 5–10 times increased risk of endometrial cancer. If given cyclically, it is given for the 1st to the 14th day of the calendar month and a withdrawal bleed will occur.

The intrauterine device (IUD) containing the progestogen levonorgestrel may also be combined with oestrogen and has the added benefits of providing contraception and managing heavy menstrual bleeding.

Micronised progesterone became available on the Australian market in 2016 and is available in oral and vaginal (pessary and gel) preparations. It has been available in Europe and the US for several decades. Large studies have indicated that it may have benefits with respect to breast safety. Mild sedation can occur and, as such, it should be taken at night.[12]

Selective oestrogen receptor modulator (SERM)[13]

The SERM bazedoxifene has been developed as an alternative to progestogen for endometrial protection. SERMs act only on oestrogen receptors, with different effects in different tissues. Bazedoxifene has an oestrogenic effect on bone and improves bone density, while exerting an anti-oestrogenic effect on the breast and endometrium. It offers superior rates of amenorrhoea compared to other MHTs and does not increase mammographic density or breast pain.

Bazedoxifene is combined with conjugated oestrogen in what is called a TSEC (tissue-selective oestrogen complex). It is suitable for use in postmenopausal women. An increased risk of VTE has been reported for both oral oestrogen and SERMs and while early studies do not reveal an additive effect on the VTE risk, the true risk remains unknown. It should not be used by women at high risk of VTE.

TSEC dose: CEE 0.45 mg + bazedoxifene 20 mg (o) daily

Tibolone

This is a selective tissue oestrogenic activity regulator with combined oestrogenic, progestogenic and androgenic properties that can be used as an excellent alternative to conventional MHT in postmenopausal women. Positive effects are on vasomotor and urogenital symptoms, sexual function, bone density and fracture risk. It is unsuitable in perimenopausal women because of an increased risk of breakthrough bleeding. It is an appropriate alternative to oestrogen therapy for women who have undergone hysterectomy. Adverse effects with breakthrough bleeding and virilisation are a concern.[10]

Dose: tibolone 2.5 mg (o) daily

Testosterone

Testosterone is usually reserved for women whose libido does not improve with tibolone and those with a premature menopause, but this indication is controversial and specialist involvement is recommended. If available, it is given as an implant of 50 mg and will last 3–12 months.

How to prescribe MHT

TABLE 105.4 presents current commonly used regimens.

Previous hysterectomy

Women do not need a progestogen and should be prescribed continuous oestrogen in either a transdermal or oral preparation. Transdermal delivery of oestrogen has a lower VTE risk.

Table 105.4 Menopausal hormonal therapy (options)	
Uterus intact	Post-hysterectomy
Transdermal O + P patch	Oral O
Transdermal O patch or gel + oral P or LNG-IUD	Transdermal O patch or gel
Oral O + oral P	Tibolone
Oral O + LNG-IUD	
Oral O + SERM (i.e. TSEC)	
Tibolone	

O = oestrogen
P = progestogen
LNG-IUD = levonorgestrel IUD
SERM = selective oestrogen receptor modulator
TSEC = tissue selective oestrogen complex
Source: Adapted from Jane and Davis, Figure 3[1]

Perimenopausal women

For women whose LMP was less than 12 months ago, the progestogen should be cyclical. Use of continuous oestrogen and progestogen too soon after the LMP can result in unpredictable breakthrough bleeding. The exception is with the use of the levonorgestrel (LNG) intrauterine system, which can be used with oral oestrogen. After 12 months of cyclical MHT, it is reasonable to transition to a continuous regimen.

Oestrogen and progesterone can be administered separately or in combined preparations. Combined cyclical preparations available in Australia are listed in TABLE 105.5).

Combined hormonal contraception is an appropriate alternative to cyclical MHT and can be used up to 50–51 years, provided there are no contraindications (see CHAPTER 99). Contraception is advisable for 12 months after the last period for women over 50 years and for 2 years for those under 50 years.

Table 105.5 Cyclical MHT preparations available in Australia[1,11]

Generic name	Daily dose*	Trade name
Oral preparations		
Oestradiol/ dydrogesterone	1 mg/10 mg, 2 mg/10 mg	Femoston
Oestradiol/ norethisterone	1 mg/1 mg, 2 mg/1 mg	Trisequens
Transdermal patch		
Oestradiol/ norethisterone	50 mcg/140 mcg, 50 mcg/250 mcg	Estalis Sequi

**Progestogen for 14 out of 28 days only*

Postmenopausal women

For women whose LMP was more than 12 months ago, continuous combined oestrogen plus progestogen therapy can be used (TABLE 105.6).

Side effects of therapy[14]

In the first 2–3 months, the woman may experience oestrogenic side effects, but these usually resolve or stabilise. Starting with a lower dose may minimise these side effects.

Premenstrual syndrome (in 15%)

Action: decrease progestogen dose *or* change to alternative progestogen

Nausea and breast symptoms

Cause: initial sensitivity to oestrogen
Action: reduce oestrogen dose, consider SERM if breast symptoms

Bleeding problems

Heavy bleeding
Action: decrease oestrogen

Unscheduled vaginal bleeding
Action: increase progestogen, consider LNG-IUD or SERM

Unscheduled vaginal bleeding occurring 3 months after initiating therapy requires formal investigation.

105

Duration of treatment[15]

Recent guidelines published by the International Menopause Society recommend that there should be no mandatory limit to the duration of MHT.

Women who are prescribed MHT should be reviewed at least annually to check on its efficacy and side effects, with treatment tailored accordingly. The mode of delivery and the type of MHT should be adjusted according to age and circumstance.

Provided contraindications do not emerge, women can continue MHT as long as it addresses therapeutic goals, symptoms and quality of life.

Vaginal dryness[11]

While vasomotor symptoms improve over time in the majority of women, genitourinary symptoms generally do not. The first-line therapy is a non-hormonal lubricant such as Replens or K-Y Gel. If these are ineffective, topical low-dose vaginal oestrogen preparations can be useful, for example:

oestrogen cream or pessary (e.g. Ovestin, Vagifem) daily at bedtime for 2–3 weeks, then once or twice weekly for maintenance

Table 105.6 Continuous MHT preparations available in Australia[1,11]

Generic name	Daily dose	Trade name
Oral preparations		
Oestradiol/drospirenone	1 mg/2 mg, 1 mg/5 mg	Angeliq 1/2, Femoston-Conti
Oestradiol/norethisterone	1 mg/0.5 mg, 2 mg/1 mg	Kliovance, Kliogest
Conjugated equine oestrogen (CEE)/ medroxyprogesterone acetate	0.625 mg/2.5 mg, 0.625 mg/5 mg	Premia
Transdermal patch		
Oestradiol/norethisterone	50 mcg/140 mcg, 50 mcg/250 mcg	Estalis Continuous

Topical oestrogen therapy is the preferred option for those women whose menopausal symptoms are limited to vaginal dryness and dyspareunia. Systemic absorption of oestrogen can occur and safety cannot be assured for women with contraindications to MHT. CO_2 Fractional Laser is an alternative treatment available for women with contraindications to topical oestrogen or for whom topical treatments have proved insufficient.

Non-hormonal therapy regimens

Lifestyle changes

Discuss triggers for hot flushes that might be avoidable, including spicy food, alcohol, coffee and emotional stressors. It is advisable to wear loose-fitting clothes and dress in layers.

Medical therapy

Non-hormonal, medical options for hot flushes include gabapentin, clonidine and antidepressants. The front-line treatments are the SSRIs and SNRIs, for example:[11]

> paroxetine 10 mg (o) daily increasing up to 20 mg daily after 1 week
> *or*
> venlafaxine 37.5 mg (o) daily, increasing to 75 mg

Complementary therapy

Options include black cohosh, red clover, soy products and other phytoestrogens (plants containing oestrogen-like compounds). Black cohosh has been linked to rare cases of abnormal liver function, hepatitis and liver failure.

The National Prescribing Service concluded that 'most complementary medicine has little evidence of efficacy and poor-quality safety data. Anecdotal evidence is particularly unreliable as hot flushes improve by up to 60% with placebo, partly due to natural fluctuation in symptoms'.[16,17]

Bioidenticals

These are mixtures of hormones prepared by compounding chemists and supplied as lozenges, troches and creams. There is inadequate data to show that these are effective or safe.

Premature ovarian insufficiency[18]

Premature ovarian insufficiency (POI) is defined as a disorder in ovarian function in any woman before the age of 40 years, irrespective of the cause. It occurs spontaneously in 1% of women before the age of 40.

Causes and associations:

- idiopathic (most common)
- genetic (10%)
  - monosomy X (Turner syndrome)
  - fragile X mutation
- iatrogenic, e.g. ovarian surgery, chemotherapy, radiotherapy
- autoimmune associations (20%), e.g. coeliac disease, diabetes, Addison's
- infection, e.g. mumps, TB, malaria, shigella
- metabolic disease, e.g. galactosaemia

Untreated POI is associated with increased incidence of osteoporosis, heart disease, cognitive impairment and premature death.

The cornerstone of treatment is MHT until the median age of menopause.

When to refer

- Symptoms insufficiently controlled with MHT
- Side effects of MHT that are not corrected by routine measures

Practice tips

- Careful pretreatment assessment is important.
- Encourage conservative management with an emphasis on lifestyle if symptoms are mild.
- Ensure the patient is informed and accepts both benefits and risks.
- Individualise hormonal therapy.
- The prime treatment for an oestrogen-deficiency disorder is oestrogen.
- Use oestrogen-only therapy for women without a uterus.
- If a uterus is present, give combined oestrogen-progestogen therapy. A SERM is a new alternative to progestogen.
- Use cyclical MHT in perimenopausal women and continuous MHT in postmenopausal women.
- Always start with a low dose of oestrogen.
- Allow about 6 months to stabilise with MHT.
- Yearly follow-up is advised.
- Problematic loss of libido can be treated with tibolone.
- Oestrogen deficiency causes vaginal dryness, which can be treated with topical oestrogen therapy.

Patient education resources

Hand-out sheets from *Murtagh's Patient Education* 7th edition:

- Menopause

References

1 Jane FM, Davis S. A practitioner's toolkit for managing the menopause. Climacteric, 2014; 17: 1–16.
2 Gold EB, Crawford SL, Avis NE et al. Factors related to age at natural menopause: longitudinal analyses from SWAN. Am J Epidemiol, 2013; 178: 70–83.
3 Burger H. Talking women: HRT and breast cancer risk. Medical Observer, 1 August 2008: 40.
4 Mazza D. *Women's Health in General Practice* (2nd edn). Sydney: Elsevier, 2011: 256–7.
5 Col NF, Guthrie JR, Politi M, Dennerstein L. Duration of vasomotor symptoms in middle-aged women: a longitudinal study. Menopause, 2009; 16 (3): 453–7.
6 Writing Group for the Women's Health Initiative Investigators. Risks and benefits of oestrogen plus progestin in healthy postmenopausal women: principal results from the Women's Health Initiative randomised controlled trial. JAMA, 2002; 288 (3): 321–33.
7 Royal Australian College of General Practitioners. HRT advice. Aust Fam Physician, 2002; 31 (8): 733–4.
8 Manson J, Aragaki A, Rossouw J et al. Menopausal hormone therapy and long-term all-cause and cause-specific mortality. The Women's Health Initiative randomized trials. JAMA, 2017; 318: 927–38.
9 Baber R. Hormone therapy and menopause: a protracted misunderstanding explained. Medicine Today, 2017; 18 (2): 23–6.
10 Vincent A, Burger H. Menopause: how to treat. Australian Doctor, 6 November 2009: 25–32.
11 Expert group for Endocrinology. In: eTG complete [Internet]. Melbourne: Therapeutic Guidelines Ltd. Available from: <www.tg.org.au>, accessed May 2018.
12 Davis S. Micronised progesterone as a component of menopausal hormone therapy. Medicine Today, 2017; 18 (1): 53–5.
13 Baber R. What's new in menopausal hormone therapy: combination oestrogen-bazedoxifene. Medicine Today, 2018: 19 (4): 47–50.
14 Baber R. The menopause: update. Medical Observer, 28 July 2006: 31–3.
15 Magraith K, Stuckey B. An update on hormone therapy for menopause. Medicine Today, 2018; 19 (1): 41–44.
16 National Prescribing Service Ltd. *Managing Menopausal Symptoms,* Review PPR 47, September 2009.
17 MacLennan AH et al. Oral oestrogen and combined oestrogen/progestogen therapy versus placebo for hot flushes. Cochrane Database Syst Rev. 2004, Issue 4. Art No. CD002978.
18 Nguyen HH, Milat F, Vincent A. Premature ovarian insufficiency in general practice: meeting the needs of women. Aust Fam Physician, 2017; 46 (6): 360–6.

Resources

The British Menopause Society <www.thebms.org.uk>
The Australian Menopause Society <www.menopause.org.au/>
Jean Hailes Foundation <www.jeanhailes.org.au>

106 Vaginal discharge

In all cases of abnormal vaginal discharge consider the possibility of the sexually transmitted infections.

Dr Stella Heley, Victorian Cytology Service, 2001

Vaginal discharge is a common complaint seen by family physicians, yet it is often difficult to solve, especially if it is recurrent or persistent. Women may complain of an increase in the amount of discharge, a change in the consistency or colour and the presence of an offensive odour. It is important to make a proper diagnosis, to differentiate between normal (physiological) and pathological discharge and to be aware of the considerable variation in secretion of vaginal fluid.

This variation extends to different age groups, with microbial causes less likely in prepubertal girls and the elderly, who more often present with dermatoses and symptoms related to reduced vaginal oestrogen.

The differential diagnoses should include consideration of normal discharge, vaginal candidiasis, bacterial vaginosis (BV), STIs, foreign body, vulval dermatoses, atrophic vaginitis and genital tract malignancy.

Table 106.1 Vaginal discharge: diagnostic strategy model

Probability diagnosis
Normal physiological discharge
Vaginitis:
- candidiasis
- bacterial vaginosis

Serious disorders not to be missed
Neoplasia:
- cancer
- fistulas

STIs/PID:
- *Chlamydia trachomatis*
- *Neisseria gonorrhoeae*
- *Mycoplasma genitalum*
- herpes simplex—types 1 and 2

Sexual abuse, esp. children
Tampon toxic shock syndrome (staphylococcal infection)
Ectopic pregnancy ('prune juice' discharge)

Pitfalls (often missed)
Atrophic vaginitis
Contact dermatitis (e.g. intravaginal pessaries and creams)
Retained foreign objects (e.g. tampons)
Erosive lichen planus
Desquamative inflammatory vaginitis
Latex allergy
Herpes simplex virus (if causes cervicitis)
Threadworms

Seven masquerades checklist
Diabetes
Drugs

Is the patient trying to tell me something?
Needs careful consideration; possible sexual dysfunction.

A diagnostic approach

A summary of the diagnostic strategy model is presented in TABLE 106.1.

Probability diagnosis

The most common causes of vaginal discharge are physiological discharge, vulovaginal candidiasis and bacterial vaginosis.

Physiological discharge

Normal physiological discharge is usually milky-white or clear mucoid and originates from a combination of the following sources:

- cervical mucus (secretions from cervical glands)
- vaginal secretion (transudate through vaginal mucosa)
- vaginal squamous epithelial cells (desquamation)
- cervical columnar epithelial cells
- resident commensal bacteria

The predominant bacterial flora are lactobacilli, which produce lactic acid from glucose derived from the epithelial cells. The lactic acid keeps the vaginal pH acidic (<4.7). Other commensal bacteria include staphylococci, diphtheroids and streptococci.

With physiological discharge there is usually no odour or pruritus.

In addition, the egg-white discharge accompanying ovulation may be noted. Normal discharge usually shows on underwear by the end of the day. Clear or white, it oxidises to a yellow or brown on contact with air. It is often increased in pregnancy and during sexual arousal. Women using the combined oral contraceptive pill may notice less discharge.

Management is largely based on reassurance and explanation.

Important causative organisms

Vulovaginal candidiasis is caused by an overgrowth of yeasts, usually *Candida albicans*, or less commonly other species such as *Candida glabrata, Candida tropicalis* and *Candida krusei.*[1] Bacterial vaginosis is a polymicrobial condition characterised by changes in the normal vaginal flora, with a reduction in key Lactobacillus species and high concentrations of anaerobic bacteria such as *Gardnerella vaginalis.*[2] *Trichomonas vaginalis* is of high prevalence in some remote Aboriginal and Torres Strait Islander communities. The comparable features are outlined in TABLE 106.2.

Serious disorders not to be missed

The 'not to be missed' group includes cancer of the vagina, cervix or uterus and STIs, including PID caused by *Chlamydia trachomatis, Neisseria gonorrhoeae* and *Mycoplasma genitalium.* Vaginal discharge is the most common presenting symptom of these STIs in women; however, they are commonly asymptomatic. Benign and malignant neoplasia anywhere in the genital tract may produce a discharge. Usually it is watery and pink or blood-stained.

Inspection should include vigilance for fistulas that may be associated with malignancy, inflammation or post-irradiation.

Pitfalls

It is common to overlook contact dermatitis caused by topical preparations. Apart from the vaginal tampon, which may be retained (knowingly or otherwise), there is a variety of preparations that can induce a sensitivity reaction. These include deodorant soaps and sprays and spermicidal creams. Ironically, the various preparations used to treat the vaginitis may cause a chemical reaction.

Seven masquerades checklist

Of this group, diabetes mellitus leading to recurrent 'thrush' and drugs causing a local sensitivity have to be considered (see TABLE 106.1).

Psychogenic considerations

This question needs to be answered, especially if the discharge is normal. The problem could be related to sexual dysfunction or it may reflect a problematic relationship, and the issue may need to be explored diplomatically. Vaginal discharge is an embarrassing problem for the patient and any discussion needs to be handled thoroughly and sensitively.

The clinical approach

History

The history is important and should include:

- nature of discharge: colour, odour, quantity
- onset and duration, relation to menstrual cycle
- irritation or itch and location
- associated dyspareunia
- pelvic or abdominal pain
- sexual history: STI risk factors, previous STIs
- use of chemicals, such as soaps, deodorants, pessaries and douches
- pregnancy possibility
- drug therapy (e.g. antibiotics, oral or topical corticosteroids)
- associated medical conditions (e.g. diabetes)

Table 106.2 Characteristics of discharge for important causes of abnormal vaginal discharge[1,3]

Infective organism	Colour	Consistency	Odour	pH (normal 4–4.7)	Associated symptoms
Candida albicans	White	Thick, lumpy (cottage cheese)	None	<4.5	Itch, soreness, redness
Trichomonas vaginalis	Yellow–green	Bubbly, profuse (mucopurulent)	Malodorous, fishy	5–6	Soreness
Bacterial vaginosis	White or grey	Watery, profuse, bubbly, homogenous	Malodorous, fishy	5–6	Irritation (sometimes)
Normal discharge	Clear–white	Varies with cycle	None	<4.5	None

Source: Weisberg[3]

Examination

Inspection in good light includes viewing the vulva, introitus, urethra, vagina and cervix. Check the vulva for erythema, excoriation, lichenification, linear fissures and atrophic changes. Look for the discharge and specific problems such as polyps, warts, prolapses or fistulas. A mucopurulent discharge appearing from the endocervix may be the clue to an STI such as *Chlamydia* or gonorrhoea. Consider bimanual pelvic examination according to history, checking for adnexal, uterine and cervical motion tenderness.

Pitfalls to keep in mind include:

- A retained tampon may be missed in the posterior fornix, so the speculum should slide directly along the posterior wall of the vagina.
- *Candida* infection may not show the characteristic discharge.
- The 'strawberry vagina' of *Trichomonas* is uncommon and bubbles may not be seen.

Acetic acid 2% may be useful in removing discharge and mucus to enable a clearer view of the cervix and vaginal walls.

Investigations[1]

- High vaginal swab for microscopy and culture
  - for *Candida* species, bacterial vaginosis
- High vaginal swab for STIs *Chlamydia trichomatis, N. gonorrhoea* and *Mycoplasma genitalium* NAAT (i.e. PCR)
  - consider *Trichmonas vaginalis* NAAT if patient from endemic region
- pH test of vaginal discharge
  - use paper with a narrow range of pH 4–7
  - result can be altered by semen, blood, cervical secretions and lubricating jelly
- Amine or 'whiff' test for BV: add a drop of 10% KOH to vaginal secretions smeared on glass slide, positive with release of fishy odour
- Wet-film microscopy of a drop of vaginal secretions (if microscope available)
- Consider PCR for herpes simplex virus if no other explanation

Preparation of a wet film

To make a wet film preparation[3] (see FIG. 106.1), place one drop of normal saline (preferably warm) on one end of an ordinary slide and one drop of 10% KOH on the other half of the slide. A sample of the discharge needs to be taken with a swab stick, either directly from the posterior fornix of the vagina or from discharge that has collected on the posterior blade of the speculum during the vaginal examination. A small amount of the discharge is mixed with both the normal saline drop and the KOH drop. A cover slip is placed over each preparation. The slide is examined under low power to get an overall impression, and under high power to determine the presence of lactobacilli, polymorphs, trichomonads, spores, clue cells and hyphae. A summary of various findings on wet film examination is presented in TABLE 106.3. Lactobacilli are long, thin Gram-positive rods; clue cells are vaginal epithelial cells that have bacteria attached so that the cytoplasm appears granular and often the entire border is obscured. They are a feature of

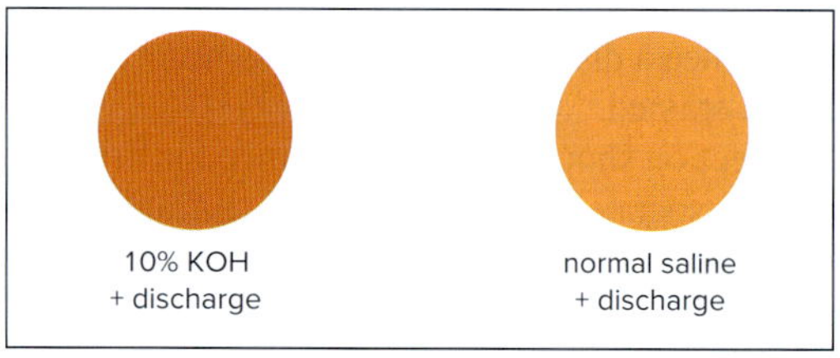

Examine for:
1 epithelial cell
2 polymorph
3 lactobacilli
4 tricomonads
5 clue cells

FIGURE 106.1 Wet film method

Table 106.3 Wet film examination

	Lactobacilli	Polymorphs	Epithelial cells	Clue cells	Other
Normal	+	None or occasional	+	–	
Candidiasis	+	None or occasional	+	–	Spores/hyphae
Trichomoniasis	Absent or scant	Numerous	+	–	Trichomonads
Bacterial vaginosis	Absent or scant	Numerous	+	2–50%	

Source: Weisberg[3]

bacterial vaginosis. Trichomonads are about the same size as polymorphs; to distinguish between the two, one needs to see the movement of the trichomonad and the beating of its flagella under high power of the microscope. Warming the slide will often precipitate movement.

Refer to FIGURE 106.2.

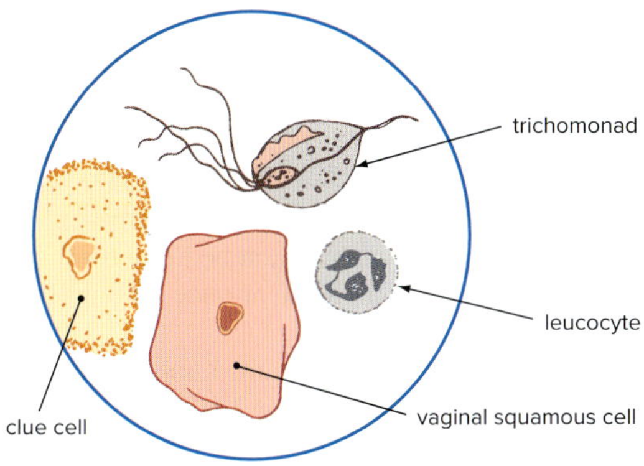

FIGURE 106.2 Relative sizes of various cells or organisms as seen in a wet smear

Vaginal discharge in children[4]

Most newborn girls have some mucoid white vaginal discharge. This is normal and usually disappears by 3 months of age. From 3 months of age to puberty, vaginal discharge is usually minimal. Vulvovaginitis is the most common gynaecological condition of childhood, the causal factors being the normal thin mucosa of the prepubescent state, moisture and irritants.

If discharge is profuse or offensive, take an intraoital swab, which may reveal organisms such as group A *Streptococcus, Haemophilus* and *Gardnerella.* An appropriate antibiotic may help in this instance. Candida infection is unusual in children from 2 years until puberty.

Sexual abuse occasionally presents as vulvovaginitis.

Vaginal discharge in the elderly

Vaginal discharge in the elderly is most commonly due to atrophic vaginitis. Other causes include foreign bodies, bacterial vaginosis and neoplasia. It is important to exclude malignancy of the uterus, cervix and vagina in the older patient.

Vulvovaginal candidiasis does not occur in healthy, non-diabetic women who have not been taking antibiotics and lack oestrogen. However, it can occur in women taking menopause hormone therapy (MHT) and topical oestrogen. In this case, stop oestrogen treatment and treat for chronic vulvovaginal candidiasis until symptoms resolve. It may then be appropriate to recommence oestrogen therapy at a lower dose or continue the usual dose, but with intermittent treatment for candida.[5]

Atrophic vaginitis

In the absence of oestrogen stimulation, the vaginal and vulval tissues begin to shrink and become thin and dry. This renders the vagina more susceptible to bacterial attack because of the loss of vaginal acidity. Rarely, a severe attack can occur with a very haemorrhagic vagina and heavy discharge:

- yellowish, non-offensive discharge
- tenderness and dyspareunia
- spotting or bleeding with coitus
- the vagina may be reddened with superficial haemorrhagic areas

Treatment

oestrogen cream or pessary (e.g. Ovestin, Vagifem) daily at bedtime for 2–3 weeks, then once or twice weekly

or

zinc and castor oil soothing cream

Note: perform a careful speculum examination.

106

Vulvovaginal candidiasis

Candida species are commensal organisms of the gastrointestinal and genital tract. Most cases of candidal vulvovaginitis are infrequent episodes resulting from sporadic increases in vaginal candida. It occurs when the vagina is exposed to oestrogen and is especially common in women aged 20–30 years and during pregnancy. It is not sexually transmissible, although sexual intercourse may be a trigger. Recurrent candidal vulvovaginitis is defined as four or more acute episodes per year.

Some 10–20% of women may be colonised with candida without signs or symptoms. Treatment is not indicated for these women.

Clinical features

- Intense vaginal and vulval pruritus
- Vulval soreness
- Vulval fissures
- Vulvovaginal erythema (brick red)
- Vaginal excoriation and oedema
- White, curd-like discharge (see FIG. 106.3)
- Superficial dyspareunia
- Dysuria

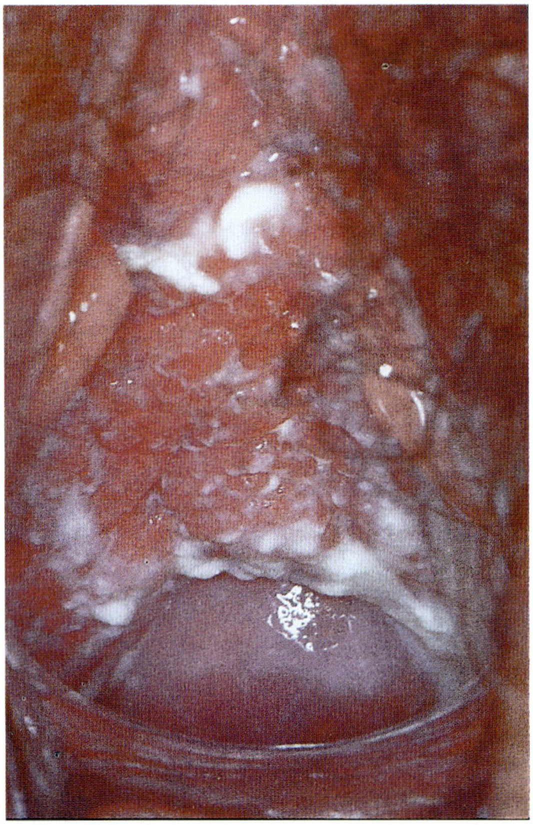

106

FIGURE 106.3 Vaginal candidiasis showing typical adherent, thick, milky-white vaginal discharge

Factors predisposing to vaginal candidiasis[6]

Endogenous

- Diabetes mellitus
- Pregnancy
- Immune deficiency, e.g. HIV

Exogenous

- Oral contraceptives (but cessation of the OCP does not usually improve candidiasis)
- MHT or topical oestrogen
- Antibiotics
- Corticosteroid therapy
- Immunosuppressants
- Orogenital/anogenital intercourse
- IUCD
- Tight-fitting jeans
- Nylon underwear
- Wet bathing suit

Treatment[5,7]

Before starting treatment, take a swab to confirm the diagnosis and determine the species of *Candida.*

For the first attack of candidiasis, it is appropriate to select one of the range of vaginal azole therapies (clotrimazole, miconazole) for 1–7 days, depending on strength. There appears to be no significant difference between azoles. Nystatin is best reserved for recurrent cases or if there is local reaction to the azoles.

Creams can be applied to the vulva if there are vulval symptoms. Combining azole therapy with a topical corticosteroid such as 1% hydrocortisone may also be useful.

Gentian violet (0.5% aqueous solution) is useful for rapid relief, if available.

Recommended initial regimen[5]

clotrimazole 1%, 2% or 10% vaginal cream, 1 applicatorful intravaginally, at bedtime for 6 nights if 1%, 3 nights if 2% or once only if 10%
or
miconazole 2% vaginal cream, 1 applicatorful intravaginally, at bedtime for 7 nights
or
clotrimazole 100 mg or 500 mg pessary intravaginally, at bedtime for 6 nights if 100 mg, once only if 500 mg

An alternative regimen, especially for recurrent infections:

nystatin vaginal cream (100 000 U per 5 g), 1 applicatorful intravaginally, at bedtime daily for 14 nights

If the patient does not tolerate vaginal therapy or prefers oral therapy, use fluconazole 150 mg (o) as a single dose

Chronic vulvovaginal candidiasis[8]

Patients with chronic vulvovaginal candidiasis are a less well-recognised and -managed group. The pathogenesis is unknown but may relate to an exaggerated immunological response to candida. Viewing the condition as a hypersensitivity reaction to the presence of candida, rather than infection, helps understanding and guides treatment. It may start at any age from menarche onwards and ceases at menopause provided MHT is not used.

The most common complaint is chronic itch with dyspareunia and pain. Vaginal discharge is common but may be absent and the typical cottage cheese exudate is not seen. Symptoms are often worse in the premenstrual week and improve during menses. Initial response to azole treatment is common but there is gradual resistance to topical therapy. Almost 95% of cases are caused by *C. albicans.*

When taking the swab, a low vaginal swab usually has a higher yield than a high vaginal swab. False negatives are common.

Treatment[5]

fluconazole 50 mg (o) once daily
or
itraconazole 100 mg (o) once daily

The time to achieve remission varies from 2 weeks to 6 months. Review treatment after 3 months. A mild topical steroid is also appropriate to use in addition.

Note: There is no evidence to support routine screening or treatment of asymptomatic partners.[1] If a male partner is symptomatic (usually balanitis in an uncircumcised male), treat with clotrimazole 1% + hydrocortisone 1% topically, 12 hourly until 2 weeks after symptoms resolve.

Candida glabrata[5]

A significant number of cases of vulvovaginal candidiasis are due to non-albicans species of *Candida. Candida glabrata* is the commonest non-albicans species, which exhibits reduced susceptibility to azoles. In resistant infections, use boric acid 600 mg (in a gelatin capsule) intravaginally at bedtime for 14 days. Do not use in pregnancy.

General advice to patients with vaginal candidiasis[5,9]

- Bathe the genital area with water and dry gently but thoroughly after showering or bathing.
- Wear loose-fitting, cotton underwear.
- Avoid wearing pantyhose, tight jeans or tight underwear.
- Do not use vaginal douches, powders or deodorants or take bubble baths.

Trichomonas vaginalis[10]

This flagellated protozoan, which is thought to originate in the bowel, infects the vagina, Skene's ducts and lower urinary tract in women and the lower genitourinary tract in men. It is easily transmitted through sexual intercourse. In Australia, trichomonas is more common in older women and women from regional and remote areas, especially Aboriginal and Torres Strait Islander. If untreated, the infection is cleared more easily in men. NAAT test is available on vaginal swab and first-pass urine.

Clinical features

- Profuse, thin discharge (grey to yellow–green in colour) (see FIG. 106.4)

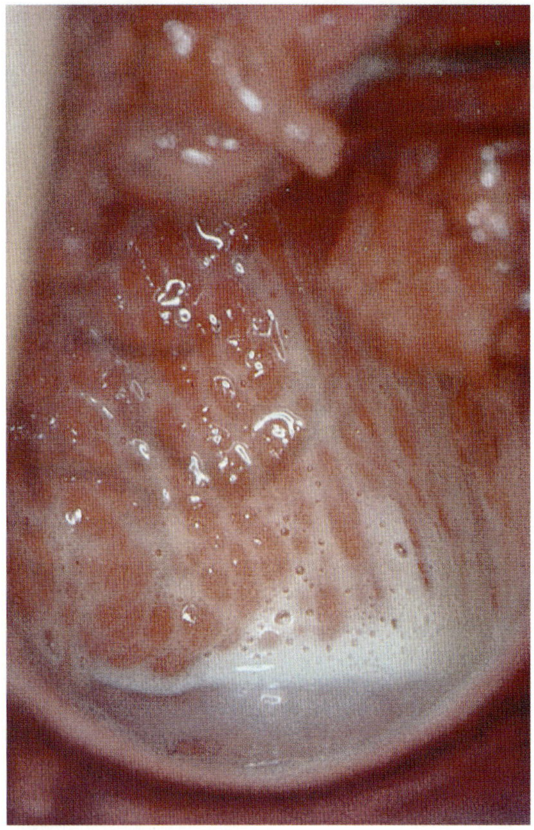

FIGURE 106.4 *Trichomonas vaginitis* showing profuse, thin, greyish discharge with erythema of the vaginal walls

106

- Small bubbles may be seen in 20–30%
- Vulval itch
- Malodorous discharge
- Dyspareunia
- Diffuse erythema of cervix and vaginal walls
- Characteristic punctate appearance on cervix

Treatment

oral metronidazole 2 g as a single dose (preferable) or 400 mg bd for 5 days (if relapse)
or
tinidazole 2 g as a single dose

- Sexual partners must be treated simultaneously
- No sexual contact is advised for 7 days after treatment for patient and partner

Bacterial vaginosis

Bacterial vaginosis is a clinical entity of mixed aetiology characterised by the replacement of the normal vaginal microflora (chiefly *Lactobacillus*) with a mixed flora (referred to as polymicrobial clinical syndrome) consisting of *Gardnerella vaginalis*, other anaerobes such as *Atopobium vaginae*, *Mobiluncus* species and *Mycoplasma hominis*. This accounts for the alkalinity of the vaginal pH.

Clinical features

- A white or grey, homogenous discharge (see FIG. 106.5)
- Malodorous
- No obvious vulvitis or vaginitis
- Liberates an amine-like, fishy odour on admixture of 10% KOH (the amine whiff test)
- Clue cells on wet preparation
- ± Dyspareunia and dysuria
- ± Pruritus (uncommon)

Note. About 50% of patients are asymptomatic.

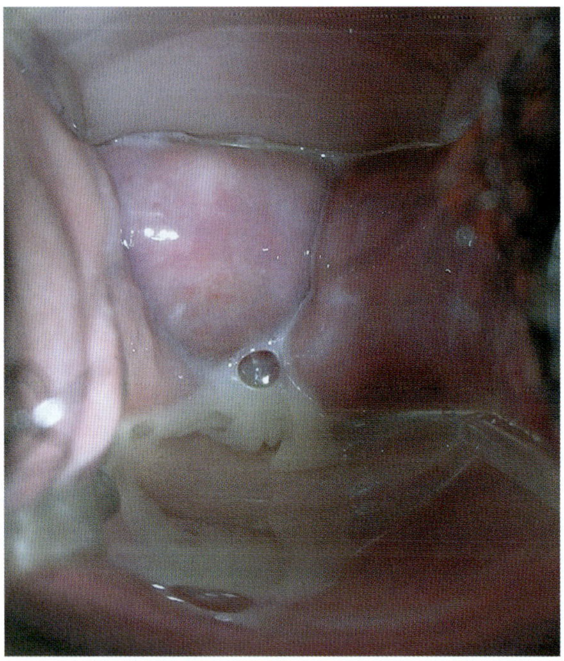

FIGURE 106.5 Bacterial vaginosis

Treatment[5]

Refer to TABLE 106.4.

If symptomatic:

metronidazole 400 mg (o) bd for 5 days (or 2 g stat)

or

0.75% vaginal gel applied at bedtime for 5 days

106

Table 106.4 Oral treatment for symptomatic bacterial vaginosis and *Trichomonas* infections

Length of treatment	Generic name	Oral dosage
1 day (statim dose)	tinidazole	500 mg × 4
	metronidazole	400 mg × 5
7 days (for recurrent)	tinidazole	500 mg daily
	metronidazole	400 mg bd

Clindamycin 300 mg (o) bd for 7 days or 2% clindamycin cream, 1 applicatorful at bedtime for 7 nights, can be used for resistant infections or during pregnancy. Treating male partners has not been recommended; however, consider screening and treating female sexual partners.[2]

Group B *Streptococcus* vaginosis[11]

Group B *Streptococcus* (*S. agalactiae*) is a commensal in up to 30% of healthy humans. It is a problem if detected in pregnant women because of the risk of serious infection in the neonate that is delivered vaginally. Other than in pregnancy, it is generally an incidental finding and should be ignored.

Rarely, Group B *Steptococcus* produces a symptomatic vulvovaginitis with an irritating discharge. However, other causes of vulvovaginitis are more common and should be considered. Suitable treatment for symptomatic patients includes clindamycin 2% vaginal cream, 1 applicatorful intravaginally at bedtime for 14 nights, and phenoxymethylpenicillin 500 mg orally, bd for 10 days.

Retained vaginal tampon

A retained tampon, which may be impacted and cannot be removed by the patient, is usually associated with an extremely offensive vaginal discharge. Its removal can cause considerable embarrassment to both patient and doctor.

Methods of removal

Using good vision the tampon is seized with a pair of sponge-holding forceps and quickly immersed under water without releasing the forceps. A bowl of water (an old plastic ice-cream container is suitable) is kept as close to the introitus as possible. This results in minimal malodour. The tampon and water are immediately flushed down the toilet if the toilet system can accommodate tampons. An alternative method is to grasp the tampon with a gloved hand and quickly peel the glove over the tampon for disposal.

Tampon toxic shock syndrome: staphylococcal infection

This rare, dramatic condition is caused by the production of staphylococcal exotoxin associated with tampon use for menstrual protection. The syndrome usually begins within 5 days of the onset of the period.

The clinical features include sudden onset fever, vomiting and diarrhoea, muscle aches and pains, skin erythema, hypotension progressing to confusion, stupor and sometimes death.

Management

Active treatment depends on the severity of the illness. Cultures should be taken from the vagina, cervix, perineum and nasopharynx. The patient should be referred to a major centre if 'shock' develops. Otherwise the vagina must be emptied, ensuring there is not a forgotten tampon, cleaned with a povidone iodine solution tds for 2 days, and flucloxacillin or vancomycin antibiotics administered.

Prevention

- Good general hygiene with care in handling and inserting the tampons.
- Change the tampon 3–4 times a day.
- Consider using an external pad at night during sleep.

When to refer

- Evidence of sexual abuse in children (to an experienced sexual assault centre)
- Recurrent, recalcitrant infections
- Presence of cancer or fistula
- Staphylococcal toxic shock syndrome

Patient education resources

Hand-out sheets from *Murtagh's Patient Education* 7th edition:

- Vaginal thrush
- Vulvovaginal irritation in children

References

1 Family Planning NSW. *Reproductive and Sexual Health: An Australian Clinical Practice Handbook* (3rd edn). Sydney: Family Planning NSW, 2016.

2 Melbourne Sexual Health Centre. MSHCG Treatment Guidelines. <www.mshc.org.au> (accessed 16/5/2018).

3 Weisberg E. Wet film examination. Aust Fam Physician, 1991; 20: 291–4.

4 The Royal Children's Hospital Melbourne. *Clinical Practice Guidelines: Prepubescent Gynaecology.* <https://www.rch.org.au/clinicalguide/guideline_index/Prepubescent_gynaecology/> (accessed 16/5/2018).

5 Expert group for Dermatology guidelines. In: eTG complete [Internet]. Melbourne: Therapeutic Guidelines Ltd. Available from <www.tg.org.au> (accessed May 2018).

6 Mackay EV et al. *Illustrated Textbook of Gynaecology* (2nd edn). Sydney: WB Saunders, Bailliere Tindall, 1992: 296–325.

7 Chute RS, Templeton DJ. Management of abnormal vaginal discharge. Medicine Today, 2009; 10 (4): 59–62.

8 Fischer G, Bradford J. *The Vulva. A Clinician's Practical Handbook.* Sydney: Family Planning NSW, 2010.

9 Watson C, Calbretto H. Comprehensive review of conventional and non-conventional methods of management of recurrent vulvovaginal candidiasis. Aust NZ J Obstet Gyn, 2007; 47 (4): 262–71.

10 Australian Sexual Health Alliance. Australian STI management guidelines for use in primary care. <www.sti.guidelines.org.au> (accessed 16/5/2018).

11 Expert group for Antibiotics guidelines. In: eTG complete [Internet]. Melbourne: Therapeutic Guidelines Ltd. Available from <www.tg.org.au> (accessed May 2018).

Resource

Mazza D. *Women's Health in General Practice* (2nd edn). Sydney: Elsevier, 2011.

107 Vulvar disorders

Genital skin is very sensitive. This sensitive organ needs protection from chemical and physical damage. The genital area is also affected by the way you feel and symptoms can appear worse at times of stress.

EXTRACT FROM PATIENT INFORMATION SHEET, 'THE DO'S AND DON'TS OF GENITAL HYGIENE', DERMATOLOGY/VULVAL DISEASES CLINIC, MERCY HOSPITAL FOR WOMEN, MELBOURNE

The dermatoses are the predominant cause of vulvar problems and this chapter focuses mainly on the important female genital skin conditions.

The vulva is that part of the female external genitalia lying posterior to the mons pubis, comprising the labia majora, labia minora, clitoris, vestibule of the vagina, vaginal opening and bulbs of the vestibule.[1]

The vaginal vestibule is an almond-shaped opening between the lines of attachment of the labia minora. The clitoris marks the superior angle and the fourchette the inferior boundary. It is approximately 4–5 cm long and 2 cm in width.[1] The four main structures that open into the vestibule are the urethra, vagina and the two secretory ducts of Bartholin's glands. The surface is composed of delicate, stratified squamous epithelium.

The genital area is affected by dermatoses found elsewhere on the skin but management is rendered more complex by the sensitivity and thinness of the skin, a tendency to superinfection, in addition to the psychological problems, including the often-resultant dyspareunia.

The vulval area, which is innervated by nerves arising from L1–2 and S2–4 nerve roots, is sensitive to noxious stimuli but the vagina is not sensitive to pain.[2] Topical creams, soaps, perfumes and other toilet products irritate the vulva easily—it is an area prone to contact dermatitis.

Clinical manifestations of vulvar disorders include itching, pain, irritation, white mucosal patches, lichenification, erosions and intertrigo[3] (see the diagnostic strategy model presented in TABLE 107.1).

Key facts and checkpoints

- If a dermatosis is suspected, check the skin on the body.
- Provoked vestibulodynia (vulvar vestibular syndrome) is a distressing, reasonably common condition that gives superficial dyspareunia. Diagnosis is by an abnormal response to light touch, even by a cotton bud.
- The vestibule can exhibit pearly papules (the equivalent of pearly penile papules) that look like tiny regular warts—they are normal.
- Approximately 20% of women carry *Candida albicans* as genital flora but less than 5% suffer from repeated or intractable clinical candidiasis.
- Not all itching and burning of the vulva and vagina is *Candida* infection. Swabs should be taken for diagnosis before committing to treatment empirically.
- The cause of vulvar irritation may be multifactorial (e.g. atopic dermatitis or *Candida* with irritant or allergic contact dermatitis from applications).
- Be alert for malignant melanoma and be aware that an area of benign pigmentation with well-demarcated edges and bluish discolouration called vulvar melanosis can develop.

Dermatitis

As expected, the various common forms of dermatitis collectively represent the prime cause of a pruritic irritating vulvar skin disorder. They classically present with itching, burning and soreness initiated by scratching leading to white plaques of lichen simplex chronicus. The manifestations can vary from symptoms without a rash to a poorly defined rash without the above symptoms.

The causes of vulvar dermatitis are:

- atopic dermatitis
- irritant contact dermatitis
- allergic contact dermatitis
- seborrhoeic dermatitis
- corticosteroid-induced dermatitis
- psoriasis

Table 107.1	Vulvar discomfort/irritation: diagnostic strategy model
Probability diagnosis Atopic dermatitis Chronic vulvovaginal candidiasis Irritant contact dermatitis (e.g. moisture with urinary incontinence or faecal soiling, panty liners, douches, bubble baths) Allergic contact dermatitis (e.g. latex, topical antimicrobials) Atrophic vaginitis Trauma—tears from vaginal intercourse, vaginal delivery	
Serious disorders not to be missed Neoplasia: • vulval intra-epithelial neoplasia • squamous cell carcinoma • Paget's disease • melanoma Provoked vestibulodynia	
Pitfalls (often missed) Psoriasis Lichen planus Lichen sclerosus Lichen simplex chronicus Aphthous ulcers Dysaesthetic vulvodynia Trichomonal vaginitis Herpes simplex virus Infestations: • threadworms • pubic lice • scabies	
Seven masquerades list Depression Diabetes Drugs Spinal dysfunction (dysaesthesia) UTI	
Is the patient trying to tell me something? Common: psychosexual problems.	

Principles of management[4]

- Take an appropriate history, including atopy, skin diseases.
- Check allergens and irritants (e.g. panty liners, soap, bubble bath, perfumed toilet paper, douches, perfumes, condoms, tea-tree oil).
- Check for heat and friction (e.g. synthetic or tight underwear, tight denim jeans, sporting costumes/tights, sweating, vigorous activity—bicycle riding).
- Check gynae-urological history (e.g. oestrogen status, faecal or urinary incontinence, vaginal discharge, 'thrush').
- Check psychosexual history (e.g. dyspareunia, partnership issues, depression).
- Carefully inspect the vulva plus the rest of the skin, scalp and nails. Look for lichenification (see TABLE 107.2).
- Appropriate investigations: vaginal swab (? *Candida albicans*), cervical screening test if due, perhaps patch testing and vulval biopsy for a rare, premalignant or suspected malignant condition, especially if thickening or textural change.

Table 107.2	Causes of common vulvar signs
White patches	Lichen simplex chronicus (lichenification)
	Lichen sclerosus
	Vitiligo
	Vulval intra-epithelial neoplasia
Erosions and ulcers	Herpes simplex or zoster
	Lichen planus
	Apthous ulcers
	Desquamative inflammatory vulvovaginitis
	Contact dermatitis
	Fixed drug reaction
	Excoriated scabies
	Crohn's disease of the vulva
Intertrigo	Atopic dermatitis
	Candida albicans
	Seborrhoeic dermatitis
	Tinea
	Erythrasma
	Psoriasis

Treatment[3,4]

- Provide supportive education and counselling.
- Correct underlying factors (e.g. tight clothes, incontinence, anal discharge, overused topical medications and cosmetics).
- Treat any secondary infection.
- Use aqueous cream moisturiser as cleanser.
- Start with potent topical corticosteroid (e.g. methylprednisolone aceponate 0.1% ointment topically until symptoms resolve) and follow with 1% hydrocortisone to prevent recurrence. Longer treatments such as 2—4 weeks are often required. Review treatment after 2 weeks.[5]

107

Psoriasis[5]

Psoriasis can affect the genital or perianal area (especially the natal cleft) and appears as a glazed, beefy red plaque without the classic scale seen elsewhere. There may be minimal or no sign of psoriasis on the skin of the body.

The main symptom is itching. It is usual to take swabs to rule out infection.

Treatment[5]

- Avoid irritants and use a soap substitute.
- First apply a potent topical steroid (e.g. methylprednisolone aceponate)—continue until resolution of rash.
- Second (when controlled) apply LPC 2% in aqueous cream daily. If not tolerated, use ichthammol 1% in aqueous cream daily.

Note: Maintenance with topical steroids—hydrocortisone 1% or resume potent agent for a flare-up.

Lichen planus[6,7]

Genital lichen planus is relatively uncommon but may affect both the vulva and vagina and can occur in association with oral lesions. It can also occur on any part of the skin, causing itchy skin rashes and nail dystrophy. Symptoms include irritation or vulval pain, dyspareunia and heavy but non-offensive vaginal discharge. Dyspareunia is usually severe.

Examination often reveals non-specific findings, ranging from subtle erythema to frank ulceration. Erosion of the mucosa surface of the introitus is a hallmark feature and may extend into the vagina and involve the cervix. If untreated, loss of the labia minor is typical and the clitoris may be buried by scar tissue.

Differential diagnoses of vulvar lichen planus include other causes of desquamative and erosive lesions, such as lichen sclerosus, pemphigus vulgaris, bullous and cicatricial pemphigoid and erythema multiforme.

A diagnostic biopsy is often difficult to obtain. Treatment is difficult and specialist input is required. Potent topical steroids provide symptomatic relief and there is a variety of treatment trials, including topical cyclosporin or oral methotrexate.[5]

Lichen sclerosus[4,5]

Also known as lichen sclerosus et atrophicus (see FIG. 107.1), this uncommon chronic inflammatory dermatosis of unknown aetiology (perhaps an autoimmune disorder) presents as well-defined white, finely wrinkled plaques that almost exclusively affect the anogenital skin, although they can occur anywhere on the body. Lichen sclerosus spares the vagina. It can run a chronic and complicated course with development of squamous cell carcinoma (SCC) in about 4% a concern. The differential diagnosis is atrophic vaginitis.

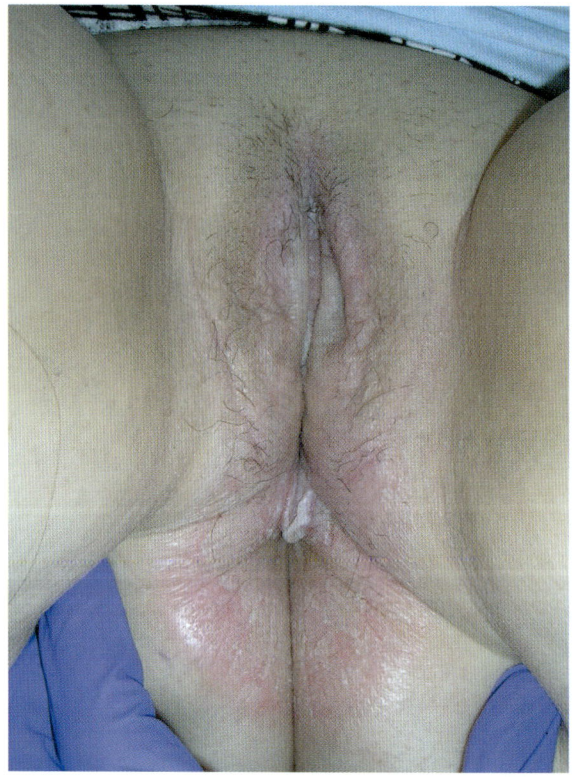

FIGURE 107.1 Lichen sclerosus et atrophicus of vulva in a 55-year-old woman. This shows white sclerotic plaques and epidermal atrophy

DxT genital pruritus + soreness + white wrinkled plaques ➜ lichen sclerosus

Clinical features

- Bimodal peak: prepubertal girls, perimenopause
- Mean age of onset in adult women is 50 years
- Pruritus is main symptom
- Soreness, burning, dyspareunia

Examination

- Variable distribution
- White wrinkled plaques
- Purpuric and ulcerated areas (due to scratching)
- May show figure of 8 pale perianal and perivaginal area

Complications if untreated

- Vulval atrophy and labial (even clitoral hood) fusion, introital stenosis
- Lifetime risk of SCC 2–6%

Management[5]

- Best in consultation with a dermatologist.
- Confirm diagnosis by biopsy (tend to avoid in children).
- Based on potent topical corticosteroids (e.g. betamethasone dipropionate 0.05% in optimised vehicle ointment applied bd until itching ceases, then daily[7]—show patients where to apply, using a mirror).
- Goal of treatment is to return the skin to a normal colour and texture, which can take up to 6 months and unlikely if scarring has already occurred.
- A lower dose topical corticosteroid can be used for maintenance as soon as the white areas have resolved.
- Long-term treatment is required in 85% of postmenopausal women.
- Lifelong surveillance with 6-monthly check-up.
- A similar topical program is used in children.
- Surgery is reserved for complications *or* SCC.

INFECTIONS

Chronic vulvovaginal candidiasis

This is different from acute candidiasis and remains difficult to treat because there may be a localised hypersensitivity to *Candida* (see CHAPTER 106).

Clinical features

- Chronic vulval itch–scratch cycle
- Burning, swelling—premenstrual exacerbation
- Dyspareunia
- Discharge not usually present
- Aggravated by courses of systemic antibiotics

Management[5]

- Swab—low vaginal—with each suspected episode, especially if discharge
- Aim for symptom remission with continuous antifungal treatment:
  - daily oral antifungals (monitor liver function tests) until symptoms clear—fluconazole 50 mg/day, or itraconazole 100 mg day (symptoms may remit in 2 weeks but often requires 6 months)
- Relieve itching with hydrocortisone 1% (do not use stronger preparations)
- Use nystatin in pregnancy

Tinea

Tinea causes an annular spreading rash with an active border that spreads from the labia to the thigh (see tinea cruris, CHAPTER 120). A problem is the development of tinea incognito from the application of topical steroids. This lacks central clearing but the active margin can be seen. Skin scrapings are necessary for diagnosis. Treatment is with a topical imidazole (avoid nystatin) or oral agents if resistant or extensive.

Pruritus vulvae

The causes of an itchy vulva to consider are:[8]

- candidiasis (rash, cottage cheese discharge)
- irritant dermatitis
  - especially if excessive sweating and tight clothing
  - sensitivity to soaps, bubble baths, cosmetics and contraceptive agents
  - overzealous washing or wiping with toilet paper
- local skin conditions:
  - psoriasis
  - dermatitis/eczema
- post-anal conditions (e.g. haemorrhoids)
- infestations:
  - threadworms (children)
  - scabies
  - pediculosis pubis
- infections (other than candidiasis):
  - *Trichomonas*
  - genital herpes, genital warts
- menopause: due to oestrogen deficiency (atrophic vaginitis)
- topical antihistamines
- vulval carcinoma
- psychological disorder (e.g. psychosexual problem, STI phobia)

If the labia minora are involved, consider lichen sclerosus. Treatment is according to the causation.

Management

This depends on the primary cause (e.g. candidiasis, incontinence), which should be treated effectively.

General measures (advice to patients)[3]

- Avoid overzealous washing.
- Take showers of no more than 5 minutes duration.
- Avoid having water too hot (lukewarm preferable).
- Use a soap substitute (e.g. aqueous cream, Cetaphil lotion) and wash it off with water only.
- Use soap alternatives (e.g. Dove, Neutrogena) for rest of body.

- Pat the skin dry after showering (avoid harsh drying).
- Do not wear tight pantyhose, tight jeans or tight underwear, or use tampons.
- Do not use vaginal douches, powders or deodorants.
- After the toilet, wipe gently with a soft, non-coloured, non-perfumed toilet paper.
- Apply a good moisturiser (e.g. Hydraderm or 5% peanut oil in aqueous cream).

Treatment

- For pruritus, apply cool moisturising cream (kept in refrigerator) when there is an urge to scratch.
- A zinc-based barrier cream or petroleum jelly may be appropriate if there is moisture irritation.
- Apply prescribed steroid ointment to the rash.

VULVOVAGINITIS IN PREPUBERTAL GIRLS

Vulvovaginitis is the most common gynaecological disorder of childhood. It can affect women of any age but is particularly common in girls, especially between the ages of 2 and 8 years. It is a type of dermatitis of the vulva and the vagina.

Mild vulvovaginitis

Symptoms of this very common problem include:

- discomfort and soreness
- vulval itching
- redness
- discharge—usually a slight yellow discharge on the underwear
- dysuria

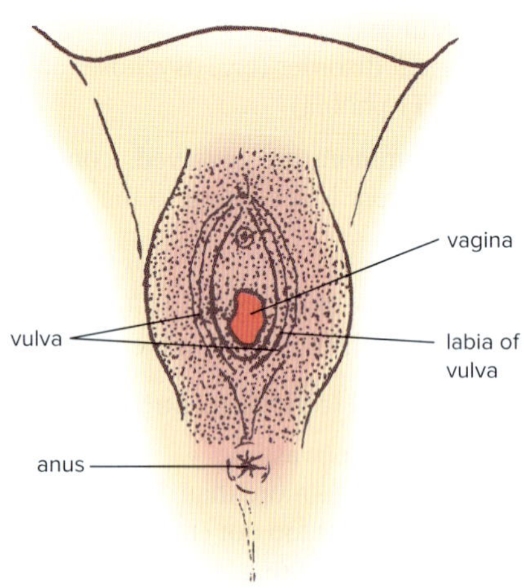

FIGURE 107.2 Typical area of inflammation of vulvovaginitis in girls

It is important not to confuse it with a urinary infection when the child is clearly uncomfortable due to stinging on urination.

The cause is usually due to a low-grade inflammation in an area with a possible underlying dermatological disorder such as atopic dermatitis, psoriasis or lichen sclerosus, leading to sensitivity to various irritants such as soaps and urine.

Affected girls are often 'atopic'.

The causal factors include:

- thin vaginal mucosa (the normal prepubescent state)
- dampness from synthetic-fibre underwear, tight clothing, wet bathers, obesity
- over- or under-wiping after passing urine
- frequent self-handling, especially with irritation
- irritants (soap residue, bubble baths, antiseptics, chlorinated water)
- 'sandbox' vaginitis: girls sitting and playing in sand or dirt may develop irritation from particulate matter trapped in the vagina

Management

- Explanation and reassurance to parents
- Avoidance of the above causal factors, especially wet bathers, synthetic underwear, bubble baths, perfumed soaps and getting overweight
- Attention to good, supervised toileting practice
- Attention to bathing and drying

It is worth soaking the child in a warm shallow bath containing half a cup of white vinegar.

Alternatively, bicarbonate of soda (10 g/10 L water) can be used.

Soothing creams such as soft paraffin creams and nappy rash creams such as zinc and castor oil cream should be applied three times daily as a short-term measure. If a powder is required, use zinc oxide (e.g. Curash). Consider an oestrogen cream.

Moderate/persistent vulvovaginitis

The symptoms may be more intense with increased itching, burning and discharge.

Important causes to consider[9]

- 'Sandbox' vaginitis
- Skin disorders, especially atopic dermatitis and lichen sclerosus (look for skin problems elsewhere on body)
- Foreign body: consider if a bloody, malodorous vaginal discharge
- Candidiasis—uncommon but consider if antibiotic therapy or possibility of diabetes

- Sexual abuse (uncommon but must not be missed)
- Pinworm infestation (*Enterobius*) (see FIG. 15.5 in CHAPTER 15)
- Sexually transmissible organisms—usually postpubertal

Examination

A careful general examination should be performed only if considered appropriate. In infants, the best examination method is to place the child on her parent's lap with the legs held well abducted. Lateral traction applied to the labia allows the hymen orifice to be examined. Look for vulval or vaginal infection.

An older child can be placed in one of two suitable positions:

1. supine, legs apart in a frog-leg position, with bottom of feet touching (generally preferred)
2. prone, knee/chest position. This allows a better view of the hymenal orifice but many children do not like this position

A rectal examination may be performed to try to feel for suspected foreign bodies in the vagina.

Taking a swab[8]

If the discharge is profuse and offensive, take an introital swab (do not take a vaginal swab). Infective vulvovaginitis in girls is often due to a group A beta-haemolytic *Streptococcus*.

Treat with an appropriate antibiotic.

Treatment of dermatitis

Most cases of vulval dermatitis will respond to short courses of 1% hydrocortisone ointment or cream, provided aggravating factors are removed.

Labial adhesions (labial agglutination)

Labial fusion is caused by adhesions considered to be acquired from vulvovaginitis after which sometimes the medial edges of the labia minora become adherent. The adhesions are certainly not present at birth. Labial fusion is regarded as a normal variant and usually resolves spontaneously in late childhood. Provided the child is able to void easily, no treatment other than reassurance is needed.

For significant adhesions, treat as follows:

- oestrogen cream once a day until resolution (usually 2–6 weeks). Once the fusion has separated, ongoing treatment with soap avoidance, topical lubricants (e.g. Vaseline) and 1% hydrocortisone
- the fusion may re-form and have to be re-treated as necessary

Occasionally, a minor surgical procedure (sometimes under general anaesthetic) to separate the labial adhesions may be required. However, such measures are not generally recommended.

VULVODYNIA

Vulvodynia describes the symptom of pain (burning, rawness or stinging) and discomfort, where no obvious cause can be found. Itch is not a feature. Causes include provoked vestibulodynia (vulvar vestibular syndrome), dysaesthetic vulvodynia and various infections (e.g. herpes simplex virus). Virtually every condition of the vulva can be painful at times; even dermatitis can become painful if scratching or splitting leads to open areas and ulceration.

Provoked vestibulodynia[2,4]

Definition

Vestibular hypersensitivity Severe vulvar or vestibular pain on touch or entry into the vagina.

Also referred to as vulvar vestibular syndrome (VVS) or vestibulitis, it is a very important disorder for the GP to be aware of in the woman with a typical history of introital dyspareunia. It is a difficult problem to treat. The characteristic feature is severe pain with vestibular touch, including attempted vaginal entry (early dyspareunia). The vestibule is very sensitive, featuring an inappropriate response to light touch. In many instances the cause of the primary condition is not apparent and a history of possible sexual abuse or other psychological provoking factors should be diplomatically elicited. Some patients can develop the problem after years of pain-free sex.[6] It is the most common cause of dyspareunia in the premenopausal female.

Secondary causes include inflammatory triggers such as irritant contact dermatitis and infection. This establishes a conditioned response.

Spontaneous resolution has been reported in up to 50% of cases. Prognosis appears to be reasonably good but depends to some extent on the premorbid traits of the patient.[3]

DxT young + nulliparous + dyspareunia → provoked vestibulodynia

Clinical features

- Delayed diagnosis (average 2–3 years)[4]
- Sexually active women in 20s and 30s

- Family history
- Pain provoked by intercourse, tampon insertion, tight underwear
- Superficial 'entry' dyspareunia
- Sexual dysfunction
- Tender vestibule on pinpoint light pressure
- Erythema (usually minute red spots) around Bartholin's duct openings (consider *Candida*)

Diagnosis

Marked tenderness to light touch of the inner vestibule with a cotton bud.

Management[4]

- Investigate and treat if suspected underlying cause
- Patient education, counselling and support
- Multidisciplinary approach often required
- Physiotherapy—rehabilitation of pelvic floor musculature by increasing awareness and increasing elasticity of the tissues of the vaginal opening
- Counselling often beneficial, especially given impact on sexual health and relationships
- Genital skin care
- Encourage use of oil-based lubricants for intercourse
- Application of lignocaine 2% gel or 5% ointment to the vestibule 10–20 minutes before intercourse

Options[10]

- Biofeedback technique
- Tricyclic antidepressants (start low, e.g. amitriptyline 10–20 mg nocte then up to 100 mg—best option)
- Gabapentinoids (e.g. pregabalin starting at 75 mg or, if not tolerated, gabapentin starting at 300 mg)
- Intralesional therapy (no more effective than other treatments):
  - triamcinolone
  - botulinum toxin
- Vestibulectomy (role uncertain and controversial)

Dysaesthetic vulvodynia[2,11]

The typical patient with this neuropathic pain problem is a middle-aged to elderly woman who presents with a constant burning pain of the labia, which typically builds up during the course of the day. Examination is often unrewarding. The underlying cause may be pudendal neuralgia (may be secondary to pudendal nerve block), referred spinal pain or simply unknown.[12]

Herpes simplex infection needs to be excluded.

Treatment options include antidepressants (TCAs and SNRIs) and gabapentinoids.

Bartholin's cyst

A Bartholin's gland swelling follows obstruction of the duct and presents as a painless vulval swelling at the posterior end of the labia majora, close to the fourchette. A simple, non-infected cyst can be left alone and may resolve spontaneously. If it becomes infected, an abscess may result, causing a painful, tender, red vulval lump. It may resolve with antibiotics or discharge spontaneously. Otherwise, drain and perform a micro and culture. The usual organism is *E. coli*. If the cyst persists and becomes large, a surgical marsupialisation procedure, which allows permanent drainage, can be performed (see FIGS 107.3A, B).

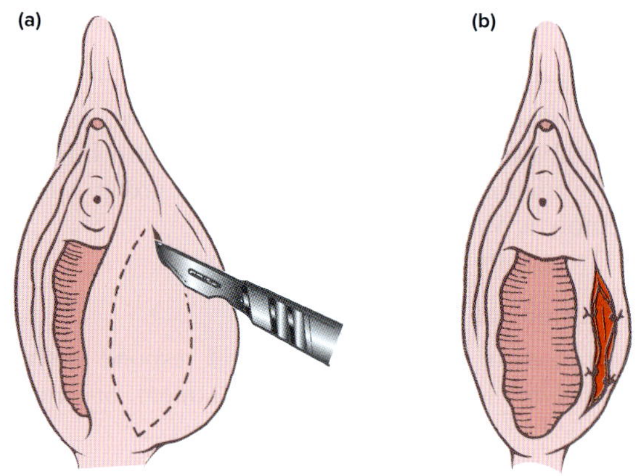

FIGURE 107.3 **(a)** Bartholin's cyst: starting the marsupialisation procedure, **(b)** postoperative appearance

> **Practice tip**
>
> - Always biopsy a focal lesion on the vulva[6]

References

1 Thomas CL (ed.). *Taber's Cyclopedic Medical Dictionary* (14th edn). Philadelphia: FA Davis, 1997: 2083, 2100.
2 Fischer G. Vulvodynia. Australian Doctor, 31 May 2002: i–viii.

3 Ang C, Sinclair R. Vulvar dermatoses: part I. Australian Doctor, 19 June 1998: i–viii.
4 Welsh BM. Vulvar dermatoses. In: *Proceedings of Dermatology Conference for General Practitioners.* Melbourne: Combined Alfred Hospital/Skin and Cancer Foundation, 2002.
5 Expert group for Dermatology guidelines. In: eTG complete [Internet]. Melbourne: Therapeutic Guidelines Ltd. Available from <www.tg.org.au>, accessed May 2018.
6 Reid R, Campion M. Vulvular disease—parts 1 and 2. Australian Doctor, 2011.
7 Fischer G, Bradford J. *The Vulva. A clinician's practical handbook.* Sydney: Family Planning NSW, 2010.
8 Farrell E. Investigating vulval itch. Medical Observer, 20 November 2009: 26.
9 Fischer G. Vulval disease in childhood. Australian Prescriber, 2005; 28: 88–90.
10 Henzell H, Berzins K. Localised provoked vestibulodynia (vulvodynia): assessment and management. Aust Fam Physician, 2015; 44 (7): 460–6.
11 Welsh BM. Management of common vulval conditions. Med J Aust, 2003; 178: 391–5.
12 Gunter J. Vulvodynia: new thoughts on a devastating condition. Obstet Gynecol Surv, 2007; 62 (12): 812–9.

Resources

International Society for the Study of Vulvovaginal Disease <www.issvd.org>

Vulval Pain Society <www.vulvalpainsociety.org>

108 Basic antenatal care

An examiner, no lover of females, thrust a femur into her hand.
'How many of these have you got?' he demanded.
'Five.'
'How do you come to that conclusion?' he asked contemptuously.
'I have two of my own, the one in my hand, and the two of my unborn child.'

ANONYMOUS ANECDOTE

Pregnancy and childbirth are very important and emotional events in the lives of women and their families. Their care during and after pregnancy is one of the most satisfying aspects of the work of the family doctor, who generally chooses breadth of knowledge rather than depth of knowledge. The changing trend towards specialisation has meant a change of role for the city practitioner and now shared obstetric care is a commonly practised routine. The quality of care that can be given in family practice is often superior to that offered in the hospital antenatal clinic, partly because of the continuing personal care offered by the family doctor.[1]

Antenatal care presents preventive medicine opportunities par excellence and is the ideal time to develop an optimal therapeutic relationship with the expectant mother. The opportunities for anticipatory guidance should be seized and education about the multitude of possible sensations during pregnancy (such as heartburn, backache, leg cramps, various fears and anxieties) should be addressed. In other words, an optimal communication system should be established between the expectant couple and the health care system.

The information presented here is a basis for the shared care strategy where family doctors share basic antenatal care with consultants and have a ready referral strategy for high-risk pregnancies.

The basic aim of antenatal care is to assess the risk of harm to mother and baby and apply the appropriate level of surveillance to minimise or eradicate harmful effects.

Preconception care

Preconception care is to be commended to the woman contemplating pregnancy and her family doctor is well placed to provide general health care and screening as well as genetic counselling.

General advice should include optimal nutrition and diet, weight control, regular exercise and discouragement of smoking, alcohol and drugs.

Ask if there are chronic conditions such as diabetes, thyroid disease, hypertension, epilepsy and thrombophilia, ensuring current management is optimal.

Folic acid (0.5 mg tablets daily) is recommended to commence at least 1 month prior to conception, continuing for the first trimester. The dose is 5 mg/day for women at increased risk, such as those on anticonvulsant medication, those with a past or family history of neural tube defects, a BMI >30, pre-pregnancy diabetes, 5-methyltetrahydrofolate deficiency or a risk of malabsorption.[2] This often comes combined with an iodine supplement (150 mcg daily), which is also recommended for women who are pregnant, breastfeeding or considering pregnancy. Examination should include blood pressure, cardiac status, urinalysis and cervical screening test (if due).

Rubella and varicella serology should be estimated and, if required, immunisation 4 weeks prior to conception should be initiated. Rubella and varicella vaccines are both live vaccines and are not recommended in early pregnancy.

Vaccinations to consider are:

- Boostrix (diphtheria, tetanus, pertussis)
- MMR (measles, mumps, rubella)
- varicella
- hepatitis B
- influenza

Genetic counselling is based on past obstetric or family history, advanced maternal age, consanguinity or high-risk racial groups (e.g. for thalassaemia or sickle cell anaemia). Screening should now be offered to all women for cystic fibrosis, spinal muscular atrophy and fragile X syndrome.

Checkpoint summary: advice to patients

- Stop smoking, recreational drugs and excessive alcohol use.
- Review current medications with your GP.
- Follow a healthy diet.
- Aim for a healthy weight.
- Take folic acid and iodine at least one month prior to conception.
- Have a good exercise routine.
- Ensure rubella and varicella immunity.
- Have a regular breast check.
- Ensure cervical screening is up to date.
- Eat freshly cooked and prepared food.
- Have a regular dental check.
- Consider genetic and family history.
- Consider health insurance cover.
- Consider and discuss future family planning.

The initial visit

It is important to calculate the expected due date if the woman knows the date of her last menstrual period and the usual length of her cycle. The use of ultrasonography from about 7 weeks gestation can help if dates are uncertain. It is often appropriate at the initial consultation to refer to the antenatal outpatient department or private obstetrician.

History checkpoints[3,4]

- Confirm pregnancy by menstrual history and by urine or serum human chorionic gonadotrophin (hCG), if necessary.
- Previous obstetric history:
  - number of pregnancies and outcomes
  - mode of previous deliveries, length and gestation, birthweight of each baby
  - complications; gestational diabetes, pre-eclampsia, cervical incompetence, fetal or neonatal abnormalities or death; pre-term or growth-restricted infants
- Medical history:
  - check for past evidence of diabetes, hypertension, cardiac, thyroid or kidney disease, iron deficiency, PCOS, STIs, mental illness and up-to-date cervical screening
- Family history:
  - features to consider are multiple pregnancies, hypertension and diabetes
- Psychosocial history:
  - this is very important and includes an assessment of the attitude towards the pregnancy and possible intimate partner violence
- Drug history:
  - includes smoking, alcohol, illicit drugs, OTC drugs and prescribed drugs
- Important points to consider:
  - establish date of confinement (see obstetric calendar in FIG. 108.1)

Examination

During the initial examination, assess the patient's general physical and mental status. Examine the following:

- basic parameters: height, weight (calculate BMI), blood pressure, heart rate, urinalysis (protein and glucose). A woman is hypertensive if the systolic BP $\geq$ 140 mmHg and/or diastolic BP is $\geq$ 90 mmHg[3]
- head and neck: teeth, gums, thyroid
- chest: including breasts/nipples
- abdomen: palpate for uterine size and listen to fetal heart (if indicated)

  Perform a cervical screening test if due.

Antenatal screening

The recommendations for antenatal screening of asymptomatic women are the source of debate, with evidence-based medicine calling into question traditional tests. TABLE 108.1 reflects the recommendations of the RANZ College of Obstetricians and Gynaecologists.[5,6] Debate continues about screening for rubella immunity, thyroid function, vitamin D and ultrasound.

Combined first trimester screening test[3]

- Maternal serum screening[7] (11–13 weeks):
  - Free β-hCG
  - PAPP-A
- Combined with nuchal translucency (i.e. nuchal fold thickness), enabling the risk of trisomy 13, 18 and 21 to be defined and compared with age-related risk
- Results may indicate very low risk (<1 in 1000), low risk (1 in 301–1000), increased risk (1 in 50–300) or high risk (>1 in 50)
- Has a sensitivity of 85% and specificity of 95%
- Risk of pre–eclampsia may be assessed and aspirin prophylaxis offered if high risk

The calculation is made from the first day of the last menstrual period																																
January	1	2	3	4	5	6	7	8	9	10	11	12	13	14	15	16	17	18	19	20	21	22	23	24	25	26	27	28	29	30	31	**January**
October	8	9	10	11	12	13	14	15	16	17	18	19	20	21	22	23	24	25	26	27	28	29	30	31	1	2	3	4	5	6	7	*November*
February	1	2	3	4	5	6	7	8	9	10	11	12	13	14	15	16	17	18	19	20	21	22	23	24	25	26	27	28				**February**
November	8	9	10	11	12	13	14	15	16	17	18	19	20	21	22	23	24	25	26	27	28	29	30	1	2	3	4	5				*December*
March	1	2	3	4	5	6	7	8	9	10	11	12	13	14	15	16	17	18	19	20	21	22	23	24	25	26	27	28	29	30	31	**March**
December	6	7	8	9	10	11	12	13	14	15	16	17	18	19	20	21	22	23	24	25	26	27	28	29	30	31	1	2	3	4	5	*January*
April	1	2	3	4	5	6	7	8	9	10	11	12	13	14	15	16	17	18	19	20	21	22	23	24	25	26	27	28	29	30		**April**
January	6	7	8	9	10	11	12	13	14	15	16	17	18	19	20	21	22	23	24	25	26	27	28	29	30	31	1	2	3	4		*February*
May	1	2	3	4	5	6	7	8	9	10	11	12	13	14	15	16	17	18	19	20	21	22	23	24	25	26	27	28	29	30	31	**May**
February	5	6	7	8	9	10	11	12	13	14	15	16	17	18	19	20	21	22	23	24	25	26	27	28	1	2	3	4	5	6	7	*March*
June	1	2	3	4	5	6	7	8	9	10	11	12	13	14	15	16	17	18	19	20	21	22	23	24	25	26	27	28	29	30		**June**
March	8	9	10	11	12	13	14	15	16	17	18	19	20	21	22	23	24	25	26	27	28	29	30	31	1	2	3	4	5	6		*April*
July	1	2	3	4	5	6	7	8	9	10	11	12	13	14	15	16	17	18	19	20	21	22	23	24	25	26	27	28	29	30	31	**July**
April	7	8	9	10	11	12	13	14	15	16	17	18	19	20	21	22	23	24	25	26	27	28	29	30	1	2	3	4	5	6	7	*May*
August	1	2	3	4	5	6	7	8	9	10	11	12	13	14	15	16	17	18	19	20	21	22	23	24	25	26	27	28	29	30	31	**August**
May	8	9	10	11	12	13	14	15	16	17	18	19	20	21	22	23	24	25	26	27	28	29	30	31	1	2	3	4	5	6	7	*June*
September	1	2	3	4	5	6	7	8	9	10	11	12	13	14	15	16	17	18	19	20	21	22	23	24	25	26	27	28	29	30		**September**
June	8	9	10	11	12	13	14	15	16	17	18	19	20	21	22	23	24	25	26	27	28	29	30	1	2	3	4	5	6	7		*July*
October	1	2	3	4	5	6	7	8	9	10	11	12	13	14	15	16	17	18	19	20	21	22	23	24	25	26	27	28	29	30	31	**October**
July	8	9	10	11	12	13	14	15	16	17	18	19	20	21	22	23	24	25	26	27	28	29	30	31	1	2	3	4	5	6	7	*August*
November	1	2	3	4	5	6	7	8	9	10	11	12	13	14	15	16	17	18	19	20	21	22	23	24	25	26	27	28	29	30		**November**
August	8	9	10	11	12	13	14	15	16	17	18	19	20	21	22	23	24	25	26	27	28	29	30	31	1	2	3	4	5	6		*September*
December	1	2	3	4	5	6	7	8	9	10	11	12	13	14	15	16	17	18	19	20	21	22	23	24	25	26	27	28	29	30	31	**December**
September	7	8	9	10	11	12	13	14	15	16	17	18	19	20	21	22	23	24	25	26	27	28	29	30	1	2	3	4	5	6	7	*October*

Or: (approximately) subtract 3 from months and add 7 to days e.g. 19/8/89
+ 7 − 3
26/5/90 Or: Naegele's rule—add 7 days, 9 months

FIGURE 108.1 Obstetric calendar to determine expected due date

Non-invasive prenatal testing (NIPT)

108

Recently, free fetal DNA testing has been available in Australia and overseas. It is performed on a maternal blood sample taken from 10 weeks gestation and allows for accurate measurement of aneuploidy of chromosomes 13, 18 and 21 (sensitivity and specificity of 99%), in addition to sex chromosomes if requested. For women who receive an increased combined first trimester screening risk result, NIPT may be an appropriate alternative prior to amniocentesis. In the event of a positive NIPT, amniocentesis or chorionic villus biopsy would usually be required for confirmation.

Visits during pregnancy

The box below is a summary of standard antenatal practice.

A common routine schedule (if all appears normal)

- Initial in first trimester: 8–10 weeks
- Up to 28 weeks: every 4–6 weeks
- Up to 36 weeks: every 2 weeks
- 36 weeks–delivery: weekly

Guidelines for screening for OGTT

- At first visit—if previous gestational diabetes or high risk
- 14—20 weeks—if above + normal initial test
- 26—29 weeks—for all other patients

Immunisations during pregnancy

- Seasonal influenza vaccine is recommended
- Pertussis booster is recommended from 28 weeks gestation

The average number of visits is 12, but the need for this many visits is being questioned—with some authorities recommending as few as six visits.

Table 108.1 Routine antenatal screening*[3,5,8]	
Recommended	Consider
First visit	
Full blood count	Serum ferritin
Blood group	Varicella serology
Rhesus and antibody screen	Haemoglobin electrophoresis (if indicated)
Rubella antibody status	
Cervical screening if due	
HBV and HCV serology	Oral glucose tolerance test (if high risk for gestational diabetes)
HIV serology (after counselling)	Vitamin D
Syphilis serology	
MSU and dipstick urine	
Discuss:	
Combined first trimester screening—11–13 weeks or NIPT	Non-invasive prenatal testing (NIPT)—from 10 weeks
Fetal anomaly scan—18–20 weeks	Protein Creatine Ration
Subsequent visits	
Oral glucose tolerance test or OGTT—26–29 weeks	Early OGTT—14–20 weeks (if high risk for gestational diabetes)
Rhesus antibodies (Rh-negative mother)—28 & 34 weeks	
FBC—36 weeks	
Genital swab for group B *Streptococcus* (GBS)—36 weeks	

A systematic review of seven RCTs found no difference in the detection of pre-eclampsia, urinary tract infection, low birthweight or maternal mortality when a schedule of reduced antenatal visits was compared with the traditional routine.[5,9] However, a sensible approach would be to plan visits according to need and circumstances in a flexible way.

For each visit, record:

- weight (to calculate gain)
- blood pressure
- uterine size/fundal height
- fetal heart (usually audible with stethoscope at 25 weeks and definitely by 28 weeks): best to have Doppler, which can detect the fetal heart from 18–20 weeks[3]
- fetal movements (if present)
- lie, presentation and position of fetus (third trimester)
- presence of any oedema
- urinalysis (protein and glucose—most clinics perform only if there is proteinuria at the first visit or if signs of hypertension, kidney disease or pre-eclampsia develop. See TABLE 108.2.

Table 108.2 Causes of proteinuria in pregnancy
Urinary tract infection
Contamination from vaginal discharge
Pre-eclampsia toxaemia
Underlying chronic kidney disease

Table 108.3	Risk factors for gestational diabetes mellitus (GDM)
High risk (1 or more)	Previous GDM
	BMI >35
	Maternal age >40 years
	Family history of diabetes (1st degree relative with diabetes or sister with GDM)
	PCOS with hyperandrogenism (clinical or biochemical)
	Indian subcontinent ethnicity
	Previous baby >4000 g
	Medications, e.g. oral corticosteroids, antipsychotics
Moderate risk (2 or more = high risk)	Maternal age 35–39 years
	BMI 25–35
	Asian, Aboriginal, Torres Strait Islander, Maori, Pacific Islander, Middle Eastern or non-white African ethnicity
	Polycystic ovarian syndrome (androgens not elevated)

Record day of first fetal movements (i.e. 'quickening') (ask patient to write down the dates):

- primigravida: 17–20 weeks
- multigravida: 16–18 weeks

Fundal height

The relative heights of the uterus fundus are shown in FIGURE 108.2. The uterus is a pelvic organ until the twelfth week of pregnancy. After this time it can be palpated abdominally. At about 20–22 weeks it has reached the level of the umbilicus and reaches

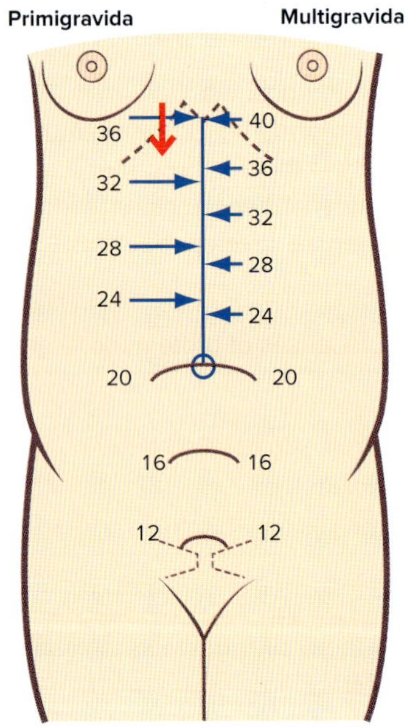

FIGURE 108.2 Fundal height in normal pregnancy (in weeks); the height of the fundus is a guide to the period of gestation. Nulliparas experience lightening at about 36 weeks when the fundal height usually reverts to the 34-week level.

the xiphisternum between 36 and 40 weeks. If the symphysis fundal height is more than 2 cm different from that expected for the gestation, the cause of this should be evaluated by ultrasound examination. Palpation of the fundal height is affected by obesity and tenseness of the abdominal wall.

108

Management of specific issues

Nutrition advice

A healthy diet is very important and should contain at least the following daily allowances:

1 Eat most:
   - fruit and vegetables (at least 4 serves)
   - cereals and bread (4–6 serves)
2 Eat moderately:
   - dairy products—3 cups (600 mL) of milk or equivalent in yoghurt or cheese
   - lean meat, poultry or fish—1 or 2 serves (at least 2 serves of red meat per week)
3 Eat least:
   - sugar and refined carbohydrates (e.g. sweets, cakes, biscuits, soft drinks)
   - polyunsaturated margarine, butter, oil and cream

Bran with cereal helps prevent constipation of pregnancy.

If the ideal diet is followed, iron, vitamin and calcium supplements should not be necessary, although most patients prefer to take OTC vitamin and mineral preparations (e.g. iron, folic acid, multivitamins, iodine). Do not diet to lose weight. It is usual to gain about 12 kg during pregnancy. Less weight gain is recommended for women who are overweight pre-conception.

Healthy environment[2]

It is appropriate to discuss measures to avoid the following infections and toxins known to be harmful in pregnancy.

Listeria

- infection in pregnancy has a fetal mortality of 30–50%
- practise good personal and food hygiene; wash hands and use fresh ingredients
- wash raw vegetables, fruit and herbs thoroughly prior to consumption
- avoid unpasteurised dairy products, soft cheeses, cold meats, pâté, raw seafood, raw egg and chilled ready-to-eat foods
- cook meat thoroughly

Mercury

- 2–3 serves/week of seafood is considered safe
- avoid regular consumption of larger fish with higher mercury levels, e.g. orange roughy, shark (flake), marlin or swordfish

Toxoplasmosis

- delegate cleaning of cat litter trays to others; if not possible, gloves should be worn during cleaning and hands washed well afterwards
- ensure litter trays are emptied daily and regularly disinfected with boiling water

Cytomegalovirus and parvovirus B19 (fifth disease)

- women who work with children or in the health care sector can further reduce risk by frequent handwashing and using gloves when changing nappies

Smoking, alcohol and other drugs

Encourage patients to stop all recreational drugs, alcohol and tobacco. Caffeine reduction is advised, with some guidelines recommending complete avoidance, while others allow for a maximum of 200 mg/day, i.e. one cup of strong espresso-style coffee, or four cups of medium-strength tea.

Other household members should also stop smoking as passive smoking may be harmful to mother and child.

There is convincing evidence that promotion of smoking cessation programs during pregnancy is effective, with improved outcomes, including reduction in preterm birth rates and low birthweight rate.[10] The fetal alcohol syndrome is a significant cause of mental impairment, so it is best to abstain.

Mothers taking illicit drugs, especially opioids and amphetamines, require identification, counselling, treatment and surveillance for the neonatal abstinence syndrome in the newborn child.

Breastfeeding

Mothers-to-be should be encouraged to breastfeed; however, their choice should be respected if that is not their wish. Give advice and relevant literature. They can be directed to a local nursing mothers' group for support and guidance if necessary.

Antenatal classes

Referral to therapists conducting such classes can provide advice and supervision on antenatal exercises, relaxation skills, pain relief in labour, infant care and breastfeeding. Enrolment with the partner is recommended.

Psychosocial and emotional stress

Antenatal visits provide an ideal opportunity to become acquainted with the patient and explore issues that help her. Provide whole-person understanding with appropriate help and reassurance where necessary. Areas to be explored include support systems, attitudes of patient and partner to the pregnancy, sexuality, expectation of labour and delivery, financial issues, and attitudes of parents and in-laws.

Mental health

The effect that pregnancy can have on mental health is variable and women with pre-existing mental illness should receive optimal support and close surveillance. Many treatments for mental illness can be safely used in pregnancy and women should be referred promptly if symptoms deteriorate.

Weight gain in pregnancy

Although a standard weight gain is given as 12 kg over 40 weeks of pregnancy, it is common for some women in Australia to gain up to 20 kg without adverse effects.[4] Encourage sensible weight control.

Normal weight gain is minimal in the first 20 weeks, resulting in a 3 kg weight gain in the first half of pregnancy. From 20 weeks onwards there is an average weight gain of 0.5 kg per week. From 36 weeks the weight gain usually levels off.[4]

Fetal movement chart

If daily fetal movements exceed 10 and the regular pattern has not changed significantly, then usually the fetus is at no risk. However, if the movements drop to fewer than 10 per day, the patient should be referred to hospital for fetal monitoring.

Vaginal bleeding in early pregnancy[12]

This is a common problem in the first trimester in particular. At least 10% of normal pregnancies will have an episode and about 15% of recognised pregnancies will miscarry. If the bleeding is light to moderate and the pain mild or absent the question is 'Can a viable pregnancy continue or is there an ectopic pregnancy or a threatened miscarriage?'

- <6 weeks: serial quantitative hCG levels should increase by at least 66% every 2 days (ultrasound usually unhelpful)
  - rises below 66% in 2 days suggest a non-viable pregnancy (consider ectopic)
  - once hCG >1500 IU/L transvaginal ultrasound should be arranged
  - gestational sac should be visualised once hCG is >1500–2000 IU/L, although variation is common
- 6–8 weeks: ultrasound is used to define an intra-uterine pregnancy and exclude an ectopic. A repeat ultrasound in 1 week may be required if viability is in doubt
- >8 weeks: normal ultrasound is reassuring since miscarriage rate is only 3% unless the amount of intrauterine blood is large

Note: Rest is not necessary for threatened miscarriage.

Be aware that an incomplete abortion can cause cervical shock (pelvic pain and fainting). Products of conception must be removed from the cervical os.

Anti-D is required only in the event of complete miscarriage.

Consider the antiphospholipid syndrome for recurrent miscarriage and arrange antibody testing (see CHAPTER 32). Refer to a specialist for full assessment if 3 consecutive miscarriages have occurred.

Nausea and vomiting in pregnancy[13]

- Nausea and vomiting occur in more than 50% of women
- Majority of cases disappear by the end of first trimester
- Mild cases can be dealt with by explanation and reassurance; it is preferable to avoid drug therapy if possible
- Simple measures:
  - small, frequent meals including ginger up to 1 g daily
  - dry crackers can be kept by the bed to consume first thing
  - a fizzy soft drink, especially ginger drinks, may help
  - ensure adequate hydration, including sucking ice chips and drinking small amounts of fluid
  - avoid stimuli such as cooking smells
  - take care with teeth cleaning
  - rest where possible, especially later in the day, as fatigue often worsens symptoms
- Medication:
  - pyridoxine (vitamin B6) 25 mg (half-tablet or full) bd or tds
  - doxylamine 25 mg tds (often sedating, consider half-tablet at night)
  - if still ineffective, add metoclopramide 10 mg tds
  - if persistent nausea and vomiting, commence ondansetron 4–8 mg tds (watch for constipation)
  - consider treating associated gastro-oesophageal reflux

Hyperemesis gravidarum

This is severe vomiting in pregnancy, which may result in severe fluid and electrolyte depletion. It occurs in about 1 in 100 pregnancies.

Associations

- Normal complication
- Hydatidiform mole
- Multiple pregnancy
- Urinary infection

Management

- Test urine—MCU (micro-culture of urine); ketones: if +ve, admit to hospital
- Ultrasound examination
- Test electrolytes, urea, LFTs
- Bed rest
- Nil orally
- Fluid and electrolyte replacement
- Pyridoxine and doxylamine as per nausea and vomiting in pregnancy
- Metoclopramide 10 mg IV → 10 mg (o) tds (if necessary); if ineffective, ondansetron 4–8 mg IV 8–12 hourly

Heartburn

Gastro-oesophageal reflux is a major source of discomfort to women in the latter half of pregnancy. Non-pharmacological treatment such as frequent small meals, avoidance of bending over and elevation of the head of the bed are the mainstays of treatment. Regular use of antacids is effective (e.g. alginate/antacid liquid—Gaviscon, Mylanta Plus—10–20 mL) before meals and at bedtime. H2-receptor antagonists or PPIs may be necessary and are considered safe.

Cramps

Pregnant women are more prone to cramp. If it develops they should be advised simply to place a pillow at the foot of the bed so that plantar flexion of the feet is avoided during sleep. Prolonged plantar flexion is the basis of the cramps. Quinine, including tonic water, should be avoided. There is no evidence that calcium supplements help cramps during pregnancy.[14]

Varicose veins

Wearing special supportive pantyhose is the most comfortable and practical management, in addition to adequate rest.

Haemorrhoids

Haemorrhoids in the later stages of pregnancy can be very troublesome. Emphasising the importance of a high-fibre diet to ensure regular bowel habit is the best management. Some women are prone to constipation in pregnancy and may require regular laxatives such as lactulose or macrogol powder. Painful haemorrhoids may be eased by the application of ice packs or perhaps haemorrhoidal ointments containing local anaesthetic, which are considered safe.

Dental hygiene

Dental problems can worsen during pregnancy so special care of teeth and gums, including a visit to the dentist, is appropriate. Continuation of cleaning with a softer brush is recommended.

Back pain

Back pain, especially low back pain, is common during pregnancy and special back care advice can help women manage this problem, which can become debilitating. Physical therapy administered by a skilled therapist can be extremely effective for pregnant patients.

Guidelines for treatment

- Keep mobilisation and manipulation to a minimum.
- Use stretching and mobilisation in preference to manipulation.
- Safeguard the SIJs in the last trimester.
- Encourage active exercises as much as possible.
- Simple paracetamol is appropriate.
- A brace may be of benefit.
- Give trigger-point injections (5–8 mL 1% lignocaine) around the SIJs if necessary.

Exercise guidelines

Exercise advice depends on the woman's fitness and exercise routine prior to pregnancy. General advice includes:

- exercise at a mild to moderate level only
- avoid overheating and dehydration
- allow for a long warm-up before exercise and a long cool-down
- choose low-impact or water exercise
- stop if there are adverse symptoms (e.g. any pain, bleeding, faintness, undue distress)
- avoid scuba diving and sky diving

Carpal tunnel syndrome

Splinting of the hand and forearm at night might be beneficial. If needed, an injection of corticosteroid into the carpal tunnel can be very effective (check drug category for risk relative to dates). Rarely, operative division of the volar carpal ligament is necessary. Most problems subside following delivery.

Hypotension

This is due to increased peripheral circulation and venous pooling. It is especially common in the first trimester. Advise to avoid standing suddenly and hot baths as these may cause syncope. Fainting may also occur when the woman lies on her back in the latter half of pregnancy (supine hypotension). It is advisable to try to lie on the left side.

Pruritus

Generalised itching (pruritus gravidarum) is usually associated with cholestasis due to oestrogen sensitivity in the third trimester. Order LFTs and, if not elevated, reassure and prescribe a soothing skin preparation (e.g. aqueous cream ± glycerol). Monitor LFTs every 1–2 weeks. If LFTs markedly abnormal or if pruritus is severe, the risk of fetal death is increased and special care and assessment is required.

Obesity[15]

Obesity is associated with increased obstetric morbidity, including difficult labour and potential anaesthetic risks. Encourage weight loss diet with the aid of a dietitian.

Breathlessness of pregnancy[16]

Consider physiological breathlessness of pregnancy in a woman with unexplained dyspnoea. It starts in the second trimester, is constant and aggravated by exercise and emotional stress. No special treatment is needed or helpful. The breathlessness usually settles 6–8 weeks after delivery.

Supplements in pregnancy

Iron

Iron is not routinely recommended for pregnant women who are healthy, following an optimal diet and have a normal blood test. Those at risk (e.g. with poor nutrition, vegan diet) will require supplementation.

Folic acid

Folic acid is advised for *all* women contemplating pregnancy, starting about a month prior to conception and continuing for the first trimester. Dose: 0.5 mg (o) daily.[12] In those at risk (as mentioned earlier in the chapter), the dose is 5 mg per day.[15]

108

Vitamin B12

Vitamin B12 is essential for the developing fetus and if deficiency is known or suspected (e.g. vegetarian/vegan diet), test and give injections of B12 if deficient.

Iodine

It is recommended, for pregnant and lactating women and those planning a pregnancy, to take 150 mcg of supplementary iodine as soon as possible by using iodised salt for cooking and a multivitamin that includes iodine.

Vitamin D

There may be a case for routine testing but it is advisable to test women who are dark-skinned, veiled and at risk.[17,18] If deficient (<25 nmol/L) or insufficient (25–50 nmol/L), aim to keep vitamin D levels >70 nmol/L with cholecalciferol 1000–2000 IU daily.[19]

Omega 3

Women who eat very little seafood should consider Omega 3 supplementation, which may be obtained from fish oil and some commercially available pregnancy supplements.

Calcium

If the woman avoids dairy in her usual diet and does not consume alternative high-calcium foods, she should take a calcium supplementation of at least 1000 mg per day.

Advice on when to seek medical help

- If contractions, unusual pain or bleeding occur before term
- If the baby is less active than usual: fetal movements should not decrease close to term
- If the membranes rupture (with fluid loss)
- The onset of regular contractions 5–10 minutes apart if >34 weeks gestation but earlier if possible premature labour occurring between 22 and 34 weeks gestation

Patient education resources

Hand-out sheets from *Murtagh's Patient Education* 7th edition:

- About your pregnancy
- Miscarriage
- Pregnancy planning

References

1. Barker JH. *General Practice Medicine.* Edinburgh: Churchill Livingstone, 1984: 76–89.
2. Royal Australian College of General Practitioners. *Guidelines for Preventative Activities in General Practice* (the Red Book; 9th edn). Melbourne: RACGP, 2016.
3. The Royal Women's Hospital (Victoria). *Clinical Practice Guidelines (Professional).* <www.thewomens.org.au> (accessed 18/5/2018).
4. Fung P, Morrison J. Obstetric share-care. Aust Fam Physician, 1989; 18: 479–84.
5. Oats JJN. Routine antenatal screening: a need to evaluate Australian practice (editorial). Med J Aust, 2000; 172: 311–12.
6. Hunt JM, Lumley J. Are recommendations about routine antenatal care in Australia consistent and evidence-based? Med J Aust, 2002; 176: 255–61.
7. The Royal Australian and New Zealand College of Obstetricians and Gynaecologists, Prenatal screening and diagnosis of chromosomal and genetic conditions in the fetus in pregnancy, 2016. <www.ranzcog.edu.au/RANZCOG_SITE/media/RANZCOG-MEDIA/Women's%20Health/Statement%20and%20guidelines/Clinical-Obstetrics/Prenatal-screening-and-diagnosis-of-chromosomal-and-genetic-conditions-(C-Obs-59)-Amended-May-2016.pdf?ext=.pdf> (accessed 18/5/2018).
8. The Royal Women's Hospital (Victoria). *Clinical Practice Guidelines.* Antenatal care schedule—routine low risk. <www.the womens.org.au>
9. Carroli G, Villar J, Piaggio G et al. WHO systematic review of randomised controlled trials of routine antenatal care. Lancet, 2001; 357: 1565–70.
10. Lumley J, Oliver S, Waters E. Interventions for promoting smoking cessation during pregnancy (Cochrane Review). In: The Cochrane Library. Issue 1, 2001. Oxford: Update Software.
11. Beischer NA, Mackay EV. *Obstetrics and the Newborn.* Sydney: Saunders, 1986.
12. Peat B. Antenatal care: common issues facing GPs in shared care. Medicine Today, 2001; June: 81–5.
13. Humphrey M. Common conditions in an otherwise normal pregnancy. In: *MIMS Disease Index* (2nd edn). Sydney: IMS Publishing, 1996: 116–20.
14. Hammer I et al. Calcium treatment of leg cramps in pregnancy. Acta Obstet Gynaecol Scand, 1981; 60: 345–7.
15. Public Affairs Committee of the Teratology Society. Teratology Public Affairs Committee Position Paper: Maternal obesity and pregnancy. Birth Defects Research (Part A), 2006; 76: 73–7.
16. Burdon J. Respiratory medicine. Check Program 395. Melbourne: RACGP, 2005: 17–8.
17. MRC Vitamin Study Research Group. Prevention of neural tube defects. Lancet, 1991; 338: 131–7.
18. Grover SR, Morley R. Vitamin D deficiency in veiled or dark-skinned pregnant women. Med J Aust, 2001; 175 (5): 151–2.
19. Ebeling PR. Routine screening for vitamin D in pregnancy: past its due date? Med J Aust, 2011; 194 (7): 234–7.

Resources

NICE <www.nice.org.uk>

NHS Fetal Anomaly Screening Programme <www.fetalanomaly.screening.nhs.uk/>

The Royal Women's Hospital <www.thewomens.org.au>

MotherSafe <www.mothersafe.org.au/>

Postnatal care

109

As concerning the bringing up, nourishment and giving of suckle to the child, it shal be beste that the mother give her child sucke her selfe, for the mothers milk is more convenient and agreeable to the infant than any other woman's or other milke.

THOMAS RAYNALDE, *THE BYRTHE OF MANKYNDE* (1540)

Education for the puerperium and caring for the baby should begin during pregnancy so that a new mother is familiar with the basic principles of motherhood, especially infant feeding.[1] The puerperium is defined as the period of approximately 42 days from the completion of the third stage to the return of the normal physiological state.

It is important to educate postpartum women on care of the baby and breastfeeding, self-care, healing of the genital tract, sexual life and contraception, nutrition and what happens to their bodies and preventive issues. The uterus involutes to non-pregnant size by 6 weeks and the cervical os should be closed by 2–3 weeks post delivery.[2]

Postnatal consultations

The two-week consultation

Mother:

- take history of birth and any perinatal complications
- check blood pressure, weight (BMI)
- assess how she is adjusting to motherhood
- look for signs/symptoms of postpartum depression
- provide encouragement and advice
- check breastfeeding

Baby:

- measure weight, height and head circumference
- routine baby examination by checking the following:
  - fontanelles
  - eyes (observation, corneal reflexes, white pupil)
  - cardiovascular examination
  - femoral pulses
  - hip tests for dislocation
  - testes fully descended
  - genitalia
  - anal region
  - skin
  - reflexes

The six-week consultation

This is basically a repeat of the previous consultation—a checklist is presented in TABLE 109.1.

Table 109.1 Checklist for postnatal check at 4–6 weeks

Mother
Enquire about vaginal discharge (lochia) and whether ceased
Ask about healing of the perineum if vaginal delivery
Check for any bowel or urinary problems
Check if breastfeeding and whether there are concerns
Check abdomen (uterus should be impalpable) and Caesarean wound if present
Check if intercourse has resumed and whether there are problems or concerns
Discuss contraception options
Advise on postnatal exercises
Discuss adequate diet, rest and personal care
Check psychological health, consider Edinburgh Postnatal Depression Scale
Consider pelvic examination, checking the perineum and pelvic floor strengths
Cervical screening test (if due)
Review antenatal screening tests for follow-up action (e.g. rubella booster)
Further follow-up if necessary
Baby
Measure weight, height and head circumference
Routine examination, e.g. check for red reflex, hips, heart sounds, testes in boys
Check growth and feeding
Complete childhood health record
Discuss immunisation schedule with parent/s

Contraception

Lactational amenorrhoea method (LAM) (CHAPTER 99) is an effective contraceptive for the first 6 months, but only if the woman remains amenorrhoeic. Because some women ovulate before their period returns, breastfeeding women are usually advised to use an additional method of contraception if they wish to avoid pregnancy.

Oral contraception

Delay to after 21 days because of the risk of thrombosis (COC) and bleeding (POP).

- The progestogen-only pill (mini pill) norethisterone 350 mcg/day
  or
  levonorgestrel 30 mcg/day
- While breastfeeding, it is safe to transfer to COC at 6 months

The POP is effective after 3 tablets have been taken. Adherence may be difficult with the POP given the strict daily 3-hour timeframe for maximum efficacy.

Etonogestrel implant (Implanon) can be inserted in the immediate postpartum period. An IUD, if used, should be fitted at or after 6 weeks.[2]

After-pains[1]

After-pains, which are more common and most intense after the second and subsequent pregnancies, are characterised by intermittent lower abdominal pains, like period pains, which are often worse during and after feeding in the first 2 weeks. They are caused by oxytocin released from the posterior pituitary, which also causes the milk ejection (let-down) reflex of nursing. Suspect endometritis if there is offensive lochia, fever and poor involution of uterus.

Treatment, after examination, is reassurance and analgesics in the form of paracetamol every 4 hours for 3 days or as long as necessary.

109

BREASTFEEDING PROBLEMS

Insufficient milk supply

Studies have shown that many women wean because of low milk supply. The problem is due mainly to lactation mismanagement such as poorly timed feeds, infrequent feeds and poor attachment. A milk ejection reflex (formerly called 'let-down reflex') is necessary to get the milk supply going. Sometimes this reflex is slow and inhibited by pain from the birth canal or breasts, stress, shyness or lack of confidence about breastfeeding. Another factor in low milk supply is the mother underestimating her production capacity. If there is insufficient supply, the baby tends to demand frequent feeds, may continually suck its hand and will be slow in gaining weight.[1] Also consider tongue tie as a cause, especially if breast attachment is affected (see CHAPTER 92).

Important factors in establishing breastfeeding:

1. positioning and attachment of the baby on the breast
2. the milk ejection reflex
3. supply and demand
4. intact milk ducts and sensory nerves
5. sufficient glandular breast tissue
6. infant being able to feed

The breasts produce milk on the principle of supply and demand. This means that the more the breasts are emptied, the more milk is produced.

Signs of low supply:

- poor weight gain
- dark, hard, infrequent stools
- <6 wet nappies per day

Advice to the mother

- Try to practise relaxation techniques.
- Put the baby to your breast as often as it demands, using the 'chest to chest, chin on breast' method.
- Feed more often than usual.
- Feed at first signs of baby's readiness to feed.
- Express after feeds if possible, because the emptier the breasts and the more nipple stimulation, the more milk will be produced.
- Make sure you get adequate rest, eat well and drink ample fluids (drink to thirst).
- If you feel more tired than expected, consider investigations: FBE, iron studies, TFTs, blood glucose and vitamin B12.

Red flag

- Beware of the sleepy baby who does not demand enough and may quietly starve.

Lactation stimulation

Lactation can be improved by more frequent breastfeeding and correct position and attachment. Consider domperidone as a galactagogue for increasing milk supply.

- domperidone 10 mg (one tablet) tds for 2–4 weeks, reducing slowly once an adequate breast-milk supply is established. Women with persistent low milk supply may increase to 20 mg three times a day (maximum 60 mg day).

Engorged breasts

Engorgement occurs when the milk supply comes on so quickly that the breasts become swollen, hard and tender. There is an increased supply of blood and other fluids in the breast as well as milk. The breasts and nipples may be so swollen that the baby is unable to latch on and suckle. Once again, lactation mismanagement is a key factor. If a newborn is attached properly and feeds often and liberally, engorgement should not happen.

Advice to the mother

- Feed your baby on demand from day 1 until the baby has had enough.
- Finish the first breast completely; maybe use one side per feed rather than some from each breast. Offer the second breast if the baby appears hungry.
- Soften the breasts before feeds or express with a warm washcloth or shower, which will help to get the milk flowing.
- Express a little milk before putting the baby to your breast (especially if the baby has trouble latching) and express a little after feeding from the other side if it is too uncomfortable.
- Massage any breast lumps gently towards the nipple while feeding.
- Apply cold packs after feeding and cool washed cabbage leaves (left in the refrigerator) between feeds. Change the leaves every 2 hours.
- Consider waking your baby for a feed if your breasts are uncomfortable or if the baby is sleeping longer than 4 hours.
- Use a good, comfortable bra.
- Take ibuprofen or paracetamol regularly for severe discomfort.

Regular feeding and following demand feeding is the best treatment for engorged breasts.

Suppression of lactation[3,4]

Women may seek suppression of lactation for a variety of reasons such as weaning the baby, not wishing to breastfeed initially, or after stillbirth.

Mechanical suppression

The simplest way of suppressing lactation once it is established is to transfer the baby gradually to a bottle or a cup over a 3-week period. The decreased demand reduces milk supply, with minimal discomfort. If abrupt cessation is required, it is necessary to avoid nipple stimulation, refrain from expressing milk and use a well-fitting bra. Use cold packs and analgesics as necessary. Engorgement will gradually settle over a 2–3 week period.

Hormonal suppression

Hormonal suppression can be used for severe engorgement but only as a last resort. It is more effective if given at the time of delivery but may produce side effects. Avoid oestrogens.

cabergoline 1 mg (o) statim (once only)

Drugs affecting lactation

Drugs that can affect lactation or a breastfed infant are listed in TABLE 109.2. Most drugs can be compatible and tolerated, but check with prescribing guidelines. Consider risk versus benefit.

Table 109.2 Drugs taken by nursing mother that can affect breastfed infant or lactation

Antibiotics:
- aminoglycosides
- chloramphenicol
- nitrofurantoin
- metronidazole
- tetracycline
- sulphonamides

Antihistamines
Antineoplastics/cytotoxics*
Benzodiazepines
Bromocriptine
Combined oral contraceptive/oestrogens
Ergotamine*
Gold salts
H_2-receptor antagonists (e.g. cimetidine, ranitidine)
Illicit drugs (e.g. cocaine, codeine combinations, cannabis, LSD)*
Lithium
Methotrexate*
Quinidine
Laxatives (e.g. senna)
Alcohol (no harmful effects unless taken in excess)
Nicotine (increased respiratory distress in infants exposed) but if necessary NRT is preferable to smoking

*Indicates contraindicated drugs

109

Nipple problems with breastfeeding

Causes of nipple trauma:

- attachment problems (most common)
- infection—bacterial, 'thrush' or viral

- vasospasm
- dermatitis (e.g. contact dermatitis)

Sore nipples[4]

Sore nipples are a common problem, thought to be caused by the baby not taking the nipple into its mouth properly, often because of breast engorgement. The problem is preventable with careful attention to the feeding position of the baby. A well-attached baby sucking strongly should not cause nipple trauma.

Advice to the mother

It is important to be as relaxed and comfortable as possible (with your back well supported) and for your baby to suck gently.

- Try to use the 'chest to chest, chin on breast' feeding position.
- Vary the feeding positions (make sure each position and attachment is correct).
- Start feeding from the less painful side first if one nipple is very sore.
- Express some milk first to soften and 'lubricate' the nipple.
- Gently break the suction with your finger before removing the baby from the breast.
- Apply covered ice to the nipple to relieve pain.
- Keep the nipples dry by exposing the breasts to the air and/or using a hair dryer on a low setting.
- Try soothing hydrogel pads inside the bra.

Note: Raynaud phenomenon, i.e. nipple vasospasm, can affect the nipple and cause painful breastfeeding. It is often mistaken for *Candida albicans* infection.

Cracked nipples

Cracked nipples are usually caused by the baby clamping on the end of the nipple rather than applying the jaw behind the whole nipple. Not drying the nipples thoroughly after each feed and wearing soggy breast pads are other contributing factors. Untreated sore nipples may progress to painful cracks.

Symptoms

At first, the crack may be so small that it cannot be seen. The crack is either on the skin of the nipple or where it joins the areola. A sharp pain in the nipple with suckling probably means the crack has developed. Feeding is usually very painful, and bleeding can occur.

Advice to the mother

Cracked nipples should heal if the baby begins to latch onto the breast fully and properly. They usually take only 1–2 days to heal.

- Follow the same rules as for sore nipples.
- Do not feed from the affected breast—rest the nipple for 1–2 feeds.
- Express the milk from that breast by hand.
- Feed that expressed milk to the baby.
- Start feeding gradually with short feeds.
- Seeking the opinion of an expert lactation consultant may be of benefit. Consider use of a nipple shield only after seeking face-to-face expert advice.
- Take paracetamol or ibuprofen just before feeding to relieve pain.

Inverted nipples

An inverted nipple is one that inverts or moves into the breast instead of pointing outwards when the baby tries to suck from it. When the areola is squeezed, the nipple retracts inwards.

Treatment[4]

The best approach is good preparation with prolonged breast contact and feeding prior to milk 'coming in' and knowledgeable helpers giving advice and confidence. If a baby continues to have ongoing problems with attachment, a nipple shield may be helpful.

MASTITIS

Mastitis, which has a high incidence (up to 20%), is basically cellulitis of the interlobular connective tissue of the breast (see CHAPTER 100). Usually restricted to lactating women, it is caused mainly by a cracked nipple or poor milk drainage. Not all mastitis is infective. Many instances are related to milk not being drained adequately and will improve if appropriate breastfeeding technique is followed. A blocked duct or ducts may be the cause. It is a serious problem and requires early treatment. Breastfeeding from the affected side can continue as the infection is confined to interstitial breast tissue and doesn't usually affect the milk supply.

Note: Mastitis must be treated vigorously—it is a serious condition. Refer to CHAPTER 100.

Bacterial mastitis

Clinical features

- A lump and then soreness (at first)
- A red, wedge-shaped, possibly tender, area
- Fever, tiredness, muscle aches and pains

Management

Prevention (in lactation).

Rule: 'Heat, rest and drain the breast'.

- Keep feeding and frequently.
- Maintain free breast drainage.
- Attend to breast engorgement and cracked nipples. If symptoms persist >24 hours or patient is unwell, commence antibiotics.[5]
- Antibiotics: resolution without progression to an abscess will usually be prevented by antibiotics:
  dicloxacillin 500 mg (o) qid for at least 5 days
  or
  flucloxacillin 500 mg (o) qid for at least 5 days
  or
  cephalexin 500 mg (o) qid for at least 5 days

  If severe cellulitis:
  flucloxacillin 2 g IV 6 hourly
- Ibuprofen or paracetamol for pain

Instructions to patients

- Keep the affected breast well drained.
- Continue breastfeeding: do it frequently and start with the sore side or begin feeding from the normal side until the milk comes and then switch to the sore side.
- Heat the sore breast before feeding (e.g. hot shower or hot washcloth).
- Cool the breast after feeding: use a cold face washer from the freezer.
- Massage any breast lumps gently towards the nipple while feeding.
- Empty the breast well: hand express if necessary.
- Get sufficient rest.
- Keep to a nutritious diet and drink ample fluids.

Breast and nipple candidiasis

Clinical features

- Painful breasts—often exquisite pain especially during and after feeding
- No fever
- Nipple pain and sensitivity
- Usually but not always bilateral
- Nipples can be pink and shiny
- ± Pink haloes around the base of the nipple
- Breasts usually normal: no heat, lumps or tender points

Note: May follow a course of antibiotics. Swabs are of limited value.

Treatment

fluconazole 150 mg (o) every second day for 3 doses[5] then oral nystatin (o) tds for 10 days
miconazole gel qid to nipple after feeds

Treat the baby with oral nystatin drops or miconazole oral gel.

Breast abscess

If tenderness and redness persist beyond 48 hours and an area of tense induration develops, then a breast abscess may have formed. It can be treated with needle aspiration or may require surgical drainage under general anaesthesia.

For a description of surgical and other management refer to CHAPTER 100.

Secondary postpartum haemorrhage[2,6]

Secondary postpartum haemorrhage is any bright bleeding from the birth canal 24 hours or more after delivery. It may vary from very slight to torrential and may occur at any time up to 6 weeks postpartum. It tends to peak at 5–10 days.

Causes

- Retained products of conception (PoC)
- Infection, especially at placental site
- Laceration of any part of the birth canal
- Coagulation disorder
- Rarely due to gestational trophoblastic disease

No cause is found in one-third of cases (i.e. idiopathic subinvolution).

Treatment

Rule: An empty and contracted uterus will not bleed.

- Investigation:
  - ultrasound (? retained PoC)
  - cervical swab for culture
  - FBE
  - beta hCG
- IV oxytocin 10 IU followed by infusion of 40 IU in Hartmann's solution
- Ergometrine 250 mcg IM or 25–50 mcg slowly IV (if continuing heavy bleeding)
- Consider misoprostol, 4 or 5 × 200 mcg tablets per rectum or otherwise by intramyometrial injection of prostaglandin F2 alpha (caution: specialist supervision)
- Exploration under general anaesthetic if blood loss >250 mL:
  - gentle blunt curettage required in the postpartum uterus (aim to prevent uterine adhesions—Asherman syndrome)
- Consider blood transfusion if Hb is <100 g/L

- Antibiotics (e.g. amoxycillin/clavulanate + metronidazole + gentamicin while awaiting culture)
- Consider Bakri balloon tamponade and uterine packing for major PPH

Note: Referral is necessary after the oxytocin/ergometrine injection. Occasionally a life-saving hysterectomy or ligation of the internal iliac arteries may be necessary.

Lochia discharge

The discharge of lochia, which is blood and sloughed-off tissue from the uterine lining, should be monitored.

Normal:

1 bloody loss = lochia rubra: 2–12 days
2 serous loss = lochia serosa: up to 20 days
3 white loss = lochia alba
4 offensive lochia = endometritis

Lochia loss persists for 4–8 weeks. Abnormal lochia rubra may indicate retained PoC or endometritis. If there is a problem, examine with a speculum and take cervical/vaginal swab.

Puerperal fever

Puerperal fever is defined as raised temperature of ≥ 38°C from day 1 to day 10. If fever, think of the three **B**s—**b**irth canal, **b**reast, **b**ladder. The cause is genital infection in about 75% of patients. Endometritis presents with offensive lochia, abdominal pain and a tender uterus. Other causes include urinary tract infection, mastitis and an intercurrent respiratory infection. Investigations include a vaginal swab for microscopy, culture and sensitivities and a midstream specimen of urine for microscopy and culture, blood culture and an FBE.

Treatment

109

amoxycillin/potassium clavulanate plus metronidazole (while awaiting sensitivities)

Beware of severe puerperal sepsis such as gram-negative septicaemia or *Clostridium welchii* septicaemia and the rare *Bacteroides fragilis*.

POSTNATAL DEPRESSIVE DISORDERS

Hormonal changes, fatigue, adjustment and physical changes can all contribute to mood changes in the postnatal period. There are three separate important problems:

1 postnatal blues
2 postnatal adjustment disorder
3 postnatal (or postpartum) depression

Postnatal blues

'The blues' is a very common problem (occurs in 80%) that arises in the first 2 weeks (usually days 3–10) after childbirth.

Clinical features

- Feeling flat or depressed
- Mood swings
- Irritability
- Feeling emotional (e.g. crying easily)
- Feeling inadequate
- Tiredness
- Sleep disturbance unrelated to baby's sleep needs
- Lacking confidence (e.g. in bathing and feeding the baby)
- Aches and pains (e.g. headache)

Fortunately, 'the blues' is a passing phase and lasts about 4–14 days. Management is based on support, reassurance and basic counselling. Contact friends and relatives to help.

Advice to the mother[3]

- Rest as much as possible.
- Accept help from others in the house.
- Talk about your concerns with a good listener.
- This is common and should improve within a week or two.

If 'the blues' lasts longer than 14 days, it is very important to contact your doctor.

Postnatal adjustment disorder

- Occurs in first 6 months
- Similar symptoms to 'the blues'
- Anxiety with handling baby
- Psychosomatic complaints
- Fearful of criticism

Treatment

- Support and reassurance
- Cognitive therapy
- Parentcraft support
- Settles with time

Postnatal depression

Some women develop a very severe depression after childbirth. Always consider it in the frequent attender. Symptoms are present for at least 2 consecutive weeks, with onset in the first few days postpartum. It should be treated as for major depression. (See CHAPTER 19 for an overview.)

- Occurs in 10–30% women
- In first 6–12 months (usually first 6 months: peaks about 12th week)
- Anxiety and agitation common
- Marked mood swings
- Poor memory and concentration
- Typical depressive features

Use the Edinburgh Postnatal Depression Scale (a score of 12 or more is significant).

Treatment

- Support, reassurance, counselling
- Group psychotherapy and support group (e.g. <www.panda.org.au>)
- Couple therapy (must involve partner)
- Postnatal depression support group
- Parentcraft support
- Hospitalisation may be necessary (especially if suicidal or infanticidal ideations)
- Medication—SSRIs (sertraline, paroxetine—agents of choice)
- Closely monitor any risk of self-harm
- Consider referral if poor response to treatment in 2 weeks

Note: Beware of puerperal psychosis with onset usually within first 2 weeks.

Postpartum psychosis

The most common postpartum psychosis is an affective disorder: mania or agitated depression. It is treatable and requires urgent attention. Symptoms that appear within the first month include unusual behaviour, agitation, delusions, hallucinations, mania and suicidal ideations.

It is rare, occurring in about 1:500 births.

Past history may be a pointer. Suspect if severe depression not responding to treatment. An important differential diagnosis is delirium with puerperal fever. Check thyroid function and organise inpatient psychiatric care. There is an increased risk of further episodes with subsequent pregnancies.

Other issues in postnatal care

Sleep deprivation

Give advice and counselling. Use the 'sleep when baby sleeps' rule. Avoid sedatives. Insomnia experienced when the baby finally sleeps should raise suspicion of postnatal depression.

Tiredness

Tiredness is very common in the first few months after delivery. It may be a presenting symptom of anaemia, depression, hypothyroidism, anxiety or depression (in particular).

Perform FBE, TFTs, iron studies, B12, blood glucose and urinalysis.

Postpartum thyroid dysfunction[6]

Postpartum thyroiditis may be misdiagnosed as postpartum depression and should always be considered in the tired, apparently depressed woman in the first 6 months after delivery. It is common in women with pre-existing autoimmune thyroid disorders and often flares up in this period. It must be differentiated from new onset or relapsing Graves disease indicated by positive anti-thyroid stimulating hormone receptor antibodies. Women who have had postpartum thyroid dysfunction are at greater risk of developing hypothyroidism within 10 years postpartum.

The initial phase of hyperthyroidism is often followed by a phase of temporary hypothyroidism, with eventual return towards normality. Beta blockers are useful during the hyperthyroidism phase, while short-term replacement with thyroxine can be required in the hypothyroid phase.

Hair loss

Increased hair shedding as telogen effluvium is common about 3–4 months after delivery. Large clumps of hair with white bulbs come out easily with combing or shampooing. Reassure that it reverts to normal in 3–6 months.

Sexual difficulties

Decreased libido is a common problem and often related to sleep deprivation, as well as hormonal changes. Decreased libido can also be due to one of the postnatal depressive disorders or to tension in adjusting to the new relationships.[2]

Dyspareunia is common, especially following an episiotomy or vaginal tear, and should be treated symptomatically and with education. Simple lubrication or vaginal oestrogens can help until perineal healing is achieved. A topical corticosteroid may be appropriate for scar tissue that appears inflamed.

Early intercourse is risky with deaths from air embolism reported in the first 2 weeks. Intercourse is not advisable in the first 6 weeks.

Elimination disorders[3]

Always enquire how the patient is coping with her bowels and urination. Simple advice such as stool softening and pelvic floor exercises will help. However, serious problems such as faecal incontinence secondary to a fistula from a third-degree tear or urinary retention due to neuropraxia of the pelvic floor can develop and need urgent attention.

Patient education resources

Hand-out sheets from *Murtagh's Patient Education* 7th edition:

- Breastfeeding and milk supply
- Establishing breastfeeding
- Mastitis with breastfeeding
- Nipple problems with breastfeeding
- Postnatal depression

References

1 Smibert J. Practical postnatal care. Aust Fam Physician, 1989; 18: 508–11.
2 The Royal Women's Hospital (Victoria). *Clinical Practice Guidelines (Professional).* Postpartum care. <www.thewomens.org.au> (accessed 20/5/2018).
3 McKenna M. Postnatal problems. In: *MIMS Disease Index* (2nd edn). Sydney: IMS Publishing, 1996: 423–5.
4 Amir L, Clements F, Walsh A. Breastfeeding. Check Program 426. Melbourne: RACGP, 2007: 2–19.
5 Expert group for Antibiotics guidelines. In: eTG complete [Internet]. Melbourne: Therapeutic Guidelines Ltd. Available from <www.tg.org.au> accessed May 2018.
6 Expert group for Endocrinology guidelines. In: eTG complete [Internet]. Melbourne: Therapeutic Guidelines Ltd. Available from <www.tg.org.au> accessed May 2018.

Part 7

Male health

110 Male health: an overview

Call it the 'M-factor', call it maleness, call it what you like—but from infancy onwards, in every age group, males are more likely to die than females.

ANDREW PATTISON[1]

In recent years, increasing attention has been focused on men's health, mainly because it became evident that the average male's lifestyle was slowly killing him. As doctors we are beginning to understand that a great proportion of male ill-health is related to behavioural and social factors.

An important statistic is the constant discrepancy in average life expectancy (ALE) between the sexes. At present in Australia, the ALE is 80.3 years for males born between 2012 and 2014 compared with 84.4 years for females.[2]

Since the beginning of the 20th century and even further back this discrepancy has continued. In 1900 the ALE for males was 55.2 years and 58.8 for females.[2] This increased to a difference of 6 years for most of the past century. However, the significant increase in ALE for both sexes has been encouraging.

Men have a significantly greater incidence of medical conditions and problems, such as cardiovascular disease, obesity, alcoholism, HIV and hypertension, as well as having higher rates of accidental death and suicide. The following comparative statistics for Australian society highlight this difference.

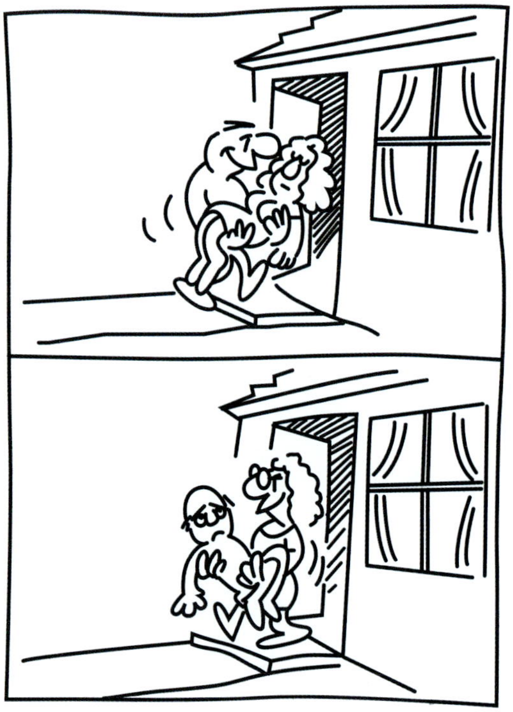

FIGURE 110.1
Source: Courtesy of Ron Tandberg

Men's health at a glance[1,2,3]

- Up to 14 years, boys are at least twice as likely as girls to die from accidental injury (e.g. motor vehicle accidents [MVAs] and drowning).
- In the 15–24 years age group, males are three times more likely to die in MVAs and three times more likely to commit suicide. The overall death rate is 3.65 times higher than for females.
- In the 25–65 age group, males are four times more likely to die from coronary artery disease, three times more likely to die in MVAs, three times more likely to commit suicide, four times more likely to die in other accidents, and twice as likely to die from cancer. The overall death rate is two times that of females.
- The figures are worse in the lower socioeconomic groups. Low-income males are nearly three times more likely to state that their overall health is poor compared to men with higher incomes.
- About 2 in 3 adult males and 1 in 4 older boys are overweight or obese.
- Roughly 1 in 4 men have a disability and almost 1 in 3 have a chronic health problem.
- Only 1 in 4 men ≥65 years get sufficient physical activity.
- An estimated 1 in 2 men (54%) have experienced sexual difficulty in the past 12 months.
- At least 4 out of 5 heroin overdose deaths occur in males.
- Aboriginal males' life expectancy is 17 years less than that of non-Aboriginal males. In the

35–45 age group, the death rate is 11 times that of non-Aboriginals.

- Workplace deaths—93% occur in males (who constitute 56% of the workforce).
- Some 46% of Australian marriages end in divorce. The majority of these are initiated by women.
- Among those convicted for acts of violence, 90% are males; 80% of the victims are males.
- In Australian schools, 90% of children with documented behavioural problems are males.

(Most of this list has been reproduced with the permission of Andrew Pattison.)

These statistics are very revealing and reflect attitudes to lifestyle. Men smoke more, drink more and indulge in greater risk-taking behaviour in general. Only 5% of men have adequate fruit and vegetable intake.[3]

Young males in particular are more likely than young females to take risks in areas such as conflict or violence, sexual behaviour, drinking, gambling and accident prevention.[4] The main causes of death by age group for Australian males are summarised in TABLE 110.1.[5]

Table 110.1 Main causes of death by age group for Australian males

Years	No. 1	No. 2	No. 3
1–14	Non-traffic accidents	Traffic accidents	Cancer
15–24	Traffic accidents	Suicide	Non-traffic accidents
25–44	Suicide	Cancer	Non-traffic accidents
45–54	Cancer	Circulatory diseases	Suicide
55–64	Cancer	Circulatory diseases	Suicide
65–74	Circulatory diseases	Cancer	Respiratory diseases
75+	Circulatory diseases	Cancer	Respiratory diseases

Prostatic disease

Ageing men find disorders of the prostate almost inevitable, as they become aware of lower urinary tract symptoms (LUTS). The usual cause of benign prostatic hyperplasia is now being managed better with α-blocking agents, such as tamsulosin and 5-alpha reductase inhibitors (such as Dutasteride), which delay the almost inevitable resection of the prostate—a procedure that provokes considerable anxiety in men. Cancer of the prostate is the second commonest cause of death from cancer in men and the third overall including both sexes, yet its management remains controversial and at times confusing, especially the screening issues (see CHAPTER 114).

Androgen deficiency[1,2]

Androgen deficiency, which affects about 1 in 200 men under 60 years of age and possibly 1 in 10 older men, is likely to be an underdiagnosed condition. About 1 in 3 cases are associated with Klinefelter syndrome, which is more common than realised, with 50% remaining undiagnosed. Androgen deficiency should be considered when the following signs and symptoms present:

- *infancy*—micropenis, small testes
- *puberty*—delayed, small testes, failure of growth of larynx or penis, failure of skin of scrotum to thicken and/or pigment, poor muscle development, poor facial, body and pubic hair, marked and persisting gynaecomastia
- *adult*—regression virilisation, mood changes, poor concentration, lethargy, hot flushes, sweats, decreased libido, decreased semen volume, gynaecomastia, osteoporotic fracture, erectile dysfunction (ED)

Androgen deficiency is an uncommon cause of ED, but men presenting with ED should be assessed for androgen deficiency (ED will be discussed in CHAPTER 116). This should be done initially through history and examination rather than a blood test, including examining the size and firmness of the testes. An orchidometer (a series of beads of various sizes to match clinical testicular size) can assist with this and can be obtained through Andrology Australia.[8]

Diagnosis is by at least two testosterone levels taken on different mornings (luteinising hormone added to the second collection if the first testosterone is low).[6] Other tests may include semen analysis (if fertility is an issue), bone density, karyotype (Klinefelter syndrome—see CHAPTER 18), FSH and iron studies (haemochromatosis).

Abnormal testosterone (for healthy males) results:[6]

- 21–35 years <10.4 nmol/L
- 70–89 years <6.4 nmol/L

Treatment under consultant guidance is with testosterone replacement with injections, gel, implants, patches or tablets.[6,7] There is no evidence that testosterone gel is a panacea.[9]

Osteoporosis in men[10,11]

While more common in women, osteoporosis still has a high prevalence in men and remains a major health concern for older men. Almost a third of Australian men >60 years of age will suffer an osteoporotic fracture.[10] Yet the identification of osteoporosis in men remains particularly poor, and this may be because it is considered a predominantly female condition. BMD testing rates for women are four times those of men.[12]

Prevention can be achieved through reducing risk factors where possible. Risk factors include poor dietary calcium, lack of weight-bearing exercise, vitamin D deficiency, hypogonadism, smoking, excess alcohol and medications (corticosteroids used for >3 months, anti-epileptics, e.g. phenytoin). Other risk factors for osteoporosis and fractures include a family history of osteoporosis, malabsorption, hyperthyroidism, hypothyroidism, hyperparathyroidism, being underweight and being at risk of falls. Men with risk factors should be screened using BMD testing. Other indications for screening include height loss, kyphosis or back pain suggesting possible vertebral fractures, low-impact fractures and possibly even high-impact fractures.[13]

Investigations can include bone densitometry, FBE, LFTs, testosterone and vitamin D. When identified, osteoporotic men should be encouraged to have adequate dietary calcium, be educated on fall-prevention strategies and encouraged to do weight-bearing exercise. Medication management options include oral bisphosphonates (first-line treatment) and calcium, vitamin D or testosterone if deficient.

Gynaecomastia

This is a 'true' enlargement of the male breasts, not to be confused with false enlargement of obese men. Gynaecomastia occurs in up to 50% of adolescent boys. Virtually no breast tissue is palpable in normal men.

If present in adult men, look for evidence of testosterone deficiency. Other causes include drugs (e.g. anabolic steroids, oestrogen, digoxin, calcium antagonists, marijuana, spironolactone, amiodarone, tricyclic antidepressants, cimetidine), liver failure, testicular feminisation syndrome and oestrogen-secreting tumours, such as adrenal carcinoma and Leydig cell tumour.

Sex-linked inherited disorders

Males bear the burden of X-linked recessive gene disorders, which always manifest as there is no normal gene on the additional X chromosome (as there is in the female) to counteract the action of the abnormal gene.

Occasionally a gene can be carried on an autosome but manifests only in one sex. An example is male-pattern baldness, manifesting as an autosomal dominant disorder in males but as a recessive disorder in females.

Examples of X-linked disorders significantly affecting males include:

- haemophilia A and B
- glucose-6-phosphate dehydrogenase deficiency
- Duchenne muscular dystrophy
- retinitis pigmentosa
- Hunter syndrome
- ocular albinism

Summary

There is an increasing emphasis on and interest in men's health. In 2008, in response to the growing awareness of men's health issues, the first Australian National Male Health Policy[14] was developed. Initiatives that have emerged from and been enhanced by this policy include programs and campaigns that focus on male mental health, work safety, male health in particular risk groups and prevention of chronic disease and injury. Examples include the Men's Sheds, Man Health and Strong Father Strong Family programs. Also available are information sources and links, resources and research on male health issues.

Many of these programs, especially those concerning mental health and psychosocial aspects such as family relationships and risk behaviour, focus on issues such as what it means to be male. Topics explored include the positives of maleness, the behaviours males should be avoiding and personal responsibility.

The GP is in an ideal position to identify, assess and manage significant health problems in males. Men's reluctance to access health services when they need them makes the GP's role all the more important. Opportunities should be grasped to discuss health issues with male patients and foster preventive issues where appropriate.

References

1 Pattison A. *The M Factor* (2nd edn). Sydney: Simon & Schuster, 2001.

2 AIHW 2016. *Australia's Health 2016*. Cat. No. AUS 199. Canberra: AIHW.

3 AIHW 2016. *The Health of Australia's Males*. Last updated 4/10/2017. Canberra: AIHW.

4 Pawlowski B, Atwal R. Sex differences in everyday risk-taking behavior in humans. Evolutionary Psychology, 2008; 6 (1): 29–42.

5 Australian Bureau of Statistics. *Causes of Death.* Canberra: ABS, 2016. Cat. No. 3303.0.

6 Expert group for Endocrinology. Male hypogonadism. In: eTG complete [Internet]. Melbourne: Therapeutic Guidelines Ltd. Available from: <www.tg.org.au>, accessed 20/11/2017.

7 Andrology Australia. *Clinical Summary Guideline 4: Androgen Deficiency,* May 2014 <www.andrologyaustralia.org/wp-content/uploads/clinical-summary-guide04_May2010.pdf> (accessed 27/1/2014).

8 Andrology Australia. The Andrology Australia orchidometer <www.andrologyaustralia.org/orchidometer/> (accessed 27/1/2014).

9 Handelsman DJ. Global trends in testosterone prescribing, 2000–2011: expanding the spectrum of prescription drug misuse. Med J Aust, 2013; 199 (8): 548–51.

10 RACGP. *Clinical Guideline for Osteoporosis Prevention, Diagnosis and Management in Postmenopausal Women and Men Over 50 Years of Age,* February 2017 (2nd edn) <www.racgp.org.au/download/Documents/Guidelines/Musculoskeletal/osteoporosis-guidelines.pdf> (accessed 22/11/2017).

11 Eisman J, Clapham S, Kehoe L. Osteoporosis prevalence and levels of treatment in primary care: the Australian Bone Care Study. J Bone Miner Res, 2004; 19 (12): 1969–75.

12 Ewald DP et al. Population rates of bone densitometry use in Australia, 2001–2005, by sex and rural versus urban location. Med J Aust, 2009; 190 (3): 126–8.

13 Mackey D et al. High-trauma fractures and low bone mineral density in older women and men. JAMA, 2007; 298 (20): 2381–8.

14 The Department of Health. National Male Health Policy, 2014 <www.health.gov.au/malehealthpolicy> (accessed 21/11/2017).

111 Scrotal pain

Acute scrotal pain in infancy and adolescence should be regarded as torsion of the testis until proved otherwise.

TEXT, PAGE 1210

Scrotal pain in males can occur in all age groups but the child or adolescent with acute scrotal pain often poses a diagnostic challenge. Serious problems include testicular torsion, strangulation of an inguinoscrotal hernia, a testicular tumour and a haematocele, all of which require surgical intervention.

Key facts and checkpoints

- Torsion of the testis is not the most common cause of acute scrotal pain in childhood and adolescence, but it is the most important.[1]
- Torsion is also a feature of young men younger than 25 years.
- Testicular pain can be referred to the abdomen.
- Torsion of the testis should form part of the differential diagnosis in a boy or young man who is vomiting and has intense pain in the lower abdominal quadrant inguinal region.
- The loss of a testicle from torsion, an avoidable problem, is a real 'time bomb' and a common reason for litigation for medical negligence.
- The clinical picture of epididymo-orchitis can mimic torsion of the testis so closely that in most boys and young men the diagnosis should be made only at surgical exploration.[1]
- An abnormality predisposing to torsion of the testis is usually present bilaterally; the opposite testis should also be fixed to prevent torsion (orchidopexy).
- Torsion must be corrected as soon as possible to reduce the chance of gangrene and loss of the testis.
- Suspect self-correcting testicular torsion in repeated episodes of severe spontaneously resolving pain. Refer for possible orchidopexy.
- Suspect abscess formation if epididymo-orchitis does not settle with a reasonable course of antibiotics. Surgical drainage may be necessary.
- A varicocele can cause testicular discomfort—examine the patient in the standing position.

The clinical approach

History

It is important to determine whether there were any pre-existing predisposing factors or history of trauma.

Key questions

- Have you noticed any burning of urine or penile discharge?
- Have you had an injury to your scrotal region such as being struck by a baseball, cricket ball or falling astride something?
- Have you travelled overseas recently?
- Have you been aware of a lump in your testicle or groin?
- Have you had an illness lately and have you noticed swelling of the glands in your neck or near your ear (i.e. screening for mumps)?
- Do you have back pain or have you injured your back?

Examination

Both sides of the scrotum must be examined and contrasted. Inguinal and femoral hernial orifices, the spermatic cord, testis and epididymis must be checked on both sides. The size, lie and elevation in the scrotum of the testis should be assessed, as should the cremasteric reflex. This is done by stroking or pinching the medial thigh, and considered positive if the testicle moves at least 0.5 cm. An absence of the ipsilateral cremasteric reflex is the most sensitive physical finding in testicular torsion but the reflex is often absent in small boys (under 2½ years) without torsion.[2]

The patient should be examined standing and supine. The scrotum and its contents are examined systematically starting with the skin, which may include sebaceous cysts or other dermatological conditions. A painful testis should be elevated gently to determine if the pain improves.

Investigations

Investigations that may help diagnose the painful testis in particular include:

- blood cell count
- urine analysis: microscopy and culture
- *Chlamydia* antigen detection tests
- ultrasound
- technetium-99m scan

Acute scrotal pain in children and adolescents—'the acute scrotum'

This problem is more likely to be encountered in the adolescent, especially after the testis enlarges at puberty (13–16 year olds).[1] A list of causes is presented in TABLE 111.1. Infants, however, can also have torsion of a testis or a testicular appendage.

Table 111.1 Causes of scrotal pain or swelling

Torsion of the testis
Torsion of a testicular appendage
Epididymo-orchitis
Mumps orchitis
Acute hydrocele
Idiopathic scrotal oedema (rare)
Haematoma/haematocele
Testicular neoplasm
Henoch–Schönlein purpura
Strangulated inguinoscrotal hernia
Scrotal skin conditions
Varicocele
Referred pain (e.g. spine, ureteric colic, abdominal aorta)

Clinical problem

A 15-year-old teenager presents with relatively acute onset of pain in his lower right abdomen and scrotum. He has vomited several times. On examination the right testicle is tender, red and swollen.

Discussion

The three main differential diagnoses of the acute scrotum in an adolescent are torsion of the testis, torsion of a testicular appendage and acute epididymo-orchitis (see FIG. 111.1). Less commonly the problem would be a haematoma or an acute hydrocele mimicking testicular torsion. This patient, however, must be regarded as having torsion of the testis until proven otherwise. Early operation with torsion is imperative because if the testis is deprived of its blood supply, infarction is inevitable and excision becomes necessary. Excluding mumps, no pre- or peripubertal youth should be diagnosed as suffering from acute epididymo-orchitis until the testis has been exposed at operation and torsion excluded.

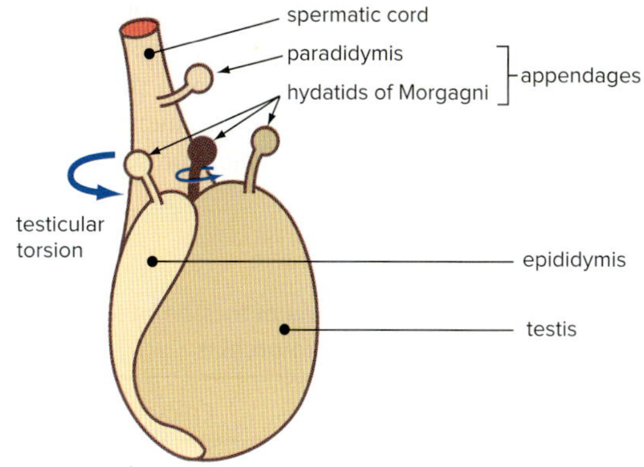

FIGURE 111.1 Illustration of torsion of the testis and an appendage: the 'black' hydatid of Morgagni is the one most likely to undergo torsion

Torsion of the testis

Torsion usually occurs because of an abnormally narrow anchoring of the testis by the testicular mesorchium posteriorly[1] and the tunica vaginalis (which normally covers only the testicle and epididymis) also covering the bottom end of the spermatic cord. This allows the testicle to have a more mobile and transverse lie, referred to as a 'bell clapper deformity', and makes it easier for the testicle to twist around upon its cord. This deformity is almost invariably present on the other testicle, so when surgical correction of the torted testis is done, orchidopexy should always be done on the other side also.

When a testicle torts, time is of the essence. One study suggests that the testicular salvage rate is 90% if detorsion occurs less than 6 hours after the onset of symptoms, but this drops to 50% after 12 hours and <10% after 24 hours.[3]

Torsion of the testis versus epididymo-orchitis

With torsion of the testicle there is pain of sudden onset, described as a severe, aching, sickening pain in the groin that may be accompanied by nausea and vomiting. With epididymo-orchitis the attack usually begins with malaise and fever and is often associated with a urinary infection. The testicle soon becomes swollen and acutely tender; however, elevation and support of the scrotum usually relieves pain in this condition (Prehn sign) while tending to increase it with a torsion. A comparison of the clinical presentations is given in TABLE 111.2.

Table 111.2 Clinical presentations of torsion of testis and acute epididymo-orchitis

	Torsion of testis	Epididymo-orchitis
Typical age	Early teens, average range 5–15 years	Young adults Elderly
Onset	Usually sudden but can be gradual	Gradual
Severity of pain	Very severe	Moderate
Associated symptoms	Vomiting Groin pain Possibly abdominal pain	Fever ± Dysuria
Examination of scrotum	Very tender and red Testis high and transverse Scrotal oedema Possibly an acute hydrocele	Swollen, tender and red; can be tender on rectal examination Possibly an acute hydrocele
Effect of gentle scrotal elevation	No change to pain or worse pain	Relief of pain
Investigations	Technetium-99m scan (if available, time permits and diagnosis doubtful)	Leucocytosis Possibly pyobacteria of urine

Radiology as a diagnostic aid

Ultrasound, particularly colour Doppler, is useful in distinguishing a cystic scrotal lump (such as a hydrocele) from a solid tumour. Its use to distinguish between a torsion and epididymo-orchitis is controversial as it cannot reliably detect changes that are diagnostic of early torsion. Since the investigation can involve unnecessary delay in treatment it is generally not recommended. A technetium-99m scan can differentiate between the two conditions: in torsion the testis is avascular, while it is hyperaemic in epididymo-orchitis.

111

At surgery the testicle is untwisted and if viable an orchidopexy is performed. A gangrenous testicle is removed (see FIG. 111.2).

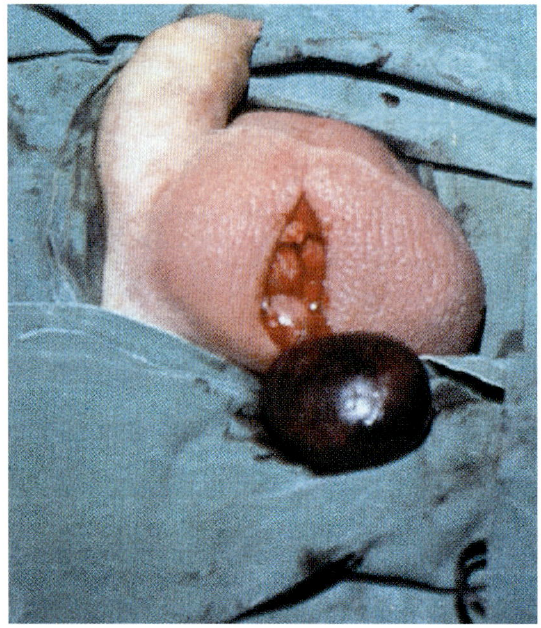

FIGURE 111.2 Torsion of the testis resulting in gangrene after 12 hours from onset of pains. The testis was excised and the other normal testis 'anchored'

Cautionary tales

Many testicles are lost because of inappropriate delays with referral for an ultrasound. The patient should be referred immediately to a surgeon or surgical centre. Teenage boys presenting with acute right iliac fossa pain, nausea and vomiting are sometimes misdiagnosed as having acute appendicitis.

Torsion of a testicular appendage

Torsion of one of the testicular appendages (most commonly the hydatid of Morgagni) accounts for 60% of cases of acute scrotal pain in children[1] (torsion of the testis accounts for 30%, and epididymo-orchitis, idiopathic and other causes comprise the remaining 10%). Vestigial remnants to the testis or the epididymis are present in 90% of the male population.[1] Torsion of a testicular appendage has a similar presentation to that of torsion of the testis but is less severe (see FIG. 111.1).

Torsion of a testicular appendage can be diagnosed by the appearance of a dark blue nodule at the upper pole of the testis called the 'blue dot sign'(provided that it is not masked by an associated hydrocele).[3] Surgical exploration may be needed to distinguish this from torsion of the testis.

Scrotal pain at various ages

Acute epididymo-orchitis

Apart from mumps, acute epididymo-orchitis is usually caused by sexually transmitted pathogens, notably *Chlamydia trachomatis* (in particular), *Mycoplasma genitalium* and *Gonococcus*, in sexually active young males and by urinary tract pathogens in older males. In older men, it usually follows urinary tract obstruction and infection or instrumentation of the lower genitourinary tract.

Investigations

Blood cell count:	leucocytosis
Urine microscopy and culture:	pyuria, bacteria and possibly *Escherichia coli* a sterile culture suggests the possibility of a chlamydial or gonorrhoeal infection[4]
NAAT/PCR:	*Chlamydia, Gonococcus, Mycoplasm genitalium*
Swabs of discharge:	*Gonococcus* (in particular)
Ultrasound:	can differentiate a swollen epididymis from a testicular tumour

Treatment

- Bed rest
- Elevation and support of the scrotum
- Analgesics
- Antibiotics[4]

Sexually active men should be treated empirically for chlamydial or gonorrhoeal infection:

use ceftriaxone 500 mg (in 2 mL of 1% lignocaine) IM (or 500 mg IV) as a single dose
plus
azithromycin 1 g (o) as a single dose
plus either
another dose of 1 g azithromycin a week later, or
doxycycline 100 mg bd for 14 days

Associated with urinary infection:

trimethoprim 300 mg (o) daily (child 4 mg/kg) for 14 days
or
cephalexin 500 mg (child 12.5 mg/kg) (o) 12-hourly for 14 days
or
amoxycillin/clavulanate 500/125 mg (child 12.5/3.1 mg/kg) (o) 12-hourly for 14 days
or (if resistance to above suspected or proven)
norfloxacin 400 mg (child 10 mg/kg up to 400 mg) (o) 12-hourly for 14 days

If severe infection, administer parenteral gentamicin + ampicillin followed by norflaxin.[5]

Orchitis

Acute orchitis is invariably due to mumps and occurs during late adolescence. Mumps orchitis has become relatively rare with vaccination. It is usually unilateral (see FIG. 111.3) but may be bilateral.

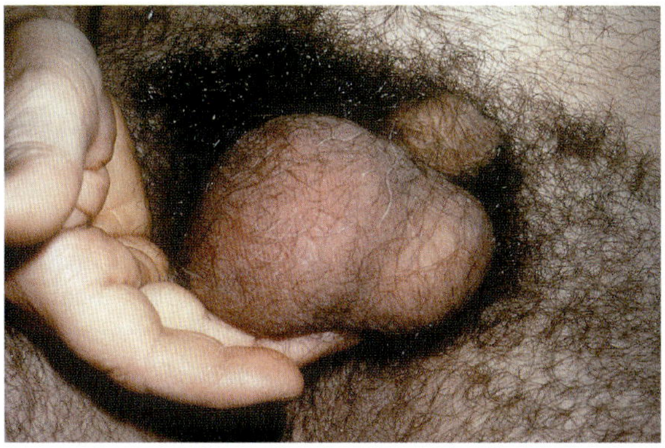

FIGURE 111.3 Mumps orchitis with a swollen, tender testicle

Testicular neoplasm

Testicular tumours can occur at all ages but are more common in young men aged 20–30 years (teratoma) and 25–40 years (seminoma). Sometimes they can mimic an acute inflammatory swelling and present with acute pain. See CHAPTER 112.

Strangulated inguinoscrotal hernia

It is possible that a supposed testicular torsion may be found to be a strangulated inguinoscrotal hernia, usually an indirect inguinal hernia extending into the scrotum. It can be detected by careful palpation of the base (neck) of the scrotum, feeling for a cough impulse and being unable to 'get above' the swelling.

Trauma and haematoceles

A diffuse haematoma into the scrotum that causes no significant problems can follow surgery to the inguinal area, a blow to this area or a fracture of the pelvis. These conditions cause extravasation of blood distally.

However, a haematocele of the tunica vaginalis can be either acute or an 'old clotted haematocele' following injury, such as a blow to the testis, or the drainage of a hydrocele. Sometimes it can arise spontaneously. All types of haematoceles require surgical exploration to exclude testicular rupture or a tumour.

Trauma to the scrotum may produce urethral injury and extravasation of urine into the scrotum. This problem requires urgent surgery.

Problems of scrotal skin

Sebaceous cysts are common and may be infected and require drainage. Less commonly, idiopathic scrotal oedema can present, usually in boys aged 5–10 years. With this condition, scrotal swelling and mild redness and tenderness begin gradually and spread, often across the midline and also possibly beyond the scrotum. Palpation reveals normal, non-tender testes but torsion needs to be excluded in some instances of the swollen red scrotum. Idiopathic scrotal oedema is believed to be allergic in origin, either localised (e.g. insect bite) or globalised as part of urticaria. It sometimes results from exposure to cold water. There may be a tender enlarged draining inguinal lymph node near the external ring.[1] Treatment includes scrotal support, analgesics and antihistamines.

Referred pain

Pain can be referred to the scrotal region from ureteric colic and quite commonly from disorders of the thoracolumbar spine, notably a disc disruption at the T12–L1 level involving the L1 nerve root. The pain therefore may be referred or radicular. In elderly men, referred pain can arise (uncommonly) from a ruptured abdominal aortic aneurysm or acute aortic dissection.

When to refer

- Any suspicion of torsion of the testis
- Sudden onset of acute scrotal pain at any age
- A history of recurrent transient testicular pain in a young man
- Presence of a tender testicular lump
- Presence of a haematocele surrounding the testis

Note: Referral should be urgent, given the critical importance of time in testicular survival.

Practice tips

- Acute scrotal pain in infancy and adolescence should be regarded as torsion of the testis until proved otherwise.
- A history of recurrent transient pain (with or without swelling of the testis) in a young person means recurrent torsion. Urgent referral is essential.
- A pitfall is the phenomenon of 'testis redux' in which the descended testis undergoes torsion, is pulled into the superficial inguinal pouch by the cremasteric reflex and then becomes fixed by oedema. Always check both testes are present in the scrotum in boys and young men with inguinal pain.
- The development of an acute hydrocele should be regarded with suspicion.
- Beware of the strangulated inguinoscrotal hernia presenting as a testicular torsion.
- Consider dissecting aneurysm in an older person presenting with testicular pain.

References

1. Hutson J, O'Brien M, Woodward A et al. *Jones' Clinical Paediatric Surgery* (6th edn). Hoboken NJ: Blackwell Publishing, 2008: 172–8.
2. Ringdahl E, Teague L. Testicular torsion. Am Fam Physician, 2006; 74: 1739–43, 1746.
3. Davenport M. ABC of general surgery in children. Acute problems of the scrotum. BMJ, 1996; 312: 435–7.
4. Expert group for Antibiotic. Genital sexually transmitted infections. In: eTG complete [Internet]. Melbourne: Therapeutic Guidelines Ltd. Available from: <www.tg.org.au>, accessed October 2017.
5. Buckley N (Chair). *Australian Medicines Handbook*. Adelaide: Australian Medicines Handbook Pty Ltd, 2016: 101.

Inguinoscrotal lumps 112

He has a rupture, he has sprung a leake.

Ben Jonson (1573–1637), *The Staple of News*

Lumps in the groin are common to both sexes but males are likely to have a greater variety of swellings in this area and several may be associated with scrotal lumps.

Lumps in the groin

The commonest swellings encountered in the groin or inguinal area are hernias and enlarged lymph nodes. The diagnosis of a hernia is usually straightforward but it must be differentiated from other swellings, including Malgaigne bulgings—these are not true hernias but diffuse swellings in both inguinal regions seen in people with poor lower abdominal musculature.[1] TABLE 112.1 lists the differential diagnoses of groin lumps.

Table 112.1 Differential diagnoses of a groin mass

Hernia—femoral, inguinal
Malgaigne bulgings
Lipoma
Undescended testis (incomplete)
Spermatic cord swelling—encysted hydrocele, lipoma
Lymph node—localised, generalised
Haematoma (post femoral artery puncture)
Neoplasm—lipoma, others
Psoas abscess
Spermatocele
Vascular anomalies: • saphenous varix • femoral aneurysm

Hernias

The commonest types of hernias in the groin are inguinal, femoral and a combination of the two. Rare hernias in the region are obturator, Spigelian (low abdominal), preperitoneal inguinal and prevascular femoral. The basic parts of a hernia are shown in FIGURE 112.1 and important anatomical landmarks in FIGURE 112.2. An indirect inguinal hernia is a hernia emerging through the deep inguinal ring, originating lateral to the inferior epigastric vessels, following the path of the spermatic cord, and which can traverse the whole length of the inguinal canal (see FIG. 112.3). It may also pass through the superficial inguinal ring into the scrotum—an inguinoscrotal hernia.

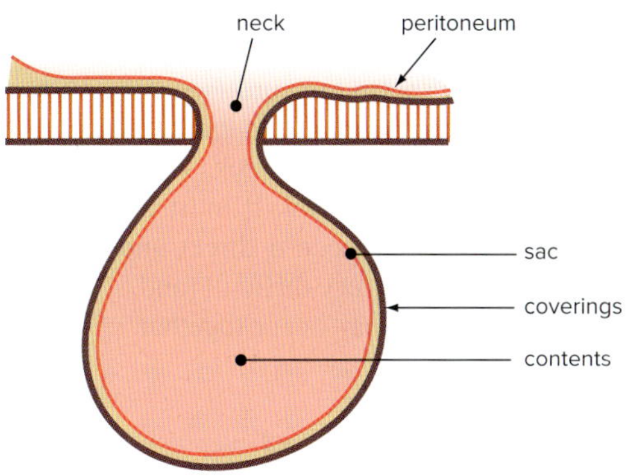

FIGURE 112.1 Basic components of a hernia

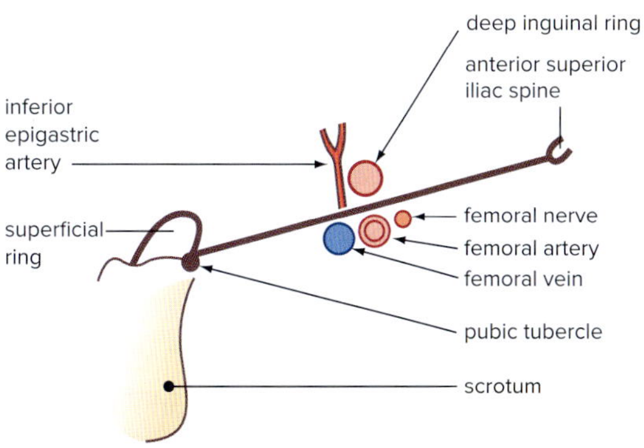

FIGURE 112.2 Key landmarks in the left inguinal region: the deep inguinal ring lies above the mid-inguinal point (between the ASIS and the pubic tubercle); the femoral artery lies below this point

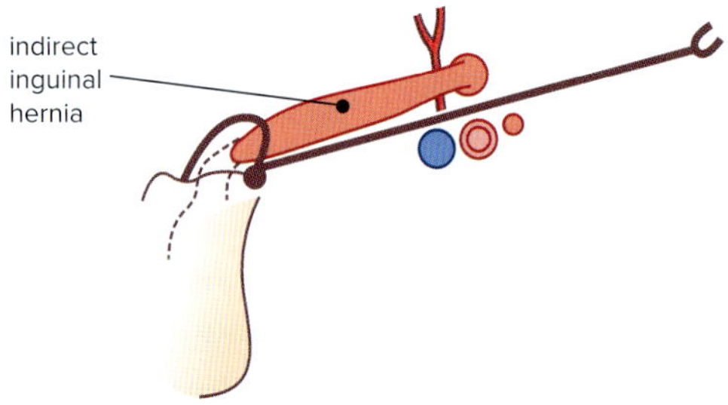

FIGURE 112.3 Left indirect inguinal hernia: it emerges lateral to the inferior epigastric artery and passes into the scrotum medial to the pubic tubercle

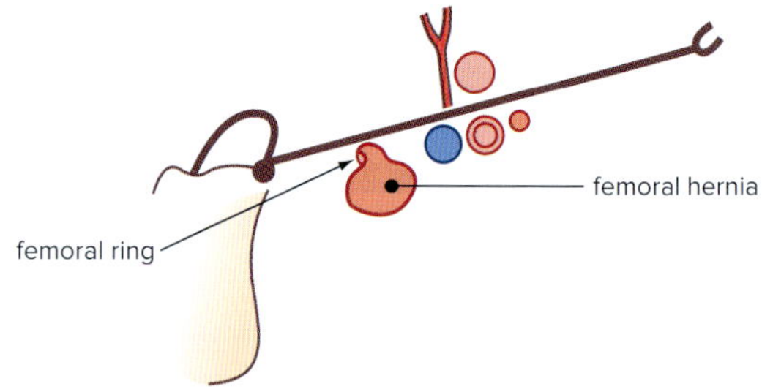

FIGURE 112.5 Left femoral hernia: its neck is lateral to the pubic tubercle and it lies below the inguinal ligament

Because of their narrow neck and oblique path in the inguinal canal, such hernias are often irreducible and can occasionally lead to strangulation of entrapped bowel.

A direct inguinal hernia originates medial to the inferior epigastric vessels and protrudes through the posterior wall of the inguinal canal, and is therefore separate from the spermatic cord (see FIG. 112.4). It is almost always seen in men and rarely descends into the scrotum. Due to a wider neck, strangulation and obstruction are most unusual. It must be emphasised that the distinction between a direct and an indirect inguinal hernia can be very difficult (and of no clinical benefit)[1] and the two may occur together.

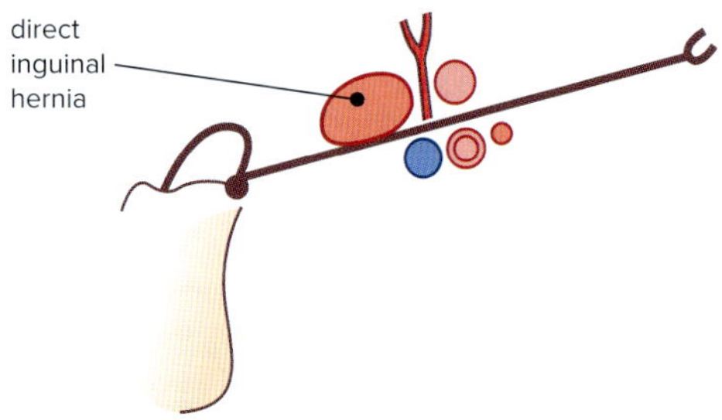

FIGURE 112.4 Left direct inguinal hernia: it emerges medial to the inferior epigastric artery and bulges forward

A femoral hernia herniates through the femoral ring (also known as the femoral canal), which is the medial component of the femoral sheath. The hernia tends to bulge forward and then upwards as it becomes larger. The neck is lateral to the pubic tubercle (see FIG. 112.5).

Femoral hernias are often small, usually occur in females and may be unnoticed by the patient. They are particularly liable to produce bowel obstruction or strangulation.

Guidelines

Acquired hernia

- Always examine the scrotum and both sides
- Frequently bilateral
- Result from muscular weakness
- Commonest—direct inguinal
- Predisposing factors:
  - age (more common with increasing age)
  - obesity
  - pregnancy
- Precipitating factors (related to above factors):
  - increased intra-abdominal pressure:
  - difficulty of micturition
  - straining at stool (constipation)
  - chronic cough (e.g. bronchitis)
  - straining or lifting heavy objects
  - nerve damage (e.g. post appendicectomy)
- Complications:
  - intestinal obstruction (see TABLE 112.2)
  - incarceration
  - strangulation
  - sliding

Table 112.2 Symptoms and signs of hernial obstruction
Colicky abdominal pain
Nausea and vomiting
Constipation and failure to pass flatus
Abdominal distension
High-pitched tinkling bowel sounds
Local tenderness and swelling of the hernia
No expansile cough impulse

Clinical features

The main symptoms and signs:

- lump
- discomfort or pain:
  - a dragging pain
  - worse after standing or walking
  - referred to testicle (indirect inguinal)
- testicular pain—referred or with compression of the spermatic cord
- expansile impulse on coughing

Note:

- A femoral hernia is easily missed in obese patients.
- Larger femoral hernias are often irreducible.
- Always attempt reduction in the recumbent position (direct hernias usually reduce easily).

Treatment

Surgery

All symptomatic hernias require repair. Those patients who are not symptomatic (a third of patients with hernias)[1] and who are medically fit should also be offered surgery. This is not so much because of the risk of strangulation (which is rare) but because most patients usually become symptomatic eventually and a watch-and-wait approach delays rather than prevents surgery.[2] Obstructed and strangulated hernias require urgent surgery. The risk of strangulation is greatest with femoral hernias, occasional with indirect inguinal hernias and very rare with direct inguinal hernias.

While generally a very safe procedure, inguinal hernia surgery complications include bruising, numbness, haematoma, infection (1–7%), recurrence and chronic pain (defined as persisting for >3 months after surgery). Chronic pain is the most serious long-term complication of hernia repair and may persist for several years. It may be severe in up to 3% of patients[1] and can require referral to pain clinics or further surgery. Laparoscopic repair is now a popular surgical option with less severe postoperative pain.[3] An increase in infertility risk and testicular atrophy on the side of the surgery has been noted but is not common.

Most patients return to work after hernia repairs in around 7 days, or 14 days for those doing strenuous work.[1]

Conservative

Asymptomatic inguinal hernias in patients with associated medical conditions, and who pose a significant operative risk, such as the frail elderly patient, can be treated with a watch-and-wait approach. Trusses have been used since ancient times to help patients with hernias, but can be difficult for a patient to manage and cannot be recommended as a definitive form of treatment.[4]

HERNIAS IN CHILDREN[5]

The most common hernias in infants are inguinal hernias and umbilical hernias.

Umbilical hernias

Clinical features

- Soft, round, skin-coloured lump in umbilicus, occurring in around 15% of infants.[6]
- May increase in size in first few months
- Not painful, not tender to palpate, easily reducible
- Swelling disappears when child asleep
- Usually gradually disappears
- Most disappear by age of 12 months[6]
- Larger ones usually disappear by age of 4 years[6]
- Consider hypothyroidism

Management

- Explanation and reassurance
- No treatment required
- Do not tape or strap (may cause strangulation and does not help)
- Refer for repair if still present at age 4 years

Inguinal hernia

Clinical features

- More common in premature infants and boys
- Present with groin lumps—may be intermittent sightings (e.g. when crying)
- May cause intermittent pain or discomfort
- If irreducible, consider possibility of strangulation

Note: Bowel strangulation is a possibility.

Management

Rules for surgical intervention:

- general rule is ASAP, especially in infants and for irreducible ones
- reducible herniae—the '6–2' rule:
  - birth–6 weeks: surgery within 2 days
  - 6 weeks–6 months: surgery within 2 weeks
  - over 6 months: surgery within 2 months

Scrotal lumps

The scrotum contains the testes and distal parts of the spermatic cords, covered by layers of fascia and the dartos muscle. The testes are invested with tunica vaginalis derived from the peritoneal cavity during their descent.[1]

Disorders of the scrotum may be acute or chronic and bilateral or unilateral. Lumps may be cystic, solid or otherwise, such as a varicocele, oedema or hernia. Solid lumps include a testicular tumour, epididymo-orchitis, and torsion of the testes. Cystic lumps include hydroceles, epididymal cysts and spermatoceles. A comparison of scrotal lumps appears in FIGURE 112.6 and TABLE 112.3. Lumps in the scrotum usually develop from deeper structures, particularly the testes and their coverings, rather than scrotal skin.

The cardinal sign of a true scrotal mass is that it is possible to palpate it from above (i.e. get above the lump) (see FIG. 112.7).

The patient usually presents with pain or a lump.

> A painless testicular lump is cancer until proven otherwise, but a testicular lump doesn't necessarily mean cancer.

Examination of the scrotum

The scrotum should be examined with the patient supine and then standing. The left testis usually hangs lower than the right. On inspection note any sebaceous cysts in the scrotal skin (common); scabies if there are very pruritic nodules; and scrotal oedema, which causes taut pitting skin. Careful palpation will elicit the relevant structures in the scrotum. Gently palpate each testis and epididymis between the thumb and the first two fingers. The spermatic cord is palpable as it enters the scrotum after passing through the superficial ring and the testis and epididymis are readily palpable.

After palpation, test for translucency of any swelling in a darkened room by shining the beam of a strong torch from behind the scrotum through the swelling. Transilluminable swellings that light up with a red glow (referred to as a 'Chinese lantern sign') include hydroceles and cysts of the epididymis. Swellings that contain blood or other tissue, such as testicular tumours and most hernias, do not transilluminate.

Unilateral scrotal swelling

It is important to determine whether the lump is inguinoscrotal or scrotal. It is scrotal if it is possible to get above the lump. If it is not possible to get above the

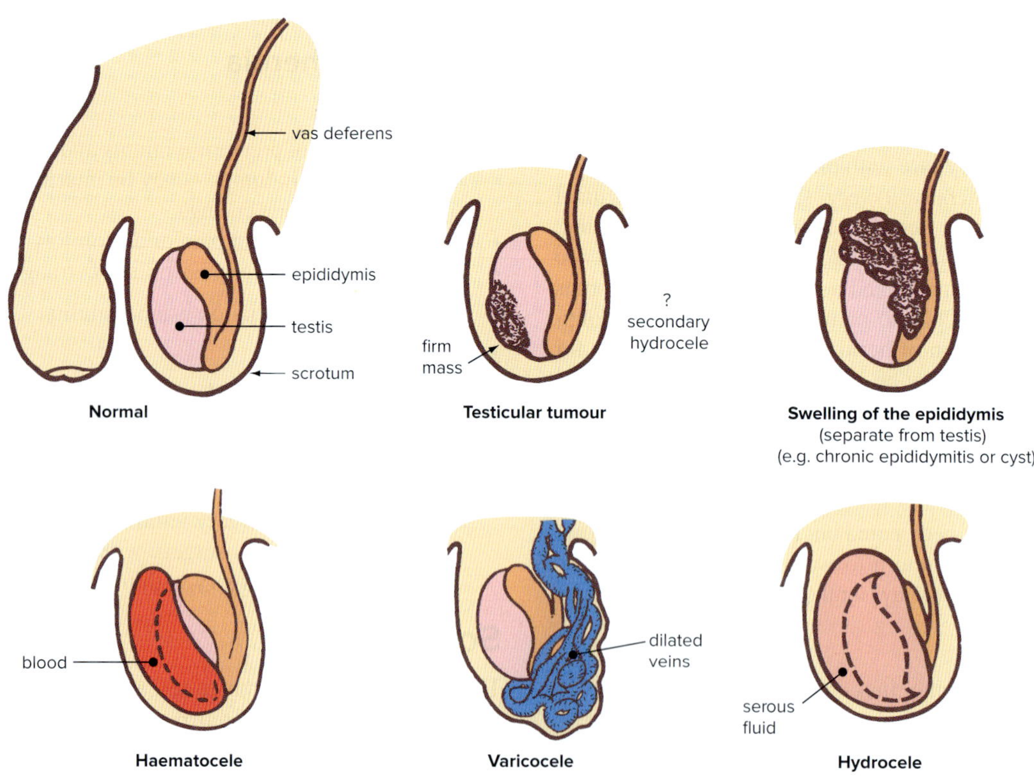

FIGURE 112.6 Basic comparison of scrotal lumps

Table 112.3 Features of scrotal lumps

	Possible clinical setting	Position	Palpation	Trans-illumination
Hydrocele	Any age Primary or secondary: • tumour • infection • torsion	Confined to scrotum Anterior: surrounds testis except posteriorly	Smooth, pear-shaped Lax or tense Testis impalpable, non-tender	Yes
Cyst of epididymis Epididymal cysts and spermatoceles clinically similar	Asymptomatic or dragging sensation	Behind and above testis	Smooth and tense Multilocular swelling Testis easily palpable Appears separate from testis	Yes
Chronic epididymo-orchitis	Non-specific Tuberculosis *Chlamydia* (Occasional associated small hydrocele)	Behind and above testis	Firm swelling Hard and craggy Normal testis	No
Varicocele	Dragging discomfort	Usually left-sided Along line of spermatic cord Above testis	Soft, like bunch of worms or grapes Collapses when patient supine and testis elevated Testis often smaller	No
Cancer	Young men 20–40 Painless lump Loss of testicular sensation	In body of testis Usually felt anteriorly May be hydrocele	Enlarged firm testis Feels heavy if large Normal epididymis (palpable)	No

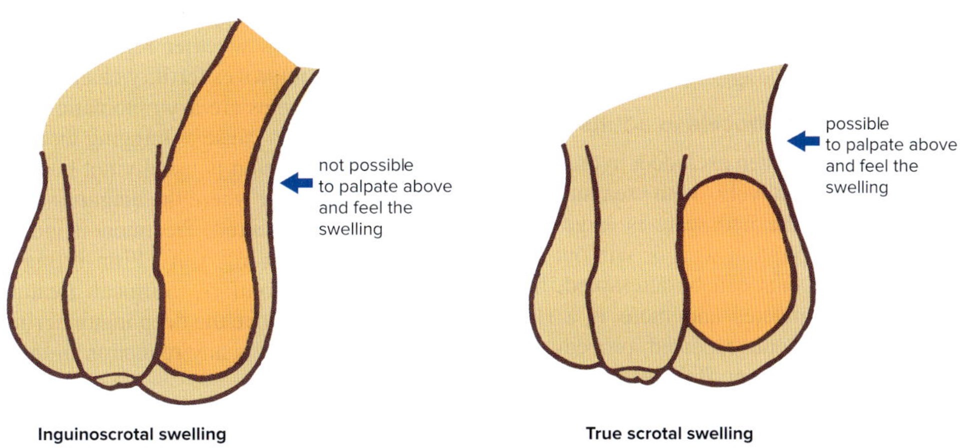

FIGURE 112.7 Difference between a true scrotal swelling and an inguinoscrotal swelling

lump then it is a large inguinal hernia or a combined hernia and hydrocele (see FIG. 112.7). This palpation should be coordinated with the cough impulse. The next feature to determine is whether the testis and/or epididymis can be palpated or whether they are obscured by a swelling.[5]

Small testes

Normal testicular size in children and adolescents is 4–14 mL or 15–35 mL in adults (this can be assessed with an orchidometer).[7,8] Length measurement is 3.5–7.5 cm in adults (average 5 cm). Small, firm testes less than 10 mL are a feature of Klinefelter syndrome.

Small soft testes indicate atrophy, which may follow mumps orchitis, oestrogen therapy, androgen deficiency or anti-androgen therapy, hypopituitarism, cirrhosis and other related conditions.

Hydrocele

A hydrocele is a collection of clear amber fluid in the tunica vaginalis and can be primary or secondary. If a hydrocele develops it is important to rule out intrascrotal disease, such as a tumour or infection. Ultrasound examination of the scrotum is helpful in assessing the state of the testis in the presence of a hydrocele. Hydroceles may be symptomless or cause dragging discomfort in the scrotum and groin.

Hydrocele in the neonate[5,9]

Hydroceles present at birth are communicating (failed closure of the processus vaginalis) or (less commonly) non-communicating, where the tunica vaginalis contains fluid, which can sometimes be loculated or cystic. Transillumination will prove that it is cystic but if the diagnosis is in doubt perform an ultrasound. Hydroceles may vary in size from day to day and can appear quite large. They do not extend proximal to the external inguinal ring so it is possible to palpate above them. There is no impulse on crying or straining. Of the 5% of those born with a hydrocele, most will resolve spontaneously within 12 months. If the hydrocele is very large or persists beyond 12 months, surgical intervention should be considered. However, surgery is the most effective long-term treatment.

Treatment of a primary hydrocele in adults

If underlying pathology has been excluded, hydroceles can be managed conservatively with reassurance and scrotal support.[10] If the hydrocele is large and uncomfortable, simple aspiration with or without the injection of sclerosing agents can be attempted, but the fluid usually reaccumulates and there is a risk of bleeding or infection with repeated procedures. However, aspiration can prevent fluid accumulation and after two or three times can often cure the problem. This sclerotherapy may be complicated by pain and inflammatory reaction to the sclerosant. Surgery is generally considered a second-line procedure after observation with or without aspiration. However surgery is the most effective long-term treatment.

> **Practice tip**
>
> Consider testicular cancer in a young man presenting with a hydrocele. Perform an ultrasound examination.

Encysted hydrocele of the cord

This is a localised fluid-filled segment of the processus vaginalis within the spermatic cord. It is palpable as a cystic lump in the upper scrotum above the testis. It characteristically moves down with traction on the testis. Treatment is not usually needed.

Epididymal cysts

These are common, often multiple, and are usually found in middle-aged/elderly men. The majority of epididymal cysts are about the size of a pea and contain a clear colourless fluid. If the cysts communicate with the vasa efferentia, a spermatocele filled with whitish fluid containing spermatozoa may form.

Epididymal cysts may be asymptomatic or they may cause discomfort and cosmetic embarrassment and if so can be excised. Fertility may be impaired in patients undergoing bilateral cyst excision.

Aspiration and injection of sclerosant agents can also be used for epididymal cysts.

Varicoceles

A varicocele is a varicosity of the veins of the pampiniform plexus (see FIG. 112.6). It is seen in 8–10% of normal males and occurs on the left side in 98% of affected patients, due to a mechanical problem in drainage of the left kidney vein. A relationship with infertility has been observed but its nature is controversial, as is whether repairing varicoceles in subfertile men improves fertility chances.[10]

Most varicoceles are asymptomatic and incidental findings. They can cause a dragging discomfort in the scrotum. Investigation is usually not necessary but an ultrasound is useful where the diagnosis is doubtful or a neoplasm is suspected. Treatment is indicated if it is symptomatic or for infertility. Firm-fitting underpants may relieve discomfort. Surgical treatment is by venous ligation, above the deep inguinal ring. Ligation is indicated if there is any reduction in the size of the left testis.

Haematoceles

These can be either acute, resulting from trauma such as a fall astride, sports injury or tapping of a hydrocele, or chronic, where there is no obvious history of injury. Haematoceles are anterior to the testis and not transilluminable. Surgical drainage is required with acute injury where there is a possibility of testicular rupture (associated urethral injury has to be considered); and a tumour has to be excluded with the chronic type. Pressure atrophy of the testis can occur with injury and is much more common if early drainage is not instigated.

Sperm granulomas

- Firm tender lumps
- Post-vasectomy—at cut end of vas

Treatment

- Leave to resolve.
- Consider NSAIDs.
- Refer for excision if symptomatic and enlarging.

Fordyce spots

These are harmless ectopic sebaceous glands 1–3 mm in diameter that appear as small raised lumps or spots of various colours (mainly red) on the shaft of the penis (Tyson's glands) or scrotum. They can be mistaken for genital warts. They are best left, but if unacceptable they can be treated with electrodissection or pulsed dye lasers or a micro-punch technique.

Testicular tumours[11,12]

A mass that is part of the testis, and solid, is likely to be a cancer. Malignant testicular tumours account for about 1–1.5% of malignant tumours in men. They mainly affect fit young men and represent the commonest cancer in men aged 15–40 years in Australia (see TABLE 112.4). Some 90–95% of testicular tumours arise from the germ cells, and for practical purposes are classified into:

- seminomas 40%
- non-seminoma germ cell tumours (NSGCT) 60%

Table 112.4 Testicular tumours

Tumour	Incidence (%)	Peak incidence (years)
Seminoma	40	25–40
Teratoma	32	20–35
Mixed seminoma/ teratoma	14	20–40
Lymphoma	7	60+
Other tumours (e.g. interstitial—Leydig, gonadoblastoma)	uncommon	variable

Clinical features

- Young men aged 15–40 years (NSGCTs peak in the third decade of life, seminomas peak in the fourth decade)
- Most common presentation is a painless lump in the body of one testis (only 1–2% present with bilateral tumours)
- Up to a quarter of men have pain at presentation
- Loss of testicular sensation
- Associated presentations (may mask tumour):
  - hydrocele
  - varicocele
  - epididymo-orchitis
  - swollen testis with trivial injury
  - gynaecomastia (teratoma)
  - back and flank pain

Risk factors

Those at high risk include those men with:

- cryptorchidism/orchidopexy (testicular dysgenesis syndrome)
- previous testicular cancer
- family history of testicular cancer (brother/father)
- Klinefelter syndrome
- infertility

Golden rules

- All solid scrotal lumps are malignant until proved otherwise and must be surgically explored.
- Beware of hydroceles in young adults.
- Tumours can mimic acute epididymo-orchitis—the so-called 'inflammatory' or 'flash fire' presentation.

If a man has a testicular lump he should visit his GP and have ultrasound screening and baseline tumour markers. If it is cancer, he should:

- be treated in a specialist centre
- undergo careful staging
- have an orchidectomy and adjunct therapy

Metastases

Testicular tumours spread by direct infiltration via the lymphatics, including retroperitoneal lymph nodes, and the bloodstream. Metastases typically occur in the para-aortic nodes and so may not be detected by abdominal palpation. They are best detected by a CT scan of the abdomen and chest. Metastases also occur in the neck, brain, liver, chest and bones.

Investigations

Investigations to aid diagnosis include:

- ultrasound of the testis should always be done as it can detect and diagnose with considerable precision underlying testicular lumps plus any invasion of the tunica

- tumour markers: α-fetoprotein and β-hCG—indicates teratomas
- lactic dehydrogenase may be elevated

Investigations for staging include:

- chest X-ray
- CT scanning of abdomen, pelvis and chest for node involvement (any spread is usually direct to the para-aortic nodes)
- lactate dehydrogenase—monitors secondary spread and indicates tumour mass

Note: Avoid scrotal needling biopsy because of the potential risk of tumour implantation in the scrotal wall. Avoid scrotal incisions for surgery.

Treatment

The initial treatment is orchidectomy through an inguinal incision with inguinal division of the spermatic cord. Further treatment then depends on the type and staging of the tumour. Early seminomas are given radiation to the ipsilateral lymph nodes or a single dose of chemotherapy. Early NSGCTs undergo active surveillance (tumour markers, CXR, CT scans) but no further treatment. More advanced disease may have further chemotherapy or radiotherapy. The results for NSGCTs in general are not as satisfactory as for seminoma, though prognosis is good for both, with current 5-year relative survival rates of 99% for localised disease (majority of presentations), 96% for regional disease and 74% for distant disease.[13] A comparison of the testicular tumours is summarised in TABLE 112.5.

Surgery should not affect the remaining testis but production of motile and functional sperm may be reduced. However, sperm production can be temporarily or permanently reduced following radiotherapy and chemotherapy. Pretreatment sperm storage may be discussed with the patient, and the psychological implications of testicular cancer need to be carefully monitored. A testicular prosthesis is an option. The GP may also play a role in coordinating appropriate active surveillance investigations.

Screening and testicular self-examination

Studies of testicular cancer have shown the benefits of early detection. However, studies to date indicate that there is insufficient evidence to screen routinely for testicular cancer in asymptomatic patients. It is recommended for those at high risk. This screening includes colour Doppler ultrasound and tumour markers. Evidence also indicates that, to date, there is little evidence to show that those performing testicular self-examination are more likely to detect early stage tumours or have better survival than those who do not.[14]

112

Table 112.5 Comparison of the common testicular cancers

	Seminoma	Non-seminoma (NSGCT)
Typical age	30–40 years	20–30 years
Incidence	40%	60%
Growth rate	Slow	Rapid
Nature	Solid	Mixed—solid + cystic
Stage at presentation	90%—stage 1	60%—stage 1
Tumour markers:		
α-FP	Never	Common
β-hCG	Occasional	Common
Treatment	Inguinal orchidectomy + radiotherapy	Stage 1: orchidectomy Relapse: chemotherapy
Sensitive to chemotherapy	+ + +	+ + +
Sensitive to radiotherapy	+ + +	±

Undescended testes (cryptorchidism)[15]

An undescended testis is one that fails to reach the bottom of the scrotum by 3 months of age despite manual manipulation. It has stopped in the normal path of descent and can occupy the intra-abdominal, inguinal canal, emergent (just outside the external ring), high scrotal and mid-scrotal positions (see FIG. 112.8). The cause of maldescent is most probably mechanical.

After the indirect inguinal hernia, it is the most common problem in paediatric surgery. The incidence at birth is 3–4%, but this falls to 1% in the first 3 months of life as testicular descent can continue, though further descent after 3 months is rare. More than two-thirds of undescended testes are located in the superficial inguinal pouch; that is, they are palpable in the groin.

The testis is usually normal at birth but may become secondarily dysplastic if left outside the scrotum.

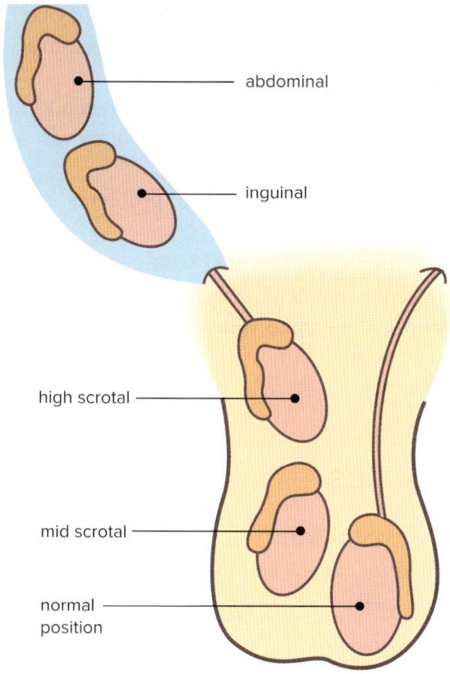

FIGURE 112.8 Undescended testis: arrested in the line of descent

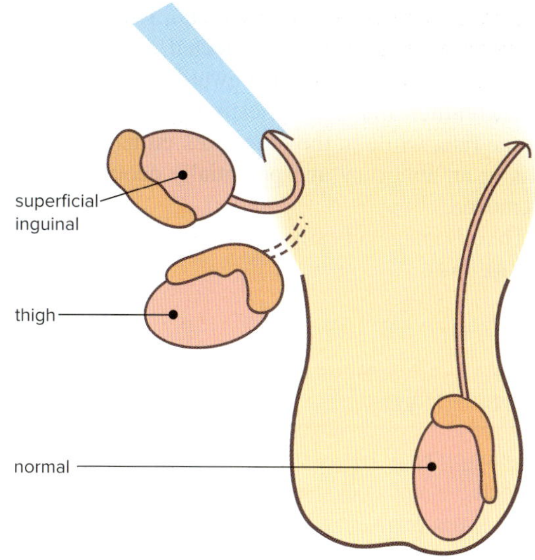

FIGURE 112.9 Undescended testis: ectopic

Retractile testis

A retractile testis is one that can be manipulated into the scrotum irrespective of the position in which it is first located. It is a common condition and requires no further investigation or treatment. The testis can be present in the scrotum under circumstances such as a warm bath but retracted out of the scrotum when cold. Cremasteric contraction is absent in the first few months after birth and is maximal between 2 and 8 years.

Ectopic testis

An ectopic testis is one that has left the normal path of descent and cannot be manipulated into the scrotum. It can be found in the perineum, upper thigh (femoral), base of the penis (prepubic), anterior abdominal wall or in the superficial inguinal pouch (see FIG. 112.9). True ectopic testes form only about 2.5% of all undescended testes.

Ascending testis

An 'ascending' testis is one that was in the scrotum in infancy but subsequently moved back to the groin because the spermatic cord failed to elongate at the same rate of body growth.

Examination[12]

The examination of the testes should take place in a warm room and relaxed environment. Begin by placing one finger on each side of the neck of the scrotum to prevent a retractile testis from being retracted when palpation is commenced with the other hand. The scrotum is then carefully palpated for a testis. If impalpable the fingertips of one hand are placed just medial to the anterior superior iliac spine and moved firmly towards the pubic tubercle where the other hand waits to entrap the testis should it appear. The diagnosis then depends on carefully determining the range of movement.

> **Practice tip**
>
> If the testis is not palpable at birth, review in 3 months. Refer for specialist evaluation if it still cannot be palpated.

The problem of non-descent

- Testicular dysgenesis and dysplasia
- Susceptible to direct trauma (if in inguinal region)
- Risk of malignant change (seminoma) is 5–10 times greater than normal

Optimal time for surgery

The optimal time for orchidopexy is 6–12 months of age. It is considered to be satisfactory as long as the testis is in the scrotum by 2 years. The production of spermatozoa is adversely affected in undescended testes from the age of 2 years onwards. Exploration for the uncommon impalpable testis is worthwhile: 50% salvage rate, while in the other 50% either there is no testis or an abnormal and potentially neoplastic testis is removed.

The advantages of early orchidopexy are summarised in TABLE 112.6.

Table 112.6	Advantages of early orchidopexy (1 year)
Provides optimal chance of fertility	
Corrects indirect inguinal hernias (coexists in 90%)	
Reduces risk of trauma	
Reduces risk of torsion	
Reduces psychological consequences	
Probably lessens the risk of malignancy (seminoma)	

Hormone injections

Injections of chorionic gonadotrophic hormones are generally not recommended. They are ineffective except for cases of borderline retractile testes.

Vasectomy

Dangerous features (caution required)

- Unmarried
- Young <35 years old
- No children
- Emotional crisis
- Spouse not involved

Postoperative

- Avoid strenuous activity and sex for 4–7 days.
- Use alternative contraception until negative semen analysis.
- First semen analysis at 3 months.
- Inform not immediately infertile.
- Need to ejaculate 20 times.

Complications[16]

- Postoperative bleeding and haematoma 4–22%
- Wound infection <1.5%
- Ongoing pain—around 10%, usually mild but can be severe
- Formation of sperm antibodies ~50%. May be a problem if subsequently requests vasectomy reversal
- Failure rate 1–2:1000 (can be from tubes not fully tied off, growing back together or a third vas deferens existing)
- Psychological and psychosexual problems

Other facts

- No difference in ejaculate appearance (sperm makes up 1% ejaculate volume) or sex drive
- No known association with prostate and testicular cancers

Practice tips

Inguinoscrotal lumps

General rules for optimal times for surgical repair in children:

- inguinal hernia—ASAP
- umbilical hernia—aged 4 years (most resolve)
- femoral hernia—ASAP
- undescended testes—6 to 12–18 months
- hydrocele—after 12 months if still large; most resolve
- varicocele—leave and review

Patient education resources

Hand-out sheets from *Murtagh's Patient Education* 7th edition:

- Hernia, inguinal
- Scrotal lumps
- Testicle: undescended
- Testicular cancer
- Testicular self-examination

References

1 Jenkins J, O'Dwyer P. Inguinal hernias. BMJ, 2008; 336: 269–72.

2 Fitzgibbons R Jr et al. The development of a clinical trial to determine if watchful waiting is an acceptable alternative to routine herniorraphy for patients with minimal or no hernia symptoms. J Am Coll Surg, 2003; 196: 737–42.

3 Memon M et al. Meta-analysis of randomised clinical trials comparing open and laparoscopic inguinal hernia repair. Br J Surg, 2003; 90: 1479–82.

4 Kingsnorth A, LeBlanc K. Hernias: inguinal and incisional. Lancet, 2003; 362: 1561–71.

5 Hutson J et al. *Jones' Clinical Paediatric Surgery* (6th edn). Hoboken NJ: Blackwell Publishing, 2008: 172–8.

6 Zendejas B, Kuchena A, Onkendi EO et al. Fifty-three-year experience with pediatric umbilical hernia repairs. J Pediatr Sur, 2011; 46 (11): 2151–6.

7 Andrology Australia. *Childhood and Adolescence Clinical Summary Guide 2. Examination of Male Genitals and Secondary Sexual Characteristics,* May 2010 <www.andrologyaustralia.org/wp-content/uploads/clinical-summary-guide02_May2010.pdf> (accessed 8/3/2014).

8 Andrology Australia. *Adulthood Clinical Summary Guide 3. Examination of Male Genitals and Secondary Sexual Characteristics,* May 2010 <www.andrologyaustralia.org/wp-content/uploads/clinical-summary-guide-03.pdf> (accessed 8/3/2014).

9 International Pediatric Endosurgery Group. *IPEG Guidelines for Inguinal Hernia and Hydrocele,* November 2009 <www.ipeg.org/hernia/> (accessed 8/3/2014).

10 Kroese A et al. Surgery or embolization for varicoceles in subfertile men. Cochrane Database. Syst Rev. 2012, Issue 10. Art No. CD000479.

11 Andrology Australia. *Clinical Summary Guide 6. Testicular Cancer, Diagnosis and Management,* May 2010 <www.andrologyaustralia.org/wp-content/uploads/clinical-summary-guide06_May2010.pdf> (accessed 8/3/2014).

12 European Association of Urology. *Guidelines on Testicular Cancer,* 2012 <www.uroweb.org/guideline/testicular-cancer/> (accessed 8/3/2014).

13 National Cancer Institute. Surveillance, Epidemiology, and End Results (SEER) Program, updated June 2013 <www.seer.cancer.gov/statfacts/html/testis.html> (accessed 8/3/2014).

14 Royal Australian College of General Practitioners, 2016. *The Guidelines for Preventive Activities in General Practice* (9th edn) <www.racgp.org.au/your-practice/guidelines/redbook/> (accessed 22/11/2017).

15 Hutson J et al. *Jones' Clinical Paediatric Surgery* (6th edn). Hoboken NJ: Blackwell Publishing, 2008: 168–71.

16 European Association of Urology. *Guidelines on Vasectomy,* 2012 <www.uroweb.org/gls/pdf/2012%20EAU%20Guidelines%20on%20Vasectomy%2061%20159.pdf> (accessed 8/3/2014).

113 Disorders of the penis

Ironically there is no organ about which more misinformation has been perpetuated than the penis.

William Masters & Virginia Johnson, *Human Sexual Response* (1970)

The most common penile disorders are those of psychosexual dysfunction and STIs, but there are many other problems and these are most often related to the foreskin.

DISORDERS AFFECTING THE FORESKIN AND GLANS

Phimosis

Phimosis is tightness of the foreskin (prepuce), preventing its free retraction over the glans penis. The foreskin is normally attached to the glans and is non-retractile in most newborns; it may remain so until puberty.[1,2] The proportion of boys with retractile foreskins is: 40% at 1 year, 90% at 4 years and 99% at 15 years.[3] Forceful retraction of the penis should be avoided until spontaneous separation occurs.[1] Once the foreskin easily retracts, the boy should learn to do this as part of normal washing, ensuring he rinses off any soap and pushes the foreskin back over the glans afterwards.[4]

'True' phimosis is caused by forceful retraction, infection or balanitis xerotica obliterans (see later in this chapter).[1,2] Indicators of true phimosis (rather than simple non-retractile foreskin) are:[3]

- foreskin not retractile by the time of established puberty
- previously retractile foreskin becomes non-retractile
- obvious ring of scar tissue at foreskin opening
- inability to visualise the urethral meatus when foreskin opening is lifted away from glans
- ballooning during and after micturition, with pinhole foreskin opening and a squirting urinary stream (though mild ballooning during micturition is common and normal)

Treatment

Inflammatory phimosis can be treated by local corticosteroid cream (e.g. 0.05% betamethasone valerate cream qid for 2–4 weeks)[3] applied generously to the tight, shiny part of the foreskin where the inner skin meets the outer skin. If the tip of the foreskin is inflamed, gently retracting it will cause the inflamed opening to 'cauliflower' up so the cream can be applied. A stronger steroid cream can be tried if this fails.

True scarring that fails to respond to steroid creams may require circumcision, though this is uncommon.[1,2] Some patients with true phimosis may have problems once they start to have intercourse and will require circumcision.

Paraphimosis

Paraphimosis occurs when a tight foreskin is forcibly retracted over the glans, gets stuck in the sulcus and cannot be pulled forward again. The glans and the foreskin distal to the tight area become swollen and painful (see FIG. 113.1) and this demands urgent resolution.[1] This problem occurs in boys aged 8–12 and the elderly, especially if a mild degree of phimosis is already present. Typically it occurs when the penis is erect or after catheterisation.

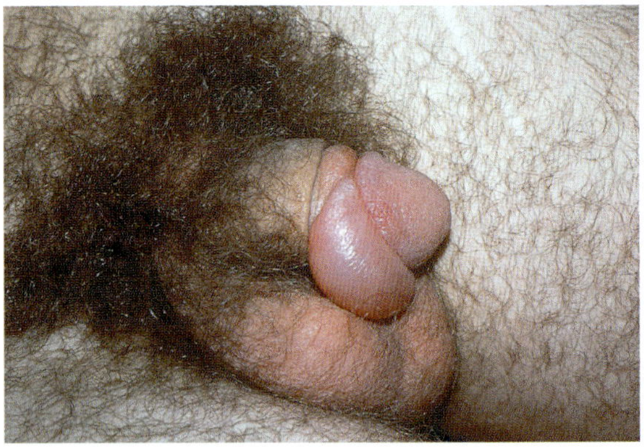

FIGURE 113.1 Paraphimosis showing retracted, swollen, oedematous foreskin

Management

Paraphimosis can usually be corrected without surgery, and urgent manual reduction should be attempted first.[3] It is usually performed without anaesthesia but a penile block (remembering never to use adrenaline in LA), systemic analgesia ± sedation or a generous application of 2% lignocaine gel or EMLA cream may be appropriate depending on the geographic location and the clinical circumstances. Local anaesthetic infiltration before manual reduction should be avoided as it increases the swelling.

Note: Do not apply ice.

Method 1: Squeeze and manual reduction A

The glans penis and oedematous tissue distal to the constricting ring of foreskin are gently squeezed for several minutes to reduce the oedema. Using a lubricating jelly, manual reduction can then be performed by trying to advance the prepuce over the glans with the index fingers while gently compressing the glans with both thumbs (see FIG. 113.2).

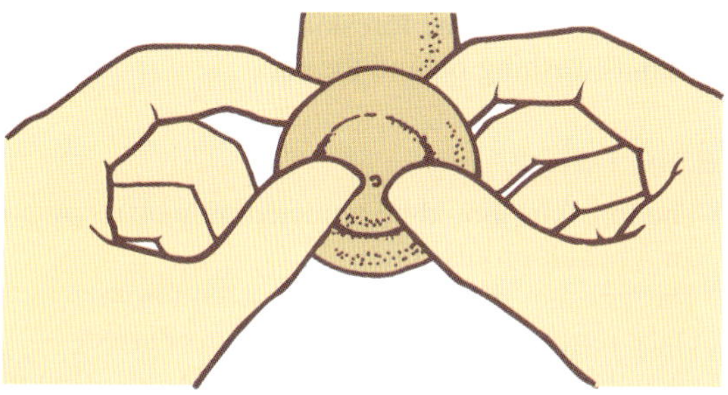

FIGURE 113.2 Acute paraphimosis: method of manual reduction

Method 2: Squeeze and manual reduction B

- Take hold of the oedematous part of the glans in the fist of one hand and squeeze firmly. A gauze swab or cool towelette will help to achieve a firm grip (see FIG. 113.3).

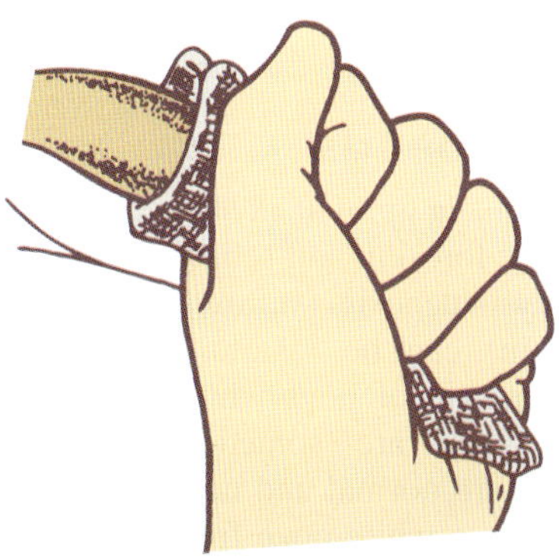

FIGURE 113.3 Acute paraphimosis: squeezing with a swab method

- Exert continuous pressure until the oedema passes under the constricting collar to the shaft of the penis.
- The foreskin can then usually be pulled over the glans.

Note: If these simpler methods are successful, educate the patient about proper foreskin management as this may prevent further attacks.

Method 3: Dorsal slit

Immediate referral is necessary if manual reduction methods fail. As an emergency, a dorsal slit incision can be made in the constricting collar of skin under local or general anaesthetic (see FIG. 113.4). The incision allows the foreskin to be advanced and reduces the swelling. Circumcision can be considered some days later when the inflammation has settled and any phimosis assessed, but a single episode of paraphimosis is not an absolute indication for circumcision.[3]

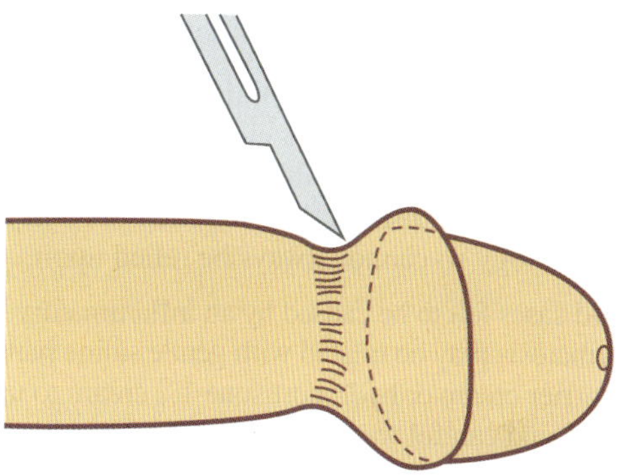

FIGURE 113.4 Acute paraphimosis: dorsal slit incision in the constricting collar of skin

Method 4: The Dundee puncture method[5]

Under a ring block local anaesthetic or general anaesthetic, make approximately 20 puncture holes in the oedematous prepuce with a 26 gauge needle (outer diameter 0.45 mm). Then, using firm but gentle pressure, express fluid from the foreskin until it is decompressed. Consider subsequent circumcision.

Balanitis (balanoposthitis)

Balanitis is inflammation of the glans; inflammation of the foreskin is called posthitis and the combination is balanoposthitis, though balanitis is the most commonly used term. Urine trapped under the foreskin converts into ammonia compounds, and an ammoniacal dermatitis (similar to that of nappy rash) causes inflammation. Other causes of inflammation include

113

irritation by soaps and other environmental substances, and trauma such as sexual activity. This inflamed area can become infected with commensal bacteria or fungi leading to infection.[1] Balanitis is common, affecting 6% of uncircumcised and 3% of circumcised males.[3]

Balanitis is actually a collection of disparate conditions with similar clinical presentation and varying aetiologies affecting a particular anatomical site.[6,7] These include:

- infections—*Candida* (the most common cause), *Streptococcus pyogenes* (uncommon but very severe), anaerobes, staphylococci, *Gardnerella*, herpes simplex
- inflammatory dermatoses—lichen sclerosis, lichen planus, psoriasis, Zoon balanitis, eczema (including irritant, allergic and seborrhoeic)
- premalignant—Bowen disease, Bowenoid papulosis, erythroplasia of Queyrat

Men presenting with balanitis should be considered for predisposing conditions such as diabetes or HIV.

Treatment

Treatment will be dependent on the cause, which will in turn be determined by the clinical picture, patient risk factors and potential culture results. Cultures can be useful, but may also pick up commensals unrelated to the aetiology so cannot always be relied upon.

- Mild cases felt to be caused by an inflammatory dermatosis may be treated with gentle saline bathing, a barrier cream or hydrocortisone 1% cream to tip of penis, and careful washing behind the foreskin.
- If there is a purulent discharge, take swabs for culture.
- Candidal balanitis is suggested by blotchy erythema with small papules that may be eroded, or dry, dull, red areas with a glazed appearance, and associated soreness ± itch.

If yeasts present:

- topical hydrocortisone + an imidazole (e.g. miconazole or clotrimazole) cream

If trichomonads present:

- metronidazole or tinidazole (oral treatment)

If bacterial infection is suspected:

- topical antibiotic ointments under the foreskin using a narrow, longish nozzle (e.g. chloramphenicol)
- severe cases caused by bacterial infection may have purulent discharge with spreading cellulitis down the penile shaft and require oral or intravenous antibiotics

Balanitis xerotica obliterans (BXO)

Thickening of the foreskin with skin pallor suggests balanitis xerotica obliterans. There is white, thickened scarring, giving an 'icing sugar' appearance to the glans. It results in progressive phimosis, typically in late childhood, usually 10–12 years. It may respond to corticosteroid cream if it is mild, but circumcision is usually indicated.

Foreskin hygiene

The normal foreskin in infants and children does not need special care and should be retracted for cleaning only after spontaneous separation of the foreskin has occurred. After this, males can practise proper hygiene by gently retracting the foreskin and washing the area as often as washing behind the ears.

Basic rules

- The foreskin should be retracted only by its owner (or a health professional)
- The foreskin should not be retracted forcibly
- Once retraction has spontaneously occurred, encourage daily retraction and gentle cleansing in the bath or shower

Instructions to patients

- During a shower or bath slide the foreskin back towards your body (see FIG. 113.5).
- Wash the end of the penis and foreskin with soap and water and then rinse off.
- After washing the area, dry the end of your penis and foreskin and then replace the foreskin.
- If the foreskin has a tendency to become irritated and smelly, slide the foreskin back sufficiently to allow free urination.

Smegma pearls

Smegma is made up of shed skin cells from the inner aspect of the foreskin and sebaceous gland excretion. Smegma cysts/deposits (yellow–white lumps beneath the foreskin) can be visible or palpable through the thin foreskin of boys whose foreskins have not retracted. They are sometimes called 'smegma pearls', and are normal and need no treatment. They can discharge a white ooze from under the foreskin. They can also be mistaken for sebaceous cysts and may cause concern for the boy or his parents, who can be reassured all is well.[1]

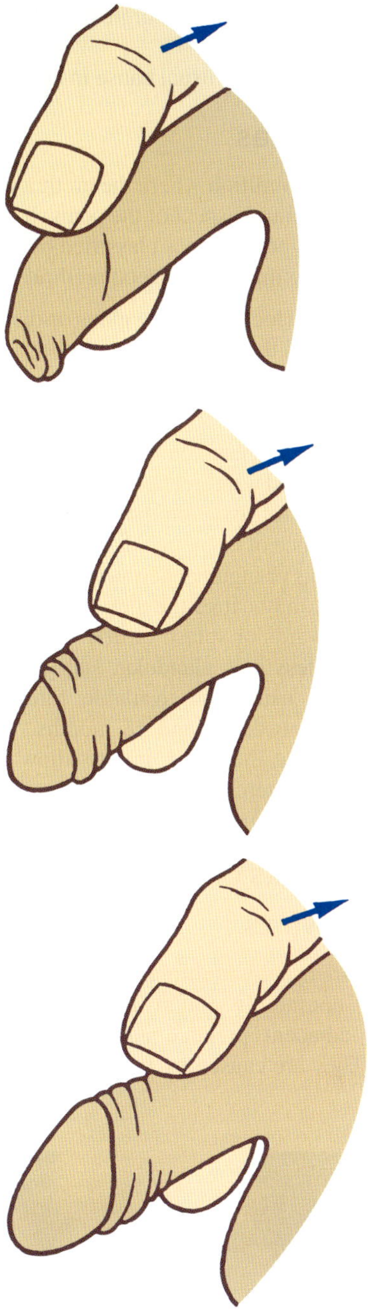

FIGURE 113.5 Foreskin hygiene: sliding foreskin back for washing

Circumcision

Circumcision is now performed in 10–20% of Australian males after peaking at 85% in the 1950s.[7] True phimosis not resolving with steroid creams, paraphimosis, recurrent balanitis, BXO or boys at high risk of UTIs are potential medical indications for circumcision. However, improved personal hygiene and better management of some of these conditions has led to a reduced medical need for circumcision. Apart from these situations and circumcision for religious reasons, circumcision for social reasons is generally discouraged. A policy statement from the Paediatric and Child Health Division of the RACP recommends against routine infant circumcision.[8]

Circumcision is generally a safe procedure but there are risks of minor complications and some rare but serious complications. In newborns, because of their small blood volume, any bleeding is of major concern and blood loss over 25 mL can be life-threatening.[1] A bleeding circumcision site can be the presentation of a coagulopathy disorder.[3] Also, because of a newborn's relatively poor immunity, septicaemia from coliform infection on the wound site is a risk. If circumcision is done, it is recommended that it be done after 6 months of age and ideally in an operating theatre under general anaesthetic and with careful surgical technique.[1]

Arguments for routine circumcision include a reduction in risk of UTIs (and their complications) in infancy, reduction of sexually transmitted infections (including HIV) and a possible reduction in the risk of penile cancer in men and cervical cancer in their female partners later in life.

Circumcision reduces the risk of UTIs by about 10-fold.[9] However, because of the low baseline risk, 111 circumcisions would be required to avoid one UTI in boys without abnormal urinary tracts.[8] The reduction in STIs including HIV has been shown to be a benefit in males in high-risk populations (such as men in Africa), but this benefit has not been consistently evident in studies in lower-risk populations such as Australia and New Zealand. While there have been some studies showing that circumcision provides a protective benefit against HPV transmission and subsequent cervical cancer risk, the introduction of HPV vaccination is likely to dramatically reduce the baseline risk of these conditions. Cancer of the penis is so rare that the overall benefit offered by circumcision would be very small, and is overshadowed by recent improved penile hygiene in men and management of phimosis. In summary, the RACP guidelines conclude the benefits do not warrant the risks in routine circumstances, but that it is reasonable for parents to weigh up the risks and benefits (after being fully informed), and to make the decision themselves with parental choice being respected.

Complications of circumcision:

- bleeding
- infection (local/septicaemia)

113

- ulceration of glans/meatus
- meatal stenosis
- penile deformity

Absolute contraindications:

- hypospadias and other congenital abnormalities (the foreskin may be a vital source of skin for subsequent repair)
- chordee (painful dorsolateral curvature of the penis during erection, which interferes with sexual intercourse)
- 'buried' penis
- sick, 'unstable' infants
- family history of bleeding
- inadequate experience of proceduralist

Frenuloplasty

A congenitally tight frenulum may lead to a tear during intercourse. Repeated bleeding occurs. Division of the frenulum and suturing in the opposite direction is preferable to circumcision.

The 'buried' penis

In the 'buried' penis syndrome (also known as the 'concealed' or 'inconspicuous' penis) the penis is not adequately exposed and looks small. There is failure of skin fixation at the base of the penis with possible excessive prepubic fat pad at the base. It is commonly seen in small children, especially chubby boys, and can cause parental concern. Manually pressing down the fat pad at the base of the penis back towards the pubic bone will allow a more reliable assessment of penile length (and often reassure the parents). This situation usually improves spontaneously over time. In adolescents and adults, a buried penis is usually associated with obesity and rarely can require surgical intervention for cosmetic or functional reasons.[10]

DISORDERS AFFECTING THE URETHRAL MEATUS

Meatal stenosis

Meatal stenosis or stricture may be congenital or acquired. It may be acquired in the circumcised child due to abrasion and ulceration of the tip of the glans. The incidence can be reduced by the application of moisturising cream for 2 weeks on the glans after circumcision.[1] Uncommon causes are direct trauma during circumcision and irritation from ammoniacal dermatitis. Meatal ulceration predisposes to meatal stenosis. It usually presents as pain during micturition or as slight bleeding on the nappy or underpants. Significant stenosis requires surgical correction by meatotomy.

Catheter trauma is the usual cause in adults.

Hypospadias

Hypospadias is a condition where the urethra opens on the underside or ventral aspect of the penis. It occurs in 1 in 350 males. Hypospadias is classified based on the location of the proximally displaced urethral orifice:[2]

- distal–anterior (located on the glans or distal shaft of the penis and the most common type)
- intermediate–middle (penile)
- proximal–posterior (penoscrotal, scrotal, perineal)

There is often associated chordee (a ventral bending of the penis associated with erection) due to a 'bowstring' effect from the lack of tissue on the ventral surface, and also a high incidence of cryptorchidism (10%) and open processes vaginalis or inguinal hernia (9–15%).[2]

Hypospadias may cause the stream of urine to be deflected downwards or splash or drip back along the penile shaft. Unless it is glandular, surgical repair is usually advised, using the available foreskin, and is usually done between 6 and 18 months.[2] Chordee may be corrected at the same time to allow eventual successful sexual intercourse. These boys should not undergo routine circumcision.

OTHER DISORDERS OF THE PENIS

Penile warts

Penile warts are usually multiple fleshy, papillomatous outgrowths, commonly found around the coronal sulcus, the adjacent prepuce and the meatus (see FIG. 113.6). They are caused by human papillomavirus

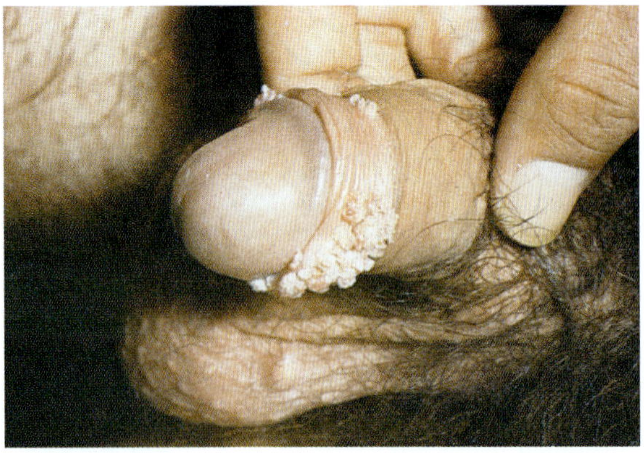

FIGURE 113.6 Penile (genital) warts caused by the human papillomavirus

and usually transmitted sexually. Look for warts within the meatus by allowing gentle dilation of the distal urethra with mosquito forceps.

Treatment is aimed at reducing any pain, bleeding, itch or embarrassment. Treatment options include:[11]

- no treatment
- self-applied treatments at home
- treatment at the surgery or a clinic

The following treatments[12] can be used with or without periodic cryotherapy:

- imiquimod 5% cream topically applied to each lesion, 3 times per week at bedtime (wash off after 6–10 hours) until the warts disappear (usually 8–16 weeks)
- podophyllotoxin 0.15% cream or 0.5% paint topically applied to each wart, twice daily for 3 days followed by a 4-day break, then repeat weekly for 4–6 cycles until the warts disappear

Pearly penile papules

These are very small, regular round lumps (actually angiofibromas) that appear on the corona of the glans of the penis (see FIG. 113.7). They are common and are often first noticed by adolescent males who should be reassured that they are normal variants. They are not premalignant and require no treatment.[13]

Fordyce spots of the penis: refer to CHAPTER 112.

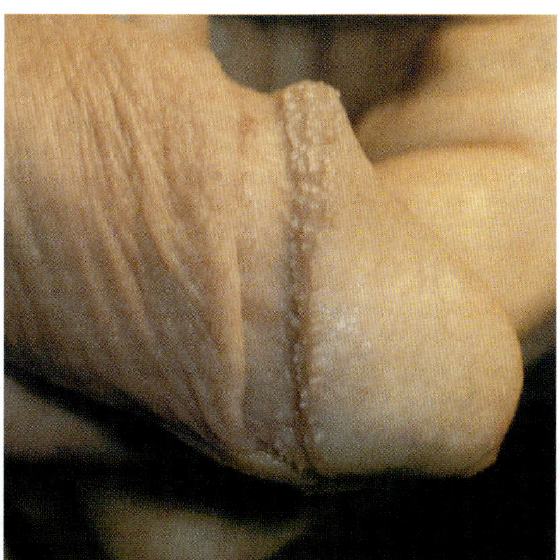

FIGURE 113.7 Pearly penile papules

Penile ulcers

A common cause of penile ulcers is trauma, related to sexual activity, to the frenulum if it is congenitally tight. Such traumatic ulcers may be slow to heal and the frenulum may need surgical division. The ulcers may resemble a venereal ulcer (e.g. syphilitic chancre or herpes simplex). Another important (although rare) cause is cancer of the penis. Various causes are listed in TABLE 113.1.

Table 113.1 Causes of penile lesions

Non-ulcerative
Balanitis:
• *Candida albicans*
• diabetes mellitus
• poor hygiene
Skin disease:
• psoriasis
• lichen planus
Fordyce spots
Venereal warts
Ulcerative
Trauma (tender)
Cancer (non-tender)
Herpes simplex (tender)
Syphilis (non-tender)
Chancroid (tender)
Granuloma inguinale (donovanosis)

Cancer of the penis

Cancer of the penis is rare, occurring in fewer than 1 in 100 000 of the male population,[14] though it can be much more common in the developing world. Some 95% of penile cancers are squamous cell carcinomas. Phimosis, smoking, multiple sexual partners and poor hygiene are the main risk factors for penile cancer.[15] There is an association with being uncircumcised and HPV infection, particularly types 16, 18 and 31.[14]

Cancer usually starts as a nodular warty growth (or ulcer) on the glans penis or in the coronal sulcus.[15] Initially it may resemble a venereal wart. Fungal balanoposthitis can be misdiagnosed as cancer. The presenting symptom may be a bloodstained or foul-smelling discharge as the lesion can be hidden by the foreskin. It is usually seen in elderly patients with poor hygiene. Associated lymphadenopathy, which is present in 50% of patients on presentation, may be infective or neoplastic. Metastases to distal sites are uncommon. Refer for management, which includes radiotherapy—usually effective.

Priapism[16]

Priapism is a persistent penile erection that continues hours beyond, or is unrelated to, sexual stimulation. It may follow penile injection. Typically, the corpora cavernosa are engorged but the corpus spongiosum and glans remain flaccid. It is a medical emergency, as it often leads to fibrosis of the cavernosal tissue and subsequent erectile dysfunction or impotence.

Subtypes of priapism include:

- Ischaemic (veno-occlusive or low flow)—this results from a failure of the detumescence mechanism (relaxation of the outflow of blood from the penis). The corpus cavernosa are rigid and tender to palpation, and the patient is in discomfort. It requires emergency treatment, and there can be subsequent penile oedema, ecchymoses and partial erections.
- Non-ischaemic (arterial or high flow)—this is from an unregulated cavernous arterial inflow. The penis is neither fully rigid nor painful. Trauma is often the cause. It does not require emergency treatment.
- Stuttering—this occurs from intermittent ischaemic priapism, and is manifested by repeated painful erections with intervening periods of detumescence. It may require emergency treatment if the events are prolonged, severe or frequent. Urologist consultation is advised.

The assessment focuses on distinguishing ischaemic from non-ischaemic. Apart from the clinical features mentioned above, cavernosal blood gases can confirm ischaemic priapism.

Duplex ultrasound can also be used, with ischaemic priapism showing little or no flow in the cavernosal arteries, and non-ischaemic showing normal to high blood flow. It can also demonstrate anatomical abnormalities such as a cavernous artery fistula in the perineum from trauma. A full blood count and film can also be part of the assessment, looking for abnormalities such as sickle cell disease, leukaemia, acute infections or platelet abnormalities. Drug screening can also be performed if suspected.

Emergency treatment for ischaemic priapism can include intracavernous injection of sympathomimetic agents such as phenylephrine as well as aspiration via a 19 or 21 gauge needle into the corpus cavernosum. If this fails, a surgical (cavernoglanular) shunt can be considered.

Peyronie disease[17]

Peyronie disease is a fibrotic process, sometimes associated with Dupuytren contracture, which affects the shaft of the penis and results in discomfort and deformity on erection. It may result from trauma while the penis is erect. It usually affects men between 45 and 60. Typically, the patient presents with painful 'crooked' erections. There is abnormal curvature of the erect penis. The penile deformity may prevent satisfactory vaginal penetration. On examination, a non-tender hard plaque may be palpable in the shaft of the penis at the point where the penis curves. Mild cases require reassurance. The problem may increase, remain static or spontaneously lessen over 1–2 years. If there is ongoing discomfort or sexual dysfunction that distresses the patient, surgical treatment by penile plication (a sutured tuck on the opposite side to straighten the deformity) may be warranted. In more severe deformities, incision and grafting of the scar or implants can be considered. Steroid injections are not recommended. Oral vitamin E has been used for treatment with unclear outcomes apart from one positive study.[18]

Chordee

Chordee is ventral or rotational curvature of the penis where the penile head usually curves upwards or downwards. It is a congenital abnormality usually caused by a ventral deficiency in the foreskin. It is usually detected soon after birth to about 18 months of age. It is often associated with hypospadias. The deformity is most apparent on erection. Early referral to a paediatric surgeon is advisable.

'Fractured' penis

A 'fractured' penis describes sudden rupture of the penile erectile tissue during intercourse, usually with a woman in the superior position, resulting in a snapping sensation with severe pain. The management is urgent urological consultation for possible surgical repair. The disruption can affect the corpus spongiosum (has a better prognosis) or the corpora cavernosa, which may be treated by drainage of the blood clot, in which case permanent erectile dysfunction is a possible complication.

Foreskin injury

Injuries to the penis are not uncommon and one is the entrapped foreskin in the trouser zipper, when attempts to free the zipper aggravate the problem. In the office, cut the zipper from the trousers (see FIG. 113.8) and

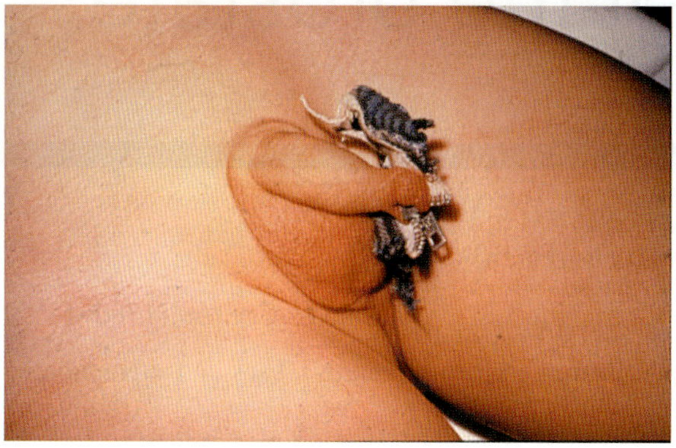

FIGURE 113.8 Entrapped foreskin in trouser zipper
Photo courtesy of Bryan Walpole

under local anaesthetic (no adrenaline), crush the zipper with pliers to open the teeth of the zipper and free the foreskin. Another method is to use a scalpel to cut the zipper immediately below the metal tag.

Erective dysfunction

Refer to CHAPTER 116.

Haematospermia

Haematospermia, which is blood in the semen, presents as a somewhat alarming symptom. It is sometimes encountered in young adults and middle-aged men. The initial step is to determine that the blood is actually in the semen and not arising from warts inside the urethral meatus or from the partner.

It usually occurs as an isolated event but can be secondary to urethral warts or prostatitis, or can occur with prostatomegaly or prostatic tumour (especially in elderly patients). If a micro-urine shows no accompanying haematuria, and prostate-specific antigen and blood pressure are normal, reassurance and a 6-week review are appropriate as spontaneous cessation of haematospermia is the rule.

Red flags for haematospermia

- Symptoms lasting longer than 4 weeks
- Palpable lesion in the prostate or along the epididymis
- Recent travel to schistosomiasis-prevalent region

Patient education resources

Hand-out sheets from *Murtagh's Patient Education* 7th edition:

- Circumcision

References

1 Hutson J et al. *Jones' Clinical Paediatric Surgery* (6th edn). Hoboken NJ: Blackwell Publishing, 2009; 179–83.

2 Tekgül S et al. European Society for Paediatric Urology. *Guidelines on Paediatric Urology,* 2013 <www.uroweb.org/wp-content/uploads/22-Paediatric-Urology_LR.pdf> (accessed 28/4/2014).

3 The Royal Children's Hospital, Melbourne. *Clinical Practice Guidelines: The Penis and Foreskin* <www.rch.org.au/clinicalguide/guideline_index/The_Penis_and_Foreskin> (accessed 28/4/2014).

4 The Royal Children's Hospital, Melbourne. Fact sheet: penis and foreskin care <www.rch.org.au/kidsinfo/fact_sheets/Penis_and_foreskin_care> (accessed 20/4/2017).

5 Hamdy FC, Hastie KH. Treatment for paraphimosis: the 'puncture' technique. Br J Surg, 1990; 77 (10): 1186.

6 Edwards S et al. 2012 European guideline for the management of balanoposthitis. First update of the original article. Int J STD AIDS, 2001; 12 (3): 68–72.

7 Melbourne Sexual Health Centre. *Guidelines: Clinical Management of Balanitis.* Melbourne: Bayside Health, 2009.

8 The Paediatrics & Child Health Division, The Royal Australian College of Physicians. Circumcision of infant males, 2010 <www.racp.edu.au/docs/default-source/advocacy-library/circumcision-of-infant-males.pdf> (accessed 20/11/2017).

9 Singh-Grewal D, Macdessi J, Craig J. Circumcision for the prevention of urinary tract infection in boys: a systematic review of randomised trials and observational studies. Arch Dis Child, 2005; 90 (8): 853–8.

10 King I et al. Buried penis: evaluation of outcomes in children and adults, modification of a unified treatment algorithm, and review of the literature. ISRN Urol, 2013; 2013: 109349 (published online 29 December 2013).

11 DermNet New Zealand Trust. Anogenital warts, 29 December 2013 <www.dermnetnz.org/viral/genital-warts.html> (accessed 22/11/2017).

12 Expert group for Antibiotic. Genital and sexually transmitted infections. In: eTG complete [Internet]. Melbourne: Therapeutic Guidelines Ltd. Available from: <www.tg.org.au>,accessed 25/11/2017.

13 DermNet New Zealand Trust. Pearly penile papules, 29 December 2013 <www.dermnetnz.org/site-age-specific/penile-papules.html> (accessed 24/11/2017).

14 American Cancer Society. Penile cancer, 6 February 2013 <www.cancer.org/cancer/penile-cancer.html> (accessed 1/4/2014).

15 Pizzocaro G et al. European Society for Paediatric Urology. *Guidelines on Penile Cancer,* 2010 <www.uroweb.org/wp-content/uploads/Penile-Cancer-2010.pdf> (accessed 1/4/2014).

16 American Urological Association. *Guideline on the Management of Priapism,* 2003 <www.auanet.org/education/guidelines/priapism.cfm> (accessed 6/4/2014).

17 Andrology Australia. Fact sheet: Peyronie's disease, August 2012 <www.andrologyaustralia.org/wp-content/uploads/Factsheet_Peyronies_2012Web2.pdf> (accessed 24/11/2017).

18 Paulis G et al. Efficacy of vitamin E in the conservative treatment of Peyronie's disease: legend or reality? A controlled study of 70 cases. Andrology, 2013; 1 (1): 120–8.

114 Disorders of the prostate

Mind and body, like man and wife, do not always agree to die together.

CHARLES COLTON (1780–1832)

The main function of the prostate gland is to aid in the nutrition of sperm and keep the sperm active. It does not produce any hormones so there is usually no alteration in sexual drive following prostatectomy.

Prostatitis

Prostatitis embraces a group of conditions with voiding discomfort and pain in the prostate referred to the perineum, low back, urethra and testes. It typically affects men aged 25–50 years. Prostatitis usually occurs in the absence of identifiable bacterial growth, when it is termed non-bacterial prostatitis. The prostate may develop acute or chronic bacterial infection. Acute bacterial prostatitis, while uncommon, can be life threatening if left untreated.[1]

Bacterial prostatitis is usually caused by urinary pathogens—*Escherichia coli* (commonest), *Enterococcus, Proteus, Klebsiella, Pseudomonas* or *Staphylococcus.* Rarely, chronic infections have been shown to be associated with *Chlamydia trachomatis.*[2]

Prostatodynia means the presence of symptoms typical of prostatitis but without objective evidence of inflammation or infection (see TABLE 114.1).

It is preferable to use the term 'prostatitis syndromes' to embrace the three terms used in TABLE 114.1.

Clinical features of acute bacterial prostatitis

Symptoms

- Fever, sweating, rigors
- Pain in perineum (mainly), back and suprapubic area
- Urinary frequency, urgency and dysuria
- Variable degrees of bladder outlet obstruction (BOO)
- ± Haematuria

Signs

- Fever
- Rectal examination: prostate exquisitely tender, swollen, firm, warm, indurated

DxT dysuria + fever + perineal pain → acute prostatitis

Complications

- Abscess
- Recurrence
- Epididymo-orchitis
- Acute retention
- Bacteraemia/septicaemia

Chronic bacterial prostatitis

Chronic bacterial prostatitis is diagnosed by a history of mild irritative voiding with perineal, scrotal and suprapubic pain. Ejaculatory pain can occur. The gland may be normal on clinical examination or tender and boggy. It should be suspected in men with recurrent UTI (see TABLE 114.2).

Table 114.1 Classification of prostatitis syndromes

	Prostatic pain	Prostatic rectal examination	Positive urine or prostate secretion culture	Positive prostatic secretion or urine white cells
Acute bacterial prostatitis	Yes	Very tender, swollen	Yes	Yes
Chronic bacterial prostatitis	Often	Normal or indurated	Occasionally	Low counts
Chronic prostatitis/chronic pelvic pain syndrome	Often	Normal	No	Nil or occasional

Table 114.2 Features of chronic bacterial prostatitis
Difficult to treat
Relapsing infection
Perineal pain
Some leucocytes in expressed prostatic secretions

Investigations

- Urine specimens and expressed prostatic secretions (EPS) obtained after prostatic massage can show excess white cells.
- Culture of the urine or ejaculate may be negative or give low counts.
- Prostatic stones (demonstrated by plain X-ray or transrectal ultrasound) may prevent successful treatment.
- Prostate-specific antigen (PSA): elevation occurs with inflammation and may cause confusion with cancer.

Treatment

Acute bacterial prostatitis[1]

For milder infection, oral treatment for 14 days with trimethoprim, cephalexin or amoxycillin/potassium clavulanate is suitable, as per treatment of cystitis. For more severe infections (as for pyelonephritis):

> amoxycillin (or ampicillin) 2 g IV 6-hourly
> *plus*
> gentamicin 4–6 mg/kg/day as a single daily dose until there is substantial improvement, when therapy may be changed to an appropriate oral agent, based on the sensitivity of the pathogen(s) isolated, for the remainder of 10–21 days, depending on clinical response.[2,3]

Urinary retention or abscess formation almost always requires endoscopic deroofing for drainage.

Chronic bacterial prostatitis

Treatment of chronic bacterial prostatitis is made difficult by uncertainty in differentiating it from non-bacterial prostatitis as cultures may grow low counts of what may be normal flora. Some 90–95% of cases of chronic prostatitis are not due to infection.[2] Avoid overtreatment with antibiotics and review regularly. Reassurance is important and it is worth suggesting frequent ejaculation and hot baths. Antibiotics should be used in patients who are culture positive with pus cells, based on culture susceptibility results. Regimes used include:[2]

> ciprofloxacin 500 mg (o) 12-hourly for 4 weeks
> *or*
> norfloxacin 400 mg (o) 12-hourly for 4 weeks
> *or*
> trimethoprim 300 mg (o) daily for 4 weeks

Chronic prostatitis/chronic pelvic pain sydrome[3]

This is the commonest and least-understood form. It is often recurrent and each episode can last several months. Recurrent antibiotic therapy is inappropriate.[2] Perform a thorough genitourinary tract investigation. The symptoms may reflect retrograde passage of urine into prostatic tissue with urate crystallisation. Management is targeted at symptom relief and can include NSAIDs, massage therapy and 5-alpha-reductase inhibitors (if BPH is present).[4] Alpha blockers, which have previously been recommended, are now considered ineffective based on a recent large randomised trial.[5] Emphasise good voiding habits. Avoid straining at the end of micturition. Encourage normal sexual activity and use stress management. Psychological counselling or a pain clinic referral may be appropriate in refractory cases.

Prostate pain syndrome is a symptomatic diagnosis, and a useful assessment tool to monitor the severity, progression and response to treatment is the International Prostate Symptom Score (IPSS).[6]

> **Practice tip**
>
> Consider bladder cancer if persistent dysuria.

Lower urinary tract symptoms (LUTS)

These symptoms can be grouped as voiding symptoms (obstructive) or storage symptoms (irritative).[7] Irritative symptoms may be caused by a bladder problem only. Obstructive symptoms are usually caused by the prostate (which can also cause irritative symptoms). The old term 'prostatism' is ill defined and best dropped.

Voiding (obstructive) symptoms

- Hesitancy
- Weak stream
- Postmicturition dribble or irregular stream
- Incomplete emptying/urinary retention
- Straining

Storage (irritative) symptoms

- Urgency
- Urge incontinence

- Frequency
- Nocturia
- Suprapubic pain

114

Bladder outlet obstruction (BOO)

Symptoms of BOO are present in most men after the age of 60 years. The commonest cause is benign prostatic hyperplasia (BPH). BPH is a histological diagnosis that, strictly, should not be used for symptoms. Only a minority of patients require surgery for relief of obstructive symptoms. Bladder outlet obstruction can also be caused by bladder neck obstruction and urethral sphincter spasm (see FIG. 114.1).

> **DxT** poor urine flow + straining to void + frequency → BOO

Clinical features of benign prostatic obstruction

- Hesitancy
- Frequency of micturition
- Urgency
- Nocturia
- Slow interrupted flow
- Terminal dribbling
- Acute retention
- Retention with overflow incontinence (less common)
- Haematuria from ruptured submucosal prostatic veins can occur
- Rectal examination usually detects an enlarged prostate

Note: Small prostate glands can also cause BOO.

The medical history should ideally include an International Prostate Symptom Score (IPSS).[8,9] The

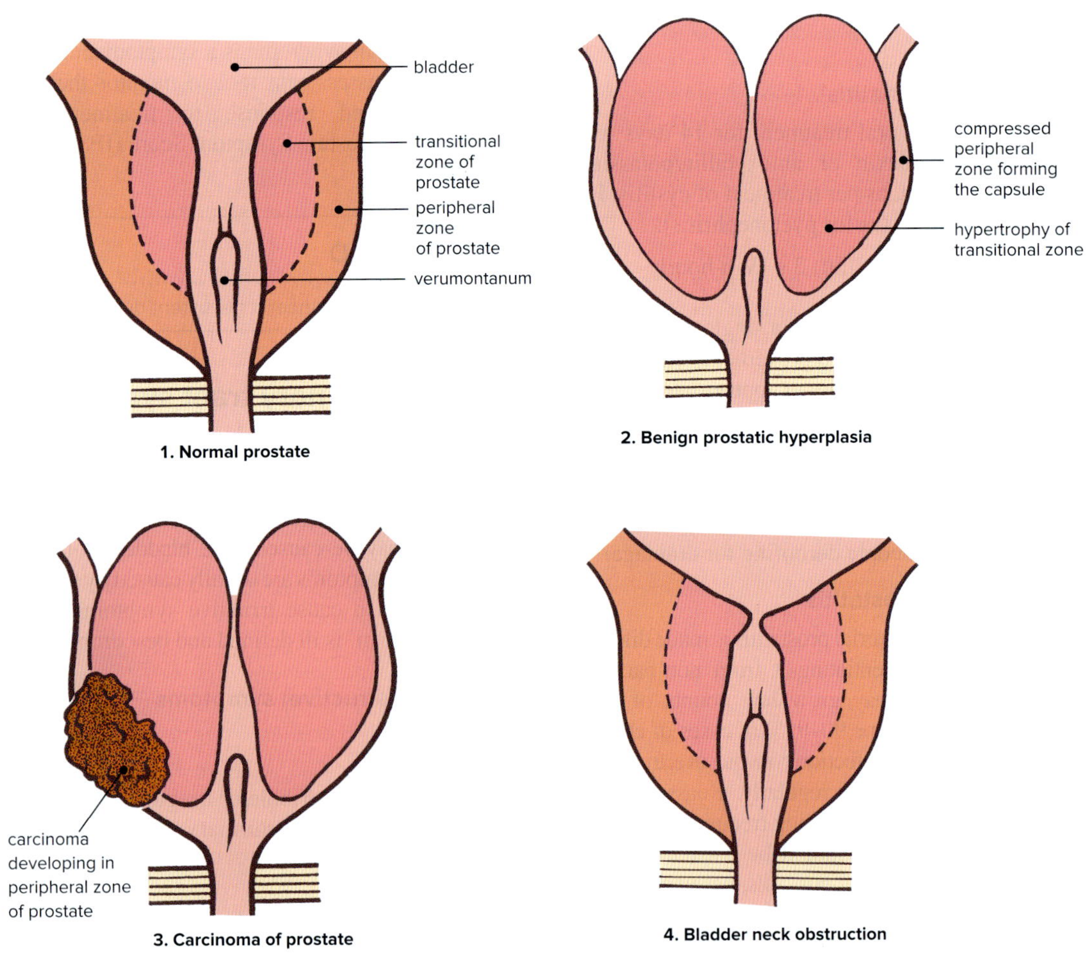

FIGURE 114.1 Diagrammatic comparison of bladder outlet obstruction

physical examination should include an abdominal examination, a digital rectal examination (DRE) and a genital examination.

Red flags for LUTS[5]

- haematuria
- incontinence, especially at night
- urinary retention
- recurrent urinary infection
- bladder calculus
- renal impairment
- hydronephrosis

Refer to a urologist.

Investigations

These include:

- midstream urine: microscopy, culture and sensitivity
- kidney function (urea, electrolytes and creatinine)
- PSA
- urinary ultrasound including a bladder residual volume
- voiding diary (frequency and volume measured for 2–3 days, and should be done in men with daytime frequency or who awaken two or more times a night to void)[7]
- urodynamic study
- urethrocystoscopy

When initial assessment demonstrates the patient having non-bothersome LUTS with or without non-suspicious prostate enlargement, and the patient does not want treatment, it is reasonable not to investigate further.[7] The patient can be reassured and reviewed as necessary. If there are bothersome LUTS, causes such as prostatic obstruction, overactive bladder or polyuria/nocturnal polyuria should be considered. Polyuria is defined as >3 L/24 hours, and nocturnal polyuria as being greater than a third of the 24-hour urine output.

If the initial assessment does reveal these or other concerns, such as an abnormal DRE/PSA, haematuria, recurrent UTI or palpable bladder, the patient should be referred to a urologist before treatment is advised.[7] Further investigations that may be organised by the urologist can include urine flow studies, cystoscopy, possibly an MRI and prostatic biopsy. A flow rate below 15 mL/s suggests obstruction and below 10 mL/s significant obstruction (see FIG. 114.2).

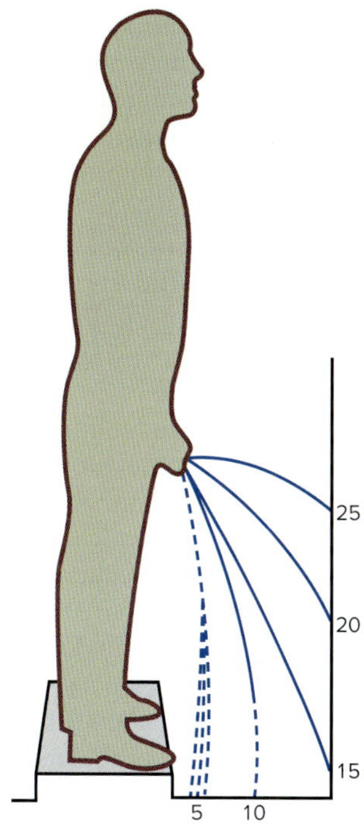

FIGURE 114.2 A visual scale of urinary flow. The numbers signify the flow rate in millilitres per second. When assessing a patient with voiding dysfunction, ask him to indicate which stream is closest to his own

Complications of prostatic obstruction

- Retention
- Urinary infection
- Bladder calculus formation
- Uraemia

Advice for patients with mild symptoms[10]

- Avoid certain drugs, especially OTC cough and cold preparations.
- Avoid or reduce caffeine and alcohol.
- Avoid highly seasoned or irritative foods.
- Avoid fluids before bedtime.
- Keep active/increase activity.

Treatment

Treatment options beyond basic management and watchful waiting (with yearly review) include medical management and surgical options.

Medical treatment

BOO patients with significant symptoms may be helped with alpha-adrenergic blocking drugs such as alfuzosin, tamsulosin, terazosin and prazosin

114

to inhibit contraction of the smooth muscle in the prostate and bladder neck. Typical doses are tamsulosin 0.4 mg daily and prazosin 0.5 mg bd, or 1 mg nocte after commencing with 0.5 mg nocte. Prazosin can be increased to a maximum of 2 mg bd. Symptoms are not improved by increasing beyond this dose. Side effects can include dizziness, and complications can occur in cataract surgery in men who have used alpha blockers, possibly due to an effect on the smooth muscle that dilates the iris (called the intra-operative floppy iris syndrome),[11] so caution needs to be used here.

The 5-alpha-reductase inhibitors (5-ARIs, e.g. finasteride, dutasteride) reduce prostatic volume by reducing testosterone conversion, and can be used in men with large prostates in association with LUTS. They are not as effective in reducing symptoms as the alpha blockers and can have sexually related side effects such as decreased libido and ejaculatory dysfunction. Urine flow improves by 3 months, plateauing at 6 months, but not to the same degree as with surgery. Two large recent studies support the combined use of alpha blockers and 5-ARIs in the medical management of BOO with large prostates.[12,13] Anticholinergic medication can also be used for symptoms caused by an overactive bladder.

Surgical management

The gold standard surgical treatment for obstruction remains transurethral resection of the prostate (TURP)[7] (see FIG. 114.3). Open prostatectomy accounts for less than 1% of benign prostatic surgery today. Surgery should be considered for men with moderate to severe symptoms who are keen on intervention and have had the risks and benefits of the procedure fully explained (including failure of relieving symptoms).

Many new surgical techniques are appearing as potential alternatives to TURP.[7] These include minimally invasive procedures that can be done as an outpatient such as transurethral needle ablation (TUNA) or transurethral incision of prostate (TUIP). These may have less risk of complications, but are not as effective at relieving symptoms as TURP and may lack sufficient durability of effect. They are sometimes considered as an option for men with anaesthetic risk or with smaller prostates. Other new surgical techniques such as Holmium laser ablation and laparoscopic and robotic prostatectomy show promise but lack robust long-term data to date. They are also dependent on operator experience and local availability.

Risks involved with TURP include a 1% risk of urinary incontinence and also decline in sexual function (both of which have been shown to be similar to watchful waiting).[14]

Absolute indications for prostatectomy include deterioration in kidney function, the development of upper tract dilatation, retention (following drainage and assessment) and bladder stones. Eighty per cent of patients have surgery for bothersome symptoms.

Postoperative guidelines for the patient

- There may be urgency even to the point of incontinence for a few days.
- Bleeding can occur intermittently for 3 weeks, so increase fluid intake.
- Avoid intercourse for 3 weeks.
- Orgasms continue but there is usually no emission with ejaculation. The semen is ejaculated back into the bladder.
- If obstructive problems recur early there may be a stricture.

Note:

- persisting postoperative frequency bothers about 15% of patients
- 10–15% reveal unsuspected cancer

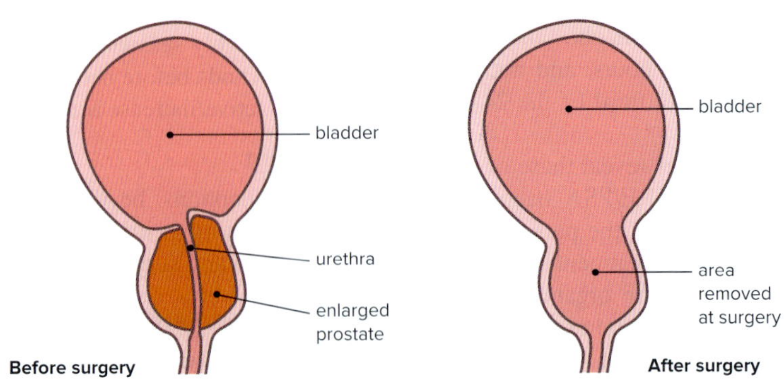

FIGURE 114.3 The process of prostatectomy

Drugs causing LUTS

Certain drugs can cause LUTS due to the effect of the drug on the bladder. It is very important for the family doctor to enquire about these drugs when evaluating such a patient. The problem is mainly an adverse effect of drugs with anticholinergic activity.

Anticholinergics

- Atropine and hyoscine compounds, for example:
  - isopropamide
  - mazindol
  - phenothiazines
  - dicyclomine
  - propantheline
  - other belladonna alkaloids
- Antidepressants:
  - especially tricyclic compounds
- Antiparkinson agents, for example:
  - amantadine
  - benzhexol
  - benztropine
  - biperiden
  - orphenadrine
  - procyclidine

Beta-adrenoceptor agonists

- Ephedrine
- Salbutamol
- Terbutaline
- OTC preparations (mainly for coughs and colds—e.g. sympathomimetics including ephedrine)

Prostate cancer

Prostate cancer is the commonest malignancy in men and the third commonest cause of death from malignant disease in Australia.[15] It is very much age dependent, with the risk increasing with age. Prostate cancer is rare before the age of 50 years, but by the age of 80 years, 80% of men have histologic carcinoma within the gland (but most are dormant).[16] The lifetime risk of being diagnosed by the age of 85 years is 1 in 5, but the risk of dying of prostate cancer by this age is 1 in 25.[15] Those men with a new diagnosis have a 92% chance of surviving for at least 5 years compared with the general population.[15] While this may sound reassuring, a younger man with a new diagnosis will have a higher risk of dying prematurely from prostate cancer as the cancer has a longer time available to progress.[17]

A family history can increase risk. The risk increases with a brother or father diagnosed with prostate cancer before the age of 65 years.[18] There is also increased risk for men with a first-degree relative with familial breast cancer (*BRCA1* or *BRCA2*).[18] Prostate cancer may be asymptomatic, even when it has extended beyond the prostate. It usually commences in the peripheral part of the gland. There are significant racial differences in the frequency that tend to change with migration, indicating that prostate cancer reflects environmental influences (and possibly dietary fat).[20]

Clinical features

Unsuspected cancers are often detected by the tumour marker PSA (a glycoprotein) or histologically after TURP. Clinical prostate cancer presents typically with rapidly progressive symptoms of lower urinary tract obstruction or of metastatic spread, especially to bone (pelvis and vertebrae).[21] Symptoms include BOO, acute retention, back or other bony pain, haematuria and uraemia, tiredness, weight loss and perineal pain.

Digital rectal examination (DRE) may reveal a nodule. Locally advanced cancer typically reveals a hard, nodular and irregular gland. The tumour may be large enough to obliterate the median sulcus. The borders may lack definition. On the other hand, with cancer, the prostate may feel normal.

Signs of abnormal prostate (DRE):

- hard lump
- asymmetry
- induration
- loss of median sulcus

Investigations

Blood analysis

- PSA:
  - can be elevated without cancer (e.g. BPH, exercise, infection, instrumentation, recent ejaculation)
  - must be tested with DRE[19]
  - is prostate specific, not prostate cancer specific

PSA guidelines (ng/mL)

Individual laboratory reference values may vary from the figures stated:

<4: normal (but in 15–25% of cancers)
4–10: intermediate
>10: strongly suggestive of cancer
>20: indicates metastatic spread

114

Other PSA parameters:[22]

- Age-specific PSA reference range:
  - 40–49 years: 0.25–2.5 ng/mL
  - 50–59 years: 0.25–3.5 ng/mL
  - 60–69 years: 0.3–5.5 ng/mL
  - 70–79 years: 0.3–7.5 ng/mL
- Free/total PSA ratio: BPH tends to have more variable PSA concentrations due to intermittent physical disturbance of the gland and subclinical prostatitis. This leads to 'showers' of inactive (non-protease) free PSA. Prostate cancer, however, constantly increases bound active PSA so the F/T PSA ratio tends to be lower (below 8%) in prostate cancer. This ratio has been suggested as being useful in men with moderately raised PSA levels (4–10 ng/mL).
- Above age-related median PSA. This has been postulated as a technique for selecting out those men who should have their PSA monitored more closely.
- The rate of PSA changes. Otherwise known as PSA kinetics, these include the 'PSA velocity' (the rate of change in PSA levels) and 'PSA doubling time' (the time taken for the PSA to double). A high velocity or a short doubling time may suggest a urology review is indicated.

The role of all of these parameters remains controversial, as does whether we should be screening for prostate cancer in low-risk men at all.

Screening

The RACGP *Guidelines for Preventive Activities in General Practice*[19] state that screening for prostate cancer is not recommended unless:

1 the man specifically asks for it *and*
2 he is fully counselled on the pros and cons

Similar recommendations have been made by other authorities.[23] The latest NH and MRC-approved guidelines are:[24]

- men should be offered the opportunity to consider and discuss the benefits and harms of PSA testing before making the decision whether or not to be tested
- the harms of PSA testing may outweigh the benefits, particularly for men aged ≥70
- men at average risk of prostate cancer who decide to undergo regular testing should be offered PSA testing every 2 years from age 50–69, and offered further investigation if the total PSA is greater than 3.0 mg/mL
- men with a family history of prostate cancer who decide to be tested should be offered PSA testing every 2 years from age 40/45–69, with the starting age depending on the strength of their family history
- digital rectal examination (DRE) is not recommended in asymptomatic men as a routine addition to PSA testing in the primary care setting but remains an important part of specialist assessment

Fully counselling a man can be challenging. A useful guide[25] on the outcomes of screening 1000 men aged 60 (with no significant family history and screened annually for 10 years) would result in the following:

- 2 men will avoid death from prostate cancer before the age of 85
- 2 men will avoid metastatic prostate cancer before the age of 85
- 85 men who do not have prostate cancer will have a biopsy
- 28 men will experience a side effect from the biopsy they consider a moderate/major problem
- 28 men will be diagnosed with prostate cancer, many of whom would have remained asymptomatic
- 25 men will undergo cancer treatment, many of whom would have remained asymptomatic
- 7–10 men will develop persistent impotence and/or urinary incontinence, and some will develop persistent bowel problems due to the treatments

Core biopsy

A urologist will consider biopsy guided by transrectal ultrasound or a transperineal approach (under general anaesthesia) if the DRE is positive or if the PSA is elevated, depending on the man's individual risk profile, clinical findings and PSA levels. A biopsy is the only certain measure of diagnosis.

Grading and staging

A good way of explaining to patients about grading and staging is to say 'the grade is how aggressive the cancer is, and the stage is how much there is and how far it has spread'.

From the biopsy, the pathologist determines the grading using the Gleason score (see TABLE 114.3 and FIG. 114.4). The score is based on the addition of the

Table 114.3 Gleason score and risk of cancer

Gleason score	Threat from cancer
2–4	Low
5–6	Moderate
7	Intermediate
8–10	High

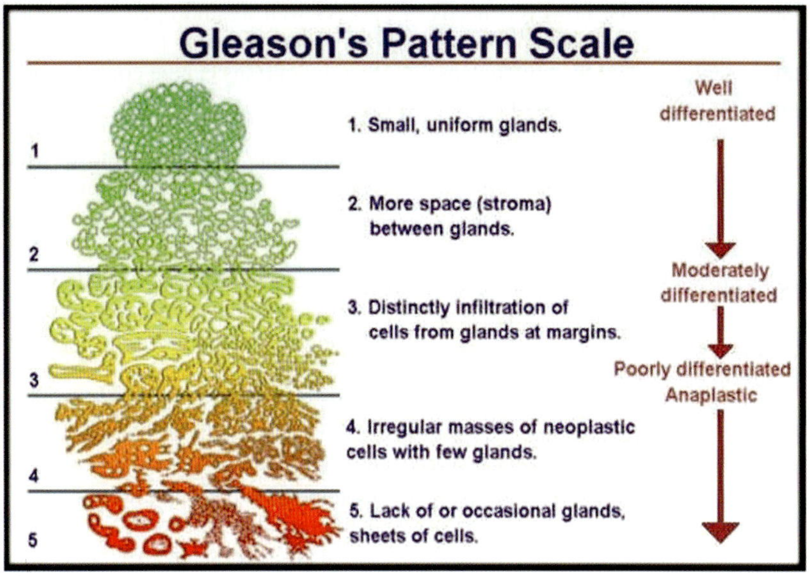

FIGURE 114.4 Gleason's pattern (grading) scale of prostate cancer [28]

grading of the 2 most common types of cells found in the samples (graded from 1, being well differentiated, to 5, most dysplastic). Therefore the lowest score possible is 2 and the highest 10. Prognosis is also determined by the ratio of the higher of the two histological scores (e.g. Gleason 7 with 80% stage 4/20% stage 3 will be worse than Gleason 7 with only 20% stage 4/80% stage 3).

Staging[26,27]

Clinical staging is based on 5 sources of information:

- the extent of the primary tumour (T category)
- whether the cancer has spread to nearby lymph nodes (N category)
- the absence or presence of distant metastasis (M category)
- the PSA level at the time of diagnosis
- the Gleason score, based on the prostate biopsy (or surgery)

Local prostate gland disease (T1–T2) is based on the DRE and transrectal ultrasound (TRUS) with T3 to T4 indicating spread beyond the capsule. Stages T1 and T2 have a good prognosis, and some T3 tumours can be cured. Whole-body radionucleide bone scanning, CT, MRI scanning and surgical pathology results also assist staging. Axial skeleton metastases are involved in 85% of patients who die of prostate cancer.[29]

After the TNM status is determined, this information is combined with the PSA and Gleason scores in what is termed *stage grouping,* from I (the least advanced) to IV (the most advanced). This will help determine treatment options and prognosis. This information can also be put into nomograms <www.nomograms.org> by either the doctor or patient to clarify the patient's status and options.

Treatment[30,31,32]

Deciding on treatment options for prostate cancer needs to take into account not only the grade and stage, but also the age and general health/life expectancy of the patient, available treatments and, importantly, patient preferences. Psychosocial support (both at the time of diagnosis and subsequently) and appropriate patient education will help make these patient preferences more clear.

Options for localised prostate cancer include radical prostatectomy, radiotherapy and no active treatment. The latter is now referred to as 'active surveillance', which means actively monitoring for changes such as a rising PSA or deteriorating biopsy results. Previously the term 'watchful waiting' was used, which was a more palliative approach used in the pre-PSA era (before 1990), which involved awaiting the appearance of symptoms or signs of local or systemic progression and then treating these as needed. Most of the evidence points to there being little difference (when the reduction in cancer risk is offset against the potential negative consequences of the interventions) in long-term outcomes between the three different approaches. This, however, needs to be put into the context of the individual patient's situation, his clinical presentation and his preferences, so active interventions may well be warranted.

Radical prostatectomy is most likely to benefit the patient with a relatively long life expectancy (>10 years), no significant surgical risk factors, a low volume stage and a low PSA and who, after being informed of the risks and benefits, prefers surgery. Approaches include radical perineal, laparoscopic and robot-assisted prostatectomy. Major complication issues include incontinence and impotence, and the risk of these will vary depending on the surgical approach and the patient's age and health.

Radiotherapy is also likely to benefit those with a long life expectancy and low-volume low PSA, who have a moderately (or worse) differentiated tumour and who, after being informed of the risks and benefits, prefer external beam or interstitial radiotherapy (brachytherapy). The main adverse reactions from external radiotherapy are faecal urgency and diarrhoea together with urine frequency. Impotence is common for up to 2 years after external beam radiotherapy.

Active surveillance is often used for those with a low life expectancy, or those who prefer to avoid the possible complications of surgery or radiotherapy. PSA monitoring is done for surveillance, or for follow-up after treatment with curative intent.

For locally advanced or metastatic disease, androgen deprivation is the cornerstone of treatment, the options being:

bilateral orchidectomy

or

daily anti-androgenic tablets, for example:

- cyproterone acetate (Androcur)
- flutamide (Eulexin)
- bicalutamide (Cosudex)
- abiraterone (Zytiga)

or

luteinising hormone releasing hormone (LHRH) agonists: depot injections of LHRH analogues, for example:

- goserelin (Zoladex)
- leuprorelin acetate (Lucrin, Eligard)

Treatment combinations for small volume metastatic prostate cancer may prolong life, for example:

- orchidectomy plus flutamide
- LHRH agonists plus flutamide or bicalutamide—LHRH agonists cause an initial surge of testosterone so a preliminary anti-androgenic agent is advised to prevent a flare in the cancer.

As well as androgen deprivation, radiotherapy to bony metastases or local disease and other adjuvant therapy options can be considered.

Complementary medicine

Among the disorders most widely promoted as benefiting from natural remedies are those of the prostate, though none has enough evidence to warrant its recommendation.[6] Herbal remedies that have been widely used include saw palmetto (*Serenoa repens*), stinging nettle (*Urtica dioica*), African prune (*Pygeum africanum*, syn. *Prunus africana*), willowherb (*Epilobium*) and cernilton.

Saw palmetto has been used widely, especially in Germany, with initial studies suggesting efficacy in LUTS consistent with BPH. However, a recent Cochrane review concludes it is not more effective than placebo.[33]

BPH has been treated with isoflavone phytoestrogens. A weak oestrogen agonist effect in males may antagonise the growth-promoting effects of androgens on the prostate. Epidemiological data indicate that in countries such as Japan where isoflavone diets are prevalent, prostatic enlargement occurs less with ageing. The most widely used source of phytoestrogens is soy protein. It is also present in lentils, chickpeas, some variations of beans and alfalfa sprouts.

A variety of nutrients may play a role in the development and progression of prostate cancer. There is evidence from some epidemiological studies that selenium, leucopenes (from tomato and tomato products), vitamin D, vitamin E, calcium and green tea in the diet protect against cancer of the prostate, though their true role remains largely unclear.[34]

References

1 Andrology Australia. Clinical Summary Guide 7: prostate disease (BPH and prostatitis—diagnosis and management), May 2010 <www.andrologyaustralia.org/wp-content/uploads/clinical-summary-guide07_May2010.pdf> (accessed 20/3/2014).

2 Expert group for Antibiotic. Urinary tract infections. In: eTG complete [Internet]. Melbourne: Therapeutic Guidelines Ltd. Available from: www.tg.org.au, (accessed 20/3/2014).

3 Buckley N (Chair). *Australian Medicines Handbook*. Adelaide: Australian Medicines Handbook Pty Ltd, 2016: 544.

4 European Association of Urology. *Guidelines on Chronic Pelvic Pain*, 2010 <www.uroweb.org/wp-content/uploads/26-Chronic-Pelvic-Pain_LR.pdf> (accessed 20/3/2014).

5 Katz DJ, Love CJ, Chung E. Lower urinary tract symptoms and benign prostatic hyperplasia: old problems, new solutions. Medicine Today, 2016; 7 (11): 14–25.

6 Nickel J et al. Alfuzosin and symptoms of chronic prostatitis—chronic pelvic pain syndrome. N Eng J Med, 2008; 359: 2663–73.

7 Litwin M et al. The National Institute of Health chronic prostatitis symptom index: development and validation of a new outcome measure. Chronic Prostatitis Collaborative Research Network. J Urol, 1999; 162: 369–75 <www.prostatitis.org/symptomindex.html> (accessed 20/3/2014).
8 American Urological Association. Management of benign prostatic hyperplasia, revised 2010 <www.auanet.org/documents/education/clinical-guidance/Benign-Prostatic-Hyperplasia.pdf> (accessed 20/3/2014).
9 Barry M et al. The American Urological Association symptom index for benign prostatic hyperplasia. The Measurement Committee of the American Urological Association. J Urol, 1992; 148: 1549.
10 Abrams P et al. Evaluation and treatment of lower urinary tract symptoms in older men. J Urol, 2009; 181: 1779.
11 Abdel-Azis S, Mamalis N. Intraoperative floppy iris syndrome. Curr Opin Opthalmol, 2009; 20: 37.
12 McConnell J et al. The long-term effect of doxazosin, finasteride, and combination therapy on the clinical progression of benign prostatic hyperplasia. N Eng J Med, 2003; 349: 2387.
13 Roehrborn C et al. The effect of dutasteride, tamsulosin and combination therapy on lower urinary tract symptoms in men with benign prostatic hyperplasia and prostatic enlargement: 2-year results from the CombAT study. J Urol, 2008; 179: 616.
14 Wasson J et al. A comparison of transurethral surgery with watchful waiting for moderate symptoms of benign prostatic hyperplasia: the Veterans Affairs Cooperative Study Group on Transurethral Resection of the Prostate. N Eng J Med, 1995; 332: 75.
15 Australian Institute of Health and Welfare. Cancer in Australia: key facts <www.aihw.gov.au/cancer/cancer-in-australia> (accessed 23/4/2014).
16 Kumar P, Clark M. *Clinical Medicine* (7th edn). London: Saunders, 2009: 674–6.
17 Baade P et al. Communicating prostate cancer risk: what should we be telling our patients? Med J Aust, 2005; 182 (9): 472–5.
18 Johns L, Heuston R. A systematic review and meta-analysis of familial prostate cancer risk. BJU Int, 2003; 91 (9): 789–94.
19 Royal Australian College of General Practitioners. *Guidelines for Preventative Activities in General Practice* (the red book) <www.racgp.org.au/your-practice/guidelines/redbook/9-early-detection-of-cancers/91-prostate-cancer/> (accessed 23/4/2014).
20 Gronberg H. Prostate cancer epidemiology. Lancet, 2003; 361: 859–64.
21 Barton S (ed.). *Clinical Evidence.* London: BMJ Publishing Group, 2001: 588–98.
22 Sikaris K. Prostate specific antigen. Aust Prescr, 2011; 34 (6): 186–8.
23 US Preventive Services Task Force. Screening for prostate cancer: US Preventive Services Task Force Recommendation Statement. Ann Intern Med, 2008; 149 (3): 185–91.
24 National Health and Medical Research Council. PSA testing for prostate cancer in asymptomatic men, information for health practitioners <www.nhmrc.gov.au/_files_nhmrc/publications/attachments/men4d_psa_testing_asymptomatic_men_140304.pdf> (accessed 23/4/2014).
25 Prostate Cancer Foundation of Australia and Cancer Council Australia PSA Testing Guidelines Expert Advisory Panel. *Draft Clinical Practice Guidelines PSA Testing and Early Management of Test-Detected Prostate Cancer.* Sydney: Cancer Council Australia <http://wiki.cancer.org.au/australia/Guidelines:PSA_Testing/Summary> (accessed 13/12/2014).
26 Prostate Cancer Foundation of Australia. How is prostate cancer graded and staged? <www.prostate.org.au/awareness/for-recently-diagnosed-men-and-their-families/partners-and-carers/diagnosis/grading-and-staging-of-prostate-cancer/> (accessed 13/12/2014).
27 American Cancer Society. Grading and staging of prostate cancer. <www.cancer.org/cancer/prostatecancer/detailedguide/prostate-cancer-staging> (accessed 23/4/2014).
28 Gleason DF. Histologic grading and clinical staging of prostatic carcinoma. In Tannenbaum M, *Urologic Pathology: The Prostate.* Philadelphia, PA: Lea and Febiger, 1977: 171–97.
29 Whitmore W. Natural history and staging of prostate cancer. Urol Clin North Am, 1984; 11 (2): 205–20.
30 Tacklind J et al. *Serenoa repens* for benign prostatic hyperplasia. Cochrane Database. Syst Rev. 2012, Issue 12. Art No. CD001423.
31 *National Health and Medical Research Council Clinical Practice Guidelines: Evidence-based Information and Recommendations for the Management of Localised Prostate Cancer* <www.nhmrc.gov.au/guidelines/publications/cp88> (accessed 23/4/2014).
32 Cancer Council Australia Advanced Prostate Cancer Guidelines Working Party. Management of locally advanced and metastatic prostate cancer. <www.cancer.org.au/health-professionals/clinical-guidelines/prostate-cancer.html> (accessed 23/4/2014).
33 Sonn G et al. Impact of diet on prostate cancer: a review. Prostate Cancer P D, 2005; 8: 304–10.
34 European Association of Urology. *Guidelines on Prostate Cancer,* 2013 <www.uroweb.org/wp-content/uploads/09_Prostate_Cancer_LR.pdf> (accessed 24/4/2014).

Part 8

Sexual health

115 The subfertile couple

You notice that the tabetic has the power of holding water for an indefinite period. He is also impotent—in fact, two excellent properties to possess for a quiet day on the river.

Dr Dunlop, Teaching at Charing Cross Hospital, 1913

Infertility is defined as the absence of conception after a period of 12 months of normal unprotected sexual intercourse.[1] The inability to conceive can be a very distressing and emotional problem for a couple, who need considerable care, empathy and relatively rapid investigation of their problem. In assessing a couple with the problem of subfertility (this term is a preferable way of describing the condition to the patients), it is appropriate to involve both partners in the consultation.

Human fertility depends on a complex series of events including:[2]

- production of gametes (sperm and oocytes) capable of fertilisation
- release of the oocyte into the fallopian tube after ovulation
- the right number of sperm have to be placed in the right place at the right time
- implantation and development of the embryo in the hormonally primed uterine mucosa
- maintenance of the growing fetus in the uterus until pregnancy is full term

As a general rule, the major factors limiting fertility are approximately one-third female, one-third male and one-third combined male and female. In addition, there are couples who fulfil the three primary fertility factors (egg, sperm and tubes) but do not conceive. This is known as unexplained (idiopathic) subfertility and accounts for 10–20% of subfertile couples.[2]

Key facts and checkpoints

- Infertility affects about 10–15% (1 in 7) of couples.[2]
- Fertility in women and men declines naturally with age.
- After the age of 32, female fertility decreases by 1.5% per year.
- Increasing female age is a common cause of decreased fertility.
- The main identifiable causes of male infertility are failure of spermatogenesis, failure of sperm delivery, impaired sperm quality and sperm autoimmunity.[2]
- Female factors include ovulation dysfunction, tubal disease, uterine disorders and peritoneal pathology.[3]
- Polycystic ovarian syndrome (PCOS) is the most common cause of ovulatory dysfunction.[4]
- In up to 20% of couples, no apparent cause is identified (idiopathic).[2]
- Assisted reproductive technology (ART) helps the majority of subfertile couples to achieve pregnancy, although success rates reduce with increasing maternal age.[5]

Physiological factors[6]

Male fertility

Fertility in the male requires:

- normal hypothalamic function producing gonadotrophin-releasing hormone (GnRH)
- normal pituitary function producing the gonadotrophin hormones—follicle stimulating hormone (FSH) and luteinising hormone (LH)
- normal seminiferous tubule and Leydig cell function
- normal sperm transport and delivery

Facts about sperm viability:

- the maximum number of viable sperm is found in the ejaculate after a 48-hour abstinence
- after entering receptive cervical mucus, sperm are capable of fertilising an egg for at least 48 hours
- sperm survive for less than 30 minutes in the vagina due to an acidic environment

Female fertility

Fertility in the female requires:

- normal function of the ovulatory cycle, which requires:
  - normal hypothalamic–pituitary function producing the hormones GnRH, FSH and LH

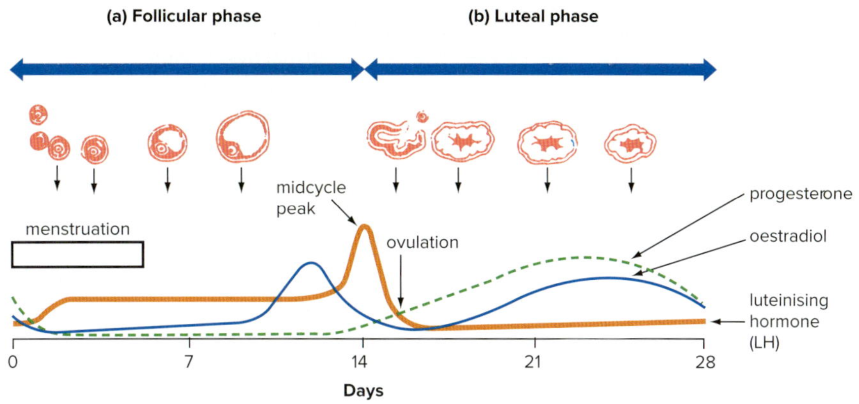

FIGURE 115.1 The normal ovulatory cycle: the midcycle peak of LH and FSH is at 14 days and ovulation occurs shortly afterwards

  - normal ovarian function with follicular response to FSH and LH (see FIG. 115.1)
  - appropriate prolactin levels (which are normally low); excessive prolactin secretion (hyperprolactinaemia) causes anovulation
- normal tubal transport and access of the ovum to incoming sperm
- receptive cervical mucus
- normal uterus to permit implantation of the fertilised ovum

Probabilities of pregnancy

About 50% of normal couples, having unprotected intercourse at least twice a week, will probably achieve pregnancy in 6 months, 85% in 1 year and 95% in 2 years.[6]

Causes of infertility

Significant causes of infertility are summarised in TABLE 115.1 and illustrated in FIGURE 115.2.

A diagnostic approach

History

Ask each partner for their age and take a general medical history, including family history, medication and drug use. Enquire about previous pregnancies in current or past relationships and outcomes.

The man

- Sexual function (problems with erections, ejaculation)
- Age of puberty
- Previous testicular problems/injury (e.g. orchitis, trauma, undescended testes, torsion)
- Past history (PH) of STIs
- PH of mumps
- PH of urethral problems
- Genitourinary surgery (e.g. hernia, vasectomy reversal)
- Occupational history (exposure to heat, pesticides, herbicides)
- Medications and drug use:
  - alcohol
  - smoking
  - chemotherapy
  - radiotherapy
  - anabolic steroids
  - aminoglycoside antibiotics
  - sulphasalazine
  - cimetidine/ranitidine
  - colchicine
  - spironolactone
  - antihypertensive agents
  - narcotics
  - phenytoin
  - nitrofurantoin
  - marijuana

The woman

- Onset of menarche
- Menstrual history
- Symptoms of ovulation (cervical mucus changes, mittelschmerz)
- Symptoms of endometriosis (dysmenorrhoea, pelvic pain, dyspareunia)
- PH of STIs and pelvic infection
- Previous IUCD use
- PH of intra-abdominal surgery (e.g. appendicitis, ovarian cyst)
- PH of genitourinary surgery

115

Table 115.1 Causes of subfertility[3]

Female factors

Ovulation dysfunction:

- hypothalamic/pituitary disorders
  - suppression of the hypothalamic-pituitary axis from stress, chronic illness, extreme exercise, malnutrition or eating disorders
  - hyperprolactinaemia
  - hypothalamic or pituitary tumours
- PCOS
- ovarian failure
  - premature ovarian failure
  - secondary to chemotherapy or radiotherapy, ovarian surgery or autoimmune disease
- other endocrine disorders
  - thyroid dysfunction
  - hyperandrogenism

Tubal disease:

- PID
- previous ectopic pregnancy
- previous tubal ligation
- tubal obstruction

Uterine abnormalities:

- fibroids
- endometrial polyps
- congenital (e.g. septate uterus, bicornate uterus)
- acquired (e.g. Asherman syndrome)

Peritoneal pathology:

- endometriosis
- adhesions
- previous peritonitis
- inflammatory bowel disease

Endometrial functional abnormalities:

- coagulation disorders or immunopathology, e.g. SLE, antiphospholipid syndrome

Male factors[7]

Pre-testicular:

- hypogonadotropic disorder (e.g. Kallman syndrome)
- hyperprolactinaemia

Testicular:

- congenital cryptorchidism (maldescent)
- inflammation (e.g. mumps orchitis, infection, trauma, torsion)
- antispermatogenic agents:
  - chemotherapy
  - drugs
  - radiation
  - heat
- Klinefelter syndrome (46 XXY)
- anti-sperm antibodies

Post-testicular:

- sexual dysfunction
- retrograde ejaculation
- obstruction:
  - vasectomy
  - congenital absence of the vas deferens, consider cystic fibrosis
  - ejaculatory duct obstruction or seminal vesicle dysfunction

Couple factors

Joint subfertility

Psychosexual dysfunction

- Medications and drug use:
  - alcohol
  - smoking, especially >20/day
  - past contraception, especially depot provera
  - anabolic steroids

Combined history

- Time trying to conceive
- Frequency and timing of intercourse
- Attitudes to pregnancy and subfertility
- Expectations for the future

Examination

A general assessment of body habitus, BMI, general health and secondary sexual characteristics should be noted in both man and woman.

The man

- Secondary sexual characteristics; note any gynaecomastia
- Genitalia
  - size and consistency of the testes—can compare to an orchidometer: normal range 15–35 mL (average 18 mL); small in Klinefelter syndrome (approx. 7–8 mL)
  - palpate epididymis and vas (present and non-tender is normal)
  - evidence of varicocele
  - PR: check prostate
  - note penis and location of urethra (always retract the foreskin for examination)

The woman

- Secondary sexual characteristics
- Thyroid status
- Note skin for acne, hirsutism
- Vaginal and pelvic examination:
  - assess uterus and ovaries (normal—present, mobile and non-tender)
  - the adnexae (any masses)

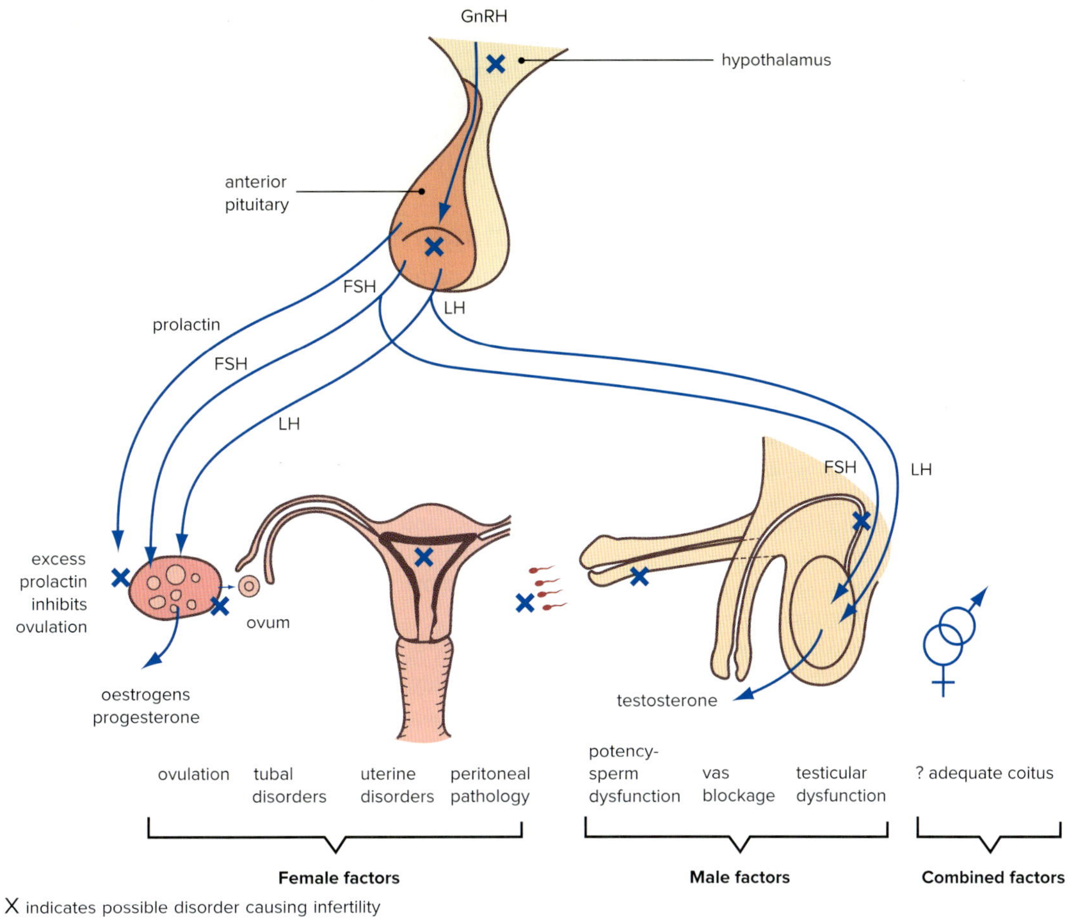

FIGURE 115.2 The major factors involved in subfertility.
Source: Adapted from Kumar and Clarke[8]

Investigations

These are usually performed after referral but the family doctor should organise initial investigations to assess where to refer (e.g. andrologist, endocrinologist, gynaecologist or fertility specialist).

Initial investigations

Male—semen analysis[7]

Collection should be made directly into a sterile container 2–3 days after sexual abstinence. If collected at home, semen should be kept at body temperature during transport to the laboratory and examined within 1 hour of collection. A repeat test in 1–3 months is indicated if the first is abnormal.[7]

- Normal values (based on WHO criteria):
  - volume ≥1.5 mL (average 2–6 mL)
  - pH ≥7.2
  - concentration ≥15 million sperm/mL
  - total sperm count ≥39 million
  - motility after 2 hours ≥32%
  - vitality ≥58%
  - normal forms ≥4%
  - leukocytes <1.0 x 10^6/ml

Female—ovulation status[3]

In most cases, regular menstrual cycles between 26 and 34 days, with appropriate variation in cervical mucus (thin at mid-cycle and thicker in the luteal phase) suggest ovulation is occurring. If ovulatory dysfunction is suspected, the following investigations are appropriate:

- serum LH, FSH and oestradiol (help identify primary hypothalamic-pituitary failure or dysfunction and primary ovarian disease; see TABLE 115.2)

115

Table 115.2 WHO classification of ovulatory dysfunction[9]

Group 1	Hypothalamic–pituitary failure	Low FSH, LH (e.g. anorexia nervosa)
Group 2	Hypothalamic–pituitary dysfunction	Normal FSH (e.g. PCOS)
Group 3	Ovarian failure	High FSH (e.g. ovarian failure)

- midluteal phase progesterone (day 21 of 28 day cycle, or 7 days before next expected period); >30 nmol/L can be used to confirm ovulation
- androgens (free testosterone, SHBG, free androgen index, 17-OH progesterone)
- thyroid function tests
- serum prolactin
- transvaginal high-resolution ultrasound (day 5–9 of cycle) for 'antral follicule count'—allows assessment of ovarian reserve, ovarian pathology or uterine structural abnormalities.
- anti-Mullerian hormone (AMH)—a predictor of ovarian function and reserve. Not essential although useful. Interpretation may be complicated and require specialist input.

Further investigations[3]

Male

If azoospermia or severe oligospermia (usually under specialist guidance):

- serum FSH level (if 2.5 times normal, indicates irreversible testicular failure)
- LH
- testosterone
- prolactin
- antisperm antibodies (in serum, semen or directly bound to sperm)
- sperm function tests
- genetic testing:
  - karyotype
  - Y chromosome microdeletions
  - cystic fibrosis gene mutation
- ultrasound of the scrotum +/− urogenital tract
- post-ejaculatory urine analsis (for retrograde ejaculation)

Female[10]

- routine preconception screening
- thyroid antibodies (TPO antibody-positive females have a higher incidence of subfertility)
- chlamydia (first-pass urine NAAT) if indicated
- consider genetic testing for fragile X gene mutation, cystic fibrosis and spinal muscular atrophy

Specialised investigations:

- hysterosalpingo-contrast-ultrasonography (Hy-Co-Sy)
- hysteroscopy/laparoscopy
- tubal dye studies

Management principles

- Both partners should be involved in management decisions since fertility is a couple's issue.
- All couples should be encouraged to optimise their general health through lifestyle changes such as weight optimisation, exercise, smoking cessation and minimised alcohol intake.
- Infertility can cause considerable emotional stress, including the taking or placing of blame by a partner and subsequent feelings of guilt. Sensitive and empathetic support is essential. This may include marital counselling.

Fertility awareness

Couples may require the following education on timing of intercourse:

- it is ideal to have intercourse every 2 days in the week before the expected time of ovulation[3]
- ova can survive up to 24 hours and sperm up to 5 days within the female genital tract
- ovulation generally occurs 14 days before menstruation
- ovulation may be identified with cervical mucus changes, when mucus becomes more slippery or like egg white
- the chance of fertilisation is best on the day of ovulation or during the time of the slippery sensation
- 2 days after ovulation, basal temperature rises slightly, around ¼–½ a degree
- recording temperature every morning for a few months can show if ovulation is regular and help predict the day of ovulation
- many women find fertility tracking websites or apps a useful aid
- urine-based ovulation detection kits are available but can be difficult to interpret
- for women with irregular periods, ovulation tracking may be of value through fertility laboratories in the treatment setting

'Fertility awareness practitioners' are available for couples interested in pursuing natural fertility methodology as an alternative to assisted reproductive technology.

Polycystic ovarian syndrome[4]

PCOS is a common condition, present in 12–18% of women of reproductive age.[11] It should be noted that it is not the same as polycystic ovaries, which occur in approximately 25% of asymptomatic, normal women.[12]

General features

Patients may present with the following:

- ovarian dysfunction—subfertility, oligomenorrhoea, anovulation
- androgen excess—acne, hirsutism and male-pattern balding
- metabolic features—upper truncal obesity, impaired glucose tolerance, dyslipidaemia, diabetes
- psychological symptoms—anxiety, depression, eating disorders

Aetiology[2]

Polycystic ovary syndrome is typically associated with insulin resistance. Insulin resistance and hyperinsulinaemia drive ovarian androgen production and suppress sex hormone–binding globulin (SHBG), leading to greater bioavailability of androgens. There is a strong hereditary basis and it is more common in Aboriginal and Torres Strait Islander and South-East Asian women. The onset can be triggered by environmental factors, particularly weight gain.

Diagnosis/investigations

Diagnosis of PCOS is made using the Rotterdam criteria, in which 2 of the following criteria are required:

- history of oligo/anovulation
- hyperandrogenism
  - clinical (hirsutism or, less commonly, male-pattern alopecia), or
  - biochemical (raised FAI or free testosterone)
- polycystic ovaries on ultrasound (at least 10 small antral follicles seen in each ovary)

Note: In young women, menstrual cycles may take up to 2 years to regulate after menarche. Irregular cycles persisting into the third year post-menarche should be investigated for PCOS.

Ultrasound is not reliable in the diagnosis of polycystic ovaries in adolescent and young women. Up to 70% of young women may have polycystic ovaries on ultrasound.

Suggested screening for all women with PCOS

- smoking history
- blood pressure
- fasting blood glucose levels
- oral glucose tolerance test (every 2 years in women with additional risk factors)
- lipid profiles

Management strategies

First-line

- lifestyle modification—weight reduction and exercise (even 5% weight loss may restore normal ovarian function)
- consider PCOS support group or psychological support

115

For women with subfertility

- screening and treat if necessary:
  - impaired glucose intolerance and diabetes mellitus
  - hyperlipidaemia
  - hypertension
- primary treatment of insulin resistance:
  - metformin
- ovulation induction—clomiphene/letrozole/gonadotrophins
- laparoscopic ovarian surgery/drilling (second-line after medical treatment)
- assisted reproductive technology (ART)

Counselling the subfertile couple[13]

The counselling of subfertile couples has to be adapted to the level reached by the couple along the infertility pathway. The needs of each couple may be very different depending on their emotional nature, their lifestyle, and their moral, religious and ethical beliefs. However, their suffering can run very deep and deserves attention, time and opportunities for free expression of feelings and concerns.

The medical counselling model developed by Colagiuri and Craig[13] (see FIG. 5.1 in CHAPTER 5) is very useful as it empowers patients to make their own decision through facilitation as opposed to the directive and advisory medical model.

The couple are provided initially with accurate and appropriate information. Anxiety is alleviated by reassurance and by dispelling myths.

The facilitation process enables the couple to ventilate any feelings of guilt, anxiety, fear, anger and sexuality. The style of questioning should aim to explore the influence that the problem has had on the couple and then the influence they have over it. These

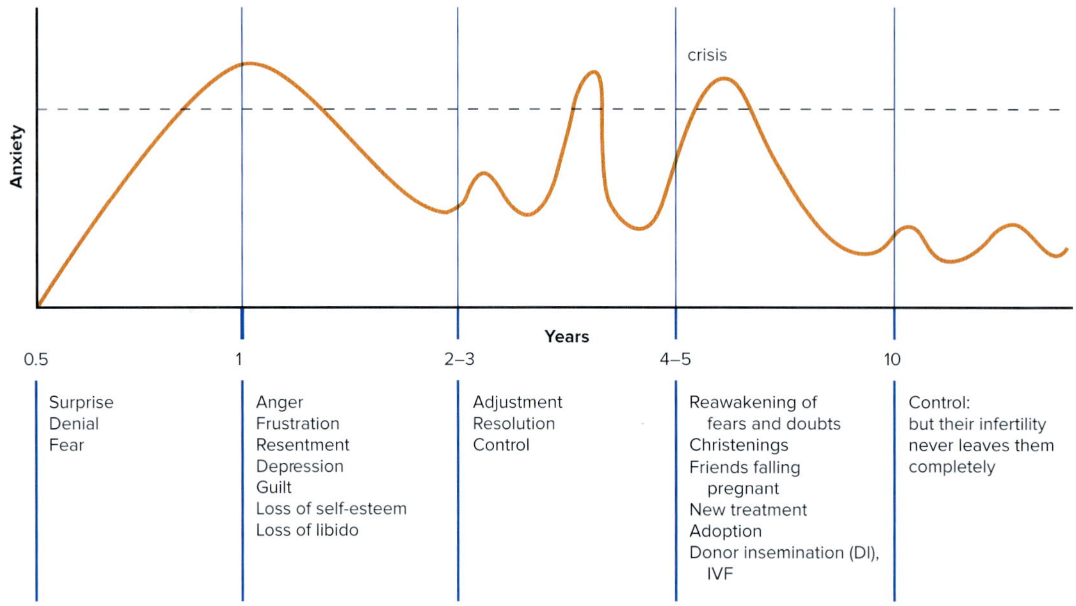

FIGURE 115.3 Emotional responses to infertility

Source: Reproduced with permission from Craig.[13]

processes then lead to decision making by the couple about further management strategies.

A graph of emotional responses to the infertility (see FIG. 115.3) can be used to help the couple explore their current and past emotional responses to their problem. Apart from helping them realise that their problem is not unique, it provides opportunities for ventilation of important feelings that can act as a basis for counselling.

Treatment[2]

Treatment options for female subfertility:

- Ovulation induction
  - metformin (for women with PCOS, use alone or with clomiphene)
  - clomiphene citrate
  - letrozole
  - gonadotrophins
    - FSH
    - LH
    - human chorionic gonadotrophin (hCG)
  - bromocryptine for hyperprolactinaemia
- Endometriosis
  - surgical ablation/excision of deposits and division of adhesions
- Surgical repair of tubal obstruction, removal of uterine septum, myomectomy and hysteroscopic resection of intrauterine adhesions are other surgical treatment options.

Treatments for male subfertility:[7]

- gonadotrophin therapy for men with hypogonadotrophic hypogonadism
- microsurgical vasovasostomy (vasectomy reversal)
- surgical correction of varicocele with oligozoospermia (role unclear)
- sympathomimetic agents (e.g. pseudoephedrine) may correct retrograde ejaculation

Assisted reproductive technology (ART)

Assisted reproductive technologies (ARTs) such as in vitro fertilisation (IVF) have revolutionised the treatment of infertility. It is estimated that more than 1.8 million ART cycles were undertaken worldwide in 2010, and that more than 6 million children have been conceived using these technologies over the last three decades.[14]

A recent study in Australia and New Zealand estimated the cumulative live birth rate of ART for all ages was 32.7% for the first complete cycle, rising to 54.3–77.2% by the eighth cycle. Success rates were significantly lower in women aged over 40, with an estimated cumulative live birth rate of 10.7% for the first complete cycle, rising to 21.0%–37.9% by the eighth cycle. IVF is rarely recommended to women aged over 44 years.[5]

Treatment options include:[12]

- IUI (intrauterine insemination with the partner's sperm)
- IVF (in vitro insemination)
  - involves the retrieval of ova, which are mixed with sperm and incubated for 2–6 days—the resultant embryo is then transferred into the uterus via the cervix
  - embryos can be frozen and stored cryogenically for up to 10 years; frozen embryos can be thawed and transferred to the uterus
- ICSI (intra-cytoplasmic sperm injection)
  - a single sperm is injected into an egg for fertilisation outside the body and then replaced into the uterus
- PGD (preimplantation genetic diagnosis)
  - recommended if a partner is affected by or carries a known genetic disease, if a couple have had multiple miscarriages or have had a number of failed embryo transfers

The role of the general practitioner

Since poor outcomes in subfertile couples are associated with delay in identification and treatment, early investigation instituted by the GP is important to expedite possible specialist involvement.

Referral is recommended after planned conception for:[3]

- 1 year if the woman is ≤35 years
- 6 months if the woman is >35 years

Consider early referral for women with amenorrhoea or oligomenorrhoea, or for couples with a known reason for infertility.

References

1 World Health Organization. WHO-ICMART revised glossary. Definition of infertility. Available from: <www.who.int/reproductivehealth/topics/infertility/definitions/en>, accessed March 2018.

2 Expert group for Endocrinology guidelines. In: eTG complete. Melbourne: Therapeutic Guidelines Ltd. Available from: <www.tg.org.au>, accessed March 2018.

3 Burns K, Smith H. The subfertile couple: a guide to investigations. Endocrinology Today, October 2016; 5(4): 6–16.

4 Boyle J, Teede H. Polycystic ovary syndrome: an update. Australian Family Physician. October 2012; 41(10): 752–6.

5 Chambers G et al. Assisted reproductive technology in Australia and New Zealand: cumulative live birth rates as measures of success. Med J Aust, 2017; 207(3): 114–8.

6 O'Connor V, Kovacs G. *Obstetrics, Gynaecology and Women's Health.* Cambridge: Cambridge University Press, 2003: 454–66.

7 Katz D, Teloken P, Shoshany O. Male infertility–the other side of the equation. Aust Fam Physician, September 2017; 46(9): 641–6.

8 Kumar PJ, Clark ML. *Clinical Medicine* (5th edn). London: Elsevier Saunders, 2003: 1028–30.

9 Illingworth P, Lahoud R. Investigation of the infertile couple 1. Medical Observer, 21 April 2006: 27–30.

10 Hunter T. Investigating fertility. O&G Magazine, Spring 2014; 6(3). Available from <www.ogmagazine.org.au/16/3-16/investigating-fertility>, accessed April 2018.

11 The Jean Hailes Foundation for Women's Health. PCOS. Available from: <https://jeanhailes.org.au/health-a-z/pcos>, accessed March 2018.

12 Family Planning NSW. *Reproductive and Sexual Health: An Australian Clinical Practice Handbook* (3rd edn). Sydney: Family Planning NSW, 2016.

13 Craig S. A medical model for infertility counselling. Aust Fam Physician, 1990; 19: 491–500.

14 Dyer S et al. International Committee for Monitoring Assisted Reproductive Technologies world report: assisted reproductive technology 2008, 2009 and 2010. *Hum Reprod*, 2016; 31: 1588–1609.

116 Sexual health

Drink, sir, provokes the desire, but it takes away the performance.

WILLIAM SHAKESPEARE (1564–1616), *MACBETH,* ACT 2, SCENE 1

Sexual health is the ability to embrace and enjoy our sexuality throughout our lives. Our sexuality is a fundamental human experience that encompasses sex, gender identities and roles, sexual orientation, eroticism, pleasure, intimacy and reproduction.[1]

Family doctors are often asked to provide advice and help for sexual concerns and are continually challenged to detect such problems presenting in some other guise. Since we deal with so much illness and prescribe so many drugs, we must be aware of the possible implications of their various effects on sexual health.

Sexual dysfunction[2]

Several studies have demonstrated that sexual concerns and problems are common, with a prevalence ranging from 20–40%. Difficult problems are summarised in TABLE 116.1. There is also evidence that health professionals do not discuss sexual concerns in consultations as often as patients would like.

Sexual dysfunction can be the bodily expression of many sorts of distress and requires consideration of biological, psychological, sociocultural and relationship factors. The unique place of general practice and the family doctor provides ideal opportunities to address the sexual concerns of patients as the family doctor often has considerable insight into the family dynamics and first-hand perspective of the individuals involved.

Table 116.1 Sexual dysfunction: difficult problems[2]

Female problems:

- lack of libido: 4 in 10 women
- orgasmic difficulties: 1 in 3 women
- painful intercourse (dyspareunia, vaginismus): 1 in 10 women

Male problems:

- lack of libido: 1 in 4 men
- erectile dysfunction: 1 in 5 men
- premature/delayed ejaculation: 1 in 4 men
- anorgasmia
- concerns about penis

Other:

- substance/medication-induced sexual dysfunction
- compulsive sexual behaviour

Opportunistic sexuality education

The family doctor has many opportunities to provide education in sexuality throughout the lifelong care of the patient and it is wise to have a strategy that matter of factly incorporates enquiries and information about sexual health.

Examples include:

- antenatal and postnatal care
- contraceptive requests
- parents concerned about their children's sex play
- serious illness—medical and surgical
- adolescent problems
- menopause

Presentation of sexual concerns

Although some patients may present directly with a complaint of sexual dysfunction, many will be less direct and use some other pretext or complaint as a 'ticket of entry' for their sexual concerns (see TABLE 116.2). Despite a seemingly terse approach

Table 116.2 How sexual issues may present in family practice[3]
Minor non-sexual complaint—'entry ticket'
Specific sexual concern
Marital or relationship problem
Non-sexual problem (as perceived by the patient)
Sexual enquiry as part of illness management
Sexual enquiry as part of total health check-up
Infertility
Menopausal symptoms

the issue must be recognised and treated with considerable importance. This may mean scheduling an appropriate time to discuss the concerns.

The effect of illness on sexual function

Doctors seldom enquire about the impact of an illness on the sexual function of patients and their partners (see TABLE 116.3). It is most appropriate to enquire about these issues with patients, e.g. the postmyocardial infarction patient, the postprostatectomy patient, the patient taking antihypertensives or other drugs (see TABLE 116.4), and the post-mastectomy or post-hysterectomy patient. Diabetes deserves special attention as more than 60% of diabetic men have reported erectile difficulties.[4]

Taking a sexual history

It is important to create a safe environment for patients to talk about their sexual behaviour and sexuality. Consider explaining why you are asking for this information and request permission to proceed. Avoid being too formal or too familiar but aim to display a wise, matter-of-fact, empathic, commonsense rapport. CHAPTER 117 covers the sexual history required when assessing for sexually transmitted infections (STIs).

Be aware that many patients will have an undisclosed history of sexual abuse.

Probing questions for a suspected sexual problem

- How are things going in your sex life?
- Do you have any difficulties with your relationship or sex life?
- Are you satisfied with the frequency and quality of your sexual experience?
- Do you have any pain or discomfort during intercourse?
- Have you had any difficulties with erections (men)?

Sexual and relationship history

A general medical history should be taken including surgical history, medication use, recreational drug and alcohol use, and smoking.

Consider the following when exploring a sexual symptom:

- What sex education did you have as a child at home or at school?
- What were your parents' attitudes to sex?

Table 116.3 Medical conditions affecting sexual performance

Cardiovascular:
- previous myocardial infarction
- angina pectoris
- peripheral vascular disease
- hypertension and its treatment

Respiratory:
- asthma
- COPD

Endocrine:
- diabetes mellitus
- thyroid dysfunction
- Cushing syndrome
- hypogonadism

Neurological:
- multiple sclerosis
- neuropathy
- spinal cord lesions
- Parkinson disease

Musculoskeletal:
- arthritis

Psychogenic:
- depression
- anxiety
- PTSD

Kidney:
- kidney failure

Urological problems:
- prostatectomy
- phimosis
- Peyronie disorder
- priapism

Hepatobiliary:
- cirrhosis

Surgical:
- vaginal repair
- hysterectomy
- others

Trauma:
- motor vehicle accidents

Cancer

Other:
- Klinefelter syndrome
- vestibulodynia

116

Table 116.4 Drugs affecting sexual arousal and function

Male	Female
Alcohol	Alcohol
Anticholinergics	Anti-androgens
Anti-epileptics	Antidepressants (selected), e.g. SSRIs
Antihistamines	Anti-epileptics
Antihypertensives	Antihypertensives (selected)
Benzodiazepines	CNS depressants
Cytotoxic drugs	Hormone contraception, e.g. combined oral contraceptive
Disulfiram	Marijuana
Marijuana	Narcotics
Narcotics	
Oestrogens	
Psychotherapeutic drugs	

- Have you experienced any upsetting or traumatic sexual experiences?
- Are you experiencing stress in any area of your life—relationship, work or home-life?
- Are you able to talk to your partner about sex?
- How was your coming-out experience (patients in same-sex relationships)?

Examination

The routine medical examination should include the basics such as urinalysis, BP measurement, genital examination and neurological where indicated.

Investigations

No particular routine tests are recommended. Tests for male erectile dysfunction (impotence) are outlined later in this chapter. Tests that may help exclude significant causes of low libido are those for diabetes, liver dysfunction, thyroid dysfunction and endocrine dysfunction. Endocrine dysfunction tests include prolactin, free testosterone, FSH, LH and oestradiol estimations. Other investigations may include pelvic ultrasonography, colposcopy or laparoscopy.

Exploring sexual myths

The acceptance of many sexual myths that have prevailed in our society may affect a couple's sexual relationship. Sexualised images in the media and pornography are a common cause of unrealistic expectations in the bedroom. These expectations can exacerbate the problem, causing disappointment and a feelings of inadequacy.

Sexual myths that could be explored include:

- men need sex, women need love
- men need more sex than women
- men must be the instigators
- sex = intercourse
- a hard erection is essential for good sex
- sufficient sexual thoughts should always make the penis erect
- both partners should achieve an orgasm every time and simultaneously
- women should be able to achieve orgasm through penetrative intercourse
- men should be ready and able to last all night
- as a person gets older there is a loss of interest in sex

Basic sexual counselling

The family doctor can learn to be an effective sex counsellor. Sex counselling can be emotionally demanding and, while good interviewing skills, interest, support and basic advice are important, additional skills are needed to be an effective counsellor.

Principles for basic sexual counselling:

- give the patient permission to talk openly about sexual matters
- allow for a relaxed exchange of information
- dispel sexual myths and correct misunderstandings
- explore the patient's anxiety and any impact on their relationship
- de-emphasise the modern-day obsession with performance and orgasm and emphasise the value of alternative forms of sexual expression (e.g. caressing, kissing, and manual and oral stimulation)
- reassure the patient that he or she is normal (where appropriate)

Inappropriate doctor behaviour is presented in TABLE 116.5.

Sexual problems can be grossly underestimated. Human beings generally have a basic craving for intimacy, touching, stroking and loving sex. Apparently harmonious relationships can lack this type of intimacy, which may lead to various psychosomatic manifestations.

Ideally the family doctor should undertake a course in sexual counselling to promote confidence in the counselling process. Patients can be taught basic methods (where appropriate) such as sensate

Table 116.5	Sexual counselling: inappropriate doctor behaviour

Overfamiliarity
Being too formal
Being too talkative
Blunt questioning
Being judgmental
Making assumptions about the other's sexuality
Imposing one's own beliefs and standards
Dogmatism
Tackling problems beyond one's experience

focus, squeeze or stop–start techniques for premature ejaculation, self-exploration using Kegel pelvic floor exercises, fantasy conditioning with books or videos, use of sex toys and behaviour modification. Complex or serious problems, especially those involving compulsive sexual behaviour, demand specialist referral.

The PLISSIT counselling model

The PLISSIT counselling model developed by Annon[5] can be used to build the skills needed to deal with sexual problems, especially if there is a psychological element.

The mnemonic PLISSIT stands for:

P = **P**ermission giving
LI = **L**imited **I**nformation
SS = **S**pecific **S**uggestion
IT = **I**ntensive **T**herapy

'Permission giving' allows patients to talk about sex, ask questions, feel guilty and so on. Their problems are shared with a reflective listening confidant.

Most medically trained people can probably provide the limited information required about sexual physiology and behavioural patterns. 'Specific Suggestion' provides ideas for self-help and may include key reference books and relevant videos. With a little support and permission, the patient can take simple action to remedy or improve a problem.

Intensive therapy, whether psychiatric or emotional, calls for deeper involvement and can be a dangerous area for the inexperienced. Referral to an appropriate practitioner is usually advisable.

Analogous roles of the penis and clitoris

An explanation of the analogous roles of the penis and clitoris (proposed by Cohen and Cohen) is a very useful strategy for educating patients and helping them to understand the relationship of intercourse and penile and clitoris stimulation with orgasm. The simple model (see FIG. 116.1) can be shown to patients

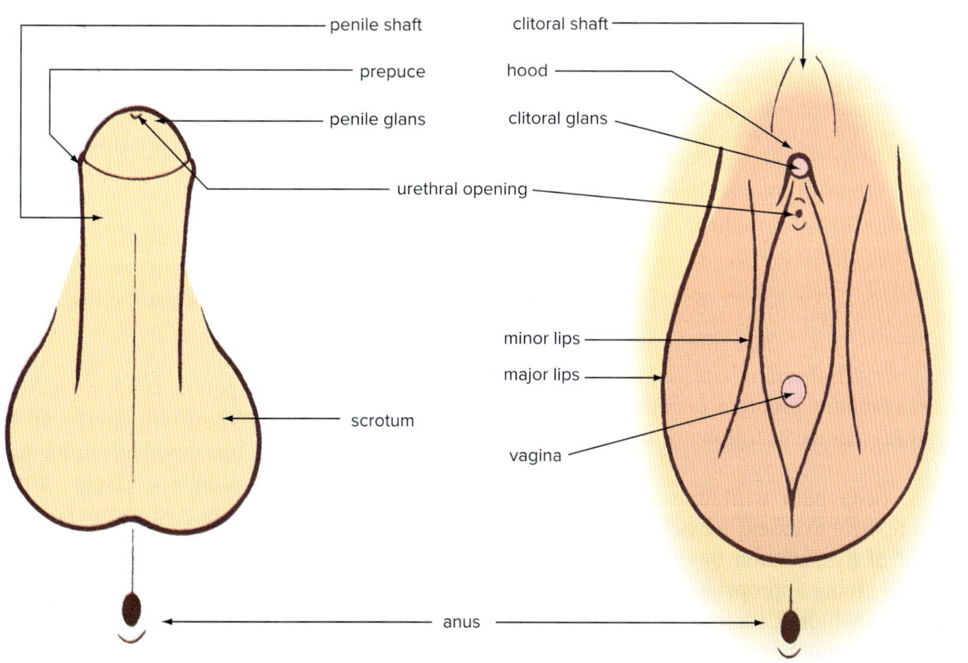

FIGURE 116.1 Analogous structures in male and female genitalia

Source: Reproduced with permission from G and M Cohen, Canadian Family Physician, 852, 31: 767–71[3]

to explain, for example, why some women are unable to achieve orgasm by intercourse alone, especially using the conventional missionary position.[3] It can readily be explained that clitoral stimulation in women is analogous to penile stimulation in men.

Female orgasmic difficulties

It is necessary to determine whether the woman has been anorgasmic or can experience orgasms from other activities such as masturbation, or manual or oral stimulation, even though she is non-orgasmic during intercourse. One-third of women may never experience orgasm, but enjoy their sexual relationships despite this.[2]

116

A common concern of women is the inability to regularly achieve orgasm through vaginal intercourse, believing there may be a physical cause. It is important to reassure that this is normal, as the majority of women are able to achieve orgasm through clitoral stimulation rather than intercourse.

The use of the Cohen model (see FIG. 116.1) is very helpful in emphasising the importance of clitoral stimulation.

Therapy includes:

- sensate focus exercises[6]
- advice on the most appropriate positions for intercourse
- permission to use:
  - books, videos
  - self-stimulation
  - vibrators

Dyspareunia

Painful intercourse is a source of considerable distress both physically and psychologically for the sufferer and also for her partner. It may be one of the 'hidden agenda' presentations with a vague complaint such as 'I am uncomfortable down below'. Tact and sensitivity is very important in management.

In particular it is helpful to keep in mind vulval vestibular syndrome, which has subtle physical signs (see CHAPTER 107). Important causes are listed in TABLE 116.6. A common problem encountered is the presence of painful scar tissue following an episiotomy, especially after the first vaginal delivery. Women who experience deep pain with intercourse need a gynaecological referral to assess for pelvic pathology.

Management of dyspareunia involves treating the organic cause and giving appropriate advice about the use of lubricants, including topical oestrogen where indicated. While this may be enough in simpler cases, it does not address the often accompanied fear of penetration,[2,7] which can continue even after the cause of dyspareunia is addressed.

Table 116.6 Important causes of dyspareunia

Pain worse on insertion
Physiological—inadequate lubrication
Vaginismus
Provoked vestibulodynia syndrome
Vaginitis in chronic candidiasis
Vulvar dermatoses (e.g. dermatitis, psoriasis, lichen planus)
Vulvovaginal atrophy (e.g. postmenopausal)
Postnatal perineal scarring
Incompletely ruptured hymen
Pain worse on deep penetration
Endometriosis
PID
Pelvic adhesions
Ovarian and uterine tumours

Vaginismus[2]

Vaginismus is the involuntary contraction of muscles around the introitus (outer third of vagina) in response to and preventing the possibility of penetration. It can be classified as primary or secondary. In primary vaginismus, tampons will probably never have been inserted. It is often related to provoked vestibulodynia (vestibular hypersensitivity—see CHAPTER 107).

A fear of penetration can be the underlying cause and may be associated with fears of internal damage, pregnancy, learned negative attitudes to sex and past sexual trauma. It is not an uncommon cause of unconsummated marriage. The problem may respond to sensitive exploration of fears and education of the anatomy and physiology. Encourage use of lubricant and a comfortable sexual position that the woman can control, usually superior.

Consider referral to specially trained physiotherapists for pelvic floor relaxation and use of vaginal trainers. Vaginal trainers can be inserted at increasing sizes for desensitisation, allowing for progressive vaginal dilation. Expert counselling is necessary if fears remain a barrier to recovery.

Lack of libido[2]

The Diagnostic and Statistical Manual of Mental Disorders, fifth edition (DSM-5) defines lack of libido in women as sexual interest/arousal disorder

(FSAD), and in men as male hypoactive sexual desire disorder (MSHDD).[8] Lack of libido is usually due to a combination of factors including relationship issues, illness, medications, drug and alcohol use, hormonal changes, stress and fatigue. Other sexual difficulties that are treated medically (e.g. erectile dysfunction) may later present with reduced libido, indicating that the underlying relationship factors have not been addressed.

Individuals or couples may benefit from basic sexual counselling from their GP, while others may request input from a sex therapist. If lack of libido is secondary to menopause, a trial of hormonal replacement therapy (HRT) may be useful. Tibolone is an HRT that has been shown to have benefit in managing loss of libido in some women.[9] Conclusive evidence in support of other drug therapies is lacking.[10]

Erectile dysfunction

Erectile dysfunction (impotence) is the inability to achieve or maintain an erection of sufficient quality for satisfactory intercourse.

Erectile dysfunction is a common problem. In an Australian study, the overall prevalence of erectile dysfunction was 61% (25% sometimes, 19% usually and 17% had complete erectile dysfunction). More than 20% of healthy men aged 60–65 years with no risk factors had moderate or complete erectile dysfunction.[4]

Traditionally, the aetiology of erectile dysfunction is classified into organic, psychogenic or mixed. In reality, however, anxiety and depression commonly accompany erectile dysfunction, irrespective of the original aetiology. Consequently, nearly all organic erectile dysfunction will eventually become 'mixed'.[11]

Causes

- psychogenic: related to stress, interpersonal or intrapsychic factors (e.g. depression, marital disharmony, performance anxiety)
- neurogenic: disorders affecting the parasympathetic sacral spinal cord (e.g. multiple sclerosis); it usually develops gradually
- vascular
- diabetes
- hypertension
- chronic kidney disease
- urological problems (e.g. Peyronie disorder, pelvic trauma and surgery)
- hormone disorder
  - androgen deficiency (e.g. testicular disease)
  - hypothyroidism
  - hyperprolactinaemia (rare) → impotence and loss of libido due to secondary testosterone deficiency
- drug-induced:
  - alcohol
  - cocaine, cannabis
  - nicotine (four times the risk by age 50)
  - antihypertensive agents
  - finesteride
- ageing
- unknown

116

> **Practice tip**
>
> Erectile dysfunction may be the first symptom of atherosclerotic disease (e.g. CAD).

History

The nature of the onset of erectile dysfunction is very important and this includes the nature of the relationship. Of particular importance is a drug history, including alcohol, nicotine, recreational drugs and pharmaceutical agents, particularly antihypertensives (beta blockers and thiazide diuretics), hypolipidaemic agents, anti-androgens (prostate cancer treatment), antidepressants, antipsychotics and H_2-receptor antagonists. Ask about nocturnal and early morning erections.

Examination

Genitourinary, cardiovascular and neurological examinations are appropriate, although may not reveal the diagnosis. A focused examination should include a rectal examination and examination of the vascular and neurological status of the lower limbs and the genitalia, especially the testicles and penis. Check the cremasteric and bulbocavernosus reflexes.

Investigations

First-line blood tests:

- morning testosterone
- TSH
- prolactin
- luteinising hormone
- fasting blood glucose

Other blood tests to consider:

- LFTs, especially GGT (alcohol effect)
- kidney function tests
- lipid studies

When the aetiology is unclear, specialist testing includes a penile duplex doppler ultrasound using an intracavernosal vasoactive agent.

116

Management

Address modifiable risk factors, including medications (if feasible), psychosocial issues and lifestyle (see NEAT, CHAPTER 7). Management should comprise appropriate patient education. The partner should be included in the discussions and general management process with an emphasis on bolstering the couple's self-image, which may have been affected by feelings of rejection or avoidance.

Psychogenic disorders

These involve psychotherapy and sex behavioural modification as outlined earlier in this chapter under Basic sexual counselling. Referral to a consultant may be appropriate.

Oral medication

PDE-5 inhibitors: the phosphodiesterase type 5 (PDE-5) inhibitors are the first-line oral medication (see TABLE 116.7). They are about 70% effective but not very effective for neurogenic ED. They do not initiate an erection but enhance whatever erection the man is capable of having. Sexual stimulation is necessary. They are contraindicated if the patient has unstable angina, recent stroke or myocardial infarction. Use with nitrates should be avoided and a nitrate should never be taken within 24 hours of use. The interaction with nitrates can result in a severe and potentially fatal hypotensive response. PDE-5 inhibitors have the potential for side effects, especially headache. Treatment is not considered a failure until a full dose has been trialled 7–8 times.[12]

Intrapenile injection[10]

Intracavernosal vasodilator injections are second-line therapy and should be supervised by an experienced practitioner.

Alprostadil intracavernosal injections:

- self-administered after supervised teaching (use a penile model if available)
- start with a lower dose, 2.5–5 mcg
- spontaneous erection in 5–20 minutes
- if prolonged erection >2 hours take 120 mg pseudoephedrine orally and have a hot shower—repeat at 4 hours if necessary (provided not hypertensive)

Vacuum constriction

Vacuum constriction devices (VEDs) may have a place in management, where pharmacological therapies have failed or are inappropriate. VEDs are often poorly tolerated in the long term due to side effects such as pain, inability to ejaculate, bruising, 'hinging' and paraesthesia.[11]

Surgery

- malleable penile prosthesis
- inflatable penile prosthesis (see FIG. 116.2)

Premature ejaculation

Premature ejaculation is defined as 'ejaculation that occurs sooner than desired' or, more precisely, as 'persistent or recurrent ejaculation, before, on or shortly after penetration and associated with significant personal distress'. In most cases, this occurs within 1 minute of vaginal penetration. It may not be clearly described by the patient so a careful history is necessary to define the problem. Ensure that the person is not suffering from erectile dysfunction. Both patient and partner may complain about the problem.

There are many approaches to treatment but they are aimed either at prolonged ejaculatory control or

Table 116.7 Phosphodiesterase type 5 inhibitors[11]

	Sildenafil (Viagra)	Tadalafil (Cialis)	Vardenafil (Levitra)
Dosage (mg)	25, 50, 100	5, 10, 20	5, 10, 20
Usual starting dose (1 hour pre i/c)	50 mg	10 mg	10 mg
Peak effect	1 hour	2 hours	1 hour
Half-life (approximately)	4 hours	18 hours	4 hours
Class side effects	Headache, nasal congestion, facial flushing, dyspepsia		
Specific side effects	Blue vision, diarrhoea	Myalgia, back pain	Visual disturbance

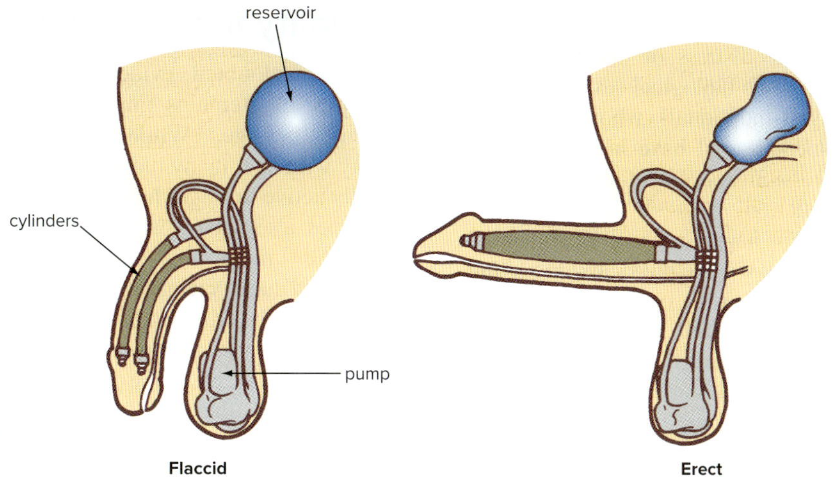

FIGURE 116.2 An inflatable prosthesis, showing positioning of the components

at satisfactory sexual activity without preoccupation with ejaculation.

Non-pharmacological treatment includes psychosexual therapy and/or behaviour therapy (including 'stop-start' techniques).

Pharmacological treatment

SSRIs have also been reported as effective—using dapoxetine 30 mg, sertraline 50 mg or paroxetine 20 mg, all about 3 hours before intercourse.[10] Some men may prefer to take SSRIs daily for managing premature ejaculation. Local anaesthetic has been suggested to reduce penile sensation, however this tends to be counterproductive as it reduces sexual pleasure.[2]

Sexual orientation and gender identity concerns[13]

For some individuals, gender identity and sexual orientation are fixed and clear, while for others it may be more fluid. It is also worth noting that identity, attraction and behaviour are not necessarily congruent. It is incumbent on the general practitioner to have a good understanding of the diversity of sex, sexuality and gender and the specific needs of the LGBTIQ (lesbian, gay, bisexual, transgender, intersex and queer) community.

Studies have found that the medical experiences of individuals identifying as LGBTIQ are 'generally poor'. Contributing factors include assumed heterosexuality, health professional discomfort, poor knowledge of LGBTIQ issues and appropriate referral networks and resources.

Definitions and facts

Lesbian: A woman who experiences an attraction to other women.

Gay: A man who experiences attraction to men. Men who have sex with men (MSM) do not always identify as gay. It can also be used as an umbrella term to describe both lesbians and gay men and perhaps bisexual people of both sexes.

Bisexual: A person who experiences attraction to their own as well as the opposite gender.

Transgender: A person whose gender identity and/or gender expression differs to their birth sex. Sexual orientation varies and is not dependent on gender identity.

Intersex: People who are born with genetic, hormonal or physical sex characteristics that are not typically 'male' or 'female'. Causes include congenital adrenal hyperplasia and androgen insensitivity syndrome. Intersex individuals can have a broad range of gender identities and sexual orientations.

Queer: A political statement as well as a sexual orientation which advocates non-binary thinking and seeing both sexual orientation and gender identity as potentially fluid.

A recent Australian sample found that 14.7% of women are same-sex attracted, 13.5% engage in same-sex behaviour, 1.2% identify as lesbian and 2.2% are bisexual; and 6.8% of men are same-sex attracted, 6.0% engage in same-sex behaviour, 1.6% are gay and 0.9% bisexual.[14]

It is estimated that up to 8% of Australians are gender diverse and individuals who are intersex constitute 1.7% of births in Australia.

Gender dysphoria[15]

Gender dysphoria is the distress or discomfort that may occur when a person's biological sex and gender identity do not align. Individuals who identify as transgender are vulnerable and have higher rates of discrimination, depression and suicidality compared with the general population.

Some patients may be happy to live in their desired gender role, but many will want to physically transition with the use of hormones, with or without surgery. Specialist referral and a multidisciplinary approach is required for those considering physical transition. Given gender identity develops in the first four years of life, young children may also require referral.

Concerns of penis size

In general practice it is not uncommon to counsel men and adolescent males for anxiety about the size of their penis. It is a manifestation of abnormal body image perception and related to the myth that a man's sexual performance depends on the size of his penis. The patient may present with minor (often trivial) non-sexual complaints as a 'ticket of entry' into the consulting room.

The average adult penis measurements are summarised in TABLE 116.8.[16,17]

Table 116.8 Average penile size (symphysis pubis to meatus)

		Flaccid	Erect
Length	centimetres	7.5–10.5	12–18
	inches	3–4	5–7
Circumference	centimetres	6–10	8–12
	inches	2.5–4	4–6

Psychological factors

It should be explained that virility and performance are not related to the size of the penis.[17] Orgasm in the female does not depend on deep vaginal penetration. Penile size was found to have little relationship to a partner's satisfaction from sexual intercourse. The vagina, which is 10 cm (4 inches) long in the unstretched state, tends to accommodate itself to the size of the penis.

Sexuality in the elderly[18]

There is undoubted evidence that sexuality, and its expression, remains important to both men and women as they age.[19] While there is a decline in sexual activity with age, many older men and women remain sexually active through their later years.

Studies also show that maintaining sexual activity is generally more important to men than women. Dyspareunia due to vaginal atrophy may be a contributing factor, for which additional lubrication, topical oestrogen or systemic hormone therapy can be of benefit.

Older people have the same needs as younger people—namely, the need for closeness, intimacy and body contact. Intercourse in the elderly may be difficult or not possible, so it may be appropriate to advise 'outercourse' which is an extension of foreplay and which provides loving body contact and intimacy. Other suggestions include planning of sexual activity, taking analgesia prior to sexual activity, alternative activities to ensure physical comfort and use of specific aids.

References

1 World Health Organization. Defining sexual health: Report of a technical consultation on sexual health, 28–31 January 2002. Geneva: WHO, 2006. Available from: <www.who.int/reproductivehealth/topics/gender_rights/defining_sexual_health.pdf>, accessed January 2018.

2 Goodwach R. Let's talk about sex. Aust Fam Physician, January/February 2017; 46(9): 14–18.

3 Cohen M, Cohen G. The general practitioner as an effective sex counsellor. Aust Fam Physician, 1989; 18: 207–12.

4 Weber MF et al. Risk factors for erectile dysfunction in a cohort of Australian men. Med J Aust, 2013; 199(2): 107–11.

5 Annon JS. *Behavioural Treatment of Sexual Problems: Brief Therapy*. Hagerstown, MA: Harper & Rowe, 1976: 45–119.

6 Ross MW, Channon-Little LD. *Discussing Sexuality*. Sydney: MacLennan & Petty, 1991: 42–66.

7 Reissing ED, Armstrong HL, Allen C. Pelvic floor physical therapy for lifelong vaginismus: A retrospective chart review and interview study. J Sex Marital Ther, 2013; 39(4): 306–20.

8 *Diagnostic and Statistical Manual* (5th edn). Washington, DC: American Psychiatric Association, 2013.

9 Family Planning NSW. *Reproductive and Sexual Health: An Australian Clinical Practice Handbook* (3rd edn). Sydney: Family Planning NSW, 2016.

10 Expert group for Endocrinology. In: eTG complete. Melbourne: Therapeutic Guidelines Ltd. Available from: <www.tg.org.au>, accessed March 2018.

11 Shoshany O, Katz D, Love C. Much more than prescribing a pill: assessment and treatment of erectile dysfunction by the general practitioners. Aust Fam Physician, September 2017; 46(9): 634–39.

12 Allan C et al. Male reproductive health. Check Program 442/443. Melbourne: RACGP, 2009: 18–30.

13 The Royal Australian College of General Practitioners. Curriculum for Australian General Practice 2016: CS16 Core skills unit. East Melbourne: RACGP, 2016.

14 Richters JD et al. Sexual identity, sexual attraction and sexual experience: the second Australian study of health and relationships. Sex Health, 2014; 11(5): 451–60.

15 Atkinson S, Russell D. Gender Dysphoria. Aust Fam Physician, November 2015; 44(11): 792–6.

16 Feldman HA et al. Impotence and its medical and psychological correlates: results of the Massachusetts male aging study. J Urol, 1994; 151: 54–61.

17 Green R. *Human Sexuality*. Baltimore: Williams & Wilkins, 1975: 22–5.

18 Yee L. Aging and sexuality. Aust Fam Physician, October 2010; 39(10): 718–21.

19 Lindau ST et al. A study of sexuality and health among older adults in the United States. N Engl J Med, 2007; 357: 762–74.

Resources

Jean Hailes Foundation <www.jeanhailes.org.au>

117 Sexually transmitted infections

He who immerses himself in sexual intercourse will be assailed by premature ageing, his strength will wane, his eyes will weaken, and a bad odour will emit from his mouth and his armpits, his teeth will fall out and many other maladies will afflict him.

MOSES BEN MAIMON (1135–1204), *MISHNEH TORAH*

Sexually transmitted infections (STIs) are a group of communicable infections, usually transmitted by sexual contact. STIs that have developed a high profile include chlamydia, the most common notifiable disease in Australia and a major cause of pelvic inflammatory disease (PID), HIV infection, syphilis and multi-drug resistant gonorrhoea. Presentations of STIs are summarised in TABLE 117.1, however most STIs are asymptomatic.

Key facts and guidelines

- In Western society most patients with STIs are in the 15–30 years age group.
- Chlamydia is detected in approximately 1 in 20 young Australians who have screening tests in general practice.[2]
- Not all STIs manifest on the genitals.
- Not all genital lesions are STIs.
- Chlamydia *trachomatis* is the commonest cause of urethritis.
- Up to 50% of men and 75% of women with *Chlamydia* may be asymptomatic.[1]
- Gonorrhoea may cause no symptoms, especially in women.
- STIs such as donovanosis, lymphogranuloma venereum and chancroid occur mainly in tropical countries.
- The presentation of STIs in children, especially vaginitis, should alert practitioners to consider sexual abuse.
- HIV infection, which is predominantly sexually transmitted, should be considered in any person at risk of STIs as well as IV drug users. It must be appreciated that it can present as an acute febrile illness (similar to Epstein–Barr mononucleosis) before going into a long asymptomatic 'carrier' phase.
- All sexually active young people aged 15–29 years should be tested annually for chlamydia with a first-pass urine or genital swab.[2]

Who is at risk of STIs?[3]

- Young people aged 15–29 years
- Men who have sex with men (MSM), especially:
  - unprotected anal sex
  - >10 partners in past 6 months
  - participate in group sex
  - use recreational drugs during sex
  - are HIV-positive
- Aboriginal and Torres Strait Islander people
- Sex workers
- People who inject drugs
- People with a past history of STIs
- People who have unprotected sex with casual partners
- People who have unprotected sex overseas
- Sexual partners of a person with an STI
- Pregnant women (more detail in CHAPTER 108)
- Neonates born to infected mothers

Practice tip

Explain and demonstrate the importance of negotiating condom use.[4]

Asymptomatic STI testing[5]

Since most STIs are asymptomatic, it is important to offer appropriate opportunistic testing to people at risk. A discrete history is also important—a detailed history and examination may serve as a barrier to proceeding to testing. Consider the following questions:

- Before we do a cervical screening test/prescribe your pill, would you also like a chlamydia test?

Table 117.1 Presentations of STIs and causative organisms[1]

Presenting condition	Causative organisms
Urethritis (male) Non-gonoccocal urethritis (NGU):	*Neisseria gonorrhoeae* *Chlamydia trachomatis* *Mycoplasma genitalium* Herpes simplex virus *Trichomonas vaginalis* *Ureaplasma urealyticum* Adenovirus
Epididymo-orchitis	*Chlamydia trachomatis* *Neisseria gonorrhoeae*
Ano-rectal syndromes (proctitis)	*Chlamydia trachomatis* (including *Lymphogranuloma venereum* or *LVG*) *Neisseria gonorrhoeae* *Mycoplasma genitalium* Herpes simplex virus
Vaginal discharge and cervicitis	*Chlamydia trachomatis* *Neisseria gonorrhoeae* *Mycoplasma genitalium* Herpes simplex virus *Trichomonas vaginalis*
PID	Polymicrobial, unidentified cause 70% *Neisseria gonorrhoeae* *Chlamydia trachomatis* *Mycoplasma genitalium*
Ano-genital ulcers	Herpes simplex virus *Treponema pallidum* (chancre) *Klebsiella granulomatis* (donovanosis) *Haemophilus ducreyi* (chancroid)
Ano-genital lumps	Pox virus (molluscum contagiosum) Human papillomavirus (genital warts) *Treponema pallidum* (condylomata lata)
Genital itch	*Phthirus pubis* (pubic lice) *Sarcoptes scabei* (scabies)
Systemic illness	Human immunodeficiency virus (HIV) Hepatitis B Hepatitis A and C (rare sexual transmission) *Treponema pallidum* (syphilis)

- It is recommended that anyone under 30 years of age who is sexually active should have an annual chlamydia test. Would you like a test today?
- I would like to ask you some questions about your sexual activity so we can decide what tests to do, is that okay?

Patients often request to be 'tested for everything' and it is important to explain that certain STIs, in particular genital warts and genital herpes, are not tested for in asymptomatic people. Genital warts is a clinical diagnosis and herpes are diagnosed on a swab of a specific lesion.

Guidelines on STI testing in asymptomatic patients are summarised in TABLE 117.2. Nucleic acid amplification tests (NAATs), such as polymerase chain reaction (PCR), should be employed on swabs in asymptomatic patients. TABLE 117.3 outlines how to test for each infection.

Table 117.2 STI testing in asymptomatic patients[6]

Who?	What infection?	How often?
Young people (age 15–29)	Chlamydia	Annually
	Hepatitis B	Confirm immune status*
Men who have sex with men (MSM)	Chlamydia	Annually, 4 monthly if higher risk
	Gonorrhoea	
	Syphilis	
	HIV	
	Hepatitis A	Confirm immune status*
	Hepatitis B	
	Hepatitis C	If HIV positive
Asymptomatic people requesting STI testing	Chlamydia	Annually
	Syphilis	Frequency according to risk
	HIV	
	Hepatitis B	Confirm immune status*
Aboriginal and Torres Strait Islander people	Chlamydia	Annually
	Gonorrhoea	
	Syphilis	
	HIV	Consider a low threshold for testing
	Hepatitis C	
	Trichomonas	Rural/remote areas
	Hepatitis B	Confirm immune status*
People who inject drugs	Chlamydia	Annually
	Gonorrhoea	
	Syphilis	
	HIV	Frequency according to risk
	Hepatitis C	
	Hepatitis A	Confirm immune status*
	Hepatitis B	
Sex workers	Chlamydia	Frequency according to risk/ requirements
	Gonorrhoea	
	Syphilis	
	HIV	
	Hepatitis B	Confirm immune status*

**Vaccinate if non-immune*

Testing after exposure[1]

Patients may present requesting STI testing following condom breakage or suspected STI exposure/contact. Post-exposure prophylaxis (PEP) for HIV or hepatitis B immunoglobulin and immunisation may be appropriate within 72 hours if moderate to high risk (more detail in CHAPTER 118). Testing should be performed, depending on risk, at the following intervals:

- HIV, syphilis and hepatitis B (if not immune)
  - baseline testing, repeat at 6 and 12 weeks
- chlamydia, gonorrhoea and trichomonas
  - initial screening with swab of any involved orifice, repeat at 2 weeks

Taking a sexual history[1,5]

A detailed sexual history may be important if a patient presents requesting STI testing or if they present with symptoms. Doctors and patients alike usually find discussing sexual matters uncomfortable, even when STI testing is requested. A skilful approach will help overcome barriers or discomfort. A non-judgmental approach and appropriate body language will facilitate patient disclosures on sensitive sexual issues.

- Are you currently in a relationship?
- How many sexual partners have you had in the past 3–12 months?
- Were these casual or regular partners?

Table 117.3 How to test in asymptomatic patients[6]

Infection	Specimen collection	Test
Females		
Chlamydia	Vaginal swab *or* first-pass urine *or* endocervical swab	Chlamydia NAAT (PCR)
Gonorrhoea	Vaginal swab *or* first-pass urine *or* endocervical swab *and* for sex workers: throat swab	Gonorrhoea NAAT (PCR)
Trichomonas	Vaginal swab *or* first-pass urine	Trichomonas NAAT (PCR)
Males		
Chlamydia	First-pass urine *and* for MSM: throat swab, rectal swab	Chlamydia NAAT (PCR)
Gonorrhoea	First-pass urine *and* for MSM: throat swab, rectal swab	Gonorrhoea NAAT (PCR)

Blood tests in females and males

Infection	Test
Syphilis	Syphilis serology
HIV	HIV Ab/Ag
Hepatitis A	Anti-HAV Ig-total
Hepatitis B	Anti-HBc Anti-HBs
Hepatitis C	HCV Ab

Note: All swabs can be self-collected except an endocervical swab, which requires collection by the clinician. First-pass urine is preferably collected at least one hour after last passing urine and does not have to be the first urine of the day.

117

- Were your sexual partners male, female or both?
- When you had sex, was it vaginal, oral or anal sex?
- Did you use condoms?
- Have you ever been diagnosed with or thought you had an STI?

For a detailed STI risk assessment:

- I'd like to ask you about some other activities that could increase someone's risk of some sexually transmitted infections and blood-borne viruses, is that okay?
- Have any of your male partners ever had sex with men?
- Have you ever been paid to have sex?
- Have you ever paid to have sex?
- Have you received any tattoos overseas?
- Have you ever injected drugs and, if so, have you ever shared needles?
- Have you ever been in jail?
- Are you a recent migrant or refugee?

Presenting conditions[1]

Urethritis in men[3]

Urethritis can be classified as gonococcal or non-gonococcal urethritis (NGU). NGU is caused most commonly by *Chlamydia trachomatis* and *Mycoplasma genitalium*, however it is common to not find any cause. Herpes simplex virus (HSV), adenovirus and *Trichomonas vaginalis* are less common causes. *Ureaplasma urealyticum* is another cause which exists as normal urethral flora.

Symptoms

The main symptoms (if present) are:

- a burning sensation when passing urine (dysuria)
- a penile discharge or leakage (clear, white or yellow)

Sometimes there is no discharge, just pain. Most often the symptoms are trivial with chlamydia.

Although a creamy pus-like discharge is typical of gonorrhoea (see FIG. 117.1), and a less obvious milky-white or clear discharge typical of chlamydia (see FIG. 117.2), it is often difficult to differentiate the causes from the discharge. In some males the only complaint is spots on the underpants or dampness under the foreskin.

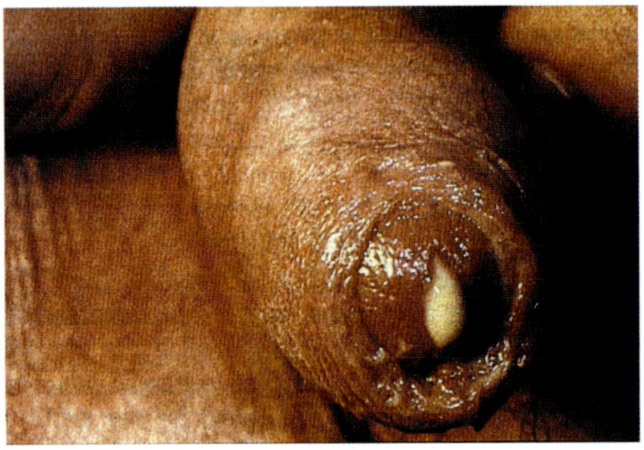

FIGURE 117.1 Gonococcal urethritis: typical purulent discharge

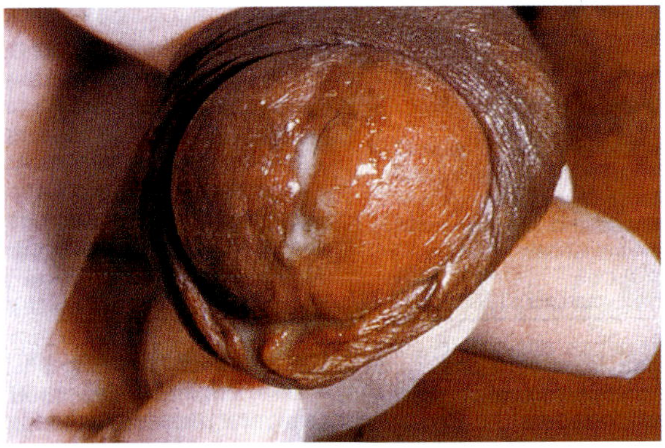

FIGURE 117.2 Chlamydia urethritis: the discharge is usually milky in colour but can also be yellow

Diagnosis

- First-pass urine (FPU) for *Chlamydia* and *Gonorrohoea* NAAT
- Urethral swab for microscopy (for NGU)

Management principles

- Given the prevalence of chlamydia in the community, it is recommended to treat with azithromycin 1 g (o) stat while waiting for other test results.
- If tests are negative and symptoms persist, consider referral for first-pass urine NAAT testing for *Mycoplasma genitalium*, HSV and adenovirus (if not available through general practice).
- Consider seeking specialist advice before treating infection other than chlamydia/gonorrhoea.
- Regardless of results, female partners are at greater risk of PID and require assessment.

Chlamydia

Incubation period

Symptoms appear 1–2 weeks after intercourse, although the incubation period can be as long as 12 weeks or as short as 5 days (compared with incubation period of gonorrhoea—about 2–3 days).

Presentation

50% of men and 75% of women are asymptomatic. Genital and anorectal infections are most common, with rare infections of the eye and oropharynx.

Infection in men can cause urethritis and lead to epididymo-orchitis. In women, infection can cause cervicitis with vaginal discharge and postcoital bleeding. Male symptoms:

- urethritis (dysuria, penile discharge)
- testicular pain
- anorectal symptoms

Female symptoms:

- dysuria
- vaginal discharge
- dyspareunia
- increased dysmenorrhoea
- pelvic pain
- anorectal symptoms

Complications

- epididymo-orchitis and secondary reduced male fertility
- chronic prostatitis
- pelvic inflammatory disease (PID)
- tubal factor infertility and ectopic pregnancy
- chronic pelvic pain
- perinatal conjunctivitis or pneumonia
- reactive arthritis +/− conjunctivitis (rare)

Treatment

For uncomplicated genital or pharyngeal infection:

doxycycline 100 mg (o) 12 hourly for 7 days
or
azithromycin 1 g (o) single dose

For anorectal infection:

doxycycline 100 mg (o) 12 hourly for 7 days if asymptomatic, 21 days if symptomatic

Sexual intercourse must be avoided until 7 days after both partners have received treatment. Reinfection rates are high so retest after 3 months.

Gonorrhoea

Gonorrhoea is most common in MSM, Aboriginal and Torres Strait Islander people living in rural and remote areas, and travellers from endemic areas.

Incubation period

Gonorrhoea has a short incubation period of 2–3 days and symptoms usually appear 2–7 days after vaginal, anal or oral sex. The incubation period can be as long as 3 weeks.

Presentation

Up to 80% of women and 10–15% of men have no genital symptoms and most people are asymptomatic in other sites, especially the pharynx, rectum and endocervix. Upper genital infection can lead to pelvic inflammatory disease in women. Gonococcal urethritis in men is characterised by a purulent urethral discharge.

Other manifestations of gonorrhoea

- epididymo-orchitis and prostatitis (males)
- urethral stricture is not uncommon in males
- perinatal conjunctivitis or pneumonia
- reactive arthritis +/− conjunctivitis (rare)

Investigations

NAATs for gonorrhoea are highly sensitive, however false positives can occur at non-genital sites. Gonococcal culture is not as sensitive but has high specificity and allows for antibiotic susceptibility testing. If an NAAT is positive, a swab should be obtained (if not already collected) for culture to determine antibiotic susceptibility prior to commencing treatment.

Treatment

Alternative treatments are not recommended because of high levels of resistance.

For uncomplicated genital, anorectal or pharyngeal infection:

ceftriaxone 500 mg IM (dissolved in lignocaine 2 mL 1%) as a single dose
plus
azithromycin 1 g (o) as a single dose

Sexual intercourse must be avoided until 7 days after both partners have received treatment. Test of cure 2 weeks after treatment is advisable.

Mycoplasma genitalium[3]

Mycoplasma genitalium should be considered in patients with persistent genital tract symptoms when chlamydia and gonorrhoea have been excluded. It has been recently identified as a cause of urethritis in men, proctitis, cervicitis and PID.

Testing has not been widely available, although access to commercial assays is increasing. NAAT can be performed on vaginal, cervical and rectal swabs or first-pass urine. Testing is only offered to asymptomatic patients if a symptomatic partner has tested positive. 117

Optimal treatment is still unclear with increasing macrolide resistance. Most people diagnosed will have been treated empirically with azithromycin 1 g (o) stat. This is likely to be effective in up to 60% of cases, however specialist advice is required if symptoms persist. Guidelines may soon change to recommend doxycyline as first-line treatment.

Anorectal syndromes (proctitis)

Proctitis is characterised by anal discharge, pain and bowel symptoms including tenesmus and constipation. The most common causes are HSV, *N. gonorrhoea* and *C. trachomatis* (particularly lymphogranuloma venerum, LGV, strains). Other causes include *M. genitalium* and non-STI causes such as inflammatory bowel disease.

It is important to perform an examination and collect swabs at the time. Request NAAT for HSV and *C. trachomatis* and culture and NAAT for *N. gonorrhoea*. LGV should be tested in the event of a positive chlamydia test, which requires the same treatment as symptomatic anorectal chlamydia infection.

Treatment should be empirical, taking into account the clinical picture and likelihood of particular STIs in the patient. Consider a combination of ceftriaxone 500 mg (IM) stat and doxycyline 100 mg (o) BD for 14–21 days, +/− antiviral therapy.[7]

Epididymo-orchitis

Epididymo-orchitis is covered in more detail in CHAPTER 111. Consider chlamydia and gonorrhoea in all sexually active men, especially men aged <35 years.

Vaginal discharge

Vaginal discharge is presented in more detail in CHAPTER 106. The most common cause of vaginal discharge in women of reproductive age is normal physiological discharge. It should be noted that vaginal thrush and bacterial vaginosis are not considered STIs, but can be associated with sex. The pathogens to consider are:

- *Candida albicans* → vaginal thrush
- *Gardnerella vaginalis* → bacterial vaginosis
- *Chlamydia trachomatis*
- *Neisseria gonorrhoeae*
- *Mycoplasma genitalum*
- *Trichomonas vaginalis* (more common in Aboriginal and Torres Strait Islander women, older women and women living in rural and remote areas)

117

Herpes simplex virus may cause vaginal discharge if HSV cervicitis is present.

Cervicitis

Cervicitis is often a forerunner to PID. The likely organisms are *C. trachomatis* or *N. gonorrhoeae*. Others causes include *M. genitalium, T. vaginalis* and HSV. If there is cervicitis only (mucopus at the cervix without uterine pain or tenderness) treat with azithromycin (o) 1 g stat.

Pelvic inflammatory disease

PID is covered in more detail in CHAPTER 103. It is not always an STI. The intra-uterine device is a possible cause. Often multiple pathogens are involved in the infection and 70% of cases have an unidentified cause.

Common pathogens are *N. gonorrhoeae, C. trachomatis* and *M. genitalium.* Swabs from the cervical os frequently underestimate the organisms involved and thus treatment needs to be directed to all possible pathogens.

Specimen collection

- endocervical swabs for NAAT and culture for *N. gonorrhoeae*
- NAAT for *C. trachomatis* and *M. genitalium*

Treatment

Therapy for PID is deliberately vigorous because the major aim is to prevent infertility and the consequent need for assisted reproductive treatment (ART) in the long term. The detailed treatment is outlined in CHAPTER 102.

Summary

Mild to moderate infection:

ceftriaxone 500 mg IM (in 2 mL of 1% lignocaine) or IV (as single dose)
plus
azithromycin 1 g as single dose
plus
metronidazole 400 mg BD for 14 days
plus
doxycycline 100 mg BD for 14 days

Severe PID: hospitalise for IV therapy

Anogenital ulcers

Most genital ulcers are herpes—any small genital ulcer that is superficially ulcerated, scabbed, red-edged, multiple and painful is invariably herpes. Consider herpes zoster if unilateral genital ulcers are present.

STI causes of anogenital ulcers include:

- Herpes simplex virus (HSV 1, HSV 2)
- *Treponema pallidum* (primary chancre)
- *Haemophilus ducreyi* (chancroid)
- *Klebsiella granulomatis* (donovanosis)

Genital ulcers due to primary syphilis and donovanosis are usually painless. Chancroid and donovanosis are rare, almost always imported infections and require specialist input if suspected. Collect a swab of the base of the ulcer or deroofed vesicle and send for NAAT testing, which is available for most causative organisms.

Genital herpes[1]

The incubation period varies from 2–12 days. A microbiological diagnosis is recommended as clinical diagnosis can be unreliable.

HSV 2 is associated with genital lesions and HSV 1 with oral lesions. HSV 1 is an increasingly common cause of a first episode of genital herpes, although recurrent genital herpes is usually caused by HSV 2.[7] Studies suggest that about 12% of Australian adults are infected with HSV 2 and 76% with HSV 1.[8] The majority of patients remain undiagnosed, with mild or asymptomatic recurrences. Once infected with HSV, the virus achieves latency in the nerve roots and is usually a lifelong infection.

Symptoms

With the first attack there is a tingling or burning feeling in the genital area. A crop of small vesicles then appears; these burst after 24 hours to leave small, red, painful ulcers. The ulcers form scabs and heal after a few days. The glands in the groin can become swollen and tender, and the patient might feel unwell and have a fever.

The first attack lasts about 2 weeks if untreated.

Males

The virus usually affects the shaft of the penis, but can involve the glans and coronal sulcus, and the anus (see FIG. 117.3). Other presenting symptoms include painful splitting of the skin, erythema with tingling/itch, urethritis and proctitis.

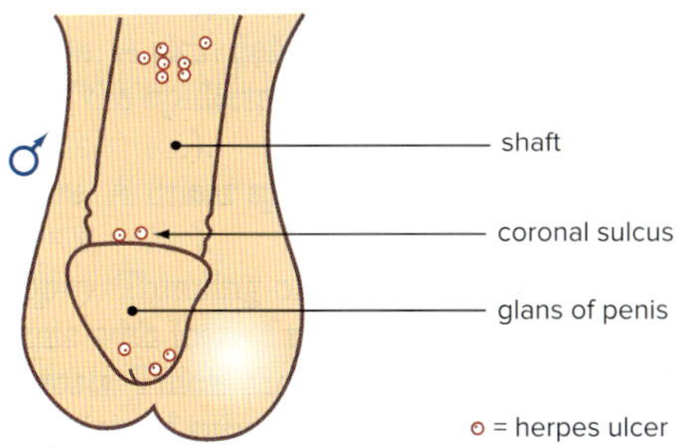

FIGURE 117.3 Usual sites of vesicles/ulcers in males

Females

Vesicles develop around the opening of and just inside the vagina, and can involve the cervix and anus (see FIG. 117.4). Passing urine might be difficult. The cervix may be the only site of lesions and these cases may be asymptomatic or present with symptoms of cervicitis including vaginal discharge. The problem could be a simple tingling around the saddle area or a scratch-like lesion on epithelium.

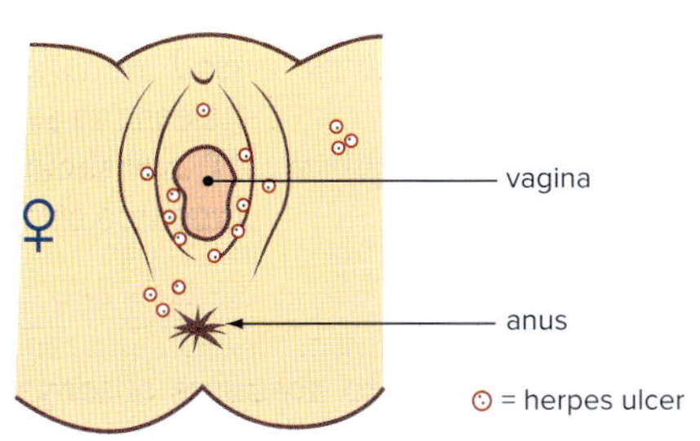

FIGURE 117.4 Usual sites of vesicles/ulcers in females

In both sexes, it can affect the buttocks and thighs. A serious but uncommon complication, especially in females, is the inability to pass urine.

Specimen collection

Take a swab from a deroofed vesicle for NAAT testing. Serological tests for HSV are not recommended.

Transmission[4]

HSV can be caught by direct contact through vaginal, anal or oral sex. Transmission of HSV 1 is usually by contact with saliva and HSV 2 is usually by sexual contact. It can appear spontaneously in people in stable relationships or years after cessation of sexual relationships. 50% of first presentations are not true primary infections.

Most HSV transmissions occur within the first few months of a relationship with asymptomatic viral shredding as the main mechanism. Combined condom use and antiviral therapy reduces the risk of transmission.

Recurrence

It is unlikely for HSV 1 to recur in the genital area. Recurrences of HSV 2 may produce prodromal symptoms prior to an outbreak, including burning, tingling or neuralgia. Fortunately, episodes become milder and less frequent over time and many will stop eventually. Emotional stress is a common trigger.

Treatment (antimicrobial therapy)

Topical treatment[3]

Pain relief can be provided in some patients with topical lignocaine 2% gel but caution is needed since it may cause sensitisation with prolonged use.

Oral treatment—first episode

For the first episode of primary genital herpes:

valaciclovir 500 mg (o) bd for 5–10 days
or
aciclovir 200 mg 8 hourly for 5–10 days

Episodic genital herpes (within 24 hours)

valaciclovir 500 mg (o) bd for 3 days
or
famciclovir 250 mg (o) 4 tablets statim, repeat in 12 hours

Suppressive treatment

Very frequent recurrences (six or more attacks annually) benefit from continuous low-dose therapy for 6 months (e.g. valaciclovir 500 mg (o) once daily). Interrupt at 6 months to evaluate.

117

Supportive treatment (advice to the patient)

- Rest and relax as much as possible. Warm salt baths can be soothing.
- Icepacks or hot compresses can help.
- Painkillers such as paracetamol or ibuprofen may give relief.
- If urination is painful, pass urine under water in a warm bath.
- Wear loose clothing and cotton underwear.

Counselling

'A chat beats medicine for herpes'. Since genital herpes is distressing and recurrent, patients are prone to feel stressed and depressed, and can be assisted by appropriate counselling and support. Sexual abstinence should be practised while lesions are active.

Syphilis

In Australia, syphilis, which has re-emerged, usually presents either as a primary lesion or through chance finding on positive serology testing (latent syphilis).

It is important to be alert to the various manifestations of secondary syphilis (refer to CHAPTER 122). The classification and clinical features of syphilis are presented in TABLE 117.4 (see also CHAPTER 29).

Transmission

- sexual intercourse (usual common mode)
- transplacental to fetus
- direct contact with open lesions (e.g. oral)

Table 117.4 Classification and clinical features of syphilis

Type	Time period	Infectivity	Clinical features
Acquired			
Early (within first 2 years of infection)			
• Primary	10–90 days, average 21	Infectious	Hard chancre Painless Regional lymphadenopathy
• Secondary	2–24 weeks after chancre (average 6)	Infectious	Coarse non-itchy maculopapular rash (usually trunk, palms and soles) Constitutional symptoms (may be mild) Condylomata lata Mucous membrane lesions
• Early latent	Months to 2 years	Infectious	No clinical features but positive serology
Late (after the second year of infection)			
• Late latent	2 years plus	Non-infectious	Risk to unborn fetus
• Tertiary (now rare)		Non-infectious	Late benign: gummas *or* Cardiovascular *or* Neurosyphilis
Congenital			
Early	Within first 2 years of life	Infectious	Stillbirth or failure to thrive Nasal infection: 'snuffles' Skin and mucous membrane lesions
Late	After second year of life	Non-infectious	Stigmata (e.g. Hutchinson teeth) Eye disease CNS disease Gummas

Management

The management of syphilis has become quite complex and referral of the patient to a specialist facility for diagnosis, treatment and follow-up is recommended.

Recommended antimicrobial therapy

Early syphilis (primary, secondary or latent) of not more than two years duration:[7]

benzathine penicillin 1.8 g IM as single dose
or
procaine penicillin 1 g IM daily for 10 days

For patients hypersensitive to penicillin:

doxycycline 100 mg (o) 12 hourly for 14 days

Note:

- sex should be avoided until ulcers are healed
- sexual contacts in the past 3 months should have treatment
- repeat serology at 3 months and then 3 monthly

Late latent syphilis: more than 2 years or indeterminate duration:

benzathine penicillin 1.8 g IM once weekly for 3 doses
or
procaine penicillin daily for 15 days

Sexual contacts in the past 6 months should have treatment. Neurosyphilis and cardiovascular and congenital syphilis are also treated with penicillin but require special regimens.

Anogenital lumps

Common pathogens:

- *Human papillomavirus* (HPV 6 and 11 account for 90%)
- *Molluscum contagiosum* (pox) virus

Uncommon:

- *Treponema pallidum*—condylomata lata

Physiological:

- Fordyce cysts, which are enlarged ectopic sebaceous glands in the mucosa, are a differential diagnosis of a genital lump

Others:

- fixed drug eruptions, aphthous ulcers, trauma, carcinoma, Crohn disease
- be aware of increased risk of HPV-related anorectal cancers in MSM.

Diagnosis

Warts and *Molluscum contagiosum* have a distinctive appearance and are readily diagnosed by inspection (see FIG. 117.5). Removal for diagnosis is usually not required. Condylomata lata are multiple lesions that resemble warts superficially but are covered by abundant exudate. They occur in secondary syphilis and leutic screen is positive.

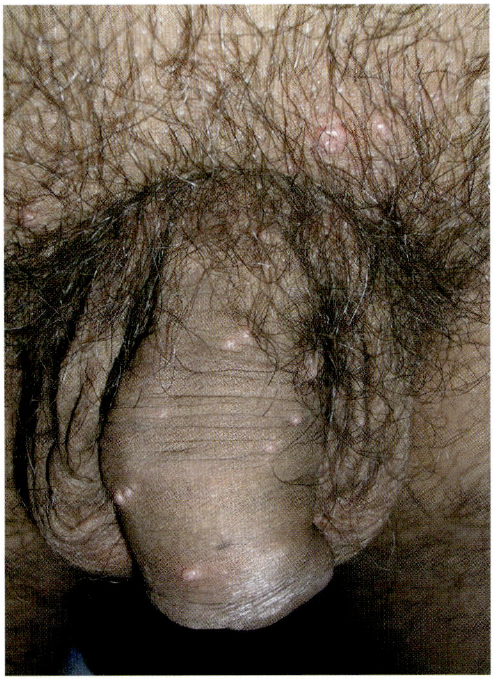

FIGURE 117.5 *Molluscum contagiosum* on and around the penis. They were on the buttocks of his female partner.

Treatment of warts

Warts may be removed by chemical or physical means, or by surgery. Treatment is cosmetic rather than curative and needs to be individualised. For small numbers of readily accessible warts the simplest treatment is:[7]

cryotherapy weekly until resolved
or
podophyllotoxin 0.5% paint or 0.15% cream:
- apply bd with plastic applicator for 3 days
- repeat in 4 days and then weekly for 4–6 cycles if necessary

Note: Paint is more suited for use on external keratinised skin. Cream is best used in perianal area, introital area and under the foreskin.
or

117

topical imiquimod 5% cream applied to each wart by the patient 3 times a week at bedtime (wash off after 6–10 hours) until the warts disappear (usually 8–16 weeks)

If warts are in the pubic region avoid shaving or waxing as this may facilitate local spread by autoinoculation of HPV into areas of microtrauma.

Treatment of *Molluscum contagiosum*[3]

These lesions often resolve spontaneously in immunocompetent patients. There are many treatment choices to provoke resolution. These include:

- cryotherapy with liquid nitrogen (for a few seconds)—can be repeated after several weeks
- podophyllotoxin 0.5% cream or paint twice daily 3 days per week for 4 weeks

Cryotherapy is usually the treatment of choice. If lesions are widespread or severe, refer for expert advice. Other destructive methods such as piercing with a needle, application of phenol or diathermy are seldom performed due to issues of pain and potential scarring.

Itch

Common pathogens:

- *Sarcoptes scabei* (scabies)
- *Phthirus pubis* (pubic lice)
- *C. albicans:*
  - vulvovaginitis—females
  - balanitis—males

C. albicans is not considered an STI but can be associated with sex. Other non-STI itchy rashes on genitals include dermatitis and psoriasis.

Diagnosis

Scabies: inspection on scraping and microscopy. Scabies is diagnosed by a very itchy, lumpy rash. It is rare to find the tiny mites, but it may be possible to find them in the burrows, which look like small wavy lines.

Pubic lice: inspection for moving lice and nits (eggs) on hair shaft.

C. albicans: swab for *Candida* culture.

Treatment

Scabies[9]

permethrin 5% cream if >6 months of age. Apply to whole body from jawline down (include every flexure and area), leave overnight, then wash off.

or

benzyl benzoate 25% emulsion left for 24 hours before washing off. Repeat after 7 days.

Wash clothing and linen after treatment and hang in sun. Repeat treatment in 7 days.The whole family and close contacts must be treated, regardless of symptoms, which can take weeks to develop. Treatment of children younger than 6 months is covered in CHAPTER 120.

Note: Persistence of the itch after treatment is common, which can take 3 weeks or more to resolve. Also prescribe a moderately potent topical corticosteroid +/– an oral antihistamine for the itch.

Pubic lice

permethrin 1% lotion: apply to pubic hair and surrounding area, leave for 20 minutes and then wash off

or

pyrethrins 0.165% with piperonyl butoxide 2% in foam base; apply as above

Shaving pubic hair is also effective. Bed clothes and underwear should be washed normally in hot water after treatment and hung in the sun to dry. Repeat the treatment after 7 days. Sometimes a third treatment is necessary. Sexual contacts and the family must be treated (young children can be infested from heavily infested parents). Where the lice or nits are attached to eyelashes, insecticides should not be used: apply white soft paraffin (e.g. Vaseline) liberally to the lashes bd for 8 days. Then remove the nits with forceps.

Extragenital STIs

Viral hepatitis

Sexual activity is a factor in the transmission of hepatitis B (in particular), hepatitis A (where faecal–oral contact is involved), hepatitis C (rare and mostly in MSM, particularly with HIV) and hepatitis D (rare, in people with hepatitis B only).

Hepatitis A vaccination is recommended to men who have sex with men and people who inject drugs.[6]

Hepatitis B

In Western societies, sexual transmission of HBV is a common mode of spread and there is a higher prevalence in men who have sex with men (MSM), inmates in correctional facilities and injecting drug users. It is also prevalent among Aboriginal and

Torres Strait Islander people living in remote areas and among people from culturally and linguistically diverse populations.

Transmission can be via:

- parenteral contact including intravenous needle sharing and non-sterile tattoo equipment
- horizontal spread via exposure to blood and bodily fluids, including semen and vaginal secretions
- vertical from mother to child (usually intrapartum or perinatal)

Even though studies have shown minute quantities of the virus can be present in saliva, tears and breast milk, they are not considered to be in high enough levels to transmit the virus.

There is no specific therapy for hepatitis B, so prevention through vaccination is important. Antiviral and immunomodulatory drugs, including entecavir, tenofovir or peginterferon alfa-2a, can be used to prevent progression to liver failure and hepatocellular carcinoma.[10]

Immunisation

Hepatitis B immunisation is provided to all Australian children and most people born from the 1990s should have received immunisation. It should be encouraged in hepatitis B marker-free people at risk of acquiring this infection. At-risk groups include Aboriginal and Torres Strait Islander people, MSM, people who inject drugs, sex workers and close contacts of persons with hepatitis B.

Hepatitis C

Sexual transmission of hepatitis C is considered rare but can occur in men who have sex with men, especially men with HIV. Over 90% of newly acquired hepatitis C infections in Australia are attributable to injecting drug use.[12]

HIV infection

Infection with HIV causes chronic immune deficiency which, if untreated, leads to acquired immunodeficiency syndrome (AIDS) after an average period of 10 years after infection.

Male-to-male sex continues to be the major HIV risk exposure in Australia, reported for 68% of HIV diagnoses in 2015, with heterosexual sex reported for 20%, both male-to-male sex and injecting drug use for 5%, and injecting drug use for 3%.[12]

HIV infection is considered in more detail in CHAPTER 27.

Pre-exposure prophylaxis (PrEP) and post-exposure prophylaxis (PEP)

Daily use of coformulated tenofovir and emtricitabine for HIV pre-exposure prophylaxis (PrEP) by populations at high risk of HIV infection is now recommended through the 2015 WHO guidelines.[13]

Post-exposure prophylaxis may be indicated when there is exposure to a known or potential HIV source. Antiretroviral treatment can be taken within 72 hours of exposure to reduce the chance of infection. Consider specialist advice, as every presentation for PEP should be assessed on a case-by-case basis.

When to refer

- Non-gonococcal urethritis:
  - if symptoms do not resolve with treatment
- Gonorrhoea:
  - if complications or symptoms do not resolve with treatment
- Syphilis:
  - early referral or discussion with a sexual health specialist/service is strongly recommended
- HIV:
  - experience in prescribing antiretroviral treatment required
- Genital warts:
  - urethral, cervical warts
  - refractory warts

Contact tracing[5]

Contact tracing is the responsibility of the infected individual but the healthcare provider also has a responsibility to initiate the process. The person infected with an STI should be advised to inform partners that they may have been exposed and should seek testing and treatment. All current partners should be treated simultaneously.

Government guidelines on contact tracing can be found at <www.contacttracing.ashm.org.au>, and include how far back to trace, which varies between conditions. In the case of a positive Chlamydia test, it is recommended to notify partners from the previous 6 months. Assistance from the local sexual health service is recommended for HIV and syphilis because it leads to more contacts being tested and treated.

There are several helpful websites including <www.letthemknow.org.au>, which assist with sending anonymous emails or text messages to contacts.

Patient-delivered partner therapy, which is when the treating clinician provides another prescription for the current partner without a consultation, remains controversial. It should be restricted to times when other means of contact tracing are likely to fail. Clinicians are advised to check with their local health department for advice on the current legislation.

Table 117.5 STIs: Twelve golden rules of management (Sexual Health Society of Victoria)

1	An STI can only be diagnosed if the possibility is considered.
2	An adequate sexual history is paramount.
3	A proper history and careful examination must precede laboratory investigations.
4	Remember the sexual partner(s)!
5	Treatment consists of the appropriate antibiotic in correct dosage for an adequate period of time.
6	A patient concerned about STIs is probably an at-risk patient.
7	Counselling and education are fundamental to STI management.
8	Penicillin will not cure NGU.
9	Not all vaginal discharges are thrush.
10	Multiple, painful genital ulcers are most often due to herpes simplex.
11	Prompt, accurate treatment of PID is necessary to preserve fertility.
12	Remember the three Cs—**C**onsent, **C**onfidentiality and **C**ounselling—of HIV antibody testing.

Good communication

Note: Tests for STIs, including the HIV antibody test, should only be performed with the patient's knowledge and consent, and after adequate counselling. An appointment should be made to give results in person, irrespective of the results.

Patient education resources

Hand-out sheets from *Murtagh's Patient Education* 7th edition:

- Chlamydial urethritis
- Gonorrhoea
- Hepatitis B
- Herpes: genital herpes
- HIV infection and AIDS
- HIV post-exposure prophylaxis
- Lice: pubic lice
- Pelvic inflammatory disease
- Warts: genital warts

References

1 Australian Sexual Health Alliance. *Australian STI management guidelines for use in primary care.* Available from: <www.sti.guidelines.org.au>, accessed March 2018.

2 Royal Australian College of General Practitioners. *Guidelines for Preventive Activities in General Practice* (9th edn). East Melbourne: Royal Australian College of General Practitioners, 2016.

3 Melbourne Sexual Health Centre. *MSHC Treatment Guidelines.* Available from: <www.mshc.org.au>, accessed March 2018.

4 Family Planning NSW. *Reproductive and Sexual Health: An Australian Clinical Practice Handbook* (3rd edn). Sydney: Family Planning NSW, 2016.

5 Bateson D et al. The who, what and from where of STIs: selective testing in asymptomatic patients. Medicine Today, 2012; 13(1): 12–21.

6 NSW STI Programs Unit. STI/HIV testing tool. Available from: <www.stipu.nsw.gov.au/wp-content/uploads/STI-HIV-Testing-Tool-online.pdf>, accessed March 2018.

7 Expert group for Antibiotic guidelines. In: eTG complete. Melbourne: Therapeutic Guidelines Ltd. Available from: <www.tg.org.au>, accessed March 2018.

8 Cunningham AL et al. Prevalence of infection with herpes simplex virus types 1 and 2 in Australia: a nationwide population based survey. Sex Transm Infect, April 2006; 82(2): 164–8.

9 Expert group for Dermatology guidelines. In: eTG complete. Melbourne: Therapeutic Guidelines Ltd. Available from: <www.tg.org.au>, accessed March 2018.

10 Expert group for Gastroenterology guidelines. In: eTG complete. Melbourne: Therapeutic Guidelines Ltd. Available from: <www.tg.org.au>, accessed March 2018.

11 Australian Government Department of Health. Fourth National Hepatitis C Strategy 2014–2017: 3–4. Available from: <www.health.gov.au/internet/main/publishing.nsf/content/A68444CDED77B3A9CA257BF0001CFD80/$File/Hep-C-Strategy2014-v3.pdf>, accessed April 2018.

12 The Kirby Institute. HIV, viral hepatitis and sexually transmissible infections in Australia Annual Surveillance Report 2016. Sydney: The Kirby Institute, UNSW, 2016: 24.

13 Wright E, Grulich A, Roy K. Australasian Society for HIV, Hepatitis and Sexual Health Medicine HIV pre-exposure prophylaxis: clinical guidelines. Journal of Virus Eradication, 2017; 3: 168–84.

Resources

Australian STI Management Guidelines for use in primary care. Australian Sexual Health Alliance 2017. <www.sti.guidelines.org.au>

Intimate parter violence and sexual assault

118

I want to tell people that family violence happens to [anybody], no matter how nice your house is, no matter how intelligent you are.

ROSIE BATTY, 2014

Intimate partner violence is defined by the World Health Organization as 'any behaviour within an intimate relationship that causes physical, psychological or sexual harm to those in the relationship'. Domestic violence emphasises the setting of the violence, whereas family violence is a broader term that includes any violence or abuse that occurs in a family, e.g. elder abuse and adolescent violence against parents.[1]

Intimate partner violence (IPV) is the most common form of violence against women. It occurs in heterosexual and homosexual relationships for both men and women; however, as intimate partner abuse is perpetrated more often against women, this chapter focuses on women (and their children) as victims of abuse.

GPs often say we do not see many patients that have experienced violence. However, it has been estimated that full-time GPs are seeing up to five women per week who have experienced some form of intimate partner abuse in the past 12 months.[2]

A major problem in dealing with IPV is that it is hidden and patients are reluctant to disclose violence when visiting medical practitioners. Another complicating factor is the fact that many patients experiencing abuse and violence may not even be aware that this is the case. Victims stress the importance of a trusting doctor–patient relationship including confidentiality and a non-judgmental attitude.

Key facts and checkpoints[4]

- In Australia, 1 in 4 women are subjected to violence or emotional abuse by an intimate partner at some time.
- Women are nearly three times more likely to have experienced intimate partner violence than men.
- Of the women who are subjected to IPV, approximately a quarter are pregnant at the time and more than half have children in their care.[5]
- Pregnancy is a high-risk time for intimate partner violence.
- Intimate partner violence is the greatest health risk factor for women aged 25–44.
- In Australia, 8 women per day are hospitalised and 1 murdered per month due to IPV.
- Alcohol is a factor in 45% of IPV incidents (i.e. neither the sole cause nor an excuse).[6]
- It is estimated that between 65% and 75% of women killed by abusive partners are killed while leaving or after leaving the relationship.[7]

Practice tip

Safety is the highest priority when working with women who are subjected to violence.

We usually think of domestic violence in terms of physical violence but it can take many forms.[3] These include:

- physical abuse
- emotional and psychological abuse
- economic/financial abuse
- social abuse (e.g. isolation)
- sexual abuse
- stalking
- use of technology to abuse, e.g. sexting
- other controlling behaviour

Possible presentations[3]

In women:

- frequent presentations of non-specific symptoms (e.g. chronic pain, headaches, functional gastrointestinal disorders, sexual dysfunction)
- psychological problems (depression, somatiform disorders, anxiety disorders, panic attacks, PTSD, suicidal ideation)

- insomnia
- eating disorders
- drug and alcohol problems
- physical injuries: usually bruising caused by punching, kicking or biting; also fractures, burns, genital trauma
- pregnancy and childbirth (e.g. unintended pregnancies, forced terminations, miscarriage, poor antenatal care, low birth weight, premature labour)—it is recommended to ask all pregnant women about violence during antenatal care

In children:

- bedwetting, sleeping disorders, anxiety, stress, depression, withdrawal
- aggressive behaviour and language
- problems at school
- chronic somatic problems and frequent presentations
- drug and alcohol abuse
- suicidal ideation in adolescence

Diagnosis

Diagnosing the problem, which is usually 'hidden', can be a challenge to the GP. It is important to set aside common assumptions about the problem and have a high index of suspicion. If you suspect domestic violence—ASK! The doctor has to take the initiative because patients rarely complain about the violence.[7] It is also the doctor's responsibility to ensure the man leaves the room to talk to the woman alone. Possible questions include:

- How are things at home?
- How are things with your partner?
- Do you get scared or frightened of your partner?
- Is there a lot of tension in your relationship?
- Do you feel your views are respected?
- Has your partner ever physically threatened or hurt you?
- Have you ever felt unsafe?

It is advised to universally screen all pregnant women for intimate partner violence.

Practice tip

Screen all pregnant women for intimate partner violence.

Barriers to communication about abuse[8]

- Concerns about confidentiality
- Perceptions about doctors:
  - do not ask directly
  - have no time
  - are not interested
- Embarrassment
- Fear of involving police/courts
- Fear of shaming family
- Fear of partner retaliation

Assessment

- Delineate the problem: pattern of violence; effect on the woman and her children; resources available to women; social/cultural environment.
- Examine and investigate presenting symptoms.
- Check for coexisting injuries (common target areas are breast, chest, abdomen and buttocks). Inspect the ears, teeth and jaw.
- Check the patient's general health status.
- Look for signs of alcohol or drug abuse.
- Keep accurate records and consider taking photographs.
- X-rays may show old fractures.

Women who are subjected to violence

Women who have been subjected to violence come from all socioeconomic and cultural groups. As a rule they enter the relationship as normal, independent and intelligent women but gradually lose self-esteem and become increasingly compliant as a coping strategy. Unfortunately, many victims are led to believe that somehow they deserve their punishment.

Groups of women at greater risk include Aboriginal and Torres Strait Islander women, young women, pregnant women, women separating from their partners, women with disability, women experiencing financial hardship and women who witnessed or were subject to violence as children.[4]

Most women simply want the violence to stop rather than leave their relationships. They are usually constrained from leaving due to financial dependance, feeling they have nowhere to go or for concerns for their children. Often the reason they stay is fear of retaliation. Women may be at various stages of change in terms of taking action in accordance with Prochaska and Di Clemente's model of change (see CHAPTER 21, FIG. 21.4) and the counsellor should be aware of this process.

Men who use violence[9]

Men who use violence come from all walks of life and social and ethnic groups. There are often no distinguishing characteristics to identify a man who will be violent towards his partner. Men who use violence tend to minimise responsibility for their use of violence, blame the victim or external factors and greatly under-report their use of violence.

Perpetrators use abuse and violence to maintain their power and control in a relationship. This is often based on community norms and expectations, along with risk factors including mental disorders, substance abuse, unemployment, poverty and coming from a family where intimate partner abuse occurred.[3] It is important to note that these risk factors are not causal.

Cycle of violence

A predictable pattern that is referred to as the 'cycle of violence' has been identified in many intimate relationships. It is controlled by the perpetrator while the victim feels confused and helpless. The cycle repeats itself with a tendency for the violence to increase in severity (see FIG. 118.1).

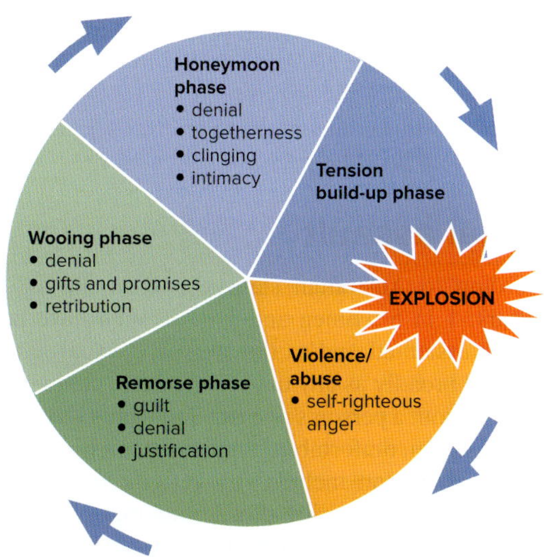

FIGURE 118.1 The cycle of IPV

Management

The key to management is initial recognition of the problem and establishment of empathic caring and support for the woman and family. It must be emphasised that men who use violence (as in most criminal activity) do not readily change their behavioural pattern and thus there is minimal prospect of the violence decreasing unless there is a dramatic reason to change. A management strategy is presented in TABLE 118.1. The immediate safety of women and any children is always the prime working rule.

Table 118.1 Management strategy for domestic violence

Suspect domestic violence, treat any physical injuries

↓

Establish the diagnosis

↓

Assess safety and initiate safety planning

↓

Establish an empathic, trusting relationship

↓

Build the victim's self-esteem and emphasise coping skills

↓

Make effective use of community resources:

- support services
- women's support group
- domestic violence resource centre (in each capital city)
- social services/police
- social workers
- private counsellors and psychologists

Useful strategies[10]

Do:

- talk to the woman alone
- believe her
- validate the decision to disclose
- provide a strong statement that violence is never okay
- reassure her that it is not her fault
- enquire about and express concern for her safety
- give information (i.e. about the course of action available to her, contacts for legal advice)
- acknowledge the complexity of the issue
- respect her right to make her own decisions
- provide follow-up and continued support

118

Harmful strategies

Don't:

- deny domestic violence
- minimise the importance of domestic violence
- blame the victim
- treat with tranquillisers
- refer to a psychiatrist
- refer to marriage guidance, but do refer to specialist counsellors
- set explicit criteria/rules (takes away victim's power yet again)

Dealing with perpetrators

It is uncommon to get the cooperation of the perpetrator in the management process. The perpetrator has to admit that they have a problem before effective counselling can begin. If they do seek help they require counselling by a skilled and experienced practitioner, as treatment will be prolonged and complex. In early intervention, the GP's role is to:[9]

- briefly assess men
- prepare them to accept a referral to a behaviour change program
- undertake alternative interventions to decrease the risk of violence if a referral is not taken up

Safety[3]

Women may not feel safe to go home and may require urgent crisis referral or an urgent safety plan. When assessing a woman's immediate safety, it is important to take the following into account:

- the woman's own assessment of her safety
- presence of risk factors in the perpetrator, including severity and duration of previous violence, history of arrest and incarceration, drug and alcohol use, access to weapons, and unemployment
- your own professional judgment

Where you reasonably believe a patient is in imminent threat of danger, you should seek their consent to report the matter to the police. Children at risk require mandatory reporting to child protection. If a violent incident develops or is imminent, it is important to assist the victim in developing a safety plan. One such plan is:

- Compile a list of emergency numbers.
- Identify family and friends who can provide support.
- Put aside emergency money.
- Pack a bag of clothing, medications and toiletries.
- Organise a safe place to store valuables and important documents.
- Identify a safe place for the woman to go to and how she will get there.
- Ask neighbours to call police if they hear any disturbance.

As a general rule the most effective intervention in arresting the violence is to arrest the violent person.[7] Consider legal interventions such as intervention orders, protection orders (AVOs) and restraining orders.

Continuing care[10]

It is important to keep in mind that the woman's ability to change her situation may be very limited. It is also important to:

- assess safety regularly, checking for escalating violence
- provide emotional support
- ensure confidentiality
- build her self-esteem by acknowledging the coping skills she has developed
- empower her to take control of decision-making: ask what she needs, explore options and present services available
- familiarise yourself with referral services and their processes:
  - domestic violence resource centres
  - relationship services
  - legal aid
  - social workers
  - social services/police
  - private counsellors and psychologists
- have information available for her to take if appropriate
- offer assistance in contacting referral services if this would be of help

Sexual assault

According to Australian statistics, since the age of 15 years, 1 in 5 women and 1 in 20 men have been sexually assaulted and/or threatened.[4] Sexual assault is defined broadly as any unwanted sexual contact that occurs without a person's consent and which makes the victim feel uncomfortable, frightened or threatened. The behaviour can include any activity from sexual harassment through to life-threatening rape.

The majority of perpetrators of sexual assault are known to their victims and a high proportion of perpetrators are current or ex-partners. For this reason, it is important to assess whether the patient is safe to return to their accommodation. Stranger assaults only make up approximately 15% of sexual assault cases.[11]

Survivors of sexual assault should be allowed to accept or decline various assessment or treatment options offered by the practitioner. Many victims do not report sexual assault to police because of fear, humiliation or shame.

Medical practitioners dealing with alleged sexual assault should familiarise themselves with the laws applicable in their state/territory. Self-care for clinicians is also of particular importance when dealing with this distressing problem.

Disclosure of sexual assault

Offer and provide privacy, safety and emotional support. Take the time to explain confidentiality and its limits, so that the patient is aware that the assault will not be discussed with the police or their family without their consent. Believe them, listen to them and be non-judgmental.

Five important things to say:

- I am sorry this happened to you.
- This is a crime—it was not your fault.
- It's good that you have talked to me about this.
- I will do what I can to help you.
- You are safe now (if applicable).

History

Most jurisdictions require that the first person who hears an allegation of sexual assault must give evidence if the complaint comes to trial, so document the exact words used.

If the patient presents following recent sexual assault, the following information will help guide management:[12,13]

- time and place of assault
- brief description of the assault (i.e. what went where)
- condom use
- details of the assailant
- preceding drug or alcohol use
- violence used and any injuries
- current contraception
- risk assessment for patient and any children
- accommodation issues

When patients disclose sexual assault that took place in the past, it is not necessary or advisable to ask all the details about what happened at the first disclosure. The patient may not be ready to tell you details and doing so may easily take them back to their trauma, leading them to decompensate. Let the patient know that you are ready to listen to more details if or when they are comfortable telling you.[14]

Management

A patient may disclose sexual assault immediately or years after the event. Management depends on when the assault occurred.

Recent sexual assault[3]

Management options include:

- forensic examination by a specialist sexual assault service, preferably within 72 hours of the assault—this is still advised if the patient is undecided about reporting the assault
- assessment and treatment of physical injuries
- emergency contraception if indicated
- testing for pregnancy or STIs according to need
- urine or blood drug testing if suspected drug-assisted sexual assault, i.e. when the patient has no memory of events and time or other suspicious circumstances—seek specialist advice
- address safety and supports at home—alternative accommodation may be required
- follow-up—patients may need to return for follow-up at 2 weeks and 3 months following STI checks
- sexual assault counselling and support groups
- ongoing support and monitoring of symptoms of trauma

118

STI testing and prophylaxis

- take swabs and/or first-pass urine for testing gonococcus and chlamydia (PCR)
- take blood for HIV, syphilis and hepatitis B
- collect swabs from the oropharynx or rectum if indicated
- give STI prophylaxis (see TABLE 118.2)—depends on type of assault and assailant; azithromycin for chlamydia prophylaxis is the most commonly used
- at 2 weeks test for chlamydia, gonorrhoea and trichomonas (depending on risk)
- at 6 and 12 weeks, test for HIV, hepatitis B and syphilis

Past sexual assault

The long-term physical and psychological consequences of sexual abuse are many, often somatic or psychological, and can have devastating consequences for the victim. Disclosure to a trusted health professional may be the first step in the healing process. A sensitive response to disclosure can be critical in this process. Offer referral to an experienced

Table 118.2 STI prophylaxis (consider)[11]

Chlamydia	1 g azithromycin (o)
Gonorrhoea (if high risk)	ceftriaxone 500 mg IM *or* where local gonococcal sensitivities permit: ciprofloxacin (500 mg orally) *or* amoxycillin (3 g orally) *and* probenecid (1 g orally)
Hepatitis B (if non-immune)	hepatitis B vaccine (dose 1)
	immunoglobulin IM (if high risk)
Syphilis (if high risk)	benzathine penicillin 1.8 g IM
Trichomonas (if high risk)	metronidazole 1 g (o)
HIV (if high risk)	consult appropriate physician

therapist or sexual assault specialist counselling service, with access to up-to-date knowledge about relevant reporting and legal processes.[14]

References

1. Long D, Lee S, Coles JY. Family violence: an illustrated guide to the terminology. Med J Aust, 2017; 207(6): 270.
2. Hegarty K, Bush R. Prevalence and associations of partner abuse in women attending general practice: A cross-sectional survey. Aust NZ J Public Health, 2002; 26(5): 437–42.
3. RACGP. *Abuse and Violence: Working with Our Patients in General Practice* (4th edn). Melbourne: The Royal Australian College of General Practitioners, 2014: 1–39.
4. Australian Institute of Health and Welfare. Family, domestic and sexual violence in Australia. Canberra: AIHW, 2018.
5. Campo M. Domestic and family violence in pregnancy and early parenthood. CFCA, December 2015: ix–xii.
6. Mouzos J, Makkai T. Women's experience of male violence: Findings from the Australian component of the International Violence Against Women survey. Canberra: Australian Institute of Criminology, 2004.
7. Hegarty K. Domestic violence: how to treat. Australian Doctor, 20 February 2009: 29–36.
8. Rodriguez MA et al. The factors associated with disclosure of intimate partner abuse to clinicians. J Fam Pract, 2001; 50(4): 338–44.
9. Hegarty K et al. Identifying and responding to men who use violence in their intimate relationships. Aust Fam Physician, April 2016; 45(4): 176–81.
10. Australian Medical Association. Supporting patients experiencing family violence. May 2015: 6–9. Available from: <https://ama.com.au/article/ama-family-violence-resource>, accessed April 2018.
11. Australian Bureau of Statistics. Personal Safety Survey. Canberra: Australian Bureau of Statistics, 2016. Available from: <www.abs.gov.au/ausstats/abs@.nsf/mf/4906.0>, accessed April 2018.
12. Mein JK et al. Management of acute adult sexual assault. Med J Aust, 2003; 178: 226–30.
13. Howlett M. Clinical assessment of sexual assault. O&G Magazine, Summer 2017; 19(4): 26–8.
14. Kinsella P, Uebergang M. Disclosures of sexual abuse: what do you do next? Aust Fam Physician, March 2015; 44(4): 122–4.

Resources

Hindmarsh E, Roberts G (eds). RACGP Manual: *Abuse & Violence, Working with Our Patients in General Practice* (The White Book) (PDFIMB).

National Sexual Assault, Domestic Family Violence Counselling Service. 1800 RESPECT (call 1800 737 732). <www.1800respect.org.au>, accessed April 2018.

Part 9

Problems of the skin

119 A diagnostic and management approach to skin problems

The skilful doctor knows by observation, the mediocre doctor by interrogation, the ordinary doctor by palpation.

CHANG CHUNG-CHING (C. 170–196 CE)

The diagnosis of skin problems depends on astute clinical skills based on a systematic history and examination and, of course, experience. If the diagnosis is in doubt, it is appropriate to refer the patient to a skilled cooperative consultant, as the referral process is an excellent educational opportunity for the GP. Another opinion from a colleague/s in a group practice is also very educative. At least, cross-referencing the skin lesion with a colour atlas facilitates the learning process.

Terminology of skin lesions

Primary lesions

- *Macule.* Circumscribed area of altered skin colour (Latin for stain) without elevation <1 cm diameter (see FIG. 119.1).
- *Patch.* Macule of >1 cm diameter (see FIG. 119.1).
- *Papule.* Palpable mass on skin surface <0.5 cm diameter (see FIG. 119.2).
- *Maculopapule.* A raised and discoloured circumscribed lesion.
- *Nodule.* Circumscribed palpable mass >0.5 cm diameter (see FIG. 119.2).
- *Plaque.* A flat-topped palpable mass >1 cm diameter.
- *Wheal.* An area of dermal oedema (can be any size), which is pale and compressible.
- *Angio-oedema.* A diffuse area of oedema extending into subcutaneous tissue.
- *Vesicle.* A fluid-filled blister <0.5 cm in diameter (see FIG. 119.3).
- *Bulla.* A vesicle >0.5 cm diameter (see FIG. 119.3).
- *Pustule.* A visible collection of pus in the skin <1 cm diameter.
- *Abscess.* A localised collection of pus in a cavity >1 cm diameter.
- *Furuncle.* A purulent infected hair follicle; includes:
  - folliculitis (small furuncles)
  - boils (larger furuncles)
- *Carbuncle.* A cluster of boils discharging through several openings.
- *Purpura.* A circumscribed deposit of blood >0.5 cm in diameter. May be macular or papular.
- *Petechiae.* Purpuric lesions <0.5 cm in diameter.
- *Ecchymosis.* Larger purpuric lesion.
- *Haematoma.* A swelling from gross bleeding.
- *Telangiectasia.* Visible dilatation of small cutaneous blood vessels.
- *Comedo.* A plug of keratin and sebum in a dilated pilosebaceous gland.
- *'Blackhead'.* An open comedo.
- *'Whitehead'.* A closed comedo.
- *Erythema.* Redness of the skin due to increased vascularity.
- *Milium.* Tiny white cyst containing keratin, from occlusion of pilosebaceous gland.
- *Papilloma.* Warty projection above the skin surface.

Secondary lesions

- *Scales.* An accumulation of excess keratin that presents as flaking.
- *Crusts (scabs).* Superficial dried secretions (serum and exudate).

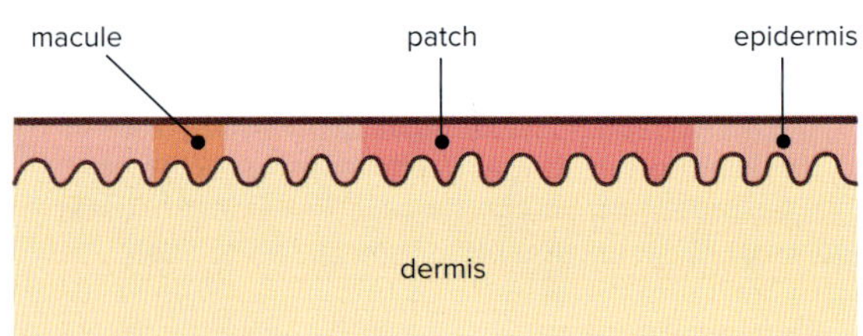

FIGURE 119.1 Macule and patch

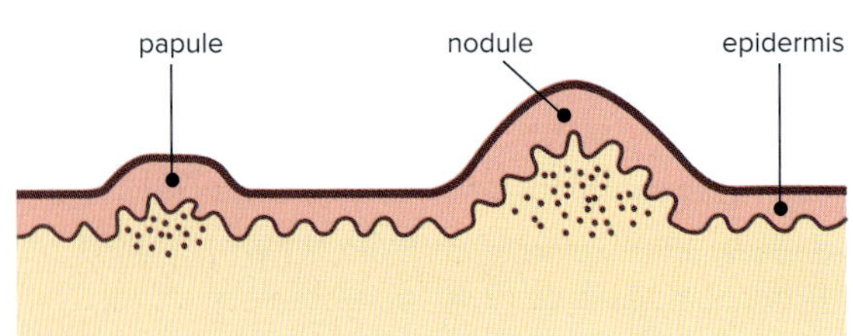

FIGURE 119.2 Papule and nodule

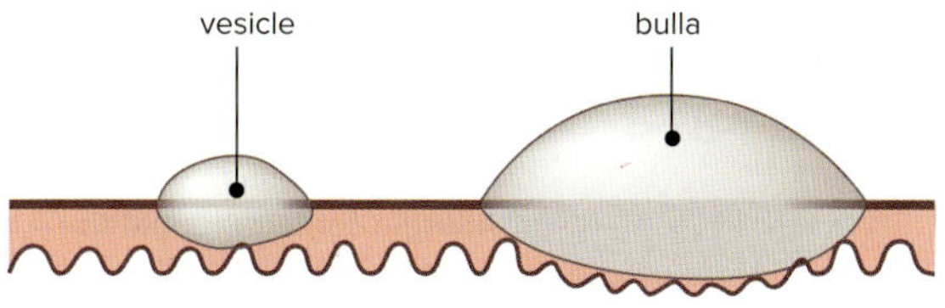

FIGURE 119.3 Vesicle and bulla

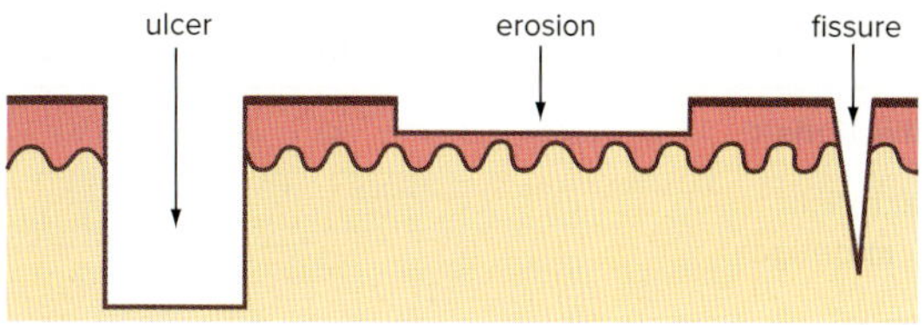

FIGURE 119.4 Ulcer, erosion and fissure

- *Ulcer.* A circumscribed deep defect with loss of all the epidermis and part or all of the dermis (see FIG. 119.4); they usually heal with scarring.
- *Erosion.* A skin defect with complete or partial loss of the epidermis; they heal without scarring (see FIG. 119.4).
- *Fissure.* A linear split in the epidermis and dermis (see FIG. 119.4).
- *Atrophy.* Thinning or loss of epidermis and/or dermis with loss of normal skin markings.
- *Sclerosis.* Thickening of the dermis with induration of subcutaneous tissue; resembles a scar but may arise spontaneously (e.g. scleroderma).
- *Scar.* A healed dermal lesion where normal structures are replaced by fibrous tissue.
- *Hypertrophic scar.* Rises above the skin surface.
- *Atrophic scar.* Settles below the skin surface.
- *Keloid.* Overgrowth of dense fibrous tissue extending beyond the original wound.
- *Excoriation.* Scratch marks causing an erosion or an ulcer (loss of epidermis).
- *Acanthosis.* Thickening of skin without accentuation of skin markings.
- *Lichenification.* Thickening secondary to chronic scratching or rubbing (in dermatitis).
- *Callus.* Localised hypertrophy of the stratum corneum.
- *Exfoliation.* Loss of epidermal keratin as large scales or sheets.
- *Keratoderma.* Thickening of skin especially stratum corneum.

A diagnostic approach

The diagnostic approach of Robin Marks[1] presented here helps to achieve order in the midst of confusion. He describes the importance of simplifying the diagnostic process by being a 'lumper' rather than a 'splitter'. Most common dermatological problems fall into one of seven categories (see TABLE 119.1). A problem that does not fit into one of these seven groups is either an unusual condition or an unusual presentation of a common condition and probably merits a consultant's opinion.

Note: TABLES 119.1 to 119.6 were prepared by Professor Robin Marks[1] and are reproduced with his permission.

Defining terms

Terms that are continually referred to in skin disease include the following:

Seborrhoeic	Yellow-brown and waxy	
Nummular	Coin-like	} (interchangeable)
Discoid	Disc-like	
Annular	Ring-like	
Circinate	Circular	
Arcuate	Curved	
Reticulate	Net-like	
Pityriasis (*pityron* = bran)	Fine, bran-like scaly desquamation or powdery	
Guttate	'Dew drop'	
Rosea	Rose-coloured	
Morbilliform	Like measles	
Morphoea	Circumscribed scleroderma or skin infiltrate	
Livido	Cyanotic discolouration	
Lichen	Any papular skin disorder resembling lichens	
Verrucous	Rough and warty	

History

The three basic questions are:[1]

1 Where is the rash and where did it start?
2 How long have you had the rash?

Note: The split into three time zone groups (see TABLE 119.2) is very useful. This question leads on to the next question regarding itch, as the patient is unlikely to tolerate an itchy eruption.

3 Is the rash itchy?
If so, is it mild, moderate or severe? The nature of the itch is very helpful diagnostically. A severe itch is one that wakes the patient at night and leads to marked excoriation of the skin, while a mild

119

Table 119.1 Common dermatological conditions

Infections

Bacterial:
- impetigo

Viral:
- warts
- herpes simplex, herpes zoster
- pityriasis rosea
- exanthemata

Fungal:
- tinea
- candidiasis
- pityriasis versicolor

Acne
Psoriasis
Atopic dermatitis (eczema)
Urticaria

Acute and chronic
Papular:
- pediculosis
- scabies
- insect bites

Sun-related skin cancer
Drug-related eruptions

itch is one that is only slightly upsetting for the patient and may not be noticeable for significant periods during the day.

Three questions the doctor must consider

1 Could this be a drug rash?
2 Has this rash been modified by treatment?
3 Do any contacts have a similar rash?

Further questions for the patient

- Do you have contact with a person with a similar eruption?
- What medicines are you taking or have you taken recently?
- Have you been exposed to anything different recently?
- Do you have a past history of a similar rash or eczema or an allergic tendency (e.g. asthma)?
- Is there a family history of skin problems?

The nature of itching[1]

The characteristics of the itch are very useful in dividing up the diagnoses: an eruption that is not itchy is unlikely to be scabies and one that is very itchy is unlikely to be a skin tumour (see TABLE 119.3).

However, nothing is absolute and variations to the rule will occur—tinea, psoriasis and pityriasis

Table 119.2 How long has the rash been present?

Acute (hours–days)	Urticaria Atopic dermatitis Allergic contact dermatitis Insect bites Drugs Herpes simplex/zoster Viral exanthemata
Acute → chronic (days–weeks)	Atopic dermatitis Impetigo Scabies Pediculosis Drugs Pityriasis rosea Psoriasis Tinea *Candida*
Chronic (weeks–months)	Psoriasis Atopic dermatitis Tinea Pityriasis versicolor Warts Cancers Skin infiltrations (such as granulomata, xanthomata)

Table 119.3 Is the rash itchy?

Very	Urticaria Atopic dermatitis Scabies, pediculosis Insect bites Chickenpox (adults) Dermatitis herpetiformis Grover disease
Mild to moderate	Tinea Psoriasis Drugs Pityriasis rosea *Candida* Stress itching/lichen simplex
Often not	Warts, tinea Impetigo, psoriasis Cancers Viral exanthemata Seborrhoeic dermatitis

versicolor are sometimes itchy and sometimes not. Chickenpox can vary from being intensely itchy, especially in adults, to virtually no itching.

Relieving or aggravating factors of the itch provide useful diagnostic guidelines; for example, Whitfield's ointment applied to an itchy eruption for a provisional diagnosis of ringworm would make the itch worse if it were due to eczema.

Examination[1]

Examine the skin in good light, preferably natural light, and ensure that any make-up is removed.

There are two basic stages in the physical examination of a rash. The first is an assessment of the characteristics of the individual lesion and the second is the distribution or pattern of the lesions.

Characteristics of the individual lesion

The single most important discriminating feature is whether it involves the dermis alone or the epidermis as well (see TABLE 119.4). If the lesion involves the epidermis there will be scaling, crusting, weeping, vesiculation or a combination of these (see FIG. 119.5). If the dermis alone is involved, the lesion is by definition a lump, a papule or a nodule (see FIG. 119.6). No lesion ever involves the epidermis without involving the dermis as well.

Other characteristics of individual lesions that must be sought are the colour, the shape and the size. It is important to feel the skin during the physical examination and to note the consistency of the lesion. Is it firm or soft? The activity of the lesion may also be useful: does it have a clearing centre and an active edge?

Distribution of the lesions

The clinician must decide whether the lesions are localised or widespread. If they are widespread, are they distributed centrally, peripherally, or both? (See TABLE 119.5.) Diagnosis is often helped when the skin lesions are in a specific area (see TABLE 119.6 and FIGS 119.7 and 119.8). Itchy papules on the penis associated with a widespread pruritus are likely to be scabies. However, care has to be taken because many misdiagnoses are made instinctively on the distribution (e.g. anything in the flexures is dermatitis or anything on the feet is tinea).

Table 119.4 Appearance of individual lesions

Epidermal	Atopic dermatitis Psoriasis Tinea Pityriasis rosea Impetigo, herpes, warts Cancers Scabies Solar keratoses
Dermal	Urticaria Insect bites, pediculosis, scabies Drugs Skin infiltrations Viral exanthemata

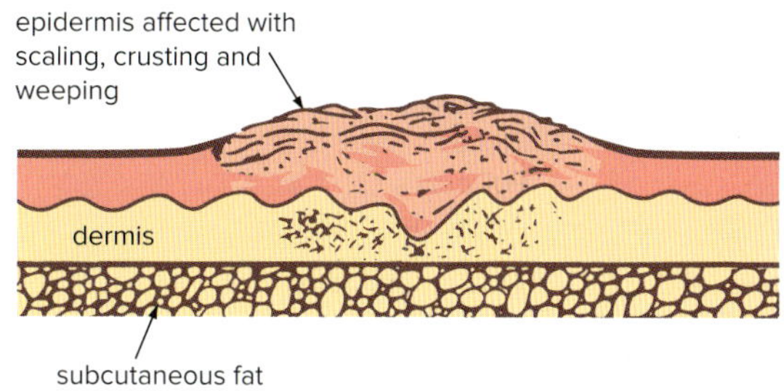

FIGURE 119.5 Epidermal skin lesion

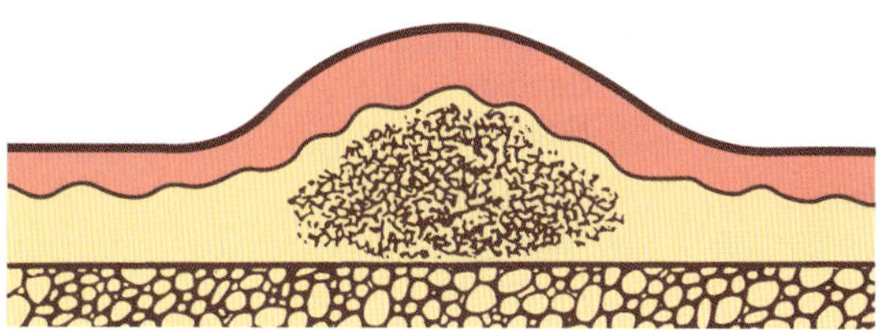

FIGURE 119.6 Dermal skin lesion

Table 119.5 Distribution of the rash

Widespread	Atopic dermatitis Psoriasis Scabies Drugs Urticaria
Central trunk (initially at least)	Pityriasis versicolor Herpes zoster Seborrhoeic dermatitis Guttate psoriasis Pityriasis rosea Viral exanthemata
Peripheral	Atopic dermatitis Herpes zoster Tinea Psoriasis Warts Insect bites

119

119

Table 119.6 Specific areas affected

Face	Rosacea Impetigo Psoriasis Atopic dermatitis Photosensitive (e.g. drugs) Herpes simplex Acne vulgaris Cancers Viral exanthemata
Scalp	Psoriasis Seborrhoeic dermatitis Pediculosis Tinea Folliculitis Atopic dermatitis
Flexures	Atopic dermatitis Psoriasis Seborrhoeic dermatitis Tinea *Candida* Pediculosis
Mouth	Aphthous ulcers Herpes simplex *Candida* Measles
Nails	Psoriasis Tinea Dermatitis
Penis	Scabies Genital herpes and warts *Candida* Psoriasis

Another feature of an eruption, which should be sought on examination, is whether the lesions are all at the same stage of evolution.

It is necessary to perform a complete physical examination as well. There is, after all, no such thing as a skin disease but rather disease affecting the skin. The clinician must always bear this in mind when managing patients complaining of a skin eruption. Disease does not affect the skin in isolation and it is unforgivable to look only at the skin and ignore the patient as a whole.

Note: In every case examine the mouth, scalp, nails, hands and feet.

Diagnostic tools

Appropriate diagnostic tools include:

- a magnifying lens
- a diascope, which is a glass slide or clear plastic spoon that is used to blanch vascular lesions in order to determine their true colour
- a 'Maggylamp', which is a hand-held fluorescent light with an incorporated magnifier; the device allows shadow-free lighting and magnification
- a dermatoscope, which is very valuable in the diagnosis of pigmented tumours but it does require skill and familiarity to achieve effective use
- Wood's light
- swabs for culture and NAAT test (PCR)
- skin scrapings or nail clippings for dermatophyte culture
- skin biopsy (even with psoriasis, etc.)

Office tests and diagnostic aids

Wood's light

Wood's light examination is an important diagnostic aid for skin problems in general practice. It has other uses, such as examination of the eye after fluorescein staining. (A low-cost, small ultraviolet light unit called 'the black light' is also available.)

Method

Simply hold the ultraviolet light unit above the area for investigation in a dark room.

Limitations of Wood's light in diagnosis

Not all cases of tinea capitis fluoresce because some species that cause the condition do not produce porphyrins as a by-product. See TABLE 119.7 for a list of the skin conditions that do fluoresce. Wood's light is really only useful for hair-bearing areas.

Porphyrins wash off with soap and water, and a negative result may occur in a patient who has shampooed the hair within 20 hours of presentation. Consequently, a negative Wood's light reading may be misleading. The appropriate way of confirming the clinical diagnosis is to send specimens of hair and skin for microscopy and culture.

Table 119.7 Skin conditions that produce fluorescence in Wood's light

Tinea capitis	Green/bright yellow (in hairs)
Erythrasma	Coral pink
Pityriasis versicolor	Pink–gold
Pseudomonas spp.	Yellowish-green
Porphyria cutanea tarda	Red (urine)

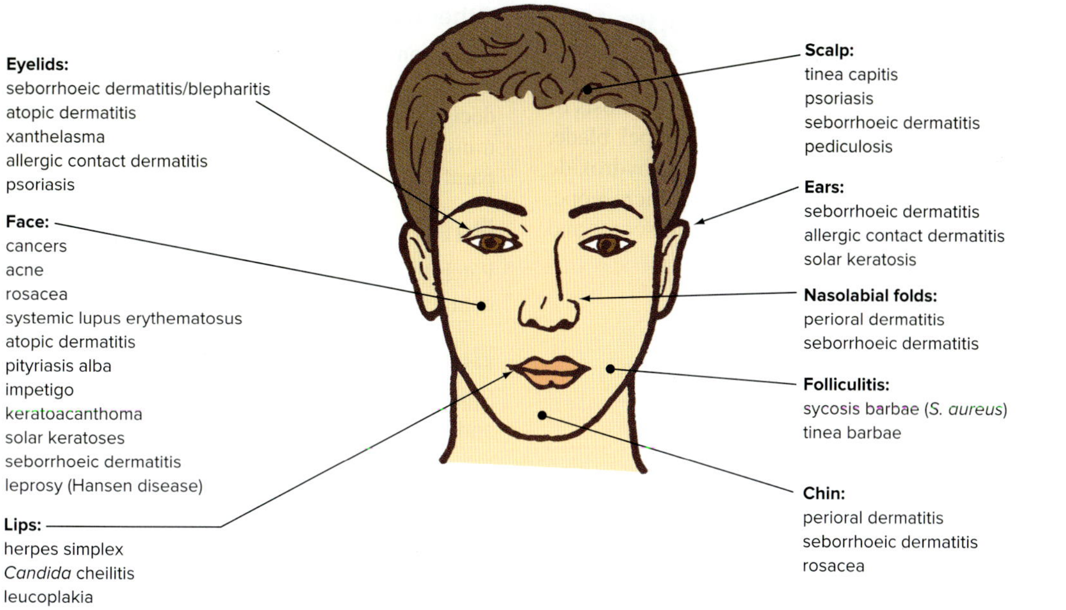

FIGURE 119.7 Typical sites on the face affected by the skin conditions indicated

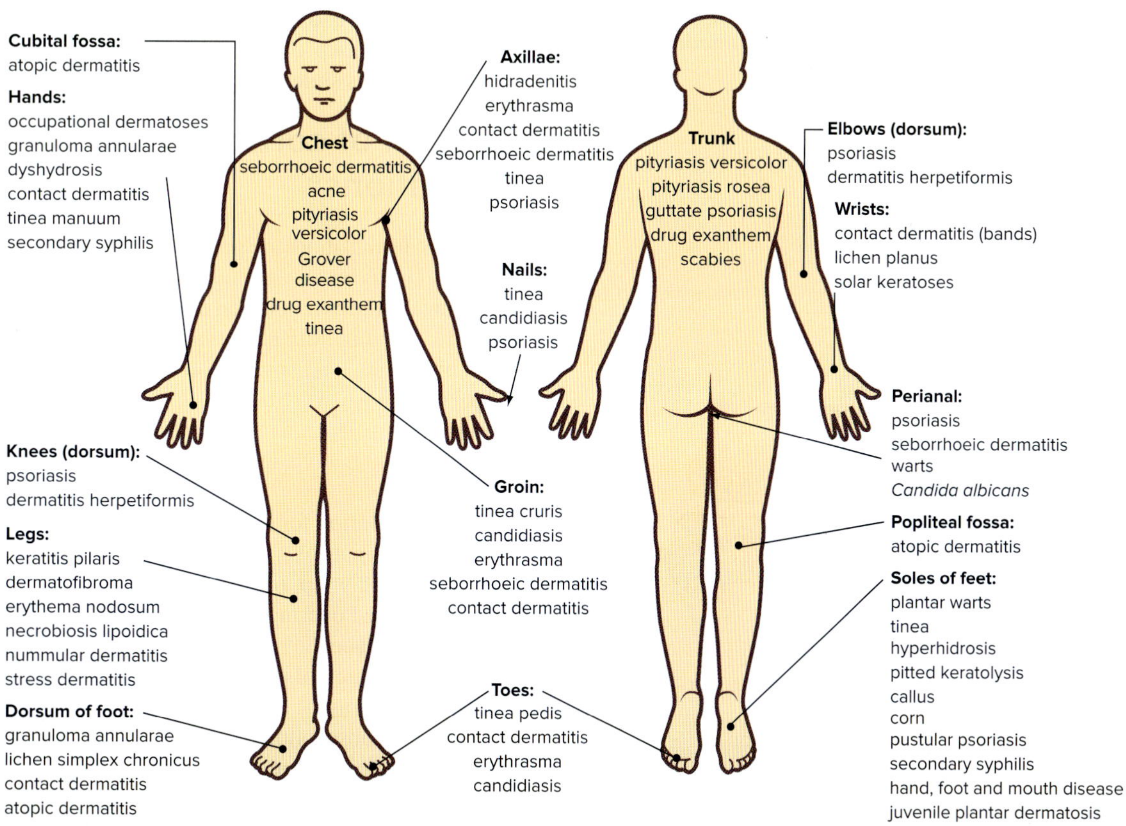

FIGURE 119.8 Typical regional location of various skin conditions

*Same conditions apply to chest and trunk

Skin scrapings for dermatophyte diagnosis

Skin scrapings are an excellent adjunct to diagnosis of fungal infections. Requirements are a scalpel blade, glass slide and cover slip, 20% potassium hydroxide (preferably in dimethyl sulphoxide) and a microscope. Skin scrapings can also be sent for microscopy and culture.

Clinical indications:

1. tinea (superficial dermatophyte infection)
2. pityriasis versicolor
3. *Candida*

Method

- Scrape skin from the active edge.
- Scoop the scrapings onto the glass microscope slide.
- Cover the sample with a drop of potassium hydroxide.
- Cover this with a cover slip and press down gently.
- Warm the slide and wait at least 5 minutes for 'clearing'.

119

Microscopic examination

- Examine at first under low power with reduced light.
- When fungal hyphae are located, change to high power.
- Use the fine focus to highlight the hyphae (see FIG. 119.9).

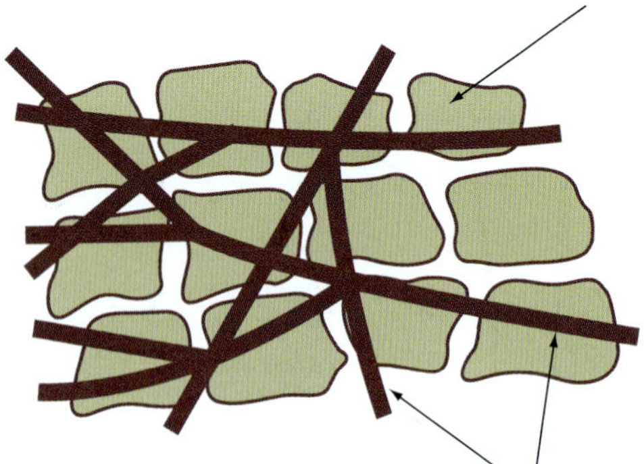

FIGURE 119.9 Diagrammatic representation of microscopic appearance of fungal hyphae

Note: Some practice is necessary to recognise hyphae.

Other uses of microscopy

Detection of the scabies mite: the burrow of the scabies mite is found (can be difficult!) and the epidermis is decisively scraped with a no. 15 scalpel blade, and transferred to a slide after adding a drop of liquid paraffin. The mite is very distinctive.

Patch testing

Patch testing is used to determine allergens in allergic contact dermatitis. Read in 48 hours.

Biopsies

Shave or punch biopsies can be useful (see FIGS 124.26 and 124.27 in CHAPTER 124).

Hair[2]

Send hair samples for microscopy and root analysis. There are two main tests:

1. the hair pull test (refer CHAPTER 126)
2. the hair pluck test

In the hair pluck test (used for tinea capitis and hair shaft disorder), a tuft of about 20 hairs is drawn out, forceps applied close to the skin of the scalp and rotated slightly prior to sharp extraction. The hair should be collected on a glass slide for counting and analysis.

Selection of corticosteroid preparations[3]

- Ointment formulations are generally more potent than creams. This is because the occlusive nature of an ointment enhances absorption of the corticosteroid.
- Creams contain more preservatives and excipients than ointments, and so are more likely to cause hypersensitivity or irritation.
- Ointments are generally recommended over creams.
- A cream base may be used for an acute weeping rash.
- Use a gel or lotion for hair-bearing areas.
- Stubborn dermatoses may benefit from occlusion, such as plastic wrap, occlusive dressings or gloves, applied overnight with appropriate securing in place.
- Choose a potency of corticosteroid appropriate to the site of the rash.
- The greatest absorption occurs through thin skin of eyelids, genitals and skin creases, where a mild corticosteroid should be used.
- The least absorption occurs through the thick skin of palms and soles, where a potent corticosteroid should be used.

- Use a moderately potent corticosteroid on the rest of the limbs and trunk.
- For *Candida* infection (e.g. secondary infection of irritant napkin dermatitis), mix 1% hydrocortisone in equal quantities with an antifungal preparation such as nystatin.

Terminology of topical skin preparations

Antipruritic agent One that relieves itching. Examples are:

- menthol (0.25%)
- phenol (0.5%)
- coal tar solution (2–10%)
- camphor (1 or 2%)

Base or vehicle A mixture of powders, water and greases (usually obtained from petroleum). The relative blending of these compounds determines the nature of the base (e.g. lotion, cream, ointment, gel or paste).

Cream A suspension of a powder in an emulsion of oil and water with the addition of an emulsifying agent. Usually applied to normal or moist skin.

Emollient A topical preparation of emulsified oils and fatty acids that is softening or soothing to the skin. It replaces natural oils in the stratum corneum. It also acts as a skin moisturiser and is therefore used on dry skin or dermatoses related to dry skin (e.g. atopic dermatitis). Examples are:

- emulsifying ointment
- sorbolene cream
- aqueous cream

Emulsion A mixture of two immiscible liquids, one being dispersed throughout the other in small droplets.

Gel A viscous substance with a greaseless, water-miscible base.

Humectant A chemical-containing agent that attracts and retains water due to its hygroscopic or osmotic properties. Examples are:

- urea 10% cream
- glycerol 10% cream

Keratolytic An agent that softens or breaks up keratin. Examples are:

- urea 10%—for xerosis or keratosis pilaris
- urea 20%—cracked palms and soles
- salicylic acid 2–10%
- alpha-hydroxy acids (e.g. lactic acid, propylene glycol)

Lotion A suspension of an insoluble powder in water. Modern lotions use an emulsifying agent, which eliminates the need to shake the lotion. An example is calamine lotion (zinc oxide 5, calamine 15, glycerine 5, water to 100).

Moisturiser An agent that increases the water content of the stratum corneum and reduces itching. Classified as:

- emollient
- humectant, and
- occlusive (e.g. white soft paraffin: Vaseline)

Ointment A suspension of a substance in an oily vehicle. Generally used for dry scaly skin.

Paint and tincture A rapidly drying liquid preparation that is very useful for intertriginous areas, especially between the toes and in the natal cleft. 'Tincture' is the preparation when alcohol is the vehicle. Example: podophyllin in tinct. benz. co. (for genital warts).

Paste Similar to ointment in composition but is more viscid. A paste consists of an ointment to which another agent, such as starch, has been added. They dry and protect.

Topical corticosteroids for chronic dermatoses

- Assure patients and parents that the benefits of topical corticosteroids outweigh the harms, and that they should not be afraid to use them.
- Once daily use is usually sufficient and encourages concordance with therapy.
- Apply liberally, not sparingly.
- Use on all areas of inflammation until the skin is perfectly clear.
- Maintain remission by using an emollient often.
- Resume topical corticosteroids promptly to control periodic flares.
- Avoid high-potency preparations on the face, in flexures and on infants.
- Corticosteroids can mask or prolong an infection.
- Adverse effects of long-term use are rare and include skin atrophy, striae, peri-oral dermatitis and steroid rosacea.

The relative clinical potency of topical corticosteroids is given in TABLE 119.8.

Skin tips

- Do no harm. Introduce the mildest possible preparation to alleviate the problem.
- Creams tend to be drying, lotions even more so.

Table 119.8 Potency ranking of the most commonly used topical corticosteroid preparations in Australia[3]

Generic name	Formulation
Group I Mild	
Desonide 0.5%	Lotion
Hydrocortisone 0.5%, 1%	Cream, ointment
Group II Moderately potent	
Betamethasone valerate 0.02%	Cream
Betamethasone valerate 0.05%	Cream, ointment
Clobetasone butyrate 0.05%	Cream
Triamcinolone acetonide 0.02%, 0.05%	Cream, ointment
Group III Potent	
Betamethasone valerate 0.1%	Cream, ointment
Betamethasone dipropionate 0.05%	Cream, ointment, lotion
Methylprednisolone aceponate 0.1%	Cream, ointment, fatty ointment, lotion
Mometasone furoate 0.1%	Cream, ointment, lotion, hydrogel
Group IV Very potent	
Betamethasone dipropionate 0.05% (in optimised vehicle)	Cream, ointment
Clobetasol propionate 0.05%	Cream*, ointment*, lotion*, shampoo

*Not available in Australia.

119

- Ointments tend to reduce dryness and have greater skin penetration. If wet—use a wet dressing (wet soaks and a lotion). If dry—use an ointment (salve).
- Occlusive dressings with plastic wraps permit more rapid resolution of stubborn dermatoses.
- Most toilet soaps are alkaline and are very drying; they should not be used on dry skin or dermatitis with dry skin. Soap substitutes include neutral soaps (Dove, Neutrogena), superfatted soaps (Oilatum) and non-soap cleanser (Cetaphil).
- Bath additives can be useful for dermatoses such as psoriasis, atopic dermatitis and for pruritus. For some people it may be better not to add it to the bath (diluting effect; accident from slipping) but to massage the oil into the dry itchy skin after the bath.
- Always give careful instructions to the patient regarding application of preparations: use a prepared handout if available.
- Alter the treatment according to the response.
- Explain the costs involved, especially where a preparation is expensive.

Rules for prescribing creams and ointments

How much?[4]

On average, 30 g of cream will cover the body surface area of an adult. The 'rule of nines', used routinely to determine the percentage of body surface area affected by burns (see FIG. 119.10), may also be used to calculate the amount of a topical preparation that needs to be prescribed.

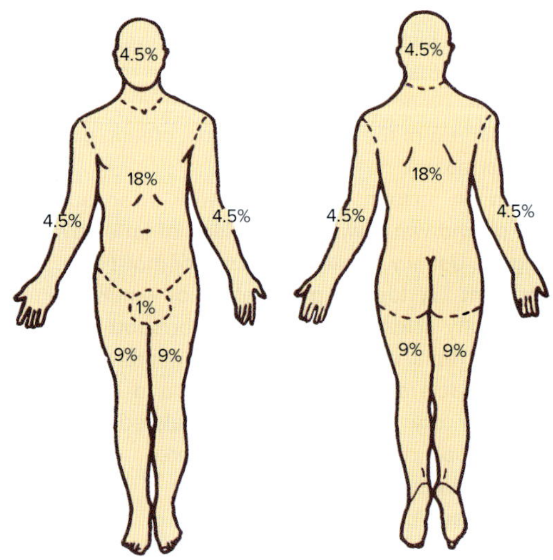

FIGURE 119.10 'Rule of nines' for body surface area

For example:

- if 9% of the body surface area is affected by eczema, approximately 3 g of cream is required to cover it
- 9 g of cream is used per day if prescribed three times daily
- a 50 g tube will last 5–6 days

One gram of cream will cover an area approximately 10 cm × 10 cm (4 square inches), and this formula may be used for smaller lesions.

Table 119.9 Suitable quantities of skin preparations for specific body areas[5] (twice daily application for 1 week)

	Creams and ointments		
	Corticosteroids	Others	Lotions
Face and neck	15–30 g	15–30 g	100 mL
Both hands	15–30 g	25–50 g	200 mL
Scalp	15–30 g	50–100 g	200 mL
Both arms	30–60 g	100 g	200 mL
Both legs	100 g	100–200 g	200 mL
Trunk	100 g	400 g	500 mL
Groin and genitalia	15–30 g	15–25 g	100 mL

TABLE 119.9 provides guidelines for approximate weekly quantities of skin preparations required to cover specific areas of the body.

Some general rules

Remember:

- that 30 g
  - will cover the adult body once
  - will cover hands twice daily for 2 weeks
  - will cover a patchy rash twice daily for 1 week
- that 200 g will cover a quite severe rash twice daily for 2 weeks

References

1 Marks R. A diagnosis in dermatology. Aust Fam Physician, 2001; 30 (11): 1028–32.

2 Marks R, Sinclair R. *A Guide to the Performance of Diagnostic Procedures used in the Management of Common Skin Diseases.* Melbourne: Skin & Cancer Foundation Publication, 2002: 25–6.

3 Expert group for Dermatology. In: eTG complete. Melbourne: Therapeutic Guidelines Ltd. Available from: <www.tg.org.au>, accessed March 2018.

4 Gambrill J. How much cream? Aust Fam Physician, 1982; 11: 350.

5 George CF et al. London: British National Formulary, Number 31, 1996; 451–6.

119

120 Pruritus

It is easy to stand a pain, but difficult to stand an itch.

CHANG CH'AO 1676

Pruritus (the Latin word for itch) is defined simply as the desire to scratch.

It is one of the most important dermatological symptoms and is usually a symptom of primary skin disease with a visible rash. However, it is a subjective symptom and diagnostic difficulties arise when pruritus is the presenting symptom of a systemic disease with or without a rash—'pruritus sine materia'. An associated rash may also be a manifestation of the underlying disease.

The broad differential diagnoses of pruritus are:

- skin disease
- systemic disease
- psychological and emotional disorders

Table 120.1	Primary skin disorders causing significant pruritus
Atopic dermatitis (eczema)	
Urticaria	
Dermatitis herpetiformis	
Grover disease	
Scabies	
Pediculosis	
Asteatosis (dry skin)	
Lichen planus	
Chickenpox	
Contact dermatitis	
Insect bites	

Physiology[1]

Itch arises from the same nerve pathway as pain, but pain and itch are distinct sensations. The difference is in the intensity of the stimulus. Unrelieved chronic itch, like unrelieved pain, can be intolerable and cause suicide. There are many similarities: both are abolished by analgesia and anaesthesia; subdued by counter-irritation, cold, heat and vibration; and referred itch occurs just like referred pain. Antihistamines that act on the H_1 receptor are often ineffective, suggesting that histamine is not the only mediator of itch.[1]

Localised pruritus

Pruritus may be either localised or generalised. Localised itching is generally caused by common skin conditions such as atopic dermatitis (see TABLE 120.1). Scratch marks are generally presented. Pruritus is a feature of dry skin. An intense, localised itch is suggestive of scabies, also known as 'the itch'.

Itching of the scalp, anal or vulval areas is a common presentation in general practice.

A careful examination is necessary to exclude primary skin disease; a detailed history and examination should be undertaken to determine if one of the various systemic diseases is responsible.

Notalgia paraesthetica is a common localised itch and/or paraesthesia (possibly also pain) in the interscapular area. It is considered to be due to pressure on spinal nerves from spinal dysfunction. It is usually relieved by physical therapy to the thoracic spine (see CHAPTER 24).[2] Pruritic rashes in children commonly include atopic dermatitis, varicella, urticaria (hives), insect bites and scabies.

Generalised pruritus[3]

Itch without rash (pruritus sine materia) may be a manifestation of systemic disease. It can accompany pregnancy, especially towards the end of the third trimester (beware of cholestasis), and disappear after childbirth. These women are then prone to pruritus if they take the contraceptive pill.[4,5]

Systemic causes are summarised in TABLE 120.2 and a summary of the diagnostic strategy model is given in TABLE 120.3.

The history may provide a lead to the diagnosis—the itching of polycythaemia may be triggered by a hot bath which can cause an unusual prickling quality that lasts for about an hour.[4] On the other hand, the itching may be caused by a primary irritant such as a bubble bath preparation.

Table 120.2 Systemic conditions that can cause pruritus

Pregnancy

Chronic kidney failure

Liver disorders:
- cholestatic jaundice, for example:
  - cancer of head of pancreas
  - primary biliary cirrhosis
  - drugs: chlorpromazine, antibiotics
- hepatic failure

Malignancy:
- lymphoma: Hodgkin lymphoma
- leukaemia, esp. chronic lymphatic leukaemia
- multiple myeloma
- disseminated carcinoma

Haematological disorders:
- polycythaemia rubra vera ('bath itch')
- iron-deficiency anaemia
- pernicious anaemia (rare)
- macroglobulinaemia

Endocrine disorders:
- diabetes mellitus
- hypothyroidism
- hyperthyroidism
- carcinoid syndrome
- hyperparathyroidism

Malabsorption syndrome:
- gluten sensitivity (rare)

Parasitic infestation:
- scabies
- ascariasis
- filariasis
- hookworm

Drugs:
- alkaloids
- aspirin/other NSAIDs
- diuretics
- ACE inhibitors
- opiates
- cocaine
- antibiotics e.g. penicillin, sulfonamides
- quinidine
- chloroquine
- CNS stimulants

Autoimmune disorders:
- polyarteritis nodosa
- sicca syndromes (e.g. Sjögren syndrome)

Neurological disorders:
- Parkinson disease
- brain tumour
- multiple sclerosis

Polyarteritis nodosa

Irritants:
- fibreglass
- others (e.g. soaps, detergents, chlorine)

Aquagenic pruritus

Xerosis (dry skin, winter itch)

HIV/AIDS

Psychological and emotional causes:
- anxiety/depression
- obsessive compulsive disorder
- psychosis
- parasitophobia

Table 120.3 Generalised pruritus: diagnostic strategy model

Probability diagnosis
Xerosis or dry skin (especially in the elderly)
Dermographism
Urticaria
Psychological/emotional[3]
Varicella (chickenpox)

Serious disorders not to be missed
Neoplasia:
- lymphoma/Hodgkin
- leukaemia: CLL
- other cancer
- HIV/AIDS

Chronic kidney failure
Primary biliary cirrhosis

Pitfalls (often missed)
Pregnancy
Tropical infection/infestation/scabies
Polycythaemia rubra vera
Polyarteritis nodosa
Lichen planus
Topical irritants (e.g. fibreglass, bubble bath)

Seven masquerades checklist
Depression
Diabetes
Drugs (several)
Anaemia (iron deficiency)
Thyroid disorders (hyper and hypo)
Spinal dysfunction (notalgia paraesthetica)

Is the patient trying to tell me something?
Quite likely: consider anxiety, parasitophobia.

Guidelines

- The prevalence of itching in Hodgkin lymphoma is about 30%. The skin often looks normal but the patient will claim that the itch is unbearable.[4]

- Pruritus due to dermographism is the most common of physical urticarias, with an exaggerated wealing tendency in response to stroking of the skin.[6]
- Pruritus can be the presenting symptoms of primary biliary cirrhosis and may precede other symptoms by 1–2 years.[3] The itch is usually most marked on the palms and soles.
- Pruritus can occur in both hyperthyroidism and hypothyroidism, especially in hypothyroidism where it is associated with the dry skin.
- Sometimes the cause is not to be found, especially in elderly patients, but is more identifiable in children.

Key history

Enquire about nature and distribution of itching. Consider pregnancy, liver disease and malignancy of the lymphatic system, particularly Hodgkin lymphoma. A careful review of any drug history is important. Note any associated general symptoms such as fever.

Key examination

- General examination of the skin, abdomen and lymphopoietic systems
- Examine for dermographism by firmly drawing a line in the patient's skin with a tongue depressor and observe for an urticarial response

Key investigations to consider

- Urinalysis
- Pregnancy test
- FBE
- ESR/CRP
- Iron studies
- Kidney function tests
- Liver function tests
- Thyroid function tests
- Random blood sugar
- Stool examination (ova and cysts)
- Chest X-ray
- Skin biopsy
- Allergy patch testing
- Lymph node biopsy (if present)
- Immunological tests for primary biliary cirrhosis (e.g. anti-mitochondrial antibodies)

Treatment

The basic principle of treatment is to determine the cause of the itch and treat it accordingly. Itch of psychogenic origin responds to appropriate therapy, such as amitriptyline for depression.[1]

If no cause is found:

- apply cooling measures (e.g. air-conditioning, cool swims)
- avoid rough clothes; wear light clothing
- avoid known irritants
- avoid overheating
- avoid vasodilatation (e.g. alcohol, hot baths/showers—keep showers short and not too hot)
- treat dry skin with appropriate moisturisers (e.g. propylene glycol in aqueous cream)
- topical treatment
  - emollients to lubricate skin
  - local soothing lotion such as calamine, including menthol or phenol (avoid topical antihistamines)
  - pine tar preparations (e.g. Pinetarsol)
  - crotamiton cream
- consider topical corticosteroids
- sedative antihistamines (not very effective for systemic pruritus)
- non-sedating antihistamines during day
- antidepressants (e.g. doxepin) or tranquillisers (if psychological cause and counselling ineffective)

PRURITIC SKIN CONDITIONS

Scabies

Scabies is a highly infectious skin infestation caused by a tiny mite called *Sarcoptes scabiei* (see FIG. 120.1). It is common in school-aged children, in closed communities such as nursing homes and in some Indigenous communities. The female mite burrows just beneath the skin in order to lay her eggs. She then dies. The eggs hatch into tiny mites that spread out over the skin and live for only about 30 days. The mite antigen, in its excreta, causes a hypersensitivity rash. Diagnosis is by microscopic examination of skin scrapings. A new IgE diagnostic test is available.

Clinical features

- Intense itching (worse with warmth and at night)
- Erythematous papular rash
- Usually on hands and wrists
- Common on male genitalia (see CHAPTER 117) (see FIG. 120.2)
- Also occurs on elbows, axillae, feet and ankles, nipples of females (see FIG. 120.3)

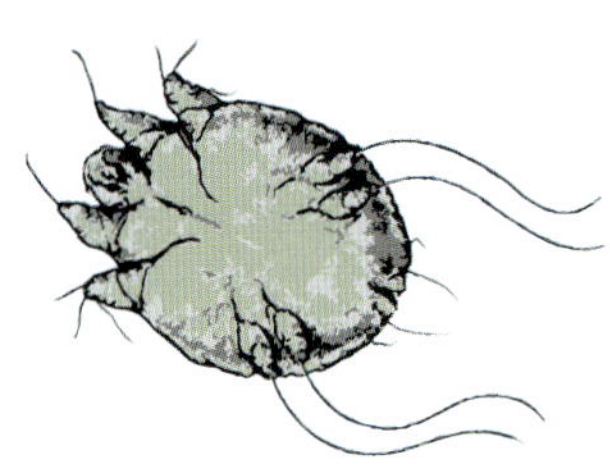

FIGURE 120.1 Scabies mite (*Sarcoptes scabiei*)

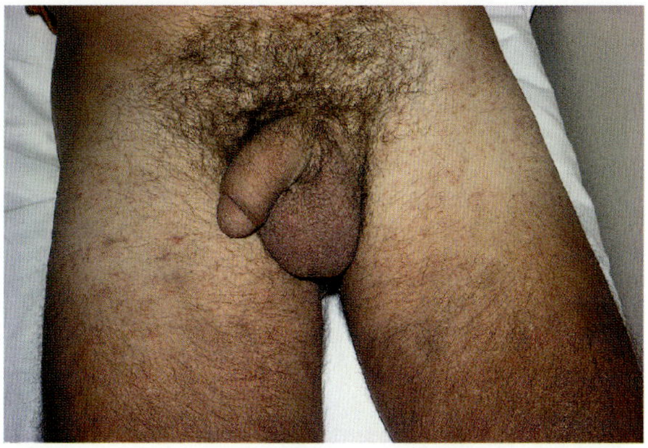

FIGURE 120.2 Genital scabies causing severe pruritus, showing bruising on the upper thighs from intense scratching

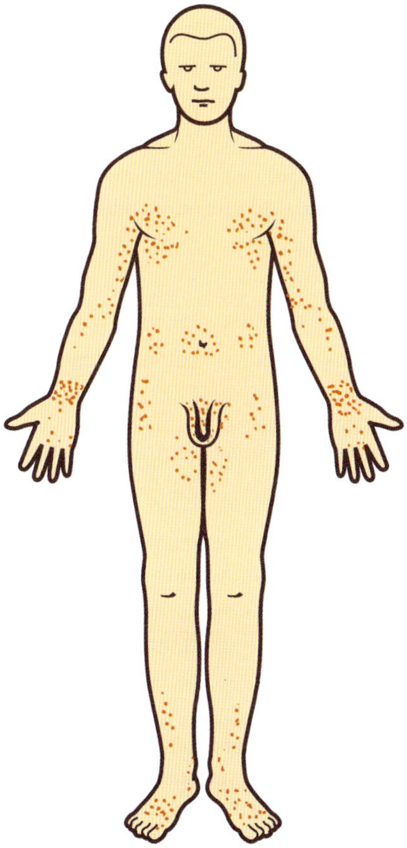

FIGURE 120.3 Typical distribution of the scabies rash

Spread

The mites are spread from person to person through close personal contact (skin to skin), including sexual contact. They may also be spread through contact with infested clothes or bedding, although this is uncommon. Sometimes the whole family can get scabies. The spread is more likely with overcrowding and sexual promiscuity.

Crusted (Norwegian) scabies

While the majority of cases have a relatively small number of mites (as few as 15), infestation with thousands or millions will cause the crusted condition of Norwegian scabies. Diagnosis is made on a scraping which reveals vast numbers of lesions. It may be encountered in nursing homes. Treatment is with ivermectin 200 mcg/kg (o) 2 doses, 7 days apart plus topical treatment. Treatment can be difficult and may require specialist input.[5]

Treatment[5]

For all ages (except children under 6 months):

- permethrin 5% cream (treatment of choice)
  or
- benzyl benzoate 25% emulsion (dilute with water if under 10 years)
- best applied to clean, cool, dry skin

- Apply to entire body from jawline down (including under nails, in flexures and genitals).
- Leave permethrin overnight, then wash off thoroughly.
- Leave benzyl benzoate for 24 hours.
- Avoid hot baths or scrubbing before application.
- Treat the whole family at the same time even if they do not have the itch.
- Wash clothing, any soft toys and bedclothes as usual in hot water and hang in sun.
- One treatment is usually sufficient but repeat scabicide treatment in 1 week for moderate and severe infections.
- For children less than 6 months use sulphur 5% cream daily for 2–3 days or crotamiton 10% cream daily for 3–5 days.

Dermatitis herpetiformis

This extremely itchy condition is a chronic subepidermal vesicular condition in which the herpes simplex-like vesicles erupt at the dermo-epidermal junction. The vesicles are so pruritic that it is unusual to see an intact one on presentation.

Some consider that it is always caused by a gluten-sensitive enteropathy. Most patients do have clinical coeliac disease.

Clinical features

- Most common in young adults
- Vesicles mainly over elbows and knees (extensor surfaces)

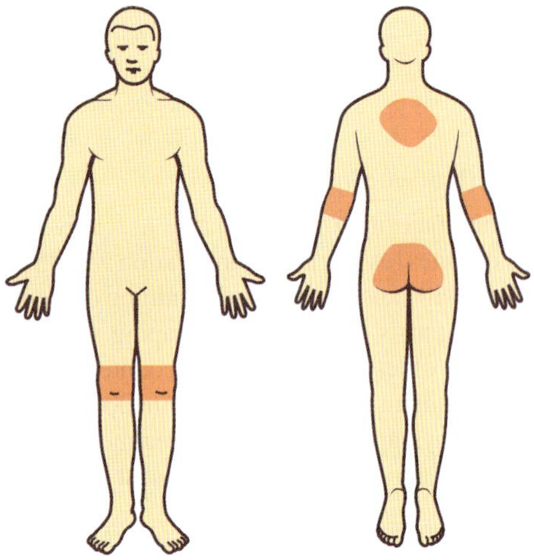

FIGURE 120.4 Typical distribution of dermatitis herpetiformis

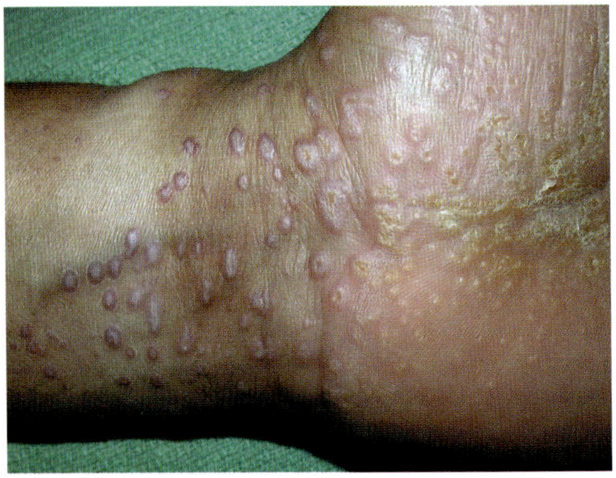

FIGURE 120.5 Lichen planus: thick, hypertropic, reddish-purple papules

120

- Also occurs on trunk, especially buttocks and shoulders (see FIG. 120.4)
- Vesicles rarely seen by doctors
- Presents as excoriation with eczematous changes
- Masquerades as scabies, excoriated eczema or insect bites
- Typically lasts for decades
- Associated with gluten-sensitive enteropathy
- Skin biopsy and immunofluorescence show diagnostic features

Treatment

- Gluten-free diet, which may suppress the condition but is slow to take effect.
- Dapsone 50 mg (o) daily, increasing up to 200 mg (o) daily with caution (usually dramatic response). Consider expert care.

Lichen planus

Lichen planus is an epidermal inflammatory disorder of unknown aetiology characterised by pruritic, violaceous, flat-tipped papules, mainly on the wrists (see FIG. 120.5) and legs. If in doubt, diagnosis is confirmed by biopsy. One differential diagnosis is a lichen planus-like drug eruption (e.g. antihypertensives, anti-malarials).

Clinical features

- Young and middle-aged adults
- 4Ps—papule, purple, polygonal, pruritic
- Small, shiny, lichenified plaques
- Symmetrical and flat-tipped
- Violaceous
- Flexor surfaces: wrists, forearms, groin, ankles
- Can affect oral mucosa— lacy white streaks (Wickham striae) or papules or ulcers
- Can affect nails, scalp and genital mucosa

Management

- Explanation and reassurance
- Cutaneous lichen planus usually resolves over 6–9 months, leaving discoloured marks without scarring
- Recurrence rare
- Asymptomatic lesions require no treatment
- Topical moderate to very potent corticosteroids (may use occlusive dressing)
- Oral prednisolone if not successful
- Intralesional corticosteroids for hypertrophic lesions
- Consider referral for expert advice

Pruritus ani

The generalised disorders causing pruritus may cause pruritus ani. However, various primary skin disorders such as psoriasis, dermatitis, contact dermatitis and lichen planus may also cause it, in addition to local anal conditions. It is covered in more detail in CHAPTER 36.

Pruritus capitis (itchy scalp)[7]

Scalp pruritus may be caused by several common skin conditions including seborrhoeic dermatitis, atopic dermatitis, psoriasis, tinea capitis, lichen simplex chronicus, contact dermatitis and pediculosis. Look for evidence of these conditions in the scalp and treat accordingly. The less severe form of seborrhoeic dermatitis is known as pityriasis capitis or dandruff.

Pruritus vulvae

Refer to CHAPTER 107.

Tinea cruris

Also known as Dhobie itch and jock itch, tinea cruris is a common infection of the groin area in young men (see FIG. 120.6), usually athletes, that is commonly caused by a tinea infection, although there are other causes of a groin rash (see TABLE 120.4). The dermatophytes responsible for tinea thrive in damp, warm, dark sites. The feet should be inspected for evidence of tinea pedis. It is transmitted by towels and other objects, particularly in locker rooms, saunas and communal showers.

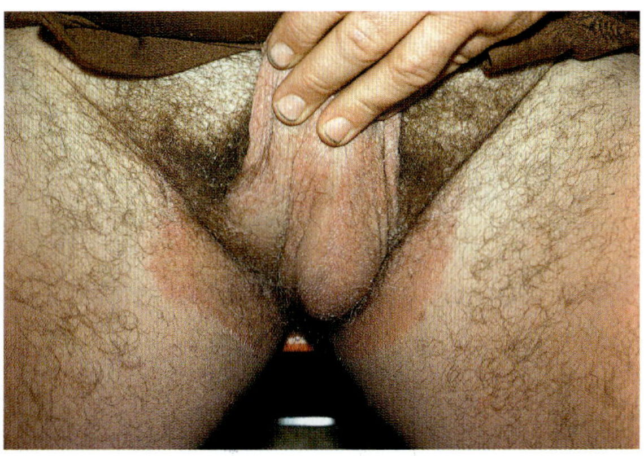

FIGURE 120.6 Tinea cruris (also known as Dhobie itch and jock itch) in a young man caused by *Trichophyton rubrum*

Table 120.4	Common causes of a groin rash (intertrigo)

Simple intertrigo

Skin disorders:
- psoriasis
- seborrhoeic dermatitis
- dermatitis/eczema

Fungal:
- *Candida*
- tinea

Erythrasma

Contact dermatitis

Clinical features

- Itchy rash
- More common in young males
- Strong association with tinea pedis (athlete's foot)
- Usually acute onset
- More common in hot months—a summer disease
- More common in physically active people
- Related to chafing in groin (e.g. tight pants, and especially synthetic jock straps)
- Scaling, especially at margin
- Well-defined border (see FIG. 120.7)

If left untreated, the rash may spread, especially to the inner upper thighs, while the scrotum is usually spared. Spread to the buttocks indicates *T. rubrum* infection.

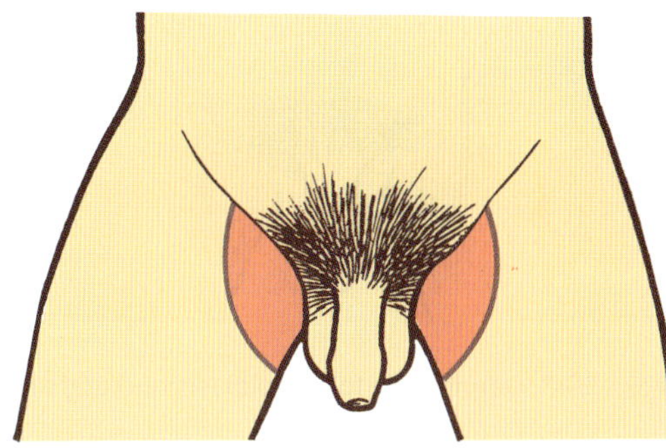

FIGURE 120.7 Dermogram for tinea cruris

Diagnostic aids

- Skin scrapings should be taken from the scaly area for preparation for microscopy (see CHAPTER 119).
- Wood's light may help the diagnosis, particularly if erythrasma is suspected.

Management

- Fastidious drying of skin folds.
- Apply topical terbinafine 1% cream or gel once or twice daily for 7–14 days or an imidazole topical preparation (e.g. miconazole or clotrimazole cream).
- Apply tolnaftate dusting powder bd when almost healed to prevent recurrence.
- If itch is severe, a mild topical hydrocortisone preparation (additional) can be used.[5]
- For persistent or recurrent eruption, use oral terbinafine for 2–4 weeks or griseofulvin for 6–8 weeks.

Candida intertrigo

Candida albicans superinfects a simple intertrigo and tends to affect patients with predisposing factors (e.g. broad-spectrum antibiotic therapy, diabetes, general debility, immune incompetence, obesity, immobility).

Clinical features

- Erythematous, macerated rash
- Occurs in flexures, submammary area and other skin folds
- Less well-defined margin than tinea (see FIG. 120.8)
- Associated satellite lesions and whitish discharge
- Yeast may be seen on microscopy

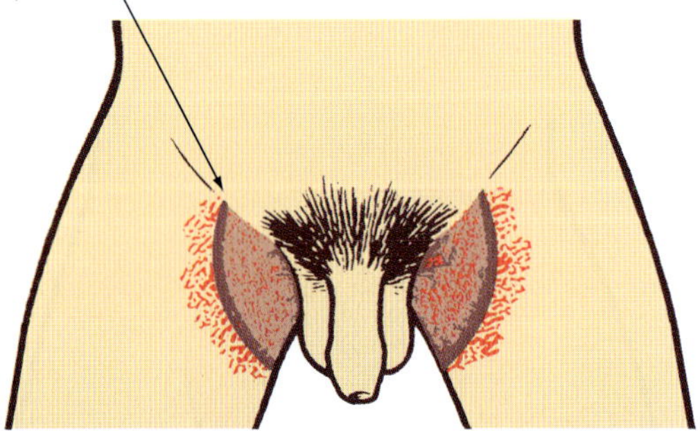

FIGURE 120.8 Dermogram for candidiasis of crural area

Treatment[5]

- Treat predisposing factors where possible.
- Apply an imidazole preparation such as miconazole 2% or clotrimazole 1%, twice daily for 2 weeks.
- Use short-term hydrocortisone cream for itch or inflammation (long-term aggravates the problem).

Erythrasma

Erythrasma, a common and widespread chronic superficial skin infection typically in a skin fold, is caused by the bacterium *Corynebacterium minutissimum,* which can be diagnosed by coral pink fluorescence on Wood's light examination. Itch is not a feature.

Clinical features

- Superficial reddish-brown scaly patches
- Enlarges peripherally
- Mild infection but tends to chronicity if untreated
- Coral pink fluorescence with Wood's light
- Common sites: groin (especially men), axillae, submammary, toe webs (see FIG. 120.9)

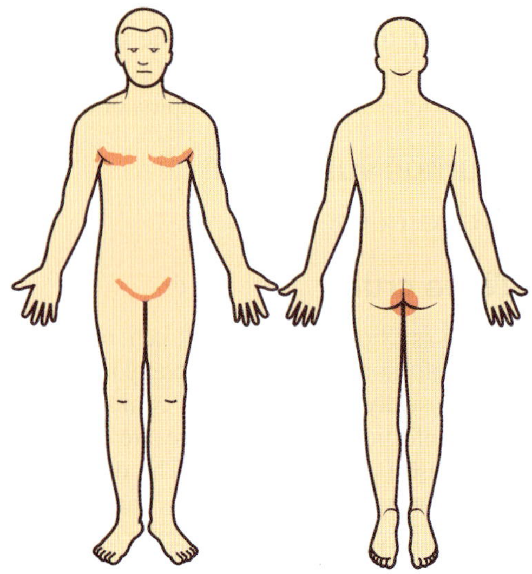

FIGURE 120.9 Typical sites of erythrasma

Treatment

- Topical imidazole e.g. miconazole or erythromycin 2% gel
- Oral roxithromycin or erythromycin
- Loose fitting clothing and antibacterial wash may prevent recurrence

Asteatotic eczema (winter itch)

This often unrecognised problem, which can be very itchy, is a disorder of the elderly. It is a form of eczema that typically occurs on the legs of the elderly (see FIG. 120.10), especially if they are subjected to considerable scrubbing and bathing. Other predisposing factors include low humidity (winter, central heating) and diuretics. The problem may be associated with a malabsorption state, hypothyroidism or drugs e.g. statins, diuretics.

Clinical features

- Dry skin
- Fine scaling and red superficial cracking
- 'Crazy paving' appearance
- Occurs on legs, especially shins
- Also occurs on thighs, arms and trunk

Treatment

Based on correcting dry skin:[8]

- Quick, cool showers (<2–3 minutes)
- Use soap-free substitutes in the shower
- Liberal use of emollients on damp skin, after the shower

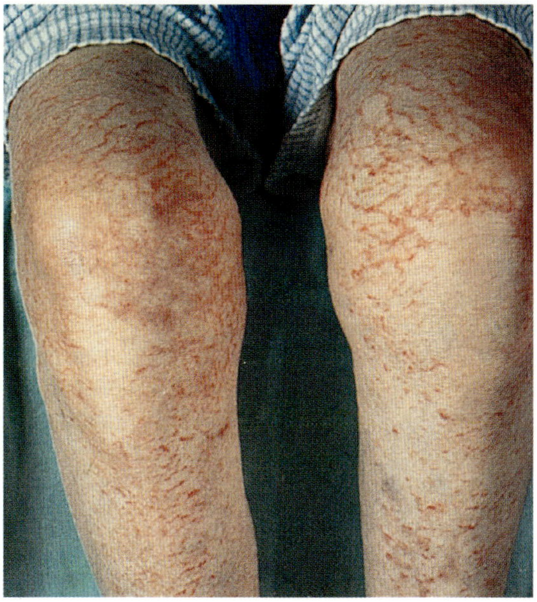

FIGURE 120.10 Asteatotic eczema (winter itch) showing the 'crazy paving' pattern with a pruritic scaling erythematous eruption on the legs of a 74-year-old man

- Avoid excessive heating in winter
- Avoid use of electric blankets
- Apply topical steroid diluted in white soft paraffin to reddened skin

'Golfer's vasculitis' (summer leg rash)[9]

This is a term used to describe an erythematous pruritic rash that appears on the legs after prolonged exercise such as golf or hiking, usually during summer months.

The rash is a red, blotchy, flat to slightly raised eruption on the lower leg. It is more common over age 50. It usually clears spontaneously within 3 days.

Brachioradialis pruritus

In this condition, itch and discomfort are limited to the outer surface of the upper limb above and below the elbow. It is often associated with sun damage, xerosis and nerve entrapment, hence the term 'golfer's itch'.[2]

Grover disease

Also known as transient acantholytic dermatosis, Grover disease produces small, firm, intensely pruritic, reddish-brown, warty papules with minimal scale, mainly on the upper trunk. It usually occurs in middle-aged to elderly men (typically 70–80 years). Trigger factors include heat, sweating, fever and occlusion, especially on photo-damaged skin. Diagnosis is by biopsy. Treatment is to relieve the itch until spontaneous resolution occurs. Effective treatments include topical (preferable) or oral corticosteroids and ultraviolet light.[3]

Cercarial dermatitis

Cercarial dermatitis (swimmer's itch) is an acute allergic dermatitis caused by contact with schistosomes in warm freshwater lakes. Skin under swimwear is often protected.

Nodular prurigo (prurigo nodularis)

These are extremely pruritic firm lumps about 1–3mm in diameter that erupt on the arms, legs and trunk. They can affect all ages and may manifest in late pregnancy. Definite diagnosis is with skin biopsy. They tend to run a long course and are difficult to treat.

Lichen simplex

Lichenification is a form of dermatitis caused by repeated scratching or rubbing, which results in epidermal thickening. Lichen simplex is the term used when no primary dermatological cause can be found. 120

Urticaria[5]

Urticaria is a common condition that mainly affects the dermis. It can be classified as acute (minutes to weeks) or chronic (lasting more than 6 weeks). It can also be classified as diffuse weal-like or papular (hives).

The three characteristic features of diffuse urticaria are:

- transient erythema, often with central pallor
- transient oedema
- transient intense itch

The most common causes are infections, especially viral URTIs, drug allergies and IgE-mediated food reactions.

Classification according to site

1. *Superficial:* affecting superficial dermis = urticaria; occurs anywhere on body, especially the limbs and trunk.
2. *Deep:* affecting subcutaneous tissue = angio-oedema; occurs anywhere but especially peri-orbital region, lips and neck.

Checklist of causes[3]

- Infections: viruses (the most common cause in children), bacteria (especially streptococcus infection), parasites, protozoa, yeasts
- C_1 esterase inhibitor deficiency (hereditary angio-oedema)—recurrent unexplained episodes of angio-oedema
- Allergies (acute allergic urticaria is dramatic and potentially very serious):
  - azo dyes
  - drugs: penicillin and other antibiotics
  - foods: eggs, fish, cheese, tomatoes, others
- Pharmacological:
  - drugs: penicillin, aspirin, codeine
  - foods: fish, shellfish, nuts, strawberries, chocolate, artificial food colourings, wheat, soy beans
  - plants: nettles, others
- Systemic lupus erythematosus
- Physical:
  - cholinergic: response to sweating induced by exercise and heat (e.g. young athletes)
  - heat, cold, sunlight
- Insect stings: bees, wasps, jellyfish, mosquitoes
- Pregnancy (last trimester), other hormonal
- Unknown (idiopathic)—80%; possible psychological factors

Investigations for chronic urticaria

- Full blood examination—look for eosinophilia of parasites
- ANA and DNA binding tests—consider SLE
- Skin prick tests

Treatment[5]

- Avoid any identifiable causes.
- Avoid salicylates and related food preparations (e.g. tartrazine).
- Consider elimination diets.
- Use oral antihistamines (e.g. cyproheptadine) or a less sedating one (e.g. cetirizine, loratadine, fexofenadine).
- Consider adding an H_2 antagonist (e.g. ranitidine 150 mg bd).
- Systemic corticosteroids (e.g. prednisolone 50 mg once daily) can relieve acute urticaria but should be avoided as high doses are required and symptoms usually return once treatment stops.[5]
- For severe urticaria with hypotension and anaphylaxis give IM adrenaline.[5]
- Use topical soothing preparation if relatively localised (e.g. crotamiton 10%, or phenol 1% in oily calamine or menthol 1% cream).
- Lukewarm baths with Pinetarsol or similar soothing bath oil.

Papular urticaria

This is a hypersensitivity to insect bites or insects in the environment, particularly seen in children aged 2–6 years. The lesions are grouped together, often as clusters of very itchy papules.

Common urticaria tends to come and go within hours but the lesions of papular urticaria persist.

The treatment for insect bites includes antipruritics and topical corticosteroids, e.g. betamethasone dipropionate 0.05% ointment or cream tds until resolved.

Flea bites

Fleas (see FIG. 120.11) cause itchy erythematous maculopapular lesions. They are usually multiple or grouped in clusters, occurring typically on the arms, forearms, leg and waist (where clothing is tight). Treat the source of infestation, particularly domestic cats and dogs. The itchy bites can be treated with an application of simple agents such as Stingose, alcohol, damp soap, anti-itch cream or a mild corticosteroid ointment.

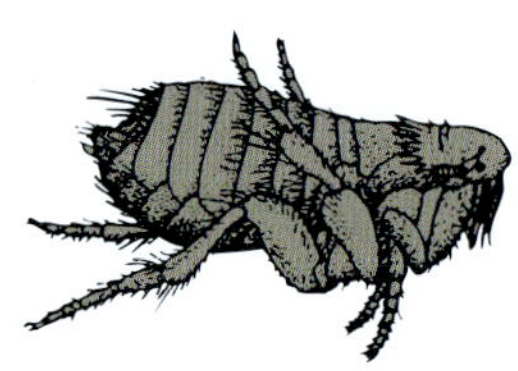

FIGURE 120.11 Flea

Bed bug bites[10]

The common bed bug (*Cimex lectularius,* see FIG. 120.12) is now a major problem related to international travel. It travels in baggage and is widely distributed in hotels, motels and backpacker accommodation. The bugs hide in bedding and mattresses. Clinically bites are usually seen in children and teenagers. The presentation is a linear group of three or more bites (along the line of superficial blood vessels), which are extremely itchy. They appear as maculopapular red lesions with possible wheals. The lesions are commonly found on the neck, shoulders, arms, torso

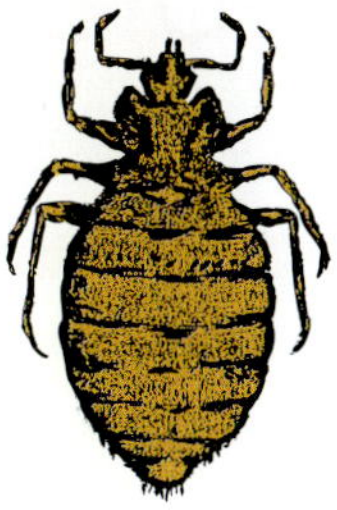

FIGURE 120.12 Bed bug

and legs. A bed bug infestation can be diagnosed by identification of rust-coloured specimens collected from the infested residence. In hotels and backpacker accommodation look for red specks in mattresses and check luggage.

Management

- Clean the lesions with antiseptic soap.
- Apply a corticosteroid ointment.
- A simple antipruritic agent may suffice e.g. calamine lotion.
- Call in a licensed pest controller.

Control treatment is basically directed towards applying insecticides to the crevices in walls and furniture. Be careful of used furniture and insist that mattresses are delivered in plastic coverings.

Sandfly bites

Refer CHAPTER 128.

When to refer

- Lichen planus
- Dermatitis herpetiformis
- Norwegian scabies

> **Practice tip**
>
> An itchy non-specific rash worse at night? Think scabies.

Patient education resources

Hand-out sheets from *Murtagh's Patient Education* 7th edition:

- Bed bug bites
- Pruritus ani
- Scabies
- Urticaria (hives)

References

1. Walsh TD. *Symptom Control.* Oxford: Blackwell Scientific Publications, 1989: 286–94.
2. Wolff K, Johnson RA et al. *Fitzpatrick's Color Atlas & Synopsis of Clinical Dermatology.* New York: McGraw-Hill, 2005: 1052–5.
3. Fry L et al. *Illustrated Encyclopedia of Dermatology.* Lancaster: MTP Press, 1981: 313–15, 485–8.
4. Hunter JAA, Savin JA, Dahl MV. *Clinical Dermatology* (3rd edn). Oxford: Blackwell Scientific Publications, 2002: 291.
5. Expert group for Dermatology. In: eTG complete. Melbourne: Therapeutic Guidelines Ltd. Available from: <www.tg.org.au>, accessed January 2018.
6. Oakley A. Dermographism. DermNet NZ. Available from: <www.dermnetnz.org/topics/dermographism>, accessed January 2018.
7. Ng J, Chong A, Foley P. The itchy scalp. Medicine Today, 2008; 9 (7): 2–9.
8. Chinniah N, Gupta M. Pruritus in the elderly—a guide to assessment and management. Aust Family Physician, 2014; 43: 710–13.
9. Australas J. Golfers vasculitis: an unusual presentation. Dermatology, 2005; 46: 11–14.
10. Bed bugs. Department of Medical Entomology, ICPMR, Westmead Hospital. Available at: <www.bedbug.org.au>.

121 Common skin problems

The power of making a correct diagnosis is the key to all success in the treatment of skin diseases; without this faculty, the physician can never be a thorough dermatologist, and therapeutics at once cease to hold their proper position, and become empirical.

LOUIS A DUHRING (1845–1913)

Skin disorders are common. They account for 10.8% of all problems[1] encountered in general practice, the most common being dermatitis/eczema, malignant skin neoplasms, solar keratoses, lacerations, warts and acne.

This chapter focuses on the common dermatoses.

Dermatitis/eczema

Dermatitis is a nonspecific inflammatory response of the skin, presenting as an erythematous rash, that is usually itchy, and sometimes scaly.[2] The terms dermatitis and eczema are often used interchangeably, with eczema referring to the process that causes dermatitis.

Dermatitis can be divided into *exogenous* causes (allergic contact, primary irritant contact, photo-allergic and phototoxic) and *endogenous,* which implies all forms of dermatitis not directly related to external causative factors. Endogenous types are atopic, nummular (discoid), vesicular hand/foot (pompholyx), pityriasis alba, lichen simplex chronicus and seborrhoeic.

Dermatitis can occur as the result of dry skin, which impairs the barrier function of the skin, making it more susceptible to irritation by soap and other contact irritants, the weather, temperature and non-specific triggers.

The meaning of atopy

The term 'atopic' refers to a hereditary background or tendency to develop one or more of a group of conditions, such as allergic rhinitis, asthma, eczema, skin sensitivities and urticaria. It is not synonymous with allergy.

An estimated 10% of the population are atopics, with allergic rhinitis being the most common manifestation.[3]

Atopic dermatitis

Features of classic atopic dermatitis:[2,4]

- itch
- usually a family history of atopy
- about 3% of infants are affected, signs appearing between 3 months and 2 years
- often known trigger factors (see TABLE 121.1) are evident

Table 121.1 Trigger factors for atopic dermatitis

Dust mite (common)
Sweating
Sand (e.g. in sandpits)
Extremes of hot and cold
Rapid temperature changes
Soap, shampoo and water/frequent washing, especially in winter
Chlorinated water
Bubble baths
Infection (viral, bacterial, fungal)
Allergy
Stress/emotional factors
Skin irritants:
- wool (e.g. sheepskin covers)
- rough clothing
- chemical disinfectants
- detergents
- petrochemical products
- pollens

Scratching and rubbing
Perfumes
Poor general health

- consider environmental allergens (e.g. dust mite, grasses, pollen, animal dander) especially if concurrent allergic rhinitis and prominent facial or periorbital involvement (usually older than 2 years)
- food allergies are rarely the main cause of the condition
- lichenification may occur with chronic atopic dermatitis
- flexures are usually involved (see FIG. 121.1)
- dryness is usually a feature

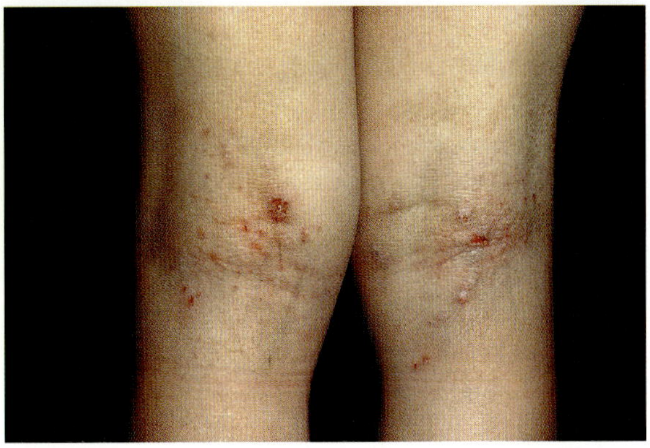

FIGURE 121.1 Atopic dermatitis in the flexures of the knees—a typical location

Criteria for diagnosis

- Itch
- Typical morphology and distribution
- Dry skin
- History of atopy
- Chronic relapsing dermatitis

Distribution

The typical distribution of atopic dermatitis changes as the patient grows older. In infants the rash appears typically on the cheeks of the face, the folds of the neck and scalp and extensor surfaces of the limbs. It may then spread to the flexures of limbs and groins (see FIG. 91.10 in CHAPTER 91). The change from infancy through to adulthood is presented in FIGURE 121.2.

During childhood a drier and thicker rash tends to develop in the cubital and popliteal fossae and on the hands and feet, which may be dry, itchy, fissured and painful. The face often clears. Refer to CHAPTER 91.

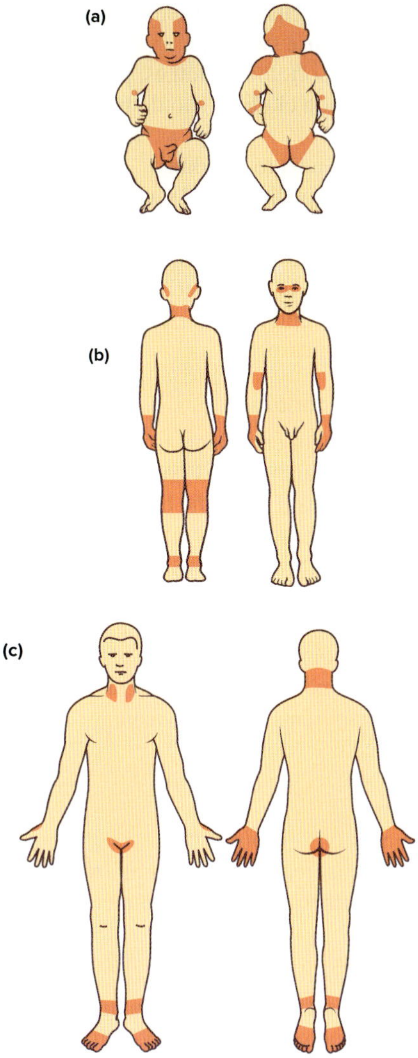

FIGURE 121.2 Relative distribution of atopic dermatitis in **(a)** infants, **(b)** children, and **(c)** typical distribution of atopic dermatitis in adults

Prognosis

It is generally correct that children tend to 'grow out of' the problem as the function of their oil and sweat glands matures. Most children go into remission or substantially improve by the time they enter primary school. A minority still have atopic dermatitis in their teenage years and then into adulthood.[2]

Management

Education and reassurance

Explanation, reassurance and support are very important. It is common for patients and parents to look for a 'cure' (particularly food allergies) and to have misplaced fear of the safety of topical corticosteroids. Emphasise that it is a chronic, relapsing condition, address allergy concerns and provide education and reassurance of the safety of topical corticosteroids.[5] Counselling is indicated where family stress and psychological factors are contributing to the problem.

Avoid irritants

- Avoid soap and perfumed products.
- Older children should have short, tepid showers.
- Avoid rubbing and scratching—keep fingernails short, consider mittens or splints at night if severe.
- Avoid overheating, particularly at night.

121

- Avoid sudden changes of temperature, especially those that cause sweating.
- Wear light, soft, loose clothes, preferably made of cotton. Cotton clothing should be worn next to the skin.
- Avoid wool next to the skin.
- Avoid dusty conditions and sand, especially sandpits.
- Consider dust mite strategies:
  - dust mite covers (premium grade) for bedding
  - wash linen in hot water >55°C
  - consider replacing fabric on chairs and changing carpet.

Improve skin condition

- Frequent use of emollients is essential to improve skin barrier function and prevent flares.
- Use a bland bath oil in the bath and a soap substitute (e.g. aqueous cream, soap-free bars, soap-free wash).
- If itch is severe, make an oatmeal bath (put half a cup of oats in a sock or stocking and add this to the bathwater).
- Apply an emollient soon after bathing.
- Apply emollients at least twice/day (choose from):
  - aqueous cream
  - sorbolene, alone or with 10% glycerine (can sting)
  - emulsifying ointment
  - paraffin creams—good in infants
  - moisturising lotions in summer

Medication[2]

Topical corticosteroids are the mainstay of therapy. The current approach is to apply them liberally until the inflamed skin is perfectly clear. Most dermatitis should clear within 7–14 days with use of the appropriate strength steroid but may require longer in severe cases. Emollients are the key to preventing flares, although periodic flares are common. When the condition flares, resume the topical corticosteroid promptly until the skin clears again.

Topical corticosteroids are available in ointments, creams and lotions. Ointments are usually the preferred option as they are more effective for dry skin and sting less. The appropriate strength corticosteroid depends on the site and the severity of the rash, see CHAPTER 119.

A general rule for recommended strength of topical corticosteroid for site:

- Face, axillae and groin—mild
- Trunk and limbs—moderately potent, potent if severe
- Hands and feet—potent

Topical corticosteroid therapy

For face, axillae and groin:

- 1% hydrocortisone ointment, daily until skin is clear
- if inadequate response, methylprednisolone aceponate 0.1% ointment or fatty ointment, daily for 7–14 days

For trunk and limbs:

- triamcinolone acetonide 0.02% ointment, daily until skin is clear
- if more severe or in the flexures, use:
  methylprednisolone aceponate 0.1% ointment or fatty ointment, daily
  or
  mometasone furoate 0.1% ointment, daily

For hands, feet, lichenified wrists and ankles:

betamethasone dipropionate 0.05% ointment, daily until skin is clear
or
betamethasone valerate 0.1% ointment, daily
or
mometasone furoate 0.1% ointment, daily

A non-steroidal alternative is pimecrolimus 1% (Elidel) cream once to twice daily as a maintenance preparation for sensitive areas e.g. face, eyelids, axillae, groin.

Oral antihistamines generally have no role in the treatment of atopic dermatitis, however, a sedating antihistamine at night is appropriate if itch prevents sleep.

Secondary infection

Atopic skin is particularly susceptible to secondary bacterial and viral infection. Skin and nasal staphylococcal carriage is also more common and may require eradication measures. Secondary infection often reduces the effectiveness of topical treatments and is a common cause of treatment failure.

Consider taking skin or nasal swabs if:

- crusting or pustules present
- dermatitis fails to respond to appropriate topical therapy.

Mupirocin 2% ointment is appropriate for localised bacterial infection, while a short course (5–10 days) of oral antibiotics is appropriate for widespread infection. For recurrent infection, consider bleach baths (sodium hypochlorite 6% solution 60 mL per bath, twice weekly).

Eczema with secondary HSV infection (eczema herpeticum) requires prompt antiviral therapy and specialist referral.

Severe dermatitis

- Expert advice usually required
- Consider occlusive dressings
- Consider wet dressings
- Consider hospitalisation
- UV band therapy as back-up
- Systemic immunosuppressants may be used for recalcitrant cases
- Oral corticosteroids are generally not recommended unless advised by a specialist

OTHER TYPES OF ATOPIC DERMATITIS

Nummular (discoid) eczema

- Chronic, red, coin-shaped plaques
- Crusted, scaling and intensely itchy
- Secondary infection common due to excoriation
- Mainly on the legs, also buttocks and trunk
- Often symmetrical (no central clearing)
- Common in middle-aged patients
- May be related to stress
- Tends to persist for months, seek expert advice

Treatment as for moderate to severe atopic dermatitis, using a potent topical corticosteroid.

Pityriasis alba

- These are white, scaly, poorly demarcated patches on the face of children and adolescents
- Very common mild condition
- More common around the mouth and on cheeks
- Can occur on the neck and upper limbs, occasionally on trunk
- It is a subacute form of atopic dermatitis
- Full repigmentation occurs eventually

Treatment

- Reassurance
- Avoid skin irritants
- Simple emollients
- May prescribe hydrocortisone 1% ointment bd for 5–7 days (rarely necessary)

Lichen simplex chronicus

- Circumscribed thick plaques of lichenification
- Caused by repeated rubbing and scratching of previously normal skin
- Due to chronic itch of unknown cause
- At sites within reach of fingers (e.g. neck, forearms, thighs, vulva, heels, fingers)
- May arise from habit

Treatment

- Explanation
- Refrain from scratching
- Potent topical corticosteroid ointment (with or without occlusion) to break the itch–scratch cycle

Dyshidrotic dermatitis (pompholyx)

- Typically in patients aged 20–40 years
- Itching vesicles usually on fingers (see FIG. 121.3)

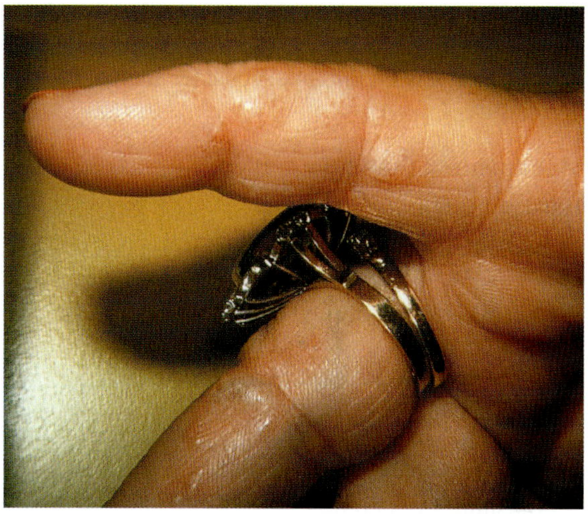

FIGURE 121.3 Pompholyx showing the typical vesicular dermatitis along the borders of the fingers. Look for associated inflammatory tinea of the feet which can precipitate it.

Photo courtesy Robin Marks

- May be larger vesicles on palms and soles
- Commonly affects sides of digits and palms
- Initial phase may be exudative as vesicles burst
- Lasts a few weeks
- Tends to recur
- Associated with atopic dermatitis, although cause is unclear
- Can be precipitated by tinea of the feet
- Possibly related to stress
- Often triggered by high humidity

Treatment

- Salt water soaks if exudative (1/2 teaspoon in 1 cup of water)
- Consider infection if exudative and treat
- Potent corticosteroids as for atopic dermatitis
- Use a cream for exudative phase, then ointment as skin dries
- Consider occlusion (e.g. damp cotton gloves)
- Oral corticosteroids (3 weeks) may be necessary

Asteatotic dermatitis

This is the common, very itchy dermatitis that occurs in the elderly, especially in the winter, with a dry 'crazy paving' pattern, especially on the legs (see CHAPTER 120).

'Asteatotic' means without moisture.

Cracked (fissured) hands/fingers

This common cause of disability is usually due to dermatitis of the hands, irritant contact dermatitis or very dry skin. It is usually part of the atopic dermatitis problem and it is important to consider allergic contact dermatitis.

Management (hand dermatitis)

Hand protection:

- avoid domestic or occupational duties that involve contact with irritants and detergents
- wear protective work gloves; cotton-lined PVC gloves
- avoid perfumed toilet soaps—use a substitute (e.g. Cetaphil lotion)
- apply emollients frequently (e.g. emulsifying ointment, glycerine-rich creams), especially after finishing work duties
- potent topical corticosteroid as for atopic dermatitis
- oral corticosteroids may be required for severe flare
- expert referral for severe cases for patch testing

121

Cracked heels

Cracked painful heels are a common problem, especially in adult women. It is a manifestation of very dry skin.

Treatment

- Soak the feet for 15 minutes in warm water containing an oil such as Alpha Keri or Derma Oil.
- Pat dry, then apply an emollient foot cream (e.g. Nutraplus—10% urea).
- Can use tissue glue (with care) to hold edges together.
- Consider surgical closure, especially if bleeding.

Contact dermatitis

Acute contact (exogenous) dermatitis can be either *irritant* or *allergic* and it is estimated that at least 70% of patients have an irritant cause. It is difficult to separate these types on clinical or histological grounds. The presence of irritant dermatitis increases the risk of developing a contact allergy.

Features:

- itchy, inflamed skin
- red and swollen
- papulovesicular
- may be dry and fissured

Irritant contact dermatitis

This is caused by primary irritants such as acids, alkalis, detergents, soaps, oils, solvents. A reaction may result from either a once-only exposure to a very irritant chemical or, more commonly, repeated exposure to weaker irritants. This is irritation, not allergy.

Allergic contact dermatitis

Caused by allergens that provoke an allergic reaction in some individuals only—most people can handle the chemicals without undue effect. It is immunologically mediated. This allergic group also includes photo-contact allergens. Approximately 4.5% of the population is allergic to nickel, which is found in jewellery, studs on jeans, keys and coins (see FIG. 121.4). Contact dermatitis is due to delayed hypersensitivity, sometimes with a long time of days to years. It is common in industrial or occupational situations, where it usually affects the hands and forearms.

Common allergens:

- ingredients/fragrances in cosmetics (e.g. perfumes, preservatives)
- topical antibiotics (e.g. neomycin)
- topical anaesthetics (e.g. benzocaine)
- topical antihistamines

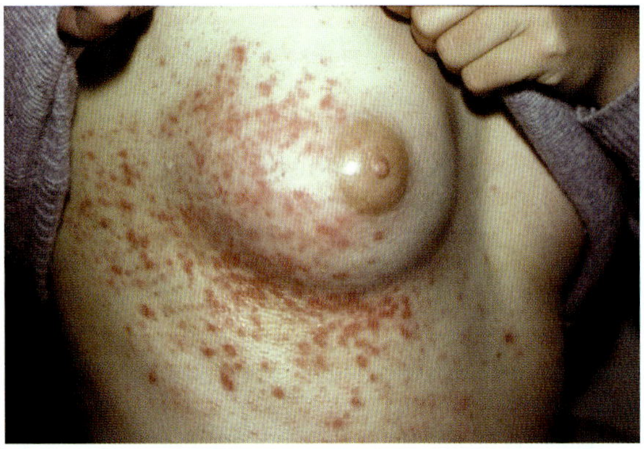

FIGURE 121.4 Contact dermatitis due to nickel-containing underwire in brassiere in 17-year-old girl with a history of eczema

- plants: *Rhus, Grevillea, Primula,* poison ivy
- metal salts (e.g. nickel sulphate, chromate)
- dyes (especially clothing dyes)
- perfumes, cosmetics
- hairdressing chemicals
- rubber/latex
- epoxy resins and glues/acrylates
- glutaraldehyde (e.g. sterilising agents)
- toluene sulfonamide compound resins: nail polish
- coral

Note: The skin of mangoes cross-reacts with *Rhus* and *Grevillea.*

Clinical features[4]

- Site and shape suggest contact
- Dermatitis ranges from faint erythema to 'water melon' face oedema
- Worse in peri-orbital region, genitalia and hairy skin; least in glabrous skin (e.g. palms and soles)
- Think of *Rhus, Grevillea* or poison ivy allergy if linear blisters on forearms and/or puffy eyes
- Improvement when off work or on holiday

Note: Can be delayed onset.

Diagnosis

- Take a thorough history; consider occupation, family history, vacation or travel history and clothes
- Review all topical applications (e.g. medicines, cosmetics) for allergic or irritant potential
- Usage test—apply products used by the patient to the cubital fossa and note development of rash
- Refer to a dermatologist for patch testing

Management

- Determine cause with vigour and remove it
- Topical corticosteroid treatment as for atopic dermatitis
- Oral prednisolone for severe cases[2] (start with 25–50 mg daily for adults for 5–7 days then gradually reduce over 2 weeks)

Seborrhoeic dermatitis

Seborrhoeic dermatitis is a very common skin inflammation that usually affects areas abundant in sebaceous glands or intertriginous areas. It is therefore common in hair-bearing areas of the body, especially the scalp and eyebrows. It can also affect the scalp, face, neck, axillae and groins, eyelids (blepharitis), external auditory meatus and nasolabial folds. The presternal area is often involved (see FIG. 121.5).

There are two distinct clinical forms: seborrhoeic dermatitis of infancy, and the adult form.

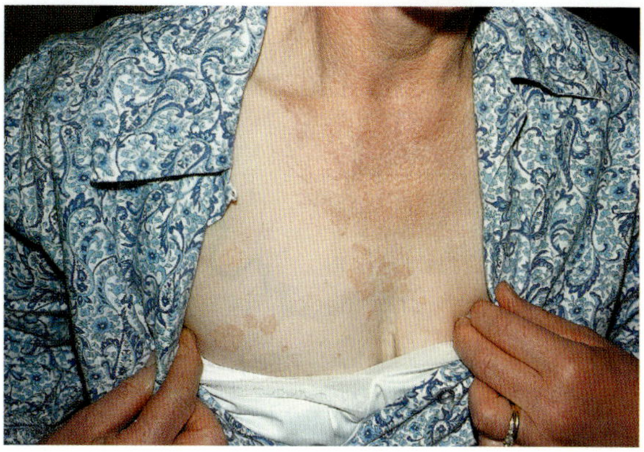

FIGURE 121.5 Seborrhoeic dermatitis in an adult showing a typical position on the chest

Studies have indicated that it may be caused by a reaction to the yeast *Malassezia* sp. It may be associated with HIV infection and Parkinson disease.

A feature of seborrhoeic dermatitis is that, unlike atopic dermatitis, it is not itchy. Seborrhoeic scale is greasy and yellowish unlike the silvery scale of psoriasis.

Treatment principles for seborrhoeic dermatitis

- Keratolytics such as salicylic acid may be used to lift the scale.
- Antiyeast treatments reduce the skin's load of *Malassezia* sp., e.g. ketoconazole, miconazole and ciclopirox.
- Topical corticosteroids target inflammation and pruritus and often used in combination.

121

Seborrhoeic dermatitis of infancy

Infantile seborrhoeic dermatitis is different from adult seborrhoeic dermatitis. In infancy, it is often known as 'cradle cap' if it affects the scalp, or nappy rash/diaper dermatitis if it involves the napkin area.

It can be difficult to differentiate the rash from that of atopic dermatitis but seborrhoeic dermatitis tends to appear very early (before atopic dermatitis), from 3–12 weeks, when androgen activity is most prevalent. Both atopic dermatitis and seborrhoeic dermatitis can present with red, scaly patches.

The different features are summarised in TABLE 121.2 and the distribution is presented in FIGURE 121.6.

In cradle cap, a flaky, scurf-like dandruff appears first, and then a yellowish, greasy, scaly crust forms. This scurf is usually associated with reddening of

121

Table 121.2 Differential diagnosis of seborrhoeic dermatitis and atopic dermatitis in infancy

	Seborrhoeic dermatitis	Atopic dermatitis (eczema)
Age of onset	Mainly within first 3 months	Usually after 2 months
Itchiness	Nil or mild	Usually severe
Distribution	Scalp, cheeks, folds of neck, axillae, folds of elbows and knees	Starts on face Elbow and knee flexures
Typical features	Cradle cap Red and yellow greasy scale	Vesicular and weeping Becomes dry and cracked
Napkin rash	Common Prone to infection with *Candida*	Less common

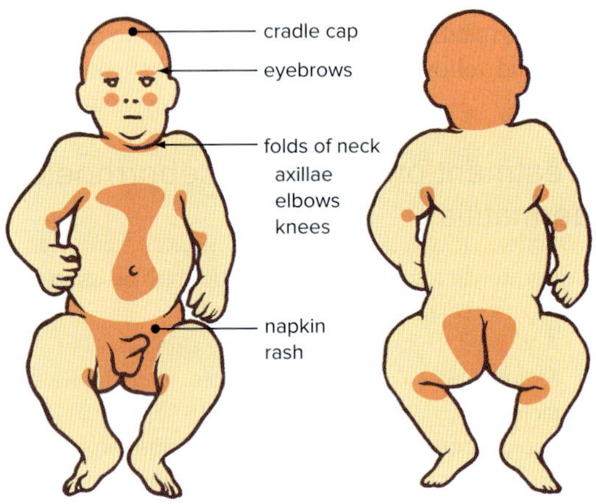

FIGURE 121.6 Seborrhoeic dermatitis: typical distribution in infants

the skin. It may resolve spontaneously within a few months (see Cradle cap, CHAPTER 91).

The dermatitis can become infected, especially in the napkin area, and this may be difficult to treat. If untreated, it often spreads to many areas of the body. It is said that cradle cap and nappy rash 'may meet in the middle'.

Treatment

Simple basic methods are:

- keep areas dry and clean
- keep skin exposed to air as much as possible
- use soap substitute (e.g. Cetaphil lotion)
- rub scales of cradle cap gently with baby oil or white soft paraffin then wash away loose scales

Medication[2]

Scalp

Infants:

- 1–2% sulphur and 1–2% salicylic acid in aqueous cream or same cream with 2% liquor picis carbonis added:
  - apply overnight to scalp, wash off next day with soap substitute
  - use 3 times a week until it clears
- Egozite cradle cap lotion (6% salicylic acid)

For persistent scalp erythema:

desonide 0.05% lotion, daily after bath

Face, flexures and trunk

desonide 0.05% lotion, bd for up to 7 days
or
hydrocortisone 1% ointment, bd for up to 7 days

Napkin area

- Mix equal parts 1% hydrocortisone with nystatin or miconazole + zinc oxide

Prognosis

Most children are clear by 18 months (rare after 2 years).

Adult seborrhoeic dermatitis

Clinical features

- Any age from teenage onwards
- The head is a common area: scalp and ears, face, eyebrows, eyelids (blepharitis), nasolabial folds (see FIG. 121.7)

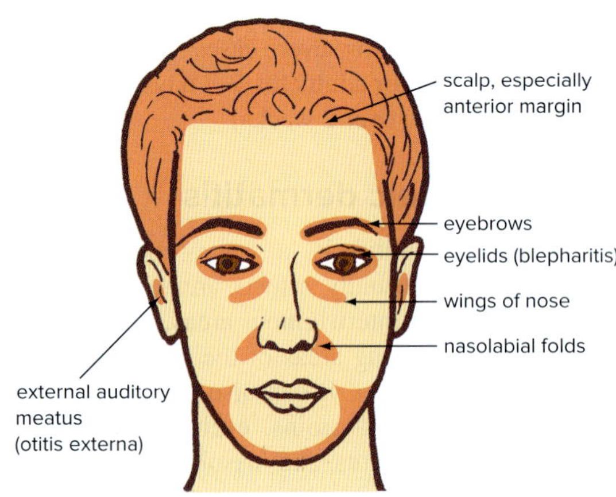

FIGURE 121.7 Seborrhoeic dermatitis: facial distribution in adults

- Other areas: centre of chest, centre of back, scapular area, intertriginous areas, especially perianal (see FIG. 121.8)

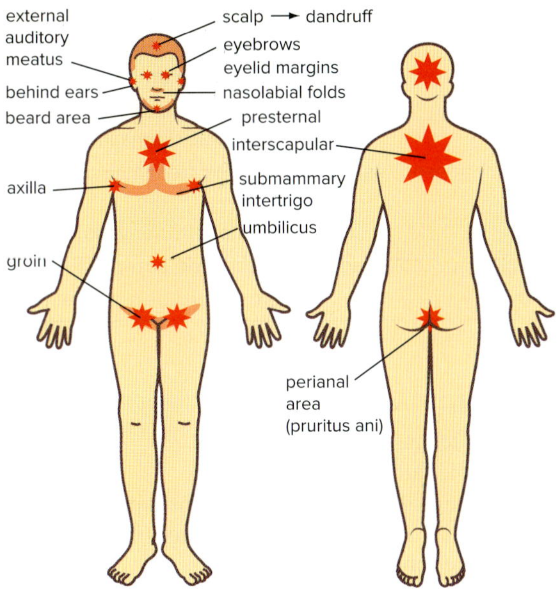

FIGURE 121.8 Seborrhoeic dermatitis: possible distribution in adults

- Pale pink, ill-defined erythematous rash characterised by loose, flaky scale
- Scale may be yellow and greasy
- Dandruff a feature of scalp area
- Worse with stress and fatigue
- It is a chronic, recurring condition

Treatment[2]

Scalp

First line treatment is an anti-yeast shampoo applied often (twice per week to daily). Shampoos often require rotation as response diminishes.
Anti-yeast shampoo options:

- ketoconazole
- ciclopirox olamine
- zinc pyrithione
- selenium sulfide

If inadequate, add a topical corticosteroid lotion for 7 nights. Options include:

- betamethasone dipropionate 0.05%
- methylprednisolone aceponate 0.1%
- mometasone furoate 0.1%

If inadequate response and especially if thick scale, add coal tar (LPC) at night, once or twice weekly and wash off the next morning with anti-yeast shampoo. Recommended topical tar preparations:

- coal tar prepared 1% emulsion or gel
- LPC 3–6% + salicylic acid 3% in aqueous cream

If all above therapies fail, use corticosteroid shampoo, clobetasol propionate 0.05%, twice weekly (use anti-yeast shampoo on the other 5 days).

Face and body

- Wash regularly using bland soap
- Combination antifungal cream and topical corticosteroid is first line:

  hydrocortisone 1% + clotrimazole 1% once or twice daily
  or
  hydrocortisone 1% + miconazole 2% cream, once or twice daily for up to 2 weeks
- If inadequate, use separate topical corticosteroids and antifungal creams:

  desonide 0.05% lotion daily for up to 2 weeks
  or
  methylprednisolone aceponate 0.1% cream daily for up to 2 weeks
  in combination with
  ketoconazole 2% or bifonazole 2% creams daily for up to 2 weeks
  or
  clotrimazole 1%, econazole 1% or miconazole 2% creams twice daily for up to 2 weeks

If treatment fails, a tar cream can be used such as LPC 1–2% (for face, flexures and groin) and LPC 3–6% (for trunk and limbs) in aqueous or sorbolene cream, once daily for up to 2 weeks.

Note: Oral antifungals are not recommended at all.

121

Psoriasis

Psoriasis (see FIG. 121.9) is a chronic, immune-mediated skin disorder of unknown aetiology which affects 2–4% of the population. It appears most often between the ages of 10 and 30 years, although its onset can occur any time from infancy to old age. It has a familial predisposition although its mode of inheritance is debatable. If one parent is affected there is a 25% chance of developing it; this rises to 65% if both parents are affected.[3]

Psoriasis is now regarded as a disorder involving activation of helper T cells in the skin. Cytokines are then released and cause skin cells to multiply faster,

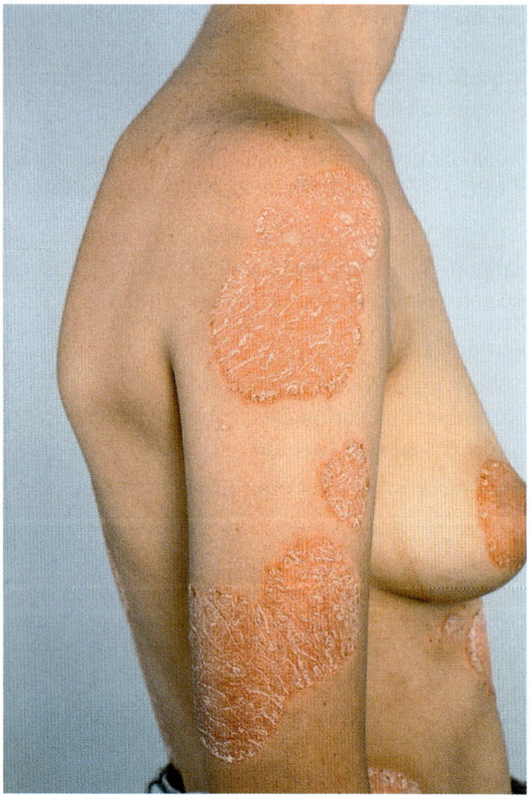

FIGURE 121.9 Psoriasis showing the typically raised pink plaques surmounted with a silvery scale

121

leading to thickening of the skin and overscaling. The new 'biological agents' intervene in this process.

Capillary dilatation explains the redness.

Be aware of association with cardiovascular disease, particularly heart disease, depressive illness, diabetes, arthritis, inflammatory bowel disease and lymphoma.[6]

Factors that may worsen or precipitate psoriasis

- Infection, especially group A *Streptococcus*
- Trauma or other physical stress
- Emotional stress
- Sunburn
- Puberty/menopause
- Drugs:
  - antimalarials (e.g. chloroquine)
  - beta blockers
  - lithium
  - NSAIDs
  - oral contraceptives

Types of psoriasis	Differential diagnosis
Infantile	Seborrhoeic dermatitis, atopic dermatitis
Plaque (commonest)	Seborrhoeic dermatitis, discoid eczema, solar keratoses, Bowen's disease
Guttate	Pityriasis rosea, secondary syphilis, drug eruption
Flexural	Tinea, candida intertrigo, seborrhoeic dermatitis
Scalp (sebopsoriasis)	Seborrhoeic dermatitis, tinea capitis
Nail	Tinea, idiopathic onycholysis
Pustular (palmoplantar)	Tinea, infected eczema
Exfoliative	Severe seborrhoeic dermatitis

The typical patient

- Older teenager or young adult
- Possible family history
- Onset may follow stress, illness or injury
- Rash may appear on areas of minor trauma—the Koebner phenomenon
- Rash improves on exposure to sun but worse with sunburn
- Worse in winter
- Itching not a feature but is present sometimes

Arthropathy

About 5% can develop a painful arthropathy (fingers, toes or a large joint) or a spondyloarthropathy (sacroiliitis).[7]

The rash

The appearance depends on the site affected. The commonest form is plaque psoriasis, which begins with red lesions that enlarge and develop silvery scaling. The commonest sites are the extensor surfaces of the elbows and knees; then the scalp, sacral areas, genitals and nails are affected (see FIG. 121.10).

Diagnosis

Psoriasis is a clinical diagnosis but biopsy may be needed for confirmation. No laboratory test (including blood testing) is available.

Principles of management

While realising there is no cure for psoriasis, the aim of treatment is to relieve discomfort, slow down the rapid skin cell division and work in consultation with a specialist to achieve these aims.[7]

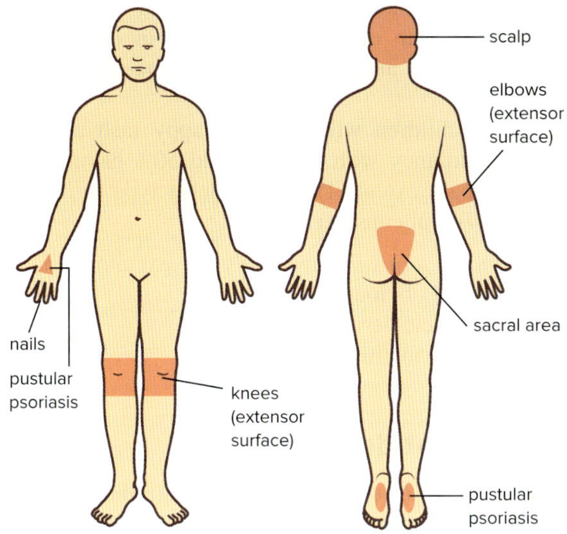

FIGURE 121.10 Psoriasis: typical skin distribution

- Provide education, reassurance and support.
- Promote general measures such as rest, and holidays, preferably in the sun.
- Promote healthy lifestyle, including balanced diet, exercise, reduced alcohol and smoking cessation.
- Advise prevention, including avoidance of skin damage and stress if possible.
- Avoid irritants and use a soap substitute.
- Recommend regular use of emollients.
- Tailor treatment (including referral) according to the degree of severity and extent of the disease.
- Shared care with a consultant is advisable.

Topical treatment options[2]

Topical agents useful for treatment of psoriasis in primary care:

- Tar preparations
  - anti-inflammatory, anti-pruritic
  - often used in combination with keratolytics (e.g. salicylic acid) to soften and lift scale
  - stinging can be avoided by using with topical corticosteroid or when symptoms mild
  - colour and odour limit concordance, apply at night
  - common preparation is liquor picis carbonis (LPC)
- Topical corticosteroids
  - most common treatment for psoriasis
  - anti-inflammatory, reduces rate of skin turnover
  - useful for flares; add tar or calcipotriol if ineffective or step down to tar alone once controlled
- Calcipotriol
  - vitamin D derivative, regulates proliferation and differentiation of keratinocytes
  - takes up to 6 weeks to take effect
  - stinging is common, reduced when used in combination with topical corticosteroid

Therapy can be monotherapy or combined therapy, e.g. tar and corticosteroids or corticosteroids and calcipotriol. Rotational therapy is often required as patients become less sensitive to one therapy over time, especially topical corticosteroids. Adding another treatment can extend disease control.

Recommended topical regimens

Chronic stable plaque psoriasis

For trunk and limb psoriasis, apply:

coal tar prepared 1% emulsion or gel, once or twice daily, for 1 month

or

LPC 6% + salicylic acid 3% cream or ointment, twice daily for 1 month

if insufficient or flare, add

moderately potent to potent topical corticosteroid ointment, daily until skin is clear (usually 2 to 6 weeks)

or if inadequate response

calcipotriol + betamethasone dipropionate 50 + 500 mcg/g ointment, daily until skin is clear (usually about 6 weeks)

Once psoriasis controlled, reduce the potency of steroid and withdraw if possible. Continue tar as maintenance therapy.

Palmoplantar psoriasis

Treat as for trunk or limb psoriasis, however higher dose of salicylic acid is required if hyperkeratotic, i.e. LPC 6% + salicylic acid 6%. Also consider earlier use of calcipotriol, given common resistance to topical therapy.

Scalp psoriasis

potent corticosteroid lotion or shampoo (as for seborrhoeic dermatitis), daily until skin is clear (usually 2 to 6 weeks)

then

coal-tar shampoo (over the counter) for maintenance

or if thickened scale, add

LPC 6% + salicylic acid 3% in aqueous cream, twice daily

if inadequate response
calcipotriol + betamethasone dipropionate 50 + 500 mcg/g gel, once daily until skin is clear (expect some response within 2 weeks)

Facial psoriasis

methylprednisolone aceponate 0.1% ointment or fatty ointment, daily for several weeks (usually 2 to 6 weeks) or 1% hydrocortisone for children
once controlled
LPC 2% + salicylic acid 2% in aqueous cream at night

Flexural (inverse) and genital psoriasis

Note that fissuring (e.g. inframammary, natal cleft) is a feature. There is little or no scale.

methylprednisolone aceponate 0.1% ointment or fatty ointment, once daily for several weeks (up to 2 weeks in children)
once controlled
LPC 2% in emulsifying ointment at night

Nail psoriasis

If patient motivated:

calcipotriol + betamethasone dipropionate 50 + 500 mcg/g ointment, in proximal nail fold and under nail, at night for up to 3 months

If onycholysis or subungual hyperkeratosis:

betamethasone dipropionate 0.05% lotion topically, twice daily under nail for up to 3 months

Expert treatments

- Dithranol topical therapy is rarely used, can stain clothes and burn unaffected skin
- Narrowband ultraviolet B phytotherapy (UV-B)
  - treatment 2–3 times a week for a few months
  - often used in combination with other therapies
- Methotrexate
  - dramatic results in severe cases
- Cyclosporin
  - symptoms quickly return when treatment stops and not recommended long term
- Acitretin is a vitamin A derivative and effective in severe intractable psoriasis (never use in females of child-bearing age)
- Biological agents
  - directed at the T cell dysfunction (i.e. immune response modifiers), e.g. efalizumab, infliximab, ustekinumab, alefacept

Nappy rash[2]

Nappy rash (or diaper dermatitis) is an inflammatory contact dermatitis occurring in the napkin area and can be a common presentation of mild or moderate underlying skin disease. It is found in children up to 2 years old and has a peak incidence from 9–12 months.[8]

Most children will develop nappy rash at some stage of infancy with an estimated 50% having it to a significant extent. The commonest type is *irritant dermatitis*, but consider also:

- *Candida albicans* (invariably present although often not obvious)
- seborrhoeic dermatitis
- atopic dermatitis
- psoriasis

Irritant dermatitis

This is a type of contact dermatitis with the erythema and scaling conforming to the napkin area. The flexures are usually spared. It is related to the activity of faecal proteases and lipases and probably not to the activity of ammonia (from urea) as previously promoted. The problem can vary from mild erythema to a severe blistering eruption with ulceration. Ultrabsorbent disposable nappies appear to be better than cloth nappies.[9] Diarrhoea is a causative factor of irritant dermatitis. If the eruption extends further than the points of contact with the nappy, an underlying skin disease such as seborrhoeic or atopic dermatitis must be suspected. Psoriasis always involves the skin folds.

Seborrhoeic dermatitis

This affects mainly the flexures of the natal cleft and groin. It is important to look for evidence of seborrhoeic dermatitis elsewhere, such as cradle cap and lesions on the face and axillae.

Atopic dermatitis

Atopic dermatitis can involve the napkin area. Pruritus is a feature and the child may be observed scratching the area. There may be evidence of atopic dermatitis elsewhere, such as on the face.

Candidiasis (monilia nappy rash)

Superinfection of intertrigo or napkin dermatitis will result in a diffuse, red, raw, shiny rash that will involve the flexures and extend beyond the napkin area as 'satellite lesions'. Candida tends to invade the skin folds and the foreskin of male babies.

Causes of nappy rash

The main predisposing factor in all types is dampness due to urine and faeces. It is far less common since the use of disposable nappies. Persistent cases often become colonised with *Candida albicans*. Other causes or aggravating factors are:

- a tendency of the baby to eczema
- a tendency of the baby to seborrhoeic dermatitis
- infection, especially *Candida* (thrush)
- rough-textured nappies
- chemicals in some baby wipes
- plastic pants (aggravates wetness)
- excessive washing of the skin with soap
- too much powder over the nappy area (avoid talcum powders)

Uncommon causes

Psoriatic nappy rash

This presents as a non-scaling eruption, primarily on the napkin area, but can extend to the flexures, trunk and limbs. The edge of the rash is sharply demarcated. The typical psoriatic scale is absent. It tends to occur in the first weeks of life. There is usually a family history.

Infections

Bacterial infections to consider include staphylococcal folliculitis, impetigo and perianal streptococcal dermatitis. Culture of the lesion will reveal the cause.

Impetigo

If there is *Staphylococcus* superinfection, bullae and pus-filled blisters will be present.

Histiocytosis X (Letterer–Siwe syndrome)

There is a similar rash to seborrhoeic dermatitis but the lesions are purpuric. In this serious syndrome the child is very ill and usually lymphadenopathy and hepatosplenomegaly may be found.

Zinc deficiency

May be more common than realised.

Management

Basic care (instructions to parents/carers):

1. Keep the area dry. Change wet or soiled nappies frequently and as soon as you notice them. Use highly absorbent disposable nappies.
2. After removing nappy, gently remove any urine or moisture with a soap substitute or warm water.
3. Wash gently with warm water, pat dry (do not rub) and then apply a barrier preparation to help protect the area. Vaseline or zinc cream applied lightly will do.
4. Expose the bare skin to fresh air wherever possible.
5. Use a soap substitute and bath oil for bathing.
6. Avoid powder and plastic pants.

Medical treatment

Some principles follow:

- The cornerstone of treatment is prevention.
- Barrier preparations should be used to protect the skin, e.g. zinc oxide (best) or white soft paraffin or a mixture of zinc oxide and castor oil or Vaseline.
- A mild topical corticosteroid is the treatment of choice.
- It is useful to add an antifungal agent.
- If infection is suspected, confirm by swab or skin scraping.
- Consider a combined steroid and antifungal agent e.g. Hydrozole.
- When nappy rash is severe, apply a stronger topical steroid for up to 7 days, e.g. methylprednisolone aceponate 0.1% ointment or fatty ointment, once daily.

  Treatment:

Atopic dermatitis	1% hydrocortisone
Seborrhoeic dermatitis	1% hydrocortisone + ketoconazole cream
Widespread (*Candida* present)	1% hydrocortisone cream mixed in equal quantities with nystatin (apply bd) or miconazole + zinc oxide (apply after nappy changes)
Psoriatic dermatitis	tar preparation, or 1% hydrocortisone
Impetigo	topical mupirocin; oral antibiotics if severe

FACIAL RASHES

Common facial skin disorders include acne, rosacea, peri-oral dermatitis and seborrhoeic dermatitis. These conditions must be distinguished from lupus erythematosus (discoid LE is more common).

Acne

Acne is inflammation of the pilosebaceous (oil) glands of the skin (see FIG. 121.11). At first there is excessive sebum production due to the action of androgen. These glands become blocked (blackheads and whiteheads) due to increased keratinisation of the sebaceous duct. A secondary bacterial infection due to *Propionibacterium acnes* in the sebum produces

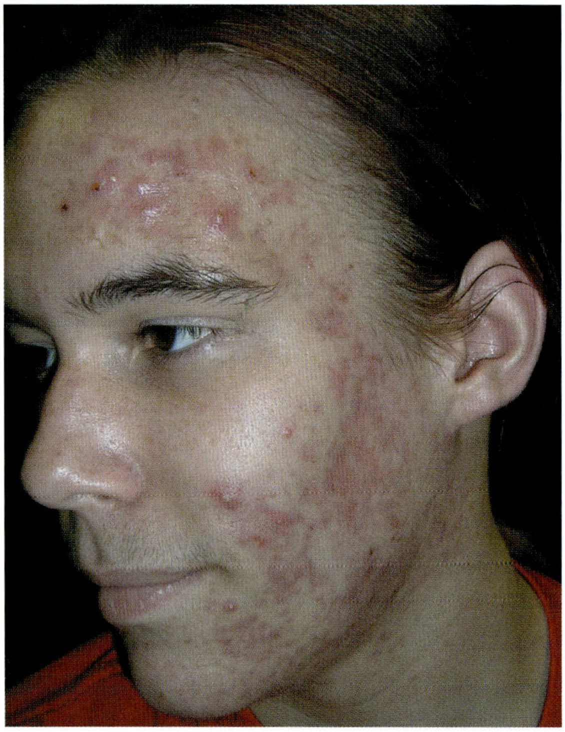

FIGURE 121.11 Facial acne showing typical nodulocystic acne, a distressing problem which has been improved greatly by the development of isotretinoin

121

lipases with the resultant free fatty acids, thus provoking inflammation characterised by red papules, pustules, nodules and cysts.

Acne usually peaks early in puberty and resolves in males during the early twenties.[2] Females are more likely to suffer ongoing acne. Consider PCOS as a causative condition.

History

In women, enquire about hirsutism and menstrual irregularity. Consider the patient's occupation (e.g chef, exposure to grease and oil exposure). Enquire about use of skin preparations—therapeutic or cosmetic, exposure to oils and drug intake.

Drugs that aggravate acne:[10]

- corticosteroids
- chloral hydrate
- iodides or bromides
- lithium
- anti-epileptics (e.g. phenytoin)
- quinine
- hormonal contraceptives (consider switching to an anti-androgenic combined oral contraceptive)

Management

Support and counselling

Adolescents hate acne; they find it embarrassing and require the sympathetic care and support not only of their doctor but also of their family. It should not be dismissed as a minor problem.

Education

People with acne should understand its pathogenesis and be given leaflets with appropriate explanations. Myths must be dispelled.

- It is not a dietary or infectious disorder.
- It is not caused by oily hair or hair touching the forehead.
- Blackheads are not dirt, and will not dissolve in hot, soapy water.

Reassure the patient that acne usually becomes less of a problem after the age of 25 years, although 15% of women and 5% of men continue to have acne as adults.

General factors

- Diet is not considered to be a causative factor but a healthy diet is encouraged.
- Special soaps and overscrubbing are unhelpful. Use a normal soap and wash gently.
- Avoid oily or creamy cosmetics and all moisturisers. Use cosmetics sparingly.
- Avoid picking and squeezing blackheads.
- Exercise, hair washing and shampoos are not of proven value.
- Ultraviolet light such as sunlight may help improve acne but avoid overexposure to the sun.

Principles of treatment[2]

1 Comedolysis: unblock the pores (follicular ducts) with keratolytics such as salicylic acid (5–10%) or benzoyl peroxide (2.5%, 5% or 10%) which also has antibacterial properties. Topical retinoids are the most effective comedolytics, e.g. tretinoin 0.025% cream or adapalene 0.1% cream or gel.
2 Decrease bacteria in the sebum with systemic antibiotics—tetracyclines or erythromycin—or with a topical antibiotic such as clindamycin.
3 Decrease sebaceous gland activity with oestrogens, spironolactone, cyproterone acetate, or isotretinoin.

Note: Oral isotretinoin is teratogenic.
Avoid concomitant use of oral and topical antibiotics.

Recommended treatment regimens

Topical regimens

Suitable for mild to moderate acne.

- Basic starting regimen is a topical retinoid in combination with benzoyl peroxide:
  - use tretinoin 0.025% cream or adapalene 0.1% cream or gel, apply each night
  - if slow response after 6 weeks, add benzoyl peroxide 2.5% or 5% gel or cream once daily (in the morning)
  - maintain for 3 months and review.
- Alternative or add-on regimens, if persistent: clindamycin HCl 600 mg in 60 mL of 70% isopropyl alcohol (e.g. ClindaTech). Apply with fingertips twice daily.

Oral antibiotics

Use for inflammatory acne: (moderate to severe papulopustular) ± trunk involvement

- doxycycline or minocycline, 50 to 100 mg per day
- erythromycin 250 to 500 mg twice daily is an alternative, especially for pregnant women
- give a minimum 12 week trial; 6 months is standard
- avoid using antibiotics alone

Other therapies

Severe cystic or recalcitrant acne (specialist care):

- spironolactone
- isotretinoin (Roaccutane): outstanding agent

Females not responding to first-line treatment:

- combined oral contraceptive pill with anti-androgenic effect (e.g. ethinyloestradiol/cyproterone acetate: Diane-35 ED)
- oral spirinolactone may be used in combination with an oral contraceptive pill as an anti-androgen (single use should be avoided due to risk of menstrual irregularity and contraindication in pregnancy)

Note: Response to any acne treatment occurs in about 8 weeks or longer.

> **Common mistakes with acne**
>
> - Not treating comedomes with a comedolytic
> - Monotherapy (e.g. antibiotics only)
> - Not using recommended combinations
> - Not using isotretinoin for cystic acne

Rosacea

Rosacea is a common persistent eruption of unknown aetiology. It is typically chronic and persistent with a fluctuant course.

Clinical features[3]

- Mainly 30–50 years
- Usually females of Celtic origin: 'the curse of the Celts'
- On forehead, cheeks, nose and chin (see FIG. 121.12 and FIG. 121.13)

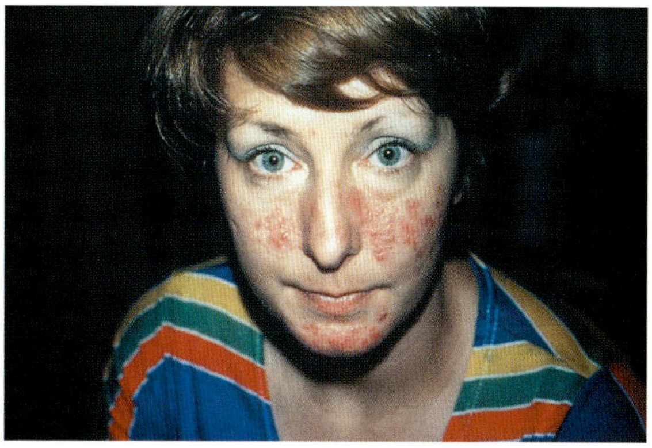

FIGURE 121.12 Rosacea: typical appearance with erythema, papules and pustules

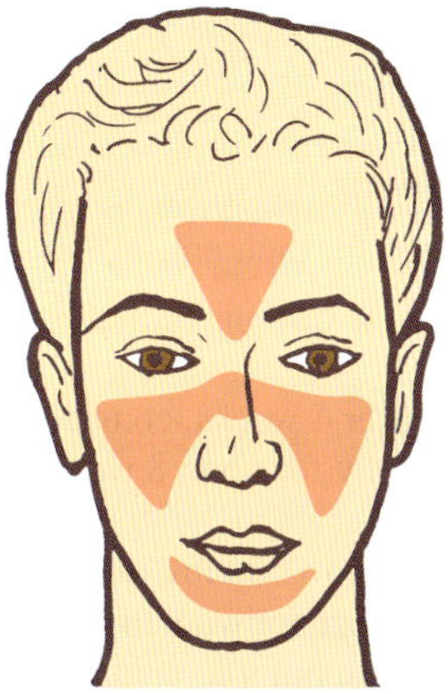

FIGURE 121.13 Rosacea: typical facial distribution

- 'Flushing and blushing' (often precedes the rash)
- Fluctuates from day to day
- Peri-orbital and peri-oral areas spared
- Vascular changes—erythema and telangiectasia
- Inflammation—papules and pustules (sterile)

121

Complications

- Blepharitis
- Conjunctivitis, rarely keratitis and corneal ulcer
- Associated rhinophyma in some cases

Management[2]

General measures

- Avoid factors that cause facial flushings (e.g. excessive sun exposure, heat, wind, alcohol, excessive exercise, hot baths, spicy foods, hot drinks—tea and coffee)
- Sun protection
- Use a gentle soap-free cleanser
- Apply green-tinted foundation to mask redness
- Avoid topical corticosteroids which can cause rebound vascular changes on cessation

Topical agents

For mild erythema and inflammatory lesions:

metronidazole 0.75% gel or cream, bd
or
azelaic acid 15% gel, once daily

Apply for 6 to 12 weeks for maximal response. Long-term treatment is usually required to prolong remission. If topical therapy is unsuccessful, add or replace with oral therapy.

For erythrotelangiectatic skin, applying a topical vasoconstrictor improves its cosmetic appearance, but the effect is temporary (about 12 hours):

brimonidine tartrate 5 mg/g gel, once daily in the morning

Systemic antibiotics

Antibiotics are used for their anti-inflammatory effect:

- Doxycycline 50 to 100 mg daily for a total of 8–10 weeks.
- If inadequate after 4 weeks, consider minocycline 50 to 100 mg daily for up to 8 weeks. Repeat for recurrences.
- Erythromycin 250 to 500 mg twice daily is an alternative for pregnant women or if doxycycline or minocycline are not tolerated.
- Low dose doxycyline or minocycline, 50 mg daily, is appropriate for longer use if symptoms recur within a month.

Laser therapy

Telangectasia, erythema and rhinophymas respond to laser therapy.

Rhinophyma

This is due to hypertrophy of the nasal sebaceous glands and is associated with older men with rosacea. Treatment options include laser ablation, shave excision or isotretinoin (see CHAPTER 59).

Peri-oral dermatitis

Clinical features

- Papular and pustular, acne-like dermatitis of lower face
- Usually young women 20–50 years
- May be seen in children and adolescents
- 'Muzzle area' distribution around mouth and on chin, sparing adjacent peri-oral area (see FIG. 121.14 and FIG. 123.15)
- Peri-orbital skin involvement is common in men
- Rash may be unilateral
- Frequently begins at the nasolabial folds
- Multiple small red macules and papules
- On a background of erythema and scaling
- Burning and irritation
- May be associated seborrhoeic dermatitis on scalp and head
- May be related to pregnancy and oral contraception
- Related to the use of creamy cosmetic products
- May be related to repeated topical corticosteroid use (may be a rebound on ceasing it)
- Peri-oral dermatitis belongs to the rosacea spectrum of disease

Treatment

- Discontinue any topical corticosteroid therapy (tends to flare initially) and all 'creamy'

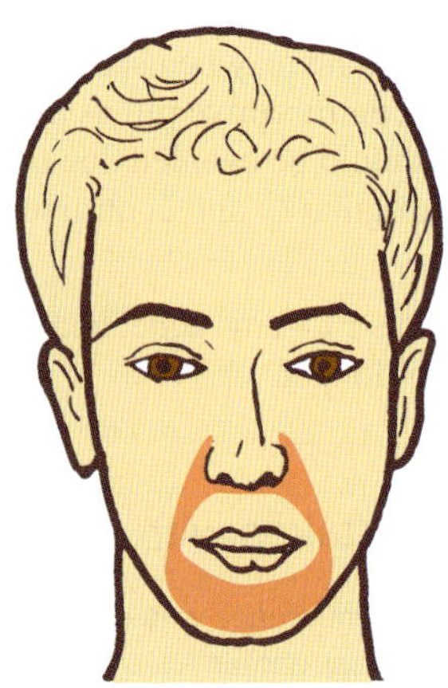

FIGURE 121.14 Peri-oral dermatitis: typical distribution

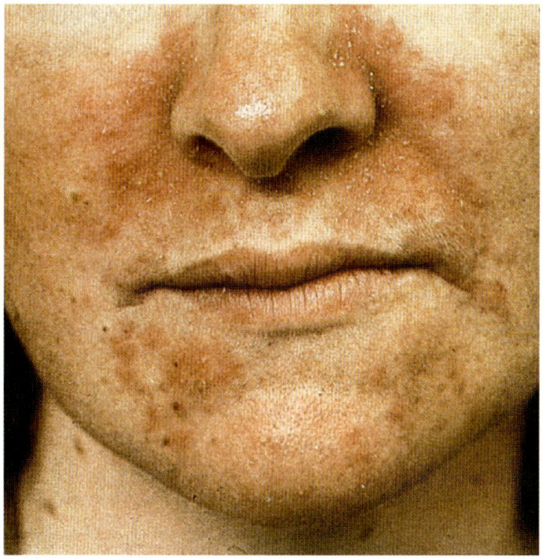

FIGURE 121.15 Peri-oral dermatitis: this eruption (which has been linked with the use of fluorinated steroid creams on the face) frequently begins in the nasolabial fold. Papules and pustules occur on a background of erythema and scaling.

preparations including cleansers, moisturisers and make-up.

- Simple treatments include cleansing with a gentle soap substitute, cold compress for irritation and use of a light emollient
- Treatment is with oral antibiotics for their anti-inflammatory properties, as for rosacea.
- Topical treatments are not as effective and may irritate: metronidazole 0.75% gel or clindamycin 1% lotion twice daily.

TINEA

Tinea (ringworm infections) is caused mainly by three major classes of dermatophytic organisms that have the ability to invade and proliferate in keratin of the skin, nails and hair.

It is most useful to perform skin scrapings and microscopy to look for encroaching septate hyphae. Confirm the diagnosis by fungal culture. Tinea cruris is presented in CHAPTER 120.

Tinea pedis (athlete's foot)

Tinea pedis is usually caused by *Trichophyton rubrum* and is the commonest type of fungal infection in humans. Candida intertrigo and interdigital maceration (alone without secondary tinea) in particular and also erythrasma, eczema and psoriasis, are important differential diagnoses.

Symptoms

The commonest symptoms are itchiness and foot odour. Sweat and water make the top layer of skin white and soggy. There is scaling, maceration and fissuring of the skin between the fourth and fifth toes and also third and fourth toes.

Advice to patients

- Keep your feet as clean and dry as possible.
- Carefully dry your feet after bathing and showering.
- After drying your feet, use an antifungal powder, especially between the toes.
- Remove flaky skin from beneath the toes each day with dry tissue paper or gauze.
- Wear light socks made of natural absorbent fibres, such as cotton and wool, to allow better circulation of air and to reduce sweating. Avoid synthetic socks.
- Change your shoes and socks daily. Spray shoes with an antifungal agent.
- If possible, wear open sandals or shoes with porous soles and uppers.
- Go barefoot whenever possible.
- Use thongs in public showers such as at swimming pools (rather than bare feet).

Treatment

Several topical antifungals can be used. Preferable to use terbinafine 1% once or twice daily for 1–2 weeks and review. If severe and spreading, prescribe oral griseofulvin (see Tinea corporis) or terbinafine for up to 6 weeks after confirming the diagnosis by fungal culture.

Castellani paint may be helpful for macerated areas.

Tinea corporis[11]

Tinea corporis (ringworm infection of the body) is usually caused by *Trichophyton rubrum* (60%) or *Microsporum canis*.[12] Strongly related to exposure to cats and dogs, while the guinea pig is a potent source of facial tinea (can present as pustular folliculitis).

Clinical features

- Spreading circular erythematous lesions (see FIG. 121.16)
- Slight scaling or vesicles at the advancing edge

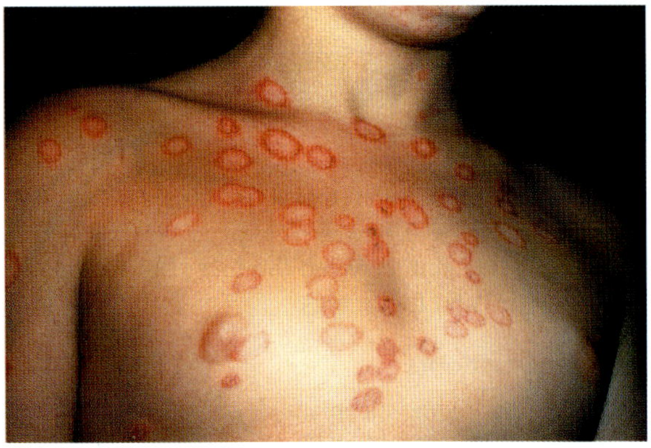

FIGURE 121.16 Multiple ringworm (tinea corporis): this 12-year-old boy presented with a two-week history of an increasing number of pruritic scaling erythematous lesions on his face, neck and upper chest. Fungal scrapings confirmed the cause as *Microsporum canis*.

Photo courtesy Robin Marks

- Central areas usually normal
- Mild itch
- May involve hair, feet and nails

Treatment

- First choice is terbinafine 1% cream or gel, once or twice daily for 1–2 weeks
- Other options include clotrimazole 1%, miconazole 2% cream, bifonazole 1% cream, ketoconazole 2% cream, applied bd for 2–4 weeks
- Oral terbinafine 250 mg or griseofulvin 500 mg daily, for up to 6 weeks if no response or widespread

Tinea capitis[2]

In Australia tinea capitis is usually due to *M. canis* acquired from cats and dogs.

Clinical features

- Usually in children (rare after puberty)
- Patches of partial alopecia
- Scaly patches
- Small broken-off hair shafts
- Hairs fluoresce yellow-green with Wood's light (not invariably, e.g. with *Trichophyton tonsurans* infection)

Treatment

terbinafine (o): adults 250 mg daily for 4 weeks; children 62.5–125 mg
or
griseofulvin (o): adults 500 mg daily; children 10 mg/kg/day (max. 500 mg) 6–8 week course

Take hair plucking and scale for culture. Treat *Trichophyton tonsurans* with terbinafine and *Microsporum canis* with griseofulvin.

Kerion

Kerion of the scalp and beard area may present like an abscess—tender and fluctuant. Usually occurs on the scalp, face or limbs. A fungal cause is possible if the hairs are plucked out easily and without pain (if painful and stuck, bacterial infection is likely).

Tinea incognito

This is the term used for unrecognised tinea infection due to modification with corticosteroid treatment. The lesions are enlarging and persistent, especially on the groins, hands and face.

The sequence is initial symptomatic relief of itching, stopping the ointment or cream and then relapse.

Tinea cruris

Refer to CHAPTER 120.

Tinea unguium (toenails and fingernails)

Refer to CHAPTER 127.

Pityriasis versicolor (tinea versicolor)[12]

Pityriasis versicolor is a superficial yeast infection of the skin (usually on the trunk) caused by *Malassezia* sp.). The old name, tinea versicolor, is inappropriate because the problem is not a dermatophyte infection. It occurs worldwide but is more common in tropical and subtropical climates.

There are two distinct presentations:

1 reddish brown, slightly scaly patches on upper trunk
2 hypopigmented area that will not tan, especially in suntanned skin

The term 'versicolor' means variable colours.

Clinical features

- Mainly young and middle-aged adults
- Brown on pale skin or white on tanned skin (see FIG. 121.17)
- Trunk distribution (see FIG. 121.18)

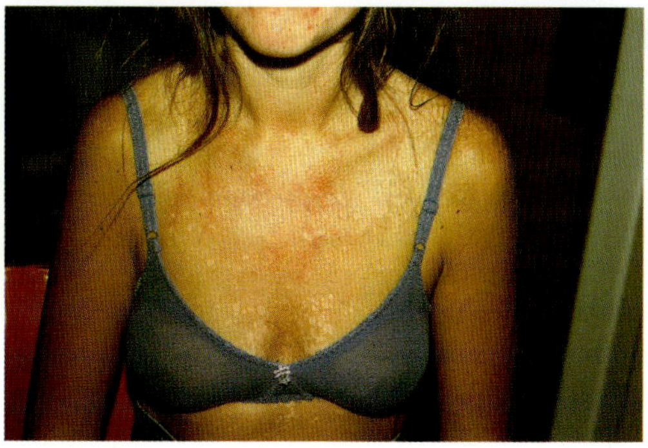

FIGURE 121.17 Pityriasis versicolor showing the hypopigmented scaly patches on a suntanned skin mainly affecting the trunk

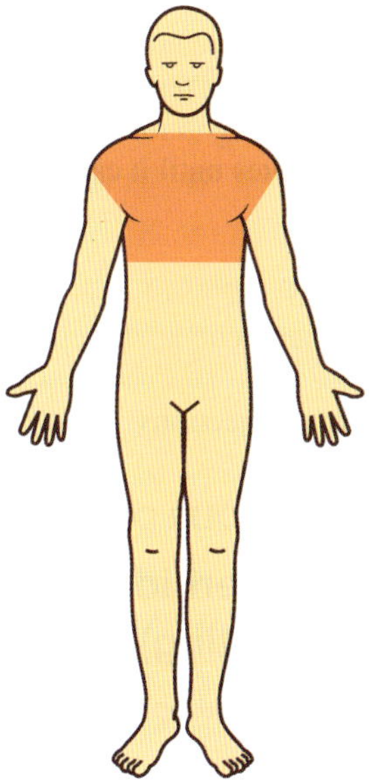

FIGURE 121.18 Pityriasis versicolor: typical truncal distribution (corresponding area on back)

- Patches may coalesce
- May involve neck, upper arms, face and groin
- Slight scaling when scratched indicates active infection
- Scales removed by scraping show characteristic short stunted hyphae with spores on microscopy
- Often recurrent, especially in summer

Differential diagnosis

Seborrhoeic dermatitis of trunk (more erythematous), pityriasis rosea, vitiligo, pityriasis alba (affects face).

Treatment[2]

econazole 1% solution to wet skin, leave overnight, for 3 nights

or

ketoconazole shampoo, once daily for 3–5 minutes and wash off, for 5 days

or

selenium sulphide 2.5% shampoo, once daily, leave on for at least 10 minutes or overnight, for 7–10 days

or (for persistent or recurrent problems)

fluconazole 400 mg orally, as a single dose

or

(for prophylaxis) itraconazole 200 mg (o) twice daily for 1 day per month for 6 months[2]

Note:

- Griseofulvin and terbinafine are inappropriate because the rash is not a fungal infection.
- Warn patients that the white patches will take a long time to disappear and that cure does not equate to disappearance. Pigment will return once there is sufficient sun to repigment the white patches.

Dry skin

Disorders associated with scaling and roughness of the skin include:

- atopic dermatitis—all types (e.g. pityriasis alba, nummular eczema, asteatotic dermatitis)
- ageing skin
- psoriasis
- ichthyotic disorders
- keratosis pilaris

Itching may be a feature of dry skin (but is not inevitable).

Aggravating factors:

- low humidity (e.g. heaters, air-conditioners)
- frequent immersion in water
- heat/hot water
- toilet soaps
- swimming in chlorinated pools

Management

- Avoid a dry home environment if possible.
- Reduce bathing.
- Bathe or shower in tepid water.
- Use a soap substitute (e.g. Dove or Neutrogena/Cetaphil lotion).
- Pat dry—avoid vigorous towelling.
- Rub in baby oil after bathing (better than adding oil to the bath).

121

- Avoid wool next to the skin (wear cotton).
- Use emollients/moisturisers (e.g. Alpha-Keri lotion, QV skin lotion, Nutraplus).

Sunburn

Sunburn is normally caused by UV-B radiation, which penetrates the epidermis and superficial dermis, releasing substances such as leucotrienes and histamines, which cause redness and pain. Severe sunburn may develop on relatively dull days because thin clouds filter UV-B poorly. Beware of solariums and the midday sun.

Clinical presentations:

Minor sunburn:	Mild erythema with minimal discomfort for about 3 days.
Moderate:	Moderate to severe erythema within a few hours; worse the following day—red, hot and moderately painful. Settles in 3–4 days with some desquamation.
Severe:	Classic signs of inflammation—redness, heat, pain and swelling. Skin develops vesicles and bullae. Systemic features develop with very severe burns (e.g. fever, headache, nausea, delirium, hypotension). May require IV fluids.

Differential diagnosis

121

- General photosensitivity: consider drugs (e.g. thiazide diuretics, tetracyclines, sulphonamides, phenothiazines, griseofulvin, NSAIDs, isotretinoin)
- Acute systemic lupus erythematosus may present as unexpectedly severe sunburn
- Photocontact dermatitis

Treatment

Oral aspirin or ibuprofen ease pain. Oil in water baths or bicarbonate of soda paste may help, and wet applications such as oily calamine lotions or simply cool compresses may give relief. Topical corticosteroids may be applied to unblistered erythematous skin, twice daily for the first 2 or 3 days. Use a moisturiser that contains aloe vera to soothe skin.

Prevention

Avoid direct exposure to summer sunlight during peak UV periods (10 am to 3 pm). Use natural shade—beware of reflected light from sand or water and light cloud. Use a sunscreen with a minimum of SPF 30. Wear broad-brimmed hats and protective clothing.

Photo-ageing/wrinkles

Prevention

- Stop smoking.
- Avoid cold, dry and windy conditions.
- Avoid exposure to the sun.
- Use an SPF 30 or more sunscreen during the day.
- Avoid soaps with perfume and alcohol.
- Wash with a 'neutral' mild soap (e.g. Neutrogena, max. twice daily) and pat dry.
- Apply a simple moisturiser immediately after the bath.

Treatment (options)

- Optimal nutrition—diet rich in fruit and vegetables
- Alpha hydroxy acid preparations (e.g. Elucent cream)
- Tretinoin (Retin-A) cream: apply once daily at bedtime (on dry skin); test for skin irritation by gradual exposure (e.g. 5 minutes at first, wash off, then 15 minutes until it can be left on overnight)
- Topical olive oil
- Lac-Hydrin (US): 12% solution may be effective alternative; other lactic acid preparations may be useful
- Botulinum toxin injections

SWEATING AND ODOUR DISORDERS

Primary hyperhidrosis (excessive sweating)[13]

This problem is usually idiopathic and prolonged.

Clinical features

- Male = female incidence
- Affects axilla, groin, soles and palms
- Onset usually around puberty
- Tends to improve after age 25 years
- Family history
- ± Bromhidrosis (malodorous perspiration)
- Usually independent of climate
- Exacerbated by stress and heat; stops during sleep

Causes (secondary/pathological)

- Fever/sepsis
- Thyrotoxicosis
- Acromegaly
- Diabetes mellitus
- Phaeochromocytoma
- Drugs: alcohol/narcotics/antidepressants

- Some neurological conditions (e.g. Parkinson)
- Malignancies especially lymphomas

Treatment[2,13]

- Avoid known aggravating factors
- First use:

  an aluminium chlorohydrate-containing antiperspirant deodorant (spray or roll on each morning) in axilla (suitable for palms and soles)
  or
  aluminium chloride hexahydrate 20% solution or spray (Driclor)—apply to affected areas at night when the area is dry (best for palms and soles, although irritation is a problem).

Additional treatments

- Iontophoresis (in specialist centres) to hands and feet.
- Injection of botulinum toxin into dermis of affected area. Proven effectiveness for axillae and palms with up to 6 months of anhydrosis.
- Oral anticholinergics (e.g. oxybutynin, propantheline) may give some benefit but are often poorly tolerated.
- Surgical sympathectomy is an option for severe, recalcitrant cases.

Body odour/bromhidrosis

Cause: poor hygiene, excessive sweating, active skin bacteria, metabolic disorders e.g. trimethylaminuria (rare)—causes fishy odour

Main focus: axillae and groin

Precautions: consider uraemia, vaginitis

Treatment

- Scrub body, especially groins and axillae, with deodorant soap at least morning and night
- Try an antibacterial surgical scrub
- Keep clothes clean, launder regularly
- Choose suitable clothes—natural fibres (e.g. cotton), not synthetics
- Use an antiperspirant deodorant
- Alternative soap—pine soap
- Diet: avoid garlic, fish, asparagus, onions, curry
- Reduce caffeine (coffee, tea and cola drinks), which stimulates sweat activity
- Consider a sugar-free diet
- Remove axillary hair
- Consider injections of botulinum toxin for excessive perspiration

Foot odour (smelly and sweaty feet)

Includes pitted keratolysis secondary to hyperhidrosis (common in teenagers).

Treatment (with options)

- Education and reassurance
- Wear cotton or woollen socks
- Aluminium chloride hexahydrate 20% solution (Driclor) or Neat Feet—apply nocte for 1 week, then 1–2 times weekly as necessary
- Shoe liners (e.g. 'Odor eaters'), charcoal inner soles
- Apply undiluted Burow's solution after a shower or bath
- Formalin 1–5% soaks every second night
- Iontophoresis
- The teabag treatment (if desperate):
  - prepare 600 mL of strong hot tea (from two teabags left in water for 15 minutes)
  - pour the hot tea into a basin with 2 L of cool water
  - soak the feet in this for 20–30 minutes daily for 10 days, then as often as required

SKIN DISORDERS OF FEET

Two conditions commonly seen in teenagers are pitted keratolysis and juvenile plantar dermatosis.

Pitted keratolysis

This common malodorous condition known as 'stinky feet' or 'sneakers feet', usually seen in 10–14-year-olds, is related to sweaty feet. It is caused by an overgrowth of bacteria that digest keratin on the feet (*Corynebacterium sp.* most common). It has a 'honeycomb' pitted appearance with maceration between the toes, resembling tinea. For mild cases no specific treatment is needed other than attending to hyperhidrosis. Otherwise, treatment includes keeping the feet dry and using clindamycin 1% lotion bd for 10 days, to remove the responsible organism. Try oral roxithromycin if topical therapy fails. Consider changing to all-leather shoes with charcoal liners. Use a drying agent to decrease sweating.

Juvenile plantar dermatosis

'Sweaty sock dermatitis' is a painful condition of weight-bearing areas of the feet. The affected skin is red, shiny, smooth and often cracked. It is rare in adults. The treatment is to avoid friction as much as possible with a barrier cream and suitable footwear, preferably with leather or open shoes and cotton socks. A simple emollient such as urea cream gives relief. Cracks can be treated with medicinal glues.

Prickly heat (miliaria/heat rash)

- Avoid sweating as much as possible.
- Keep the skin dry and cool (e.g. fan, air-conditioner).
- Dress in loose-fitting cotton clothing.
- Attend to bedding—cotton sheets, no plastic underlay.
- Reduce activity.
- Avoid frequent bathing and overuse of soap.
- Dilute topical steroid cream bd.

Treatment

lotion: salicylic acid 2%, menthol 1%, chlorhexidine 0.5% in alcohol or calamine lotion

or

Egozite (infants), Isophyl (adults)

If severe: hydrocortisone 1% + clotrimazole 1% cream (brief spells only).

Prevention

- Ego Prickly Heat powder

CHILBLAINS AND FROSTBITE

Chilblains (perniosis)

These are localised inflammatory reactions, caused by prolonged exposure to cold, usually on toes and fingers (see FIG. 121.19) but also on heels, nose, ears and thighs (horse riding).

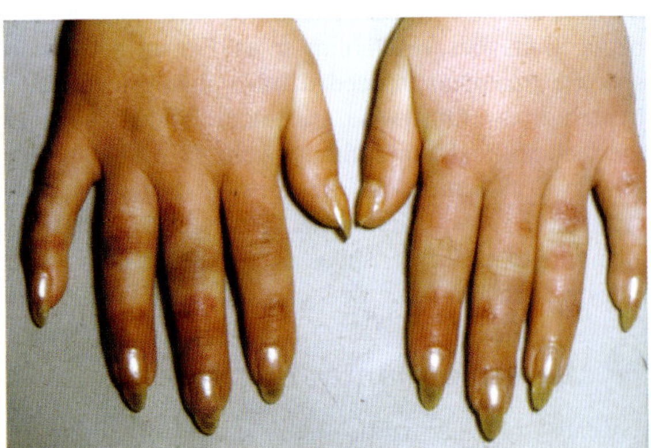

FIGURE 121.19 Chilblains (perniosis) showing erythematous purplish swellings on fingers

Precautions

- Think Raynaud phenomenon.
- Protect from trauma and secondary infection.
- Do not rub or massage injured tissues.
- Do not apply heat or ice.
- Wear warm gloves and socks.

Differences between chilblains and Raynaud phenomenon:

- chilblains are intermittent without a pattern
- itchy at the onset
- patchy appearance (can be more generalised)
- Raynaud has two or three phases including a 'dead white' phase with line of demarcation
- it is significant if it extends to the MCP joints

Treatment

- Elevate affected part
- Warm gradually to room temperature

Drug treatment

- Potent topical corticosteroid (see TABLE 119.9 in CHAPTER 119) twice daily
- If severe and recurrent, apply glyceryl trinitrate vasodilator spray or 0.2% ointment or patch sparingly once daily (use plastic gloves and wash hands for ointment), although weak supportive evidence

Other treatment

- Drink rum at night
- Nifedipine CR 30 mg (o) once daily (if very severe)
- UVB therapy weekly for 4–6 weeks prior to cold weather

Frostbite

Treatment depends on severity.

Precautions

- Watch for secondary infection, tetanus, gangrene.

Treatment

- Elevate affected limb
- Rewarm in water just above body temperature 40°C (104°F) or use body heat (e.g. in axillae)
- Avoid thawing or refreezing
- Surgical debridement
- Don't debride early (wait until dead tissue dried)
- Don't drink alcohol or smoke
- For blistering, apply warm water compresses for 15 minutes every 2 hours

Drug treatment

- Analgesics

Patient education resources

Hand-out sheets from *Murtagh's Patient Education* 7th edition:

- Atopic dermatitis (eczema)
- Body odour
- Contact dermatitis
- Dry skin
- House dust mite management
- Nappy rash
- Pityriasis rosea
- Psoriasis
- Ringworm (tinea)
- Rosacea and perioral dermatitis
- Seborrhoea in infants
- Sunburn
- Sweaty and smelly feet
- Tinea pedis

References

1 Britt H, Miller GC, Charles J. General practice activity in Australia 2009–11. BEACH data. Sydney: Australian Institute of Health and Welfare and the University of Sydney, December 2010.

2 Expert group for Dermatology. In: eTG complete. Melbourne: Therapeutic Guidelines Ltd. Available from: <www.tg.org.au>, accessed April 2018.

3 Berger P. *Skin Secrets.* Sydney: Allen & Unwin, 1991: 93–170.

4 Brown P. Dermatitis/eczema. In: *MIMS Disease Index* (2nd edn). Sydney: IMS Publishing, 1996: 142–4.

5 Smith S, Dixit S, Fischer G. Childhood atopic dermatitis: Overcoming parental anxiety. Medicine Today, 2013; 14 (6): 47–52.

6 Tritton SM, Cooper A. Management of psoriasis. Update. Medical Observer, 30 November 2007: 27–30.

7 Howard A, Gamboni S. Psoriasis: how to treat. Australian Doctor, 18 January 2013: 17–24.

8 Gallachio V. Nappy rash. Aust Fam Physician, 1988; 17: 971–2.

9 Aldridge S. Nappy rash. Australian Paediatric Review, 1991; 2 (1): 2.

10 Sullivan J, Preda V. A clinically practical approach to acne. Medicine Today, 2008; 9 (1): 47–56.

11 Gin D. Tinea infections. In: *MIMS Disease Index* (2nd edn). Sydney: IMS Publishing, 1996: 511–13.

12 Hunter JAA, Savin JA, Dahl MV. *Clinical Dermatology* (3rd edn). Oxford: Blackwell Scientific Publications, 2002: 159–60.

13 Perera E, Sinclair M. Hyperhidrosis and bromhidrosis— a guide to assessment and management. Aust Fam Physician, 2013; 42 (5): 266–9.

Resources

DermNet NZ: the dermatology resource <www.dermnetnz.org>
Therapeutic Guidelines: eTG Complete <www.tg.org.au>

122 Acute skin eruptions

They say love's like the measles—all the worse when it comes late in life.

DOUGLAS JERROLD (1803–57)

The sudden appearance of a rash, which is a common presentation in children (see CHAPTER 93), usually provokes patients and doctors alike to consider an infectious aetiology, commonly of viral origin. However, an important cause to consider is a reaction to a drug.

A knowledge of the relative distribution of the various causes of rashes helps with the diagnostic methodology. Many of the eruptions are relatively benign and undergo spontaneous remission. Fortunately, the potentially deadly rash of smallpox is no longer encountered.

The diagnostic model is outlined in TABLE 122.1.

A diagnostic approach

The diagnostic approach to skin eruptions presupposes a basic knowledge of the causes; a careful history and physical examination should logically follow.

The history should include:

- site and mode of onset of the rash
- mode of progression
- drug history
- constitutional disturbance (e.g. pyrexia, pruritus)
- respiratory symptoms
- herald patch?
- diet—unaccustomed food
- exposure to irritants
- contacts with infectious disease
- bleeding or bruising tendency

The examination should include:

- skin of whole body
- nature and distribution of rash, including lesion characteristics
- soles of feet
- nails
- scalp
- mucous membranes
- oropharynx
- conjunctivae and the lymphopoietic system (? lymphadenopathy ? splenomegaly)

Laboratory investigations may include:

- a full blood examination
- syphilis serology
- Epstein–Barr mononucleosis test
- HIV test
- rubella haemagglutination tests (x 2)
- viral and bacterial cultures

Dermatological manifestations of systemic disease

- Painful red nodules
  - erythema nodosum
- Photosensitive rash
  - dermatomyositis (inflamed muscles + rash)—cause unknown, malignancy known association
  - systemic lupus erythematosis
- Palpable purpura
  - vasculitis—primary or secondary (e.g. sepsis), various causes
- Painful ulceration
  - pyoderma granulosum

  Causes
  - inflammatory bowel disease
  - rheumatoid arthritis
  - haematological malignancies

Acute skin eruptions in children

The following skin eruptions (some of which may also occur in adults) are outlined in CHAPTER 93.

- Measles
- Rubella
- Viral exanthem (fourth disease)
- Erythema infectiosum (fifth disease)
- Roseola infantum (sixth disease)
- Kawasaki disease
- Varicella
- Impetigo

Table 122.1 Acute skin eruptions: diagnostic strategy model

Probability diagnosis

Hand, foot and mouth disease
Erythema infectiosum (slapped cheek disease or fifth disease)
Roseola infantum (sixth disease)
Other viral exanthema (e.g. enterovirus)
Pityriasis rosea
Impetigo
Folliculitis (e.g. pseudomonas, staphylococcus)
Varicella (chickenpox)
Herpes zoster (shingles)
Herpes simplex
Urticaria
Drug reaction (see TABLE 122.4)

Serious disorders not to be missed

Vascular/vasculitis:

- Henoch–Schönlein purpura
- Stevens–Johnson syndrome/toxic epidermal necrolysis
- other vasculitides e.g. polyarteritis nodosa

Infection:

- purpura of meningococcus, typhoid, other sepsis
- scarlet fever
- primary HIV infection
- secondary syphilis
- measles
- rubella (in pregnancy)

Other:

- erythema nodosum

Pitfalls (often missed)

- guttate psoriasis
- Epstein–Barr virus (EBV) mononucleosis
- arbovirus infection (e.g. dengue, Ross River fever, Barmah Forest virus, Japanese encephalitis)
- scabies
- Kawasaki disease
- eczema herpeticum
- zoonoses (e.g. listeriosis, Q fever)

Rarities:

- filovirus diseases (e.g. Ebola, Marburg virus)
- erythema multiforme

Pityriasis rosea

Pityriasis rosea is a common but mild acute inflammatory skin disorder. The cause is thought to be a viral agent (possibly human herpes virus 6 or 7).

Clinical features

- Any age, mainly older children and young adults
- Preceding oval or round herald patch (1–2 weeks); can have 2–3, but none in 20% (can be mistaken for ringworm)
- Oval, salmon-pink or copper-coloured eruption 0.5–2 cm
- Coin-shaped patches with scaly margins 1–2 cm
- Follows cleavage lines of skin (see FIGS 122.1 and 122.2) with 'Christmas tree' pattern on back
- On trunk ('T-shirt' distribution)
- Occurs also on upper arms, upper legs, lower neck, face (rare) and axillae
- Patients not ill
- Itch varies from nil to severe (typically minor itching)
- Scale is on inner aspect of active border

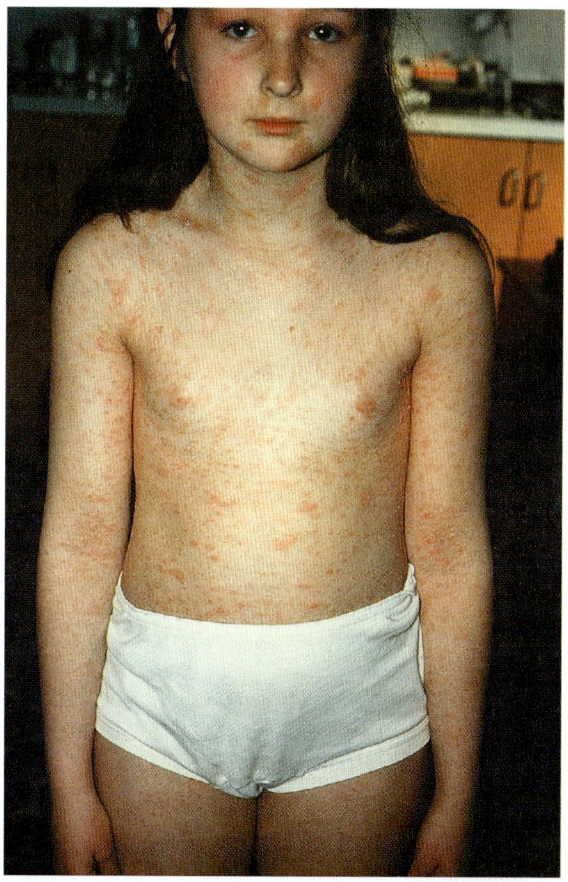

FIGURE 122.1 Pityriasis rosea in a 10-year-old child showing the salmon pink scaly eruption following skin cleavage lines—the 'Christmas tree' pattern

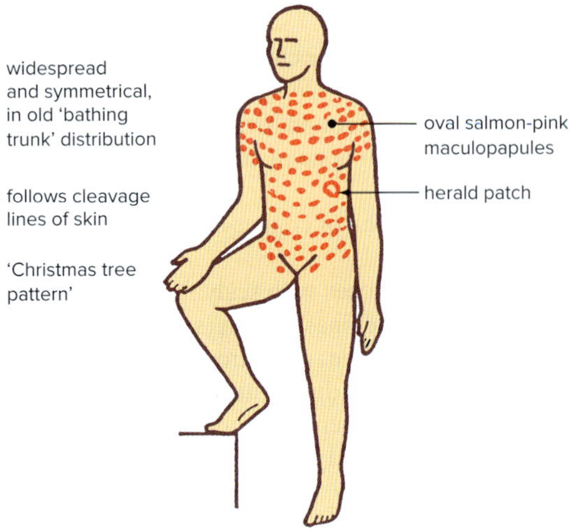

FIGURE 122.2 Pityriasis rosea: typical distribution

Differential diagnosis

Herald patch: tinea corporis/discoid eczema.

Generalised rash: seborrhoeic dermatitis (slower onset), guttate psoriasis, drug eruption (see TABLE 122.2), secondary syphilis.

Table 122.2 Drugs that cause eruptions suggestive of pityriasis rosea[1]

Main drugs:

- captopril
- gold salts
- penicillamine

Others:

- arsenicals
- barbiturates
- bismuth
- clonidine
- metoprolol
- metronidazole

122

Prognosis

A mild, self-limiting disorder with spontaneous remission in 2–10 weeks (average 2–5). It does not appear to be contagious. Recurrence is rare.

Management

- Explain and reassure with patient education handout.[2]
- Bathe and shower as usual, using a neutral soap (e.g. Neutrogena).
- Use a soothing bath oil (e.g. QV Bath Oil).
- For a bothersome itch, apply mild topical corticosteroid ointment or calamine lotion with 1% phenol or menthol 1% in aqueous cream.
- For a severe itch, use a potent topical corticosteroid once or twice daily.
- UV therapy is good but, like psoriasis, sunburn must be avoided. Expose the rash to sunlight or UV therapy (if florid) three times a week, with care.

Secondary syphilis

The generalised skin eruption of secondary syphilis varies and may resemble any type of eruption from psoriasiform to rubelliform to roseoliform. The rash usually appears 6–8 weeks after the primary chancre.

Clinical features (rash)

- Initially faint pink macules
- Then becomes maculopapular
- Can involve whole body (see FIG. 122.3)
- Palms and soles involved
- Dull red in colour and round
- More prolific on flexor surfaces
- Symmetrical and relatively coarse
- Asymptomatic

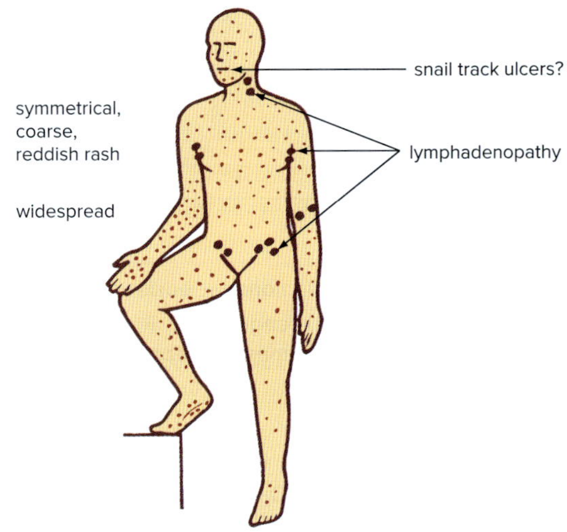

FIGURE 122.3 Secondary syphilis: typical features

Associations (possible)

- Mucosal ulcers: 'snail track'
- Lymphadenopathy
- Patchy hair loss
- Condylomata lata

Treatment

- As for primary syphilis (see CHAPTER 117)

Primary HIV infection

A common manifestation of the primary HIV infection is an erythematous, maculopapular rash, although other skin manifestations such as a roseola-like rash and urticaria can occur.

Clinical features

- Symmetrical
- May be generalised
- Lesions 5–10 mm in diameter
- Common on face and/or trunk
- Can occur on extremities including palms and soles (see FIG. 122.4)
- Non-pruritic

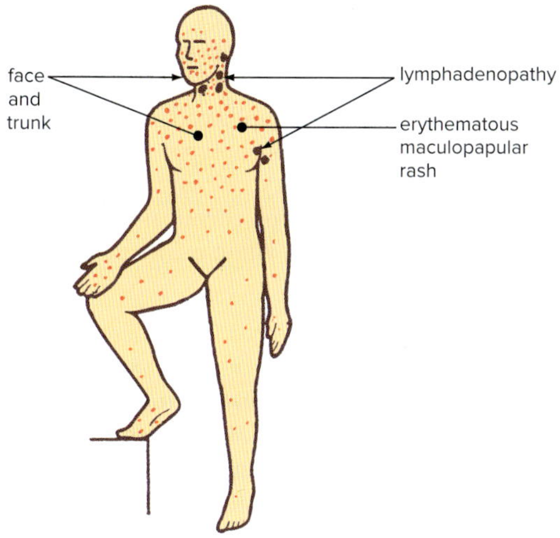

FIGURE 122.4 Primary HIV infection: typical features

Note: mimics glandular fever

If such a rash accompanied by an illness like glandular fever occurs, HIV infection should be suspected and specific tests ordered.

Guttate psoriasis

Guttate psoriasis is the sudden eruption of small (2–10 mm in diameter), very dense, round, red papules of psoriasis on the trunk (see FIGS 122.5 and 122.6). The rash may extend to the proximal limbs.

It is usually seen in children and adolescents and often precipitated by a streptococcal throat infection.

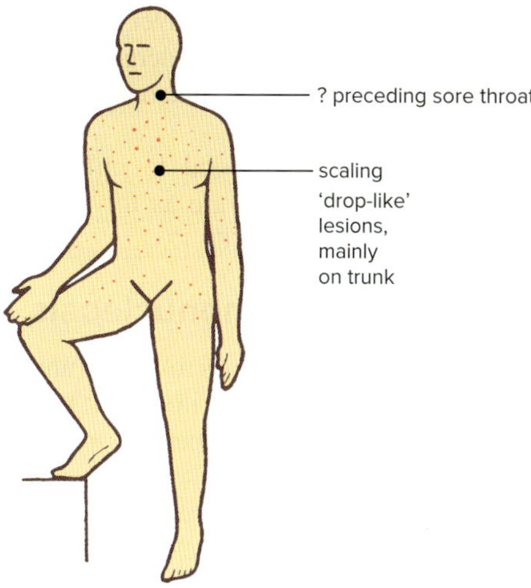

FIGURE 122.5 Guttate psoriasis: small, drop-like lesions, mainly on trunk

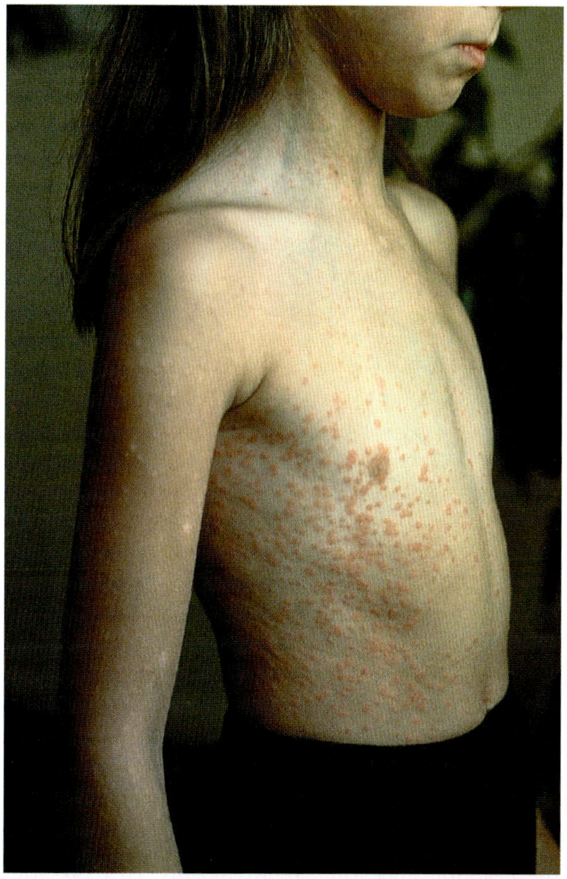

FIGURE 122.6 Guttate psoriasis in a child showing the small dense, round erythematous papules of psoriasis on the trunk

122

The rash soon develops a white silvery scale. It can persist for up to 6 months. It may undergo spontaneous resolution or enlarge to form plaques, which may become chronic.

Plaques are likely to respond to milder topical treatments. Treatment options are as for psoriasis of the trunk and limbs (see CHAPTER 121).

Epstein–Barr mononucleosis

The rash of EBM is almost always related to antibiotics given for tonsillitis (see FIG. 28.3 in CHAPTER 28). The primary rash, most often non-specific, pinkish and maculopapular (similar to that of rubella), occurs in about 5% of cases only. The secondary rash, which can be extensive and sometimes has a purplish-brown tinge, is most often precipitated by one of the penicillins (see FIG. 122.7):

- ampicillin 90–100% association
- amoxycillin 90–100% association
- penicillin up to 50%

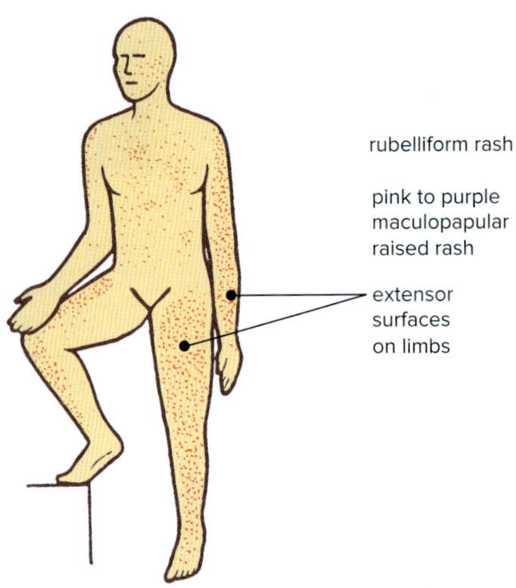

FIGURE 122.7 Epstein–Barr mononucleosis: typical rash induced by penicillin, amoxycillin or ampicillin

122

DRUG ERUPTIONS

A rash is one of the most common side effects of drug therapy, which can precipitate many different types of rash; the most common is exanthematous, also described as toxic erythema (see TABLE 122.3). Most drug-evoked dermatoses have an allergic basis with the eruption appearing approximately 10 days after administration, though much sooner if previously sensitised.[3] The most common drugs that cause skin eruptions are summarised in TABLE 122.4.

Table 122.3 Most common types of drug eruptions[3,4]

Toxic erythema/exanthematous
Urticaria/angioedema
Erythema multiforme
Eczematous dermatitis
Fixed drug reaction
Photosensitivity

Others:

- acneform
- psoriasiform
- lichenoid
- pigmentation
- erythema nodosum
- Stevens–Johnson syndrome/toxic epidermal necrolysis
- vasculitis/purpuric
- pigmentary
- exfoliative

The most important fact to realise about drug reactions is that their appearances are so variable—they may mimic almost any cutaneous disease and, in addition, create unique appearances of their own. Genetic factors appear to be implicated in predisposition to drug reactions e.g. HLA phenotype.

When taking a history it is appropriate to enquire about medications or chemicals that may be overlooked such as aspirin, vitamins, toxins, laxatives and medicated toothpaste.

Toxic erythema

The maculopapular erythematous eruption is either morbilliform or scarlatiniform. It is more pronounced on the trunk than on the limbs and face but may become confluent over the whole body (see FIG. 122.8).

Drugs that typically cause toxic erythema include:

- antibiotics:
  - penicillin/cephalosporins
  - sulphonamides
- thiazides
- carbamazepine
- barbiturates
- allopurinol
- gold salts

Photosensitivity

Several antibiotics increase the sensitivity of the skin to UV light and may lead to a rash with a distribution according to sunlight exposure. The photosensitive rash may be erythematous, resembling sunburn; eczematous; or vesiculobullous.

Table 122.4 The most common drugs that cause skin eruptions

Antimicrobials:	Penicillin/cephalosporins* Sulphonamides* Tetracyclines Nitrofurantoin Streptomycin Griseofulvin Metronidazole Antiretroviral agents Trimethoprim Dapsone
Diuretics:	Thiazides Frusemide
Anti-epileptics:	Carbamazepine* Phenytoin Lamotrigine Phenobarbitone
Tranquillisers:	Phenothiazines Barbiturates Chlordiazepoxide
Anti-inflammatory and analgesics:	Gold salts Aspirin/salicylates Codeine/morphine Pyrazalones (e.g. BTZ) Other NSAIDs*
Hormones:	Combined oral contraceptive Stilboestrol Testosterone
Others:	Phenolphthalein Immunoglobulins Amiodarone Cytotoxic drugs Quinidine/quinine Bromides and iodides Sulphonylureas Allopurinol* Warfarin Amphetamines

* Often severe

Typical drugs:

- tetracyclines
- sulphonamides/sulphonylureas
- thiazides and frusemide
- phenothiazines
- retinoids
- amiodarone
- griseofulvin
- antiretrovirals
- antihistamines, especially promethazine
- antimalarials
- psoralens

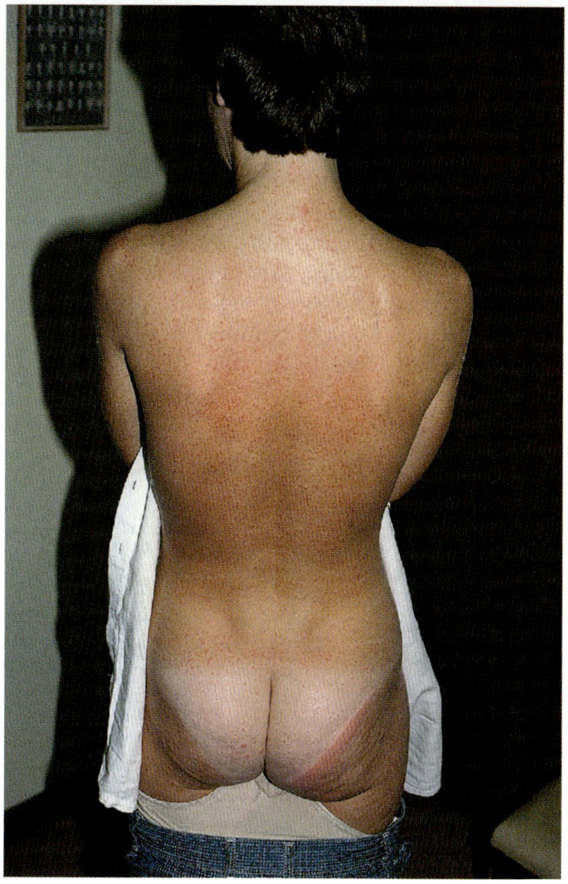

FIGURE 122.8 Toxic erythema: maculopapular erythematous scarlatiniform eruption caused by amoxicillin

122

Fixed drug eruption

The mechanism of fixed drug eruption is unknown. The most commonly affected areas are the face, hands and genitalia. The lesions, which are usually bright red but can have other characteristics, are fixed in site and appearance within hours of the drug's administration.

Typical drugs:

- NSAIDs
- sulphonamides
- phenolphthalein
- tetracyclines
- penicillins
- salicylates
- combined oral contraceptive pill
- barbiturates
- quinine

Treatment of any drug reaction

The important aspect of management is to recognise the offending agent and withdraw it. The rash should be treated according to its nature.

There is a therapeutic impulse to prescribe antihistamines but they should be reserved for the treatment of urticarial drug eruptions. They may actually delay healing in purpuric, erythematous and vesiculobullous reactions. Antihistamines may act as allergens and show cross-sensitivity with phenothiazines, sulphonamides and topical antihistamines.

TABLE 122.5 lists drugs with the highest skin reaction rates.

Table 122.5 Drugs with the highest skin reaction rates[4]
Penicillin and derivatives
Sulphonamides*
Trimethoprim*
Thiazide diuretics
Allopurinol*
Dapsone*
NSAIDs, esp. piroxicam*
Nevirapine*, abacavir*
Barbiturates
Quinidine
Anti-epileptics (phenytoin, lamotrigine*)
Blood products
Gold salts

* Severe reactions

122

ERYTHEMA

Erythema multiforme

Erythema multiforme is a hypersensitivity reaction affecting the skin and mucosal surfaces. It is usually triggered by viral infection, most commonly herpes simplex virus (HSV).

Clinical features

- Mainly in children, adolescents, young adults
- Symmetric
- Erythematous papules
- Mainly backs of hands, palms, forearms and face (see FIG. 122.9)
- Also on feet and toes, mouth
- Occasionally on trunk and genitalia
- Polymorphic

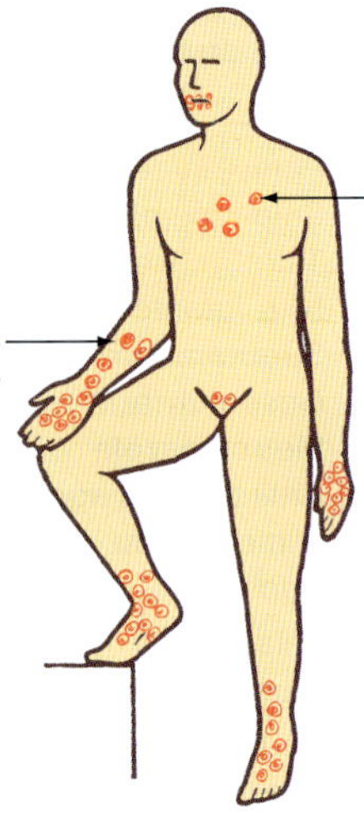

FIGURE 122.9 Erythema multiforme: typical distribution

- Vesicles and bullae may develop
- Self-limiting (up to 2 weeks)

Causes and associations

Associations include:

- unknown 50%
- herpes simplex virus 33%
- other infections: *Mycoplasma* pneumonia, tuberculosis, *Streptococcus*, HIV, adenovirus
- drugs 10%:
  - barbiturates
  - penicillin
  - sulphonamides
  - phenothiazines
  - anti-epileptics e.g. phenytoin

Stevens–Johnson syndrome/toxic epidermal necrolysis

Stevens–Johnson syndrome (SJS) and toxic epidermal necrolysis (TEN) are now believed to be variants of the same condition, distinct from erythema multiforme. It is a rare and unpredictable reaction to medication which is severe and often fatal. Onset is usually sudden, with fever, sheet-like skin, mucosal loss and constitutional symptoms. Inpatient treatment and cessation of the causative drug are required.

Causes

- Beta lactams (penicillins, cephalosporins)
- Sulphonamides

- Anti-epileptics e.g. phenytoin (known genetic factors)
- NSAIDs
- Allopurinol

Erythema nodosum

Erythema nodosum is characterised by the relatively sudden onset of bright red, raised, tender nodules on the shins, knees and ankles (see FIG. 29.1, CHAPTER 29). It is an acute, inflammatory, immunological reaction in the subcutaneous fat. The nodules may also appear on the thighs and the arms. Adult females are typically affected. An arthritic reaction can affect the ankles and knees. It is often associated with recent infection and illness.

Causes/associations

- Sarcoidosis (commonest known cause)
- Infections:
  - streptococcal infections e.g. strep throat
  - viral infections (e.g. hepatitis B)
  - tuberculosis
  - leprosy
  - chlamydia infection
  - fungal infections
  - bacterial gastroenteritis
- Inflammatory bowel disorders (e.g. Crohn)
- Drugs:
  - sulphonamides
  - tetracyclines
  - oral contraceptives
  - bromides and iodides
- Malignancy (e.g. lymphoma, leukaemia)
- Pregnancy
- Unknown (about 40%), perhaps autoimmune

Investigations

Tests include FBE, ESR/CRP, chest X-ray (the most important), streptococcal serology (e.g. ASOT) and Mantoux test.

Treatment

Identify the cause if possible. Rest, leg elevation and NSAIDs (e.g. ibuprofen 400 mg (o) bd) for the acute stage. Systemic corticosteroids speed resolution if severe episodes.

- prednisolone 0.75 mg/kg (o) up to 25 mg once daily for 2 weeks, then reduce

Prognosis

There is a tendency to settle spontaneously over 3–8 weeks. The lesions may recur.

HERPES ZOSTER

Herpes zoster (shingles) is caused by reactivation of varicella zoster virus (acquired from the primary infection of chickenpox) in the dorsal root ganglion. The term comes from the Greek *herpes* (to creep) and *zoster* (a belt or girdle). Shingles is from the Latin *cingere* (to gird) or *cingulum* (a belt). In most instances the reason for reactivation is unknown, but occasionally it is related to an underlying malignancy, usually leukaemia or a lymphoma, to immunosuppression, or to a local disease or disturbance of the spine or spinal cord, such as a tumour or radiotherapy.

The incidence is 3.4 cases per 1000 population per year. A person of any age can get herpes zoster but it is more common in people over 50 years.

Clinical features

The main features are:

- the condition is preceded by several days of radicular pain with hyperaesthesia
- unilateral patchy rash in one or two contiguous dermatomes (see FIG. 122.10)
- intense erythema with papules in affected skin
- later crusting and separation of scabs after 10–14 days, often with depigmentation
- regional lymphadenopathy

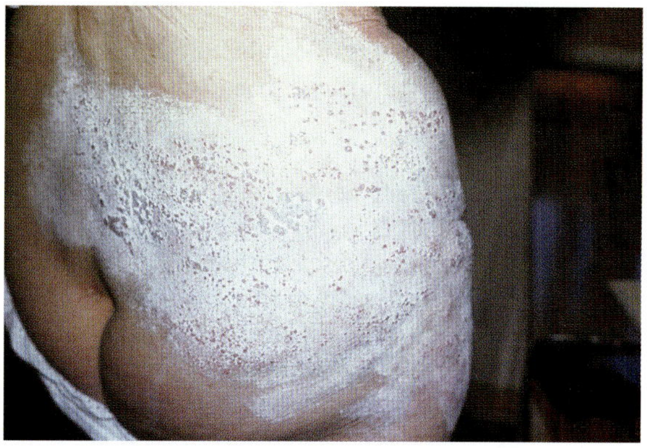

FIGURE 122.10 Herpes zoster (shingles) involving the L2 nerve root in a 63-year-old woman presenting with low back and groin pain. Calamine lotion has been applied to soothe the discomfort.

Distribution

Any part of the body may be affected, but thoracic and trigeminal dermatomes are the most common. It follows the distribution of the original varicella rash (worse on the face and trunk).

Cranial nerve involvement

The trigeminal nerve—15% of all cases:

- ophthalmic branch—50% affects nasociliary branch with lesions on tip of nose and eyes (conjunctivae and cornea)
- maxillary and mandibular—oral, palatal and pharyngeal lesions

The facial nerve: lower motor neurone facial nerve palsy with vesicles in and around external auditory meatus (notably posterior wall)—the Ramsay–Hunt syndrome.

Complications

- Rare: meningoencephalitis
- Uncommon: motor paralysis
- Common:
  - postherpetic neuralgia; increased incidence with age and debility, with duration greater than 6 months:

less than 50 years	1%
50–59 years	7%
60–69 years	21%
70–79 years	30–50%

  - the neuralgia resolves within 1 year in 70–80% of these patients but in others it may persist for years
  - eye complications of ophthalmic zoster including keratitis, uveitis and eyelid damage

Management

- Provide appropriate detailed explanation and reassurance. Dispel myths: namely, explain that it is not a dangerous disease; the patient will not go insane or die if the rash spreads from both sides and meets in the middle.
- Explain that herpes zoster is only mildly contagious, however people can acquire chickenpox after exposure to a person with the disorder. It is advisable to avoid contact with those who have never had chickenpox, are not immunised and people who are immunocompromised or undergoing chemotherapy. Consider giving varicella zoster immunoglobulin to immunocompromised contacts who have no history of varicella.
- *Treating the rash:* Instruct the patient to avoid overtreating the rash, which may become infected. Calamine lotion may be soothing but removal of the calamine can be painful. For a hot, painful rash, to remove crusts and exudate, bathe the lesions with saline three times daily. A drying lotion (e.g. menthol in flexible collodion) is most soothing and suitable. Cover the lesions in a light, non-adherent padded dressing.

Oral medication[5]

Analgesics such paracetamol with or without codeine should be first-line therapy ± tricyclic antidepressants.

Antiviral therapy with a guanine analogue may reduce the duration of the disease in all people.

Optimal indications—patients:

- treated within 72 hours of onset of vesicles
- who are >50 years of age
- who are immunocompromised
- with acute severe pain
- with involvement of special areas (e.g. eye, perineum)

Dose (e.g. herpes ophthalmicus):

famciclovir 250 mg 8 hourly (o) for 7 days
or
valaciclovir 1000 mg 8 hourly (o) for 7 days
or
aciclovir 800 mg (child: 20 mg/kg) (o) 5 times daily for 7 days

Note: increase dose in immunocompromised patients.

Corticosteroids

For severe pain, consider prednisolone 50 mg (o) mane for 7 days then taper.

Prevention

- Varicella zoster vaccine (Zostavax).

Postherpetic neuralgia[6]

This pain, mostly encountered in the elderly, is usually severe, varying in quality from paroxysmal stabbing pain to burning or aching. Spasms of pain upon light brushing of the skin are a feature.

Treatment is difficult and a careful 'trial and error' approach can be used until appropriate evidence from scientific trials establishes the optimal treatment.

Treatment options[7]

- Basic analgesics: paracetamol 1 g (o) 6–8 hourly
- TENS as often as necessary (e.g. 16 hours/day for 2 weeks)
  plus
- Oral medication:
  - tricyclic antidepressants, for example: amitriptyline 10–25 mg (o) nocte, increasing to a maximum 75–100 mg nocte

or

- pregabalin (for lancinating pain) 75 mg (o) nocte initially, increasing the dose gradually to maximum tolerated dose (up to 300 mg bd)

or

- gabapentin 100–300 mg (o) daily (nocte) initially, increasing as tolerated to maximum 2400 mg

- Topical medication (trial for a few days):

  lignocaine 5% ointment or 10% gel

  or

  lignocaine 5% patch to painful area

Evidence-based medicine

Systematic reviews confirm that oral antiviral agents (as above) are beneficial for preventing postherpetic neuralgia while tricyclic antidepressants and gabapentin are beneficial for relieving the established condition.[8]

Physical treatments

- Local corticosteroid and anaesthetic injections.
- Nerve blocks (e.g. supraorbital nerve).
- Excision of painful skin scar is no longer recommended.

Herpes simplex[6]

Herpes simplex is a common infection caused by the large DNA herpes simplex virus (HSV), which can cause a vesicular rash anywhere on the skin or mucous membranes (see FIG. 122.11). There are two major antigenic strains of HSV:

- HSV I, which commonly involves the lips and oral mucosa
- HSV II, which basically affects the genitalia (common in adolescents and young adults)

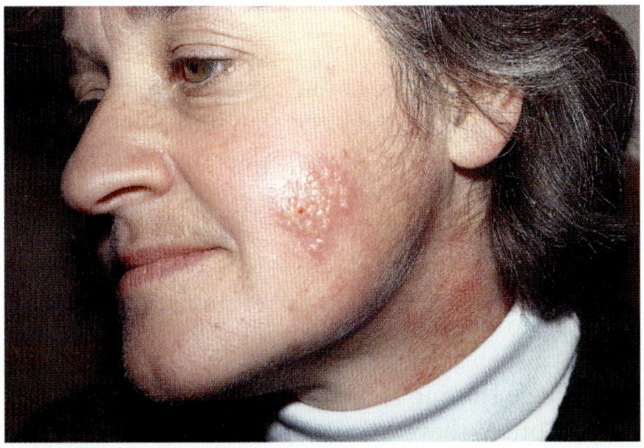

FIGURE 122.11 Acute eruption of herpes simplex on the face—a recurrent problem in this person

Epidemiology

HSV has a worldwide distribution and is spread orally or genitally by infected secretions. Primary HSV infection is usually a disease of childhood, characteristically causing acute gingivostomatitis in a preschool child (see CHAPTER 72).

TABLE 122.6 summarises the major manifestations of HSV and the possible complications.

Table 122.6 Herpes simplex virus: manifestations and complications

Examples of manifestations
Herpes labialis (synonyms: fever blisters, cold sores)
Keratoconjunctivitis, including dendritic ulcer
Genital infection
Other areas of skin such as buttocks
Complications
Eczema herpeticum
Erythema multiforme (3–14 days postinfection), often recurrent
Myeloradiculopathy with genital herpes
Pneumonia
Encephalitis

Recurrent infection

Recurrences range from weeks to months and appear due to reactivation rather than re-infection. The cause is not clear but there are several known precipitating factors. These are fever, sunlight, respiratory infections, menstruation, emotional stress, local trauma and, with genital lesions, sexual intercourse.

Fatalities

HSV infections can be potentially fatal. Reactivated HSV can cause a focal destruction encephalitis. The untreated case fatality rate is as high as 70%, but this can be greatly reduced with the use of aciclovir. Neonates exposed to HSV can develop fatal disseminated infection. In compromised patients the infection can be severe.

Diagnosis

If the clinical picture is uncertain swab of vesicle fluid for PCR can aid diagnosis.

Genital herpes

See CHAPTER 117.

Herpes labialis (classic cold sores)

The objective is to limit the size and intensity of the lesions.

Treatment

At the first sensation of the development of a cold sore:

- apply an ice cube to the site for up to 5 minutes every 60 minutes (for first 12 hours)
- topical applications include:

 lignocaine 2% with or without chlorhexidine 0.05% gel topically, every 3 hours
 or
 idoxuridine 0.5% preparations (e.g. Virasolve) applied hourly
 or
 povidone–iodine 10% cold sore paint: apply on swab sticks 4 times a day until disappearance
 or
 aciclovir 5% cream 5 times daily for 4 days
 or
 penciclovir 1% cream for 4 days

 Note: Corticosteroids are contraindicated.

Oral medication

For a severe primary attack:

 aciclovir 400 mg (child: 10 mg/kg up to 400 mg) 8 hourly for 5 days or until resolution
 or
 famciclovir or valaciclovir

Prevention

122 If exposure to the sun precipitates the cold sore, use an SPF 30 or more sun protection lip balm, ointment or Solastick. Zinc sulphate solution can be applied once a week for recurrences. Oral aciclovir 200 mg bd or valaciclovir 500 mg daily for 6 months (then review), can be used for severe and frequent recurrences.[8]

Advice to the patient

Herpes simplex is contagious. It is present in saliva and can be spread in a family by the sharing of drinking and eating utensils and toothbrushes, or by kissing. It is most important not to kiss an infant if you have an active cold sore.

FOLLICULITIS[5]

Folliculitis, which is infection in and around hair follicles, can be superficial or deep. Responsible organisms include bacteria (most common) but consider dermatophytes and yeasts (e.g. *Candida albicans, Malassezia*).

Superficial folliculitis

This usually presents as mild itchy pustules on an erythematous base on any part of hair-bearing skin, particularly in hot weather in a patient who is often a chronic carrier of *S. aureus*. A swab supports diagnosis. Management involves removal of the cause and the application of an antiseptic wash, such as triclosan 1%, chlorhexidine or povidone–iodine. If *S. aureus* is identified consider mupirocin 2% ointment or cream topically, twice daily for 5 days. Occasionally oral flucloxacillin may also be required.

Bacterial folliculitis[3]

A generalised acute erythematous maculopapular rash can be a manifestation of bacterial folliculitis, typically caused by *S. aureus* or *Pseudomonas aeruginosa.*

Pseudomonas folliculitis can cause confusion, the typical features being:

- rapidly spreading rash
- mainly on trunk, buttocks and thighs, especially axillae and groin
- itchy
- small pustules surrounded by circular red–purple halo
- follows immersion in a hot spa bath or tub

Treatment is based on the sensitivity of the cultured organisms (e.g. ciprofloxacin). Many cases resolve spontaneously in 1–2 weeks.

Folliculitis of trunk from spa baths

'Hot tub folliculitis' is caused by *P. aeruginosa* (usually) in poorly chlorinated water maintained at temperatures 37–40°C.

Treatment is with ciprofloxacin 500 mg (o) bd for 7 days.

Pseudofolliculitis[5]

Folliculitis barbae is a chronic inflammatory disorder caused by a foreign-body reaction to the hair shaft. It is not an infection but a complication of hair removal techniques. It is common in men with curly hair and in the groin area. It tends to recur.

Management

- Prior to shaving, wash the skin with warm water and a soap substitute.
- Change shaving habits: avoid close shaving; shave less often; shave in direction of hair growth; shave on relaxed skin (i.e. do not pull the skin taut) and use good-quality blades.

- Consider laser hair removal if appropriate.
- Permanently stopping hair removal techniques is the best treatment.
- If persistent, use benzoyl peroxide 5% gel or solution topically, twice daily.
- If no response after 6 weeks, add clindamycin–benzoyl peroxide + clindamycin 5% + 1% gel topically, once daily.

Deep folliculitis

Deep forms are usually very tender and painful. Examples are styes, boils (furuncles) and carbuncles.

Boil (furuncle)

This is an *S. aureus* infection of a hair follicle and may occur in any hair-bearing site. The painful red nodule enlarges, becomes fluctuant and develops a necrotic centre, which discharges a core of thick yellow pus tinged with blood (with associated relief of pain).

Treatment (adults)

- (According to swabs) di(flu)cloxacillin 500 mg or cephalexin 500 mg (orally, 6 hourly for 5–7 days) or clindamycin 450 mg (8-hourly for 5 days)

Boils—recurrent

- Obtain swabs
- 3% hexachlorophene body wash daily
- Mupirocin to the lesions and nares
- Antibiotics (as above)—according to swabs

Carbuncle

This is a cluster of small abscesses involving a group of adjoining hair follicles and discharging pus from several points. Common sites are the back of the neck, the shoulders, buttocks or over the hips. Treatment is as for a boil.

Stye of eye

- Apply heat with direct steam from a thermos onto the closed eye or by a hot compress (helps spontaneous discharge).
- Perform lash epilation to allow drainage (incise with a size 11 blade if epilation doesn't work).
- Only use topical antibiotic ointment (e.g. chloramphenicol) if infection is spreading locally, and systemic antibiotics if distal spread noted by pre-auricular adenitis.

Patient education resources

Hand-out sheets from *Murtagh's Patient Education* 7th edition:

- Herpes simplex (cold sores)
- Herpes zoster (shingles)
- Pityriasis rosea

References

1 Hunter JAA, Savin JA, Dahl MV. *Clinical Dermatology* (3rd edn). Oxford: Blackwell Scientific Publications, 2002: 64.
2 Murtagh J. *Patient Education* (7th edn). Sydney: McGraw-Hill, 2016.
3 Thomas RM. Drug eruptions. Med Int, 1988; 49: 2038–42.
4 Expert group for Dermatology. In: eTG complete. Melbourne: Therapeutic Guidelines Ltd. Available from: <www.tg.org.au>, accessed April 2018.
5 Expert group for Antiobiotic. In: eTG complete. Melbourne: Therapeutic Guidelines Ltd. Available from: <www.tg.org.au>, accessed April 2018.
6 Dwyer DE, Cunningham AL. Herpes simplex and varicella zoster virus infection. Med J Aust, 2002; 177: 267–72.
7 Expert group for Neurology. In: eTG complete. Melbourne: Therapeutic Guidelines Ltd. Available from: <www.tg.org.au>, accessed April 2018.
8 Lancaster T, Warehain D, Yaphe J. Postherpetic neuralgia. In: Barton S (ed.), *Clinical Evidence* (Issue 7). London: BMJ Publishing Group, 2002: 739–45.

123 Skin ulcers

An ulcer, which occurring at any of the vital parts of the body secretes a copious quantity of pus and blood, and refuses to be healed, even after a course of proper and persistent medical treatment, is sure to have a fatal determination.

SUSHRUTA-SAMHITA (5TH CENTURY BCE)

An ulcer is a localised break in the epidermal tissue of the surface of the skin or mucous membrane as a result of trauma, pressure, infection; they are associated with an underlying pathology. This applies particularly to leg ulcers. Ulcers are commonly found on the legs and feet, on areas exposed to the sun, and over bony prominences on the sacrum and heels. They may be clean, sloughy or necrotic.

The national morbidity survey (UK) showed that 2–3 per 1000 patients per annum consulted their GP with 'chronic ulcers of the skin'.

Key facts and checkpoints[1,2]

- The great majority of leg ulcers are vascular in origin due to arterial insufficiency or venous hypertension or to a combination of the two i.e. mixed ulcers.
- If clinical findings don't provide the diagnosis, ordering the ankle-brachial index (ABI) is essential if pulses are not palpable to exclude arterial disease. Duplex Doppler ultrasound is the key investigation for both venous and arterial disease.
- Most ulcers are multifactorial:
  1. venous + obesity + immobility (often with osteoarthritis) + poor compliance, or
  2. venous + arterial + trauma + infection
- Identify and treat any intrinsic or extrinsic factors impairing wound healing.
- High-stretch compression bandages are better than short-stretch compression bandages, which are mainly used in lymphoedema, and multilayer is best.
- Elastic bandages are better than non-elastic bandages.
- Venous surgery can improve outcomes—newer methods use non-surgical foam injections and lasers.
- A moist environment delivered by modern dressings provides a physiological environment for wound healing.
- Adequate wound debridement is essential to remove necrotic material and slough, and enable healing to commence and progress.
- It is important to consider biopsy as hypergranulation that does not respond quickly to topical treatment with hypertonic saline, silver nitrate and compression bandaging may be an SCC.
- Diabetic ulcers may be either neuropathic, which are mostly caused by pressure damage due to sensory neuropathy, or ischaemic due to loss of peripheral arterial circulation.
- Autoimmune diseases are the underlying cause of vasculitic wounds. They result from damage caused by circulating antibodies often seen in RA, lupus and scleroderma. They are very painful and difficult to heal without the use of immunosuppressants.
- Accurate diagnosis of the ulcer is vitally important for management decisions.
- Bacterial swabs are unhelpful because all chronic ulcers will become colonised with both Gram-positive and Gram-negative bacteria.

The clinical approach

It is useful to keep in mind the various causes of ulcers (see TABLE 123.1). The commonest causes or types are venous and ischaemic ulcers of the leg, pressure ulcers (decubitus) and trauma. It is important not to misdiagnose malignant ulcers, including 'Marjolin ulcer', which is a squamous cell carcinoma (SCC) developing in unstable chronic scars or ulcers (e.g. burns, venous ulcers, tropical ulcers) of long-standing duration. Amelanotic melanoma is a specific trap.

History

A careful history helps determine the cause of the ulceration. Relevant history includes previous deep venous thrombosis or pulmonary embolism, diabetes, rheumatoid arthritis, inflammatory bowel disease,

Table 123.1 Types and causes of skin ulcers

Traumatic

Decubitus (related to trauma—pressure injury)

Vascular:

- Venous
  - varicose veins
  - post thrombophlebitis
- Arterial insufficiency
- Skin infarction (thrombolytic ulcer)
- Vasculitis
  - rheumatoid arthritis, SLE, scleroderma

Infective:

- Tropical ulcer
- Tuberculosis
- *Mycobacterium ulcerans* (Buruli ulcer)
- Post cellulitis
- Chronic infected sinus

Malignant:

- Squamous cell carcinoma
- Marjolin ulcer (SCC) in long-standing ulcer
- Basal cell carcinoma (rodent ulcer)
- Malignant melanoma
- Ulcerating metastases

Neurotrophic:

- Peripheral neuropathy (e.g. diabetes)
- Peripheral nerve injuries (e.g. leprosy)

Haematological:

- Polycythaemia
- Spherocytosis
- Sickle cell anaemia

Miscellaneous:

- Artefactual
- Medications e.g. nicorandil, nicotine
- Pyoderma gangrenosum inflammatory ulcer
- Insect and spider bites

chronic skin ulcers and arterial insufficiency, including a history of intermittent claudication and ischaemic rest pain.

A drug history is important, considering especially beta blockers and ergotamine, which can compromise the arterial circulation, corticosteroids and NSAIDs, which affect healing, and nifedipine, which tends to aggravate ankle oedema.

Examination[3]

Any ulcer should be assessed for the following characteristics:

- site
- shape
- size
- edge—consider consistency
- floor
- base
- discharge
- surrounding skin:
  - colour (? signs of inflammation)
  - sensitivity
- mobility in relation to underlying tissue
- regional lymph nodes

Site of ulcer

Venous ulcers typically occur on the medial side of the leg in relation to incompetent perforating veins in the traditional gaiter area (see FIG. 123.1).

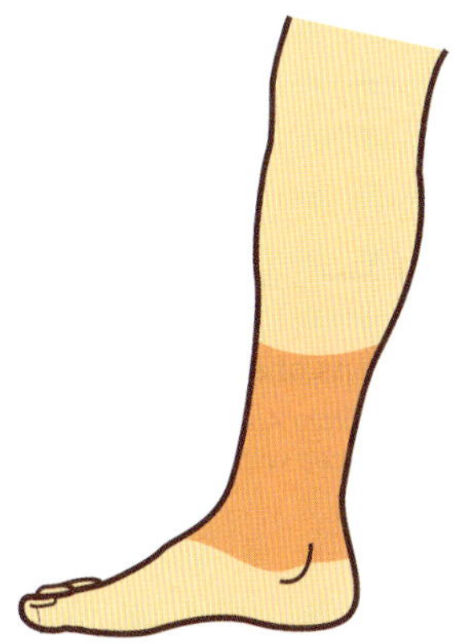

FIGURE 123.1 Area typically affected by varicose eczema and ulceration (the 'gaiter' area)

Ischaemic ulcers tend to occur on the lateral side and anterior part of the leg and the foot.

Trophic ulcers, which are associated with neuropathy, occur on parts subject to repeated pressure and trauma, such as the ball of the foot or the pulps of the fingers.

Postsolar keratoses

Solar-induced ulcers, such as SCCs and BCCs, occur on such parts exposed to the sun. It should be noted if the ulcer is related to old scars, including burns and chronic ulcers.

Size, shape and edge

The classic appearances of various ulcers are presented in FIGURE 123.2. These are general guidelines only. Infective ulcers due to *Mycobacterium* species and pressure injury tend to have an undermined edge while a trophic ulcer is punched out and typically round in surface shape. A raised firm ulcer edge may indicate malignancy.

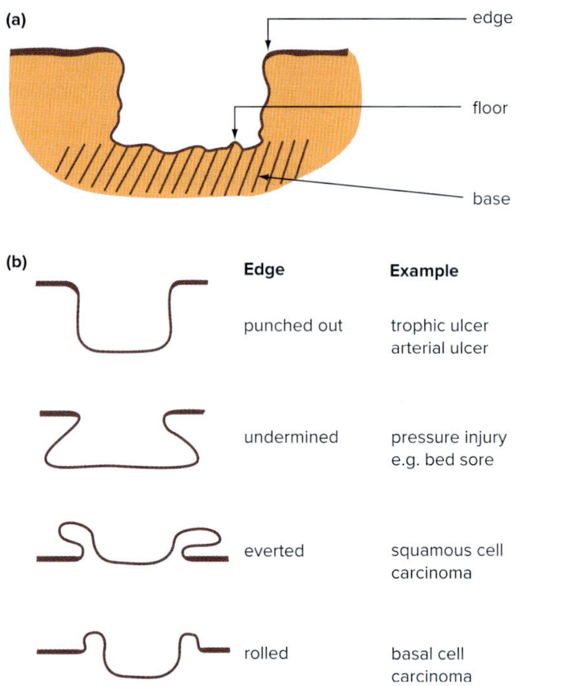

FIGURE 123.2 **(a)** Parts of an ulcer, **(b)** types of ulcer.

Source: Davis et al. *Symptom Analysis and Physical Diagnosis* (2nd edn), page 309. Reproduced with permission from Pergamon Press

Floor of the ulcer

The floor or base of the ulcer provides useful clinical information. A dry or extended base or necrotic eschar in the floor implies ischaemia. Venous ulcers on the other hand are often superficial and tend to have fibrinous exudate and ooze, sometimes purulent fluid.

Colour guide:

- black—necrosis, ischaemia
- yellow—slough
- red—granulation
- pink—epithelium

123

Investigations

The following should be considered, according to the clinical findings:[4]

- full blood count
- ESR/CRP
- random blood sugar/HbAIc (known diabetes)
- kidney function tests
- rheumatoid factor tests
- duplex Doppler ultrasound
- swab for specific organisms
- biopsy, especially if SCC suspected (be careful of biopsy if melanoma: amelanotic melanomas are a trap); also accurately identify an infective organism

Lower limb ulceration

The most common causes of lower limb ulceration are venous disease, arterial disease, mixed venous and arterial, and diabetes.

Differentiating between leg ulcers (85%) and foot ulcers (15%) is very important since they present two very different problems.[3] According to the survey by Stacey, venous disease is present in two-thirds of leg ulcers, while arterial disease occurs in 28% (see TABLE 123.2). Ulceration on the foot frequently has an arterial aetiology (72%), with many of these patients also having diabetes, whereas venous disease is present in only 6%.[5]

Table 123.2 Causes of chronic ulceration of the leg and foot[5]

	%
The leg	
Venous disease	52
Mixed venous and arterial disease	15
Arterial disease	13
Others	20
The foot	
Arterial disease	72
Mixed venous and arterial disease	2
Venous disease	4
Others	22

The differential characteristics are presented in TABLE 123.3.

A general examination, including the leg, is very important. This includes examining the venous drainage (CHAPTER 66), the arterial pulses and the sensation of the leg, and checking for the presence of diabetes.

Appropriate investigations (if required) include:

- full blood count
- blood sugar
- duplex Doppler ultrasound for arterial circulation

To swab or not to swab

A routine ulcer swab is not considered to be of significant value. If specific organisms such as *Mycobacterium ulcerans* are suspected, then cultures are necessary. Biopsy is considered to be accurate.

Table 123.3 Comparison of typical features of venous and arterial ulceration of the leg

	Venous	Arterial
Site	Around ankle and lower third of leg (gaiter area) Just above medial and lateral malleoli	Distal to ankle Over pressure points on toes, side of foot, metatarsal heads
Pain	Nil to mild	Usually moderate to severe
Oedema	Pitting oedema usually present	Usually absent
Ulcer features	'Ragged' edge Often superficial Ooze + + +	'Punched out' Often deep, involving deep fascia Dry
Associated limb features	Varicosities Leg warm, red, oedematous Varicose dermatitis Haemosiderin deposits Atrophie blanche	'Cold' extremities Ischaemic changes Diminished or absent peripheral pulses Thin, shiny, dry skin Poor perfusion
History	Limb oedema Past DVT Failed graft	Peripheral vascular disease—claudication, rest pain Diabetes Smoker
ABI	>0.9	<0.5–0.7

Source: Based on a table prepared by Dr Denise Findlay; reproduced with permission

Measurement of ankle/brachial pressure index

To plan management of a leg ulcer, it is ideal to determine the blood flow with hand-held Doppler ultrasound. Measure ankle and brachial systolic pressures and then determine the ABI, which is the ankle pressure divided by the brachial pressure. Typical levels are:[4]

Normal range	0.91–1.3
Normal	>0.9 (venous ulcer)
Ischaemic	<0.5 (arterial ulcer)
Claudicant	0.5–0.9 (mixed arterial–venous ulcer, significant ischaemia if <0.8)

The ability to determine the cause of the ulceration and thus treat accordingly, especially with pressure dressings, has been a major advance in management. An ABI <0.8 warrants caution in applying any compression; <0.4 demands urgent referral.

General rule: Low compression 0.7–0.8; no compression <0.7.

Arterial (ischaemic) ulcers

Ischaemic ulcers are generally localised to the most peripheral areas below the ankle joint (see FIG. 123.3), such as the tips of the toes and the point of the heel, or to pressure points such as the heels, malleoli or head of the first metatarsal.

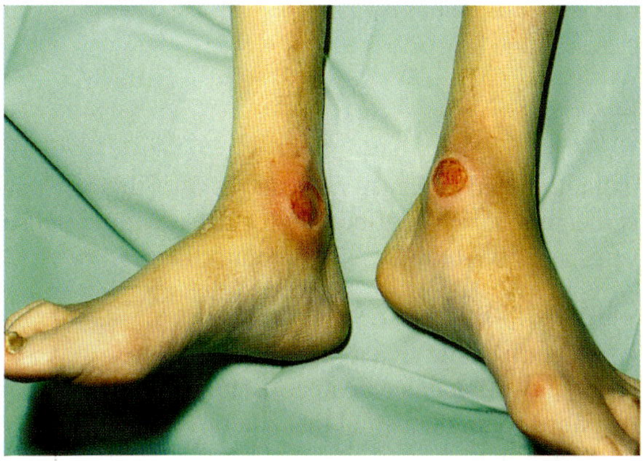

FIGURE 123.3 Ischaemic 'arterial' ulcers in an elderly woman with a long history of intermittent claudication and a recent history of nocturnal ischaemic rest pain in the feet. The ulcers healed after reconstruction for arterial obstruction. Photo courtesy Terry Devine

Clinical features

- Painful
- Punched out
- Minimal granulation tissue

Management is directed towards reperfusion.

Venous ulceration

Venous ulceration (synonyms: 'varicose', 'stasis' and 'gravitational' ulcers) accounts for the majority of leg ulcers. Chronic venous insufficiency is one of the most common medical problems in the elderly, with an estimated incidence of 5.9%.[6]

The problem is invariably secondary to deep venous thrombophlebitis. The subsequent chronic venous hypertension produces trophic changes such as hyperpigmentation (see FIG. 123.4), fibrotic thickening,

123

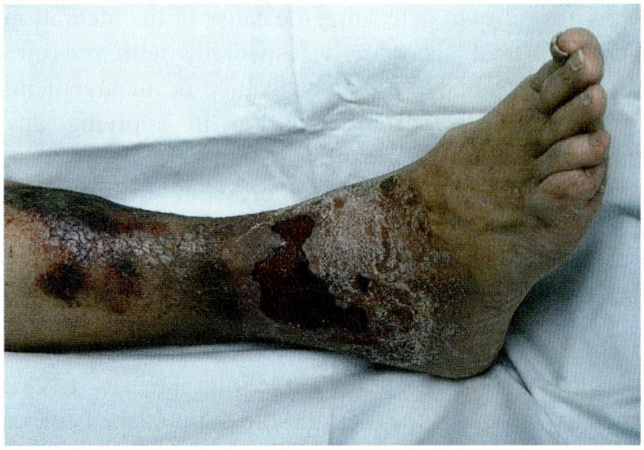

FIGURE 123.4 Venous ulceration in an elderly patient with postphlebitic varicose 'eczema'. Venous pigmentation, dermatitis, atrophy and calcification of the subcutaneous tissues are present.

Photo courtesy Terry Devine

induration and oedema. The end point of this process is ulceration, which affects 3% of those with varicose veins and 30% of those with trophic changes.[7]

Clinical features[8]

- Occur in same area as venous eczema
- Shallow (but can reach periosteum)
- More common medial than lateral
- Sometimes circumferential
- Granulating floor sometimes with surrounding inflammation—may be cellulitis
- Notoriously slow in healing without adequate compression
- Generally not tender but can be painful
- Associated pain is usually relieved by raising the leg

123

On examination, superficial varicosities are usually but not invariably present. Pitting oedema may be present early but with time fibrosis and firm induration develop. Other clinical features include dermatitis (eczema), punctate capillary proliferation, haemosiderin, hyperpigmentation and 'atrophie blanche' (porcelain white scar with rim of telangiectasia).[8]

Management (venous leg ulcers)

A major advance in the management of venous ulcers has been the finding that wounds heal better in an occluded or semi-occluded state.[9] A moist environment also aids healing. The dressing will control the wound environment. The main treatment is graduated compression at 20–40 mmHg. See TABLE 123.4.

Table 123.4 Wound management principles

The good	The bad
Hydration	Dryness
Washing with water or saline	Excess antiseptics
Insulation protection	Exposure to air
	Scabs, crust, slough
Dressings	
Compression (venous)	Dry dressings
Hydrogel	Gauze packing
Foams	Tulles
Minimal changes	Oedema/ lymphoedema

Principles of optimal management

- Explanation about the cause, and promotion of patient compliance
- Promoting clean granulation tissue to permit healing (see TABLE 123.4)
- Meticulous cleansing and dressing (avoid soaps and sensitising preparations)
- Prevention and control of infection—antibiotics indicated only if cellulitis (cephalexin or erythromycin): if infection is confirmed NOT where inflammation is present (as in most venous ulcers)
- Firm elastic compression bandage—use a minimal stretch bandage from base of toes to just below the knee. The degree of compression depends on the blood flow and is proportional to it
- Bed rest with elevation (if severe, 45–60 minutes twice a day and at night): ensure legs are elevated higher than the heart
- Encourage early ambulation and exercise
- Appropriate modification of lifestyle including weight reduction, smoking cessation (NB)
- Good nutrition includes a healthy balanced diet with ample protein and complex carbohydrates
- Be aware of drugs that can adversely affect healing (see TABLE 123.5)

Note: Firm compression is the single most important factor in the healing of venous ulcers.[2,7] Options include elastic stockings, elastic bandages, zinc paste bandages (Unna's boots) and legging orthoses.[11]

Cleansing/debridement agents

There are many cleansing agents, including:

- N saline, surfactants e.g. QV wash and warm tap water

Table 123.5	Drugs that can hamper healing[10]
Nicotine/smoking	
Corticosteroids	
Cytotoxic agents	
Aspirin/NSAIDs	
Antibiotics	
Beta blockers	
Hydrourea	

As a rule, avoid antiseptics, which destroy cells, although cadexomer iodine, which is a slow-release form of iodine, is non-toxic to tissues, reduces bacterial load and clears odorous slough. However, wash off iodine solution after 5 minutes. Iodosorb is a low-dose iodine dressing appropriate for infected, contaminated wounds, particularly a diabetic wound. A good combination is normal saline cleansing followed by IntraSite Gel for debridement, covered with a foam dressing. Strong salt dressings (e.g. Mesalt or Curasalt) are very good for cleaning contaminated, infected wounds and hypergranulation but need changing daily and to be covered by a very absorbent overlying dressing.

Hydrogels such as IntraSite Gel, which have been found to be effective at debridement (including black necrotic areas), have generally replaced enzyme dressings.

Lymphoedema[12]

This is not pitting oedema but a reduction in the function of the lymph vessels to drain extracellular fluid.

Primary lymphoedema is caused either by malformation of the lymph vessels or by damage from bacteria, fungi, parasites, insects, chemicals, radiotherapy or surgery. Secondary lymphoedema is caused by primary malignancy or intralymphatic propagation of a tumour. Lymphoedema results in major changes to the skin such as thickening of the skin, build-up of scale and keratin and worsening hyperkeratosis, producing a warty appearance.

Wounds are common in lymphoedema. They are managed by treating the wound environment with appropriate dressing, but the main treatment is significant compression with either specially developed garments or inelastic bandages. Difficult cases should be referred to a specialist lymphoedema clinic.

A simple clinical test for determining a lymphoedema component in a swelling of the lower leg is the Stemmer's sign test. This test is performed by lifting and pinching the skin at the dorsum of the second toe on each foot. A positive Stemmer's sign results when the skin cannot be lifted and pinched together. The test is negative for lymphoedema when the skin can be pinched and lifted. A positive Stemmer's sign *always indicates lymphoedema, but a negative sign does not always rule out lymphoedema.*

Wound dressing[9,13]

There are six main types of modern wound dressings: films, hydrogels, hydrocolloids, alginates, foams and hydroactives (foam-like)—all expensive. Films, hydrogels and hydrocolloids increase the wound moisture whereas alginates and foams absorb exudate. The more traditional dressings such as tulle gras, non-adherent pad dressings and saline soaks have little use. A lightweight cohesive bandage or a lightweight tubular bandage can be used to hold non-adherent dressings in place.

General rules:[10]

- allow 2–3 cm of dressing greater than the wound
- place one-third above and two-thirds below the wound
- remove when 'strike-through' occurs
- remove with care in older patients
- remove under the shower if necessary
- when in doubt, DO NOT HARM: use foam and gel combinations

Medicated occlusive bandages

There are several suitable occlusive paste bandages for ambulant patients, which ideally should be left on for 7–14 days. These contain zinc oxide. Examples include Flexi-Dress, Gelocast and Zipzoc (which are zinc paste bandages with no preservatives).

Patch testing for an allergic response should be performed for a few days beforehand.

Bandages

Bandages have two main uses:

- retention: to keep a dressing in place
- compression: to assist venous return

High-stretch compression bandages are best.
Method of application:

- spiral application from toes with figure 8 around ankles, then spiral to knee
- 50% overlap
- constant tension provides graduated compression (Laplace's Law)

Pitfalls and other factors to be considered

- Treat the primary cause by surgery or other means (e.g. varicose veins, vascular insufficiency).
- If oedema, elevate legs and prescribe diuretics. An ulcer will not heal in the presence of significant ankle oedema.
- Clarify the cause of oedema, which may be due to medication e.g. calcium channel blockers.
- Be careful of allergy to local applications (e.g. zinc).
- Be careful of irritation from local applications (e.g. antibiotics). Antibiotic-impregnated dressings are not generally recommended.
- Avoid heavy packing of the wound.
- Consider grafting (pinch skin or split thickness).
- Consider oxpentifylline (Trental 400) for chronic occlusive arterial disease and venous disease.[8]

Post-healing and prevention of ulcers

- Encourage preventive measures, such as regular walking, good nutrition, no smoking, elevation of leg when resting, great care to avoid trauma.
- Apply emollients for varicose eczema.
- Wear a compression-grade elastic stocking for varicose ulcers (e.g. Jobst Fast-Fit, Jobst Venoscan).

A recommended treatment routine for a leg ulcer is presented in TABLE 123.6. It is desirable (for the outpatient) to leave the dressings and bandages in place for 1 week, perhaps 2 weeks, depending on the state of the dressing.

Principles of management for chronic ulcers are summarised in TABLE 123.7.

Table 123.6 A recommended leg ulcer treatment method

Clean with normal saline

- If slough, apply IntraSite Gel
- Dressing: non-adherent e.g. Allevyn; Melolin
- Occlusive paste bandage—e.g. zinc oxide (7–14 days), from base of toe to just below knee, plus compression bandage
  or
  Compression bandage (e.g. Eloflex) to just below knee
- Consider Tubigrip stockinette cover

Table 123.7 Principles of management of chronic ulcers[14]

Ulcer type	Major management principles
Venous	Control venous insufficiency: • compression bandage • improve calf muscle pump action (ambulation, exercises) • vertical leg drainage
Arterial	Vascular assessment for surgical intervention
Mixed venous/ arterial	Vascular assessment for surgical intervention
Pressure	Eliminate or reduce pressure

Decubitus ulcer (pressure injury)

123

Pressure injuries tend to occur in immobile patients, especially those who are unconscious, paralysed or debilitated. The cause is skin ischaemia from sustained pressure over a bony area, particularly the heels, sacrum, hips and buttocks. Poor general health, including anaemia, is a predisposing factor.

The classification of pressure injuries is based on the level of tissue damage and depths of the wound:

- Stage 1: non-blanching erythema
- Stage 2: partial thickness (superficial) ulceration
- Stage 3: full thickness ulceration
- Stage 4: deep full thickness—skin loss with extensive tissue loss

Unstageable: deep tissue injury.

Clinical features

- Preliminary area of fixed erythema at pressure site
- Relatively sudden onset of necrosis and ulceration
- Ulcer undermined at edges
- Possible rapid extension of ulcers
- Necrotic slough in base

Prevention

- Good nursing care including turning patient every 2 hours
- Regular skin examinations by the nursing and medical staff
- Special care of pressure areas, including gentle handling
- Special beds, mattresses (e.g. air-filled ripple) and sheepskin to relieve pressure areas
- Good nutrition and hygiene
- Control of urinary and faecal incontinence
- Avoid the donut cushion
- Avoid soaps

Treatment[13]

The most important principle is early intervention including relief of pressure, friction and shear. Use above prevention measures, plus:

- clean base with warm water or saline solution and a surfactant (applied gently via a syringe)
- general guidelines for dressings:
  - deep ulcers—alginates (e.g. Algisite M, Kaltostat)
  - shallow ulcers—hydrocolloids (e.g. DuoDERM, CGF)
  - dry or necrotic ulcers—hydrogels (e.g. IntraSite, Purolin gel)
  - heavy exudative ulcers—foams (e.g. Lyofoam, Lyofoam extra, Allevyn, Cutinova Cavity)
- give vitamin C, 500 mg bd
- give antibiotics for spreading cellulitis (otherwise of little use)
- for non-healing large pressure wounds, apply negative pressure therapy
- review patient's nutritional status as it impacts on both formation of pressure injury and slow healing
- healing is usually satisfactory but, if not, surgical intervention with debridement of necrotic tissue and skin grafting may be necessary; this is very effective if the patient can cope

Undressing wounds

Removal of dressings from ulcerated wounds is very important. The contact layer should be removed slowly to prevent detachment of fragile epithelial surface cells and trauma to healthy granulation tissue.[15]

Role of honey

Honey has been advocated for centuries for healing ulcers. A particular type, Medihoney, is marketed. It provides moist healing and has antibacterial properties. Care has to be taken with over-moisturisation and maceration. Its role is still somewhat controversial as is the application of sugar, cromoglycate powder, maggots and hyperbaric oxygen.

Trophic ulcers

Trophic ulcers are due to neuropathy causing loss of sensation (invariably diabetic) and usually follow an injury of which the patient was unaware (see FIG. 123.5).

A feature is a deep, punched-out lesion (similar to ischaemic ulcers) over pressure points. A common site is the ball of the foot under the first metatarsal head, but the heel or a bunion may also be affected.

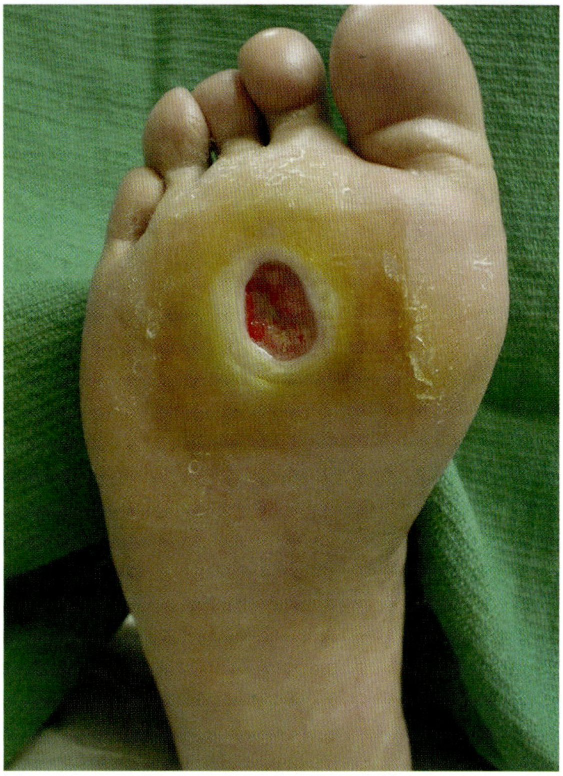

FIGURE 123.5 Neuropathic ulcer under the third metatarsal of the right foot in a patient with diabetes

The ulcers may extend to the bone and into joints. They are prone to secondary infection.

Treatment is based on controlling the diabetes and clearing infection with appropriate antibiotics, but referral for surgical management is usually essential.

Mycobacterium ulcerans (Buruli ulcer)

Buruli ulcer (also known as a Bairnsdale or Daintree ulcer) is caused by *Mycobacterium ulcerans* and usually begins as a painless papule or nodule that forms a necrotic ulcer over weeks to months. An undermined edge is a classic feature.

It occurs in specific geographic locations, namely coastal Victoria, Far North Queensland and the tropical regions of Central and West Africa.

There is a current epidemic in coastal Victoria, where possums are believed to be a reservoir. All age groups may be affected, including children.

Early referral to an infectious diseases unit is recommended, with 8 to 12 weeks of oral antibiotics (usually rifampicin and clarithomycin) required, along with specialist wound care. Surgical debridement of the ulcer may also be necessary.

DERMATITIS ARTEFACTA AND NEUROTIC EXCORIATIONS

These self-inflicted ulcerated or erosive skin lesions have a psychological basis.

Dermatitis artefacta

In this condition, patients deny self-trauma and may have deep-seated psychological problems, or they may be malingering or manipulative for secondary gain.

Neurotic excoriations

These lesions, which are usually identical to the artefactual lesions, are caused by patients who admit to scratching, picking or digging at their skin (FIG. 123.6). It occurs at times of stress and treatment is seldom successful. Treatment consists of counselling with CBT, a trial of antidepressants and topical antipruritics such as:

coal tar solution (liquor picis carbonis) and menthol in sorbolene cream

or

menthol (0.5%) or phenol (1.0%) in aqueous cream

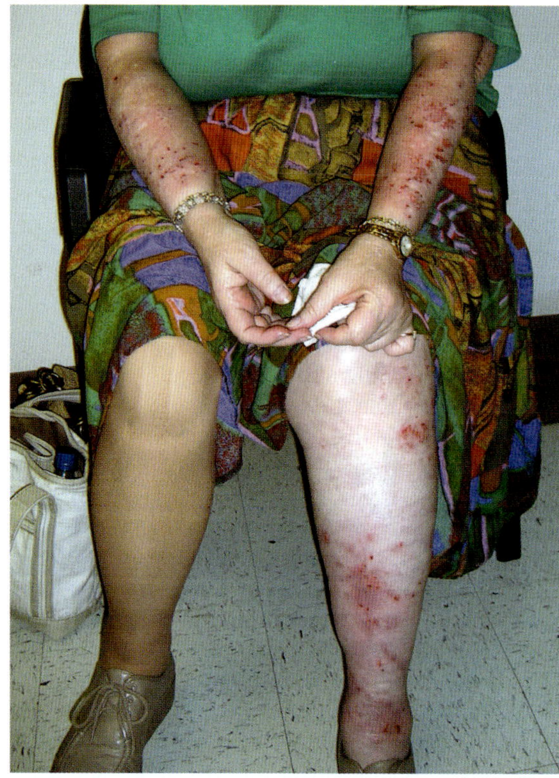

FIGURE 123.6 Neurotic excoriations (neurodermatitis) seen on three of four extremities. The fourth extremity is a prosthetic leg.[16]

Practice tips

Principles of treatment[10]

- Occluded and moist wounds heal faster.
- Maintain moist wound environment.
- Control exudate and debris (remove excess—leave enough to allow cellular regeneration).
- Maintain/improve circulation.
- Insulate and protect.

123

Patient education resources

Hand-out sheets from *Murtagh's Patient Education* 7th edition:

- Pressure sores (bed sores)

References

1. Kelly R. Leg ulcers and wound healing. In: *Dermatology Conference Notes.* Melbourne: Combined Alfred Hospital/Skin and Cancer Foundation, 2002: 29.
2. Sussman G. Ulcer dressing and management. Aust Fam Physician, 2014; 43 (9): 588–92.
3. Davis A, Bolin T, Ham J. *Symptom Analysis and Physical Diagnosis* (2nd edn). Sydney: Pergamon Press, 1990: 380–9.
4. Moulds R (Chair). Therapeutic Guidelines: Ulcer and Wound Management (Version 1). Therapeutic Guidelines Ltd, 2012 (eTG Complete).
5. Australian Wound Management Association and the New Zealand Wound Care Society. *Australian and New Zealand Clinical Practice Guideline for Prevention and Management of Venous Leg Ulcers.* Osborne Park, WA: Cambridge Publishing, 2011.
6. Beauregard S, Gilchrest BA. A survey of skin problems and skin care regimens in the elderly. Arch Dermatol, 1987; 123: 1638–43.

7 Fry J, Berry HE. *Surgical Problems in Clinical Practice.* London: Edward Arnold, 1987: 115–17.
8 Weller C, Evans S. Venous leg ulcer management in general practice—practice nurses and evidence based guidelines. Aust Fam Physician, 2012; 41 (5): 331–7.
9 Fitzpatrick JE. Stasis ulcers: update on a common geriatric problem. Modern Medicine Australia, 1990; June: 81–8.
10 Sussman G. An introduction to chronic wounds and their management. Proceedings Monash University Update Course. Melbourne: Monash University, 2009: 1–28.
11 Vernick SH, Shapiro D, Shaw FD. Legging orthosis for venous and lymphatic insufficiency. Arch Phys Med Rehab, 1987; 68: 459–61.
12 Rockson SG. Update on the biology and treatment of lymphedema. Curr Treat Options Cardiovasc Med, April 2012; 14 (2): 184–92.
13 Sussman G, Weller C. Wound dressing products update. J Pharm Prac Res, 2006; 36 (4) 318–24.
14 Findlay D. Wound management and healing in general practice. Annual Update Course notes. Melbourne: Monash University, 1996; 13–16.
15 Rowland J. Pressure ulcers: a literature review and a treatment scheme. Aust Fam Physician, 1993; 22: 1819–27.
16 Usatine RP, Saldan-Arragui MA. Excoriations and ulcers and legs. J Fam Pract. 2004, 53(9), 713–16.

Resources

Grey JE, Enoch S, Harding KG. ABC of wound healing: wound assessment. BMJ, 4 February 2006; 332 (7536): 285–8.
Australian Wound Management Association. Pan Pacific Clinical Practice Guideline for the Prevention and Management of Pressure Injury. Osborne Park, WA: Cambridge Publishing, 2012.

124 Common lumps and bumps

It will never get well if you pick it.

AMERICAN PROVERB

Lumps and bumps are very common presentations and the skin a very common site for neoplastic lesions. Most of these lesions only invade locally, with the notable exception of malignant melanoma. Pigmented skin tumours thus demand very careful consideration, although only a very few are neoplastic. The optimum time to deal with the problem and cure any skin cancer is at its first presentation. The family doctor thus has an important responsibility to screen these tumours and is faced with two basic decisions: the diagnosis and whether to treat or refer.

Most skin lumps are benign and can be left in situ, but the family doctor should be able to remove most of these lumps if appropriate and submit them for histological verification. The main treatment options available in family practice are: biopsy, cryotherapy, curette and cautery, excision or intralesional injections of corticosteroid.[1] A list of common and important lumps is presented in TABLE 124.1.

Table 124.1 Important lumps and their tissue of origin[3]

Skin and mucous membranes

Fibroepithelial polyp (skin tag)

Epidermoid (sebaceous) cyst

Implantation cyst

Sebaceous hyperplasia

Mucocele

Hypertrophic scar and keloid

Warts and papillomas

Pox virus lumps:
- molluscum contagiosum
- orf
- milker's nodules

Seborrhoeic keratoses

Granuloma annularae

Dermatofibroma

Solar keratosis/actinic keratosis

Keratoacanthoma

Malignant tumours:
- basal cell carcinoma
- squamous cell carcinoma
- Bowen disease
- malignant melanoma
- Kaposi sarcoma
- secondary tumour

Subcutaneous and deeper structures

Lipoma

Neurofibroma

Lymph node (see CHAPTER 61)

Pseudoaneurysm

Musculoskeletal:
- ganglion
- bursae

Skin cancer

The three main skin cancers are the non-melanocytic skin cancers—basal cell carcinoma (BCC) and squamous cell carcinoma (SCC)—and melanoma. The approximate relative incidence is BCC 80%, SCC 15–20%, and melanoma less than 5%.[2] The incidence of non-melanocytic skin cancer, which is increasing 2.5 times as fast as other cancers, is approximately 800 new cases per 100 000 population per year, and 25 per 100 000 for melanoma. About 80% of skin cancer deaths are due to melanoma and the rest mainly due to SCC.[2]

A diagnostic approach to the lump

As with any examination, the routine of look, feel, move, measure, auscultate and transilluminate should be followed.

The lump or lumps can be described thus:

- number
- site
- shape—regular or irregular
- size (in metric units)
- position
- consistency (very soft, soft, firm, hard or stony hard)
- solid or cystic

- mobility
- surface or contour
- special features:
  - attachments (superficial/deep)
  - exact anatomical site
  - relation to anatomical structures
  - relation to overlying skin
  - colour
  - temperature (of skin over lump)
  - tenderness
  - pulsation (transmitted or direct)
  - impulse
  - reducibility
  - percussion
  - fluctuation (? contains fluid)
  - bruit
  - transilluminability
  - special signs: slipping sign, emptying sign of cavernous haemangioma
  - spread: local, lymphatic, haematogenous
  - regional lymph nodes
  - ? malignancy (is it primary or secondary?)

Relation of the lump to anatomical structures[3]

The question 'In what tissue layer is the lump situated?' needs to be addressed.

- Is it in the skin? The lump moves when the skin is moved (e.g. epidermoid cyst).
- Is it in subcutaneous tissue? The skin can be moved over the lump. The slipping sign: if the edge of the lump is pushed, the swelling slips from beneath the finger (e.g. lipoma).
- Is it in muscle? The lump is movable when the muscle is relaxed but on contraction of the muscle this movement becomes limited.
- Is it arising from a tendon or joint? Movement of these structures may cause a change in the mobility or shape of the tumour.
- Is it in bone? The lump is immobile and best outlined with the muscles relaxed.

LUMPS OF THE SKIN AND MUCOUS MEMBRANES

Fibroepithelial polyps

Synonyms: skin tags, acrochordon, benign squamous papilloma, soft fibroma.

Clinical features

- Benign skin overgrowth
- Pedunculated soft fibroma
- Increased incidence with age
- Commonest on neck, axillae, trunk, groins
- No malignant potential
- Can be irritating or unsightly to patient

Management

- Can leave or remove
- To remove:

  snip off with scissors or bone forceps (see FIG. 124.1)
  or
  tie base with fine cotton or suture material
  or
  diathermy or electrocautery of base
  or
  apply liquid nitrogen (see FIG. 124.2)

  These methods do not require local anaesthetic.

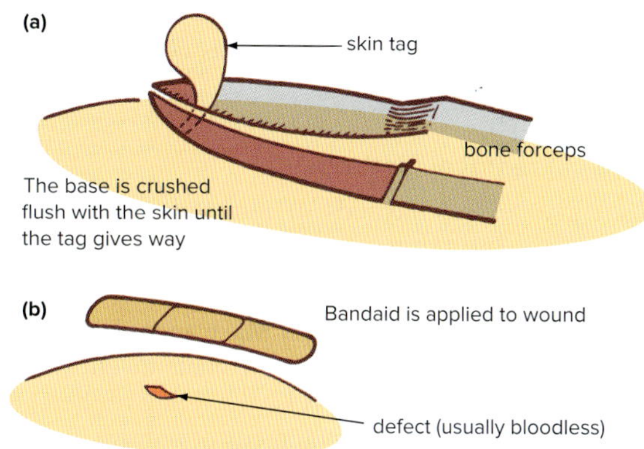

FIGURE 124.1 Removal of skin tag using bone forceps

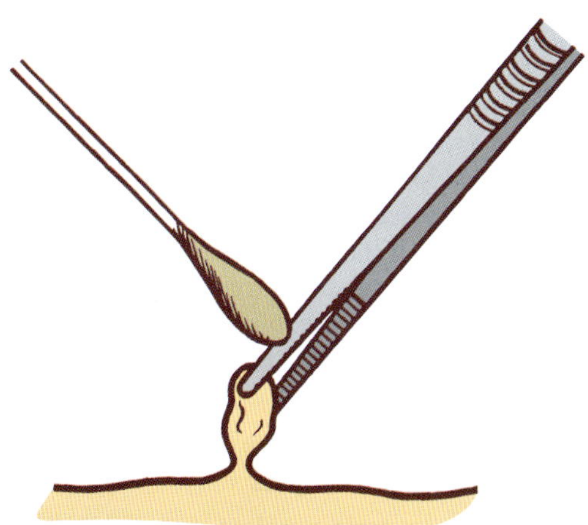

FIGURE 124.2 Removal of skin tag by liquid nitrogen: a cotton bud soaked in liquid nitrogen is applied to the forceps, which grasp the tag firmly

Epidermoid (sebaceous) cyst

Synonyms: 'pilar' cyst, keratinous cyst, wen, epidermoid cyst, sebaceous cyst (similar in appearance).

Clinical features

- Firm to soft regular lump (usually round)
- Fixed to skin but not to other structures (see FIG. 124.3a)
- Move with the skin
- Found in hair-bearing skin mainly on scalp—then face, neck, trunk, scrotum
- Contains sebaceous material
- Usually fluctuant
- May be a central punctum containing keratin
- Tendency to inflammation

Management

If before puberty—think of polyposis coli. Can leave if small and not bothersome.

Surgical removal methods

There are several methods of removing epidermoid cysts after infiltrating local anaesthetic over and around the cyst. These include:

- *Method 1: Incision into cyst* Make an incision into the cyst to bisect it, squeeze the contents out with a gauze swab and then avulse the lining of the cyst with a pair of artery forceps or remove with a small curette.
- *Method 2: Incision over cyst and blunt dissection* Make a careful skin incision over the cyst, taking care not to puncture its wall. Free the skin carefully from the cyst by blunt dissection. When it is free from adherent subcutaneous tissue, digital pressure will cause the cyst to 'pop out'.
- *Method 3: Standard dissection* Incise a small ellipse of skin to include the central punctum over the cyst (see FIG. 124.3b). The objective is to avoid rupture of the cyst. Inserting curved scissors (e.g. McIndoe's scissors), free the cyst by gently opening and closing the blades (see FIG. 124.3c). Bleeding is not usually a problem. Send the cyst for histopathology.

124

Treatment of infected cysts

Incise the cyst to drain purulent material. When the inflammation has resolved completely the cyst should be removed by method 1 or method 3 (see above).

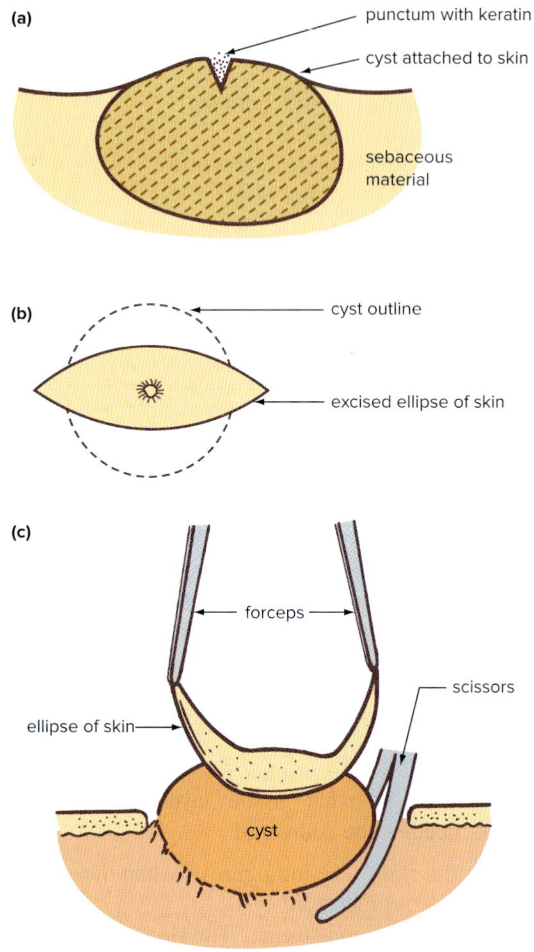

FIGURE 124.3 **(a)** Configuration of a sebaceous cyst; **(b), (c)** standard dissection of a large sebaceous cyst

Implantation cyst

Synonym: implantation dermoid.

Clinical features

- Small cystic swelling
- May be tender
- Usually follows puncture wounds
- Especially on finger pulp (e.g. hairdressers, sewers)
- Contains mucus

Management

- Incision removal (similar to epidermoid cyst)

Mucocele

A mucous retention cyst.

Clinical features

- A benign tumour
- Cyst containing mucus
- Appears spontaneously
- Common on lips and buccal mucosa
- Smooth and round
- Yellow or blue colour

Management

- Incision removal

Hyperplastic scarring

Hypertrophic scar

A hypertrophic scar is simply a lumpy scar caused by a nodular accumulation of thickened collagen fibres. It does not extend beyond the margins of the wound and regresses within a year but sometimes can be permanent.

Keloid

A keloid is a special type of hyperplastic scar that extends beyond the margins of the wound.

Clinical features

- Firm, raised, red–purple, skin overgrowth
- Common on ear lobes, chin, neck, shoulder, upper trunk
- Hereditary predisposition (e.g. dark-skinned person)
- Follows trauma, even minor (e.g. ear piercing)
- May be burning or itchy and tender

Management of scarring

- Prevention (avoid procedures in keloid-prone individuals).
- Compression and silicone dressings
- Intradermal injection of corticosteroids in early stages (2–3 months) or intralesional cytotoxics (e.g. fluorouracil) or X-ray treatment of surgical wounds within 2 weeks of operation.[4]
- Consider re-excision of hypertrophic scarring

Warts and papillomas

Warts are skin tumours caused by the human papillomavirus (HPV). The virus invades the skin, usually through a small abrasion, causing abnormal skin growth. Warts are transmitted by direct or fomite contact and may be autoinoculated from one area to another.[5]

Clinical features

- Average incubation period—4 months
- Increased incidence in children and adolescents
- Peak incidence around adolescence
- Occurs in all ethnicities at all ages
- About 25% resolve spontaneously in 6 months[5] and 70% in 2 years
- Present as various types

Types of warts

These include common warts, plane warts, filiform warts (fine elongated growths, usually on the face and neck), digitate warts (finger-like projections, usually on scalp), genital and plantar warts (see FIG. 124.4).

Common warts

These are skin-coloured tumours with a rough surface, found mainly on the fingers, elbows and knees.

Plane warts

These are skin-coloured, small and flat, occurring in linear clusters along scratch lines (see FIG. 124.5). They mainly occur on the face and limbs. They are difficult to treat because they contain very few virus particles. They are prone to Koebner phenomenon, which is seeding when a scratch passes through a plane wart.

Treatment options

Topical applications:[5]

- salicylic acid—for example: 5–20% in flexible collodion (apply daily or bd) or 16–17% salicylic acid + 16–17% lactic acid
- formaldehyde 2–4% alone or in combination
- podophyllotoxin 0.5% for anogenital warts—it is good on mucosal surfaces but does not penetrate normal keratin
- cytotoxic agents (e.g. 5-fluorouracil: very good for resistant warts such as plane warts and periungual warts)
- the immunomodulator, imiquimod

124

Cryotherapy

Carbon dioxide (−56.5°C) or liquid nitrogen (−195.8°C) destroys the host cell and stimulates an immune reaction.

Note:

- excessive keratin must be pared before freezing
- the results are often disappointing

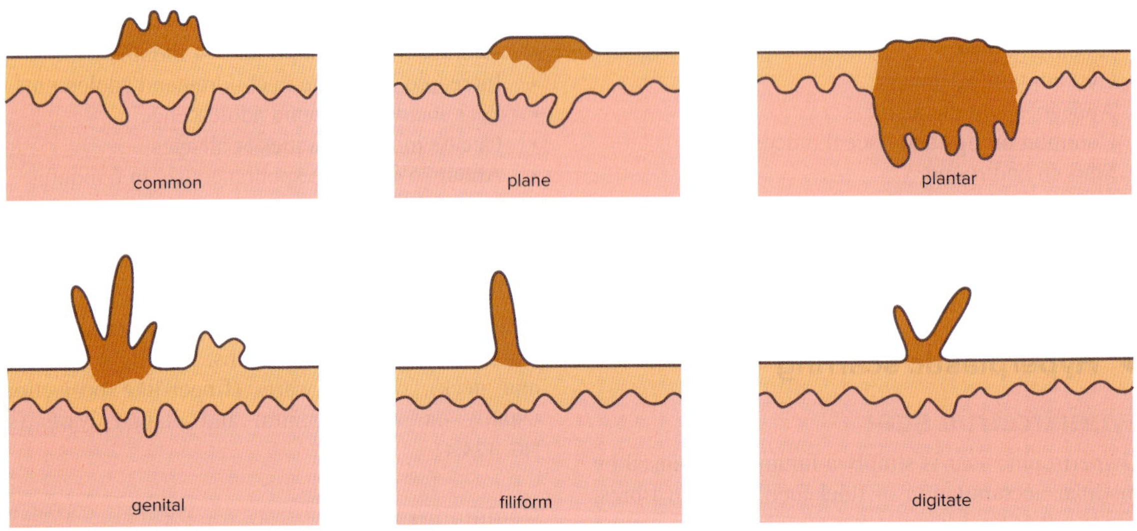

FIGURE 124.4 Configuration of various types of warts

Curettage

A most common treatment; some plantar warts can be removed under LA with a sharp spoon curette. The problem is a tendency to scar, so avoid over a pressure area such as the sole of the foot.

Electrodesiccation

A high-frequency spark under LA is useful for small, filiform or digitate warts. A combination of curettage and electrodesiccation is suitable for large and persistent warts.

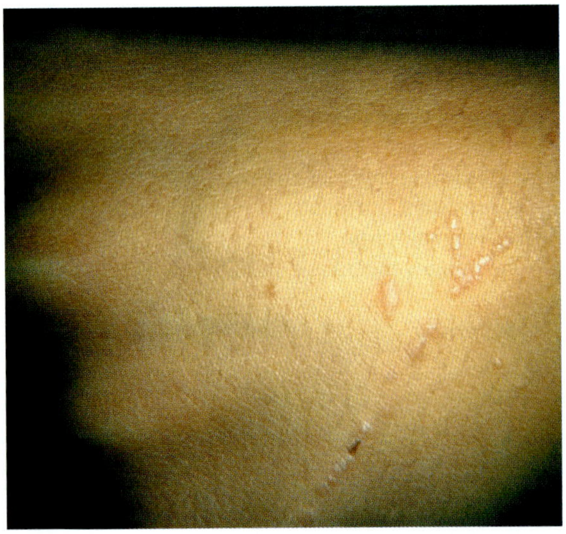

FIGURE 124.5 Plane warts on the dorsum of the hand

124

Vitamin A and the retinoids

- Topical retinoic acid (e.g. tretinoin 0.1% cream—Retin-A) is effective on plane warts
- Systemic oral retinoid, acitretin (Neotigason) for recalcitrant warts (with care)

Medication

- Consider cimetidine

Specific wart treatment

The method chosen depends on the type of wart, its site and the patient's age.

- *Plantar warts:* refer to CHAPTER 68
- *Genital warts:* podophyllotoxin 0.5% paint or imiquimod (best for penile warts, see CHAPTER 117)
- *Filiform and digitate warts:* liquid nitrogen or electrodissection
- *Plane warts:* liquid nitrogen; salicylic acid 20% co (e.g. Wartkil); consider 5-fluorouracil cream or tretinoin 0.05% cream (Retin-A)
- *Common warts:* a recommended method:
  1. Soak the wart/s in warm soapy water.
  2. Rub back the wart surface with a pumice stone.
  3. Apply keratolytic paint (only to the wart; protect the surrounding skin with Vaseline). The paints: formalin 5%, salicylic acid 12%, acetone 25%, collodion to 100%.[4]

Do this daily or every second day.
Carefully remove dead skin between applications

or (preferable applications)
(adult) 16% salicylic acid, 16% lactic acid in collodion paint (Dermatec, Duofilm), apply once daily until wart cleared
(children) 8% salicylic acid, 8% lactic acid in collodion
Combined method: salicylic acid 70% paste in linseed oil. Leave 1 week then pare and freeze (cryotherapy).

- *Periungual warts (fingernails):* consider 5-fluorouracil or liquid nitrogen with care. Always use a paint rather than ointment or paste on fingers.
  Specialised treatment includes bleomycin, immunotherapy (e.g. topical diphencyprone—DPCP) and cantharidin

Pox virus lumps

Skin tumours can be caused by pox viruses, some of which result from handling infected sheep, cows and monkeys and other animals such as deer. Hence they are usually found in sheep shearers, farmers and zookeepers.

Molluscum contagiosum

This common pox virus infection can be spread readily by direct contact, including sexual contact (see CHAPTER 117). The incubation period is 2–26 weeks.

Clinical features

- Common in school-aged children
- Single or multiple (more common)
- Shiny, round, pink-white papule (see FIG. 124.6)
- Hemispherical up to 5 mm

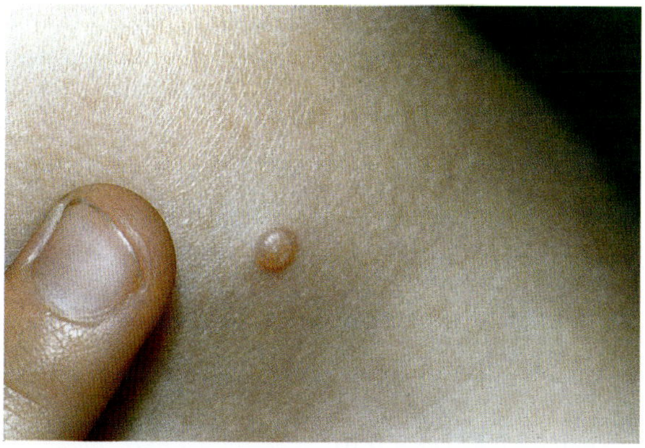

FIGURE 124.6 Molluscum contagiosum with the round, pink, pearly appearance and central punctum

- Central punctum gives umbilical look
- Can be spread by scratching

Management

They are difficult to treat. Avoid using the bath—they spread to other body parts and those sharing the bath. Showering is preferable. There is a case for simply reassuring the family and waiting for spontaneous resolution.

Treatment options

- Liquid nitrogen with care (a few seconds following topical anaesthetic) then dry dressings for 2 weeks
- Pricking the lesion with a pointed stick soaked in 1% or 2.5% phenol
- Application of 15% podophyllin in Friar's Balsam (compound benzoin tincture)
- Application of 30% trichloracetic acid
- Application of imiquimod 0.1% cream tds for 6 weeks
- Destruction by electrocautery or diathermy
- Ether soap and friction method
- Lifting open the tip with a sterile needle inserted from the side (parallel to the skin) and applying 10% povidone–iodine (Betadine) solution (parents can be shown this method and continue to use it at home for multiple tumours)
- If more localised, covering with a piece of Micropore or Leucosilk tape—change every day after showering (may take a few months). This method also prevents spread
- For large areas, aluminium acetate (Burow's solution 1:30) applied bd can be effective

Note: The extract of the *Cantharis beetle* (cantharidin) (prepared as Cantharone) if available is reportedly very effective.

Orf

Orf is due to a pox virus and presents as a single papule or group of papules on the hands of sheep-handlers after handling lambs with contagious pustular dermatitis. The papules change into pustular-like nodules or bullae with a violaceous erythematous margin. It clears up spontaneously in about 3–4 weeks without scarring and usually no treatment is necessary.

> **Practice tip for orf**
>
> Rapid resolution (days) can be obtained by an intralesional injection of triamcinolone diluted 50:50 in normal saline.[6]

Milker's nodules (pseudo cowpox)

In humans 2–5 papules appear on the hands about 1 week after handling cows' udders or calves' mouths. It is caused by a parapoxvirus. The papules enlarge to become tender, grey nodules with a necrotic centre and surrounding inflammation (see FIG. 124.7). The patient can be reassured that the nodules are a self-limiting infection and spontaneous remission will occur in 5–6 weeks without residual scarring. One infection gives lifelong immunity.

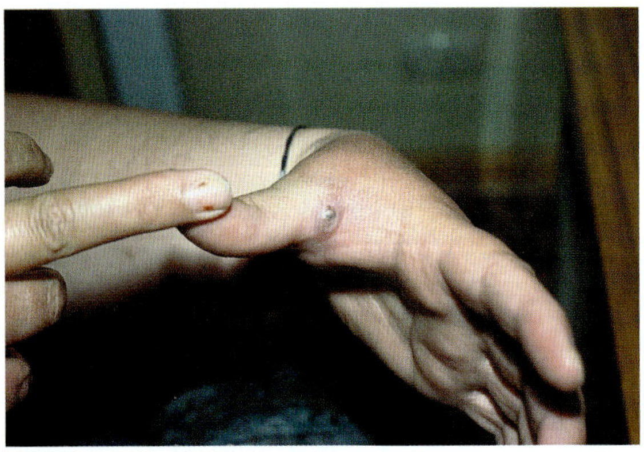

FIGURE 124.7 Milker's nodule in a person who milks cows showing the grey nodule with the necrotic centre

Practice tip for milker's nodule

Rapid resolution (days) can be obtained by an intralesional injection of triamcinolone diluted 50:50 in normal saline.[6]

Seborrhoeic keratoses

Synonyms: seborrhoeic warts, senile warts, senile keratoses (avoid these terms).

Clinical features

- Very common
- There is a variety of subtypes
- Increasing number and pigmentation with age >40 years
- Sits on skin, appears in some like a 'sultana' pressed into the skin (i.e. well-defined border)
- Has a 'pitted' surface (see FIG. 124.8)
- May be solitary but usually multiple
- Common on face and trunk, but occurs anywhere
- Usually asymptomatic
- Usually causes patients some alarm (confused with melanoma)

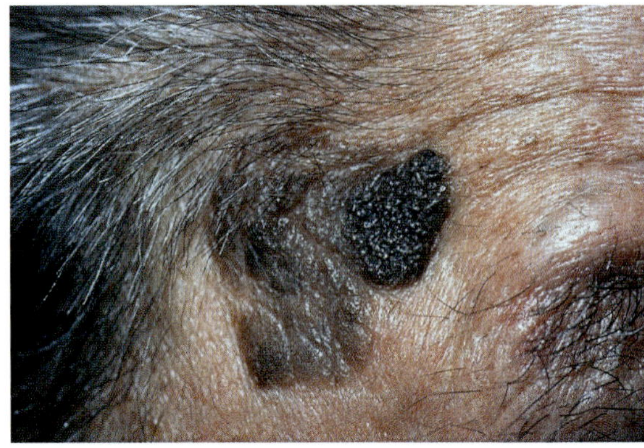

FIGURE 124.8 Seborrhoeic keratosis in a 70-year-old man. The large pigmented warty mass appears to sit on top of the skin.

Photo courtesy Robin Marks

Management

- Usually nil apart from reassurance
- Does not undergo malignant change
- Can be removed for cosmetic reasons
- Light cautery to small facial lesions or ablative laser therapy
- Freezing with liquid nitrogen (especially if thin) decolours the tumour
- 10% (or stronger) phenol solution applied carefully—repeat in 3 weeks
- Apply trichloroacetic acid to surface: instil gently by multiple pricks with a fine-gauge needle, twice weekly for 2 weeks
- May drop off spontaneously
- If diagnosis uncertain, remove for histopathology

Stucco keratoses

This subtype of seborrhoeic keratoses comprises multiple, non-pigmented (often white), small, friable keratoses over the lower legs. They can be treated with a topical keratolytic such as 3–5% salicylic acid in sorbolene.

Granuloma annularae

Granuloma annularae are a common benign group of papules arranged in an annular fashion.

Clinical features

- Most common among children and young adults
- Firm papules grouped in a 'string of pearls' pattern (see FIG. 124.9)
- Dermal nodules
- May be associated with minor trauma

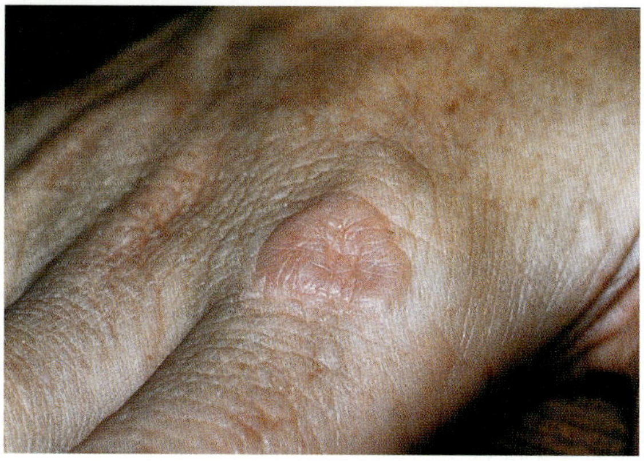

FIGURE 124.9 Granuloma annularae: this pearly papular tumour was longstanding on this finger. After taking a small biopsy, 20 mg of methylprednisolone acetate was injected into the tumour.

- Associated with diabetes
- Usually on dorsum or sides of fingers (knuckle area), backs of hands, the tops of feet, elbows and knees

Management[7]

- Check urine/blood for sugar
- Give reassurance (they usually subside in a year or so)
- Cosmetic reasons:
  - first-line: potent topical corticosteroids ± occlusion, apply bd for minimum of 4–6 weeks
  - if ineffective: intradermal injection into the extending outer margin of triamcinolone 10% or similar corticosteroid (dilute equal volume with N saline); can repeat at 6-weekly intervals if effective

Dermatofibroma

Synonyms: sclerosing haemangioma; histiocytoma.

This is a common pigmented nodule arising in the dermis due to a proliferation of fibroblasts, believed to develop as an abnormal response to minor trauma including insect bites. The nodule gives a characteristic button-like feel and dimpling when laterally compressed (pinched) from the side with the fingers.

Clinical features

- Usually multiple
- Firm, well-circumscribed nodules
- Oval, 0.5–1 cm in diameter
- Freely mobile over deeper structures
- Slightly raised in relation to skin
- Mainly on limbs, especially legs
- May itch
- Mainly in women
- Variable colour, pink or brown, tan or grey or violaceous
- Characteristic 'dimple' sign on pinching margins

Treatment

- Reassurance
- Simple excision if requested

Solar keratoses[7]

Solar keratoses (actinic keratoses or sun spots) are reddened, adherent, scaly hyperkeratotic thickenings occurring on light-exposed areas. They represent intra-epidermal keratinocytic dysplasia with a potential for malignant change, especially on the ears.

Clinical features

- Sun-exposed fair skin
- Mainly on face, ears, scalp (if balding), forearms, dorsum of hands (especially) (see FIG. 124.10)
- Vary in size from 2–20 mm in diameter
- Dry, rough, adherent scale
- Usually asymptomatic
- Discomfort on rubbing with towel
- Scale can separate to leave oozing surface
- A small proportion undergo malignant change

Management[7]

- Can disappear spontaneously
- Liquid nitrogen

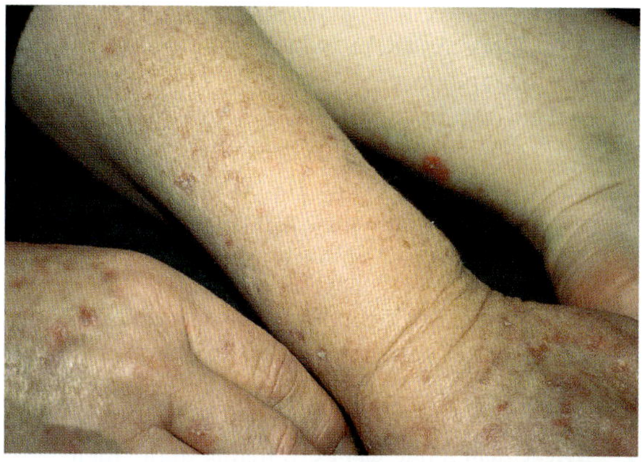

FIGURE 124.10 Solar keratoses showing the reddened, scaly thickenings on sun-exposed areas. Biopsy of one of the lesions proved SCC.

- Topical field treatment for patients with multiple solar keratoses or who cannot tolerate repeated cryotherapy:
  5-fluorouracil 5% cream daily for 3–4 weeks on face or 3–6 weeks on arms and legs
  or
  imiquimod, once daily 3 times a week for 3-4 weeks (for one to three cycles with 4-week spells between cycles)
  or
  ingenol mebutate 0.015% gel topically on face or scalp, once daily for 3 consecutive days
  or
  ingenol mebutate 0.05% gel topically on trunk or limbs, once daily for 2 consecutive days
- Surgical excision for suspicious and ulcerating lesions
- Tenderness on lateral pressure requires a biopsy to exclude SCC
- Biopsy if doubtful

Topical field treatments cause severe inflammation that can last up to several weeks; warn the patient and show them the expected erythema using patient information handouts. Fluorouracil is most commonly used due to its lower cost but causes inflammation for several weeks. Ingenol produces dramatic erythema and vesiculation within 24–48 hours, but the skin heals in approximately 7 days.

> **Terminology**
>
> **Solar keratoses** 'sun spots'
> **Solar lentigines** 'age spots' or 'liver spots'

Keratoacanthoma

Keratoacanthomas (KA), which are rapidly evolving tumours of keratinocytes, occur singly on light-exposed areas. They are now considered a low-risk variant of SCC.[7] The major problem is differentiation from SCC, especially if on the lip or ear. The relative growth rates of three types of skin tumours are shown in FIGURE 124.11.

Clinical features

- Rapidly growing lesion on sun-exposed skin
- Raised crater with central keratin plug (see FIGS 124.12 and 124.13)
- Grows to 2 cm or more
- Arises over a few weeks, remains static, then spontaneously disappears after about 4–6 months; can leave a big scar
- Can be confused with SCC

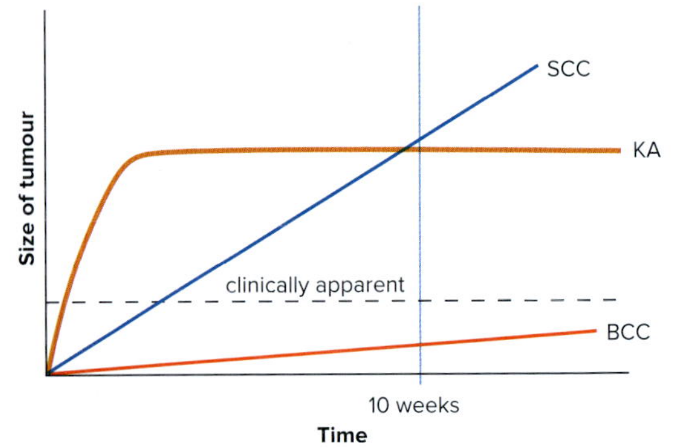

FIGURE 124.11 Relative growth rates of three types of skin tumours: keratoacanthoma, squamous cell carcinoma and basal cell carcinoma

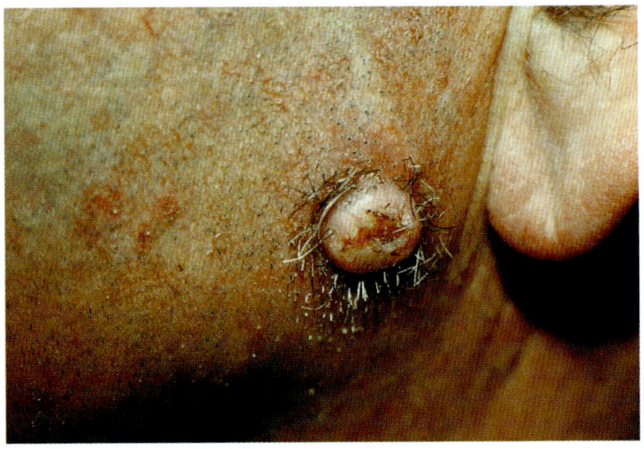

FIGURE 124.12 Keratoacanthoma: this tumour, with its central plug, appeared suddenly on the face of a 63-year-old man. It may be confused with squamous cell carcinoma. Surgical excision is appropriate treatment.

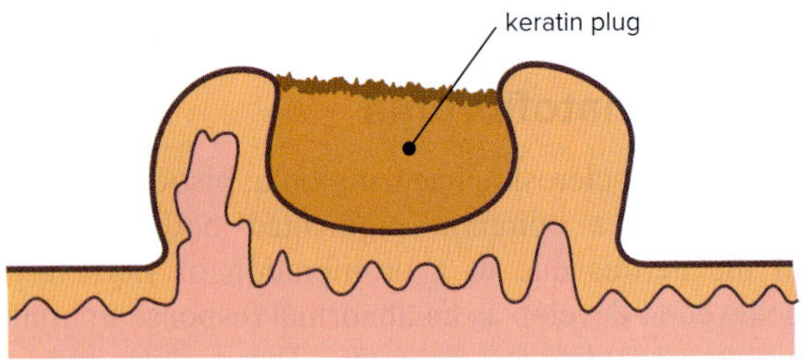

FIGURE 124.13 A typical keratoacanthoma

Management

- Remove by excision—perform biopsy
- If clinically certain—curettage/diathermy
- Treat as SCC (by excision) if on lip/ear

The recommended treatment is surgical excision and histological examination. Ensure a 2–3 mm

124

margin for excision. Most patients will not tolerate a tumour for 4–6 months on an exposed area such as the face while waiting for a spontaneous remission. Also, if it is an SCC, a potentially lethal cancer has remained in situ for an unnecessarily long period.

Sebaceous hyperplasia

Sebaceous hyperplasia presents as single or multiple nodules on the face, especially in older people. The nodules are small, yellow–pink, slightly umbilicated and are found in a similar distribution to BCCs, for which they may be mistaken. There is no need for surgical excision. Cryotherapy or fine wire diathermy achieves good results.

Basal cell carcinoma[8]

Clinical features

- Most common skin cancer (80%)
- Age: usually >35 years
- More frequent in males
- Mostly on sun-exposed areas: face (mainly), neck, upper trunk, limbs (10%) (see FIG. 124.14)
- May ulcerate easily = 'rodent ulcer'
- Slow-growing over years
- Has various forms: nodular, pigmented, ulcerated, etc.
- Stretching the skin demarcates the lesion, highlights pearliness and distinct margin
- Does not metastasise via lymph nodes or bloodstream
- Local spread is a problem (see FIG. 124.15)
- Can spread deeply if around nose, eye or ear

Clinical types

1. Cystic nodular—translucent or pale grey
2. Ulcerated—nodular BCC that has necrosed centrally
3. Pigmented—usually spotted, may be all black
4. Superficial—erythematous scaly patch, may be misdiagnosed as eczema or psoriasis
5. Morphoeic (fibrotic)—scar-like, poorly defined margin
6. Common: pearly edge, telangiectasia, ulcerated (see FIG. 124.16)
7. Basi-squamous—mixed BCC & SCC

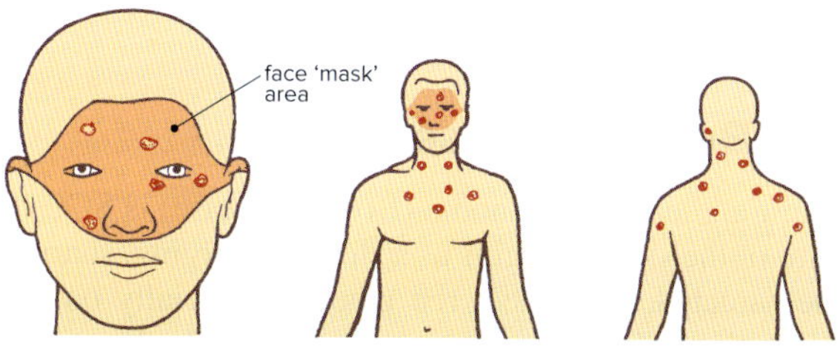

FIGURE 124.14 Typical areas in which basal cell carcinomas occur

Red flag pointer for BCC

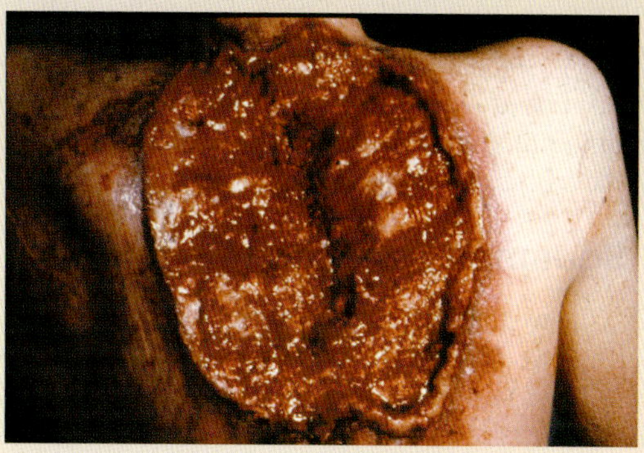

FIGURE 124.15 Grossly neglected basal cell carcinoma on back

Photo courtesy Robin Marks

Management[8]

- Simple elliptical excision (3–4 mm margin) is best.
- If not excision, do biopsy before other treatment.
- Radiotherapy is an option, especially in frail people.
- Mohs micrographic surgery—a form of surgical treatment suitable for large or recurrent tumours or those in a site when maximal normal tissue needs to be preserved.
- Photodynamic therapy—response rate is >90% for nodular and superficial BCCs.

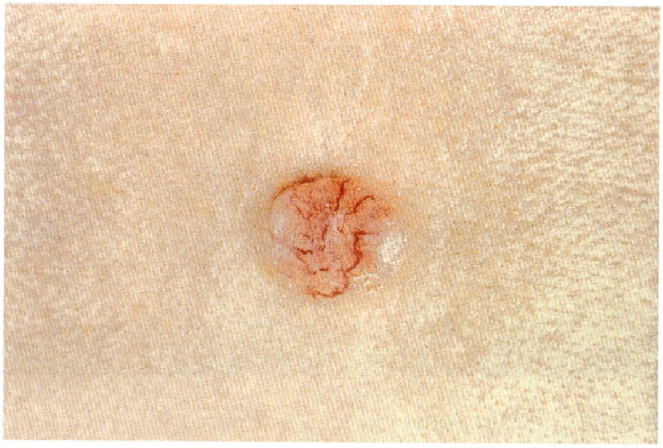

FIGURE 124.16 Basal cell carcinoma showing a pearly nodular appearance with telangiectatic vessels

- Cryotherapy is suitable for well-defined, histologically confirmed, superficial tumours at sites away from head and neck. Use judiciously and infrequently.

Note: For proven BCC but not on nose and around eyes, imiquimod may be an option. To biopsy a BCC, do a shave biopsy, not a punch biopsy.

Squamous cell carcinoma[7]

SCC is an important malignant tumour of the epidermis; it is also found on sun-exposed areas, especially in fair-skinned people. It tends to arise in premalignant areas such as solar keratoses, burns, chronic ulcers, leucoplakia and Bowen disease, or it can arise de novo. Keratoacanthoma is a variant.

Note: Although BCC and SCC are related to cumulative sun exposure, they are not always found in sun-exposed areas.

Clinical features

- Usually >50 years
- Initially firm thickening of skin, especially in solar keratosis
- Surrounding erythema
- The hard nodules soon ulcerate (see FIG. 124.17)
- Occurs on the hands and forearms and the head and neck (see FIG. 124.18)

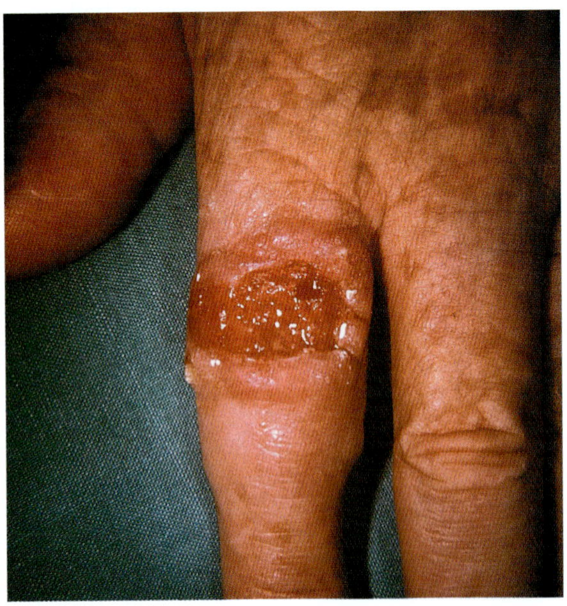

FIGURE 124.17 Squamous cell carcinoma. This recurrent, non-healing lesion on the index finger of a 58-year-old man had raised hard edges and was fixed to tendon and bone. Treatment was by surgical amputation of the finger.

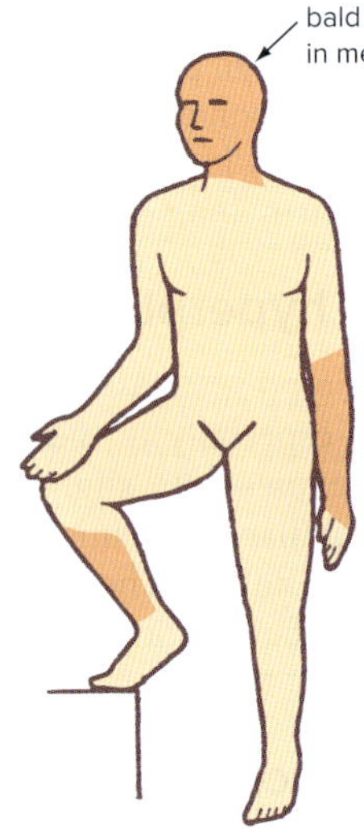

FIGURE 124.18 Common sites of squamous cell carcinoma

- Ulcers have a characteristic everted edge
- Capable of metastases (especially those on lips and ears) and may involve regional nodes
- SCCs of ear, lip, oral cavity, tongue and genitalia are serious and need special management

Management

- Early excision of tumours <1 cm with a 3–5 mm margin, to deep fat level.
- Referral for specialised surgery and/or radiotherapy if large, in difficult site or lymphadenopathy.
- SCCs of the ear and lip, which have considerably more malignant potential, can be excised by wedge excision.
- There is no alternative to surgery if the SCC is over cartilage—central nose or helix.

Note: Surgery is the treatment of choice for most tumours; cryotherapy, imiquimod and curettage are not.

Radiotherapy is an optional treatment in a biopsy-proven tumour where surgery is not feasible or will cause unacceptable morbidity.

Bowen disease[7]

Intra-epidermal carcinoma (Bowen disease) is SCC in situ of the skin. It begins as a slowly enlarging, sharply demarcated, thickened, red plaque, especially on the lower legs of females. It may resemble solar keratosis, dermatitis, or a patch of psoriasis. It remains virtually unchanged for months or years. It may become very crusty, ulcerate or bleed. It has a potential for malignant change since it is a full thickness SCC in situ.

Management

- Biopsy first for diagnosis
- Wide surgical excision if small
- Skin grafting may be required
- Cryotherapy by double freeze thaw technique
- Topical therapy with fluorouracil 5% cream or imiquimod 5% cream are options, but referral to a consultant is advisable

Note: Biopsy a single patch of suspected psoriasis or dermatitis not responding to topical steroids.

LUMPS ON EARS

Lumps on ears, especially on the helix, demand close attention. SCCs that arise here have up to 17 times the ability to metastasise and demand early wedge resection.

Causes of ear lumps include:

- solar keratosis
- BCC
- SCC
- keratoacanthoma
- gouty tophi
- chondrodermatitis nodularis helicis

Chondrodermatitis nodularis helicis[9]

This lump, which is not a neoplasm, presents as a painful nodule on the most prominent part of the helix or antihelix of the ear (see FIGS 124.19 and 124.20). It is seen more often in men while it is found more often on the antihelix in women. It appears to be caused by pressure between the head and the pillow at night. Histologically a thickened epidermis overlies inflamed cartilage. It looks like a small corn, is tender, and affects sleep if that side of the head lies on the pillow. It can be treated initially by cryotherapy or an intralesional injection of triamcinolone. Most resolve if the patient sleeps on the opposite side. If cryotherapy fails, wedge resection under local anaesthetic is an effective treatment.

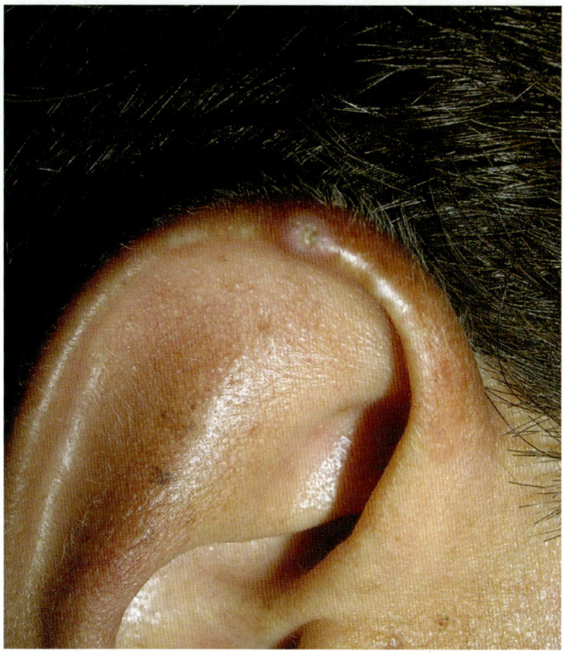

FIGURE 124.20 Chondrodermatitis nodularis helicis on the right ear in a 44-year-old man

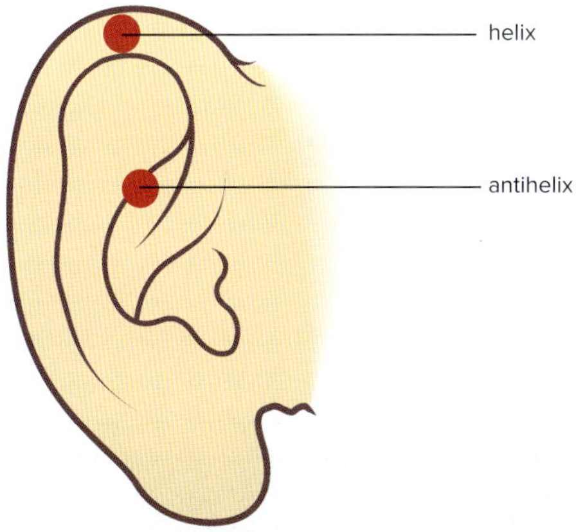

FIGURE 124.19 Typical sites of chondrodermatitis nodularis helicis

Malignant melanoma

These are usually enlarging pigmented lesions with an irregular, notched border. Refer to CHAPTER 125 on pigmented skin lesions.

Secondary tumour

These complex tumours may metastasise from the lung, melanoma or bowel and may arise in surgical scars (e.g. for breast cancer).

Kaposi sarcoma[10]

Kaposi sarcoma is a tumour of vascular and lymphatic endothelium that is related to human herpes virus type 8. There are three types:

- 'classic' or 'sporadic' form of primary tumour seen mostly in elderly males of central or eastern European origin

- 'endemic' form seen in males from Central Africa
- immunosuppressed-related form commonly associated with AIDS. Widespread lesions affect skin, bowel, oral cavity and lungs

Kaposi sarcoma presents as brownish-purple papules on the skin and mucosa (any organ).

Treatment is with radiotherapy, immunotherapy or chemotherapy.

LUMPS OF SUBCUTANEOUS AND DEEPER STRUCTURES

Lipoma

Lipomas are common benign tumours of mature fat cells situated in subcutaneous tissue.

Clinical features

- Soft and may be fluctuant
- Well defined; lobulated (see FIG. 124.21)
- Rubbery consistency
- May be one or many
- Painless
- Most common on limbs (especially arms) and trunk
- Can occur at any site

Management

- Reassurance about benign nature
- Removal for cosmetic reasons or to relieve discomfort from pressure. Use surgical excision or punch biopsy

Surgical excision

Many lipomas can be enucleated using a gloved finger, but there are a few traps: some are deeper than anticipated, and some are adjacent to important structures such as large nerves and blood vessels. Others are tethered by fibrous bands, and can recur. Recurrence is also possible if excision is incomplete.

Caution: Lipomas on back (don't shell out easily). If >5 cm consider referral.

Note: Ultrasound is good at assessing depth of lipoma. CT scan or MRI will help diagnose and define.

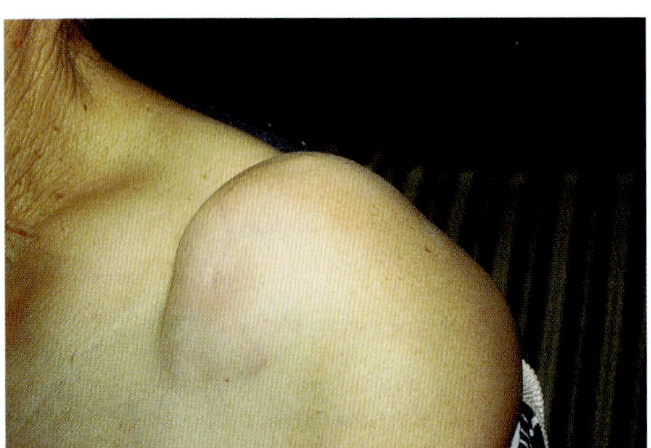

FIGURE 124.21 Lipoma: this 66-year-old woman had a long-standing soft, fluctuant, rubbery lump of 18 years. It was surgically removed for cosmetic reasons

Neurofibroma

These benign tumours are firm (sometimes soft), painless, subcutaneous lumps often aligned lengthwise in the long axis of a limb in relation to peripheral nerves (see FIG. 124.22). The lumps are more mobile from side to side than along the long axis. Some are tender to pressure with associated pain and paraesthesia on the nerve distribution.

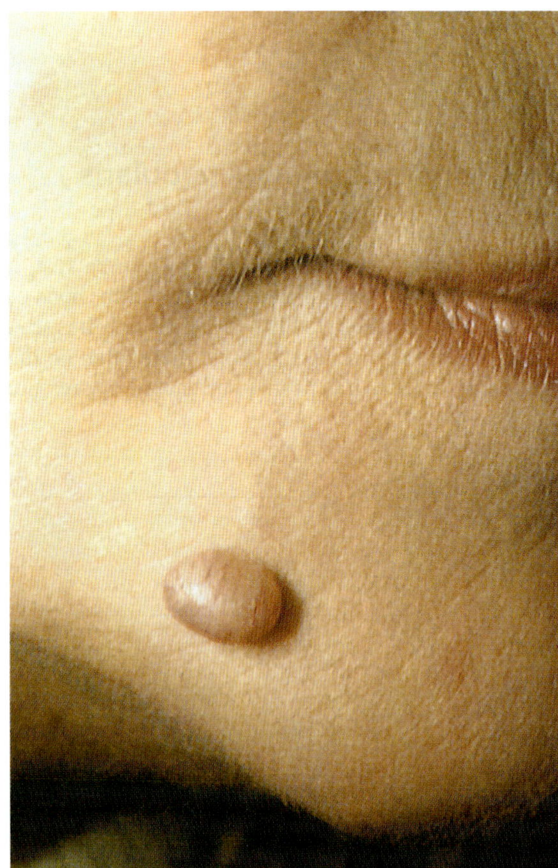

FIGURE 124.22 Neurofibroma. This mobile firm subcutaneous lump was tender to firm pressure.

124

Bursae

Bursae are cystic sacs between the skin and an underlying bony prominence or sacs of gelatinous fluid that separate and aid gliding of adjacent tendons and ligaments.

Pseudoaneurysm[11]

A pseudoaneurysm is a sac-like dilatation of the arterial wall (but not all three layers of the wall). It presents as an expanding subcutaneous nodule located close to a superficial artery. It can form after blunt or penetrating trauma that injures the vessel, leading to a haemorrhage into the vessel wall. Investigate with ultrasound and manage with caution. Refer to a vascular surgeon for surgical management.

Ganglion

Ganglia are firm cystic lumps associated with joints or tendon sheaths.

Clinical features

- Deep subcutaneous lumps
- Around joints or tendon sheaths (see FIG. 124.23)
- Mostly around wrists, fingers, dorsum of feet
- Immobile, fixed to deep tissues
- Translucent
- Contain viscid gelatinous fluid
- Associated with arthritis and synovitis
- May disappear spontaneously
- Recurrences common

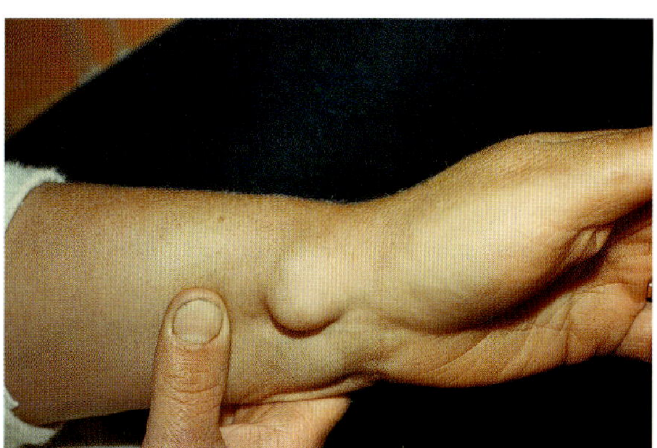

FIGURE 124.23 Ganglion of wrist—firm, immobile and translucent. It was eventually treated by aspiration of gelatinous fluid followed by infusion of 40 mg methylprednisolone acetate.

Management

- Can be left—wait and see
- Do not 'bang with a Bible'
- Needle aspiration and steroid injection
  or
  surgical excision (can be difficult)
- Suture compression technique: a larger gauge catgut suture is inserted through the middle of the ganglion and firmly tied over it. Side pressure may express the contents through the needle holes. Remove the knot 12 days later.

Injection treatment of ganglia

Ganglia have a high recurrence rate after treatment, with a relapse rate of 30% after surgery. A simple, relatively painless and more effective method is to use intralesional injections of long-acting corticosteroid, such as methylprednisolone acetate.[12]

Method

1. Insert a 21 gauge needle attached to a 2 mL or 5 mL syringe into the cavity of the ganglion.
2. Aspirate some (not all) of its jelly-like contents, mainly to ensure the needle is in situ.
3. Keeping the needle exactly in place, swap the syringe for an insulin syringe containing up to 0.5 mL of steroid.
4. Inject 0.25–0.5 mL (see FIG. 124.24).
5. Rapidly withdraw the needle, pinch the overlying skin for several seconds and then apply a light dressing.
6. Review in 7 days and, if still present, repeat the injection using 0.25 mL of steroid.

Up to six injections can be given over a period of time, but 70% of ganglia will disperse with only one or two injections.[9] Be aware of possible subsequent hypopigmentation of overlying skin, especially in people with darker skin.

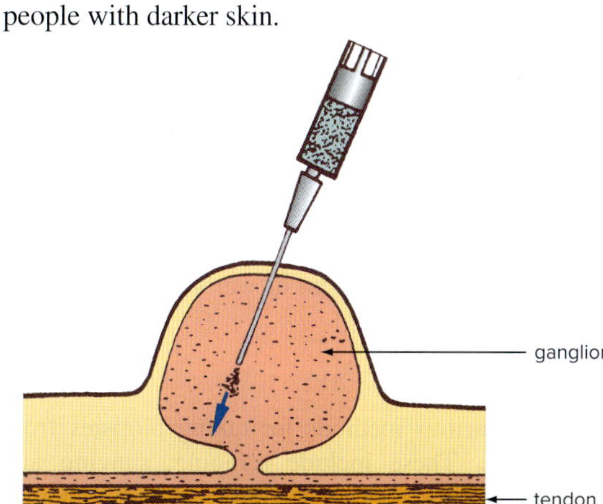

FIGURE 124.24 Injection treatment of ganglion

124

Some preferred therapeutic options

Liquid nitrogen therapy

Ideally, liquid nitrogen is stored in a special large container and decanted when required into a small thermos flask or spray device.

The easiest method of application to superficial skin tumours (see TABLE 124.2) is via a ball of cotton wool rolled rather loosely on the tip of a wooden applicator stick. The ball of cotton wool should be slightly smaller than the lesion, to prevent freezing of the surrounding skin.

Table 124.2 Superficial skin tumours suitable for cryotherapy

Warts (plane, periungual, plantar, anogenital)
Skin tags
Seborrhoeic keratoses
Molluscum contagiosum
Sebaceous hyperplasia
Solar keratoses

Method (basic steps)

1. Inform the patient what to expect.
2. Pare excess keratin with a scalpel.
3. Use a cotton wool applicator slightly smaller (not larger—see FIG. 124.25a) than the lesion.
4. Immerse it in nitrogen until bubbling ceases.
5. Gently tap it on the side of the container to remove excess liquid.
6. Hold the lesion firmly between thumb and forefinger.
7. Place applicator vertically (see FIG. 124.25b and FIG. 124.25c) on tumour surface.
8. Apply with firm pressure: do not dab.
9. Freeze until a 2 mm white halo appears around the lesion.

Explain likely reaction to patient, such as the appearance of blisters (possibly blood blisters). The optimal time for retreatment of warts is in 2–3 weeks (not longer than 3 weeks).

124

Biopsies

There are various methods for taking biopsies from skin lesions. These include scraping, shaving and punch biopsies, all of which are useful but not as effective or safe as excisional biopsies.

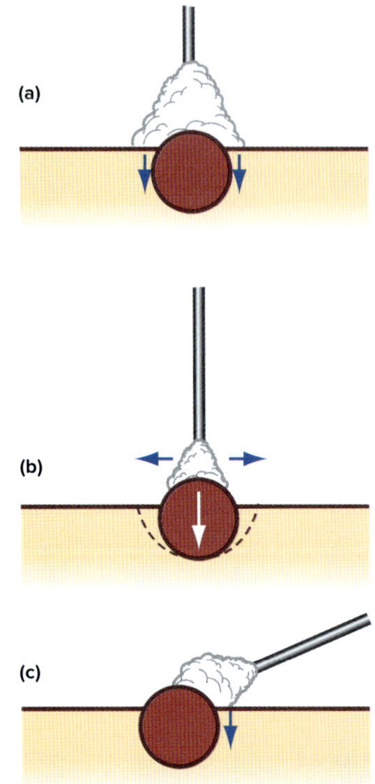

FIGURE 124.25 Application of liquid nitrogen with cotton wool applicator: **(a)** applicator too large, **(b)** correct size and approach of applicator, **(c)** correct size but wrong position of applicator

Shave biopsies

This simple technique is generally used for the tissue diagnosis of premalignant lesions and some malignant tumours, but not melanoma.

Method

1. Infiltrate with LA.
2. Holding a number 10 or 15 scalpel blade horizontally, shave off the tumour just into the dermis (see FIG. 124.26).
3. Diathermy may be required for haemostasis.

The biopsy site usually heals with minimal scarring.

Punch biopsy

This biopsy (see FIG 124.27) has considerable use in general practice where full-thickness skin specimens are required for histological diagnosis. (Good quality disposable biopsy punches are available from Dermatech Laboratories.)

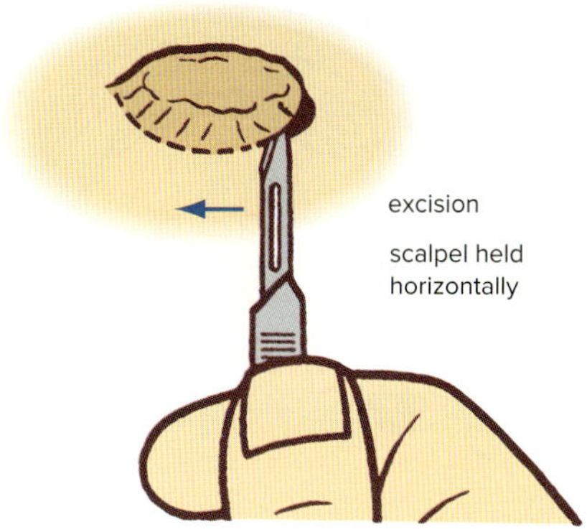

FIGURE 124.26 Shave biopsy

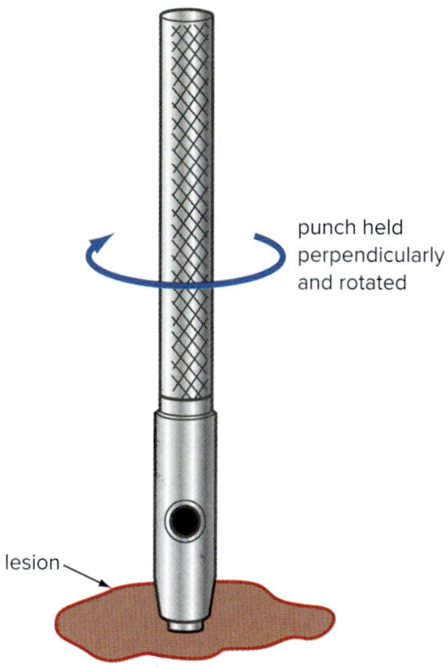

FIGURE 124.27 Punch biopsy

Steroid injections into skin lesions

Suitable lesions for steroid injections are:

- plaque psoriasis
- granuloma annularae
- hypertrophic scars (early development)
- keloid scars (early development)
- alopecia areata
- chondrodermatitis nodularis helicis
- lichen simplex chronicus
- necrobiosis lipoidica
- hypertrophic lichen planus
- orf and milker's nodules

Triamcinolone is the appropriate long-acting corticosteroid (10 mg/mL). It may be diluted in equal quantities with saline.

Method

1. The steroid should be injected into the lesion (not below it).
2. Insert a 25 or (preferably) 27 gauge needle, firmly locked to a small insulin-type 1 mL syringe, into the lesion at the level of the middle of the dermis (see FIG. 124.28).
3. High pressure is required with some lesions (e.g. keloid).
4. Inject sufficient steroid to make the lesion blanch.
5. Several sites will be needed for larger lesions, so preceding LA may be required in some instances. Avoid infiltration of steroid in larger lesions: use multiple injections.

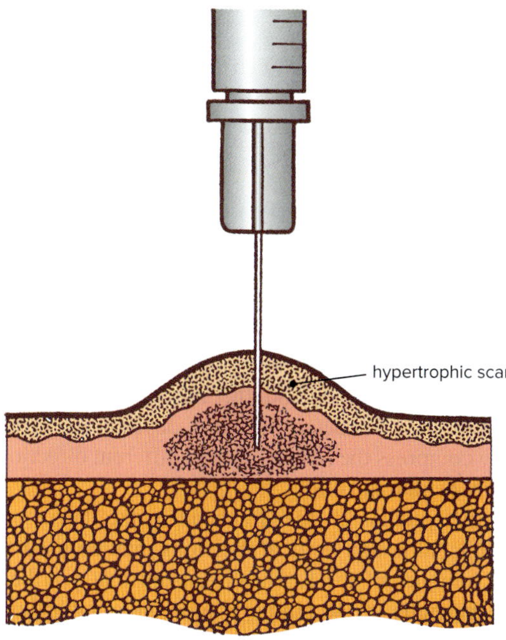

FIGURE 124.28 Injection of corticosteroid into mid-dermis

Elliptical excisions

Small lesions are best excised as an ellipse. Generally, the long axis of the ellipse should be along the skin tension lines identified by natural wrinkles.

The intended ellipse should be drawn on the skin (see FIG. 124.29). The placement will depend on such factors as the size and shape of the lesion, the margin required (usually 3 mm) and the skin tension lines.

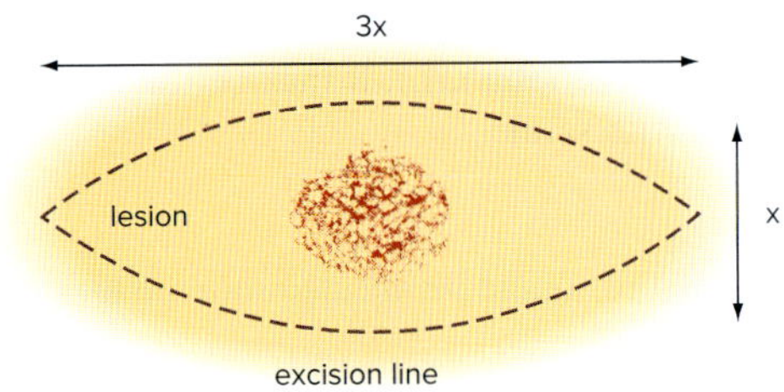

FIGURE 124.29 Ellipse excision

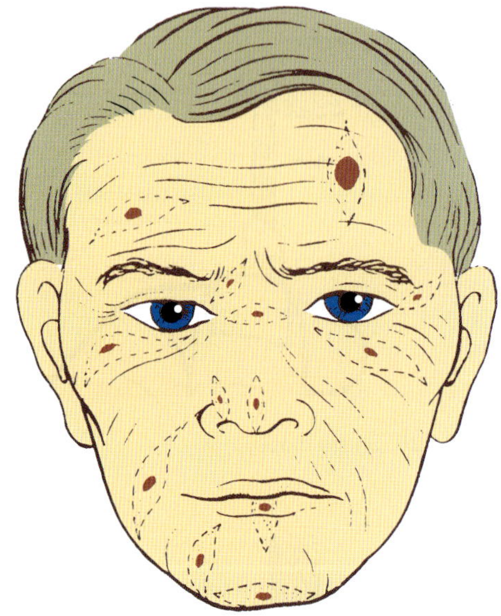

FIGURE 124.30 Recommended lines for excisions on face

Source: Adapted from JS Brown, *Minor Surgery: A Text And Atlas.* London: Chapman & Hall, 1986

General points[9]

- The length of the ellipse should be three times the width.
- This length should be increased (say, to four times) in areas with little subcutaneous tissue (dorsum of hand) and high skin tension (upper back).
- A good rule is to obtain an angle at each end of the excision of 30° or less.
- These rules should achieve closure without 'dog ears'.

Excisions on the face

It is important to select optimal sites for elliptical excisions of tumours of the face. As a rule it is best for incisions to follow wrinkle lines and the direction of hair follicles in the beard area. Therefore, follow the natural wrinkles in the glabella area, the 'crow's feet' around the eye, and the nasolabial folds (see FIG. 124.30). To determine non-obvious wrinkles, gently compress the relaxed skin in different directions to demonstrate the lines.

For tumours of the forehead make horizontal incisions, although vertical incisions may be used for large tumours of the forehead. Ensure that you keep your incisions in the temporal area quite superficial, as the frontal branch of the facial nerve is easily cut.

124

When to refer[9]

Referral should be considered for:

- uncertainty of diagnosis
- suspicion of melanoma
- tumours larger than 1 cm
- recurrent tumours, despite treatment
- incomplete excised tumours, especially with poor healing
- doubts about appropriate treatment
- recommended treatment beyond skills of practitioner
- frequent multiple tumours (e.g. organ transplant patients)
- SCC on the lip or ear
- infiltrating or scar-like morphoeic BCC, particularly those on the nose or around the nasal labial fold
- cosmetic concerns, such as lesions in the upper chest and upper arms where keloid scarring is a potential problem

Key points

- Uncomplicated small tumours are best removed by an elliptical excision with a 3 mm margin for BCC and a 4 mm margin for SCC.
- Caution should be used in the management of tumours on the face, including the ears and lips.

Patient education resources

Hand-out sheets from *Murtagh's Patient Education* 7th edition:

- Fatty tumour (lipoma)
- Molluscum contagiosum
- Seborrhoeic keratoses
- Skin cancer
- Warts

References

1 Paver R. The surgical management of cutaneous tumours in general practice. Modern Medicine Australia, 1991; March: 43–51.
2 Marks R. Skin cancer. In: *MIMS Disease Index* (2nd edn). Sydney: IMS Publishing, 1996: 469–72.
3 Davis A, Bolin T, Ham J. *Symptom Analysis and Physical Diagnosis* (2nd edn). Sydney: Pergamon Press, 1990: 302–6.
4 de Launey WE, Land WA. *Principles and Practice of Dermatology* (2nd edn). Sydney: Butterworths, 1984: 280–1.
5 Berger P. Warts: how to treat them successfully. Modern Medicine Australia, 1990; August: 28–32.
6 Reddy J. Intralesional injection for orf: a practice tip. Aust Fam Physician, 1993; 22: 65.
7 Expert group for Dermatology. In: eTG complete. Melbourne: Therapeutic Guidelines Ltd. Available from: <www.tg.org.au>, accessed March 2018.
8 Telfer NR, Colver GB, Bowers PW. Guidelines for the management of basal cell carcinoma. BJ Dermatology, 2008; 159: 35.
9 Sinclair R. Skin cancer and benign lesions. Australian Doctor, 7 Sept 2012; 25–32.
10 Wolff K, Johnson RA. *Fitzpatrick's Color Atlas & Synopsis of Clinical Dermatology* (5th edn). New York: McGraw-Hill, 2006: 536–8.
11 Murrell DF. Pseudoaneurysm. Medical Observer, 11 July 2008: 38.
12 La Villa G. Methylprednisolone acetate in local therapy of ganglion. Clinical Therapeutics, 1986; 47: 455–7.

Resource

Hayes M. *Skin Cancer, Melanoma and Mimics.* Brisbane: Skin Cancer Books, 2013.

125 Pigmented skin lesions

The skin calls for the faculty of close observation and attention to detail.

Louis A Duhring (1845–1913), valedictory address, University of Pennsylvania Medical School

The management of pigmented skin lesions is a constant concern for all practitioners and requires careful evaluation based on the natural history of these lesions and the increasing incidence of malignant melanoma in particular.

Most pigmented lesions are benign and include simple moles or melanocytic naevi, seborrhoeic keratoses, freckles and lentigines. Reassurance is all that is necessary in the management of these problems.

However, one-third of all melanomas arise in pre-existing naevi, many of which are dysplastic, and it is the recognition and removal of such naevi that is so important in the prevention of melanoma.[1]

Malignant melanoma is doubling in incidence each decade, which is an alarming statistic considering the public education programs about the hazards of sun exposure. Of equal interest is the fact that the cure rate for melanoma is also increasing, reflecting earlier diagnosis and treatment. The most important factor in management is early detection. It is most appropriate for GPs to acquire skills in dermoscopy, which significantly improves diagnostic accuracy for melanoma.[2]

A classification of pigmented skin lesions is given in TABLE 125.1.

Key facts and checkpoints

- The incidence of melanoma is greatest in white Caucasians and increases with proximity to the equator.
- The early diagnosis and treatment of melanoma profoundly affects the prognosis.
- Melanoma is extremely rare before puberty.
- Currently the greatest rate of increase is in men >55 years.
- Most people have 5–10 melanocytic naevi on average.
- Multiple dysplastic naevi carry a higher risk of malignant change, which may occur in young adults. Such patients require regular observation (with photography).

Table 125.1 Classification of pigmented skin lesions

Non-melanocytic
Pigmented basal cell carcinoma
Seborrhoeic keratoses
Solar keratoses
Dermatofibroma
Pyogenic granuloma
Foreign body granuloma
Talon noir (black heel)
Tinea nigra
Becker naevus
Melanocytic
Non-melanoma
Freckles
Lentigines
Naevi:
1. congenital
2. acquired:
— junctional → compound → intradermal
— halo
— blue
— Spitz
— dysplastic
Melanoma
1. Lentigo maligna (Hutchinson melanotic freckle)
2. Superficial spreading melanoma
3. Nodular melanoma
4. Acral lentiginous melanoma

Pyogenic granuloma

Synonyms: granuloma, granuloma telangiectaticum, acquired haemangioma.

A pyogenic granuloma is a 5–10 mm soft vascular lesion (without pus) due to a proliferation of capillary vessels. It is considered to be an abnormal reaction to minor trauma (see FIG. 125.1).

Clinical features

- Common in children and young adults
- Usually on hands and face
- Bright red 'raspberry'-like lesion
- Raised, sometimes pedunculated
- Friable—bleeds easily

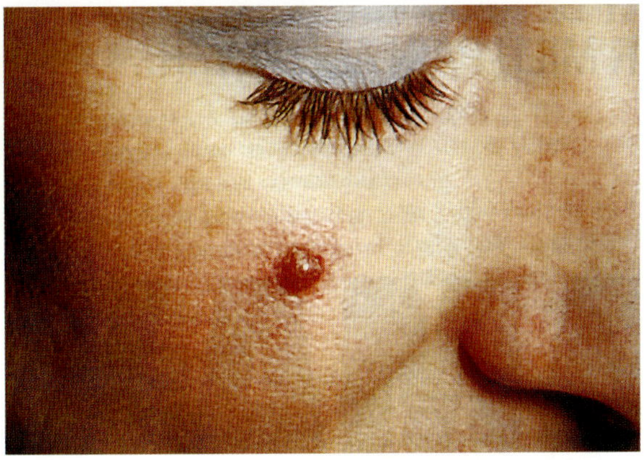

FIGURE 125.1 Pyogenic granuloma showing bright red, friable tumour on face. It followed a puncture from a spiky plant in the garden.
Photo courtesy Robin Marks

Beware of misdiagnosing pyogenic granuloma for a nodular melanoma.

Management

It must be distinguished from amelanotic melanoma or anaplastic SCC. Shave biopsy or curettage with electrocautery of base. The specimen must be sent for histological examination. They are prone to recur.

Talon noir ('black heel')

Talon noir is a black spotted appearance on the heel and is common in sportspeople. A similar lesion (probably smaller) is often found on the other heel.

'Black heel' is formed by small petechiae caused by the trauma of the sharp turns required in sport: shearing stress on the skin of the heel produces superficial bleeding. The diagnosis can be confirmed by gentle paring of the callus to reveal the multiple small petechial spots in the epidermis; these are then pared away. If there is doubt about the diagnosis (malignant melanoma is the main differential diagnosis), the lesion should be excised.

Tinea nigra

Tinea nigra is characterised by solitary black macular lesions on the palm or sole. The simple technique of taking skin scrapings to reveal fungal elements will allow easy differentiation from malignant melanoma.

Becker naevus

Becker naevus is a faint, brown, diffuse pigmented area with a component of coarse hairs and is usually found on the shoulder and upper trunk. It occurs mainly in boys around puberty. It is not a birthmark, it is benign and reassurance is appropriate.

Freckles

Freckles are small, brown flat macules (usually <0.5 cm), coloured by excessive epidermal melanin without any increase in the number of naevus cells (melanocytes). They occur mainly on light-coloured skin and tend to darken in summer and fade in winter. Cosmetic improvement can be achieved through the use of sunscreens.

Lentigines

Lentigines are small, rounded, brown to black macular areas ranging from 1 mm to 1 cm or more across. They are very common and may appear in childhood as a few scattered lesions, often on areas not exposed to the sun. In the elderly, lentigines often develop on sun-damaged skin, usually on the backs of the hands (so-called 'liver spots') and on the face.

Unlike freckles they have increased numbers of melanocytes.

Management

- Treatment is usually unnecessary. Liquid nitrogen or excision can be used for cosmetically unacceptable lesions. Sunscreens are needed to prevent further darkening of existing lesions.
- Otherwise, rather than use 'fade cream', use fresh lemon juice. Squeeze lemon juice (½ lemon) into a small bowl and apply the juice to the spots daily. Continue for 8 weeks.
- Apply tretinoin 0.05% cream daily at night, if necessary.
- Laser for severe cases.

Congenital melanocytic naevi

These moles are present at birth and are sometimes large.

Clinical features

- Variable colour—brown to black
- Sometimes hairy and protruding
- Increased risk of malignant change (especially in larger ones)

Common acquired naevi

These are the common moles for which an opinion is so often sought. The moles are localised, benign

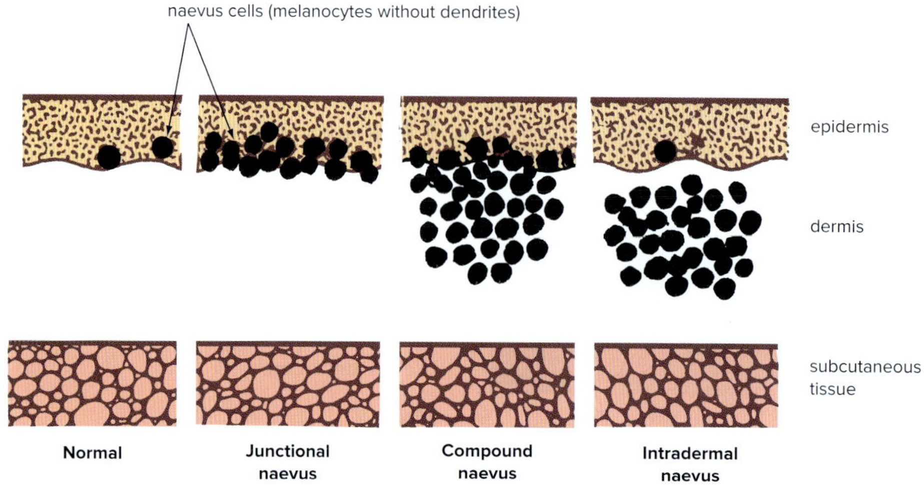

FIGURE 125.2 Comparison of melanocyte (naevus cell) distribution in various common acquired naevi

proliferations of naevus cells. There may be a sharp increase in numbers during pregnancy. New lesions appear less frequently after the age of 20 years. The types are junctional, compound and intradermal. Naevi in children are usually the junctional type with proliferating naevus cells clumped at the dermo-epidermal junction. With time the naevus cells 'move' into the dermis. A compound naevus has both junctional and dermal elements. With maturation all the naevus cells move into the dermis. Refer to FIGURE 125.2.

Clinical features

Junctional

- Usually <5 mm
- Circular-shaped macules
- May be slightly elevated
- Colour usually brown to black
- May be 'fuzzy' border

Most naevi of the palms, soles and genitals are junctional but there is no evidence to support the traditional view that naevi in these sites have more malignant potential.[2]

Compound

- Dome-shaped, slightly raised pigmented nodules
- Up to 1 cm in diameter
- Colour varies from light to dark brown/black, but lighter than junctional naevi (see FIG. 125.3)
- Most are smooth but surface can be rough or verrucoid
- Larger ones may be hairy, especially after puberty
- Become 'flesh'-coloured in time

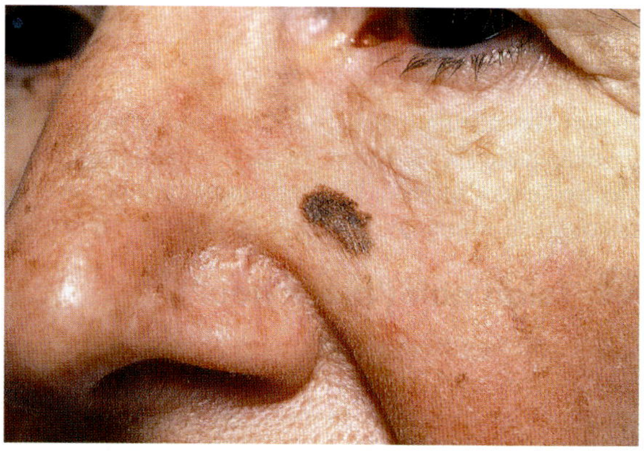

FIGURE 125.3 Compound naevus. This pigmented lesion, which was benign, has been present since birth. At puberty there is often a rapid increase in size and colour.
Photo courtesy Robin Marks

Intradermal

- Look like compound but less pigmented
- Often skin-coloured
- May evolve to pink or brown senile nodules or to soft, pedunculated tags

Malignant potential of common acquired melanocytic naevi

- *Junctional:* have significant potential to undergo malignant change (as long as junctional activity is present)
- *Compound:* very rarely undergo malignant change
- *Intradermal:* these are totally benign lesions

Management

- Provide appropriate reassurance.
- Observe.
- If lesion is changing or there is uncertainty, perform surgical excision (2 mm margin) for histopathology.

Halo naevus

A halo naevus consists of a depigmented halo around a central melanocytic naevus (see FIG. 125.4). It is the result of an autoimmune reaction. The central naevus gradually involutes. It tends to occur around puberty. Multiple halo naevi are often seen on the trunk of adolescents.

Caution: A halo can occur around a melanoma.

Management

Measure the lesion. Reassure and do nothing, as it usually disappears over the next few years; if doubtful at all, remove and obtain histological diagnosis.

Blue naevus

A blue naevus presents as a solitary, slate-grey–blue dermal lesion. Blue naevi usually present in childhood and adolescence on the lower back and buttocks and the limbs, especially dorsa of the hands and feet. Malignant change is rare. They are often excised for cosmetic reasons.

Spitz naevus (benign juvenile melanoma)

Spitz naevi are also called benign juvenile melanomas or spindle cell naevi.

Clinical features

- Solitary pigmented or erythematous nodules
- Often appear in children, usually 4–8 years
- Develop over 1–3 months
- Well-circumscribed, dome-shaped lesions

Management

Surgical excision is treatment of choice (because of rapid growth and best 'reassurance' policy).

Dysplastic melanocytic naevi

These are large, irregular moles that appear predominantly on the trunk in young adults (see FIG. 125.5). They can be familial or sporadic and are markers of an increased risk of melanoma, rather than necessarily being premalignant lesions. Even so, melanoma may arise within these lesions more frequently than would be expected by random chance.[3]

They are considered to be intermediate between benign naevi and melanoma.

Clinical features

- Age: adolescence onwards
- Large >5 mm (variable size)
- Most common on trunk
- Irregular and ill-defined border
- Irregular pigmentation
- Background redness
- Variable colours—brown, tan, black, pink, red
- Variation of colours within the naevus
- Most are stable and do not progress to melanoma

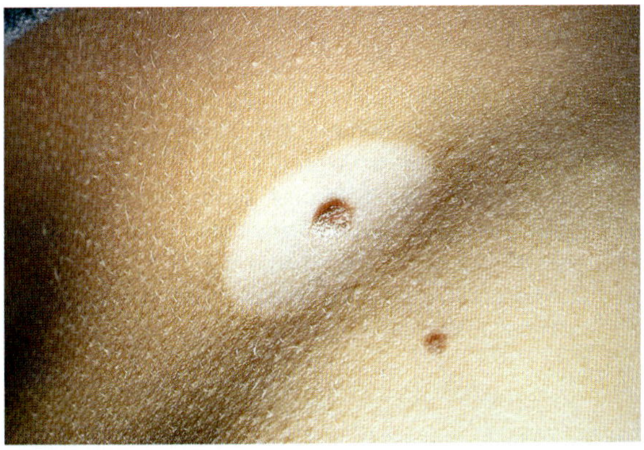

FIGURE 125.4 Halo naevus in a child. The central lesion is usually a benign pigmented naevus.
Photo courtesy Robin Marks

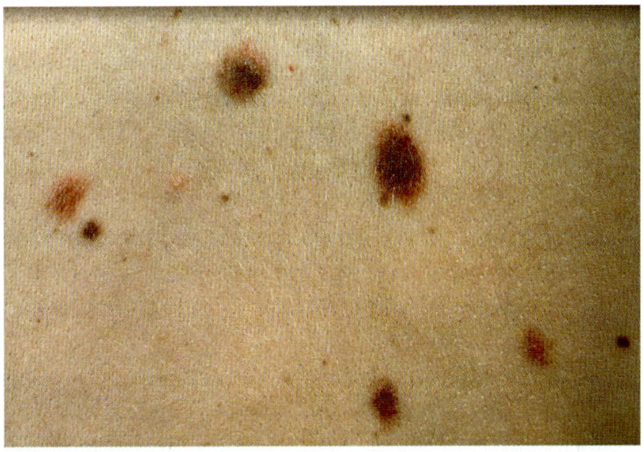

FIGURE 125.5 Dysplastic melanocytic naevi. These lesions may have ill-defined borders and irregular pigmentation.
Photo courtesy Robin Marks

Dysplastic naevus syndrome

The presence of multiple, large, irregular pigmented naevi, mainly on the trunk, presents a difficult management problem, especially if there is a family history of melanoma. The lifetime risk of melanoma may approach 100% for such patients.

Management

Use a follow-up program (similar to excised early melanoma) of 6 monthly review for 2 years (3-monthly if family history of melanoma) and yearly thereafter, provided no lesions become malignant during the first 2 years. During this time the patient and family should become well versed in surveillance. Apart from measurement, good professional-quality photographs of areas of the body including total body photography or specific lesions of concern may also be helpful.

Any suspicious lesions should be excised for histological examination.

Advice to patients

To decrease your chances of getting a melanoma, you should protect yourself from the sun. These rules should be followed.

- Try to avoid direct sunlight when the sun is at its strongest (from 10 am to 3 pm).
- Always wear a broad-brimmed hat and long-sleeved shirt in the sun.
- Use an SPF 30 or more sunscreen on exposed skin and renew the sunscreen regularly.
- Sunbaking might give you a good tan but it is also going to increase your chances of getting a melanoma, so you should avoid it.

Melanoma

Melanomas are malignant tumours derived from melanocytes, with the skin being the most common site.

The early diagnosis of melanoma is vital to outcome. Thickness of a melanoma when it is removed is the major factor determining prognosis: it is vital to detect melanomas when they are in the thin stage and look like an unusual freckle.

In Australia, only about 30% of melanomas develop in pre-existing melanocytic naevi (moles).[2,3] The majority arise in apparently normal skin. Initially the tumour tends to spread laterally in many cases and it should be removed at this stage when it is easily cured. An irregular border or margin is suggestive of the tumour.

Risk factors

- History of previous melanoma (fivefold)
- Presence of many moles (50 or more), especially atypical dysplastic naevi
- Family history (one or more members, especially first-degree relatives)
- History of many sunburns
- Sun sensitive skin/fair complexion
- Patient age and sex: increasing age and male
- Tanning (including solarium) treatments
- History of multiple non-melanoma skin cancers

Clinical features

- Typical age range 30–50 years (average 40 years)
- Can occur anywhere on the body—more common: lower limbs in women, upper back in men
- Often asymptomatic
- Can bleed or itch

Warning signs

The sign of major importance is a recent change in a 'freckle' or mole:

- change in size—at edge or thickening
- change in shape
- change in colour—brown, blue, black, red, violet, white, including combinations
- change in surface
- change in the border
- bleeding or ulceration
- other symptoms (e.g. itching)
- development of satellite nodules
- lymph node involvement

Red flag pointers for melanoma[4]

- New or changing lesion (see preceding change list)
- Rapidly growing nodule of any colour
- Non-healing lump or ulcer
- The 'ugly duckling' syndrome: a prominent pigment lesion that stands out from any other
- A lesion that concerns the patient
- Dermoscopic changes on follow-up or poor dermoscopic–clinical correlation

Types

Lentigo maligna[3]

Lentigo maligna (Hutchinson melanotic freckle) is a slow-growing form of intra-epidermal melanoma that occurs on areas exposed to light (usually the face), predominantly in older patients (see FIG. 125.6). If allowed to remain, it may become invasive and the prognosis will be similar to that for other invasive melanomas. These lesions have all the variations in size, shape and colour of superficial melanomas. Dermoscopic features include an annular-granular pattern, asymmetric follicular pigmented openings and rhomboidal structures.[4] Lentigo maligna should be excised.

Superficial spreading melanoma

Like lentigo maligna, the initial growth is in a lateral or radial intra-epidermal manner, rather than in an invasive downward or vertical manner (see FIG. 125.7). It exhibits a striking colour variation. Through a dermatoscope there is typically a range of colours with architectural disorder, radial streaming, branched streaks, pseudopods, peripheral black dots and blue-white structures.[4] It accounts for 70% of melanomas. It can be detected early by biopsy—shave is preferred to punch (less sampling error). Excisional biopsy is preferable.

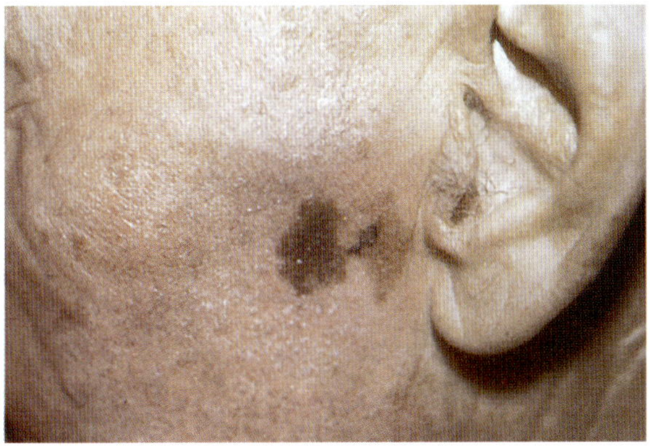

FIGURE 125.6 Lentigo maligna in a 72-year-old man. Excision is recommended as it is a form of intra-epidermal melanoma.

Photo courtesy Robin Marks

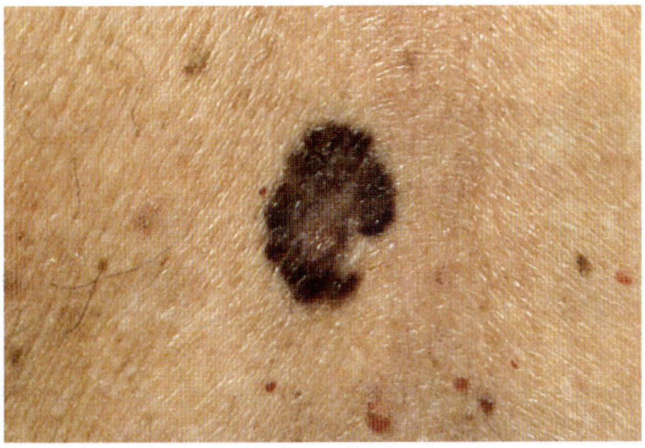

FIGURE 125.7 Superficial spreading melanoma with an irregular border which has altered and variable colours. Requires excision.

Photo courtesy Robin Marks

Nodular melanoma

Nodular melanomas account for 20% of melanomas, are aggressive and invasive, and have no radial growth phase. They are typically found on the trunk and limbs of young to middle-aged individuals (see FIG. 125.8). It may have a 'blueberry'-like nodule. Prognosis is determined by thickness at the time of excision. Dermatoscopy is usually less useful.

The early nodular melanoma problem[4,5]

Nodular melanoma can present a diagnostic dilemma since the ABCD rule (see later in this chapter) often does not apply. The mnemonic EFG, standing for 'Elevated', 'Firm' and 'Growing for more than 1 month', is more appropriate. Early melanomas tend to be symmetrical, non-pigmented, even in colour, of small diameter and to grow vertically.

They are often mistaken for a haemangioma or a pyogenic granuloma. If one is suspicious, refer early to a specialist/specialist clinic.

Acral lentiginous melanoma

These typically occur on palms, soles and distal phalanges (see FIG. 125.9). They have a poorer prognosis than other types. They occur mainly in people with dark skin.

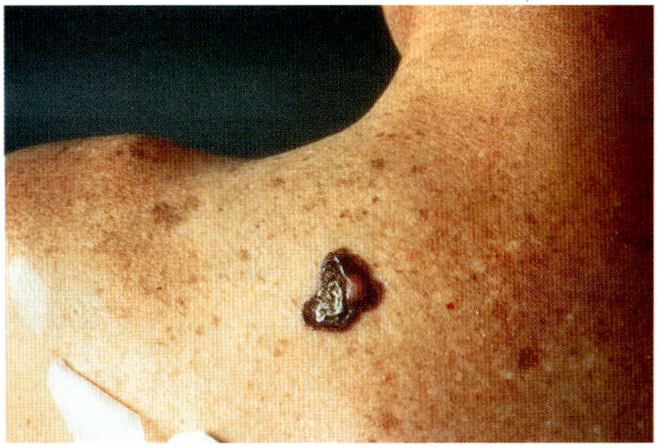

FIGURE 125.8 Nodular melanoma on the back. It has no radial growth phase and because it grows vertically can be readily misdiagnosed. The ABCD rule often does not apply but this lesion shows variable colours and an irregular border.

Photo courtesy Robin Marks

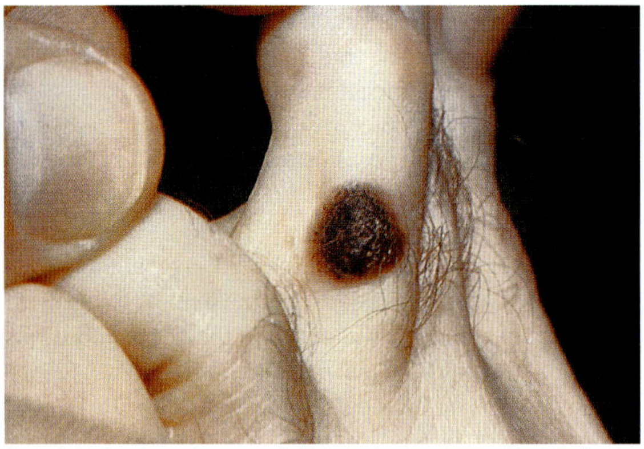

FIGURE 125.9 Acral lentiginous melanoma. A 30-year-old man presented with a 'mole' on his toe that had become 'lumpier'. This type of melanoma, which occurs on the distal areas of the limbs, begins as a spreading pigmented, macule before developing into a nodule surrounded by a pigmented halo (as shown).
Photo courtesy Robin Marks

Desmoplastic melanoma[4]

This is a rare and aggressive subtype of melanoma. They are often subtle clinically and sometimes scar-like. Most are non-pigmented.

Variations

Amelanotic melanomas are flesh-coloured papules that increase in size or change shape. These lesions can be extremely difficult to diagnose and the poor prognosis associated with them is due to late diagnosis rather than an increased malignancy.

The features and associations of melanoma subtypes are presented in TABLE 125.2.

Prognosis

Determinants of prognosis include:[3]

- thickness (Breslow classification)
- level or depth (worse in level IV or V) (see FIG. 125.10)

Table 125.2 Features and associations of melanoma subtypes[5,6]

Melanoma subtype	Frequency %	Radial growth phase	Location	Average age	Occupation profile
Superficial spreading	70	+	Trunk (back), limbs (legs)	Middle-aged	Indoor worker
Nodular	20	–	Trunk, limbs	Middle-aged	Indoor worker
Lentigo maligna	7.5	+	Head, neck	Elderly	Outdoor worker
Acral lentiginous	2.5	+	Palms, soles mucosae	Not known	Not known

Source: Reproduced with permission of J Kelly[5,6]

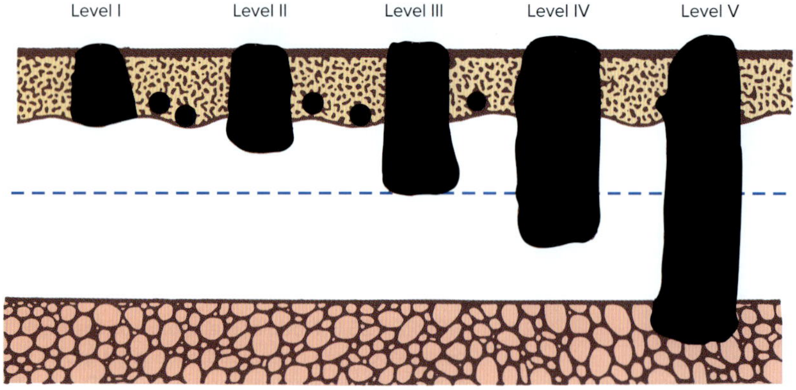

FIGURE 125.10 Assessment of tumour level: the levels of melanoma invasion

- site (worse on head and neck, trunk)
- sex (worse for men)
- age (worse >50 years)
- amelanotic melanoma
- ulceration

Vertical growth is associated with invasion and the prognosis worsens with depth. The chance of cure is greater than 90% if a melanoma is removed when it is less than 0.75 mm thick.[3] If the lesion is allowed to invade to a thickness of 4 mm or more, the likelihood of a cure is reduced to less than 30%.[3]

The influence of tumour thickness on 5-year survival rates is shown in TABLE 125.3.

Table 125.3 The diagnostic model for a presenting problem

Range of tumour thickness (mm)	Level (Clark)	5-year survival rates %
0	I	
<0.76	II	95
0.76–1.5	III	70–98
1.51–4.0	IV	55–85
>4.0	V	30–60

Source: Reproduced with permission of J Kelly[6]

Staging is based on the tumour level (depth) shown in FIGURE 125.10:

- level I—confined to the epidermis (in situ)
- level II—tumour cells extend into the superficial (papillary) dermis
- level III—tumour cells fill up the superficial dermis
- level IV—tumour cells extend into the deeper (reticular) layer
- level V—invasion of subcutaneous tissue

Differential diagnosis

There are several common skin lesions that may be mistaken for melanoma.[1] They are:

- haemangioma (thrombosed)
- dermatofibroma (sclerosing haemangioma)
- pigmented seborrhoeic keratosis
- pigmented BCC
- junctional and compound naevi
- blue naevi
- dysplastic naevi
- lentigines

Facilitating early diagnosis of melanoma

An adequate light source without shadows is essential. Refer to CHAPTER 119 for use of the 'Maggylamp' and the dermatoscope, which is a very important and useful adjunct to diagnosis.

Clinical examination of the skin[1]

It is important to examine the entire skin and not just the lesion presented by the patient. Comparison of pigmented skin lesions is very helpful in differentiating between benign and malignant. One satisfactory routine is:

- Starting at the head, examine the hairline, backs of ears, neck, back, and backs of the arms. Pull down the underwear to expose the buttocks; examine the backs of the legs.
- With the patient facing you, examine the anterior hairline, the front of the ears, the forehead, cheeks and neck, moving downwards to the anterior chest. Move bra straps as required to achieve complete coverage. Then examine the abdomen, pulling down the underwear to examine as far as the pubic hairs.
- Then examine the anterior surfaces of the legs. The 'Maggylamp' is very useful for this examination.

After scanning the entire skin surface and comparing and contrasting naevi, specific lesions may be examined with the dermatoscope. Compare suspicious lesions with similar lesions elsewhere on the patient's skin.

Applying the ABCDE system[1]

A = **A**symmetry
Melanoma is almost always asymmetrical. Most non-melanoma lesions are symmetrical, oval or round.

B = **B**order
The border of the melanoma is usually well defined, especially in the more malignant, compared with the dysplastic naevus, which is almost always indistinct with a fading-out 'shoulder' effect. The border of the melanoma is irregular while most benign lesions have a regular edge.

C = **C**olour
The classic blue–black colour is helpful but the *variety* of colours present in most melanomas is the most helpful. Magnification usually visualises greys, whites, violets, reds, oranges and shades of brown

interspersed in the darker blue–black pigmentation. Early melanomas developing in dysplastic naevi tend not to have this deep pigmentation.

D = **D**iameter

The majority of melanomas when first seen are at least 7 mm in diameter, especially if arising from a pre-existing naevus. However, it is possible to diagnose small nodular melanomas <5 mm.

E = **E**volution and/or **E**levation

Elevation indicates invasion and is a sign of more advanced disease and a flat lesion may become raised.

> **Practice tip**
>
> Not all melanomas are black and black may not be present in some melanomas.

Diagnosis by exclusion

In the diagnostic process consider the lesions outlined in the differential diagnosis and check out the various characteristics. Haemangiomas may have an emptying sign when pressed with a finger. Pigmented BCCs can be difficult if they are fully pigmented but this is uncommon. The characteristic pearly-grey look and the telangiectasia are usually still visible on magnification with the 'Maggylamp'. The most useful feature of dysplastic naevi is that they are usually multiple and lesions for comparison can generally be found elsewhere. Dysplastic naevi also have greater breadth and height and often a darker nodule in the centre—the 'target' sign. A small but significant number of melanomas are undiagnosable.

Pitfalls in diagnosis of melanoma

- Nodular melanoma
- Small melanoma
- Amelanotic melanoma
- Regressing melanoma
- Rapidly growing melanoma

Management points for naevi and melanomas

- Do not inject local anaesthetic directly into the lesion.
- Incisional biopsy of a melanoma or suspicious mole is best avoided.
- Accurate clinical diagnosis, with the definitive treatment performed in one stage, is optimal, rather than excision biopsy with follow-up surgery.

Management tips[1]

- The solitary dysplastic naevus has no significant malignant potential.
- Multiple excision of naevi is not justified.
- If in doubt, perform excision biopsy with a margin of 2 mm. Refer to FIGURE 125.11 for the protocol for a suspicious lesion.

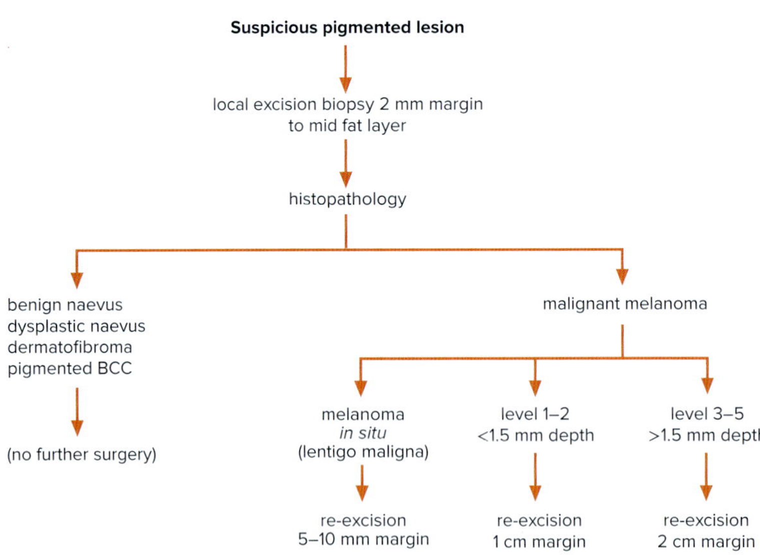

FIGURE 125.11 Plan for management of a suspicious pigmented lesion

- If melanoma is strongly suspected, referral to a consultant is necessary.
- Beware of the pigmented BCC—it is easily missed but it usually has a shiny surface.
- Do not freeze a pigmented lesion—take a biopsy.

Guidelines for excision margins[4,7] (Breslow thickness)

- Suspicious lesion—margin 2 mm
- Melanoma *in situ*—margin 5–10 mm
- Melanoma <1 mm thick—margin 1 cm
- Melanoma 1–4 mm thick, minimum margin 1 cm and maximum 2 cm
- Melanoma >4 mm thick, margin 2 cm (minimum)

Counselling

An encouragingly positive and supportive approach can realistically be taken for most patients, as the overall survival for melanoma in Australia is around 90%.[8]

Even with tumours greater than 4 mm thickness, 50% of patients will survive.

Follow-up

Follow-up tends to be based on the tumour thickness:[1]

- 1 mm—6 monthly review for 2 years
- 1–2 mm—4 monthly for 2 years, 6 monthly for next 2 years, then yearly for 10 years
- >2 mm—review by both specialist and GP, regularly, for 10 years

The first site of metastasis is usually the lungs, so a yearly chest X-ray is advisable. Refer to a multidisciplinary melanoma unit or oncologist when metastases are suspected.

Practice tips[9]

- Excision biopsy with 2 mm margin is appropriate whenever possible.
- Wider excision is then based on the Breslow thickness.
- Sentinel lymph node biopsy for tumours >1 mm thickness provides accurate prognostic information.

References

1 McCarthy W. The management of melanoma. Aust Fam Physician, 1993; 22: 1177–86.
2 Roberts H, Haskett M, Kelly J. Melanoma: clinical features and early diagnostic techniques. Medicine Today, May 2006; 7 (5): 39–47.
3 Marks R. Skin cancer. In: *MIMS Disease Index* (2nd edn). Sydney: IMS Publishing, 1996: 469–72.
4 Expert group for Dermatology. In: eTG complete. Melbourne: Therapeutic Guidelines Ltd. Available from: <www.tg.org.au>, accessed March 2018.
5 Kelly J. Nodular melanoma—no longer as simple as ABC. Aust Fam Physician, 2003; 32 (9): 702–9.
6 Kelly J. Malignant melanomas—how many have you missed? Med J Aust, 1996; 164: 431–6.
7 Sladden MJ et al. Updated evidence-based clinical practice guidelines for the diagnosis and management of melanoma: definitive excision margins for primary cutaneous melanoma. Med J Aust 2018: 208(3): 132–42.
8 English D et al. *Cancer Survival Victoria 2007*. Melbourne: Cancer Epidemiology Centre, Cancer Council Victoria, 2007: 40.
9 Thompson JF, Scolyer RA, Kefford RF. Melanoma: a management guide for GPs. Aust Fam Physician, 2012; 41 (7): 470–3.

126 Hair disorders

Look it's only death. It's not like losing your hair.

HAROLD BRODKEY UPON LEARNING HE HAD AIDS, *NEW YORKER MAGAZINE* 1994

The hair of our scalp is referred to as our crowning glory and the threat of hair loss in both sexes provokes extraordinary anxiety bordering on grief in some people. It behoves us as medical practitioners to treat the patient presenting with 'I'm losing my hair' with appropriate support and understanding. Likewise, the problem of hirsutism provokes similar anxiety and concerns about body image. Interestingly, women present with hair loss more than men.

Key facts and checkpoints

- There are two types of hair: terminal hair, which is coarse and well pigmented, and vellus hair, which is fine, soft and relatively unpigmented.
- Alopecia is a generic term for hair loss.
- Hair loss (alopecia) generates considerable anxiety and the fear of total hair loss should be addressed with the patient and a realistic prognosis given.
- Androgenic alopecia is the most common cause of human hair loss, affecting 50% of men by age 40 and up to 50% of women by age 60.[1] Other common causes are alopecia areata, seborrhoeic dermatitis and tinea capitis (see TABLE 126.1).
- In telogen effluvium, the traumatic event has preceded the hair loss by about 2 months (peak loss at 4 months).
- Although severe stress could precipitate alopecia areata, day-to-day stressors are not considered to be a trigger. Stress seems to be a consequence of alopecia rather than the cause of it.[2]
- Hair loss can be patchy or diffuse where it involves the entire scalp.
- Patchy loss—alopecia areata and trichotillomania.
- Generalised loss—telogen effluvium, systemic disease, drugs (see TABLE 126.2).
- Alopecia areata has a poor prognosis if it begins in childhood, if there are several patches and there is loss of eyebrows or eyelashes.
- Scarring alopecia can be an indicator of lupus erythematosus or lichen planus.

Table 126.1 Hair loss: diagnostic strategy model

Probability diagnosis
Androgenetic alopecia (male pattern baldness) Alopecia areata Telogen effluvium (incl. postpartum) Anagen effluvium (esp. cytotoxic therapy) Seborrhoeic dermatitis Scars (e.g. trauma, burns)
Serious disorders not to be missed
Infection: • tinea capitis/kerion • bacterial folliculitis • secondary syphilis • post-febrile state • cutaneous leishmaniasis Cancer: • treatment for cancer Other: • systemic disease (e.g. lupus)
Pitfalls (often missed)
Rarities: Heavy metal poisoning Nutritional: • severe dieting • malnutrition • zinc/iron deficiency
Seven masquerades checklist
Drugs (cytotoxics, anticoagulants, antiepileptics, amphetamines, anti-thyroid agents, various hormones, cessation OCP) Thyroid/other endocrine (hypothyroidism)
Is the patient trying to tell me something?
Emotional stress → telogen effluvium; trichotillomania

The normal hair growth cycle

An understanding of the process of normal hair growth is necessary to comprehend and evaluate hair disorders. Each follicle progresses quite independently through regular cycles of growth and shedding (see FIG. 126.1).

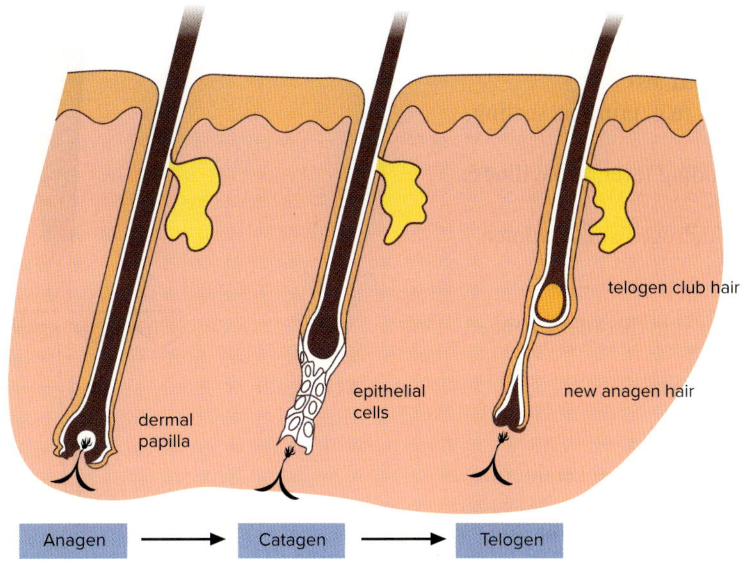

FIGURE 126.1 The normal hair cycle

Table 126.2 Causes of diffuse hair loss
Androgenetic alopecia
Telogen effluvium
Postpartum telogen effluvium
Alopecia areata (diffuse type)
Drugs—cytotoxics and others
Hypothyroidism
Nutritional: • iron deficiency • severe dieting • zinc deficiency • malnutrition
Post-febrile state
Anagen effluvium

The three phases of follicular activity are:[3]

1. Anagen phase—the active growth phase of hair production.
   - The dermal papilla stimulates division of epithelial cells that produce the hair shaft.
   - The hair shaft grows 1 cm per month.
   - It lasts for about 2.5–5 years on the scalp (average 1000 days).
   - It lasts 1–2 months on eyebrows and eyelashes and 6–9 months in the axilla and pubis.
   - It varies between individuals.
2. Catagen phase—a short transition phase from active growth to inactivity (the involutional stage).
   - The base of the hair becomes club-shaped.
   - It lasts for only about 2 weeks.
3. Telogen phase—the resting (dormant) phase of the cycle at the end of which the club hair with its non-pigmented bulb is shed.
   - This lasts 2–4 months (average 100 days).
   - The percentage of hairs in telogen varies from site to site—10% in scalp to 60–80% in pubic hair.[1]
   - The hair is anchored in the follicle but does not grow longer.
   - The follicle then re-enters anagen.

Thus every 3–5 years every hair on the scalp is shed and replaced.

Some facts on hair numbers[3]

- Hair growth is asynchronous (i.e. continuous production and shedding).
- Humans produce 1 km of hair a month.
- About 50–100 hairs are shed daily without a reduction in density.
- The scalp contains, on average, 100 000 hair follicles.
- The hair follicle is subject to melanocytic activity.
- At least 25% of hair must be shed before a noticeable loss of density occurs.
- Hair loss counts consistently above 100 per day indicate excessive hair loss.
- Significant hair loss tends to block the shower drain or be visible all over the pillow.

Key history

- Onset, duration, quantity and rate of loss
- Localised or generalised loss
- Associated symptoms (e.g. pruritus, scaling, pustules)
- Systems review including fever, acute illness, surgery, stressors
- Symptoms of hyperandrogenism in women (e.g. hirsutism, acne)
- Endocrine features
- Past history including skin disorders, cancer, thyroid disorders
- Family history of hair loss

Key examination

- General review with emphasis on endocrine system and examination of scalp
- Look for exclamation mark hair, 'white bulb' hair, state of bald patch (clean, scaly, scarred or inflamed) and the unusual pattern of trichotillomania

Key investigations

Consider:

- FBE/ESR
- pituitary hormones (FSH/LH/prolactin)
- hair pull test
- trichogram
- scalp biopsy
- skin scrapings and hair sample for fungal microscopy and culture

Alopecia areata, alopecia totalis and alopecia universalis

Alopecia areata is a disorder of the hair follicle causing a sudden onset of localised or diffuse hair loss. It is thought to be an autoimmune disorder that has a genetic susceptibility (20% have a positive family history). Men and women are affected equally, with the disorder most commonly occurring in the first two decades of life.[4] The hairs are affected during the growth phase, resulting in cessation of anagen.

DxT patch of complete hair loss + clean scalp + exclamation-mark hairs ➜ alopecia areata

Clinical features

- Complete hair loss (small patch or diffuse)
- Pigmented hairs often lost first
- Clean normal scalp

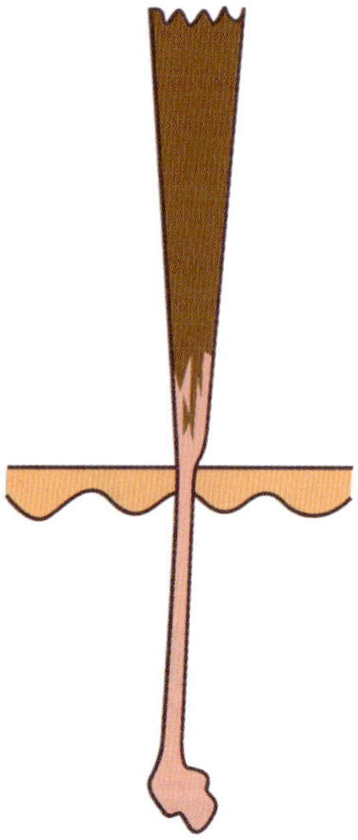

FIGURE 126.2 Exclamation-mark hair (a feature of alopecia areata)

- No or minimal inflammation
- Exclamation-mark hairs, especially around the periphery (see FIG. 126.2)

Associations

- Loss of facial (beard in men) or body hair
- Nail changes—dystrophy or pitting

Alopecia areata[2]

An unpredictable pattern of remission and relapse is characteristic. Patches may:

- regrow hair spontaneously (up to 50% within 12 months if a single patch)
- stay the same for many months
- enlarge and coalesce with other patches

The prognosis is poorer with more widespread involvement and younger age of onset (<5 years of age).

Localised patches

Treatment options include:

- topical potent corticosteroid (especially in children), e.g. betamethasone dipropionate 0.05% cream or lotion, once or twice daily for 3–4 months
- intralesional steroids—triamcinolone 10 mg/mL or betamethasone acetate/phosphate 5.7 mg/mL bd (caution needed on face—risk of cutaneous atrophy). Multiple injections required.
- topical minoxidil 5% bd (for 4 or more months) only when hair growing

Extensive area (>50% loss)

Treatment options include:

- Counselling
- Alopecia areata support group
- Use of cosmetic aids (e.g. eyebrow tattoos, wigs, hair pieces, scarves) and camouflage
- Topical steroids not recommended—ineffective
- Topical immunotherapy or systemic immunosuppresion under specialist care may help
- Systemic steroids only for active and progressive cases: prednisolone 0.75 mg/kg (o) daily for 3–4 weeks, then taper off over 2 months

Alopecia totalis

- This is where the alopecia extends over the total scalp.
- There is, at best, a 50% chance of hair recovery in a fit adult but only a very small chance in childhood.

Alopecia universalis

- This is where the alopecia involves the eyebrows and eyelashes as well. Recovery is rare.

Scarring alopecia[3]

In this condition, the hair follicles are damaged and if the follicular openings cannot be seen with a magnifying lens, regrowth of hair cannot be expected. Thus, the process is irreversible and a scalp biopsy is essential to determine the diagnosis. Apart from obvious causes such as trauma, severe burns, a carbuncle and scalp ringworm with kerion, the causes of scarring alopecia are as follows.

- Lichen planopilaris—this is a variant of lichen planus that produces small follicular papules in the scalp that tend to heal with scarring and destruction of hair follicles; treatment, which is difficult, includes corticosteroids, antimalarials and etretinate[3]
- Discoid lupus erythematosus—this gives a similar picture to the former and tends to be treated in a similar manner
- Folliculitis decalvans—a chronic folliculitis of the scalp, probably as a response to staphylococci on the scalp; treated with long-term tetracyclines
- Pseudopelade—a slowly progressive, non-inflammatory, scarring condition causing patchy areas of hair loss without any obvious preceding skin disease

Telogen effluvium[5]

Telogen effluvium, which is increased shedding of hairs in the telogen phase, is one of the most common causes of diffuse hair loss and can be triggered by a variety of stressors.

It is worth noting that follicular matrix cells have a high metabolic rate second only to haematological tissue and stress can result in shunting into premature telogen with cessation of anagen.[3]

An obligatory delay occurs between the 'insult' or precipitating event and the onset of hair shedding because the hair follicle cycles through catagen and telogen—approximately 2–3 months when the club hairs with white bulbs of telogen are shed.

Greater than 25% of hair must be lost before there is a perceptible thinning and in this disorder up to 50% loss is common.

DxT stressful event + 2–3 month gap to diffuse hair loss + 'white bulbs' → telogen effluvium

Patients usually complain of large clumps of hairs with white bulbs coming out with gentle tugging on combing or shampooing (this can exceed 150 hairs per day compared with the normal average of 50–100 hairs).

Stress precipitants of acute telogen effluvium

- Any severe stress
- Childbirth (common)
- High fever
- Weight loss, especially crash dieting
- Trauma—surgical or accidental
- Oral contraceptive pill (OCP) cessation
- Perimenopause
- Malnutrition
- Haemorrhage

Course of telogen effluvium

If uncomplicated, spontaneous recovery can be expected in 6–9 months so reassurance with explanation is usually all that is required. If it persists longer than 6 months, consider the chronic idiopathic form or an unmasked androgenetic alopecia. However, if there is concern about non-recovery and the stress factors are corrected, topical minoxidil 5% lotion (2% if too irritant) twice daily for a minimum of 4 months is an option.[2] Referral to a specialist is advised for relapsing episodes or incomplete recovery.

Chronic telogen effluvium[6]

This occurs usually in perimenopausal and postmenopausal women. It may be primary and idiopathic or secondary to hypothyroidism, hyperthyroidism, malnutrition or cancer. The feature is episodes of dramatic hair shedding that recover but recur weeks to months later and last up to several days. It does not result in obvious balding—it is self-limiting and does not usually need treatment.

Anagen effluvium

This is hair loss during the anagen phase and is typically seen in association with cancer chemotherapy and radiotherapy to the scalp, which results in immediate metabolic arrest. Hair loss is diffuse, involving the whole scalp. Anagen hair shafts are identified by their long and pigmented hair bulb. The follicle may remain in anagen, leading to a quick recovery, or move into telogen, thus delaying growth by about 3 months.

Drug-induced alopecia

Drugs are a very important cause of alopecia (see TABLE 126.3). They may cause telogen effluvium, anagen effluvium or accelerate androgenetic alopecia.

Drugs tend to cause telogen effluvium but cancer chemotherapy, radiation to the scalp, thallium/mercury/arsenic and colchicine in high dosage cause anagen effluvium. Acceleration of androgenetic alopecia is caused by hormone therapy, namely the OCP, danazol, testosterone and anabolic steroids.

Androgenetic alopecia (male pattern baldness)

This is the most common form of alopecia, which is age related and is genetically determined in addition to being androgen dependent. The key androgen is dihydrotestosterone, which is produced from testosterone by 5α reductase. The typical pattern of hair loss is recession of the frontotemporal hair with progression to the crown, with some men losing hair quickly and others more slowly. In others the pattern is unpredictable. The typical male pattern is shown in FIGURE 126.3.

Alopecia affects 30% of men by age 30 and 50% by age 50.

Androgenetic alopecia in women

- In women, the pattern of hair loss is different from men.
- Diffuse thinning occurs, usually on the top of the head (the crown). The front hairline usually remains but in some women this can recede with bitemporal loss (see FIG. 126.4).
- Although hair loss can appear in men and women as early as the 20s, it may not appear before the age of 50 in women.
- Some women notice a short period of considerable hair loss but this may be followed by a long stable period of no loss. Total loss of hair rarely occurs in women.

Table 126.3 Drug-induced causes of alopecia generally from prolonged use[1,2]

Cytotoxic agents/thallium

Amphetamines

Anticoagulants: heparin, warfarin

Anti-epileptics: phenytoin, sodium valproate, carbamazepine

Anti-inflammatories: indomethacin, gold, penicillamine, salicylate

Antigout agents: allopurinol, colchicine

Antihelminthic agents: albendazole/mebendazole

Antiparkinson: levodopa, bromocriptine

Antithyroid agents/thyroxine/iodine/carbimazole

Cardiovascular agents:
- amiodarone
- statins, clofibrate
- selected ACE inhibitors
- selected beta blockers

Cimetidine

Gentamicin

Hormones: OCP, androgens, danazol

Interferon

Lithium

Vitamin A derivatives/retinoids: Roaccutane

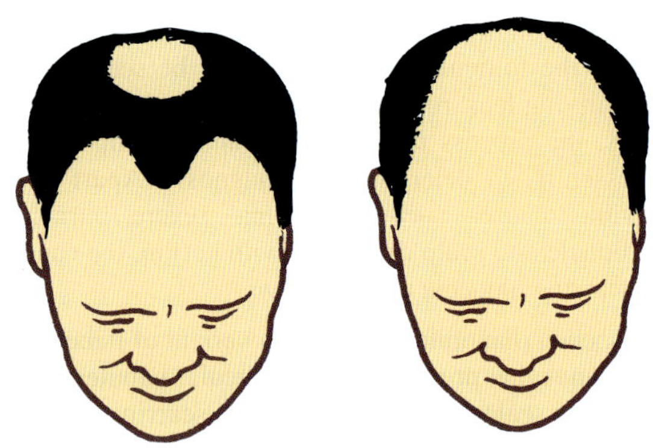

FIGURE 126.3 Typical male pattern baldness

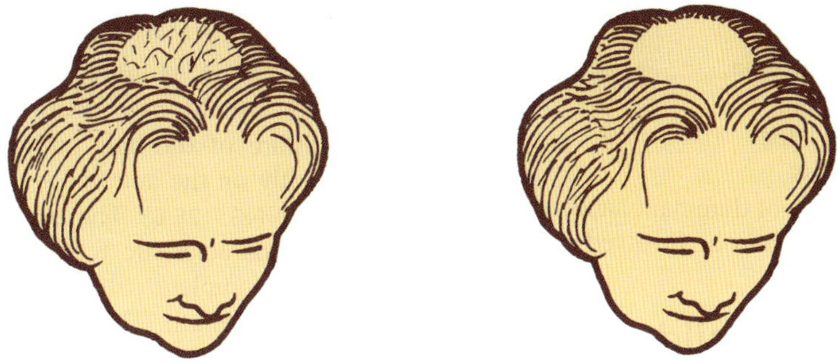

FIGURE 126.4 Typical female pattern baldness

- It may be unmasked after an episode of diffuse hair loss such as after childbirth or an acute illness.
- Hair loss may be accelerated by conditions associated with androgen excess (e.g. polycystic ovarian syndrome), however, fewer than 5% of women with androgenic alopecia will have elevated serum androgens.[2]

Treatment (men)

It is appropriate to counsel men to accept their balding as part of a natural ageing process. This includes cutting the hair short to make it look better cosmetically. If baldness is not acceptable, some options include wearing a toupee, a wig or other hair substitute or having a hair transplant operation. However, with hair transplantation, the new hair is often just as likely to disappear as the original hair.

Medical treatments are generally expensive and improvements are only sustained for the duration of treatment, so it is important to explore the patient's expectations when discussing treatment options.

Available medications[2]

- Minoxidil 5%, 1 mL applied once or twice daily to the scalp for at least 6–12 months. The results vary from good to no change. Reassure the patient that it is normal for hair shedding to increase in the first 4–6 weeks of minoxidil treatment.
- Finasteride 1 mg tablet taken daily for a minimum of 2 years. There is a risk of sexual dysfunction (e.g. erectile dysfunction, reduced libido) and gynaecomastia (rare), which tend to resolve with time or cessation. Rare reports of persistent sexual dysfunction after stopping finasteride have been published. Mental health problems have also been noted.
- For severe cases, use topical minoxidil and oral finasteride as combination therapy.

Treatment (women)

Physical treatments/hair styling

This includes the use of wigs, hair transplantation and camouflage. Wigs can be worn on the whole head or on the bald spot, or fibres can be interwoven into the remaining hairs.

Camouflage can be used either by having the existing hair bleached by a skilled hairdresser or by colouring the scalp the same colour as the hair. Mascara can be lightly brushed into the roots of the hair at receding hairlines or along gaps.

Medications[1]

minoxidil 5% topical application bd for at least 6–12 months (to assess efficacy) although one large trial has approved its effectiveness generally in women[7]

or

spironolactone 50 to 100 mg daily, increasing to 200 mg daily if no apparent benefit after 6 months; monitor blood pressure, kidney function and liver biochemistry

Spironolactone is contraindicated in pregnancy and side effects include postural hypotension, polyuria and irregular menses. Concurrent use with the combined oral contraceptive pill is appropriate to control menses and for contraception in women of reproductive age.

As for men, these drugs tend to prevent further loss and, if effective, need long-term use.

Trichotillomania (hair pulling)

This is patchy hair loss caused by deliberate plucking or twisting of hair shafts. It is reasonably common in young children, where it may be of little significance, simply being a 'habit'. In older children and adults it may be an obsessive compulsive disorder often associated with stress.[3]

Clinical features

- Incomplete patchy alopecia
- Hairs of different length
- Hairs broken and twisted
- Strange pattern of loss
- Tends to occur on side of dominant hand
- Eyelashes or eyebrows may be involved

Hair disorders in children

Loose anagen (growing hair) syndrome[8]

This is a disorder of the hair follicle characterised by the ability to pluck anagen hairs painlessly from the scalp by gentle pulling. It presents as very thin, wispy new hair growth. It is an autosomal dominant trait.

Clinical features

- Thin wispy hair with tatty ends
- More common in girls; can affect boys
- Onset in early childhood—usually <5 years
- Large clumps easily pulled out at play
- Light microscopy of hair shafts aids diagnosis

DxT fair females under 5 + thin wispy hair + easy loss with pulling → loose anagen syndrome

Outcome

- Spontaneous improvement with age
- Usually normal hair by teens

Treatment

- Reassurance and explanation
- Gentle hair care

Traction alopecia

Traction alopecia is thinning of the hair seen in female children and young women due to very tight hairstyles, as with ponytails, excessive hair rolling and hair braiding in particular. The bald areas that show short broken hairs and sometimes scarring are found in areas of maximal tug. The most common type is 'marginal alopecia' found in the forehead and sides at the hair edges (see FIG. 126.5). Patients should be advised to cease the procedure. Rollers that cause traction can be replaced by those that heat.

Trichotillomania[8]

This occurs in children typically between 4 and 10 years, usually as a nocturnal habit; parents may be unaware of the hair pulling. The affected areas are usually on the anterior and temporal areas of the head (see FIG. 126.6). The areas are never completely bald. A characteristic feature is an irregular-shaped area of incomplete patchy alopecia containing hairs of different length. The variable length is due to the fact that some hairs will not break with pulling while others will break at varying distances from the scalp surface. There may be associated follicular pustules.

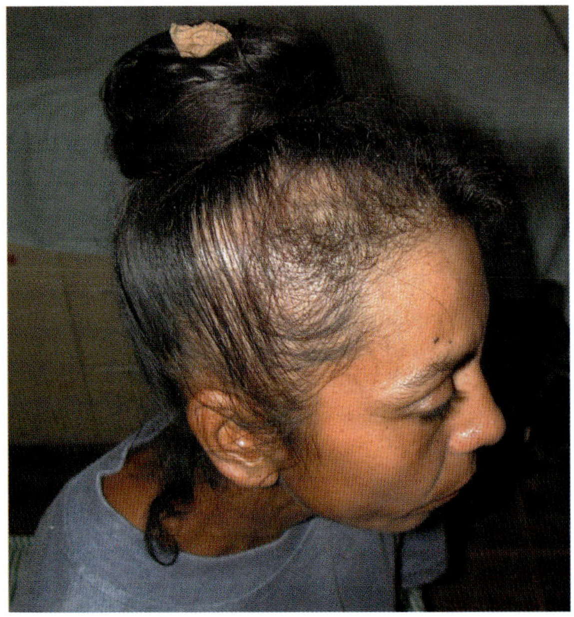

FIGURE 126.5 Traction alopecia in an adult from pulling the hair up in a tight bun

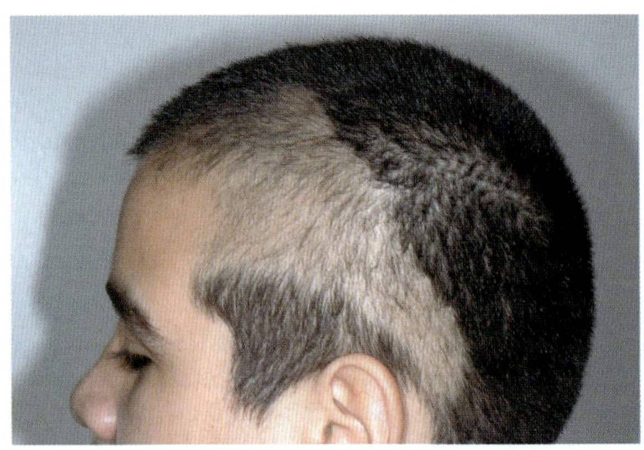

FIGURE 126.6 Trichotillomania in an 11-year-old boy. Note the incomplete patchy hair loss and unusual pattern.

However, scrapings should be taken to exclude a particular type of tinea capitis (black dot ringworm) caused by *Trichophyton tonsurans*. The management is similar to thumb sucking or nail biting with a low-key approach. It does not imply a significant psychological problem.

Localised alopecia areata

This can also occur in children. Most childhood cases resolve spontaneously but it can progress to total hair loss or recurrent alopecia can occur. Regrowth decades later is a possibility. Treatment with potent topical steroids for 12 weeks or so may help.

Tinea capitis

This is a dermatophyte infection that produces an area of incomplete, 'unclean' alopecia with various degrees of scaling and inflammation of the scalp surface. A boggy swelling (kerion) can develop in severe cases. Important dermatophyte carriers include pet puppies, kittens and rabbits. Wood's light examination will be positive in only 50% of cases. Confirm diagnosis with scalp scrapings for microscopy and culture.

Office procedures

The following procedures can be useful in determining diagnosis and prognosis.

The hair-pull test[3]

In this simple method, 50–100 hairs are grasped between thumb and forefinger and gently pulled proximal to distal. This is repeated 6–8 times and should yield a total of 2–5 telogen hairs, which can be analysed. More than eight hairs per pull is abnormal.

Trichogram

Twenty to 50 hairs are extracted by a short, sharp pull with artery forceps. The anagen-to-telogen ratio is calculated. The ratio is decreased in telogen effluvium because of the increased numbers of hairs in telogen.

Scalp biopsy

This differentiates between scarring and non-scarring alopecia and also between alopecia areata and trichotillomania.

Light microscopy of hair shafts

Light and/or electron microscopy is indicated if a hair shaft defect is suspected. Skin scrapings and hair samples are taken for fungal microscopy and culture.

Hirsutism

Hirsutism is growth in the female of excess, coarse, terminal pigmented hair in androgen-dependent sites, namely in a male sexual pattern (e.g. upper lip, beard area and back; see FIG. 126.7).

Most cases are due to idiopathic hirsutism, which may follow ethnic or familial factors, or to polycystic ovarian syndrome. Other causes include adrenal hyperplasia, virilising adrenal tumours, Cushing syndrome, virilising ovarian tumours and certain medications.

The diagnostic strategy model is presented in TABLE 126.4 and followed by the key features.

Table 126.4 Hirsutism in women: diagnostic strategy model

Probability diagnosis
Constitutional (physiological or familial)
Polycystic ovarian syndrome (PCOS)
Serious disorders not to be missed
Cancer/tumour:
• virilising ovarian tumour
• adrenal tumours (cancer and adenoma)
• ectopic (paraneoplastic) hormone production (e.g. lung cancer, carcinoid)
Pitfalls (often missed)
Postmenopausal
Rarities:
• porphyria cutanea tarda
• congenital adrenal hyperplasia
• gonadal dysgenesis
Seven masquerades checklist
Drugs (many incl. phenytoin, danazol, minoxidil, anabolic steroids, cyclosporin, corticosteroids, phenothiazines, interferon α, penicillamine)
Thyroid/other endocrine (prolactinaemia, Cushing syndrome, acromegaly, hypothyroidism)

Key history

History of age and rate of onset, extent and activity of the hair. Menstrual history, family history and past medical history including endocrine disorders and drugs, especially those listed above.

Key examination

- General inspection including distribution and character of the hair growth, endocrine abnormalities (e.g. Cushing syndrome), skin, abdomen and breasts

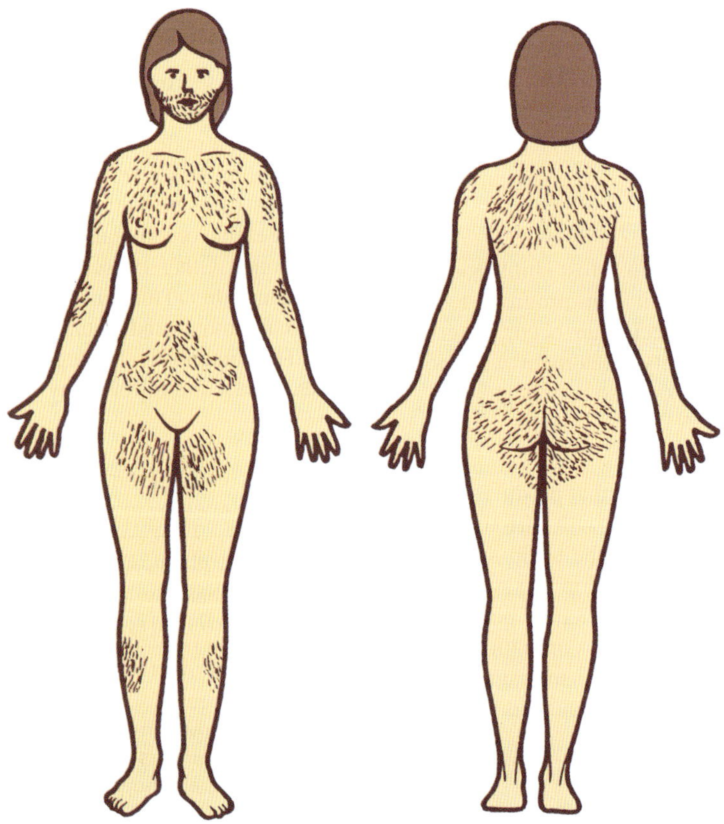

FIGURE 126.7 Areas prone to hirsutism

- Note other features of virilisation, specifically androgenic alopecia, acne, deepening of the voice and clitoromegaly (if indicated)

Key investigations

- Consider pituitary hormones (e.g. FSH, LH, ACTH, TSH, prolactin)
- Androgens (e.g. serum testosterone, SHBG, DHEAS, 17-OH progesterone)
- Pelvic ultrasound (polycystic ovaries)
- Urinary porphyrins
- Imaging of pituitary and adrenal regions

Routine investigation is not required unless hirsutism is severe, is of sudden onset or there are other features of virilisation.

Hirsutism of reasonably sudden onset is an important marker for serious underlying pathology. It is important to exclude adrenal or ovarian pathology.

For patients with severe hirsutism and regular menses, serum testosterone, DHEAS and early morning 17-hydroxyprogesterone levels should be measured. If menses are irregular, measure follicle stimulating hormone, luteinising hormone and serum prolactin.

Appropriate investigations include pelvic ultrasound to diagnose polycystic ovaries and serum testosterone and dehydroepiandrostenedione (DHEA), which indicates an adrenal cause of androgen excess if elevated.

> **Red flags**
>
> - Virilisation
> - Abrupt onset of hirsutism
> - Pelvic or abdominal mass

Principles of management

- Exclude underlying adrenal or ovarian pathology.
- Support the patient to achieve an acceptable body image through appropriate advice and referral.
- Recommend appropriate cosmetic measures, which include bleaching, waxing, depilatory creams or shaving.

- Do not pluck hairs, especially around the lips and chin—plucking stimulates hair growth but shaving appears to have no effect.
- Laser may also help but seems to be most suitable for dark hair on a light skin and provides temporary removal, lasting up to 9 months.

Pharmaceutical options[9]

These include either suppression of ovarian and/or adrenal androgen production (oral contraception or dexamethasone) or inhibition of androgen action at the hair follicles (spironolactone and cyproterone acetate).

If the woman is of reproductive age and has no immediate wish for fertility, use:

combined oral contraceptive pill (COCP): ethinyloestradiol + cyproterone or drosperinone

Cyproterone and drosperinone have anti-androgenic properties. Other COCPs may also be useful because they increase SHBG production and reduce ovarian androgen production.

Anti-androgenic drugs:[1]

spironolactone 100–200 mg (o) daily (takes 6–12 months to respond)

For women who are premenopausal or perimenopausal, use:

cyproterone acetate 10–100 mg (o) daily for 10 days of each menstrual cycle plus an COCP

Cyproterone used alone usually leads to hypo-oestrogenism. Therefore, it should be combined with oestrogen unless this is contraindicated. Alternative oestrogen combination regimens are required for postmenopausal women.

Topical eflornithine HCl 11.5% (Vaniqa) cream for topical use on facial hair and hair under the chin is a newer preparation that slows hair regrowth. Apply thinly twice a day.

Hypertrichosis

Hypertrichosis is the increased growth of fine vellus or downy hair over the body that may either be generalised (usually) or localised. It is non-androgen dependent hair and does not respond to anti-androgen therapy. The cause is generally unknown—it may be primary or constitutional where it is usually apparent prior to puberty and where it is evenly distributed over the back and limbs. Prepubertal hypertrichosis is commonly familial but a positive family history is not always determined.

An important cause of secondary hypertrichosis is drugs. Drugs that are implicated include phenytoin, minoxidil, cyclosporin, interferon alpha and corticosteroids, both systemic and topical.

It is also associated with an underlying neoplasia, such as stomach cancer, when it is termed hypertrichosis lanuginosa acquisita or 'malignant down'.

Other causes include anorexia nervosa, the menopause, systemic illness, starvation and a few rare syndromes (e.g. Cornelia de Lange syndrome). Treat the underlying cause, otherwise treatment is only necessary if it concerns the patient. Physical hair removal techniques are appropriate for hair that is non-androgen dependent.

SCALY SCALP DISORDERS

Dandruff

Dandruff (pityriasis capitis) is mainly a physiological process, the result of normal desquamation of scale from the scalp. It is most prevalent in adolescence and worse around the age of 20.

If it is persistent with heavy scaling, seborrhoeic dermatitis and scalp psoriasis, which is distinguished by palpable plaques, are likely causes.

Dandruff and seborrhoeic dermatitis are related conditions on a continuum of severity. They are caused mainly by the fungal genus *Malassezia*, such as *M. globosa*, which produces lipases that break down sebum. They both have a common pathogenesis and are chronic recurring conditions presenting with scaling and a varying degree of itch. More importantly, they all respond to similar treatments.

Treatment

Shampoos:

- zinc pyrithione (e.g. Dan-Gard, Head and Shoulders)
  or
- selenium sulphide (e.g. Selsun)

Method: massage into scalp, leave for 5 minutes, rinse thoroughly—twice weekly.

Treatment of persistent or severe dandruff:

- coal tar plus salicylic acid compound (Sebitar) shampoo
  or
- T Gel/Ionil T plus shampoo

Method: as above, followed by Sebi Rinse or ketoconazole (Nizoral) shampoo. If persistent, especially itching, and Nizoral shampoo is ineffective, use a corticosteroid (e.g. betamethasone scalp lotion).

Dry hair

Advice to patients

- Don't shampoo every day.
- Use a mild shampoo (labelled for 'dry or damaged hair').
- Use a conditioner.
- Have hair cut regularly to remove split or frayed ends.
- Avoid heat (e.g. electric curlers, hair dryers).
- Wear head protection in hot winds.
- Wear a rubber cap when swimming.

Oily hair

Advice to patients

- Shampoo daily with a 'shampoo for oily hair'.
- Massage the scalp during the shampoo process.
- Leave the shampoo on for at least 5 minutes.
- Avoid hair conditioners.
- Avoid overbrushing.
- Attend to lifestyle factors: relaxation and balanced diet are important.

Patient education resources

Hand-out sheets from *Murtagh's Patient Education* 7th edition:

- Dandruff
- Hair loss in women
- Hirsutism
- Male pattern baldness

References

1. Cargnello S, Sheil R. Hair loss and hirsutism: how to treat. Australian Doctor; 21 November 2003: 31–8.
2. Expert group for Dermatology. In: eTG complete. Melbourne: Therapeutic Guidelines Ltd. Available from: <www.tg.org.au>, accessed March 2018.
3. Cargnello J. I think I'm losing my hair. Aust Fam Physician, 1997; 26: 683–7.
4. Grinzi P. Hair and nails. Aust Fam Physician, 2011; 40(7): 476–84.
5. Sinclair R, Yazdabadi A. Common hair loss disorders. Update. Medical Observer, 4 September 2009: 25–7.
6. Whiting DA. Chronic telogen effluvium: increased scalp hair shedding in middle aged women. J Am Acad Dermatol, 1996; 35: 889–906.
7. Lucky AW et al. A randomised placebo-controlled trial of 5% and 2% topical minoxidil solutions in the treatment of female pattern hair loss. J Am Acad Dermatol, 2004; 50: 541–53.
8. Thomson K, Tey D, Marks M (ed.). *Paediatric Handbook* (8th edn). Oxford: Wiley-Blackwell, 2009: 284–5.
9. Expert group for Endocrinology. In: eTG complete. Melbourne: Therapeutic Guidelines Ltd. Available from: <www.tg.org.au>, accessed March 2018.

Nail disorders 127

A physician should wear white garments, put on a pair of shoes, carry a stick and an umbrella in his hand, and walk about with a mild and benignant look as a friend of all created beings. He should be cleanly in his habits and well shaved, and should not allow his nails to grow.

SUSHRUTA-SAMHITA (5TH CENTURY BCE)

Making a diagnosis of abnormal nails for a concerned patient can be quite simple for a few obvious conditions. However, in many cases the diagnosis can be elusive when we are not familiar with classic patterns that are seen so infrequently. The diagnostic process can be facilitated by learning the basic anatomy and function of the nail, as well as characteristic patterns, which are presented with the aid of diagrams in this chapter. There are, in fact, only a limited number of ways in which injury, infection and inflammation can present in a nail.[1]

The main nail problems encountered in general practice are trauma, onychomycosis, infection, ingrowing toenails, paronychia and psoriasis. Fungal nail infection and psoriasis are the commonest causes of nail dystrophy. Damage to the nail from trauma or disease results in nail dystrophy. The problem of nail changes due to onychotillomania, be it from excessive nail biting, picking or cleaning, should be suspected from the history and examination.

The examination should include a general inspection of the skin including in the webbing of the toes, looking for evidence of a skin disorder such as psoriasis, atopic eczema, lichen planus and tinea.

Key facts and checkpoints

- The growth rate of nails varies between individuals: fingernails average 0.5–1.2 mm per week while toenails grow more slowly.[2]
- An avulsed or totally dystrophic nail will take up to 9 months to regrow.
- It takes approximately 6 weeks to grow a new cuticle.
- Beau's lines associated with a severe acute illness take about 3 months to appear.
- Do not confuse chronic paronychia with onychomycosis. The former affects the nail folds, the latter mainly affects the distal nail.
- Nail clippings for culture and histology may be the only way to differentiate between nail dystrophy and onychomycosis.
- Not all white crumbly nails are caused by a fungus.
- Suspect melanoma in any subungual pigmented lesion. Do not confuse with subungual haematomas, which 'grow out' with the nail. They usually present as a longitudinal pigmented streak. Beware of amelanotic melanoma, which may mimic chronic paronychia or a pyogenic granuloma.[2,3] Any suspicion necessitates early referral.
- Various dermatoses and connective tissue disorders can affect the nails—psoriasis, lichen planus, lupus erythematosus, scleroderma, bullous pemphigoid, Darier disease (keratosis follicularis).[4]
- Clubbing of the fingers is basically an abnormality of the fingertips—look for evidence of major pulmonary or cardiac disease.
- Significantly bitten or traumatised nails may be a symptom of a major anxiety disorder—explore psychogenic issues.

A summary of causes of abnormal nails is presented in TABLE 127.1.

Key history

Enquire about a history of severe stress or illness and possible onychotillomania, be it excessive nail biting, picking or cleaning. Ask whether the hands are frequently in wet work (e.g. dishwashing, soaps and detergents) or dirt.

Key examination

Careful examination of nails: look for associated skin disease (e.g. psoriasis, atopic dermatitis, tinea pedis, lichen planus).

Key investigations

- Nail clippings for culture and histology
- FBE and ESR
- Consider LFTs

Table 127.1 Abnormal nails: diagnostic strategy model (modified)

Probability diagnosis
Fungal infection: onychomycosis
Onycholysis
• trauma to nail bed
• trauma from biting
• trauma from habit picking
Onychogryphosis
Paronychia
Psoriasis
Serious disorders not to be missed
Melanoma
Iron deficiency: koilonychia
Liver disease: leuconychia
Endocarditis: splinter haemorrhages
Chronic kidney failure: white bands, half-and-half nail
Glomus tumour
Bowen disorder/SCC
Pitfalls (often missed)
Atopic dermatitis
Lichen planus
Pyogenic granuloma (usually with ingrowing toenails)[3]
Drug effects (e.g. tetracycline)
Pseudomonas infection
Connective tissue disorders (e.g. SLE)
Arsenic (Mees stripes)

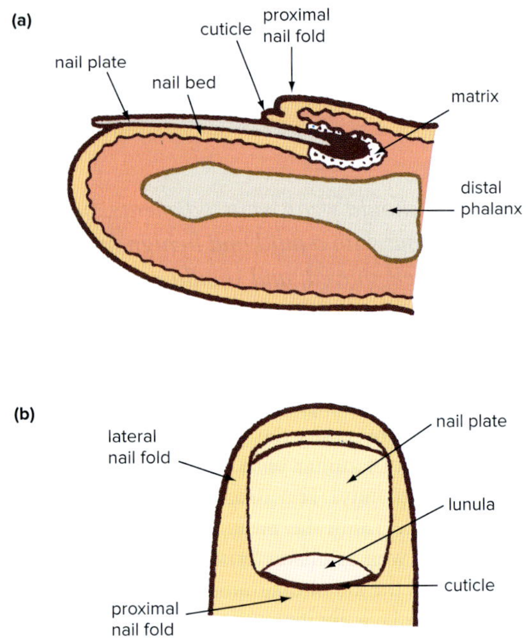

FIGURE 127.1 Normal anatomy of the nail. Diagram of the nail apparatus: **(a)** lateral section view, **(b)** dorsal surface view

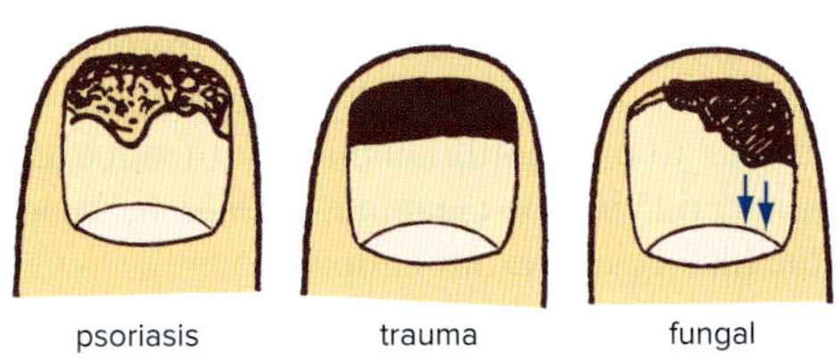

FIGURE 127.2 Lifting of the nail plate (onycholysis)

Anatomy and function of the nail

The basic nail unit (apparatus) consists of the nail matrix, the proximal and lateral nail folds, the cuticle and the nail plate (see FIG. 127.1). The hard keratin of the nail plate is formed in the nail matrix. The matrix, which contains germinal epithelium, lies in an invagination of the epidermis (the nail fold) and is protected by a waterproof seal formed by the cuticle. The matrix runs from the proximal end of the nail fold to the cuticle.

The nail bed closely approximates the distal phalanx. The nail has an important functional and cosmetic role. It enhances fine touch and motor skills for picking up fine objects, such as a pin from a flat surface, not possible without fingernails.

Nail disorders and their causes[1]

Lifting of the nail plate (onycholysis)

See FIGURE 127.2.

Causes

- Trauma
- Factitious (self-induced)
- Tinea
- Psoriasis
- Photosensitivity, usually tetracyclines
- Others (e.g. warts, lichen planus)
- Hyperthyroidism
- Nail destruction:
  - squamous cell carcinoma
  - melanoma
  - lichen planus

Thickening of the nail plate

Causes

- Developmental
- Trauma
- Tinea
- Psoriasis (see FIG. 127.3)
- Onychogryphosis
- Age-related changes

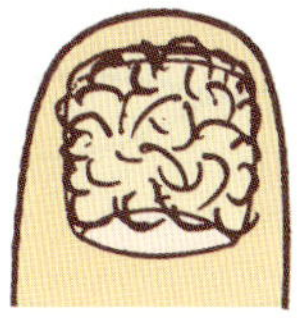

FIGURE 127.3 Psoriasis

Thinning of the nail plate

Causes

- Trauma—wear and tear (repeated water immersion)
- Artificial fingernails—application and removal
- Lichen planus
- Peripheral vascular disease (impaired peripheral circulation)
- Twenty-nail dystrophy, usually children
- Brittle nails

Pitting of the nail plate

See FIGURE 127.4.

Causes

- Psoriasis
- Alopecia areata
- Atopic dermatitis

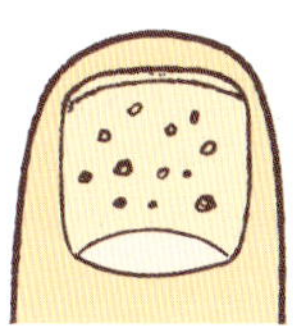

FIGURE 127.4 Pitting of the nail plate

Longitudinal marks in the nail plate

See FIGURE 127.5.

Causes (grooved)

- Myxoid cyst
- Angiofibroma
- Ageing

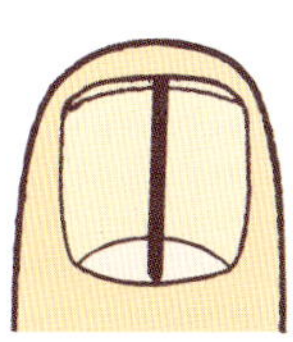

FIGURE 127.5 Longitudinal marks in the nail plate

Causes (central single stripe)

- Darier disease
- Hereditary/congenital
- Mechanical trauma

Horizontal grooves in nail plate

Causes

- Beau's lines (from acute illness) (see FIG. 127.6)
- Habit tic (picking cuticle of thumb nail) (see FIG. 127.7)
- Atopic dermatitis
- Raynaud phenomenon

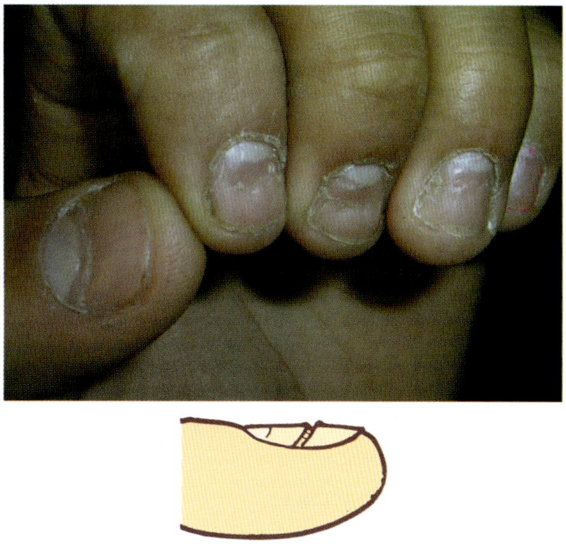

FIGURE 127.6 Beau's lines in nails following an episode of acute cholecystitis a few months earlier

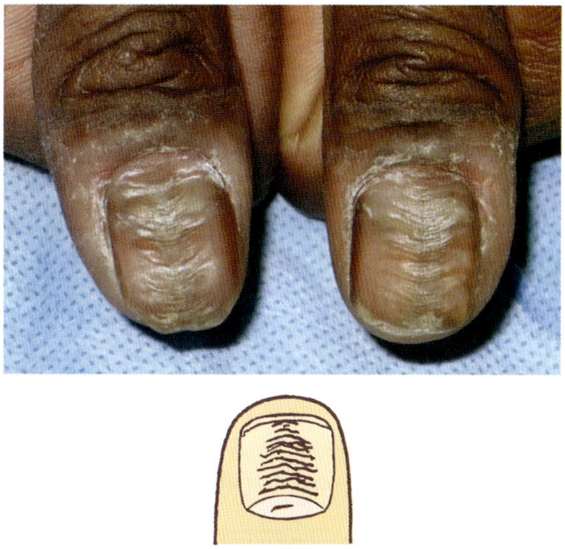

FIGURE 127.7 Habit tic: horizontal grooves on thumb nails

127

Horizontal single white lines or band

Causes

- Chemotherapy
- Arsenic poisoning
- Kidney failure

Lamellar splitting (onychoschizia)

See FIGURE 127.8.

Causes

- Trauma—repeated wetting and drying (e.g. housework)

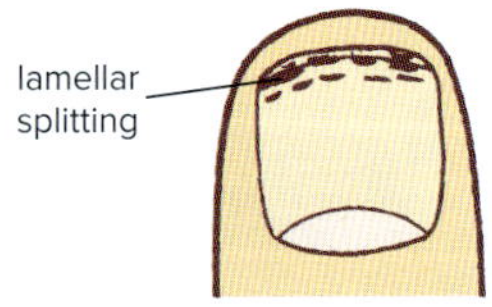

FIGURE 127.8 Lamellar splitting

Abnormal curvature

Causes

Spoon nails: koilonychia

See FIGURE 127.9.

- Idiopathic (most cases, esp children)
- Hereditary
- Trauma
- Iron deficiency
- Haemochromatosis

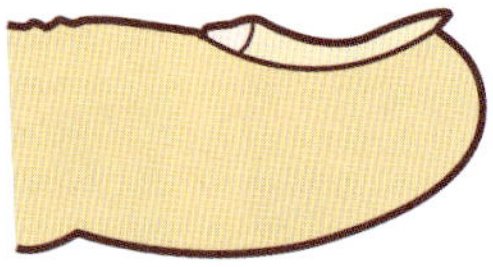

FIGURE 127.9 Spoon nails (koilonchya)

Overcurvature

- Hereditary pincer nail

Clubbing

See FIGURE 127.10.

- Hereditary/congenital
- Lung disease (e.g. cancer, pulmonary fibrosis, sepsis)
- Heart disease (e.g. congenital cyanotic, SBE)
- Liver disease (e.g. cirrhosis)
- Gastrointestinal disorders (e.g. Crohn disease)

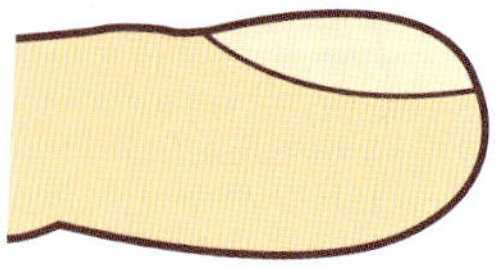

FIGURE 127.10 Clubbing

Splinter haemorrhages

See FIGURE 127.11.

Causes

- Minor trauma (e.g. manual workers)
- Bacterial endocarditis

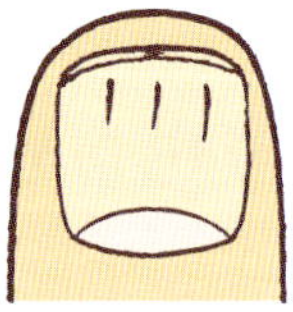

FIGURE 127.11 Splinter haemorrhages

Discolouration of the nail plate

- White:
  - striate leuconychia (usually trauma)
  - liver cirrhosis
  - hypoalbuminaemia (total whiteout)
- Red:
  - splinter haemorrhages
  - kidney failure
  - polycythaemia
  - CO poisoning
  - glomus tumour
- Brown:
  - fungal infection
  - cigarette staining
  - drugs—gold, chlorpromazine
  - Addison disease
  - psoriasis (‘oil stain’ patches)
  - melanoma
- Black:
  - haematoma
  - melanoma
  - racial pigmentation
  - naevus
  - minocycline
  - cytotoxic drugs (transverse bands)
- Green:
  - *Pseudomonas* infection
  - *Aspergillus* infection

- Blue:
  - antimalarials
  - argyria
- Yellow:
  - yellow nail dystrophy (? respiratory illness)
  - fungal infections
  - psoriasis
  - slow growth
  - tetracyclines
- Half (pale proximal) and half (brown or red distal) (i.e. half-and-half nails)
  - kidney failure (chronic)
  - liver cirrhosis
  - trauma (biting, splits, splinters)

Swelling of the proximal nail folds (paronychia)

- Trauma (e.g. biting)
- Manicure (retracting the cuticles)
- *Candida* infection
- Staphylococcal infection
- Herpetic whitlow

Swelling of the lateral nail folds

- Ingrowing toenails
- Retinoids
- Overcurvature of the nail plate

Tumours of the nail fold

Benign:
- myxoid (mucus) cyst
- warts
- periungual fibroma

Malignant:
- squamous cell carcinoma
- melanoma

Destruction of the nail apparatus

- Trauma
- Lichen planus
- Melanoma
- Bowen disease
- Squamous cell carcinoma

Onycholysis[1]

Onycholysis refers to the separation of the nail plate from the underlying nail bed and is a sign rather than a disease. This separation creates a subungual space with an air interface that gathers unwanted debris, such as dirt and keratin. It is usually seen in fingernails but it can develop in toenails from rubbing against shoes. Adverse local reactions to agents such as formaldehyde and resins in polishes or nail glues can distort nails.

Self-induced trauma is a common cause from obsessive manipulation, including meticulous cleaning and frequent manicuring.

The band of discolouration at the end of the separated nail is usually in a straight line compared with other causes such as psoriasis and tinea. Tinea may be distinguished from other causes by white or yellow streaks or 'spears' travelling proximally in the nail.

Greenish discolouration indicates invasion by *Pseudomonas pyocyanea* or *Aspergillus.*

Management[5]

First exclude psoriasis, tinea (check toe webbing) and trauma (check history).

Fingernails

- Keep nails as short as possible
- Avoid insertion of sharp objects under nails for cleaning out debris
- Apply tape (Micropore or similar) over free edge for months, until healed
- Avoid unnecessary soaps and detergents—wear gloves for housework, gardening, etc.
- Keep hands out of water
- Use a mild soap and shampoo
- First-line treatment especially if mild infection is white vinegar soaks, diluted 1:1 with water—10 minutes two times daily for 3–4 weeks.[6]

Toenails

- Exclude fungal infection (clinical tinea pedis)—culture
- Improve footwear to avoid any rubbing

Pharmaceutical treatment

- Daily application of an imidazole (e.g. clotrimazole) or terbinafine
- Potent topical corticosteroids in lotion form may be useful
- For *Pseudomonas* infection soak the nails in vinegar or Milton's solution and/or gentamicin sulphate cream
- If *Candida albicans* confirmed, best to use oral treatment, e.g. fluconazole or itraconazole[6]

Refer difficult and unresponsive cases to a dermatologist.

127

Psoriasis of nails

Psoriasis can have many manifestations, such as pitting, onycholysis, discolouration, splinter haemorrhages, distal subungual hyperkeratosis (which can resemble warts) and severe total nail dystrophy (often with arthropathy). Psoriasis can closely mimic onychomycosis, which should be excluded by fungal culture and histology before commencing presumed tinea therapy.

There is no effective topical therapy for psoriasis of the nails but a trial of a potent corticosteroid lotion may help selected cases. Intralesional steroid injections, which are painful and require multiple treatments, can help. Successful treatment of the skin does not help the nails.

Onychomycosis (fungal nail infection)

Key facts and checkpoints

- Affects 3–5% of population and 40% over 60 years[1]
- Classified as superficial, distal or proximal
- Toenails affected more commonly than fingernails
- The most common form is distal lateral subungual caused by *Trichophyton mentagrophytes* var. *interdigitale* (typical of toe web space tinea and responds well to terbinafine) or by *Trichophyton rubrum* (common on sole of foot and more resistant)
- Superficial white onychomycosis is also common, and is usually confined to the toenails with small superficial white plaques with distinct edges and caused by *Trichophyton mentagrophytes* var. *interdigitale*
- Total dystrophic onychomycosis—whole nail affected, thickened, opaque and yellow brown (caused by *Trichophyton* sp.)
- *Candida albicans* and other fungi are not a common factor
- Diagnosis—always confirm by culture and histology of the distal nail plate clippings placed in formalin. Positive in 60–80% of cases

Treatment[5,6]

In most cases it is not a major clinical problem and no treatment is a reasonable plan. Regular nail clipping is important. The antifungal treatment of choice for all types of toenail tinea is:

terbinafine 250 mg (o) daily for 12 weeks (cures 70–80% of cases); 6 weeks for fingernails

An alternative is itraconazole 200 mg (o) bd for the first week of each month for 2 months for fingernails; 3–4 months for toenails.

Tips

No improvement apart from the proximal part of the nail will be noticed after months because it takes 12 months or more for the toenail to grow.

Mark the base of the dystrophic nail with a scalpel blade or black ink to assess progress.

Topical treatment for superficial or distal nail involvement[7]

amorolfine 5% (Loceryl) nail lacquer 1–2 times weekly after filing (fingernails: 6 months; toenails: 9–12 months)

or

miconazole tincture daily until resolution

or

ciclopirox lacquer daily until resolution

A systematic review found poor evidence for the effectiveness of topical therapy for onychomycosis.[8]

Consider twice-daily applications of tea-tree oil indefinitely for tinea pedis and tinea unguium.

PARONYCHIA

Acute paronychia

This is a painful condition that is mainly due to bacterial infection, especially *Staphylococcus aureus*.

Management

Uncomplicated with localised pus:

- simple elevation of nail fold or puncture the fold—close to drain pus
- advice on hygiene
- antibiotics not usually necessary
- if not responding to drainage, use (di)flucloxacillin
- exclude diabetes

Complicated with subungual extension:

- small vertical incision alongside the nail, or
- removal of nail in part or totally
- exclude diabetes

Chronic paronychia

Clinical features

- Painless
- A form of traumatic nail dystrophy
- Loss of cuticle fundamental to diagnosis

Causes

- Excessive manipulation of cuticles (e.g. by manicurists)

- Occupational (e.g. chefs, housewives, nurses, fishmongers)
- Frequent contact with water, detergents and chemicals
- Habit tic—picking the nail fold

Note:

- Secondary infection with *Candida* common but not basic cause.
- The damaged cuticle permits access of water and grit to the nail matrix and causes inflammation of the proximal nail fold.

Management[4,5]

- Culture organisms
- Exclude diabetes
- Basic nail care advice:
  - keep hands dry (avoid wet work if possible)
  - wear cotton-lined gloves when washing dishes (for max. of 15 minutes)
  - minimise contact with water, soap, detergents, lipid solvents and other irritants
  - never pick, push back or manicure cuticles
  - never insert anything beneath cuticle for cleaning
  - wear cotton gloves in garden
  - use a mild soap and shampoo

Medications[5]

For *Candida* (if cultured):

tincture miconazole 2% bd for 7 days
or
clotrimazole topical preparations

For *Staphylococcus* (if cultured):

Bactroban topical ointment

Topical medications to nail folds (especially if persistent exudate):
4% thymol in alcohol (SVR) qid
or
10% sulphacetamide in alcohol

Vaseline (to waterproof) can be applied frequently (5–10 times daily) when it is dry and without exudate.
Very potent topical corticosteroids are helpful.
Refer unresponsive cases.

Atopic dermatitis

- Avoid irritants: special soaps, wear gloves for dishwashing
- Good nail hygiene
- Apply potent topical steroids to proximal nail fold

Lichen planus

This commonly presents in the nail with atrophy of one or more nails. The nail plate is predisposed to breaking and splitting as it thins. If advanced, a pterygium arising from the proximal nail fold grows as the nail matrix is destroyed and eventually total loss of the nail may occur.

Biopsy of the nail matrix is recommended before treatment.

Intralesional steroids into the proximal nail fold are the treatment of choice if seen prior to destruction of the nail unit. Otherwise a trial of prednisolone 25 mg (o) daily for 4 weeks, reducing the dose gradually over 1–2 weeks, may induce temporary remission.

Twenty-nail dystrophy

This is an uncommon disorder seen in preschool or pre-adolescent children with thinning and roughening of all or almost all 20 nails. It may be a prodrome to psoriasis, lichen planus or alopecia areata but it tends to be a self-limiting condition and most cases resolves over 2–3 years.[4]

It is reported to respond well to the very potent topical steroid, clobetasol.

Brittle nails

The nails break easily, usually at their distal end. Brittle nails are age related and are usually caused by local physical factors, such as repeated water immersion, and exposure to chemicals, such as detergents, alkalis and nail polish removers and also hypothyroidism and digital ischaemia. Systemic causes such as deficiency of iron and vitamins are not considered to be a common factor.

Calcium does not contribute to the hardness of nails and calcium deficiency does not cause brittle nails.[4] No cosmetic applications appear to be helpful.

Management[4]

- Avoid excessive hydration and trauma
- Wear rubber gloves with cotton liners for wet work
- Massage Vaseline or nail creams (e.g. Eulactol or NeoStrata) into the nail several times daily
- Nail polishes and hardeners (preferably without formalin) may give a good cosmetic result

Nail apparatus melanoma

Clinical features[5]

- Rare but potentially fatal
- Responsible for 2–3% of all melanomas

- All age groups but especially in seventh decade
- Affects all ethnic groups in all climates
- Presents as a longitudinal pigmented streak in the nail (see FIG. 127.12)
- Hutchinson sign (pigmentation of the proximal nail fold) may be present
- Usually diagnosed late
- Mortality >50%
- Median survival <12 months after diagnosis
- Early recognition and referral may result in a cure

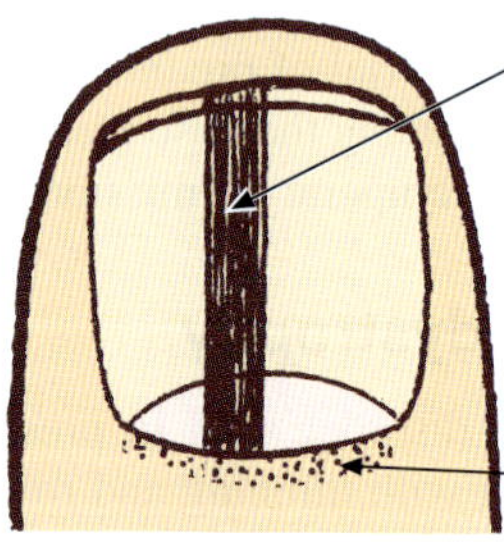

FIGURE 127.12 Longitudinal pigmented streak: sign of nail apparatus melanoma

Management

- All cases require a longitudinal nail biopsy for diagnosis
- If confirmed, treatment is based on Breslow thickness and level of invasion
- Level 1 or in situ—removal of whole nail apparatus
- Invasive melanoma—amputation of distal phalanx

Glomus tumours

Glomus tumours are those mysterious little tumours that occur beneath the nail plate and can give paroxysms of sharp pain.

They are small purplish lesions that are exquisitely tender to touch and activate with changes in temperature. They may not be visible but may be revealed when the nail bed is blanched with gentle pressure. Imaging may be needed for diagnosis. Treatment is surgical.

Onychogryphosis

Onychogryphosis, or irregular thickening and overgrowth of the nail, is commonly seen in the big toenails of the elderly and appears to be related to pressure from footwear (see FIG. 127.13). It is really a permanent condition. Simple removal of the nail by avulsion is followed by recurrence some months later. Softening and burring of the nail gives only temporary relief, although burring sometimes provides a good result.

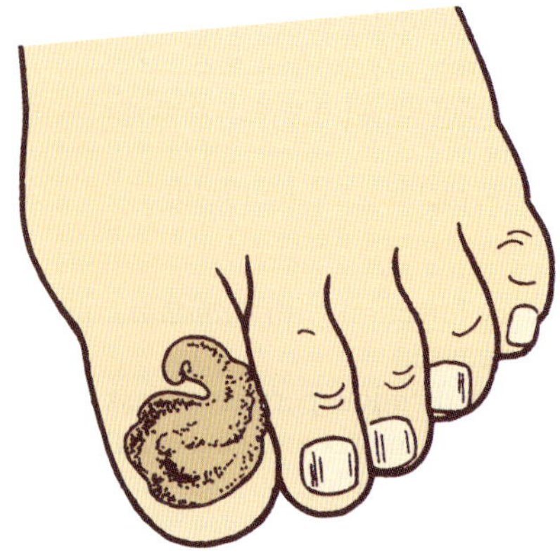

FIGURE 127.13 Onychogryphosis

The powder from burring can be used as culture for fungal organisms. Permanent cure requires ablation of the nail bed after removal of nail.

Two methods of nail ablation are:[6]

1 total surgical excision
2 cauterisation with phenol (with care)

Ingrowing toenails

Refer to section in CHAPTER 68.

Periungual warts

These are similar to other warts and fortunately rarely spread under the nail to the nail bed. Caution is needed with treatment.

Cryotherapy must be used with caution to avoid damage to the nail matrix—otherwise it is usually safe but often ineffective. Consider wart paints under occlusion.

Subungual haematoma[9]

The small, localised haematoma

There are several methods of decompressing a small localised haematoma under the fingernail or toenail that causes considerable pain. The objective is to release the blood by drilling a hole in the overlying nail with a hot wire or a drill/needle.

Treatment

Method 1: the sterile needle

Simply drill a hole by twisting a standard disposable hypodermic needle (21 or 23 gauge) into the selected

127

site. Some practitioners prefer drilling two holes to facilitate the release of blood.

Method 2: the hot paper clip

Take a standard, large paper clip and straighten it. Heat one end (until it is red hot) in the flame of a spirit lamp. Immediately transfer the hot wire to the nail, and press the point lightly on the nail at the centre of the haematoma. After a small puff of smoke, an acrid odour and a spurt of blood, the patient will experience immediate relief (see FIG. 127.14).

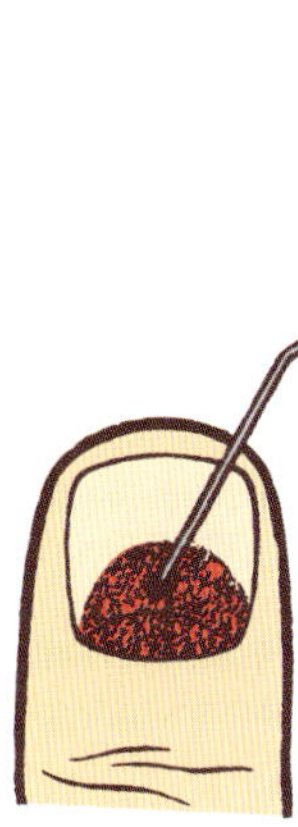

FIGURE 127.14 Treatment of subungual haematoma. The point of a heated end of a paper clip is pressed lightly on the nail at the centre of the haematoma.

Method 3: electrocautery

This is the best method. Simply apply the hot wire of the electrocautery unit to the selected site (see FIG. 127.15). It is very important to keep the wire hot at all times and to be prepared to withdraw it quickly, as soon as the nail is pierced. It should be painless.

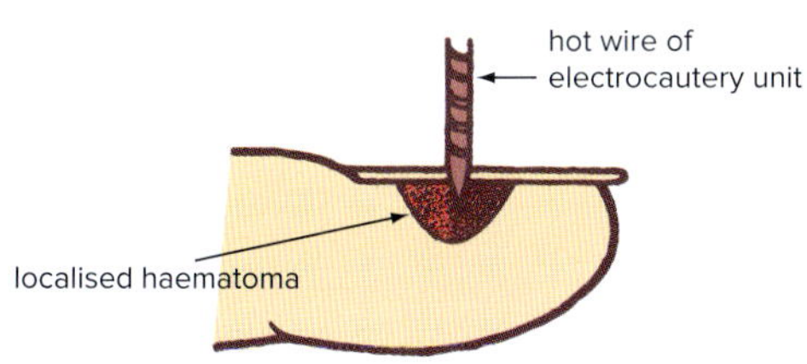

FIGURE 127.15 Electrocautery to subungual haematoma

Important precautions

- Reassure patients that the process will not cause pain; they may be alarmed by the preparations.
- The hot point must quickly penetrate, so go no deeper than the nail. The blood under the nail insulates the underlying tissues from the heat and, therefore, from pain.
- The procedure is effective for a recent traumatic haematoma under tension. Do not attempt this procedure on an old, dried haematoma as it will be painful and ineffective.
- Advise the patient to clean the nail with spirit or an antiseptic and cover with an adhesive strip to prevent contamination and infection.
- Advise the patient that the nail will eventually separate and a normal nail will appear in 6–9 months.

The large haematoma

Where blood occupies the total nail area, a relatively large laceration is present in the nail bed.

Treatment

To permit a good, long-term functional and cosmetic result it is imperative to remove the nail and repair the laceration (see FIG. 127.16).

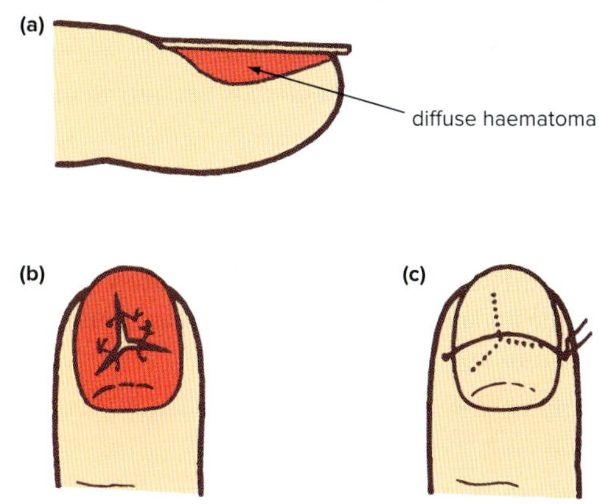

FIGURE 127.16 Treating the diffuse haematoma: **(a)** the diffuse haematoma, **(b)** sutures to laceration, **(c)** fingernail as splint

Method

- Apply digital nerve block to the digit.
- Remove the nail.
- Repair the laceration with 4/0 plain catgut.
- Replace the fingernail, which acts as a splint, and hold this in place with a suture for 10 days.

Myxoid pseudocyst

There are two types of digital myxoid pseudocysts (also known as mucous cysts) appearing in relation to the distal phalanx and nail in either fingers or toes (more common) (see FIG. 127.17). One type occurs in relation to, and often connecting with, the distal

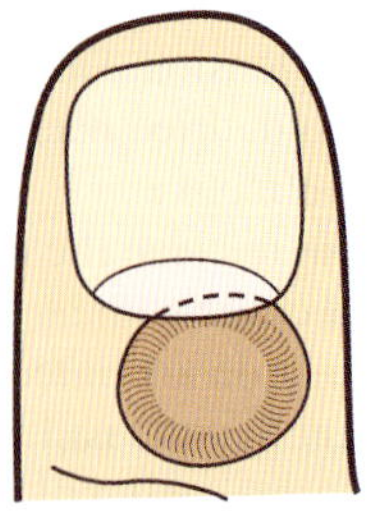

FIGURE 127.17 Myxoid pseudocyst: typical position of the cyst

interphalangeal joint and the other occurs at the site of the proximal nail fold. The latter (more common) is translucent and fluctuant, and contains thick clear gelatinous fluid, which is easily expressed after puncture of the cyst with a sterile needle. Osteoarthritis of the DIP is associated with leakage of myxoid fluid into the surrounding tissue to form the cyst.

Some pseudocysts resolve spontaneously. If persistent and symptomatic attempt:[9]

repeated aspiration (aseptically) at 4–6 weekly intervals
or
cryosurgery
or
puncture, compression, then infiltration intralesionally with triamcinolone acetonide (or similar steroid)

They tend to persist and recur; if so, refer to surgery for total excision of the proximal nail fold and/or ligation of the communicating stalk to the DIP or (preferably) microscopic dissection to the capsule defect and capsule repair.

Patient education resources

Hand-out sheets from *Murtagh's Patient Education* 7th edition:

- Nail disorders

References

1. Sinclair R. There is something wrong with my nail. Aust Fam Physician, 1997; 26: 673–81.
2. Hunter JA, Savin JA, Dahl MV. *Clinical Dermatology*. Oxford: Blackwell Scientific, 1989: 70.
3. Grinzi P. Hair and nails. Aust Fam Physician, 2011; 40 (7): 471–84.
4. Byrne M, Howard A. Common nail disorders: how to treat. Australian Doctor, 31 October 2005: 38–40.
5. Sinclair R. Treating common nail problems. Aust Fam Physician, 1997; 26: 949–2.
6. Expert group for Dermatology. In: eTG complete. Melbourne: Therapeutic Guidelines Ltd. Available from: <www.tg.org.au>, accessed March 2018.
7. Thai K. Nail disease: is it fungal and how should it be managed? Medicine Today, 2014; 15(6): 35–47.
8. Crawford F, Hart D et al. Topical treatments for fungal infections of the skin and nails of the foot. Cochrane Database Syst Rev. 2000; (2): CD001434.
9. Murtagh J. *Practice Tips* (7th edn). Sydney: McGraw-Hill, 2016.

Part 10

Accident and emergency medicine

128 Emergency care

When Elisha arrived, he went alone into the room and saw the boy lying dead on the bed. He closed the door and prayed to the Lord. Then he lay down on the boy, placing his mouth, eyes and hands on the boy's mouth, eyes and hands. As he lay stretched out over the boy, the boy's body started to get warm—the boy sneezed seven times and then opened his eyes.

II KINGS 4: 32–5 (A MIRACLE OR SUCCESSFUL ARTIFICIAL RESUSCITATION?)

Definition of the emergency

Emergency: 'An event demanding immediate medical attention'.

The GP must be available and organised to cope with the medically defined emergency when it comes. Emergency care outside the hospital represents one of the most interesting and rewarding areas of medical practice. City doctors will have to modify their degree of availability, equipment and skills according to the availability of paramedical emergency services, while others, especially remote doctors, will need total expertise and comprehensive equipment to provide optimal circumstances to save their patients' lives.

The immediate approach to a specific emergency differs from normal, less urgent medical practice. The usual method of history and examination is replaced with a technique of rapid assessment and immediate management. In fact, the primary diagnosis is sometimes possible on the information available over the telephone, or during the first few seconds of surveying the patient.

An obvious yet important concept is that of 'time criticality', which implies that certain patients are at high risk of a critical outcome of deterioration if there is significant delay in appropriate management. A classic example in general practice would be acute coronary syndromes.

Refer also to childhood emergencies (see CHAPTER 96).

Key facts and checkpoints

- The most common emergency calls in a survey of a typical rural general practice[1] were accidents and violence (51%), abdominal pain (10%), dyspnoea (7%), chest pain (6%), syncope/blackout (5%), other acute pain (5%).
- The prevalence of emergency calls was 2.6 per 1000 population per week.
- The most common specific conditions in this study[1] were lacerations (19%), fractures (11%), injuries from transport accidents (11%), asthma (4%), ischaemic heart pain (3.5%), appendicitis (3%).
- The most common causes of sudden death were myocardial infarction (67%), accidents (10%), cerebrovascular accidents (7%), pulmonary embolism (6%), suicide (4%).
- The main vital emergency procedures were cardiopulmonary resuscitation, intubation and ventilation, intravenous access (including venous cutdown), intravenous (or rectal) dextrose and arrest of haemorrhage.

Principles of management

The important principles of management of the emergency call can be summarised as follows:

1. The practitioner must be aware of life-threatening conditions.
2. The practitioner should be prepared mentally and physically.
3. PLAN, EQUIP and PRACTISE.
4. Chest pain/collapse/myocardial infarction (collectively) represents *the* premium emergency call.
5. Beware of children with respiratory distress and traumatic injuries.
6. The most saveable patients are those with blood loss. Hence IV fluids for intravascular volume expansion are essential.
7. The necessary basic skills to cope with most emergencies involve DRSABCD—danger, response, send for help, airway, breathing, circulation, defibrillator.
8. Have the equipment and the skills to handle body fluids potentially contaminated with blood-borne viruses.

9 Seventy per cent of cardiac arrests occur in the home, so the availability of a portable defibrillator is important.

Vital basic skills

1 Rapid intravenous access
2 Cardiopulmonary resuscitation, including upper airway relief, intubation and ventilation, treatment of cardiac arrhythmias and defibrillation
3 Cricothyroidotomy
4 Arrest of haemorrhage
5 Knowledge of usage of common emergency drugs

Alarming symptoms and signs

- unconsciousness
- convulsions
- chest pain in an adult, especially associated with pallor and sweating
- pallor and sweating in any patient with pain, collapse or injury
- collapse, especially at toilet
- significant haemorrhage
- breathlessness, including asthma
- the agitated patient threatening homicide or suicide (take a police officer for company)

Don't forget the value of oxygen

Ideally, the doctor who attends emergency calls should carry an oxygen delivery unit or at least rely on the simultaneous arrival of an ambulance with resuscitation equipment. Remember, oxygen is a treatment for hypoxia, not for breathlessness; a pulse oximeter is very useful. Most cases require a high flow rate of 8–10 L/minute.

Medical emergencies typically requiring high-flow oxygen:[2]

- acute pulmonary oedema
- acute anaphylaxis
- cardiopulmonary arrest
- collapse
- status epilepticus
- shock, sepsis
- major haemorrhage, major trauma

Medical emergencies where oxygen should be used with caution, unless oximetry confirms hypoxia:[2]

- underlying COPD—however, in the above medical emergency scenarios, start with high flow during urgent phase, but reduce after reassessment
- myocardial infarction—high-flow oxygen may increase infarct size
- stroke
- obstetric emergencies—may harm the fetus if the mother is not hypoxaemic

Twelve golden rules

Here are 12 important rules for the diagnostic approach to the emergency call.

1 Always consider the possibilities of hypoglycaemia and opioid overdosage in the unconscious patient.
2 Consider intra-abdominal bleeding first and foremost in a patient with abdominal pain who collapses at the toilet.
3 Acute chest pain represents myocardial infarction until proven otherwise.
4 Exclude meningitis and septicaemia in a child with a rapid onset of drowsiness and pallor.
5 Consider a ruptured intra-abdominal viscus in any person, especially a child, with persistent post-traumatic abdominal pain.
6 Consider acute anaphylaxis in patients with a past history of allergies.
7 Consider substance use and organic causes for patients with acute psychosis or bizarre behaviour.
8 Consider ectopic pregnancy in any woman of child-bearing age presenting with acute abdominal pain.
9 If a patient is found cyanosed, always consider upper-airway obstruction first.
10 Beware of the asthmatic who is cyanosed with a 'silent chest' and tachycardia.
11 Consider ventricular fibrillation or other arrhythmia in an adult with sudden collapse or dizziness.
12 Consider subarachnoid haemorrhage in anyone with a sudden onset of severe headache.

Important medical emergencies in adults

This section includes summarised protocols for management of emergencies. Further detail is available on websites such as the medical blog Life in the Fast Lane (<https://lifeinthefastlane.com/>).

Acute anaphylaxis and anaphylactic reactions

Common causes: bee stings, wasp stings, other bites (e.g. imported red fire ants, jack jumper ants), parenteral antibiotics (especially penicillin), food reactions (e.g. peanuts, fish). See FIGURE 128.1.

Other causes: allergic extracts, blood products, antivenom, radiological contact materials, anaesthetic agents, NSAIDs.

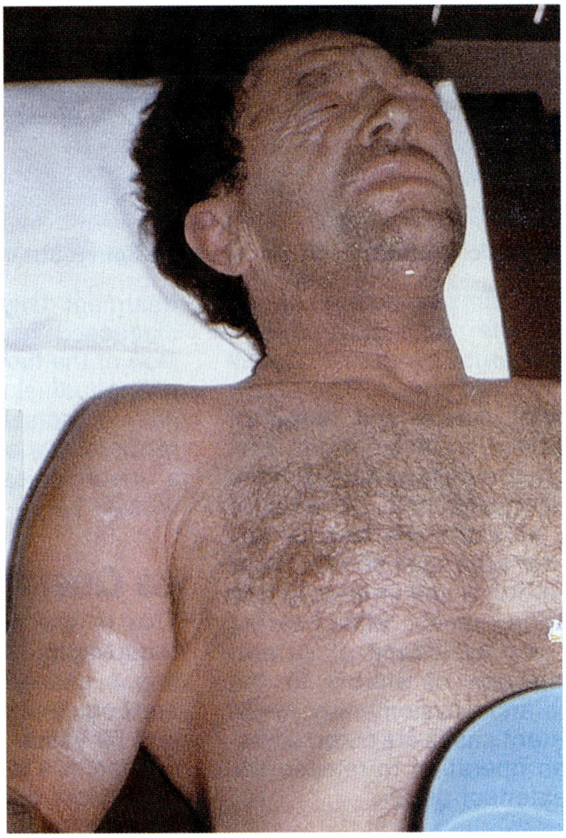

FIGURE 128.1 Acute anaphylaxis with respiratory difficulty caused by a European wasp sting

The onset of anaphylaxis from exposure is usually rapid—typically 10–20 minutes. The early administration of adrenaline saves lives. The diagnosis is basically a clinical one.[3]

Symptoms

- Skin: pruritus—generalised, palate, hands, feet, urticaria, angio-oedema
- Respiratory: wheeze, stridor
- Nausea and vomiting, abdominal pain, diarrhoea
- Hypotension: syncope, collapse
- Palpitations

Note: The early danger symptom is itching of the palms of hands and soles of the feet.

Differential diagnosis: syncope

Refer to the adult anaphylaxis kit in CHAPTER 80.

First-line treatment (adults)[3,4]

- Call for help
- Remove cause (e.g. bee sting) if possible. Lay the patient down
- Oxygen 8 L/min (by face mask)
- Adrenaline 0.5 mg (1:1000) IM best given in mid antero-lateral thigh (mg = mL of 1:1000 adrenaline)

  Set up IV access.
- If no rapid improvement:
  - repeat IM adrenaline every 3–5 minutes
  - set up adrenaline infusion: 1 mg adrenaline to 1000 mL N saline (i.e. 1 mL = 1 mcg adrenaline) bolus of 50 mcg (= 50 mL) can be given as required (best with ECG monitor)
- Set up additional IV line (preferably two 'wide bore' lines) and infuse crystalloid solution (e.g. N saline 1–2 L) with bolus (20 mL/kg) over 1–2 min
- Salbutamol aerosol inhalation (or nebulisation if severe), especially if wheeze/stridor
- Consider promethazine (25 mg) IV and hydrocortisone (250 mg) IV
- Admit to hospital (observe at least 4 hours)
- Discharge on promethazine 25 mg tds + prednisolone 50 mg/day for 3 days. Provide an adrenaline autoinjector

Angio-oedema and acute urticaria

Acute urticaria and angio-oedema are essentially anaphylaxis limited to the skin, subcutaneous tissues and other specific organs. They can occur together.

Treatment

- Uncomplicated cutaneous swelling—antihistamines e.g. diphenhydramine or promethazine 50 mg (o) *or*

  25 mg IM if more severe or prednisolone 25–50 mg (o) as a single dose
- Upper respiratory involvement

  adrenaline 0.3 mg SC or IM or 5 mg nebulised

Acute cardiogenic pulmonary oedema

Keep in mind the mnemonic LMNOP (lasix, morphine, nitrates, O_2, CPAP).

- Keep the patient propped up in bed with legs over side
- Oxygen by mask or intranasally (8 L/min)
- Glyceryl trinitrate (nitroglycerin) 300–600 mcg sublingual (tablet or spray); can use IV nitrates (if BP >100 mmHg)
- Insert IV line (large bore cannula)
- Frusemide 40 mg IV, increasing to 80 mg IV as necessary (or twice the patient's normal oral dose)

- Morphine 1–2.5 mg IV—but caution: reserve for chest pain and anxiety
- CPAP (continuous positive airway pressure)—for unresponsive cases or BiPAP (if available)—in ambulance, ED or CCU

Give amiodarone 3–5 mg/kg loading dose IV infusion if rapid atrial fibrillation.

Note: Keep in mind underlying cause e.g.:

- myocardial infarction (? silent)
- arrhythmia
- cardiomyopathy
- anaemia

Severe asthma[4]

Severe asthma is a life-threatening condition that is resistant to standard treatment. It requires intensive medication because of marked obstruction to the air passages, due to severe smooth muscle spasm and inflammation, producing mucosal oedema and mucous impaction. Beware the 'silent chest'. (Refer to CHAPTER 82.)

Initial treatment (summary)

- Oxygen 8 L/min by mask to maintain SpO_2 >95%
- Salbutamol 12 puffs (adult) in a spacer (4 × 4 × 4 rule)

  or
- Continuous nebulised 0.5% salbutamol by face mask, using 8 L/min oxygen for nebulisation

  Insert IV line
- hydrocortisone 250 mg IV or IM

If poor response:

- add ipratropium 500 g into the salbutamol nebuliser
- magnesium sulphate 2 g (25–100 mg/kg) IV over 20 minutes
- adrenaline 0.5 mg 1:1000 SC or IM or 1:10 000 IV

If not responding, exhausted and moribund:

- intubation with intermittent positive pressure ventilation (IPPV)
- hydration with IV fluids

Opioid respiratory depression[4]

- Attend to airway (e.g. pocket mask and bag)
- naloxone 0.4 mg IV boluses titrated to clinical effect

Beware of recurrence of respiratory depression or neurogenic pulmonary oedema from excess naloxone.

Refer to CHAPTER 75.

Severe hypoglycaemia (confirm by blood glucose around 3 mmol/L or less)

128

glucagon 1 mL (=1 mg) IM or SC (most practical option)
then oral glucose if able to swallow—can repeat glucagon
or
50% dextrose 20 mL IV through securely positioned cannula, large vein (if IV line difficult, administer rectally by pressing the nozzle of a large syringe into the anus and injecting slowly)

Myocardial infarction/unstable angina

Refer to CHAPTER 40.

First-line management

- Insert IV line
- Glyceryl trinitrate (nitroglycerin) 300 mcg (½ tab) SL or spray, unless BP <90 mmHg or pulse <50/min
- Aspirin 300 mg (½ or 1 tab)
- Morphine 1 mg per minute IV until pain relief (up to 15 mg)—usually 2.5–10 mg (lower dose if elderly/frail)
- ECG (set up by an assistant)
- CPAP or BiPAP (if available)
- Arrange ambulance and hospitalisation

Hyperventilation

Calm the patient with a firm but reassuring voice. Remove them from anxiety-provoking stimuli such as panicking bystanders. Consider the possibility of an alternative diagnosis causing hypoxia.

Status epilepticus and serial seizures

Status epilepticus = repeated convulsions (usually >5 minutes) without regaining consciousness after initial tonic–clonic seizure. Significant mortality at >30 minutes.
Serial seizures = repeated convulsions after regaining consciousness.

Management

(Refer to CHAPTER 84.)

- Lie patient on side

128

- Ensure adequate oxygenation: attend to airway (e.g. Guedel tube); give oxygen 8 L/min (check blood sugar)
  If persisting >5 minutes: (summarised)
  midazolam 5–10 mg IM or IV over 2–5 minutes (lorazepam, if available, has stronger evidence)
  or
  midazolam 5–10 mg buccally (tear top off plastic ampoule,[5] slowly drip into patient's mouth between gums and cheek—with syringe or from ampoule)
  or
  midazolam 5–10 mg intranasally—1–3 drops at a time into alternate nostrils
  repeat once in 15 minutes (if necessary)
  or
  diazepam 0.05 mg/kg/minute IV until the seizures cease or respiratory depression begins (beware of respiratory depression and other vital parameters): usually 10–20 mg bolus in adult
  When seizures cease, follow immediately with:
  phenytoin 15–20 mg/kg IV over 30 minutes
  or
  sodium valproate 10 mg/kg by slow IV infusion
  Other drugs to consider:
  phenobarbitone, thiopentone

Electric shock

Facts

- Direct current (DC) from welding machines or lightning produces more electrolyte tissue damage and burns than does AC (domestic supply).
- Injuries occur at sites distant from entry or exit.
- Severe muscle contractions can cause bone fracture or posterior dislocation of the shoulder.
- Household shocks tend to cause cardiac arrest (ventricular fibrillation), and myocardial damage is common.
- Ischaemic necrosis of a limb or digit is possible.
- Apparently minor initial injuries may be very misleading (see FIG. 128.2).
- Neurological deficits and psychoneurotic sequelae are common in survivors.

Principles of management

- Attend to DRSABC (see FIG. 128.7). 'Danger' must always come first.
- Make the site safe: switch off the electricity. Use dry wool to insulate rescuers.
- 'Treat the clinically dead'.
- Give a precordial thump in a witnessed arrest.
- Consider a cervical collar (? cervical fracture).

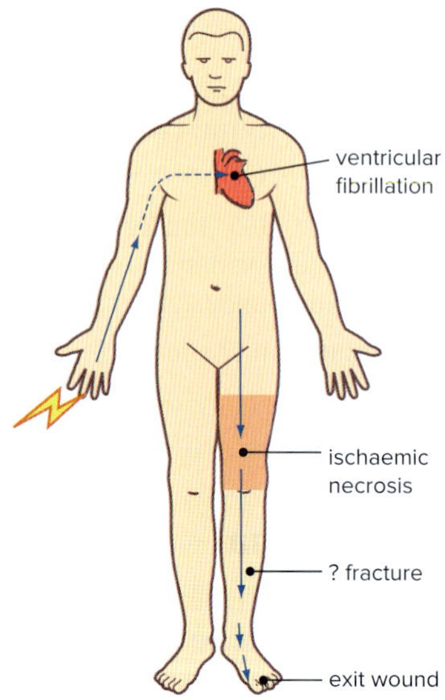

FIGURE 128.2 Effect of electric shock passing through the body

Bystander CPR and prolonged respiratory support for electric shocks and lightning strike can be lifesaving.

- Provide basic cardiopulmonary resuscitation, including defibrillation (as required).
- Carefully examine the whole body, especially the limbs.
- Consider:
  - X-ray of limbs or spine as appropriate
  - checking for myoglobinuria and kidney failure
  - tetanus and clostridial prophylaxis
- Get expert help—intensive care unit, burns unit.

Lightning strike

Prevention (during an electrical storm)

- Don't shelter under trees or tall objects ('splash effect'—see FIG. 128.3).[6]
- Stay indoors—shelter in a building or closed car.
- Avoid using phone.
- Avoid holding metal objects (e.g. golf clubs).
- Keep as low to ground as possible (e.g. curl up in a ditch).
- Avoid being in a group.

Clinical effects

- Burn injury: the 'flashover' phenomenon—clothing disintegrates

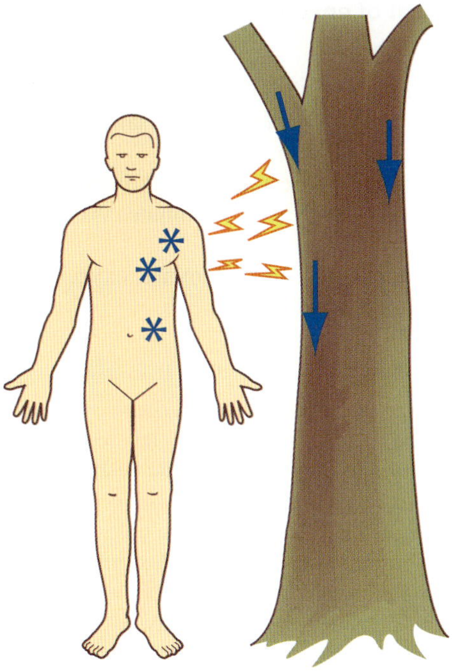

FIGURE 128.3 'Splash effect', where current jumps from a path of higher resistance, such as a tree

- Blast injury: ruptured spleen, subdural, ruptured eardrum
- Electrical injury as for household shock (uncommon)

Petrol and solvent sniffing

Substances commonly sniffed include petrol, glues, spirit-based paints, paint spray cans and other aerosols. Refer to drug and alcohol services wherever possible.

The three main acute problems are:

1. shaking and fitting: give midazolam IV or IM or diazepam IV (as for convulsions)
2. agitation/aggressive behaviour, self-harm: try to calm patient in a well-lit room; sedate with diazepam; give haloperidol for hallucinations or delusions
3. general debilitation: this may include acute infections (e.g. chest infection), anaemia, malnutrition

Near-drowning[4]

Near-drowning is survival after asphyxia from submersion in a liquid medium. Hypoxia is the final common pathway in drowning or near-drowning, whether by water aspiration (wet drowning) or by glottic closure (dry drowning).

The rules to remember are that victims can respond to resuscitation after considerable immersion time (up to 30 minutes) and that mouth-to-mouth resuscitation should always be attempted, even if pulseless or with fixed, dilated pupils. The usual routine of basic life support and CPR applies. All symptomatic patients should receive high-flow oxygen and ideally CPAP or BiPAP. Those requiring intubation should receive positive end expiratory pressure (PEEP) in an in-patient facility.

Artificial surfactant given via an endotracheal tube is supported by some evidence in children, but not (yet) in adults.[7]

There is no significant difference in outcome and management between salt-water and fresh-water drowning. Hypothermia should be attended to with warming, such as a hot-air blanket if available and warm fluids.

Epistaxis

Refer to CHAPTER 59.

Migraine

Refer to CHAPTER 56.

Bites and stings

Bites and stings from animals, spiders and insects are common in Australia and the US but fatal bites are uncommon.

Snake bites

Snake bites are more common and severe in those handling snakes and in those trying to kill the snake, particularly while inebriated. Snakes are more aggressive when mating or sloughing their skin (about four times a year). They strike for one-third of their length at 3.5 metres/second. Over 70% of bites are on the legs. Sea snakes are not a major problem in Australian waters.

First aid

1. Keep the patient as still as possible.
2. Do not wash, cut, apply ice, manipulate the wound or use a tourniquet.
3. Immediately bandage the bite site firmly (same tightness as for sprained ankle). A 15 cm elasticated or crepe bandage is ideal: it should extend above the bite site for 15 cm (e.g. if bitten around the ankle, the bandage should cover the leg up to the knee).

4 Splint the limb to immobilise it: a firm stick or slab of wood would be ideal.
5 Transport to a medical facility for definitive treatment. Do not give alcoholic beverages or stimulants.

Note: A venom detection kit is used to examine a swab of the bitten area or a fresh urine specimen, but only to identify the snake species involved.

The bandage can be cautiously removed when the patient is safely under medical observation. Observe for symptoms and signs of envenomation.

Antivenom for most venomous Australian snakes in addition to a polyvalent vaccine is available.

Envenomation

Not all patients become envenomated and the antivenom should not be given unless there is evidence of this. Envenomation is more likely when the snake has a clear bite, such as in snake handlers, barefooted people or those who have placed their hands in burrows.

Apart from non-specific systemic effects (as listed) there may be major organ effects according to the type of snake and its toxin. These include coagulopathy, neurotoxicity, myolysis and kidney damage.

Important early symptoms of snake bite envenomation include:

- nausea and vomiting (a reliable early symptom)
- abdominal pain
- excessive perspiration
- severe headache
- dizziness, blurred vision
- difficulty speaking or swallowing
- coagulation defects (e.g. haematuria)
- tender lymphadenopathy

The greatest danger is respiratory obstruction and failure or unexpected catastrophic bleeding (e.g. intracerebral haemorrhage).

Refer to FIGURE 128.4 for detailed effects.

Investigations and observation

- Careful observations (e.g. vital signs, conscious state)
- Test all urine for blood and protein
- FBE, serum electrolytes, LFTs, KFTs
- Watch for coagulopathy (e.g. spitting and coughing blood, bleeding from wounds/IV site, haematuria)
- Serial whole blood clotting time (a plain glass tube): normal <5–8 min, >15 min significant
- Coagulation screen—APTT and PT or INR
- Venom detection kit: wound site (best) or urine (not always indicator)

Treatment of envenomation

See note 2 (below).

- Reassure patient at all times
- Set up a slow IV infusion of N saline
- Keep adrenaline on standby
- Dilute the specific antivenom (1 in 10 in N saline) and infuse slowly over 30 minutes via the tubing of the saline solution
- Have adrenaline, antihistamines, oxygen and steroids on standby
- Monitor vital signs
- Provide basic life support as necessary

Note 1: The use of prophylactic adrenaline is controversial and some authorities reserve it for a reaction to the antivenom. It is best avoided with brown snake envenomation and with coagulopathy.

Note 2: Do not give antivenom unless clinical signs of envenomation or biochemical signs (e.g. positive urine, or abnormal clotting profile).

Note 3: One ampoule is usually sufficient.

Spider bites[4]

The toxin of most species of spider causes only localised pain, redness and swelling, but the toxin of some, notably the deadly Sydney funnel-web spider (*Atrax robustus*), can be rapidly fatal.

Rule: a bite from a large black spider should be managed initially as for a funnel-web spider, particularly within a 160 km radius of Sydney.

First aid

- Sydney funnel-web: as for snake bites
- Other spiders: apply an ice pack, do not bandage

Treatment

1 Sydney funnel-web

Signs of envenomation (in order):

- muscle fasciculation—limb → tongue/lip
- marked salivation or lacrimation
- piloerection
- dyspnoea
- neurological symptoms (e.g. disorientation, coma)

Treatment of envenomation

- specific antivenom (usually 4–8 vials)
- admit to a hospital critical care area
- resuscitation and other supportive measures

2 Other spider bites

The toxins of most species of spiders cause only localised symptoms, but the venom of a select few,

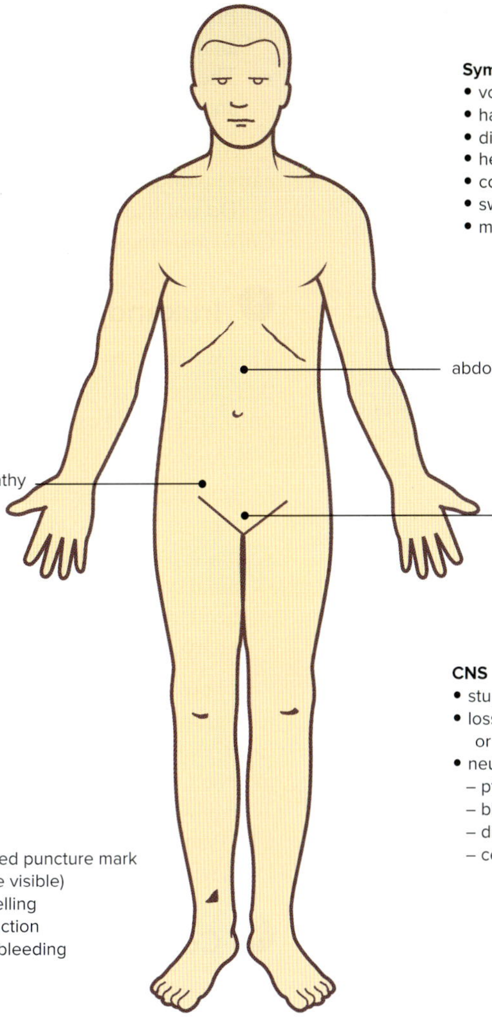

FIGURE 128.4 How to recognise snake bite envenomation

namely the red-back spider of Australia (*Latrodectus hasseltii*) and the related black widow spider of the US (*Latrodectus mactans*), can cause envenomation. This is rarely fatal but is more serious in the young, the frail and the elderly. The bite wounds are prone to infection.

Treatment of envenomation; ice, analgesia.

- antivenom exists, but rarely needed, IM or IV

Bee stings

First aid

1. Scrape the sting off sideways with a fingernail or knife blade. Do not squeeze it with the fingertips.
2. Apply 20% aluminium sulphate solution (Stingose) or methylated spirits.
3. Apply ice to the site.
4. Rest and elevate the limb that has been stung.

If anaphylaxis, treat as outlined earlier.

Preventive measures (if hypersensitive)

- Avoid bees (and wasps) if possible.
- Immunotherapy to honey bee (or wasp) venom. There is no cross-allergy between the honey bee, the 'yellow jacket' (*Vespula*) wasp and the paper wasp. For the bee, use pure venom antigen. However, *Vespula* requires specific hyposensitisation.
- Immunotherapy should be offered to those:
  - with a history of asthma who have had a single severe reaction to a bee sting
  - who have had a minimum of three stings with serial crescendo reactions
  - occupationally exposed who manifest severe reactions

– with elevated venom-specific IgE (RAST) antibodies, or positive venom prick tests

Centipede and scorpion bites

The main symptom is pain, which can be very severe and prolonged. Scorpions found in Australasia usually cause only minor systemic symptoms.

First aid[8]

1 Apply local heat (e.g. hot water with ammonia—household bleach).
2 Clean site.
3 Local anaesthetic (e.g. 1–2 mL of 1% lignocaine) infiltrated around the site.
4 Consider opioids—morphine or fentanyl—for pain.
5 Check tetanus immunisation status.

Box jellyfish or sea wasp (*Chironex fleckeri*)[4]

This is the most dangerous jellyfish in Australian waters and has been responsible for at least 80 extremely painful and sudden deaths.[5] Death can occur in minutes due to cardiopulmonary failure, especially in children. There can be up to 180 metres of stinging tentacles. The sting gives a 'frosted ladder' appearance. The jellyfish is limited to tropical waters north of the Tropic of Capricorn (Exmouth in west to Gladstone in east) and is found in coastal waters during the summer.

Prevention

- Avoid swimming, paddling and wading in 'jellyfish alert' areas in unsafe months.
- Otherwise, use a 'stinger suit'.

Treatment[3]

- Remove the victim from the water to prevent drowning.
- Immediately remove tentacles.
- Pour vinegar liberally (up to 2 L) over sting site and surrounding area.
- Use a cold pack for small stings and ice massage for large areas.
- Check respiration and pulse.
- Start immediate cardiopulmonary resuscitation if necessary.
- Gain IV access; give oxygen and up to 5 mL inotropes if necessary.
- Give box jellyfish antivenom by IV injection for major stings (may need at least 6 ampoules if patient remains in cardiac arrest).
- Provide pain relief if required (ice, lignocaine and analgesics—fentanyl or morphine).
- The use of IV magnesium is supported only by anecdotal evidence.[9]

Note: A delayed reaction can occur—the stings can cause pain after weeks (oral steroids are used).

Do not use pressure immobilisation bandaging for *Chironex* stings.

Irukandji syndrome[4]

This is caused by *Carukia barnesi,* a tiny box jellyfish that can penetrate safety nets for *Chironex,* and possibly other species of box jellyfish. Initially a mild sting with a delayed severe syndrome (usually after 30 minutes):

- severe generalised back, abdominal and muscle pain and muscle cramps
- chest pain, sweating and anxiety
- anxiety, restlessness, 'impending doom' feeling
- headache, nausea, vomiting
- tachycardia, hypertension

There is no specific first aid or antivenom but resuscitation measures may be needed as death can occur from pulmonary oedema or cardiac arrest. Measures include morphine or fentanyl 5 mg IV every 5 minutes as required, blood pressure control (e.g. phentolamine, CPAP and oxygen for pulmonary oedema) and possibly IV magnesium (minimal evidence for this).[9]

Common jellyfish stings[4]

These include bluebottle (*Physalia* species) and others that cause intense local pain (up to an hour or more) and linear skin redness. Systemic effects are uncommon.

Treatment

- Wash the sting site with sea water.
- Remove any tentacles with gloved hands or water.
- Immerse affected site in hot water at 45°C for 20 minutes. This is quite hot, so check tolerance to temperature on other limb.
- Vinegar is not helpful.

Stinging fish[4]

The sharp spines of the stinging fish have venom glands that can produce severe pain if they spike or even graze the skin. The best known of these is the stonefish. Others include bullrout, catfish, sea-urchins and crown of thorns (may need an X-ray). The toxin is usually heat-sensitive. Stingrays cause a gash wound with possible superinfection.

Envenomation

- Intense pain
- Localised swelling
- Bluish discolouration

Treatment

- Clean the wound—consider exploration.
- Bathe or immerse the affected part in very warm to hot (45°C, not scalding) water—this may give instant relief.[4]
- Give simple analgesics.
- If pain persists, give a local injection/infiltration of lignocaine 1% or even a regional block. If still persisting, consider morphine IV or fentanyl IV.
- A specific stonefish antivenom is available. Best given IV by slow infusion in CCU.

Mollusc bite (blue-ringed octopus, cone shell)[4]

Mollusc venoms usually cause numbness or paraesthesia but can be rapidly fatal if prolonged muscular weakness leads to respiratory paralysis.

Treatment

- Apply compression bandage to bite site (usually hand/arm).
- Immobilise the limb.
- Arrange transport (preferably by ambulance) to a medical facility.
- Observe for respiratory paralysis—ensure adequate ABC.

Sandfly (biting midges) bites

For some reason, possibly the nature of body odour, the use of oral thiamine has been suggested to prevent sandfly bites. Evidence is scarce.

Dose: thiamine 100 mg orally, daily

Other bites and stings

This includes bites from ants, wasps and mosquitoes.

First aid

1 Wash the site with large quantities of cool water.
2 Apply vinegar (liberal amount) or aluminium sulphate 20% solution (Stingose) to the wound for about 30 seconds.
3 Apply ice for several minutes.
4 Use soothing anti-itch cream or 5% lignocaine cream/ointment if very painful.

Medication is not usually necessary unless an acute allergic reaction develops.

The embedded tick[4]

Some species of ticks can be very dangerous to human beings, especially to children. In Australia, tick paralysis is confined to the eastern seaboard. Be careful in children 1–5 years—they are usually found in the scalp behind the ears. As it is impossible to distinguish between dangerous and non-dangerous ticks, early removal is mandatory. The tick should be totally removed—do not leave the mouthparts behind. Do not attempt to grab the tick by its body and tug. This is rarely successful in dislodging the tick, and may inject more toxin into the host.

As an office procedure, many practitioners grasp the tick's head as close to the skin as possible with fine forceps or tweezers, and pull the tick out sideways with a sharp rotatory action. This is acceptable, but not as effective as the methods described here.

First aid outdoor removal method

- Loop a strong thin thread (as a half-hitch lasso) around the tick's head as close to the skin as possible, and pull sharply with a twisting motion. Suitable materials include strong silk sutures or dental floss.
- A pyrethrin-based spray is often used.

Office procedure

- Infiltrate a small amount of local anaesthetic into the skin around the site of embedment.
- With a number 11 or 15 scalpel blade, make the necessary very small excision, including the mouthparts of the tick, to ensure total removal (see FIG. 128.5).

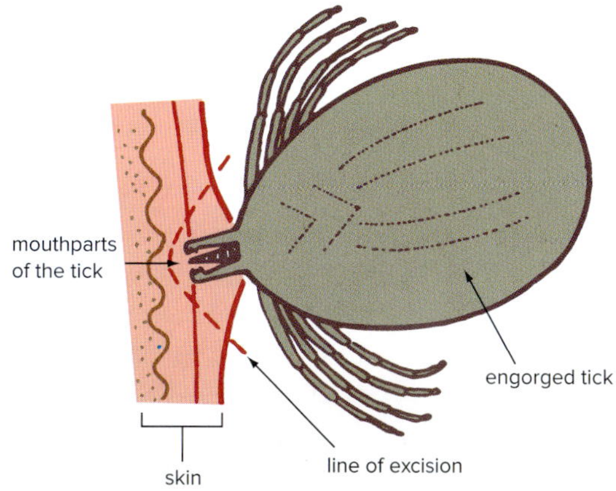

FIGURE 128.5 Removing the embedded tick

128

- If the tick body has already been removed, the skin containing the mouthparts is easily excised using a 2 or 3 mm punch biopsy blade.
- The small defect can usually be closed with a bandaid (or Steri-Strips), rather than a suture.
- Careful observation is needed after removal.

Human bites and animal bites

These bites can cause problems of suppurative infection and management in general. They are outlined in CHAPTER 132.

Vital emergency skills

Cardiopulmonary resuscitation

Cardiopulmonary arrest (CPA) It is essential that all doctors are familiar with the protocol for instituting basic life support in such an eventuality. Sick patients do visit our offices daily and the potential for sudden collapse, including a cardiac arrest, is ever present. About 75% of arrests are due to ventricular fibrillation and more than 75% of victims have severe coronary artery disease.[10] After 3 minutes of CPA (unconsciousness, no pulse, no respiration) there is an increasing risk of permanent cerebral dysfunction.

Important causes of sudden death are outlined in TABLE 128.1.[11]

The ABC basic life support for cardiac arrest should be followed, but DRSABCD is best. The S (send for help) should include sending for a defibrillator, because the final D (defibrillation) is urgent—thc outcome appears to be directly related to the speed of defibrillation. The 'chain of survival' principle for a victim of out-of-hospital cardiac arrest is presented in FIGURE 128.6.

Table 128.1 Causes of sudden death

Cardiac arrhythmias:
- ventricular fibrillation (75%)
- ventricular tachycardia
- torsade de pointes VT (? drugs)
- sick sinus syndrome
- severe bradycardia

Sudden pump failure:
- acute myocardial infarction
- cardiomyopathy

Cardiovascular rupture:
- myocardial rupture
- dissecting aneurysm of aorta
- subarachnoid haemorrhage

Acute circulatory obstruction:
- pulmonary embolism

Others:
- aortic stenosis
- pulmonary hypertension
- mitral valve prolapse
- electrolyte abnormalities
- glue sniffing

Basic life support[12]

FIGURE 128.7 represents a logical DRSABCD plan for the adult patient who collapses or is found apparently unconscious.

1 Shake and shout at the patient.
2 Check breathing.
3 Check pulse (feel carotid adjacent to thyroid cartilage).
4 Call for help (if no pulse). Ring 000 (112 also works on mobile services—the international standard number).

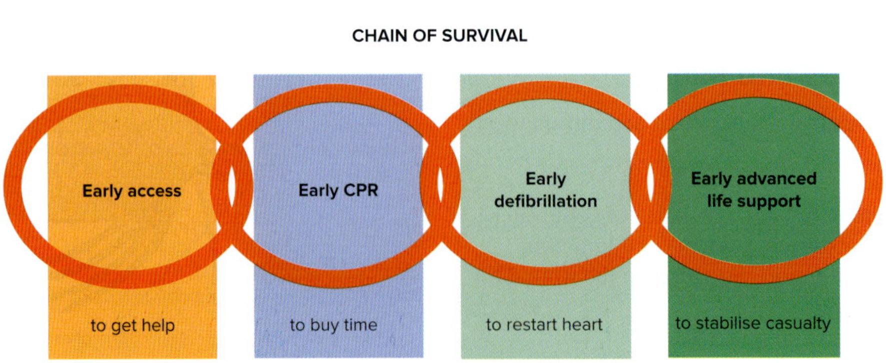

FIGURE 128.6 The chain of survival for a victim of out-of-hospital cardiac arrest

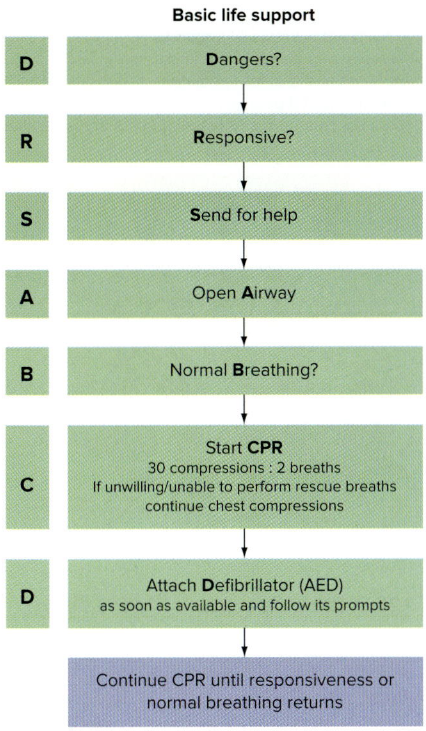

FIGURE 128.7 Basic life support algorithm

Source: Adapted from Australian Resuscitation Council material

5 Finger sweep oropharynx (clear it).
6 Place victim on back on firm surface.
7 Thump precordium (if arrest witnessed).
8 Tilt head back (to maximum).
9 Lift chin (use airway if available).
10 Commence basic life support:
   - rescue breaths (RBs)—2 strong breaths
   - external chest compressions (no pause)—30 compressions
   - continue alternating 30 compressions (at rate of 100 beats/min) with 2 strong breaths

Attach automated external defibrillator (if necessary).

Note: The ratio of 30:2 with one or two rescuers is favoured. Some authorities recommended continuous compression only. This is most appropriate for the untrained resuscitator.

The basic schedule for cardiopulmonary resuscitation is presented in TABLE 128.2.

Method of rescue breathing/ventilation

With the victim's head in the 'sniffing the morning air' position (head totally tilted back and chin pulled forward) the rescuer takes a deep breath and seals his or her lips around the mouth or nose of the victim. Pinch the victim's nose if using mouth-to-mouth resuscitation. Five full breaths are given within 10 seconds (see FIG. 128.8 and FIG. 128.9). Rescue breathing/ventilation (also called expired air resuscitation—EAR) is the only method of artificial respiration that successfully ventilates the patient.[10] If the chest does not move easily, obstruction is present. If available, a sucker should be used to clear the oropharynx. Firmly fitting dentures should be left in place as they make artificial respiration easier. A Resuscitube or Laerdal pocket mask (which should be in the doctor's bag) is ideal for EAR; it saves mouth-to-mouth contact and probably improves the efficacy of ventilations.

External chest compression

Evidence supports the need to maintain cardiac compression following a cardiac arrest. This should be commenced on any person who is not responsive and not breathing normally.

Compressions are safely performed by finding the xiphisternal notch then placing the broad heel of one hand over the lower half of the sternum (in adults) with

Table 128.2 Basic schedule for CPR

	Infant <1 year	Child	Adult
Compression (rate per min)	100–120	100–120	100–120
Depth of compression (cm)	2–3	3–4	4–5
Position of compression	Centre sternum	Centre sternum	4 cm above xiphisternum
Method	2 fingers	1 hand	2 hands
Ventilation (rate per minute)	20	16	12
Head tilt	Nil	Mid	Full

Note: Check the International Liaison Committee on Resuscitation (ILCOR) guidelines <www.ilcor.org>.

For optimal airway patency:

1 Clear foreign matter from mouth: use finger sweep from airway: blow between shoulder blades; consider a Heimlich manoeuvre

2 Lay patient supine on flat, firm surface (A). Note how the soft tissue of the pharynx can obstruct the airway by falling backwards.

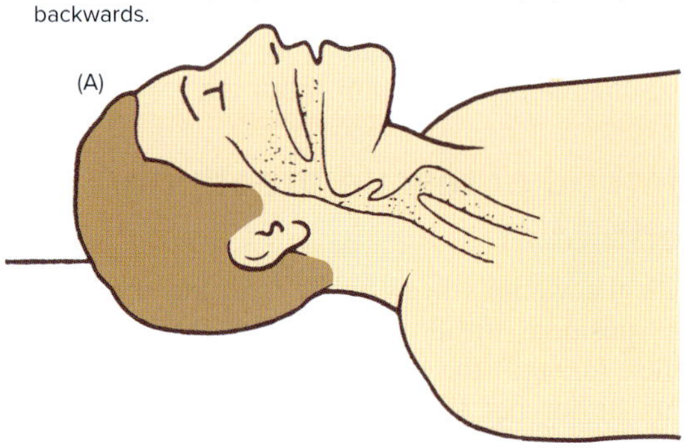

3 In order to overcome this, apply a head tilt (B) plus a chin lift (C) or jaw thrust manoeuvre.
(*Note:* avoid excessive movement of the neck if spinal injury is suspected, but clearing the airway has first priority.)

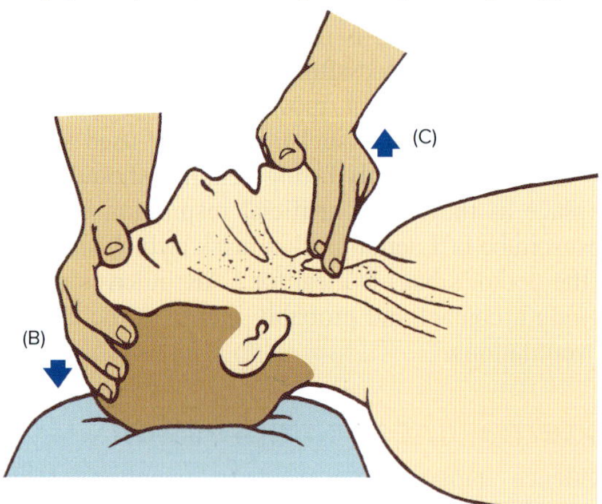

Slight flexion of the neck with small cushion

FIGURE 128.8 Basic life support: A = Airway

the heel of the second hand placed over the first with the fingers interlocked. Remember to keep the arms and elbows straight as the sternum is rhythmically depressed for 4–5 cm or one-third of chest length. Try to keep to this position as 'wandering' causes fractured ribs or worse. The fingers must be kept off the chest.

Maintain the compression for 0.5 seconds, then relax—compressions should be smooth, regular and uninterrupted.

Check pupil size and reaction to light and the carotid or femoral pulse. The compressions should ideally produce an impulse in the femoral pulse. Another person can check for carotid or femoral pulsation during CPR.

Rescue breathing:

1 Five full breaths within 10 seconds.
2 Observe rise of chest, not of abdomen.
3 Look, listen and feel for exhalation.
4 Check the carotid pulse.
5 If no pulse, commence full cardiopulmonary resuscitation.

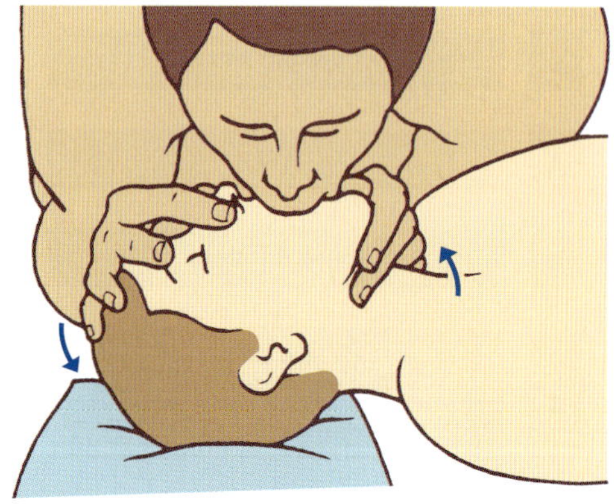

FIGURE 128.9 Basic life support: B = Breathing

Maintenance of CPR

Consider ceasing CPR if there is no improvement in 30 minutes. Exceptions where prolonged CPR can be successful are cold water drowning, electrical injuries, marine envenomation, snake bite and certain poisonings (e.g. cyanide and organophosphate).

Advanced cardiac life support

Advanced life support depends on the availability of skilled personnel and appropriate equipment.

Optimal initial support involves:

- airway management
- endotracheal intubation (otherwise bag and oxygen)
- ECG monitoring
- intravenous access (large peripheral or central vein)

Optimal initial therapy involves:

- defibrillation
- oxygen
- cardioactive drugs, especially adrenaline

If an ECG recording is unavailable the best course of action is:

- defibrillation
- if unsuccessful, adrenaline IV; repeat every 3 minutes

Consider anti-arrhythmic agents—amiodarone, lignocaine, magnesium.

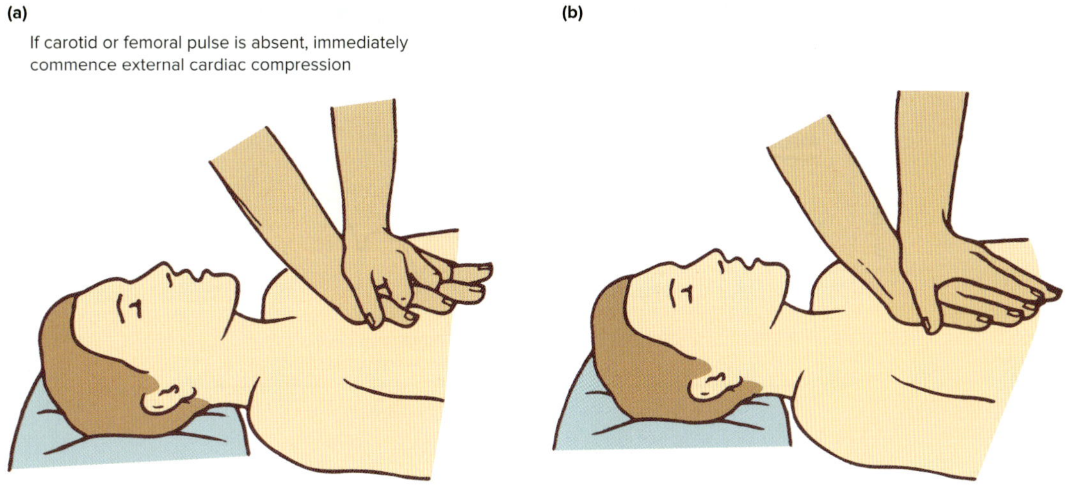

External cardiac compression with fingers locked **(a)**, and with fingers extended **(b)**. Heel of one hand placed on lower sternum 2 finger breadths above the xiphoid sternal junction. Heel of second hand placed on first. Ensure fingers don't exert pressure. The patient should be lying on a firm surface, the operator level with shoulder.

FIGURE 128.10 Basic life support: C = Circulation

Advanced life support: defibrillation[12,13]

- Minimise interruptions to chest compressions.
- Give a single shock instead of stacked shocks (single shock strategy) for ventricular fibrillation/pulseless ventricular tachycardia.
- Where the arrest is witnessed by a health care professional and a manual defibrillator is available, then up to three shocks may be given (stacked shock strategy) at the first defibrillation attempt.
- Biphasic defibrillation (usually biphasic at 360 joules)—where specific devices have been identified to be efficacious at other energy levels these should be used if known. *However*, where the health care professional is unsure of the energy level recommended for a specific device, a default energy level of 200 J should be used without delay.
- After each defibrillation attempt give 2 minutes of CPR before checking rhythm and pulse.

For defibrillation, two paddles or pads should be placed correctly on the chest wall, using one of two positions:

- one to right of upper sternum (under right clavicle) and the other over the apex of the heart (see FIG. 128.11)
- one over anterior wall of chest and the other under tip of left scapula

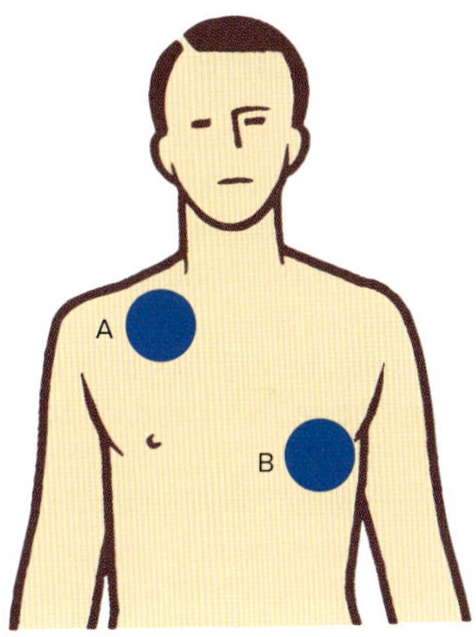

FIGURE 128.11 Standard position of two paddles for defibrillation: A under right clavicle, B under left breast

Hairs on the chest should be shaved to accommodate the paddles.

Urgent intravenous access

It is preferable to aim for transcutaneous cannulation of veins initially so a peripheral line should be introduced into a vein in the cubital fossa. Several lines may be required with massive blood loss.

Alternative routes:

- central venous cannulation: most doctors should be able to cannulate the external jugular vein with a standard cannula

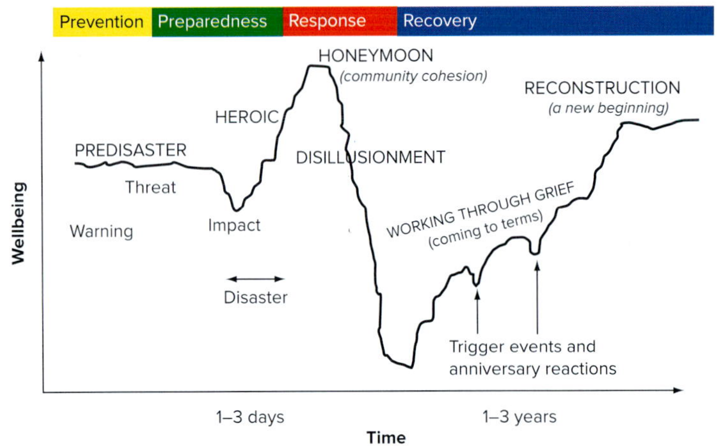

FIGURE 128.12 Phases of disaster: a storyline of disasters over time shows both the phases of disaster and prevention/preparedness/response/recovery (PPRR)[15]

Source: Reproduced in adapted form after modification from RJ Ursano et al;[15] *Training Manual for Human Services Workers in Major Disasters* (2nd edn). Washington DC: Department of Health and Human Services, Substance Abuse and Mental Health Services Administration, 2000; and RJ Ursano et al.: page 8[15]

- peripheral venous cutdown
- intraosseous infusion (see CHAPTER 96)

Disaster medicine

The frequency of disasters and the number of people affected by them are increasing. This is due to a number of factors, including increased media coverage, global movement of populations, and human habitation in more disaster-prone areas.

Disaster management is a crucial, rapidly expanding discipline in the world of general practice. 'The World Medical Association recommends that disaster medicine training be included in the curricula of university and postgraduate courses in medicine'.[14]

Disaster situations 'from the medical standpoint . . . are characterised by an acute and unforeseen *imbalance* between the capacity and *resources* of the medical profession and the *needs* of survivors who are injured, or whose health is threatened, over a given period of time'.[15]

Disaster management differs relative to the time of disaster impact, with four phases to be considered: prevention, preparedness (disaster impact), response and recovery (PPRR). Management also varies depending on the hazard that caused the disaster: for example, bushfire, flood, heatwave, drought, nuclear accident or terrorism.

Key facts and checkpoints

- Preparedness:
  - Evidence shows that preparedness helps in recovery.[16]
- Response:
  - It is valuable for GPs to maintain an up-to-date vulnerable patients list.
  - Maintenance of business-as-usual is the most crucial GP response.
- Recovery:
  - May take days, weeks, months, years or decades.
  - Most people recover with limited to no assistance, and the temptation to insist upon psychological therapy for all should be resisted.
- Self-care:
  - GPs could be considered a vulnerable group during a disaster in their community.

A systematic approach

It is useful to consider a GP's role according to the four phases of disaster, PPRR. In order to do this a general practice would benefit from an emergency response plan or disaster plan.[17]

During the acute event, emergency response systems, including fire, ambulance and police services, work with GPs to provide the most benefit, and to minimise the risk of potential harm to themselves, the patients or other responders.

In an isolated area, the GP may be the only respondent for a considerable time. In this situation triage and improvisation are important.

Recovery

In the first weeks

There is distress, denial and disbelief, lasting days to weeks. Most people will recover. Some will require minimal support; a few will require greater support.

In order to reduce distress due to a traumatic experience, psychological first aid (PFA) aims to improve short-term and long-term functioning. It is evidence-informed and endorsed by the World Health Organization (WHO) and the Australian Red Cross.[18] Such first aid opens the door for some to go on to more significant counselling, but this more formal therapy should not be 'thrust upon' everyone by well-meaning authorities.

Psychological first aid (PFA)

PFA requires no psycho-education. It involves:

- ensuring individuals are physically safe, with shelter and basic human needs met
- comforting and quietly listening to what individuals want to say. It is *not* asking individuals to talk about what happened, or telling them it is good for them to talk about it
- connecting individuals with loved ones or friends
- orientating individuals to goals to improve the sense of efficacy—small, practical, achievable tasks assist the return to normal routine[18]

GPs who are already part of the community have a significant head start when it comes to offering PFA. PFA is not *critical incident stress debriefing,* which has not been shown to be useful, and may even be harmful to some individuals.

In the following weeks, months and years

As mentioned above, most patients and families will recover unassisted. Physical and mental health effects of a disaster may coexist in the aftermath.[19] A key element is surveillance for deterioration of chronic conditions, emerging mental and physical health conditions,[19] and increased substance use.

Supporting children is best done by supporting their parents[20] and by assisting them to return to a normal routine.[21] Recurrent viewing of the event on media is not recommended.

Disasters divide lives in two; for some the effects may endure for decades, or span generations, depending on the characteristics of the individuals, the families and the disaster.[22]

References

1 Murtagh J. The anatomy of a rural practice. Aust Fam Physician, 1981; 10: 564–7.

2 O'Driscoll B et al. British Thoracic Society guideline for oxygen use in adults in healthcare and emergency settings. BMJ Open Respiratory Research, 2017;4:e000170.

3 Mehr S, Kemp A. Anaphylaxis. Update. Medical Observer, 2 October 2009: 24–5.

4 Moulds R (Chair). *Therapeutic Guidelines: Toxicology and Wilderness* (Version 2). Melbourne: Therapeutic Guidelines Ltd, 2012.

5 Buckley N (Chair). *Australian Medical Handbook.* Adelaide: Australian Medicines Handbook Pty Ltd, 2013: 660–5.

6 Crocker B, Thomson S. Lightning injuries. Patient Management, 1991; November: 51–5.

7 Macintosh I, Austin S. Management of drowning in children. J Paediatr Child Health, 2017; 9: 415–19.

8 Isbister G, Bawaskar H. Scorpion envenomation. NEJM, 2014; 5: 457–63.

9 Rathbone J et al. Review article: Role of magnesium sulphate in the management of Irukandji syndrome: a systematic review. Emerg Med Australas, 2017; 29: 9–17.

10 Kumar PJ, Clarke MC. *Clinical Medicine* (5th edn). London: Bailliere Tindall, 2003: 781–2.

11 Papadakis MA, McPhee SJ. *Current Medical Diagnosis and Treatment* (52nd edn). New York: The McGraw-Hill Companies, 2013: 392–3.

12 Jacobs IG (Chair). New changes to resuscitation guidelines. Australian Resuscitation Council, 2006. <www.resus.org.au>

13 American Heart Association in collaboration with the International Liaison Committee on Resuscitation. Guidelines 2000 for cardiopulmonary resuscitation and emergency cardiovascular care: international consensus on science, part 3: adult basic life support. Resuscitation, 2000; 46 (1–3): 29–71.

14 World Medical Association. A Statement on Medical Ethics in the Event of Disasters. 57th WMA General Assembly, October 2006.

15 Ursano RJ, Fullerton CS, Weisaeth L et al. Individual and community responses to disasters. In: Ursano RJ et al (eds), *Textbook of Disaster Psychiatry.* Cambridge: Cambridge University Press, 2007: 8.

16 Bissell RA, Pinet L, Nelson M et al. Evidence of the effectiveness of health sector preparedness in disaster response: the example of four earthquakes. Family & Community Health, Jul-Sep 2004; 27 (3): 193–203.

17 RACGP. Emergency Response Planning Tool 2013 (accessed 4 January 2104). <www.erpt.racgp.org.au>

18 World Health Organization (WHO). *Psychological First Aid: Guide for Field Workers.* Geneva: World Health Organization, 2011.

19 Freedy JR, Simpson WM Jr. Disaster-related physical and mental health: a role for the family physician. Am Fam Physician, 2007; 75 (6): 841–6.

20 MacDonald E, Olesen S, Harris A et al. *Guide for Health Professionals Working in Primary Care.* ACATLGN, 2010.

21 Wooding S, Raphael B. Psychological impact of disasters and terrorism on children and adolescents: experiences from Australia. Prehosp Disaster Med, Jan–Mar 2004; 19 (1): 10–20.

22 Raphael B. *NSW Health: Disaster Mental Health Manual,* 2012.

129 The doctor's bag and other emergency equipment

Almost everyone who goes to bed counts upon a full night's rest: like a picket at the outposts, the doctor must be ever on call.

Karl F Marx (1796–1877)

GPs who perform home visits and nursing home visits require the traditional doctor's bag that includes the basic tools of trade: drugs (including those for emergency use), stationery and various miscellaneous items. Country doctors will by necessity use their bag for more emergency home and roadside calls. These recommended contents are simply a guide for cross-checking.

Essential requirements for the bag

- Sturdiness
- Lockable (e.g. combination lock)
- Ready interior access
- Uncluttered
- Disposable single-use items
- Light, portable equipment
- Regular checks to ensure non-expired drugs
- Storage in a cool place (not boot of car)

Traditionalists may prefer the Gladstone bag, whose style confers a sense of time-honoured assurance. Pragmatists may opt for a fishing tackle box: far from elegant, but the sight of those organised compartments emerging during a crisis can calm the nerves.

Stationery (checklist)

- Practice letterhead and envelopes
- Prescription pads
- Sickness/off-work certificates
- X-ray, pathology referral forms
- Accounting and Medicare forms
- Dangerous drugs record books
- Continuation notes
- Tie-on labels for emergencies
- Recommendation forms (to psychiatric/mental hospitals)
- Pens

Many of these items will increasingly be replaceable by a portable computer connected to a virtual 'paperless' office.

Miscellaneous items

- Quick reference cards:
  - the doctor's bag checklist[1]
  - dosage details of drugs, all age groups
- Handbook of emergency medicine

Many details can be stored on a smartphone, including drug dosage apps, local maps and local emergency phone numbers.

Equipment

- Sphygmomanometer (aneroid)
- Stethoscope
- Pulse oximeter
- Diagnostic set (auriscope + ophthalmoscope)
- Tongue depressors
- Tourniquet
- Small needle disposal bottle
- Scissors
- Syringes 2, 5, 10 mL
- Needles 19, 21, 23, 25 gauge
- Scalp veins (butterfly) needles
- IV cannulae 16, 18, 20 gauge
- Alcohol swabs
- Micropore tape
- Thermometer
- Spacer (e.g. Volumatic, for asthma)
- Artery forceps
- Urine testing sticks
- Pathology specimen bottles
- Skin swabs, throat swabs
- Torch
- Patellar hammer
- Oral airway (e.g. Revivatube, Resuscitube—FIG. 129.1, Guedel)
- Laerdal pocket mask (FIG. 129.2)
- Scalpel (disposable)
- Examination gloves

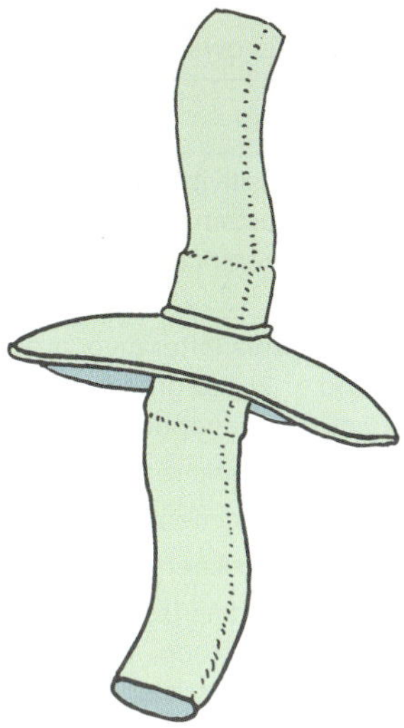

FIGURE 129.1 The two-way Resuscitube

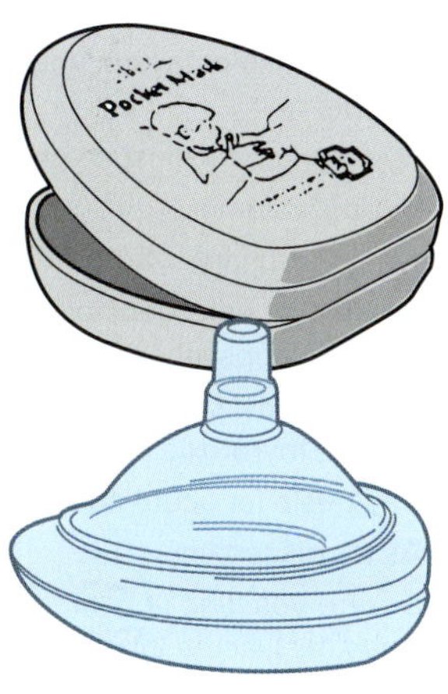

FIGURE 129.2 The Laerdal pocket mask

Drugs

Drugs (oral)

- Samples of commonly used:
  - analgesics
  - antibiotics
  - antidiarrhoeal agents
  - anti-emetics
  - antihistamines
  - sedatives
- Glyceryl trinitrate (although sublingual tablets deteriorate after opening)
- Soluble aspirin (for myocardial infarction)
- Sumatriptan

Drugs (sprays)

- Glyceryl trinitrate
- Salbutamol aerosol

Drugs (topical)

- Anaesthetic eyedrops

Drugs (injectable)

Refer to TABLE 129.1.

A study of 512 Queensland GPs revealed the range of emergency equipment and essential drugs carried.[4] The most common emergencies were acute asthma, psychiatric emergencies, seizures, hypoglycaemia, anaphylaxis, impaired consciousness, shock, poisoning and overdose. The drugs used most were adrenaline, benztropine, diazepam, glucagon, haloperidol, hydrocortisone, naloxone and salbutamol (inhaler).

The issue of what drugs to carry is always an interesting intellectual exercise. It could reduce to just a few items such as adrenaline, diazepam, naloxone and morphine.[5] Doctors who are called to manage emergencies more frequently and in more remote locations generally prefer a broader range of drugs, which requires increased checking of stocks.

Drugs (suppositories)

- Indomethacin

The country doctor's bag

Rural doctors, especially in isolated areas, usually carry additional equipment in their motor vehicles when called to the scene of an accident or other emergency. The equipment will vary according to geographic factors, the ambulance service and the special interests and enthusiasm of the practitioner.

Storage of drugs

The main issues are safe storage of opioid drugs, avoidance of overheating (keep <25°C), accessibility in emergencies and careful recording of Schedule 8 drugs in a register. Diphtheria and tetanus vaccines should be stored in a refrigerator.

Emergency drugs

The value of emergency drugs for the doctor's bag continues to be debated. Essential drugs are highlighted in TABLE 129.1. One challenging paper suggests that drugs such as penicillin, diazepam, haloperidol, chlorpromazine, frusemide and tramadol be replaced.[2] The options recommended as more appropriate would be ceftriaxone or cefotaxime (for severe infections),

129

Table 129.1 Drugs available on PBS (except those marked #) <www.pbs.gov.au/browse/doctorsbag>[2,3]

Drug	Presentation	Indications
Adrenaline*	1 mg/mL (1:1000)	Hypersensitivity reactions and anaphylactic shock, asthma†, ventricular asystole, croup, ventricular fibrillation (to assist CPR)
Atropine sulphate	0.6 mg/1 mL	Bradycardia (after myocardial infarction), 2nd or 3rd degree heart block, ureteric colic†, organophosphate poisoning
Benztropine*	Cogentin 2 mg/2 mL	Acute dystonic reactions
Benzylpenicillin*	3 g with 10 mL water	Meningococcaemia, pneumonia (adults)
Ceftriaxone#	2 g powder with 10 mL solvent	Meningococcaemia, septicaemia
Dexamethasone	4 mg/1 mL	Severe asthma (esp. elderly), moderate to severe croup, anaphylaxis, acute Addisonian crisis
Diazepam*	10 mg/2 mL	Status epilepticus and other convulsions such as eclampsia, sedation in acute anxiety and severe tension headache, psychiatric emergencies including acute alcohol withdrawal
Frusemide*	Lasix 20 mg/2 mL	Left ventricular failure, acute pulmonary oedema
Glucagon*	1 mg + 1 mL solvent	Hypoglycaemia (insulin or oral therapy)
Glucose#	50% (500 mg/mL in 50 mL)	Hypoglycaemia
Glyceryl trinitrate*	Spray 400 mcg/dose	Acute coronary syndrome
Haloperidol*	Serenace 5 mg/1 mL	Psychiatric emergencies such as severe agitation, psychoses; migraine
Hydrocortisone sodium succinate*	100 or 250 mg/2 mL	Anaphylaxis, severe asthma, Addisonian crisis, thyrotoxic crisis, acute allergies
Methoxyflurane	3 mL pack with inhaler	Analgesia for acute pain
Midazolam#	5 mg/1 mL	As for diazepam
Metoclopramide* or	Maxolon 10 mg/2 mL	Severe vomiting (e.g. Meniere syndrome, gastritis), acute labyrinthitis, migraine
Prochlorperazine	Stemetil 12.5 mg/mL	
Morphine sulphate*	15 mg/1 mL or 30 mg/1 mL	Acute pulmonary oedema, relief of severe pain (e.g. cardiac pain, colic)
Naloxone (more than one ampoule)*	Narcan 0.4 mg/mL	Opiate respiratory depression
Oxytocin	10 units/1 mL	Postpartum haemorrhage
Promethazine*	Phenergan 50 mg/2 mL	Acute allergic conditions (see FIG. 129.3), anti-emetic†
Salbutamol*	MD inhaler and/or nebuliser solution	Bronchial asthma, other bronchospasm
Tramadol	100 mg/2 mL	Moderate to severe pain
Water	5 mL	diluent

*Essential drugs

†May be useful as an alternative drug

#Drugs not supplied as PBS doctor's bag items

All drugs listed are injectable except salbutamol inhaler

Note: The author recommends the 'Minijet' syringe packs for ideal emergency use. The range includes naloxone 5 mL, aminophylline, atropine, adrenaline, dextrose, lignocaine, isoprenaline, sodium bicarbonate

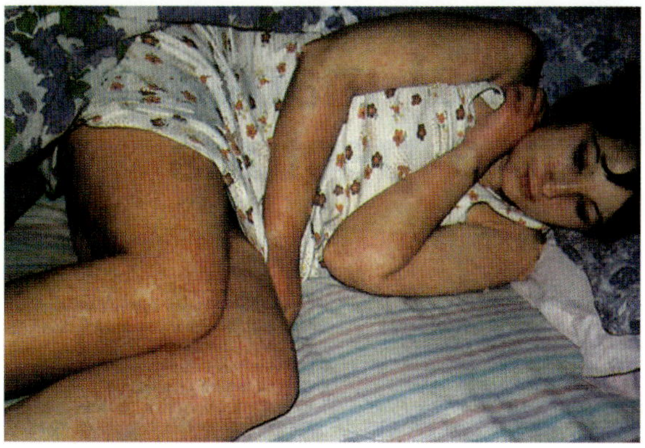

FIGURE 129.3 Home visit to a 25-year-old woman with acute urticaria caused by an upper respiratory viral infection. She was given 25 mg promethazine IM for severe pruritus and vomiting

midazolam, olanzapine and amiodarone, while CPAP or BIPAP is preferable to frusemide for acute ventricular failure.

Medical emergencies in general practice—a management proposal

Note: Using basic equipment and doctor's bag (mainly adult dosages)

Don't forget:

- **Secure IV line (may need rapid bolus N saline)**
- **Oxygen (where recommended)**
- **Measure vital signs**

Acute cardiogenic pulmonary oedema (ventricular failure)	Frusemide 40–80 mg IV (or twice usual dose) Glyceryl trinitrate 1 dose (spray) Consider (especially if chest pain)—morphine 2.5–5 mg IV
Acute anaphylaxis	Adrenaline 0.3–0.5 mg (1:1000) IM, repeat every 3 minutes as necessary or set up adrenaline infusion (see CHAPTER 128) If no rapid improvement: • salbutamol inhalation • IV fluids • ? hydrocortisone/glucagon
Angio-oedema and acute urticaria	Promethazine 25 mg IM
Asthma	Salbutamol 6 (<6 years)–12 (adults) puffs by spacer Hydrocortisone 200 mg IV If severe: • adrenaline 0.3–0.5 mg 1:1000 IM or SC or infusion
Croup (severe)	Dexamethasone 0.15 mg/kg IM or prednisolone 1 mg/kg (o)
Epilepsy (seizure)	Diazepam 5–20 mg IV or midazolam 0.2 mg/kg IM
Opiate respiratory depression	Naloxone HCl 0.4 (or 0.2) mg IV + 0.4 mg IM
Acute coronary syndrome	Aspirin 300 mg soluble tab Glyceryl trinitrate spray or tablets (max. 3) If pain, morphine sulphate 2.5–5 mg IV + metoclopramide
Hypoglycaemia	Glucagon 1 mg/mL SC, IM or IV, then sweet drink or 20–30 mL 50% glucose IV
Migraine (severe)	Prochlorperazine 12.5 mg IV *or* Metoclopramide 10 mg IV ± dihydroergotamine IV or IM *or* Haloperidol 5 mg IM or 1V
Cluster headache	100% oxygen 6 L/min for 15 minutes Metoclopramide 10 mg IV
Movement disorders (from antipsychotic medication)	Benztropine 1–2 mg IV or IM
Meningococcaemia	Benzylpenicillin 60 mg/kg IV
Ureteric colic	Morphine 10–15 mg IM or IV ± metoclopramide Indomethacin suppository
Vertigo (acute)	Prochlorperazine 12.5–25 mg IM or promethazine 25 mg IM
Vomiting	Prochlorperazine 12.5 mg IM or IV or metoclopramide 10 mg

Practice tips

- Check your doctor's bag every month for drugs that may be expired, damaged or in short supply (your practice nurse can do this).[3]
- Replace any used drugs or materials the day after use.
- Always have your bag handy but don't carry it in the car in hot weather. It is best to be able to grab it from a safe, accessible spot when you leave for an emergency.
- Security is an issue. Drugs of addiction (tramadol and morphine) may be kept separate and then taken from their secure place when their use is anticipated (e.g. myocardial infarction, severe biliary or kidney colic). Tramadol appears to be a satisfactory alternative but beware of the serotonin syndrome.
- Keep a spare kit in your surgery if you or your assistants or locums perform a lot of emergency work.
- Familiarise yourself with the layout of your bag so that using it in urgent circumstances is efficient.
- Use a large intravenous cannula wherever possible if rapid infusion is required.

References

1 Hogan C. Home visits, emergencies and use of the doctor's bag. Medical Observer, 28 April 2000: 73–5.
2 Holmes J. Time to restock the doctor's bag. Aust Prescriber, 2012; 35: 7–9.
3 Baird A. Emergency drugs in general practice. Aust Fam Physician, 2008; 37 (7): 541–6.
4 Johnston CL et al. Medical emergencies in general practice in south-east Queensland: prevalence and practice preparedness. Med J Aust, 2001; 175: 99–103.
5 Murtagh J. The doctor's bag. What do you really need? Aust Fam Physician, 2000; 29 (1): 25–8.

Stroke and transient ischaemic attacks

130

A mild attack of apoplexy may be called death's retaining fee.

GILLES MÉNAGE (1613–92)

Glossary of terms

Stroke A focal neurological deficit lasting longer than 24 hours caused by intracerebral haemorrhage or infarction.

Stroke in evolution An enlarging neurological deficit, presumably due to infarction, which increases over 24–48 hours.

Transient cerebral ischaemic attack (TIA) A transient episode of neurological dysfunction caused by focal brain, spinal cord or retinal ischaemia without infarction.[1]

Key facts and checkpoints

- Stroke is the second most common (10–12%) cause of death in the Western world. Most are ischaemic (thrombotic or embolic), but 15–20% are haemorrhagic.
- A stroke or TIA must be considered a medical emergency.
- One in 10 patients with a TIA is likely to have a stroke shortly afterwards—usually within 2 weeks and most within 48 hours. The risk is greatest if older than 60, symptoms last more than 10 minutes and there is weakness or a speech impediment with the TIA.[2]
- Clinical assessment (including neurological examination) investigations and treatment should be commenced quickly.
- The best approach to stroke management is aggressive attention to primary and secondary prevention.
- The main risk factors for stroke are atrial fibrillation, hypertension, smoking, age and diabetes.
- Cardiac disease can be a source of emboli.
- Most patients with a stroke or TIA require urgent imaging to find the cause and guide treatment.
- Ideally, patients should be referred to a stroke unit ASAP—within 3 hours.
- Order a CT or MRI scan on all patients with suspected TIAs and strokes (if not referring to a stroke unit): if normal, repeat within 7 days (CT scans unreliable after 7 days). Such imaging is required to differentiate between ischaemia and haemorrhage.
- Consider the possibility of a cryptogenic stroke,[1] especially from a patent foramen ovale (PFO) (in 20–25% of population and responsible for 50% of cryptogenic strokes) in relatively young people presenting with a stroke: this leads to paradoxical emboli (from veins to the brain). PFOs may be detected by echocardiography and sealed with a percutaneous closure device, although this is not routine.
- Consider the possibility of endocarditis if there is a heart murmur.
- Keep in mind atherosclerotic disease of the aortic arch as a source of cerebral embolism.
- The place of carotid endarterectomy for asymptomatic carotid stenosis remains controversial. It should be seriously considered if the stenosis is severe, the risk of surgery is low (3% risk of major stroke), the team has proven expertise and the patient is medically fit with a good life expectancy.[1]
- Carotid artery stenting for the treatment and prevention of stroke is an evolving procedure.

Modifiable risk factors for cerebrovascular disease[2]

Major: hypertension, smoking, cardiovascular disease, atrial fibrillation (especially valvular), diabetes.

Others: cardiac failure, dyslipidaemia, obesity, alcohol excess, oral contraception, migraine, stress.

Control of risk factors is the key approach to management. Control of hypertension, including systolic hypertension in the elderly, and smoking cessation are vital factors for reduction of the incidence of stroke. A meta-analysis of 14 randomised trials showed that a reduction of blood pressure of

5–6 mmHg is associated with about 40% reduction in stroke incidence.[1]

130

Stroke

Facts[1]

- Stroke is the third most common cause of death in Australia.
- About one-third of people who have a stroke will die within 1 month.
- About 50% of ischaemic strokes are preceded by TIAs.
- Symptomatic carotid artery stenosis is the major risk factor for stroke.
- Thromboembolism from vascular disease outside the brain causes 70% of strokes and 90% of TIAs.
- Such sources are atheromatous plaques within the carotid or vertebral systems or cardiac causes (e.g. postmyocardial infarction).
- Echocardiography is an important investigation with TIAs since LV dysfunction and the size of the left atrium are the strongest independent predictors of thromboembolism.

Pathophysiological groups of cerebral infarction

The three main groups are:

- single penetrator or small vessel disease (lacunar syndrome)—probably due to in situ small vessel disease
- cardio–emboli (heart to artery embolism)
- large vessel artery-to-artery embolic infarcts (see TABLE 130.1)

Differential diagnosis ('stroke mimics')

- Syncope
- Seizure (and subsequent Todd paresis)
- Migraine
- Cerebral tumour and other space-occupying lesions
- Hypoglycaemia
- Hyponatraemia
- Delirium
- Head injury
- MELAS syndrome
- Medically unexplained (e.g. somatisation)

Table 130.1 Types and incidence of stroke[2]

Stroke subtype	Frequency (%)
Haemorrhagic stroke:	
• primary intracerebral	10
• subarachnoid haemorrhage	5
Ischaemic stroke:	
• large vessel (artery-to-artery embolism)	30
• cardio–embolic	20
• small vessels (lacunar infarcts)	15
• uncertain type	15
• rare (e.g. venous infarction)	5

Diagnostic guidelines

- Sudden stroke is typical of embolism.
- The clinical picture depends on the vessel involved.
- In young people <50 years consider PFO.
- With cerebral haemorrhage the stroke evolves steadily, often over hours: the putamen (50%) is the commonest site.
- Lacunar CVAs:
  - small, deep infarcts
  - pure motor hemiplegia most common effect
  - lack of cortical signs
  - the neurological deficit may progress over 24–36 hours
  - outcome usually good
- Investigate all, including SAH, with CT scans or MRI (may need a lumbar puncture for SAH diagnosis). MRI is preferred if available.
- Carotid duplex Doppler ultrasound scan can accurately determine atherosclerotic narrowing of the extracranial carotid circulation.

Pitfalls

- Mistaking visual or sensory migraine equivalents in young adults for TIAs
- Mistaking a CVA for labyrinthitis (rare over 50 years)
- Failure to perform carotid duplex Doppler ultrasound or CT scan before starting aspirin for TIA or small stroke (because of missing small haemorrhage, unsuspected tumour or a subdural)
- Diagnosing small stroke as a lacuna (may be a stroke in evolution)

Management

The development of an acute stroke or TIA is a medical emergency and admission to a stroke unit (if available) as soon as possible is advised. Care in a stroke unit gives the patient the greatest chance of independent survival.[3]

Immediate

- Stabilise ventilation—consider intubation and oxygen.
- Exclude head trauma.
- Obtain urgent CT or MRI scan (non-contrast CT scan is emerging investigation of choice).

- Treat any seizures.
- Treat any hypoglycaemia.

General

- Investigate, including carotid duplex Doppler ultrasound (for carotid territory symptoms).
- Treat hypertension (systolic >140) vigorously—it carries a six times increased risk of stroke.
- Give IV fluid, electrolyte and nutritional support (nil orally until swallowing has been assessed).
- Good nursing care is the cornerstone of management.
- Physiotherapy and speech therapy.
- Vigorous rehabilitation.
- Clot extraction for intracerebral haemorrhage: consider urgent surgical evacuation for haematomas of the posterior fossa (cerebellum) and cerebral white matter.[1] Shunt insertion may be needed. No medical therapy is of proven value.
- SAH: requires urgent referral (vasospasm and rebleeding are the main causes of morbidity and mortality):
  - nimodipine ± surgery
- Ischaemic stroke: give aspirin 150–300 mg (o) daily within 48 hours if CT scan/MRI has excluded cerebral haemorrhage or other blood-thinning agents are not used. Early intervention within 3–4.5 hours (ideally) of onset with tissue plasminogen activator (tPA). Recent trials indicate improved outcomes with tPA (but not with streptokinase). However, there appears to be a 5–7% risk of intracerebral haemorrhage[1] and slight increase in incidence of death in the first few days.

The usual thrombolytic tPA therapy is alteplase 0.9 mg/kg up to 90 mg IV over 1 hour, with 10% of the dose given as an initial bolus[1] or tenecteplase. Withhold aspirin for 24 hours.

Note: Avoid steroids, mannitol, haemodilution and anticoagulation in acute stroke.[4]

Transient ischaemic attacks

Clinical features

- Sudden onset and short duration (<60 minutes)
- Usually complete clinical recovery in less than 24 hours
- Consciousness usually preserved
- Ninety per cent usually in anterior circulation
- Carotid TIAs—unilateral features
- Vertebrobasilar TIAs—often have bilateral or crossed features

130

A comparison of the main clinical features of carotid (anterior circulation) ischaemia and vertebrobasilar (posterior circulation) ischaemia is presented in FIGURE 130.1. The carotid circulation accounts for 80% of TIAs.

Differential diagnoses of TIAs are presented in TABLE 130.2.

Some ischaemic syndromes

- Transient monocular blindness (amaurosis fugax)
- Transient hemisphere attacks
- The 'locked-in' syndrome

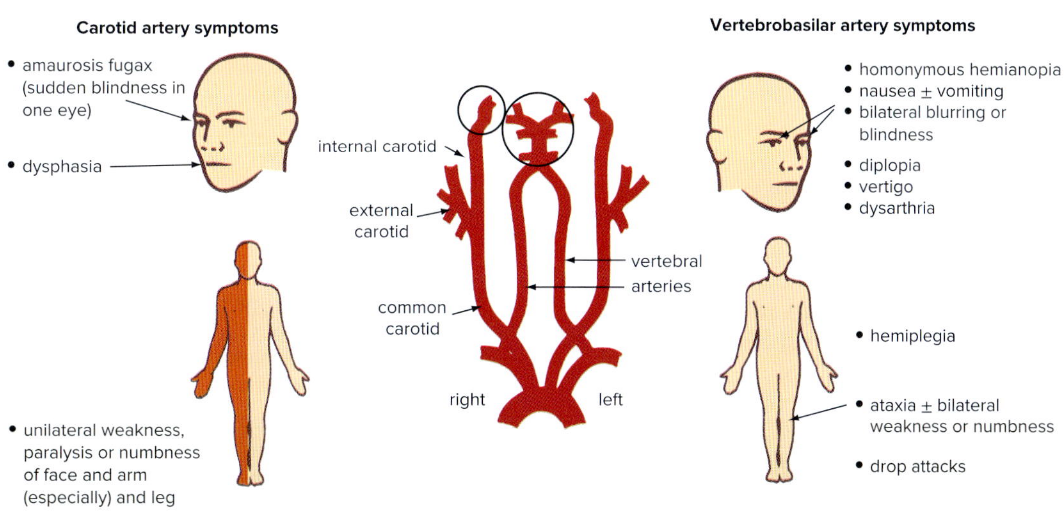

FIGURE 130.1 Cerebral arterial circulation with some important clinical features of carotid and vertebrobasilar ischaemia

Source: Reproduced with permission from C Kenna and J Murtagh, *Back Pain and Spinal Manipulation,* Sydney: Butterworth, 1989

Table 130.2 Differential diagnosis of TIAs

Classic migraine (with aura)
Unusual migraine variants:
- hemiplegic
- ophthalmoplegic
- retinal

Focal epileptic seizures:
- complex partial
- simple partial

Multiple sclerosis
Transient global amnesia
Syncope

Intracranial structural lesions:
- arteriovenous malformation
- tumour

Vestibular disorders:
- acute labyrinthitis

Benign paroxysmal positional vertigo
Meniere syndrome
Hypoglycaemia
Adverse drug reactions
Toxic reactions

Peripheral nerve lesions:
- carpal tunnel syndrome
- Bell palsy

Psychological conditions:
- anxiety/hyperventilation
- panic attacks
- somatisation

- Vertebrobasilar:
  - bilateral motor loss
  - crossed sensory and motor loss
  - diplopia
  - bilateral blurring or blindness

Amaurosis fugax

This is the sudden transient loss of vision in one eye (like a 'curtain or shade' coming from above or below) due to the passage of an embolus through the retinal vessels from ipsilateral carotid vessel disease. It is a feature of a TIA in the carotid artery circulation and is often the first clinical evidence of carotid stenosis.[5] About 20% of all TIAs present as amaurosis fugax.[6] Amaurosis fugax may forewarn of the development of hemiparesis or blindness and should be considered a matter for urgent attention and rectification. Give aspirin immediately. Carotid endarterectomy may be required for high grade stenosis.

Differential diagnosis of transient amaurosis fugax

- thromboembolic phenomena
- vasospasm
- temporal arteritis
- blood—sickle cell, polycythaemia
- retinal—haemorrhage, venous thrombosis, detachment
- optic neuritis
- vitreous floaters

Transient hemisphere attack (usually middle cerebral artery)

- Affects motor or sensory or both
- Usually face and arm (more than leg)
- Dysphasia common

The 'locked-in' syndrome

In this syndrome, which may be transient or persistent, patients remain conscious and aware of their dilemma but are unable to speak or move the limbs, particularly the arms. It may be possible to communicate with patients using eye responses to commands. The cause is invariably a lesion in the brain stem.

Significance of TIAs

- Five years after a TIA, 22–51% (average 1 in 3) patients (without treatment) will have a stroke.[5,7] This figure may be higher for those with ipsilateral high-grade (70% or more) carotid stenosis.
- The highest risk is in the first 6 months.
- A carotid artery TIA has more serious prognostic significance. Such patients are at high risk of developing a stroke that is potentially preventable.
- Referral for investigation is appropriate.
- All patients should have a carotid duplex Doppler ultrasound and CT scan or MRI at presentation.
- Cardiac status should be addressed because of an association with myocardial infarction.

ABCD2 stroke risk tool[6]

This screening tool is useful as a predictor for risk of stroke in the first 7 days of a TIA.

A = **A**ge ≥ 60 years (1 point)
B = **B**P ≥ 140 systolic or ≥ 90 diastolic (1 point)
C = **C**linical features: any unilateral limb weakness (2 points), speech impairment without weakness (1 point)

D1 = **D**uration: ≥ 60 minutes (2 points), 10–59 minutes (1 point), <10 minutes (0 points)
D2 = **D**iabetes: 1 point

Maximum 7 points
Scores: 0–3 = 1% risk of stroke at 2 days; 4–5 = 4% risk of stroke at 2 days; 6–7 = 8% risk of stroke at 2 days.

Variants on this tool include ABCD3.

Investigations[8]

- A CT scan, 12–lead ECG and carotid imaging are essential investigations in the first hours of a suspected TIA
- Blood tests, echocardiography, MRI and Holter or bedside cardiac monitoring are likely to improve diagnosis
- Carotid duplex Doppler ultrasound for carotid territory symptoms
- Transoesophageal echocardiography

Management

- All high-risk patients admitted to a stroke unit or specialist TIA clinic: urgent attention for atrial fibrillation and carotid artery stenosis
- Aim to minimise the risk of a major stroke
- Determine cause and correct it (if possible)
- Early neurorehabilitation
- Advise cessation of smoking and treat hypertension (if applicable)
- Anti-platelet therapy (especially for carotid ischaemia):

  aspirin 100–300 mg (o) daily (gives 30% protection from stroke or death after TIA)[9]
  or
  clopidogrel 75 mg (o) daily (or clopidogrel + aspirin)
  or
  dipyridamole CR + aspirin 200 mg/25 mg (o) bd (shows better outcomes than aspirin alone)[10]
  or
  ticlopidine (only if others unsuitable)

Antiplatelet therapy reduces the relative risk of stroke, myocardial infarction or vascular death by 22% (95% confidence interval 14–30%) in people with an ischaemic stroke or TIA due to arterial disease, compared with no treatment.[2]

- Anticoagulation therapy: warfarin:
  - for vertebrobasilar ischaemia (with increasing frequency of TIAs)
  - for failed anti-platelet therapy
  - use direct oral anticoagulants (DOACs) for non-valvular atrial fibrillation >65 years of age
- Carotid endarterectomy has been proven to have a place in the management of carotid artery stenosis; the decision depends on the expertise of the unit. There is no evidence that surgery is appropriate for asymptomatic patients, nor for symptomatic patients with a stenosis less than 50%. Symptomatic patients benefit from surgery particularly for stenoses greater than 70%.[11,12] If the stenosis is >90%, refer immediately. Greater than 75% stenosis is associated with a 2% per annum rate of ipsilateral ischaemic stroke.[1]
- Percutaneous transluminal angioplasty (stenting). Carotid artery stenting for the treatment and prevention of stroke should be restricted to those who are unsuitable for carotid endarterectomy.[11]

130

Guiding rules for carotid artery stenosis

70–99%—intervention
50–69%—'grey area': refer
<50%—observe

Atrial fibrillation[1,13]

- The main source of cardio–embolic infarction
- Increased with risk factors—hypertension, previous embolism and recent CHF (previous 3 months)
- With non-valvular AF, annual risk of CVA is 2.5% (no risk factors) to 17.6% (2 + risk factors)
- Risk of stroke about 6 times that of other people
- Intermittent AF can also be a risk

Management

- People with AF aged under 65 with no other risk factors do not require anticoagulant therapy.[14]
- Valvular disease: warfarin—target INR 2–3
- Non-valvular AF: calculate the risk-benefit ratio for anticoagulant therapy.
- Do not offer aspirin monotherapy solely for stroke prevention to people with AF.[14]

Selecting antithrombotic therapy in non-valvular AF is assisted by the $CHADS_2$ index, a validated tool (see TABLE 130.3). Many guidelines use a variation, the CHA_2DS_2-VASc score.

Table 130.3 CHADS$_2$ criteria and stroke risk[13] (for carotid and vertebral arteries)

CHADS$_2$ criteria	Points	Stroke risk	Recommended therapy
Previous stroke or TIA	2	High (2–6)	Warfarin (INR 2–3) or DOACs
Age ≥75 years	1	Moderate (1)	Warfarin or DOACs, but bleeding risk may outweigh benefit
Hypertension	1	Low (0)	Nil
Diabetes mellitus	1		
Heart failure	1		

130

Cerebral venous thrombosis[2]

This rare cause of stroke may present as an acute or chronic cerebrovascular disorder. It should be suspected particularly in women in the postpartum period presenting with severe headache or focal neurological defects. Diagnosis is by MRI. In the acute phase, treatment is by anticoagulation with heparin followed by warfarin for approximately 6 months.

Indications for carotid duplex Doppler ultrasound

- Bruit in neck
- TIAs if diagnosis uncertain
- Crescendo TIAs (two or more in 1 week and longer lasting)
- Internal carotid artery symptoms
- Hemispheric stroke
- Prior to major vascular surgery (e.g. CABG)

Stroke in children

Stroke in children is relatively uncommon. Causes include paradoxical embolus (e.g. PFO), cerebral vasculopathy (e.g. vasculitis), arterial dissection and metabolic disease. The most common clinical presentation of stroke in childhood is acute hemiparesis due to involvement of the carotid distribution.[1] Investigation includes immediate brain MRI or CT scan, transthoracic echocardiography, thrombophilia factors (e.g. V Leiden) and urine homocysteine. Consider also sickle-cell disease. Initial treatment within 48 hours and after imaging is aspirin 2–5 mg/kg up to 300 mg orally daily.

When to refer

- Refer immediately to a stroke unit
- Suspicion of SAH
- Carotid artery stenosis on carotid duplex Doppler ultrasound scan
- Cerebellar haemorrhage on CT scan
- Stroke in a young patient <50 years (consider PFO and other, less common causes)

Key checkpoints

Proven strategies

Three proven strategies to improve outcome of acute stroke (level I evidence):

- management in a stroke unit
- giving IV tPA within 3 hours of ischaemic stroke
- giving antiplatelet agents ASAP and within 48 hours of ischaemic stroke

First aid for stroke

Is it a stroke?
Think **FAST**
↓
Face (ask person to smile)
Arms (raise both arms)
Speech (speak a simple sentence)
Time (within 3 hours)
then, if yes
Refer to stroke unit ASAP
Don't give aspirin

Patient education resources

Hand-out sheets from *Murtagh's Patient Education* 7th edition:

- Stroke

References

1 Moulds R (Chair). *Therapeutic Guidelines: Neurology* (Version 3). Melbourne: Therapeutic Guidelines Ltd, 2011; 175–201.
2 Claiborne Johnston S et al. Short-term prognosis after emergency department diagnosis of TIA. JAMA, 2000; 284: 2901–6.

3 Stroke Unit Trialists' Collaboration. Organised inpatient (stroke unit) care for stroke (Cochrane Review). In: The Cochrane Library. Issue 3, 2004. Chichester, UK: John Wiley & Sons Ltd.
4 Lindley RI, Landau P. Early management of acute stroke. Australian Prescriber, 2004; 27: 120–3.
5 Kumar PJ, Clark ML. *Clinical Medicine* (7th edn). London: Elsevier Saunders, 2009: 767–93.
6 Rothwell PM et al. A simple score (ABCD) to identify individuals at high early risk of stroke after transient ischaemic attack. Lancet, 2005; 366: 29–36.
7 Joff R. Diagnosis and treatment of transient ischaemic attacks. Modern Medicine Australia, 1994; 37 (8): 18–23.
8 Worthington J. How to investigate patients following a TIA. Medicine Today, 2013; 14 (2): 13–21.
9 Leicester J. Stroke and transient cerebral ischaemic attacks. In: *MIMS Disease Index* (2nd edn). Sydney: IMS Publishing, 1996: 487–9.
10 Halkes PH et al. ESPRIT study group. Aspirin + dipyridamole versus aspirin alone after cerebral ischaemia of arterial origin: a randomised controlled trial. Lancet, 2006; 367: 1665–73.
11 Stroke Foundation. *Clinical Guidelines for Stroke Management 2017.* Melbourne, Australia.
12 North American Symptomatic Carotid Endarterectomy Trial (NASCENT). N Engl J Med, 1991; 325: 445–53.
13 Connolly S et al. Clopidogrel plus aspirin versus oral anticoagulation for atrial fibrillation in the Atrial fibrillation Clopidogrel Trial with Irbesartan for prevention of Vascular Events (ACTIVE W): a randomised controlled trial. Lancet, 2006; 367: 1903–12.
14 NICE Clinical Guideline. Atrial fibrillation: management. National Institute for Health and Care Excellence (UK), 2014.

Resources

National Stroke Foundation, Australia. *Clinical Guidelines for Stroke Management,* 2013. <www.strokefoundation.com.au>

European Society of Cardiology Guidelines <www.escardio.org>

131 Thrombosis and thromboembolism

Thrombosis is an ugly thought;
Dicumarol and heparin,
Statistics show, prevent most ills
Like thrombus of the coronary, infarction of the heart
And tests are made so many times
That arms turn blue and blood runs thin

David Littman, 'The Good Old Days', *N Engl J Med*, 1965

A thrombus is defined as a clot formed in the circulation from the constituents of the blood, whereas emboli are fragments of thrombus that break off and block vessels downstream. Almost half of adult deaths in Western countries are due to thrombosis of coronary or cerebral arteries, or to pulmonary embolism.[1] A thrombus is the result of a cascade of events involving platelets, RBCs, coagulation factors and the vessel wall.

Conditions predisposing to thrombosis:

- thrombophilia
- thrombocytosis (platelets)
- polycythaemia rubra vera

Thrombophilia[2]

Thrombophilia refers to a disorder of haemostasis in the form of a primary coagulopathy leading to a tendency to thrombosis. This should be considered in patients with major unprecipitated venous thromboembolism with or without a strong family history of venous thrombosis. Several causes can be tested, both inherited and acquired:

- inherited:
  - factor V Leiden gene mutation (activated protein C resistance)
  - prothrombin gene mutation
  - protein C deficiency
  - protein S deficiency
  - antithrombin deficiency
- acquired:
  - antiphospholipid antibodies (anticardiolipin or anti-ß$_2$ GPI)
  - elevated homocysteine level
  - lupus anticoagulant

The above factors can all be measured in the laboratory with specific genetic tests, coagulation or antibody-based tests. Other acquired causes (regarded as risk factors) include malignancy, oral contraceptives, HRT, immobilisation, obesity, smoking, pregnancy and major surgery. Most DVTs do not require investigation for an underlying cause, but consideration should be given to screening patients who have had an unprovoked DVT. Refer to a haematologist if thrombophilia is proven or suspected. Of particular interest is factor V Leiden, which occurs in about 4% of Caucasians; the relative risk of venous thrombosis is increased three to seven times in heterozygotes and 80 times in homozygotes.[2]

Indications for investigation

- Recurrent or unusual thrombosis
- Arterial thrombosis <30 years
- Skin necrosis, especially on warfarin
- Recurrent fetal loss
- Familial thromboembolism

Venous thromboembolism

A feature of venous thrombosis is that it develops in normal vessels, with key factors being stasis and increased coagulability, including thrombophilia. The classic example is deep venous thrombosis of the leg veins. Another poorly recognised thrombosis is axillosubclavian venous thrombosis, which is associated with pulmonary embolism in 30% of cases.[3]

Other sites of deep vein thrombosis are the pelvic/ovarian veins, which should be suspected in a person at risk with pelvic pain and swollen upper thighs, mesenteric venous thrombosis and cerebral sinus thrombosis, which are usually due to thrombophilia.

Deep venous thrombosis

Past history is very important.

Risk factors

- Family history
- Thrombophilia
- History of previous thromboembolism
- Drugs (e.g. OCP, tamoxifen, HRT)
- Malignancy (watch idiopathic DVT)
- Increasing age; age >40
- Varicose veins
- Significant illness, esp. heart failure and cancer
- Other chronic illness
- Recent surgery
- Major/orthopaedic surgery
- Immobility
- Long flights
- Pregnancy/puerperium
- Obesity
- Dehydration

There is an up to 20% association with pulmonary emboli, of which 30% may be fatal. DVT may be asymptomatic, but usually causes tenderness in the calf. DVT may present with painless unilateral leg swelling. Because of the potentially serious consequences from untreated thromboembolism, it is essential to objectively confirm or exclude clinically suspected disease.

Examination

May be low-grade fever.

Examine both legs. Look for:

- swelling of calf and thighs
- asymmetry
- erythema
- superficial veins

Feel for:

- warmth
- tenderness (gently squeeze calves)
- pitting oedema

Don't test Homan's sign (pain on sharp dorsiflexion of foot) as it may dislodge a thrombus.

Refer to Wells criteria (e.g. <www.nice.org.uk/guidance/cg144/chapter/guidance#terms-used-in-this-guidance> or <www.mdcalc.com/wells-criteria-for-dvt/>).

Investigations

- Duplex ultrasound: accurate for above-knee thrombosis; improving for distal calf
- Should be repeated in 1 week if initial test normal
- Contrast venography: reserved if ultrasound doubtful

Note:

- MRI appears to be very accurate for DVT, but is not yet available generally.
- The plasma D-dimer can help to 'rule out' thrombosis. Where the clinical probability of venous thrombosis is low, a normal D-dimer effectively excludes the diagnosis. However, where clinical probability is high, appropriate imaging with Doppler ultrasound or a lung scan should be performed. A raised D-dimer is non-specific and does not help with diagnosis.

Treatment[3,4]

Provide education and counselling. Admit to hospital (usually 5–7 days)—can treat as an outpatient. Drugs used in the treatment of thromboembolism are summarised in general format in TABLE 131.1.

- Collect blood for APTT, international normalised ratio (INR) and platelet count
- Check renal function
- LMW heparin e.g. enoxaparin or dalteparin

  or

  unfractionated heparin (UFH) 330 U/kg, SC loading dose then 250 U/kg bd SC (or monitor with APTT)

  or

  UFH 5000 U bolus IV then infusion in N saline (12 500 U over 12 hours)
  - monitor with APTT after 4–8 hours then for 5–7 days

  or

  fondaparinux SC, according to weight e.g. 50–100 kg: 7.5 mg SC daily
- Oral anticoagulant (warfarin) for 3 months (or 6 months if unprovoked)
  commence on day 1 or 2, usually 5 mg nocte for 2 nights and then according to INR monitoring (max. 30 mg in 3 days)
- Do not give aspirin
- Mobilisation within the limits of pain, tenderness and swelling
- Class II graded compression stocking to affected leg in proximal DVT associated with significant swelling. The stocking may be above or below the knee depending on the extent of the swelling.

Long term: complete resolution 50–80% at 6 months and almost 100% by 12 months.

Table 131.1 Drugs employed in thrombotic disorders

Antiplatelet

Aspirin
Clopidogrel
Dipyridamole
Prasugrel
Ticagrelor
Ticlopidine
Glycoprotein IIb/IIIa inhibitors (e.g. abciximab)

Anticoagulants

Heparin:

- unfractionated/standard
- low molecular weight
    - dalteparin
    - enoxaparin
    - danaparoid

Vitamin K antagonists:

- phenindione
- warfarin

Clotting factor inhibitors:

- direct thrombin inhibitors[5]
    - bivalirudin (IV use)
    - dabigatran (oral)
    - lepirudin (IV use)
- factor Xa inhibitors
    - apixaban (oral)
    - fondaparinux (SC use)
    - rivaroxaban (oral)

Thrombolytics

Alteplase
Reteplase
Streptokinase
Tenecteplase
Urokinase

Prevention

Surgery

- Early ambulation
- LMW heparin or new anticoagulants for orthopaedic (for 14–35 days) or other high-risk surgery (for 1 week or until fully mobile) See TABLE 131.1
- Graded pressure elastic stockings
- Physiotherapy
- Pneumatic compression (especially in high-risk patients where heparin is contraindicated)
- Electrical calf muscle stimulation during surgery

Prolonged travel/immobilisation

- Keep hydrated—ample water.
- Avoid or restrict alcohol and coffee.
- Exercises—3–4 minutes per hour (e.g. walking, calf contraction—e.g. foot pumps, see FIG. 131.1, ankle circles, knee lifts).
- Injections—LMWH just prior to flying and on arrival for those at high risk. Use a prophylactic dose (e.g. enoxaparin 40 mg or dalteparin 5000 U—both SC injections twice daily).

Pulmonary embolism[6]

Refer to CHAPTER 40 for more detail on the clinical features and management of pulmonary embolism. CT pulmonary angiography is very specific and appears to be as sensitive as V/Q scanning for embolism, and is currently the preferred first-line investigation. The basis of treatment is LMW heparin and warfarin, as for DVT.

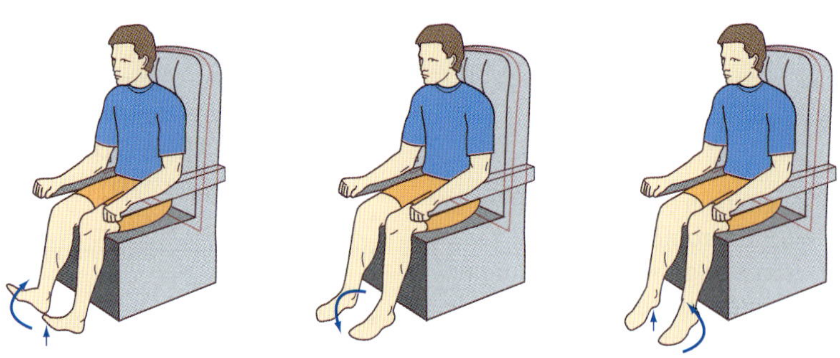

FIGURE 131.1 Foot pump exercises to prevent DVT during prolonged air travel

1 Start with the feet flat and both heels on the floor, lift the feet (toes up) as high as you can.
2 Return the feet to the flat position, pressing them firmly on the floor.
3 Lift the heels high, keeping the balls of the feet on the floor.

Continue this up-and-down movement for at least 30 seconds. Repeat often.

Arterial thromboembolism

The common serious manifestations of this are myocardial infarction, stroke, occlusion of the arterial system of the lower limbs and 'eye' embolism (e.g. central retinal artery thrombosis). Emboli originate from the left side of the heart, the carotid arteries or the iliac arteries. Atrial fibrillation is an important predisposing factor.

Preventing systemic embolism in atrial fibrillation[6]

Atrial fibrillation (AF) accounts for about 15% of ischaemic strokes caused by systemic embolism of cardiac thrombi. This risk gradually increases with age. Use of warfarin or DOAC reduces the annual incidence of stroke during AF from 4.5% to 1.4%—a risk reduction of almost 70%. The decision to use it or an antiplatelet agent is a difficult one and should be made in consultation with a cardiologist. Although aspirin reduces stroke rate by about 20% in patients with AF when compared with no treatment, it has half the effectiveness of warfarin/DOACs and is less able to prevent severe strokes. As a general rule, all patients with AF should start on warfarin or an appropriate DOAC unless <65 years old or have a major contraindication to its use. It is not indicated in patients with lone AF who are less than 60 years of age with no risk factors. If using warfarin, start with a low dose (e.g. 2–4 mg) and maintain an INR of 2–3 with regular checks. Anticoagulant therapy is also required to prevent embolism after cardioversion.

Drug treatment of thrombotic disorders

The direct oral anticoagulants (DOACs)[5]

The term DOAC is replacing NOAC as, over time, these medications become less 'novel'. These alternatives to warfarin are currently indicated for thromboprophylaxis in non-valvular atrial fibrillation and post-hip and knee replacement surgery. Rivaroxaban is also approved for treatment and secondary prevention of DVT and PE. They need less monitoring than warfarin, but so far only dabigatran has an effective antidote (idarucizumab). Intracranial bleeding is less likely with DOACs compared with warfarin. Caution for use is required in renal impairment and they are contraindicated in patients with renal failure. This requires measurement of creatinine clearance (not eGFR, which does not allow for weight).

Warfarin

Warfarin is an oral agent used in the treatment and prevention of venous thromboembolism, unlike the antiplatelet drugs which have little or no benefit and are recommended in arterial disease. Before prescribing warfarin, the risk of bleeding should be evaluated and discussed with each patient. Indications for warfarin treatment are outlined in TABLE 131.2.

Table 131.2 Warfarin anticoagulation

Indications
Prosthetic cardiac valves
Deep venous thrombosis, pulmonary thromboembolism
Atrial fibrillation (selected cases)
Postoperatively in lower limb orthopaedic surgery (low dose)
Postcoronary bypass surgery (selected cases)
Thrombosis in antiphospholipid antibody syndrome
Contraindications
Active bleeding
History of intracranial haemorrhage
Uncontrolled hypertension
Liver disease with impaired synthetic function—based on INR
Pregnancy

131

Actions[4]

- Antagonises vitamin K.
- Depresses factors VII, IX and X (half-life of 30–40 hours) and prothrombin.
- Achieves full anticoagulation effect after 5–7 days.
- Prothrombin time (INR ratio) of 2–3 times normal control indicates therapeutic effect.
- The INR is a good indicator of effectiveness and risk of bleeding.
- Duration of effect is 4–5 days after cessation.
- It can cause thrombocytopenia.
- Antidote is vitamin K ± plasma or prothrombin complex concentrate.

Initiation of warfarin treatment[7,8]

An estimate of the patient's final steady dose is made. The patient is commenced on this dose and the INR monitored daily and the dose altered accordingly.

- Measure INR first to establish baseline.
- Generally warfarin is commenced on same day or day after heparin is commenced.
- Heparin can be ceased when INR >2 for 2 consecutive days.

- Typical loading dose is 5–10 mg (o) daily (usually 5 mg) for 2 days (avoid dose >30 mg over 3 days without INR).
- Adjust the dosage according to an INR table (eTG Complete: Therapeutic Guidelines Ltd <www.tg.org.au>) from the third day. Some pathology laboratories offer patients this personalised adjustment service.
- Establish the INR in the therapeutic range, usually 2–3 (average 2.5).
- Maintenance dose is usually reached by day 5.
- The INR reflects the warfarin dose given 48 hours earlier.
- Warfarin is best taken in the evening and INR measured in the morning.

Note:

- Warfarin should be discontinued at 3 months following a first episode of a non-extensive venous thromboembolic event that occurred in the setting of a major, transient risk factor.[9]
- Watch for potential drug interactions.

Recommended target INR values are given in the box.

Recommended INR target values

Prevention of DVT	2.0–3.0
Treatment of DVT or PE	2.0–3.0
Preventing systemic embolism:	2.0–3.0
• atrial fibrillation	
• post myocardial infarction	
• tissue heart valve	
• valvular heart disease	
Mechanical prosthetic heart valve	2.5–3.5
Prevent recurrence of MI	2.0–3.0
Antiphospholipid antibody syndrome thrombosis	2.0–3.0

Overdosage of warfarin

Signs of warfarin overdosage include:

- unexpected bleeding after minor trauma
- epistaxis
- spontaneous bruising
- unusually heavy menstrual bleeding
- gastrointestinal bleeding

Management of overdosage[10]

1 Urgent measurement of INR is required.
2 If the only evidence of overdosage is a small increase of the INR above the therapeutic range, cessation of warfarin for 1 to 2 days followed by a continuation at a lower dose is appropriate.
3 If the INR is markedly elevated (>5.0) consider giving oral vitamin K e.g. 10 mg tablet.
4 If bleeding is minor, transient action as in point 2 is still appropriate.
5 If bleeding is persistent, or severe, or involves closed body cavities (such as pericardium, intracranial, fascial compartment), urgent admission to hospital is essential. The anticoagulation may need to be reversed by administering oral or parenteral vitamin K. Infusion of fresh frozen plasma and/or prothrombin complex concentrate (best option) may also be necessary.

Drug interactions

There are so many potential interactions between warfarin and other drugs that the following general principles should be applied:

1 Maintain the simplest possible drug regimens. Avoid polypharmacy.
2 Aspirin is contraindicated while the patient is on warfarin because of the combined antiplatelet and anticoagulation effects. The risk of gastrointestinal bleeding is also increased. Other NSAIDs should also be avoided (see TABLE 131.3).
3 If the patient's drug regimen must be altered during warfarin therapy, then the INR should be followed closely until stable.

Advice to the patient

- Keep to a consistent diet.
- Do not take aspirin or liquid paraffin.
- Always mention that you take warfarin to any doctor, dentist or chemist you are consulting.
- Remember to take tablets strictly as directed and have your blood tests.
- Report signs of bleeding, such as black motions, blood in urine, easy bruising, unusual nose bleeds, heavy periods, 'purple toes'.

Note: Give the patient the information sheet about risks.

Bleeding while on heparin

- Recheck APTT
- Cease or reduce heparin
- Admit patient—alert laboratory and haematologist

Antidotes:

- protamine sulphate will reverse (use with caution)
- fresh frozen plasma
- clotting factors (as guided by consultant)

Table 131.3 Some important drug interactions with warfarin

Effects on warfarin activity	Drug
↑ Increased	Allopurinol Amiodarone Anabolic steroids Antibiotics (broad spectrum) Antifungals Aspirin—salicylates (high doses) Chloral hydrate Cimetidine Clofibrate Gemfibrozil Metronidazole Miconazole NSAIDs, including COX-2 inhibitors Paracetamol (large doses) Phenytoin Proton-pump blockers Quinidine/quinine Ranitidine SSRIs Sulphonamides Tamoxifen Thyroxine Herbal medicines: • dong quai • papaya • St John's wort
↓ Decreased	Antacids Antihistamines Barbiturates Anti-epileptics (e.g. carbamazepine) Cholestyramine (reduced absorption) Griseofulvin Haloperidol Oestrogen/oral contraceptives Rifampicin Vitamin C
Increased or decreased	Alcohol Chloral hydrate Diuretics Ranitidine

Practice tips for warfarin[11]

- Consider avoiding use if patient compliance is likely to be poor.
- The INR result reflects the warfarin dose administered 48–72 hours earlier.
- Advise and encourage patient to keep a record in an 'anticoagulant diary' of drug dosage and INR results.
- An unacceptable INR is >5.0.
- Discontinue therapy if skin necrosis or 'purple toes syndrome' occurs.

131

References

1 Kumar P, Clark M. *Clinical Medicine* (7th edn). London: Elsevier-Saunders, 2009: 465.
2 Joseph J. *Thrombophilia.* Common sense pathology. RCPA, 2004.
3 Moulds R (Chair). *Therapeutic Guidelines: Cardiovascular* (Version 5). Melbourne. Therapeutic Guidelines Ltd, 2012.
4 Buckley N (Chair). *Australian Medicines Handbook.* Adelaide: Australian Medicines Handbook Pty Ltd, 2016: 327–338.
5 Brieger D, Curnow J. Anticoagulation: a GP primer on the new anticoagulants. Aust Fam Physician, 2014; 43 (5): 254–9.
6 Gallus AS. Anticoagulation: how to treat. Australian Doctor, 4 March 2005: 29–36.
7 Walker ID et al. *Guidelines on Oral Anticoagulation* (3rd edn). Br J Haematol, 1998; 101: 374–87.
8 Gallus AS. Consensus guidelines for warfarin therapy—recommendations from the Australasian Society of Thrombosis and Haemostasis. Med J Aust, 2000; 172: 600–5.
9 Boutitie F et al. Influence of preceding length of anticoagulant treatment and initial presentation of venous thromboembolism on risk of recurrence after stopping treatment: analysis of individual participants' data from seven trials. BMJ, 2011; 342: d3036.
10 Baker R et al. Australian and NZ consensus guidelines for warfarin reversal. Med J Aust, 2004; 181 (9): 492–7.
11 Campbell P, Roberts R, Eaton V et al. Managing warfarin therapy in the community. Australian Prescriber, 2001; 24: 86–9.

132 Common skin wounds and foreign bodies

The variety of foreign bodies which have found their way into the rectum is hardly less remarkable than the ingenuity displayed in their removal.
A turnip has been delivered PR by the use of obstetric forceps.
A stick firmly impacted has been withdrawn by inserting a gimlet into its lower end.
A tumbler, mouth downwards, has several times been extracted by filling the interior with a wet plaster of Paris bandage, leaving the end of the bandage extruding, and allowing the plaster to set.

BAILEY AND LOVE, *SHORT PRACTICE OF SURGERY*, 1943

Injuries to the skin, including simple lacerations, abrasions, contusions and foreign bodies, are among the commonest problems encountered in general practice. To manage these cosmetically important injuries well is one of the really basic and enjoyable skills of our profession.

Key facts and checkpoints

- Keep a well-prepared treatment room with good, sterile instruments and dressings, and an assistant who facilitates their management.
- With lacerations, check carefully for nerve damage, tendon damage and arterial damage.
- In wounds caused by glass, beware of slivers—explore carefully and X-ray (or high-resolution ultrasound) if in doubt.
- Beware of electrical or thermal wounds because marked tissue necrosis can be hidden by slightly injured skin.
- Beware of roller injuries such as car wheels.
- Beware of pressure gun injuries such as oil and paint. The consequences can be disastrous.
- Beware gravel rash wounds, where retained fragments of dirt and metal can leave a 'dirty', tattoo-like effect in the healed wound.
- Avoid suturing the tongue, and animal and human bites, unless absolutely necessary.
- Keep diagrams or photographs of wounds in your medical records.
- Have a management plan for medical needle-stick injuries.

Contusions and haematomas

A contusion (bruise or ecchymosis) is the consequence of injury causing bleeding in subcutaneous or deeper tissue while leaving the skin basically intact. It might take weeks to resolve, especially if extensive.

A haematoma is a large collection of extravasated blood that produces an obvious and tender swelling or deformity. The blood usually clots and becomes firm, warm and red; later (about 10 days) it begins to liquefy and becomes fluctuant.

Principles of management

- Explanation and reassurance
- **RICE** (for larger bruises/haematomas) for 48 hours
  R = **R**est
  I = **I**ce (for 20 minutes every 2 waking hours)
  C = **C**ompression (firm elastic bandage)
  E = **E**levation (if a limb)
- Analgesics: paracetamol
- Avoid needle aspiration (some exceptions)
- Avoid massage
- Local heat may be applied after 72 hours
- Consider possibility of bleeding disorder if bleeding is out of proportion to the injury

PROBLEMATIC HAEMATOMAS

Some haematomas in certain locations can cause deformity and other problems.

Haematoma of nasal septum[1]

Refer CHAPTER 59.

Haematoma of the pinna[1]

When trauma to the pinna causes a haematoma between the epidermis and the cartilage, a permanent deformity known as 'cauliflower ear' may result. The haematoma, if left, becomes organised and the normal contour of the ear is lost.

The aim is to evacuate the haematoma as soon as practical and then to prevent it reforming. One can achieve a fair degree of success, even on haematomas that have been present for several days.

Method

Under aseptic conditions insert a 25 gauge needle into the haematoma at its lowest point and aspirate the extravasated blood (see FIG. 132.1A). Apply a padded clamp to the haematoma site and leave on for 30–40 minutes (see FIG. 132.1B). Generally, daily aspiration and clamping are sufficient to eradicate the haematoma completely.

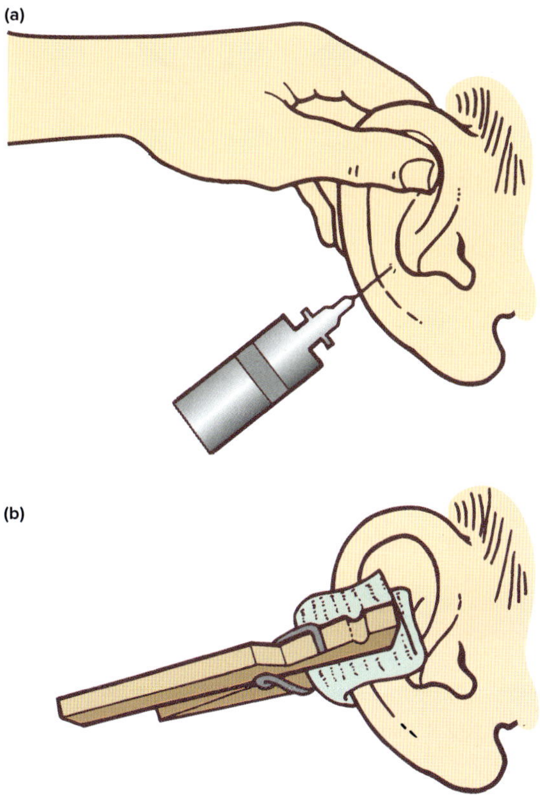

FIGURE 132.1 Treatment of haematoma of the pinna

Subungual haematomas

These important haematomas are discussed in CHAPTER 127.

Abrasions

Abrasions vary considerably in degree and potential contamination. They are common with bicycle, motorcycle and skateboard accidents. Special care is needed over joints such as the knee or elbow.

Rules of management

- Clean meticulously, remove all ground-in dirt, metal, clothing and other material.
- Scrub out dirt with sterile normal saline under anaesthesia (local infiltration or general anaesthesia for deep wounds).
- Treat the injury similarly to a burn.
- When clean, apply a protective dressing (some wounds may be left open).
- Use paraffin gauze and non-adhesive absorbent pads such as Melolin.
- Ensure adequate follow-up.
- Immobilise a joint that may be affected by a deep wound.

132

Lacerations

Lacerations vary enormously in complexity and repairability. Very complex lacerations and those involving nerves or other structures should be referred to an expert.

Principles of repair

- Good approximation of wound edges minimises scar formation and healing time.
- Pay special attention to debridement.
- Avoid deep layers of suture material in a contaminated wound—consider drainage.
- Inspect all wounds carefully for damage to major structures such as nerves and tendons and for foreign material:
  - shattered glass wounds require careful inspection and perhaps plain X-ray or ultrasound
  - high-energy wounds (e.g. motor mowers) are prone to have metallic foreign bodies and associated fractures
- Consider X-rays of wounds to look for foreign objects or fractures (compound fractures).
- Trim jagged or crushed wound edges, especially on the face.
- All wounds should be closed so that opposite layers line up.
- Avoid leaving dead space.
- Do not suture an 'old' wound (greater than 8 hours) if it is contaminated: leave 4 days before suturing (unless

infected). You may need to excise a thin section off each edge to obtain a new healing surface.

- Take care in poor healing areas, such as backs, necks, calves and knees, and in areas prone to hypertrophic scarring, such as over the sternum, chest or shoulder.
- Use atraumatic tissue-handling techniques, with minimal handling of wound edges.
- Everted edges heal better than inverted edges.
- A suture is too tight when it blanches the skin between the thread—loosen it.
- Avoid tension on the wound, especially in fingers, lower leg, foot or palm.
- A finer scar and better result is obtained by using a large number of fine sutures rather than fewer thick sutures more widely spread.
- Avoid haematoma.
- Apply a firm pressure dressing when appropriate, especially with swollen skin flaps.
- Consider appropriate immobilisation for wounds. Many wound failures are due to lack of immobilisation from a volar slab on the hand or a back slab on the leg.

132

Practical aspects

Suture material

See TABLE 132.1.

Table 132.1 Selection of suture material (guidelines)

Skin	Nylon 6/0	Face
	Nylon 3/0	Back, scalp
	Nylon 5/0	Elsewhere
Deeper tissue (dead space)	Catgut 4/0 Dexon/Vicryl 3/0 or 4/0	Face Elsewhere
Subcuticular	Monofilament absorbable e.g. Monocryl 4/0	
Small vessel ties	Plain catgut 4/0	
Large vessel ties	Dexon/Vicryl	

- Monofilament nylon sutures are generally preferred for skin repair.
- Use the smallest calibre compatible with required strains.
- The synthetic, absorbable polyglycolic acid or polyglactin sutures (Dexon, Vicryl) are stronger than catgut of the same gauge, but are not as suitable as catgut on the face or subcuticularly.

Instruments

Examples of good-quality instruments:

- locking needle holder (e.g. Crile–Wood 12 cm)
- skin hooks
- iris scissors
- toothed forceps

Holding the needle

The needle should be held about two-thirds of the way back from the tip; it can distort if held right near the back end (see FIG. 132.2). Tougher tissues may require grasping the needle at its centre.

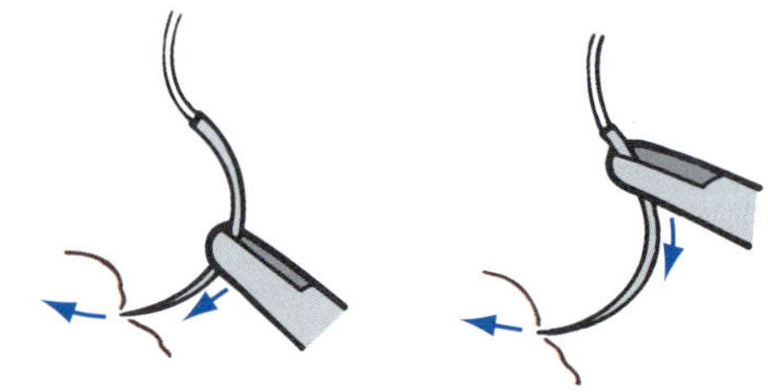

FIGURE 132.2 Holding the needle

Dead space

Dead space should be eliminated to reduce tension on skin sutures. Use buried, absorbable sutures to approximate underlying tissue. This is done by starting suture insertion from the fat to pick up the fat/dermis interface so as to bury the knot (see FIG. 132.3).

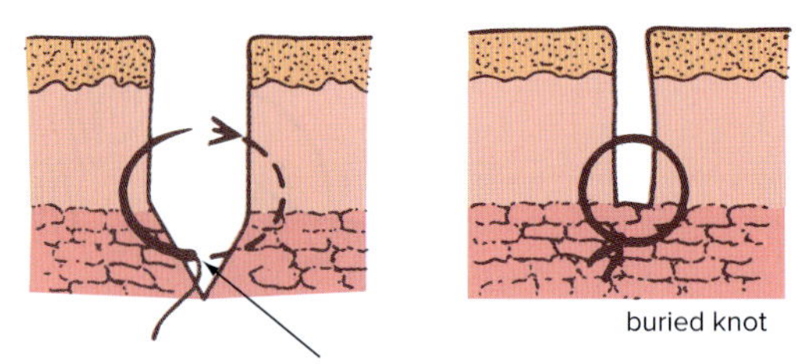

FIGURE 132.3 Eliminating dead space

Everted wounds

Eversion is achieved by making the 'bite' in the dermis wider than the bite in the epidermis (skin surface) and making the suture deeper than it is wide. Shown are:

- simple suture (see FIG. 132.4A)
- vertical mattress suture (see FIG. 132.4B)

The mattress suture is the ideal way to evert a wound.

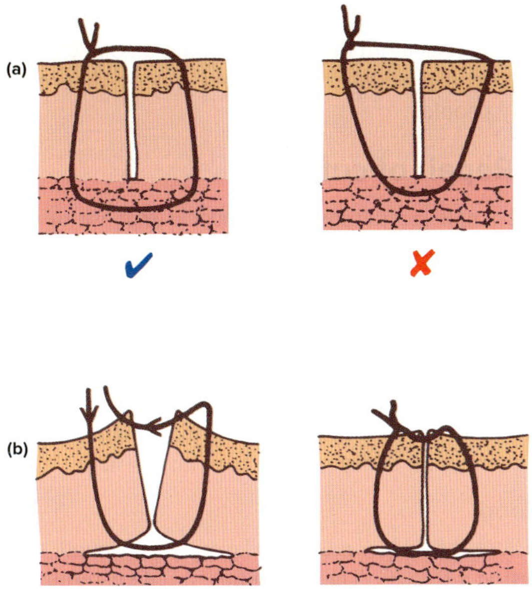

FIGURE 132.4 Everted wounds: **(a)** correct and incorrect methods of making a simple suture, **(b)** vertical mattress suture

Number of sutures

One should aim to use a minimum number of sutures to achieve closure without gaps but sufficient sutures to avoid tension. Place the sutures as close to the wound edge as is reasonably possible.

Practice tips

- Have the patient lie down for suturing and the parents of children sit down.
- Avoid using antibiotic sprays and powders in simple wounds—resistant organisms can develop.
- Consider tetanus and gas gangrene prophylaxis in contaminated and deep necrotic wounds.
- Give a tetanus booster if the patient has not had one within 5 years for dirty wounds or within 10 years for clean wounds.
- Give tetanus immunoglobulin if patient is not immunised and the wound is grossly contaminated.
- Never send head-wound patients home before thoroughly washing their hair and carefully examining for other lacerations.
- Any laceration in the cheek, mandible or lower eyelid may damage the facial nerve, parotid duct or lacrimal duct respectively.
- When a patient falls onto glass it takes bone to halt its cutting path. Assume all structures between skin and bone are severed.

SPECIAL TECHNIQUES FOR VARIOUS WOUNDS

The three-point suture

In wounds with a triangular flap component, it is often difficult to place the apex of the flap accurately. The three-point suture is the best way to achieve this while minimising the chance of strangulation necrosis at the tip of the flap.

Method

1. Pass the needle through the skin of the non-flap side of the wound.
2. Then pass it through the subcuticular layer of the flap tip at exactly the same level as the reception side.
3. Finally, pass the needle back through the reception side so that it emerges well back from the V flap (see FIG. 132.5).

Triangular flap wounds on the lower leg

132

Triangular flap wounds below the knee are a common injury and are often treated incorrectly. Similar wounds in the upper limb heal rapidly when sutured properly, but lower limb injury will not usually heal at first intention unless the apex of the flap is given special attention.

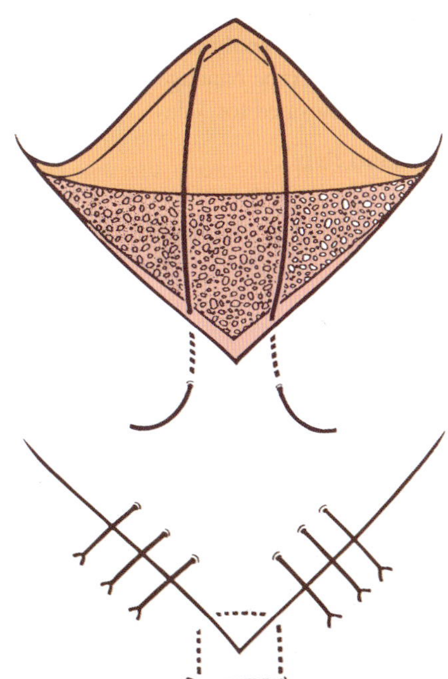

FIGURE 132.5 The three-point suture

132

Proximally based flap

A fall through a gap in floorboards will produce a proximally based flap; a heavy object (such as the tailboard of a trailer) striking the shin will result in a distally based flap.

Often the apex of the flap is crushed and poorly vascularised; it will not survive to heal after suture.

Treatment methods (under infiltration with LA)

1. Preferred method: to attempt to salvage the distal flap, scrape away the subcutaneous tissue on the flap and use it as a full-thickness graft.
2. An alternative is to excise the apex of the flap, loosely suture the remaining flap and place a small split-thickness graft on the raw area (see FIG. 132.6).

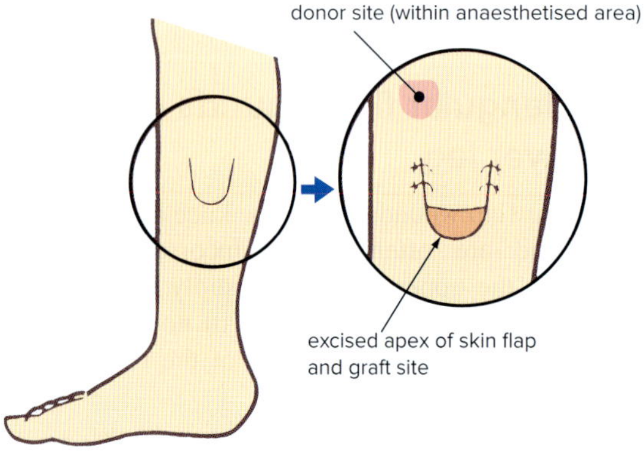

FIGURE 132.6 Triangular flap wound repair: proximally based flap

For both methods apply a suitable dressing and strap firmly with a crepe bandage. The patient should rest with the leg elevated for 3 days.

Distally based flap

See FIGURE 132.7. This flap, which is quite avascular, has a poorer prognosis. The same methods as for the proximally based flap can be used. Trimming the flap and using it as a full thickness graft has a good chance of repair in a younger person but a poor chance in elderly people.

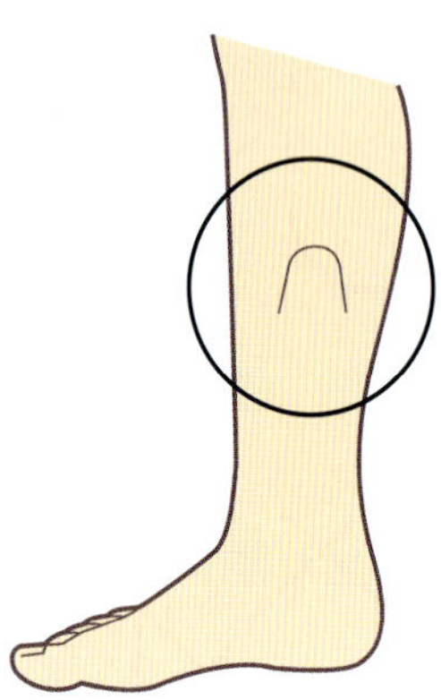

FIGURE 132.7 Triangular flap wound repair: distally based flap

Repair of cut lip

While small lacerations of the buccal mucosa of the lip can be left safely, more extensive cuts require careful repair. Local anaesthetic infiltration may be adequate, although a mental nerve block is ideal for larger lacerations of the lower lip.

For wounds that cross the vermilion border, meticulous alignment is essential. It may be advisable to pre-mark the vermilion border with gentian violet or a marker pen. It is desirable to have an assistant.

Method

1. Close the deeper muscular layer of the wound using 4/0 CCG. The first suture should carefully appose the mucosal area of the lip, followed by one or two sutures in the remaining layer.
2. Next, insert a 6/0 monofilament nylon suture to bring both ends of the vermilion border together. The slightest step is unacceptable (see FIG. 132.8). This is the key to the procedure.
3. Close the inner buccal mucosa with interrupted 4/0 plain catgut sutures.
4. The outer skin of the lip (above and below the vermilion border) is closed with interrupted nylon sutures.

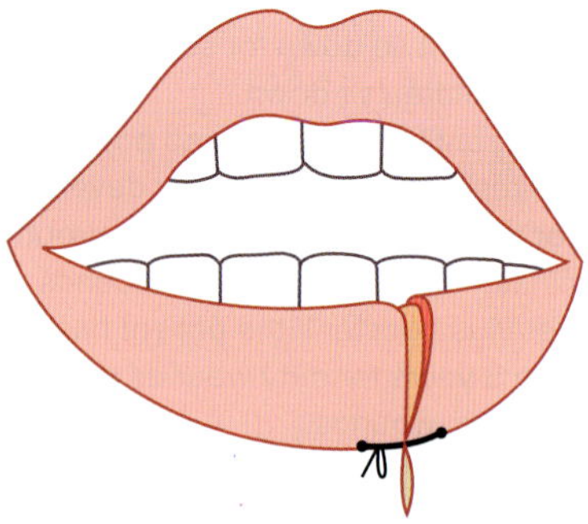

FIGURE 132.8 The lacerated lip: ensuring meticulous suture of the vermilion border

Post-repair

1. Apply a moisturising lotion (or petroleum jelly) along the lines of the wound.
2. Remove nylon sutures in 3–4 days (in a young person) or 5–6 days (in an older person).

Repair of lacerated eyelid

General points

- Preserve as much tissue as possible.
- Do not shave the eyebrow.
- Do not invert hair-bearing skin into the wound.
- Ensure precise alignment of wound margins.
- Tie suture knots away from the eyeball. If necessary, leave suture ends long and tape the strands away from the eye.

Method

1 Place an intermarginal suture behind the eyelashes if the margin is involved.
2 Repair conjunctiva and tarsus with 6/0 catgut.
3 Then repair skin and muscle (orbicularis oculi) with 6/0 nylon (see FIG. 132.9).

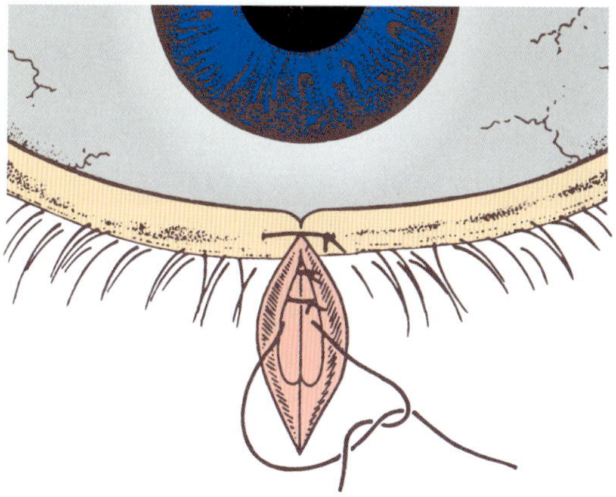

FIGURE 132.9 The lacerated eyelid

Repair of tongue wound

Wherever possible, it is best to avoid repairs to tongue wounds because these heal rapidly. However, large flap wounds to the tongue on the dorsum or the lateral border may require suturing. The best method is to use buried catgut sutures.

Method

1 Get patient to suck ice for a few minutes, then infiltrate with 1% lignocaine and leave for 5–10 minutes.
2 Use 4/0 or 3/0 catgut sutures to suture the flap to its bed, and bury the sutures (see FIG. 132.10).

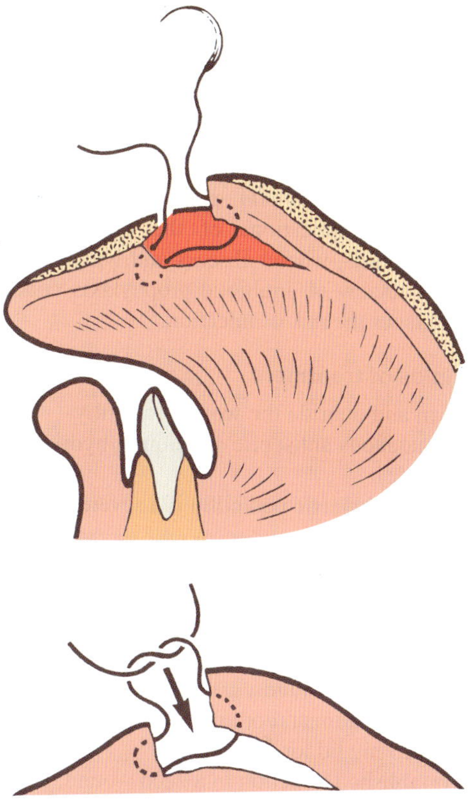

FIGURE 132.10 Repair of tongue wound

It should not be necessary to use surface sutures. If it is, 4/0 silk sutures will suffice.

Instruct the patient to rinse the mouth regularly with salt water until healing is satisfactory.

The amputated finger

In this emergency situation, instruct the patient to place the severed finger directly into a fluid-tight sterile container, such as a plastic bag or sterile specimen jar. Then place this 'unit' in a bag containing iced water with crushed ice.

Note: Never place the amputated finger directly in ice or in fluid such as saline. Fluid makes the tissue soggy, rendering microsurgical repair difficult.

Care of the finger stump

Apply a simple, sterile, loose, non-sticky dressing and keep the hand elevated.

132

132

Bite wounds

Human bites and clenched fist injuries

Human bites and clenched fist injuries can present a serious problem of infection. Beta-lactamase-producing anaerobic organisms in the oral cavity (e.g. Vincent's) can penetrate the damaged tissue and form a deep-seated infection. *Streptococcus* species, staphylococcal organisms and *Eikenella corrodens* are common pathogens. Complications of the infected wounds include cellulitis, wound abscess and lymphangitis. A Cochrane review of antibiotic prophylaxis concluded that it reduces the risk of infection.[2]

Principles of treatment

- Clean and debride the wound carefully (e.g. aqueous antiseptic solution or hydrogen peroxide).
- Give prophylactic penicillin if a severe or deep bite.
- Avoid suturing if possible.
- Tetanus toxoid (although minimum risk).
- Consider rare possibility of HIV and hepatitis B or C infections.
- For high-risk wounds, give procaine penicillin 1.5 g IM statim and/or amoxycillin/clavulanate 875/125 mg bd for 5 days.[3]
- If established infection in a deep wound, take a swab and give metronidazole 400 mg (o) bd for 14 days plus either cefotaxime 1 g IV 8 hourly or ceftriaxone 1 g IV daily for 14 days.

Dog bites

Non-rabid

Dog bites typically have poor healing and carry a risk of infection with anaerobic organisms, including tetanus, staphylococci and streptococci. Puncture and crush wounds are more prone to infection than laceration. Up to 25% of dog bite wounds become infected, with the first signs appearing in about 24 hours.[4]

Principles of treatment (see FIG. 132.11):

- Clean and debride the wound with aqueous antiseptic, allowing it to soak for 10–20 minutes.
- Aim for open healing—avoid suturing if possible (except in 'privileged' sites with an excellent blood supply such as the face and scalp).

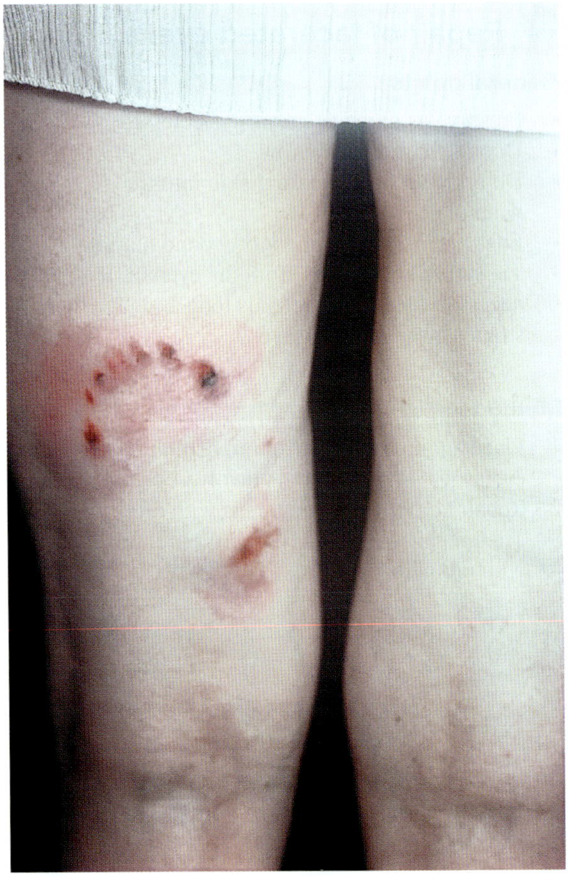

FIGURE 132.11 Dog bite treated by sterile dressing and anti-tetanus vaccination

- Apply non-adherent, absorbent dressings (paraffin gauze and Melolin) to absorb the discharge from the wound.
- Tetanus prophylaxis: immunoglobulin or tetanus toxoid.
- A 2008 Cochrane review found no evidence supporting prophylactic antibiotics for dog or cat bites.[2] Small wounds presenting within 8 hours that do not involve joints or tendons do not require antibiotics.
- However, for a severe or deep bite, give prophylactic penicillin: 1.5 million units procaine penicillin IM statim, then orally for 5–10 days. An alternative is amoxycillin/clavulanate for 5–7 days. Use this antibiotic for 7–10 days for an established infection (depending on swab).[4]
- Inform the patient that slow healing and scarring are likely.

Rabid or possibly rabid dog (or other animal)

Not currently applicable in Australia (see CHAPTER 15).

- Wash the site immediately with detergent or saline (preferable) or hydrogen peroxide or soap (if no other option).
- Do not suture.
- If rabid:
  - human rabies immune globulin (passive)
  - antirabies vaccine (active)
- Uncertain: capture and observe animal, consider vaccination.

Cat bites

Cat bites have the greatest potential for suppurative infection, with *Pasteurella multocida* being the most common organism. The same principles apply as for the management of human or dog bites. For deep or delayed wounds, use amoxycillin + clavulanate for prophylaxis for 5 days. For infection, swab the wound but start with metronidazole + doxycycline or ciprofloxacin.[3] It is important to clean a deep and penetrating wound. Another problem is cat-scratch disease, presumably caused by a Gram-negative bacterium, *Bartonella henselae.*

Clinical features of cat-scratch disease

- An infected ulcer or papule pustule at bite site (30–50% of cases) after 3 days or so[5]
- 1–3 weeks later: fever, headache, malaise, regional lymphadenopathy (may suppurate)
- Intradermal skin test positive
- Benign, self-limiting course usually not requiring antibiotic treatment
- Sometimes severe symptoms for weeks, especially in immunocompromised
- For lymphadenopathy unresolved after 1 month, or significant morbidity, treat with erythromycin or roxithromycin for 10 days[3]

Water-related wound infections[3]

These complex infections may require expert advice.

Coral cuts

Wounds from coral cuts are at risk of serious infection with *Vibrio* organisms (marine pathogens) or *Streptococcus pyogenes.* Such wounds require cleaning with antiseptics, debridement, dressing and antibiotic cover with doxycycline 100 mg bd or cephalexin 500 mg bd for 7 days.

Fish tank/swimming pool granuloma

Due to *Mycobacterium marinum*, which causes a localised papular or nodular skin lesion, usually in people who clean aquaria or swimming pools. Diagnosis is by biopsy and culture (acid-fast bacilli).

Treatment: single lesion excision (may suffice). May need antibiotic therapy e.g. clarithromycin (o) bd for 3–4 months plus rifampicin for severe or unresponsive infection. Seek expert advice.

Aeromonas species wound infections

From fresh or brackish water or mud exposure to open wounds. Treat with ciprofloxacin for 14 days.[3]

Shewanella putrefaciens

From salt or brackish water, particularly legs with vascular compromise. Causes severe cellulitis with necrosis, even sepsis. Treat with ciprofloxacin or meropenem/imipenem.

Scalp lacerations in children

If lacerations are small but gaping use the child's hair for the suture, provided it is long enough.

Method

Make a twisted bunch of the child's own hair on each side of the wound. Tie a reef knot and then an extra holding knot to minimise slipping. Ask an assistant to drop compound benzoin tincture solution (Friar's Balsam) on the hair knot. Leave the hair 'suture' long and get the parent to cut the knot in 5 days.

Forehead and other lacerations in children

Despite the temptation, avoid using reinforced paper adhesive strips (Steri-Strips) for children with open wounds. They will merely close the dermis and cause a thin, stretched scar. They can be used only for very superficial epidermal wounds in conjunction with sutures.

Adhesive glue for wound adhesion

A tissue adhesive glue can be used successfully to close superficial smooth and clean skin wounds, particularly in children. Commercial preparations such as Histoacryl, Dermabond and Epiglu (active ingredient enbucrilate) are available. SuperGlue also serves the purpose although sterility and toxicity have to be considered. The glue should be used only for superficial, dry, clean and fresh wounds. No gaps are permissible with this method; glue in the wound will block healing. Avoid glues if possible.

Wound anaesthesia in children

Consider topical anaesthetic preparations for wound repair in children. They include lignocaine and prilocaine mixture (EMLA cream) and adrenaline and cocaine (AC) liquid. Use the latter with caution.

Some practitioners use an ice block to freeze the lacerated site, with or without a little lignocaine dripped into the wound. The child is asked to hold the ice while a suture is rapidly inserted.

Removal of skin sutures

Suture marks are related to the time of retention of the suture, its tension and position. The objective is to remove the sutures as early as possible, as soon as their purpose is achieved. The timing of removal is based on common sense and individual cases. Silk and other polyfilament sutures are more reactive and should be removed early. After suture removal, it is advisable to support the wound with Micropore skin tape/Steri-

Strips for 1–2 weeks, especially in areas of skin tension.

Method

1 Use good light and have the patient lying comfortably.
2 Use fine, sharp scissors that cut to the point, or a disposable suture cutter blade, and a pair of fine, non-toothed dissecting forceps that grip firmly.
3 Cut the suture close to the skin below the knot with scissors or blade (see FIG. 132.12A).
4 Gently pull the suture out towards the side on which it was divided—that is, always towards the wound (see FIG. 132.12B).

(a)

(b)

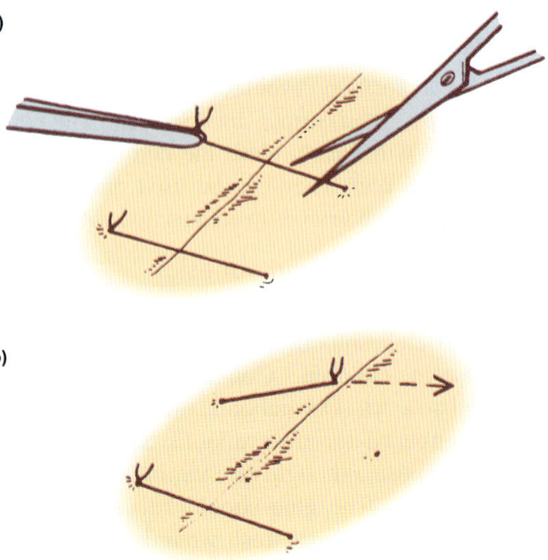

FIGURE 132.12 Removal of skin sutures: **(a)** cutting the suture, **(b)** removal by pulling towards wound

When to remove non-absorbable sutures

For removal of sutures after non-complicated wound closure in adults, see TABLE 132.2.

Table 132.2 Time after insertion for removal of sutures

Area	Days later
Scalp	6
Face	3 (or alternate at 2, rest 3–4)
Ear	5
Neck (anterior)	4 (or alternate at 3, rest 4)
Chest	8
Arm (including hand and fingers)	8–10
Abdomen	8–10 (tension 12–14)
Back	12
Inguinal and scrotal	7
Perineum	2
Legs	10
Knees and calf	12
Foot (including toes)	10–12

Note: Decisions need to be individualised according to the nature of the wound and health of the patient and healing. In general, take sutures out as soon as possible. One way of achieving this is to remove alternate sutures a day or two earlier and remove the rest at the usual time. Steri-Strips can then be used to maintain closure and healing.

Additional aspects

In children, tend to remove 1–2 days earlier. Allow additional time for backs and legs, especially the calf. Nylon sutures can be left in longer because they are less reactive. Alternate sutures may be removed earlier (e.g. face in women).

Burns[5,6]

Management depends on extent and depth (burns are classified as superficial or deep—otherwise first, second or third degree).

First degree burns are superficial and involve only the epidermis, causing pain, redness and swelling. A scald, which is a burn caused by moist heat, is an example. Healing proceeds quickly.

Second degree or partial skin thickness burns cause the epidermis to blister and become necrotic with subsequent serous ooze.

In *third degree* or full thickness burns, there is deep necrosis and perhaps anaesthesia from destroyed nerve endings. If extensive (>9% of body surface area) and deep there is a possibility of hypovolaemia and shock.

A major burn, which is a medical emergency, is an injury of more than 20% of the total body surface for an adult and 10% for a child.

First aid

The immediate treatment of burns, especially for smaller areas, is immersion in cool to cold, running water such as tap water, for a minimum of 20 minutes. Do not disturb charred adherent clothing but remove wet clothing.

Chemical burns should be liberally irrigated with water. Apply 1 in 10 diluted vinegar to alkali burns and sodium bicarbonate solution for acid burns.

Refer the following burns to hospital:

- >9% surface area, especially in a child (see 'rule of nines', CHAPTER 119) The patient's hand size equals approximately 1%.[7]
- >5% in an infant
- all deep burns
- burns of difficult or vital areas (e.g. face, hands, perineum/genitalia, feet)
- burns with potential problems (e.g. electrical, chemical, circumferential)
- suspicion of inhalational injury

Always give adequate pain relief. During transport, continue cooling by using a fine-mist water spray.

Treatment

1 *Very superficial—intact skin.* Can be left with application of a mild antiseptic only (e.g. aqueous chlorhexidine). Review if blistering.

2 *Superficial—blistered skin.* Apply a dressing to promote epithelialisation (e.g. hydrocolloid sheets, hydrogel sheets) covered by an absorbent dressing *or* (best option) a retention adhesive material (e.g. Fixomull, Mefix, Hypafix) with daily or twice daily cleaning of the serous ooze and reapplication of outer stretch bandage. Fixomull can be left in place for up to 2 weeks.

Guidelines to patient for retention dressings

- First 24 hours: keep dry. Pat dry any ooze coming through the dressing with a clean tissue.
- From day 2: wash over dressing twice daily. Use gentle soap and water, rinse then pat dry. Do not soak. Rinse only. Do not remove the dressing as it may cause pain and damage to the wound. If the wound becomes red, hot or swollen, or if pain increases, return to the clinic.
- From day 7: return to the clinic for removal of the dressing. Two hours prior to coming into the clinic, soak the dressing with olive oil then cover with cling wrap (e.g. GLAD Wrap).

Note: Dressing must be soaked off with oil (e.g. olive, baby, citrus or peanut). Debride 'popped blisters'. Only pop blisters that interfere with dermal circulation.

3 *Deep burns.* If considerable ooze, apply the following in order:

- SoloSite gel, Solugel or similar
- non-adherent neutral dressing (e.g. Melolin)
- layer of absorbent gauze or cotton wool (larger burns)

Change every 2–4 days with analgesic cover. Surgical treatment, including skin grafting, may be necessary.

The Alfred Hospital publishes excellent burns guidelines at <www.vicburns.org.au>.

Exposure (open method)

- Keep open without dressings (good for face, perineum or single surface burns)
- Renew coating of antiseptic cream every 24 hours

Dressings (closed method)

- Suitable for circumferential wounds
- Cover area with non-adherent tulle (e.g. paraffin gauze)
- Dress with an absorbent, bulky layer of gauze and wool
- Use a plaster splint if necessary

Burns to hands

For superficial blistered burns to the hand or similar 'complex' shaped parts of the body apply strips of the retention stretch adhesive dressings as described above. They conform well to digits. Apply an outer bandage. At 7 days, soak the dressings in oil for 2 hours prior to coming in to the clinic.

FOREIGN BODIES

Penetrating gun injuries

Injuries to the body from various types of guns present decision dilemmas for the treating doctor. The following information represents guidelines, including special sources of danger to tissues from various foreign materials discharged by guns.

132

Gunshot wounds

Airgun

The rule is to remove subcutaneous slugs but to leave deeper slugs unless they lie within and around vital structures (e.g. the wrist). A special common problem is that of slugs in the orbit. These often do little damage and the ophthalmologist may decide to leave them alone.

0.22 rifle (the pea rifle)

The same principles of management apply but the bullet must be localised precisely by X-ray. Of particular interest are abdominal wounds, which should be observed carefully, as visceral perforations can occur with minimal initial symptoms and signs.

0.410 shotgun

The pellets from this shotgun are usually dangerous only when penetrating from a close range. Again, the rule is not to remove deep-lying pellets—perhaps only those superficial pellets that can be palpated.

Pressure gun injuries

Injection of grease, oil, paint and similar substances from pressure guns (see FIG. 132.13) can cause very serious injuries, requiring decompression and removal of the substances.

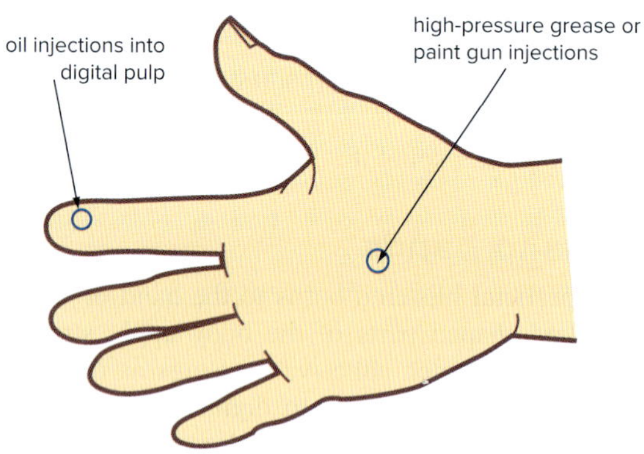

FIGURE 132.13 Dangerous accidental injections into the hand

Grease gun and paint gun

High-pressure injection of paint or grease into the hand requires urgent surgery if amputation is to be avoided. There is a deceptively minor wound to show for this injury, and after a while the hand feels comfortable. However, ischaemia,[1] chemical irritation and infection can follow, with gangrene of the digits, resulting in, at best, a claw hand due to sclerosis. Treatment is by immediate decompression and meticulous removal of all foreign material and necrotic tissue.

Oil injection

Accidental injection of an inoculum in an oily vehicle into the hand also creates a serious problem with local tissue necrosis. Such injections are common on poultry farms during fowl-pest injections. If injected into the digital pulp, this may necessitate amputation.

Splinters under the skin

The splinter under the skin is a common and difficult procedural problem. Instead of using forceps or making a wider excision, use a disposable hypodermic needle to 'spear' the splinter (see FIG. 132.14) and then use it as a lever to ease the splinter out through the skin.

A 'buried' wooden foreign body can be detected by ultrasound.

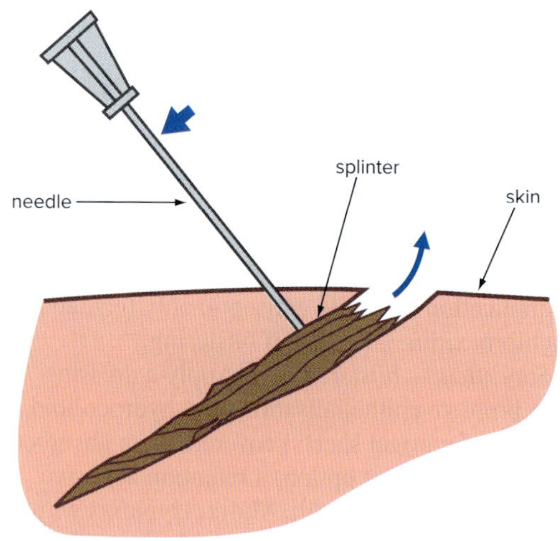

FIGURE 132.14 Removal of splinters in the skin

Embedded fish hooks

Two methods of removing fish hooks are presented here, both requiring removal in the reverse direction, against the barb. Method 2 is recommended as first-line management.

Method 1

1 Inject 1–2 mL of LA around the fish hook.
2 Grasp the shank of the hook with strong artery forceps.
3 Slide a D11 scalpel blade in along the hook, sharp edge away from the hook, to cut the tissue and free the barb (see FIG. 132.15).
4 Withdraw the hook with the forceps.

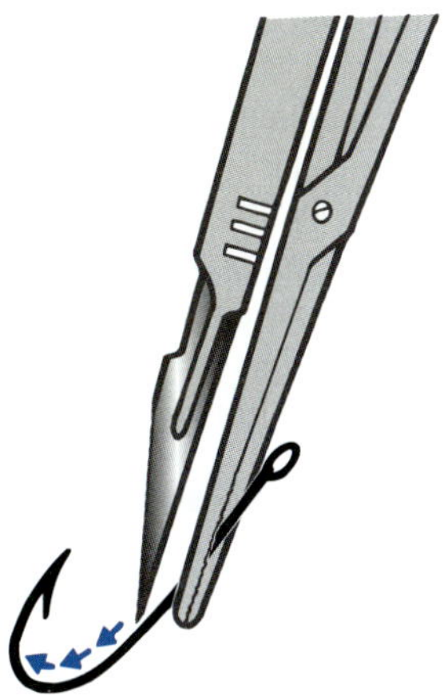

FIGURE 132.15 Removal of fish hook by cutting a path in the skin

Method 2

This method, used by some brave fishermen, relies on a loop of cord or fishing line to forcibly disengage and extract the hook intact. It requires no anaesthesia and no instruments—only nerves of steel, especially for the first attempt.

1 Take a piece of string about 10–12 cm long and make a loop. One end slips around the hook, the other hooking around one finger of the operator.
2 Depress the shank with the other hand in the direction that tends to disengage the barb.
3 At this point give a very swift, sharp tug along the cord.
4 The hook flies out painlessly in the direction of the tug (see FIG. 132.16). Wear safety goggles!

Note: You must be bold, decisive, confident and quick—half-hearted attempts do not work.

For difficult cases, some local anaesthetic infiltration may be appropriate. Instead of a short loop of cord, a long piece of fishing line double looped around the hook and tugged by the hand, or flicked with a thin ruler in the loop, will work.

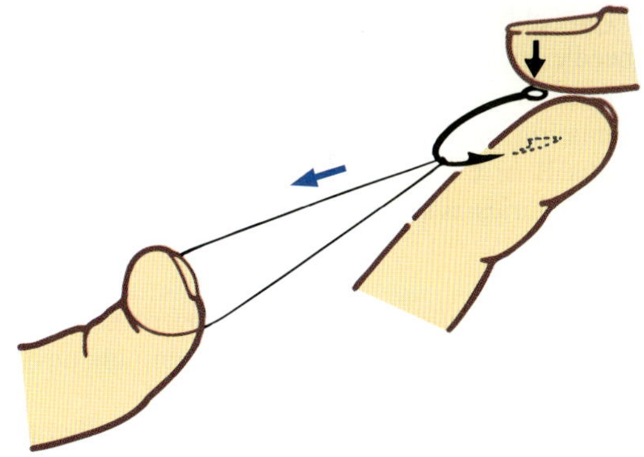

FIGURE 132.16 Fisherman's method of removing a fish hook intact

Needle-stick and sharps injuries

Accidental skin puncture by contaminated 'sharps', including needles (with blood or bloodstained body fluids), is of great concern to all health care workers. Another problem that occurs occasionally is the deliberate inoculation of people such as police by angry, sociopathic individuals. A needle-stick accident is the commonest incident with the potential to transmit infections such as HIV and hepatitis B, C or D. The part of the venipuncture that is most likely to cause the accident is the recapping or resheathing of the needle. This practice should be discouraged.

Infections transmitted by needle-stick accidents are summarised in TABLE 132.3. The risk from a contaminated patient is greatest with hepatitis (10–30%), while the risk of seroconversion or clinical infection after a needle-stick injury with HIV-positive blood is very

Table 132.3 Infections transmitted by needle-stick accidents

Viruses
HIV
Hepatitis B, C, D
Herpes simplex
Herpes varicella zoster
Bacteria
Streptococcus
Staphylococcus
Syphilis
Tetanus
Tuberculosis
Other
Malaria

low (probably about 1 in 300).[8] In children injured by needle stick incidentally in the community (e.g. at the beach or park), there are no published reports of transmission of a blood-borne virus such as HIV or hepatitis B or C.[9] The risk of tetanus, especially for outdoor injuries, is significant and should be addressed.

Prevention

- Avoid physically struggling with overdose victims or high-risk patients for lavage or venipuncture.
- Do not recap needles.
- Dispose of needles immediately and directly into a leak-proof, puncture-proof sharps container.
- Avoid contact with blood.
- Wear protective gloves (does not prevent sharps injury).

Postexposure prophylaxis

Postexposure prophylaxis (PEP) must be considered for high-risk exposure such as hollow blood-containing needles, deep injury and high viral load or late-stage HIV infection of the source.[3] Although in most instances of sharps injuries PEP is not justified, do seek expert advice.

Management[10]

- Wash affected site with soap and water without scrubbing. Also wash or irrigate any areas of skin, eye/conjectiva or other mucous membrane exposed to blood or body fluids.
- Do not suck or squeeze wound.
- Encourage bleeding.
- Reassure the patient that the risk of viral infection is very low.
- Obtain information about and blood from the sharps victim and the source person (source of body fluid). A known carrier of hepatitis B surface antigen or an HIV-positive source person will facilitate early decision making.

Note: It takes 3 months to seroconvert with HIV so the patient may be infected but negative on initial tests.

Consider the exposed person's wishes after discussing the risks/benefits of treatment including adverse effects.

Known hepatitis B carrier source person

- If injured person is immune—no further action
- If non-vaccinated and non-immune:
  - give hyperimmune hepatitis B gammaglobulin within 48 hours
  - commence course of hepatitis B vaccination within 24 hours

Known hepatitis C carrier source person[10]

- The recipient needs to have follow-up HCV antibody tests at 1 and 6 weeks and ALT levels at 4–6 months.
- There is no effective immunoprophylaxis available. Consider early therapy should seroconversion occur.

Known HIV-positive source person[10]

Refer to consultant about relative merits of drug prophylaxis (ART) and serological monitoring. A case control study by the US Centers for Disease Control and Prevention indicated that giving zidovudine following a needle-stick injury decreases the rate of HIV seroconversion by 79%.[11]

HIV postexposure prophylaxis consists of 2–3 antiretroviral medications administered for 28 days. Seek advice urgently, because prophylaxis is ideally commenced within 2 hours of exposure.

Unknown risk source person

Take source person's blood (if consent is given) and sharps victim's blood for hepatitis B (HBsAg and anti-HBs) and hepatitis C and HIV status tests. Commence hepatitis B vaccination if not vaccinated.

Note: Informed consent for testing and disclosure of test results for involved person should be obtained.

Tetanus prophylaxis

Tetanus is a very serious disease but completely preventable by active immunisation. Immunisation should be universal, as per the childhood and adult immunisation program. However, all patients with wounds should be assessed for their tetanus status and managed on their merits. For severe wounds, the possibility of gas gangrene should also be considered.

Tetanus-prone wounds:

- compound fractures
- penetrating injuries
- foreign bodies
- extensive crushing
- delayed debridement
- severe burns
- pyogenic infection

For the primary immunisation of adults, tetanus toxoid (available combined with diphtheria and, often, pertussis) is given as two doses 6 weeks apart, with a third dose 6 months later. Booster doses of tetanus toxoid are given as an adolescent and at age 50. Give a booster dose at the time of major injury unless it is less than 5 years since the previous dose.[12]

Table 132.4 Guide to tetanus prophylaxis in wound management[3]

Time since vaccination	Type of wound	Tetanus toxoid	Tetanus immunoglobulin
History of 3 or more doses of tetanus toxoid			
<5 years	All wounds	No	No
5 to 10 years	Clean minor wounds	No	No
	All other wounds	Yes	No
>10 years	All wounds	Yes	No
Uncertain vaccination history or less than 3 doses of tetanus toxoid			
	Clean minor wounds	Yes	No
	All other wounds	Yes	Yes

Passive immunisation

Passive immunisation, in the form of tetanus immunoglobulin 250 units by IM injection, is reserved for non-immunised individuals or those of uncertain immunity wherever the wound is contaminated or has devitalised tissue. It should be given as soon as possible, on the day of injury. Wounds at risk include those contaminated with dirt, faeces/manure, soil, saliva or other foreign material; puncture wounds; and wounds from missiles, crushes and burns.

The guide is outlined in TABLE 132.4.

References

1 Hansen G. *Practice Tips.* Aust Fam Physician, 1982; 11: 867.

2 Medeiros I, Saconato H. Antibiotic prophylaxis for mammalian bites. Cochrane Database Syst Rev. 2001; updated 2008, Issue 2. Art No. CD001738.

3 Moulds R (Chair). *Therapeutic Guidelines: Antibiotic* (Version 15). Melbourne: Therapeutic Guidelines Ltd, 2017.

4 Broom J, Woods ML. Management of bite injuries. Australian Prescriber, 2006; 29: 6–8.

5 Papadakis MA, McPhee SJ et al. *Current Medical Diagnosis and Treatment* (52nd edn). New York: The McGraw-Hill Companies, 2013: 1549–53.

6 Moulds R (Chair). *Therapeutic Guidelines: Toxicology and Wilderness* (Version). Melbourne: Therapeutic Guidelines Ltd, 2008: 253–69.

7 Rhodes J et al. The surface area of the hand and the palm for estimating percentage of total body surface area: Results of a meta-analysis. Br J Dermatol, 2013; 169: 76–84.

8 Trevillyan JM, Denholm JT, Spelman D. Managing community needlestick injuries. Medicine Today, 2009; 10 (9): 80–3.

9 Royal Children's Hospital, Melbourne, Australia. Clinical Practice Guideline on needle stick injury. <www.rch.org.au/clinicalguide/index.cfm> (accessed April 2018).

10 Buckley N (Chair). *Australian Medicines Handbook.* Adelaide: Australian Medicines Handbook Pty Ltd, 2013: 189–90.

11 Cardo D et al. A case-control study of HIV seroconversion in health care workers after percutaneous exposure. New Engl J Med, 1997; 337: 1485–90.

12 Australian Technical Advisory Group on Immunisation (ATAGI). *The Australian Immunisation Handbook* (10th edn). Canberra: Australian Government Department of Health, 2017.

133 Common fractures and dislocations

The broken bone, once set together, is stronger than ever.

John Lyly (1554–1606)

Common fractures and dislocations usually apply to the limbs, the shoulder girdle and the pelvic girdle and their management requires an early diagnosis to ensure optimum treatment and to prevent complications. Early diagnosis depends on the physician being vigilant and on having knowledge of the less common conditions so that a careful search for the diagnosis can be made.

The diagnosis is dependent on a good history followed by a careful examination, good-quality X-rays appropriate to the injury (e.g. stress view) and, if necessary, special investigations. The family doctor should develop the habit of looking at a patient's X-rays. Such a back-up to the radiologist's report can help avoid missed diagnoses.

The usual rule is: if in doubt, X-ray. However, in response to over-ordering of X-rays in many circumstances where a fracture is very unlikely, handy algorithms have been developed, such as the Ottawa Ankle and Knee rules and the Canadian C-spine Rule.[1]

There are many pitfalls involved in managing fractures and dislocations. Many injuries, such as fractures of the arm and hand, may seem trivial but can lead to long-term disability. This chapter presents guidelines to help avoid these pitfalls.

Key facts and checkpoints

- A fracture usually causes deformity but may cause nothing more than local tenderness over the bone (e.g. scaphoid fracture, impacted fractured neck of femur).
- The classic signs of fracture are:
  - pain
  - tenderness
  - loss of function
  - deformity
  - swelling/bruising
  - (crepitus)
- X-ray examination of the upper limb should include views of joints proximal or distal to the site of the injury, and X-rays in both AP and lateral planes.
- If an X-ray is reported as normal but a fracture is strongly suspected, one option is to splint the affected limb for about 10 days and then repeat the X-ray.
- As a rule, displaced fractures must be reduced whereby bone ends are placed in proper alignment and then immobilised until union occurs.
- Fractures prone to loss of position should be monitored radiologically, particularly in the first 1–2 weeks following reduction.
- Bone union is assessed clinically by reduced pain at the fracture site and reduced fracture mobility. It is assessed radiologically by X-ray features such as trabecular continuity across the fracture site and bridging callus.
- Non-union is caused by such factors as inadequate immobilisation, excessive distraction, loss of healing callus, infection or avascular necrosis.
- Stiffness of joints is a common problem with immobilisation in plaster casts and slings, so the joints must be moved as early as possible. Early use is possible if the fracture is stable.
- A dislocation is a complete disruption of one bone relative to another at a joint.
- A subluxation is a partial displacement such that the joint surfaces are still in partial contact.
- A sprain is a partial disruption of a ligament or capsule of a joint.
- Always consider associated soft-tissue injuries such as neuropraxia to adjacent nerves, vascular injuries and muscle compartment syndromes.
- The key strategy of most reduction manoeuvres is traction, especially for dislocations. This may be supplemented with translation or leverage.
- A stress fracture is an incomplete fracture resulting from repeated small episodes of trauma, which individually would be insufficient to damage the bone. Stress fractures, especially in the foot, are most likely to result from sport, ballet, gymnastics and aerobics. These overuse injuries were initially described as 'march' fractures in military recruits with rapidly increased exercise levels.[2]

- Typical stress fractures (with their usual cause) include:
  - navicular (sprinting sports, football)
  - metatarsal neck (running, walking, basketball, jumping)
  - base of fifth metatarsal (dancing)
  - femur—neck or shaft (distance running)
  - ulna (weight-lifting)
  - distal radial and ulnar epiphyses (gymnastics)
  - talus (running)
  - proximal tibia (running, football)
  - lumbar spine
  - medial tibia (running, football)
  - distal phalanges (guitar playing)
  - cervical spinous process (gardening)
  - lumbar vertebrae—pars interarticularis (fast bowling)
  - spiral humerus (throwing sports)
  - rib—1st (weight-lifting)
  - rib—8th (tennis)

Easily missed fractures: red flags

- Supracondylar fracture in children
- Elbow fractures in children, especially lateral humeral condyle
- Trampoline injuries in children
- Scaphoid fracture
- Scapholunate dislocation
- Skull fractures, especially temporal
- Talar dome fractures
- All intra-articular fractures
- Avascular heads of humerus and femur

Testing for fractures[3]

This method describes the simple principle of applying axial compression for the clinical diagnosis of fractures of bones of the forearm and hand, but also applies to bones of the limbs.

Many fractures are obvious when applying the classic methods of diagnosis but it is sometimes more difficult if there is associated soft-tissue injury from a blow or if there is only a minor fracture such as a greenstick fracture of the distal radius.

A soft-tissue injury of the forearm will, like a fracture, show pain, tenderness, swelling and possibly loss of function. It will not, however, be painful if the bone is compressed axially—that is, in its long axis. Therefore, asking about pain while compressing the bone from end to end (avoiding any direct pressure on the traumatised area) is a useful way to highlight a fracture.

Walking is another method of applying axial compression; pain makes walking very difficult in the presence of a fracture in the weight-bearing axis or pelvis.

Method

1. Grasp the affected area both distally and proximally with your hands.
2. Compress along the long axis of the bones by pushing in both directions, so that the forces focus on the affected area (fracture site, see FIG. 133.1A). Alternatively, compression can be applied from the distal end with stabilising counterpressure applied proximally (see FIG. 133.1B).
3. The patient will accurately localise the pain at the fracture site.

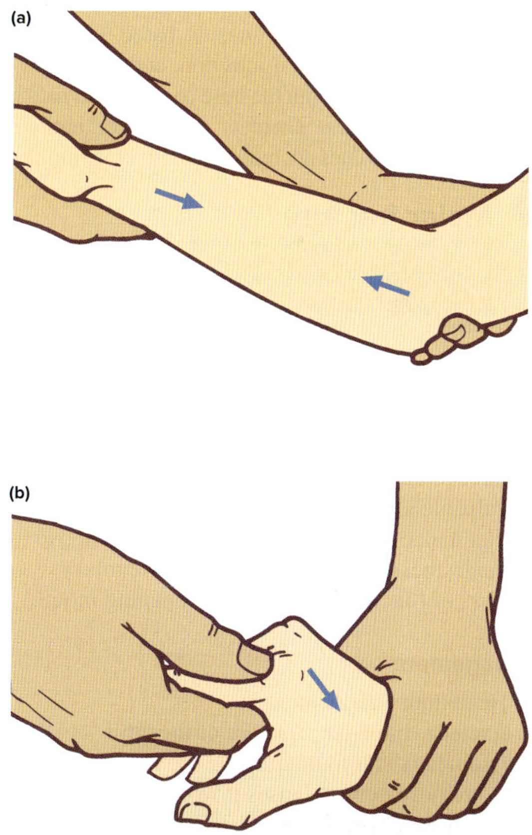

FIGURE 133.1 Testing for fractures: **(a)** axial compression to detect a fracture of the radius or ulna bones, **(b)** axial compression to detect a fracture of the metacarpal

133

Treatment of head, spine and chest fractures

INJURIES OF THE SKULL AND FACE

Skull fractures

Closed fractures without any neurological symptoms do not require active intervention. Depressed fractures may require elevation of the depressed fragment. Compound fractures of the vault require careful evaluation and referral. Special care is required over the midline as manipulation (usually by elevation) of any depressed fragment can tear the sagittal sinus, causing profuse and fatal bleeding. Beware of the associated extradural or subdural haematoma (see CHAPTER 75).

Base of skull fractures

These fractures are difficult to diagnose on radiography but their presence is indicated by bleeding from the nose, throat or ears, or by 'raccoon eyes'. CSF may be observed escaping, especially through the nose, if the dura is also torn.

133

Treatment of basal fractures is based on looking for and treating intracranial infection, and avoidance of excessive interference with the nose or ear; avoid packing and nasogastric tubes. There is no role for antibiotic prophylaxis as this does not reduce the risk of meningitis.[4]

Malar fracture

A fractured zygomaticomaxillary complex (malar) is a common body contact sports injury or injury resulting from a fight. See FIGURE 133.2.

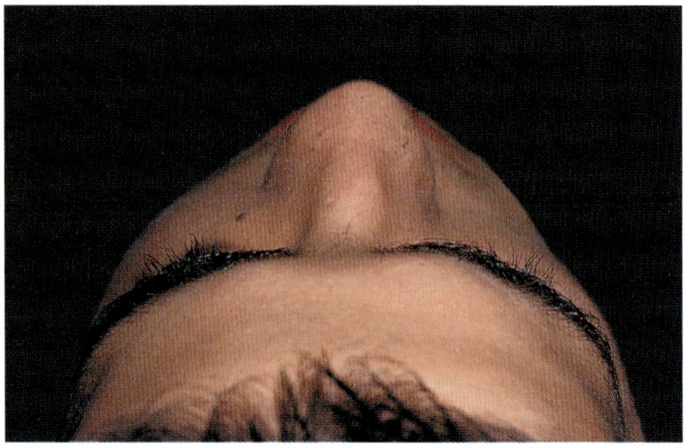

FIGURE 133.2 Fractured malar (right) showing circumocular haematoma and depression of the infraorbital margin

Used with permission from Knoop KJ, Stack LB, Storrow AB, Thurman RJ (eds): *The Atlas of Emergency Medicine*, 4th ed. New York: McGraw-Hill, 2016. Photo contributor: Edward S. Amrhein, DDS

Clinical features

- Swelling of cheek
- Circumocular haematoma
- Subconjunctival haemorrhage
- Palpable step in infraorbital margin
- Flat malar eminence when viewed from above
- Paraesthesia due to infraorbital nerve injury
- Loss of function (i.e. difficulty opening mouth)

Management

- Head injury assessment
- Exclude 'blow-out' fracture of the orbit
- Exclude ocular trauma:
  - remove contact lenses if worn
  - check visual acuity
  - check for diplopia
  - check for hyphaema
  - check for retinal haemorrhage
- Persuade patient not to blow nose (can cause surgical emphysema)
- If fracture displaced, refer for reduction under general anaesthesia

Reduction methods

- Elevation by temporal or intraoral approach—healing can be expected in 3–4 weeks
- Some require interosseous wiring or plating or pinning

Fracture of mandible

A fracture of the mandible follows a blow to the jaw. The patient may have swelling (which can vary from virtually none to severe), pain, deformity, inability to chew, malalignment of the jaw and teeth and drooling of saliva. Intraoral examination is important as submucosal ecchymosis in the floor of the mouth is a pathognomonic sign.

A simple office test for a suspected fractured mandible is to ask patients to bite on a wooden tongue depressor (or similar firm object). Ask them to maintain the bite as you twist the spatula. If they have a fracture they cannot hang onto the spatula because of the pain.[5]

X-rays:

- AP views and lateral obliques
- an orthopantomogram provides a global view

First aid management

- Check the patient's bite and airway
- Remove any free-floating tooth fragments and retain them
- Replace any avulsed or subluxed teeth in their sockets

Note: Never discard teeth.

- First aid immobilisation with a four-tailed bandage, which can be made by splitting a bandage from both ends, leaving an intact central area to support the chin (see FIG. 133.3)

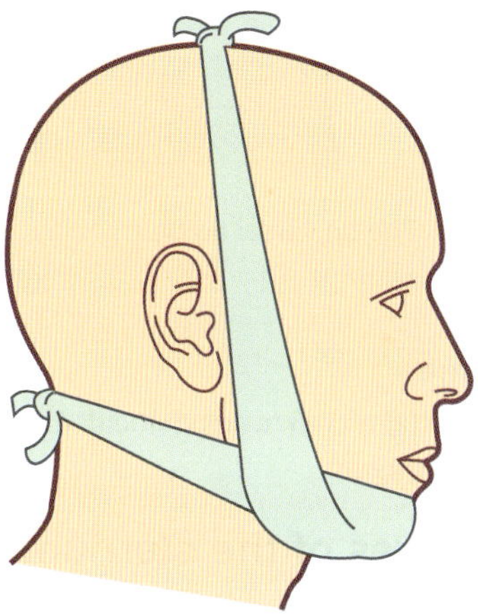

FIGURE 133.3 Immobilisation of a fractured mandible in a four-tailed bandage

Treatment

Refer for possible internal fixation.

A fracture of the body of the mandible will usually heal in 6–12 weeks (depending on the nature of the fracture and fitness of the patient).

Dislocated jaw

The patient may present with unilateral or bilateral dislocation. The jaw will be 'locked' and the patient unable to articulate or close the mouth. It is very distressing.

Method of reduction

- Get the patient to sit upright with the head against the wall. Wear protective gloves, if available.
- Wrap a handkerchief or cloth around both thumbs and place the thumbs over the lower molar teeth, with the fingers firmly grasping the mandible on the outside.
- Firmly thrusting with the thumbs, push downwards towards the floor (see FIG. 133.4).

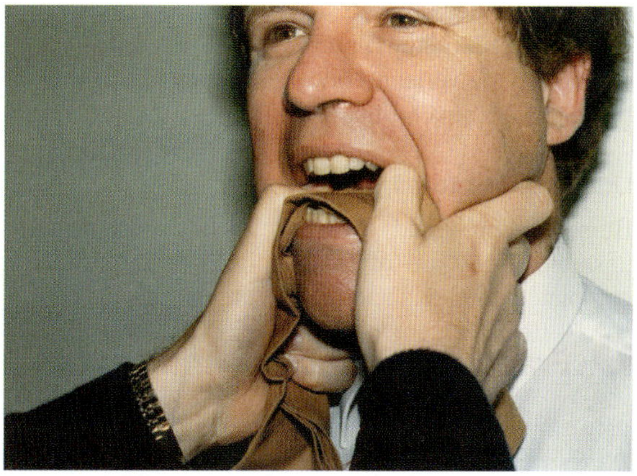

FIGURE 133.4 Method of reduction of a dislocated jaw by downward traction on the mandible

This action invariably reduces the dislocation, but the reduction can be reinforced by the fingers rotating the mandible upwards as the thumbs thrust downwards.

INJURIES OF THE SPINE

Cervical fractures, especially of the atlas (C1), axis (C2) and odontoid process, require early referral with the neck immobilised in a cervical collar, in a supine position. A hard collar is preferred, but a soft collar with sandbags on either side of the head to prevent movement will suffice.

Thoracolumbar fractures

Fractures or fracture dislocations of the thoracic and lumbar vertebrae, without neurological deficit, are classified as either stable or unstable. Due to the forces involved, these fractures often coexist with other injuries.

Stable fractures

- Compression fractures of vertebral body with <50% loss of vertical height
- Minor fractures
- Laminar fractures

Treatment: a custom-fitted back brace is worn, usually for 6–12 weeks, with physiotherapy involvement to restore function.

Special problems:

- retroperitoneal haematoma
- paralytic ileus
- associated kidney rupture with L1 fractures
- underlying vertebral body pathology in the elderly (e.g. myeloma or metastases)

Unstable fractures

Burst fractures and shearing fractures are usually unstable. They are often associated with partial or complete paraplegia and require urgent referral.

Fractures of sacrum and coccyx

133

No treatment apart from symptomatic treatment is required. Manual reduction per rectum can be attempted for significant forward displacement of the coccyx. Advise the use of a rubber ring or special cushion (such as a Sorbo cushion) when sitting. Consider excision of the coccyx for persistent discomfort.

INJURIES OF THE THORACIC CAGE

Fractured rib

Clinical features

- Pain over the fracture site, especially with deep inspiration and coughing
- Localised tenderness and swelling
- Pain in the site upon whole-chest compression (rib springing)
- X-ray confirms diagnosis and excludes underlying lung damage (e.g. pneumothorax). There is a high incidence of false negative fractures on X-ray, so caution is necessary.
- Suspect splenic, hepatic and kidney trauma with lower rib fractures

Treatment

A simple rib fracture can be extremely painful. The first treatment strategy is to prescribe analgesics, such as paracetamol, and encourage breathing within the limits of pain. An intercostal nerve block is effective in the acute situation, but is very temporary. An elastic rib belt with Velcro fastening has often been used for single or double rib fractures, although the evidence for effectiveness is scanty (see FIG. 133.5).

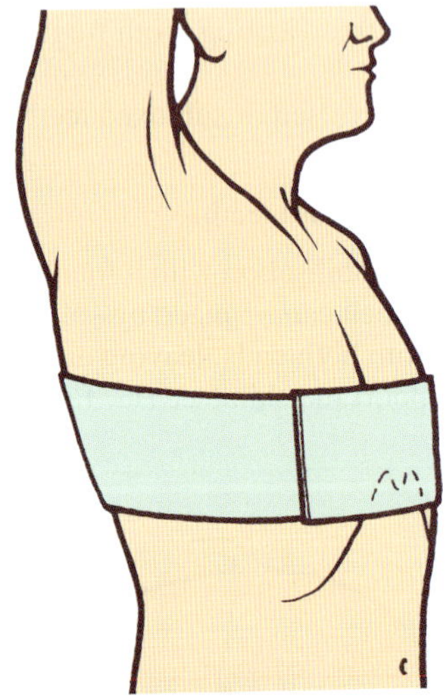

FIGURE 133.5 The universal rib belt

Healing time

Healing may take 3–6 weeks; local discomfort may persist much longer.

Fractures of the sternum

These are treated symptomatically with analgesics but careful evaluation of thoracic injuries, including cardiac tamponade or myocardial contusion, is essential. A significantly depressed fracture should be referred. An ECG is advisable.

Treatment of limb fractures

To properly reduce any displaced fracture, the following steps must be taken (see FIG. 133.6A).[6]

1. Disimpact the fragments, usually by increasing the deformity.
2. Re-establish the correct length of the bone.
3. Re-establish the correct alignment by proper reduction of the fracture.
4. Stabilise the bone in an acceptable position for as long as it takes to heal.

The above steps will only be achieved with adequate anaesthesia, analgesia and relaxation. Maintenance of the reduction depends upon the

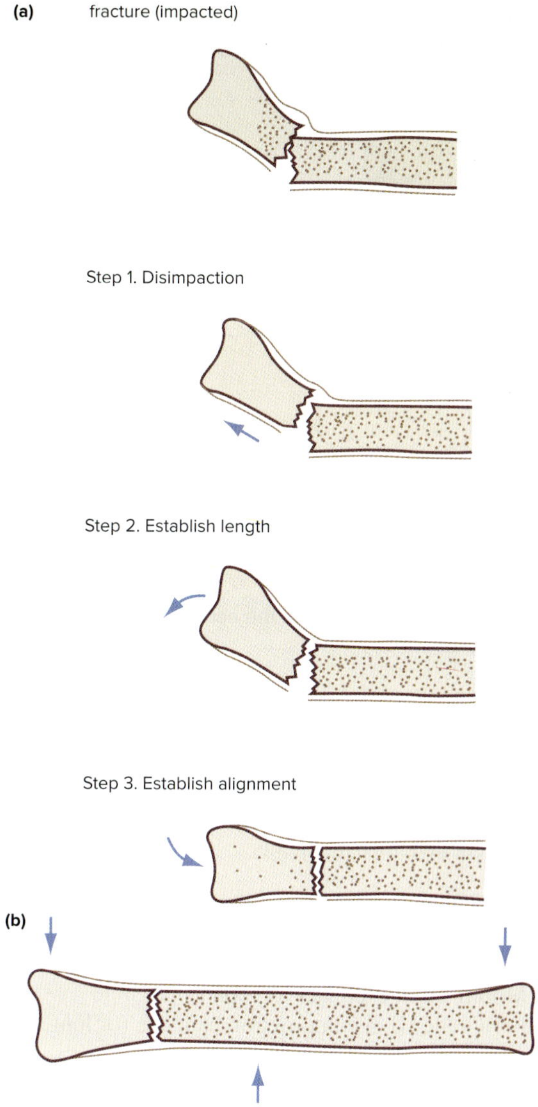

FIGURE 133.6 **(a)** Principles of reduction of fractured bones, **(b)** Principles of moulding to maintain reduction: the arrows indicate the three point pressure areas required to maintain reduction

moulding, which utilises the intact periosteal bridge to hold the fracture fragments in a reduced position. FIGURE 133.6B illustrates the principle of moulding to maintain reduction.[6]

Orthopaedic problems that cause difficulties in diagnosis and management are outlined in TABLE 133.1.

Table 133.1 Important orthopaedic problems that cause difficulties in diagnosis and management[7]

Shoulders
Posterior dislocation of the shoulder
Recurrent subluxations
Unstable surgical neck fractures of humerus
The avascular humeral head
Elbow
Supracondylar fractures with forearm ischaemia
Fracture of the lateral humeral condyle in children
Fractured neck of radius in children
The Monteggia fracture with dislocation of radial head
Wrist
Scaphoid fractures
Scapholunate dislocation
The unstable Colles fracture
Fingers
Phalangeal fractures
Intra-articular fractures
Penetrating injuries of the MCP joint
Gamekeeper's thumb (MCP joint)
The hip
Developmental dysplasia of the hip
Septic arthritis
Slipped capital femoral epiphysis
Subcapital fractures
Stress fractures of the femoral neck in athletes
Impacted subcapital femoral neck fracture in the elderly
Foot and ankle
Talar dome lesions
Stress fractures of the navicular
Intra-articular fractures

Fractures of the clavicle

This fracture typically follows a history of a fall onto the outstretched hand or elbow, although it may also occur with a direct blow to the clavicle or the point of the shoulder. The patient has pain aggravated by shoulder movement and usually supports the arm at the elbow and clasped to the chest. The most common fracture site is at the junction of the outer and middle thirds, or in the middle third. Consider the possibility of neurovascular injury.

Treatment

- St John's elevated sling to support arm—for 3 weeks
- Figure-of-eight bandage (used mainly for severe discomfort)
- Early active exercises to elbow, wrist and fingers
- Active shoulder movements as early as possible

Special problem

Type II fracture at the lateral end of the clavicle that is displaced: this fracture, which usually occurs in elderly patients following low energy injuries,[8] is often subject to delayed or non-union. The line of fracture passes through the conoid and trapezoid ligaments. Consider referral for open reduction.

Healing time

Healing time is 4–8 weeks.

The appropriate use of slings for fracture-dislocations is presented in TABLE 133.2.

Table 133.2 Appropriate use of slings for fracture–dislocations

Collar and cuff	Fractured shaft of humerus
Broad arm sling (hand horizontal)	Fractured forearm Fractured scapula
St John's high sling (hand points at opposite shoulder)	Fractured clavicle Fractured neck of humerus Subluxed acromioclavicular joint Dislocated acromioclavicular joint Subluxed sternoclavicular joint

133

Fractures of the scapula

Fractures of the scapula may include:

- body of scapula: due to a crushing force, considerable blood loss, may be rib fractures
- neck of scapula (may involve joint)
- acromion process (due to a blow or fall on the shoulder)
- coracoid process (due to a blow or fall on the shoulder)

Treatment

- Broad-based triangular sling for comfort
- Early active exercises for shoulder, elbow and fingers as soon as tolerable
- A large glenoid fragment usually requires surgical reduction because of potential glenohumeral joint instability

Healing time

Healing takes several weeks to months.

DISLOCATIONS OF THE SHOULDER AND CLAVICLE

Acromioclavicular joint dislocation/subluxation

A fall on the shoulder, elbow or outstretched arm can cause varying degrees of separation of the acromioclavicular (AC) joint, causing the lateral end of the clavicle to be displaced upwards (see FIG. 133.7).

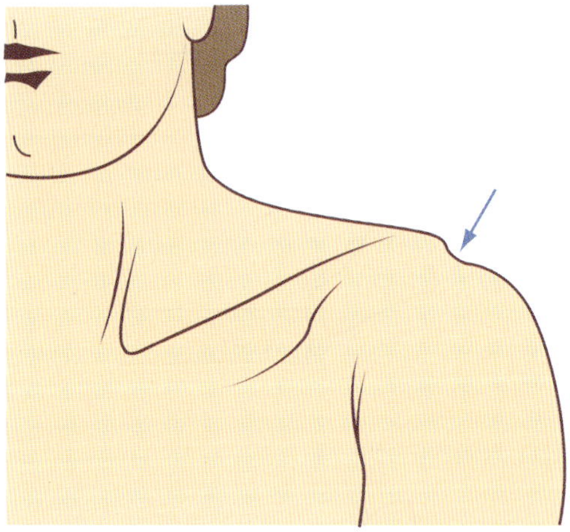

FIGURE 133.7 Subluxation of the acromioclavicular joint: typical appearance

- Grades I, II: partial separation, involving tearing of the AC capsule and ligaments
- Grade III: complete tearing, also affecting the coracoclavicular ligaments

Treatment

- Analgesics
- St John's high sling (suitable for all injuries)
- Mobilisation exercises as soon as possible
- For Grade III, a compression bandage (or long straps of adhesive low-stretch strapping) with padding at pressure points—elbows, clavicle and coracoid. The clavicle should be manipulated into its correct position and the forearm elevated: applying pressure from above (clavicle) and below (elbow) to achieve compression, apply a bandage over the outer end of the clavicle and round the elbow joint, which is flexed to 90°. The bandage or strapping is worn for 2–3 weeks.[8] Many patients are unable to tolerate this method of treatment. Skin irritation or blisters are common. This occurs particularly with adhesive strapping and the deformity commonly requires correction after the removal of the bandage or strapping. The same effect may be achieved with an orthotic device known as a Kenny-Howard sling or brace.
- The issue of internal fixation versus conservative treatment for a complete dislocation is

controversial in that the bulk of patients treated conservatively have minimal residual symptoms. However, a significant minority have residual symptoms in the form of AC joint pain and traction effects on the brachial plexus due to loss of scapular suspension. The patients most likely to have these symptoms are those with high grades of separation, involvement of the dominant shoulder and participation in employment or sports that place heavy physical demands on the shoulder girdle. If there is disruption of the suspensory ligaments of the clavicle, surgical reduction and stabilisation is the preferred option.[8] If in doubt, refer within the first few weeks of injury for consideration of the pros and cons of conservative versus surgical treatment.

Sternoclavicular joint dislocation/ subluxation

This uncommon injury is caused by a fall or very heavy impact on the shoulder, causing the medial end of the clavicle to move forwards or anterior (making it prominent) or backwards.[9] Plain X-rays are difficult to interpret and a CT scan is the ideal diagnostic method.

Special problem

A special problem is backward (inward) displacement of the clavicular end with danger to major blood vessels and the trachea. This is one of the few potentially life-threatening orthopaedic injuries. Urgent referral for reduction is essential, especially if stridor or venous obstruction is present. A first aid measure is to place a sandbag between the shoulders with the patient supine and to extend the abducted arm on the affected side.[10] Closed reduction can usually be achieved under anaesthesia. The reduction is nearly always stable.

Treatment

Forward subluxation or dislocation, unlike posterior dislocation, is nearly always unstable and resists attempts at maintaining closed reduction. Despite the persistence of a medial clavicular swelling, most patients need a sling for only 1–2 weeks and the bulk of their pain settles over the following months. Surgery is generally indicated only for an unusually painful and chronic anterior sternoclavicular dislocation.

Dislocation of the shoulder

Dislocations of the shoulder joint can be caused by an impact on the arm by falling directly on the outer aspect of the shoulder, or by a direct violent impact, or by a forceful wrenching of the arm outwards and backwards.

Types of dislocation

- Anterior (forward and downward)—95% of dislocations
- Posterior (backward)—diagnosis often overlooked
- Recurrent anterior dislocation (recurrent posterior dislocation extremely rare)

Anterior dislocation of the shoulder

Management

AP and lateral X-rays should be undertaken to check the position and exclude an associated fracture. The arm should be assessed for the presence of neurological injury before reduction. Reduction can be achieved under general anaesthesia (easier and more comfortable) or with intravenous morphine ± diazepam/midazolam. A variety of methods can be used for anterior dislocation; two are described below. Satisfactory analgesia and patient relaxation are vital to the success of any of the methods.

Kocher method

(See FIG. 133.8.)

- Elbow flexed to 90° and held close to the body
- Slowly rotate arm laterally (externally)
- Adduct humerus across the body by carrying point of elbow while simultaneously applying longitudinal traction along the line of the humerus
- Rotate arm medially (internally)

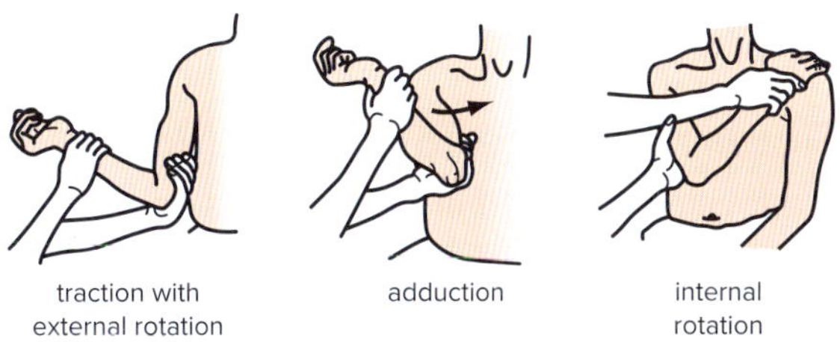

FIGURE 133.8 Kocher method for a dislocated shoulder

Hippocratic method

Apply traction to the outstretched arm by a hold on the hand with countertraction from stockinged foot in the medial wall of the axilla. This levers the head of the humerus back. It is a good method if there is an associated avulsion fracture of the greater tuberosity.

Postreduction

- Reduction is complete if the hand can rest comfortably on the opposite shoulder.
- Confirm reduction by X-ray in two planes and again assess for unsuspected fractures (e.g. glenoid rim or greater tuberosity fractures).
- Keep the arm in a sling for 2 weeks.
- Apply a swathe bandage to the chest wall.
- After immobilisation, begin pendulum and circumduction exercises.
- Combined abduction and lateral rotation should be avoided for 3 weeks.

Posterior dislocation of the shoulder

This is the most commonly misdiagnosed major joint dislocation.[7] Posterior dislocation most often follows an epileptic seizure or electrical shock. The postictal patient with a painful shoulder has a posterior dislocation of the shoulder until proven otherwise. Less often this injury is caused by a fall onto the outstretched hand with the arm internally rotated or by a direct blow to the front of the shoulder. If any doubt persists about the diagnosis, a CT scan is appropriate.

The shoulder contour may look normal, but the major clinical sign is painful restriction of external rotation, which is usually completely blocked. Beware of the problem of pain in the shoulder after a convulsion. An 'axillary shoot through' X-ray view should be routinely ordered following shoulder trauma.

Reduction of posterior dislocation

Using appropriate analgesia or anaesthesia, apply traction to the shoulder in 90° of abduction (with the elbow at right angles) and laterally (externally) rotate the limb. Referral for reduction is advisable.

Recurrent anterior dislocation

Acute anterior shoulder dislocation may tear or stretch the anterior capsular ligaments from their bony origin. This may predispose to recurrent anterior dislocation or subluxation. (Recurrent posterior instability is rare.)

A simple procedure for reducing recurrent anterior dislocation is as follows.

- Get the patient to sit comfortably on a chair with legs crossed.
- The patient then interlocks hands and elevates the upper knee so that the hands grip the knee.
- The knee is gradually lowered until its full weight is taken by the hands. At the same time the patient has to concentrate on relaxing the muscles of the shoulder girdle. This method usually effects reduction without the use of force.

Recurrent dislocation often requires definitive surgery, depending on the frequency of dislocations and the degree of apprehension between episodes.

The Bankart lesion

Teenagers and young adults who sustain a traumatic dislocation of the shoulders tend to have the Bankart lesion, which is avulsion of the anteroinferior capsulolabral complex, leading to a high rate of recurrent dislocation. This should be considered for an arthroscopic anterior stabilisation.

Pitfalls

- Nerve injury, especially axillary (circumflex) nerve
- A fractured neck of the humerus, especially in the elderly, may mimic a dislocation
- Associated fractures (greater tuberosity, head of radius, glenoid) may require internal fixation
- Great difficulty with some reductions (this is often related to inadequate analgesia; the use of excessive force may result in fracture)
- Failing to X-ray all suspected dislocations before and after reduction; failing to obtain an axillary view to show posterior displacement or fractures of the humerus or glenoid

FRACTURES OF THE HUMERUS

Fractured greater tuberosity of humerus

Treat with a combination of immediate mobilisation and rest in a sling unless grossly displaced, when surgical reduction is advisable. Shoulder stiffness can be a disabling problem, so early movement is encouraged, with review in 7 days. This fracture should be monitored by X-ray within 2 weeks after injury. Undetected displacement may lead to mechanical impingement against the acromion. This fracture may also be an indication of the patient having had a transient glenohumeral dislocation.

Fractured surgical neck of humerus

This usually occurs in the elderly due to a fall onto the outstretched hand. The fragments may be impacted. The greater tuberosity may also be fractured. Watch out for associated dislocation. In adolescents, fracture–separation of the upper humeral epiphysis occurs.

Treatment (no displacement or impaction)

- Triangular sling
- When pain subsides (10–14 days), encourage pendulum exercises in the sling
- Aim for full activity within 8–12 weeks post-injury

Displaced fractures may require internal fixation. Severely comminuted fractures may predispose to post-traumatic osteoarthritis or humeral head avascular necrosis. Consider referral with a view to prosthetic hemiarthroplasty.

Healing

Union usually occurs in 4 weeks and consolidation at 6 weeks.

Pitfalls with fractures of the surgical neck

Minimally displaced fractures of the surgical neck of the humerus are usually managed conservatively, but overzealous early mobilisation can lead to non-union.[10] If there is a communication of this fracture with joint fluid, movement washes away the fracture haematoma and leads to the development of true pseudoarthrosis. Judicious early immobilisation will avert this complication.

The cardinal fracture management rule is: 'First ensure that stability of the fracture is sufficient to allow healing before prescribing rehabilitation exercises or early use of the extremity'.[7] However, prolonged immobility can cause its own problems. Hand and elbow exercises should commence early, and gentle shoulder 'pot stirring' at around 2–3 weeks.

The management of various humeral fractures is summarised in FIGURE 133.9.

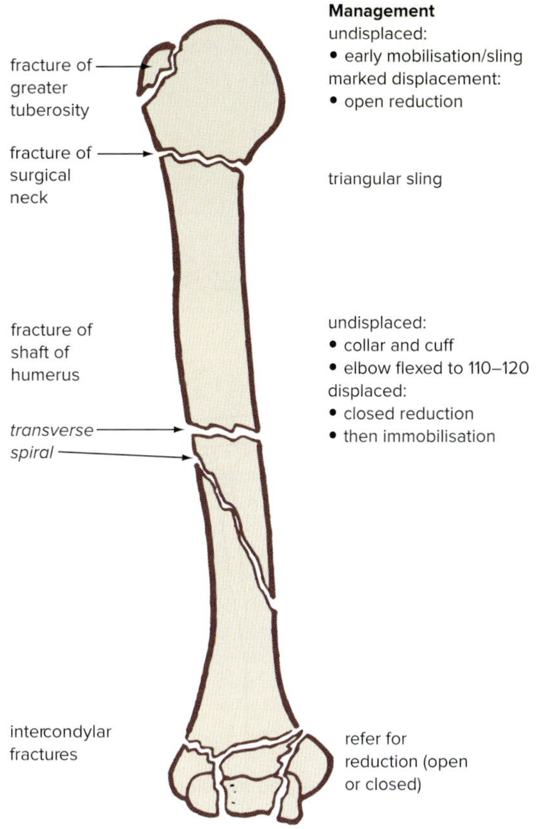

FIGURE 133.9 Various fractures of the humerus in adults

Fracture of shaft of humerus

Humeral shaft fractures may be:

- spiral—due to a fall on the hand
- transverse or slightly oblique—fall on elbow with arm abducted
- comminuted—heavy blow

Caution: watch for radial nerve palsy.

Treatment

- Perfect bony opposition is not necessary; some overriding is acceptable but distraction of the fragments is not.
- Undisplaced fracture: collar and cuff with elbow flexed to 110–120°.
- Significantly displaced humeral shaft fractures may require manipulation under anaesthetic. However, the vast majority of shaft fractures realign to a satisfactory extent under gravitational effects in a sling once muscle spasm and oedema have subsided. A U-shaped hanging cast or slab enhances the gravitational effect and assists splintage.

Intercondylar fractures in adults

Intercondylar fractures, which may be T-shaped or Y-shaped, are usually caused by a fall on the point of the elbow, which drives the olecranon process upwards, splitting the condyles apart. Fractures involving the joint can cause long-term problems of post-traumatic osteoarthritis and joint stiffness. Referral for reduction (closed or open) is appropriate.

INJURIES OF THE ELBOW AND FOREARM

Fractures and avulsion injuries around the elbow joint in children

Potentially severe deforming injuries include:

- supracondylar fractures
- fracture of the lateral humeral condyle

- fracture of medial humeral epicondyle (see FIG. 133.10)
- fracture of neck of radius

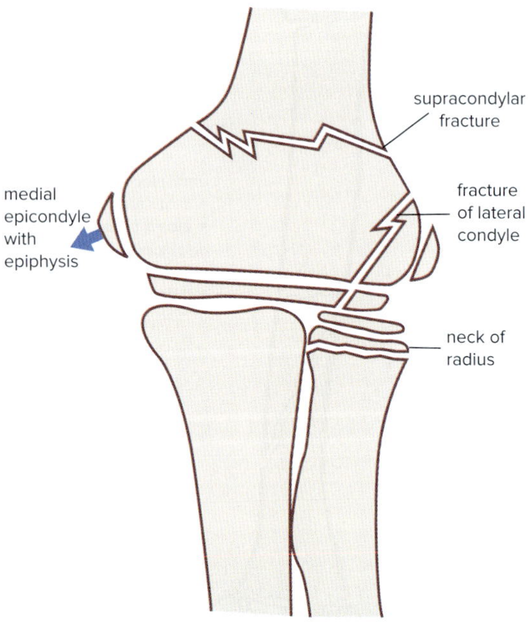

FIGURE 133.10 Fractures and avulsion injuries around the elbow joint in children

Fractures around the elbow in children require referral to consultants experienced in radiology and fracture management.

Supracondylar fractures with forearm ischaemia

Supracondylar fractures represent about half of all elbow fractures in children and most are extension fractures following falls onto the outstretched arm.

Pressure of the displaced bony fragments causes impingement on the brachial artery, which can lead to impending forearm flexor compartment ischaemia and muscle death. Severe forearm pain is the most significant and important sign of ischaemia. Neuropraxia of the median, radial or ulnar nerves is common. These injuries almost invariably recover.

This diagnosis must always be assumed in displaced supracondylar fractures in children. Thus, it is the GP's responsibility to ensure treatment is expedited. The brachial and radial pulses should be assessed carefully.

The fracture is reduced by hyperflexion of the elbow during traction (after lateral displacement has been corrected), and then immobilisation in collar and cuff and stockinet vest. The fully flexed elbow with the usually intact posterior periosteal hinge provides fracture stability. Plaster casting is unnecessary and some would suggest contraindicated because of the significant risk of ischaemic contracture. Circulatory status requires monitoring in the first 24 hours following injury. The collar and cuff should be used for 6 weeks. The invariably stiff elbow quickly resolves without a need for formal therapy.

Fracture of the lateral humeral condyle

Fractures of the lateral humeral condyle also result from a fall onto the outstretched arm in children (see FIG. 133.10). The fracture line passes vertically or obliquely through the lateral condyle and thus crosses the distal humeral growth plate. It occurs in an age group prior to the appearance of the epiphysis of the lateral epicondyle. Pain and swelling over the lateral elbow, but without the gross deformity of a supracondylar fracture of the humerus, could make one suspect this injury. The fracture is commonly overlooked on X-ray. Comparison views of the opposite elbow are particularly helpful in diagnosing this injury.

Recognition of the fracture and early open reduction and internal fixation with wires are vital to reduce the risk of premature plate closure. Such growth plate disturbance may result in a progressive valgus deformity of the elbow and the late development of an ulnar nerve palsy.

The Salter–Harris classification of epiphyseal injuries (FIG. 133.11), which is widely used, has therapeutic and prognostic implications. Most of these injuries heal well but some have the potential for growth arrest or asymmetrical bone growth, leading to deformity and permanent disability, especially type V. Types I and II (the most common) have an excellent prognosis but type III and IV require precise reduction.[11]

Fracture of the medial humeral epicondyle

This problem occurs typically in adolescents following a fall onto the outstretched hand. The medial epicondyle may be avulsed by massive flexor pronator muscle contraction together with abduction stresses on the forearm. Avulsion of the epicondyle occurs in the young patient before the epiphysis is united. If displaced, this fracture is best treated by open reduction

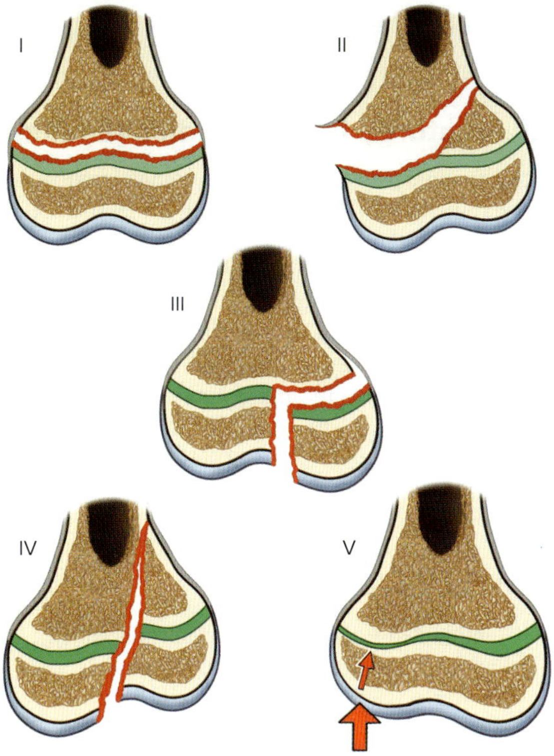

FIGURE 133.11 Salter–Harris classification of growth plate fractures. V represents compression of the growth plate (green in the figure) as shown by the region arrowed

Source: Brukner and Khan's Clinical Sports Medicine, 4th edn McGraw-Hill, Sydney, 2009.

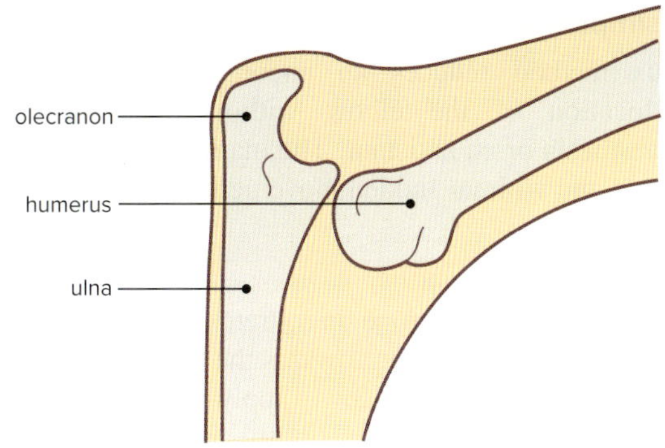

FIGURE 133.12 Dislocated elbow: uncomplicated posterior dislocation

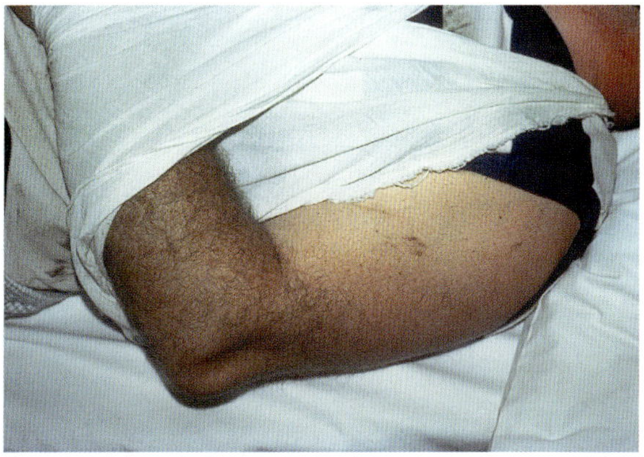

FIGURE 133.13 Dislocated elbow showing posterior displacement of the ulna and radius, with the typical deformity

and internal fixation. Untreated injuries commonly result in non-union, elbow pain and restricted elbow extension.

Fractured neck of radius

This fracture is caused by a child falling on to the outstretched hand. The fracture line is transverse and is situated immediately distal to the epiphysis.

The degree of tilt is critical. Up to 15° of tilt is acceptable but, beyond that, reduction (preferably closed) will be necessary. The head of the radius must never be excised in children.

Dislocated elbow

A dislocated elbow is caused by a fall onto the outstretched hand, forcing the forearm backwards to result in posterior and lateral displacement (see FIGS 133.12 and 133.13). The peripheral pulses and sensation in the hand must be assessed carefully. It may result in vascular injury to the brachial artery or injury to the median and ulnar nerves. Check the function of the ulnar nerve before and after reduction.

Treatment

Attempt reduction with patient fully relaxed under anaesthesia. It is important to apply traction to the flexed elbow while allowing it to extend (to approximately 20–30° of flexion) to enable correction of the lateral displacement and then the posterior displacement.

Follow-up

Encourage early mobilisation with gentle exercises in between resting the elbow for 2–3 weeks in a collar and cuff with the elbow flexed above 90°, avoiding passive movements. A plaster cast should not be used because of the risk of ischaemic necrosis of muscle. This will minimise the possibility of myositis ossificans. Recurrent dislocation of the elbow is uncommon.

A simple method of reduction

This method reduces an uncomplicated posterior dislocation of the elbow without the need for anaesthesia or an assistant. The manipulation must be gentle and without sudden movement.

Method

1. The patient lies prone on a stretcher or couch, with the forearm dangling towards the floor.
2. Grasp the wrist and slowly apply traction in the direction of the long axis of the forearm (see FIG. 133.14).
3. When the muscles feel relaxed (this might take several minutes), use the thumb and index finger of the other hand to grasp the olecranon and guide it to a reduced position, correcting any lateral shift.

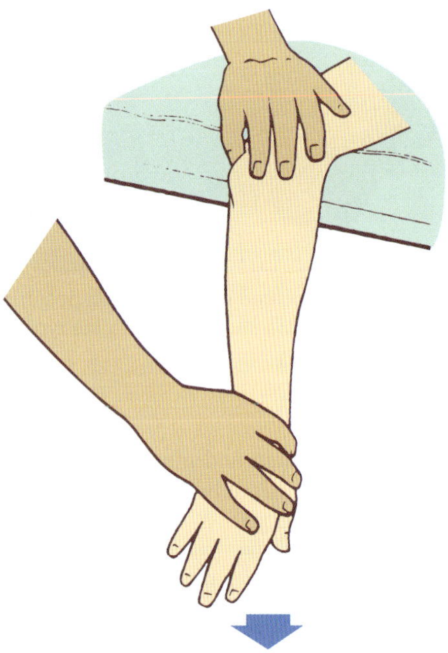

FIGURE 133.14 Dislocated elbow: method of reduction by traction on the dependent arm

Pitfalls

- Incomplete reduction: ulna articulates with capitellum and not the trochlea
- Injury to ulnar nerve (spontaneous recovery usually occurs after 6–8 weeks)
- Associated fractures (e.g. coronoid process), which may cause instability

'Pulled' elbow

See CHAPTER 64.

Fractured head of radius (adults)

If the fracture is very slight and undisplaced, treat conservatively with the elbow at right angles in a collar and cuff until the pain subsides sufficiently to allow flexion/extension and pronation/supination exercises.

Elbow stiffness is a major problem even after apparently trivial radial head fractures. Early mobilisation is vital. Excision of the radial head should be considered for highly comminuted fractures that limit the ability to mobilise the elbow early or predispose to post-traumatic osteoarthritis. Associated distal radio-ulnar joint or wrist injuries are often overlooked.

Fractured olecranon

- Comminuted fracture (with little displacement): sling for 3 weeks and active movements
- Transverse (gap) fracture: open reduction with screw or wire

Monteggia fracture–dislocation of the radial head

Fractures of the proximal third of the ulna with dislocation of the radial head (Monteggia fracture–dislocation) (see FIG. 133.15) have a history of mismanagement during treatment. The radial head dislocation is easily overlooked.

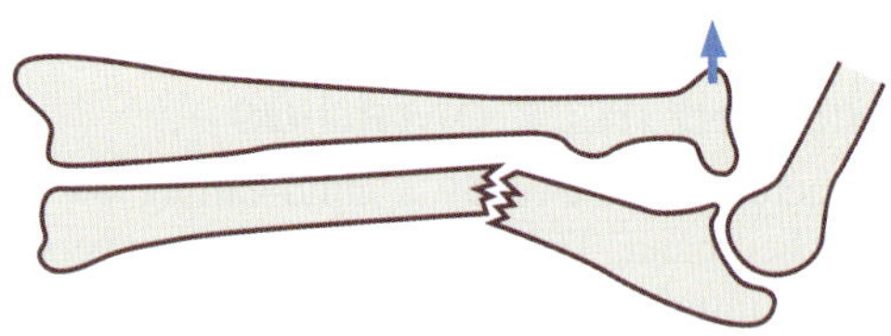

FIGURE 133.15 Monteggia fracture–dislocation of the radial head; it is important not to miss a dislocated head of radius with a fracture of the proximal third of the ulna

Redislocation or subluxation of the radial head is common.

Since surgical intervention is advisable, referral of displaced forearm fractures for early surgery is recommended. Surgical plating of the ulnar shaft maintains the radial head in a reduced position. Follow-up X-rays are mandatory to ensure that there has not been a late redislocation of the radial head.

Fracture–dislocation in the lower forearm (Galeazzi injury)

This injury is usually caused by a fall on to the hand and is a combination of a fractured radius (at the junction of its middle and distal thirds) and subluxation of the distal radio-ulnar joint. The patient should be referred, as open reduction is often required.

Fractures of the radius and ulna shafts

General features

In adults, it is more common to break both forearm bones. Displaced fractures of both bones require perfect reduction, which can generally only be achieved by surgical reduction and plating. Less-than-satisfactory reduction interferes with normal pronation and supination. A fracture of one bone alone is uncommon and usually caused by a direct blow. For a fracture of one bone alone, look for evidence of an associated dislocation of the other forearm bone. In children, greenstick fractures are common. Fractured radial shafts tend to slip and ulnar fractures heal slowly. Dislocation of the head of the radius or inferior radio-ulnar joint can be missed if X-rays do not include the elbows and wrist joints. The rule is to X-ray the joints above and below any injury.

Reduction

- A greenstick fracture is readily straightened by firm pressure.
- A complete fracture (spiral or transverse) is reduced by traction and rotation.
- A slight overlap and angulation is permissible in children, but perfect reduction is essential in adults.
- A plaster cast should include both the elbow and the wrist joints.

Healing time: (adults) spiral fracture—6 weeks; transverse fracture—12 weeks.

INJURIES OF THE WRIST

Colles fracture of lower end of radius

Colles fractures rival clavicular in being the most common of all fractures. A Colles is a supination fracture of the distal 3 cm of the radius, caused by a fall onto the outstretched hand.

Clinical features

- Usually an elderly woman
- Osteoporosis is common
- Fall on dorsiflexed hand
- Fracture features:
  - impaction
  - posterior displacement and angulation
  - lateral displacement and angulation
  - supination
  - dinner fork deformity (see FIG. 133.16)

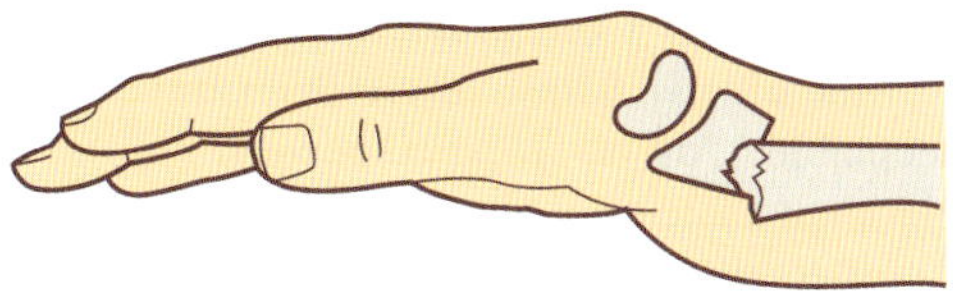

FIGURE 133.16 Dinner fork deformity of Colles fracture: a fracture of the distal head of the radius showing impaction and posterior displacement and angulation

Treatment

- If minimal displacement—below-elbow plaster for 4 weeks, then a crepe bandage
- If displaced: meticulous reduction under anaesthesia:
  - set in flexion 10°, ulnar deviation 10° and pronation (see FIG. 133.17)
  - below-elbow plaster 4–6 weeks (6 weeks maximum time)
  - unstable fractures may require an above-elbow cast initially with the forearm in pronation
  - check X-ray at 10–14 days; position may be lost as swelling subsides and plaster becomes loose

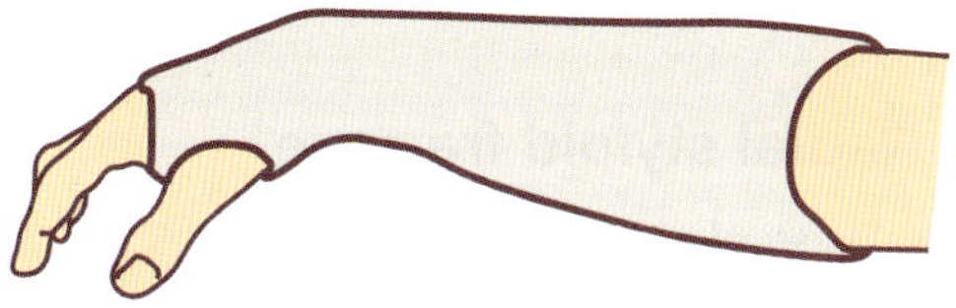

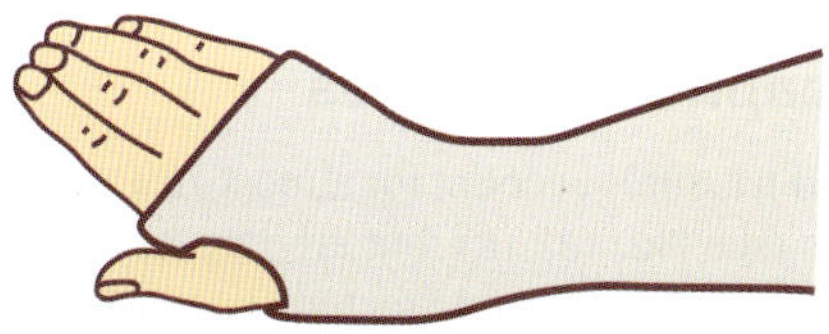

FIGURE 133.17 Ideal position of the forearm in a Colles plaster: note ulnar deviation, slight flexion and pronation

133

Problems associated with Colles fracture:

- watch for ruptured extensor pollicus longus tendon
- stiffness of the elbow, MCP joints and IP joints
- discomfort at inferior radio-ulnar joint due to disruption
- regional pain syndrome

Pitfall: the unstable Colles fracture[7]

With the advent of modern imaging techniques and power equipment it has become a simple procedure to pin unstable Colles fractures percutaneously, even in the elderly. Thus, severe deformities are now unacceptable. An early percutaneous pin is much simpler than a late osteotomy. Colles fractures deserve more respect than they received in the past.

Remember the basic classification into intra-articular and extra-articular fractures. Restoring reasonable joint surface alignment is an important part of the treatment and fortunately is usually relieved with simple traction under local or general anaesthesia.

133

Smith fracture of lower end of radius

This is often referred to as a 'reverse Colles'. It is caused by a fall onto the back of the hand. The lower fragment is flexed and impacted on the upper fragment. It is reduced and immobilised for 6 weeks in a cast as for Colles fracture but with the wrist extended. Unstable fractures may require an above-elbow cast initially with the forearm in supination.

Ulna styloid fracture

Treat symptomatically. Delayed union or non-union is common, but rarely symptomatic.

Radial styloid fracture

Undisplaced: plaster slab for 3 weeks.
Displaced: closed reduction and plaster slab for 6 weeks. If this fails—open reduction.

Scaphoid fractures

Scaphoid fractures account for almost 75% of all carpal fractures (see FIG. 133.18), but are rare in children and the elderly.[11] A scaphoid fracture is caused typically by a fall onto the outstretched hand.

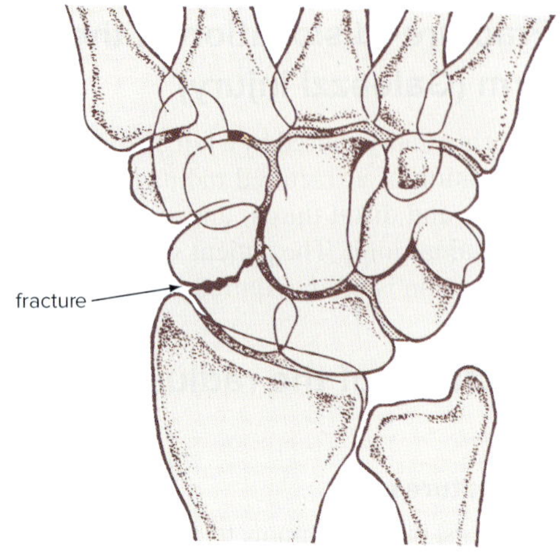

FIGURE 133.18 Typical appearance of a fractured scaphoid

Features

- Pain on lateral aspect of wrist
- Tenderness in the anatomical snuffbox (the key sign)
- Swelling in and around the snuffbox
- Pain or clicking on movement of the wrist
- Pain on axial compression of the thumb towards the radius

There is a 20% rate of false positive reporting of scaphoid radiographs and clinical confirmation of the diagnosis is mandatory.[12]

If a scaphoid fracture is highly suspected in the presence of a normal X-ray of wrist, immobilise the wrist in a scaphoid plaster for 10 days (ensure 1st MCP joint is immobilised), remove it and then re-X-ray. Isotopic bone scan may be indicated in cases where suspicion of fracture is high despite normal X-rays. For undisplaced and stable fractures, 6–8 weeks in a below-elbow scaphoid cast usually suffices (see FIG. 133.19). Displaced fractures of the scaphoid require reduction (either open or closed) and, if unstable, internal fixation.

All scaphoid fractures require late X-ray evaluation of treatment to diagnose non-union before they become symptomatic from late degenerative changes. Early bone grafting of a non-union can prevent fragment collapse and radioscaphoid degenerative changes.

Pitfall

The fracture may not be apparent on routine wrist X-rays. Request lateral, antero-posterior and specific scaphoid views.

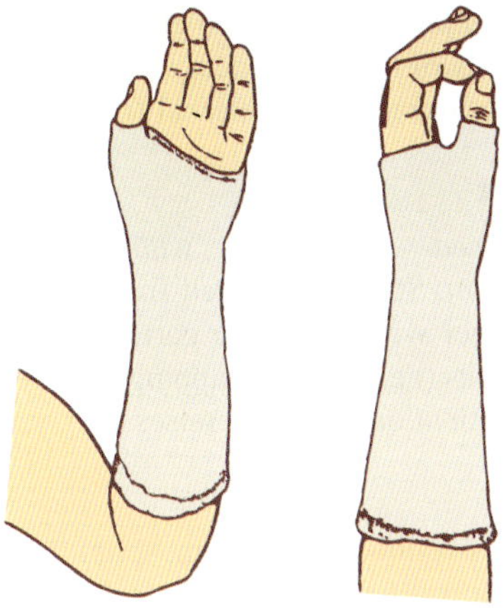

FIGURE 133.19 Appearance of the scaphoid plaster. Note that the first MCP joint is enclosed, with 2–5 MCP joints free.

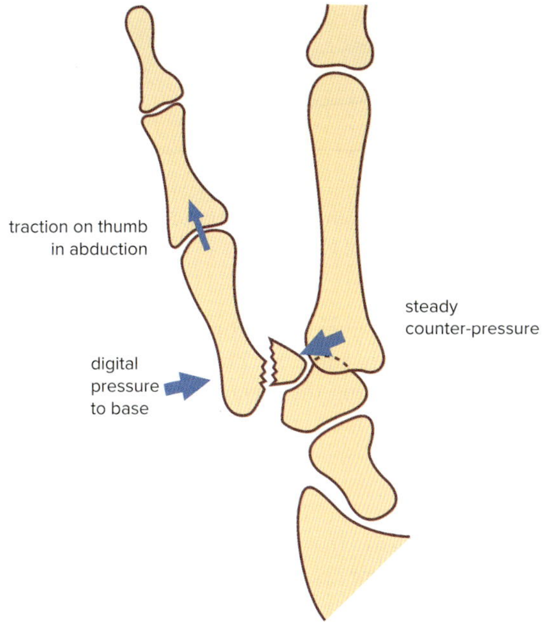

FIGURE 133.20 Method of reduction of a Bennett fracture–dislocation of the first carpometacarpal joint

Scapholunate dissociation

This not uncommon carpal injury results from disruption of the scapholunate interosseous ligament and palmar radiocarpal ligaments. It results in a gap appearing between the scaphoid and lunate bones (the so-called 'Terry Thomas' sign on plain AP X-rays of the wrist) and the scaphoid rotating into a vertical position on lateral X-rays. It is associated with pain in the wrist on dorsiflexion. Median nerve compression may occur after wrist or carpal dislocations.

Early diagnosis with referral simplifies treatment. This injury has been recognised only in recent times.

INJURIES OF THE HAND

The management of hand fractures is all about restoring function. A single stiff or deformed joint can have a lifelong impact on hand function.

Thumb fractures

The thumb's special function renders injuries more difficult than other digits. Fractures well clear of the joints in the proximal and distal phalanges are treated in a similar way to other digits. However, intra-articular injuries are more common and internal fixation is more likely on the thumb than other digits.[13]

Bennett fracture

This is a fracture–dislocation of the first carpometacarpal joint. The larger fragment of the first metacarpal dislocates proximally and laterally (see FIG. 133.20).

Treatment

Under anaesthesia, the thumb is reduced using the forces indicated (see FIG. 133.20). A scaphoid plaster is applied with the thumb in the open grasp position. If anatomical reduction cannot be achieved by closed means, then open reduction and internal fixation is indicated. Percutaneous pinning with wires under X-ray control is also commonly used to hold an anatomical reduction.

Gamekeeper's (or skier's) thumb

This problematic injury of the metacarpophalangeal joint is presented in more detail in CHAPTER 64.

Metacarpal fractures

Metacarpal fractures can be stable or unstable, intra-articular or extra-articular, and closed or open. They include the 'knuckle' injuries resulting from a punch, which is prone to cause a fracture of the neck of the fourth and fifth metacarpal. As a general rule, most metacarpal (shaft and neck) fractures are treated by correcting marked displacements with manipulation (under anaesthesia) and splinting with a below-elbow, padded posterior plaster slab that extends up to the dorsum of the proximal phalanx and holds the metacarpophalangeal joints in a position of function (see FIG. 133.21).

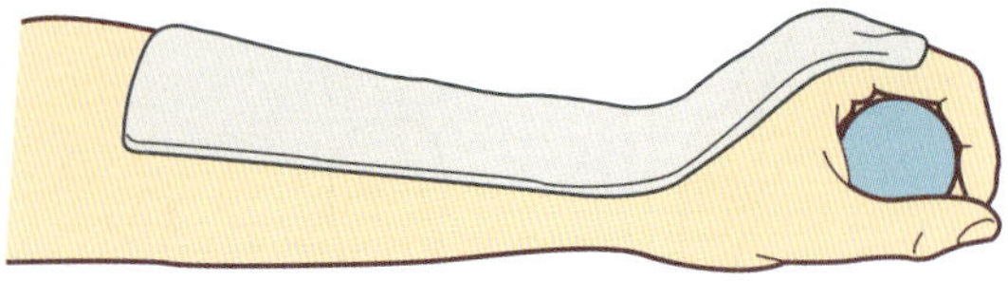

FIGURE 133.21 Fracture of the metacarpal: showing position of function with posterior plaster slab and the hand gripping a roll of felt padding

There is often a tendency for metacarpal fractures to rotate and this must be prevented. This is best achieved by splinting the metacarpophalangeal joints at 90°, which corrects any tendency to malrotation. If there is gross displacement, shortening or rotation then surgical intervention is indicated. A felt pad acts as a suitable grip. The patient should exercise the free fingers vigorously. Remove the splint after 3 weeks and start active mobilisation.

Phalangeal fractures

133

These fractures result from either direct trauma causing a transverse or a comminuted fracture, or a torsional force causing an oblique fracture. The tendency to regard fractures of phalanges (especially middle and proximal phalanges) as minor injuries (with scant attention paid to management and particularly to follow-up care) is worth highlighting. These fractures require as near-perfect reduction as possible, careful splintage and, above all, early mobilisation once the fracture is stable—usually in 2–3 weeks.

Nevertheless, overzealous mobilisation can be as dangerous as prolonged immobilisation. Early operative intervention should be considered if the fracture is unstable.

Angulation is usually obvious but it is most important to check for rotational malalignment, especially with torsional fracture. A simple method is to get the patient to make a fist of the hand and check the direction in which the nails are facing. Furthermore, each finger can be flexed in turn and checked to see if the fingertips point towards the tubercule of the scaphoid (palpable halfway along the base of the thenar eminence and 1.5 cm distal to the distal wrist crease).

The phalanges

- *Distal phalanges:* usually crush fractures; generally heal simply unless intra-articular. Disturbance of nail growth is common.
- *Middle phalanges:* tend to be displaced and unstable—beware of rotation.
- *Proximal phalanges:* of the greatest concern, especially of the little finger; intra-articular fractures usually need internal fixation.

Treatment

Non-displaced phalanges with no rotational malalignment. Strap the injured finger to the adjacent normal finger with an elastic garter or adhesive tape for 2–3 weeks (i.e. 'buddy strapping') (see FIG. 133.22). Start the patient on active exercises.

or

If pain and swelling is a problem, splint the finger with a narrow dorsal or anterior slab (a felt-lined strip of malleable aluminium can be used).

An alternative is to bandage the hand while the patient holds a tennis ball or appropriate roll of bandage in order to maintain appropriate flexion of all interphalangeal joints.

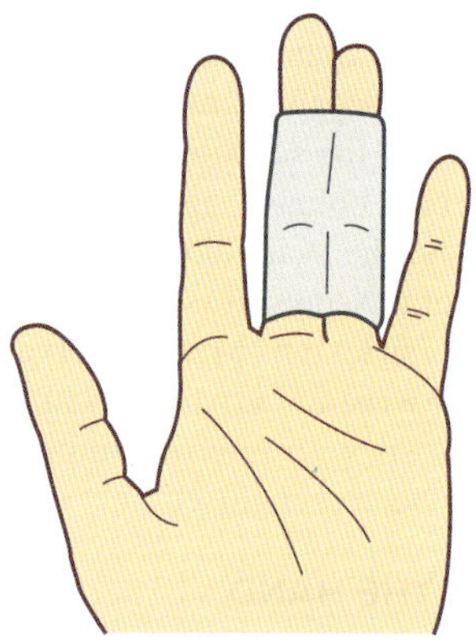

FIGURE 133.22 Treatment of non-displaced phalanges by 'buddy strapping': the fractured finger is strapped to an adjacent healthy finger. A thin gauze between the two fingers reduces irritation.

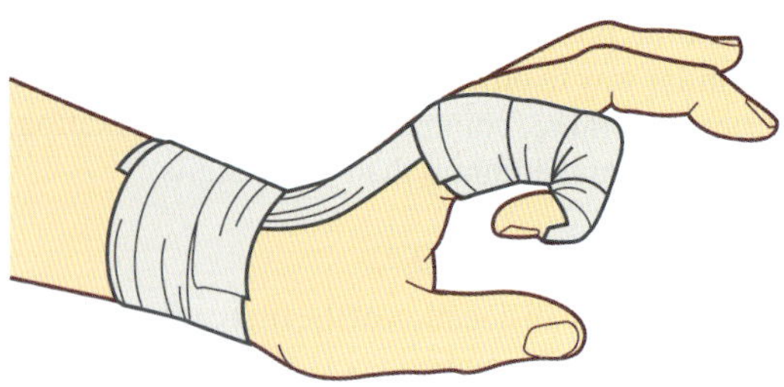

FIGURE 133.23 Method of splinting a phalangeal fracture of the index finger by a posterior plaster slab

Displaced phalangeal fractures (usually proximal and middle). With suitable anaesthesia, correct the deformity by traction and direct digital pressure. Maintain correction by splintage for 2–3 weeks. Ensure flexion at the interphalangeal joints with a dorsal padded plaster slab from above the wrist to the base of the fingernail (see FIG. 133.23).

Intra-articular phalangeal fractures

Intra-articular phalangeal fractures are a great problem to manage as subsequent stiffness of even a single interphalangeal joint can be a significant disability. Subsequent degenerative changes are common.

These fractures often occur in association with subluxation or dislocation of the joint. Reduction and fixation of the fracture may be an integral part of restoring joint stability. Displaced intra-articular phalangeal fractures, especially with joint instability, require referral.

Mallet finger

Refer to CHAPTER 64.

Penetrating injuries to the hand

Assessing these injuries requires a careful history and examination. The pugilist who sustains a seemingly minor cut over a 'knuckle' may have a tooth-penetrating injury to the metacarpophalangeal joint. In the flexed position, the dorsal hood is drawn over the joint. The point of penetration of the hood retracts as the finger extends and 'locks' saliva into the joint. This injury invariably results in a severe septic arthritis unless aggressively treated with surgical debridement and high-dose antibiotics. Given the common occurrence of oral pathogens, antibiotic cover should include anaerobic organisms.

Refer to CHAPTER 132.

Dislocated fingers

In most cases, the distal part dislocates dorsally.

For dislocated fingers, immediate reduction is advisable. Test for an associated fracture and X-ray if appropriate. General anaesthesia may be necessary for reduction of a dislocated thumb.

Simple reduction of a dislocated interphalangeal joint

This method employs the principles of using the patient's body weight as the distracting force to achieve reduction of the dislocation. It is relatively painless and very effective.

Method

1 Face the patient, both in standing positions.
2 Firmly grasp the distal part of the dislocated finger. A better grip is achieved by wrapping simple adhesive tape around the end of the finger.
3 Ask the patient to lean backward, while maintaining the finger in the fixed position (see FIG. 133.24).
4 As the patient leans back, sudden, painless reduction should spontaneously occur. Otherwise under a ring block or sedation apply traction and push the proximal phalangeal head dorsally. Splint the joint for 3 weeks to allow soft-tissue healing.

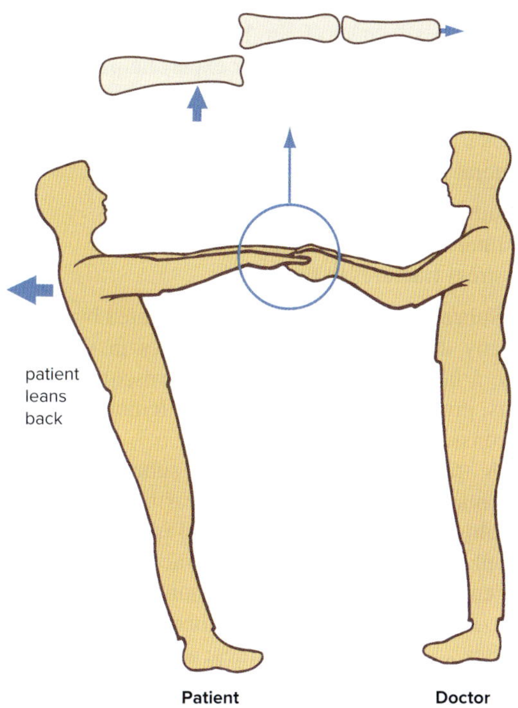

FIGURE 133.24 Reduction of a dislocated finger

Pitfalls

- Instability—torn collateral ligaments: unstable in lateral direction
- Interposed volar plate—postreduction full flexion absent
- Fractures of base of phalanx
- Extensor mechanism rupture (e.g. buttonhole deformity at PIP joint or mallet finger deformity at DIP joint)

These problems may need surgical reduction.

133

INJURIES TO THE PELVIS AND HIP

Fractures of the pelvis

Fractures of the pelvic ring are either:

1 stable: a single fracture
2 unstable: a break at two sites or association with disruption of the symphysis pubis or sacroiliac articulation

Treatment

Stable pelvic fracture:

- symptomatic, especially analgesics
- bed rest as pain symptoms dictate
- attempt walking with an aid as soon as comfortable

Unstable fractures: these are usually serious with possible associated visceral damage or blood loss. Patients should be referred for expert help.

Femoral fractures

Femoral neck fractures include:

- subcapital fractures
- intertrochanteric fractures
- stress fractures in the young

Subcapital fractures are usually treated by pinning. Greatly displaced subcapital fractures in the elderly have a high risk of femoral head avascular necrosis. Thus, prosthetic replacement of the femoral head may be considered as a primary option.

A trap can be the impacted subcapital fracture that may allow partial weight-bearing, thus making radiological investigation essential in elderly patients complaining of hip pain. The fracture may not be evident on plain X-rays. If suspicion of fracture is still high, a bone scan should be performed.

Beware of the teenage athlete who complains of hip pain after running. Exclude a slipped upper femoral epiphysis and then a stress fracture. A technetium-99m bone scan will detect the fracture. A stress fracture may displace without warning, posing a serious risk of femoral head avascular necrosis. Thus, stress fractures must be considered for prophylactic pinning.

A summary of the management of other femoral fractures is presented in FIGURE 133.25.

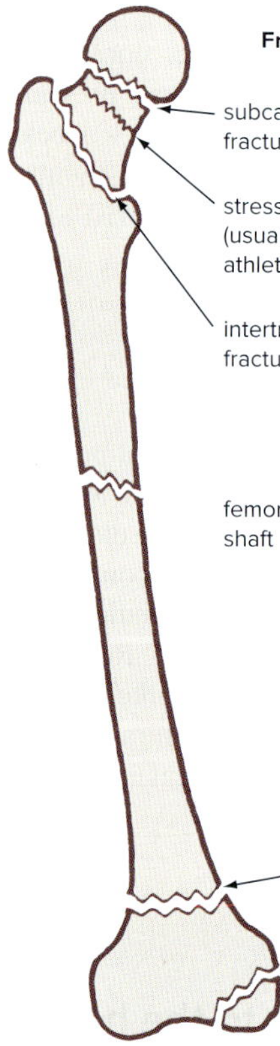

FIGURE 133.25 Management of basic fractures of the femur

Posterior dislocation of the hip

This causes a very painful shortened leg, which is held adducted, medially rotated and slightly flexed. Be careful of sciatic nerve damage. Early reduction within hours minimises the risk of avascular necrosis of the femoral head.

Management

- Adequate analgesia
- X-rays to confirm diagnosis and exclude associated fracture
- Reduction of the dislocated hip under relaxant anaesthesia
- Follow-up X-ray to confirm reduction and exclude any fracture not visible on the first X-ray
- Intra-articular bone fragments need to be excluded by CT scanning

Note: Femoral neurovascular injury may occur in the rare cases of anterior dislocation of the hip.

INJURIES OF THE LOWER LIMBS

Patella dislocation and subluxation

An acute dislocation needs to be reduced as a medical emergency.

The dislocated patella, which occurs mainly in children and young adults, especially girls, is always displaced laterally (see FIG. 133.26), often

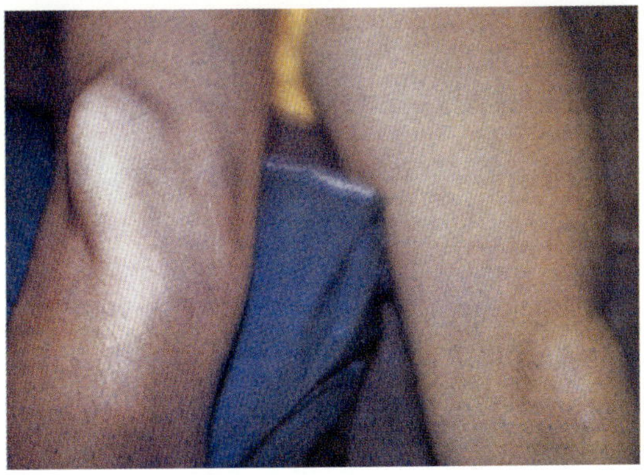

FIGURE 133.26 Dislocated patella showing lateral displacement

following a rotational and valgus force. The patient may feel the patella dislocate and it may sometimes reduce spontaneously. It may be associated with an osteochondral injury on the medial facet of the patella or the lateral femoral condyle. There is often a tense joint effusion, especially in the presence of an osteochondral fracture. Predisposing factors include valgus knees, a small mobile patella, a laterally placed tibial tuberosity, a shallow patellofemoral groove and ligamentous laxity. Immediate reduction can be attempted by gently flexing the hip to relax the quadriceps, placing the thumb under the lateral edge of the patella and pushing it medially as the knee is extended. This may be attempted without anaesthesia or by using morphine and intravenous diazepam as a relaxant.

X-rays with anteroposterior, lateral, skyline and intracondylar views should be taken to exclude an associated osteochondral fracture.

The usual RICE treatment should be given initially and crutches provided. Rest of the injured knee is achieved using a knee splint with the knee held in extension and crutches for 4 weeks.

Weight-bearing is permitted when the swelling has subsided and the patient is gradually taken off the crutches. Introduce quadriceps exercises with the knee in extension.

Patellar subluxation is when the patella is mobile and does not actually dislocate, but results in episodic pain and feelings of instability. Physiotherapy and appropriate splinting for sporting activities is helpful before surgical stabilisation is considered.

Recurrent dislocations/subluxations in young females (14–18 years) require surgery—combined tibial tubercle transfer with lateral release of the capsule. Immediate surgery in the acute phase is undertaken only in the presence of haemarthrosis with an osteochondral fracture.

Fractures of the patella

- Fractures without displacement: walking plaster cylinder 4 weeks
- Displaced single transverse fracture: surgical reduction with Kirschner wires
- Displaced and comminuted fracture: refer to consider patellectomy

Fractures of both tibia and fibula

The nature and management of these fractures vary considerably. Some fractures are caused by blunt injuries, such as a blow from a motor car bumper, while twisting forces cause a spiral fracture of both bones at different levels. As a general rule, referral of patients to a specialist is necessary, especially where soft-tissue damage is significant. Management of fractures with minimal soft-tissue damage can be summarised thus:

- no or minimal displacement: full-length cast as for isolated fracture of tibia
- displacement: reduction under general anaesthesia, then application of cast as above (meticulous alignment essential)
- period of immobilisation: adults 16 weeks, children 8 weeks

133

Fracture of fibula[11]

An isolated fracture of the fibula is usually due to stress or to a direct blow. The patient is generally able to stand and move the knee and ankle joints. However, most spiral fractures are associated with injuries of the ankle or knee. The ankle in particular should be examined and X-rayed.

Treatment is usually with analgesics to control the pain and no more than a crepe bandage or a walking stick is necessary. A below-knee walking plaster for about 3 weeks will help those with severe discomfort.

Fracture of the tibial shaft

A fracture of the tibia alone is uncommon in adults but more common in children, due to a twisting injury. Reduction may not be necessary in some patients. Many can be reduced to a satisfactory position in the anaesthetised patient by letting the fractured leg hang over the edge of the table with the knee at a right angle.

A padded cast from the groin to the metatarsal necks is applied with the knee joint at 10° of flexion, and the ankle at a right angle. This should be maintained for 3–4 months.

Toddler's fracture[11]

Toddler's fracture is a hairline spiral fracture of the tibia that is common in children aged 1–2 years. They may present with failure to weight-bear after minimal or no known trauma. The fracture may not be seen on X-ray. A backslab for 4 weeks may relieve discomfort.

Fracture around the ankle

The ankle is one of the areas liable to fractures. The commonest mechanism is forceful inversion of the foot, which can cause fracture of the fibula on a level with the joint line and tearing of the lateral collateral ligament. Other injuries can also occur, such as fracture of the medial malleolus and tearing of the tibiofibular syndesmosis. At least three views on X-ray are needed: AP, lateral and a half oblique 'mortise' view.

Undisplaced, uncomplicated fractures are treated with a plaster cast from just below the knee to the toes for 6–8 weeks. The foot must be plantigrade (i.e. with the foot at 90° to the leg and neither in varus nor in valgus).[11] Fractures treated in plaster need X-ray monitoring. Unsuspected displacement may occur as swelling subsides and the plaster loosens. Occult displacement of the fracture leading to mal-union will predispose to ankle osteoarthritis. Fractures that are displaced or cause instability of the ankle joint require surgery to achieve stability followed by a longer period of immobilisation.

Ankle/talus/subtalar joint dislocations

These dislocations may result in vascular compromise. The stretched overlying skin may rapidly necrose. Refer early.[10]

Stress fractures of the foot

Stress fractures of the navicular, calcaneus and metatarsal bones can be found in otherwise healthy people from the age of 7 onwards. Long-distance runners and high-performance athletes are also susceptible.

Clinical features

- Localised pain during weight-bearing activity
- Localised tenderness and swelling (not inevitable)
- Plain X-rays are necessary but show no fracture in about 50% of cases;[8] X-rays can be repeated in 2–3 weeks if a fracture is suspected
- A nuclear bone scan may confirm the diagnosis

Navicular

This hitherto unrecognised stress fracture has become apparent with the advent of CT scanning, which shows up the fracture better than nuclear scanning. It is seen in athletes involved with running sports and presents as poorly localised midfoot pain. Plain X-ray is usually normal. The fracture, like the scaphoid fracture, is difficult to manage since delayed union and non-union are common. Cast immobilisation for 8 weeks may avoid the need for an operation.

Metatarsal bones

The second metatarsal is probably the most common site of all for stress fracture because it is invariably the largest metatarsal and absorbs a greater load than the others.

Treatment

- Rest is the basis of treatment
- Resting the foot with crutches for 6 weeks provides optimal healing
- Healing usually takes 6–8 weeks
- Gradual resumption of activity

Lisfranc joint injury (midfoot sprain)[14]

This is basically a dislocation of the tarsometatarsal joints of the foot. The spectrum ranges from partial strains with no displacement to complete tears with separation of the first and second metatarsal bones (FIG. 133.27). Causes range from low-energy compression and twisting to high-energy crush forces. Diagnosis is usually confirmed by weight-bearing plain X-rays. Treatment depends on the degree of stability. Surgical reduction and fixation is required if there is evidence of instability.

Fractures of the toes

Most toe injuries are easy to treat but, like the fingers, the great and little toes demand special attention. Intra-articular injuries of the great toe (unless undisplaced) should be treated by internal fixation.

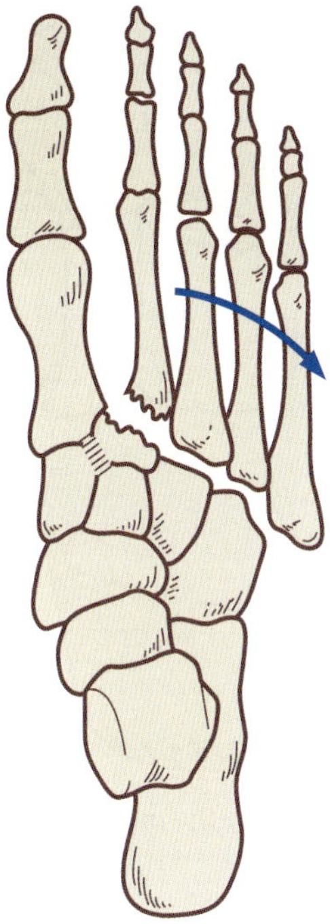

FIGURE 133.27 Lisfranc dislocation at midfoot joints—this severe case shows fracture of the base of the second metatarsal.

'Buddy strapping' can be used for many uncomplicated fractured phalanges of the toes, which tend to angulate and rotate more readily and are often harder to control than finger fractures. Strapping them to their adjacent toes on both sides simultaneously tends to counteract this problem.

Like the little finger, the little toe is injured by forceful abduction and if allowed to heal in that position may leave difficulties in wearing shoes.[11]

Approximate average immobilisation times for various fractures are given in TABLE 133.3.

Dislocation of toes

Dislocations occur mainly at the metatarsophalangeal joint and are rare; they require special care because of the strong tendons crossing the joint. Perfect reduction of the dislocated great toe is essential and it should be supported by a below-knee plaster cast extending beyond the toes. Temporary internal fixation with a Kirschner wire or open ligamentous repair may be required.[12]

Table 133.3 Healing of uncomplicated fractures (adults)

Fracture	(Approximate) average immobilisation time (weeks)
Rib	3–6 (healing time)
Clavicle	4–8 (2 weeks in sling)
Scapula	weeks to months
Humerus:	
• neck	3–6
• shaft	8
• condyles	3–4
Radius:	
• head of radius	3
• shaft	6
• Colles	4–6
Radius and ulna (shafts)	6–12
Ulna—shaft	8
Scaphoid	8–12
Metacarpals:	
• Bennett fracture	6–8
Other MCs	3–4
Phalanges (hand):	
• proximal	3
• middle	2–3
• distal	2–3
Pelvis	rest in bed 2–6
Femur:	
• femoral neck	according to surgery
• shaft	12–16
• distal	8–12
Patella	3–4
Tibia	12–16
Fibula	0–6
Both tibia and fibula	16
Pott fracture	6–8
Lateral malleolus avulsion	3
Calcaneus:	
• minor	4–6
• compression	14–16
Talus	12
Tarsal bones (stress fracture)	8
Metatarsals	4
Phalanges (toes)	0–3
Vertebrae	
• spinous process	3
• transverse process	3
• stable vertebrae	3
• unstable vertebrae	9–14
• sacrum/coccyx	3

Important principles:
- children under 8 years usually take half the time to heal
- have a check X-ray in 1 week (for most fractures)
- radiological union lags behind clinical union

Note: immobilisation times vary considerably, depending on factors such as trauma degree and soft-tissue injuries.

133

Analgesia and relaxation

For the reduction of dislocations, analgesia and relaxation are appropriate. Resuscitation facilities and an experienced practitioner are required to handle this procedure. All drugs should be given intravenously and titrated to achieve the desired effect. Adverse effects include respiratory depression and hypotension.[10] The choice of agents is presented in TABLE 133.4.

Table 133.4 Analgesic and relaxant/sedative agents

	IV dose	Antidote
Relaxant/sedative agent		
Diazepam	0.1–0.2 mg/kg (5–10 mg)	Flumazenil
Midazolam	0.05–0.1 mg/kg (2–5 mg)	Flumazenil
Analgesic agent		
Fentanyl	1–2 mcg/kg (50–100 mcg)	Naloxone
Morphine	0.1–0.2 mg/kg (5–15 mg)	Naloxone

133

Plastering tips

Plaster of Paris

The bucket of water

- Line the bucket with a plastic bag for easy cleaning.
- The water should be deep enough to allow complete vertical immersion.
- Use cold water for slow setting.
- Use tepid water for faster setting.
- Do not use hot water: it produces rapid-setting and brittle plaster.

The plaster rolls

- Do not use plaster rolls if water has been splashed on them.
- Hold the roll loosely but with the free end firm and secure (see FIG. 133.28).
- Ensure that the centre of the plaster is fully wet.
- Drain surface water after removal from the bucket.
- Gently squeeze the roll in the middle: do not indent.

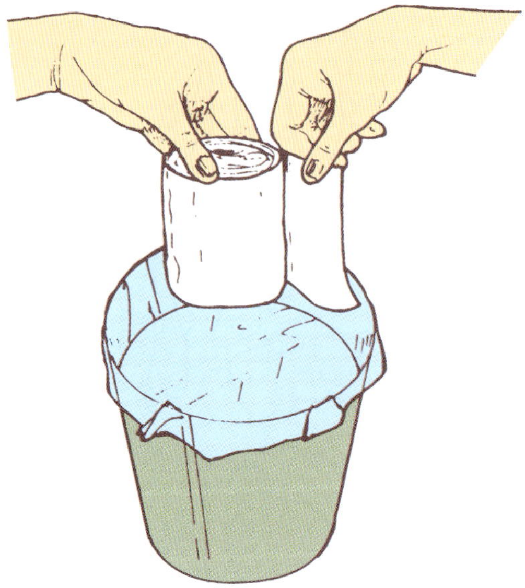

FIGURE 133.28 Holding the plaster roll

Padding

- Use Velband or stockinette under the plaster.
- With Velband, moisten the end of the roll in water to allow it to adhere to the limb.
- For legs, make extra padding around the ankle and heel.
- Avoid multiple layers of padding.

Method

- Use an assistant to support the limb where possible (e.g. hold the arm up with fingers of stockinet).
- Lay the bandage on firmly but do not pull tight.
- Lay it on quickly.
- Overlap the bandage by about 25% of its width.

Note: It is good practice to review the patient the next day.

Patient education resources

Hand-out sheets from *Murtagh's Patient Education* 7th edition:

- Plaster cast instructions

References

1 Stiell I. The Ottawa Rules. <www.theottawarules.ca> (accessed 22/5/2018).
2 Aweid B et al. Stress fractures. Trauma, 2013; 15 (4): 308–21.
3 Brentnall E. Diagnosing a fracture. Aust Fam Physician, 1990; 19: 948.

4 Ratilal B et al. Antibiotic prophylaxis for preventing meningitis in patients with basilar skull fractures. Cochrane Database Syst Rev. 2011. Issue 8. Art No. CD004884.

5 Brentnall E. Spatula test for fracture of mandible. Aust Fam Physician, 1992; 21: 1007.

6 McMenimen PJ. Management of common fractures of the upper limb. Aust Fam Physician, 1987; 16: 783–91.

7 Young D, Murtagh J. Pitfalls in orthopaedics. Aust Fam Physician, 1989; 18: 645–60.

8 Bokor D. Management of outer clavicle fractures and acromioclavicular joint dislocations. Medicine Today, April 2009; 10 (4): 67–70.

9 Peterson L, Renström P. *Sports Injuries: Their Prevention and Treatment.* Sydney: Methuen, 1986: 179–81.

10 Mohammed KD, Sonnabend DH. A GP's guide to the reduction of dislocations. Modern Medicine Australia, 1996; 39 (2): 100–8.

11 Mead HJ. Paediatric limb fractures and dislocations: how to treat. Australian Doctor, 26 October 2007: 35–42.

12 McRae R, Esser M. *Practical Fracture Treatment* (4th edn). Churchill Livingstone Elsevier, 2002: 201–5.

13 Carter G. Fractures and dislocations of fingers and toes. Aust Fam Physician, 1993; 22: 310–17.

14 Brukner P, Khan K. *Brukner & Khan's Clinical Sports Medicine.* Sydney: McGraw-Hill Australia, 2009; 856–7.

Resources

Apley AG, Solomon L. *Apley's System of Orthopaedics and Fractures* (9th edn). London: Hodder Education, 2010.

O'Connor S, Talley, N. *Clinical Examination: A Systematic Guide to Physical Diagnosis* (7th edn). Chatswood: Elsevier, 2014.

Part 11

Health of specific groups

134 The health of Aboriginal and Torres Strait Islander peoples

'Closing the Gap' is a long-term ambitious framework that builds on the foundation of respect and unity provided by the 2008 National Apology to the Aboriginal and Torres Strait Islander Peoples. It acknowledges that improving opportunities for Indigenous Australians requires intensive and sustained effort from all levels of government, as well as private and not-for-profit sectors, communities and individuals.'

COUNCIL OF AUSTRALIAN GOVERNMENTS (COAG) 2008

The major health challenge in Australia (and several other developed countries) is the health status of its Indigenous peoples, which continues to be significantly worse than that of other Australians.

The 2017 AIHW figures estimated the average life expectancy for Aboriginal and Torres Strait Islander males was 69.1 years (a gap of 10.6 years compared with other Australians) and 73.7 years for women (a gap of 9.5 years).[1]

The commonest cause of death is cardiovascular disease, especially ischaemic heart disease which causes about 57% of these deaths.[2] The contrast with other Australians is most marked at 25–54 years. Diseases of the circulatory system, injury and poisoning, respiratory illness and neoplasms continue to be important causes of death. Deaths from infectious diseases and genitourinary disorders continue to occur at much higher rates than among other Australians.

One in nine adults have type 2 diabetes—a prevalence 3.3 times higher at any age than the general population.[3]

Records written by early settlers indicated that the Indigenous people appeared to be in good health, probably better than the majority of new arrivals transported from England. The total Aboriginal population has been estimated as 750 000 in 1788. It fell to about 70 000 in the 1930s after 150 years of exposure to white civilisation. Significant causes were deaths at the hands of the settlers (recorded as approximately 20 000) and infectious disease.

The main diseases that decimated the population were smallpox (two severe epidemics: 1789 and 1829–30), influenza, TB (very severe), pneumonia, measles, varicella, whooping cough, typhoid and diphtheria. The Aboriginal and Torres Strait Islander population is now estimated to be 700 000.

The level of infant and maternal mortality continues to be a concern. After great reductions in infant mortality rates in the 1970s, there has been a levelling off, with rates remaining 3–5 times higher than those of other Australians. Despite some improvement, we all need to work to close the gap, and general practice is an ideal setting to embrace this.[4,5]

It is important to understand that Aboriginal and Torres Strait Islander people have a diverse range of different cultures, with each group needing a special understanding of its cultural issues. This understanding is best gleaned from local community members and groups.

Practitioners working in primary health care in rural and remote areas in Central and Northern Australia are advised to use the *CARPA Standard Treatment Manual*.[6]

Key facts and checkpoints

- Consider the importance of cultural issues at each consultation.
- If assistance is required with a cultural issue, consider involving an indigenous health worker in the consultation. Such health workers are a vital part of the team.
- Always consider multiple medical conditions in the sick person.
- Remember the importance of opportunistic screening for relatively common conditions:
  - type 2 diabetes (9% prevalence urban, 21% rural)
  - hypertension
  - kidney function (eGFR, ACR)
  - other cardiovascular risk factors (smoking, dyslipidaemia, Group A streptococcus infection)
  - hepatitis B (2% prevalence urban, 8% rural)
  - STI urine screening (men and women)
  - cervical screening
  - anaemia in children
  - hearing loss in children

- Screening investigations to consider include:
  - blood sugar (finger-prick test)
  - serum lipids
  - urea and electrolytes
  - hepatitis B serology
  - BMI
  - urine dipstick and ACR
- Cervical cancer is 6–8 times more common in Aboriginal and Torres Strait Islander women.
- Other common cancers are lung and liver.
- Appropriate skin care is a key to Indigenous health, with prevention, early detection and treatment of skin infection being important to reduce the burden of invasive infection in children.
- Approximately 50% of children have chronic tympanic membrane perforations, with very significant consequences for language development and school achievement.
- The incidence of end-stage kidney failure is 10 times that of non-Indigenous Australians.
- Some extra childhood immunisations are recommended (see schedule), e.g. in some regions, BCG vaccination is recommended for newborn children.
- Influenza and pneumococcal vaccines are recommended for adults over 50 years.
- The prevalence of asthma is higher (16.5%) compared with other Australians (10.2%).
- Depressive illness, as in the general community, is a significant concern. Suicide is far more common than in other Australians, by a factor of 2.7 for males and 1.7 for females.
- Alcohol use is a serious health and community problem. Although non-drinking is more common in this population, so too is binge drinking.
- Another drinking problem is kava, a drink made from a plant native to the Pacific Islands. Its effects are similar to alcohol and benzodiazepines, with marked muscle relaxation.[4,6] Excessive use causes acute and long-term problems.
- Prevention, early detection and appropriate treatment of skin infection is key to Aboriginal and Torres Strait Islander health.

National survey

The first national survey of the health of Aboriginal and Torres Strait Islander peoples took place in 1994, and the most recent survey (2012–13) found that around 40% consider their health to be good or excellent.[3]

The 2012–13 survey highlighted the following disorders:

- asthma
- ear and hearing problems
- diabetes
- hypertension
- kidney disorders
- heart disease
- skin disorders
- eye problems, including trachoma
- nutritional status (especially obesity)
- substance abuse (e.g. alcohol, marijuana, petrol sniffing)
- dental problems (a reversed trend of dental caries)[7]
- psychological distress and family stressors

According to BEACH data, the seven most common problems managed at encounters with Aboriginal and Torres Strait Islander patients were (in order) respiratory infections, diabetes, hypertension, depression/anxiety, asthma, immunisation, otitis media.[8]

The low health status of Aboriginal and Torres Strait Islander peoples has many underlying causes, and should be understood in terms of the social determinants of health; these are what Professor Sir Michael Marmot calls the 'causes of the causes'.[9] Many of these stem from historical dispossession, poverty and intergenerational trauma. Determinants include geographical isolation, high population mobility, unemployment, poor housing, low education attainment, temperature extremes in central Australia, increased exposure to infectious diseases, especially in subtropical areas, and a lack of appropriate service deliveries. 134

Poor living conditions including overcrowding contribute to poor health outcomes, such as substance abuse, domestic violence, other social dysfunction and child malnutrition. Other environmental health issues, such as lack of adequate shelter, lack of basic amenities such as clean running water and adequate sewage disposal facilities, and lack of refrigeration, all impact on health.

Associated comorbidities of children admitted to the infectious diseases ward of the Royal Darwin Hospital[10] included dehydration (50%), malnutrition (60%), hypokalaemia (70%), iron deficiency (90%), anaemia (25%), pneumonia (24–32%), chronic suppurative otitis media (37%), urinary tract infection (10%) and scabies (25%).

Priority health problems have been identified by the National Aboriginal Health Strategy and are summarised in TABLE 134.1.

Aboriginal and Torres Strait Islander culture and the doctor–patient relationship

An understanding of Aboriginal and Torres Strait Islander cultural issues is fundamental to successful

Table 134.1 Priority Indigenous health problems

Clinical
Diabetes
Cardiovascular disease
Injury (and youth suicide)
Kidney disease
STIs
Mental health
Poor nutrition
Ear infections
Women's problems
Socioeconomic
Education of Indigenous children (particularly in rural and remote areas)
Housing
Water supply
Alcohol and substance misuse
Domestic violence and sexual abuse
Child abuse
Gambling
Unemployment

134

management outcomes. Doctors should realise that, while examining Indigenous patients, they are themselves being examined. Failure to bridge the cultural divide leads to frustration on both sides: the patient has little faith in the promise of health gains, and the clinician cannot understand why his or her supposedly clear instructions are not being carried out.[11]

Arguably, the most important step after dealing with the presenting complaint is encouraging the patient to feel welcome enough to want to return. Managing chronic health issues is a marathon, not a sprint. A single visit to a brilliant specialist is less useful than ongoing interaction with a generalist local clinician who is culturally sensitive and applies basic, evidence-based treatment according to the patient's needs and preferences.

Handy communication hints include:

- Allow extra consultation time.
- Don't be afraid of pauses during conversation.
- Avoid jargon; recheck the patient's understanding.
- For complex explanations, use images.
- Be aware of your body language, including eye contact.
- Be humble and listen; you don't have all the answers!

Doctors who work in Aboriginal or Torres Strait Islander communities (see FIG. 134.1) must appreciate and respect the local culture and be aware of its significance to health and behaviour.

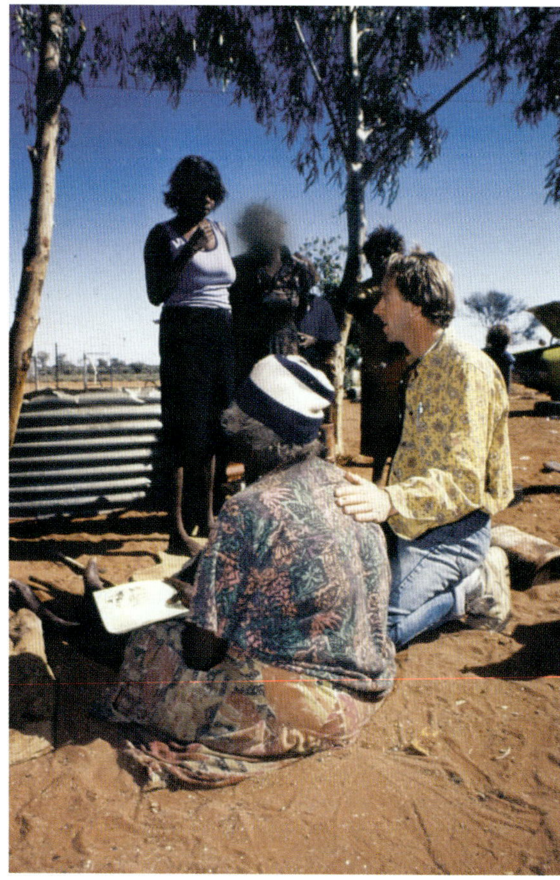

FIGURE 134.1 Doctor on an outback home visit in Central Australia

Courtesy Alice Springs Rural District Department of Health and Community Services

Many patients feel more relaxed during the consultation if accompanied by a relative or friend, who can provide support and help them interpret your medical advice later.

Women's business

'Women's business' can be defined as the range of experience and knowledge that is the exclusive preserve and domain of Indigenous women. It encompasses issues about menstruation, pregnancy, childbirth and contraception.[12] Such matters may traditionally not have been discussed directly but were conveyed indirectly through stories, ceremonies and songs. For more traditional women it is taboo to talk about women's health issues to male doctors or male health workers, or to be physically examined by them. Doing so may cause shame and embarrassment.[13]

Men's business

Similarly, the cultural issue of men's business needs to be understood and respected. This applies to manhood initiation rites, circumcision, sexuality and sexually transmitted infections.

Sorry business

'Sorry business' is the process of grieving, and this needs to be clearly understood. There is a cultural obligation for mourners to grieve the death of a relative in a special way, sometimes for many days or weeks. Mourners may change their appearance and avoid any mention of the deceased person's name or any portrayal of his or her likeness. The place where the person died may be deserted for a certain time (which can impact on medical clinics) and then ceremonially 'smoked out'.

Common problems in children[14]

Aboriginal and Torres Strait Islander children suffer the same spectrum of health problems as children in developing countries and Indigenous communities throughout the world, and the infant mortality rate remains high. The major problems are malnutrition, diarrhoeal disease, skin infections and respiratory tract infection. Common problems are presented in TABLE 134.2.

Acute respiratory tract infections are a common reason for admission to hospital. Bacterial pneumonias occur more commonly than in non-Indigenous children and usually present late. Chronic upper respiratory tract disease is typical in younger children and mucopurulent nasal discharge is present in most preschool children.

Chronic suppurative otitis media, which is almost universal in preschool children, is often refractory to treatment and can lead to significant hearing impairment in many children. It can develop without apparent preceding acute otitis media and may be related to poor nutrition and anaemia. The basic treatment is ear toilet with povidone–iodine solution, followed by dry mopping with rolled toilet paper/tissue 'spears', or initial use of the 'spears' followed by acetic acid drops.

Skin infection and infestation are almost as prevalent as respiratory tract disease. Scabies is endemic and occasionally reaches epidemic proportions. It can be a very debilitating problem and can present in very young infants, in the first few weeks of life.[14]

Table 134.2 Common clinical problems in children

Perinatal
Low birthweight
Asphyxia
Infections
Preschool
Failure to thrive
Malnutrition
Anaemia
Respiratory infection
Diarrhoeal disease
Hepatitis B
Skin infection/infestation (incl. scabies)
Urinary tract infection
Meningitis
Joint and bone infection
Chronic suppurative otitis media
Later childhood and adolescence
Bacterial and viral infections
Parasitic infestation
Streptococcal infection:
• rheumatic fever
• glomerulonephritis
Trauma
Substance abuse
Obesity
Chronic suppurative otitis media

Anaemia, usually iron deficiency, is found in at least 25% of children in remote regions. Apart from reduced intake, intestinal loss from hookworm and other parasitic infection is an important factor. Treatment includes deworming in addition to iron supplements.

Diarrhoeal disease is a very common reason for hospital admission. Causes of infective gastroenteritis include rotavirus, bacteria including *Shigella*, *Salmonella* and *Campylobacter*, and parasites such as *Giardia lamblia*, *Strongyloides* and *Cryptosporidium.*

Other important and serious problems encountered more frequently in Aboriginal and Torres Strait Islander children include bacterial meningitis (especially *Haemophilus influenzae*), septic arthritis and osteomyelitis, pyomyositis, *Streptococcus pyogenes* infections with associated glomerulonephritis and rheumatic fever, urinary tract calculi, urinary tract infection (especially at 6–18 months of age), hepatitis B and petrol sniffing (see CHAPTER 128).

Appropriate levels of immunisation in these communities will have enormous health benefits.

134

Poliomyelitis, diphtheria, pertussis, tuberculosis and *H. influenzae* are now rare and it is hoped that hepatitis B, varicella and HPV infections will be drastically reduced.

Specific disorders requiring attention

The GP attending Aboriginal and Torres Strait Islander patients should develop special skills in the diagnosis and management of the following health concerns:

- diabetes mellitus, frequently with hypertension and kidney disease
- trauma
- substance abuse, including alcohol and smoking
- ear and eye infections
- respiratory disorders—URTIs and LRTIs, asthma
- skin disorders (e.g. fungal infections, impetigo, leg ulcers, cellulitis, boils)
- parasitic infestations (e.g. scabies, lice)
- gastrointestinal infections (e.g. *Campylobacter* enteritis, giardiasis, *Shigella*)
- sexually transmitted infections
- psychosocial dysfunction
- bites and stings
- severe infections (e.g. meningitis, rheumatic fever, septicaemia)
- hepatitis B
- tropical diseases (where applicable)
- worm infestation (e.g. strongyloides)

However, the general management of medical disorders follows the principles and treatment guidelines outlined in this book. Antibiotic and other treatment guidelines for rural and remote communities are most useful.[6]

Cardiovascular disease[2,15]

Cardiovascular disease is a major cause of continuing high rates of mortality and morbidity, particularly ischaemic heart disease, but also rheumatic heart disease and stroke. Mortality from ischaemic heart disease is almost twice that of the non-Indigenous population overall and 6–8 times higher in those aged 25–64 years. Reasons for this include high smoking rates (2.6 times the rate for others)[3], type 2 diabetes (3.3 times the rate), obesity and low rates of physical activity. Rheumatic heart disease is 64 times as common in the Northern Territory Aboriginal population compared to the Australian average.[16]

Targets for secondary prevention of cardiovascular disease and diabetes mellitus are as presented in CHAPTER 20.

Ear infections[6]

Otitis externa and otitis media with its acute and chronic complications are major health problems in Aboriginal and Torres Strait Islander children, especially in rural and remote regions. Acute otitis media should be treated early and aggressively with antibiotics to (somewhat) reduce the risk of chronic suppurative otitis media, which is very difficult to cure once established. Check carefully for a perforation, which may affect management.

Treatment guidelines[17]

• Acute otitis media	Amoxycillin (50 mg/kg/day, in divided oral doses for 7 days) or procaine penicillin (IM). If no response, consider amoxycillin 90 mg/kg/day or amoxycillin/clavulanate or cefaclor or azithromycin. Review in 4–7 days
• Acute suppurative otitis media	Oral antibiotics (as above, but for 14 days) + dry mop ear using tissue 'spears' prior to each application of antibiotic ear drops
• Chronic suppurative otitis media	Wash with povidone–iodine 5% solution using a 20 mL syringe with plastic tubing 1, 2 or 3 times daily (if available), then dry mop with rolled tissue spears. Teach this method to family members. If available, suction kits are useful. Then instil ciprofloxacin 2–4 drops qid until the ear is dry, especially in the presence of a perforation of the tympanic membrane
• Otitis externa	Gently clean out debris with tissue spears followed by acetic acid 0.25%; insert Kenacomb or Sofradex drops or ointment 12-hourly on a gauze wick (if no perforation), otherwise ciprofloxacin with hydrocortisone drops 12 hourly
• Acute mastoiditis	Parenteral IM or IV flucloxacillin/dicloxacillin ± gentamicin IM or IV and hospitalisation

Eye infections[6]

Treatment guidelines

- *Peri-orbital cellulitis and penetrating eye trauma.* Arrange evacuation to hospital; if critically ill or delay in transfer give empirical treatment with ceftriaxone IM or IV once daily. Add gentamicin IM or IV as single dose for a child <3 months or patients with other risk factors such as diabetes.
- *Conjunctivitis.* Consider two swabs if indicated (for microculture and *Chlamydia PCR*). If not viral, apply topical chloramphenicol eye drops or ointment.
- *Neonatal gonococcal ophthalmia and Chlamydia infection.* Refer to CHAPTER 51.
- *Gonococcal conjunctivitis.* (Particularly if lots of pus, or in neonates) give ceftriaxone 1 g IM (children; 50 mg/kg/dose).
- *Trachoma.* These patients have 'scratchy' eyes and watery discharge ± red eye (see FIG. 134.2):
  - if over 6 kg and not pregnant: azithromycin (o) as single dose
  - if under 6 kg or pregnant: erythromycin or roxithromycin (o) for 21 days
  - check and treat household contacts
  - check routinely for 'follicles' of trachoma

Skin and soft-tissue infections

Skin infections are the commonest presenting problem in many clinics.[18,19] These include a high incidence of scabies and tinea corporis (ringworm), boils and carbuncles, infected wounds, impetigo and cellulitis. A notably serious complication of skin infections is post-streptococcal glomerulonephritis secondary to *S. pyogenes* infection. Scabies is the most common skin infestation and commonly starts as an itchy rash with pinhead papules in the web spaces of the fingers.

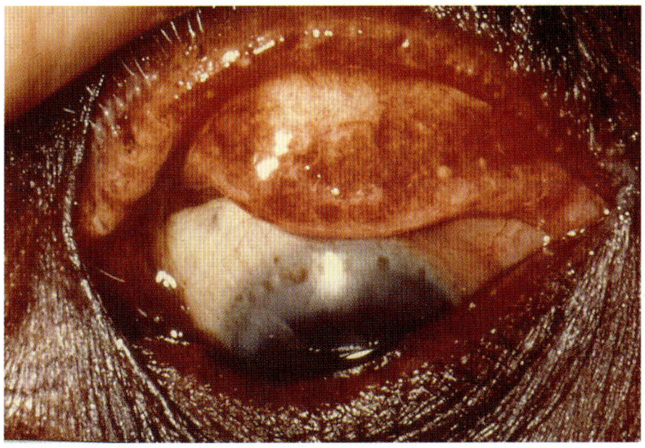

FIGURE 134.2 Trachoma showing conjunctival follicles and papillae, subconjunctival scarring, including conjunctivalisation of the meibomian orifices, paramarginal sulcus formation and, on the cornea, a 2 mm vascular pannus and Herbet's pits

Photo taken from the 1980 grading manual prepared by Fred Hollows and Hugh Taylor for workers in the National Trachoma and Eye Health Program (courtesy Dr David Tamblyn)

Recommended treatment (in summary)[6,19]

Impetigo and other skin sores

- Soak and remove crusts with saline or soap and water or povidone–iodine or potassium permanganate (Condy's crystals) solution
- Antibiotic treatment (if required)

  benzathine penicillin, IM, statim dose
  or
  flucloxacillin/dicloxacillin (o) or cephalexin (o) or co-trimoxazole (o) for 3–7 days

Cellulitis (mild–moderate) and erysipelas

As for impetigo, above
or
procaine penicillin IM daily for 5 days
or
benzathine penicillin IM on days 1 and 3 or daily for 3–5 days

If no improvement: flu/dicloxacillin (as below) plus probenecid

Boils, carbuncles, abscesses, bullous impetigo (*Staphylococcus aureus* infections)

Flu/dicloxacillin (o) 6 hourly for 5–10 days

Suppurative wound infections

- Use local measures such as aseptic dressings and topical antiseptics
- If necessary, add flu/dicloxacillin (as above); consider clindamycin

Tinea corporis (ringworm)

- Use benzoic acid ointment, Whitfield's ointment or one of the imidazole preparations: apply 1–3 times daily for 4–6 weeks or for 1 week after rash resolves
- Systemic agents (e.g. griseofulvin (o) once daily) may be necessary

Scabies

- Apply permethrin 5% cream or benzyl benzoate 25% emulsion (see CHAPTERS 117 and 120). Treat household members.

- For children less than 2 months use:
  sulphur 5% cream for 2–3 days
  or
  crotamiton 10% cream daily for 3–5 days
- For infected scabies, use flu/dicloxacillin or erythromycin

Pityriasis versicolor (white spot)

Refer to CHAPTER 121.

GABHS INFECTIONS

Group A beta-haemolytic *Streptococcus* (GABHS) infections are a significant problem, causing diseases such as pharyngotonsillitis, impetigo, cellulitis, otitis media and scarlet fever. Two important immunological reactions to the streptococcus toxin are acute rheumatic fever and post-streptococcal glomerulonephritis (PSGN).[2]

Acute rheumatic fever

Rheumatic fever and its effects are a serious cause of cardiovascular morbidity and mortality in Aboriginal and Torres Strait Islander peoples, who have the highest rate of acute rheumatic fever of any ethnic group in the world, with an incidence of 250–300 per 100 000 children.[20] It is a classic hallmark of overcrowding,
134 poverty and lack of hygiene, all of which facilitate streptococcal infection (see CHAPTER 35 for clinical features).

Treatment is with benzathine penicillin (IM).

Acute glomerulonephritis

There is an association between PSGN (see CHAPTER 76) and streptococcal skin and throat infections. Impetigo is the more frequent antecedent to PSGN. A study based on the fact that the Aboriginal and Torres Strait Islanders have an incidence of end-stage kidney failure 10 times greater than the general population found that people with a history of PSGN in childhood had a risk of overt albuminuria more than six times that of a control group.[21] There is no simple treatment of PSGN and preventing streptococcal infection remains the most important control strategy. Penicillin is beneficial in preventing spread during epidemics.

COMMUNICABLE DISEASES

Communicable diseases remain a problem, with an up to 10-fold increase over the non-Indigenous population for diseases such as hepatitis A, hepatitis B, meningococcal disease, *Salmonella*, *Chlamydia* and tuberculosis.[3]

Tuberculosis

The rate of TB in Aboriginal and Torres Strait Islanders is 10–15 times higher than for other people in the Northern Territory.[2] This is related to poverty, overcrowding, malnutrition and homelessness. Early diagnosis and treatment is the key to its control. This includes detection of latent TB infection in those at risk and strategies to prevent transmission in acute cases. BCG immunisation in high-risk groups is a key preventive strategy and is recommended for newborns from high-risk communities (see CHAPTER 29).

Leprosy (Hansen disease)

Leprosy (see CHAPTER 15) has been endemic in Northern Australia for over 100 years, although the incidence is reducing. Control strategies include early diagnosis of new cases, treatment with multidrug therapy, monitoring of treatment to ensure its completion, and prevention of nerve function impairment (NFI). NFI is monitored by a brief voluntary muscle and sensory test. If detected early, it responds to anti-inflammatory medication such as prednisolone.

BCG vaccination, used to prevent TB, has probably had a protective efficacy against leprosy of approximately 50%.[2]

Worm infestations

Intestinal helminths are common in tropical northern Australia. Symptoms may include diarrhoea and abdominal pain with or without distension. Anaemia is common with hookworm infestation. Refer to CHAPTER 15 for more information.

Treatment[6]

- Hookworm, roundworm, threadworm—pyrantel embonate or mebendazole or albendazole
- Whipworm—mebendazole or albendazole
- Strongyloidiasis—albendazole or thiabendazole
- Cutaneous larva migrans—albendazole or thiabendazole

Community worm program. In selected communities a worm eradication program is recommended for children between the ages of 6 months and 12 years with either pyrantel embonate or albendazole.

Sexually transmitted infections

In the discussion and management of STIs, it is important to be aware of the significance of men's and women's 'business'; that is, the cultural sensitivities regarding specific gender feelings and issues, which need to be observed. For some women, it is inappropriate for a male doctor to discuss such issues with them but appropriate for a female doctor, nurse or health worker to do so. The same taboo may apply for a female health worker discussing STIs with a male patient.

STI screening consists of counselling, taking blood for RPR, hepatitis B and HIV, and a first-void urine sample for *Gonococcus*, *Chlamydia* and *Trichomonas* PCR (NAAT). Anyone who presents with an STI symptom such as a discharge or skin lesion should additionally have urethral/cervical swabs for *Gonococcus* and *Chlamydia*, ulcer swabs, viral media swab if suspected herpes, 'snip' biopsy (where appropriate) for Donovanosis or malignancy, and urine for MCU. Women can take their own tampon swabs instead of a cervical swab if preferred. All sexually active females under 25 years should be screened opportunistically for *Chlamydia* (in particular) and gonorrhoea. Follow-up after therapy and contact tracing, screening, treatment and notification are all necessary.

Specific treatment[6]

Refer also to CHAPTER 117.

Urethritis and cervicitis

azithromycin 1 g (o) as single dose
plus
amoxycillin 3 g (o) + probenecid 1 g (o)—
single dose (but use ceftriaxone 500 mg (IM) in penicillin-resistant areas)

Genital sores

Herpes simplex, syphilis and Donovanosis are much more common than chancroid and lymphogranuloma venereum. Serology for syphilis is essential. Advise to avoid sex and for males to use condoms until treatment is completed and lesions well healed.

Syphilis

benzathine penicillin 1.8 g IM as single dose, if infected less than 2 years ago. If >2 years or unsure, repeat same dose weekly for 2 further injections.

Donovanosis (granuloma inguinale)

azithromycin 0.5–1 g (o) once daily for 7 days
or
1 g (o) once weekly for 4 weeks
(if not pregnant or breastfeeding); if so, give erythromycin or roxithromycin

Herpes simplex

See CHAPTER 117.

Genital warts

See CHAPTER 117.

Pelvic inflammatory disease

If sexually acquired, it is usually due to *Neisseria gonorrhoeae* or *Chlamydia trachomatis* (less likely). For treatment, see CHAPTER 103.

Vaginal infections

Refer to CHAPTERS 106 and 117 for treatment. *Trichomonas vaginalis* is usually sexually transmitted, while *Candida albicans* and bacterial vaginosis are not.

Communication tips[22]

- Don't assume English is a first language, particularly in remote areas.
- Don't assume a nod means understanding and/or agreement to treatment.
- Check hearing as chronic ear infections can impair it.
- Appreciate the different family network, particularly the tendency of grandmothers and aunts to care for children.
- Don't assume a broken appointment means the patient will not return for treatment. Often family and cultural duties take precedence.
- Be aware of cultural sensitivity.
- Don't touch a patient, particularly of the opposite sex, without seeking permission and explaining what you are doing.
- Be aware that patients may not be comfortable with direct questions about their family and health.
- Don't be too stern or authoritative during a consultation.
- Ensure receptionists and other staff understand the cultural sensitivities involved.
- Be accepting, respectful and non-judgmental.

Practice tips

- Anaemia is common in Indigenous children—be on the lookout for it. Consider giving pyrantel embonate or mebendazole in a hookworm endemic area.
- Asthma is common—consider it in coughing children.
- In children with failure to thrive, consider insufficient food, urinary tract infection, GIT infection or parasites and recurrent illness.

continued

continued

- Beware of diarrhoea in children—attend to fluid and electrolyte replacement.
- Think pelvic inflammatory disease in a woman of child-bearing age presenting with abdominal pain. Be watchful for penicillinase-producing *Neisseria gonorrhoeae* (although it remains uncommon in Indigenous communities).
- Consider the possibility of rheumatic fever or glomerulonephritis with *S. pyogenes* throat infection and treat with an optimal course of antibiotics (e.g. single injection of benzathine penicillin).
- In tropical areas, consider diseases such as melioidosis, dengue and Ross River infection.
- Promote immunisation programs.
- In the fitting or aggressive patient, alcohol withdrawal is the commonest cause, but the possibility of petrol sniffing should also be considered.
- Kidney failure is common: look for it if proteinuria, diabetes, hypertension, general debility or recurrent infections.
- Serum creatinine measures are also useful. A level of <150 mmol/L is regarded as a safe limit for kidney function.
- Consider urine albumin–creatinine ratio (ACR) testing in adults to detect and monitor early kidney disease. As kidney disease has a progressive nature, regular monitoring is important.[18] Kidney function must be monitored at least annually.
- Donovanosis (granuloma inguinale), which can be chronic and progressive, presents initially as raised beefy nodules or sores. Microscopy of scrapings or snip or pinch biopsy will confirm the diagnosis.[18]
- Medroxyprogesterone acetate (Depo-Provera) and Implanon are very useful contraceptive agents but always adhere to guidelines for informed consent.
- Because adherence to medication may be a problem with some patients, once-a-day therapy is recommended where possible.
- Point-of-care laboratory equipment (HbA1c, urine ACR) is very helpful for monitoring diabetic patients as it can be used in remote communities by trained health workers.

References

1 Australian Institute of Health and Welfare. Deaths. Web report, 2017. <www.aihw.gov.au/reports/life-expectancy-death/deaths-in-australia/contents/life-expectancy> (accessed 24/5/2018).

2 Couzos S, Murray R. *Aboriginal Primary Health Care: An Evidence-based Approach* (2nd edn). Melbourne: Oxford University Press, 2003.

3 Australian Bureau of Statistics. *Australian Aboriginal and Torres Strait Islander Health Survey: Biomedical Results, 2012–13.* Available from: <http://www.abs.gov.au/ausstats/abs@.nsf/mf/4727.0.55.003>.

4 Senior T, Hindmarsh E et al. Aboriginal and Torres Strait Islander Health. RACGP Check Unit 473, 2011.

5 Wakeman J, Stothers K. Aboriginal and Torres Strait Islander health: general practice embraces its significant role to close the gap (Editorial). Aust Fam Physician, 2014; 43: 1–2, 7.

6 Central Australian Rural Practitioners Association. *CARPA Standard Treatment Manual* (7th edn). Alice Springs: CARPA, 2017. <https://www.remotephcmanuals.com.au/#> (accessed 22/5/2018).

7 Jamieson LM, Sayers SM, Roberts-Thomson KF. Clinical oral health outcomes in young Australian adults compared with national-level counterparts. Med J Aust, 2010; 192: 558–66.

8 Charles J, Britt H, Knox S. Encounters with Indigenous patients in Australian general practice. Aust Fam Physician, 2005; 34 (10): 810–11.

9 Marmot M. Social determinants and the health of Indigenous Australians. Med J Aust, 2011; 194 (10): 512–13.

10 Ruben AR, Walker A. Malnutrition among rural Aboriginal children in the Top End of the Northern Territory. Med J Aust, 1995; 162: 400–3.

11 Coleman J. Health communication with Aboriginal and Torres Strait Islanders. In: Groves M, Fitzgerald, J, eds, *Communication Skills in Medicine.* Melbourne: IP Communications, 2010.

12 O'Connor M. Women's business. Aust Fam Physician, 1994; 23: 40–4.

13 National Aboriginal Health Strategy Working Party. *A National Aboriginal Health Strategy.* Canberra: Department of Aboriginal Affairs, 1989: 193.

14 Walker A. Common health problems in Northern Territory Aboriginal children. Aust Fam Physician, 1994; 23: 55–62.

15 Walsh WF. Editorial: Cardiovascular health in Indigenous Australians: a call for action. Med J Aust, 2001; 175: 351–2.

16 Australian Institute of Health and Welfare (AIHW). Rheumatic heart disease and acute rheumatic fever in Australia: 1996–2012, Cardiovascular Disease Series. Cat. No. CVD 60. Canberra, 2013.

17 Darwin Otitis Guidelines Group. Recommendations for clinical care guidelines on the management of otitis media in Aboriginal and Torres Strait Islander populations. Canberra: Office for Aboriginal and Torres Strait Islander Health, DOHA, 2010.

18 Marquardt T. Managing skin infections in Aboriginal and Torres Strait Islander children. Aust Fam Physician, 2014; 43: 1–2, 17–19.

19 Marley J (Chair). *Therapeutic Guidelines: Dermatology* (Version 3). Melbourne: Therapeutic Guidelines Ltd, 2009 (eTG Complete).

20 Mashford L (Chair). *Therapeutic Guidelines: Rheumatology* (Version 1). Melbourne. Therapeutic Guidelines Ltd, 2006: 201–7.

21 Atkins RC. How bright is their future? (Editorial). Med J Aust, 2001; 174: 489–90.

22 Ryan K. Skill with Indigenous patients: cultural issues. Australian Doctor, 9 March 2001: 66–7.

Refugee health

135

A refugee is a person who owing to a well founded fear of being persecuted for reasons of race, religion, nationality, membership of a particular social group or political opinion is outside the country of his nationality and is unable or owing to such fear is unwilling to avail himself of the protection of that country.

THE UNITED NATIONS CONFERENCE OF PLENIPOTENTIARIES ON THE STATUS OF REFUGEES AND STATELESS PERSONS 1951[1]

The health of refugees is a special challenge for GPs, who are in an ideal opportunistic position to treat these disadvantaged people with their many mental and physical health problems.[2] About 13 000 refugees settle in Australia each year with the majority from Southern and South-East Asia, the Middle East and Saharan Africa. Refugees, especially refugee children, arrive with a variety of medical problems that may escape detection unless appropriate screening is undertaken. Many problems are asymptomatic, latent or occult and may be considered inconsequential by the affected person or guardian. Studies conducted in New South Wales[3] show that there is a high rate of diseases of personal and public health significance in a sample of children from refugee-specific clinics. Most of the children in the study had disorders that were asymptomatic. The study identified 25% with anaemia, 27% serology positive for schistosomiasis, and 16% with current or recent malaria, while 69% were hepatitis B non-immune, 25% were tuberculin skin test positive and 20% had low vitamin D levels.[3]

Predeparture screening[4]

Refugees, like other migrants, have to meet predetermined health criteria to be granted a permanent visa. The basic medical requirements are:

- history and examination
- chest X-ray if ≥ 11 years of age
- HIV and syphilis tests if ≥ 15 years of age
- hepatitis B test if pregnant or an unaccompanied minor
- malaria-rapid antigen test, tuberculosis (mantoux or interferon gamma)
- tests for intestinal helminths (worms)
- MMR immunisation ≤ 30 years

Applicants are offered treatment for most disorders. However, active TB precludes the granting of a visa. An additional 'fitness to fly' predeparture assessment is usually performed prior to travel. However, because of the high prevalence of both acute and chronic infective diseases and the inconsistencies of screening results, it is likely that many illnesses remain undiagnosed or untreated upon arrival in their new country.

Communication issues

Good communication with refugees and their families is fundamental to good outcomes. This involves appropriate rapport, understanding of and interest in their problems. A professional interpreter is the best tool available when dealing with a patient whose language is unfamiliar,[4] and the national Translating and Interpreting Service provides GPs with a free phone interpreter in many circumstances. It is important to emphasise that confidentiality will be respected. Non-verbal communication is obviously an important strategy and includes empathetic nodding, listening and friendliness. Be aware of the financial restraints of refugees, especially when a family needs treatment, and arrange for investigation, specialist referral and treatment in a public hospital setting. In the authors' experience, refugees have a predilection for investigations and injections and these factors need to be tactfully weighed when explaining restrained management approaches (see FIGS 135.1 and 135.2).

Medical assessment

All refugees should be offered a comprehensive health assessment, ideally within one month of arrival in Australia. Common presenting problems are summarised in TABLE 135.1.

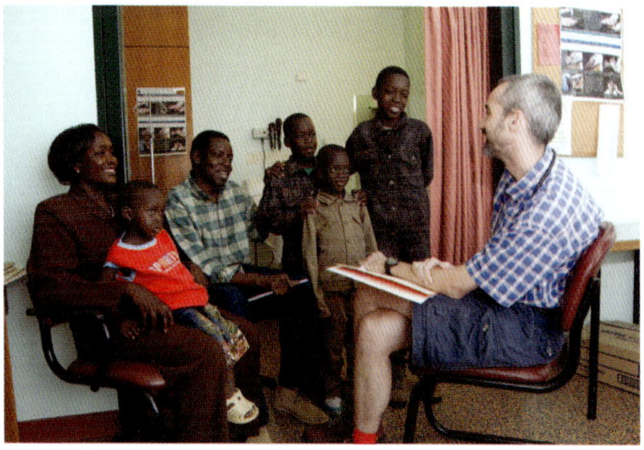

FIGURE 135.1 Initial health contact with a refugee family
Photo courtesy of Dr Joshua Davis

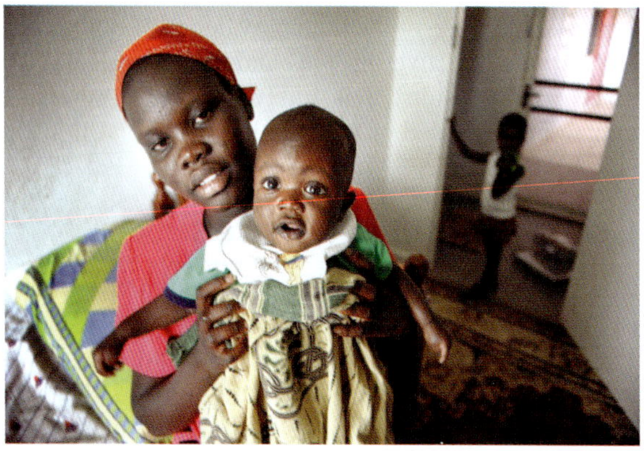

FIGURE 135.2 African refugee family at home
Photo by Newspix/Jay Town

135

Table 135.1 Common presenting problems[4]
Psychological and behavioural disorders
Anaemia, especially iron deficiency
Oro-dental disease
Intestinal parasites
Malaria
Helicobacter pylori infection/peptic ulcer disease
Vitamin deficiencies, especially vitamin D, B12
Disorders of special senses: skin, eyes, ears
Chronic disease

History

The usual approach should be followed but with an additional emphasis on the person's background and reasons for migration including any time in refugee camps, exposure to violence, torture, trauma and other forms of abuse including sexual trauma. The following checklist is recommended.[5]

- Presenting problem/s
- Family history including haemoglobinopathy or other genetic disorders
- Migration history
- Past history including tropical diseases
- Developmental history
- Immunisation
- Diet, with emphasis on vitamin intake
- Drug history, including drugs of addiction—especially IV use; smoking
- Mental health and history of trauma, behavioural issues in children
- Basic general life drives: appetite, weight, energy, sleep, mood, sex

Examination

- General: growth, weight, BMI, percentile charts
- Skin: note any rash, BCG scars, pallor, jaundice
- Hearing and vision
- Oro-dental
- Cardiovascular
- Respiratory
- Lymphopoietic: note any lymphadenopathy or hepatosplenomegaly
- Genitourinary: note any genital mutilation
- Urinalysis

Screening (recommended investigations)[5,6,7]

- FBE, ESR, CRP
- Electrolytes, KFTs, LFTs
- TB: chest X-ray, Mantoux tuberculin sensitivity test, interferon gamma release assay (IGRA)
- Malaria: thick and thin blood films, plasmodium rapid antigen test
- Blood-borne viruses: HIV, hepatitis B, hepatitis C
- STIs: syphilis, PCR for *Chlamydia* and *Gonococcus*
- Helminths: *Strongyloides* serology, faeces microscopy (ova/cysts/parasites)
- Schistosomiasis serology

Consider: iron studies, serum vitamin A, D and B12, and serum electrophoresis for haemoglobinopathy screen.

Specific common issues

A summary of special issues for refugees is presented in TABLE 135.2.

Table 135.2 Special issues for refugees

Social isolation and displacement
Tropical/third world diseases (e.g. helminths, malaria, schistosomiasis)
Infections (TB, hepatitis B and C, HIV)
Sexual and reproductive health
Female genital mutilation
Dental health
Nutritional deficiencies (e.g. rickets, vitamin B12)
Childhood growth and development
Immunisation status
Chronic medical problems
Specific genetic disorders

Psychological issues[7]

Predictably these traumatised people experience a wide range of psychological sequelae, particularly loneliness/isolation, post-traumatic stress disorder with anxiety and depression. They experience the whole gamut of the usual life-stage conditions, financial concerns and gender-related issues that we encounter in everyday general practice. However, these problems are compounded possibly by cultural differences and poor language skills if they come from a non-English-speaking background. Effective communication and counselling skills are required to tease out, identify and manage any psychological disorders. Psychological distress often presents as physical symptoms such as headaches, chest pains and upper gastrointestinal discomfort.

Many refugees seem to manage very well with the transition, feeling relief to be in a safe and supportive environment.

According to one refugee children's group, children and adolescents may exhibit disorders such as:[5]

- behavioural problems
- aggression
- acting out
- running away
- poor concentration and school performance
- somatic complaints
- self-harming or suicidal ideation
- anxiety, phobias or depression

A recommended tool for assessing children's psychological well-being is the *Strength and Difficulties Questionnaire*, available online at <www.sdqscore.org>.

Vitamin D deficiency[5]

This is a prevalent problem, particularly in children, for a variety of reasons, including poor dietary intake, dark skin, relocation to higher latitudes and low levels in breast milk. Those undergoing rapid growth, particularly infants and adolescents, are at greatest risk of insufficiency. Most children will be asymptomatic but check for signs of rickets (see CHAPTER 9) and deficiency such as leg bowing, delayed walking, bone and muscle aches and weakness. Blood levels of 25-OH vitamin D <50 nmol/L require treatment—a particular problem for families in meeting the costs of treatment.

Vitamin B12 deficiency[8]

It is important to recognise and treat vitamin B12 deficiency early to prevent permanent neurological changes. The problem can get overlooked in the complexity of multiple issues in refugees. It should be considered in the same context as any other vitamin and mineral deficiency such as vitamin D.

Helicobacter pylori infection

Besides dietary deficiency the other major risk factor in developing countries is *Helicobacter pylori* infection with figures indicating that up to 90% of the population is infected[5] (see CHAPTER 47). This infection should be considered in any adult with symptoms suggestive of peptic ulcer disease or any child with chronic abdominal pain, other GIT symptoms and failure to thrive. Consider a helicobacter breath test and triple therapy.

Haemoglobinopathies[5]

Genetic disorders such as sickle-cell disease (Africa), α and β thalassaemia and glucose-6-phosphate dehydrogenase (G6PD) (latter two Mediterranean, Africa and South-East Asia in particular) are over-represented in refugee populations (see CHAPTER 18). Affected people may be asymptomatic carriers or symptomatic, with symptoms including haemolysis precipitated by infection, cold, hypoxia, drugs and antioxidants. Look for skeletal abnormalities and hepatosplenomegaly on examination and screen with appropriate tests if clinically indicated.

Hepatitis B

Routine hepatitis B vaccination does not occur in endemic areas of Asia and Africa. The rate of infection there is at least eight times higher than the background infection rate of 0.9% in the general Australian population.[5] In particular, those coming from refugee camps are highly susceptible to the spread of hepatitis B. Those with active infection may be asymptomatic, so screening (HBsAg, HBsAb, HBcAb) and subsequent management are important health issues for the refugees and the community. See CHAPTER 58.

Malaria

Malaria is a common infection in endemic regions where most African and South-East Asian refugees originate. Children under 5 years are at most risk and although predeparture testing should detect infected people, some may manifest the disease after arrival. The diagnosis is made on three separate thick and thin blood films but one single test supplemented with a rapid antigen test may be a practical way of detecting the disease (see CHAPTER 15). Treatment should be directed by an experienced consultant.

Schistosomiasis

Schistosomiasis (see CHAPTER 15) is a blood trematode often encountered in African refugees; it is usually acquired in childhood from swimming in contaminated freshwater. Approximately 200 million people are infected worldwide. Many of those infected are asymptomatic while chronic infection may manifest as gastrointestinal symptoms (e.g. diarrhoea, nausea, abdominal pain), failure to thrive/weight loss, respiratory symptoms such as chronic cough, and urinary symptoms that include haematuria. Detecting eggs in the stool or urine may be difficult but serology has high sensitivity and specificity. Eosinophilia, which often correlates with duration, is a feature. If positive, a renal tract ultrasound is advisable and the patient should be referred to a renal physician. Treatment of the infection is with praziquantel.

135

Strongyloides (human threadworm)

Strongyloides (see CHAPTER 15) is a common infestation in refugees with a prevalence of up to 11% in some groups.[5] It can survive asymptomatically for decades but may present with recurrent abdominal pain and watery diarrhoea, failure to thrive/weight loss, and skin and respiratory symptoms (similar to schistosomiasis). Diagnosis is by identifying larvae in concentrated stool (see FIG. 135.3), which can be elusive, and by eosinophilia and serology, which has good sensitivity and specificity. Treatment with ivermectin or albendazole can be complex and consultant help is advisable.

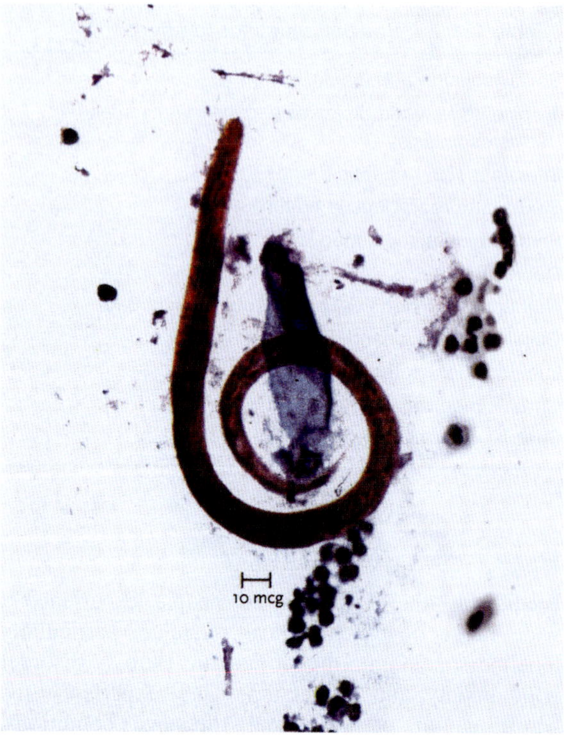

FIGURE 135.3 *Strongyloides stercoralis* ova and parasite in stool

Tuberculosis[6]

Tuberculosis (see CHAPTER 29) is a major health problem in the countries of origin of refugees. Most of those infected are asymptomatic and may go undiagnosed unless properly screened. It is important to detect those (particularly children) with latent infection and non-pulmonary disease. Investigations include a chest X-ray, tuberculin skin test (Mantoux) and an IGRA (check if Medicare rebatable). It is recommended that all refugees should have a clinical assessment by a specialist chest clinic within 2 months of arrival. Special issues include:

- status of IGRA test, including ability to predict subsequent active TB
- HIV and TB
- multidrug-resistant TB

Both TB and HIV are reportable conditions in Australia and their management is specialised.

Immunisation

Immunisation catch-up is a difficult area of management for all doctors treating refugees. Written records are the only reliable form of documentation but immunity from past immunisations cannot be taken for granted. It is advisable to follow formal catch-up guidelines, which are summarised in TABLE 135.3.

Table 135.3 Catch-up immunisation schedule for newly arrived refugees[9]

Vaccine type	Age	Number of doses	Notes
MenCCV	>12 months	1	
DTPa	<10 years	4	If 4th dose given <3.5yo, needs 5th dose
	>10 years	3	
MMR	born <1966	2	
IPV (polio)	<4 years	4	
	≥4 years	3	
Hepatitis B	<11 years	3	Paed form
	11–15 years	2	Adult form
	≥ 16 years	3	Adult form
Hib	2–11 months	2 or 3	Then booster
	12–59 months	1	Then booster
13vPCV (pneumococcus)	<7 months	3	
	7–11 months	2	
	12–59 months	1	
HPV (papilloma)	12–18 years	3	Both female & male
BCG	Varies	1	Check criteria
Varicella	18 months –13 years	1	
	14 onwards	2	
MenC	Any	1	ACWY is 4-valent meningococcal
ACWY	15–19 years	1	
Rotavirus	<6 months	2 or 3	Regime differs with brand

For specific details about minimum dosing interval availability and funding refer to the catch-up schedule (see Resources).

These guidelines are available in the latest edition of *The Australian Immunisation Handbook* (see Resources).

Rehabilitation

A huge challenge facing refugees is the so called 'settlement issue' as they confront the complexities of adjusting to a totally new way of life with their various physical, psychological and social problems. The settling process is a source of considerable stress as new arrivals, many with large families, are likely to move house several times in their first few years.

The general practitioner is ideally placed to act as an advocate for the rehabilitation of his or her patients and family. Of course, GPs from a similar background have an advantage, but special skills are required to understand the issues and to gain access to available rehabilitation and support services (see Resources). Resources are also provided by the RACGP.

Key recommendations (Australasian Society for Infectious Diseases)[6]

- All refugees should be offered a comprehensive health assessment, ideally within 1 month of arrival in Australia.
- This should include:
  - screening for and treatment of the following conditions: tuberculosis, brucellosis, malaria, blood-borne viral infections, schistosomiasis, helminth infection and sexually transmitted infections
  - testing for and treatment of other infections (e.g. *Helicobacter pylori*) as indicated by clinical assessment
  - assessment of immunisation status, and catch-up immunisations where appropriate.
- The assessment can be undertaken by a GP or within a multidisciplinary refugee health centre.
- An appropriate interpreter should be used when required.
- The initial assessment should take place over at least two visits: the first for initial assessment and investigation, and the second for review of results and treatment/referral.
- Psychological, dental, nutritional, reproductive and developmental health issues should also be addressed at the post-arrival health assessment.

135

Practice tips

- It is helpful to become familiar with the clinical features of the relevant tropical diseases.
- It is also advisable to learn about the significant cultural and religious customs of the ethnic groups you are likely to encounter.

continued

continued

- Important diseases that 'must not be missed' include malaria, tuberculosis, schistosomiasis, HIV, typhoid fever, meningoencephalitis and severe psychological illness such as psychosis and major depression, especially with suicide risk.
- Be aware of pseudo 'neutropenia' since some people, especially of African origin, have a different reference range for neutrophil counts.[4]
- Doctors should consider their own safety in dealing with people coming from a theatre of violence who may be subject to vicarious trauma (also known as secondary traumatic stress).[4]
- The use of professional interpreter services is a vital component of sound communication skills.
- A multidisciplinary health care team will help meet the needs of practitioners in addressing most problems, especially complex ones.
- Practitioners have a useful range of resources including refugee clinics in each state, chest clinics, torture and trauma services, and immunisation advice.

References

1 United Nations High Commissioner for Refugees. Basic facts (online). <www.unhrc.org>
2 Harris M, Zwar N. Refugee health. Aust Fam Physician, 2005; 34 (10): 825–9.
3 Raman S, Wood N et al. Matching health needs of refugee children with services: how big is the gap? Aust NZ J Public Health, 2009; 33 (5): 466–70.
4 Smith M. Refugee health. Medical Observer. Update. 5 June 2009: 24–6.
5 Koh A, Zwi K, Walls T. Newly arrived refugee children. Australian Doctor, 30 January 2009: 21–8.
6 Murray RJ, Davis JS, Burgner DP. The Australasian Society for Infectious Diseases guidelines for the diagnosis, management and prevention of infections in recently arrived refugees: an abridged outline. Med J Aust 2009; 190: 421–5.
7 Benson J, Phillips C, Gardner J et al. Multicultural health. RACGP Check Unit 477, 2011.
8 Benson J, Maldari T, Turnbull T. Vitamin B12 deficiency. Why refugee patients are at risk. Aust Fam Physician, 2010; 39 (4): 215–7.
9 The Royal Children's Hospital Melbourne. Catch-up immunisation in refugees (updated February 2018). Available at <www.rch.org.au/immigranthealth/clinical/Catchup_immunisation_in_refugees/> (accessed 24/5/2018).

Resources

Victorian Department of Health. Quick Guide. Catch-up immunisation for Victoria. March 2010. <www.health.vic.gov.au/immunisation>

Murray RJ, Davis JS, Krause V et al. Diagnosis, management and prevention of infections in recently arrived refugees. Australasian Society for Infectious Diseases.

Australian Government Department of Health and Ageing. *Australian Immunisation Handbook*. <immunise.health.gov.au/>

Appendix I Percentile charts: infant girls

INFANT GIRLS

NAME BIRTH DATE NO.

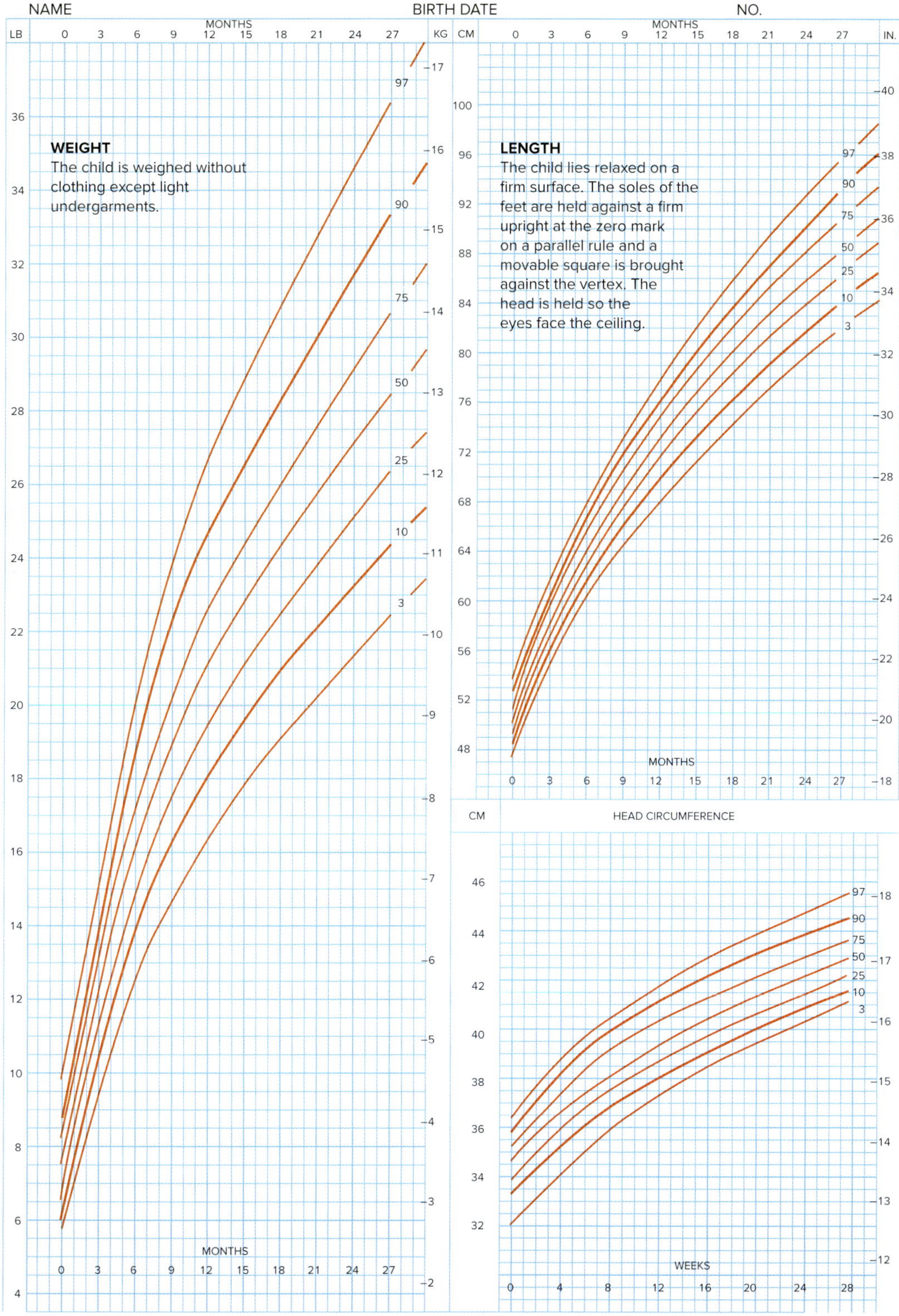

Appendix II Percentile charts: infant boys

INFANT BOYS

NAME BIRTH DATE NO.

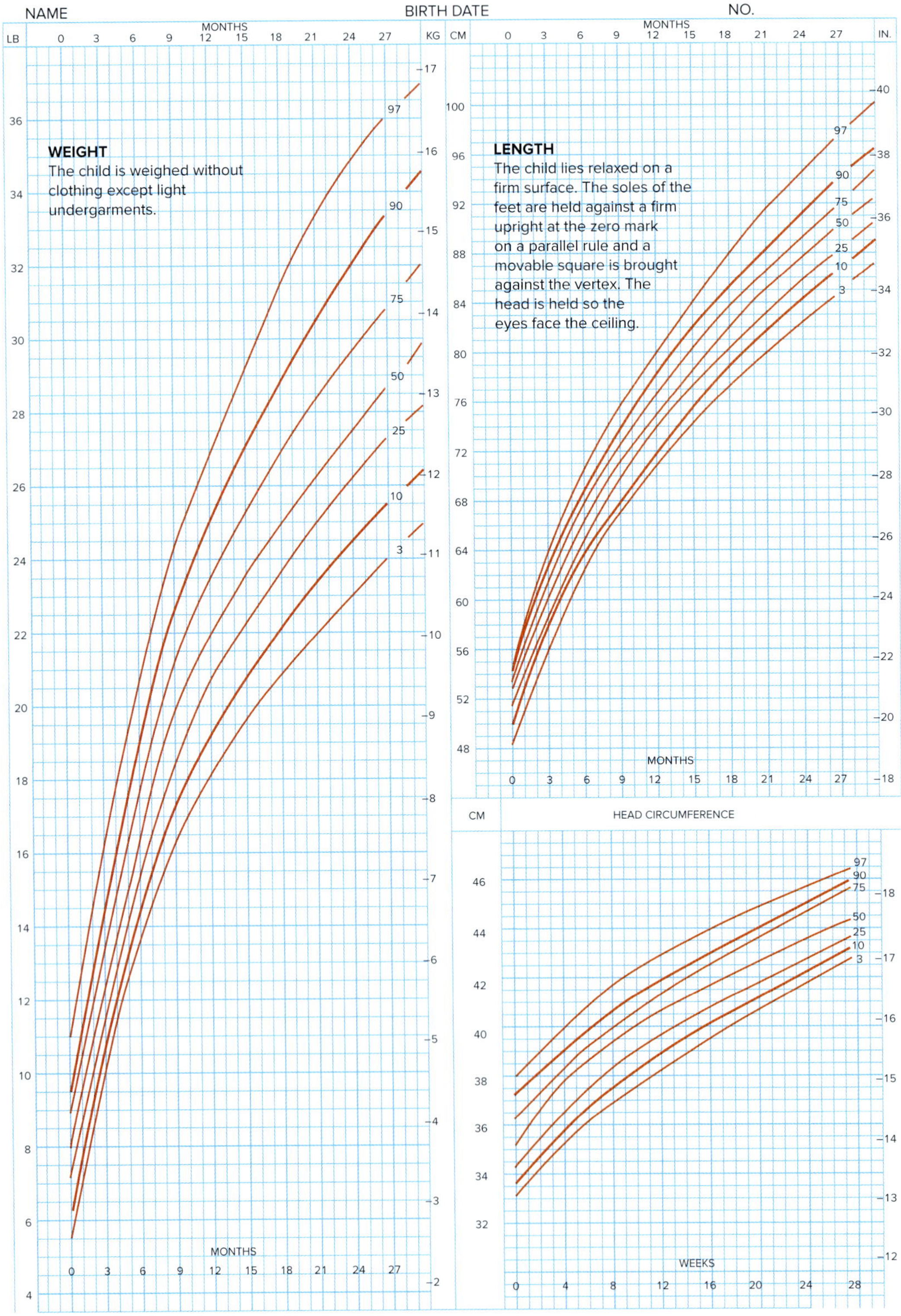

Appendix III Percentile charts: girls

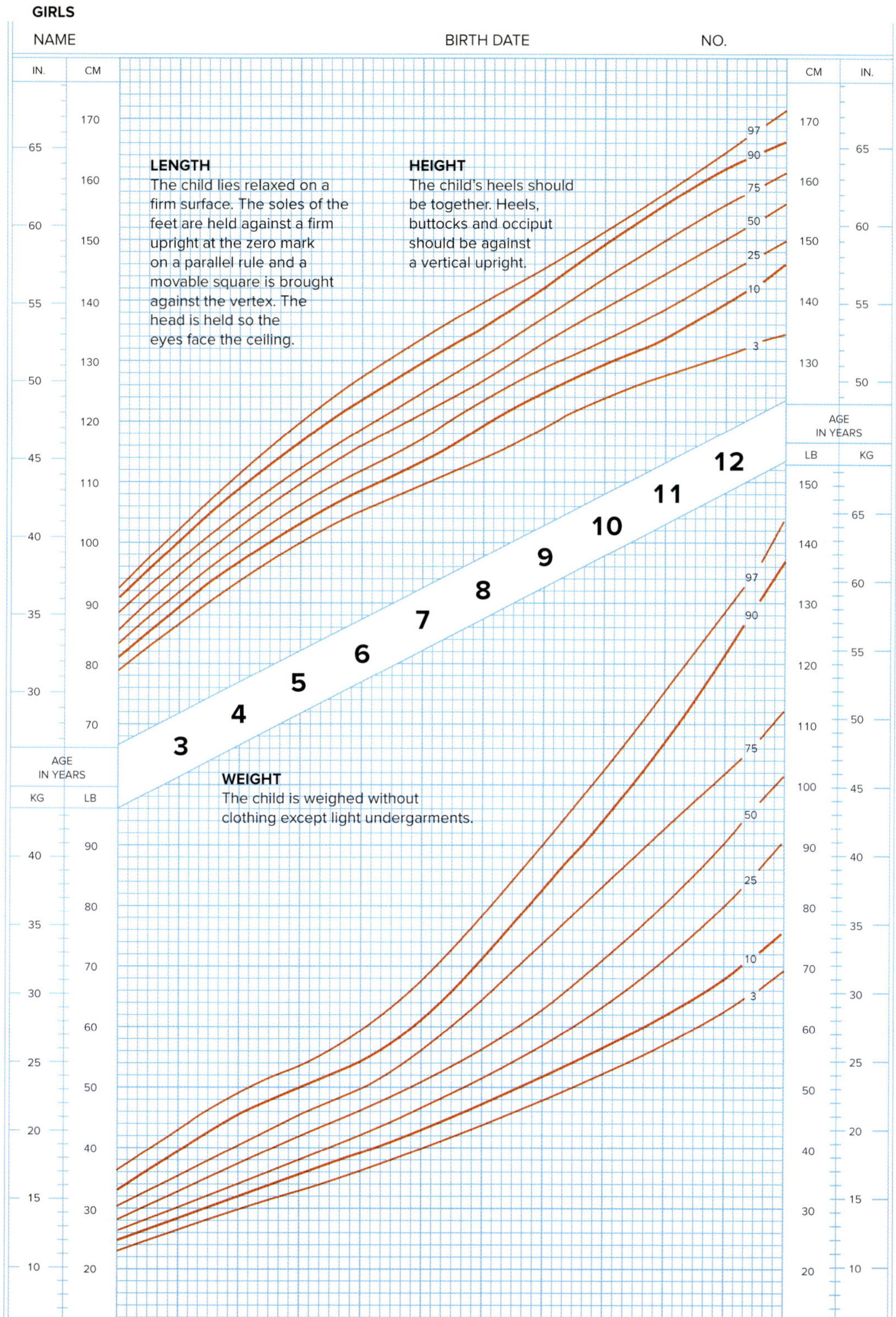

Appendix IV Percentile charts: boys

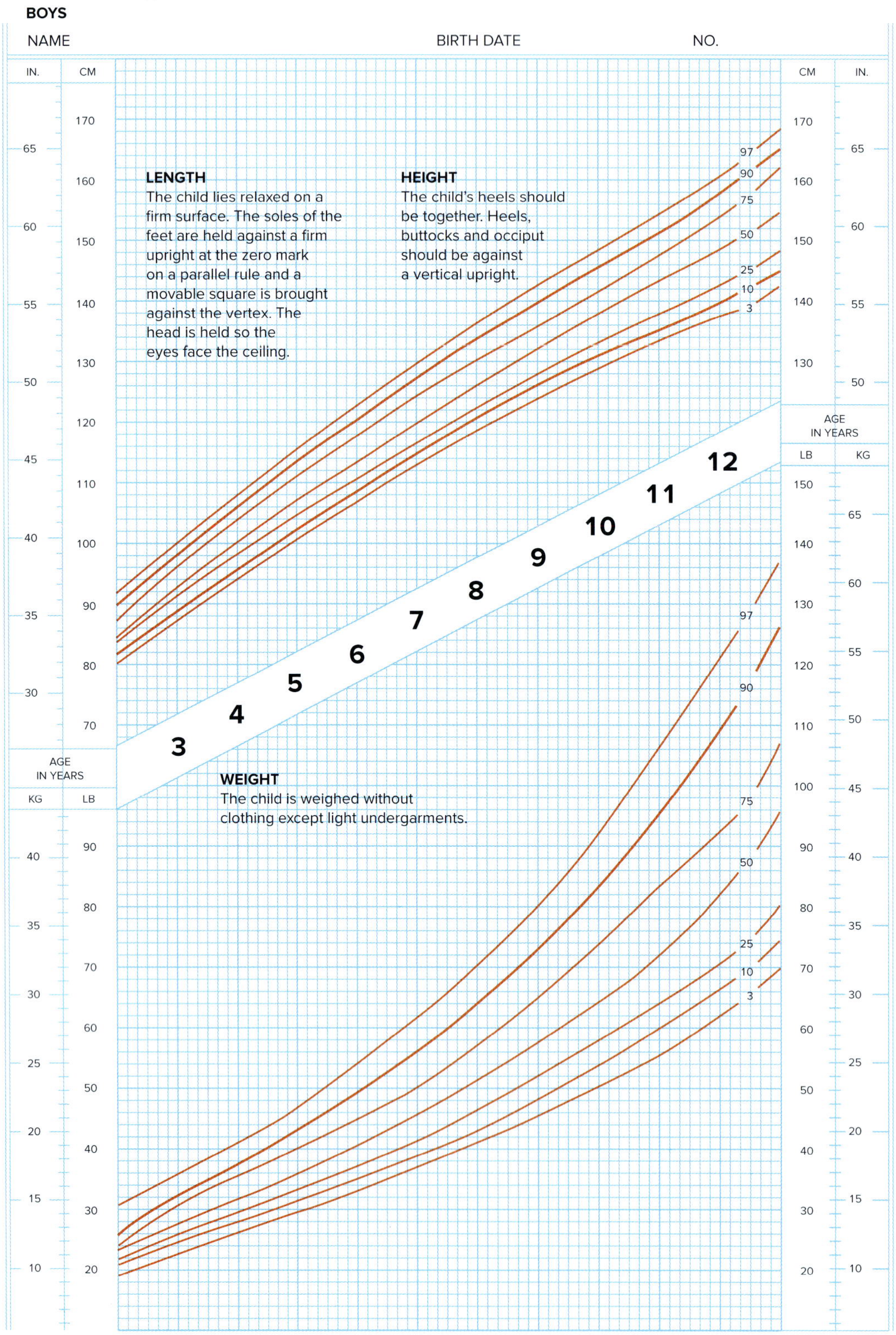

Appendix V The Australian Nutrition Foundation: weight for height chart

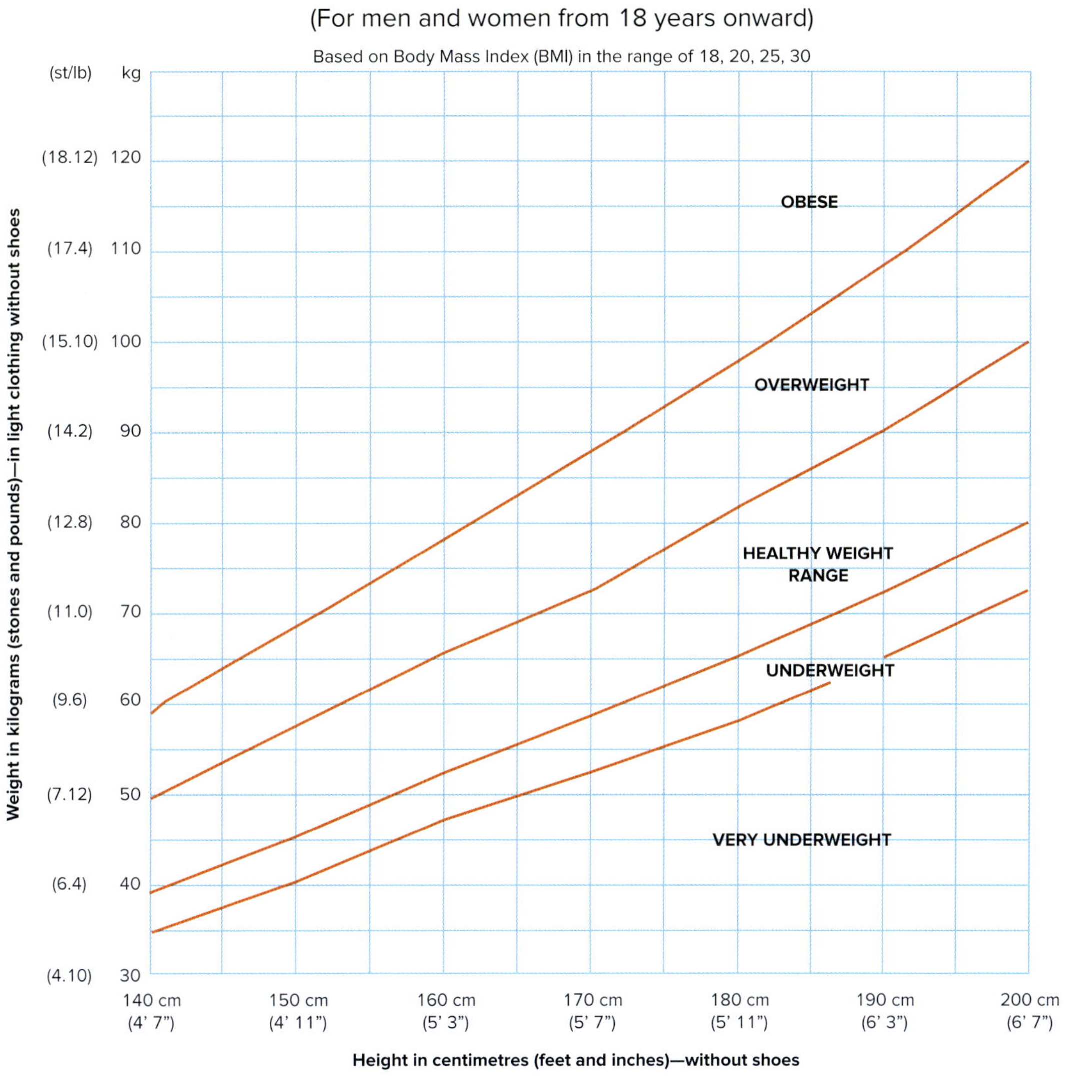

Index

Page numbers in **bold** indicate sections or extensive treatment of a topic.
Page numbers in *italics* indicate figures or tables.
Entries starting with numbers precede the alphabetical sequence, excepting numbers preceding the names of chemicals, which are ignored in filing. For example: 5-fluorouracil files as fluorouracil.

C

E

G

H

J

K

P

Q

R

S

W